Haynes-Glasscock-Shambaugh Surgery of the Ear

Alex D. Sweeney • George B. Wanna
Matthew L. Carlson • Elizabeth L. Perkins
Editors

Haynes-Glasscock-Shambaugh Surgery of the Ear

Seventh Edition

Springer

Editors
Alex D. Sweeney
Department of Otolaryngology—Head and Neck Surgery
Baylor College of Medicine
Houston, TX, USA

George B. Wanna
Department of Otolaryngology—Head and Neck Surgery
Icahn School of Medicine at Mount Sinai
New York, NY, USA

Matthew L. Carlson
Department of Otolaryngology—Head and Neck Surgery
Mayo Clinic
Rochester, MN, USA

Elizabeth L. Perkins
Department of Otolaryngology—Head and Neck Surgery
Vanderbilt University Medical Center
Nashville, TN, USA

ISBN 978-3-032-18263-0 ISBN 978-3-032-18264-7 (eBook)
https://doi.org/10.1007/978-3-032-18264-7

This work was supported by Vanderbilt University

This Springer imprint is published by the registered company Springer Nature Switzerland AG
The registered company address is: Gewerbestrasse 11, 6330 Cham, Switzerland

Preface

The publication of this book's seventh edition is bittersweet. Since the sixth edition, our world has changed in a number of notable ways. The *SARS-CoV-2* pandemic, in particular, was an unimaginable tragedy, and it's hard to move forward without considering what we have lost. We would like to dedicate the introduction of the seventh edition to our friend, mentor, and a namesake of the book itself, Dr. Michael E. Glasscock, III.

After a prestigious and multifaceted career, Dr. Glasscock died in 2018. In the end, he left us as he lived—on his own terms. As was noted in his obituary, which was published in the journal that he founded, "In his room were pictures of his family, his mentors, his fellows, his helicopter, his Texas ranch, and the many books he authored. All testaments to a man well-loved and a life well-lived."[1]

We are lucky to have been influenced by Mike, and we can think of no greater honor to his legacy than publishing the seventh edition of Glasscock & Shambaugh's Surgery of the Ear in a manner that will be freely accessible to anyone in the world with an Internet connection. We have no doubts that this is what Mike would have wanted.

Also, on the theme of things Mike would have wanted, we have made another special change to this edition of the book. The best evidence of Mike's legacy as an educator is found in those he trained to become educators themselves. Though Mike's own light has extinguished, his training lineage will eternally illuminate our path as surgeons. In this vein, the editors of the seventh edition met recently, and amid a discussion on the challenges of publishing a book through the pandemic, we were inspired by the notion that we have all been profoundly influenced, personally and professionally, by one of Mike's trainees in particular—Dr. David S. Haynes. David's gifts as a surgeon, clinician, and educator have become self-evident throughout his career, and his generosity and humanism have made him an unparalleled figure in our collective experience. Through these attributes, David has not only carried on Mike's legacy in Neurotology but built upon it in a spectacular fashion. As such, we did not feel appropriate publishing the newest edition of this book without recognizing David.

Welcome to the seventh edition of Haynes, Glasscock, Shambaugh's "Surgery of the Ear".

Alex D. Sweeney, M.D.

[1]Haynes DS. Michael E. Glasscock, III, MD.: Obituary 1933–2018. *Otology & Neurotology*. 2018. 39: 667–668.

Acknowledgement

This book is dedicated to our wonderful **families**, **mentors**, **departments**, and **trainees**—without whom, nothing would be possible.

We are deeply grateful to **Herbert O. and Vineta Christopher**, whose generous gift has made it possible to offer this book as open access, free of charge to all. Their support enables the global sharing of knowledge, fosters collaboration, and contributes to the advancement of healthcare worldwide.

To our chapter **authors** and **associate editors**: we sincerely appreciate your time, patience, and invaluable expertise.

We would like to acknowledge **George Card**, whose drawings were a foundation of the illustration program for this book series.

We also extend our appreciation to the **Brown Foundation** and the **Dorothy L. McGee Endowment** for their generosity, which played a vital role in bringing this book to life.

Editors

Alex D. Sweeney, MD
Editor in Chief

Brown Foundation Associate Professor, former Dorothy L. McGee Endowed Chair
Vice Chair of Clinical Affairs and Director of the Neurotology Division and Neurotology Fellowship Program
Bobby R. Alford Department of Otolaryngology—Head and Neck Surgery
Baylor College of Medicine

Adjunct Associate Professor at the Baylor College of Medicine Department of Neurosurgery, Texas Children's Hospital Department of Surgery, and University of Houston Department of Communication Sciences and Disorders

Matthew L. Carlson, MD
Professor of Otolaryngology and Neurologic Surgery
Division Chair, Otology and Neurotology
Medical Director, Cochlear Implant Program
Program Director, Neurotology and Lateral Skull Base Surgery Fellowship
Mayo Clinic, Rochester

George Wanna, MD, MHCM, FACS
Professor of Otolaryngology—Head and Neck Surgery
Professor of Neurosurgery
Ichan School of Medicine at Mount Sinai

Chair, Department of Otolaryngology
New York Eye and Ear Infirmary of Mount Sinai and Mount Sinai Beth Israel

Executive Vice Chairman of the Department of Otolaryngology—Head and Neck Surgery
Mount Sinai Health System

Elizabeth L. Perkins, MD
Assistant Professor of Otolaryngology—Head and Neck Surgery
Assistant Professor of Neurosurgery
Vanderbilt University Medical Center

Consulting Editor

David S. Haynes, MD, MMHC
Professor of Otolaryngology—Head and Neck Surgery and Neurosurgery
Neurotology Division Chief and Fellowship Program Director
Vanderbilt University Medical Center

Chief Experience Officer
Vanderbilt University Medical Center

Associate Editors

Michael H. Freeman, MD
Virginia Ear, Nose and Throat

John Marinelli, MD
Mayo Clinic School of Medicine
Department of Otolaryngology—Head and Neck Surgery

Zachary G. Schwam, MD
Icahn School of Medicine at Mount Sinai
Department of Otolaryngology—Head and Neck Surgery

Benjamin D. Lovin, MD
University of Virginia School of Medicine
Department of Otolaryngology—Head and Neck Surgery

Contents

Contributors

Dunia Abdul-Aziz, M.D. Department of Otolaryngology—Head and Neck Surgery, Massachusetts Eye and Ear and Massachusetts General Hospital, Boston, MA, USA

Department of Otolaryngology—Head and Neck Surgery, Harvard Medical School, Boston, MA, USA

Meredith E. Adams, M.D. Department of Otolaryngology—Head and Neck Surgery, University of Michigan, Ann Arbor, MI, USA

Oliver F. Adunka, M.D., M.B.A. Department of Otolaryngology—Head and Neck Surgery, The Ohio State University Wexner Medical Center, Columbus, OH, USA

Yuri Agrawal, M.D., M.P.H. Department of Otolaryngology—Head and Neck Surgery, University of Colorado, Boulder, CO, USA

Syed Ahsan, M.D. Otology/Neurotology, Kaiser Permanente—Southern California, Department of Otolaryngology Head & Neck Surgery, University of California, Irvine, Irvine, CA, USA

Kyle Allen, M.D., M.P.H. Tampa Bay Hearing and Balance Center, Tampa, FL, USA

Jennifer Alyono, M.D., M.S. Department of Otolaryngology—Head and Neck Surgery, Stanford University, Stanford, CA, USA

Emily Ambrose, M.D. Department of Otolaryngology—Head and Neck Surgery, University of Colorado Anschutz Medical Campus, Aurora, CO, USA

Stephanie Moody Antonio, M.D. Department of Otolaryngology—Head and Neck Surgery, Eastern Virginia Medical School, Norfolk, VA, USA

Eric N. Appelbaum, M.D. Wellstar Medical Group, Marietta, GA, USA

Alexandra M. Arambula, M.D. Department of Otolaryngology—Head and Neck Surgery, Case Western Reserve University/University Hospitals Cleveland Medical Center, Cleveland, OH, USA

Moisés Arriaga, M.D. Department of Otolaryngology—Head and Neck Surgery, Louisiana State University School of Medicine, New Orleans, LA, USA

Our Lady of the Lake Hearing and Balance Center, Baton Rouge, LA, USA

Eric E. Babajanian, M.D. Spokane Ear, Nose and Throat, Spokane, WA, USA

Seilesh Babu, M.D. Department of Neurotology, Michigan Ear Institute, Henry Ford Health System, Novi, MI, USA

Emily Bacalao, M.D. Department of Otolaryngology—Head and Neck Surgery, University of Colorado Anschutz Medical Campus, Aurora, CO, USA

Michael Baddour, M.D. Department of Otolaryngology—Head and Neck Surgery, Emory University, Atlanta, GA, USA

Renee M. Banakis Hartl, Au.D., M.D. Department of Otolaryngology—Head and Neck Surgery, University of Michigan School of Medicine, Ann Arbor, MI, USA

Manohar Bance, M.B., Ch.B., M.Sc. Otology and Skull Base Surgery, University of Cambridge, Cambridge, UK

Anna Bareiss, M.D. Department of Otolaryngology—Head and Neck Surgery, College of Medicine, University of Arkansas for Medical Sciences, Little Rock, AR, USA

Gregory J. Basura, M.D., Ph.D. Department of Otolaryngology—Head and Neck Surgery; Division of Otology—Neurotology/Skull Base Surgery, University of Pittsburgh Medical Center/University of Pittsburgh, Pittsburgh, PA, USA

Marc L. Bennett, M.D., M.M.H.C. Department of Otolaryngology—Head and Neck Surgery, Vanderbilt University Medical Center, Nashville, TN, USA

Jason A. Beyea, M.D., Ph.D. Department of Otolaryngology, Queen's University School of Medicine, Kingston, ON, Canada

Dennis I. Bojrab, M.D. Department of Neurotology, Michigan Ear Institute, St. John Providence Hospital and Medical Centers, Novi, MI, USA

Joseph T. Breen, M.D. Department of Otolaryngology—Head and Neck Surgery, Mayo Clinic, Jacksonville, FL, USA

Kevin B. Brown, M.D., Ph.D. Department of Otolaryngology—Head and Neck Surgery, University of North Carolina, Chapel Hill, NC, USA

Craig A. Buchman, M.D. Department of Otolaryngology—Head and Neck Surgery, University of Utah, Salt Lake City, UT, USA

Matthew L. Bush, M.D., Ph.D., M.B.A. Department of Otolaryngology—Head and Neck Surgery, University of Kentucky Medical Center, Lexington, KY, USA

Michael W. Canfarotta, M.D. Department of Otolaryngology—Head and Neck Surgery, Vanderbilt University Medical Center, Nashville, TN, USA

John P. Carey, M.D. Department of Otolaryngology—Head and Neck Surgery, Johns Hopkins University School of Medicine, Baltimore, MD, USA

Matthew L. Carlson, M.D., M.B.A. Department of Otolaryngology—Head and Neck Surgery, Mayo Clinic, Rochester, MN, USA

Geoffrey C. Casazza, M.D. Department of Otolaryngology—Head and Neck Surgery, University of Utah School of Medicine, Salt Lake City, UT, USA

Stephen P. Cass, M.D., M.P.H./M.S.P.H. Department of Otolaryngology—Head and Neck Surgery, University of Colorado Anschutz Medical Campus, Aurora, CO, USA

Adam M. Cassis, M.D. Arizona Hearing and Balance, Chandler, AZ, USA

Alexander Chern, M.D. Department of Otolaryngology—Head and Neck Surgery, Johns Hopkins University School of Medicine, Baltimore, MD, USA

Garret W. Choby, M.D. Department of Otolaryngology—Head and Neck Surgery, University of Pittsburgh, Pittsburgh, PA, USA

Department of Neurologic Surgery, University of Pittsburgh, Pittsburgh, PA, USA

Maura K. Cosetti, M.D. Department of Otolaryngology—Head and Neck Surgery, Icahn School of Medicine at Mount Sinai, New York, NY, USA

Benjamin T. Crane, M.D., Ph.D. University of Rochester School of Medicine, Strong Memorial Hospital, Rochester, NY, USA

Francis X. Creighton Jr, M.D. Department of Otolaryngology—Head and Neck Surgery, Johns Hopkins University School of Medicine, Baltimore, MD, USA

Roberto A. Cueva, M.D. Southern California Permanente Medical Group, San Diego, CA, USA

University of California, San Diego, CA, USA

Nicholas L. Deep, M.D. Department of Otolaryngology—Head and Neck Surgery, Division of Otology and Neurotology, Mayo Clinic, Phoenix, AZ, USA

Charles C. Della Santina, M.D., Ph.D. Department of Otolaryngology—Head and Neck Surgery, Johns Hopkins University School of Medicine, Baltimore, MD, USA

Nicholas A. Dewyer, M.D. Department of Otolaryngology—Head and Neck Surgery, University of Arizona College of Medicine, Tucson, AZ, USA

John L. Dornhoffer, M.D. Department of Otolaryngology—Head and Neck Surgery, University of Arkansas for Medical Sciences, Little Rock, AR, USA

C. Eduardo Corrales, M.D. Otology, Neurotology and Skull Base Surgery, Harvard Medical School, Division of Otolaryngology, Brigham and Women's Hospital, Boston, MA, USA

Susan D. Emmett, M.D., M.P.H. Department of Otolaryngology—Head and Neck Surgery, College of Medicine; Department of Epidemiology, Fay W. Boozman College of Public Health; and Center for Hearing Health Access, University of Arkansas for Medical Sciences, Little Rock, AR, USA

Mana Espahbodi, M.D. Department of Otolaryngology—Head and Neck Surgery, University of Utah School of Medicine, Salt Lake City, UT, USA

Caleb J. Fan, M.D. Department of Neurotology, Michigan Ear Institute, St. John Providence Hospital and Medical Centers, Novi, MI, USA

J. Michael Fitzpatrick, Ph.D. Professor Emeritus of Computer Science, Computer Engineering, Electrical Engineering, Radiology, and Neurosurgery, Vanderbilt University, Nashville, TN, USA

Michael H. Freeman, M.D. Department of Otolaryngology—Head and Neck Surgery, Vanderbilt University Medical Center, Nashville, TN, USA

Wanda Fussell, M.D. Department of Neurotology, Michigan Ear Institute, St. John Providence Hospital and Medical Centers, Novi, MI, USA

Bruce J. Gantz, M.D. Department of Otolaryngology—Head and Neck Surgery, University of Iowa Hospitals and Clinics, Iowa City, IA, USA

Paul W. Gidley, M.D. Department of Head and Neck Surgery, UT MD Anderson Cancer Center, Houston, TX, USA

Michael B. Gluth, M.D. Ear Sciences Centre, University of Western Australia and Ear Science Institute Australia, Perth, WA, Australia

Justin S. Golub, M.D., M.S. Department of Otolaryngology—Head and Neck Surgery, Columbia University Vagelos College of Physicians and Surgeons, New York, NY, USA

NewYork-Presbyterian/Columbia University Irving Medical Center, New York, NY, USA

Jamie J. Van Gompel, M.D. Department of Neurologic Surgery, Mayo Clinic, Rochester, MN, USA

Samuel P. Gubbels, M.D. Department of Otolaryngology—Head and Neck Surgery, University of Colorado School of Medicine, Aurora, CO, USA

Richard K. Gurgel, M.D., M.S.C.I. Department of Otolaryngology—Head and Neck Surgery, University of Utah School of Medicine, Salt Lake City, UT, USA

Courtney D. Hall, P.T., Ph.D. James H. Quillen Veteran's Affairs Medical Center, Auditory and Vestibular Research Enhancement Award Program, Mountain Home, TN, USA

Department of Physical Therapy, East Tennessee State University, Johnson City, TN, USA

Ophir Handzel, M.D. Department of Otolaryngology—Head and Neck Surgery, Harvard Medical School, Boston, MA, USA

Marlan R. Hansen, M.D. Department of Otolaryngology—Head and Neck Surgery, University of Iowa Hospitals and Clinics, Iowa City, IA, USA

H. Ric Harnsberger, M.D. Department of Radiology, University of Utah, Salt Lake City, UT, USA

Jeffrey P. Harris, M.D., Ph.D. Department of Otolaryngology—Head and Neck Surgery, University of California San Diego Medical Center, San Diego, CA, USA

VA Healthcare System, San Diego, CA, USA

Michael S. Harris, M.D. Division of Otology and Neurotologic Skull Base Surgery, Department of Otolaryngology and Communication Sciences, Medical College of Wisconsin, Milwaukee, WI, USA

Jonathan L. Hatch, M.D. Department of Otolaryngology—Head and Neck Surgery, Medical University of South Carolina, Charleston, SC, USA

David S. Haynes, M.D., M.M.H.C. Department of Otolaryngology—Head and Neck Surgery, Vanderbilt University Medical Center, Nashville, TN, USA

Sukwoo Hong, M.D. International Fellow in Neurosurgery and Otorhinolaryngology, Department of Neurologic Surgery, Mayo Clinic, Rochester, MN, USA

Andrew T. Huang, M.D. Bobby R. Alford Department of Otolaryngology—Head and Neck Surgery, Baylor College of Medicine, Houston, TX, USA

Mikayla Huestis, M.D. Department of Otolaryngology—Head and Neck Surgery, Eastern Virginia Medical School, Norfolk, VA, USA

Jacob B. Hunter, M.D. Department of Otolaryngology—Head and Neck Surgery, Thomas Jefferson University School of Medicine, Philadelphia, PA, USA

Brandon Isaacson, M.D. Department of Otolaryngology—Head and Neck Surgery, University of Texas Southwestern Medical Center, Dallas, TX, USA

Kenneth C. Iverson, M.D. Division of Pediatric Otolaryngology, Department of Otolaryngology – Head and Neck Surgery, University of Kentucky Medical Center, Lexington, KY, USA

Robert Jackler, M.D. Department of Otolaryngology—Head and Neck Surgery, Stanford University, Stanford, CA, USA

Abraham Jacob, M.D. Center for Neurosciences, Tucson, AZ, USA

Jeffery Jacob, M.D. Department of Neurologic Surgery, Henry Ford Health System, Novi, MI, USA

Danny Jandali, M.D. Department of Otolaryngology—Head and Neck Surgery, Duly Health and Care, Glen Ellyn, IL, USA

Jeffrey R. Janus, M.D. Department of Otolaryngology—Head and Neck Surgery, Mayo Clinic, Jacksonville, FL, USA

Nicole T. Jiam, M.D. Department of Otolaryngology—Head and Neck Surgery, University of California San Francisco School of Medicine, San Francisco, CA, USA

Evan Jones, M.D. Bobby R. Alford Department of Otolaryngology—Head and Neck Surgery, Baylor College of Medicine, Houston, TX, USA

Sagar Kansara, M.D. Bobby R. Alford Department of Otolaryngology—Head and Neck Surgery, Baylor College of Medicine, Houston, TX, USA

Emily Kay-Rivest, M.D. Department of Otolaryngology—Head and Neck Surgery, McGill University, Montreal, QC, Canada

Elizabeth A. Kelly, M.D. Department of Otolaryngology, Boys Town National Research Hospital, Omaha, NE, USA

Bradley W. Kesser, M.D. Department of Otolaryngology—Head and Neck Surgery, University of Virginia School of Medicine, Charlottesville, VA, USA

Rihan Khan, M.D. Department of Radiology, Dartmouth-Hitchcock Medical Center, Lebanon, NH, USA

Daniel E. Killeen, M.D. Department of Otolaryngology—Head and Neck Surgery, University of Texas Southwestern Medical Center, Dallas, TX, USA

Arvind Kumar, M.D. Department of Otolaryngology—Head and Neck Surgery, University of Illinois – Chicago, Chicago, IL, USA

Department of Otolaryngology—Head and Neck Surgery, Northwestern University, Chicago, IL, USA

Robert F. Labadie, M.D., Ph.D. Department of Otolaryngology—Head and Neck Surgery, Medical University of South Carolina (MUSC), Charleston, SC, USA

Kenneth H. Lee, M.D., Ph.D. Department of Otolaryngology—Head and Neck Surgery, University of Texas Southwestern Medical Center, Dallas, TX, USA

Samuel C. Levine, M.D. Department of Otolaryngology—Head and Neck Surgery, University of Minnesota, Minneapolis, MN, USA

Charles J. Limb, M.D. Department of Otolaryngology—Head and Neck Surgery, University of California San Francisco School of Medicine, San Francisco, CA, USA

Kenny F. Lin, M.D. Department of Otolaryngology—Head and Neck Surgery, Houston Methodist Hospital, Houston, TX, USA

Nathan R. Lindquist, M.D. Bobby R. Alford Department of Otolaryngology—Head and Neck Surgery, Baylor College of Medicine, Houston, TX, USA

Michael J. Link, M.D. Department of Neurological Surgery, Mayo Clinic, Rochester, MN, USA

Philip D. Littlefield, M.D. Otology & Neurotology, Sharp Rees-Stealy Medical Group, San Diego, CA, USA

Benjamin Lovin, M.D. Department of Otolaryngology—Head and Neck Surgery, University of Virginia College of Medicine, Charlottesville, VA, USA

Lawrence R. Lustig, M.D. Department of Otolaryngology—Head and Neck Surgery, Columbia University Irving Medical Center, New York, NY, USA

Alexander Malone, M.D. Florida ENT and Allergy, Tampa, FL, USA

Nauman F. Manzoor, M.D. Department of Otolaryngology—Head and Neck Surgery, Virginia Commonwealth University, Richmond, VA, USA

John P. Marinelli, M.D. Department of Otorhinolaryngology—Head and Neck Surgery, Mayo Clinic, Rochester, MN, USA

R. Mark Wiet, M.D. Otology, Neurotology, and Lateral Skull Base Surgery, Neurotology and Skull Base Surgery, Northwestern Medicine Regional Medical Group, Central Dupage Hospital, Winfield, IL, USA

Landon Massoth, M.D. Department of Otolaryngology—Head & Neck Surgery, University of Oklahoma Health Sciences Center, Oklahoma City, OK, USA

Bradford J. May, Ph.D. Department of Otolaryngology—Head and Neck Surgery, Johns Hopkins University School of Medicine, Baltimore, MD, USA

Devin L. McCaslin, Ph.D. Department of Otolaryngology—Head and Neck Surgery, Division of Audiology, University of Michigan, Ann Arbor, MI, USA

John T. McElveen Jr, M.D. Carolina Ear & Hearing Clinic, PC, Raleigh, NC, USA

Carolina Ear Research Institute, Raleigh, NC, USA

Sean O. McMenomey, M.D. Department of Otolaryngology—Head and Neck Surgery, New York University School of Medicine, NYU Langone Health, New York, NY, USA

Beth N. McNulty, M.D. Division of Otology, Neurotology, and Cranial Base Surgery, Department of Otolaryngology—Head and Neck Surgery, University of Kentucky Medical Center, Lexington, KY, USA

Theodore R. McRackan, M.D., M.S.C.R. Department of Otolaryngology—Head and Neck Surgery, Medical University of South Carolina, Charleston, SC, USA

Cliff A. Megerian, M.D. Department of Otolaryngology—Head and Neck Surgery, University Hospitals Cleveland Medical Center, Cleveland, OH, USA

Rahul Mehta, M.D., M.S. University of Mississippi Medical Center, Jackson, MS, USA

Aaron C. Moberly, M.D. Division of Otology and Neurotology, Department of Otolaryngology—Head and Neck Surgery, Vanderbilt University Medical Center, Nashville, TN, USA

Peter J. Morone, M.D., M.S.C.I. Department of Neurological Surgery, Vanderbilt University Medical Center, Nashville, TN, USA

Sarah E. Mowry, M.D. Department of Otolaryngology—Head and Neck Surgery, University Hospitals Cleveland Medical Center, Cleveland, OH, USA

Albert Mudry, M.D., Ph.D. Department of Otolaryngology—Head & Neck Surgery, Stanford University School of Medicine, Stanford, CA, USA

Thomas Muhleman, M.D. Ascentis Healthcare, Kansas City, KS, USA

Ashley M. Nassiri, M.D., M.B.A. Department of Otolaryngology—Head and Neck Surgery, University of Colorado School of Medicine, Aurora, CO, USA

Department of Otorhinolaryngology—Head and Neck Surgery, Mayo Clinic, Rochester, MN, USA

Brian A. Neff, M.D. Department of Otolaryngology—Head and Neck Surgery, Mayo Clinic, Rochester, MN, USA

James L. Netterville, M.D. Department of Otolaryngology—Head and Neck Surgery, Vanderbilt University Medical Center, Nashville, TN, USA

Christopher Ian Newberry, M.D. Department of Otolaryngology—Head and Neck Surgery, University of Utah School of Medicine, Salt Lake City, UT, USA

Rhode Island ENT Physicians, Inc., Brown University, Providence, RI, USA

Brendan P. O'Connell, M.D. Charlotte Eye, Ear, Nose and Throat, Charlotte, NC, USA

Steven R. Otto, M.A. House Clinic and House Ear Institute, Los Angeles, CA, USA

Lorne S. Parnes, M.D. Department of Otolaryngology—Head and Neck Surgery, Schulich School of Medicine and Dentistry, Western University, London Health Sciences Centre-University Hospital, London, ON, Canada

Akash Patel, M.D. Department of Neurosurgery, Baylor College of Medicine, Houston, TX, USA

Neil S. Patel, M.D. Department of Otolaryngology—Head and Neck Surgery, University of Utah, Salt Lake City, UT, USA

Stanley Pelosi, M.D. Department of Otolaryngology—Head and Neck Surgery, Long Island Jewish Medical Center, New Hyde Park, NY, USA

Angela Peng, M.D. Bobby R. Alford Department of Otolaryngology—Head and Neck Surgery, Baylor College of Medicine, Houston, TX, USA

Myles L. Pensak, M.D. Department of Otolaryngology—Head and Neck Surgery, University of Cincinnati College of Medicine, Cincinnati, OH, USA

Enrique R. Perez, M.D. Department of Otolaryngology—Head and Neck Surgery, Icahn School of Medicine at Mount Sinai, New York, NY, USA

Archana Podury, M.D. Department of Otolaryngology—Head and Neck Surgery, University of California, San Diego, San Diego, CA, USA

Dennis S. Poe, M.D., Ph.D. Department of Otolaryngology—Head and Neck Surgery, Boston Children's Hospital, Harvard Medical School, Boston, MA, USA

Alicia M. Quesnel, M.D. Department of Otolaryngology—Head and Neck Surgery, Harvard Medical School, Boston, MA, USA

William J. Riggs, Au.D. Department of Otolaryngology—Head and Neck Surgery, The Ohio State University Wexner Medical Center, Columbus, OH, USA

Alejandro Rivas, M.D. Department of Otolaryngology—Head and Neck Surgery, Case Western Reserve University/University Hospitals Cleveland Medical Center, Cleveland, OH, USA

Daniel S. Roberts, M.D., Ph.D. Division of Otolaryngology—Head and Neck Surgery, University of Connecticut School of Medicine, Farmington, CT, USA

Joseph P. Roche, M.D. Department of Otolaryngology—Head and Neck Surgery, University of Cincinnati, Cincinnati, OH, USA

Douglas S. Ruhl, M.D. Otology & Neurotology, Department of Otolaryngology—Head & Neck Surgery, Madigan Army Medical Center, Tacoma, WA, USA

Robert Saadi, M.D. Department of Otolaryngology—Head and Neck Surgery, University of Arkansas for Medical Sciences, Little Rock, AR, USA

Hitomi Sakano, M.D., Ph.D. Department of Otolaryngology—Head and Neck Surgery, University of Texas Southwestern Medical Center, Dallas, TX, USA

Peter L. Santa Maria, M.D., Ph.D. Department of Otolaryngology—Head and Neck Surgery, University of Pittsburgh, Pittsburgh, PA, USA

Firas K. Sbeih, M.D. University of Central Florida College of Medicine, Orlando, FL, USA

Lisa A. Schimmenti, M.D. Department of Clinical Genomics, Mayo Clinic, Rochester, MN, USA

Christopher A. Schutt, M.D. Department of Neurotology, Michigan Ear Institute, Henry Ford Health System, Novi, MI, USA

Zachary G. Schwam, M.D. Department of Otolaryngology—Head and Neck Surgery, Icahn School of Medicine at Mount Sinai, New York, NY, USA

Marc S. Schwartz, M.D. Department of Neurological Surgery, University of California—San Diego, San Diego, CA, USA

Michael D. Seidman, M.D. Otologic/Neurotologic/Skull Base Surgery, Wellness and Integrative Medicine, Advent Health, Orlando, FL, USA

Otolaryngology—Head and Neck Surgery, University of Central Florida, Orlando, FL, USA

Department of Otolaryngology—Head and Neck Surgery, University of South Florida, Tampa, FL, USA

Maroun T. Semaan, M.D. Department of Otolaryngology—Head and Neck Surgery, University Hospitals Cleveland Medical Center, Cleveland, OH, USA

Rosh K. Sethi, M.D., M.P.H. Department of Otolaryngology—Head and Neck Surgery, Harvard Medical School, Boston, MA, USA

Dana Farber Cancer Center, Boston, MA, USA

Clough Shelton, M.D. Department of Otolaryngology—Head and Neck Surgery, University of Utah School of Medicine, Salt Lake City, UT, USA

Neil T. Shepard, Ph.D. Department of Otolaryngology—Head and Neck Surgery, Division of Audiology, University of Michigan, Ann Arbor, MI, USA

Yuki Shinya, M.D., Ph.D. Research Fellow in Neurosurgery and Otorhinolaryngology, Department of Neurologic Surgery, Mayo Clinic, Rochester, MN, USA

Tanya Singh, M.D. University of Central Florida College of Medicine, Orlando, FL, USA

Jeffrey P. Staab, M.D. Departments of Psychiatry and Psychology, and Otorhinolaryngology—Head and Neck Surgery, Mayo Clinic, Rochester, MN, USA

Hinrich Staecker, M.D., Ph.D. Department of Otolaryngology—Head and Neck Surgery, University of Kansas Health System, Kansas City, KS, USA

Barry Strasnick, M.D. Department of Otolaryngology—Head and Neck Surgery, Eastern Virginia Medical School, Norfolk, VA, USA

Lara E. Strotheide, Au.D. Department of Otolaryngology—Head and Neck Surgery, Emory University Medical Center, Atlanta, GA, USA

Daniel Q. Sun, M.D. Department of Otolaryngology—Head and Neck Surgery, University of Cincinnati, Cincinnati, OH, USA

Alex D. Sweeney, M.D. Department of Otolaryngology—Head and Neck Surgery, Baylor College of Medicine, Houston, TX, USA

Hiroki Takeda, M.D. Department of Otolaryngology—Head and Neck Surgery, University of Colorado School of Medicine, Aurora, CO, USA

Andrew J. Thomas, M.D. Department of Otolaryngology—Head and Neck Surgery, University of Utah School of Medicine, Salt Lake City, UT, USA

J. Thomas Roland Jr, M.D. Department of Otolaryngology—Head and Neck Surgery, NYU Langone Health, New York, NY, USA

Reid C. Thompson, M.D. Department of Neurological Surgery, Vanderbilt University Medical Center, Nashville, TN, USA

Roksolyana Tourkevich, M.D. Center for Neurosciences, Tucson, AZ, USA

Henri Traboulsi, M.D. Texas Children's Hospital Department of Surgery, Division of Otolaryngology, Houston, TX, USA

Bobby R. Alford Department of Otolaryngology—Head and Neck Surgery, Baylor College of Medicine, Houston, TX, USA

Kiley Trott, M.D. Department of Otolaryngology—Head and Neck Surgery, Thomas Jefferson University School of Medicine, Philadelphia, PA, USA

Betty S. Tsai Do, M.D. The Permanente Medical Group, Kaiser Permanente, Walnut Creek, CA, USA

Debara L. Tucci, M.D., M.S., M.B.A. National Institute of Deafness and other Communication Disorders, National Institutes of Health, Bethesda, MD, USA

Omar Ungar, M.D. Department of Otolaryngology—Head and Neck Surgery, Harvard Medical School, Boston, MA, USA

Esther X. Vivas, M.D. Department of Otolaryngology—Head and Neck Surgery, Emory University Medical Center, Atlanta, GA, USA

Peter Volsky, M.D. Department of Otolaryngology—Head and Neck Surgery, Eastern Virginia Medical School, Norfolk, VA, USA

Teresa G. Vos, M.D. Department of Otolaryngology—Head and Neck Surgery, University of North Carolina, Chapel Hill, NC, USA

J. Walter Kutz Jr, M.D. Department of Otolaryngology—Head and Neck Surgery, University of Texas Southwestern Medical Center, Dallas, TX, USA

George B. Wanna, M.D., M.H.C.M. Department of Otolaryngology—Head and Neck Surgery, Icahn School of Medicine at Mount Sinai, New York, NY, USA

Bryan K. Ward, M.D. Department of Otolaryngology—Head and Neck Surgery, Johns Hopkins University School of Medicine, Baltimore, MD, USA

Athanasia Warnecke, M.D., Ph.D. Department of Otorhinolaryngology, Hannover Medical School, Hannover, Germany

De'Andre A. Warren, M.D. Department of Otolaryngology—Head and Neck Surgery, Case Western Reserve University/University Hospitals Cleveland Medical Center, Cleveland, OH, USA

Peter A. Weisskopf, M.D. Division of Otology and Neurotology, Departments of Otolaryngology and Neurosurgery, Mayo Clinic, Phoenix, AZ, USA

D. Bradley Welling, M.D., Ph.D. Department of Otolaryngology—Head and Neck Surgery, Massachusetts Eye and Ear, Harvard Medical School, Boston, MA, USA

Department of Otolaryngology—Head and Neck Surgery, Harvard Medical School, Boston, MA, USA

Stephen J. Wetmore, M.D., M.B.A. Department of Otolaryngology—Head and Neck Surgery, West Virginia University School of Medicine, Morgantown, WV, USA

Cameron C. Wick, M.D. Department of Otolaryngology—Head and Neck Surgery, University Hospitals Cleveland Medical Center, Cleveland, OH, USA

Richard Wiet, M.D. Department of Otolaryngology—Head and Neck Surgery, Rush University Medical Center, Chicago, IL, USA

Clinical Otolaryngology and Neurosurgery, Feinberg School of Medicine, Northwestern University, Chicago, IL, USA

David Wilde, M.D. Bobby R. Alford Department of Otolaryngology—Head and Neck Surgery, Baylor College of Medicine, Houston, TX, USA

Eric P. Wilkinson, M.D. Idaho Ear Clinic, Meridian, ID, USA

Peng You, M.D. Department of Otolaryngology—Head and Neck Surgery, Schulich School of Medicine and Dentistry, Western University, London Health Sciences Centre-University Hospital, London, ON, Canada

Samy Youssef, M.D., Ph.D., M.Sc. Department of Neurosurgery, University of Colorado Anschutz Medical Campus, Aurora, CO, USA

Part I

Scientific Foundations

1 The History of Modern Otologic and Neurotologic Surgery

Albert Mudry

The introduction of anesthesia with ether and chloroform in the 1840s and the setting up of asepsis (sterilization), antisepsis (disinfection), and arterial clamps in the 1860s opened up a completely new surgical era with the possibility to operate for more than only a few minutes with fewer surgical complications. In parallel, medication for pain relief became synthetized, thus rendering post-operative care more successful and affordable for the patients [1]. It was the beginning of safer and more effective surgery, allowing operative otology to definitively engage in its modern development from the 1870s and finally enlarge its field of expertise in the surrounding structures since the 1960s. Friedrich Bezold (Fig. 1.1), who inspired George Shambaugh Jr. (Fig. 1.2), the father of this book, wrote in 1906: "Our therapeutic actions are mostly of surgical nature as in most of the well-developed specialties. But the danger of an incompetent operator who does not know the variations is much greater here than in any other region […] It requires, therefore, years of practice to gain an accurate judgment and use the many points gained by the examination, which is equally true of the many delicate operations that have to be performed in this way" [4]. The roots of ear surgery can be found in antiquity [5]. Its progressive evolution is related to different factors, notably the development of instruments improving the quality of vision in the ear, the growth of knowledge regarding ear anatomy and pathology, the invention of various small surgical instruments, and the ingenuity of man [6]. It is impossible to describe the modern history of surgical otology and neurotology in a few pages. Only the great steps, exemplified by the main actual operations, will be presented [7].

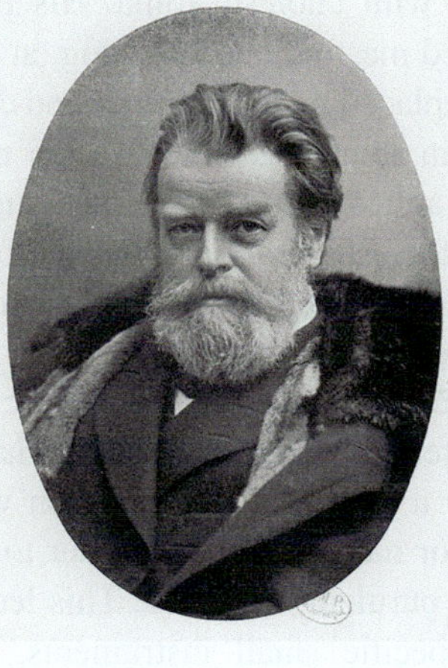

Fig. 1.1 Friedrich Bezold [2]. (Courtesy of Albert Mudry MD, PhD)

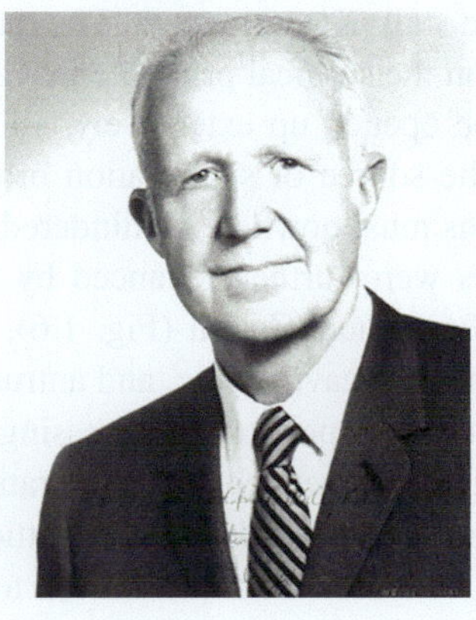

Fig. 1.2 George Shambaugh Jr. (Reprinted with permission from Rubin W. George Shambaugh [3])

Mastoidectomy

In the 1850s, surgery of the ear was limited to the auricle (trauma and tumors), artificial tympanic membrane perforation and the first attempts to develop a tympanostomy tube, and extraction of foreign bodies and polyps. The number of

A. Mudry (✉)
Department of Otolaryngology—Head & Neck Surgery, Stanford University School of Medicine, Stanford, CA, USA
e-mail: amudry@stanford.edu

A. D. Sweeney et al. (eds.), *Haynes-Glasscock-Shambaugh Surgery of the Ear*, https://doi.org/10.1007/978-3-032-18264-7_1

instruments was thus limited. Nevertheless, some surgeons started to surgically open the mastoid area in cases of inflammation of the mastoid area and the internal part of the ear. William Wilde described his postauricular incision known as "Wilde's incision" [8]. Another was Anton von Tröltsch who wrote: we "should again draw attention to a discredited and forgotten operation, the opening of the mastoid, and help to give it the place it deserves in surgery" [9]. In 1873, Hermann Schwartze (Fig. 1.3) published an extensive description of his experience in the treatment of mastoid disease [11]. He laid down clear indications for surgery: mastoid infection which had failed to settle by conventional anti-inflammatory means within a week; postaural, external ear canal or cervical abscess formation; postaural fistulae and chronic middle ear suppuration with cholesteatoma. His principle was to open the diseased mastoid antrum using, at first, a trephine. This was later replaced by the hammer and chisel (the gouge was introduced in about 1890). His earlier mastoidectomies were "funnelled antrostomies," the idea being to always have a direct vision of the surgical field. Later, a full cortical mastoidectomy was introduced but it soon became apparent that, although the operation was good for acute mastoiditis, the original claims for the treatment of chronic middle ear disease and cholesteatoma were not substantiated. Thus, there grew a need for a more radical operation with notably the removal of one or more ossicles in order to bring about the cessation of the purulent otorrhoea. This led to the production of some specific small instruments. In 1889, Ernst Küster (Fig. 1.4) [13] recommended the removal of the posterior meatal wall and Ernst von Bergmann [14], the removal of the outer attic wall. Küster wrote: "The rational treatment must be based on the surgical principle that a diseased bony cavity should be opened up extensively, all diseased tissue removed, and the source of suppuration brought clearly to the light. The pus must nowhere be hindered in its outflow." These principles were further advanced by Ludwig Stacke (Fig. 1.5) and Emmanuel Zaufal (Fig. 1.6), who sought to combine the tympanic cavity, attic, and antrum into one cavity which facilitated inspection and dressing. There was no fundamental difference between their operations except that Stacke [17] worked backwards from the attic to the antrum and Zaufal [18] forwards from the antrum to the attic. Otto Körner suggested a modification of the radical operation that consisted of removing the upper posterior wall of the auditory canal and the outer wall of the antrum, leaving some of the outer attic wall in order to preserve the malleus and incus. Schwartze, in 1893, also extended his own simple mastoidectomy to include removal of the posterior and superior meatal walls and middle ear contents. The set of instruments largely expended to complete such an operation, and the operation room was specifically arranged. One of the problems with the earlier cases of radical mastoidectomy was that after healing, the cavity became inaccessible from the ear canal. To overcome this, the meatoplasty was devised by

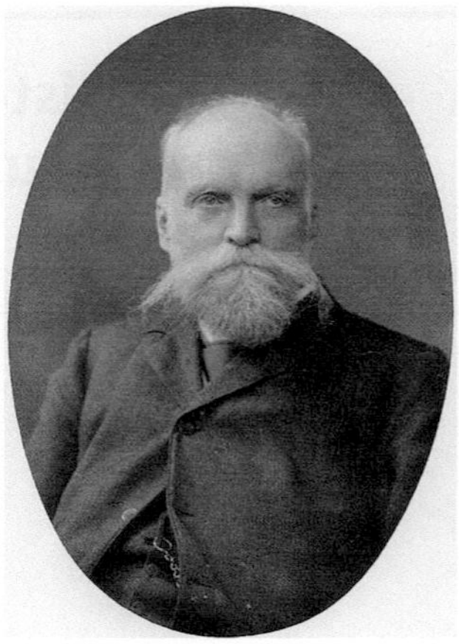

Fig. 1.3 Hermann Schwartze [10]. (Courtesy of Albert Mudry MD, PhD)

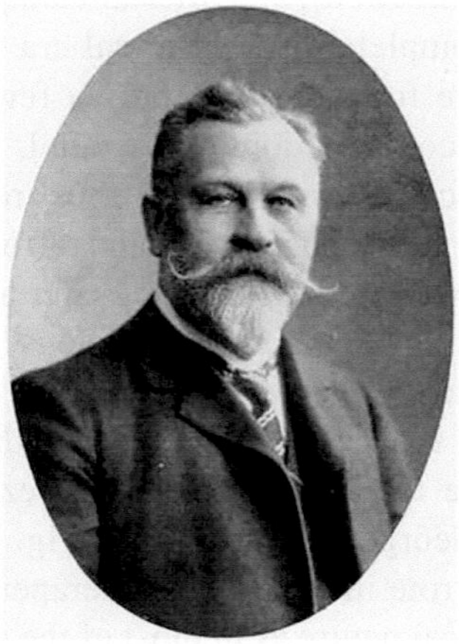

Fig. 1.4 Ernst Küster [12]. (Courtesy of Albert Mudry MD, PhD)

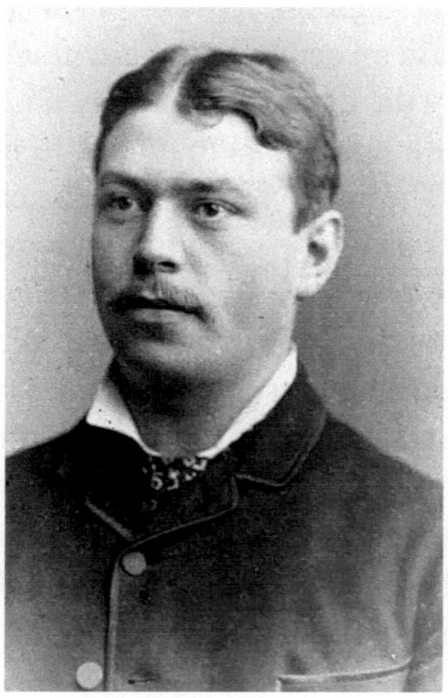

Fig. 1.5 Ludwig Stacke [15]. (Courtesy of Albert Mudry MD, PhD)

Stacke, Schwartze, Rudolf Panse (Fig. 1.7), and others. The enlarged meatus gave good access to the cavity and enabled closure of the postaural wound by primary suture. Before meatoplasty, it was quite common for a deliberate postaural

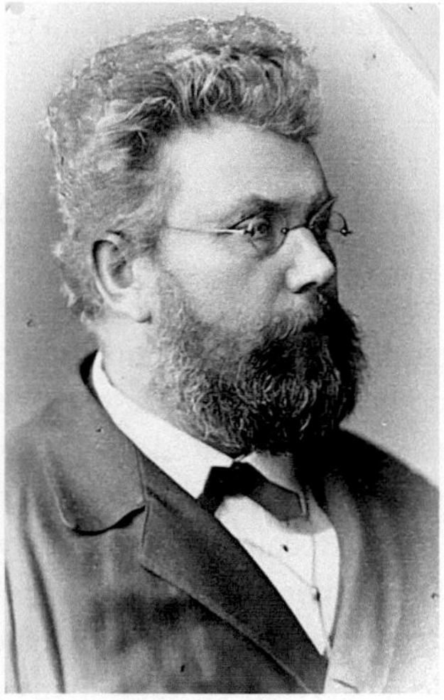

Fig. 1.6 Emmanuel Zaufal [16]. (Courtesy of Albert Mudry MD, PhD)

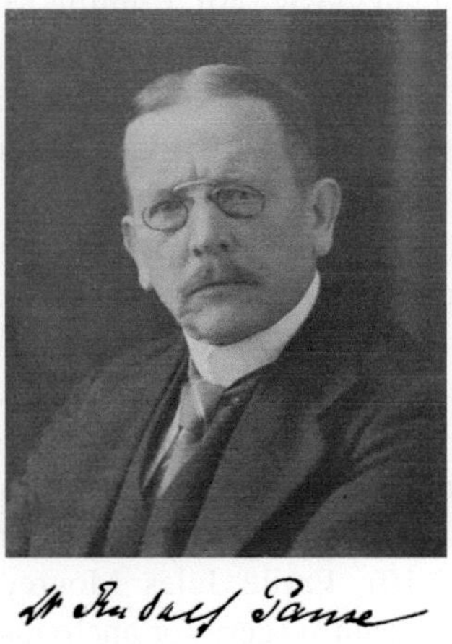

Fig. 1.7 Rudolf Panse. (Reprinted with permission from Zange J [19])

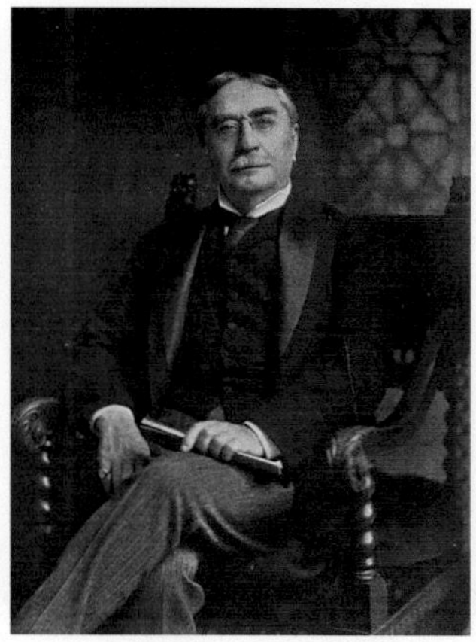

Fig. 1.8 Daniel Benett St John Roosa. (Reprinted with permission from Jackler RK et al. [28])

fistula to be created to facilitate dressing of the mastoid cavity. There followed a period of a few years during which time many ears were automatically subjected to the radical operation and patients suffered from often unnecessary hearing loss. The same men who first advocated the radical procedure were themselves the first to attempt to save the ossicles and hence the hearing. They thus initiated the phase of conservatism aimed at the preservation of the middle ear function in those cases with only atticoantral disease and otherwise healthy middle ears. The incisions of these early mastoid operations were mostly postauricular. Fritz Thies claimed that the endaural approach to radical mastoidectomy was his invention [20] but the earliest record of an endaural incision is credited to Johannes Kessel in 1885 [21]. In 1910, Gustav Bondy [22] described his endomeatal atticoantrostomy, the "Bondy's operation", which became largely used in the first part of the twentieth century. It resembles that of the classical radical mastoidectomy, but it differs, in that the ossicles and intact pars tensa of the tympanic membrane are left in place. At the beginning of the twentieth century, the great lines of the various types of mastoid surgery were described and the first foot-drills were introduced, notably by William Macewen to prepare his transmastoidal route to the brain [23]. They were in relation with the encountered pathology, notably acute mastoiditis, cholesteatoma, and chronic otitis media. It is at this moment that the first books dealing exclusively with mastoid and ear surgery are published. Frederick Whiting explains why: "The great interest in the importance of the modern mastoid operation appear to furnish adequate reason for the elaboration of the subject by monograph, since, owing to lack of space, the most voluminous of recent textbooks does not attempt the minutiae of detail which are indispensable to the beginner in his lack of experience; such special departments of a specialty are, in fact, beyond the capacity of any work not encyclopedic in its character" [24]. By the 1930s, the essential indications for mastoid surgery were established. In the 1950s, canal wall-up techniques were notably introduced by Claus Jansen to preserve anatomy and function as much as possible [25].

Myringoplasty

Promotion of healing of a perforation in the tympanic membrane by cautery destruction of the edges of the perforation was first mentioned in 1848 by Wilde [26]. Tröltsch proposed to use zinc powder in 1862 [27]. It was Daniel Benett St John Roosa (Fig. 1.8) who promoted the technique with silver nitrate in 1873 [29]. Trichloracetic acid was introduced by Okuneff in 1895 [30]. This cautery technique continued to be episodically used during the twentieth century. At the same time various artificial tympanic membranes, like a "paper patch," were proposed, notably by Joseph Toynbee (Fig. 1.9) [32]. The surgical repair of perforation of the tympanic membrane was first described in 1878 as a "myringoplasty" by Emil Berthold, who used a thick skin graft from the forearm after having previously made "free the margin

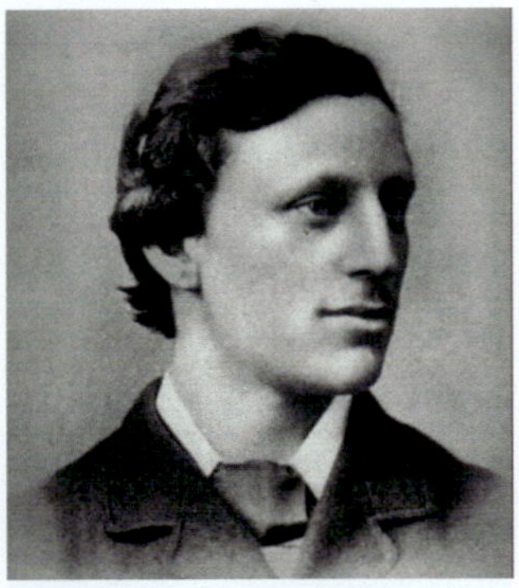

Fig. 1.9 Joseph Toynbee. (Reprinted with permission from Mudry A [31])

around the perforation" [33]. At approximately the same time, Edward Talbot Ely, better known for his interest in the surgery of prominent auricles [34], described an operation where "the edges of the perforation were freshened by scarping, and a piece of skin laid over it" [35]. A controversy originated about the priority of this operation. Berthold practiced this technique at least for 10 years [36], but this operation remained confidential and was finally condemned in 1902 [37]. Myringoplasty means surgery confined to the tympanic membrane itself. There is no manipulation of the ossicles, and the drum head is not lifted from its position in the ear canal. At the same time, in cases of chronic ear discharge, Kessel proposed to cut out the remnants of the tympanic membrane and to take out the malleus and incus to improve the power of regeneration of the tympanic membrane. He remarked that in one patient, the healing process of the tympanic membrane, which was cut out four times, covered the stapes, and the hearing was improved. In the contralateral ear, Kessel kept the anterior part of the tympanic membrane, which he used to cover a part of the middle ear [21].

Mobilization and Extraction of the Stapes

Confronted with the anchylosis of the stapes, Kessel demonstrated in pigeons, in 1876, that opening of the oval window did not necessarily result in destructive damage to the inner ear as was generally feared. He proposed to extract the stapes (later named stapedectomy) to improve hearing in these cases [38]. Because the results were not good, Kessel went a step further, in 1878, in mobilizing the stapes by applying pressure to its head in various directions [39]. At the end of the nineteenth century, many otologists were practising stapes mobilization. In 1888, Emile Boucheron reported 60 mobilizations, with the best results in those cases with early ankylosis [40]. Camille Miot reported, in 1890, 200 stapes mobilizations [41], with results considered as good. There were no deaths or labyrinthine complications in his series. Clarence Blake described a case in 1892 [42] where he had removed the stapes, which resulted in an improvement in the patient's hearing and in 1893 Frederick Lafayette Jack reported a series of cases of extraction of the stapes with specifically designed instruments [43]. Kessel's mobilization was practised by many other surgeons and most of the results, which were not all reported, were disappointing and sometimes disastrous, not only to hearing but also to life. This prompted Adam Politzer (Fig. 1.10), Emile Jules Moure, and Vincenze Cozzolino to condemn surgery for anchylosis of the stapes in 1894 [45]. The situation was made worse in 1900 when Friedrich Siebenmann [46] and Ricardo Botey [47] rejected all forms of surgery for deafness [48].

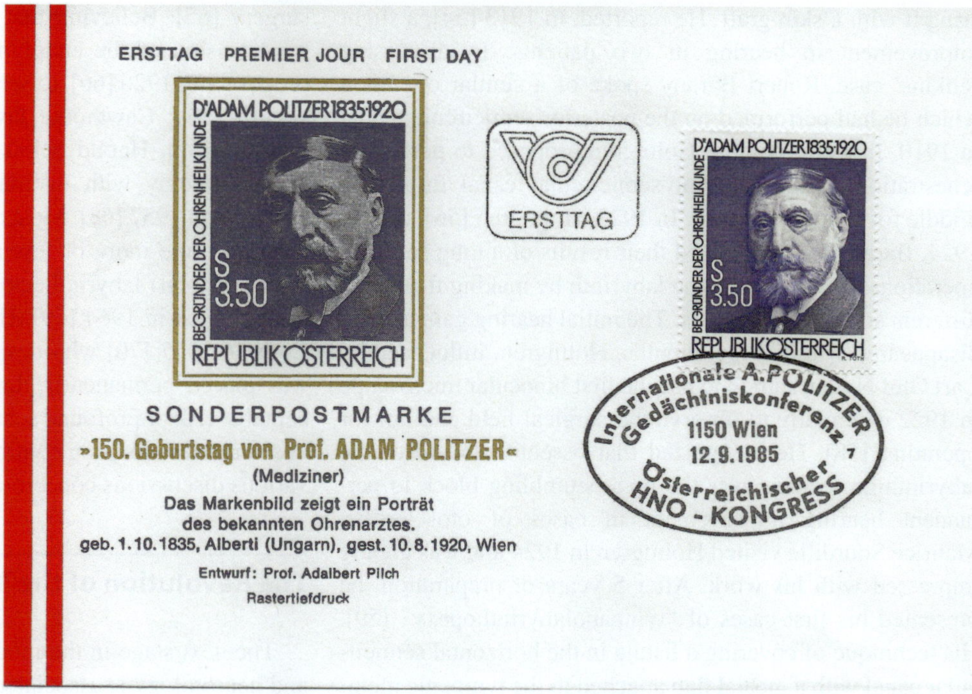

Fig. 1.10 Adam Politzer portrait on a first day cover letter in 1985. (Reprinted with permission from Mudry A and Young JR. [44])

Drainage of Otologic Brain Abscesses

At the same time that advances in surgery of the temporal bone were being made, attention was being successfully directed to the management of the intracranial complications of mastoid infection, which were predominant causes of mortality and morbidity of mastoiditis. Meningitis and subdural abscess were lethal but brain abscess, extradural abscess and lateral sinus thrombosis were conditions that were becoming amenable to surgery. Ernst von Bergmann proposed an extradural subtemporal approach through the middle fossa to approach brain abscess and Macewen a mastoidal route at the end of the nineteenth century. William Arbuthnot Lane [49] and Charles Ballance [50] established a treatment of sinus thrombosis in ligating the internal jugular vein at the turn of the 1890s. During the early part of the twentieth century, there was some controversy as to whether intracranial pus should be drained via a mastoidectomy or separately via a craniotomy. In general, these abscesses were drained via the mastoid, the technique being to follow the discharging tract intracranially and to open the abscess cavity with a trocar and cannula. It was the first step of extension of surgical otology in its surrounding structures. Körner was particularly interested in this topic and described the various ways of drainage of these abscesses [51]. "Suppuration in the temporal bone," wrote Ballance in 1919, "does not differ from suppuration in other bones, and it is only natural that progress in its treatment should have been in part the work of those in practice as general surgeons and in part the work of such aural surgeons who, though devoting themselves to special practice, are inspired with the spirit of surgery" [52]. This is the first step where the otologist meets and shares competence with the neurosurgeon. Despite the benefits of the first antibacterial therapy, otitis media remained the most frequent cause of brain abscess in the 1940s. Thereafter, with the production of new antibiotics, the incidence decreased abruptly.

Fenestration of the Semicircular Canal

In the first part of the twentieth century, stapes surgery and more generally surgery for deafness continued to remain condemned by the majority of otologists. Nevertheless, a number of chance observations were made which encouraged further attempts to relieve deafness in otosclerosis without touching the stapes. Karl Adolf Passow, in 1897, made a window in the promontory and covered it with the tympanic membrane [53]. His patient noted a slight improvement in hearing. Ballance related an earlier case in which he had discovered a fistula into the lateral semicircular canal during the course of mastoid surgery. He covered it with a skin graft and was gratified that not only was the patient free of vertigo but also that there had been an improvement in hearing. He attempted to repeat the process in other cases but never had the same outcome. George Jenkins believed that otosclerosis was caused by hypersecretion of labyrinthine fluids and thus attempted to decompress the labyrinth by making a window into the lateral semicircular canal and covering it with a skin graft. He reported, in 1913 [54], a slight improvement in hearing in two patients. In discussing Jenkins' case, Robert Barany spoke of a similar operation which he had performed on the posterior semicircular canal in 1910. In 1917, Gunnar Holmgren proposed to perform a fenestration of the superior semicircular canal through a middle fossa approach [55]. In 1923, Holmgren [56], and, in 1924, Barany [57] published their results of a long series of operations to decompress the labyrinth by making fistulae in different semicircular canals. The initial hearing gain usually disappeared within a few months. Holmgren, influenced by Carl Olof Nylen, started to use the first binocular microscope in 1922 essentially to observe the surgical field and not for operating [58]. He recognized that osseous closure of the labyrinthine window was the great stumbling block to permanent hearing improvement in cases of otosclerosis. Maurice Sourdille visited Holmgren in 1924 and was greatly impressed with his work. After 5 years of preparation, he presented his first cases of "tympanolabyrinthopexy" [59]. His technique of covering a fistula in the horizontal semicircular canal with a meatal flap attached to the tympanic membrane was initially performed in three stages, later reduced to two, in order to avoid infection and labyrinthitis. Julius Lempert was inspired by the technique which he followed closely but performed the operation endaurally, with an ophthalmic binocular loupe and in one stage. He called this the "fenestration operation" and published his first successful results in 1938 [60]. Lempert found that the incus was not needed, as Sourdille had insisted, "to carry sound across the mobile incus from the tympanic membrane to the horizontal canal window" and by removing it he was able to create a larger fenestra, which he called the "fenestra nov-ovalis" as it resembled in size the oval window which it replaced. In 1938, Shambaugh Jr. became Lempert's pupil. He chose from the outset to use the binocular-operating microscope and self-retaining retractor allowing continuous irrigation and suction in order to endochondralize the fenestra and to remove all bone dust particles [61]. These two factors greatly reduced the tendency toward osteogenic closure of the fenestra. This operation became outdated at the end of the 1950s.

Surgery for Menière's Disease

In 1874, Jean Martin Charcot put forward the idea that perhaps transection of the VIII nerve might arrest the symptoms of vertigo [62]. Robert Henry Parry reported the first successful intracranial section of the VIII nerve in 1904. For the first time, he used the middle fossa approach to the cerebellopontine angle and the internal auditory canal. The same year, William Milligan [63] and Richard Lake [64] opened the horizontal semicircular canal and vestibule through the mastoid. Walter Eduard Dandy was a great supporter of this surgery [65]. Believing that Menière's disease was due to hypertension of the endolymphatic sac, George Portmann proposed, in 1926 [66], to surgically open the endolymphatic sac. In 1947, Cawthorne favored horizontal canal labyrinthotomy [67]. Harald Schuknecht introduced oval window labyrinthotomy with instillation of streptomycin into the vestibule in 1957 [68]. Most of these techniques used a transmastoid route more or less associated with a translabyrinthine (or total) labyrinthectomy. Sacculotomy was initiated by Izak Fick in 1964 [69]. His idea was extended by Thane Cody in 1967 [70] who designed a stainless steel tacit that was placed permanently through the footplate with unacceptable risk of profound sensorineural deafness. These various surgeries are often controversial and remain a subject of various discussions concerning their potential success.

The Revolution of the Microscope

The next stage in the modern history of surgical otology and neurotology is associated with the radical change in the management of acute disease brought about by the introduction of antibiotics and the reappraisal of surgical techniques made possible by the use of the Zeiss OPMI 1 operating microscope and the general use of the electrical drill in the 1950s. It had a revolutionary impact on surgery of the ear. In 1959, Shambaugh Jr., wrote: "No branch of medical science has been altered more profoundly, advanced more rapidly and benefited so greatly by sulfonamide and antibiotic therapy than has surgery of the ear. In the short span of two decades fatalities from otitis media and its intracranial complications have been reduced tenfold and the simple mastoid operation for acute suppuration has become a rarity, while reconstructive operations on the hearing mechanism have begun to write a brilliant chapter in the advancement of medical science" [71]. William House (Fig. 1.11) adds: "I can remember taking 4 or 5 hours to do a radical mastoid with

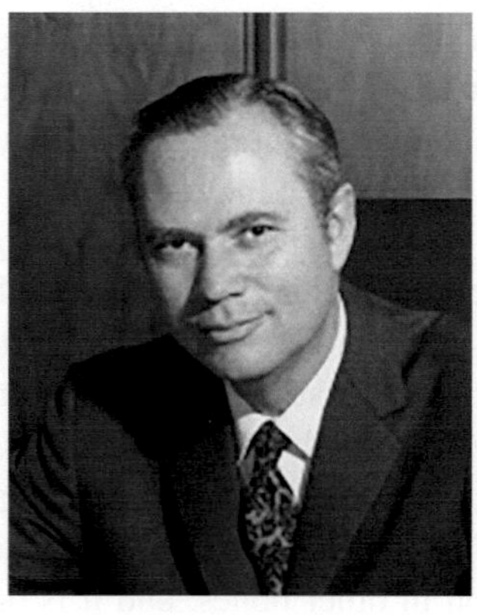

Fig. 1.11 William House. (Reprinted with permission from Berliner KI [72])

the headlight and loops, the two hands on the drill, and the squirt and suck technique, which was the way that mastoid surgery was done. But times were changing" [73]. In the 1960s, an air-driven hand piece replaced the conventional, belt-driven hand piece, giving more flexibility in the used speed, allowing each step of a mastoidectomy to be done with different sizes of drills. These changes allowed the passage from "normal surgery" to "microsurgery" of the ear and led to the publication of new otology and neurotology surgical books and special trades catalogues of specific instruments. It was the ideal time chosen by Shambaugh Jr. to publish the first edition of his *Surgery of the ear*, which became, through its first six editions, a classic text studied by generations of ear surgeons.

Tympanoplasties

The mechanics of the fenestrated ear remained obscure until Gyorgy von Békésy and Arthur Juers began to study the problem. Juers, in 1948, noted that the drum membrane of the fenestrated ear had to be intact "to protect the round window somewhat from sound pressure" [74]. In 1950, Hallowell Davis and Theo Walsh defined the residue of unrestored conductive loss after successful fenestration as being "due to loss of the impedance-matching mechanism of the drum membrane, ossicular chain and the oval window" [75]. Thus, the two basic principles of tympanoplasty were defined, namely, "sound protection for the round window" and "sound-pressure transformation for the oval window." Following these concepts, Walter Moritz, in 1950 [76], first described the use of pedicled skin flaps to construct a closed middle ear cavity in cases of chronic suppuration in order to provide shielding of the round window. This idea was quickly taken up by Fritz Zöllner in 1951 [77] and Horst Wullstein in 1952 [78]. The latter advocated the use of free skin grafts, either from the meatus or from postaural skin and described his famous five types of tympanoplasty. Wullstein introduced the term tympanoplasty in 1952 [79]. The grafts were used to repair the tympanic membrane and close the tympanic cavity and were positioned as free "onlay" grafts over the membrane remnant or whatever elements of the ossicular chain remained after surgical excision of the disease (types 1–3). If only a mobile footplate remained, this was left exteriorized and the skin graft was positioned so as to create a round window baffle (type 4). If the stapes was fixed by tympanosclerosis or otosclerosis, a fenestration was performed (type 5). At the beginning, Wullstein started using free retroauricular skin grafts of three quarters thickness, while Zöllner preferred the retroauricular pedicular type. In 1953, Wullstein changed to full-thickness and Zöllner, in 1954, abandoned the pedicle on realizing that it was of no value in the nutrition of the transplant. At the same time, Max Edward Pohlman already suggested the use of an artificial tympanic membrane called the "Korogel insert." It consisted of a tube closed at one end and made of a flexible plastic material in different sizes and shapes to fit the individual ear [80]. Following the technique introduced by Siegfried Unterberger in 1954 [81], Zöllner also used fascia lata from 1956, and Simson Hall recommended autologous cheek mucosa in 1958. After the first attempt by Urban Örtegren in 1958 [82], Hans Heermann made the use of temporalis fascia very popular [83] as did Lloyd Stoors [84], both in 1961. Claros Domenech [85], and Ettore Bocca [86] introduced autologous periosteum in 1959. John Shea [87], and Harold Tabb [88] independently described, in 1960, the use of vein graft, Shea using the "underlay" technique for the first time. Jordan Ringenberg, described the use of ear lobe fat in 1962 [89], Jansen used cartilage [90] and perichondrium [91] in 1963, and Victor Goodhill promoted tragal perichondrium in 1964 [92]. The best take rates reported were between 70% and 90%, and the most widely used grafting substance was temporalis fascia. Homograft (allogenous) material started with amniotic membrane [93] in 1954, skin [94] in 1958, cornea [95] in 1958, dura mater [96] in 1961, peritoneum [97] in 1961, perichondrium [98] in 1962, pericardium [99] and vein [100] in 1963, aortic valve [101] in 1965, and temporalis fascia in 1970 [102]. The majority of these materials were only used by a few surgeons and for a short period of time. The first homograft tympanic membrane was inserted by Ned Chalat in 1964 [103] and the "en bloc" homograft tympanic membrane with ossicles was reported by Christian Betow in the same year [104]. The technique was then popularized by Jean Marquet [105].

Alongside the reconstruction of the tympanic membrane in tympanoplasties was also the reconstruction of the ossicular chain, often named "collumellisation." Many different materials have been proposed up to the present day. Michel Portmann had already used homograft ossicles in 1959, and he too promoted homograft drum and ossicle complexes. Heinz Utech used cartilage for ossicular reconstruction in 1960 [106]. Carlo Zini made homograft ossicles from teeth [107]. Homograft ossicles results in the large series were comparable to the use of other more readily obtainable tissues. Overall, though, the technique has not gained wide acceptance, despite the availability of material through tissue banks created by Michel Portmann and Guy Lacher, Dietrich Plester, Gilbert Sedee, Ugo Fisch (Fig. 1.12), Rodney Perkins, and Mansfield Smith. Attention then turned toward the use of heterograft nasal cartilage and other implant materials at the end of the 1950s [109], such as polyethylene, stainless steel wire, Teflon, proplast, and ceramic, as means of reconstructing the ossicular chain. It led to much creativity and ingenuity to build up a continuity between the ossicles. The concepts of total ossicular replacement prosthesis (TORP) to produce a columella from the tympanic mem-

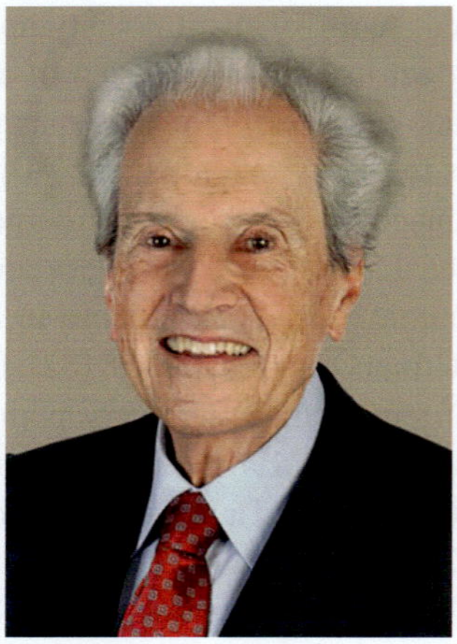

Fig. 1.12 Ugo Fisch. (Reprinted with permission from Mudry A and Huber A [108])

brane to the oval window and partial ossicular replacement prosthesis (PORP) from the stapes head to the tympanic membrane were introduced in the early 1970s. David Austin, in 1971 [110], presented his classification of the anatomical defects found in the ossicular chain in 1151 consecutive ears with chronic suppurative otitis media and proposed a number of ingenious ways of sculpturing autologous or allogeneic malleus head or incus to restore ossicular continuity. In conjunction with all these tympano-plastic techniques was the introduction and use of non-absorbable plastic sheeting, such as polyethylene, Teflon, and Silastic to prevent adhesions and help maintain an aerated middle ear. Absorbable substances such as Gelfoam and Gelfilm were advocated originally by Wullstein in 1960 [111]. Regularly new types, and with new material, of PORP and TORP were developed. Until now, none of them has definitively become the standard.

Stapedectomy and Stapedotomy

In 1947, Terence Cawthorne [67], and, in 1949 [112], Gino Cornelli reintroduced stapedectomy; the former covered the oval window with a tympanomeatal flap, which produced little hearing improvement, whilst the latter achieved better hearing results, simply by opening the oval window after removal of the stapes, in 41 cases. Samuel Rosen by chance rediscovered stapes mobilization in 1952 when he was palpating the stapes to assess its degree of fixation prior to proceeding to a fenestration operation under local anaesthesia [113]. He was surprised by the sudden restoration of the patient's hearing. There was less postoperative vertigo, a normal ear canal and drum, and an initial hearing improvement in about 70% of cases [114]. In most of these, though, the hearing gain gradually reduced, and a lasting improvement was only achieved in about 25% of patients. Stapes mobilization rapidly enjoyed worldwide popularity and was an important advance in the surgical treatment of otosclerosis. Various modifications to the operation were made, including the anterior crurotomy mobilization described by Milos Basel [115] and Edmund Prince Fowler [116] in 1956. Two years later, the scene changed again with the reintroduction of stapedectomy by Shea [117]. He removed the whole stapes, covered the open oval window initially with "a thin slice of connective tissue" and replaced the stapes with a nylon replica. He later used a short length (4.5 mm) of fine polythene tubing, placed between the incus and vein, which replaced connective tissue. Shea thus established the two important principles: the oval window should be sealed and the ossicular continuity restored. Many modifications followed. They were the fat wire prosthesis by Harold Schuknecht [118], the Gelfoam wire prosthesis by Howard House of Los Angeles [119], the operation of anterior crurotomy with removal of the footplate, and replacement of the posterior crus to rest on a vein graft (interposition) described by Michel Portmann [120], the stainless steel by Manford McGee [121], and the Teflon wire by Frederick Guilford [122]. Shea in 1962 introduced the idea of making a limited opening in the stapes footplate (stapedotomy) through which he placed a Teflon piston [123]. Stapes surgery experience grew throughout the world, and large series were published. Progressively, various types of pistons were developed by different schools of otological surgery [124].

Vestibular Schwannoma Surgery

The internal auditory meatus is, in a sense, the meeting point between the territories of the neurosurgeon and the otologist. Even if brain abscesses of otological origin opened this area to the otologist, it is the surgery of vestibular schwannoma which definitively associated these two specialties to become neurotology. In 1900, Carl Sternberg [125] suggested that, on the basis of postmortem appearances, a tumor of the VIII nerve in the internal auditory canal might be favorable for operative removal. During those early years of the century, though the surgery of cerebral tumors was in considerable disrepute, due largely to the publication of von Bergmann's discouraging views on the subject, the first operations upon undoubted acoustic tumors in any considerable number began to be undertaken [126], and in 1903, Victor Horsley appears to have had a series of six cases, at least one of which made an unusually perfect recovery [127]. Already in 1894, Ballance successfully removed a tumour from the posterior fossa, but Harvey Cushing later doubted that the tumour was an acoustic neuroma and thought that it was more likely to have been a meningioma. He therefore attributed the first removal of an acoustic neuroma in 1895 to Thomas Annandale [128]. The mortality and morbidity of the early cases was high, due to late presentation, poor anaesthesia and haemorrhage, usually related to the anterior inferior cerebellar artery, which resulted from the commonly used technique of finger enucleation. Fedor Krause, in 1903, reported on 83.8% operative mortality using the unilateral suboccipital approach [129]. This was reduced dramatically in Cushing's first report in 1917 to 30% in his first 30 operations and later to 4% in his 1932 report. Cushing used a bilateral suboccopital approach to the posterior fossa, which allowed not only a wide decompression but also the opportunity to explore both sides because it was not always possible to determine the exact location of the lesion preoperatively. Radiology enabled Salomon Eberhard Henschen to describe widening of the opening of the internal auditory canal as a diagnostic sign [130]. In 1911, Cushing invented silver clips to arrest haemorrhage. Walter Dandy introduced ventriculography in 1918 [131] and pneumoencephalography a year later [132]. These diagnostic procedures enabled accurate preoperative localization of intracranial masses and allowed to choose the best route possible for the extraction of the tumour. Dandy favoured total removal of acoustic tumours via a unilateral suboccipital approach and performed his first such case in 1917. Only a year after Krause's paper on the suboccipital approach, Panse in 1904 proposed that an approach through the labyrinth might allow removal of an acoustic neuroma as large as a hen's egg [133]. He defined the anatomical limits of that exposure as the lateral sinus, the jugular bulb, the carotid artery, and the temporal lobe. The facial nerve he thought should be sacrificed but he did concede that with certain tumours it might be possible to reroute the nerve by mobilizing it from the geniculate ganglion to the stylomastoid foramen. Franciscus Hubertus Quix is usually credited with the first removal of an acoustic neuroma by the translabyrinthine approach in 1912 [134]. He predicted that the translabyrinthine approach could bring a small acoustic neuroma within the province of the otologist. This hope was quickly dampened by Cushing who warned that "while the otologist doubtless will be the first to recognize and diagnose these cases [...] there is no possible route more dangerous or difficult than this one [...] proposed by Panse"; Ballance merely dismissed the technique as "objectionable for obvious reasons." One of the principal causes of mortality in the suboccipital approach was the disturbance of the anterior inferior cerebellar artery. Sterling Bunnell performed the first successful intratemporal suture of the facial nerve in 1927 [135] and the first successful grafting within the temporal bone in 1930 [136]. Most neurosurgeons were nevertheless reluctant to advise surgery unless the tumour was so large as to be causing pressure on the brainstem or raised intracranial pressure. It was in this climate in 1956 that William House was persuaded to operate on acoustic neuromas. He had sent a young fireman, in whom he had diagnosed an acoustic neuroma, to a neurosurgeon. The young man died 3 days postoperatively. The following year, two further cases were referred for neurosurgery and although both survived they suffered facial palsies. After preliminary study, William House and John Doyle, the neurosurgeon, performed the first middle cranial fossa approach to the internal auditory meatus using an operating microscope in 1960 [137]. The first few tumours were only partially removed. William House worked on the trans-labyrinthine approach using temporal bones and, following a controversy with Doyle, performed the first operation alone. In July 1963, William Hitselberger replaced Doyle, and the first otologist/neurosurgeon team was formed. This was the model which over 25 years spread around the world. William House published his first 47consecutive translabyrinthine cases in 1964 [138]. There were no fatalities, and the majority of patients had preservation of their facial nerve function. The success of these cases was largely due to a policy of early diagnosis, and surgery depended also on advances in diagnostic techniques in the fields of audiology and radiology, as well as on the microsurgical skills of the otologist and neurosurgeon. In 1964, the technique of meatocisternography was introduced [139], using contrast medium and polytomography to define the contents of the internal auditory meatus. Robert Rand and Theodore Kurze, in 1965, were among the first neurosurgeons to apply microsurgical techniques to acoustic neuroma removal via the suboccipital transmeatal route [140]. This route has in the last part of the twentieth century regained popularity with otologists as in suitable cases it is possible to remove the tumour and preserve hearing such as Mansfield Smith, Ray Miller, and Dale Cox, in 1973 [141]. Derald Brackmann wrote: "The goal of acoustic tumor surgery is to accomplish a total tumor removal without increasing the neurological deficit. The ultimate extension of this concept is the preservation of hearing. The middle cranial fossa and suboccipital approaches offer the possibility of accomplishing this ideal" [142]. Neurotology was born, and Los Angeles became its mecca. William House has trained otologists from all over the world and has not only changed the outlook for those patients suffering from cerebellopontine angle tumours [143] but also opened the whole field of microsurgical skull base surgery which has been in turn developed and popularized by Fisch who described most of the usual approaches [144] and others. This development was accelerated with the invention of computer tomography followed by magnetic resonance imaging in the 1970s and 1980s.

Auditory Implants

The first auditory implant was performed by André Djourno and Charles Eyriès in 1957. They inserted a single copper wire near a small segment of the eighth cranial nerve of a

50-year-old man who was totally deaf [145]. It enabled him to perceive speech rhythm. This report stimulated others and in particular two groups in California: William House and the Doyle brothers, and Blair Simmons and Robert White. In 1961, William House with John Doyle implanted two subjects with a single gold electrode placed in the scala tympani. One of these was later replaced with a multiple electrode system. Simmons implanted a six-electrode device in 1964 and found that the patient was able to hear a wide range of sounds [146]. The patient suffered an unforeseen complication of loss of vision due to retinitis pigmentosa, which greatly affected his progress as he was unable to lipread. Caution was advised by the leading otologists of the day and further clinical work was effectively stopped for several years. In 1969, William House again implanted a further patient, this time with a six-electrode system developed by his new collaborator Jack Urban [147]. Success with this case led to further implants and the technique became established as a means of alleviating total deafness. Other groups in San Francisco (Robert Schindler, Michael Merzenich and Robert Michelson) [148], France (Claude Henri Chouard) [149], Germany (Paul Banfai) [150], and Austria (Kurt Burian) [151] began clinical work in the 1970s. In Australia, Graeme Milbourne Clark used a prototype 10-electrode system in 1978 which was initially complex [152]. It was the first commercialized implant. Ellis Doueck and his group, in London, pioneered the extracochlear implant in 1977 [153]. Cochlear implants are now produced commercially and are nationally approved for clinic use. William House was the first to use a cochlear implant in a prelingually deaf child in 1980.

The idea to implant a vibrator percutaneously into the mastoid bone to stimulate it directly, began in Göteborg with Per-Ingvar Brånemark and Anders Tjellström in the 1960s. In 1977, they implanted the first Baha™ (bone anchored hearing aid) [154]. In 1981 and in the same spirit, Jack Hough, of Oklahoma City, developed a fully implantable bone conduction device, without much success [155]. In the 1990s, the Baha™ became a worldwide-used implant.

Lasers, Endoscopes, and Computers

In 1980, Rodney Perkins [156] and Joseph Di Bartholomeo [157] were the first to use a laser argon in ear surgery to perform the fenestration of the footplate during stapedotomy. In 1989, Herbert Silverstein tested the KTP laser [158] and George Lesinski the CO_2 [159]. A few years later, Rudolf Häusler tested the erbium:YAG [160]. Progressively, largely accepted for stapedotomy, use of some of these lasers was then disputably enlarged to myringotomy, coagulation of the membranous labyrinth for benign positional vertigo, and stabilizing prostheses by making holes into the incus or malleus.

The first comprehensive description of endoscopy in the cerebellopontine angle was provided by Eugène Doyen in 1917 [161]. He described an endoscopic technique for selective fifth nerve section in trigeminal neuralgia. Another description of this technique was given by Werner Prott in 1974 [162], advocating a transmastoid retrolabyrinthine approach. Transtympanic middle ear endoscopy was initially reported by Yasuya Nomura in 1982 [163]. In 1993, Kevin McKennan described second-look endoscopic inspection of mastoid cavities through a small postauricular incision [164]. At the same time, Jean-Marc Thomassin reported operative ear endoscopy for mastoid cavities and designed an instrument set to be used in these settings [165]. The main discussions concerned the possible indications and limits of such a surgical otological technique. The next step was to use the endoscope in neurotology [166]. This development of endoscopic ear surgery results from the limitations of the microscope line-of-sight visualization, so that the structures behind or to the side of obstructions cannot be seen. It was the first step in the transformation of the traditional "funnel technique" of methodological and progressive identification of key anatomical landmarks *en route* to the surgical target to the "tunnel technique." The next step is to use image-guided systems of surgical navigation whereupon it is possible to virtually see the vital anatomic landmarks via interactive imaging rather than by direct surgical exposure.

Conclusion

I hope that this short history of modern surgical otology and neurotology will encourage readers to explore the treasures of our past, in a spirit of fun and with pleasure. It will undoubtedly bring forward new ideas and projects for the continuing development and improvement of this marvelous specialty.

References

1. Mudry A. Some thoughts about the history of otorhinolaryngology, head and neck surgery (OHNS). Hist Otorhinolaryngol. 2016;1:59–79.
2. Bezold F. Galarie hervorragender Arzte und Naturforscher. Munchen: Lehmann; 1903.
3. George Shambaugh RW. 90 and on the way to 100-what a role model! Otolaryngol Head Neck Surg. 1994;110(3)
4. Bezold F. Lehrbuch der Ohrenheilkunde. Wiesbaden: Bergmann; 1906. p. 6.
5. Mudry A. The history of otology. *A tribute to Adam Politzer*. Asuncion: Wayenborgh; 2015.
6. Fisch U, Mörgeli C, Mudry A. Mikroskop und Ohr. *Der Weg zur Mikrochirurgie*. Zürich: Medizinhistorisches Museum; 2012.

7. Weir N, Mudry A. Otorhinolaryngology: an illustrated history. 2nd ed. Ashford: Headley; 2013.
8. Wilde W. Practical observations on aural surgery. London: Churchill; 1853. p. 237–8.
9. Tröltsch A. Ein Fall von Anbohrung des Warzenfortsatzes bei Otitis interna mit Bemerkungen ueber diese Operation. Virchow Arch Path Anat. 1861;21:295–314.
10. Schwartze H. Galarie hervorragender Arzte und Naturforscher. Munchen: Lehmann; 1910.
11. Schwartze H, Eysell A. Ueber die künstliche Eröffnung des Warzenfortsatzes. Arch Ohrenheil. 1873;7:157–87.
12. Küster E. Galarie hervorragender Arzte und Naturforscher. Munchen: Lehmann; 1909.
13. Küster E. Ueber die Grunsätze der Behandlung von Eiterungen in starrwandigen Höhlen, mit besonderer Berücksichtigung des Empyems der Pleura. Leipzig/Berlin: Thieme; 1889.
14. Bergmann E. Surgical treatment of diseases of the brain, 1890, Reprint. New York: Gryphon; 1994. p. 866–7.
15. Stacke L. Album of von Troltsch 25th Jubilee, collected in 1886.
16. Zaufal E. Album of von Troltsch 25th Jubilee, collected in 1886.
17. Stacke L. Indicationen, betreffend die Excision von Hammer und Amboss. Arch Ohrenheil. 1890;31:201–15.
18. Zaufal E. Technik der Trepanation des Proc. Mastoid Nach Küster'schen Grundsätzen. Arch Ohrenheil. 1890;30:291–4.
19. Zange J. Rudolf Panse zum Gedachtnis. Archiv fur Ohren-, Nasen-un Kehlkopfheilkunde. 1943;152:102–4.
20. Thies F. Diskussion. Verh Dtsch Otol Ges. 1908;52–54.
21. Kessel J. Ueber die Otorrhoe und ihre Behandlung. XXII Wissenschaftliche Rundschau. Arch Ohrenheil. 1885;22:286.
22. Bondy G. Totalaufmeislung mir Erhaltung von Trommelfell und Gehörknöchelchen. Monatsschr Ohrenheilk. 1910;44:15–23.
23. Macewen W. Pyogenic infective diseases of the brain and spinal cord. Glasgow: Maclehose; 1893. p. 304.
24. Whiting F. The modern mastoid operation. Philadelphia: Blakiston; 1905. p. ix.
25. Jansen C. Die Erhaltung des äusseren Gehörganges bei der Radikaloperation und eine neue Art der Tympanoplastik. Zentralbl HNO. 1962;74:36.
26. Wilde W. Contribution to aural surgery part III. Inflammatory affections of the membrana tympani and middle ear. *Dublin Quart.* J Med Sci. 1848;5(1):82–111.
27. Tröltsch A. Die Krankheiten des Ohres, ihre Erkenntniss und Behandlung. Würzburg: Stahel; 1862. p. 195.
28. Jackler RK, Alyono JC, Mudry AC. The American Otological Society at its sesquicentennial: insights into the society's formative years. Otol Neurotol. 2018;39(4S Suppl 1):S1–9.
29. Roosa St John DB. A practical treatise on the diseases of the ear. New York: Wood; 1873, p.377.
30. Okuneff WN. Ueber die Anwendung des Acidum trichloraceticum bei chronischen eitrigen Entzundungen des Mittelohres. Monatsschr Ohrenheil. 1895;29:1–14.
31. Mudry A. The making of a career: Joseph Toynbee's first steps in otology. J Laryngol Otol. 2012;126(1):2–7.
32. Toynbee J. On the use of an artificial membrana tympani, in cases of deafness, dependent upon perforation or destruction of the natural organ. London: Churchill; 1853.
33. Berthold E. Ueber Myringoplastik. Wien Med Blaetter. 1878;26:627–30.
34. Ely ET. An operation for prominence of the auricles. Arch Otol. 1881;10:97–9.
35. Ely E. Skin-grafting in chronic suppuration of the middle ear. Arch Otol. 1880;9:343–5.
36. Berthold E. Die ersten zehn Jahre der Myringoplastik nebst Angaben verbesserter Methoden zur Heilung von alte. Berlin: Hirschwald; 1889.
37. Gomperz B. De l'amélioration des troubles de l'audition, suites d'otites suppurées. Ann Mal Oreille Larynx. 1902;28:297–326.
38. Kessel J. Über die Durchschneidung des Steigbügelmuskels beim Menschen und über die Extraction des Steigbügels resp. der Columella bei Thieren. Arch Ohrenheil. 1876;11:199–217.
39. Kessel J. Ueber das Mobilisiren des Steigbügels durch Ausschneiden des Trommelfelles, Hammers und Ambosses bei Undurchgängigkeit der Tuba. Arch Ohrenheil. 1878;13:69–88.
40. Boucheron E. La mobilisation de l'étrier et son procédé opératoire. Union Med Paris. 1888;46:412–3.
41. Miot C. De la mobilisation de l'etrier. Rev Laryngol Otol Rhinol. 1890;10:113–30.
42. Blake CJ. Operation for removal of the stapes. Box M & S J. 1892;127:469.
43. Jack FL. Removal of the stapes in chronic catarrhal and in chronic suppurative otitis media. In: Burnett C, editor. System of diseases of the ear, nose, and throat. Vol. I. Philadelphia: Lippincott; 1893. p. 465–80.
44. Mudry A, Young JR. Otitis media with effusion: Politzer's 100 year legacy. Int J Pediatr Otorhinolaryngol. 2020;136:110160.
45. Gradenigo G. Compte rendu XIe congrès de médecine international tenu à Rome du 29 mars au 5 avril 1894. Ann Mal Oreille Larynx. 1894;20:498–519.
46. Siebemann F. Traitement chirurgical de la sclérose otique. Ann Mal Oreille Larynx. 1900;26(2):467–74.
47. Le BR. traitement chirurgical de la sclérose otique. Ann Mal Oreille Larynx. 1900;26(2):129–40.
48. Anonymous. XIIIe congrès international de médecine Paris, 2-9 août 1900. Ann Mal Oreille Larynx. 1900;26(2):401–34.
49. Lane WA. Five cases of the middle ear complicated by suppuration in its vicinity. BMJ. 1889;1(1479):997–8.
50. Ballance C. On the removal of pyaemic thrombi of the lateral sinus. Lancet. 1890;135(3481):1057–61.
51. Körner O. Lehrbuch der Ohrenheilkunde. Wiesbaden: Bergmann; 1906. p. 195–217.
52. Ballance C. Essays on the surgery of the temporal bone, vol. 2. London: Macmillan; 1919.
53. Passow KA. Diskussion. *Verhandl Dtsch Otol Ges.* 1897;143–144.
54. Jenkins GJ. Otosclerosis: certain clinical features and experimental operative procedures. In: Transactions of the XVIIth International Congress of Medicine, London, vol. 16; 1913. p. 609.
55. Holmgren G. Till otosclerosens kirurgiska behandling. Nordisk Tidskrift Oto-Lar. 1917;2:217–25.
56. Holmgren G. Some experiences in surgery for otosclerosis. Acta Otolaryngol. 1923;5:460–6.
57. Barany R. Die Indikationen zur Labyrinthoperation. Acta Otolaryngol. 1924;6:260.
58. Holmgren G. Operations on the temporal bone, carried out with the help of the lens and the microscope. Acta Otolaryngol. 1922;4:386–93.
59. Sourdille M. Résultats primitifs et secondaires de quatorze cas de surdité opérés pour otospongiose. Rev Laryngol. 1930;51:595.
60. Lempert J. Improvement of hearing in cases of otosclerosis: new one-stage surgical technique. Arch Otolaryngol. 1938;28:42–97.
61. Shambaugh G Jr. Fenestration operation for otosclerosis. Acta Otolaryngol. 1949;Suppl 129:1–100.
62. Charcot JM. Vertigo ab aure laesa (maladie de Ménière). Gaz Hôp (Paris). 1874;47:73–4.
63. Milligan W. Ménière's disease, a clinical and experimental inquiry. J Laryngol Rhinol Otol. 1904;19:440.
64. Lake R. Removal of the semicircular canals in a case of unilateral aural vertigo. Lancet. 1904;1:1567–8.
65. Dandy WE. The surgical treatment of Ménière's disease. Surg Gynec Obst. 1941;72:421–5.
66. Portmann G. Le traitement chirurgical des vertiges par l'ouverture du sac endolymphatique. Presse Méd. 1926;104:1635–7.

67. Cawthorne T. Ménière's disease. Ann Otol Rhinol Laryngol. 1947;56:18–38.
68. Schuknecht H. Ablation therapy in the management of Ménière's disease. Acta Otolaryngol Suppl. 1957;132:1–42.
69. Fick IA. Decompression of the labyrinth. Arch Otolaryngol. 1964;79:447–58.
70. Cody DT, Simonton KM, Hallberg OE. Automatic repetitive decompression of the saccule in endolymphatic hydrops (tack operation). Preliminary report. Laryngoscope. 1967;77(8):1480–501.
71. Shambaugh GE. Surgery of the ear. Philadelphia: Saunders; 1959. p. V.
72. Berliner KI. In Memoriam: William F. House, D.D.S., M.D., the "Father of Neurotology" 1923–2012. Otol Neurotol. 2013;34(3):386–7.
73. House WF. Forty years of ear after ear, year after year. Otolaryngol Head Neck Surg. 1996;114:717–9.
74. Juers AL. Observations on bone conduction in fenestration cases. Ann Otol Rhinol Laryngol. 1948;57:28–40.
75. Davis H, Walsch TE. The limits of improvement of hearing following the fenestration operation. Laryngoscope. 1950;60:273–95.
76. Moritz W. Hörverbessernde Operationen bei chronisch-entzündlichesn Prozessen beider Mittelohren. Z Laryngol Rhinol Otol. 1950;29:578–83.
77. Zöllner F. Die Radikal-Operation mit besonderem Bezug auf die Hörfunktion. Z Laryngol Rhinol Otol. 1951;30:104–11.
78. Wullstein H. Operationen am Mittelohr mit Hilfe des freien Splatlappentransplantates. Arch Ohr Nas Kehlkopfheilk. 1952;161:422–35.
79. Wullstein HL. Die Eingriffe zur Gehörverbesserung. In: Uffenorde W, editor. Anzeige und Ausführung der Eingriffe an Ohr, Nase und Hals. 2nd ed. Stuttgart: Thieme; 1952. p. 227–58.
80. Pohlman ME. The artificial ear drum. Ann Otol Rhinol Laryngol. 1951;60:117–21.
81. Unterberger S. Zur Paukenplastik. Monatsschr Ohrenheilk Laryngol. 1955;89(1):41–2.
82. Örtegren U. Trumhinneplastik. Forhandl Sven Otolaryngol Foren. 1958;59:16–8. (Swedish)
83. Heermann H. Trommelfellplastik mit Fasciengewebe vom Musculus temporalis nach Begradigung der vorderen Gehörganswand. HNO. 1961;9:136–7.
84. Storrs LA. Myringoplasty with the use of fascia grafts. Arch Otolaryngol. 1961;74:45–9.
85. Claros-Domenech A. Cent tympanoplasties pratiquées à l'aide d'une greffe libre de membrane périostique. Rev Laryngol (Bordeaux). 1959;80:917–21.
86. Bocca E, Cis C, Zernotti E. L'impiego di lembr liberi di periostio nella timpanoplastica. Arch Ital Otol. 1959;70(Suppl 40):205–11.
87. Shea J. Vein graft closure of eardrum perforation. Arch Otolaryngol. 1960;72:445–7.
88. Tabb GH. Closure ofperforations of the tympanic membrane by vein grafts. Laryngoscope. 1960;70:271–86.
89. Ringenberg JC. Fat graft tympanoplasty. Laryngoscope. 1962;72:188–92.
90. Jansen C. Cartilage tympanoplasty. Laryngoscope. 1963;73:1288–302.
91. Jansen C. On the use of perichondrium in tympanoplasty. Arch Ohr Nas Kehlkopfheilk. 1963;182:610–4.
92. Goodhill V, Brockman SJ. Tympanoplasty with perichondral graft. Arch Otolaryngol. 1964;79:131–7.
93. Schrimpf WJ. Repair of tympanic membrane perforations with human amniotic membrane; report of fifty-three cases. Ann Otol Rhinol Laryngol. 1954;63:101–15.
94. Burian K. Vergleichende klinische Untersuchungen an autoplastischen und konservierte homoioplastischen Hauttransplantaten bei je 75 Fällen von Tympanoplastik. Arch Ohr Nas Kehlkopfheilk. 1958;171:116–9.
95. Holewinski J. A trial of covering the tympanic membrane with a corneal graft. Otolaryngol Pol. 1958;12:349–50. (Polish)
96. Proebrazhensky YB. The employment of preserved dura mater graft in tympanoplasty. Vestn Otorinolaring. 1961;23:60–6. (Russian)
97. Birch DA. Preliminary communication: myringoplasty performed with a peritoneum homograft. J Laryngol Otol. 1961;75:922–3.
98. Jansen C. Die Erhaltung des äusseren Gehörgangs bei der Radikaloperation une eine neue Art der Tympanoplastik. Zentralblatt HNO. 1962;74:36.
99. Trombetta A. Perforation of tympanic membrane and tympanoplasty. Arch Otolaryngol. 1963;77:81–4.
100. Nickel AL. The use of homologous vein grafts in otolaryngology. Laryngoscope. 1963;73:919–25.
101. Cornish CB. Use of freeze-dried aortic valve homografts in aural surgery. Lancet. 1965;1(7392):943.
102. Hildmann H, Steinbach E. Experimentelle Untersuchungen zur Verträglichkeit von Fascientransplantaten. Arch Ohr Nas Kehlkopfheilk. 1970;196:133–6.
103. Chalat NJ. Tympanic membrane transplant. Harper Hosp Bull. 1964;22(janv–febr):27–34.
104. Betow K. 20 years of experience with homografts in ear surgery. J Laryngol Otol Suppl. 1982;5:1–28.
105. Marquet J. Reconstructive micro-surgery of the ear drum by means of a tympanic membrane homograft. Acta Otolaryngol. 1966;62:459–64.
106. Utech H. Bessere Endhörergebnisse bei der Tympanoplastik durch Veränderungen der Operationstechnik. Z Laryngol Rhinol Otol. 1960;39:367–71.
107. Zini C. Homotransplantation de dent en tympanoplastie. Rev Laryngol (Bordeaux). 1970;91:258–61.
108. Mudry A, Huber A. In Memoriam: Ugo Fisch March 3, 1931 to December 12, 2019. Otol Neurotol. 2020;41(5):574–6.
109. Harrison W, Shambaugh G Jr, Kaplan J, Derlacki EL. Prosthetics in the middle ear. Arch Otolaryngol. 1959;69:661–6.
110. Austin DF. Ossicular reconstruction. Arch Otolaryngol. 1971;94:525–35.
111. Wullstein H. Tympanoplasty. The problem of the free graft and the mucous membrane graft. Arch Otolaryngol. 1960;71:363–8.
112. Cornelli G. Tecnica e risultati della apertura del vestibulo labirintico attraverso la finestra ovale nella terapia della otosclerosi. Revista L'Ospedale Maggiore. 1949;2:55–62.
113. Rosen S. Palpation of stapes for fixation. Arch Otolaryngol. 1952;56:610–5.
114. Rosen S. The development of stapes surgery after five years. Arch Otolaryngol. 1958;67:129–41.
115. Bazek M, Fowler EP Jr. Anatomical factors in stapes mobilization operations. Arch Otolaryngol. 1956;63:589.
116. Fowler E. Anterior crurotomy. Acta Otolaryngol. 1956;46:319–88.
117. Shea J. Fenestration of the oval window. Ann Otol Rhinol Laryngol. 1958;67:932–51.
118. Schuknecht HF, Oleksiuk S. The metal prosthesis for stapes ankylosis. Arch Otolaryngol. 1960;71:287–95.
119. House HP. Footplate surgery in otosclerosis. J Laryngol Otol. 1962;76:73–86.
120. Portmann M. Interposition: surgical procedure for stapes ankylosis. In: Schuknecht H, editor. Otosclerosis. International. Symposium, Detroit 1960. Boston: Little Brown; 1962. p. 429–45.
121. McGee TM. Techniques and experiences with stapedectomy and metal implant. In: Schuknecht H, editor. Otosclerosis. International. Symposium, Detroit 1960. Boston: Little Brown; 1962. p. 489–95.
122. Guilford FR. Experiences in the surgery of otosclerosis. In: Schuknecht H, editor. Otosclerosis. International. Symposium, Detroit 1960. Boston: Little Brown; 1962. p. 523–41.

123. Shea J, Sanabria F, Smyth G. Teflon piston operation for otosclerosis. Arch Otolaryngol. 1962;76:516–21.
124. Fritsch M, Naumann IC. Phylogeny of stapes prosthesis. Otol Neurotol. 2008;29:407–15.
125. Sternberg C. Beitrag zur Kenntnis der sogenannten Geschwülste des Nervus acusticus. Zeitschr Heilk. 1900;21:163–86.
126. Cushing H. Tumors of the nervus acusticus and the syndrome of the cerebellopontine angle. Philadelphia/London: Saunders; 1917. p. 10–3.
127. Stewart T, Holmes G. Symptomatology of cerebellar tumors; a study of forty cases. Brain. 1904;27:522–91.
128. Gibson G. Remarks on the results of surgical measures in a series of cerebral cases. Edinburgh Med J. 1896;41:689–92.
129. Krause F. Zur Freilegung der hinteren Felsenbeinfläche und des Kleinhirns. Beitr Klin Chir. 1903;37:728–64.
130. Henschen F. Die Akustikustumoren eine neue Gruppe radiographisch darstellbarer Hirntumoren. Fortschr Geb Rontgenstr Nuklearmed. 1912;18:207–15.
131. Dandy WE. Ventriculography following the injection of air into the cerebral ventricles. Ann Surg. 1918;68:5–11.
132. Dandy WE. Roentgenography of the brain after the injection of air into the spinal canal. Ann Surg. 1919;70:397–403.
133. Panse R. Ein Glioms des Akusticus. Arch Ohrenheil. 1904;61:251–5.
134. Quix FH. Ein Fall von translabyrintharisch operiertem tumor acusticus. Verhandl Deutsch Otol Gesell. 1912;21:245–55.
135. Bunnell S. Suture of the facial nerve within temporal bone, with a report of the first successful case. Surg Gynecol Obstet. 1927;45:7–12.
136. Bunnell S. Surgical repair of the facial nerve. Arch Otolaryngol. 1937;25:235–59.
137. House WF. Surgical exposure of the internal auditory canal and its contents through the middle cranial fossa. Laryngoscope. 1961;71:1363–85.
138. House WF. Report of cases. Arch Otolaryngol. 1964;80:617–67.
139. Scanlan RL. Positive contrast medium (lophendylate) in diagnosis of acoustic neuroma. Arch Otolaryngol. 1964;80:698–706.
140. Rand RW, Kurze TL. Micro-neurosurgical resection of acoustic tumors by a transmeatal posterior fossa approach. Bull Los Angel Neurol Soc. 1965;30:17–20.
141. Smith MFW, Miller RN, Cox DJ. Suboccipital microsurgical removal of acoustic neurinomas of all sizes. Ann Otol Rhinol Laryngol. 1973;82:407–14.
142. Brackmann DE. Middle cranial fossa approach. In: House WF, Luetje CM, editors. Acoustic tumors. Volume II: management. Baltimore: University Park Press; 1968. p. 15.
143. House WF, Luetje CM. Acoustic tumors. 2 vols. Baltimore: University Park; 1979.
144. Fisch U, Mattox D. Microsurgery of the skull base. Suttgart/New York: Thieme; 1988.
145. Djourno A, Eyries C, Vallancien B. De l'excitation électrique du nerf cochléaire chez l'homme, par induction à distance, à l'aide d'un micro-bobinage inclus à demeure. C R Soc Biol (Paris). 1957;151:423–5.
146. Simmons FB. Electrical stimulation of the auditory nerve in man. Arch Otolaryngol. 1966;84:2–54.
147. House W. Cochlear implants. Ann Otol Rhinol Laryngol. 1976;85(Suppl 27):1–93.
148. Michelson RP. The results of electrical stimulation of the cochlea in human sensory deafness. Ann Otol Rhinol Laryngol. 1971;80:914–9.
149. Chouard CH, Mac Leod P. Implantation of multiple electrodes for rehabilitation of total deafness: preliminary report. Laryngoscope. 1976;86:1743–51.
150. Banfai P, Hortmann G, Wustrow F. Erste Beobachtung nach einer Cochlear-Implant-Operation. HNO. 1978;26(11):377–80.
151. Burian K. Klinische Erfahrungen mit der Elektrostimuation des Hörorgans. Arch Otorhinolaryngol. 1979;223(1):139–66.
152. Clark GE, Pyman BC, Bailey QR. The surgery for mulit-electrode cochlear implantations. J Laryngol Otol. 1979;93:215–23.
153. Doueck E. A new approach to the cochlear implant. Proc R Soc Med. 1977;70(6):379–83.
154. Tjellström A, Lindström J, Hallen O, Albrektsson T, Branemark PI. Osseointegrated titanium implant in the temporal bone. Am J Otol. 1981;2:304–10.
155. Hough J, Himelick T, Johnson B. Implantable conduction hearing device: Audiant bone conductor. Ann Otol Rhinol Laryngol. 1986;95:498–504.
156. Perkins R. Laser stapedotomy for otosclerosis. Laryngoscope. 1980;90:228–41.
157. Di Bartholomeo JR, Ellis M. The argon laser in otology. Laryngoscope. 1980;90:1786–96.
158. Silverstein H, Rosenberg S, Jones R. Small fenestra stapedotomies with and without KTP laser: a comparison. Laryngoscope. 1989;99:485–8.
159. Lesinski EG, Stein JA. CO_2 laser stapedotomy. Laryngoscope. 1989;99(6 Pt 2 Suppl 46):20–4.
160. Häusler R, Schär PJ, Pratisto H, Weber HP, Frenz M. Advantages and dangers of erbium laser application in stapedotomy. Acta Otolaryngol. 1999;119:207–13.
161. Doyen E. Surgical therapeutics and operative techniques, vol. I. London: Baillière, Tindall & Cox; 1917. p. 599–602.
162. Prott W. Möglichkeiten einer Endoskopie des Kleinhirnbrückenwinkels auf transpyramidalem-retrolabyrinthärem Zugangweg – Cisternoskopie. HNO. 1974;22:337–41.
163. Nomura Y. Effective photography in otolaryngology, head and neck surgery: endoscopic photography of the middle ear. Otolaryngol Head Neck Surg. 1982;90:395–8.
164. McKennan KX. Endoscopic "second-look" mastoidoscopy to rule out residual epitympanic / mastoid cholesteatoma. Laryngoscope. 1993;103:810–4.
165. Thomassin JM, Korchia D, Doris JMD. Endoscopic-guided otosurgery in the prevention of residual cholesteatoma. Laryngoscope. 1993;103:936–43.
166. Rosenberg SI, Silverstein H, Willcox TO. Endoscopy in otology and neurotology. Am J Otol. 1994;15:168–72.

Embryology and Developmental Anatomy of the Ear

2

Michael W. Canfarotta, Rosh K. Sethi, and C. Eduardo Corrales

Development of the External, Middle, and Inner Ear

Auricle

Development of the auricle begins by the fourth week of gestation and is derived from the first (mandibular) and second (hyoid) branchial arches. By the sixth week, 6 cartilaginous-filled structures fuse around the ear canal to form the hillocks of His. The growth and maturation of the six hillocks ultimately give rise to the tragus (1), helical crus (2), ascending helix (3), upper portion of scapha, horizontal helix, and antihelix (4), descending helix, middle portion of the scapha, and antihelix (5), and the inferior helix and antihelix (6) [1] (Fig. 2.1). At birth, the overall size of the ear is generally two-thirds of the adult size [3] and reaches adult size by the age of 6 years [4]. Failure of fusion may result in the formation of preauricular pits, sinuses, or clefts [5].

Abnormal development can additionally give rise to anotia, cryptotia, and microtia.

External Auditory Canal

The external auditory canal begins to develop from the first branchial cleft by 4 weeks gestation and a pit is formed by ectodermal proliferation. An epithelial core canalizes from medial to lateral by 28 weeks. Failure of this process can result in membranous or bony stenosis or atresia. A more detailed overview of microtia and atresia is provided in Chap. 33.

Tympanic Membrane

The tympanic membrane is formed in three layers by the invagination and fusion of the first branchial cleft (ectoderm) laterally and the first pharyngeal pouch (endoderm) medially, resulting in epidermal and mucosal layers, respectively. The fibrous middle layer is derived from mesenchyme of neural crest origin and is surrounded by ossification centers of the tympanic ring. The tympanic ring elements fuse by the tenth week, except for a defect that is later observed as the notch of Rivinus. The tympanic ring serves to support the tympanic membrane and is postulated to function in the inhibition of inward epithelial migration. Failure of the latter may lead to congenital cholesteatoma formation at the junction of the first and second branchial arches [6]. The tympanic membrane is nearly adult size at birth but is more horizontally oriented until approximately 3 years of age, when it reaches adult angulation [7].

Tympanic Cavity

Around the third week of gestation, the middle ear cavity begins to appear as the tubotympanic recess, which is an outpouching of the first pharyngeal pouch. Expansion of this pouch begins inferiorly within the tympanic cavity and subsequently envelopes the ossicles, continues to the epitympanum and mastoid antrum by 22 weeks, and ultimately forms an open tympanic space by 8 months [8]. Mastoid pneumatization continues through 5 years postnatally and the growth rate slows until it reaches an adult size, generally by age

M. W. Canfarotta (✉)
Department of Otolaryngology—Head and Neck Surgery, Vanderbilt University Medical Center, Nashville, TN, USA

R. K. Sethi
Department of Otolaryngology—Head and Neck Surgery, Harvard Medical School, Boston, MA, USA

Dana Farber Cancer Center, Boston, MA, USA

C. E. Corrales (✉)
Otology, Neurotology and Skull Base Surgery, Harvard Medical School, Division of Otolaryngology, Brigham and Women's Hospital, Boston, MA, USA
e-mail: ccorrales@bwh.harvard.edu

A. D. Sweeney et al. (eds.), *Haynes-Glasscock-Shambaugh Surgery of the Ear*, https://doi.org/10.1007/978-3-032-18264-7_2

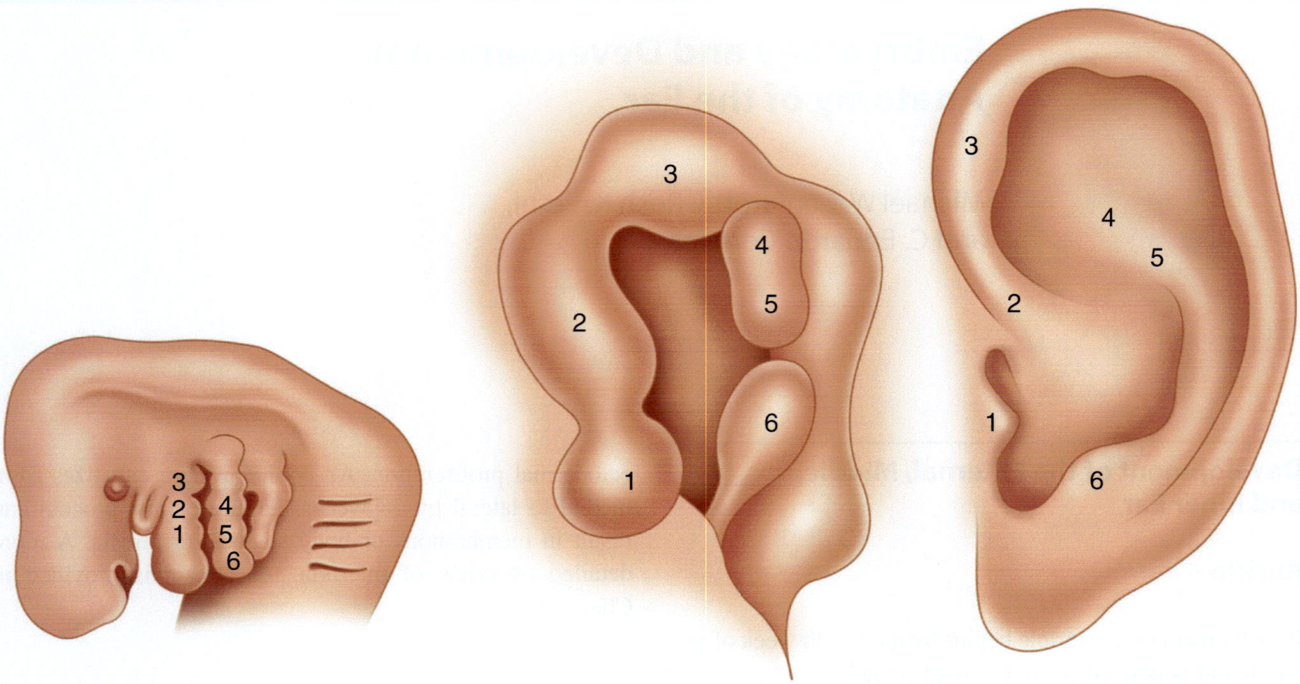

Fig. 2.1 Development of the auricle. (**a**) The six hillocks of His develop from the first (numbers 1–3) and second (numbers 4–6) branchial arches (11 mm embryo). (**b**) 15 mm embryo stage. (**c**) Numbered hillocks corresponding to the developed anatomy of the adult auricle. (Adapted from Levine H [2])

10 in females and age 15 in males [9]. In the neonate, the mastoid tip is not fully developed and expands over time, which is an important consideration during postauricular approaches to the mastoid and middle ear in children, as the facial nerve can be found in a more lateralized position.

Ossicular Chain

The ossicular chain functions by transferring sound energy from the tympanic membrane to the fluid-filled inner ear. Development of the ossicles begins at 4 weeks and is dependent upon the neural crest mesenchyme of the first (Meckel's cartilage, mandibular arch) and second (Reichert's cartilage, hyoid arch) branchial arches. A notable exception is the vestibular surface of the stapes footplate and its annular ligament, which arise from the otic capsule. The ossicles have attained adult size by 15 weeks. Ossification begins shortly after and is generally complete by 30 weeks. The stapes begins to develop its ring shape by 10 weeks and encircles the stapedial artery (artery associated with the second arch), which typically regresses during development. The "dual-arch" theory suggests that the head of the malleus and body and short process of the incus develop from the first arch, whereas the manubrium of the malleus, long process of the incus, stapes superstructure, and tympanic surface of the stapes footplate is derived from the second arch [10] (Fig. 2.2). The tensor tympani muscle is innervated by the mandibular branch of the trigeminal nerve, which are both first branchial arch derivatives. Similarly, the stapedius muscle is innervated by the facial nerve, which are both second branchial arch derivatives. The embryologic origin of the ossicular chain can be simplified such that the portions of the ossicles typically visible through the tympanic membrane on otoscopy are derived from the second branchial arch.

Congenital anomalies of the middle ear can occur due to disruptions during the development of the first and second branchial arches. Major abnormalities are associated with ear canal atresia, an absent or rudimentary tympanic membrane, and malformed middle ear anatomy, while minor abnormalities are generally confined to the middle ear with a normal tympanic membrane [12]. Ossicular chain abnormalities typically present with a 40–60 dB conductive hearing loss in childhood, and these can include fixation of the malleus or incus, absent or hypoplastic ossicles, fusion or misarticulation of ossicles, and ankylosis of the stapes.

In the case of a suspected congenital ossicular chain abnormality, an exploratory tympanotomy can be considered, but it is critical to counsel families on possible findings and outcomes associated with ossiculoplasty, particularly as congenital conductive hearing loss can also be managed conservatively with hearing aids. Ossiculoplasty can provide a safe and effective treatment option for isolated malleus or incus abnormalities [13]. Ankylosis of the stapes footplate can occur congenitally and is associated with a non-progressive maximal conductive hearing loss. This pathology can be challenging to

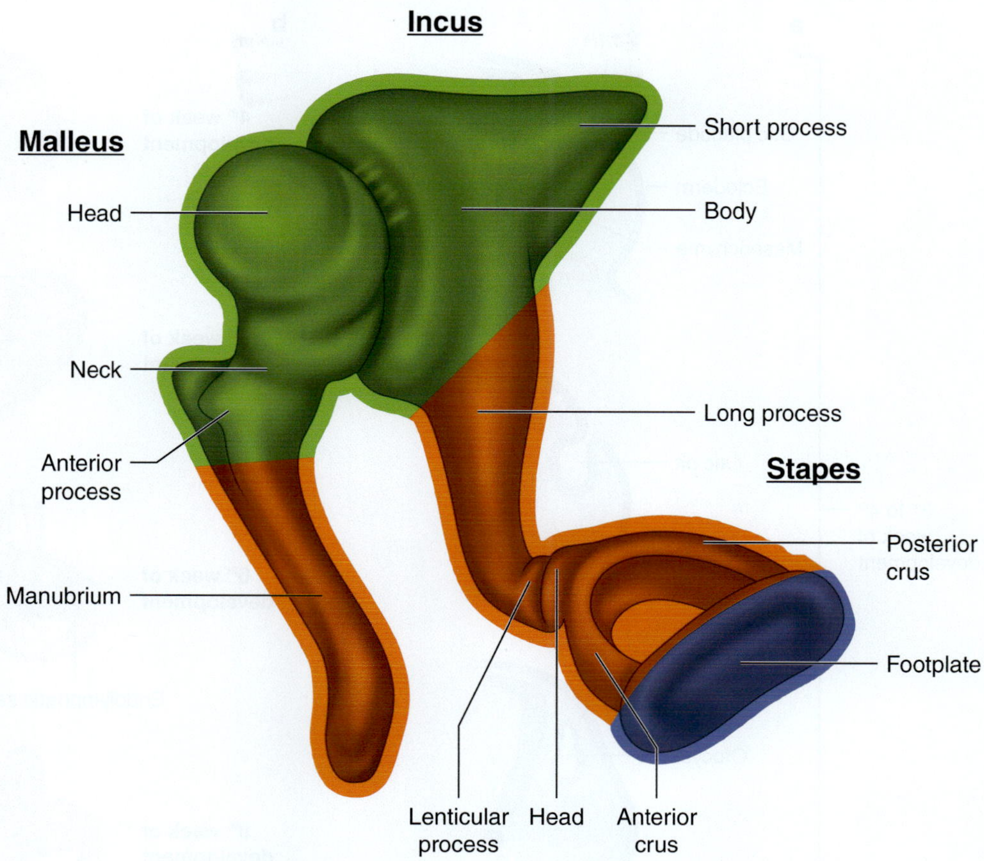

Fig. 2.2 Adult anatomy and embryologic origin of the ossicular chain. The ossicular chain develops from contributions from three different embryologic sources: (1) first branchial arch (green), (2) second branchial arch (orange), and (3) otic capsule (blue). (Adapted from Nolan J and Rivera AL [11])

differentiate from juvenile otosclerosis, which is typically progressive in nature. Congenital stapes footplate fixation is thought to occur due to the arrest or maldevelopment of the annular ligament of the oval window, likely after the tenth week of gestation [14]. Computed tomography of the temporal bone in congenital stapes footplate fixation is generally normal, but an absent or hypoplastic pyramidal eminence and stapedial tendon should raise suspicion [15]. Timing for stapedectomy in this patient population is controversial because surgical intervention does carry a risk for profound sensorineural hearing loss [16]. Some have suggested postponing surgery until at least the age of 5 years to reduce the risk related with recurrent otitis media [16, 17] while others recommend delaying intervention until the child can be involved in the consent process [18]. Nonetheless, with careful patient selection, stapedectomy can provide a safe and effective treatment option for patients with congenital stapes footplate fixation in the hands of an experienced surgeon [19].

Inner Ear

Development of the inner ear begins during the third week of gestation as the otic placode, which is a thickening of ectoderm on the lateral surface of the cephalic end of the embryo. By the fourth week, the placode invaginates to become a closed sac surrounded by mesoderm, referred to as the otocyst (Fig. 2.3a). In subsequent weeks, the otocyst continues to lengthen and the ventral portion becomes the cochlear duct and saccule while the dorsal portion forms the semicircular canals, utricle, and endolymphatic duct. This developmental process is illustrated in Fig. 2.3b. In the fifth week, the lower pole of the saccule lengthens and becomes the cochlear duct. Following this, the semicircular canals develop with first the superior, then posterior, and lastly lateral canal, which are distinct by the end of the sixth week. The cochlear duct continues to elongate and generally reaches 2.5 turns by the eighth week.

Epithelial cells within the cochlear duct differentiate to form the organ of Corti during the seventh week, with an inner ridge forming the osseous spiral lamina and an outer ridge forming the inner and outer hair cells. Mesenchyme that surrounds the membranous labyrinth differentiates into cartilage and ultimately becomes the otic capsule. This cartilage undergoes vacuolization in the tenth week to form perilymphatic spaces of the scala tympani and scala vestibuli. The tunnel of Corti is complete around 21 weeks and becomes functional, at least within the basal turn [1].

The otic capsule forms from the cartilaginous structure surrounding the labyrinth, with ossification beginning during the

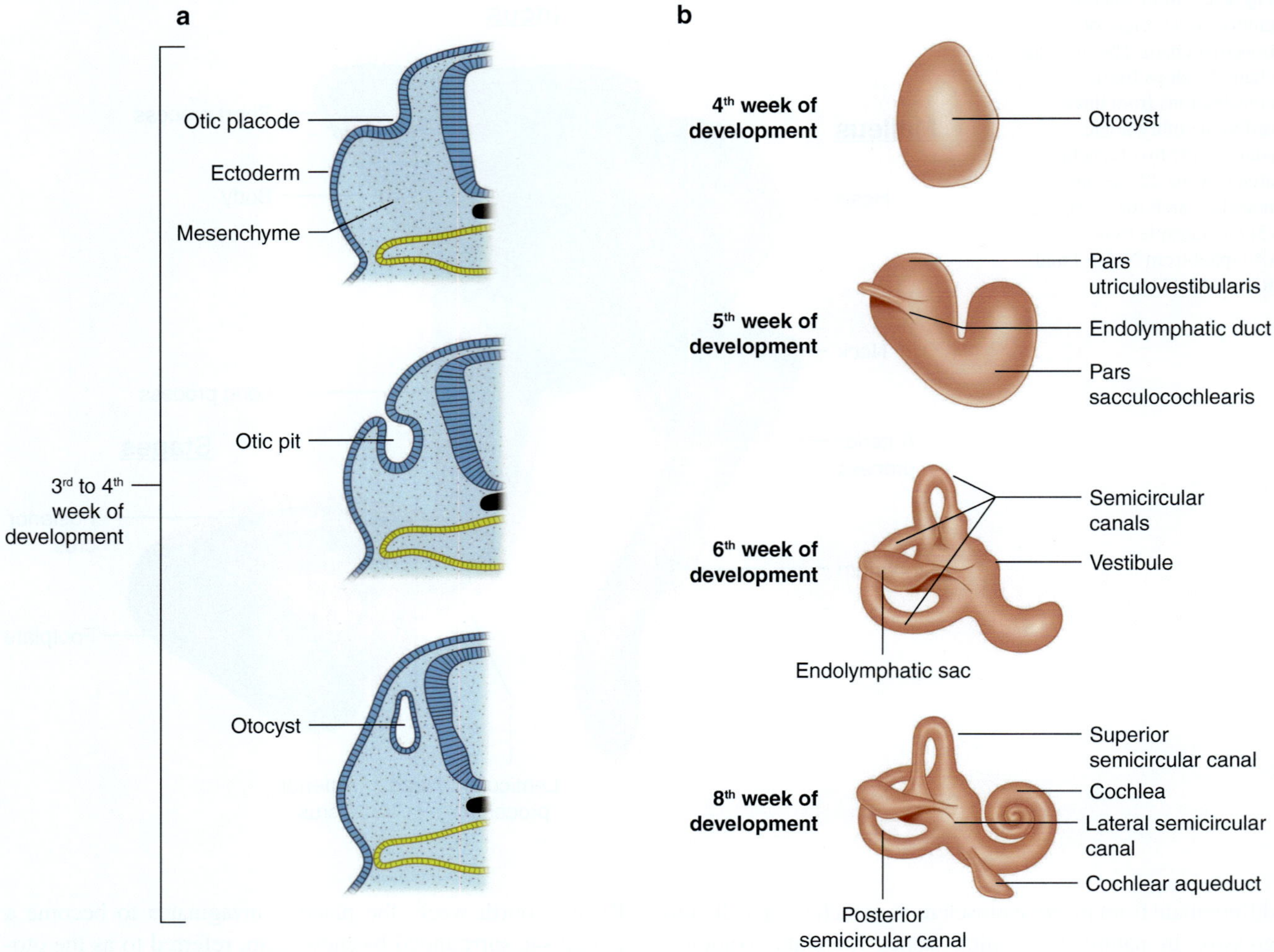

Fig. 2.3 Development of the inner ear. (**a**) The otocyst develops from the invagination of the otic placode during the third and fourth week. (**b**) From the fourth to eighth week, the otocyst lengthens to form a ventral portion containing the cochlear duct and saccule and dorsal portion containing the semicircular canals, utricle, and endolymphatic duct. (Adapted from Dhanasingh A [20])

eighth week from 14 centers. The developing stapes abuts the cartilaginous otic capsule during the ninth week and forms the oval window. The rim of the otic capsule and footplate remain cartilage, and the annular ligament forms at the interface. The round window also does not ossify but rather becomes a fibrous tissue boundary between the cochlear duct and middle ear. Ossification of the otic capsule near the round window occurs between the eighteenth and twenty-sixth weeks. The tympanomeningeal or Hyrtl's fissure is a patent connection between the fossula of the round window and posterior cranial fossa present during development [21]. Incomplete ossification of this fissure can result in a congenital CSF leak [22].

Along with the facial nerve, the vestibulocochlear nerve develops from the facioacoustic primordium in the third week of gestation. The vestibulocochlear ganglia arise from the ectoderm of the otocyst. During otocyst development, the vestibulocochlear ganglion divides into a superior division to innervate the superior and lateral ampullae of the semicircular canals and utricle, as well as an inferior division to innervate the posterior ampulla and saccule. The remainder of the nerve fibers become the spiral ganglion and follow the spiral growth of the cochlea to innervate hair cells.

Inner ear abnormalities occur due to aberrant or arrested development and can be divided into defects that affect the osseous and membranous labyrinth or the membranous labyrinth alone. The most common membranous defect observed in cases of congenital hearing loss occurs with incomplete development of the caudal portion of the otocyst resulting in cochleosaccular dysplasia, which was first described by Scheibe in 1892 [23]. This malformation is described by complete or partial absence of the organ of Corti with collapse of the cochlear duct and saccule and degeneration of the stria vascularis, yet normal development of the vestibular system, which occurs at an earlier stage. A milder form involving the cochlear basal turn is referred to as Alexander dysplasia. Earlier defects in development occur less frequently and can result in complete membranous labyrinthine dysplasia (Bing-Siebenmann).

Combined membranous and osseous cochlear malformations generally occur due to arrested development between the third and eighth weeks. Dependent upon the timing of arrest, this can result in the following malformations:

- Week 3 (early): *Michel's deformity*, or complete labyrinthine aplasia, is characterized by absence of inner ear structures including the internal auditory canal.
- Week 3 (late): *Rudimentary otocyst* occurs from developmental arrest slightly later and presents as a millimeter-sized round or ovoid cavity without an associated internal auditory canal.
- Week 4: *Common cavity* presents as a lack of differentiation between the vestibular and cochlear portion of the otocyst and the size of the cavity can be variable yet differs from rudimentary otocyst as it is generally connected with the internal auditory canal at its center.
- Week 5: *Incomplete partition type I* is characterized by a cystic cochlea with absent modiolus and interscalar septa and is accompanied by a dilated vestibule.
- Week 5 and 6: *Cochlear aplasia* is the absence of the cochlea with either a normal labyrinth or dilated vestibule. *Cochlear hypoplasia* occurs due to arrest slightly later in development and is subdivided into four groups but generally characterized by small external dimensions with various internal architectural deformities [24].
- Week 7: *Incomplete partition type II* (*Mondini deformity*) is defined by an apical modiolar defect with a cystic cochlear apex, dilated vestibule, and enlarged vestibular aqueduct.

Congenital inner ear malformations and associated auditory rehabilitation options are discussed in further detail in Chaps. 19 and 49.

Malformations of the semicircular canals can occur in the presence of a normal cochlea. Dysplasia or aplasia of the lateral semicircular canal is generally the most common finding, as it is the last canal to develop, and is the most specific abnormality of CHARGE syndrome, though many different otologic anomalies may be coexistent [25].

Development of the Facial Nerve

The facial nerve is developmentally derived from the second branchial arch and provides motor innervation to the muscles of facial expression, stylohyoid, posterior belly of the digastric, and stapedius, as well as sensory innervation to the anterior two-thirds of the tongue for taste sensation via special visceral afferent fibers of the chorda tympani nerve. The course of the facial nerve is complex, and understanding the development of the intratemporal portion can be beneficial for the neurotologic surgeon to identify anatomic variations.

Facial nerve development starts as the facioacoustic primordium during the third week of gestation and divides into cranial nerves VII and VIII by 5 weeks. During the fourth week, the chorda tympani nerve enters the mandibular arch and terminates near the mandibular nerve to become the lingual nerve and supply taste sensation to the anterior two-thirds of the tongue. In the sixth week, the greater superficial petrosal nerve develops from the ventral surface of the geniculate ganglion. The nerve to stapedius subsequently develops during the seventh week [26].

The fallopian canal is a bony canal through which the facial nerve traverses within the temporal bone. It begins proximally at the meatal foramen in the internal auditory canal and ends distally at the stylomastoid foramen. It is composed of three distinct segments: (1) labyrinthine, (2) tympanic, and (3) mastoid. Between each segment is a genu, with the first developing from the nerve being pushed forward by the developing otic capsule. During the tenth week, the facial nerve forms a second genu in the middle ear. The distal portion of the nerve continues inferiorly from the second genu, and the distal or mastoid segment is more anteriorly positioned than seen in adults. The fallopian canal first develops as a sulcus within the cartilaginous otic capsule and passes posteriorly from the geniculate ganglion, lying superior to the developing stapes, and turns inferiorly near the developing round window. Ossification begins by the sixteenth week and is partially complete by the twenty-sixth week gestation. During this time, the nerve is pulled posteriorly by the developing tympanic ring.

Aberrant development may result in abnormal positioning or variations of the facial nerve and fallopian canal. Congenital malformations of the outer and middle ear are commonly associated with anterior and lateral displacement of the nerve, and in as many as 50% of atretic ears, the facial nerve can be abnormal [27]. Given the close association of the facial nerve and otic capsule during development, anterior displacement of the nerve can result in the inability of the developing stapes to meet the otic capsule, leading to a rudimentary stapes formation [28]. Similarly, although the embryologic mechanism is unknown, the facial nerve may also bifurcate around the stapes [29]. In perhaps the most clinically relevant variant, the tympanic segment of the nerve can be dehiscent in up to 55% of cases [30], which may be due to failure of fusion of two ossification centers within the middle ear.

Development of Sensory Nerves of the Ear

Sensory innervation to the eustachian tube, middle ear, and medial aspect of the tympanic membrane is supplied by Jacobson's nerve, which is a branch of the glossopharyngeal nerve. During development, this is formed from a ventral offshoot of the geniculate ganglion that reaches the glossopharyngeal ganglion during the seventh to eighth weeks. Clinically, this forms the tympanic plexus along the cochlear promontory, which can be the site of origin for glomus tympanicum tumors arising from paraganglion cells. By 13 weeks, communicating branches fuse from the dorsomedial aspect of the facial nerve to the superior ganglia of the vagus and glossopharyngeal nerves, forming Arnold's nerve (auricular branch of vagus), which traverses the tympanomastoid fissure to supply sensation to the posterior aspect of the external auditory canal. The nervus intermedius, a sensory branch of the facial nerve, travels between the main trunk and vestibulocochlear nerve and joins the motor root at the geniculate ganglion, additionally supplying sensation to the posterior aspect of the external auditory canal. Decreased sensation in this region, referred to as the Hitselberger's sign, has been associated with pathology of the cerebellopontine angle, including vestibular schwannomas [31]. Lateral to the external auditory meatus, the concha is also supplied by the nervus intermedius and Arnold's nerve. The anterior aspect of the external auditory canal, tragus, and superior helix are supplied by the auriculotemporal nerve, which is a sensory branch of the mandibular division of the trigeminal nerve. Neural development of the auriculotemporal nerve is intimately associated with the middle meningeal artery, as two roots of the mandibular nerve course around the artery. These roots subsequently join deep to the lateral pterygoid muscle and then travel between the neck of the mandible and sphenomandibular ligament, where the nerve divides to form auricular and temporal components. Nerve trunks of the cervical plexus form during the fourth week of gestation, and the second and third cervical nerves form the great auricular nerve to supply sensation to the lobule, antihelix, and helix.

Development of Arterial Supply to the Temporal Bone and Ear

The embryologic development of the vascular system begins at approximately 3 weeks as the primitive heart becomes recognizable. Six aortic arches subsequently develop during the third and fourth week. The first arch (mandibular artery) generally involutes around 4 weeks, and the second arch (hyostapedial artery) later in development. The third arch becomes the internal carotid artery, the fourth arch becomes the aortic arch on the left and brachiocephalic artery on the right, the fifth arch completely involutes, and the sixth arch becomes the pulmonary arteries.

Development of the internal carotid artery is illustrated in Fig. 2.4. The role of the mandibular artery is unclear [33], but some suggest that it is a precursor to the Vidian artery in the

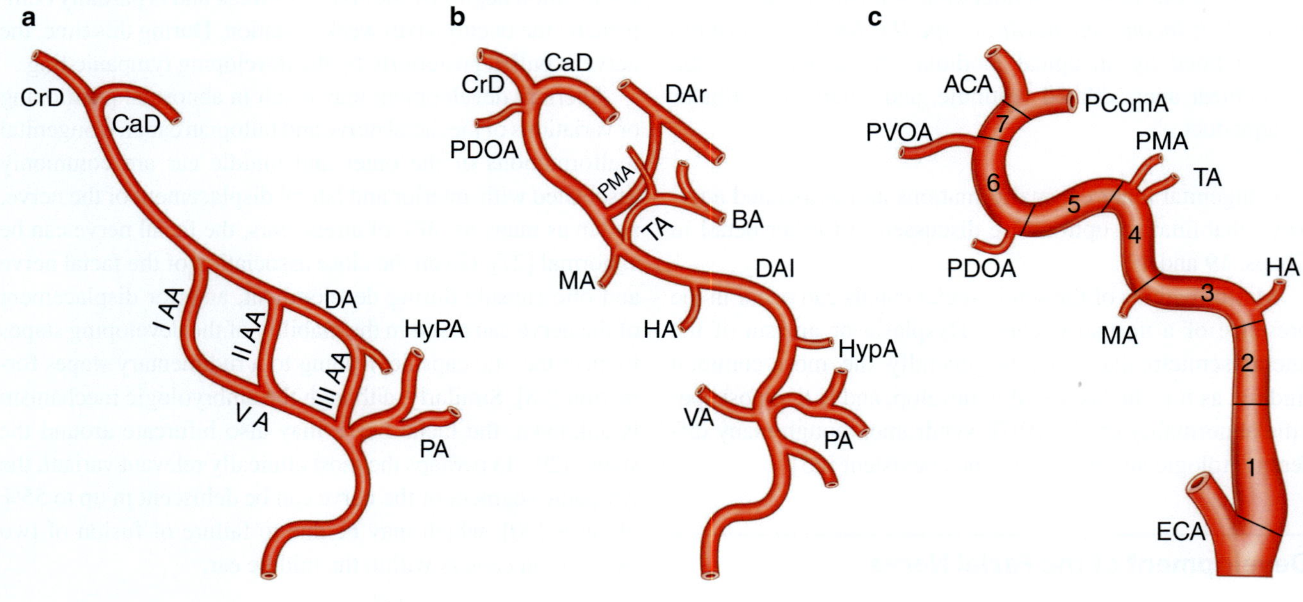

Fig. 2.4 Embryologic development of the internal carotid artery. (**a**) The dorsal and ventral aorta (DA and VA) are linked by three aortic arches (I–III AA). (**b**) The hypoglossal artery (HypA) and proatlantal artery (PA) ultimately contribute to the formation of external carotid artery (ECA) branches. The VA regresses while the DA forms embryonic arteries, (**c**) which later develop into 7 segments of the internal carotid artery. The *cervical segment* (1) derives from III AA. The *ascending intrapetrous segment* (2) derives from the DA, II AA, and III AA. The *horizontal petrous segment* (3) is divided by the hyoid artery (HA), which is the dorsal remnant of II AA. The *intracavernous ascending segment* (4), which is divided by the mandibular artery (MA, remnant of I AA), derives from the dorsal remnant of I AA and primitive maxillary artery (PMA), connecting the left and right dorsal aorta (DAl and DAr). The trigeminal artery (TA) is a branch of this segment and serves as a primitive connection between the cavernous internal carotid artery and basilar artery (BA). The *horizontal intracavernous segment* (5) traverses from the PMA to the primitive dorsal ophthalmic artery (PDOA). The *clinoid segment* (6) traverses between the PDOA and primitive ventral ophthalmic artery (PVOA). Lastly, the *terminal segment* (7) traverses between the PVOA and primitive internal carotid artery bifurcation into the anterior cerebral artery (ACA) and posterior communicating artery (PComA). (Adapted from Bonasia S and Robert T [32])

adult [34]. The hyoid artery elongates rapidly between the seventh and nineteenth weeks and gives rise to the stapedial artery after passing through the developing stapes, and it is important for the ultimate development of dural, facial, and orbital arteries.

The stapedial artery branches to form the supraorbital and maxillomandibular arteries. The supraorbital artery follows the ophthalmic root of the trigeminal nerve to allow for development of orbital branches and the middle meningeal artery. The maxillomandibular artery exits the cranial cavity through the foramen spinosum. Around the eighth week, the maxillomandibular and supraorbital arteries are annexed by the ventral pharyngeal and ophthalmic artery, respectively. This results in the adult configuration of the middle meningeal artery arising from the internal maxillary artery with backflow and regression of the stapedial artery proximal to the stapes, which becomes the superior tympanic branch of the middle meningeal artery. When the proximal portion of the maxillomandibular artery regresses instead of the proximal stapedial artery, this results in an absent or reduced size of the foramen spinosum. In this scenario of a persistent stapedial artery, the middle meningeal artery arises from the stapedial artery instead of the internal maxillary artery. Persistent stapedial arteries can present with conductive hearing loss, pulsatile tinnitus, or can be incidentally found during middle ear surgery. There is some concern regarding cauterization of the vessel due to the risk of hearing loss, facial palsy, and hemiplegia [35], but some have reported successful ablation without sequelae [36, 37].

The adult vasculature of the middle ear is ultimately supplied by the carotico-tympanic artery (branch of the petrous internal carotid artery and remnant of the embryologic hyostapedial artery), the superior tympanic artery (branch of the middle meningeal artery), inferior tympanic artery (branch of the ascending pharyngeal artery), anterior tympanic artery (branch from either the internal maxillary, superficial temporal, or external carotid artery), and stylomastoid artery (branch of the external carotid or occipital artery) (Fig. 2.5).

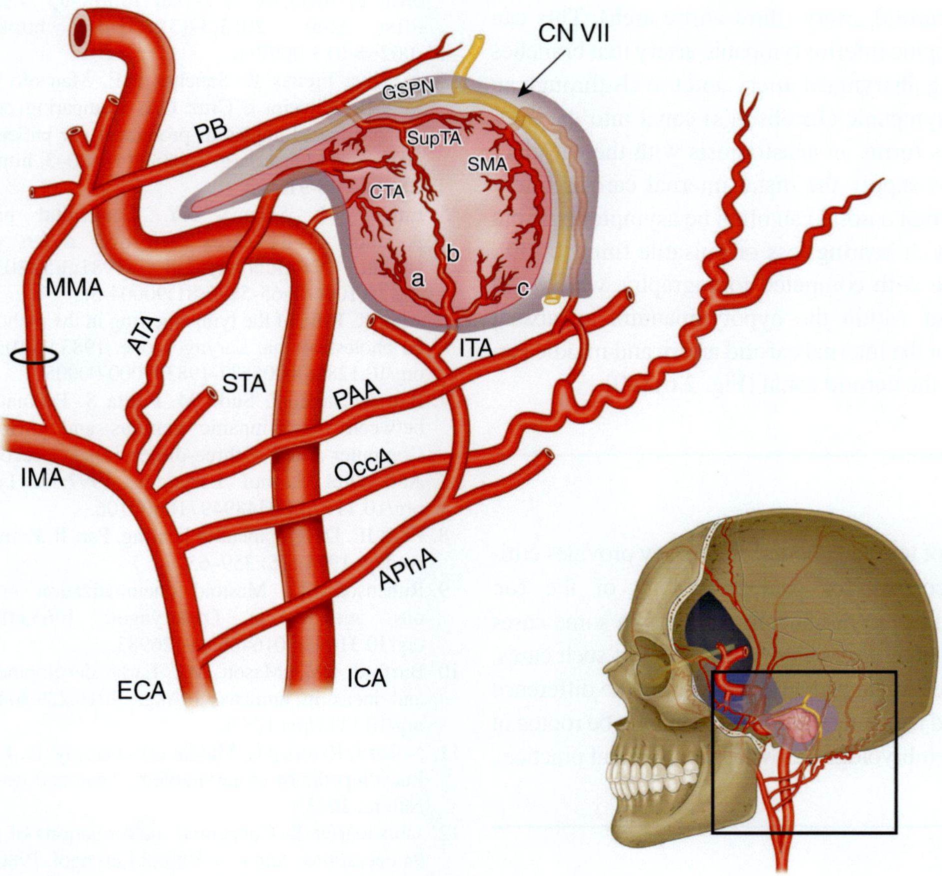

Fig. 2.5 Illustration of arterial supply to the middle ear. The middle ear is supplied by the (1) anterior tympanic artery (ATA), which branches from the internal maxillary artery (IMA) after it bifurcates from the superficial temporal artery (STA); (2) superior tympanic artery (SupTA) that branches from the petrous branch (PB) of the middle meningeal artery (MMA) and courses with the greater superficial petrosal nerve (GSPN); (3) stylomastoid artery (SMA), which either branches from the posterior auricular artery (PAA) or occipital artery (OccA) and enters the fallopian canal with the facial nerve (CN VII); (4) inferior tympanic artery (ITA), which is a branch of the anterior division of the ascending pharyngeal artery (APhA) and enters the tympanic cavity through Jacobson's canal to form anterior (**a**), middle (**b**), and posterior branches; and (5) carotico-tympanic artery (CTA), which originates from the petrous internal carotid artery (ICA). (Adapted from Bonasia S and Robert T [32])

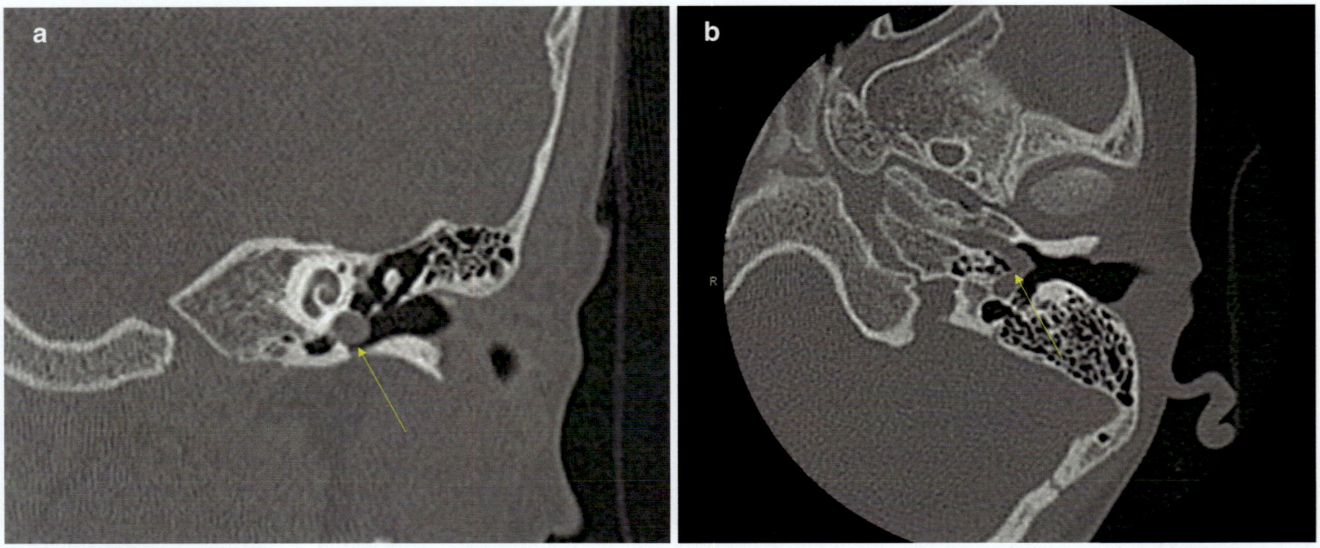

Fig. 2.6 (**a**) Coronal and (**b**) Axial computed tomography images of a left ear with an aberrant carotid artery (yellow arrow) abutting the malleus and the tympanic membrane. (Courtesy of Alex D. Sweeney, MD)

An aberrant carotid artery results from agenesis of the cervical internal carotid artery (third aortic arch). This can result in a hypertrophic inferior tympanic artery that branches from the ascending pharyngeal artery and travels through an enlarged inferior tympanic (Jacobson's) canal into the middle ear space. This forms an anastomosis with the caroticotympanic artery to supply the distal internal carotid artery flow [38]. An aberrant carotid can often be asymptomatic but can also present with hearing loss or pulsatile tinnitus [39]. Diagnosis is made with computed tomography, which will show enhancement within the hypotympanum, an absent bone plate between the internal carotid artery and middle ear, and/or absence of the carotid canal (Fig. 2.6) [40].

Conclusions

An understanding of temporal bone embryology provides critically important context for pathophysiology of the ear. Structural deformities are not uncommon, and in some cases can lie insidiously until discovered later in life. In such cases, as well as cases seen in the pediatric population, the difference between a good and bad outcome could potentially be rooted in the application of embryologic knowledge to clinical practice.

References

1. Sulik KK, Cotanche DA. Embryology of the ear. In: Toriello HV, Reardon W, Gorlin RJ, editors. Hereditary hearing loss and its syndromes. Oxford University Press; 2004.
2. Levine H. Cutaneous carcinoma of the head and neck: management of massive and previously uncontrolled lesions. Laryngoscope. 1983;93(1):87–105.
3. Purkait R. Progression of growth in the external ear from birth to maturity: a 2-year follow-up study in India. Aesth Plast Surg. 2013;37(3):605–16. https://doi.org/10.1007/s00266-013-0097-1.
4. da Silva Freitas R, Sanchez ME, Manzotti MS, Baras F, Ono MC, de Oliveira e Cruz GA. Comparing cephaloauricular and scaphaconchal angles in prominent ear patients and control subjects. Aesth Plast Surg. 2008;32(4):620–3. https://doi.org/10.1007/s00266-008-9160-8.
5. Emery PJ, Salama NY. Congenital pre-auricular sinus. A study of 31 cases seen over a ten year period. Int J Pediatr Otorhinolaryngol. 1981;3(3):205–12. https://doi.org/10.1016/0165-5876(81)90004-5.
6. Aimi K. Role of the tympanic ring in the pathogenesis of congenital cholesteatoma. Laryngoscope. 1983;93(9):1140–6. https://doi.org/10.1288/00005537-198309000-00005.
7. Ikui A, Sando I, Sudo M, Fujita S. Postnatal change in angle between the tympanic annulus and surrounding structures. Computer-aided three-dimensional reconstruction study. Ann Otol Rhinol Laryngol. 1997;106(1):33–6. https://doi.org/10.1177/000348949710600106.
8. Peck JE. Development of hearing. Part II. Embryology. J Am Acad Audiol. 1994;5(6):359–65.
9. Rubensohn G. Mastoid pneumatization in children at various ages. Acta Otolaryngol. 1965;60:11–4. https://doi.org/10.3109/00016486509126983.
10. Burford CM, Mason MJ. Early development of the malleus and incus in humans. J Anat. 2016;229(6):857–70. https://doi.org/10.1111/joa.12520.
11. Nolan J, Rivera AL. Middle ear anatomy. In: Kountakis SE, editor. Encyclopedia of otolaryngology, head and neck surgery. Springer Nature; 2013.
12. Jahrsdoerfer R. Congenital malformations of the ear. Analysis of 94 operations. Ann Otol Rhinol Laryngol. 1980;89(4 Pt 1):348–52. https://doi.org/10.1177/000348948008900410.
13. Vincent R, Wegner I, Derks LS, Grolman W. Congenital ossicular chain malformations with mobile stapes in children: results in 17 cases. Laryngoscope. 2016;126(3):682–8. https://doi.org/10.1002/lary.25351.
14. Lindsay JR, Sanders SH, Nager GT. Histopathologic observations in so-called congenital fixation of the stapedial

footplate. Laryngoscope. 1960;70:1587–602. https://doi.org/10.1288/00005537-196012000-00001.
15. Nassiri AM, Benson JC, Doerfer KW, et al. Absent pyramidal eminence and stapedial tendon associated with congenital stapes footplate fixation: intraoperative and radiographic findings. Am J Otolaryngol. 2021;42(6):103144. https://doi.org/10.1016/j.amjoto.2021.103144.
16. House JW, Sheehy JL, Antunez JC. Stapedectomy in children. Laryngoscope. 1980;90(11 Pt 1):1804–9. https://doi.org/10.1288/00005537-198011000-00007.
17. De la Cruz A, Angeli S, Slattery WH. Stapedectomy in children. Otolaryngol Head Neck Surg. 1999;120(4):487–92. https://doi.org/10.1053/hn.1999.v120.a89626.
18. Kempfle JS, Remenschneider AK. Management of congenital conductive hearing loss. Oper Tech Otolaryngol Head Neck Surg. 2024:26–36.
19. Carlson ML, Van Abel KM, Pelosi S, et al. Outcomes comparing primary pediatric stapedectomy for congenital stapes footplate fixation and juvenile otosclerosis. Otol Neurotol. 2013;34(5):816–20. https://doi.org/10.1097/MAO.0b013e318280db7b.
20. Dhanasingh A. Embryology of inner ear malformation types and its radiological relevance. In: Li Y, editor. Cochlear implantation for common cavity deformity. Springer Nature; 2022.
21. Spector GJ, Lee D, Carr C, et al. Later stages of development of the periotic duct and its adjacent area in the human fetus. Laryngoscope. 1980;90(5 Pt 2):1–31. https://doi.org/10.1288/00005537-198005001-00001.
22. Lovin BD, Appelbaum EN, Makoshi L, Whitehead WE, Sweeney AD. Spontaneous congenital perilabyrinthine cerebrospinal fluid fistulas. Ann Otol Rhinol Laryngol. 2021;130(12):1360–8. https://doi.org/10.1177/00034894211007242.
23. Scheibe A. A case of deaf-mutism, with auditory atrophy an anomalies of development in the membranous labyrinth of both ears. Arch Otolaryngol. 1892:12–22.
24. Sennaroğlu L, Bajin MD. Classification and current management of inner ear malformations. Balkan Med J. 2017;34(5):397–411. https://doi.org/10.4274/balkanmedj.2017.0367.
25. Sanlaville D, Verloes A. CHARGE syndrome: an update. Eur J Hum Genet. 2007;15(4):389–99. https://doi.org/10.1038/sj.ejhg.5201778.
26. Sataloff RT. Embryology of the facial nerve and its clinical applications. Laryngoscope. 1990;100(9):969–84. https://doi.org/10.1288/00005537-199009000-00011.
27. Cressman WR, Pensak ML. Surgical aspects of congenital aural atresia. Otolaryngol Clin N Am. 1994;27(3):621–33.
28. Lambert PR. Congenital absence of the oval window. Laryngoscope. 1990;100(1):37–40. https://doi.org/10.1288/00005537-199001000-00009.
29. Nager GT. Pathology of the ear and temporal bone. Philadelphia: Lippincott Williams & Wilkins; 1993. p. 147–74.
30. Baxter A. Dehiscence of the fallopian canal. An anatomical study. J Laryngol Otol. 1971;85(6):587–94. https://doi.org/10.1017/s0022215100073849.
31. Hitselberger WE, House WF. Acoustic neuroma diagnosis. External auditory canal hypesthesia as an early sign. Arch Otolaryngol. 1966;83(3):218–21. https://doi.org/10.1001/archotol.1966.00760020220007.
32. Bonasia S, Robert T. Arterial supply of the middle ear. In: Robert T, Bonasia S, Bojanowski MW, editors. Anatomy of cranial arteries, embryology and variants. Springer Nature; 2023.
33. Padget DH. The development of cranial arteries in the human embryo. Contrib Embryol. 1948:205–62.
34. Lasjaunias P, Bereinstein A, Ter Brugge KG. Surgical neuroangiography. Berlin: Springer; 2001.
35. Hogg ID, Stephens CB, Arnold GE. Theoretical anomalies of the stapedial artery. Ann Otol Rhinol Laryngol. 1972;81(6):860–70. https://doi.org/10.1177/000348947208100619.
36. Govaerts PJ, Marquet TF, Cremers WR, Offeciers FE. Persistent stapedial artery: does it prevent successful surgery? Ann Otol Rhinol Laryngol. 1993;102(9):724–8. https://doi.org/10.1177/000348949310200914.
37. Hitier M, Zhang M, Labrousse M, Barbier C, Patron V, Moreau S. Persistent stapedial arteries in humans: from phylogeny to surgical consequences. Surg Radiol Anat. 2013;35(10):883–91. https://doi.org/10.1007/s00276-013-1127-z.
38. Lasjaunias P, Santoyo-Vazquez A. Segmental agenesis of the internal carotid artery: angiographic aspects with embryological discussion. Anat Clin. 1984;6(2):133–41. https://doi.org/10.1007/BF01773165.
39. Windfuhr JP. Aberrant internal carotid artery in the middle ear. Ann Otol Rhinol Laryngol Suppl. 2004;192:1–16. https://doi.org/10.1177/00034894041130s301.
40. McElveen JT, Lo WW, el Gabri TH, Nigri P. Aberrant internal carotid artery: classic findings on computed tomography. Otolaryngol Head Neck Surg. 1986;94(5):616–21. https://doi.org/10.1177/019459988609400515.

Anatomy of the Temporal Bone and Skull Base with Surgical Implications

3

Jennifer Alyono and Robert Jackler

Introduction

While the temporal bone is a highly complex anatomical structure because its viscera are locked rigidly in bone, its surgically crucial relationships tend to be more predictable than for most other organs. Mastery of these relationships is central to safe and effective surgery of the ear and skull base. In this chapter, our goal is to overview the relevant temporal bone anatomy as this knowledge is fundamental to subsequent mastery of procedural anatomy involving step-wise surgical technique. Contrary to common belief, the temporal bone got its name not because the "temple" is the seat of the soul but rather the passage of time. The name derives from the observation that aging of a man is first noted by the appearance of gray hair in this region. Petrous refers to "stony hard," a description which refers to the density and hardness of the structure, especially its deeper structures. The term petrous pyramid is a misnomer as the structure does not possess four surfaces converging to a point but is rather a roughly triangular shaped elongated ridge. The mastoid got its name from the "breast-like" shape of its tip. The naming conventions of structures of the temple bone and its viscera reveal the colorful history of discovery and discoverers, over many centuries [12, 13].

In our original illustrations, we build upon the work of the many anatomists and surgeons before us who have described and illustrated the ear through careful observation and dissection. Notable works in surgical anatomy of the ear include those of Albert Tuttle [17], Arthur Cheatle [4], Barry Anson and James Donaldson [6], Aina Julianna Gulya and Harold Schuknecht [7], and Albert Rhoton [14]. Our illustrations are enriched by the modern ability to visualize the three-dimensional relationships of the temporal bone through high-resolution imaging. Close collaboration between artist and surgeon, in this instance over a three-decade period, has been critical for achieving informative and accurate illustrations of important anatomical features and their complex relationships. We are grateful to medical illustrator Christine Gralapp for the excellence of her craft.

The original illustrations which appear in this chapter (Figs. 3.1, 3.2, 3.3, 3.4, 3.5, 3.6, 3.7, 3.8, 3.9, 3.10, 3.11, 3.12, 3.13, 3.14, 3.15, 3.16, 3.17, 3.18, 3.19, 3.20, 3.21, 3.22, 3.23, 3.24, 3.25, 3.26, 3.27, 3.28, 3.29, 3.30, 3.31, 3.32, 3.33, 3.34, 3.35, 3.36, 3.37, 3.38, 3.39, 3.40, 3.41, 3.42, 3.43, 3.44, 3.45, 3.46, 3.47, 3.48, 3.49, 3.50, 3.51, 3.52, 3.53, 3.54, and 3.55) are available online for non-commercial, educational use as part of an atlases of otology and neurotology maintained by Stanford Otolaryngology-Head & Neck Surgery (https://skullbasesurgeryatlas.stanford.edu, https://otosurgeryatlas.stanford.edu) Many of the illustrations are also available in print form [10].

The ear is composed of three components: the external, middle, and inner ear. The external ear includes the pinna and external auditory canal. The middle ear includes the tympanic cavity and ossicles and is connected to the nasopharynx through the Eustachian tube. The inner ear includes the cochlea, semicircular canals, and vestibule. The temporomandibular joint (TMJ) is a synovial articulation between the temporal bone and mandible, located anterior to the ear canal [11]. Published with permission from Robert Jackler, MD who maintains copyright ownership and right to future use.

J. Alyono (✉) · R. Jackler
Department of Otolaryngology—Head and Neck Surgery, Stanford University, Stanford, CA, USA
e-mail: jalyono@stanford.edu

A. D. Sweeney et al. (eds.), *Haynes-Glasscock-Shambaugh Surgery of the Ear*, https://doi.org/10.1007/978-3-032-18264-7_3

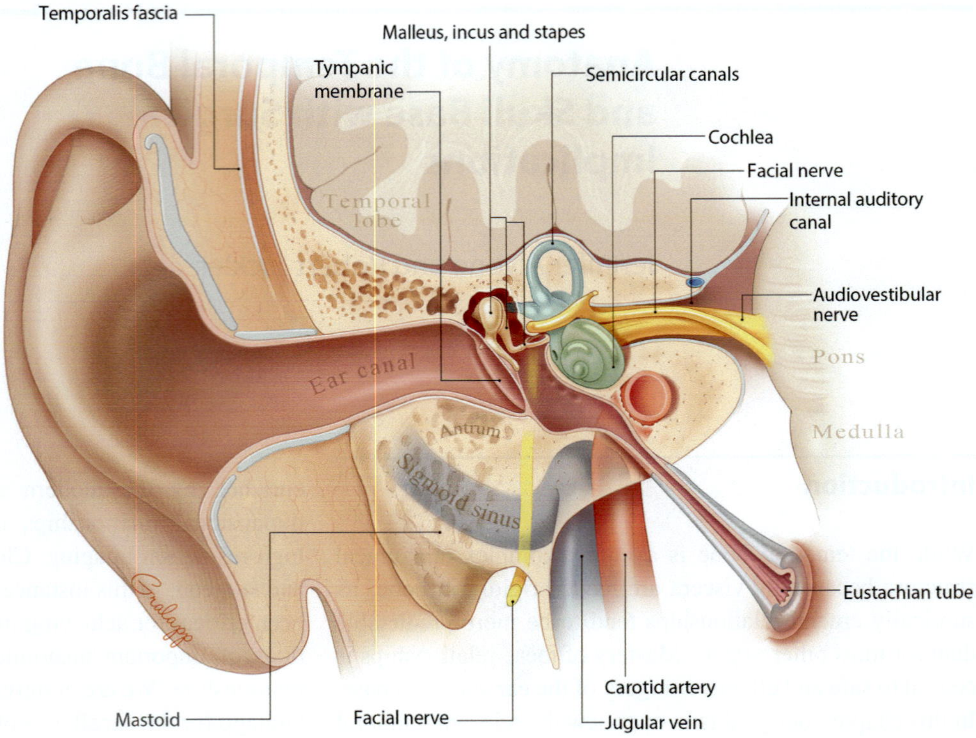

Fig. 3.1 Coronal schematic of the ear

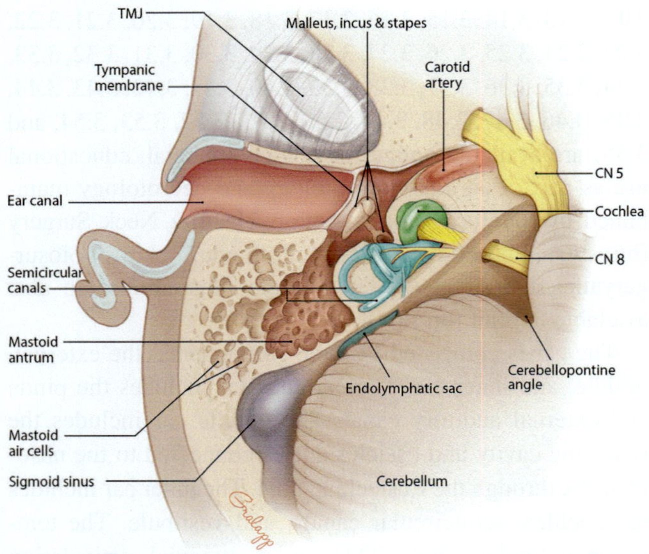

Fig. 3.2 Axial schematic of the ear. (Published with permission from Robert Jackler, MD who maintains copyright ownership and right to future use)

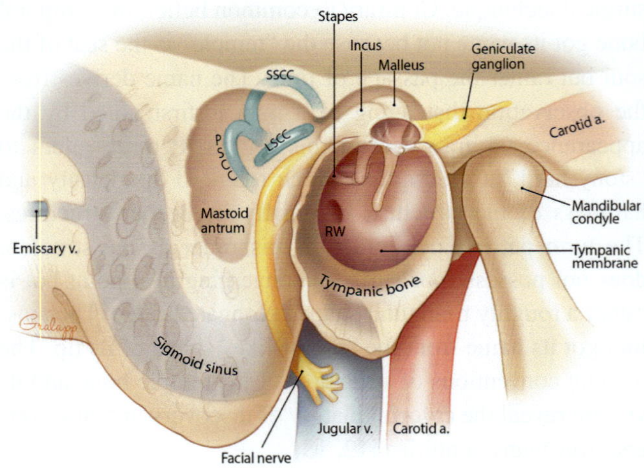

Fig. 3.3 Lateral schematic of the ear. LSCC Lateral semicircular canal, PSCC posterior semicircular canal, SSCC superior semicircular canal, RW round window. (Published with permission from Robert Jackler, MD who maintains copyright ownership and right to future use)

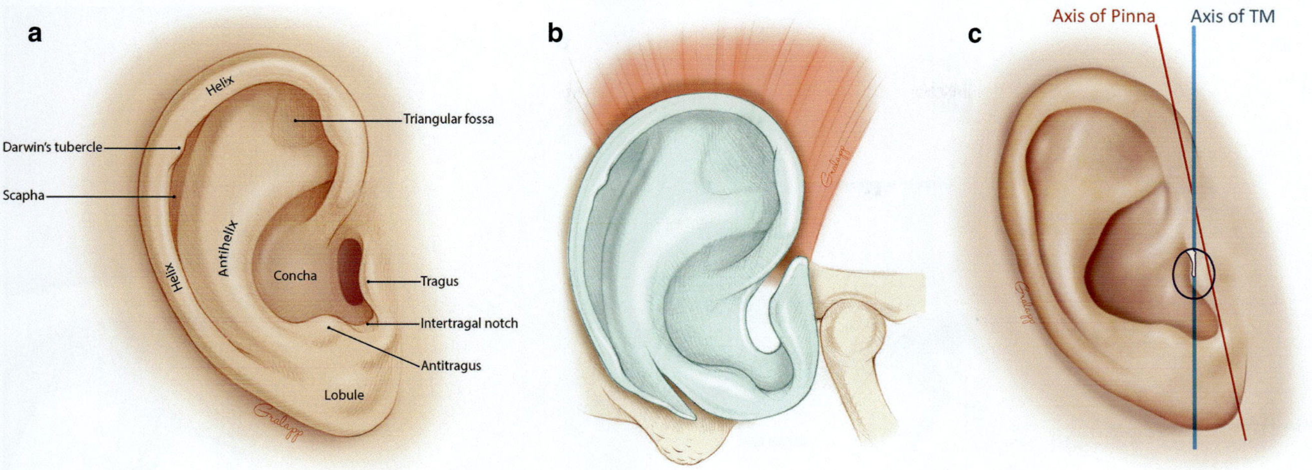

Fig. 3.4 External surface (**a**) and cartilaginous anatomy (**b**) of the pinna. The pinna aids in sound amplification and localization. Its shape is determined by the configuration of the underlying elastic cartilage framework. The incisura, important in meatoplasty and endaural approaches, is the interval between the anterior crus of the helix and the superior aspect of the tragus. (**c**) Note the axis of the pinna is not in the vertical plane, as is the tympanic membrane, but 15–20° rotated posteriorly. (Published with permission from Robert Jackler, MD who maintains copyright ownership and right to future use)

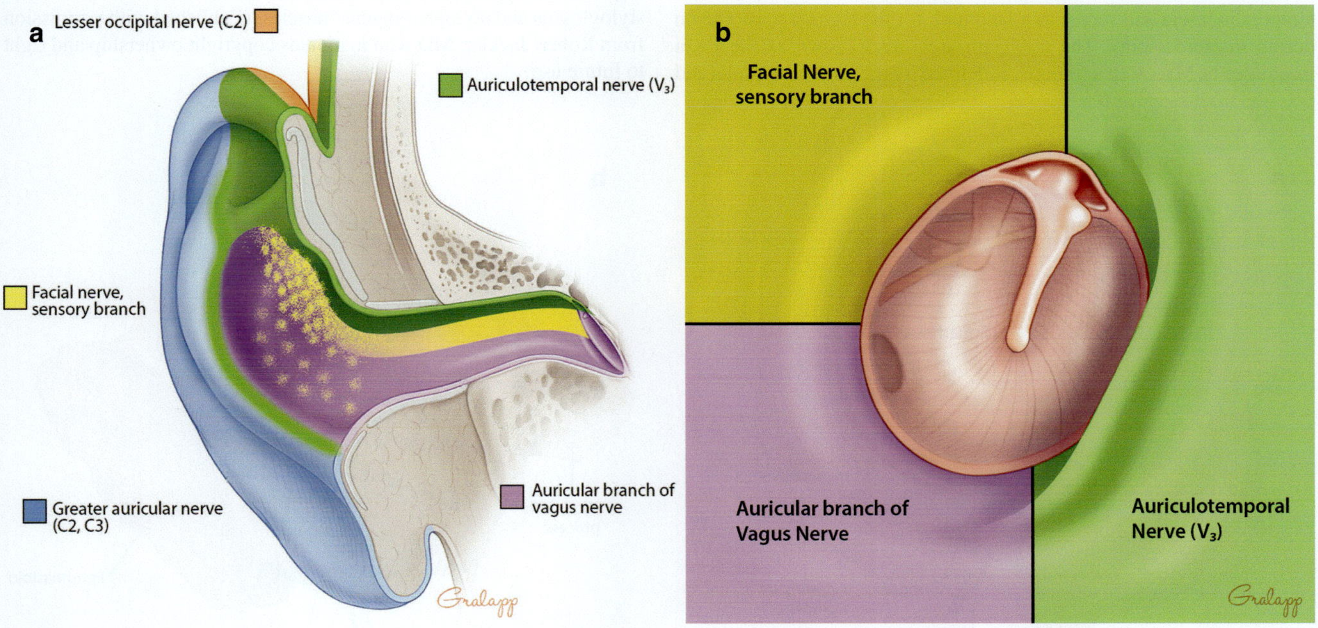

Fig. 3.5 Sensory innervation to the pinna (**a**) and ear canal (**b**) is provided by the auriculotemporal nerve (V3), lesser occipital nerve (C2), greater auricular nerve (C2, C3), auricular branch of the vagus nerve (Arnold's nerve), and sensory branches of the facial nerve. Hitselberger sign, or hypesthesia of the concha, results from dysfunction of the sensory branches of the facial nerve [8]. Arnold's reflex, or cough with manipulation of the external auditory canal, results from stimulation of the auricular branch of the vagus nerve [2]. The tympanic branch of the glossophyangeal nerve (Jacobsen's nerve) provides sensation to the middle ear. (Published with permission from Robert Jackler, MD who maintains copyright ownership and right to future use)

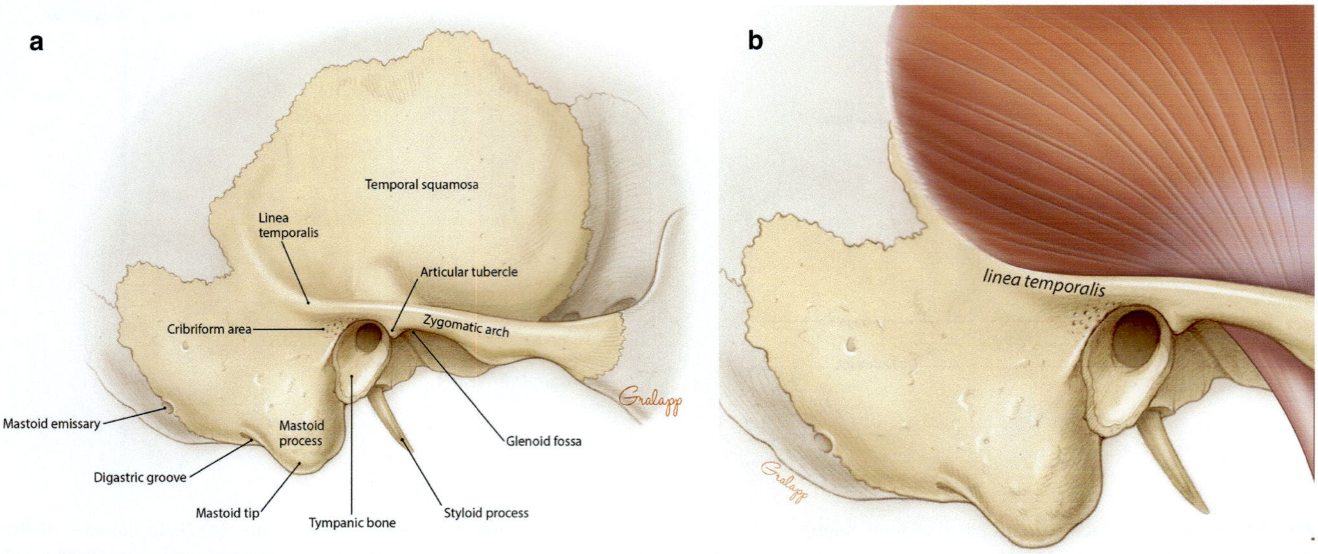

Fig. 3.6 Temporal bone surface anatomy (**a**) and attachment of the temporalis muscle (**b**). The temporalis muscle is one of the muscles of mastication. Fan-shaped, it spans the temporal squamosa and extends medial to the zygomatic arch, before inserting on the coronoid process of the mandible. The linea temporalis serves as the attachment of the temporalis fascia and serves as a landmark for the tegmen mastoideum during mastoidectomy. The cribiform area, also known as the fossa mastoidea or Macewen's triangle, is defined by the linea temporalis and the posterosuperior margin of the ear canal. The mastoid process serves as the attachment for the sternocleidomastoid, splenius capitus, longissimus capitis, and posterior belly of the digastric muscles. The styloid process arises anterior to the stylomastoid foramen and gives attachment to the stylohyoid and stylomandibular ligaments as well as the styloglossus and stylopharyngeus muscles. (Published with permission from Robert Jackler, MD who maintains copyright ownership and right to future use)

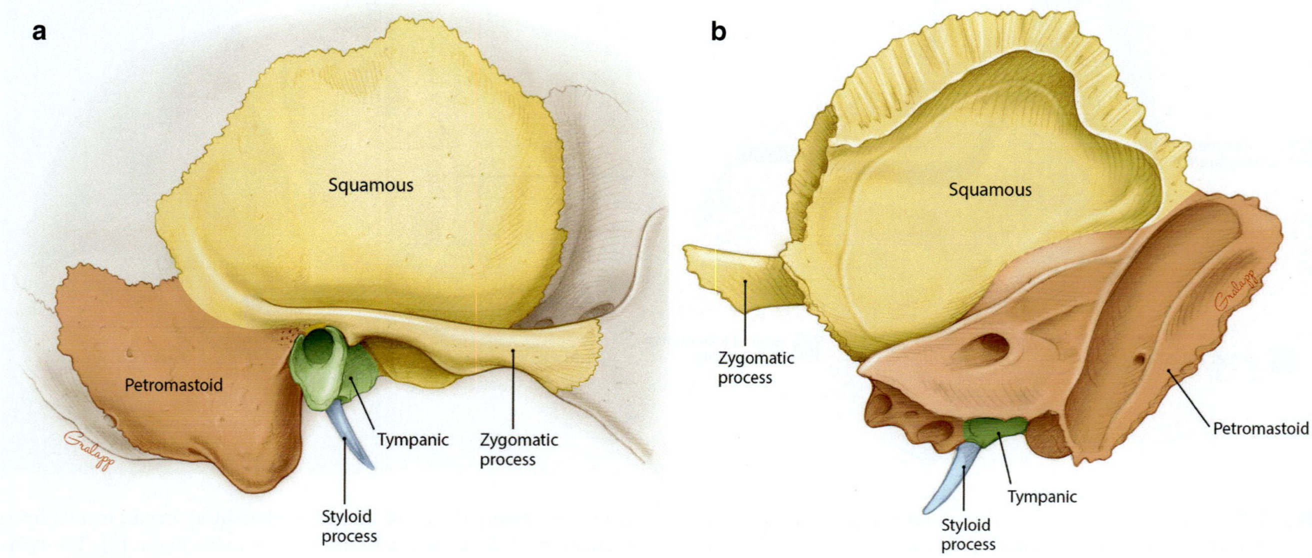

Fig. 3.7 Lateral (**a**) and medial (**b**) views of the temporal bone. The temporal bone is composed of squamous, petromastoid, tympanic, and styloid portions. The tympanic portion forms the anterior, inferior, and posterior walls of the external auditory canal; it is an incomplete ring such that it is open superiorly. The squamous portion serves as the lateral wall of the middle fossa and interfaces with the parietal bone superiorly along the squamosal suture. This suture continues anteriorly as the sphenosquamosal suture where the squamous portion interfaces with the sphenoid bone. The zygomatic process arises from the inferolateral squamous portion to interface with the zygomatic bone along the temporozygomatic suture. The occipitomastoid suture runs between the mastoid portion of the temporal bone and the occipital bone. A sulcus for the middle meningeal artery can be seen along the medial surface of the squamous portion. (Published with permission from Robert Jackler, MD who maintains copyright ownership and right to future use)

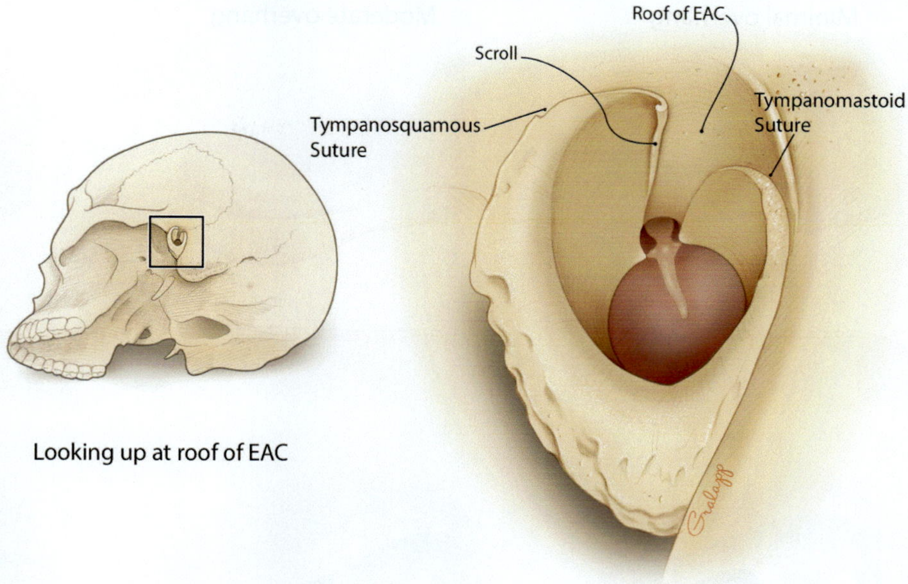

Fig. 3.8 The tympanic portion of the temporal bone forms two suture lines: the tympanosquamous suture anterosuperiorly and the tympanomastoid suture posteroinferiorly. The scroll is a curled edge of the tympanic bone at the tympanosquamous suture line. Elevation of the ear canal skin and periosteum at these suture lines often requires sharp dissection. Removal of the scroll is needed to provide an unobscured view of the epitympanum. (Published with permission from Robert Jackler, MD who maintains copyright ownership and right to future use)

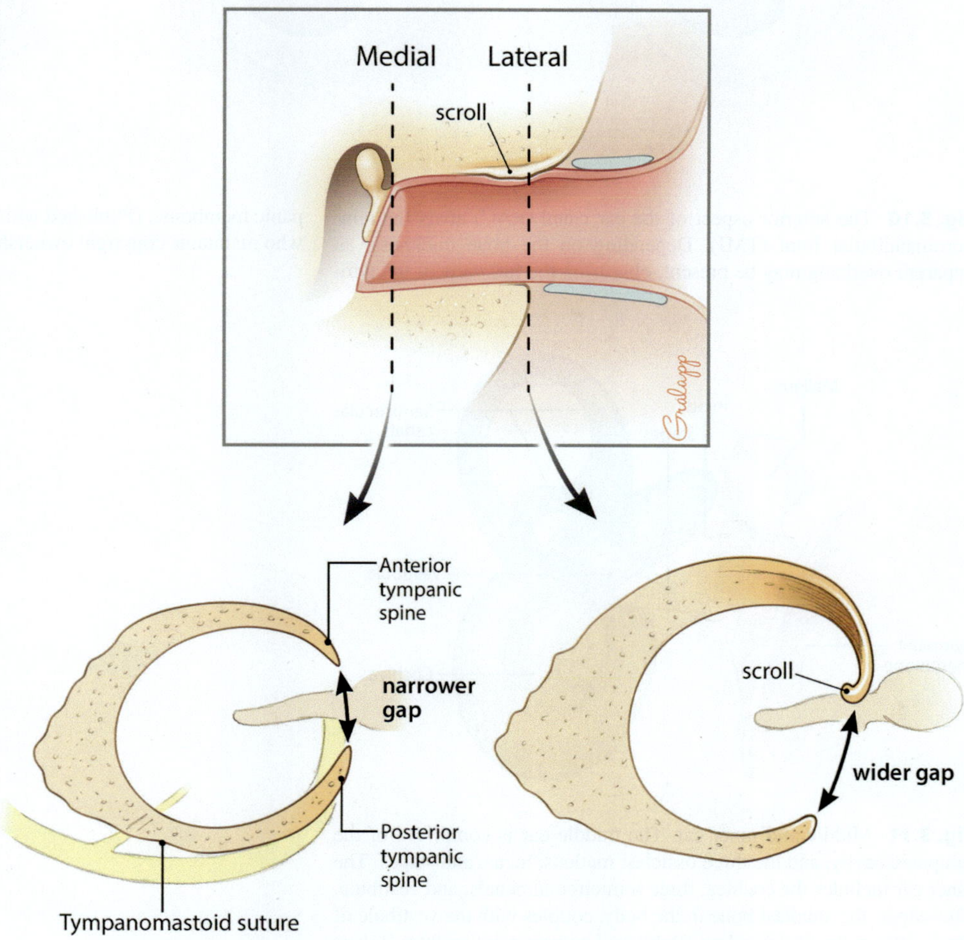

Fig. 3.9 The tympanic bone has a different shape at the annular level and at the bony cartilage junction. The scroll exists only laterally. Also of note, the tympanic membrane is tilted such that the anteroinferior canal is longer than the posterosuperior. (Published with permission from Robert Jackler, MD who maintains copyright ownership and right to future use)

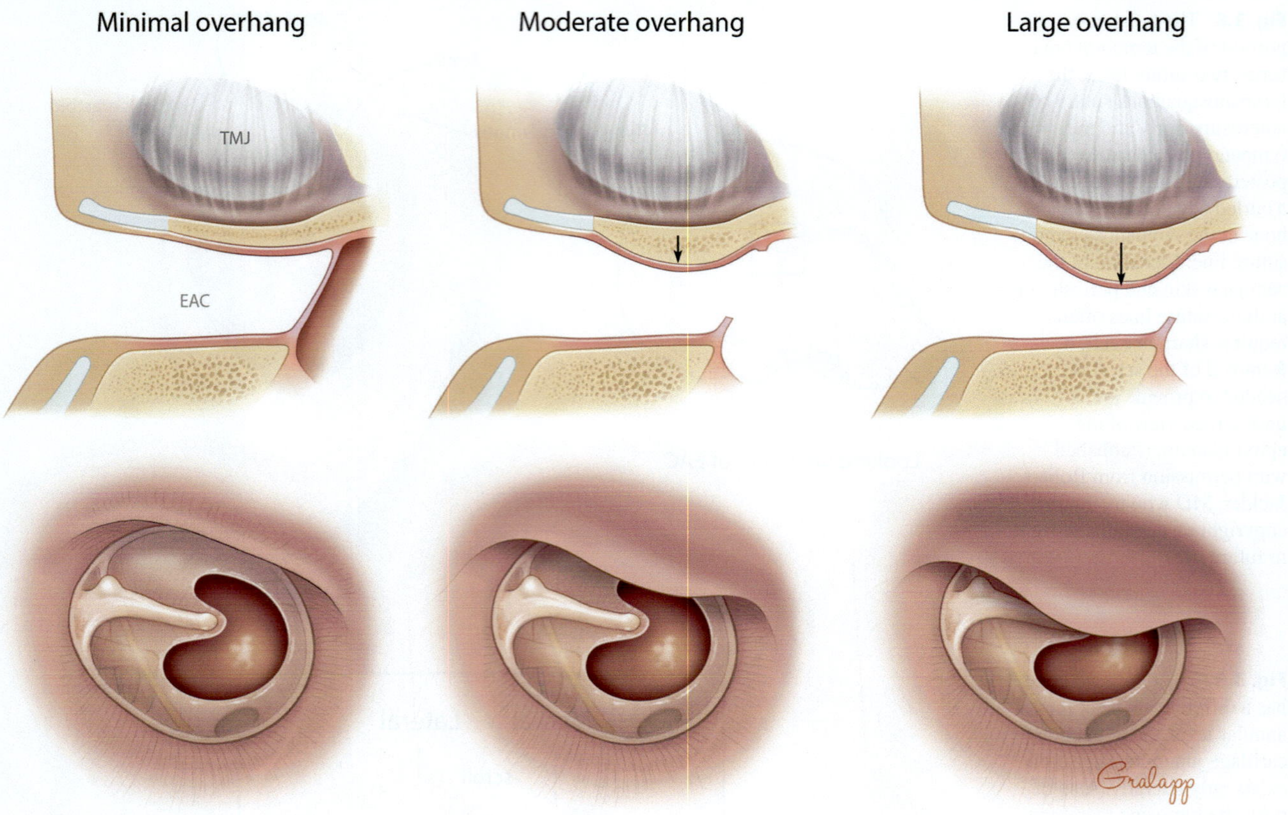

Fig. 3.10 The anterior aspect of the ear canal (EAC) abuts the temporomandibular joint (TMJ). Depending on the bone thickness, an apparent overhang may be present, obscuring the full view of the tympanic membrane. (Published with permission from Robert Jackler, MD who maintains copyright ownership and right to future use)

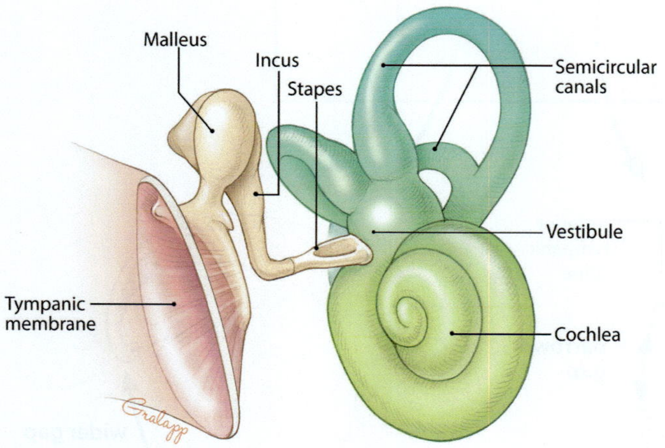

Fig. 3.11 Middle and inner ear. The middle ear is comprised of the tympanic cavity, and the three ossicles: malleus, incus, and stapes. The inner ear includes the cochlea, three semicircular canals, and vestibule. The stapes, the smallest bone in the body, couples with the vestibule of the cochlea at the oval window. (Published with permission from Robert Jackler, MD who maintains copyright ownership and right to future use)

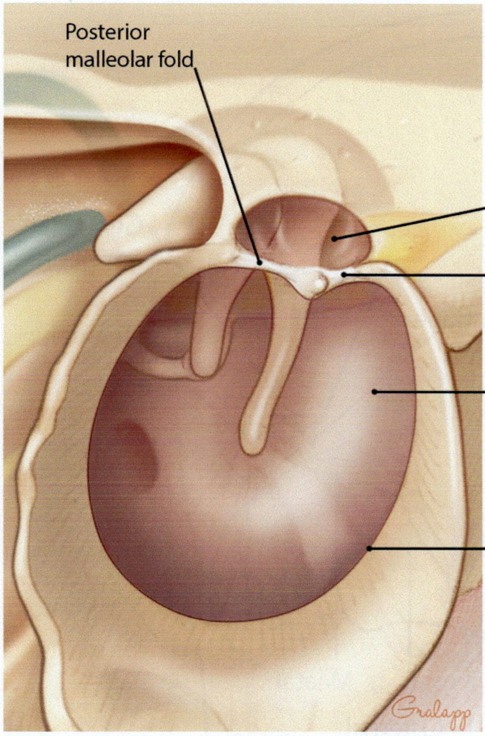

Fig. 3.12 Three layers comprise the tympanic membrane: a lateral squamous epithelium, a medial mucosal epithelium, and a middle fibrous layer called the pars propria. The tympanic membrane is divided into the pars tensa inferiorly and the pars flaccida superiorly. The tympanic membrane couples with the ossicular chain through its attachment to the manubrium of the malleus. The notch of Rivinus is a gap in the tympanic ring superiorly. The anterior and posterior malleolar folds arise from the lateral process of the malleus and attach to the ends of the bony annulus. The epitympnaum, or attic, is the portion of the middle ear superior to the bony annulus, while the hypotympanum is inferior. The mesotympanum lies medial to the pars tensa. Within the epitympanum, medial to the pars flaccida and lateral to the neck of the malleus, is Prussak's space. This subspace of the epitympanum is notable as the location where pars flaccida acquired cholesteatomas form. (Published with permission from Robert Jackler, MD who maintains copyright ownership and right to future use)

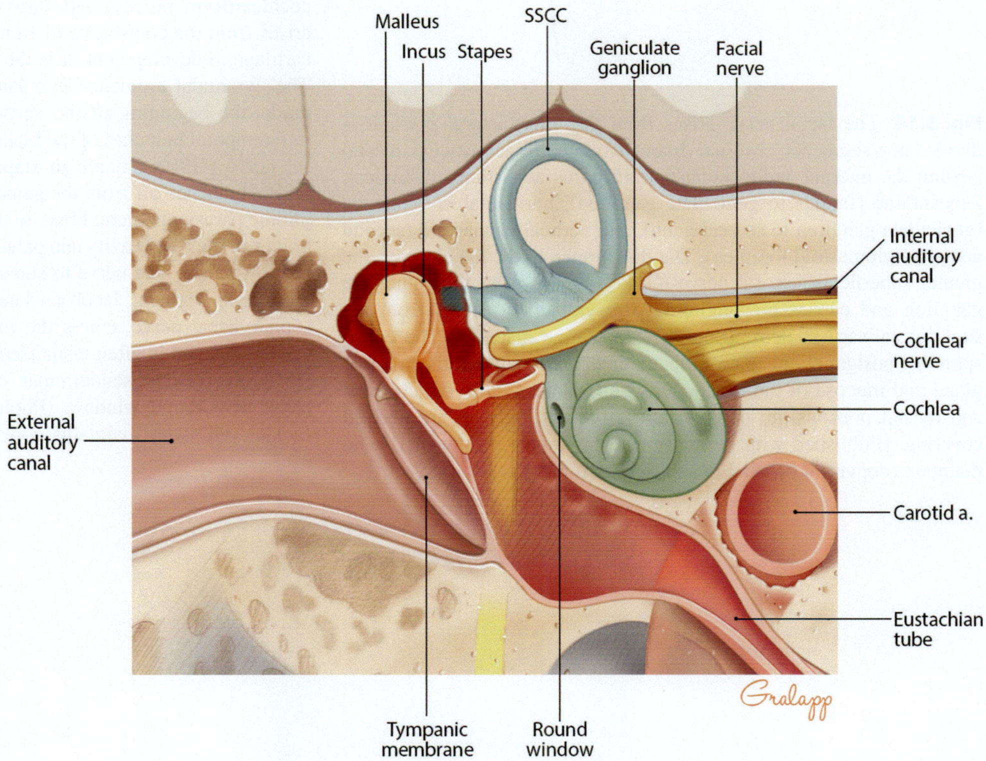

Fig. 3.13 The protympanum, the portion of the tympanic cavity located anterior to the tympanic membrane, includes the orifice to the Eustachian tube. The epitympanum contains the head of the malleus and the body and short process of the incus. SSCC Superior semicircular canal. (Published with permission from Robert Jackler, MD who maintains copyright ownership and right to future use)

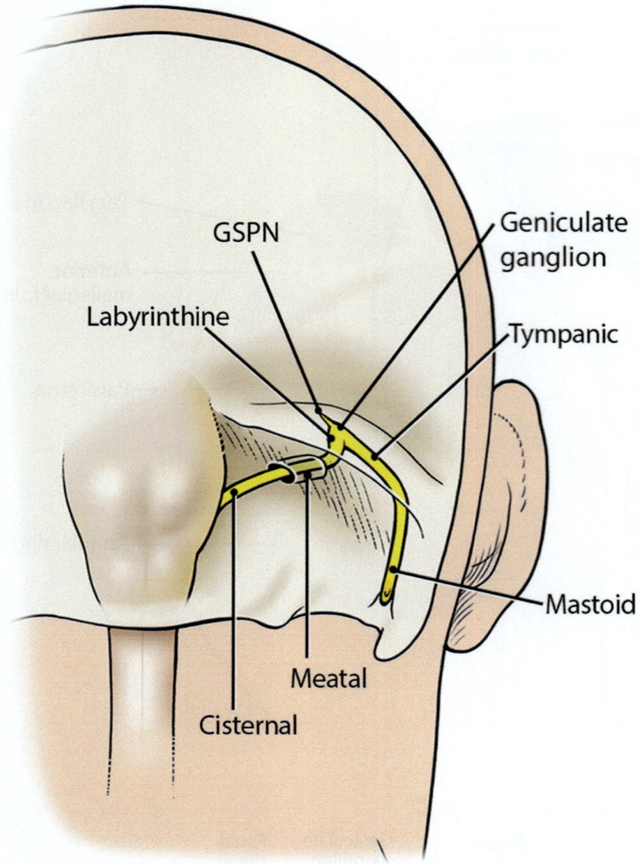

Fig. 3.14 The facial nerve arises from the lower lateral pons. It is divided into segments: cisternal (brainstem to porus acousticus), meatal (within the internal auditory canal from porus acousticus to fundus), labyrinthine (fundus to geniculate ganglion), horizontal or tympanic (geniculate ganglion to second genu), and vertical or mastoid (second genu to stylomastoid foramen). The first branch of the facial nerve, the greater superficial petrosal nerve (GSPN), arises from the geniculate ganglion and carries preganglionic parasympathetic fibers from the superior salivary nucleus to the sphenopalatine ganglion. The corresponding postganglionic parasympathetic fibers synapse at the lacrimal gland and mucosa of the nasal cavity and palate. Within the cisternal and meatal portions, no perineurium is present, only an arachnoidal covering. (Published with permission from Robert Jackler, MD who maintains copyright ownership and right to future use)

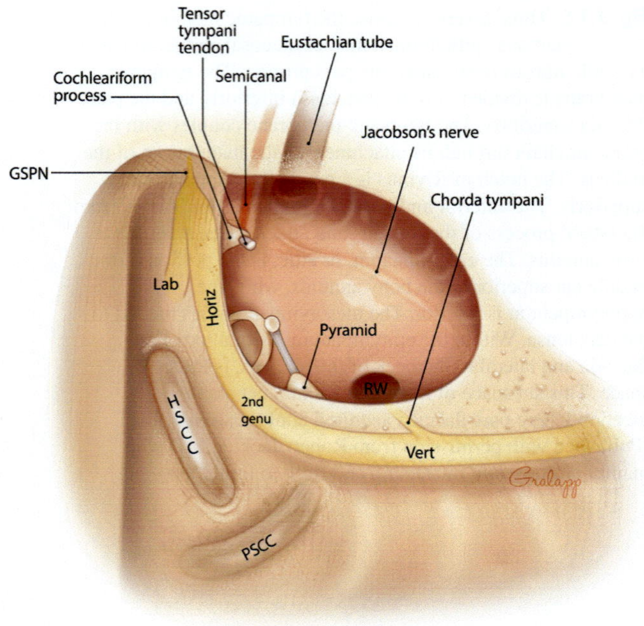

Fig. 3.15 The intratemporal facial nerve lies within a bony channel called the Fallopian canal. The labyrinthine segment (Lab) is the shortest, narrowest segment. The geniculate ganglion, also known as the first genu, is dehiscent on the middle fossa floor in 25% of ears. The horizontal (Horiz) segment traverses the middle ear floor superior to the cochleariform process and stapes. As the horizontal fallopian canal arises from the confluence of Reichert's cartilage and the otic capsule cartilage in development, it is the segment most commonly dehiscent. The pyramidal eminence is a landmark for the second genu, which marks the beginning of the vertical (Vert) segment. There are three intratemporal branches of the facial nerve: the greater superficial petrosal nerve (GSPN), nerve to stapedius muscle, and chorda tympani. GSPN branches off from the geniculate ganglion and contains preganglionic parasympathetic fibers to the lacrimal gland and mucous membranes of the nasal cavity and palate, as well as afferent taste fibers from the soft palate. The nerve to stapedius and chorda tympani arise from the vertical segment. Jacobsen's nerve, the tympanic branch of the glossopharyngeal nerve, enters the middle ear via the inferior tympanic canaliculus and is often visualized overlying the cochlear promontory. HSCC Horizontal semicircular canal, PSCC posterior semicircular canal, RW round window. (Published with permission from Robert Jackler, MD who maintains copyright ownership and right to future use)

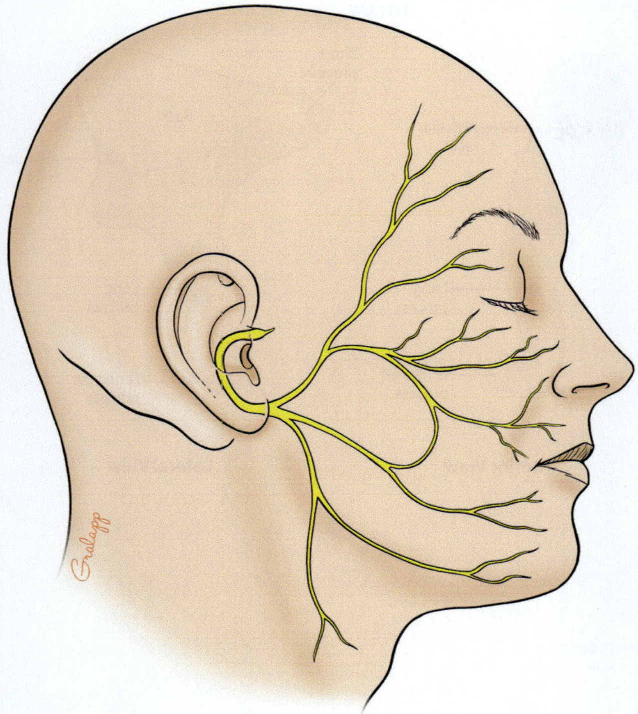

Fig. 3.16 The facial nerve exits the temporal bone at the stylomastoid foramen and then traverses the parotid gland to provide innervation to the muscles of facial expression in five terminal branches: temporal, zygomatic, buccal, marginal mandibular, and cervical. (Published with permission from Robert Jackler, MD who maintains copyright ownership and right to future use)

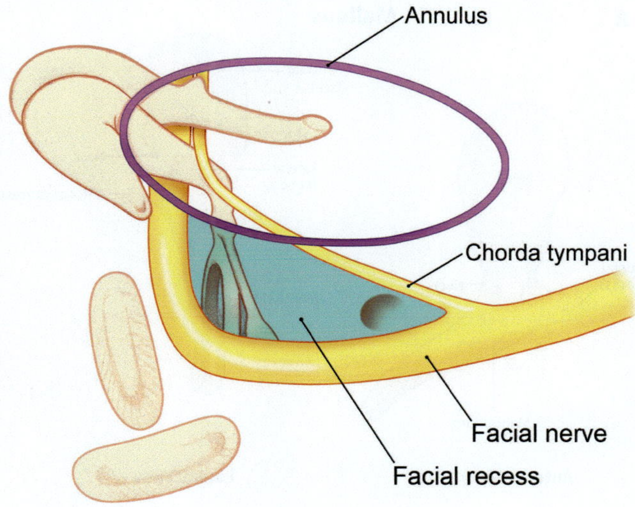

Fig. 3.17 The anatomical relations of the facial recess (blue shading) include the chorda tympani nerve, which branches from the mastoid segment of the facial nerve. It crosses deep to the tympanic annulus, lateral to the incus, and deep to the malleus before exiting the skull via the petrotympanic fissure. The chorda tympani nerve provides afferent taste sensation for the anterior two thirds of the tongue and efferent parasympathetic innervation of the submandibular and sublingual salivary glands. The facial recess provides a surgical path to the middle ear via the mastoid. It is bounded by the facial nerve posteriorly, chorda tympani anteriorly, and incudal buttress superiorly. (Published with permission from Robert Jackler, MD who maintains copyright ownership and right to future use)

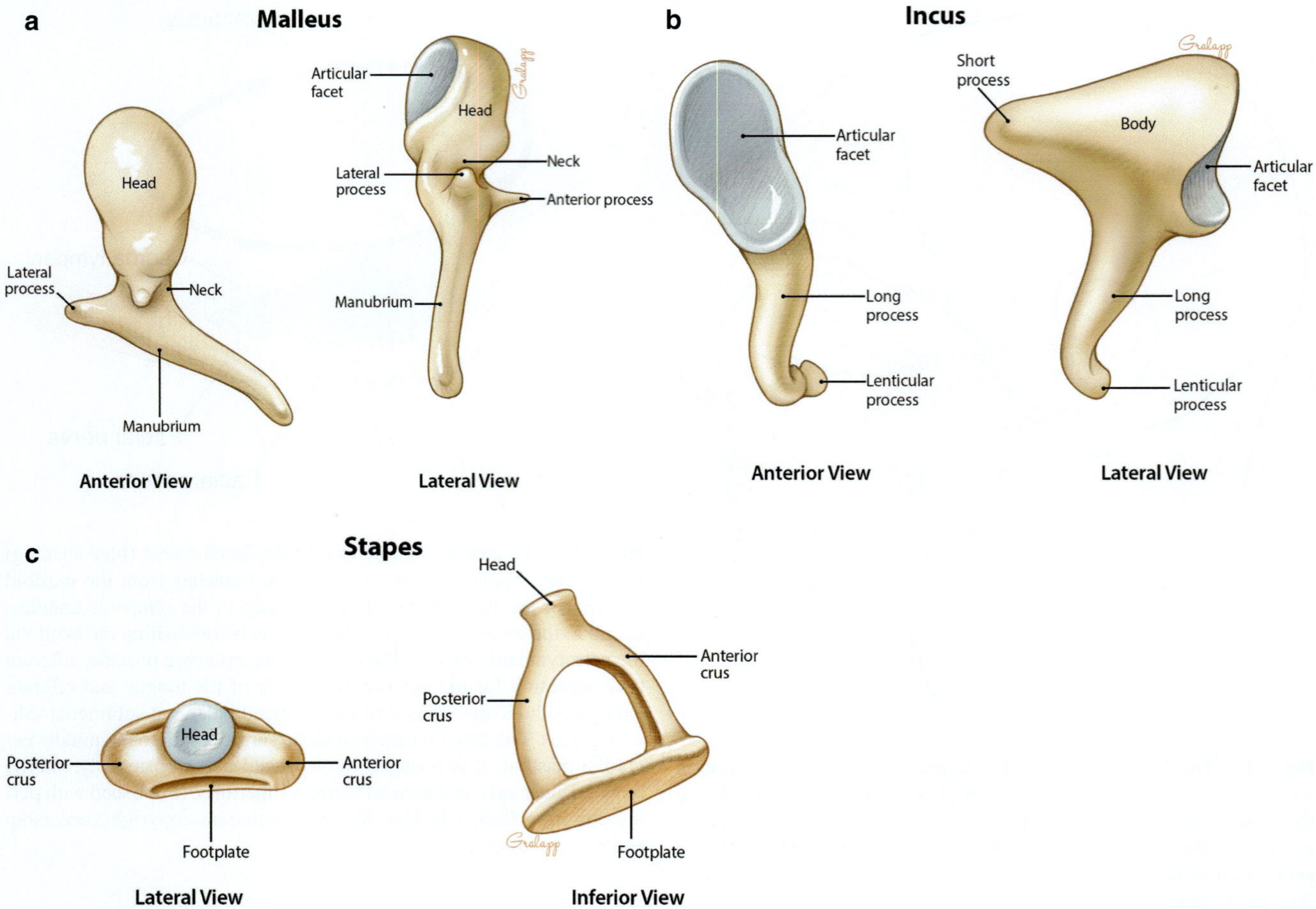

Fig. 3.18 Malleus (**a**), incus (**b**), and stapes (**c**). The three ossicles, or middle ear bones, act as a lever arm to amplify sound as it is conducted from the tympanic membrane to the oval window. The manubrium and lateral process of the malleus attach to the tympanic membrane. The head of the malleus, and the body and short process of the incus are located in the epitympanum, while the remainder of the ossicular components are in the mesotympanum. The head of the stapes articulates with the lenticular process of the incus. The footplate of the stapes is held in place by the annular ligament at the oval window. The stapedial tendon inserts on the posterior aspect of the stapes head. The tensor tympani tendon inserts on the medial aspect of the malleus manubrium. (Published with permission from Robert Jackler, MD who maintains copyright ownership and right to future use)

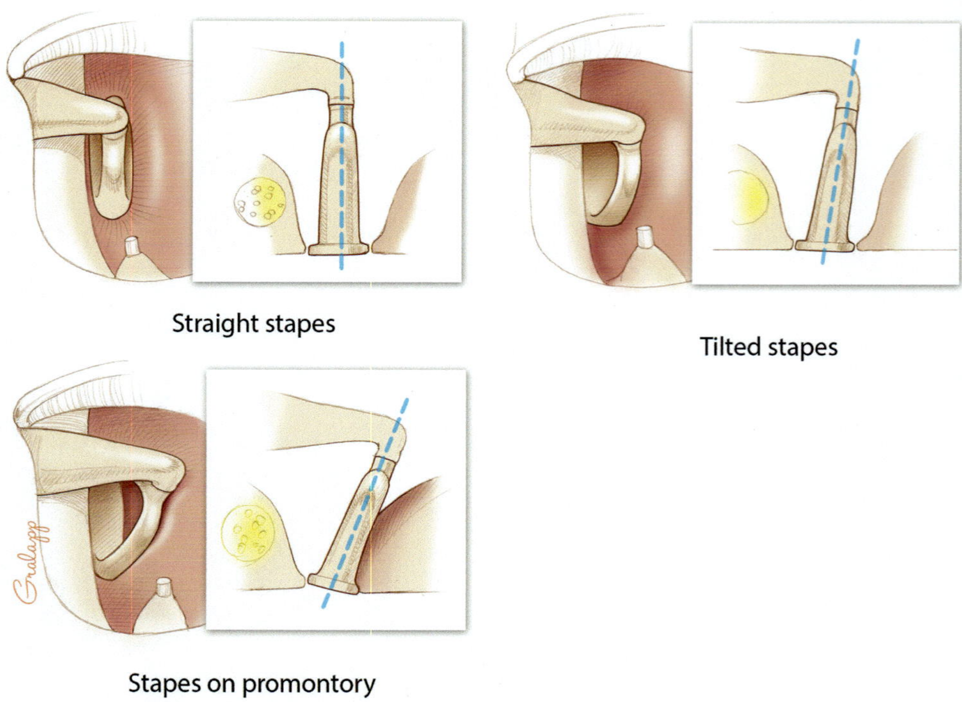

Fig. 3.19 The orientation of the stapes superstructure varies and may be upright or tilted inferiorly toward the promontory or even leaning against it. (Published with permission from Robert Jackler, MD who maintains copyright ownership and right to future use)

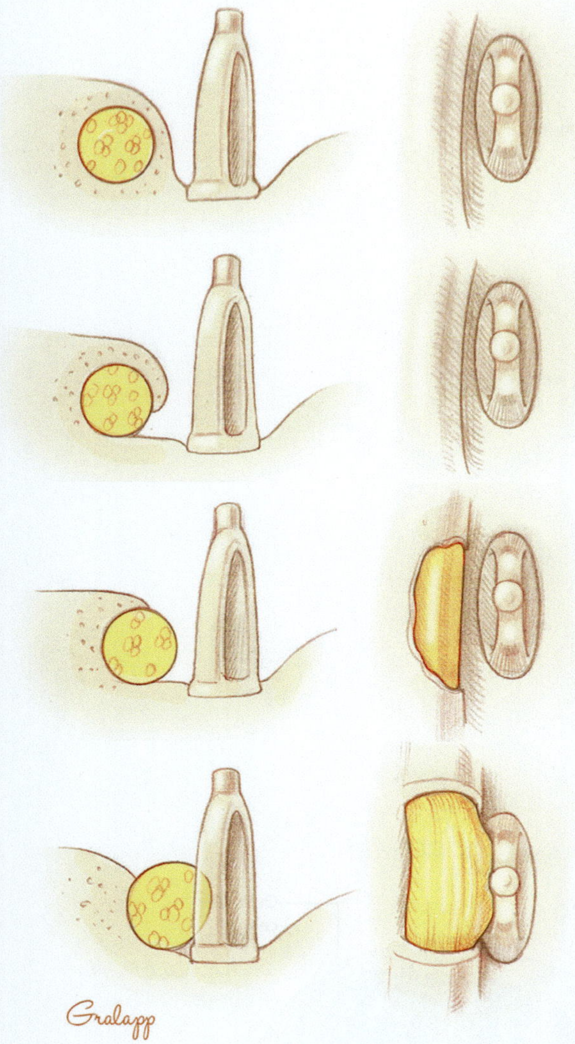

Fig. 3.20 The facial nerve is situated immediately superior to the oval window and stapes. The nerve is usually dehiscent on its lower surface, out of the surgeon's line of sight. Occasionally, it lies fully dehiscent including its lateral surface. Rarely the facial nerve may prolapse from its canal and even impinge on the stapes arch. In such cases, the surgeon must determine if a patient's conductive hearing loss is due to stapes fixation or merely from the facial nerve leaning on the crura. (Published with permission from Robert Jackler, MD who maintains copyright ownership and right to future use)

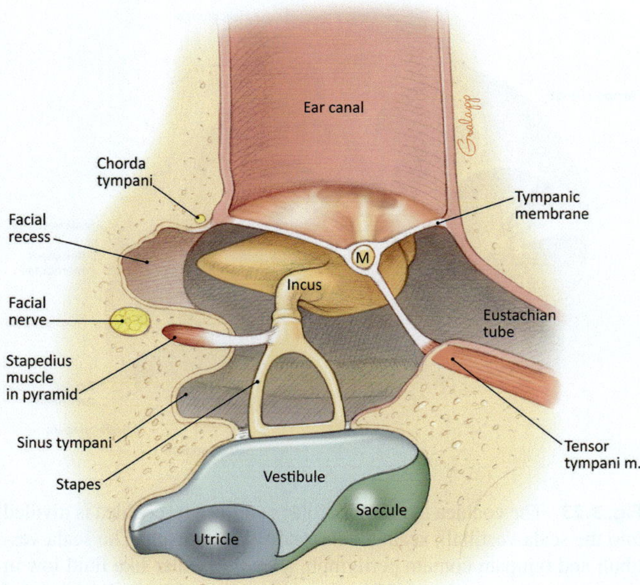

Fig. 3.21 The anatomy of the posterior tympanic spaces. The facial recess lies laterally between the tympanic membrane and pyramidal ridge containing the facial nerve at its base. The sinus tympani lies deep to the facial nerve and is of variable depth. The normal relationship of the utricle and saccule to the footplate is also illustrated. The distance from footplate to the utricle is approximately 2 mm while the space to the saccule is about 1.25 mm, measurements which may be substantially reduced in endolymphatic hydrops. M Malleus. (Published with permission from Robert Jackler, MD who maintains copyright ownership and right to future use)

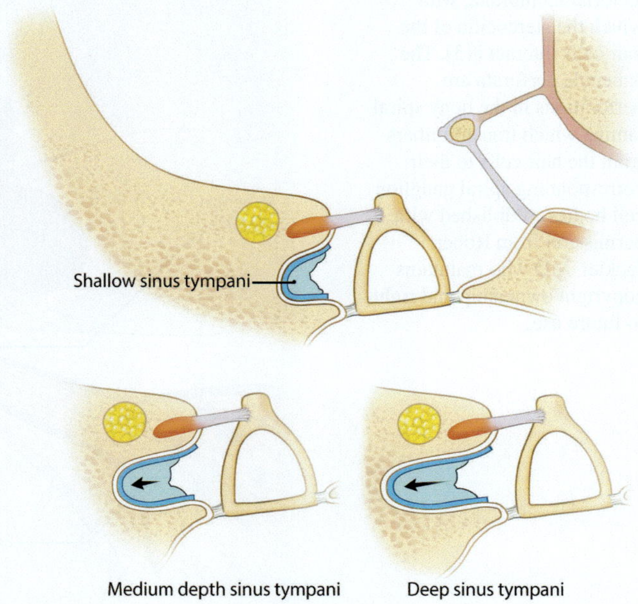

Fig. 3.22 The posterior extension, or depth, of the sinus tympani is variable (A). Historically, it has been known as a frequent site of residual cholesteatoma. With the advent of endoscopic otologic techniques, surgical inspection of the sinus tympani has been improved [1]. (Published with permission from Robert Jackler, MD who maintains copyright ownership and right to future use)

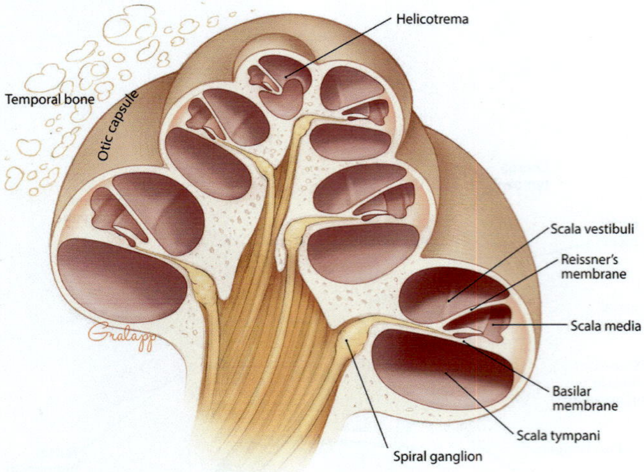

Fig. 3.23 The cochlea in mid-modiolar section. The cochlea is divided into the scala vestibuli, scala media, and scala tympani. The scala vestibuli and tympani contain perilymph, an extracellular-like fluid low in potassium concentration and high in sodium. The scala media, bounded by the basilar and Reissner's membranes, contains endolymph. Endolymph is an intracellular-like fluid high in potassium and relatively low in sodium. Perilymph of the scala vestibuli communicates with that of the scala tympani at the helicotrema, at the apex of the cochlea. (Published with permission from Robert Jackler, MD who maintains copyright ownership and right to future use)

Fig. 3.24 The organ of Corti is comprised of sensory outer and inner hair cells, supporting Deiters', Hensen's, and Claudius cells, and the tectorial membrane, with which the stereocilia of the hair cells interact [13]. The habenula perforata are perforations in the bony spiral lamina which transmit fibers from the hair cells to their corresponding spiral ganglion cell bodies. (Published with permission from Robert Jackler, MD who maintains copyright ownership and right to future use)

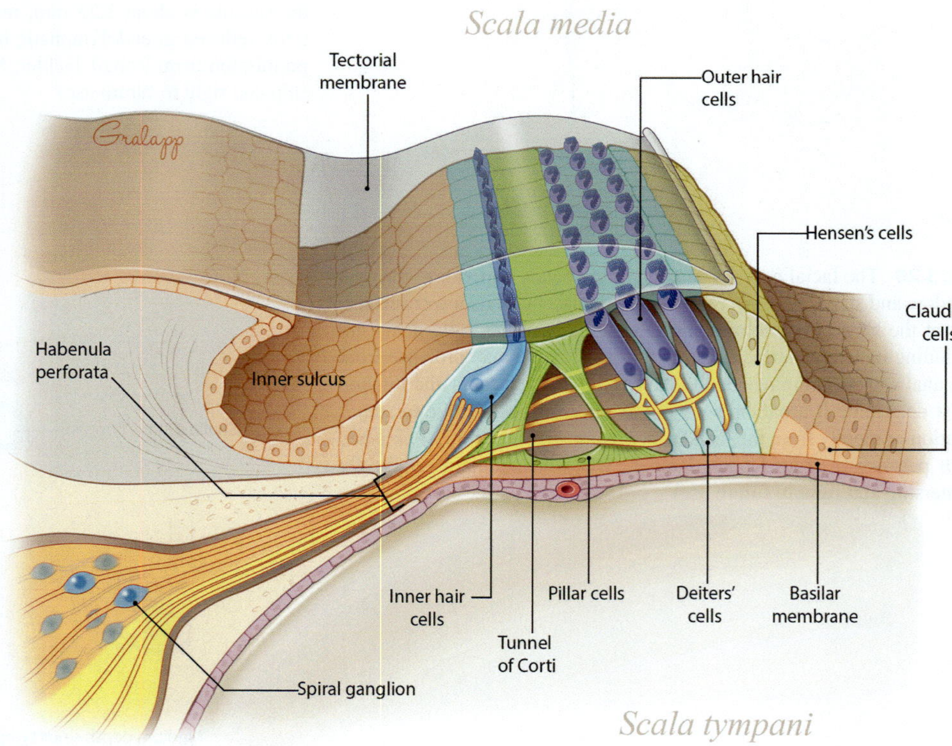

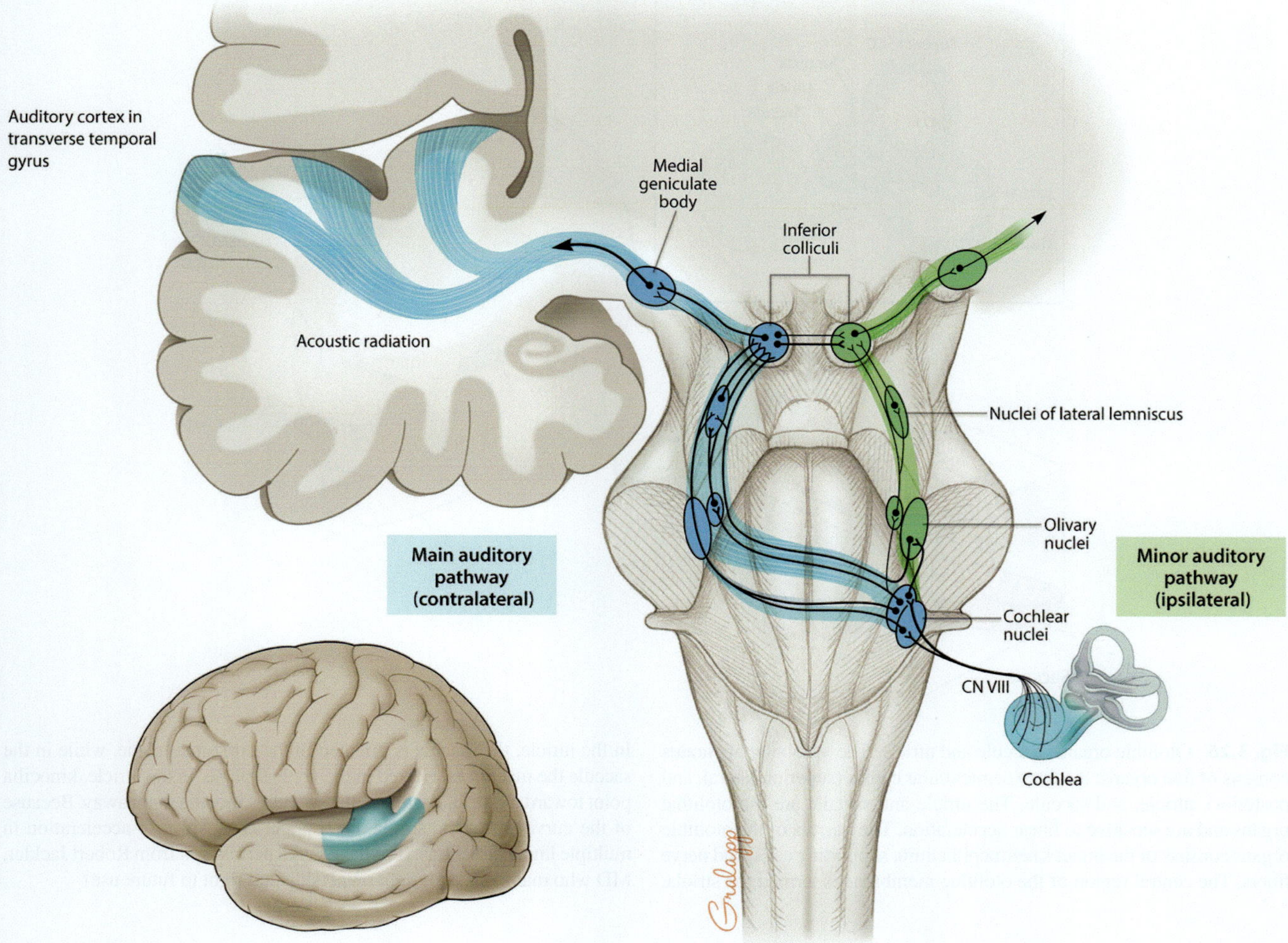

Fig. 3.25 Central auditory afferent pathways. The auditory nerve afferent fibers synapse first at the spiral ganglion in the modiolus and then at the cochlear nucleus. From the cochlear nucleus, the majority of fibers cross to contralateral superior olivary nuclei, while a minority remain ipsilateral. From the olivary complex in the pons, the signal ascends to the lateral lemniscus, then inferior colliculus, to the medial geniculate body of the thalamus, finally projecting to the auditory cortex. The auditory cortex is located in the transverse temporal gyrus of the temporal lobe, just inferior to the Sylvian fissure. (Published with permission from Robert Jackler, MD who maintains copyright ownership and right to future use)

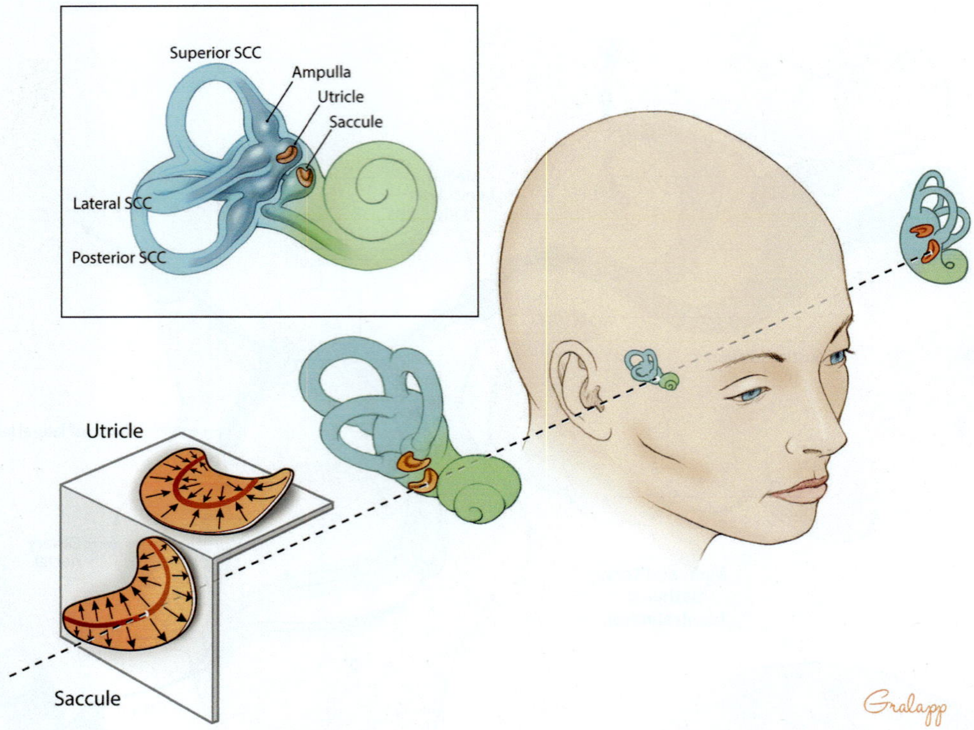

Fig. 3.26 Otolithic organs: Saccule and utricle. The vestibular apparatus consists of five organs: the three semicircular canals (superior, lateral, and posterior), utricle, and saccule. The utricle and saccule are the otolithic organs and are sensitive to linear acceleration. The macula of the otolithic organs consists of the organ's neuroepithelium, supporting cells, and nerve fibers. The central region of the otolithic membrane is termed the striola. In the utricle, the macula is oriented in the horizontal plane, while in the saccule the macula is oriented in the vertical plane. In the utricle, kinocilia point toward the striola, while in the saccule, kinocilia point away. Because of the curvature of the striola, each organ is sensitive to acceleration in multiple linear directions. (Published with permission from Robert Jackler, MD who maintains copyright ownership and right to future use)

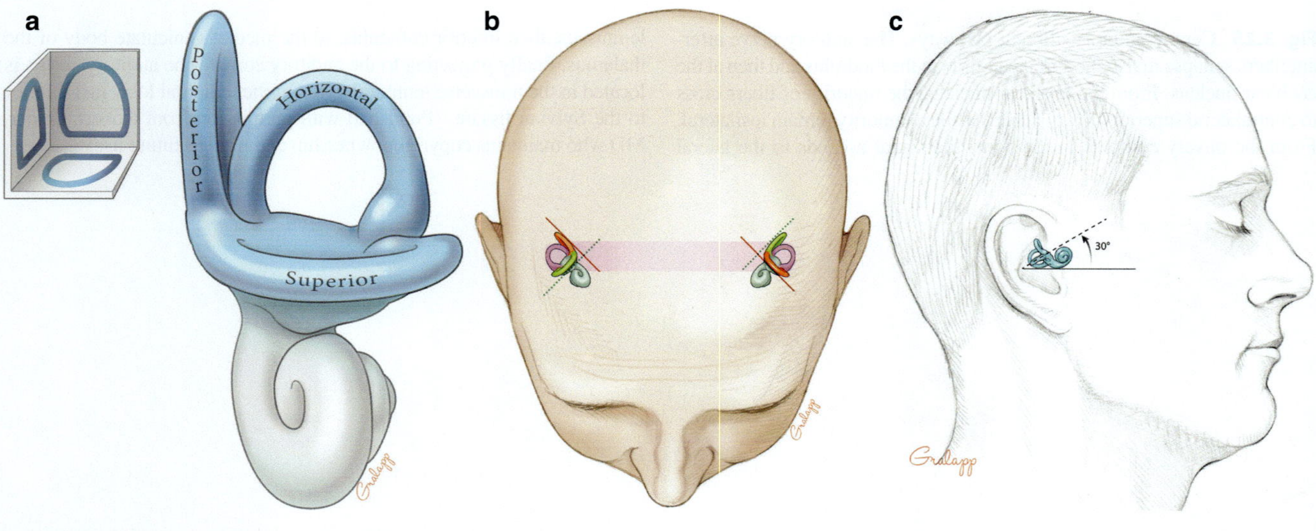

Fig. 3.27 Orientation of semicircular canals. (**a**) The three semicircular canals sense angular acceleration and are mutually perpendicular. (**b**) The lateral semicircular canals are co-planar, while the posterior and opposite superior canals are co-planar. (**c**) The lateral semicircular canals are oriented at a 30°_tilt from horizontal. Published with permission from Robert Jackler, MD who maintains copyright ownership and right to future use

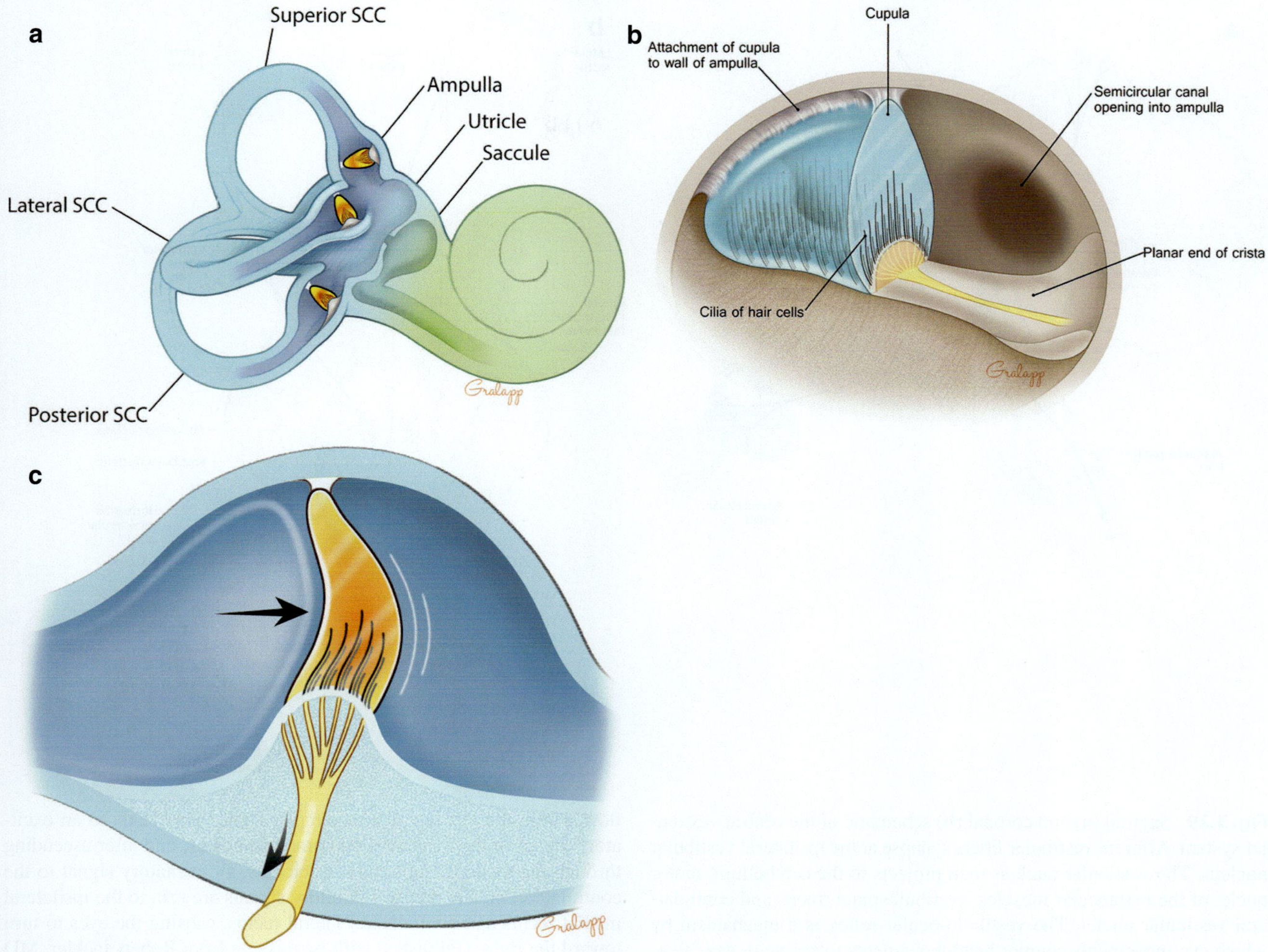

Fig. 3.28 Each semicircular canal has a dilated bulbous end, called the ampulla. The ampulla contains the sensory epithelium and the cupula (a gelatinous mass into which the hair cell stereocilia extend). As the endolymphatic fluid within the semicircular canals is displaced with head movement, this deforms the cupula, displacing the attached hair bundles. (Published with permission from Robert Jackler, MD who maintains copyright ownership and right to future use)

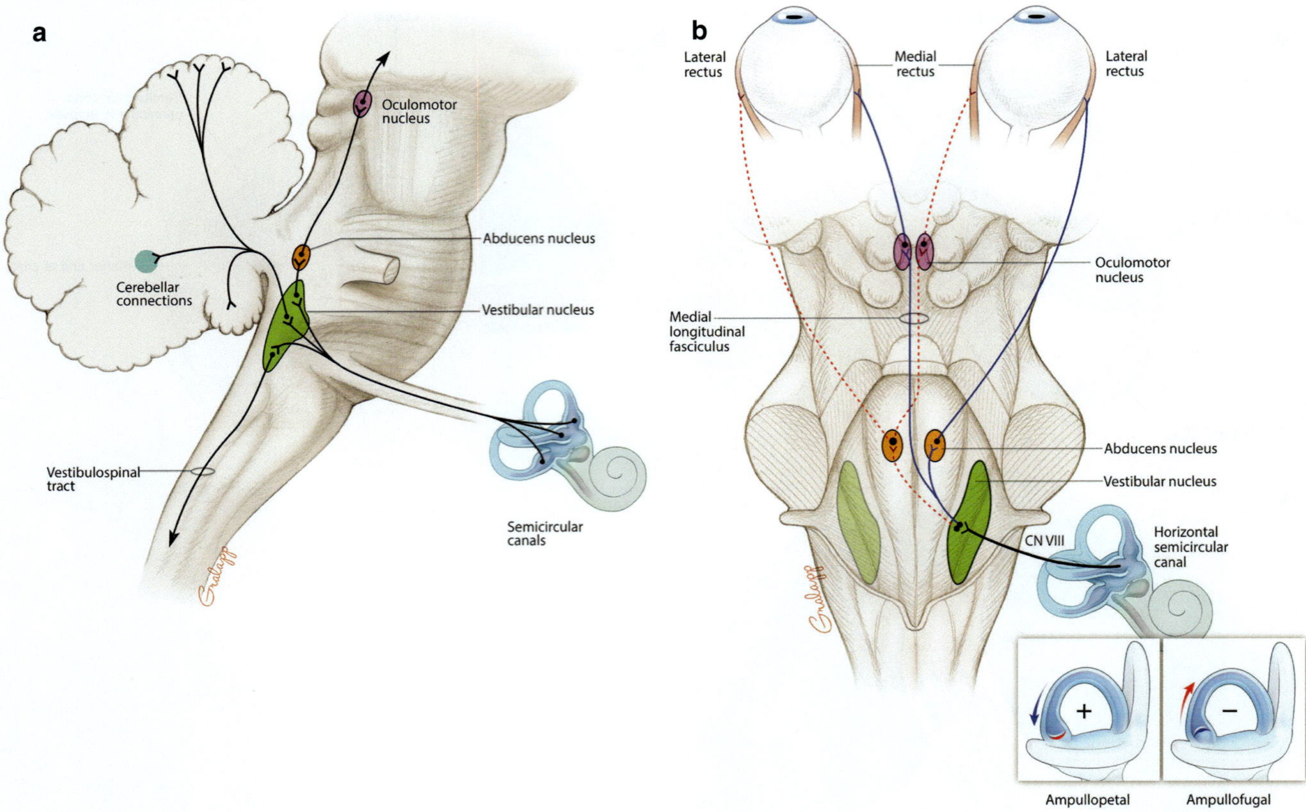

Fig. 3.29 Sagittal (**a**) and coronal (**b**) schematic of the central vestibular system. Afferent vestibular fibers synapse at the ipsilateral vestibular nucleus. The vestibular nucleus then projects to the cerebellum, motor nuclei of the extraocular muscles, vestibulospinal tracts, and contralateral vestibular nuclei. The vestibulo-ocular reflex is a mechanism by which eye movements counter head movements to maintain gaze fixation. For example, turning the head toward the left causes ampullopetal flow within the left lateral semicircular canal. This leads to an excitatory signal to the ipsilateral oculomotor nucleus, and after ascending through the medial longitudinal fasciculus, an excitatory signal to the contralateral medial rectus. Inhibitory signals are sent to the ipsilateral medial rectus and contralateral lateral rectus, causing the eyes to turn toward the right. (Published with permission from Robert Jackler, MD who maintains copyright ownership and right to future use)

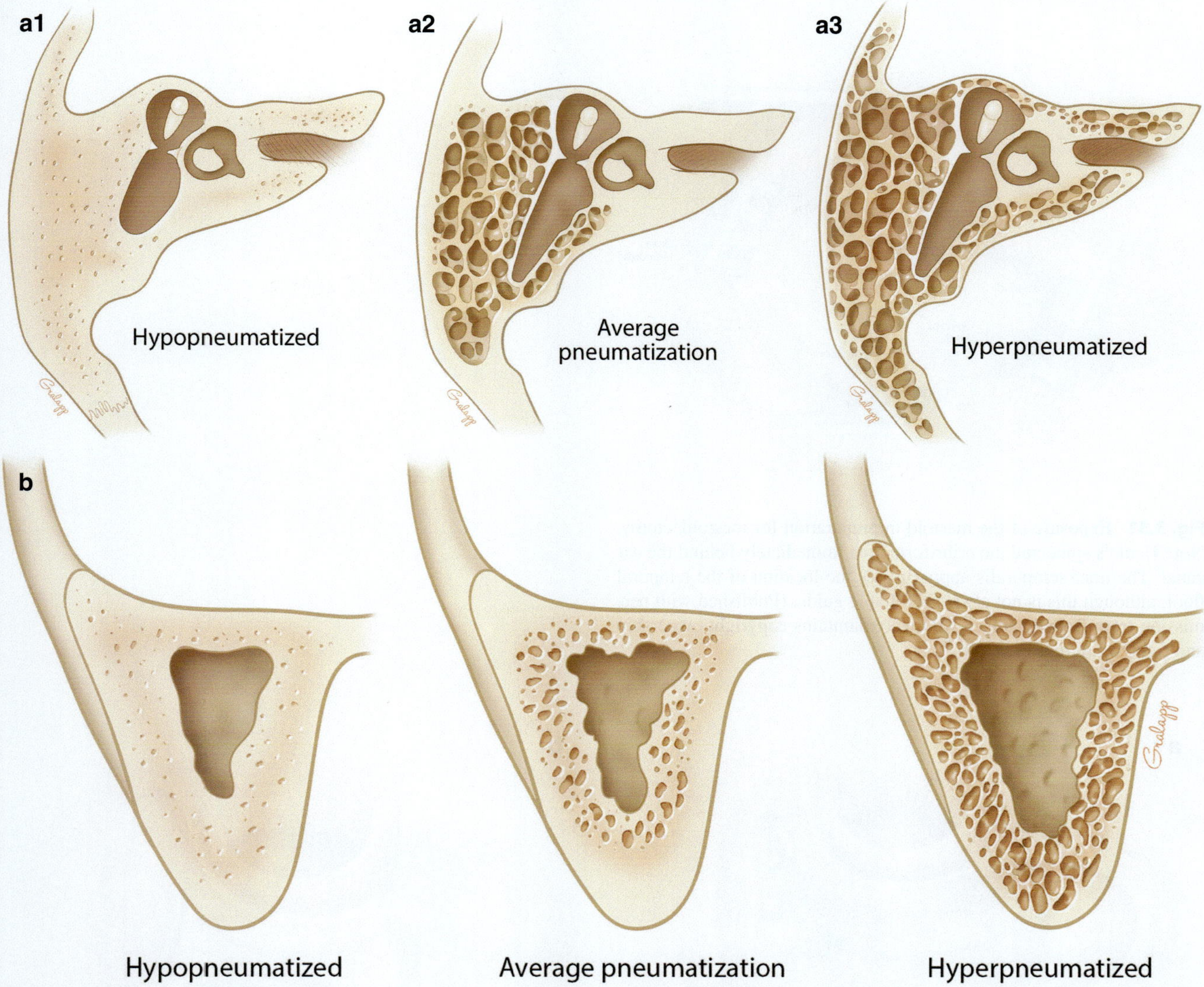

Fig. 3.30 Variation in mastoid pneumatization in axial (**a**) and coronal (**b**) view. Pneumatization of the antrum, the largest mastoid air cell, remains relatively constant, even in a hypopneumatized temporal bone. In extensively pneumatized temporal bones the cell tracts may extend into the root of the zygoma, medially into the petrous apex, and posterior to the sigmoid sinus. (Published with permission from Robert Jackler, MD who maintains copyright ownership and right to future use)

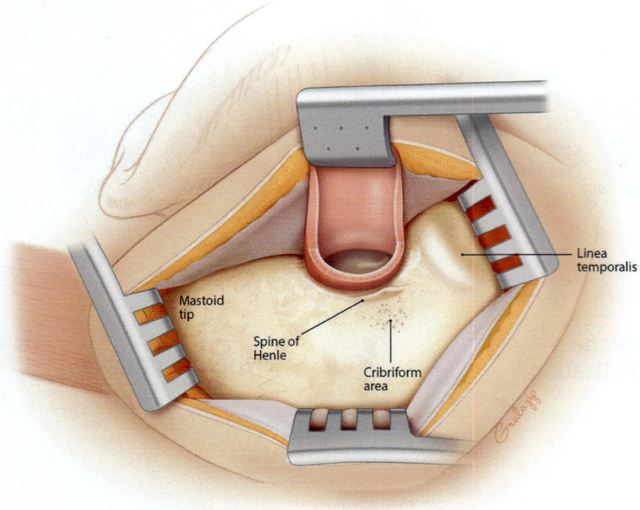

Fig. 3.31 Exposure of the mastoid in preparation for mastoidectomy. Note Henle's spine and the cribriform area immediately behind the ear canal. The linea temporalis approximates the location of the temporal floor, although this is not always a reliable guide. (Published with permission from Robert Jackler, MD who maintains copyright ownership and right to future use)

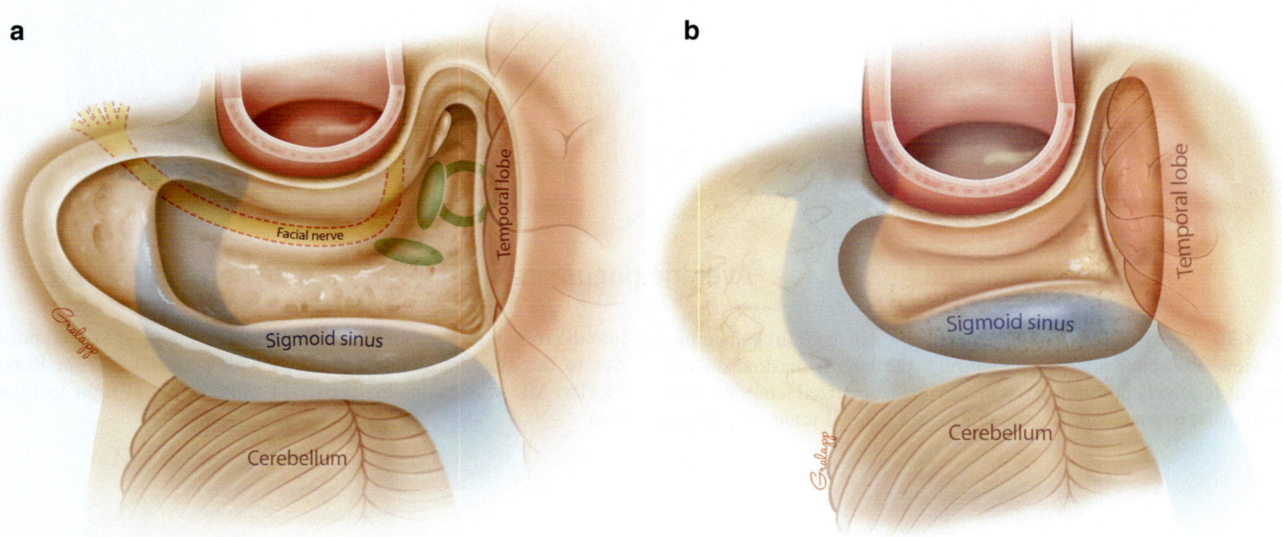

Fig. 3.32 Mastoid relationships in a normally pneumatized and hypopneumatic ear following mastoidectomy. In a normally pneumatized mastoid (**a**), the tegmen mastoideum, sigmoid sinus and ear canal are delineated superiorly, posteriorly, and anteriorly, respectively. The incus and malleus can be seen in the epitympanum through the antrum. The lateral semicircular canal serves as a critical landmark for the facial nerve, which lies at the same depth and immediately below. In a hypopneumatic mastoid (**b**), the tegmen mastoideum is low-lying, such that the temporal lobe lies in a relatively inferior position. The sigmoid sinus and posterior fossa are also positioned more anteriorly, collectively creating a smaller mastoid cavity. (Published with permission from Robert Jackler, MD who maintains copyright ownership and right to future use)

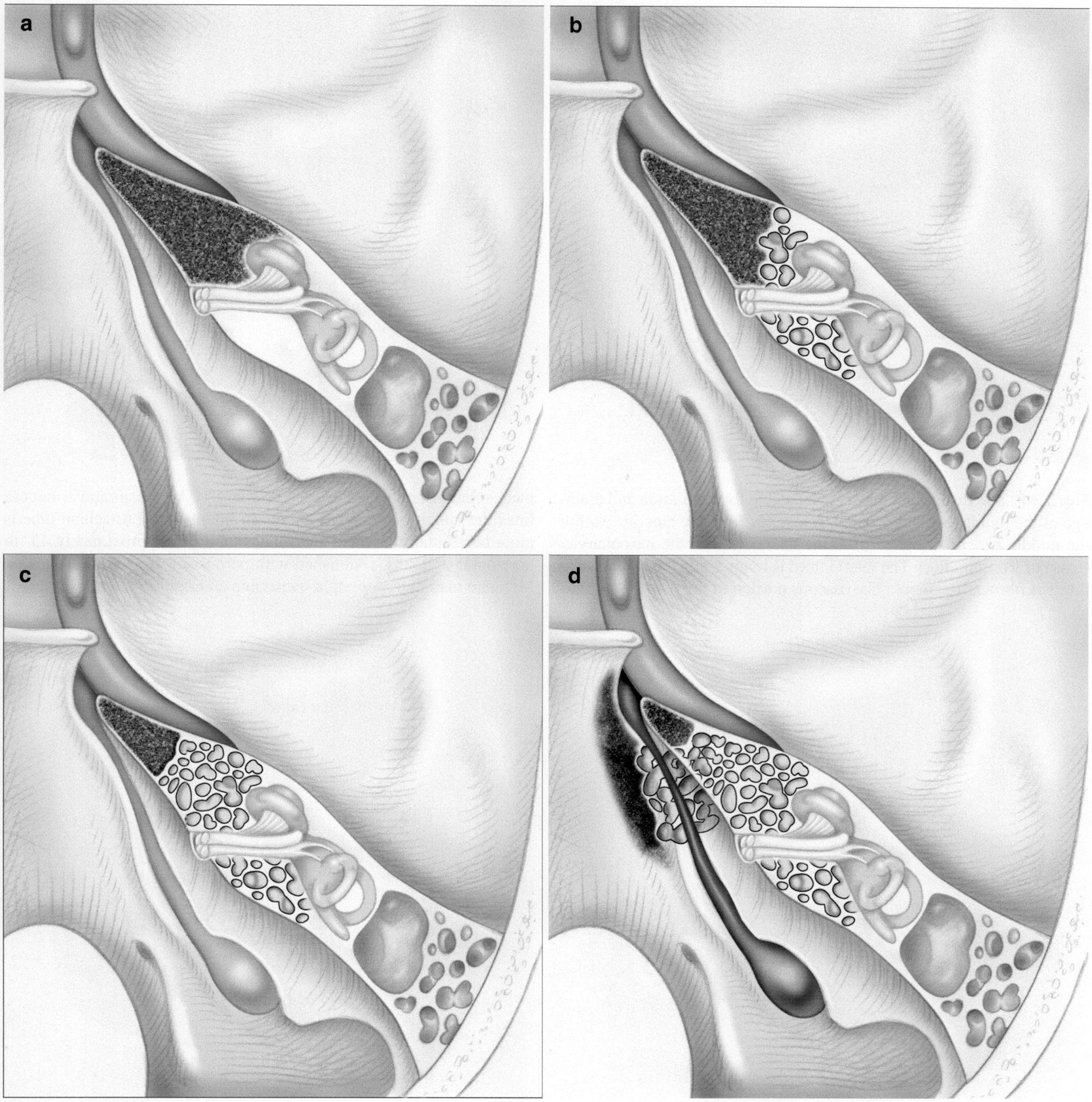

Fig. 3.33 The petrous apex is variably pneumatized (**a**–**d**), and is filled with bone marrow when air cells are not present. In exceptionally well-pneumatized petrous apices (**d**), pneumatization may extend to the petroclival junction, predisposing one to cholesterol granuloma [9]. (Published with permission from Robert Jackler, MD who maintains copyright ownership and right to future use)

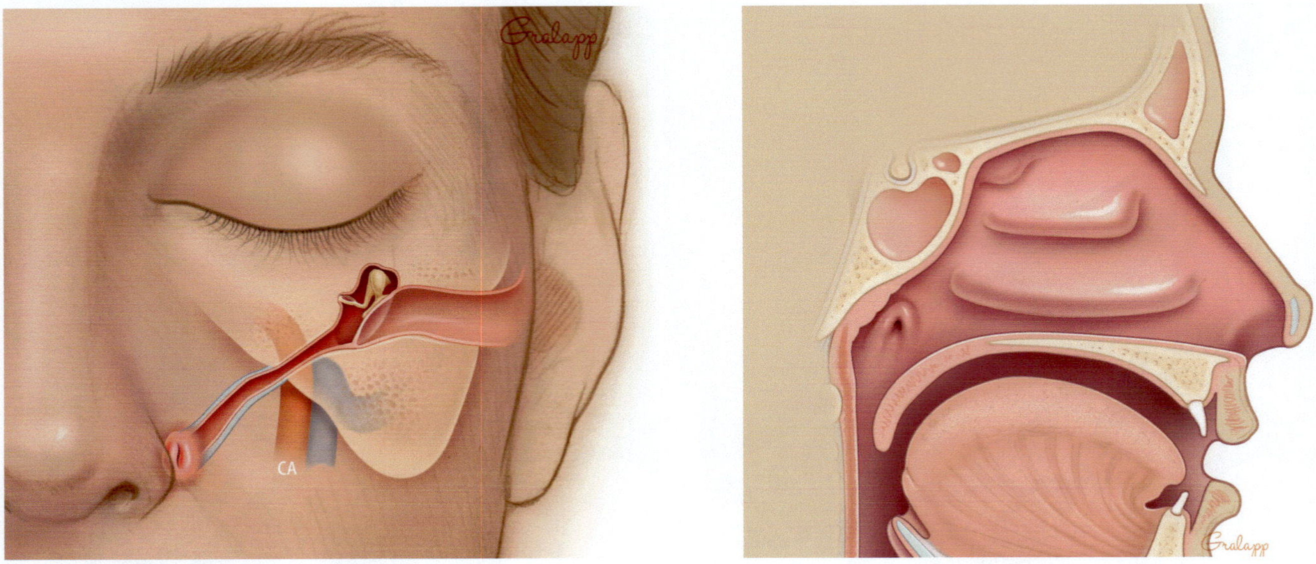

Fig. 3.34 The Eustachian tube is responsible for ventilation and drainage of the middle ear and mastoid. It extends from the anterior wall of the middle ear (protympanum) to the lateral wall of the nasopharynx (fossa of Rosenmüller). The lateral third is bony, while the medial two-thirds is fibrocartilaginous. The osseous portion of the tube has an intimate relationship with the carotid artery (CA). Respiratory mucosa lines the length of the tubal lumen. In infants, the Eustachian tube is more horizontally oriented and rotates until it is approximately 45° to horizontal in adults. (Published with permission from Robert Jackler, MD who maintains copyright ownership and right to future use)

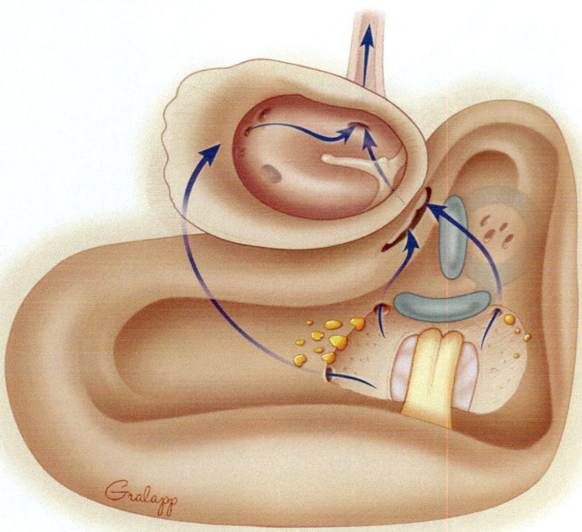

Fig. 3.35 In cases of extensive pneumatization, cell tracts may pass around and even through the semicircular canals. In this illustration, routes of CSF leakage after neurotologic surgery are traced. The perilabyrinthine tracts enable CSF flow to reach the middle ear via the fossa incudis. An alternative direct pathway to the middle ear passes inferior to the cochlea. All routes traverse the final common pathway via the Eustachian tube. (Published with permission from Robert Jackler, MD who maintains copyright ownership and right to future use)

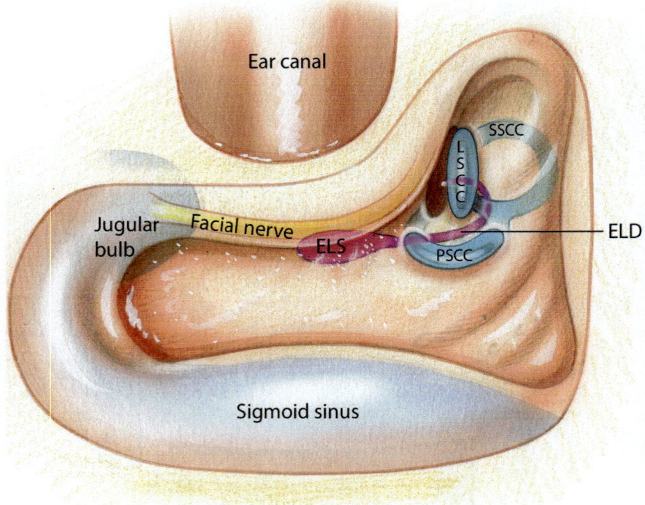

Fig. 3.36 The endolymphatic duct lies in a bony canal known as the vestibular aqueduct and arises from the deep aspect of the vestibule and pursues a "J" shaped course en route to its sac. The aqueduct crosses behind the common crus of the posterior and superior semicircular canals (SSCC) en route to its operculum into the posterior cranial fossa. Surgical exposure of the endolymphatic sac (ELS) involves removing bone posterior to the descending facial nerve, inferior to the posterior semicircular canal (PSCC), anterior to the sigmoid sinus, and superior to the jugular bulb. LSCC Lateral semicircular canal. (Published with permission from Robert Jackler, MD who maintains copyright ownership and right to future use)

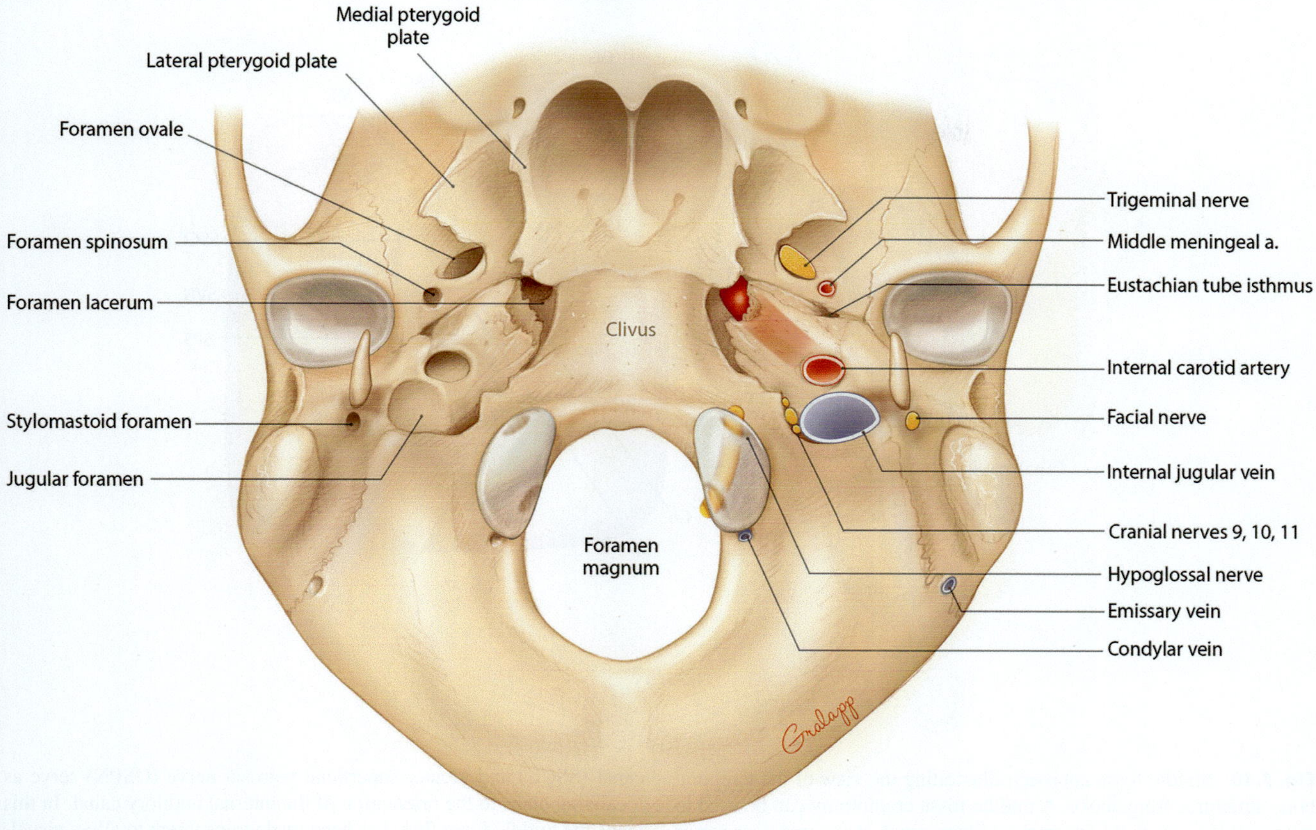

Fig. 3.37 Osseous anatomy of the cranial base as seen from below. (Published with permission from Robert Jackler, MD who maintains copyright ownership and right to future use)

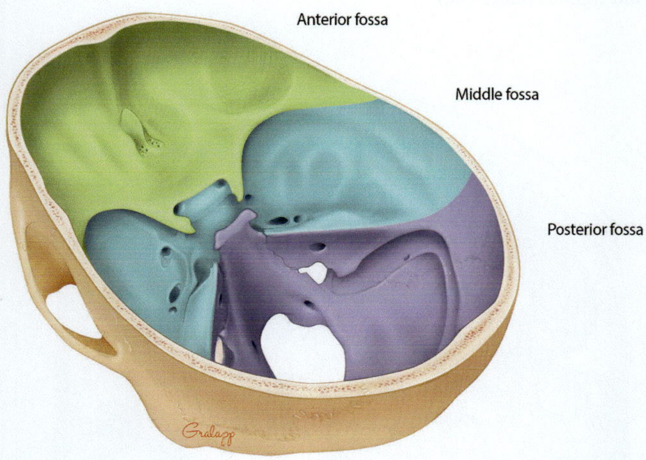

Fig. 3.38 Oblique view of the cranial base. The skull base is divided into three fossae: anterior, middle, and posterior. (Published with permission from Robert Jackler, MD who maintains copyright ownership and right to future use)

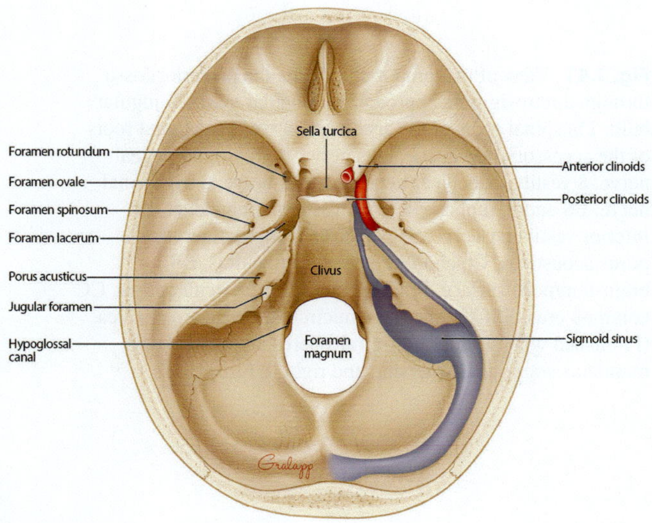

Fig. 3.39 Cranial base as seen from above. (Published with permission from Robert Jackler, MD who maintains copyright ownership and right to future use)

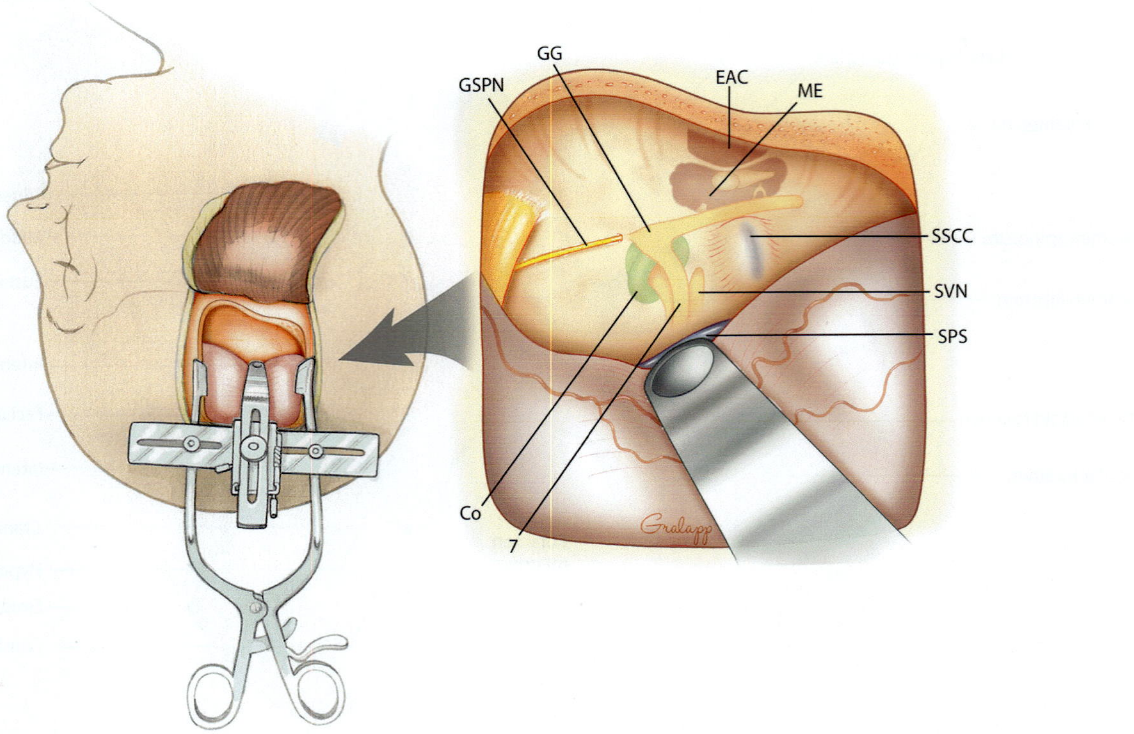

Fig. 3.40 Middle fossa approach illustrating the view of the temporal bone structures from above. A middle fossa craniotomy can be used to approach lesions of the internal auditory canal, decompress or repair the perigeniculate facial nerve, repair tegmen or superior semicircular canal dehiscences, or address lesions of the petrous apex. In this example, dural elevation off of the anterior face of the petrous pyramid has been completed and a retractor placed behind the crest of the petrous pyramid. The arcuate eminence overlying the superior semicircular canal (SSCC) and greater superficial petrosal nerve (GSPN) serve as localizing clues to the orientation of the internal auditory canal. In this view, the middle fossa floor has been made transparent to allow visualization of the petrous contents. EAC External auditory canal, ME middle ear, SVN superior vestibular nerve, SPS superior petrosal sinus, 7 facial nerve, Co cochlea, GG geniculate ganglion. (Published with permission from Robert Jackler, MD who maintains copyright ownership and right to future use)

Fig. 3.41 View of the temporal bone via the posterior fossa through a retrosigmoid approach. JV Jugular vein, JB jugular bulb, 11s spinal roots of the accessory nerve, 11c cranial roots of the accessory nerve, 10 vagus nerve, 9 glossopharyngeal nerve, 8 vestibulocochlear nerve, 7 facial nerve, 5 trigeminal nerve, ES endolymphatic sac, VA vestibular aqueduct, IV inferior vestibular nerve, SV superior vestibular nerve, PA porus acousticus, Ch choroid plexus, Fl flocullus, BS brainstem/pons surface, PSCC posterior semicircular canal, CC common crus, SSCC superior semicircular canal, Co cochlea. (Published with permission from Robert Jackler, MD who maintains copyright ownership and right to future use)

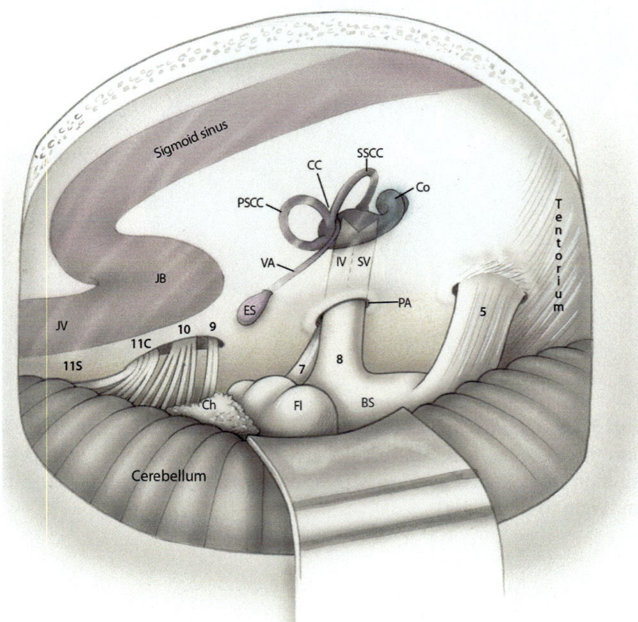

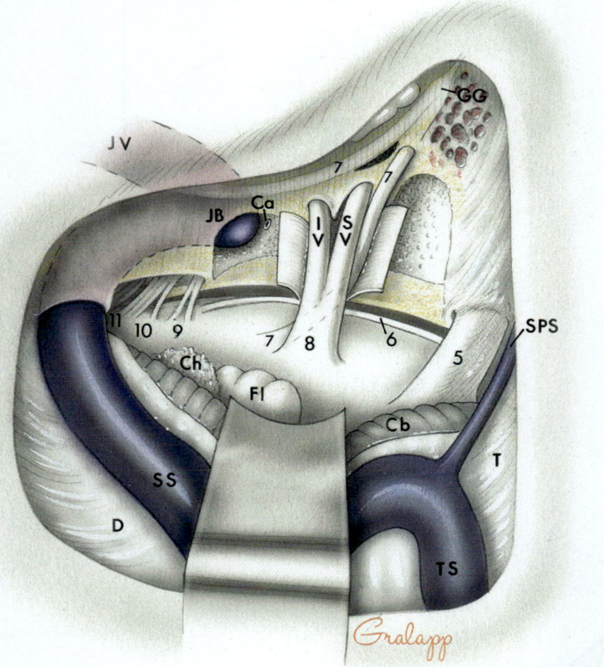

Fig. 3.42 View of the posterior fossa from the translabyrinthine approach. JV Jugular vein, JB jugular bulb, SS sigmoid sinus, TS transverse sinus, SPS superior petrosal sinus, 11 accessory nerve, 10 vagus nerve, 9 glossopharyngeal nerve, 8 vesitbulocochlear nerve, 7 facial nerve, 6 abducens nerve, 5 trigeminal nerve, IV inferior vestibular nerve, SV superior vestibular nerve, GG geniculate ganglion, Ch choroid plexus, Fl flocullus, Ca cochlear aqueduct, Cb cerebellum, D posterior fossa dura. (Published with permission from Robert Jackler, MD who maintains copyright ownership and right to future use)

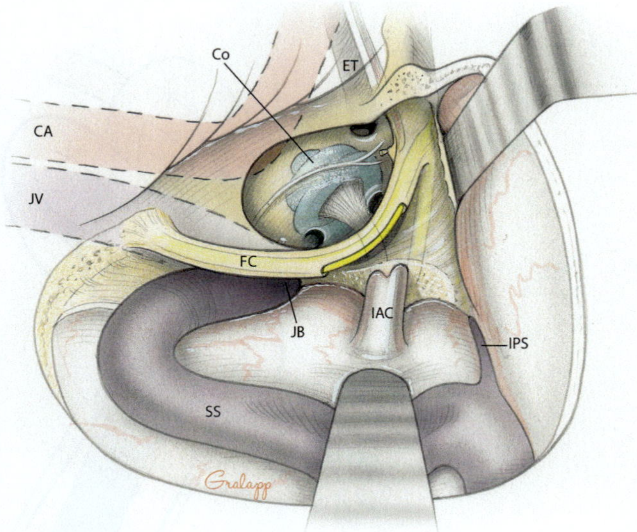

Fig. 3.43 A transparent view through the floor of the middle ear demonstrates the relationships between the cochlea (Co), jugular bulb (JB), and carotid artery (CA). The fallopian (FC) and the internal auditory (IAC) canals have been skeletonized. JV Jugular vein, SS sigmoid sinus, IPS inferior petrosal sinus, ET Eustachian tube. (Published with permission from Robert Jackler, MD who maintains copyright ownership and right to future use)

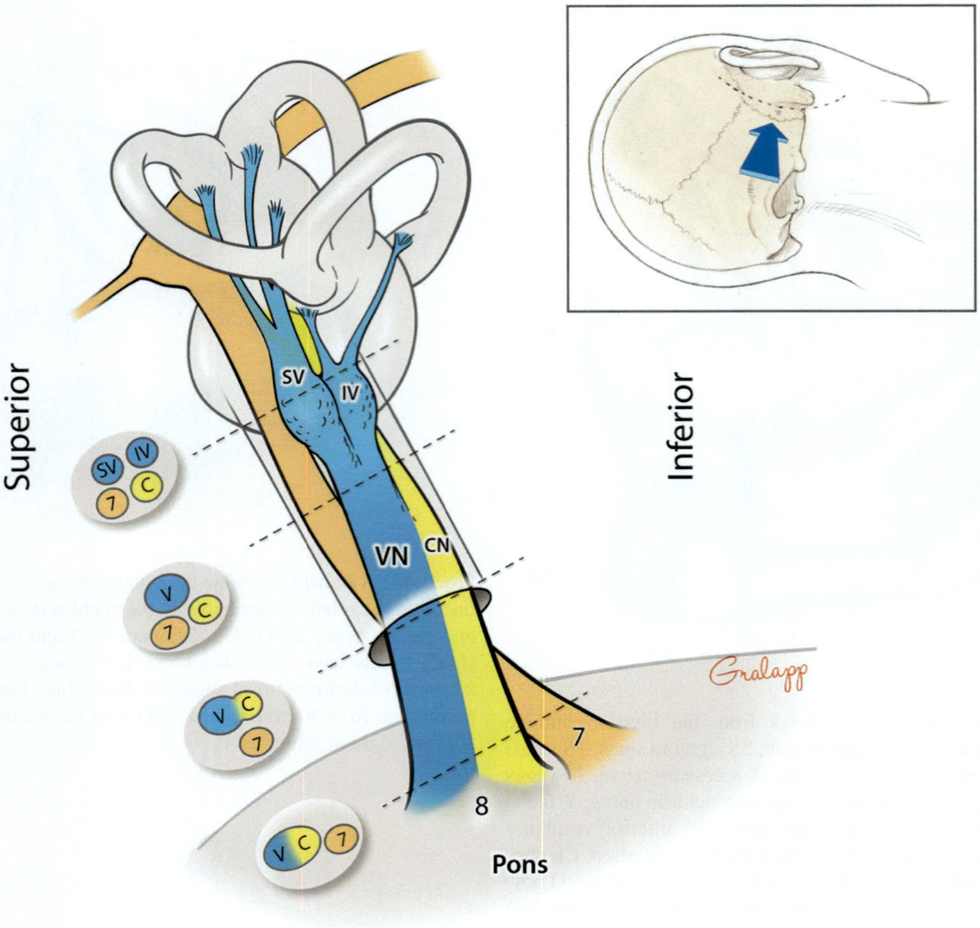

Fig. 3.44 Posterior view of the internal auditory canal and cerebellopontine angle as seen from a retrosigmoid perspective. The seventh and eighth cranial nerves traverse the internal auditory canal from their origin at the pons. The facial nerve (7) begins anteroinferior to the origin of the eighth nerve (8) at the brainstem, rotating to become anterosuperior at the canal's lateral boundary, known as the fundus. The eighth nerve fibers split into vestibular (VN) and cochlear (CN) components, which rotate 90° from the porus (medial opening to the canal) to the fundus [16]. At the brainstem, the cochlear fibers are inferior to the vestibular fibers, but become anterior to the vestibular nerve at the fundus. The vestibular nerve further splits into superior (SV) and inferior (IV) vestibular nerves. The cell bodies for the first-order vestibular afferent neurons are found in the vestibular (Scarpa's) ganglia, found at the distal SV and IV nerves. The superior vestibular nerve innervates the lateral semicircular canal, superior semicircular canal, and utricle. The inferior vestibular nerve innervates the saccule, and also gives off the singular nerve to innervate the posterior semicircular canal. The glial-Schwann sheath junction, also known eponymously as the Obersteiner-Redlich zone, represents the transition point along the nerve from central to peripheral myelin. Though variable in location, this zone is typically found at or medial to the porus [3]. While historically vestibular schwannomas have been thought to arise from this transition zone, more recent evidence suggests most schwannomas arise more distally [15]. (Published with permission from Robert Jackler, MD who maintains copyright ownership and right to future use)

Fig. 3.45 Orientation of nerves at the fundus of the internal auditory canal. A Anterior, P posterior, S superior, I inferior, SV superior vestibular nerve, IV inferior vestibular nerve, 7 facial nerve, C cochlear nerve, VC vertical crest also known eponymously as "Bill's Bar," TC transverse crest. It is important to emphasize that the orientation of the nerves at the fundus varies as the bundles traverse their course towards the pons. (Published with permission from Robert Jackler, MD who maintains copyright ownership and right to future use)

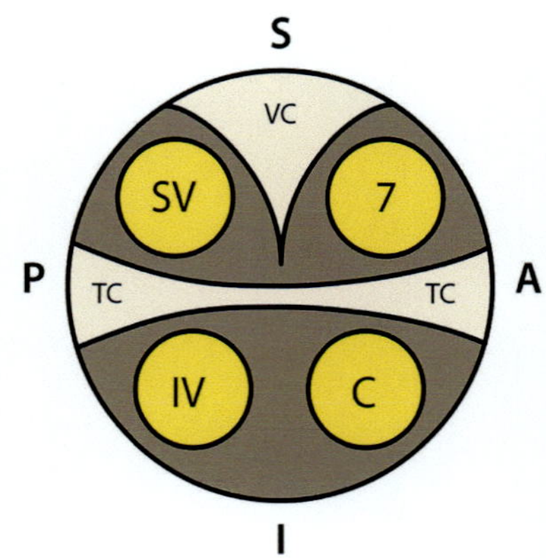

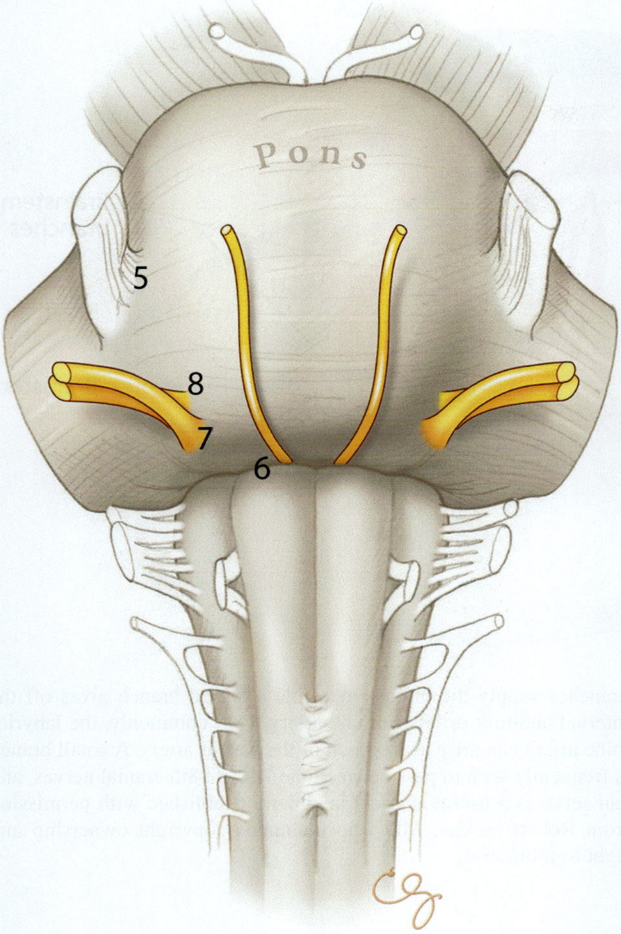

Fig. 3.46 Ventral perspective of the pons and medulla illustrating the anatomical relationships of the cranial nerves. Note that the facial nerve (7) enters the lower lateral pons inferior to the eighth (8) nerve. 5 Trigeminal nerve, 6 abducens nerve [5]. (Published with permission from Robert Jackler, MD who maintains copyright ownership and right to future use)

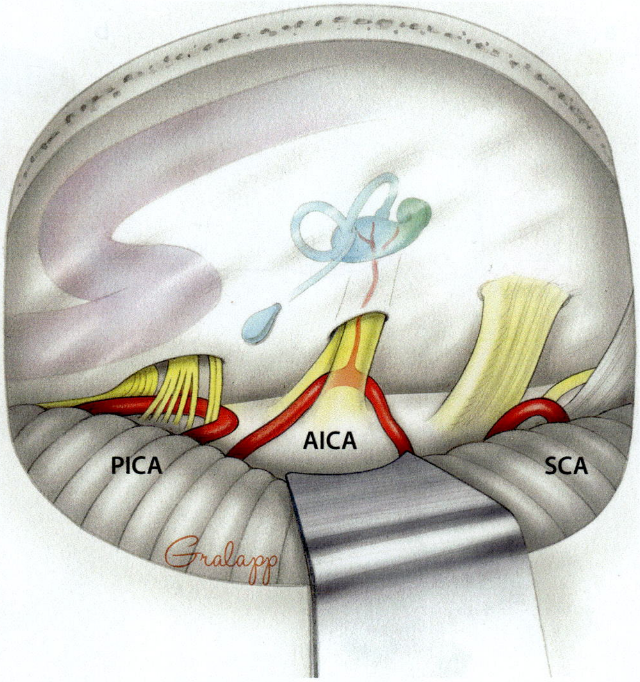

Fig. 3.47 Arterial supply to the cerebellum includes the posterior inferior cerebellar artery (PICA), anterior inferior cerebellar artery (AICA), and superior cerebellar artery (SCA). The SCA arises from the basilar artery near its terminal bifurcation. The PICA is often the largest branch of the vertebral artery. Its anterior medullary segment passes near the hypoglossal nerve rootlets, while its lateral and tonsillomedullary segment passes near the origins of the 9th, 10th, and 11th cranial nerves. (Published with permission from Robert Jackler, MD who maintains copyright ownership and right to future use)

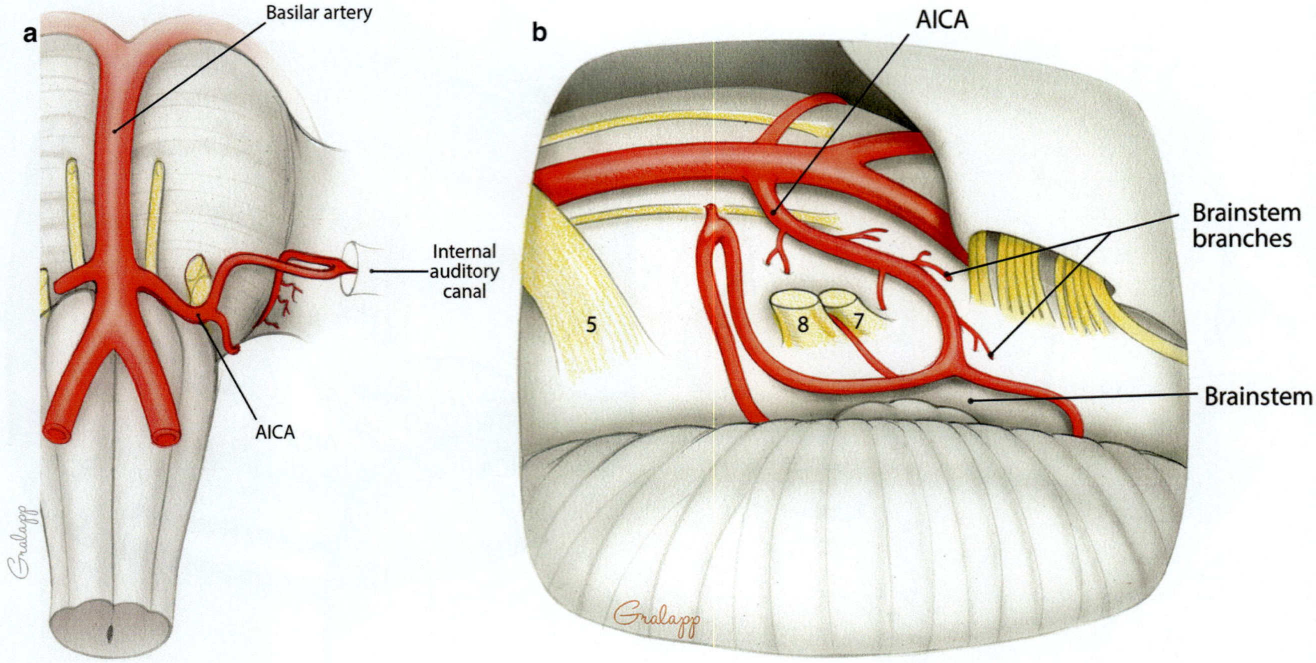

Fig. 3.48 Frontal (**a**) and lateral (**b**) views of the brainstem and vertebrobasilar system. Paired vertebral arteries merge to form a single midline basilar artery, supplying the spinal cord, brainstem, cerebellum, and occipital lobes. The anterior inferior cerebellar artery (AICA) most commonly branches from the basilar artery, but may also arise more inferiorly at the vertebrobasilar junction, or even less frequently, from the vertebral artery. Proximal penetrating AICA branches supply the brainstem, while a lateral branch gives off the internal auditory or labyrinthine artery. Less commonly, the labyrinthine artery can arise as a branch of the basilar artery. A small branch is frequently seen to pass between the 7th and 8th cranial nerves, and can serve as a useful surgical landmark. (Published with permission from Robert Jackler, MD who maintains copyright ownership and right to future use)

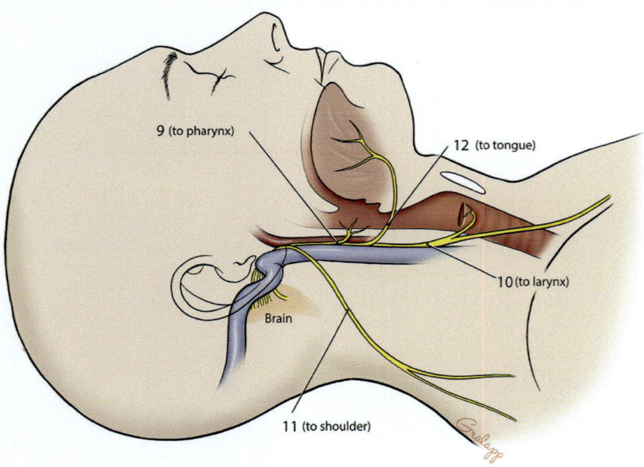

Fig. 3.49 Cranial nerves 9, 10, and 11 as well as the internal jugular vein pass through the jugular foramen. Cranial nerve 12, which passes through the hypoglossal canal, is another important neural consideration in surgeries involving the jugular foramen. (Published with permission from Robert Jackler, MD who maintains copyright ownership and right to future use)

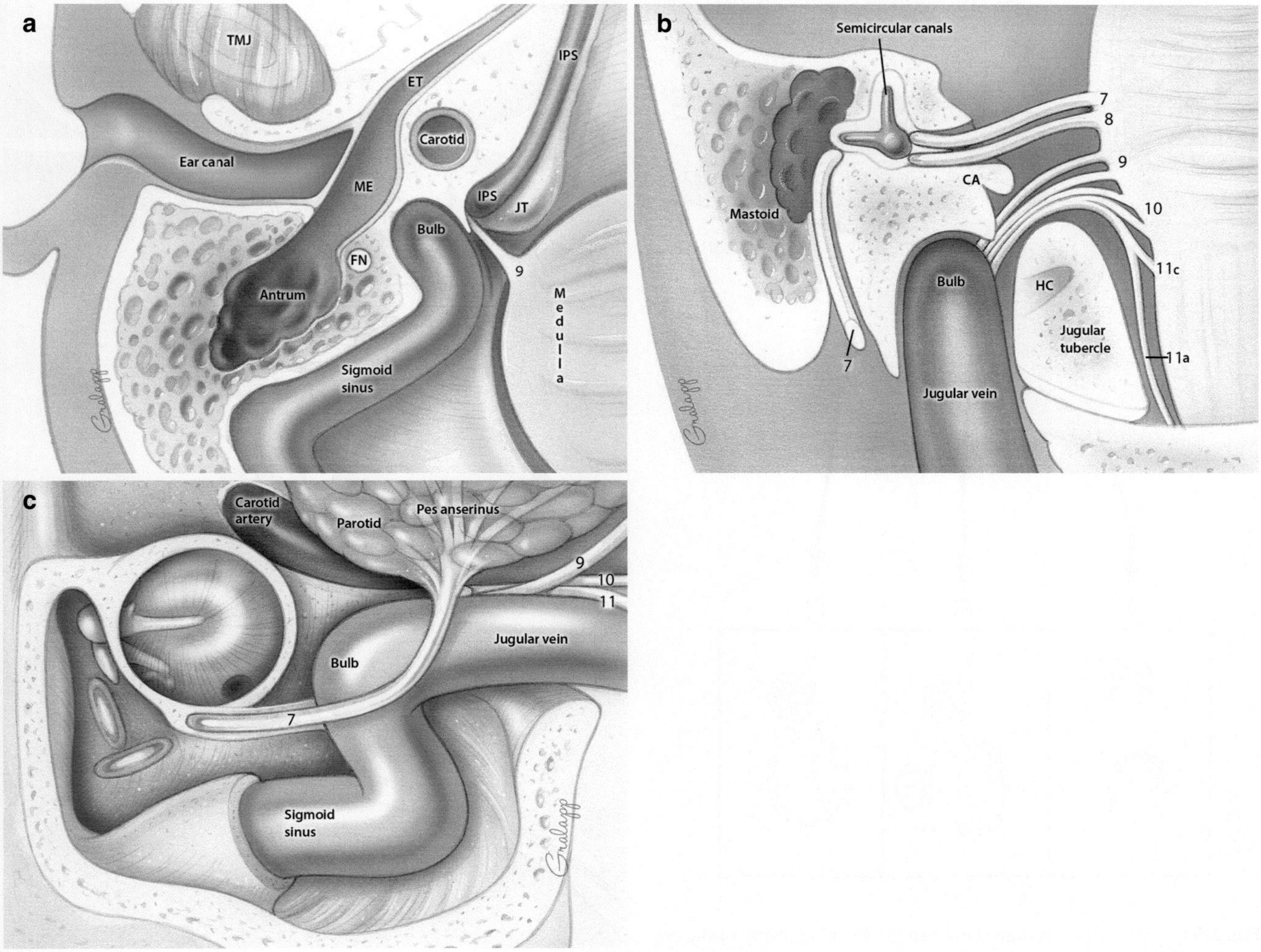

Fig. 3.50 Axial (**a**), coronal (**b**), and lateral (**c**) views of the jugular foramen region. The jugular foramen is divided into two parts by a fibrous or bony septum called the jugular spine into the anteromedial pars nervosa and the posterolateral pars vascularis. The pars nervosa contains the inferior petrosal sinus and CN 9, while the pars vascularis contains the jugular bulb and cranial nerves 10 and 11. The jugular tubercle, part of the occipital bone, forms the roof of the hypoglossal canal. The jugular vein is separated from the carotid anteriorly by a thin ridge of bone called the carotid ridge. TMJ Temporomandibular joint, ET Eustachian tube, ME middle ear, FN facial nerve, IPS inferior petrosal sinus, JT jugular tubercle, 7 facial nerve, 8 vestibulocochlear nerve, 9 glossopharyngeal nerve, 10 vagus nerve, 11c cranial root of the accessory nerve, 11a spinal root of the accessory nerve, HC hypoglossal canal, CA cochlear aqueduct. (Published with permission from Robert Jackler, MD who maintains copyright ownership and right to future use)

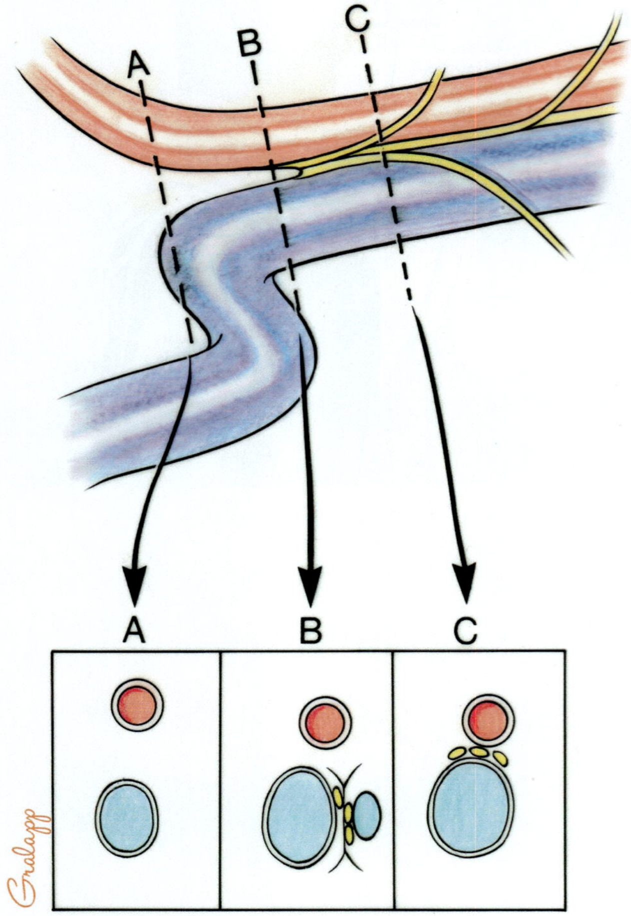

Fig. 3.51 Axial cross-sections demonstrate the relationship of the cranial nerves to the jugular vein and carotid artery in a jugular foramen approach. (**a**) The lower cranial nerves lie below the plane of the jugular bulb. Here, there is relatively wide bony separation between the vein and carotid artery. (**b**) The lower cranial nerves are aligned in the fibro-osseous septum between the jugular vein and inferior petrosal sinus at the level of the mid-jugular foramen. (**c**) Extracranially, the lower cranial nerves are narrowly sandwiched between the carotid and jugular vein. (Published with permission from Robert Jackler, MD who maintains copyright ownership and right to future use)

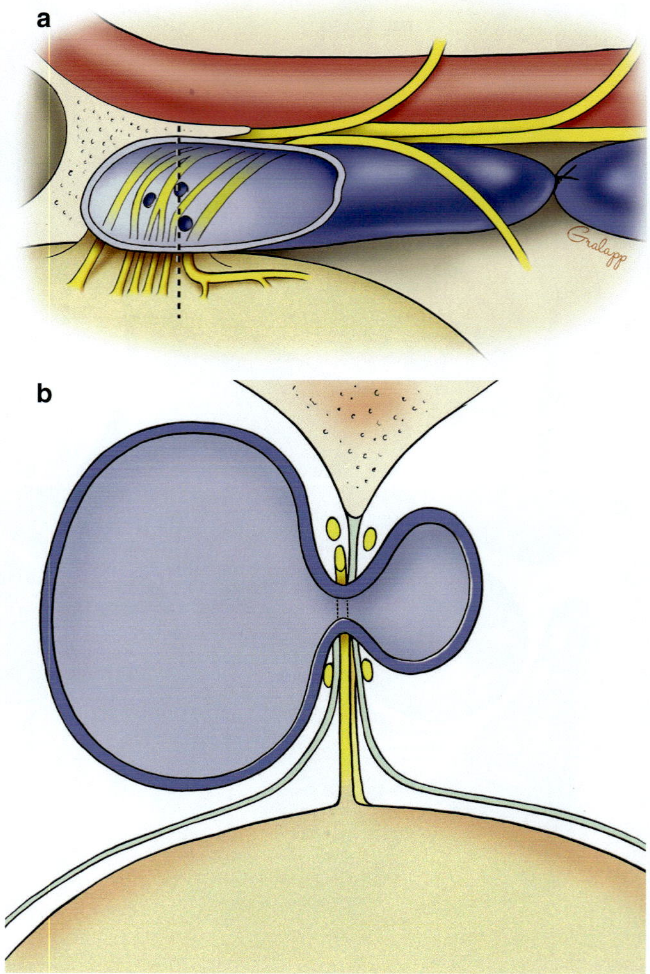

Fig. 3.52 Detail of the neurovascular relationships of the jugular foramen in lateral (surgical) (**a**) and axial (**b**) views. The dashed line marks the level of the axial view. The lower cranial nerves turn 90° from their root entry zone to their exit out of the jugular foramen. Several perforations connect the medial jugular vein to the lateral aspect of the inferior petrosal sinus. When jugular foramen tumors penetrate the medial pars nervosa, it is often through these perforations that the tumor can involve the inferior petrosal sinus. (Published with permission from Robert Jackler, MD who maintains copyright ownership and right to future use)

a

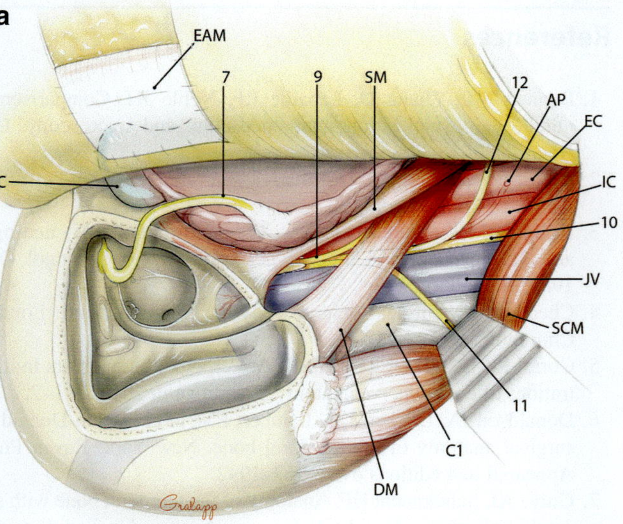

b

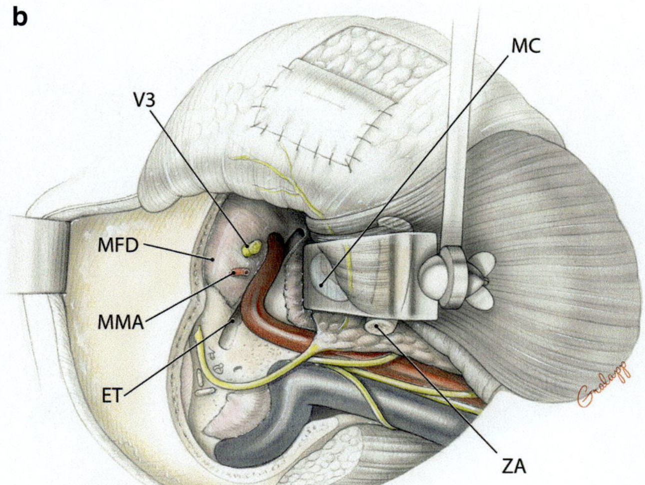

Fig. 3.53 (**a**) In this exposure of the jugular foramen, the facial nerve has been rerouted anteriorly, and the canal wall taken down. Neither maneuver is required for most jugular foramen tumors. The sternocleidomastoid muscle is retracted posteriorly, while the digastric and stylohyoid muscles have been reflected anteriorly. Note the lateral process of C1, which serves as a surgical landmark for the vertebral artery as it exits the vertebra's foramen transversarium to enter the brainstem. MC Mandibular condyle, EAM external acoustic meatus, 7 facial nerve, 9 glossopharyngeal nerve, 10 vagus nerve, 11 accessory nerve, 12 hypoglossal nerve, SM styloid muscle, AP ascending pharyngeal artery, EC external carotid, IC internal carotid, JV jugular vein, SCM sternocleidomastoid muscle, C1 transverse process of C1, DM digastric muscle. (**b**) Surgical view following a postauricular infratemporal fossa type B approach. The carotid artery has been exposed along its horizontal portion, allowing access to the apical petrous bone and clivus. ET Eustachian tube, MMA middle meningeal artery, MFD middle fossa dura, V3 third division of trigeminal nerve, MC mandibular condyle, ZA zygomatic arch. (Published with permission from Robert Jackler, MD who maintains copyright ownership and right to future use)

a

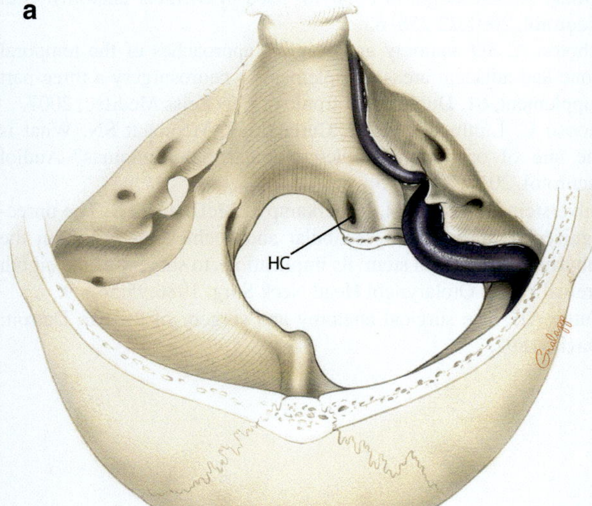

b

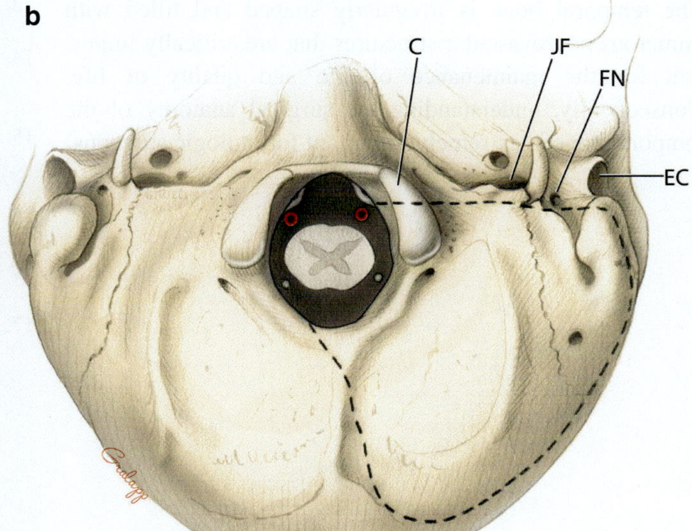

Fig. 3.54 Bone removal in a far lateral approach to the foramen magnum as seen from above (**a**) and below (**b**). The anterior limits of bony removal are the ear canal (EC), facial nerve (FN), and jugular foramen (JF). A portion of the occipital condyle (C) is removed. HC Hypoglossal canal. (Published with permission from Robert Jackler, MD who maintains copyright ownership and right to future use)

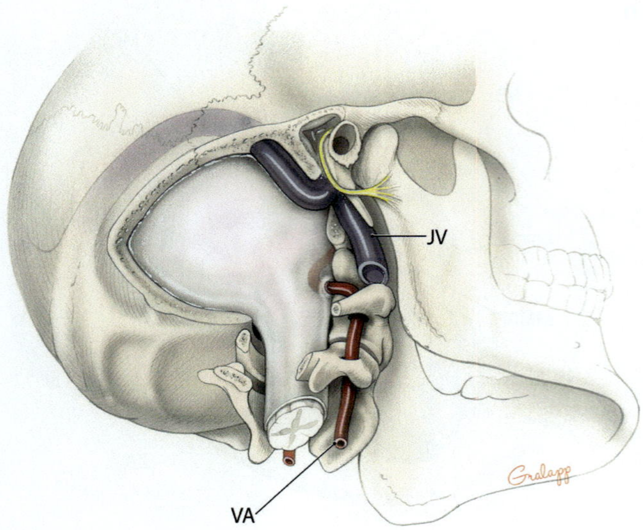

Fig. 3.55 In this posterolateral view of a far lateral approach, laminectomy of the first three cervical vertebrae has been performed, allowing increased cervical exposure. The vertebral artery (VA) can be seen passing through the foramen transversarium of the cervical vertebrae. JV Jugular vein. (Published with permission from Robert Jackler, MD who maintains copyright ownership and right to future use)

Conclusions

The temporal bone is irregularly shaped and filled with numerous neurovascular structures that are critically important for the maintenance of life and quality of life. Consequently, understanding the surgical anatomy of the temporal bone is extremely important for otologic surgeons.

References

1. Bennett ML, Zhang D, Labadie RF, Noble JH. Comparison of middle ear visualization with endoscopy and microscopy. Otol Neurotol. 2016;37:362–6.
2. Bloustine S, Langston L, Miller T. Ear-cough (Arnold's) reflex. Ann Otol Rhinol Laryngol. 1976;85:406–7.
3. Bridger MW, Farkashidy J. The distribution of neuroglia and Schwann cells in the 8th nerve of man. J Laryngol Otol. 1980;94:1353–62.
4. Cheatle AH. Surgical anatomy of the temporal bone. London: Churchill; 1907.
5. Corrales CE, Jackler RK, Mudry A. Perpetuation of errors in illustrations of cranial nerve anatomy. J Neurosurg. 2016;28:1–7.
6. Donaldson JA, Duckert LG, Lambert PM, et al. Anson-Donaldson surgical anatomy of the temporal bone. New York: Raven Press. Appeared in 4 editions over 1967–1992.
7. Gulya AJ, Schuknecht HF. Anatomy of the temporal bone with surgical implications. New York: Informa. Appeared in 3 editions over the years 1995–2007.
8. Hitselberger WE, House WF. Acoustic neuroma diagnosis. External auditory canal hypesthesia as an early sign. Arch Otolaryngol. 1966;83:218–21.
9. Jackler RK, Cho M. A new theory to explain the genesis of petrous apex cholesterol granuloma. Otol Neurotol. 2003;24:96–106.
10. Jackler RK. Atlas of skull base surgery and neurotology. 2nd ed. New York: Thieme; 2009.
11. Jackler RK, Gralapp C, Mudry A. Revisiting Max Brödel's 1939 classic coronal illustration of the ear. Otol Neurotol. 2014;35:555–60.
12. Lustig LR, Jackler RK, Mandelcorn R. The history of otology through its eponyms I: anatomy. Am J Otol. 1998;19:371–38.
13. Mudry A. The origin of eponyms used in cochlear anatomy. Otol Neurotol. 2001;22:258–63.
14. Rhoton A. 3D anatomy and surgical approaches of the temporal bone and adjacent areas, Supplement to neurosurgery a three-part supplement, 61. Dublin: Medtronic & Carl Zeiss Meditec; 2007.
15. Roosli C, Linthicum FH Jr, Cureoglu S, Merchant SN. What is the site of origin of Cochleovestibular Schwannomas? Audiol Neurotol. 2012;17:121–5.
16. Silverstein H, Norrell H, Haberkamp T, McDaniel AB. The unrecognized rotation of the vestibular and cochlear nerves from the labyrinth to the brain stem: its implications to surgery of the eighth cranial nerve. Otolaryngol Head Neck Surg. 1986;95:543–9.
17. Tuttle AH, The surgical anatomy and surgery of the ear. Detroit: Davis, 1892.

Middle Ear Mechanics in Otology

4

Manohar Bance

Introduction

Every surgeon, when operating on the middle ear, is essentially performing mechanical engineering by manipulating a lever to maximize acoustic power transfer from the external ear canal through the middle ear to the inner ear. Pathology that results in conductive hearing loss also affects this mechanical lever function. Many ear surgeons would appreciate sufficient background in middle ear mechanics to understand the interventions they routinely perform and the effects of pathology on the engineering principles involved. The basic science literature in this area is often inaccessible without a basic grasp of some fundamental concepts about the physics of the middle ear.

While not addressed in this chapter, it is worth remembering that otologists tend to ignore the contributions of the external ear canal to hearing because its length and shape are not usually manipulated for hearing results. Not only do the resonances of the pinna and ear canal help sound localization, the conchal resonances increase sound pressure at the entrance to the ear canal by up to 10 dB, and ear canal resonances reach up to 20 dB at 2700 Hz [1, 2]. In selected frequencies, these effects may be as large as middle ear pressure gains.

Clearly, middle ear reconstruction is not easy. Otherwise, predictably good results would be the norm, and in reality, they certainly are not [3]. Most work on middle ear mechanics has been performed on normal middle ears in cadaveric temporal bones, and much of the data reviewed here are from such experiments. In practice, however, surgeons deal with abnormal middle ears due to scarring, poor ventilation, and fluid, which can dominate postoperative hearing results through their mechanical effects. In fact, much of middle ear surgery is a balance between hearing outcomes and achieving stability of the middle ear (e.g. "propping up" prostheses, large cartilage grafts to reconstruct the scutum), the latter of which can come with an acoustic/mechanical price.

In the following section, we will review some basic concepts in acoustics and mechanics.

Decibels (dB)

Many numbers in otology are expressed in dB, which behave very differently from the linear number systems that are used in everyday life. A decibel is the log of a *ratio* of the *measured number* divided by a *reference number*. Different types of dBs simply have different reference numbers. For instance, dB SPL uses a fixed sound pressure as its reference and is $20*\text{Log}_{10}$ of the ratio [sound pressure in pascals/reference pressure of 0.00002 pascals]. dB HL (hearing level), which is used on audiograms, replaces the reference of 0.00002 pascals with a sound pressure level that an "average healthy" person can hear for each frequency. Decibels grow and shrink on a log scale, so an increase of 6 dB SPL is actually a doubling in sound pressure, and +20 dB is tenfold change in sound pressure. Increasing from 0 to +20 dB SPL is a tenfold increase, and going from +20 dB to +40 dB SPL is another tenfold increase again from the first increase (100× original), a much bigger arithmetic change than the first +20 dB. The actual linear arithmetic change for a given dB increase depends on the level where the measurement is starting. If the measured number is smaller than the reference, then the ratio will be less than 1, and the log of numbers less than 1 is negative. dB values can be positive as well as negative. Decibels have the advantage of being symmetric, in that +20 dB is a ten-fold increase in SPL, and −20 dB is a ten-fold decrease in SPL.

The non-linearity of decibels is important to appreciate, as otologists may not think that a 6 dB improvement is much change in hearing (and in fact, human loudness perception seems to work more on a log than linear scale), while it is

M. Bance (✉)
Otology and Skull Base Surgery, University of Cambridge, Cambridge, UK
e-mail: mlb59@cam.ac.uk

A. D. Sweeney et al. (eds.), *Haynes-Glasscock-Shambaugh Surgery of the Ear*, https://doi.org/10.1007/978-3-032-18264-7_4

actually a doubling in sound pressure. Hence, a hearing aid producing 6 dB more SPL requires twice as much power, and a 20 dB increase in hearing level is actually a ten-fold increase in acoustic power reaching the cochlea.

Vibrations

If a mass is disturbed from rest and is connected to restoring forces (generically "springs"), then it will be pulled back to its original position. Because masses have inertia, they will overshoot this initial point on their return until their motion is reversed again by the springs, again overshooting in the opposite direction and, in turn, causing a to-and-fro motion (Fig. 4.1).

Essentially, energy is being exchanged between the mass and the springs. This back-and-forth movement is a vibration, and if we plot the displacement of a part of the system against time, we will plot a sine wave. Air is one such mass spring system (supplying both the mass and the springs by its compliance), and acoustic sound is a manifestation of this vibration. A sinusoid can be characterized by three features: its amplitude, its frequency, and its phase. Figure 4.1 shows these generically. The phase is always relative to some other time varying signal (i.e. it leads or lags the other signal in time). Physicists often plot displacement, velocity, or acceleration of such a system. Velocity leads displacement by 90°, (i.e. velocity is minimal when the mass is at rest at the ends of its displacement cycle), and acceleration leads velocity by 90° again. Typically, in the ear, we tend to plot the phase of the vibration velocity (rather than displacement or acceleration) relative to the force that is causing the forced vibration, which is the sound pressure. This phase can tell us important information about the mechanics of the system, as described below.

If vibrations have phase, then how they interact when added depends on their relative phases. For instance, vibrations can reflect the edges of structures and meet oncoming vibrations, and if they are in phase (0 or 360°), they will sum, and if they are out of phase (180°), they will cancel each other out. This will cause nodes of high vibration and antinodes of low vibration amplitude on structures, unless the frequency is so low that the whole structure is vibrating as just one part of the wave and moving together (in-phase motion). If all parts move in phase and with the same amplitude, then this is called rigid body vibration (e.g. the skull at low frequencies in bone conduction hearing). Essentially, all structures will break up into vibrating subunits at high frequencies, and at what frequency this happens is dependent on the mechanical properties of the structure.

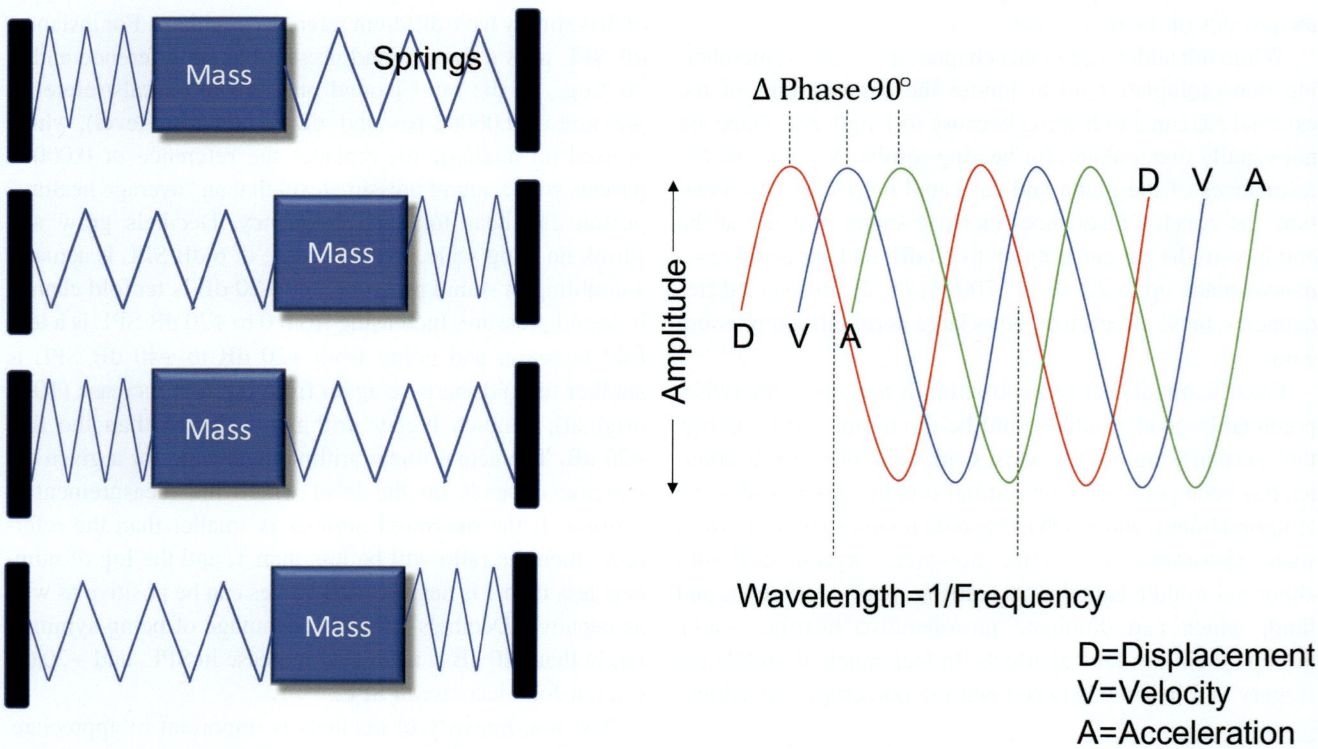

Fig. 4.1 A simple mass spring system exchanges energy between potential energy of the springs and kinetic energy of the mass. Its motion is tracked by a sine wave, in which displacement lags velocity by 90° and velocity lags acceleration by 90°

Mass-Spring Systems and Impedance

A simple vibrator is often modelled as a mass-spring system (Fig. 4.1). How rapidly it vibrates (its frequency) depends on the amount of the mass and the strength of the springs. Masses have inertia, which "fights" multiple reversals of direction/second at higher frequencies, and thus, are easier to vibrate at low frequencies. Conversely, springs are easier to vibrate at high frequencies. This "reluctance" to vibrate is called impedance, which has two components: reactance (mass and stiffness reactance) and resistance. Resistance converts energy to heat and dampens vibrations that otherwise might be excessive. In the ear, friction is generally not as useful because it dampens wanted vibrations. With the reactive component of impedance, the energy is not lost, but rather is stored either in the spring's deformation or in the kinetic energy of the mass. In practical terms, it still opposes vibration if it is acting against the direction the mass is moving. However, unlike resistance, the impedance depends on the vibration frequency with which we are trying to drive the system. At some frequency, the stored energy is efficiently transferred between the springs and masses and causes movement in the same direction as the mass is moving, resulting in a dramatic increase in vibration velocity. This is the resonance frequency of the system (Fig. 4.2). Most systems are stiffness dominated at low frequencies (i.e. adding more stiffness increases their impedance much more than adding mass), and mass dominated at high frequencies. A purely stiffness dominated system will double its vibration velocity (halve its impedance) for every doubling in frequency (6 db/octave slope). A purely mass dominated system behaves conversely.

One way to look at a system to determine if it is stiffness or mass dominated is to look at the phase of the vibration velocity with respect to the phase of the pressure. Vibrating systems are usually described by velocity phase rather than by acceleration or displacement phase. At low frequencies, when the system is purely stiffness dominated, spring deformation (displacement, which lags velocity by 90°) rather than velocity is in phase with the force applied (pressure), as $F = -kx$ (Hooke's law, where k is the spring constant, F is force and x is displacement), making it so the velocity phase actually leads the pressure phase by 90° ($\pi/2$). At high frequencies (mass dominated), the vibration is in phase with acceleration (which leads velocity by 90°), according to the equation $F = ma$ (where m = mass, a = acceleration), making it so the velocity phase lags behind the pressure phase by −90° (see Fig. 4.2). At resonance, where mass and stiffness are balanced, the phase of velocity and pressure is 0, and impedance is only due to resistance. Other things can also cause a phase lag beyond mass, such as delays in the system; therefore, a phase lag doesn't always imply a mass dominated system.

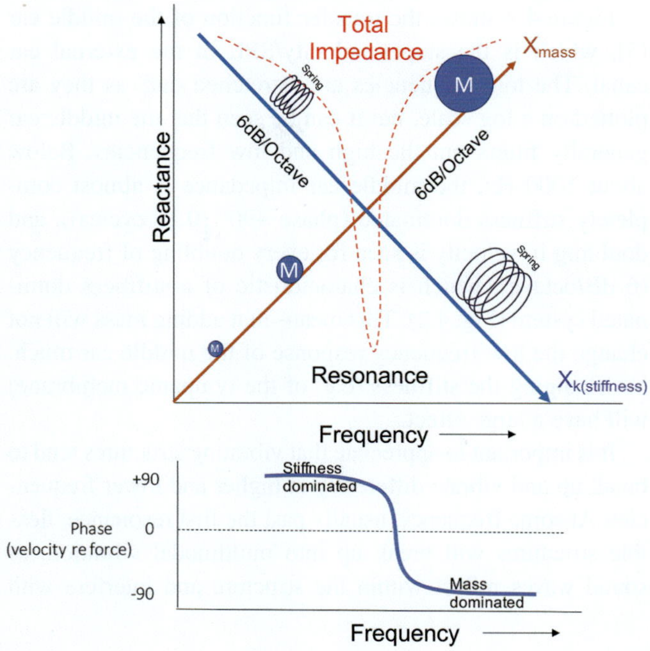

Fig. 4.2 Mass reactance increases with increasing frequency at 6 dB/octave, and stiffness reactance decreases by the same amount. The dashed line indicates total impedance, which shows a dramatic drop at the resonance frequency when mass and stiffness impedance are equal. Below the resonance frequency, the system is stiffness dominated (velocity leads sound pressure by +90°) and above resonance the velocity lags sound pressure by 90°

An important concept is that, although springs show higher impedance (i.e. larger resistance to vibration) at low frequencies, if we are trying to vibrate a mass by applying force through a spring, the spring will not vibrate much at low frequencies and will instead transfer the force to the mass. At higher frequencies, the spring has lower impedance, will vibrate more, and will transfer less of the force to the mass. Hence, compliances tend to absorb higher frequencies and transmit lower frequencies. This concept is important in areas like transcutaneous bone conduction devices, in which the skin absorbs higher frequencies, or in cases where there is softening of the incudo-stapedial joint or a fibrous fracture of the malleus, which can present with a high frequency conductive hearing loss [4].

More Complex Vibrating Systems

Figures 4.1 and 4.2 show simple mass spring systems, but it is important to note that most real systems are much more complicated and have many resonances. Also, while Fig. 4.2 shows a sharp resonance for a simple mass-spring system, in the ear, there is considerable damping, and with overlapping resonances, the ear shows a much broader band-pass type of response.

Figure 4.3 shows the transfer function of the middle ear [5], which is the stapes velocity/SPL in the external ear canal. The low frequencies are "stretched out" as they are plotted on a log scale, but it can be seen that the middle ear generally filters out the high and low frequencies. Below about 1000 Hz, the middle ear impedance is almost completely stiffness dominated (phase +90° (0.25 cycles)), and doubling in velocity is seen for every doubling of frequency (6 dB/octave), which is characteristic of a stiffness dominated system (Fig. 4.2). This means that adding mass will not change the low frequency response of the middle ear much, but changing the stiffness (e.g. of the tympanic membrane) will have a large effect.

It is important to appreciate that vibrating structures tend to break up and vibrate differently at higher and lower frequencies. At some frequency, usually past the first resonance, flexible structures will break up into multimodal vibration, as sound waves reflect within the structure and interfere with each other. Figure 4.4a demonstrates this concept for a simple string or rod. In flexible drum-like structures like the tympanic membrane (TM), the 3D vibration modes can become complex. Figure 4.4b shows real TM movements over one cycle at 396 Hz, and although all parts do not move the same amount, they move in the same direction at the same time (in-phase). Figure 4.4c shows the same TM at 4000 Hz, and it can be seen that the TM breaks up into subunits that vibrate at different amplitudes and phases. This concept has very important implications for the middle ear. First, as we will see below, the main lever action of the middle ear becomes less efficient, and second, at high frequencies, the area next to the umbo determines its movement, rather than the whole TM, making it so that damping this area will affect malleus movements more than damping other parts of the TM that are effectively decoupled from it. This concept also stipulates that, at low frequencies, changing one part of the TM affects the overall motion of TM because everything is moving in phase.

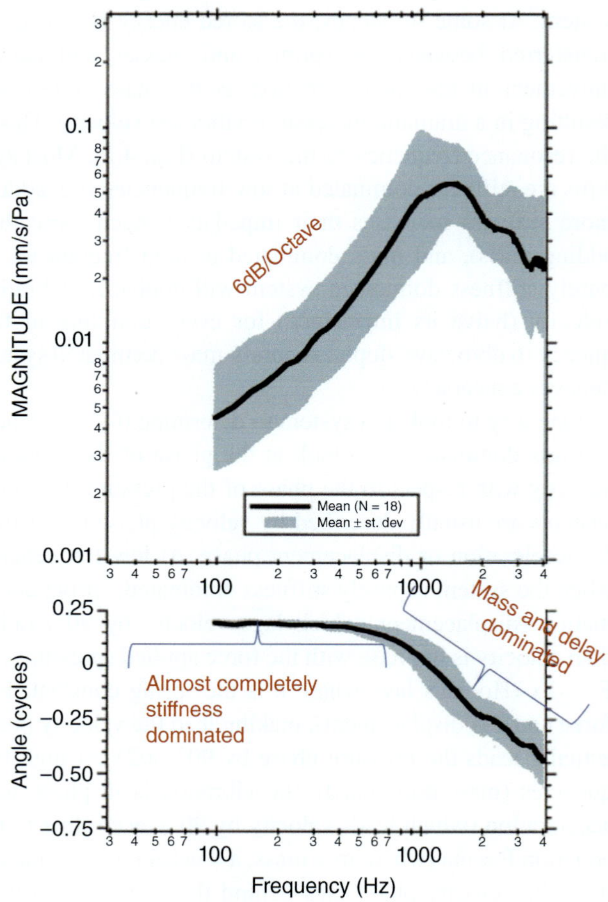

Fig. 4.3 Middle ear transfer function, i.e., stapes velocity external ear canal (EAC) pressure. The top panel is the mean (black line) and standard deviation (shaded), and the bottom panel is the phase relationship of stapes velocity to EAC pressure. In the lower frequencies, there is a phase lead of approximately 0.25 cycles (90°). The lower frequencies show characteristics of being stiffness dominated. (Adapted from Voss et al. with permission [5])

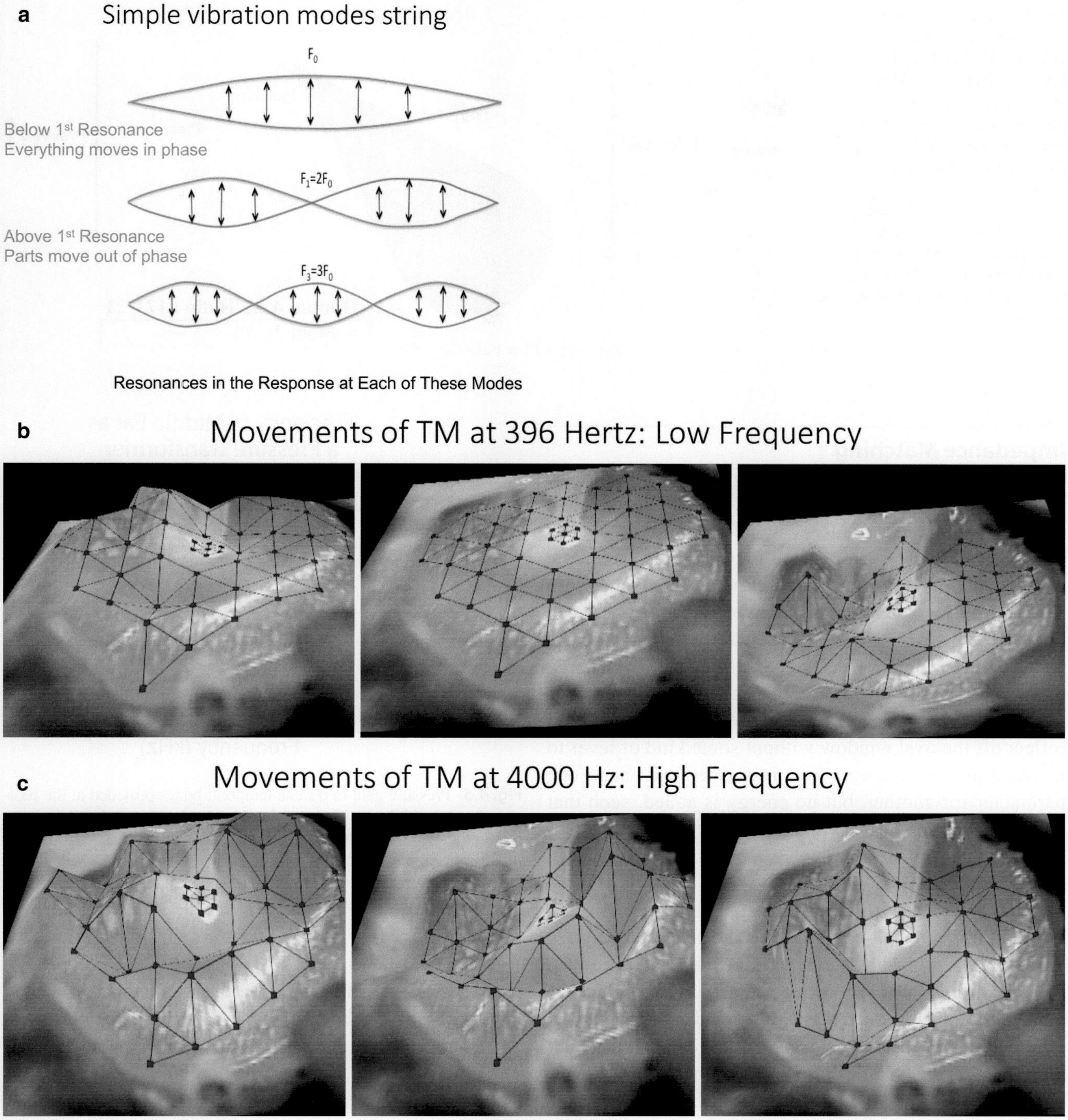

Fig. 4.4 (**a**) shows the multimodal vibration modes on a simple 2D structure, a string. The first fundamental frequency F_O is decided by the length of the string. The 2nd (F_1) and 3rd (F_2) resonant mode frequencies are integer multiples of $F_{O,}$ as reflections from the ends interfere with wave motion from the origin. (**b**) shows vibration modes measured and animated from a real human TM at 396 Hz over one cycle. It can be seen that although different parts show displacement at different amplitudes, during the vibration cycle, all parts move in phase. (**c**) shows the TM vibration modes over one cycle for 4000 Hz. It can be seen that different parts of the TM break up into differently vibrating modes, each moving out of phase with other parts

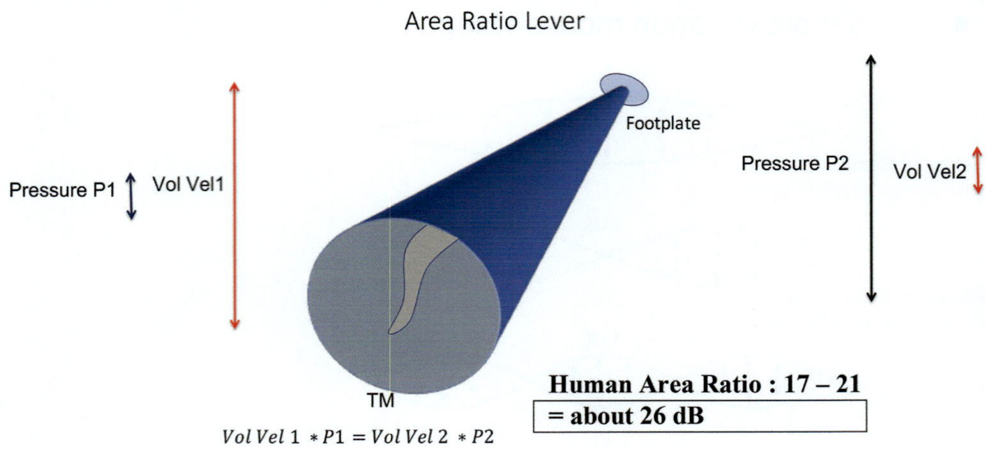

Fig. 4.5 The human area ratio lever. The volume velocity (Vol Vel 1) and Pressure (P1) at the TM are interchanged for increased pressure (P2) and decreased volume velocity (Vel Vel2) at the stapes footplate. The product of volume velocity and pressure at the TM and the footplate is unchanged. The human area ratio is about 20 to 1 from TM to footplate, which is about 26 dB gain in pressure

Impedance Matching

When trying to transfer energy from one medium to another, the amount of energy being transferred depends on the relative properties of the two mediums. Acoustic energy can only be propagated, reflected or changed into heat, and better matching of acoustic impedances between two mediums leads to more efficient energy transfer. A fundamental problem with the ear is that acoustic energy in air is not well matched to drive the impedance load of cochlear fluids and membranes. Most energy would reflect off the oval window without some kind of lever to increase pressure. Levers or transformers exchange one parameter for another, but no energy is added, such that the gain made possible by the middle ear is a gain in pressure at the footplate or inner ear, rather than a gain in total energy.

In the middle ear, the most important impedance matching function (although not perfect) is the area ratio between the size of the tympanic membrane and oval window (a variation on the hydraulic press principle) seen in Fig. 4.5. While other types of levers, such as the "ossicular lever" due to different lengths of the incus and malleus [6] and the catenary lever [7] due to the curved shape of the TM, may exist, they are not important contributors to pressure gain in the human middle ear. In this area ratio kind of lever, large volume velocity and low pressure at the TM are exchanged for large pressure and low volume velocity at the oval window (Fig. 4.5).

The TM area in humans is about 66 mm^2, and the footplate area is about 3.2 mm^2 [8], which creates a ratio of about 20:1, correlating with a roughly 26 dB increase in pressure. However, the TM is not an ideal piston at high frequencies, because it breaks up into multimodal vibrations as seen in Fig. 4.5, so that the effective lever ratio is much less than 26 dB at higher frequencies. In a classic experiment, Kurokawa and Goode [9] measured how much extra sound pressure was needed to vibrate the stapes footplate at equivalent amplitudes with and without the middle ear (Fig. 4.6) and found that the gain provided by the middle ear was roughly 20–25 dB at lower frequencies (which is almost exactly what we might predict from the area ratios) but was much less at higher frequencies where the TM breaks up into multimodal vibrations.

Aibara et al. [10] actually measured the pressure in the vestibule and calculated the pressure gain from the external ear canal to the inner ear (Fig. 4.7). The pressure transfer function in the inner ear is a bandpass that is best between 1 and 3 kHz, where the middle ear is most efficient. While it might be expected that the gain would be 20 dB lower in the lower frequencies in Fig. 4.7 without the middle ear, based on Fig. 4.6, some of the annular ligament impedance impacts the low frequency pressure gain from the middle ear to the vestibule.

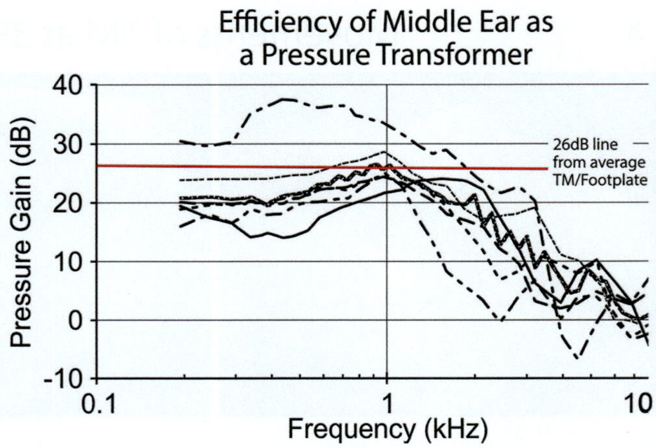

Fig. 4.6 Pressure gain in 6 fresh temporal bones provided at the footplate by the middle ear, as determined by the increase in EAC pressure required to achieve the same stapes displacement with and without the middle ear in place. It can be seen that the middle ear adds substantial gain at low frequencies below about 800 Hz, but above this frequency, the efficiency of the pressure gain transformer drops rapidly. (Adapted with permission from Kurokawa and Goode [9])

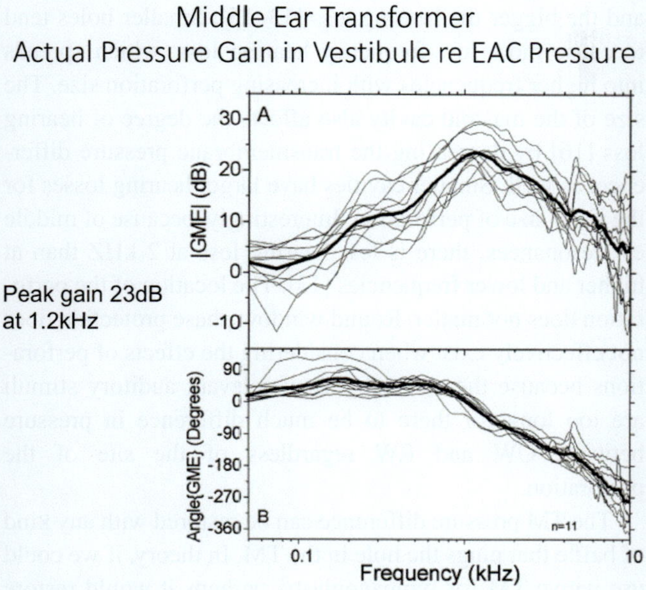

Fig. 4.7 Actual pressure gain measured in the vestibule relative to EAC pressure. The pressure gain is a bandpass between 0.5 and about 3 kHz. The upper panel is the magnitude, and the lower panel the phase of the gain. (Adapted from Aibara et al. with permission [10])

Fig. 4.8 The cochlea is represented schematically as a rolled-out tube. The size of the sinusoids represents the pressure. The EAC pressure is augmented at the oval window (OW), by about 20 dB, and attenuated at the round window (RW), by the middle ear. The pressure difference between these two windows drives the basilar membrane vibrations

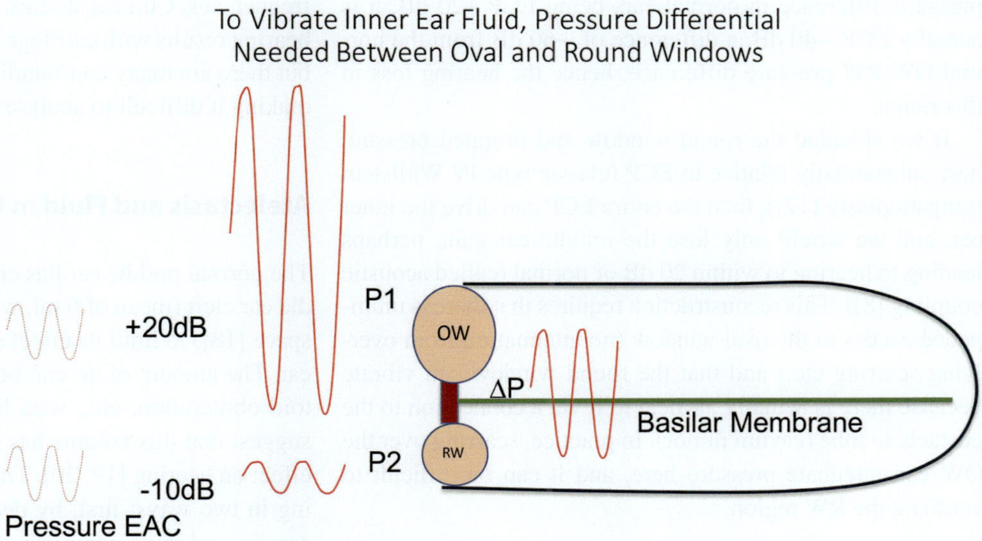

No middle ear surgery can restore normal hearing without recreating this lever ratio. It is important to appreciate that a vibrating TM is the engine of impedance matching. If there is middle ear fluid, the TM is thickened, or the TM has a perforation which acts as a pressure shunt, then normal hearing is impossible.

Oval Window (OW) and Round Window (RW) Pressure Difference

The driving force for basilar membrane vibration is not pressure at the OW, but the difference between OW and RW pressure (Fig. 4.8). Thus, we can manipulate this driving force by either increasing pressure at the oval window or by decreasing pressure at the round window.

Since the normal middle ear increases external canal pressure (ECP) by about 20–26 dB (10 to 20×) at the oval window relative to ECP, this factor dominates the OW-RW pressure difference. Dropping the pressure at the round window to a 1/10 of the ECP wouldn't change the absolute pressure difference much. For instance, if the ECP was 100 pressure units (PU), and middle ear pressure gain increased it to 2000 PU (+26 dB), then the difference between the OW and RW pressure wouldn't be much affected if we dropped the pressure at round window to 10 PU or left it at 100 PU. Hence, in the normal ear, hearing is dominated by the pressure gain at the oval window, and shielding at the round window is not very important. This has been termed ossicular coupling [11].

Middle Ear Pathology and Reconstruction

Acoustic Coupling

If we were to lose the middle ear totally, we might expect a loss of about 20–30 dB (the gain of the middle ear). In fact, we get a hearing loss of about 60 dB. Again, this is because we need to consider not just the loss of pressure gain at the OW but the change in the difference of pressures between the OW and RW. With the middle ear missing, the pressure is almost the same at the oval and round windows. Actually, there is a small difference, which is about 1/100th of the external canal pressure (−40 dB). So instead of the windows pressure difference in normal ears being ECP +20 dB, it is actually ECP −40 dB, a difference of −60 dB from the normal OW-RW pressure difference, hence the hearing loss in this range.

If we shielded the round window and dropped pressure here substantially relative to ECP (classic type IV Wullstein tympanoplasty [12]), then the entire ECP can drive the inner ear, and we would only lose the middle ear gain, perhaps leading to hearing to within 20 dB of normal (called acoustic coupling [8]). This reconstruction requires that there is unimpeded access to the oval window (no attenuation from overlying scarring etc.) and that the round window can vibrate because there is actually air next to it via a connection to the eustachian tube (cavum minor). In practice, scarring over the OW can attenuate pressure here, and it can be difficult to ventilate the RW region.

TM Perforations

A hole in the TM decreases the area ratio for the lever in Fig. 4.5, but even in the low frequency region where the TM is actually an efficient piston, halving the area would only decrease the pressure gain by 6 dB. In practice, we get 20–30 dB hearing losses from a perforation of this size [13]. Much of the hearing loss is because the perforation creates a pressure shunt that decreases trans-membrane pressure, particularly at the lower frequencies where wavelengths are very long. The consequence is similar pressure on both sides of the TM. The larger the hole, the bigger the pressure shunt, and the bigger the hearing loss [13–15]. Smaller holes tend to cause more low frequency hearing loss, which spreads into higher frequencies with increasing perforation size. The size of the mastoid cavity also affects the degree of hearing loss [16] by decreasing the transmembrane pressure difference, as well. Smaller cavities have larger hearing losses for the same size of perforation. Interestingly, because of middle ear resonances, there is less hearing loss at 2 kHZ than at higher and lower frequencies [13]. The location of the perforation does not matter. Round window phase protection does not effectively exist when considering the effects of perforations because the wavelengths of relevant auditory stimuli are too long for there to be much difference in pressure between OW and RW regardless of the site of the perforation.

The TM pressure difference can be restored with any kind of baffle that plugs the hole in the TM. In theory, if we could use native TM for tympanoplasty, perhaps it would restore normal hearing. However, in reality, the material we choose for repair doesn't just create a baffle, it also loads the TM and changes the function of the rest of the TM. Our own work suggests that higher frequencies are more affected by massive and stiff reconstructions, such as cartilage, than the low frequencies. Clinical studies, however, seem to show similar hearing results with cartilage and fascia reconstructions [17], but there are many confounding factors in clinical outcomes, making it difficult to analyse this one variable.

Atelectasis and Fluid in the Middle Ear

The normal middle ear has enough compliant air in the middle ear cleft (mean of 6 ml, with about 2 ml in the middle ear space [18]) to limit its effect on the impedance of the middle ear. The amount of air can be substantially reduced by mastoid obliteration, etc., with little effect on hearing. Models suggest that this volume has to fall by 90% or so to have an effect on hearing [19, 20]. The effect of fluid can affect hearing in two ways: first, by decreasing the volume of middle ear air, and thus increasing stiffness, which causes low frequency hearing loss; second, by mass loading, the TM as fluid volume increases, causing high frequency hearing loss [19].

Middle Ear Ossicular Reconstruction

It is difficult to talk about middle ear reconstruction without specifying exactly where one end of the connector is compared to the other end in the middle ear, and one of the confusing aspects of middle ear reconstruction is that its classification is varied, inconsistent, and imprecise. The literature is full of various meanings from terms such as Type

III ossiculoplasty, Partial Ossicular Replacement Prosthesis (PORP) and Total Ossicular Replacement Prosthesis (TORP), which don't specify where the connection is laterally. Essentially, middle ear reconstruction can also be classified along a scheme similar to the distinction between ossicular coupling and acoustic coupling described above. The main distinguishing feature is whether the attempt is to increase pressure at the OW or just provide access to the OW and protect the RW (i.e., pressure reduction RW).

Based on this, Table 4.1 is a schema for classifying ossicular reconstruction.

Vector of Reconstruction

At any joint, there can be forces causing translation or rotation (Fig. 4.9).

Efficient transduction through the middle ear primarily requires piston-like translations of the stapes footplate. If the joint between a prosthesis and remaining ear structures

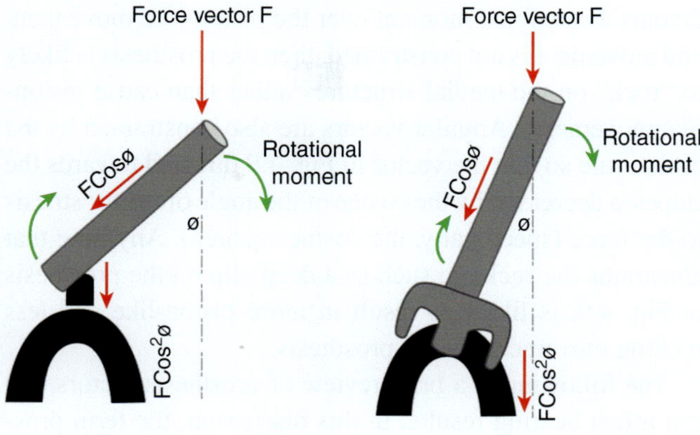

Fig. 4.9 Two situations are represented. On the left, there is marked angulation of the prosthesis on the stapes head, resulting in more rotational moment, and less of a piston-like force vector transmitted by the prosthesis. This causes rocking and rotation of the prosthesis, rather than driving the stapes into the vestibule. The force in the direction of the stapes footplate is determined by the cosine of the angle to the force vector. On the right, a more in-line reconstruction is represented, with much larger piston-like force transmission, and less rotational movements. Also, the rotational movement is constrained by the cup which grasps the head of the stapes

Table 4.1 Classification of middle ear hearing reconstruction techniques

A. Pressure Gain Reconstruction to OW (PGROW): Area Ratio Pressure Gain Reconstructed		
This reconstruction type tries to regain ossicular coupling. It requires an intact and vibrating TM, ventilated middle ear, and good coupling from the TM to medial structures connected to the inner ear.		
In general, the lateral and medial and mid prosthesis interface/stabilizers should be specified, e.g., medial +/− footplate shoe, lateral +/− cartilage overlay, mid-shaft +/− cartilage, or other stabilizers. The most commonly used are in bold face.		
(I) Direct connection TM to residual ossicles		
a) Direct connection incus onto TM		(D-IOT- Wullstein type 2)
b) Direct connection stapes head onto TM		**(D-SHOT-Wullstein type 3)**
(II) Connectors between TM and residual ossicles		
Connecting	*Acronym*	*Current terminology or examples*
Stapes Head onto TM	**SHOT**	**PORP**
Stapes Head onto Malleus	**SHOM**	**PORP**
Stapes Head onto Incus	SHOI	E.g. Cement, Applebaum
Stapes Head onto Both	SHOTM	PORP
TM and Malleus		
Stapes Head to Artificial or Relocated Malleus	SHOAM	PORP to relocated malleus
Stapes Footplate onto TM	**FOT**	**TORP**
Stapes Footplate onto Malleus	**FOM**	**TORP**
Stapes Footplate onto Incus	FOI	E.g. stapes piston on mobile footplate
Stapes Footplate onto Both TM and Malleus	FOTM	
Stapes Footplate onto relocated or artificial malleus	FOAM	E.g. TORP to relocated malleus
Vestibule to TM	VOT	TORP with stapedotomy
Vestibule to Malleus	VOM	Malleostapediopexy
Vestibule to Incus	**VOI**	**Standard stapedotomy**
Vestibule to Both TM and Malleus	VOB	
Vestibule to Artificial or Relocated Malleus	VOAM	Rarely used
Incus to TM	IOM	Rarely used
Incus to Malleus	IOT	E.g. cementing IM joint, rarely used
B. Planned Drop Round Window Pressure (PDRoWP)		
This is similar to acoustic coupling. It requires unimpeded access without scarring to the OW and a ventilated RW niche, so that the RW membrane can vibrate.		
PDRoWP-FP: Stapes footplate access (Wullstein type 4)		
PDRoWP -V: Inner ear access with removal of stapes footplate (Wullstein type 5b)		
PDRoWP -HC: Inner ear access with lateral canal fenestration (Wullstein type 5a)		

favours a rotational moment over the piston-like movement, and movement is not constrained, then the prosthesis is likely to "rock" on the medial structures rather than cause piston-like movements. Angular vectors are also constrained by the cosine rule so that the vector in Fig. 4.9 directed towards the stapes is decreased by the cosine of the angle of the prosthesis to the force (specifically, the cosine squared). Anything that constrains the rocking, such as a deep clip on the prosthesis in Fig. 4.9, is likely to result in more piston-like and less rocking movements of the prosthesis.

The following is a brief review of prosthesis factors that can affect hearing results. In this discussion, the term prosthesis also includes biologic materials such as cartilage and bone, as well as allografts.

Rigidity As mentioned earlier, compliances can attenuate transmission of high frequencies. Almost all prostheses are rigid enough to transmit the vibration forces applied to them accurately without dissipating them in flexion or compression within the material, which is more of a concern with prostheses such as cartilage that might soften with time. As mentioned earlier, when trying to drive a load through a spring, compliances tend to absorb higher frequencies, so that we might expect a reduction in the high frequency function with a very soft prosthesis. We previously demonstrated that placing a very soft material between the prosthesis and the TM could have a similar slight reduction in high frequency responses [21]. However, even soft materials are likely to transmit low frequencies relatively well, which might account for the anecdotal reports of "cholesteatoma" conduction in which pathology bridges the gap between the stapes head and the TM.

Mass The middle ear is not clearly mass dominated in any part of the normal auditory range. However, masses that are in this range and are used for reconstruction can have a small effect on frequencies above 4 kHz, as we [22] and others [23] have shown. This means that mass is not a large factor in prosthesis design, or in using sculpted bone, etc., but larger prostheses designs are likely to contact other structures in the middle ear and experience damping. With time, they may actually adhere to the structures they contact.

Another factor to consider with larger masses is that they may be more easily dislodged by the inertial forces caused by head trauma or high accelerations.

Tension Tension has a large effect on low frequency transmission in the middle ear, as we [24, 25] and others [26] have consistently shown. Tension increases stiffness of the tympanic membrane and the annular ligament and decreases the low frequency response of the middle ear. As mentioned earlier (Fig. 4.3), the middle ear is almost completely stiffness dominated in the low frequencies, and it is not surprising that tension has a major effect in this frequency range. When reading the literature, care has to be taken when considering comparisons between prostheses of different shapes, as many differences are dominated by the effect the shape has on tension when placed in the ear, rather than the prosthesis itself. In practice, the least amount of tension can lead to the prosthesis being unstable, and some tension is needed to hold the prosthesis firmly in place.

Prosthesis Head Size We have shown [27] that prosthesis head size had little effects on function of a PORP type prosthesis, within the range tested. Too big a head size will increase tension in the TM if it has to be "wedged," which can affect the low frequency response. Too small of a head size might only sample one area of the TM that has decreased motion when the TM undergoes multimodal vibration at high frequencies (Fig. 4.4). Therefore, it would be useful to have a head size large enough to average over many vibration modes (much as the malleus does normally). Essentially, a head size over 3–4 mm accomplishes this task. Much larger sizes can be used to stabilize the TM, but also may be difficult to place.

Stapes Head Versus Footplate Connection A recurring debate occurs around whether it is best to reconstruct to the stapes head or to the footplate, with at least some of the clinical literature favouring the stapes head [3]. This perception is likely confounded by the more advanced pathology that is often associated with loss of the stapes suprastructure. However, middle ear experiments, including those done by our group, do not seem to show any mechanical advantage between a reconstruction from the TM to the footplate (FOT in Table 4.1), versus the TM to the stapes head (SHOT in Table 4.1) [28]. Experiments were carefully designed to keep the FOT and SHOT in the same vertical vector. Clinically, reconstructions to the footplate may have different angulations than those to the stapes head, and rotational vectors (Fig. 4.9) are easier to constrain on the stapes head than on the footplate, by putting deep clips or drilling an acetabulum into the prosthesis, which may account for the variability in clinically reported outcome measures between SHOT and FOT reconstructions.

When reconstructing to the malleus rather than to the TM (FOM and SHOM in Table 4.1), some investigators [29]) have actually found worse results in reconstructing to the stapes head (SHOM) than to the footplate (FOM), but the results of these reconstructions are confounded by the large differences in angulation between these two types of reconstruction when connecting to the malleus, unlike in FOT and SHOT reconstructions. Differences may well be dominated by this angulation, which varies from ear to ear.

Reconstruction to the TM Versus to the Malleus Again, there is substantial clinical debate around this issue. While there may be a role for the malleus as a pressure gain device [7] through the catenary lever principle, its role in the human ear is not clear. Certainly, it is possible that better results are seen clinically in reconstructions to the malleus (FOM or SHOM) than to the TM (FOT OR SHOT) because the malleus acts as a stabilizer in the long term, rather than any mechanical advantage. We compared reconstructions from the stapes head to the TM and to the malleus (SHOM and SHOT) and found a slight advantage to the SHOM below 2 kHz [24], although it is quite possible that this was confounded by the changes in angulation and tension that reconstruction to the malleus and tympanic membrane incur. Others have tried to reconstruct with cement [30] from the footplate to the malleus or TM to remove tension effects and have found no difference in transfer function of the middle ear from these two types of reconstruction.

Placement on the Footplate The optimal location of the prosthesis on the footplate has been sparsely studied. Vlaming and Feenstra [31] found no difference between anterior and central footplate sites, whereas another study [32] showed that the footplate centre was the best site, with the anterior not quite as good and posterior footplate least effective. In general, the centre is likely to cause the least amount of rocking movements of the footplate, which are less effective at generating inner ear fluid pressure.

Stapedotomy

Stapedotomy differs from other middle ear reconstructions, in that, apart from the fixed stapes footplate, the anatomy and physiology of the middle ear are normal. Theoretically, this should mean that normal impedance matching and hearing can be achieved. As might be expected, stiffening of the annular ligament initially causes a conductive hearing loss in the low frequencies where the annular ligament stiffness has the most effect, which then progresses into the higher frequencies as the fixation progresses, a common and well-recognized clinical progression.

It can be confusing thinking only in terms of pressure gain when considering the mechanics of stapedotomy reconstruction. At first consideration, having a very small point only 0.4–0.6 mm in diameter should increase the pressure gain by the area ratio principle even more than in the normal ear. However, hearing is ultimately related to the volume velocity of fluid that the stapes footplate is able to produce. Having a large increase in pressure distributed over a small area actually decreases the total volume velocity of inner ear fluids. There is an optimal area of the footplate for maximizing impedance matching to produce the most volume velocity, and it is likely larger than 0.4 mm. Lumped parameter simple mathematical models [20] seem to suggest that the normal footplate is about the ideal size and that a 0.4 mm piston will perform worse by about 5 dB than a 0.6 mm piston, and 10 dB worse than a 0.8 mm piston in the low frequencies. We have shown similar results empirically in a temporal bone model [33], finding that between 500 and 4000 Hz performance was better by 2–3 dB when using a 0.6-mm-diameter piston compared with a 0.4-mm-diameter piston, and increased again by 2–4 dB when using a 0.8 mm piston.

Clinically, however, a systematic review [34] did not find any compelling difference in clinical results between studies using different sized pistons. Again, factors such as the size of the fenestra, the effective piston diameter caused by scar moving with the piston, and test-retest variations in audiometry will add variability to the clinical results.

Conclusions

While this chapter has focused on the principles of mechanical transfer of energy through the middle ear, it is important to remember that multiple, hearing-relevant parameters are being manipulated by the surgeon or by the disease process. Hence, individual effects that might each result in a 5 dB drop in hearing level can interact non-linearly to produce a larger hearing loss than the sum of their individual contributions.

It is also important for surgeons to appreciate that many surgical principles are a compromise between hearing efficacy and long-term stability of the reconstruction. For instance, large pieces of cartilage may be used to reconstruct the TM, which have less than ideal vibration characteristics, in order to prevent recurrent retraction pockets or cholesteatoma. Similarly, a prosthesis may be stabilized by soft tissue that clearly causes some damping but improves the long-term stability of the reconstruction.

Surgeons must remember that, as soon as they finish operating, the body physiology and pathophysiology takes over. Consequently, reconstructions should be planned for the eventual state of the middle ear, not the state at the time of surgery. For instance, if middle ear ventilation is extremely unlikely, then a FOM or FOT columella from the stapes footplate is unlikely to work, and other hearing options might be considered.

References

1. Shaw EA. Transformation of sound pressure level from the free field to the eardrum in the horizontal plane. J Acoust Soc Am. 1974;56(6):1848–61.
2. Shaw EA, Teranishi R. Sound pressure generated in an external-ear replica and real human ears by a nearby point source. J Acoust Soc Am. 1968;44(1):240–9.

3. Merchant SN, et al. Toynbee Memorial Lecture 1997. Middle ear mechanics in normal, diseased and reconstructed ears. J Laryngol Otol. 1998;112(8):715–31.
4. Chien W, et al. Isolated fracture of the manubrium of the malleus. J Laryngol Otol. 2008;122(9):898–904.
5. Voss SE, et al. Acoustic responses of the human middle ear. Hear Res. 2000;150(1–2):43–69.
6. Ichirō Kirikae, The structure and function of the middle ear. 1960, Tokyo: University of Tokyo Press.
7. von Helmholtz H. The mechanism of the ossicles of the ear and membrana tympani. Pfluger Archiv fur Physiologie. 1868:1.
8. Wever E, Lawrence M. Physiological acoustics. Princeton: Princeton University Press; 1954.
9. Kurokawa H, Goode R. Sound pressure gain produced by the human middle ear. Am J Otol. 1995;113:349–55.
10. Aibara R, et al. Human middle-ear sound transfer function and cochlear input impedance. Hear Res. 2001;152(1–2):100–9.
11. Peake WT, Rosowski JJ, Lynch TJ 3rd. Middle-ear transmission: acoustic versus ossicular coupling in cat and human. Hear Res. 1992;57(2):245–68.
12. Wullstein HL. The surgical restoration of hearing in chronic otitis media and its audiological basis. Ann Otol Rhinol Laryngol. 1958;67(4):952–63.
13. Lerut B, et al. Functional correlations of tympanic membrane perforation size. Otol Neurotol. 2012;33(3):379–86.
14. Voss SE, et al. Middle-ear function with tympanic-membrane perforations. II. A simple model. J Acoust Soc Am. 2001;110(3 Pt 1):1445–52.
15. Voss SE, et al. Middle-ear function with tympanic-membrane perforations. I. Measurements and mechanisms. J Acoust Soc Am. 2001;110(3 Pt 1):1432–44.
16. Voss SE, et al. How do tympanic-membrane perforations affect human middle-ear sound transmission? Acta Otolaryngol. 2001;121(2):169–73.
17. Jalali MM, et al. Comparison of cartilage with temporalis fascia tympanoplasty: a meta-analysis of comparative studies. Laryngoscope, 2016.
18. Molvær O, Vallersnes F, Kringlebotn M. The size of the middle ear and the mastoid air cells. Acta Otolaryngologica. 1978;85:24–32.
19. Ravicz M, Rosowski J, Merchant S. Mechanisms of hearing loss resulting from middle-ear fluid. Hear Res. 2004;195:105–30.
20. Rosowski JJ, Merchant SN. Mechanical and acoustic analysis of middle ear reconstruction. Am J Otol. 1995;16(4):486–97.
21. Morris DP, Bance M, Van Wijhe RG. How do cartilage and other material overlay over a prosthesis affect its vibration transmission properties in ossiculoplasty? Otolaryngol Head Neck Surg. 2004;131(4):423–8.
22. Bance M, Morris DP, Van Wijhe R. Effects of ossicular prosthesis mass and section of the stapes tendon on middle ear transmission. J Otolaryngol. 2007;36(2):113–9.
23. Nishihara S, Aritomo H, Goode RL. Effect of changes in mass on middle ear function. Otolaryngol Head Neck Surg. 1993;109(5):899–910.
24. Bance M, et al. Comparison of the mechanical performance of ossiculoplasty using a prosthetic malleus-to-stapes head with a tympanic membrane-to-stapes head assembly in a human cadaveric middle ear model. Otol Neurotol. 2004;25(6):903–9.
25. Morris DP, et al. Optimum tension for partial ossicular replacement prosthesis reconstruction in the human middle ear. Laryngoscope. 2004;114(2):305–8.
26. Yamada H, Goode RL. A self-adjusting ossicular prosthesis containing polyurethane sponge. Otol Neurotol. 2010;31(9):1404–8.
27. Bance M, et al. How does prosthesis head size affect vibration transmission in ossiculoplasty? Otolaryngol Head Neck Surg. 2007;137(1):70–3.
28. Alian WA, et al. Prosthetic reconstruction from the tympanic membrane to the stapes head or to the stapes footplate? A laser Doppler study. J Otolaryngol Head Neck Surg. 2012;41(2):84–93.
29. Murugasu E, Puria S, Roberson JB Jr. Malleus-to-footplate versus malleus-to-stapes-head ossicular reconstruction prostheses: temporal bone pressure gain measurements and clinical audiological data. Otol Neurotol. 2005;26(4):572–82.
30. Shimizu Y, Goode RL. Effect of absence of malleus on ossiculoplasty in human temporal bones. Otolaryngol Head Neck Surg. 2008;139(2):301–6.
31. Vlaming MS, Feenstra L. Studies on the mechanics of the reconstructed human middle ear. Clin Otolaryngol Allied Sci. 1986;11(6):411–22.
32. Asai M, Huber AM, Goode RL. Analysis of the best site on the stapes footplate for ossicular chain reconstruction. Acta Otolaryngol. 1999;119(3):356–61.
33. Wegner I, et al. The effect of piston diameter in stapedotomy for Otosclerosis: a temporal bone model. Otol Neurotol. 2016;37(10):1497–502.
34. Wegner I, et al. A systematic review of the effect of piston diameter in stapes surgery for otosclerosis on hearing results. Laryngoscope. 2016;126(1):182–90.

Auditory Physiology: Inner Ear

5

Gregory J. Basura

Cochlear Anatomy

Location and Labyrinth

The mammalian inner ear containing the cochlea consists of contiguous spaces within the temporal bone that contains the otic capsule or bony labyrinth. The bone that comprises the otic capsule is touted as some of the hardest in the human body. The inner ear serves important functions involving hearing and balance. Within the bony labyrinth lies a series of interconnected soft tissue ducts and spaces known as the membranous labyrinth (Fig. 5.1). The term 'canal' is often reserved to describe structures within the bony labyrinth, while a 'duct' typically denotes membranous channels. The membranous labyrinth is divided into inferior (cochlear duct and saccule of the vestibule) and superior (utricle of the vestibule and three semicircular [horizontal, superior/anterior and posterior] canals with respective ampullae) divisions [1]. The organ of Corti (sensory organ of hearing) is housed within the cochlear duct [2–4].

Following conversion of extraneous sound energy into frank vibrations of the middle ear lateral ossicular chain (malleus and incus), the entry point of converted sound energy into vibrational stimulation of the inner ear occurs at the first inner ear window: the stapes-oval window interface overlying the inner ear vestibule. The height of the cochlea is approximately 5 mm with an overall length of 34 mm that spans 2 and ¾ turns [1]. At the basal end of the cochlea, adjacent and within 2 mm of the oval window, is the second inner ear window, the round window niche, and round window membrane that opens to the middle ear. The two windows of the cochlea allow for effective propagation of a traveling wave of the inner ear fluids that ultimately stimulates hair cell activity across the length of the cochlea from the wider base (portion closest to the oval window) to the more narrowed apex (portion furthest from the oval window; Fig. 5.2).

The bony cochlea is coiled around a central axis point, the modiolus, that consists of thinned bone that allows for passage of auditory nerve fibers that coalesce from hair cell synapses into the auditory nerve that traverses the internal auditory meatus and canal to the brainstem [5, 6]. The modiolus typically points in an antero-lateral and inferior direction in an orientation not too dissimilar from the external auditory canal [1]. Extending from the modiolus, the central osseous spiral lamina partitions the cochlea into an upper *scala vestibuli* and lower *scala tympani*. The two bony laminae and the osseous spiral lamina provide an attachment for a vital component of the membranous labyrinth known as the basilar membrane. The organ of Corti sits on top of the basilar membrane, a structure that also helps constitute the membranous cochlear duct (third cochlear compartment known as the *scala media*) and provides the lower border of the membranous labyrinth (Fig. 5.1). Together, the organ of Corti and the associated basilar membrane are collectively referred to as the cochlear partition. A second soft tissue boundary (Reissner's membrane) extends across the width of the cochlear canal to define the vestibular border of the cochlear duct. The *scala media*, retains the shape of the cochlea and contains many of the neural elements of hearing [7]. Figure 5.1 shows a cross section of the membranous labyrinth that is bounded by Reissner's membrane superiorly and the basilar membrane inferiorly. It is bordered on the lateral side by the outer cochlear wall and the spiral ligament. The lateral wall of the membranous labyrinth is lined by the stria vascularis a vascularized structure that helps to maintain the metabolic environment within the endolymphatic fluid or endolymph within the *scala media* [8]. The *scala media* separates the *scala tympani* and *scala vestibuli* for most of the length of the cochlea as the compartments coil and converge at the narrowed apex known as the helicotrema [8].

G. J. Basura (✉)
Department of Otolaryngology—Head and Neck Surgery; Division of Otology—Neurotology/Skull Base Surgery, University of Pittsburgh Medical Center/University of Pittsburgh, Pittsburgh, PA, USA
e-mail: basuragj@upmc.edu

A. D. Sweeney et al. (eds.), *Haynes-Glasscock-Shambaugh Surgery of the Ear*, https://doi.org/10.1007/978-3-032-18264-7_5

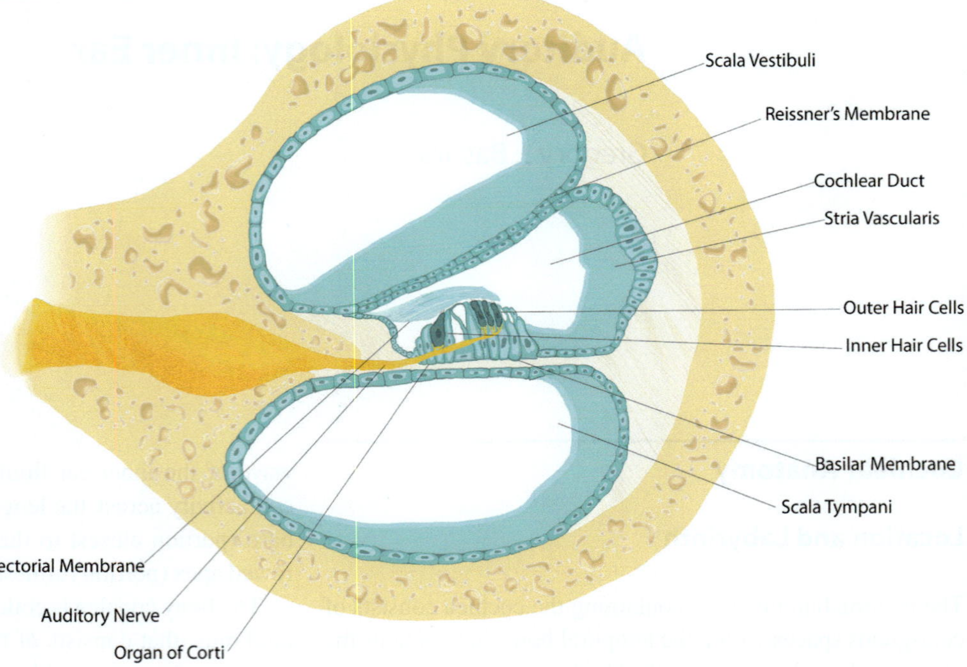

Fig. 5.1 Cross-section of the cochlea demonstrating the relationships of the membranous compartments. Note the Organ of Corti seated on the basilar membrane within the scala media

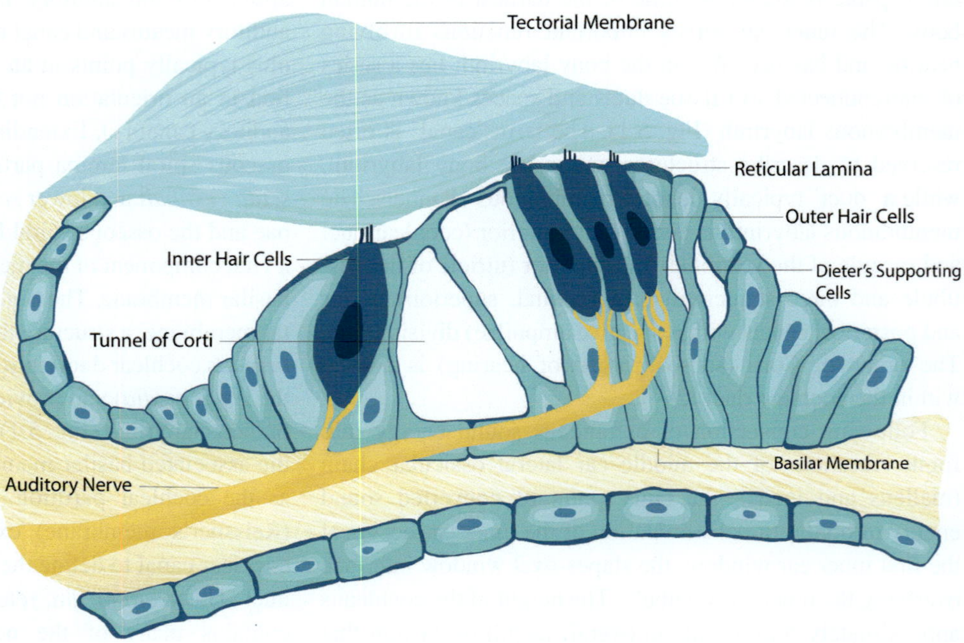

Fig. 5.2 High magnification of the Organ of Corti. Note the relationship of the Inner Hair cells to the Outer Hair cells

Anatomically, the spiral lamina and basilar membrane share an inverse relationship with the spiral lamina being wider at the base and narrowed at the apex, while the basilar membrane is typically more narrowed at the base and wider at the apex [8–10]. This anatomic disparity is touted to contribute to the frequency specificity of basilar membrane motion. Basilar membrane stiffness and thickness decreases from base to apex [11], while in a radial dimension, the basilar membrane is much stiffer than in the longitudinal direction [12].

When sound traverses the external ear canal and middle ear structures, it results in stapes vibrations at the oval window and fenestra vestibuli, which are then transmitted to the basilar membrane via the endolymphatic and perilymphatic fluids being displaced and propagated from cochlear base to apex across the basilar membrane. The inner ear fluid wave travels across the *scala vestibuli* around the helicotrema and across the *scala tympani* to the round window. A pressure gradient is created due to the fluid pressure in *scala vestibuli* being greater than that in the *scala tympani*, which causes the cochlear partition to vibrate. Some perilymph fluid is eventually shunted between the basal turn of the *scala tympani* to the *scala media* of the jugular fossa and cerebrospinal fluid of the subarachnoid space via the cochlear aqueduct [13].

Organ of Corti and Inner Ear Fluids

The organ of Corti is an epithelial-based structure that runs the length of the basilar membrane within the *scala media* [14]. Located medially and seated on top of the osseous spiral lamina is the periosteal spiral limbus that attaches to Reissner's membrane and helps to form the tectorial membrane; an acellular collagen-based gelatinous structure that lies over the inner (IHC) and outer hair cells (OHCs) [15]. Two regions above the organ of Corti constitute the tympanic surface of the tectorial membrane (Fig. 5.2). Along the radial border of the tectorial membrane is Hardesty's membrane that attaches directly to stereocilia of the OHCs [16–18], while the stereocilia of the IHCs are mostly untethered but may be contacted by a thickened region known as Hensen's stripe [17, 18]. Basilar membrane displacement following mechanical forces in relation to the tectorial membrane results in mechano-transduction or shearing force between the stereocilia of the hair cells and the tectorial membrane. This process leads to the generation of an electrical signal following resultant stereocilia deflection on the hair cells [19]. The cochlea is quite sensitive since even the slightest displacement of the hair cells will provoke a neural response [20, 21]. The variability in function between IHC and OHCs reflects the nature and variety of the nerve fibers innervating each cell type [22]. As a result, IHCs are involved primarily with sensory function [23], while the OHCs are traditionally involved with mechanical feedback [24, 25].

The pillars of Corti, forming the tunnel of Corti, lie between the rows of IHCs and OHCs (Fig. 5.2). On the lateral side are three rows of OHCs that are anchored inferiorly by supporting Deiter's cells that along with the superior aspects of OHCs form an interwoven matrix that supports the hair cells. This matrix, or reticular lamina, also forms a protective barrier from endolymph in the *scala media*; a fluid and electrolyte composition that is toxic to hair cells [7]. Within the organ of Corti, a row of flask-shaped IHCs extends along the axial border of the basilar membrane. Columnar OHCs occupy a more radial position and contribute to greater than 75% of the sensory cells within the cochlea [12]. The IHC and OHCs not only differ in position and morphology but functionally IHCs are directly correlated with basilar membrane vibration velocity, while OHCs are correlated with basilar membrane displacement potentials [16, 23].

The fluid configuration within the cochlea is critical to achieve an optimal basilar membrane traveling wave and resultant cellular depolarization leading to synaptic activity [26–28]. Between the osseous and membranous labyrinth resides perilymphatic fluid or perilymph; a fluid concentration low in potassium and high in sodium that is like cerebrospinal fluid and blood serum. This fluid is found within the *scala vestibuli* and *scala tympani*. Within the *scala media* lies endolymphatic fluid or endolymph; a fluid with high potassium and low sodium typical of concentrations found in the intra-cellular compartments. This concentration is maintained, in part, by the stria vascularis and the planum semilunatum (near cristae), dark vestibular cells and from the perilymph across the labyrinth membranes. The longitudinal flow of endolymph is estimated to be quite slow (0.004–0.007 mm/min) as it runs from the stria vascularis to the *scala media* to the ductus reuniens and saccule and eventually to the endolymphatic sac. The electrolyte composition of endolymph in the *scala media* that is maintained, in part, by the stria vascularis creates an endocochlear potential or an electrochemical gradient that is approximately +60 to +100 mV in relation to perilymph.

The basilar membrane is tonotopically organized and anatomically the stiffness of the membrane decreases from the base to the apex as the width also increases across the length of the cochlea. To achieve sound specific perception, the inner ear traveling wave of the basilar membrane vibrates optimally and with maximal amplitude at the frequency dependent location that is commensurate with the frequency of the presented sound [29, 30]. Cochlear hair cell stimulation following basilar membrane displacement to a traveling wave stimulates adjacent nerve fibers that are organized according to frequencies that they are most sensitive to (Fig. 5.3). This tonotopic organization reveals lower frequencies travel further to the apex (apical turn) of the cochlea and high frequencies are retained at the base (basal turn). The anatomic organization and tonotopic arrangement of the inner ear allows for the parsing of complex sounds into narrow frequency bands (Fig. 5.3). The resultant "characteristic" or "best" frequency is that frequency that a hair cell is most sensitive to at that location within the cochlea.

Hair Cell Function

There are approximately 3500 IHCs organized in a single row on the medial (modiolar) side on the tunnel of Corti and 12,000 OHCs arranged in three rows on the lateral (strial) side. The primary purpose of the IHC and OHCs is to transduce mechanical displacement of the basilar membrane into resultant electrochemical signals. As mentioned, the cribriform walls of the modiolus form a porous floor to allow for passage of small nerves from the ganglion for the spiral auditory nerve. The ganglion is enclosed in Rosenthal's canal. In contrast to IHCs that are attached to afferent nerve fibers, OHCs are primarily connected to efferent fibers [22, 23].

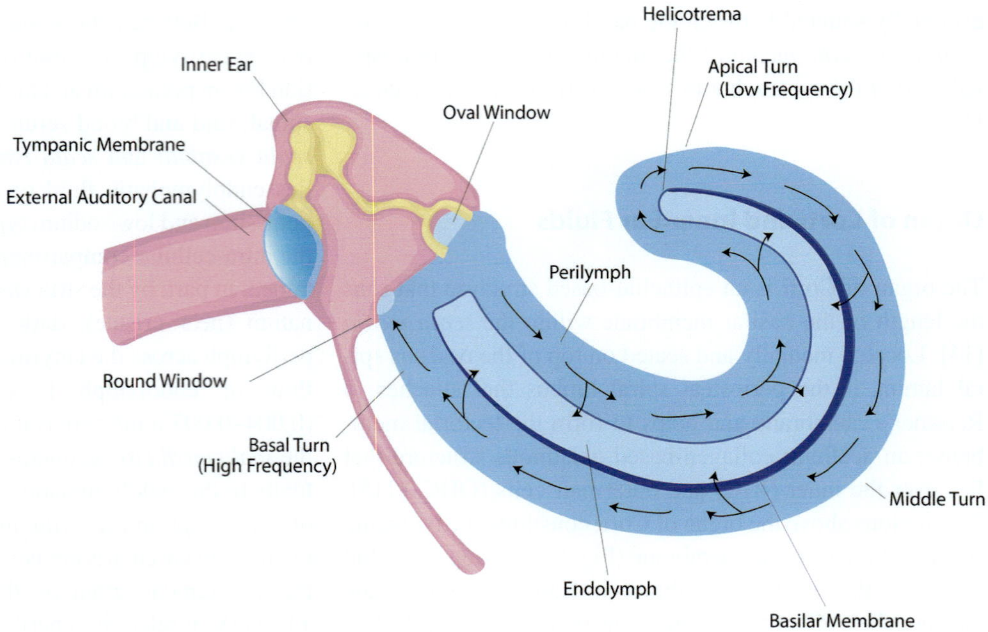

Fig. 5.3 Cartoon schematic of the unrolled cochlea showing the direction (arrows) of the inner ear traveling fluid wave following mechano-transduction of sound energy at the stapes-oval window interface. Note the tonotopic organization of the cochlear where high frequency sound is registered at the basal turn with low frequency registration at the apex

Myelinated cochlear nerve fibers extend radially from the spiral ganglion canal to the IHCs. Unmyelinated nerve fibers cross the lumen of the tunnel of Corti between the IHCs and OHCs [18].

Neural signals then propagate down the auditory nerve which exits the cranial cavity via the internal acoustic meatus to the central auditory pathways [31]. Figure 5.2 presents a schematic of the IHC and OHCs. The apical region of each hair cell includes a cuticular plate that in association with supporting cells forms the reticular lamina. Hair cells do not possess true stereocilia and rather have the equivalent of microvilli that contain an actin core [31]. The filaments rooted in the cuticular plate project through the reticular lamina and reside adjacent to kinocilium to deflect secondary to mechanical forces. Rows of stereocilia are found on hair cells with at least two on each individual IHC and three or more on OHCs with the longest stereocilia on the lateral (strial) side and the shortest on the medial (modiolar) side [8]. The longest projections are on OHCs that contact the tectorial membrane that leads to deflection with basilar membrane excursion. Connecting stereocilia to each other are filamentous cross-links and from the tips of the shortest stereocilia to the sides of the tallest by tip-links. This anatomic configuration assures that stereocilia stay connected and move as a single unit when the longer stereocilia are deflected.

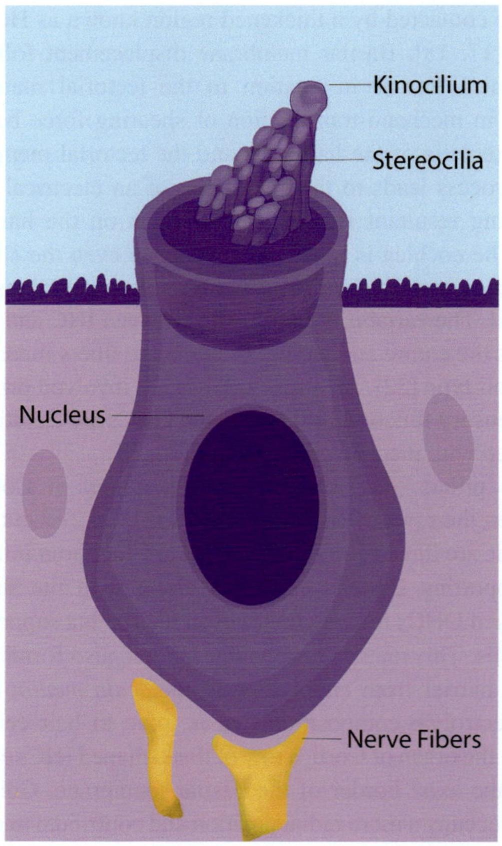

Fig. 5.4 Schematic showing a high magnification of an Inner Hair Cell. Note the flask shape and the large intra-cellular organelles to accommodate high metabolic demands. On the apical surface of the cell are stereocilia that with deflection toward (positive) the tallest kinocilium causes mechanically gated ion channels to open with a subsequent influx of potassium and calcium

The IHCs arranged in a single row are flask-shaped, being wider at the bottom and narrower at the top and retain only afferent synapses (Fig. 5.4). These cells are equipped for increased metabolic activity and as such have increased numbers of mitochondria and Golgi bodies [8]. While they are highly metabolic, IHCs are considered passive transducers within the auditory system [32]. Their stereocilia do not

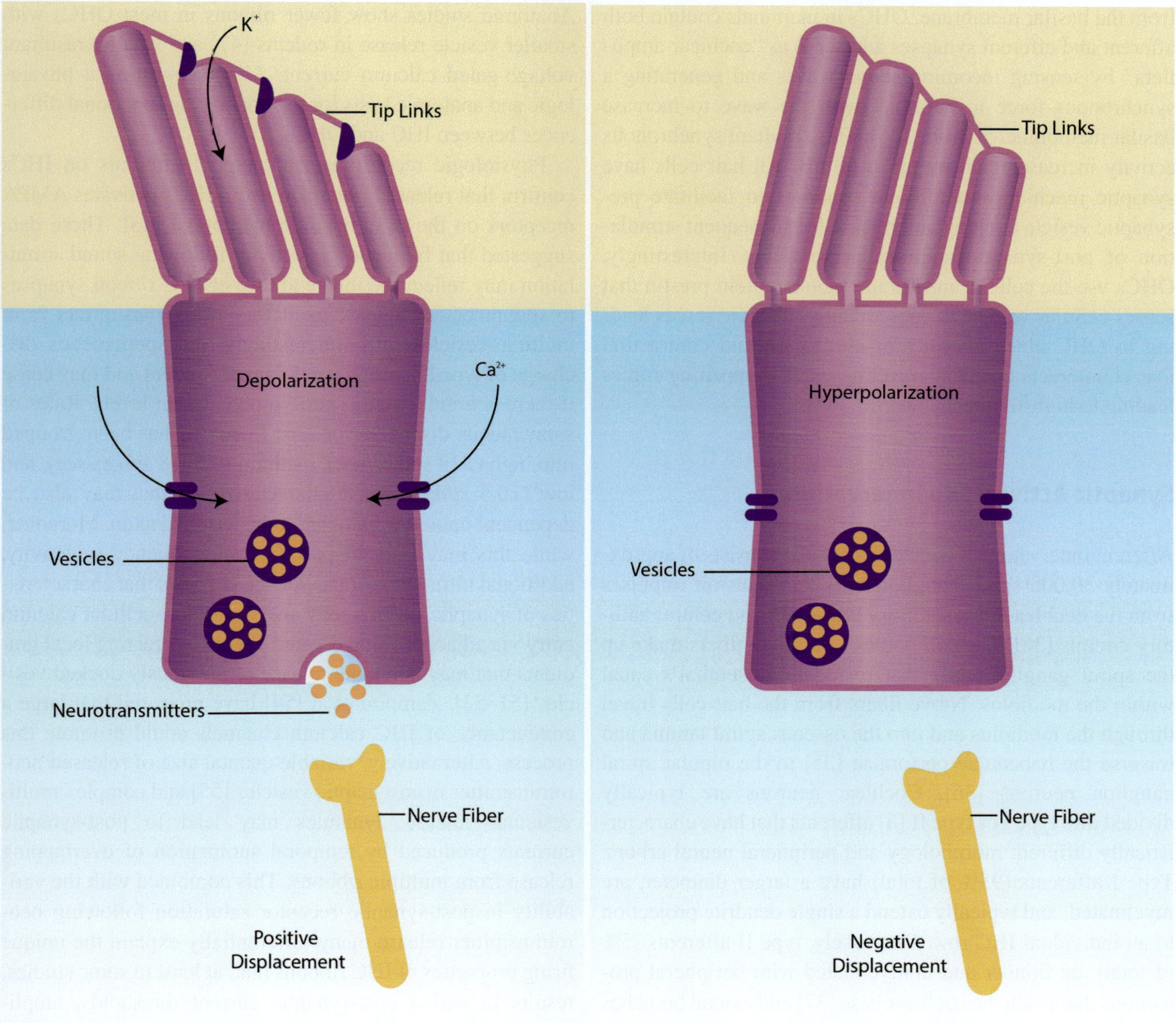

Fig. 5.5 Schematic showing the relationship of stereocilia to the kinocilium leading to cellular depolarization or hyperpolarization. Note that when the hair bundle is tipped toward the kinocilium potassium and subsequent voltage-gated calcium channels open resulting in cellular depolarization (positive deflection) and synaptic propagation. When tipped away (negative deflection), channels are closed leading to cellular hyperpolarization

attach or extend into the tectorial membrane, and they are deflected by fluid in between the reticular lamina and the tectorial membrane. Stereocilia, when deflected toward the tallest kinocilium (positive deflection) causes the tip links to stretch that leads to the opening of stretch-sensitive cationic channels. The large electrochemical gradient created by the cochlear potential allows for a sizeable influx of cationic current from potassium and calcium ions. The resultant and subsequent opening of voltage-gated calcium channels leads to cellular depolarization [32] and eventual synaptic propagation of electrical activity (Fig. 5.5). The resultant calcium currents that are mediated by the voltage-gated channels lead to excitatory neurotransmitter (glutamate) release and postsynaptic stimulation of the auditory nerve. Conversely, bending of stereocilia away from the kinocilium (negative deflection) results in relaxation of the tip links and continued closure of potassium and calcium channels and a resultant hair cell hyperpolarization. The process of cellular depolarization and hyperpolarization is a critical step leading to the conversion of mechanical sound stimuli following traveling wave propagation into a useable electrochemical signal.

Conversely, OHCs are cylindrical and are arranged in three rows and contain microfilaments and microtubules along the lengths of the cells [33, 34]. This anatomy, orientation, and resultant motile property results in significantly tuned, frequency-specific activity even when stimulated from the basilar membrane. OHCs in mammals contain both afferent and efferent synapses and serve as "cochlear amplifiers" by sensing incoming sound waves and generating a synchronous force in harmony with the wave to increase basilar membrane vibration [35]. This resultant synchronous activity increases gain by up to 60 dB. All hair cells have synaptic machinery at afferent synapses to facilitate pre-synaptic vesicle docking and release for subsequent stimulation of post-synaptic auditory nerve fibers. Interestingly, OHCs use the cellular membrane motor protein prestin that senses cellular voltage to subsequently generate forces leading to OHC electromotility or elongation and contraction that counteracts cochlear traveling wave dampening forces leading to high-frequency hearing [33].

Synaptic Activity and Innervation

Afferent innervation of cochlear hair cells consists of approximately 30,000 spiral ganglion cells that transmit impulses from the cochlea to the auditory brainstem and central auditory circuits [36]. The cell bodies of afferent fibers make up the spiral ganglion cells that reside in Rosenthal's canal within the modiolus. Nerve fibers from the hair cells travel through the modiolus and into the osseous spiral lamina and traverse the habenulae perforatae [35] to the bipolar spiral ganglion neurons [36]. Cochlear neurons are typically divided into type I or type II [8] afferents that have characteristically different morphology and peripheral neural arbors. Type I afferents (95% of total) have a larger diameter, are myelinated, and typically extend a single dendrite projection to an individual IHC row. Conversely, type II afferents (5% of total) are thinner and unmyelinated with peripheral projections that reach the cochlear base [37] and extend branches to multiple OHCs [38, 39].

Each IHC is innervated by approximately 20 type I afferent neurons that largely transmit acoustic information to central auditory circuits about signal/sound intensity, frequency and timing [40]. Frequency selectivity reflects isolated IHC innervation along the cochlear tonotopic axis. Specific patterns of neuro-transmitter release onto afferent dendrites [41, 42] are thought to be required to achieve effective frequency selectivity as evidenced by documented patterns of multiple-vesicle release from IHC ribbon synapses [43–45]. Elegant physiologic measurements of cellular capacitance taken from hair cells with postsynaptic afferent recordings have provided critical information about hair cell ribbon synapse physiology and neurotransmitter release from both IHC and OHCs. Currently, more basic science data exist for type I afferent to IHC synapses along the tonotopic axis [46] than for type II afferents. As a result, predictions about neurotransmitter release that corresponds to synaptic vesicle number per ribbon in mammals can be made [47, 48]. Anatomic studies show fewer ribbons in most OHCs with smaller vesicle release in rodents [47] and smaller resultant voltage-gated calcium currents [49]; suggesting a physiologic and anatomic basis for the underlying functional differences between IHC and OHCs.

Physiologic recordings from type I afferents on IHCs confirm that released glutamate from IHCs activates AMPA receptors on the post-synaptic membrane [43]. These data suggested that frequency selectivity following sound stimulation may reflect the innate ability of IHC ribbon synapses to spontaneously release excitatory neurotransmitters from multiple-vesicles [50]. Interestingly, the spontaneous discharge of type I neurons is calcium dependent and may cease if there is a reduction in perilymph calcium levels. Rates of spontaneous discharge for type I neurons has been grouped into high (>18 spikes/sec), medium (0.5–18 spikes/sec), and low (<0.5 spikes/sec); a characterization that may also be dependent upon the diameter of the terminal axon. Moreover, while this may only in part explain frequency selectivity, additional ultra-structural evidence suggests that characteristics of synaptic ribbons may also limit intra-cellular calcium entry via adjacent voltage-gated channels, creating local gradients that may stimulate release of previously docked vesicles [51–53]. Zampini et al [54] have proposed that large a conductance of IHC calcium channels could promote this process. Alternatively, variable quantal size of released neurotransmitter from synaptic vesicles [55] and complex multi-vesicular release dynamics may lead to post-synaptic currents produced by temporal summation of overlapping release from multiple ribbons. This combined with the variability in post-synaptic receptor saturation following neurotransmitter release many differentially explain the unique firing properties of IHC ribbons that, at least in some studies, results in varied post-synaptic current thresholds, amplitudes, and dynamic range [56, 57]. Regardless of the variation in explanations in underlying mechanism, many observations have agreed that the rate of synaptic vesicle fusion and ultimate neurotransmitter release from hair cell ribbons is strongly calcium-dependent. As a result, neurotransmitter release may increase or decrease based simply on calcium influx variability, yet it has been shown that the peak timing of neurotransmitter release remains constant at different release rates [58]. This finding supports the idea of phase-constancy following acoustic stimulation where the intensity of afferent firing is at best frequency [59].

The remaining 5% of fibers are considered type II and are structurally smaller and may be myelinated or unmyelinated [60]. These fibers synapse directly onto OHCs and a single fiber diverges to form branches that synapse with multiple other OHCs. Many investigators have described the pre-synaptic structures of OHCs [61–63] that retain from 25 synaptic ribbons per OHC [64] versus the often observed 20 or greater found on a typical IHC. Synaptic ribbons on OHCs are slightly taller and thinner with half as many fused synaptic vesicles as found on IHCs, yet direct comparison in the apical turn of juvenile rodent cochlea revealed no significant differences in synaptic ribbon size and only a 23-fold difference in the numbers of synaptic vesicles [63]. Interestingly, despite being fewer in number, the size of synaptic vesicles at OHCs ribbons are more heterogeneous [65]. As a result, the overall strength of neuro-transmission from each OHC is low, with an estimated single synaptic vesicle released once for every four maximal pre-synaptic stimuli [63]. Despite that finding, Weisz et al [66] demonstrated effective and rapid glutamate release from OHCs following pre-synaptic stimulation and when stimulated sequentially revealed that at least 10 OHCs were pre-synaptic to a given type II afferent for an overall release probability from each OHC onto type II afferents at 0.25 vesicles per action potential. When compared to the synaptic dynamics of IHCs where each action potential lead to the release of 40–50 synaptic vesicles at a single synaptic contact [43, 48] suggests that these synaptic dynamic differences may, in part, provide bases for the well-documented functional differences between IHC and OHCs.

Functional Differences Between IHC and OHCs

Differences between IHC and OHC function are rooted, in part, in the above-described type I and type II cochlear afferent configurations that are differentiated by innervation patterns, synaptic dynamics, and ultra-structural morphology. As a result, type I afferents aligned with IHCs encode primarily sound/signal content, while the function of type II afferents aligned with OHCs is not completely clear. Specific to OHCs are efferents that originate from the olivocochlear bundle (Rasmussen's bundle) to provide central inhibition of hair cell activity via descending inputs [67]. These inputs arise from the brainstem and synapse on OHCs. The complete purpose of these inputs is currently unclear, yet they are implicated in assisting in understanding speech in environments with high background noise. The finding of weaker synaptic dynamics as compared to IHCs does highlight diminished sound encoding by these cells as higher levels of neurotransmitter release are required to exceed the action potential threshold in type II afferents [68]. Interestingly, despite different functions and functional strength, Brown et al [69] has suggested that since type I and II afferents essentially project to similar regions of the brainstem cochlear nuclei that combined sound intensity and frequency might co-activate both afferents. The close (750 μm) proximity of synaptic zones between type I and type II afferents may lead to type II afferent activation to sound intensities significant enough to maximally displace basilar membranes. Despite differences in synaptic strength, dynamics and vesicle size, and release properties, both hair cell types express synaptotagmin IV and otoferlin two proteins touted to be involved in calcium-dependent cellular capacitance [47, 70]. However, functional differences between IHC and OHCs may reflect many structural and anatomic findings such as the vesicular glutamate transporter (VGlut3) that is essentially absent from OHCs, yet is necessary for neural transmission in IHCs [71]. Moreover, a substantial disparity in voltage-gated calcium channels associated with OHC ribbons in the rodent cochlea has been reported as compared to IHCs [72]. Taken together, these data suggest that the combination of various innervation patterns, synaptic dynamics, and ultra-structural morphology help differentiate IHCs and OHCs.

Conclusions

The anatomic, cellular, and physiologic properties of the inner ear all play a critical role in the effective transduction of mechanical sound energy into an electrochemical signal that is processed by the central auditory pathways. Effective conversion and propagation of sound energy requires mechanical displacement of the inner ear fluids and the basilar membrane that culminates in the release of excitatory neurotransmission at hair cell synapses and the auditory nerve. Cochlear hair cell stimulation following basilar membrane displacement to a traveling wave stimulates adjacent nerve fibers that are organized according to frequencies that they are most sensitive to. Tonotopic arrangement of the inner ear allows for the parsing of complex sounds into narrow frequency bands for optimal sound processing. Current and future studies are designed to better understand the molecular aspects of normal sound processing as it relates to pathologic circumstances that include sudden, progressive and genetic hearing loss, and how to approach regain of function.

Acknowledgments The author would like to thank Miss Taylor Forrest for drafting and creating all of the figures/illustrations for this chapter.

References

1. Toth M, Alpar A, Boden G, et al. Surgical anatomy of the cochlea for cochlear implantation. Ann Anat. 2006;188:363–70.
2. Curthoys IS, Markham CH, Curthoys EJ. Semicircular duct and ampulla dimensions in cat, Guinea pig and man. J Morphol. 1977;151:17–34.
3. Fleischer G. Hearing in extinct cetaceans as determined by cochlear structure. J Paleontol. 1976;50:133–52.
4. Geisler JH, Luo Z-X. The petrosal and inner ear of Herpetocetus sp. (Mammalia: Cetacea) and their implications for the phylogeny and hearing of archaic mysticetes. J Paleontol. 1996;70:1045–66.
5. Kermack KA, Mussett F. The ear in mammal-like reptiles and early mammals. Acta Palaeontol Pol. 1983;28:147–58.

6. Jorgenson JM, Locket NA. The inner ear of the echidna Tachyglossius aculeatus: the vestibular sensory organs. Proc Biol Sci. 1995;260:183–9.
7. Lim DJ. Cochlear anatomy related to cochlear micromechanics: a review. J Acoust Soc Am. 1980;67:1686–95.
8. Harada Y, Tagashira N, Takunida M, et al. Three-dimensional ultrastructure of cochlea: a review. Adv Otorhinolaryngol. 1990;45:49–68.
9. Wever EG, McCormick JG, Palin J, et al. Cochlea of the dolphin, Tursiops truncatus: the basilar membrane. Proc Natl Acad Sci U S A. 1971;68:2708–11.
10. Webster DB, Webster M. Morphological adaptations of the ear in the rodent family Heteromyidae. Am Zool. 1980;20:247–54.
11. Naidu RC, Mountain DC. Basilar membrane tension calculations for the gerbil cochlea. J Acoust Soc Am. 2007;121:994–1002.
12. Echteler SM, Fay RR, Popper AN. Structure of the mammalian cochlea. In: Fay RR, Popper AN, editors. Comparative hearing: mammals. New York: Springer-Verlag; 1994. p. 134–71.
13. Su WY, Marion MS, Hinojosa R, et al. Anatomical measurements of the cochlear aqueduct, round window membrane, round window niche, and facial recess. Laryngoscope. 1982;92:483–6.
14. Kimura RS. The ultrastructure of the organ of Corti. Int Rev Cytol. 1975;42:173–222.
15. Lim DJ. Functional structure of the organ of Corti: a review. Hear Res. 1986;22:117–46.
16. Dallos P, Billone MC, Durrant JD, et al. Cochlear inner and outer hair cells: functional differences. Science. 1972;177:356–8.
17. Hoshino T. Contact between the tectorial membrane and the cochlear sensory hairs in the human and the monkey. Arch Otorhinolaryngol. 1977;217:53–60.
18. Raphael Y, Altschuler RA. Structure and innervation of the cochlea. Brain Res Bull. 2003;60:397–422.
19. Hudspeth AJ. How the ear's works work. Nature. 1989;341:397–404.
20. Rhode WS, Geisler CD. Model of the displacement between opposing points on the tectorial membrane and reticular lamina. J Acoust Soc Am. 1967;42:185–90.
21. Corey DP, Hudspeth AJ. Kinetics of the receptor current in bullfrog saccular hair cells. J Neurosci. 1983;3:962–76.
22. Eybalin M. Neurotransmitters and neuromodulators of the mammalian cochlea. Phys Rev. 1993;73:309–73.
23. Fettiplace R, Hackney CM. The sensory and motor roles of auditory hair cells. Nat Rev Neurosci. 2006;7:19–29.
24. Dallos P. The active cochlea. J Neurosci. 1992;12:4575–85.
25. Fettiplace R. Active hair bundle movements in auditory hair cells. J Physiol. 2006;576:29–36.
26. Guinan JJ, Salt A, Cheatham MA. Progress in cochlear physiology after Bekesy. Hear Res. 2012;293:12–20.
27. Anniko M, Wroblewski R. Ionic environment of cochlear hair cells. Hear Res. 1986;22:279–93.
28. Waltner JG, Raymond S. On the chemical composition of the human perilymph and endolymph. Laryngoscope. 1950;60:912–8.
29. Schratzenstaller B, Janssen T, Alexiou C, et al. Confirmation of G. von Bekesy's theory of paradoxical wave propagation along the cochlear partition by means of bone-conducted auditory brainstem responses. ORL J Otorhinolaryngol Relat Spec. 2000;62:1–8.
30. Zhang Y, Kim CK, Lee KJB, et al. Resultant pressure distribution pattern along the basilar membrane in the spiral shaped cochlea. J Biol Phys. 2007;33:195–211.
31. Roberts WM, Howard J, Hudspeth AJ. Hair cells: transduction, tuning, and transmission in the inner ear. Annu Rev Cell Biol. 1988;4:63–92.
32. Wangemann P. K+ cycling and the endocochlear potential. Hear Res. 2002;165:1–9.
33. Brownell WE. Outer hair cell electromotility and optoacoustic emissions. Ear Hear. 1990;11:82–92.
34. Dallos P. The role of outer hair cells on cochlear function. Prog Clin Biol Res. 1985;176:207–30.
35. Spoendlin H. Anatomy of cochlear innervation. Am J Otolaryngol. 1985;6:453–67.
36. Meyer AC, Moser T. Structure and function of cochlear afferent innervation. Curr Opin Otolaryngol Head Neck Surg. 2010;18:441–6.
37. Berglund AM, Ryugo DK. Hair cell innervation by spiral ganglion neurons in the mouse. J Comp Neurol. 1987;255:560–70.
38. Brown MC. Morphology of labeled afferent fibers in the guinea pig cochlea. J Comp Neurol. 1987;260:591–604.
39. Jagger DJ, Housley GD. Membrane properties of type II spiral ganglion neurones identified in a neonatal rat cochlear slice. J Physiol. 2003;552:525–33.
40. Young ED. Neural representation of spectral and temporal information in speech. Philos Trans R Soc Lond B Biol Sci. 2008;363:923–45.
41. Fuchs PA. Time and intensity coding at the hair cell's ribbon synapse. J Physiol. 2005;566:7–12.
42. Moser T, Neef A, Khimich D. Mechanisms underlying the temporal precision of sound coding at the inner hair cell ribbon synapse. J Physiol. 2006;576:55–62.
43. Glowatzki E, Fuchs PA. Transmitter release at the hair cell ribbon synapse. Nat Neurosci. 2002;5:147–54.
44. Wittig JH Jr, Parsons TD. Synaptic ribbon enables temporal precision of hair cell afferent synapse by increasing the number of readily releasable vesicles: a modeling study. J Neurophysiol. 2008;100:1724–39.
45. Rutherford MA, Chapochnikov NM, Moser T. Spike encoding of neuro- transmitter release timing by spiral ganglion neurons of the cochlea. J Neurosci. 2012;32:4773–89.
46. Johnson SL, Forge A, Knipper M, Munkner S, Marcotti W. Tonotopic variation in the calcium dependence of neurotransmitter release and vesicle pool replenishment at mammalian auditory ribbon synapses. J Neurosci. 2008;28:7670–8.
47. Johnson SL, Franz C, Knipper M, Marcotti W. Functional maturation of the exocytotic machinery at gerbil hair cell ribbon synapses. J Physiol. 2009;587:1715–26.
48. Beutner D, Moser T. The presynaptic function of mouse cochlear inner hair cells during development of hearing. J Neurosci. 2001;21:4593–9.
49. Knirsch M, Brandt N, Braig C, Kuhn S, Hirt B, Munkner S, Knipper M, Engel J. Persistence of Ca(v)1.3 Ca2þ channels in mature outer hair cells supports outer hair cell afferent signaling. J Neurosci. 2007;27:6442–51.
50. Siegel JH. Spontaneous synaptic potentials from afferent terminals in the guinea pig cochlea. Hear Res. 1992;59:85–92.
51. Roberts WM. Localization of calcium signals by a mobile calcium buffer in frog saccular hair cells. J Neurosci. 1994;14:3246–62.
52. Graydon CW, Cho S, Li GL, Kachar B, von Gersdorff H. Sharp Ca(2)(þ) nanodomains beneath the ribbon promote highly synchronous multivesicular release at hair cell synapses. J Neurosci. 2011;31:16637–50.
53. Matthews G, Sterling P. Evidence that vesicles undergo compound fusion on the synaptic ribbon. J Neurosci. 2008;28:5403–11.
54. Zampini V, Johnson SL, Franz C, Knipper M, Holley MC, Magistretti J, Russo G, Marcotti W, Masetto S. Fine tuning of CaV1.3 Caþ2 channel properties in adult inner hair cells positioned in the most sensitive region of the Gerbil Cochlea. PLoS One. 2014;9:113750.
55. Chapochnikov NM, Takago H, Huang CH, Pangrsic T, Khimich D, Neef J, Auge E, Gottfert F, Hell SW, Wichmann C, Wolf F, Moser T. Uni- quantal release through a dynamic fusion pore is a candidate mechanism of hair cell exocytosis. Neuron. 2014;83:1389–403.
56. Keen EC, Hudspeth AJ. Transfer characteristics of the hair cell's afferent synapse. Proc Natl Acad Sci. 2006;103:5537–42.

57. Schnee ME, Castellano-Munoz M, Ricci AJ. Response properties from turtle auditory hair cell afferent fibers suggest spike generation is driven by synchronized release both between and within synapses. J Neurophysiol. 2013;110:204–20.
58. Goutman JD. Transmitter release from cochlear hair cells is phase locked to cyclic stimuli of different intensities and frequencies. J Neurosci. 2012;32:17025–35.
59. Rose JE, Brugge JF, Anderson DJ, Hind JE. Phase-locked response to low- frequency tones in single auditory nerve fibers of the squirrel monkey. J Neurophysiol. 1967;30:769–93.
60. Anson BJ, Warpeha RL, Rensink MJ. The gross and macroscopic anatomy of the labyrinths. Ann Otol Rhinol Laryngol. 1968;77:583–607.
61. Siegel JH, Brownell WE. Presynaptic bodies in outer hair cells of the chinchilla organ of Corti. Brain Res. 1981;220:188–93.
62. Simmons DD, Liberman MC. Afferent innervation of outer hair cells in adult cats: II. Electron microscopic analysis of fibers labeled with horseradish peroxidase. J Comp Neurol. 1988;270:145–54.
63. Weisz CJ, Lehar M, Hiel H, Glowatzki E, Fuchs PA. Synaptic transfer from outer hair cells to type II afferent fibers in the rat cochlea. J Neurosci. 2012;32:9528–36.
64. Fujikawa T, Petralia RS, Fitzgerald TS, Wang YX, Millis B, Morgado-Diaz JA, Kitamura K, Kachar B. Localization of kainate receptors in inner and outer hair cell synapses. Hear Res. 2014;314:20–32.
65. Sobkowicz HM, Rose JE, Scott GE, Slapnick SM. Ribbon synapses in the developing intact and cultured organ of Corti in the mouse. J Neurosci. 1982;2:942–57.
66. Weisz C, Glowatzki E, Fuchs P. The postsynaptic function of type II cochlear afferents. Nature. 2009;461:1126–9.
67. Nieuwenhuys R. Anatomy of the auditory pathways, with emphasis on the brain stem. Adv Otorhinolaryngol. 1984;34:25–38.
68. Weisz CJ, Glowatzki E, Fuchs PA. Excitability of type II cochlear afferents. J Neurosci. 2014;34:2365–73.
69. Brown MC, Berglund AM, Kiang NY, Ryugo DK. Central trajectories of type II spiral ganglion neurons. J Comp Neurol. 1988;278:581–90.
70. Beurg M, Safieddine S, Roux I, Bouleau Y, Petit C, Dulon D. Calcium- and otoferlin-dependent exocytosis by immature outer hair cells. J Neurosci. 2008;28:1798–803.
71. Akil O, Seal RP, Burke K, Wang C, Alemi A, During M, Edwards RH, Lustig LR. Restoration of hearing in the VGLUT3 knockout mouse using virally mediated gene therapy. Neuron. 2012;75:283–93.
72. Roberts WM, Jacobs RA, Hudspeth AJ. Colocalization of ion channels involved in frequency selectivity and synaptic transmission at presynaptic active zones of hair cells. J Neurosci. 1990;10:3664–84.

Neurophysiology: The Central Auditory System

6

Nicole T. Jiam, Bradford J. May, and Charles J. Limb

Introduction

The auditory nervous system is an elaborate neural system that governs sound representation. This elegant and exquisitely tuned circuitry allows a listener to choose to attend or ignore sensory information that he or she receives in the face of competing stimuli and suboptimal listening conditions—almost without conscious effort. Yet, a listener's ability to determine whether an acoustic event is worthwhile is also derived from the auditory system's intrinsic and enormously intricate capacity to extract multiple cues from sound. Despite the fact that sound frequently evolves on several dimensions (e.g., pitch, loudness, location) over the span of milliseconds, a listener is able to recognize the changes and maintain attention during its acoustic transformation. Indeed, the central auditory system is a remarkable neural network capable of undefined levels of auditory information processing. The purpose of this chapter is to provide the reader with an overview of central auditory processing and the functional characteristics that define each subcenter. This chapter reviews how sound is represented by the central auditory system; beginning from the cochlear nucleus to the auditory cortex. We characterize each major auditory nucleus involved in sound-driven activity and summarize the neuroanatomy and neurophysiology of auditory pathways and cortex that give way to sound perception in normal hearing listeners. Within each section, we introduce relevant studies that demonstrate the clinical implications of auditory nuclei.

N. T. Jiam · C. J. Limb (✉)
Department of Otolaryngology—Head and Neck Surgery, University of California San Francisco School of Medicine, San Francisco, CA, USA
e-mail: nicole.jiam@ucsf.edu; charles.limb@ucsf.edu

B. J. May
Department of Otolaryngology—Head and Neck Surgery, Johns Hopkins University School of Medicine, Baltimore, MD, USA
e-mail: bmay@jhu.edu

Methodology to Study Auditory Processing and Disorders

The animal model is a common method used to study central auditory processing. Cats and nonhuman primates are the most frequently used animal models and, in many ways, have shaped our current understanding of the central auditory system (Fig. 6.1) [1]. While much of our knowledge on the auditory system has been derived from nonhuman species, experimental animals are limited as a model system in studying higher cognitive processes such as the human auditory cortex. As a result, our continual understanding of human auditory function is much more reliant on indirect measures of neural activity, such as functional neural imaging. The obvious difficulties of studying in vivo human auditory function are further complicated by large heterogeneity among individual auditory anatomy and physiology. Within the existing literature, cytoarchitectonic and chemoarchitectonic methods have been used in anatomical studies to define subregions of the auditory cortex and neural circuitry involved in the central auditory system. Investigators have also found success in using physiological approaches based on receptive field properties, determination of bandwidths, spectral bandwidths of target neurons, and temporal response qualities. To a certain extent, our current understanding of the auditory system has been largely shaped by approaches that subdivide the central auditory system into subunits. The inevitable outcome from this approach is that we know a great deal more about each individual subunit than its relationship with one another or with other sensory systems. In other words, this approach makes it difficult to understand the whole brain model for acoustic processing. For these reasons, broad brain mapping strategies (e.g., functional magnetic resonance imaging (fMRI), functional near-infrared spectroscopy (fNIRS)) are increasingly more common tools used in studying how auditory regions interact with nonauditory regions. Electroencephalography (EEG) and magnetoencephalography (MEG) are two neuroimaging techniques that uniquely provide excellent temporal

A. D. Sweeney et al. (eds.), *Haynes-Glasscock-Shambaugh Surgery of the Ear*, https://doi.org/10.1007/978-3-032-18264-7_6

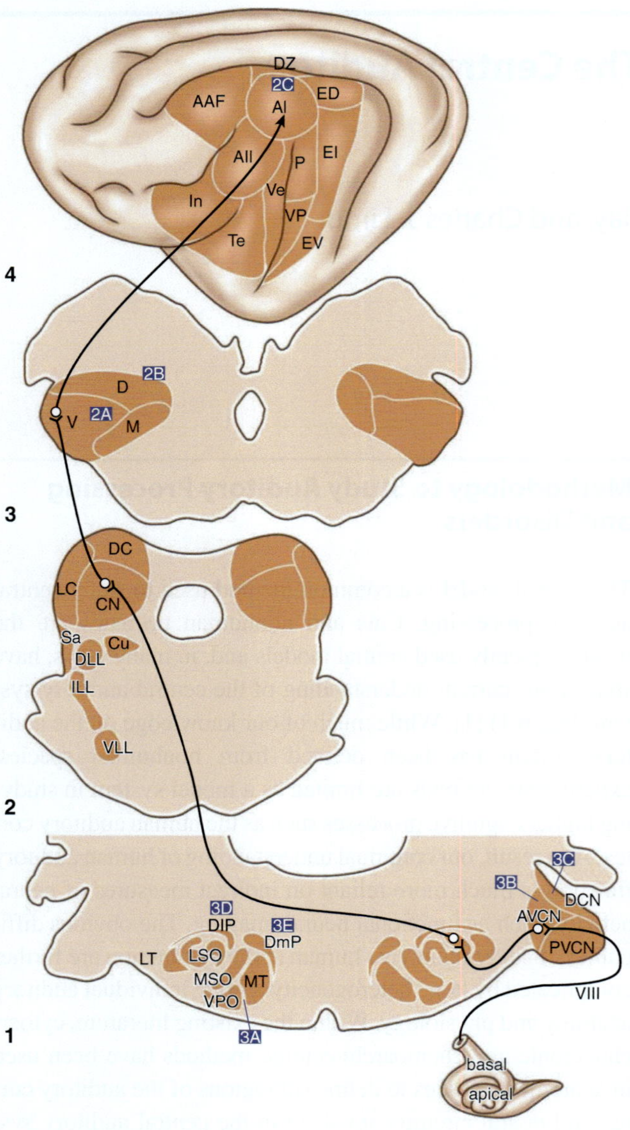

Fig. 6.1 The central auditory pathway. Key nuclei in the feline auditory system and elements of the lemniscal pathway from the medulla (1), midbrain (2), thalamus (3), and auditory cortex (4). (Figure and caption adapted from Lee et al. [1] Licensed under CC-BY 4.0)

resolution on a millisecond time-scale. EEG measures electrical signals provided by a group of neurons, whereas MEG measures the concurrent magnetic signals induced by these electric signals. There are limitations to both techniques. Electric signals are attenuated by the skull, limiting accurate EEG source-localization. However, MEGs are much less accessible and much more expensive to use.

Cochlear Nucleus

As previously described, sounds are broken into constituent frequency components within the cochlea, and each individual auditory nerve fiber corresponds to a particular area of the cochlea in a tonotopic fashion. Approximately 30,000 auditory nerve fibers carry the ascending peripheral information toward the cochlear nucleus [2]—what many regard as the first nucleus involved in central auditory processing [3]. Early anatomic descriptions of the auditory brainstem [4] and cellular morphology led to the understanding that the cochlear nucleus can be effectively divided into two functional components: the ventral and dorsal subdivisions. The ventral cochlear nucleus (VCN) provides the primary afferent input to the superior olive, lateral lemniscus, and inferior colliculus (ICC). Each of these structures regulate the selective coding of both local (e.g., phase, level of individual frequency components) and global properties (e.g., amplitude modulations of the spectral envelope) of sound. Projections to the VCN bifurcate into an ascending branch toward the anterior VCN and a descending branch toward the posterior VCN and dorsal cochlear nucleus (DCN), with approximately a ratio of two VCN neurons per auditory nerve fiber [5]. Again, the systematic arrangement of the projections reflects the tonotopic organization recapitulated in the cochlea's frequency map. However, the VCN has multiple terminal fields, which transform the previously one-dimensional frequency map into two-dimensional frequency laminas for sound encoding.

In the VCN, there are anatomically defined neuronal populations that are regionally organized [5]. These include the spherical bushy cells (anteriorly located), the globular bushy cells (intermediately located), and the octopus cells (posteriorly located). Multipolar cells are not only the most structurally diverse neurons but also the most dispersed neurons within the VCN. Our understanding of these basic physiological properties arose from early intracellular experiments that used labeling materials, such as horseradish peroxidase, to track cellular migration within the cochlear nucleus [6].

Previous studies have ablated projections exciting the VCN via the trapezoid body [7, 8]. As expected, the effect was deafness, akin to removal of the cochlea or the auditory nerve. Unilateral lesions to the VCN result in sound localization impairments due to a lack of binaural information. Without VCN inputs, particularly in the early stages of development, sound-driven patterns of neural connectivity are disrupted in the cochlear nucleus [9]. These synapses may be rescued in part by swift intervention to restore input (e.g., cochlear implantation or hearing aid amplification) to the VCN, and will consequentially inhibit the hypertrophic effect on sound processing [10]. In noise-exposed animal studies, VCN bushy cells become more excitable and exhibit hyperacusis-like firing patterns—suggesting that this functional component of the central nervous system may be an important contributor to hyperacusis [11].

While the VCN representations are linear, narrowly tuned, and distributed, dorsal cochlear nucleus (DCN) representations are nonlinear, broadly tuned, and integrative. The DCN is a center for multisensory integration [12] and is thought to be involved with acousticomotor behaviors and pinna-based sound localization [13]. Here, principal output neurons are bipolar in appearance and deliver excitatory information to the apical dendrites and the cell bodies of the vestibular, cerebellar, and somatosensory nuclei [14]. This three-layered structure receives descending inputs from outside the nucleus and local target neurons from the outer molecular layer via mossy fibers. This information converges onto granule cells which are small cell bodies scattered along the outer molecular layer [15]. The axons of granule cells traverse the DCN to excite pyramidal cells (otherwise known as fusiform cells) or inhibit local interneurons called the cartwheel cells [5]. In addition to its input from the granule and cartwheel cells, pyramidal cells sometimes receive inputs from the auditory nerve fibers and other inhibitory sources in the deep layer. Similar to the VCN, the tonotopic organization demonstrated in the cochlea is preserved within the DCN. The deep layer of the DCN is comprised of giant cell and vertical cells [16]. Giant cells are similar to pyramidal cells in their physiological properties and are ideal for encoding the spectral shape of complex sounds [17]. However, unlike pyramidal cells, giant cell dendrites do not reach the molecular layer where parallel fibers lie. Vertical cells, on the other hand, are inhibitory interneurons.

In DCN processing, biologically relevant spectral information is provided by the head-related transfer function (HRTF) [18, 19]. This filter shape illustrates the directional effects of the head and the pinna on a free-field stimulus as it propagates to the ear drum. This sort of information is crucial for accurate localization of sound source elevation. Type IV neurons are responsible for encoding spectral cues for sound localization by driving the HRTF-related discharge rates in the DCN. Because type IV neurons have nonlinear spectral integration properties, these neurons can respond selectively to spectral shapes as opposed to solely the magnitude to individual frequency components [20].

Although the mechanisms have not yet been fully elucidated, the most widely accepted physiological model for tinnitus remains neural hyperactivity. As it stands, tinnitus may be a reflection of a disruption in DCN processing [21]. Studies have suggested that spontaneous discharge rates in the DCN increases with aging or with metaplasticity as a result of transient exposure to loud noise [22]. Unfortunately, the neural hyperactivity runs the risk of activating the very same neural pathways as an auditory stimulus, resulting in the perception of a phantom sound [23, 24]. In studies with guinea pigs, it was found that DCN bimodal plasticity is stimulus timing-dependent [25, 26]. The investigators, in addition to several other authors, suggest that tinnitus may be related to abnormal cross-modal plasticity of somatic-auditory interactions [26–29].

More recently, DCN-mediated representation of complex sounds was evaluated using rats with moderate high-frequency hearing loss following acoustic trauma [30]. Following acoustic trauma, there was a transient degradation in the tuning of auditory nerve fibers and a loss of inhibitory inputs in DCN. The authors report that even after several months, the quality of spectral representation remained poor in post-trauma neurons (Fig. 6.2) [8, 30]. Additional experiments have attempted to characterize DCN processing disorders by sectioning the ascending axonal projections of pyramidal cells and giant cells—otherwise known as the dorsal acoustic stria (DAS). Unlike lesions to the pathways affecting the VCN, DAS abnormalities have little effect on basic perceptual hearing such as absolute thresholds in quiet and background noise [8]. Significant deficits are observed, however, in tasks that require identification of sound source elevation [31, 32]. For instances, cats are normally able to make reflexive head movements toward sudden, unexpected sounds and their accuracy in sound-guided response approaches the performance levels of humans. Although cats with bilaterally lesioned DAS are somewhat able to compensate for directional hearing impairments in the horizontal dimension (using binaural cues from the ventral pathways toward the superior olivary complex), they perform poorly with any task involving the vertical dimension [31].

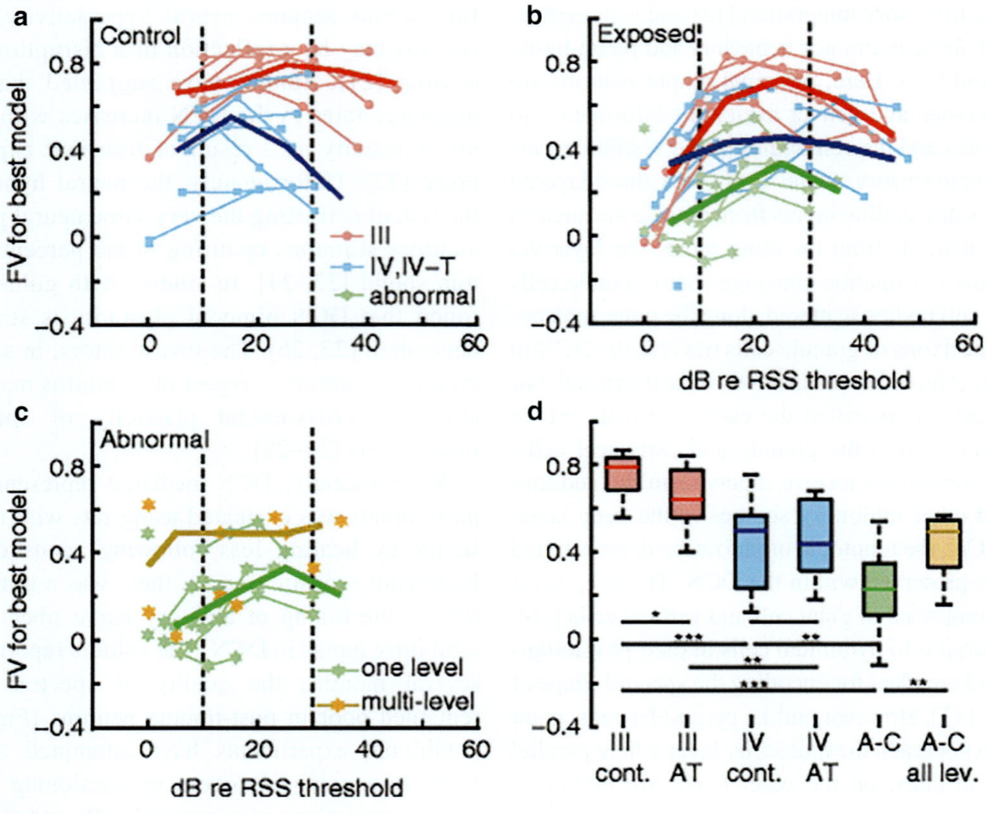

Fig. 6.2 Acoustic trauma reduces the accuracy of the spectral representation in DCN neurons. (**a**) fv for model fits to data in control animals, plotted against sound level. The heavy lines are median values in 10 dB bins. (**b**) fv for model fits to data in exposed animals, plotted against sound level (**c**) fv for model fits to data for abnormal neurons (types A, B, C, N = 4, 3, 3). Green plots are repeated from (**b**) for fits at single sound levels and gold plots are fits to multiple sound levels simultaneously; for the multi-level fits, only one data point is plotted for each neuron, at the highest sound level. The gold line is the population median as usual. (**d**) Box plots summarizing the distributions of fv in various neuron types (III, IV/IV-T, and abnormal) for control (cont) and exposed (AT) animals. The fv value for each neuron is its median value between 10 and 30 dB re threshold. Ranksum statistical comparisons are summarized by the horizontal lines with significance: $*P < 0.1$; $**P < 0.01$; $***P < 0.001$. (Reproduced with permission [30])

Auditory Brainstem Pathways and Physiology

Within the ventral brainstem and near the trapezoid body lies the superior olivary complex. The superior olivary complex is made up of three nuclei: the medial superior olive (MSO), the lateral superior olive (LSO), and the medial nucleus of the trapezoid body (MNTB). Ascending pathways from the VCNs converge in the superior olivary complex to provide binaural information regarding any interaural discrepancies in time (e.g., interaural time differences, ITDs) and sound pressure levels (interaural level differences, ILDs). Based on its input, the superior olivary complex has the ability to modulate cochlear sensitivity and cochlear nucleus inhibitory interactions via descending efferent pathways.

Olivocochlear feedback pathways play a pivotal role in hearing protection, selective attention, and listening in noise [33–35]. The neural circuitry of the olivocochlear reflex is comprised of auditory nerve fibers, postero-ventral cochlear nucleus neurons, and medial olivocochlear fibers. Medial olivocochlear (MOC) projections provide bilateral feedback to the outer hair cells in the cochleae [36]. A MOC-driven hyperpolarization of outer hair cells reduces cellular sensitivity to depolarizing currents from the mechanical activation of the basilar membrane. The MOC neurons also provide feedback to the granule cells of the cochlear nucleus, reducing cochlear nucleus sensitivity via a dynamic self-tuning system [37]. In mammals, the olivocochlear system is also constituted by pathways between the auditory cortex to the cochlea [38–41]. As such, cortical descending pathways, from pyramidal neurons located in layers V and VI of the auditory cortex [42], also activate the olivocochlear reflex and produce a suppression of cochlear responses. Dragicevic et al. [43] used auditory cortex electrical microstimulation in adult chinchillas to evaluate auditory cortical mechanisms driving cochlea sensitivity and the olivocochlear reflex circuit and found that these peripheral modulations appear to be comprised of two functionally different efferent pathways. Audiometric assessments on people with sectioned vestibular nerves and animal studies of olivocochlear function revealed that a loss in olivocochlear feedback impairs selective listening, particularly in the presence of competing streams of auditory information [44, 45].

In most mammals, the MSO is a two-dimensional sheet composed of bipolar dendritic fields. The lateral bipolar dendrites receive input from the ipsilateral VCN and the medial bipolar dendrites receive input from the contralateral VCN [46]. High security endbulb synapses between spherical bushy cells and bipolar neurons and subthreshold oscillations mediated by voltage-gated Na+ channels preserve the timing and frequency tuning of the auditory signal [47, 48]. As expected, this precisely timed delivery allows for the MSO to play an important role in the temporal comparison of sound-evoked discharge rates between two ears. Binaural timing differences provide essential information for azimuthal (left-right) sound localization. Additionally, the MSO is involved with spatial masking releases where competing auditory information (e.g., multiple speakers at a cocktail party) is distilled into separate and distinct auditory objects. This process is also known as auditory streaming and reduces signal interference by as much as 20 decibels. It is thought that individuals with unilateral hearing aids or cochlear implants struggle with complex speech perception because they lack access to binaural cues that are vital for directional hearing in difficult listening environments [49].

The LSO is composed of bipolar cells that traverse across the hila of the nucleus. Similar to the MSO, it receives inputs from the same spherical bushy cell population—but only from the ipsilateral cochlear nucleus [50]. Contralateral inhibitory inputs from the cochlear nucleus are provided by globular bushy cells via the MNTB [46]. As a result of this configuration, monaural responses to contralateral stimuli have an inhibitory effect. Unlike the MSO, the LSO is responsible for using the magnitude of sound energy interference (from the upper torso, head, and outer ear) to compute ILDs and not timing. The lower frequency limit for the sound shadow is dependent on the shape of the head such that larger mammals typically interface with lower frequency cues because their heads attenuate longer acoustic wavelengths [51]. Bilateral projections from ILD-sensitive LSO neurons ascend through the lateral lemniscus to the central nucleus of the inferior colliculus (ICC).

The ICC consists of a central core of sound processing neurons, the central nucleus (tonotopic core), and a surrounding belt of polysensory nuclei with less robust sound-driven responses (nontonotopic belt). The tonotopic organization of the central auditory system continues to be preserved within the central nucleus along its dorsal-ventral axis; high frequency information is sent in the contralateral direction and low-frequency information is carried in the ipsilateral direction toward the midbrain [52]. The resulting effect is an ICC with representation of both contralateral low and high frequency information. Other anterograde tracing studies demonstrated that excitatory inputs from ITD-sensitive MSO neurons and ILD-sensitive LSO neurons are anatomically segregated within the ICC [53]. A unilateral lesion in the ICC or a higher structure in the central auditory system will manifest as localization deficits from the contralateral sound field [54]. The proposed mechanism for selective lateralized distribution of ascending olivary inputs to the central nucleus is through the acoustic chiasm. Therefore, any lesion to the lateral lemniscus should produce similar effects.

Previous immunohistologic experiments also revealed that the ICC has both excitatory and inhibitory effects on the medial geniculate body (MGB) [55]. In fact, a characteristic component of the ICC is its sensitivity to excitatory and inhibitory signals. When excitatory signals from the brainstem are reduced in number or strength, the ICC may grow silent. On the other hand, a loss of tonic inhibition from the brainstem may result in abnormally hyperactive neurons.

High neuronal activity in the ICC has been suggested to be a causal factor in tinnitus, hyperacusis, loudness recruitment, and audiogenic seizures. Several immunocytochemical animal studies have reported a loss of GABA in the ICC with age [56]. A decrease in GABAergic transmission in the presence of upregulated glutamate contributes to a number of audiological disorders that occur with presbycusis [57]. In fact, it has been suggested that this loss of central inhibition induces tinnitus by producing lasting and stronger responses to auditory stimuli or spontaneous activity in the absence of sound [58, 59]. The ICC is a major player in auditory and nonauditory networks. As such, the ICC has been identified as a potential culprit in inducing tinnitus because of its well-established physiological vulnerability to central inhibition [60]. Audiogenic seizures are also thought to arise from the ICC. This theory is largely based on animal studies of epilepsy and insensitivity to GABA inhibition [61]. Rats that appear to be more vulnerable to epilepsy seem to require larger amounts of GABA in order to suppress the discharges in response to auditory stimulation. Consistent with this observation, GABA antagonists (e.g., bicuculline) can induce epileptiform activity in normal neurons.

Thalamus

The auditory thalamus, otherwise known as the MGB, receives input from the central nucleus of the ICC. Based on cytoarchitectural structure and patterns of neural connectivity, the MGB is frequently referred to as three different regions: a ventral principal cell area, a medial magnocellular area, and a structurally diverse dorsal area [62, 63]. The ventral division of the MGB receives most of its input from the large tufted cells from the ICC, local inhibitory neurons (e.g. small stellate cells) [64], and descending projections from the auditory cortex. The dorsal and medial regions of the MGB receive diffusely tuned and polysensory inputs from multiple brainstem nuclei. Like the midbrain, tonotopy is preserved within the ventral region of the MGB. Physiological properties found in the midbrain are also reflected in the MGB. For example, many neurons in the ventral division are tuned in frequency, level, and time. Although the MGB responds to acoustic stimuli presented to either ear, there seems to be preference for one ear. Similar to the midbrain, low-frequency neurons are sensitive to ITD cues in binaural sounds, and high-frequency neurons are particularly responsive to ILD information [65]. Anatomical and functional abnormalities of the MGB have deleterious effects on an individual's ability to process rapidly changing speech sounds [66]. These deficits have been implicated by studying aberrant thalamic anatomy in cadaveric dyslexic brains [67]. Normal brains typically have symmetrically sized MGBs, whereas the left MGB is often smaller in dyslexic brains because of a decrease in large projection neurons. Of note, the left ventral MGB has been shown to be largely involved with recognizing speech in noisy environments as opposed to quiet environments [68] and its cortical target is an important player in speech processing - the left hemisphere of the cerebral cortex [69]. Thalamic abnormalities among people with language impairments have also been reported in electrophysiological studies [70]. People with dyslexia generally demonstrate less mismatch negativity in tasks involving rapid speech changes. It has been suggested that this observation arises from an inability to process rapid change and detection of a deviant stimulus from a repeating background. In a prior animal study, implanted electrodes demonstrated the association between the observed mismatch negativity and activity in the extralemniscal divisions of the MGB [71].

Most of the excitatory outputs from this region are directed towards the cellular layer IV of A1 (the primary auditory field) [72]. Additionally, the ventral region of the MGB receives descending feedback arising from the cortex and limbic systems to condition ascending representations before they reach the auditory cortex. This complex circuitry also allows cognitive factors such as learning, attention, and state of arousal to stimulate a subpopulation of thalamic neurons while suppressing others [65, 73]. The impact of corticofugal feedback on sound processing has been studied in anesthetized cats using single-unit activity recordings in the ventral division of the MGB [74]. When large areas of A1 are silenced by cryogenic blockade, neurons in the ventral division of the MGB have reduced spontaneous rates, increased signal-to-noise ratios, and changes in frequency tuning. These findings suggest that the primary auditory cortex has both excitatory and inhibitory effects on the auditory thalamus. A similar study involving the MGB of mustached bats found that neural responses to frequencies are heightened in both magnitude and selectivity when frequency-related regions in the auditory cortex are stimulated. Pharmacological inhibition of the auditory cortex, however, prevents the effect [75].

Auditory Cortex

The auditory cortex receives all its acoustic information from the thalamus and is responsible for integrating parallel streams of information into fully enriched auditory representations. This is in direct contrast to the auditory brainstem where complex sounds are extracted and distilled into individual features. The final higher order transformations are acoustic representations that are shaped not only by its perceptual inputs but also by a listener's experience, the biological context, and the behavioral state. Although our understanding of the auditory system remains relatively limited, it is fairly established that much of the human auditory cortex is centered along the superior temporal gyrus (planum polare, Heschl's gyrus, and planum temporale). The primary auditory field (A1) is the first region involved in cortical processing for sound and receives much of its input directly from the ventral subdivision of the thalamus [76, 77]. Functionally, the A1 appears to play an important role in auditory identification and integration of the spectral and temporal qualities of sound. Histologically, the A1 is comprised of densely packed small cells in layer IV, heavily myelinated fibers, and abundant levels of cytochrome oxidase [78]. There are three main areas—A1, rostral (R), and rostrotemporal (RT) regions—that comprise the auditory core [78]. Each of these areas are activated in a parallel fashion and possess distinctive neural connections to other areas of the cortex. In fact, much of the transverse temporal gyrus, also known as Heschl's gyrus, consists of the auditory core.

There is a cytoarchitecturally distinct belt that surrounds the auditory core. This region of the auditory cortex receives much of its input from the dorsal (MGD) and medial nuclei (MGM) of the thalamus. Ventral to the belt lies the parabelt [79]. Its main function is to process polysensory information. Like the belt, the parabelt receives input from the MGD, MGM, and nonauditory regions near the superior temporal sulcus. Processed auditory information from the parabelt and belt regions is sent to the temporal, parietal, and frontal lobes—which suggests a role in auditory memory and visuospatial representation [80]. Where there is dysfunction between non-auditory and auditory connectivity, however, auditory disorders may arise. An auditory hallucination is a paracusia that involves perceiving sounds in the absence of an auditory stimulus. In 1978, Feinberg [81] suggested that the malfunctioning of a basic feed-forward system, otherwise known as the corollary discharge mechanism [82, 83], may underlie auditory hallucinations. Several EEG studies in schizophrenic patients and healthy controls have supported this line of thought by demonstrating a smaller N100 amplitude during talking than listening in healthy controls— demonstrating aberrations in the corollary discharge system [84–87]. Relatedly, functional connectivity, as measured by EEG coherence between frontal and temporal lobes in the gamma band, was significantly higher during talking than listening in healthy controls versus unaffected in schizophrenic patients [88]. These findings again suggest that there is failure to dampen auditory responsiveness to self-generated speech in patients who hallucinate [85]. Although there is little consistency among the current literature regarding the frequency of neural activity invoked by auditory hallucinations and the mechanisms behind these auditory disorders, there is relatively more certainty regarding the location of the activity invoked. Event-related potentials (ERPs) elicited by probes during auditory hallucination compared to non-hallucination have demonstrated left temporal lobe activation [89]. Similarly, a number of structural and functional magnetic resonance imaging studies have identified the left superior temporal cortex as an important player in auditory hallucinations [90–93].

On the other end of the spectrum, high levels of multisensory connectivity can result in remarkable feats in sound processing and production. In an fMRI study of jazz improvisation, a high-level task requiring spontaneous activity, there were increased medial prefrontal and temporal activities and a decrease in dorsolateral prefrontal activity among professional musicians [94]. Later, McPherson et al. [95] used fMRI to study piano improvisation among 12 professional jazz pianists in response to emotional cues. The study demonstrated that activity in the prefrontal cortex and other brain networks associated with creativity is highly modulated by emotional context (Fig. 6.3) [95]. More recently, an fMRI study on music-evoked fear and joy demonstrated that fear stimuli evoked higher network centrality in the auditory association cortex as compared to joy stimuli—highlighting emotion-characteristic hubs within the auditory cortex and the role it plays in the emotional processing of sounds [96]. Altogether, these findings suggest that creative states of sound production and processing may involve multisensory processes that span both auditory and non-auditory regions.

In many ways, music serves as an excellent tool to advance our understanding of higher level auditory function. This complex acoustic stimulus is arguably the most difficult auditory percept for a listener to perceive, derive meaning, and experience emotions. Additionally, it is well established that the human cortex is uniquely specialized for the process-

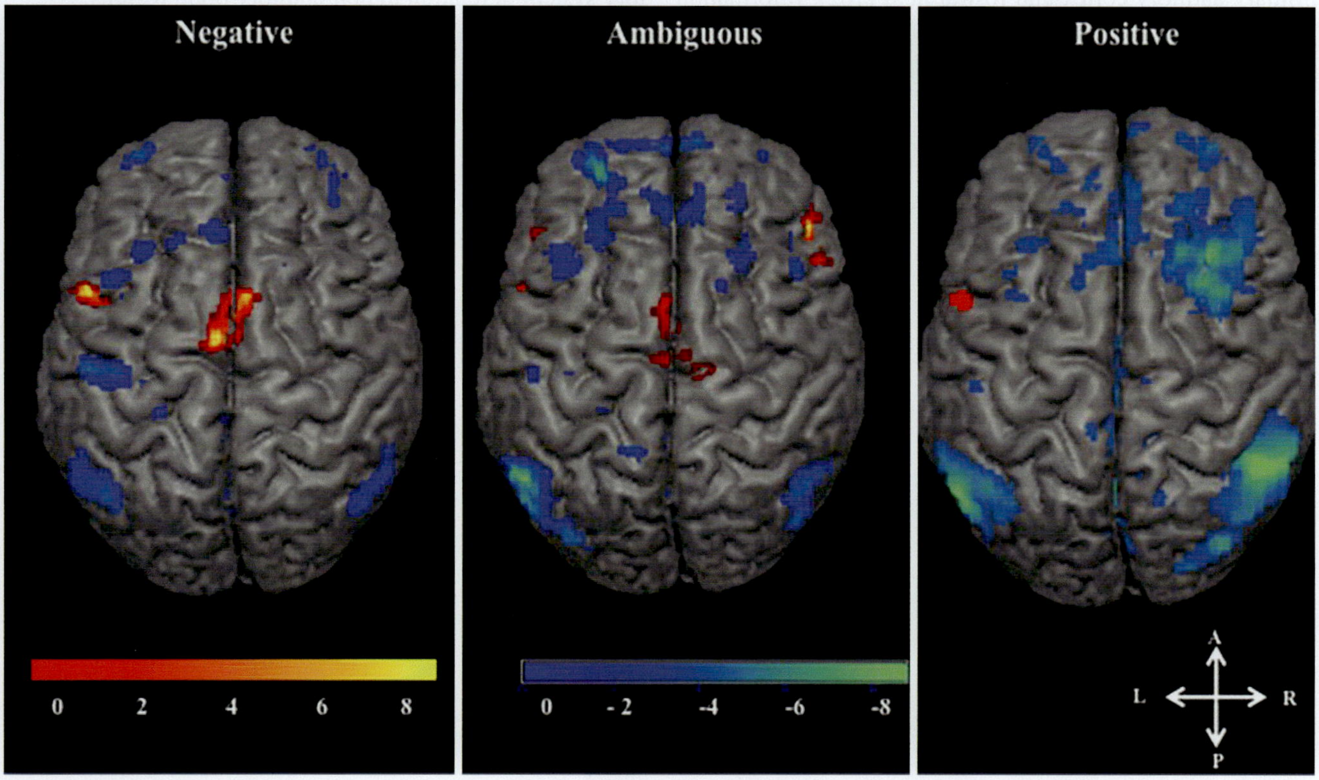

Fig. 6.3 Three-dimensional surface projections of activations and deactivations during improvisation for different emotion conditions. The scale bar shows the range of t-scores; the axes demonstrate anatomic orientation. Abbreviations: A anterior, P posterior, R right, L left. (Figure and caption reproduced from McPherson et al. [95] Licensed under CC-BY 4.0)

ing of music. This discernment stems from a number of observations including a population code within the human auditory cortex that can differentiate between changes in pitch and timbre [97, 98], an exquisite sensitivity to spectral versus temporal context and processing [99], and dual-pitch processing mechanisms [100]. As such, elucidating the processing mechanisms and basic auditory circuitry by which the brain is able to achieve the remarkable feat will lend itself to a much more comprehensive and deeper understanding of multimodal interactions between the brainstem, temporal lobe, and nonauditory centers behind sound.

In hearing, a fundamental perceptual ability is the auditory object [98]. Similar to the visual system, it is thought that the auditory cortex possesses parallel cortical processing streams that allow for acoustic signals to be identified (what is it?) and localized (where is it?). Unlike the visual system, however, auditory-object perception is highly reliant on temporal structure processing. Kraus and Nicol [101] posited that, for spoken language, sound's identity and the semantic meaning of the words undergo separate processing streams akin to the visual "what" and "where" pathways. In this hierarchical processing model, auditory information is processed in parallel pathways specialized for the extraction of spatial and non-spatial components of the auditory stimulus. In non-human primate studies, it is thought that the ventral processing pathway (auditory-object extraction) begins in the primary auditory cortex and rostral field [102]. Information from these core areas is delivered to the anterior lateral belt region and later, the ventral lateral prefrontal cortex (Fig. 6.4) [98]. fMRI human imaging data also supported this model of spatial versus non-spatial processing [103, 104]. Later, Lomber and Malhotra [105] conducted the first behavioral study of the auditory "what" and "where" pathways by using reversible cooling deactivation in selective cat non-A1 regions. They found that bilateral deactivation of the posterior auditory fields resulted in poor sound localization, whereas bilateral deactivation of the anterior auditory field inhibited pattern discrimination. Using intracranial recordings, electrocortical stimulation, and surgical ablation of the human primary auditory cortex, Hamilton et al. [106] demonstrated that speech response latency and receptive field analyses occur in parallel and distinct information processes in the auditory cortex. These study findings support an auditory cortical model where the identification of an acoustic stimulus and spatial localization of a sound are processed in separate streams. As with many of the other auditory nuclei, there is still very little understanding of how the classical auditory cortex interacts with other brain regions (e.g., prefrontal cortex, hippocampus) [107, 108]. We do not yet understand the roles that these brain regions play in auditory processing and the neural mechanisms that formulate these interactions. Therefore, future studies and continual advancements in techniques are needed to better understand the auditory system in relation to non-auditory brain regions.

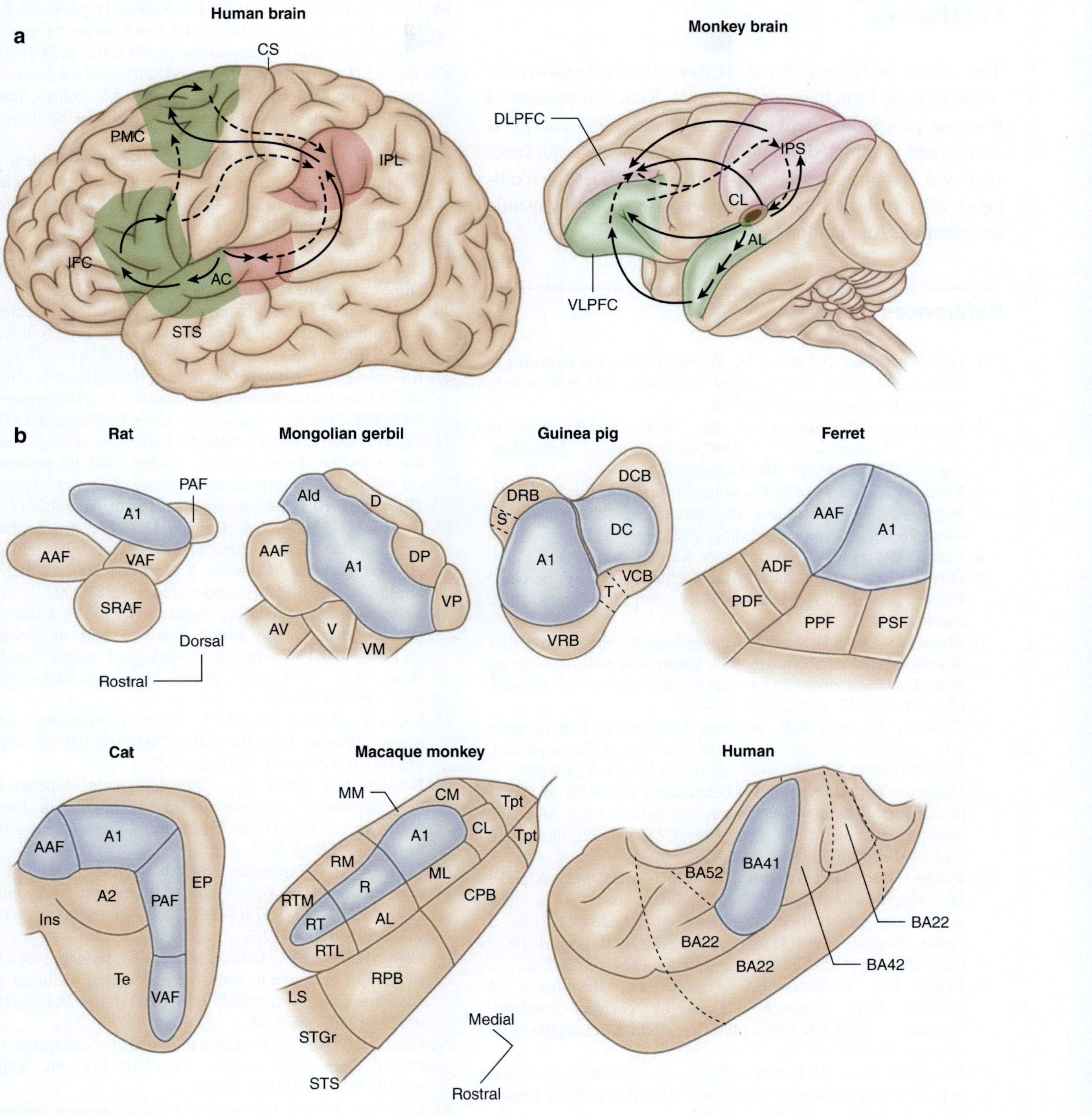

Fig. 6.4 Dual pathways of information flow in the auditory system and the organization of the auditory cortex (**a**) Information processing in the primate auditory system is hypothesized to occur in two streams: The 'dorsal' stream (red), which may preferentially analyze space and motion, are involved in audiomotor processing and the 'ventral' stream (green) are preferentially involved in auditory-object processing. Solid arrows indicate feedforward projections, and dashed arrows indicate feedback projections. (**b**) A schematic representation of the organization of the auditory cortex (AC) in different species. The lemniscal auditory thalamocortical projection terminates in the 'core' regions of the AC (blue shading), including the primary auditory cortex (A1). Solid lines indicate boundaries between auditory fields, and dashed line indicate anatomical boundaries. Abbreviations: A2 secondary auditory cortex, AAF anterior auditory field, ADF anterior dorsal field, Ald dorsal region of the primary auditory field, AL anterolateral belt, AV anteroventral field, CL caudolateral belt region of the AC, BA41 Brodmann area 41, CM caudomedial area, CPB caudal parabelt, CS central sulcus, D dorsal field, DC dorsocaudal field, DCB dorsocaudal belt, DLPFC dorsolateral prefrontal cortex, D P dorsoposterior field, DRB dorsorostral belt, E P ectosylvian posterior auditory region, IFC inferior frontal cortex, Ins insula, IPL intraparietal lobule, IPS intraparietal sulcus, LS lateral sulcus, ML mediolateral belt, MM mediomedial belt, PAF posterior auditory field, PDF posterior dorsal field, PMC premotor cortex, PPF posterior pseudosylvian field, PSF posterior suprasylvian field, RM rostromedial belt, RPB rostral parabelt, RTL rostrotemporal lateral belt, RTM rostrotemporal medial belt, SRAF suprarhinal auditory field, STGr superior temporal gyrus rostral to the parabelt, STS superior temporal sulcus, T transitional belt area, Te temporal, Tpt temporal lobe association cortex, V ventral field, VAF ventral auditory field, VCB ventrocaudal belt, VLPFC ventrolateral prefrontal cortex, VM ventromedial field, V P ventroposterior field, VRB ventrorostral belt. (Adapted from Bizley et al. [98], Hackett [109] and Rauschecker et al. [110])

Conclusions

The central auditory pathway is more than a highway for sound passing from the ear to the brain. Rather, it consists of multiple processing steps through which sound energy is refined and interpreted. As our understanding of brain functions and systems neuroscience increases, so does the likelihood of novel and targeted diagnostic and therapeutic interventions for audition.

References

1. Lee CC, Kishan AU, Winer JA. Wiring of divergent networks in the central auditory system. Front Neuroanat. 2011;5:46. https://doi.org/10.3389/fnana.2011.00046.
2. Rasmussen AT. Studies of the viiith cranial nerve of man. Laryngoscope. 1940;50(1):67–83. https://doi.org/10.1288/00005537-194001000-00008.
3. Rhode WS, Greenberg S. Physiology of the cochlear nuclei. In: Popper AN, Fay RR, editors. The mammalian auditory pathway: neurophysiology. Springer-Verilog; 1992. p. 94–152.
4. LdN R. The primary acoustic nuclei. Raven Press; 1981.
5. Osen KK. Cytoarchitecture of the cochlear nuclei in the cat. J Comp Neurol. 1969;136(4):453–84. https://doi.org/10.1002/cne.901360407.
6. Rhode WS, Oertel D, Smith PH. Physiological response properties of cells labeled intracellularly with horseradish peroxidase in cat ventral cochlear nucleus. J Comp Neurol. 1983;213(4):448–63. https://doi.org/10.1002/cne.902130408.
7. Casseday JH, Neff WD. Auditory localization: role of auditory pathways in brain stem of the cat. J Neurophysiol. 1975;38(4):842–58. https://doi.org/10.1152/jn.1975.38.4.842.
8. Masterton RB, Granger EM, Glendenning KK. Role of acoustic striae in hearing: mechanism for enhancement of sound detection in cats. Hear Res. 1994;73(2):209–22. https://doi.org/10.1016/0378-5955(94)90237-2.
9. Ryugo DK, Pongstaporn T, Huchton DM, Niparko JK. Ultrastructural analysis of primary endings in deaf white cats: morphologic alterations in endbulbs of Held. J Comp Neurol. 1997;385(2):230–44. https://doi.org/10.1002/(sici)1096-9861(19970825)385:2<230::aid-cne4>3.0.co;2-2.
10. Ryugo DK, Kretzmer EA, Niparko JK. Restoration of auditory nerve synapses in cats by cochlear implants. Science. 2005;310(5753):1490–2. https://doi.org/10.1126/science.1119419.
11. Martel DT, Shore SE. Ventral cochlear nucleus bushy cells encode hyperacusis in Guinea pigs. Sci Rep. 2020;10(1):20594. https://doi.org/10.1038/s41598-020-77754-z.
12. Ansorge J, Wu C, Shore SE, Krieger P. Audiotactile interactions in the mouse cochlear nucleus. Sci Rep. 2021;11(1):6887. https://doi.org/10.1038/s41598-021-86236-9.
13. Kanold PO, Young ED. Proprioceptive information from the pinna provides somatosensory input to the cat dorsal cochlear nucleus. J Neurosci. 2001;21(19):7848–58. https://doi.org/10.1523/jneurosci.21-19-07848.2001.
14. Adams JC, Warr WB. Origins of axons in the cat's acoustic striae determined by injection of horseradish peroxidase into severed tracts. J Comp Neurol. 1976;170(1):107–21. https://doi.org/10.1002/cne.901700108.
15. Manis PB. Responses to parallel fiber stimulation in the Guinea pig dorsal cochlear nucleus in vitro. J Neurophysiol. 1989;61(1):149–61. https://doi.org/10.1152/jn.1989.61.1.149.
16. Kane ES, Puglisi SG, Gordon BS. Neuronal types in the deep dorsal cochlear nucleus of the cat: I. Giant neurons. J Comp Neurol. 1981;198(3):483–513. https://doi.org/10.1002/cne.901980308.
17. Young ED, Davis KA. Circuitry and function of the dorsal cochlear nucleus. In: Oertel D, Fay RR, Popper AN, editors. Integrative functions in the mammalian auditory pathway. Springer-Verlag; 2002. p. 160–206.
18. Musicant AD, Chan JC, Hind JE. Direction-dependent spectral properties of cat external ear: new data and cross-species comparisons. J Acoust Soc Am. 1990;87(2):757–81. https://doi.org/10.1121/1.399545.
19. Rice JJ, May BJ, Spirou GA, Young ED. Pinna-based spectral cues for sound localization in cat. Hear Res. 1992;58(2):132–52. https://doi.org/10.1016/0378-5955(92)90123-5.
20. Yu JJ, Young ED. Linear and nonlinear pathways of spectral information transmission in the cochlear nucleus. Proc Natl Acad Sci. 2000;97(22):11780–6. https://doi.org/10.1073/pnas.97.22.11780.
21. Kaltenbach JA. Summary of evidence pointing to a role of the dorsal cochlear nucleus in the etiology of tinnitus. Acta Otolaryngol Suppl. 2006;556:20–6. https://doi.org/10.1080/03655230600895309.
22. Tagoe T, Deeping D, Hamann M. Saturation of long-term potentiation in the dorsal cochlear nucleus and its pharmacological reversal in an experimental model of tinnitus. Exp Neurol. 2017;292:1–10. https://doi.org/10.1016/j.expneurol.2017.02.011.
23. Brozoski TJ, Bauer CA, Caspary DM. Elevated fusiform cell activity in the dorsal cochlear nucleus of chinchillas with psychophysical evidence of tinnitus. J Neurosci. 2002;22(6):2383–90. https://doi.org/10.1523/jneurosci.22-06-02383.2002.
24. Kaltenbach JA, Afman CE. Hyperactivity in the dorsal cochlear nucleus after intense sound exposure and its resemblance to tone-evoked activity: a physiological model for tinnitus. Hear Res. 2000;140(1–2):165–72. https://doi.org/10.1016/s0378-5955(99)00197-5.
25. Shore S, Zhou J, Koehler S. Neural mechanisms underlying somatic tinnitus. Prog Brain Res. 2007;166:107–23. https://doi.org/10.1016/s0079-6123(07)66010-5.
26. Koehler SD, Shore SE. Stimulus timing-dependent plasticity in dorsal cochlear nucleus is altered in tinnitus. J Neurosci. 2013;33(50):19647–56. https://doi.org/10.1523/jneurosci.2788-13.2013.
27. Cacace AT. Expanding the biological basis of tinnitus: crossmodal origins and the role of neuroplasticity. Hear Res. 2003;175(1–2):112–32. https://doi.org/10.1016/s0378-5955(02)00717-7.
28. Levine RA, Nam EC, Oron Y, Melcher JR. Evidence for a tinnitus subgroup responsive to somatosensory based treatment modalities. Prog Brain Res. 2007;166:195–207. https://doi.org/10.1016/s0079-6123(07)66017-8.
29. Herraiz C. Assessing the cause of tinnitus for therapeutic options. Expert Opin Med Diagn. 2008;2(10):1183–96. https://doi.org/10.1517/17530059.2.10.1183.
30. Li Y, Ropp TJ, May BJ, Young ED. Dorsal cochlear nucleus of the rat: representation of complex sounds in ears damaged by acoustic trauma. J Assoc Res Otolaryngol. 2015;16(4):487–505. https://doi.org/10.1007/s10162-015-0522-z.
31. Sutherland DP, Masterton RB, Glendenning KK. Role of acoustic striae in hearing: reflexive responses to elevated sound-sources. Behav Brain Res. 1998;97(1–2):1–12. https://doi.org/10.1016/s0166-4328(98)00008-4.
32. May BJ. Role of the dorsal cochlear nucleus in the sound localization behavior of cats. Hear Res. 2000;148(1–2):74–87. https://doi.org/10.1016/s0378-5955(00)00142-8.
33. Winslow RL, Sachs MB. Effect of electrical stimulation of the crossed olivocochlear bundle on auditory nerve response to tones in noise. J Neurophysiol. 1987;57(4):1002–21. https://doi.org/10.1152/jn.1987.57.4.1002.

34. Buño W. Auditory nerve fiber activity influenced by contralateral ear sound stimulation. Exp Neurol. 1978;59(1):62–74. https://doi.org/10.1016/0014-4886(78)90201-7.
35. Liberman MC. Rapid assessment of sound-evoked olivocochlear feedback: suppression of compound action potentials by contralateral sound. Hear Res. 1989;38(1–2):47–56. https://doi.org/10.1016/0378-5955(89)90127-5.
36. de Venecia RK, Liberman MC, Guinan JJ Jr, Brown MC. Medial olivocochlear reflex interneurons are located in the posteroventral cochlear nucleus: a kainic acid lesion study in Guinea pigs. J Comp Neurol. 2005;487(4):345–60. https://doi.org/10.1002/cne.20550.
37. Brown MC, Liberman MC, Benson TE, Ryugo DK. Brainstem branches from olivocochlear axons in cats and rodents. J Comp Neurol. 1988;278(4):591–603. https://doi.org/10.1002/cne.902780410.
38. Malmierca MS, Ryugo DK. Descending connections of the auditory cortex to the midbrain and the brainstem. In: CE WJaS, editor. The auditory cortex. Springer; 2011. p. 189–208.
39. Robles L, DP. The senses: a comprehensive reference. In: Basbaum II KA, Shepherd GM, Westheimer G, Albright TD, Masland RH, Dallos P, Oertel D, Firestein S, Beauchamp GK, Bushnell MC, Kaas JH, Gardner E, editors. Efferent system. Academic Press; 2008. p. 413–45.
40. Saldaña E, Feliciano M, Mugnaini E. Distribution of descending projections from primary auditory neocortex to inferior colliculus mimics the topography of intracollicular projections. J Comp Neurol. 1996;371(1):15–40. https://doi.org/10.1002/(sici)1096-9861(19960715)371:1<15::Aid-cne2>3.0.Co;2-o.
41. BR Schofield. Central descending auditory pathways. In: Ryugo DK RR Fay, Popper AN, ed. Auditory and vestibular efferents. Springer; 2010:261–290.
42. Bajo VM, Moore DR. Descending projections from the auditory cortex to the inferior colliculus in the gerbil, Meriones unguiculatus. J Comp Neurol. 2005;486(2):101–16. https://doi.org/10.1002/cne.20542.
43. Dragicevic CD, Aedo C, León A, et al. The olivocochlear reflex strength and cochlear sensitivity are independently modulated by auditory cortex microstimulation. J Assoc Res Otolaryngol. 2015;16(2):223–40. https://doi.org/10.1007/s10162-015-0509-9.
44. Micheyl C, Collet L. Involvement of the olivocochlear bundle in the detection of tones in noise. J Acoust Soc Am. 1996;99(3):1604–10. https://doi.org/10.1121/1.414734.
45. Rajan R. Effect of electrical stimulation of the crossed olivocochlear bundle on temporary threshold shifts in auditory sensitivity. II. Dependence on the level of temporary threshold shifts. J Neurophysiol. 1988;60(2):569–79. https://doi.org/10.1152/jn.1988.60.2.569.
46. Cant NB, Casseday JH. Projections from the anteroventral cochlear nucleus to the lateral and medial superior olivary nuclei. J Comp Neurol. 1986;247(4):457–76. https://doi.org/10.1002/cne.902470406.
47. Smith PH, Joris PX, Yin TC. Projections of physiologically characterized spherical bushy cell axons from the cochlear nucleus of the cat: evidence for delay lines to the medial superior olive. J Comp Neurol. 1993;331(2):245–60. https://doi.org/10.1002/cne.903310208.
48. Bondy BJ, Haimes DB, Golding NL. Physiological diversity influences detection of stimulus envelope and fine structure in neurons of the medial superior olive. J Neurosci. 2021;41(29):6234–45. https://doi.org/10.1523/jneurosci.2354-20.2021.
49. Blamey PJ, Maat B, Başkent D, et al. A retrospective multicenter study comparing speech perception outcomes for bilateral implantation and bimodal rehabilitation. Ear Hear. 2015;36(4):408–16. https://doi.org/10.1097/aud.0000000000000150.
50. Cant NB. The cochlear nucleus: neuronal types and their synaptic organization. In: Webster DB, Fay RR, editors. The mammalian auditory pathway: neuroanatomy. Springer-Verlag; 1992. p. 66–116.
51. Mills AW. On the minimum audible angle. J Acoust Soc Am. 1958;30(4):237–46. https://doi.org/10.1121/1.1909553.
52. Glendenning KK, Masterton RB. Acoustic chiasm: efferent projections of the lateral superior olive. J Neurosci. 1983;3(8):1521–37. https://doi.org/10.1523/jneurosci.03-08-01521.1983.
53. Loftus WC, Bishop DC, Saint Marie RL, Oliver DL. Organization of binaural excitatory and inhibitory inputs to the inferior colliculus from the superior olive. J Comp Neurol. 2004;472(3):330–44. https://doi.org/10.1002/cne.20070.
54. Jenkins WM, Masterton RB. Sound localization: effects of unilateral lesions in central auditory system. J Neurophysiol. 1982;47(6):987–1016. https://doi.org/10.1152/jn.1982.47.6.987.
55. Winer JA, Saint Marie RL, Larue DT, Oliver DL. GABAergic feedforward projections from the inferior colliculus to the medial geniculate body. Proc Natl Acad Sci USA. 1996;93(15):8005–10. https://doi.org/10.1073/pnas.93.15.8005.
56. Caspary DM, Milbrandt JC, Helfert RH. Central auditory aging: GABA changes in the inferior colliculus. Exp Gerontol. 1995;30(3–4):349–60. https://doi.org/10.1016/0531-5565(94)00052-5.
57. Caspary DM, Ling L, Turner JG, Hughes LF. Inhibitory neurotransmission, plasticity and aging in the mammalian central auditory system. J Exp Biol. 2008;211(Pt 11):1781–91. https://doi.org/10.1242/jeb.013581.
58. Bauer CA, Brozoski TJ, Holder TM, Caspary DM. Effects of chronic salicylate on GABAergic activity in rat inferior colliculus. Hear Res. 2000;147(1–2):175–82. https://doi.org/10.1016/s0378-5955(00)00130-1.
59. Mossop JE, Wilson MJ, Caspary DM, Moore DR. Downregulation of inhibition following unilateral deafening. Hear Res. 2000;147(1–2):183–7. https://doi.org/10.1016/s0378-5955(00)00054-x.
60. Meikle MB, Vernon J, Johnson RM. The perceived severity of tinnitus. Some observations concerning a large population of tinnitus clinic patients. Otolaryngol Head Neck Surg. 1984;92(6):689–96. https://doi.org/10.1177/019459988409200617.
61. Faingold CL. Role of GABA abnormalities in the inferior colliculus pathophysiology - audiogenic seizures. Hear Res. 2002;168(1–2):223–37. https://doi.org/10.1016/s0378-5955(02)00373-8.
62. Rioch D. Studies on the diencephalon of carnivora part I. The nuclear configuration of the thalamus, epithalamus, and hypothalamus of the dog and cat. J Comp Neurol. 2004;49. https://doi.org/10.1002/cne.900490102.
63. Morest DK. The neuronal architecture of the medial geniculate body of the cat. J Anat. 1964;98(Pt 4):611–30.
64. Andersen RA, Roth GL, Aitkin LM, Merzenich MM. The efferent projections of the central nucleus and the pericentral nucleus of the inferior colliculus in the cat. J Comp Neurol. 1980;194(3):649–62. https://doi.org/10.1002/cne.901940311.
65. Suga N, Zhang Y, Yan J. Sharpening of frequency tuning by inhibition in the thalamic auditory nucleus of the mustached bat. J Neurophysiol. 1997;77(4):2098–114. https://doi.org/10.1152/jn.1997.77.4.2098.
66. Tallal P. Auditory temporal perception, phonics, and reading disabilities in children. Brain Lang. 1980;9(2):182–98. https://doi.org/10.1016/0093-934x(80)90139-x.
67. Galaburda AM, Menard MT, Rosen GD. Evidence for aberrant auditory anatomy in developmental dyslexia. Proc Natl Acad Sci USA. 1994;91(17):8010–3. https://doi.org/10.1073/pnas.91.17.8010.

68. Mihai PG, Tschentscher N, von Kriegstein K. Modulation of the primary auditory thalamus when recognizing speech with background noise. J Neurosci. 2021;41(33):7136–47. https://doi.org/10.1523/jneurosci.2902-20.2021.
69. Wada JA, Clarke R, Hamm A. Cerebral hemispheric asymmetry in humans. Cortical speech zones in 100 adults and 100 infant brains. Arch Neurol. 1975;32(4):239–46. https://doi.org/10.1001/archneur.1975.00490460055007.
70. Kraus N, McGee TJ, Carrell TD, Zecker SG, Nicol TG, Koch DB. Auditory neurophysiologic responses and discrimination deficits in children with learning problems. Science. 1996;273(5277):971–3. https://doi.org/10.1126/science.273.5277.971.
71. Kraus N, McGee T, Littman T, Nicol T, King C. Nonprimary auditory thalamic representation of acoustic change. J Neurophysiol. 1994;72(3):1270–7. https://doi.org/10.1152/jn.1994.72.3.1270.
72. Winer JA, Diamond IT, Raczkowski D. Subdivisions of the auditory cortex of the cat: the retrograde transport of horseradish peroxidase to the medial geniculate body and posterior thalamic nuclei. J Comp Neurol. 1977;176(3):387–417. https://doi.org/10.1002/cne.901760307.
73. Taylor JA, Hasegawa M, Benoit CM, et al. Single cell plasticity and population coding stability in auditory thalamus upon associative learning. Nat Commun. 2021;12(1):2438. https://doi.org/10.1038/s41467-021-22421-8.
74. Villa AE, Rouiller EM, Simm GM, Zurita P, de Ribaupierre Y, de Ribaupierre F. Corticofugal modulation of the information processing in the auditory thalamus of the cat. Exp Brain Res. 1991;86(3):506–17. https://doi.org/10.1007/bf00230524.
75. Zhang Y, Suga N. Modulation of responses and frequency tuning of thalamic and collicular neurons by cortical activation in mustached bats. J Neurophysiol. 2000;84(1):325–33. https://doi.org/10.1152/jn.2000.84.1.325.
76. Luethke LE, Krubitzer LA, Kaas JH. Cortical connections of electrophysiologically and architectonically defined subdivisions of auditory cortex in squirrels. J Comp Neurol. 1988;268(2):181–203. https://doi.org/10.1002/cne.902680205.
77. Kaas JH, Hackett TA, Tramo MJ. Auditory processing in primate cerebral cortex. Curr Opin Neurobiol. 1999;9(2):164–70. https://doi.org/10.1016/s0959-4388(99)80022-1.
78. Hackett TA, Preuss TM, Kaas JH. Architectonic identification of the core region in auditory cortex of macaques, chimpanzees, and humans. J Comp Neurol. 2001;441(3):197–222. https://doi.org/10.1002/cne.1407.
79. Hackett TA, Stepniewska I, Kaas JH. Subdivisions of auditory cortex and ipsilateral cortical connections of the parabelt auditory cortex in macaque monkeys. J Comp Neurol. 1998;394(4):475–95. https://doi.org/10.1002/(sici)1096-9861(19980518)394:4<475::aid-cne6>3.0.co;2-z.
80. Hackett TA, Stepniewska I, Kaas JH. Prefrontal connections of the parabelt auditory cortex in macaque monkeys. Brain Res. 1999;817(1–2):45–58. https://doi.org/10.1016/s0006-8993(98)01182-2.
81. Feinberg I. Efference copy and corollary discharge: implications for thinking and its disorders. Schizophr Bull. 1978;4(4):636–40. https://doi.org/10.1093/schbul/4.4.636.
82. Sperry RW. Neural basis of the spontaneous optokinetic response produced by visual inversion. J Comp Physiol Psychol. 1950;43(6):482–9. https://doi.org/10.1037/h0055479.
83. von Holst E, Mittelstaedt H. Das Reafferenzprinzip: Wechselwirkungen zwischen Zentralnervensystem und Peripherie. Naturwissenschaften. 1950;37(20):464–76. https://doi.org/10.1007/BF00622503.
84. Ford JM, Gray M, Faustman WO, Roach BJ, Mathalon DH. Dissecting corollary discharge dysfunction in schizophrenia. Psychophysiology. 2007;44(4):522–9. https://doi.org/10.1111/j.1469-8986.2007.00533.x.
85. Ford JM, Roach BJ, Faustman WO, Mathalon DH. Synch before you speak: auditory hallucinations in schizophrenia. Am J Psychiatry. 2007;164(3):458–66. https://doi.org/10.1176/ajp.2007.164.3.458.
86. Ford JM, Mathalon DH, Heinks T, Kalba S, Faustman WO, Roth WT. Neurophysiological evidence of corollary discharge dysfunction in schizophrenia. Am J Psychiatry. 2001;158(12):2069–71. https://doi.org/10.1176/appi.ajp.158.12.2069.
87. Ford JM, Mathalon DH, Kalba S, Whitfield S, Faustman WO, Roth WT. Cortical responsiveness during inner speech in schizophrenia: an event-related potential study. Am J Psychiatry. 2001;158(11):1914–6. https://doi.org/10.1176/appi.ajp.158.11.1914.
88. Ford JM, Mathalon DH. Corollary discharge dysfunction in schizophrenia: can it explain auditory hallucinations? Int J Psychophysiol. 2005;58(2–3):179–89. https://doi.org/10.1016/j.ijpsycho.2005.01.014.
89. van Lutterveld R, Sommer IE, Ford JM. The neurophysiology of auditory hallucinations - a historical and contemporary review. Front Psych. 2011;2:28. https://doi.org/10.3389/fpsyt.2011.00028.
90. Allen P, Larøi F, McGuire PK, Aleman A. The hallucinating brain: a review of structural and functional neuroimaging studies of hallucinations. Neurosci Biobehav Rev. 2008;32(1):175–91. https://doi.org/10.1016/j.neubiorev.2007.07.012.
91. Barta PE, Pearlson GD, Powers RE, Richards SS, Tune LE. Auditory hallucinations and smaller superior temporal gyral volume in schizophrenia. Am J Psychiatry. 1990;147(11):1457–62. https://doi.org/10.1176/ajp.147.11.1457.
92. Diederen KM, Neggers SF, Daalman K, et al. Deactivation of the parahippocampal gyrus preceding auditory hallucinations in schizophrenia. Am J Psychiatry. 2010;167(4):427–35. https://doi.org/10.1176/appi.ajp.2009.09040456.
93. Dierks T, Linden DE, Jandl M, et al. Activation of Heschl's gyrus during auditory hallucinations. Neuron. 1999;22(3):615–21. https://doi.org/10.1016/s0896-6273(00)80715-1.
94. Limb CJ, Braun AR. Neural substrates of spontaneous musical performance: an fMRI study of jazz improvisation. PLoS One. 2008;3(2):e1679. https://doi.org/10.1371/journal.pone.0001679.
95. McPherson MJ, Barrett FS, Lopez-Gonzalez M, Jiradejvong P, Limb CJ. Emotional intent modulates the neural substrates of creativity: an fMRI study of emotionally targeted improvisation in jazz musicians. Sci Rep. 2016;6:18460. https://doi.org/10.1038/srep18460.
96. Koelsch S, Skouras S, Lohmann G. The auditory cortex hosts network nodes influential for emotion processing: an fMRI study on music-evoked fear and joy. PLoS One. 2018;13(1):e0190057. https://doi.org/10.1371/journal.pone.0190057.
97. Allen EJ, Burton PC, Olman CA, Oxenham AJ. Representations of pitch and timbre variation in human auditory cortex. J Neurosci. 2017;37(5):1284–93. https://doi.org/10.1523/jneurosci.2336-16.2016.
98. Bizley JK, Cohen YE. The what, where and how of auditory-object perception. Nat Rev Neurosci. 2013;14(10):693–707. https://doi.org/10.1038/nrn3565.
99. Malone BJ, Beitel RE, Vollmer M, Heiser MA, Schreiner CE. Spectral context affects temporal processing in awake auditory cortex. J Neurosci. 2013;33(22):9431–50. https://doi.org/10.1523/jneurosci.3073-12.2013.
100. Bendor D, Osmanski MS, Wang X. Dual-pitch processing mechanisms in primate auditory cortex. J Neurosci. 2012;32(46):16149–61. https://doi.org/10.1523/jneurosci.2563-12.2012.
101. Kraus N, Nicol T. Brainstem origins for cortical 'what' and 'where' pathways in the auditory system. Trends Neurosci. 2005;28(4):176–81. https://doi.org/10.1016/j.tins.2005.02.003.

102. Tian B, Reser D, Durham A, Kustov A, Rauschecker JP. Functional specialization in rhesus monkey auditory cortex. Science. 2001;292(5515):290–3. https://doi.org/10.1126/science.1058911.
103. Alain C, Arnott SR, Hevenor S, Graham S, Grady CL. "What" and "where" in the human auditory system. Proc Natl Acad Sci USA. 2001;98(21):12301–6. https://doi.org/10.1073/pnas.211209098.
104. Maeder PP, Meuli RA, Adriani M, et al. Distinct pathways involved in sound recognition and localization: a human fMRI study. NeuroImage. 2001;14(4):802–16. https://doi.org/10.1006/nimg.2001.0888.
105. Lomber SG, Malhotra S. Double dissociation of 'what' and 'where' processing in auditory cortex. Nat Neurosci. 2008;11(5):609–16. https://doi.org/10.1038/nn.2108.
106. Hamilton LS, Oganian Y, Hall J, Chang EF. Parallel and distributed encoding of speech across human auditory cortex. Cell. 2021;184(18):4626–4639.e13. https://doi.org/10.1016/j.cell.2021.07.019.
107. Sugihara T, Diltz MD, Averbeck BB, Romanski LM. Integration of auditory and visual communication information in the primate ventrolateral prefrontal cortex. J Neurosci. 2006;26(43):11138–47. https://doi.org/10.1523/jneurosci.3550-06.2006.
108. Teki S, Kumar S, von Kriegstein K, et al. Navigating the auditory scene: an expert role for the hippocampus. J Neurosci. 2012;32(35):12251–7. https://doi.org/10.1523/jneurosci.0082-12.2012.
109. Hackett TA. Information flow in the auditory cortical network. Hear Res. 2011;271(1–2):133–46.
110. Rauschecker JP, Scott SK. Maps and streams in the auditory cortex: nonhuman primates illuminate human speech processing. Nat Neurosci. 2009;12(6):718–24.

7 Vestibular Physiology

Bryan K. Ward and Yuri Agrawal

Introduction

Intact vestibular sensation is critical for maintaining balance, seeing clearly, and navigating the world. For the classic Aristotelian senses of hearing, smell, vision, taste, and touch, our brain relies on their input for awareness of external stimuli. Vestibular sensation, on the other hand, provides the brain with information on movements of the head and body in space and permits navigation. Some have proposed the vestibular system is a sixth sense. The vestibular system, however, is one among many self-monitoring senses that are now recognized. While people enjoy vestibular stimulation in forms like dancing, amusement rides, or even rocking to sleep as a child, we seldom can point to our favorite vestibular stimulus, like we can for a good meal or favorite piece of music. The functions of the vestibular system go unnoticed in daily activities. We are more likely to pay attention when the system goes awry, causing vertigo and disorientation. This chapter will review the basic anatomy and physiology of the vestibular system as well as provide a general approach for evaluating patients with dizziness and balance problems.

Anatomy of the Vestibular System

The vestibular system consists of five end organs: three semicircular canals (superior, lateral and posterior) and two otoconial end organs (utricle and saccule) Fig. 7.1. Each ear has two vertical semicircular canals (superior [or anterior] and posterior) and a lateral (or horizontal) semicircular canal. The vertical canals fuse at the common crus, and all canals open into the vestibule. The vertical canals are approximately coplanar with a canal of the opposite ear (right anterior canal with the left posterior canal, RALP, and left anterior canal with the right posterior canal, LARP), Fig. 7.2a. The lateral semicircular canals are roughly parallel to Earth when sitting upright, but pitched upward approximately 20° from Reid's horizontal plane (the line between the inferior orbital rim and external auditory canal, Fig. 7.2b) [22]. The saccule and utricle are nearly planar structures, with the saccule oriented vertically and the utricle horizontally.

These five vestibular end organs are located within the dense otic capsule of the temporal bone. Early anatomists marveled at the maze-like appearance to the bony semicircular canals and vestibule and called this organ the labyrinth. The labyrinth is divided into an outer bony labyrinth and an inner membranous labyrinth. The membranous labyrinth is a fibrous epithelial core tube floating within the fluid-filled hull of the bony labyrinth and tethered to its walls by collagen fibers.

The division between bony and membranous labyrinth creates two potential spaces: a perilymph compartment between the bony and membranous labyrinth and an endolymph compartment within the membranous labyrinth. Perilymph fills the perilymph space and has an ionic composition similar to cerebrospinal fluid (CSF). The perilymph space communicates intracranially with the subarachnoid space via the cochlear aqueduct, accounting for its similar ionic composition to CSF. Endolymph fills the endolymph space within the membranous labyrinth and is a potassium rich fluid, more akin to intracellular fluid. The membranous labyrinth communicates with the endolymphatic sac via the endolymphatic duct inside the vestibular aqueduct.

The labyrinthine artery supplies blood to the vestibular end organs. This artery is most commonly a terminal branch of the anterior inferior cerebellar artery (AICA) and sends separate branches to the cochlea and the vestibular system shortly after entering the labyrinth. The anterior vestibular

B. K. Ward
Department of Otolaryngology—Head and Neck Surgery, Johns Hopkins University School of Medicine, Baltimore, MD, USA

Y. Agrawal (✉)
Department of Otolaryngology—Head and Neck Surgery, University of Colorado, Boulder, CO, USA
e-mail: yuri.agrawal@cuanschutz.edu

A. D. Sweeney et al. (eds.), *Haynes-Glasscock-Shambaugh Surgery of the Ear*, https://doi.org/10.1007/978-3-032-18264-7_7

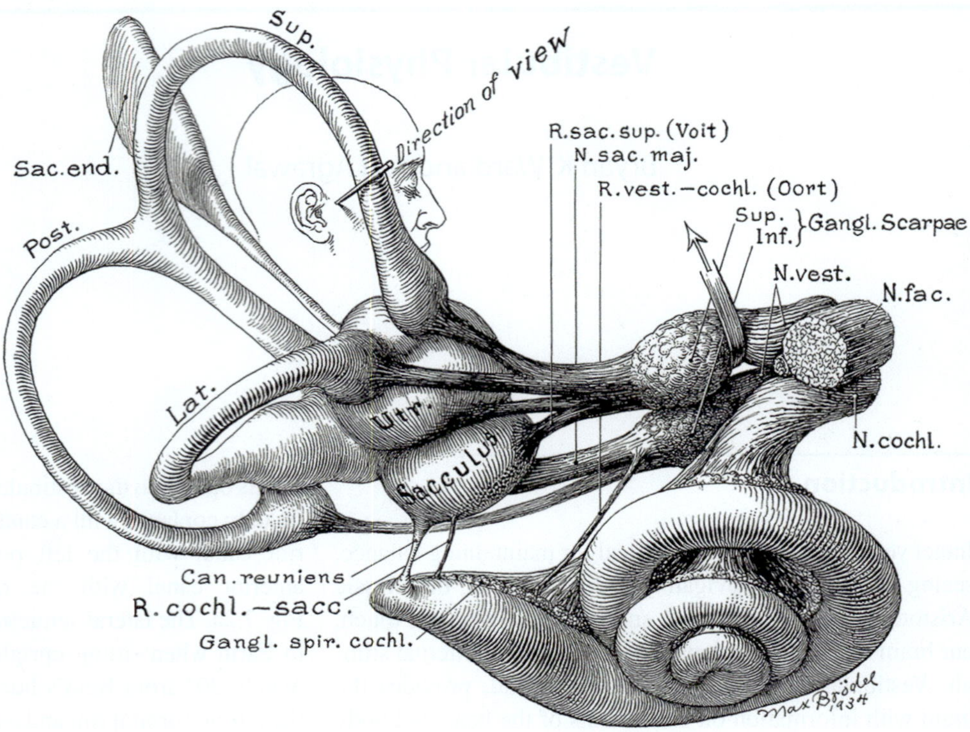

Fig. 7.1 Anatomy of the labyrinth. The anatomic structures shown include the utricle (Utr.), Sacculus, anterior or superior semicircular canal (Sup.), posterior semicircular canal (Post.), and horizontal or lateral semicircular canal (Lat.). The superior vestibular nerve innervates the lateral and anterior semicircular canals and the utricle. The inferior vestibular nerve innervates the posterior semicircular canal and the saccule. The cell bodies for the vestibular nerves are located in Scarpa's ganglion (Gangl. Scarpae). (Illustration courtesy of the Max Brödel Archives, Department of Art as Applied to Medicine, Johns Hopkins University School of Medicine)

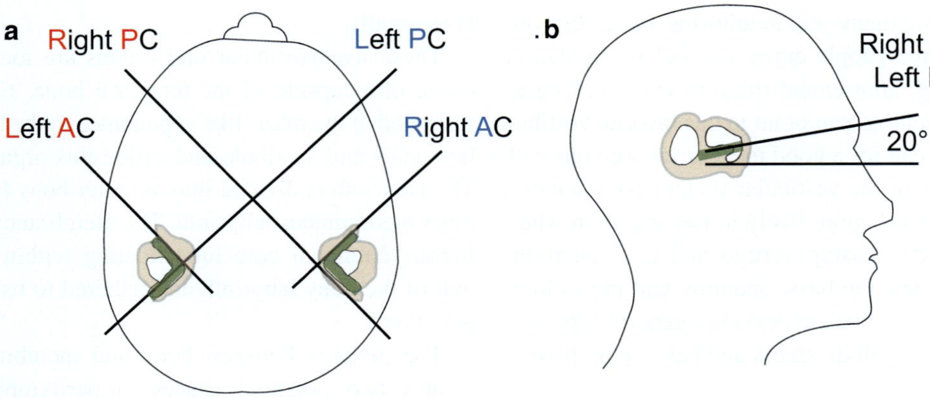

Fig. 7.2 Orientation of the semicircular canals with respect to the skull. (**a**), The right posterior canal (PC) and left anterior (or superior) canal (AC) are approximately coplanar, as are the left posterior canal and right anterior canal. These planes are sometimes referred to as LARP, left anterior, right posterior, and RALP, right anterior, left posterior. (**b**), the lateral (or horizontal) semicircular canal (LC) is oriented pitched upward approximately 20° from Reid's horizontal plane (inferior orbital rim to the external auditory canal). (Adapted by Bryan Ward from Barber HO, Stockwell CW. Manual of Electronystagmography. St Louis: Mosby; 1976. ©Bryan Ward. Used with permission)

artery supplies the superior and lateral canal ampulla and utricle. The common cochlear artery branches into cochlear and vestibulocochlear arteries; the latter subsequently branches into the posterior vestibular artery and primarily supplies the posterior semicircular canal and saccule [67]. The vestibular end organs are innervated by two vestibular nerves: the superior and inferior vestibular nerves. The cell bodies for these predominantly bipolar neurons are within Scarpa's ganglion. Each vestibular nerve has approximately 25,000 neurons [70]. The superior vestibular nerve innervates the utricle, lateral, and superior semicircular canals, as well as a tiny anterior portion of the saccule via Voit's nerve. The inferior vestibular nerve innervates the majority of the saccule and the posterior semicircular canal. A small nerve branch of the inferior vestibular nerve called the posterior ampullary nerve travels through the singular canal to innervate the posterior semicircular canal and is of historical importance as posterior ampullary nerve section was performed for recalcitrant posterior semicircular canal benign paroxysmal positional vertigo (BPPV). Today, posterior canal BPPV is managed with repositioning maneuvers or rarely by surgical plugging of the posterior semicircular canal in cases refractory to physical therapy.

Similar to in the cochlea, the vestibular system's primary functional unit is the hair cell (Fig. 7.3). The hair cell is a mechanoreceptor that translates vibration into a neural signal. The apical ends of hair cells contain stereocilia arranged in a bundle of 50–100 stereocilia and 1 kinocilium, increasing in length in an ascending pattern toward a kinocilium at one end. This arrangement provides each hair cell with polarity. Protein filaments called tip links connect or 'link' to the apical ends of stereocilia [50]. These serve two purposes: (1) they mechanically connect adjacent stereocilia so that a shear force moves the bundle as a unit and (2) as the hair cells are displaced toward the kinocilium, mechanically gated ion channels open, resulting in potassium ion influx into the hair cells. This potassium influx triggers calcium to enter the basal end of the hair cell and increases the release of glutamate neurotransmitter into the synapse. Consequently, the firing rates of the primary vestibular afferent nerves increase [72]. If the stereocilia are displaced away from the kinocilium, the channels close, hyperpolarizing the hair cell and increasing the threshold to trigger an action potential; thereby decreasing the firing rate of the afferent nerve (Fig. 7.4).

The context or environment in which a hair cell exists primarily determines the stimulus to which a particular hair cell best responds. This contributes to why, despite similar basic

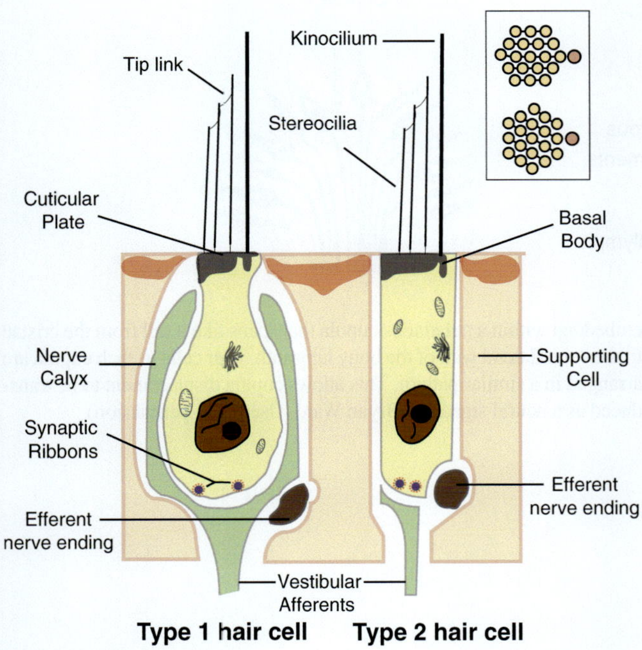

Fig. 7.3 There are two hair cell types in the mammalian labyrinth (type 1 and type 2). Anatomic components of the hair cell are shown. Hair cell stereocilia are arranged in a bundle pattern (inset) with the stereocilia increasing in height toward a single kinocilium [14]. Different patterns of hair cell bundles have been described [8]. (©Bryan Ward. Used with permission)

structure, hair cells can respond to an enormous range of stimuli from very low-frequency stimuli of fractions of a cycle per second in the vestibular system to beyond 100,000 cycles per second in bat echolocation [25]. In the vestibular system, this context also allows the hair cells of the semicircular canals to respond to angular acceleration (rotation) of the head, whereas those of the otoconial organs respond to linear acceleration (translation) or head tilt.

The hair cells of the semicircular canals are located within dilated portions of the canals called the ampullae. The hair cells are within the membranous labyrinth and arranged in rows along the surface of the sensory epithelium called the crista ampullaris or crest, a saddle-shaped structure along one wall of the membranous labyrinth (Fig. 7.5). Semicircular canal afferents enter the labyrinth through the cristae. The apical ends of the hair cells are embedded within a gelatinous cupula that spans the ampullae like a sail. This arrangement allows displacement of a cupula to couple with displacement of its hair cells. In the semicircular canals, the hair cells are aligned in a consistent pattern ascending toward the kinocilium all in the same direction. Displacement of a cupula therefore displaces the hair cells of that crista in the same direction, uniformly either exciting or inhibiting associated afferents of that semicircular canal.

The utricle and saccule are otoconial end organs. Just as for the semicircular canals, the sensory components of these organs are surrounded by endolymph within the membranous labyrinth. The utricle is oriented in a predominantly horizontal plane (parallel to the Earth when the head is upright, Fig. 7.6a) and the saccule is in a vertical or sagittal plane (Fig. 7.6b). Homologous to the cristae of the semicircular canals, the sensory portion of the otoconial organs is called the macula, a multi-layered structure of glycoproteins, proteoglycans, and calcite (limestone) crystals that sit atop the hair cells (Fig. 7.6c) [49, 56]. The most superficial layer is called the otoconial layer: a loose fibrous network interspersed with hexagonal crystals of calcium carbonate called otoconia. In fish, this layer is organized as a single large crystal or stone of calcium carbonate called an otolith, whereas in mammals it is seen as a diffuse sheet of smaller otoconia. The second layer is the gelatinous layer, which has a dense sheet of cross-linked filaments that allows coupling between the otoconial layer and the looser columnar layer [49]. The apical ends of hair cells are embedded within this gelatinous matrix. As the otoconial membrane (otoconia and gelatinous layer) moves during head movements, hair cells are deflected, affecting the firing rates of the primary vestibular afferents. Unlike in the cristae of the semicircular canals, however, the hair cells of the maculae are not uniformly arranged. The hair cells of the utricle and saccule are aligned oppositely on either side of a dividing line called the striola. For the saccule, the kinocilium are facing away from the striola, whereas for the utricle, the kinocilium are facing the striola [84].

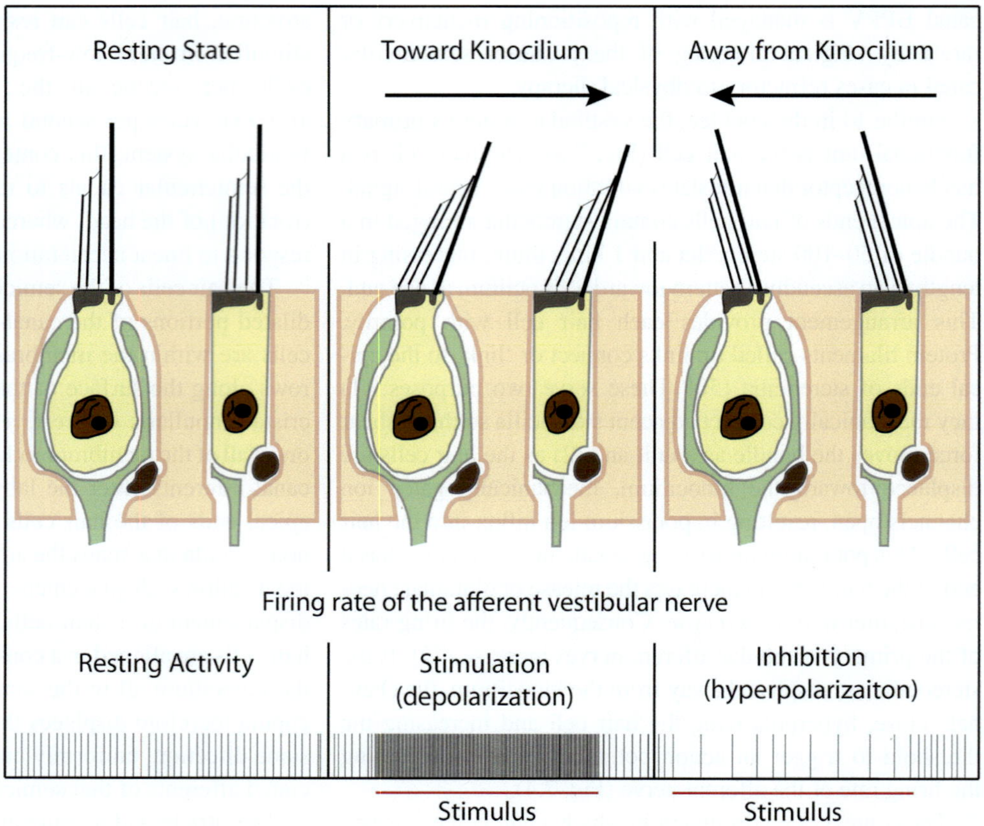

Fig. 7.4 Afferent firing rate of an individual vestibular nerve afferent fiber as a function of the stereocilia displacement. With displacement of the hair cell bundle toward the kinocilium, afferent firing rate increases, and with displacement of the bundle away from the kinocilium, afferent firing rate decreases. (©Bryan Ward. Used with permission)

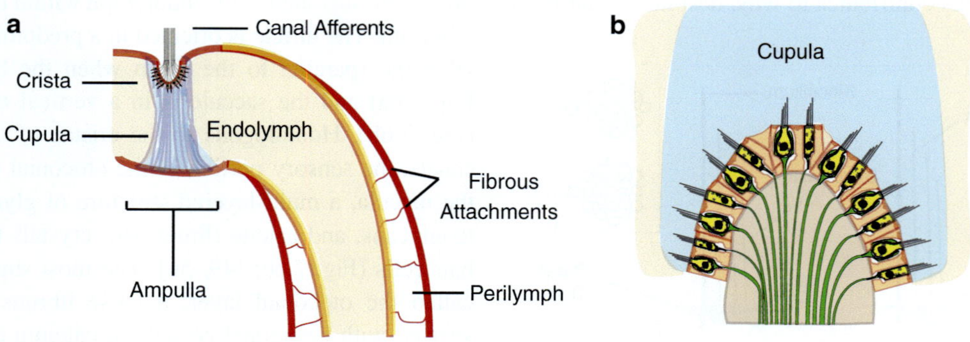

Fig. 7.5 Structure of the semicircular canals. (**a**) The membranous labyrinth is anchored to the walls of the bony labyrinth by fibrous collagen filaments. The endolymph filled membranous labyrinth is dilated at the ampulla of each semicircular canal. (**b**) Hair cells line the cristae and are embedded within a gelatinous cupula that spans like a sail from the cristae to the contralateral wall of the bony labyrinth. Hair cells in each cupula are arranged in a similar pattern. This allows cupula displacement to be transduced as a neural signal. (©Bryan Ward. Used with permission)

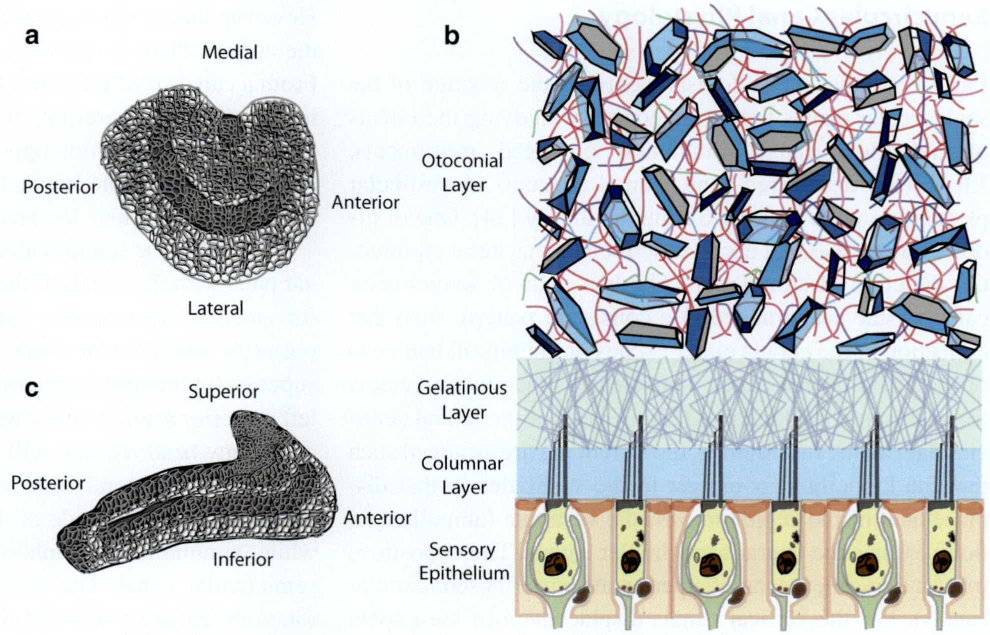

Fig. 7.6 Structure of the otoconial organs. The orientation of the right utricle is shown in (**a**) and the right saccule in (**b**). (**c**) The otoconial membrane has three layers: an otoconial layer comprised of otoconia and connecting filaments, a gelatinous layer in which the kinocilium insert, and a columnar layer. Shearing movement of the columnar layer is transmitted by the gelatinous layer, a dense mesh of randomly oriented fibers. This provides rigidity for all directions of movement. (©Bryan Ward. Used with permission)

Neurophysiology

Mammalian vestibular hair cells have two flavors: type 1 and type 2 (Fig. 7.2). Type 1 vestibular hair cells are phylogenetically younger than type 2 and are enveloped by a calyx, an axon of a primary vestibular afferent. These type 1 calyx hair cells are located more in the central areas of the semicircular canal cristae and near the striola of the utricle and saccule [26, 28]. Type 2 bouton hair cells are located more in the periphery. The type 1 hair cells primarily synapse on primary vestibular afferents with an irregularly spaced discharge pattern. The type 2 hair cells primarily communicate with synapses that have afferents that discharge with a regularly spaced pattern. Some vestibular afferents synapse on both type 1 and type 2 hair cells and are called dimorphic afferents. Dimorphic afferents can have either regular or irregular discharge patterns and tend to discharge regularly when in the periphery and irregularly when in the central areas of the crista or near the striola. Vestibular afferents with regular and irregular discharge patterns have a range of unique properties that can translate to clinical observations. Gentamicin, for instance, preferentially affects the type 1 hair cells that are associated with irregularly discharging afferents [60]. These afferents are thought to primarily encode information about the timing of head movements, for instance, during complex stimuli such as keeping one's gaze fixed during walking [47]. They are also more sensitive to high frequency stimuli and electrical currents. These irregular afferents also are preferentially lost with aging [5] or with chronic metabolic conditions like type 2 diabetes mellitus [66]. On the other hand, regularly firing vestibular afferents (associated with type 2 hair cells) are thought to better encode the fidelity of a head movement signal but are less sensitive to more complex stimuli [77].

In the absence of a stimulus, vestibular afferents maintain a baseline neural discharge or firing rate that can be either increased with excitation or decreased during inhibition (Fig. 7.4) [59]. The system is therefore bidirectional, allowing it to maintain linear responses over a wide range of different frequency stimuli and to eliminate a stimulus threshold. Finally, it provides constant input to the vestibular nucleus. The brain is continuously comparing the firing rates of each side's vestibular afferents, with differences interpreted as head movement. When the vestibular nuclei identify an asymmetry in firing rate between the two sides, the brain interprets this difference as a head rotation toward the side with increased firing rate. For prolonged asymmetries, such as during an attack of Menière's disease or vestibular neuritis, nystagmus is generated that persists until either the brain adapts to the new asymmetry or the stimulus resolves. Vertigo or the sense of rotation also occurs but adapts separately from the activity in the vestibular nucleus.

The vestibular system contains efferent nerve fibers that originate in the brainstem and project bilaterally to synapse on any of the vestibular end organs. There are several hypotheses of the functional role of efferents, but generally their function in human vestibular physiology is unknown.

Vestibular Physiology

The semicircular canals detect head angular (rotational) acceleration and the otoconial end organs detect head linear acceleration (translation) as well as head tilt.

Semicircular Canal Physiology

Early vestibular physiologists identified the function of the semicircular canals first in pigeons. By studying the effects of individual canal stimulation on head movements, J.R. Ewald discovered fundamental concepts in vestibular physiology upon which we continue to rely [24]. One of his observations was that each semicircular canal has a preferential direction of stimulation. The hair cells of semicircular canal cristae are arranged in a consistent pattern, such that deflection of the cupula either excites or inhibits all hair cells of the crista of that canal. This creates polarization vectors for each semicircular canal (Fig. 7.7a). For the lateral semicircular canals, for instance, the stereocilia are arranged such that the kinocilium is closest to the vestibule, so that displacement of the cupula *toward* the vestibule (ampullopetal flow) excites the lateral semicircular canals. The opposite is true for the vertical canals (superior and posterior semicircular canals). For the vertical canals displacement of the cupula *away* from the vestibule (ampullofugal flow) is excitatory. While this arrangement may seem counterintuitive, it allows for a simple rule: head rotation in the plane of each semicircular canal and toward that side is maximally excitatory to that semicircular canal.

To further understand how semicircular canals are preferentially excited by a head rotation in that plane and toward that side, it is helpful to consider what occurs in the cupula during a head rotation. As the head turns or rotates, both the labyrinth and head rotate in the same direction in a space-fixed reference frame (i.e., when looking at the head from above, both seem to be moving through space (Fig. 7.8).

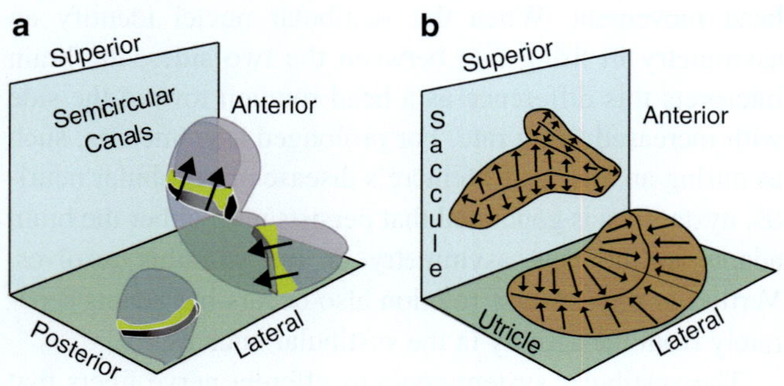

Fig. 7.7 Force polarization vectors for the cristae and maculae. (**a**) The semicircular canal cristae are polarized in a uniform direction, with forces directed away from the vestibule preferentially stimulating the anterior (superior) and posterior semicircular canals (ampullofugal flow) and those directed toward the vestibule stimulating the lateral semicircular canal (ampullopetal flow). (**b**) In the utricular macula the kinocilia are directed toward the striola, whereas in the saccule they are directed away from the striola. (©Bryan Ward. Used with permission)

However, due to viscosity of the endolymph and elasticity of the cupula, there is relatively less movement of the cupula. From a canal-fixed reference frame (i.e., if one was standing in the cupula), therefore, it appears the cupula is being deflected in the direction opposite the head rotation. It is this *relative motion* of the cupula that the brain uses to determine the direction to which the head is rotating.

Recall that the semicircular canals are organized as coplanar pairs with the canals of the opposite ear. The left superior (or anterior) semicircular canal is coplanar with the right posterior semicircular canal (LARP plane) and the right superior (or anterior) semicircular canal is coplanar with the left posterior semicircular canal (RALP plane), Fig. 7.2. As a result, any head rotation will excite one side and inhibit the other. For the lateral semicircular canals, horizontal head rotations toward the side of the canal stimulates that canal, while simultaneously inhibiting the contralateral lateral semicircular canal. The superior canal is excited by head rotations that are downward and to the side in the plane of the canal, and the posterior canal is excited by head rotations that are upward and to the side in the plane of that canal. For each of these head rotations, there is a contralateral canal that is being inhibited during the head rotation.

Another of Ewald's observations was that excitation provides stronger stimuli to semicircular canals than inhibition. This asymmetry in sensitivity to excitation and inhibition occurs because of the resting firing rate of vestibular afferents described above. If we assume that a baseline firing rate for a vestibular nerve afferent at rest is approximately 100 spikes per second [27], this rate can increase to several hundred spikes per second during excitation, but can only decrease to zero during inhibition. This creates an imbalance such that excitation imparts a greater vestibular stimulus than inhibition.

The above principles of semicircular canal physiology are known as Ewald's laws and can be seen during clinical head impulse testing. If a clinician wants to assess the function of a specific semicircular canal, one can ask the patient to keep his gaze fixed on a target (e.g., the examiner's nose) and then deliver a head impulse (high acceleration, low amplitude head rotation) in the plane of the semicircular canal being tested. During the head impulse, the firing rate of semicircular canal afferents for the tested canal increase, whereas those of the contralateral side decrease to "inhibitory cutoff" or approximately zero firing rate. When delivered at the appropriate velocity (at least 200° per second), the clinical head impulse test isolates the function of the semicircular canal in the plane being stimulated with a head rotation.

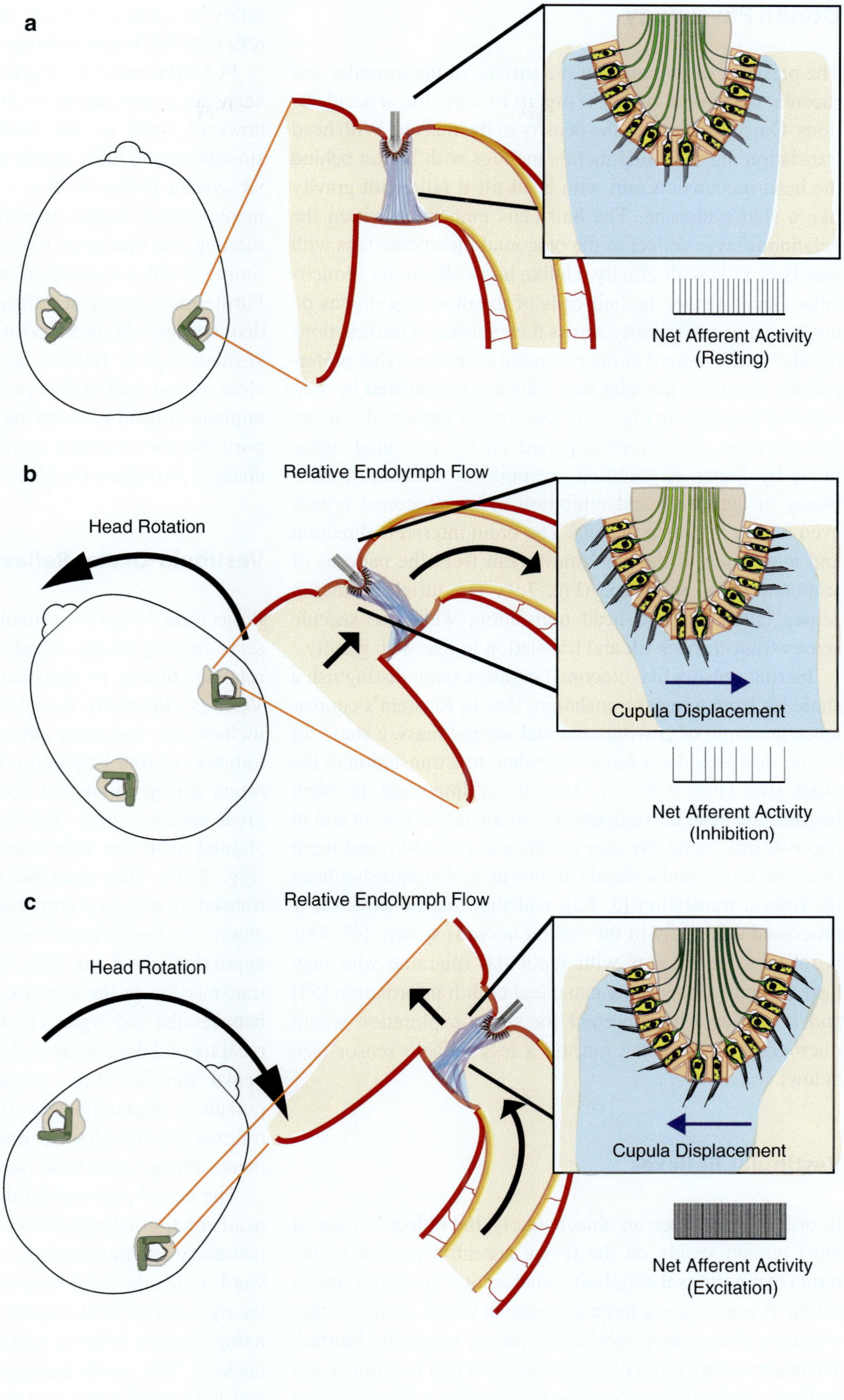

Fig. 7.8 Physiology of the semicircular canals. At rest, vestibular afferents maintain resting discharge activity (**a**). In a head frame of reference, during a head angular acceleration (head rotation), the head with the labyrinth and endolymph rotate to either the left (**b**) or to the right (**c**). Due to inertia, there is relative endolymph flow in the opposite direction that induces deflection of the lateral semicircular canal cupula. From a cupula frame of reference, the cupula is either deflected in an inhibitory direction (**b**), resulting in decreased vestibular afferent discharge, or an excitatory direction (**c**), resulting in increased vestibular afferent discharge. (©Bryan Ward. Used with permission)

Otolith Physiology

The presence of otoconia on the surface of the utricular and saccular maculae allow these organs to sense linear accelerations. Otoconia increase the density of the macula. With head translation the otoconial membrane lags with inertia behind the head movements and with head tilt it falls with gravity like a slab avalanche. The hair cells embedded within the gelatinous layer deflect as the otoconial membrane lags with inertia or falls with gravity. Unlike hair cells in the semicircular canal cristae, the hair cells of the otoconial organs do not have uniform polarity across their surface. The directions of relative movement of the otoconial membrane that preferentially stimulate macular hair cells are represented by sensory force vectors in Fig. 7.7b. Despite the pattern of sensory force vectors, the forces imparted on the otoconial membrane by linear acceleration are uniform, creating a symphony of activation and inhibition in the otoconial organs even within the same macula. The brain interprets direction and magnitude of the head movement from the patterns of stimulation and inhibition (Fig. 7.9). The utricle primarily senses lateral tilt and head translation, while the saccule senses front-to-back tilt and translation in line with gravity.

Inertial sensors like otoconial organs cannot distinguish a static tilt from a linear translation. Due to Einstein's equivalence principle of gravitational and inertial mass, a static tilt to one side provides a force equivalent to a translation to the other side (Fig. 7.9b, c). This is an important problem because the head movements are completely different and in opposite directions. We now understand that additional input from the semicircular canals allows us to distinguish a head tilt from a translation [3, 62], and that this information is processed separately in the central nervous system [4]. This is relevant for patients with vestibular migraine who may have difficulty integrating canal and otolith information [53] and is particularly important for space exploration where microgravity makes the macula a less reliable sensor (see below).

Vestibular Reflexes

In order for us to see an object clearly, the object of interest must remain steady on the fovea, a central portion of the retina that permits the highest visual acuity. Small deviations off the fovea creates a large decrease in visual acuity, so that when an object moves across the retina, it appears blurred. There are several types of eye movements that function to get an image to the fovea or to keep it there. Saccades (rapid eye movements that take the eyes from one point to another) and quick vergence (rapid movement of both eyes to either a near or far target) are two types of eye movements that bring objects to the fovea. Smooth pursuit (a visually induced reflex to track a moving object) and the vestibulo-ocular reflex (VOR) keeps an image on the fovea once it is there.

For slow-moving objects, smooth pursuit adequately keeps an object steady on the fovea. For faster movements, however, such as the head movements during walking, smooth pursuit fails, and we need a faster reflex. The vestibular system primarily drives fast reflexes. For quick movements such as those imposed on the head during walking or running, the eyes must move with the appropriate speed and timing in order to compensate for the movement of the head. Furthermore, postural reflexes are needed to adjust for sudden changes in head position. The vestibulo-ocular and vestibulo-spinal reflexes are critical for maintaining both clear vision and stable posture during both planned and unplanned head movements. Increasing evidence also supports that the vestibular system is involved in rapidly sensing changes in posture for blood pressure control.

Vestibulo-Ocular Reflexes

Projections from the vestibular system to oculomotor nuclei serve to keep images steady on the fovea while the head is rotating, tilting, or translating through space. The angular VOR is classically recognized as a three-neuron arc that includes the vestibular afferent, an interneuron, and an oculomotor neuron. Its purpose is to keep an image fixed on the retina during an angular head rotation, and it does so with great accuracy [80]. The extraocular muscles are roughly aligned with the orientations of the semicircular canals (Fig. 7.10). This contributes to any head rotation rapidly translating into an accurate eye rotation. The angular VOR is among the fastest human reflexes, with a response latency of approximately 8 ms [20]. The rate limiting step in neural transmission is the synapse. There are only three neurons between the end organ's highly sensitive hair cell mechanoreceptor and the corresponding fast contractions of the extraocular muscles. For comparison, the latency of smooth pursuit is approximately 100 ms [17]. Visually induced reflexes are too slow to provide compensatory eye movements during quick head movements.

The neural pathway for the angular VOR for a horizontal head rotation (the three-neuron arc) and appropriate compensatory eye movement is shown in Fig. 7.11. For a rightward horizontal head rotation, there is relative excitation of the right lateral semicircular canal afferents and an accompanying increase in firing activity at the right medial vestibular nucleus. This sends excitatory projections to the contralateral left lateral rectus and the ipsilateral right medial rectus via the medial longitudinal fasciculus, while simultaneously inhibiting the contralateral left medial rectus and the ipsilateral right lateral rectus (not shown). The net result is a vestibular-induced eye movement to the left. For a rightward

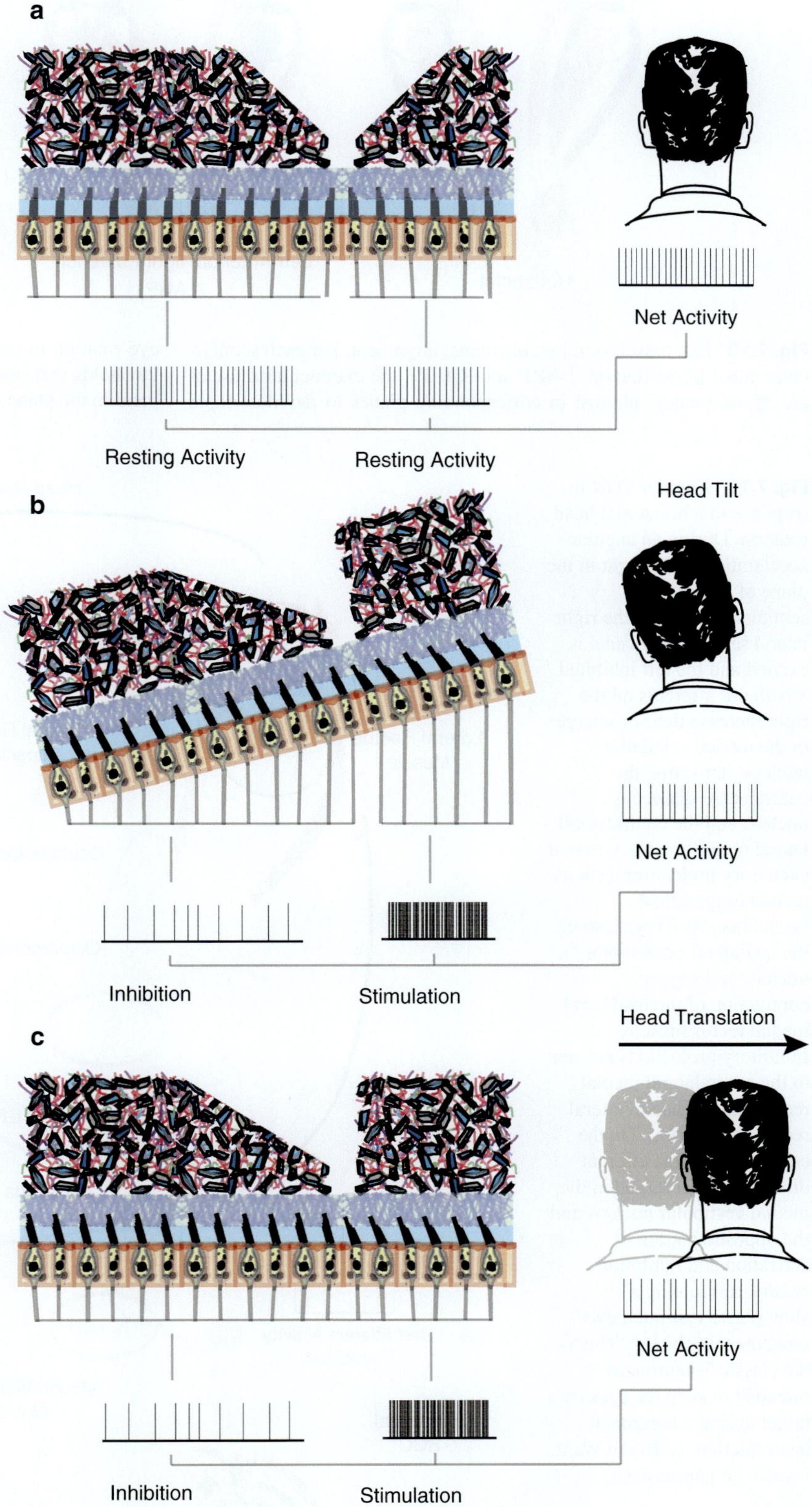

Fig. 7.9 Physiology of the otoconial organs (**a**) At rest there is a baseline firing rate of otolithic afferents of the utricle (shown) and saccule. With left head tilt (**b**) the otoconial membrane falls with gravity, resulting in a portion of the hair cells being deflected in an excitatory direction and others deflected in an inhibitory direction. This information is synthesized in the vestibular nucleus. (**c**) If a person translates to the right, the same net force is transmitted to the otoconial membrane, resulting in the same activity as a head tilt to the left (**b**). The brain uses input from the semicircular canals to distinguish a head tilt from a translation. (©Bryan Ward. Used with permission)

head rotation, the eyes should drift to the left in order to keep the object stable on the fovea. Since the semicircular canals are coplanar, the mirror image occurs on the contralateral side. The same rightward head rotation leads to inhibition of the left lateral semicircular canal, resulting in inhibition of the left medial rectus and right lateral rectus. The end physiological outcome is the same when considering one or both sides in this example; nevertheless, it is important to recall that for any head movement one side is being excited, while the other is being inhibited. Although excitation is stronger

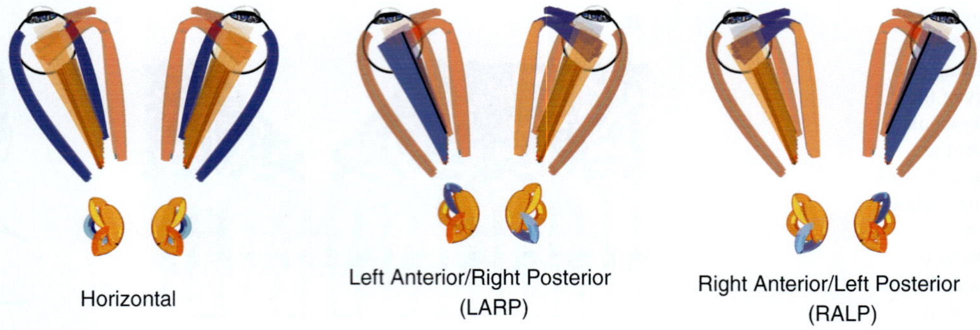

Fig. 7.10 Eye muscle-semicircular canal alignment. For each semicircular canal plane (lateral, LARP and RALP), the extraocular muscles are approximately aligned in corresponding planes to facilitate rapid eye rotation in response to head rotation and supporting Ewald's first law holds that stimulation of a semicircular canal causes an eye movement in the plane of that canal. (©Bryan Ward. Used with permission)

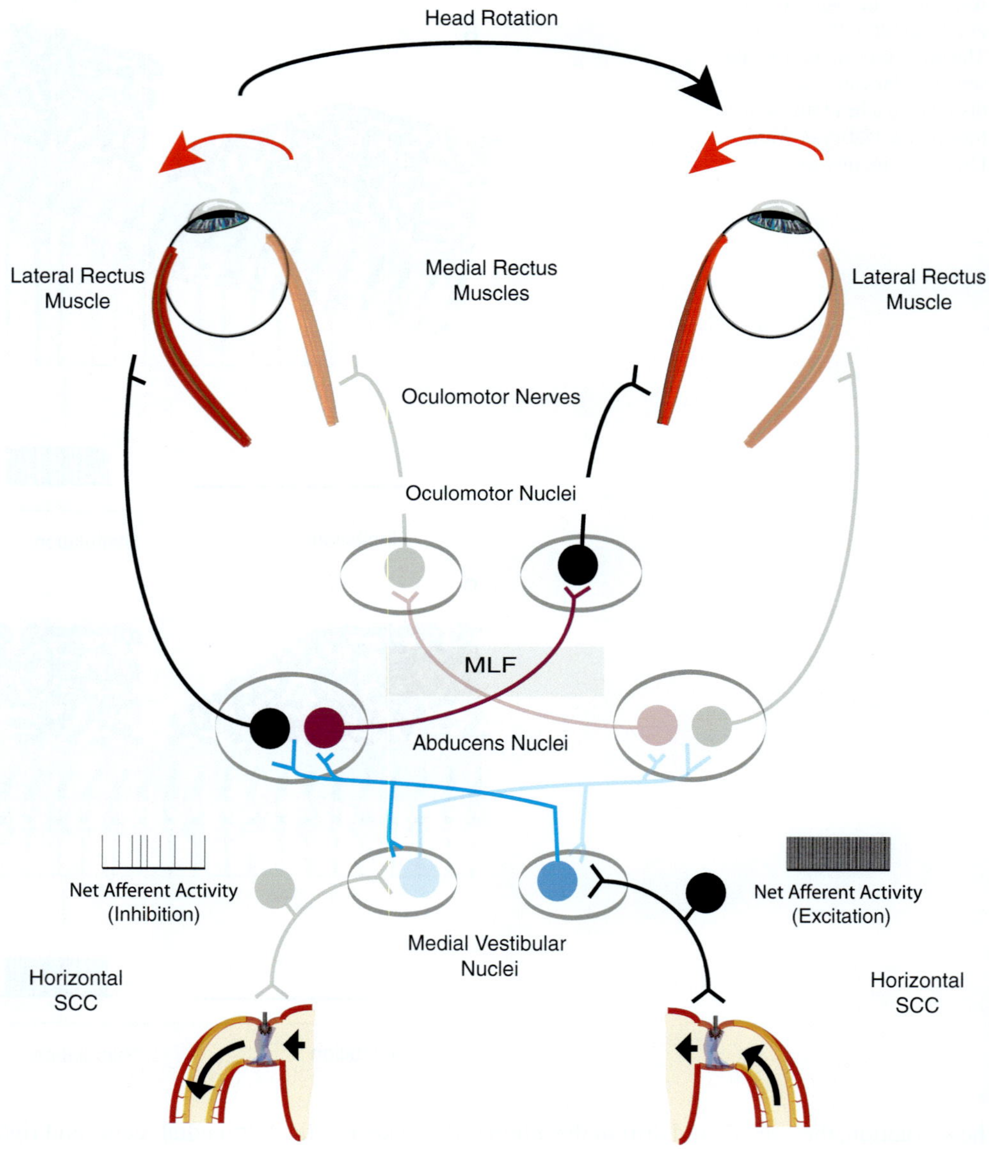

Fig. 7.11 Angular VOR in response to a horizontal head rotation. During an angular acceleration to the right in the plane of the lateral semicircular canals, the right lateral semicircular canal is excited and the left inhibited. Vestibular afferents on the right increase their discharge in the medial vestibular nucleus, activating the contralateral abducens nucleus and the contralateral lateral rectus muscle. Crossed excitatory projections (via the medial longitudinal fasciculus, MLF) synapse in the ipsilateral oculomotor nucleus and trigger contraction of the ipsilateral medial rectus muscle. Inhibitory projections are sent to the contralateral medial rectus and ipsilateral lateral rectus (not shown). On the contralateral side, afferent discharge is decreased in the medial vestibular nucleus and the opposite pattern of activation and inhibition occurs, reinforcing a slow-phase vestibular eye movement to the left. This is the classic 3-neuron arc intended to keep the eyes on a target during a horizontal head rotation. (©Bryan Ward. Used with permission)

than inhibition, the inhibitory contribution from the contralateral side accounts for why patients with loss of vestibular function on one side can still generate a VOR response to some slower head rotations ipsilateral to their lesioned side. This same push-pull pathway also exists for the vertical canals, with their neural projections ending on extraocular muscles that align with the vertical canals that are being stimulated or inhibited during the head rotation (Fig. 7.10).

The most common way clinicians assess vestibular function in patients with balance and dizziness disorders is by quantifying the VOR. The *gain* of the VOR is a ratio of the amount of eye movement relative to the amount of head movement. If the VOR is functioning perfectly, this value should be 1.0, i.e., the eye movement should perfectly account for the head movement. Normally the VOR performs well (with a gain close to 1.0) over a broad frequency range between 0.02 and 25 Hz. Even small time delays of the VOR (more than 2–3° per second) can lead to an unstable image on the retina [15]. When a patient has bilateral loss of vestibular function, objects in his vision can appear to bounce during head movements. This movement of the visual scene during head movements is called oscillopsia and is a common complaint of patients who have lost inner ear balance function on both sides. This occurs because visually triggered eye movements are too slow to adequately compensate for any mismatch between the visual scene and the fovea. Oscillopsia is less common in patients with vestibular loss on one side, but can occur during high velocity head rotations toward the deficient side.

In addition to responding to angular rotations, the eyes must be able to respond to translational or linear movements and head tilt. The linear VOR compensates for these movements and is mediated by responses initially sensed by the otoconial organs. When tilting or rolling the head to the side, the eyes make a compensatory rotation or torsional movement in the opposite direction called ocular counter roll. When the head translates, both target distance and location of the target in the visual field are important for the eye movement response. The closer the target of interest, the larger the eye movement must be in order to compensate for the head movement (Fig. 7.12). For near targets, the eyes also must move in a disconjugate manner to keep the target fixed on the fovea during the movement. The translational VOR is slightly slower than the angular VOR, but still faster than visually induced eye movements [73].

Vestibulo-Spinal Reflexes

Information from the vestibular, visual, and proprioceptive systems are combined to keep us upright. The vestibular system drives vestibulospinal reflexes and postural control strategies to compensate for perturbations to posture. The pioneering studies of the vestibular physiologists Flourens

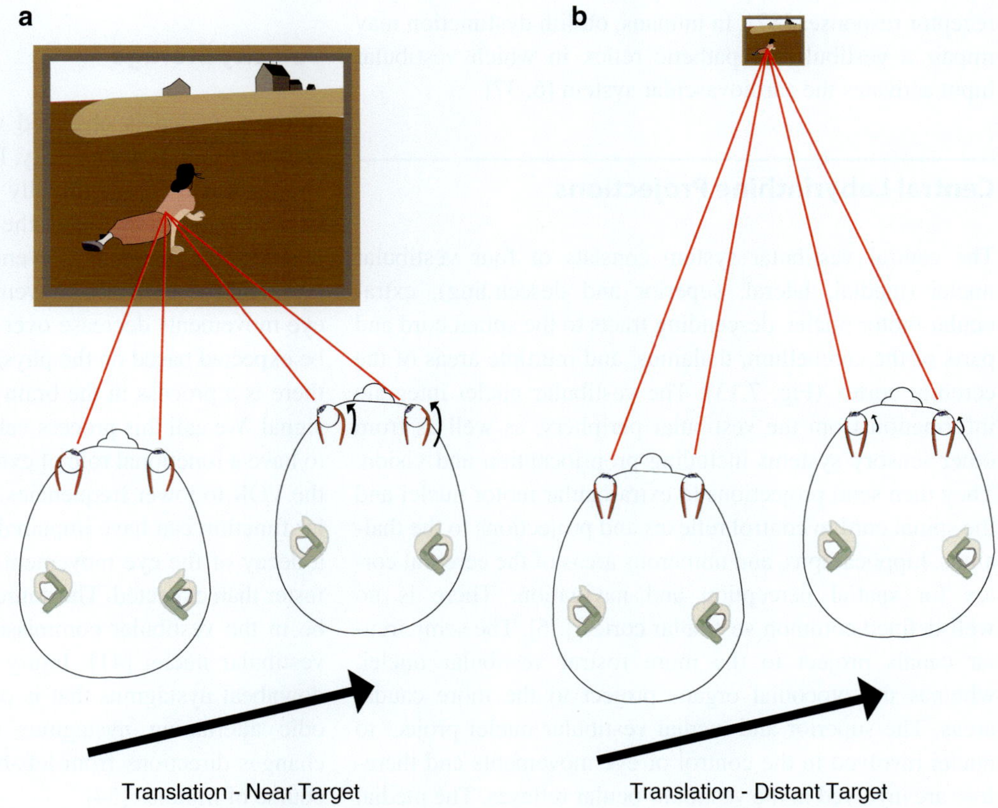

Fig. 7.12 Linear vestibulo-ocular reflex. The linear VOR is mediated by the otoconial organs and depends on both target distance and location within the visual field. When the head translates to the right while viewing a near target (**a**) the eyes must rotate by a greater amount than for a distant target (**b**) near the horizon where little eye rotation is needed to keep the target on the fovea. Similarly, when moving forward nearer a target, the eyes must rotate in a disconjugate way (i.e., each eye rotates by a different amount). (©Bryan Ward. Used with permission)

[30] and Ewald [24] first identified the core principles of vestibular physiology by studying the vestibulocollic reflexes in pigeons. They observed head movements in the planes of the stimulated semicircular canals. We sometimes see this phenomenon in patients with superior canal dehiscence syndrome where head movements occasionally occur in the plane of the superior semicircular canal in response to tones or pressure changes. Vestibulocollic and other vestibulospinal reflexes help to keep the head and body steady in space during movements such as walking [35].

The vestibular system helps maintain postural tone [14]. Drop attacks in Menière's disease are thought to be related to sudden changes in postural tone due to altered input from the otolith organs [81]. The cervical vestibular-evoked myogenic potential (VEMP) relies on a vestibulospinal reflex in which inhibitory projections are activated when the saccule is stimulated by a loud low-frequency sound. VEMPs are most commonly recorded from the sternocleidomastoid muscle, but these inhibitory reflexes can also be recorded in more distal extensors including the triceps and soleus muscles, among others.

The vestibular system also assists in regulating autonomic function. Patients often develop transient autonomic abnormalities after vestibular lesions including nausea, vomiting, and sometimes sweating, diarrhea, and palpitations [88]. While orthostatic hypotension is believed to be most commonly of cardiovascular origin, growing evidence supports that otolithic inputs contribute to the control of blood pressure during changes in posture, prior to the initiation of baroreceptor responses [87]. In humans, otolith dysfunction may impair a vestibulo-sympathetic reflex in which vestibular input activates the cardiovascular system [6, 37].

Central Labyrinthine Projections

The central vestibular system consists of four vestibular nuclei (medial, lateral, superior and descending), extraocular motor nuclei, descending tracts to the spinal cord and parts of the cerebellum, thalamus, and multiple areas of the cerebral cortex (Fig. 7.13). The vestibular nuclei integrate information from the vestibular periphery, as well as from other sensory systems including proprioception and vision. They then send projections to extra-ocular motor nuclei and the spinal cord to control reflexes and projections to the thalamus, hippocampus, and numerous areas of the cerebral cortex for spatial perception and navigation. There is no well-defined common vestibular cortex [36]. The semicircular canals project to the more rostral vestibular nuclei, whereas the otoconial organs project to the more caudal areas. The superior and medial vestibular nuclei project to nuclei involved in the control of eye movements and therefore are involved in the vestibulo-ocular reflexes. The medial vestibular nucleus also is the source for the medial vestibulospinal tract. There are numerous commissural interconnections between the vestibular nuclei.

The cerebellum is critical for adaptive behavior of vestibular reflexes and for compensating after a vestibular injury. The vestibular nuclei are the only non-cerebellar nuclei to receive direct projections from the cerebellar cortex. This has led several anatomists to consider them "displaced" cerebellar nuclei. The flocculonodular lobe of the cerebellum, known as the archicerebellum, is one of the oldest portions of the cerebellum. The principal components include the centrally located nodulus and uvula, the paraflocculus, and the flocculus (Fig. 7.13 *inset*). The paraflocculus or cerebellar tonsils can be impacted during chiari malformation. The flocculus can often be seen during retrosigmoid approaches to a cerebello-pontine angle mass. The flocculus/paraflocculus have a role in controlling the neural (velocity-to-position) integrator circuits described below [89]. The nodulus and uvula influence low-frequency vestibular input and assist in resolving the tilt/translation problem described above [86]. The centrally located vermis and fastigial nucleus control tone and both have abundant projections to the vestibular nucleus.

The vestibular system also projects to numerous areas of the cerebral cortex. There are projections to the hippocampus and people with vestibular disorders have difficulties with visuospatial information processing. This may account for some of the more amorphous symptoms patients with vestibular conditions may mention such as "brain fog."

Velocity Storage

A phenomenon is observed when you rotate someone in darkness at constant velocity. In this circumstance, the semicircular canal cupula initially displaces, and then returns to its resting position. When the cupula returns to its original position, the person will eventually no longer sense a rotation, and the VOR eye movements will cease; however, the eye movements decrease over time slower than what would be expected based on the physics of the cupula. This implies there is a process in the brain that perseverates the velocity signal. We call this process velocity storage and it is thought to have a functional role of extending the frequency range of the VOR to lower frequencies. Patients with loss of vestibular function can have impaired velocity storage, resulting in a decay of the eye movement response to a rotation that is faster than expected. The source of this process is thought to be in the vestibular commissural neurons that connect the vestibular nuclei [41]. Injury to the nodulus can result in downbeat nystagmus that is positional and can create periodic alternating nystagmus (PAN) in which nystagmus changes directions from left-beating to right-beating in the course of minutes [54].

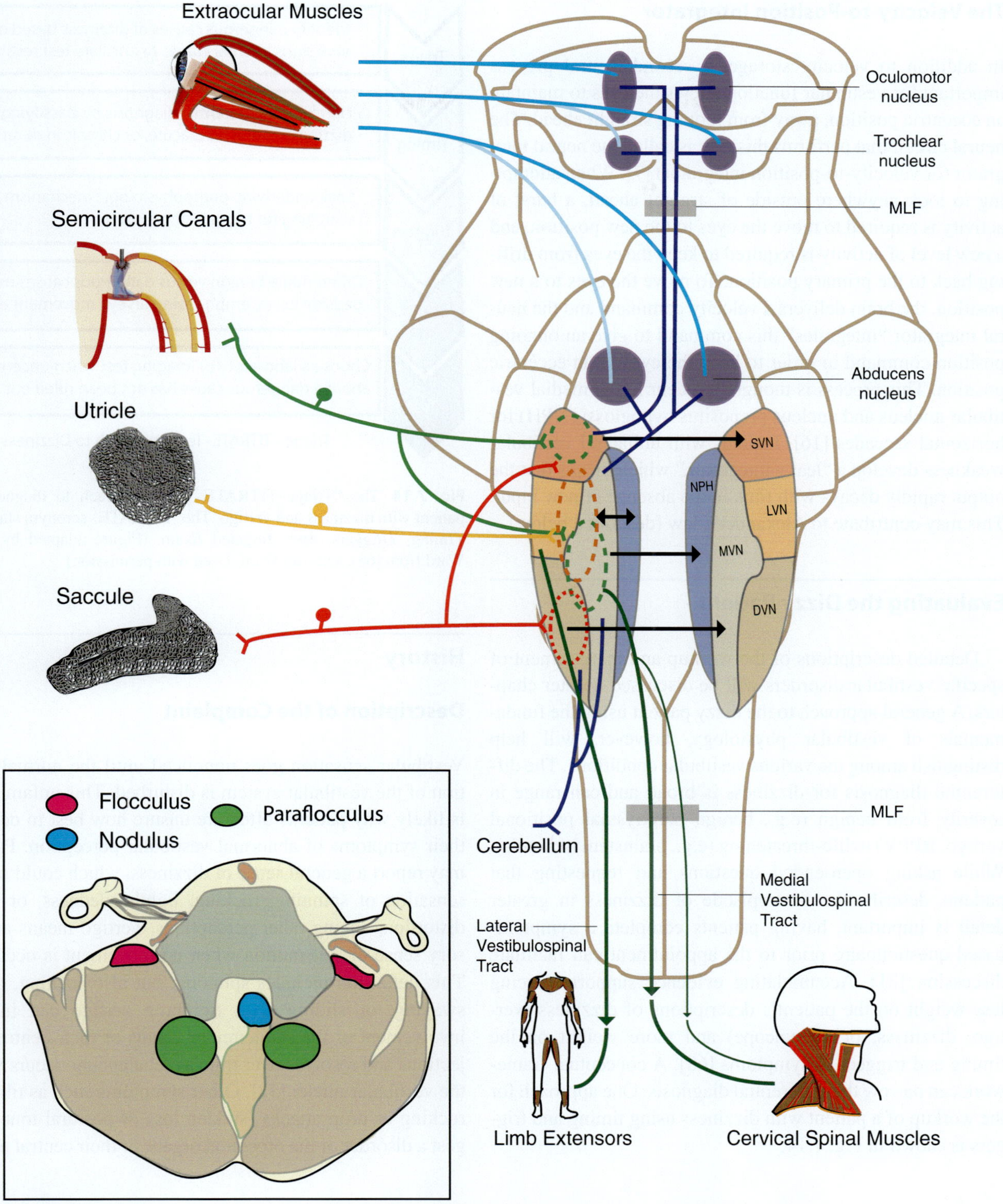

Fig. 7.13 Central projections from the vestibular periphery. The semicircular canals, utricle, and saccule project to the ipsilateral vestibular nuclei (superior vestibular nucleus, SVN, lateral vestibular nucleus, LVN, medial vestibular nucleus, MVN, and descending vestibular nucleus, DVN). Signals from the vestibular nuclei communicate with the contralateral vestibular nucleus via vestibular commissural pathways (black arrow, site of velocity storage). The nucleus prepositus hypoglossi (NPH) is the location of the neural integrator for horizontal eye movements (bidirectional arrow). Ascending projections communicate with extraocular motor neurons for the VOR and via the thalamus to the hippocampus and cortex (not shown). Descending projections via the medial and lateral vestibulospinal tracts control vestibulospinal reflexes. The cerebellum (inset) as shown on an axial MRI receives signals from the vestibular nucleus. The vestibulocerebellum consists of the flocculus, paraflocculus, and nodulus/uvula. MLF, medial longitudinal fasciculus. (©Bryan Ward. Used with permission)

The Velocity-to-Position Integrator

In addition to velocity storage, a second central process important for vestibular function allows the eyes to maintain an eccentric position, away from looking straight ahead. The neural circuit that performs this task is called the neural integrator (or velocity-to-position integrator) [7]. When attempting to look anywhere outside of straight ahead, a burst of activity is required to move the eyes to the new position, and a new level of activity is required to keep the eyes from drifting back to the primary position. To move the eyes to a new position, the brain delivers a velocity command and the neural integrator "integrates" this command to give an ongoing position command in order to keep the eyes in an eccentric position. This process is thought to occur in the medial vestibular nucleus and nucleus prepositus hypoglossi (NPH) for horizontal saccades [16]. Patients with unilateral vestibular weakness develop a "leaky integrator," which means that the output rapidly decays with time in the absence of new input. This may contribute to Alexander's law (described below).

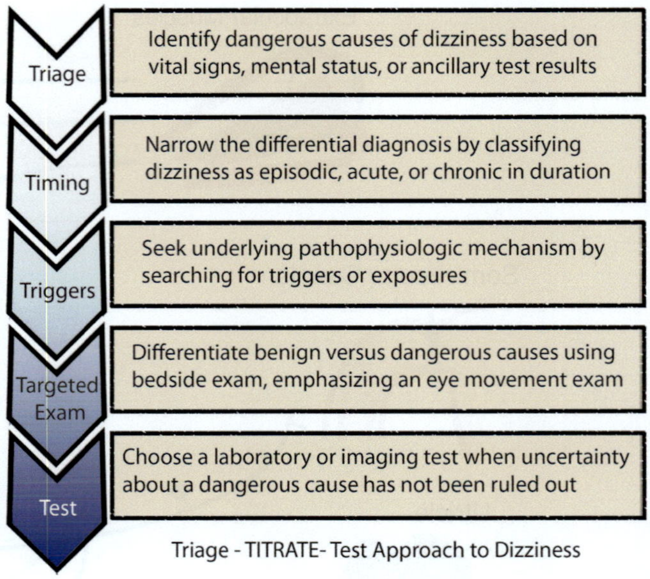

Fig. 7.14 The "Triage–TITRATE–Test" approach to diagnosing a patient with dizziness and vertigo. The 'TITRATE' acronym stands for *TI*ming, *TR*iggers, *A*nd, *T*argeted *E*xam. (Figure adapted by Bryan Ward from [68]. ©Bryan Ward. Used with permission)

Evaluating the Dizzy Patient

Detailed descriptions of the workup and management of specific vestibular disorders will be discussed in later chapters. A general approach to the dizzy patient using the fundamentals of vestibular physiology, however, will help distinguish among the various vestibular conditions. The differential diagnosis for dizziness is broad and can range in severity from benign (e.g., benign paroxysmal positional vertigo, BPPV) to life-threatening (e.g., brainstem ischemia). While asking open-ended questions and requesting that patients describe the first episode of dizziness in greater detail is important, having patients complete a symptom-based questionnaire prior to the appointment can facilitate discussion [31]. Accumulating evidence supports placing less weight on the patient's descriptions of dizziness (vertigo, dizziness, or presyncope) and more weight on the timing and triggers of symptoms [68]. A conceptual framework can narrow the differential diagnosis. One approach for the workup of a patient with dizziness using timing and triggers is shown in Fig. 7.14.

History

Description of the Complaint

Vestibular sensation goes unnoticed until the normal function of the vestibular system is disturbed. This unfamiliarity is likely why patients often are unsure how best to describe their symptoms of abnormal vestibular perception. Patients may report a general sense of dizziness, which could mean a sensation of spinning, rocking, lightheadedness, or visual distortion, among other perceptions. Vertigo means an illusory sense of self-motion when no movement is occurring. This definition includes spinning, but also rocking, tilting, swaying, or sliding [10]. Spinning vertigo can indicate involvement of the semicircular canals or their central projections and resolves over time as rebalancing occurs within the vestibular nuclei [38]. Other symptoms such as tilting or rocking or drop attacks (sudden loss of postural tone) suggest a disorder of the otoconial organs or their central projections. More general sensations of disequilibrium or fear of falling can have vestibular causes, but also problems with proprioception or musculoskeletal weakness. Presyncope may occur with anxiety, cardiovascular disease, or autonomic dysfunction. As mentioned above, qualitative descriptions do not often correlate well to a diagnosis [68]. Syncope or loss of consciousness, however, should prompt a workup for cardiovascular causes or seizures.

Timing of the Initial Episode

Descriptions of events around the time of the first episode may suggest contributing factors, for instance, onset of symptoms around a motor vehicle accident or head trauma (temporal bone fracture or traumatic brain injury), stapes surgery (perilymph fistula or misplaced prosthesis), or hospital infection (ototoxicity). The duration of symptoms during an episode is critical for obtaining a history from a patient with dizziness. In some conditions like benign paroxysmal positional vertigo is short-lasting (typically less than 1 min), whereas others like an episode of Menière's disease or vestibular neuritis last hours. Episodes of vestibular migraine can last minutes to days, while in other conditions like bilateral vestibulopathy symptoms are chronic rather than episodic.

Precipitating Factors

Vertigo can occur spontaneously, but oftentimes is triggered or temporally associated with a preceding event. Ask patients to identify any repetitive or reproducible triggers. Orthostatic dizziness occurs after arising from a supine or sitting position and may indicate orthostatic hypotension or postural orthostatic tachycardia syndrome (POTS). Other triggers can include head positions (i.e., after achieving a head position), head movements (i.e., time-locked to the head movement), or movements in the visual scene. Some visual scene movements can induce a sense of self-motion in people without vestibular disorders called *vection*. A common example is the illusory backward movement one can experience, for instance, when sitting on a stopped train and seeing out of one's peripheral vision a neighboring train beginning to move forward.

Sounds or changes in pressure as in a Valsalva maneuver can also induce vertigo in some patients. Sounds that induce vertigo in association with nystagmus is called Tullio phenomenon and pressure applied to the external ear canal that induces vertigo and nystagmus is called Hennebert sign. Both findings should prompt clinicians to consider a third mobile window syndrome like superior semicircular canal dehiscence syndrome. Sometimes chemical triggers such as certain foods or beverages (e.g., sharp cheeses, red wine, etc.), medications, weather, or hormonal changes can lead a clinician to consider a diagnosis of vestibular migraine. Other rarer precipitating factors include prolonged passive motion like on a cruise ship (mal de débarquement), heights, exercise, or deep-sea diving.

Associated Symptoms

Visual symptoms, particularly during head movements, can be associated with vestibular disorders. Oscillopsia is a false sense that the world is oscillating. Patients describe that when moving the head, the world appears to bob or shake. With bilateral vestibulopathy (e.g., after systemic gentamicin or streptomycin ototoxicity), the VOR cannot compensate for head movements and the patient is unable to maintain fixation on a target during even minor head movements. This greatly impairs one's ability to read during walking or driving and should tip off the clinician to search for peripheral vestibular impairment. If patients describe "visual lag" after a head movement, there may be a deficit in part of the labyrinth. For example, when a patient with a plugged semicircular canal performs a fast head movement in the plane of that canal, the VOR can fail to keep the eyes on target for fast head movements in that plane and toward the plugged side.

The presence of aural fullness and changes in hearing or tinnitus around the time of vertigo is part of the diagnosis of Menière's disease [58]. Sweating, palpitations, and dyspnea can be associated with panic attacks. Some central causes of vertigo are associated with a number of other neurologic findings. Headaches or visual changes are often associated with vestibular migraine. Vertebrobasilar insufficiency can cause associated dysarthria, paresthesia, or diplopia. Facial numbness or weakness, ataxia, dysphagia, or hoarseness, in association with dizziness or vertigo can indicate a cerebellopontine angle tumor, or if occurring together and acutely, could represent ischemia of the lateral medulla (Wallenberg syndrome). Changes in vision associated with oscillopsia and imbalance could reflect Cogan's syndrome.

Other Medical Conditions

Many medications taken for conditions such as epilepsy, hypertension, cardiac arrhythmias, and hyperglycemia can induce dizziness symptoms that mimic a vestibular disorder. Hypoglycemia is common and can cause dizziness. Psychiatric disorders such as generalized anxiety disorders, panic disorders, agoraphobia (fear of particular locations or situations that induce panic), or acrophobia (fear of heights) can induce dizziness and vertigo. Chronic ear disease including cholesteatoma can lead to peripheral vestibular disorders, particularly if there is a fistula in the lateral semicircular canal. In children, otitis media has been linked to dizziness as well [18]. Other common conditions including diabetes mellitus, thyroid disease, anemia, autoimmune diseases, and cardiovascular disease can cause dizziness symptoms.

Family History

Several vestibular conditions such as migraine and Menière's disease can be familial [19]. Some familial bilateral vestibular loss syndromes have been identified, and as the cerebellum is involved in control of vestibular function, there are also neurologic conditions that affect the cerebellum such as spinocerebellar ataxia 6 and episodic ataxia syndromes that can cause vertigo symptoms [33].

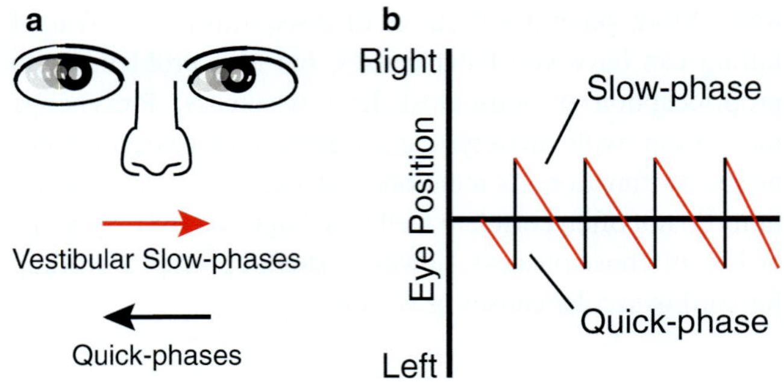

Fig. 7.15 Jerk nystagmus. Nystagmus due to vestibular stimulation has a slow-phase and a quick-phase. (**a**) The eyes slowly drift to the left and rapidly reset to the right. (**b**) If the horizontal position of the pupil is tracked over time, this generates a "sawtooth" pattern of jerk nystagmus, with a slow-phase and quick-phase. Nystagmus is often defined as the observed quick-phase (e.g., right-beating), but the slow-phases are the vestibular components. (©Bryan Ward. Used with permission)

Physical Exam

The otolaryngologist must evaluate whether the cause of a patient's dizziness is peripheral (i.e., with its origins in the labyrinth and vestibular nerves), or central (at the level of the brainstem or above). There are two general categories of the bedside vestibular exam: evaluating for static vestibular imbalance and dynamic vestibular imbalance. In performing a clinical examination of the vestibular system, much of the assessment relies on inspecting the eyes. The static components are observed without performing any provocative maneuvers. These include interpreting the pattern of spontaneous nystagmus if present as well as assessing for proper alignment of the eyes. The dynamic components require participation and are observed after the examiner perturbs the patient's vestibular system. These dynamic components include assessing for the presence of head-shaking nystagmus, appropriate eye movement responses to head impulse testing, and positional nystagmus.

Assessing Static Vestibular Imbalance

Nystagmus

Nystagmus (Greek for nod off, sleepiness) is the back and forth beating of the eyes. When nystagmus has two different components—one slow and one fast—we call it jerk nystagmus (Fig. 7.15). The slow-phase component of nystagmus is the part that is due to the vestibular system. Nystagmus is often described as referring to the fast or quick phase (e.g., right-beating or left-beating) because the quick phase is the more obvious component on exam. This is unfortunate because it is more useful to understand nystagmus by describing the slow phase, the component of nystagmus that is driven by the vestibular afferents. By knowing the direction of the slow-phase eye movements, we can deduce what part of the labyrinth is being stimulated. Recall that for a peripheral vestibular stimulus, the eyes move in the plane of the stimulated semicircular canal. If the physiology above is understood, it is much easier to interpret the nystagmus.

For example, in a patient when a left vestibular schwannoma is removed, a spontaneous nystagmus develops immediately after emerging from anesthesia. We expect the vestibular system on the side of surgery is no longer providing information to the brainstem. Spontaneous nystagmus therefore results from imbalance in vestibular input. The left labyrinth that underwent surgery no longer provides input to the vestibular nuclei, and the brainstem is therefore receiving an imbalanced signal between the two sides, with relatively greater signal coming from the contralateral right ear. The brain interprets this imbalance as a head rotation to the side of the non-operated ear. We therefore observe a mixed horizontal-torsional nystagmus.

We expect this pattern of nystagmus by thinking about what components of the vestibular system remain. In this case, the contralateral lateral semicircular canal input tells the patient's brain she must be rotating to that side. For a rotation to the right ear, the appropriate compensatory reflex is a vestibular-induced eye movement directed toward the surgical side (slow phase), followed by a resetting (quick phase) that is directed away from the side of surgery. The contralateral posterior canal provides a vertical (slow-phase down or upbeating) and torsional component (slow-phase top-pole of the eyes rolling to the left), and the contralateral superior canal provides a vertical (slow-phase up or downbeating) and torsional component (slow-phase top-pole of the eyes rolling to the left)

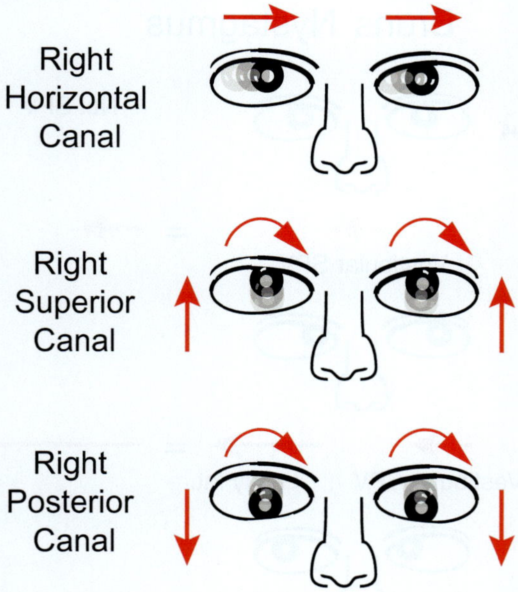

Fig. 7.16 Slow-phase eye movements generated by sustained excitation of the individual semicircular canals. Excitation of the right lateral semicircular canal generates a horizontal nystagmus with leftward slow phases. Excitation of the right superior semicircular canal generates an upward and torsional eye movement (counterclockwise with respect to the patient, i.e., superior poles of the eyes move leftward with intorsion of the right eye and extorsion of the left eye). Excitation of the right posterior canal results in downward and torsional slow-phase eye movements. Note that the torsional eye movements are the same direction for the superior and posterior canals on the same side. (©Bryan Ward. Used with permission)

(Fig. 7.16). If these are combined, there is an unopposed horizontal component, the vertical components cancel, and the torsional components sum. This is why we observe a mixed horizontal-torsional nystagmus for a peripheral vestibular lesion.

A nystagmus of peripheral origin can be suppressed by visual fixation. This means that when looking at a patient's eyes in room light and asking them to fixate on a target, any nystagmus is likely to be suppressed unless it is robust. In our example above, a spontaneous nystagmus may be seen in visible light only for a few hours after surgery. To bring out the nystagmus, the eyes should be examined with Frenzel lenses (high-diopter glasses, which allow the examiner to see the patient's eyes clearly but minimize the patient's ability to fixate) or in darkness with infrared light using video-oculography goggles. Some observations that should alert the clinician that there may be a central cause of nystagmus include pure vertical and pure torsional nystagmus, regardless of direction of gaze. A mixed horizontal-torsional nystagmus is commonly peripheral (acute unilateral loss as described above) and a mixed vertical-torsional nystagmus is consistent with BPPV and superior canal dehiscence syndrome.

Alexander's Law

A unique pattern of nystagmus occurs in patients with an acute unilateral vestibular loss in which the intensity of the nystagmus varies depending on whether the patient is looking toward or away from the direction of the nystagmus quick phase. If the nystagmus intensifies when looking in the direction of the quick phase and is relatively suppressed when looking in the direction of the slow phase, the nystagmus obeys Alexander's law (Fig. 7.17). When attempting to maintain the gaze eccentrically, the eye needs a signal to keep the eye in place. The brain integrates the saccade velocity in order to maintain a position signal and overcome the elastic recoil of the extraocular muscles. The anatomic substrate in the brain that does this calculation to maintain eccentric eye position is called the neural integrator. It is helpful to imagine that the eyes *want* to maintain a neutral position and that brainstem circuitry must function normally to keep the eyes in a different position. Gaze-evoked nystagmus is a commonly encountered finding on extreme lateral gaze, even among normal adults and is thought to be related to the interaction between this natural recoil and the neural integrator. During an acute unilateral vestibular loss, the neural integrator is thought to become 'leaky', meaning that its gaze holding ability is compromised, so that when trying to maintain a lateral gaze, the eyes drift to center. When this process is combined with spontaneous nystagmus, the nystagmus quick phases add to the quick phases of the gaze-evoked nystagmus (looking in the direction of the quick phases) and subtract when looking in the other direction. Immediately after a peripheral vestibular lesion, Alexander's law is observed. As the brain adapts to the spontaneous nystagmus by rebalancing the discharge in the vestibular nuclei, peripheral nystagmus is not observed with visual fixation.

Bruns' nystagmus can be seen in patients with a combination of a unilateral vestibular loss *and* a cerebellar insult. This can, for example, be seen in patients with a large vestibular schwannoma [57] or in patients who had surgery to remove a posterior fossa lesion and have ischemia to the ipsilateral cerebellum. The result is a problem with gaze-holding from the cerebellar injury with the usual leaky integrator effect of Alexander's law after a unilateral vestibular impairment. When the patient looks toward the intact side, the functioning labyrinth and the leaky neural integrator add to generate slow phases toward the side with less function (Fig. 7.17). When the patient looks to the side with less function, however, the effect of the leaky neural integrator is stronger than the vestibular signal, resulting in slow phases to the intact side and fast phases toward the pathologic side.

There are different forms of nystagmus that have central origins in addition to some of those mentioned above. *End-point* nystagmus can occur in normal individuals when they direct their gaze to the extreme limit of range of motion.

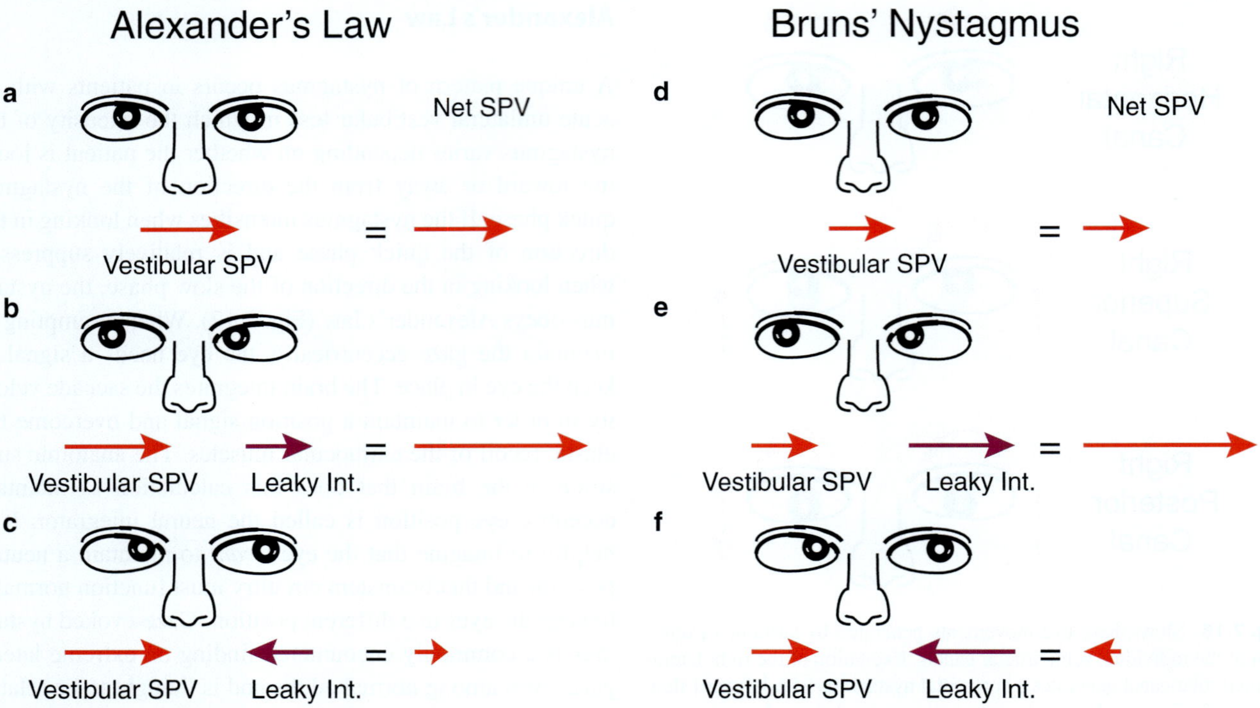

Fig. 7.17 Alexander's Law and Bruns' Nystagmus. After a unilateral loss of vestibular function, a central process called the 'leaky integrator' contributes to the observed eye motion by allowing the eye to drift back to center, regardless of its position. The combination of this drift back to center and the eye movement due to the unilateral vestibular loss causes the nystagmus to be more obvious when looking in the direction of the quick-phase (i.e., away from the lesion). In the example above, there is a left unilateral loss of vestibular function. When the eyes are looking straight ahead (**a**), only the vestibular slow-phase velocity (SPV) contributes to the eyes drifting to the left and beating to the right. When the eye looks in the direction of the quick phase (**b**), the drift back to the center due to the leaky integrator adding to the vestibular SPV and the nystagmus increases in intensity. When the eyes look in the direction of the slow phase (**c**), the leaky integrator causes the eyes to drift right, opposing the SPV, and decreasing the intensity of nystagmus. Bruns' nystagmus is a variation of this in which the intensity of the leaky integrator exceeds that of the vestibular slow-phase velocity, such that the effect is the same when looking straight ahead (**d**) and in the direction of the quick phases (**e**), but when looking in the direction of the slow-phases, the nystagmus direction appears to reverse (**f**). (©Bryan Ward. Used with permission)

Other forms of gaze-evoked nystagmus can occur with alcohol consumption or some medications [1]. In *pendular nystagmus,* the eyes drift back and forth like a pendulum, without any quick phases, and this can be attributed to brainstem pathology. In *periodic alternating nystagmus*, a jerk nystagmus is observed that changes direction approximately every 2 min and is attributed to pathology in the cerebellar nodulus and uvula. It is thought to be related to interference with cerebellar inhibition of vestibular circuitry [54] and can be treated with baclofen. *Congenital nystagmus* as the name implies is present shortly after birth. Characteristically, it worsens with attempts at fixation and in light and diminished in darkness, contrary to what occurs in vestibular nystagmus. Other forms of central nystagmus are described in detail elsewhere [55].

In summary, the otolaryngologist can distinguish a peripheral nystagmus from a central nystagmus based on a few key bedside findings. If the nystagmus increases when visual fixation is removed, if there is a combination of horizontal and torsional components to the nystagmus, and if the intensity increases when looking in the direction of the quick phase, this indicates a *peripheral* vestibular lesion. If, on the other hand, the nystagmus cannot be suppressed with fixation and is pure vertical or torsional, and does not obey Alexander's law, clinicians should think of *central* causes of nystagmus.

Ocular Alignment

Assessing for ocular misalignment, skew deviation, or a head tilt is also important for distinguishing peripheral from central causes of dizziness and vertigo. The balanced input from the utricle on both sides tells the brain we are upright. With a sudden loss of function on one side, the net activity is an imbalance in utricular input that causes the person to imagine he is tilting his head to the contralateral remaining side. The person subconsciously attempts to compensate for this perceived tilt, and these compensatory maneuvers can be observed on bedside exam. In response to unilateral loss of utricular input, the appropriate compensatory maneuvers are to: (1) perform a torsional eye movement with the top-pole of the eyes rotating away from the functioning side, (2) elevate the eye ipsilateral to the side that is functioning and depress the eye on the contralateral side, and (3) to roll or tilt the head in order to compensate for the perceived tilt. This combination of findings is called the ocular tilt reaction. Subjectively, the patient may feel that either he or the world is tilted and would be inaccurate if trying to set a line upright with respect to gravity. He may complain of vertical diplopia (one object on top of another).

We can test for a skew by having the patient fix his gaze on our nose and covering one of the patient's eyes, then the other. If a skew is present, we should observe that one eye moves upward and the other downward as we alternate covering each eye (Fig. 7.18). A combination of head tilt and skew can sometimes be seen in patients who have recently undergone surgery for a vestibular schwannoma, but the brain often quickly compensates by central mechanisms, and so the behaviors rapidly become subtle. As a result, if an otolaryngologist sees a skew, she should be concerned that the patient might have a central lesion. Wallenberg or lateral medullary syndrome, for instance, results from a posterior inferior cerebellar artery (PICA) stroke and causes skew due to ischemia of the caudal vestibular nuclei. A patient who undergoes surgery for a vestibular schwannoma and has an obvious skew or a Bruns' nystagmus may have cerebellar or brainstem ischemia.

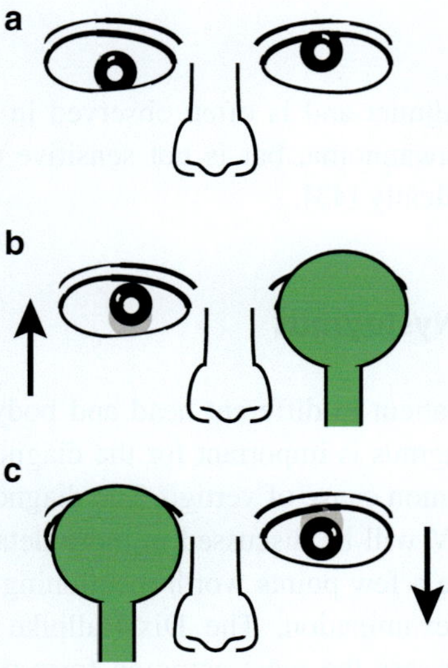

Fig. 7.18 Test of skew. The alternate eye cover test can detect a skew deviation. The eyes are vertically misaligned (**a**), but this may not be obvious at initial evaluation. The examiner occludes one eye (**b**) and then moves it to the contralateral eye (**c**) while assessing for a vertical corrective movement to suggest vertical misalignment of the eyes. (©Bryan Ward. Used with permission)

Assessing Dynamic Vestibular Imbalance

Bedside Clinical Head Impulse Test (HIT)

Described in greater detail above, the clinical head impulse test (or head thrust test) has emerged in recent years as a highly valuable clinical test of vestibular function that is easy to adopt and should be used routinely by otolaryngologists as a screen of vestibular function [39]. The test allows the examiner to isolate the function of each of the six semicircular canals [21]. To perform the test, the examiner has the patient look at a target (for instance, the tip of her nose) while performing a brief, high acceleration rotation in the plane of the semicircular canal being tested. In a patient with intact vestibular function, his eyes should remain fixed on the examiner's nose during the entire head movement. If the patient's eyes drift off the target during the head movement and make a quick saccade back to the target, this indicates a deficiency of vestibular function for the semicircular canal in the plane that is being tested (Fig. 7.19). For example, if a patient is unable to maintain his gaze on the target during a rapid head impulse rotating to the right, it suggests failure of the vestibulo-ocular reflex of the right lateral semicircular canal. For clinical head impulse testing of the vertical canals, we recommend rotating the patient's head 45° to align the vertical semicircular canals with the plane being assessed and to rotate the head up and down to assess either the RALP (right anterior-left posterior) canal planes or the LARP (left anterior-right posterior) canal planes, respectively. When the head is aligned in the RALP plane, a downward head rotation will assess function of the right anterior semicircular canal and an upward rotation will assess function of the left posterior semicircular canal. If the patient was instructed to maintain his gaze on a target during an unpredictable head movement, the eyes should remain fixed upon that target, so long as vestibular sensation is intact. While this clinical head impulse test is a useful screening tool, newer quantitative tests (video head impulse testing) are also available and becoming widely adopted.

Post Head-Shaking Nystagmus

When patients have an imbalance in dynamic vestibular function, a post head-shaking nystagmus can develop when the eyes are observed without visual fixation (using Frenzel lenses or video-oculography with infrared lighting). To perform the test, the examiner positions the patient's head with

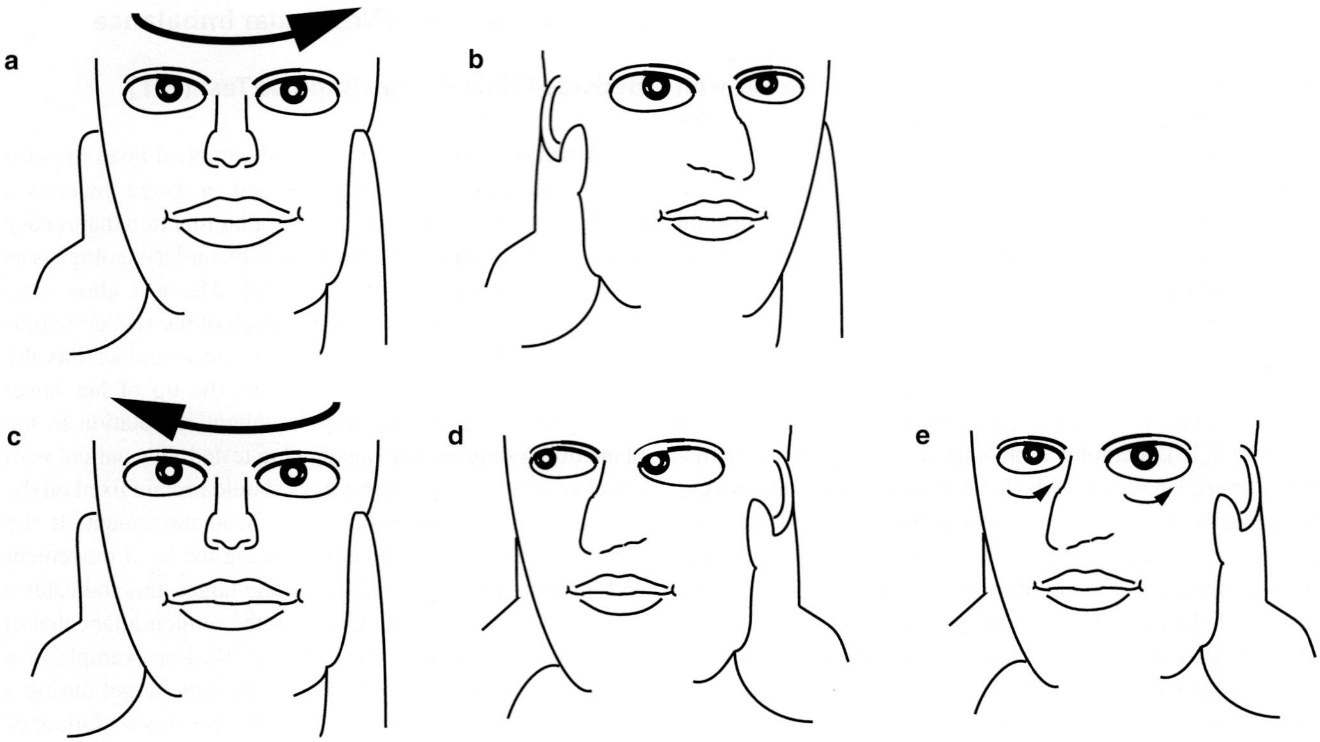

Fig. 7.19 Clinical head impulse test. The upper panels demonstrate a normal functioning left lateral semicircular canal and the lower panels a hypofunctioning right lateral semicircular canal. The patient is asked to keep their gaze fixed on the examiner's nose (**a**). With brief, high acceleration, low-amplitude head rotations to the left, the eyes remain fixed on the target (**b**). With rapid head rotation to the right (**c**), however, the eyes drift off target with the head movement (**d**) and quickly refix on the examiner's nose (**e**), demonstrating a 'refixation saccade' and indicating weakness of the right lateral semicircular canal. (©Bryan Ward. Used with permission)

nose pitched downward (chin-to-chest) approximately 20° to align the lateral semicircular canal parallel with the Earth. The examiner then shakes the patient's head horizontally for 20 cycles (approximately 30° and a rate of 2 Hz), abruptly stops, and observes the eyes for nystagmus. In patients with intact, symmetric vestibular function, no nystagmus (or one or two beats) should be observed; however, in patients with asymmetric vestibular function, a brisk nystagmus is observed after completing the head rotations [29].

When the head is rotated with high velocity to both sides in patients with asymmetric vestibular function, there is an asymmetry in the peripheral input. It is thought that the activity accumulates centrally within the velocity storage mechanism and that the nystagmus observed reflects discharge of that accumulated activity [29]. For instance, in a patient with a compensated right unilateral vestibular loss, a brisk horizontal nystagmus should be observed with slow-phases directed to the right (i.e., beating to the intact left ear). During the test, each head rotation stimulates the remaining left lateral semicircular canal (with little stimulation on the right). When the head suddenly stops moving, the velocity storage perseverates the signal, and the clinician observes eye movements consistent with a rotation toward the intact ear. Post head-shaking nystagmus is a useful clinical adjunct and is often observed in patients with vestibular schwannoma, but is not sensitive enough to be used diagnostically [43].

Positional Nystagmus

Placing the patient in different head and body positions to observe nystagmus is important for the diagnosis of BPPV, the most common cause of vertigo. The diagnosis and treatment of BPPV will be discussed in more detail later, however, there are a few points worth mentioning pertaining to the bedside examination. The Dix-Hallpike maneuver is designed to assess the most common form of BPPV (that affects the posterior semicircular canal). It is performed by rotating the patient's head 45° toward the side being tested and placing the patient supine with the head hanging off the head of the table, below the plane of the table by about 20° . The eyes are examined for an upbeat and torsional nystagmus [52]. The nystagmus is often robust enough to observe in visible light, however, removing fixation can assist in making the eye movements more apparent. The nystagmus observed as a result of BPPV has some characteristic features [9]. There is a latency of up to 30 s (typically less than

10 s) after placing the patient in the position before the onset of nystagmus and vertigo, the nystagmus is transient (about 15 s), and it decreases with repeat testing. Some patients can have positional nystagmus that does not obey these characteristic features. The vertigo occurs during the head movement, not after, the nystagmus has no latency or persists while the patient is in the tested position. This can indicate that the positional nystagmus has a central origin.

Importantly, if the nystagmus has the characteristic latency and transient nystagmus of BPPV, understanding the peripheral vestibular physiology can identify the affected canal, as the eyes move in the plane of the canal being stimulated, regardless of the patient's gaze direction. If the patient looks toward the ear that is being tested (the down ear), the nystagmus will be more torsional, if they look toward the ear that is up, the nystagmus will be more vertical, and in central gaze it will be a mixture of horizontal and vertical. No matter the direction of gaze, the eye is attempting to rotate in the plane of the posterior semicircular canal being stimulated.

BPPV can also affect the other semicircular canals. The lateral semicircular canal is the second most common and can be tested by placing the patient supine and rolling their head 90° to the right and observing for a horizontal nystagmus and then rolling their head to the left and observing for nystagmus. Characteristically, nystagmus will be observed in both positions, with the fast phases either beating toward the Earth (geotropic) or beating away from the Earth (apogeotropic). The nystagmus can last longer than for posterior canal BPPV. The direction reflects which limb of the lateral semicircular canal the debris is occupying. To determine which ear is affected, when the patient is lying on the side in which the nystagmus is most intense, the fast phase will be directed toward the affected ear. So for geotropic lateral canal BPPV, on the side with strongest nystagmus, the affected ear is the one that is closer to the Earth. For apogeotropic lateral canal BPPV, on the side with the stronger nystagmus, the affected ear is the ear that is up. Due to Ewald's second law, nystagmus will be more intense for the lateral canal for ampullopetal flow (i.e., toward the ampulla or cupula), and we can use the intensity of the nystagmus to determine the side affected. Treatment for lateral canal BPPV will be discussed in Chap. 54.

Rarely the superior semicircular canal is affected by BPPV and can be diagnosed in the Dix-Hallpike position. This is likely uncommon because the otoconial debris is gravity-dependent, and any debris in the superior semicircular canal is likely to fall to a more dependent canal with head movements. The direction of the eye movements should determine whether the superior or posterior semicircular canal is involved. The eyes should rotate in the direction of the affected superior semicircular canal, regardless of gaze direction (slow phase up and down beating, with a torsional component). Due to the rarity of superior (or anterior) canal BPPV and to the more likely possibility that downbeat nystagmus represents a central finding, a central source of positional downbeat nystagmus should be sought before assuming this diagnosis. Central downbeating nystagmus will be downbeat in all directions of gaze. Some potential causes include Chiari malformation, vertebrobasilar insufficiency, multiple sclerosis, lithium, and anticonvulsants. Central positional nystagmus can be seen in asymptomatic humans [61], as well as in vestibular migraine [71]. If downbeat nystagmus is observed, otolaryngologists should refer the patient to a neurologist.

Examination of Posture and Gait

The vestibular system sends projections to spinal musculature and controls spinal reflexes that assist the VOR. When an external force is applied to the neck or body, neck and limb extensor muscles react in order to compensate for the perturbation. As a result, impairment of the vestibular system can affect vestibulospinal reflexes and these impairments can be identified on bedside exam. Patients with vestibular hypofunction can have abnormalities of gait, posture, or head tilt. Simply examining a patient's gait can be helpful for a range of neurologic conditions, including vestibular weakness. Patients with mild bilateral vestibular hypofunction may have normal gait, but those more severely affected or with comorbid cerebellar ataxia will have a wide base of support and may sway when walking. Patients with a vestibular asymmetry may drift to the affected side when walking [46]. Observing the patient's response to external perturbations, during walking by gentle shove, can identify impaired vestibulospinal reflexes. The Fukuda stepping test is a test in which the patient marches in place with the eyes closed for 30 s [32]. Rotation can indicate acute vestibular asymmetry, but may not be sensitive for chronic vestibular asymmetry [42].

Standing balance is a combination of vestibular, proprioceptive, and visual inputs. There are therefore overlapping conditions that affect these other systems that can produce similar findings. The Romberg test is a test of standing balance that when modified can be used to systematically assess each of these three primary components in balance. In the classic Romberg test, the examiner assesses body sway when a patient stands with the feet together and with eyes either open or closed [76]. Closing the eyes eliminates vision, leaving proprioception and vestibular inputs. A failure here suggests impaired proprioception. If the patient stands on a thick foam pad (limiting proprioception), the vestibular system is further challenged [2]. There have been several modifications of the Romberg, including horizontal head shaking during eyes closed that have been purported to be more sensitive to vestibular impairment [74]. Although the amount of vestibular sensation that is isolated in these tests is controversial, the tests are sensitive to proprioceptive impairment and appear to be for vestibular impairment as well.

Other Tests

Vestibular diagnostics will be discussed in Chap. 13. There are several ancillary bedside tests, however, that may be helpful in particular cases. Dynamic visual acuity is a functional test of the semicircular canals that can be performed in the clinic. The clinician obtains a value for static visual acuity by asking the patient to read a Snellen eye chart with their head still and records the value for the line representing the best visual acuity the patient can identify. This test is best performed with the patient wearing their glasses or contact lenses and viewing a distant eye chart. The examiner rotates the patient's head back-and-forth in the horizontal plane at a frequency of approximately 2 Hz while the patient identifies which line on the Snellen eye chart she can accurately read while the head is moving. The difference between the static visual acuity and the visual acuity with head movement represents the patient's dynamic visual acuity. Recall that in order to see clearly, an object must remain fixed on the fovea and that the VOR serves this function for quick, unpredictable head movements. Dynamic visual acuity therefore assesses the degree of retinal slip due to poor function of the vestibular system and is a test of oscillopsia. Normal subjects lose approximately one to two lines of visual acuity during head movements, whereas patients with vestibular impairment can lose four or more lines of visual acuity during head rotation.

Assessing a patient's eye movements in response to performing a nose-pinch Valsalva, tragal compression, or with sound played to one ear can help identify superior semicircular canal dehiscence syndrome [64], particularly if the eye movement response is in the plane of the affected superior semicircular canal. Asking a patient to hyperventilate for 30 s can bring out hyperventilation-induced nystagmus, a finding present in some patients with vestibular paroxysmia (vascular compression syndrome of the eighth cranial nerve [78]) or a small vestibular schwannoma [63]. Hyperventilation reduces the partial pressure of CO_2 in the blood and cerebrospinal fluid, increasing the pH, and altering the binding of extracellular calcium to albumin. This leads to increased rates of discharge and conduction via the vestibular nerves that are partially demyelinated from a neighboring blood vessel of tumor. Smooth pursuit and VOR cancellation can be useful in identifying CANVAS syndrome (cerebellar ataxia, neuropathy, and vestibular areflexia [79], and vibration over the mastoid can identify a vestibular asymmetry [69].

Vestibular Physiology in Everyday Life

Patients may ask about several common experiences of vertigo and dizziness that occur in day-to-day life that are explained with an understanding of the above vestibular physiology.

Motion Sickness

Motion sickness is a common complaint of people traveling in cars, boats, planes, or any other form of transit and has been recognized at least as long as the earliest forms of written text [44]. It appears to be produced predominantly from artificial motion, and therefore was recognized as seasickness before modern transportation [65]. Symptoms include pallor, nausea, vomiting, sweating, and drowsiness. Nearly anyone with a functioning vestibular system can become motion sick in the right circumstances. The psychologist William James noted that patients without vestibular function did not experience motion sickness [48], and this led to a popular early belief that the only use for vestibular function was to induce dizziness [40].

The common underlying stimulus that promotes motion sickness is sensory conflict. This sensory conflict can be among different senses such as vision and vestibular or different sensors in the same sensory organ (e.g., otoconial organ and semicircular canal inputs). Differences in the expected sensory input and the actual sensory input can also induce motion sickness. This is likely why similar past experiences or repeat exposures are less likely to induce symptoms of motion sickness. Seasickness is induced by movements of the vessel that differs from one's perception in the cabin, and the sensory conflict theory provides an explanation for why viewing the horizon can help alleviate symptoms. Commonly, when one returns to land after being at sea, he can experience a rocking sensation that typically dissipates in hours. In an extreme form, this can become chronic, and this chronic rocking sensation after motion is known as mal de débarquement (bad disembarkation) syndrome.

Alcohol Nystagmus

Acute intoxication with alcohol can cause a peripheral vestibular nystagmus and vertigo that is positional. Although most of the effects of alcohol are central, affecting ion channels and neurotransmitters, people can experience a peripheral head position-dependent vertigo and nystagmus with excessive alcohol consumption [11]. Positional alcohol nystagmus is thought to be due to alcohol diffusing into the cupula of the labyrinth, creating a cupula that is alternatively less, and then more buoyant relative to the surrounding endolymph due to the progressive diffusion and metabolism of alcohol (Fig. 7.20a). As a result, the semicircular canals that usually detect angular rotation become sensitive to gravity as the cupula either floats or sinks with head position. The mixed signals between the semicircular canals indicating rotation and the otolith organs indicating the head still can induce motion sickness.

MRI-Induced Vertigo

People working around strong magnetic fields like those in magnetic resonance imaging (MRI) machines often report transient sensations of vertigo. Since the vertigo or sense of rotation is transient, these experiences were thought to be the result of head movements through a magnetic field. It turns out, however, if you look at a subject's eyes when they are lying still in the MRI and are not fixating (i.e., in darkness), they have constant horizontal nystagmus the entire time they are in a magnetic field of at least 1.5 T [83]. This occurs regardless of whether any MR images are being obtained. This magnetic vestibular stimulation is the result of interactions between strong static magnetic fields and the constant flow of ions through inner ear endolymph that sustains the resting discharge. The interaction creates a constant force called a Lorentz force that presses on the cupula of the semicircular canals [75] (Fig. 7.20b). The Lorentz force causes a constant displacement of the cupula of the semicircular canals, creating an effect similar to constant acceleration [82]. The effect scales with magnetic field strength, but is not harmful, except for inducing transient dizziness and nausea.

Acrophobia

Acrophobia or fear of heights spans a spectrum from a formal diagnosis of acrophobia, which affects approximately 5% of the population [23], to visual height intolerance, which occurs in about one-third of people [45]. We learned that standing balance relies on a combination of vision, proprioception, and vestibular signals. Nearly all people develop unstable posture at heights. The greater the height (capping at approximately 20 m), the less visual feedback people have available for maintaining posture, and the more they rely on vestibular and proprioceptive cues. As a result, body sway increases during standing [85]. Body position has a significant impact on a subject's perception of height intolerance, such that lying on one's stomach and looking over an edge reduces symptoms (Fig. 7.20c). This suggests that body sway at heights due to limited sensory cues promotes anxiety and enhances the experience of height intolerance. Some with visual height intolerance, however, continue to place greater weight on visual cues. Patients with acrophobia, for instance, keep their gaze fixed on the horizon, widen their gait, and stiffen their muscles, leading to increased sway [13]. This increased reliance that our brain places on vestibular and proprioceptive cues for maintaining balance at heights is also a good reason why patients with vestibular disorders should avoid heights.

Amusement Rides

As kids, we often enjoy spinning in circles and experiencing the after effects (and observing others experiencing them). If a child spins for a prolonged period in one direction and then quickly stops, they experience a strong sense of rotation and disrupted gait. The reason for this feeling is that, when we rotate at constant angular velocity, the cupula eventually resumes a stationary position. As described above, the semicircular canals detect angular acceleration, and at constant angular velocity, acceleration is zero, so eventually the cupula returns to its original position. Abruptly stopping causes a temporary deflection of the cupula in the other direction. This induces a feeling that we are rotating in a direction opposite the one in which we were spinning, and our gait is disrupted as vestibulospinal tracts try to compensate for the vestibular asymmetry. This forms the basis of the vestibular contribution to feelings that we experience after amusement rides and playground equipment, as well as rotational chair testing, in which we can observe the decay of nystagmus in response to a step in constant angular velocity. Rotational chair testing will be discussed further in Chap. 13.

Space Exploration

While not a common encounter for the practicing otologist, people exposed to microgravity environments will become increasingly prevalent as commercial space exploration expands. The unique environments of microgravity pose problems for humans who have evolved to navigate a world with fixed gravity [51]. When astronauts leave the gravity of Earth and enter an environment of weightlessness, their otoconia organs no longer have a net gravitational vector. As a result, astronauts can become disoriented and develop motion sickness or strange illusions of tilting or inversion (i.e., being upside down). They also lose the ability to detect a static head tilt, as their otoconial organs now can only detect translation (Fig. 7.20d). This impairs a person's ability to determine upright and causes them to become especially dependent on visual cues. Fortunately, the brain can adapt to these changes; nevertheless, transitions among environments with different gravity can induce dizziness and motion sickness.

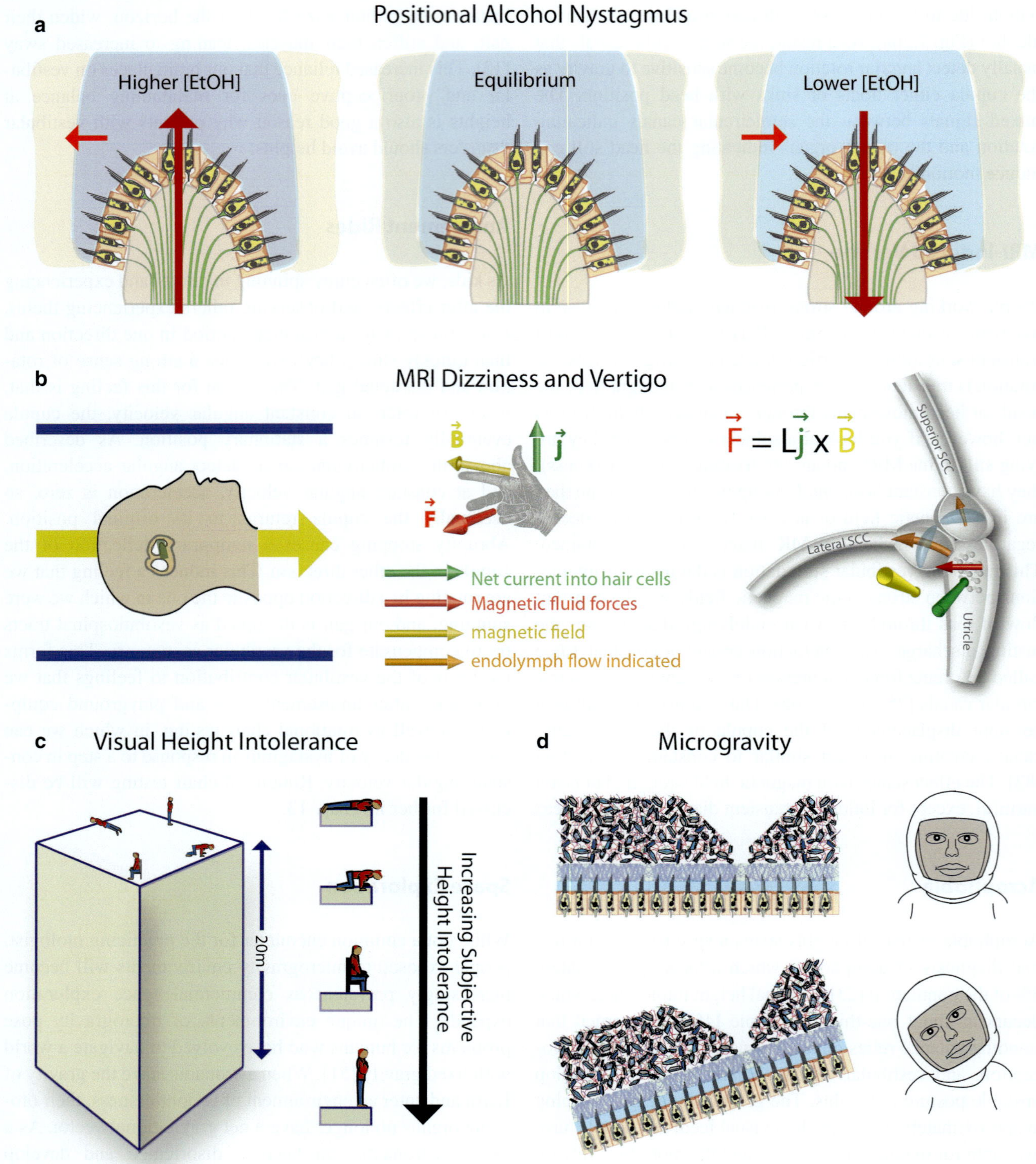

Fig. 7.20 (**a**) Mechanism of positional alcohol nystagmus depends on relative density of the endolymph and cupula. Lower density alcohol (EtOH) first perfuses the cupula due to vascular supply and slowly equilibrates with the endolymph space (middle panel) before becoming more concentrated in the endolymph as the alcohol is absorbed. Whenever there is a density difference between the cupula and endolymph, the cupula becomes displaced with head position [34]. (**b**) Magnetic vestibular stimulation occurs due to the interactions between the ionic currents entering the hair cells (*j*) and the static magnetic field of an MRI (*B*). This creates a Lorentz force (*F*) that displaces the cupula and induces nystagmus and vertigo [82]. The direction of the force is represented by the right-hand rule. (**c**) The intensity of subjective height vertigo peaks at approximately 20 m and is dependent on body position. Upright stance is least stable and induces greatest subjective height vertigo [12]. (**d**) In low gravity environments like space, there is no net gravitational vector. The otoconial organs function similar to on Earth, but in this environment an astronaut's ability to detect head tilt makes them more visually dependent. (©Bryan Ward. Used with permission)

Conclusion

The vestibular system allows head acceleration to be sensed, processed, and accommodated. It is a critical part of human physiology, without which, motion intolerance would result.

References

1. Abel LA, Parker L, Daroff RB, Dell'Osso LF. End-point nystagmus. Invest Ophthalmol Vis Sci. 1978;17(6):539–44.
2. Agrawal Y, Carey JP, Hoffman HJ, Sklare DA, Schubert MC. The modified romberg balance test: normative data in U.S. adults. Otol Neurotol. 2011;32(8):1309–11.
3. Angelaki DE, McHenry MQ, Dickman JD, Newlands SD, Hess BJ. Computation of inertial motion: neural strategies to resolve ambiguous otolith information. J Neurosci Off J Soc Neurosci. 1999;19(1):316–27.
4. Angelaki DE, Yakusheva TA. How vestibular neurons solve the tilt/translation ambiguity. Comparison of brainstem, cerebellum, and thalamus. Ann N Y Acad Sci. 2009;1164(May):19–28.
5. Anniko M. The aging vestibular hair cell. Am J Otolaryngol. 1983;4(3):151–60.
6. Aoki M, Sakaida Y, Tanaka K, Mizuta K, Ito Y. Evidence for vestibular dysfunction in orthostatic hypotension. Exp Brain Res. 2012;217(2):251–9.
7. Arnold DB, Robinson DA. The oculomotor integrator: testing of a neural network model. Exp Brain Res. 1997;113(1):57–74.
8. Bagger-Sjöbäck D, Takumida M. Geometrical Array of the vestibular sensory hair bundle. Acta Otolaryngol. 1988;106(5–6):393–403.
9. Bhattacharyya N, Gubbels SP, Schwartz SR, Edlow JA, El-Kashlan H, Fife T, Holmberg JM, et al. Clinical practice guideline: benign paroxysmal positional vertigo (update). Otolaryngol Head Neck Surg. 2017;156(3_suppl):S1–47.
10. Bisdorff A, Von Brevern M, Lempert T, Newman-Toker DE. First consensus document of the committee for the classification of vestibular disorders of the B Arany society. J Vestib Res. 2009;19:1–13.
11. Brandt T. Positional and positioning vertigo and nystagmus. J Neurol Sci. 1990;95(1):3–28.
12. Brandt T, Arnold F, Bles W, Kapteyn TS. The mechanism of physiological height vertigo. I. Theoretical approach and psychophysics. Acta Otolaryngol. 1980;89(5–6):513–23.
13. Brandt T, Kugler G, Schniepp R, Wuehr M, Huppert D. Acrophobia impairs visual exploration and balance during standing and walking. Ann N Y Acad Sci. 2015;1343(April):37–48.
14. Brodal A, Pompeiano O, Walberg F, Andkhson PJ, Peble TL, Carpenter MB. The vestibular nuclei and their connections, anatomy and functional correlations. J Neuropathol Exp Neurol. 1964;23(2):345–6. http://insights.ovid.com/jnen-neuropathology-experimental-neurology/jnexn/1964/04/000/vestibular-nuclei-connections-anatomy-functional/14/00005072.
15. Burr DC, Ross J. Contrast sensitivity at high velocities. Vis Res. 1982;22(4):479–84.
16. Cannon SC, Robinson DA. Loss of the neural integrator of the oculomotor system from brain stem lesions in monkey. J Neurophysiol. 1987;57(5):1383–409.
17. Carl JR, Gellman RS. Human smooth pursuit: stimulus-dependent responses. J Neurophysiol. 1987;57(5):1446–63.
18. Casselbrant ML, Villardo RJM, Mandel EM. Balance and otitis media with effusion. Int J Audiol. 2008;47(9):584–9.
19. Cha Y-H, Kane MJ, Baloh RW. Familial clustering of migraine, episodic vertigo, and ménière's disease. Otol Neurotol. 2008;29(1):93–6.
20. Collewijn H, Smeets JB. Early components of the human Vestibulo-ocular response to head rotation: latency and gain. J Neurophysiol. 2000;84(1):376–89.
21. Cremer PD, Halmagyi GM, Aw ST, Curthoys IS, McGarvie LA, Todd MJ, Black RA, Hannigan IP. Semicircular canal plane head impulses detect absent function of individual semicircular canals. Brain. 1998;121(Pt 4):699–716.
22. Santina D, Charles C, Potyagaylo V, Migliaccio AA, Minor LB, Carey JP. Orientation of human Semicircular canals measured by three-dimensional multiplanar CT reconstruction. J Assoc Res Otolaryngol. 2005;6(3):191–206.
23. Depla MFIA, ten Have ML, van Balkom AJLM, de Graaf R. Specific fears and phobias in the general population: results from The Netherlands mental health survey and incidence study (NEMESIS). Soc Psychiatry Psychiatr Epidemiol. 2008;43(3):200–8.
24. Ewald JR. Physiologische Untersuchungen ueber das Endorgan des Nervus Octavus. J.F. Bergmann; 1892.
25. Fenton MB, Bell GP. Recognition of species of insectivorous bats by their echolocation calls. J Mammal. 1981;62(2):233–43.
26. Fernández C, Baird RA, Goldberg JM. The vestibular nerve of the chinchilla. I. Peripheral innervation patterns in the horizontal and superior Semicircular canals. J Neurophysiol. 1988;60(1):167–81.
27. Fernandez C, Goldberg JM. Physiology of peripheral neurons innervating Semicircular canals of the squirrel monkey. II. Response to sinusoidal stimulation and dynamics of peripheral vestibular system. J Neurophysiol. 1971;34(4):661–75.
28. Fernández C, Goldberg JM, Baird RA. The vestibular nerve of the chinchilla. III. Peripheral innervation patterns in the utricular macula. J Neurophysiol. 1990;63(4):767–80.
29. Fetter M, Zee DS, Koenig E, Dichgans J. Head-shaking nystagmus during vestibular compensation in humans and rhesus monkeys. Acta Otolaryngol. 1990;110(3–4):175–81.
30. Flourens P. Recherches expérimentales sur les propriétés et les fonctions du système nerveux dans les animaux vertébrés. Balliere; 1842.
31. Friedland DR, Tarima S, Erbe C, Miles A. Development of a statistical model for the prediction of common vestibular diagnoses. JAMA Otolaryngol Head Neck Surg. 2016;142(4):351–6.
32. Fukuda T. The stepping test: two phases of the labyrinthine reflex. Acta Otolaryngol. 1959;50(2):95–108.
33. Gazquez I, Lopez-Escamez JA. Genetics of recurrent vertigo and vestibular disorders. Curr Genomics. 2011;12(6):443–50.
34. Goldberg JM, Wilson VJ, Cullen KE, Angelaki DE, Broussard DM, Büttner-Ennever JA, Fukushima K, Minor LB. The vestibular system in everyday life. In: The vestibular system: a sixth sense. New York: Oxford Academic; 2012a. p. 2–20.
35. Goldberg JM, Wilson VJ, Cullen KE, Angelaki DE, Broussard DM, Büttner-Ennever JA, Fukushima K, Minor LB. The vestibulospinal system and postural control. In: The vestibular system. New York: Oxford University Press; 2012b.
36. Guldin WO, Grüsser O-J. Is there a vestibular cortex? Trends Neurosci. 1998;21(6):254–9.
37. Hallgren E, Migeotte P-F, Kornilova L, Delière Q, Fransen E, Glukhikh D, Moore ST, et al. Dysfunctional vestibular system causes a blood pressure drop in astronauts returning from space. Sci Rep. 2015;5(December):17627.
38. Halmagyi GM, Cremer PD. Assessment and treatment of dizziness. J Neurol Neurosurg Psychiatry. 2000;68(2):129–34.
39. Halmagyi GM, Curthoys IS, Cremer PD, Henderson CJ, Todd MJ, Staples MJ, D'Cruz DM. The human horizontal Vestibulo-ocular reflex in response to high-acceleration stimulation before and after unilateral vestibular neurectomy. Exp Brain Res. 1990;81(3):479–90.
40. Hobhouse E. Aural Vertigo. Lancet. 1924;203(5251):821–2.

41. Holstein GR, Martinelli GP, Wearne S, Cohen B. Ultrastructure of vestibular commissural neurons related to velocity storage in the monkey. Neuroscience. 1999;93(1):155–70.
42. Honaker JA, Boismier TE, Shepard NP, Shepard NT. Fukuda stepping test: sensitivity and specificity. J Am Acad Audiol. 2009;20(5):311–4. quiz 335.
43. Humphriss RL, Baguley DM, Moffat DA. Head-shaking nystagmus in patients with a vestibular schwannoma. Clin Otolaryngol Allied Sci. 2003;28(6):514–9.
44. Huppert D, Benson J, Brandt T. A historical view of motion sickness-A plague at sea and on land, also with military impact. Front Neurol. 2017;8(April):114.
45. Huppert D, Grill E, Brandt T. Down on heights? One in three has visual height intolerance. J Neurol. 2013;260(2):597–604.
46. Ishikawa K, Edo M, Yokomizo M, Terada N, Okamoto Y, Togawa K. Analysis of gait in patients with peripheral vestibular disorders. ORL J Otorhinolaryngol Relat Spec. 1994;56(6):325–30.
47. Jamali M, Chacron MJ, Cullen KE. Self-motion evokes precise spike timing in the primate vestibular system. Nat Commun. 2016;7(October):13229.
48. James W. The sense of dizziness in deaf-mutes. Am Ann Deaf Dumb. 1882;28(2):102–17.
49. Kachar B, Parakkal M, Fex J. Structural basis for mechanical transduction in the frog vestibular sensory apparatus: I. The otolithic membrane. Hear Res. 1990;45(3):179–90.
50. Kachar B, Parakkal M, Kurc M, Zhao Y, Gillespie PG. High-resolution structure of hair-cell tip links. Proc Natl Acad Sci USA. 2000;97(24):13336–41.
51. Karmali F, Shelhamer M. Neurovestibular considerations for sub-orbital space flight: a framework for future investigation. J Vestib Res. 2010;20(1):31–43.
52. Kim J-S, Zee DS. Benign paroxysmal positional vertigo. New Engl J Med. 2014;370(12):1138–47.
53. King S, Wang J, Priesol AJ, Lewis RF. Central integration of canal and otolith signals is abnormal in vestibular migraine. Front Neurol. 2014;5(November):233.
54. Leigh RJ, Robinson DA, Zee DS. A hypothetical explanation for periodic alternating nystagmus: instability in the optokinetic-vestibular system. Ann N Y Acad Sci. 1981;374:619–35.
55. Leigh RJ, Zee DS. The neurology of eye movements. Oxford University Press; 2015.
56. Lim DJ. Otoconia in health and disease. Ann Otol Rhinol Laryngol. 1984;93(4_suppl):17–24.
57. Lloyd SKW, Baguley DM, Butler K, Donnelly N, Moffat DA. Bruns' nystagmus in patients with vestibular schwannoma. Otol Neurotol. 2009;30(5):625–8.
58. Lopez-Escamez JA, Carey J, Chung W-H, Goebel JA, Magnusson M, Mandalà M, Newman-Toker DE, et al. Diagnostic criteria for Menière's disease. J Vestib Res. 2015;25(1):1–7.
59. Lowenstein O, Sand A. The activity of the horizontal semicircular canal of the dogfish Scyllium canicula. J Exp Biol. 1936;13(4):416–28.
60. Lyford-Pike S, Vogelheim C, Chu E, Della CC, Santina, and John P. Carey. Gentamicin is primarily localized in vestibular type I hair cells after intratympanic administration. J Assoc Res Otolaryngol. 2007;8(4):497–508.
61. McAuley JR, Dickman JD, Mustain W, Anand VK. Positional nystagmus in asymptomatic human subjects. Otolaryngol Head Neck Surg. 1996;114(4):545–53.
62. Merfeld DM, Zupan L, Peterka RJ. Humans use internal models to estimate gravity and linear acceleration. Nature. 1999;398(6728):615–8.
63. Minor LB, Haslwanter T, Straumann D, Zee DS. Hyperventilation-induced nystagmus in patients with vestibular schwannoma. Neurology. 1999;53(9):2158–68.
64. Minor LB, Solomon D, Zinreich JS, Zee DS. Sound- and/or pressure-induced vertigo due to bone dehiscence of the superior Semicircular Canal. Arch Otolaryngol Head Neck Surg. 1998;124(3):249–58.
65. Money KE. Motion sickness. Physiol Rev. 1970;50(1):1–39.
66. Myers SF, Ross MD. Morphological evidence of vestibular pathology in long-term experimental diabetes mellitus. II. Connective tissue and neuroepithelial pathology. Acta Otolaryngol. 1987;104(1–2):40–9.
67. Nabeya D. A study in the comparative anatomy of the blood-vascular system of the internal ear in Mammalia and in homo (Japanese). Practica Otologica (Kyoto). 1923;16:1–120.
68. Newman-Toker DE, Edlow JA. TiTrATE: A novel, evidence-based approach to diagnosing acute dizziness and vertigo. Neurol Clin. 2015;33(3):577–99. viii.
69. Nuti D, Mandalà M. Sensitivity and specificity of mastoid vibration test in detection of effects of vestibular neuritis. Acta Otorhinolaryngol Ital. 2005;25(5):271–6.
70. Park JJ, Tang Y, Lopez I, Ishiyama A. Age-related change in the number of neurons in the human vestibular ganglion. J Comp Neurol. 2001;431(4):437–43.
71. Polensek SH, Tusa RJ. Nystagmus during attacks of vestibular migraine: an aid in diagnosis. Audiol Neurootol. 2010;15(4):241–6.
72. Precht W. Vestibular mechanisms. Annu Rev Neurosci. 1979;2:265–89.
73. Ramat S, Zee DS. Ocular motor responses to abrupt interaural head translation in normal humans. J Neurophysiol. 2003;90(2):887–902.
74. Reicke N. The Romberg head-shake test within the scope of equilibrium diagnosis. HNO. 1992;40(6):195–201.
75. Roberts DC, Marcelli V, Gillen JS, Carey JP, Della Santina CC, Zee DS. MRI magnetic field stimulates rotational sensors of the brain. Curr Biol. 2011;21(19):1635–40.
76. Rogers JH. Romberg and his test. J Laryngol Otol. 1980;94(12):1401–4.
77. Sadeghi SG, Chacron MJ, Taylor MC, Cullen KE. Neural variability, detection thresholds, and information transmission in the vestibular system. J Neurosci Off J Soc Neurosci. 2007;27(4):771–81.
78. Strupp M, Lopez-Escamez JA, Kim J-S, Straumann D, Jen JC, Carey J, Bisdorff A, Brandt T. Vestibular paroxysmia: diagnostic criteria. J Vestib Res. 2016;26(5–6):409–15.
79. Szmulewicz DJ, Waterston JA, MacDougall HG, Mossman S, Chancellor AM, McLean CA, Merchant S, Peter Patrikios G, Halmagyi M, Storey E. Cerebellar ataxia, neuropathy, vestibular areflexia syndrome (CANVAS): A review of the clinical features and video-oculographic diagnosis. Ann N Y Acad Sci. 2011;1233(September):139–47.
80. Tabak S, Collewijn H, Boumans LJ, van der Steen J. Gain and delay of human Vestibulo-ocular reflexes to oscillation and steps of the head by a reactive torque helmet. I. Normal subjects. Acta Otolaryngol. 1997;117(6):785–95.
81. Tumarkin A. The otolithic catastrophe: a new syndrome. Br Med J. 1936;2(3942):175–7.
82. Ward BK, Otero-Millan J, Jareonsettasin P, Schubert MC, Roberts DC, Zee DS. Magnetic vestibular stimulation (MVS) as a technique for understanding the Normal and diseased labyrinth. Front Neurol. 2017;8(April):122.
83. Ward B, Zee D. Dizziness and Vertigo during MRI. N Engl J Med. 2016;375(21):e44.
84. Wersäll J, Bagger-Sjöbäck D. Morphology of the vestibular sense organ. In: Kornhuber HH, editor. Vestibular system part 1: basic mechanisms. Springer Berlin Heidelberg; 1974. p. 123–70. Handbook of sensory physiology, 6/1.
85. Wuehr M, Kugler G, Schniepp R, Eckl M, Pradhan C, Jahn K, Huppert D, Brandt T. Balance control and anti-gravity muscle activity during the experience of fear at heights. Physiol Rep. 2014;2(2):e00232.

86. Yakusheva T, Blazquez PM, Angelaki DE. Frequency-selective coding of translation and tilt in macaque cerebellar nodulus and uvula. J Neurosci Off J Soc Neurosci. 2008;28(40):9997–10009.
87. Yates BJ, Bolton PS, Macefield VG. Vestibulo-sympathetic responses. Compr Physiol. 2014;4(2):851–87.
88. Yates BJ, Bronstein AM. The effects of vestibular system lesions on autonomic regulation: observations, mechanisms, and clinical implications. J Vestib Res. 2005;15(3):119–29.
89. Zee DS, Yamazaki A, Butler PH, Gücer G. Effects of ablation of flocculus and paraflocculus of eye movements in primate. J Neurophysiol. 1981;46(4):878–99.

8 Genetics in Otology and Neurotology

Lisa A. Schimmenti

Foundations of Human Hearing Genetics

The genetic basis of hearing impairment results from alterations in gene expression in the specific cell types required for the detection of sound [1]. There are well over two hundred genes associated with hearing loss, and this number increases monthly [2–4]. At the time of writing, the standard genetic method for identifying the basis of hearing loss is by Targeted next-generation sequencing of approximately 150–200 known genes that are associated with both syndromic and non-syndromic hearing loss [5]. Targeted next- generation sequencing can identify the basis of hereditary hearing loss in approximately 40–60% of affected patients with congenital or childhood onset hearing loss [5–9] and provides a more streamlined method to query genes with potentially causative variants.

DNA sequence variants in hearing loss genes are classified according to their potential role in causation of hearing loss. Genetic variants that are likely to cause hearing loss are classified as pathogenic or likely pathogenic. Genetic variants that are unlikely to cause hearing loss are classified as benign or likely benign. Genetic variants that do not meet criteria for being neither benign nor pathogenic are classified as "variants of unknown significance". The term "mutation" is used less and less frequently to describe a DNA sequence change as the term lacks specificity and holds a negative connotation for patients affected by a condition [10]. Thus, for this chapter, the terms "pathogenic variant" or "likely pathogenic variant" will be used to describe a DNA sequence change that is causative of a condition. Furthermore, it is important to understand the nature of the heredity of hearing loss and whether a pathogenic variant is typically inherited as a dominant, recessive, or both, as well as X-linked or through mitochondria.

L. A. Schimmenti (✉)
Department of Clinical Genomics, Mayo Clinic, Rochester, MN, USA
e-mail: Schimmenti.Lisa@mayo.edu

The Role of Proteins in Cellular Function

The concepts of heredity hearing loss categorized into dominant and recessive patterns hold more meaning by considering the biology of each specific protein and its role within the cells of the cochlea to perform basic tasks of receiving sound input and transmitting that input to the central nervous system. Imagine an inner hair cell of the cochlea and cells surrounding it in the organ of Corti. This amazing structure is incredibly complex. Not only do the cells of the organ of Corti need to complete the tasks of every other cell to survive and make energy, these cells have several specialized roles to detect sound, transport ions, and maintain structural integrity [1].

For example, hair cells have projections called stereocilia tethered to one another through proteins called tip links composed of protocadherin 15 (PCDH15) and cadherin 23 (CDH23). Stereocilia respond to sound by deflection toward the tallest stereocilia on the apex of the hair cell permitting mechanotransduction of positively charged ions and in so doing, set forth a cascade of cellular events that culminate in the release of neurotransmitters at the base of the cell to stimulate the afferent nerve contacts below [11, 12]. But when specific proteins that contribute to a hair cell are absent or their structure is sufficiently compromised due to pathogenic variants in the genes that encode these proteins, the cell may not be capable of transmitting sound input, or in many situations, the cell's survival is imperiled, leading to decreased sound detection. This is also true of other cell types within the organ of Corti that rely upon accurate protein expression to survive and transduce sound signals [1].

The Cellular Basis of Dominant and Recessive Inheritance

We are made of millions of cells, and in each cell, there is a nucleus containing nearly identical deoxyribonucleic acid (DNA). This DNA is packaged into chromosomes. Humans

A. D. Sweeney et al. (eds.), *Haynes-Glasscock-Shambaugh Surgery of the Ear*, https://doi.org/10.1007/978-3-032-18264-7_8

have a haploid set of 23 chromosomes and a complete or diploid set of 46 chromosomes comprised of 44 autosomes and two sex chromosomes. A typical biologic male has 46 chromosomes with two of those chromosomes being an X and Y, and a typical biologic female has two X chromosomes.

Each person receives one haploid set of chromosomes from each parent, and thus, we receive one copy of each autosomal gene from each parent. Each copy of the gene is called an allele. Thus, each cell has two alleles of nearly every gene (except for the X and Y chromosome in a male), one maternally and the other paternally contributed.

The Central Dogma of Molecular Biology states that genes, made of DNA, are transcribed to messenger ribonucleic acid (mRNA), and this mRNA is translated to protein by the successive addition of amino acids in accordance with a triplet nucleotide code [13]. Sequence variants in DNA may result in abnormalities of a protein product through loss or gain of nucleotides (called insertions or deletions), abnormalities in mRNA splicing, the presence of an early stop codon (called a nonsense variant), substitution of a different amino acid that would be typically found in a given protein at a given position (called a missense variant) or loss of large swaths, spanning thousands of base pairs of genomic DNA, that include coding sequence (copy number variants). Some missense variants, early stop codons or insertion/deletions are benign and do not significantly impact protein function while others are pathogenic and can be associated with a disease or condition [10].

While we have all been trained to think about dominant and recessive genes in terms of inheritance patterns only, there is often confusion that results from this paradigm. For some proteins, having one normal copy of its gene is sufficient to allow a cell to function normally. Thus, for recessive conditions, pathogenic variants are present in *both* copies of the gene to have the condition. This explains why carriers of a recessive pathogenic variant are not affected, as they have a normal copy of the gene along with the abnormal copy of the gene. For other proteins, having a pathogenic variant in only one copy of its gene results in harm to the cell and would be sufficient to cause a condition. This is typical for dominant conditions. For some proteins, depending upon the *type* of variant that occurs within that protein, they can function as a dominant or a recessive.

To summarize, a dominant condition is one that results from having a pathogenic variant in one copy of a gene whereas a recessive condition results from having a pathogenic variant in both copies of the gene. Thus, for all genes, we have two alleles, one from each parent. For hearing loss to be associated with a recessive condition, both alleles must have an identified pathogenic variant. The term bi-allelic is used to describe the presence of pathogenic variants in both copies or alleles of a gene. For a dominant form of hearing loss, only one allele must have an identified pathogenic variant.

Hearing Genetics: The Big Picture

For over 60% of deaf or hard of hearing children, there is an identifiable genetic cause [1]. For 70% of individuals who are deaf or hard of hearing, hearing loss will be the only condition, and this is called non-syndromic hearing loss. For 30% of individuals who are deaf or hard of hearing, their hearing loss will be part of a constellation of clinical findings and is called syndromic hearing loss. Thus, for the majority of deaf or hard of hearing individuals, there will be a genetic basis of hearing loss and for a third of individuals with genetic hearing loss, the hearing loss will be part of a syndrome (Fig. 8.1).

There are over 400 forms of syndromic hearing loss [14]. Usher syndrome, a condition characterized by congenital hearing loss followed by retinitis pigmentosa, is found in 4–11% of deaf or hard of hearing individuals [15]. Branchio-oto-renal syndrome, a condition characterized by abnormalities of the pinna, ear tags or pits, branchial arch remnants, and sometimes renal anomalies that can lead to end stage kidney disease, has a prevalence of less than 1% of deaf/hard of hearing individuals [16]. Pendred syndrome, the association of hearing loss with enlarged vestibular aqueduct and thyroid goiter, is the second-most common cause of sensorineural hearing loss [17]. Thus, all patients will present with hearing loss, but it is difficult to detect that a syndromic cause of hearing loss is present, a priori, and it is clinically difficult to determine if a child who is deaf or hard of hearing has a syndromic or non-syndromic form of hearing loss. For individuals with syndromic hearing loss, genetic testing may be the only way to determine if a deaf/hard of hearing individual is at risk for a syndrome prior to the onset of other symptoms (Fig. 8.1).

Recessive Pathogenic Variants Associated with Hearing Loss

To date, the majority of genes associated with congenital hearing loss are inherited in an autosomal-recessive manner. Autosomal-recessive inheritance requires pathogenic variants in both copies of the gene, one from each parent, to have a condition.

Curated lists of hearing loss genes can be identified through ClinGen [18] and the Hereditary Hearing Loss Homepage [4]. The phenotype most typically associated with recessive hearing loss is congenital onset bilateral sensorineural hearing loss, but there are few exceptions. The highest prevalence of recessive hearing loss can be found in infants with congenital profound sensorineural hearing loss [19, 20].

The genes associated with recessive hearing loss as of August 2024 are catalogued in Fig. 8.2. Curated genes that

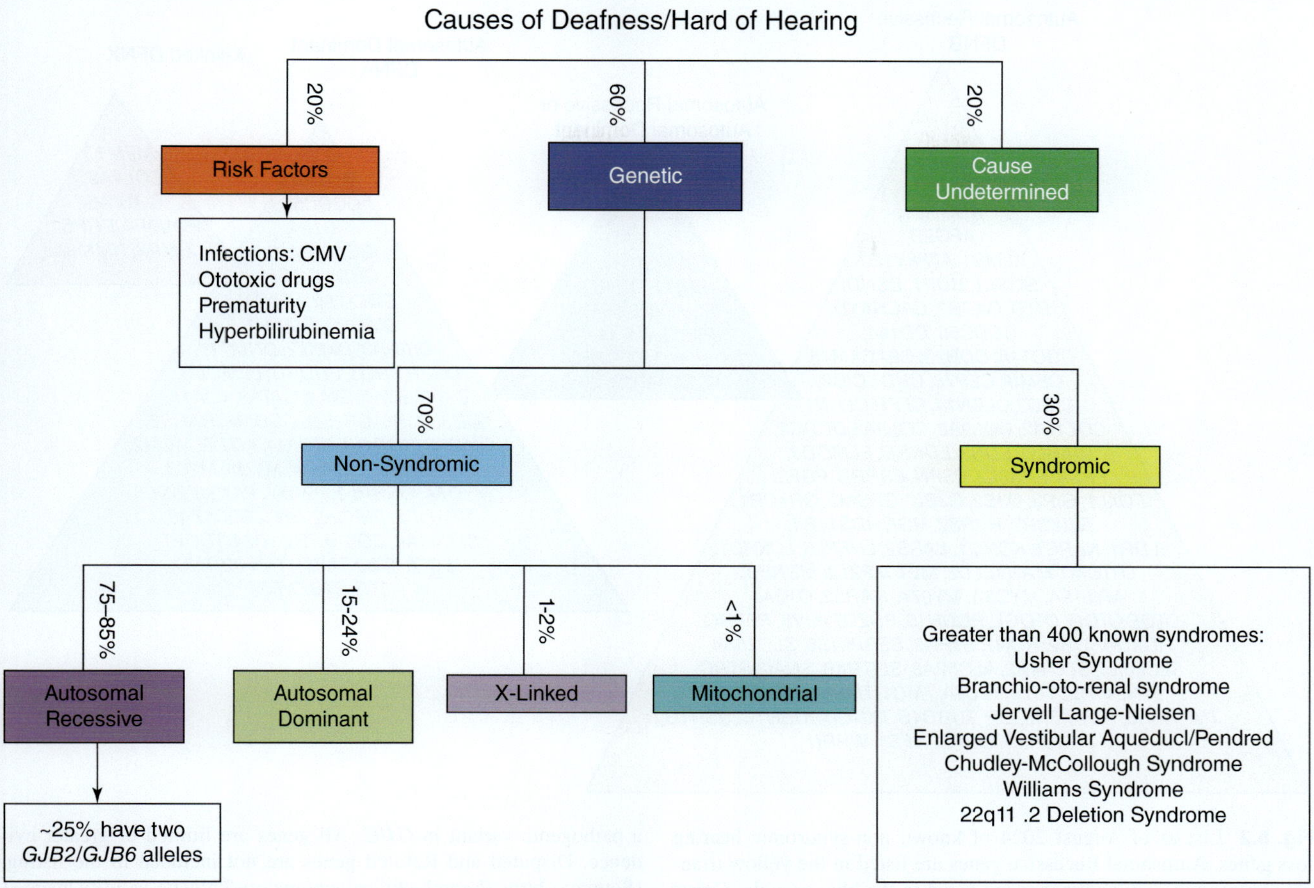

Fig. 8.1 Flow chart showing causes of hearing loss overall with a breakdown of genetic hearing loss divided by syndromic and non-syndromic forms. (Adapted from *Neurogenetics for the Practitioner.* Ed. Pastores GM. Elsevier. 2024)

have been associated with hearing loss are noted. This list is dynamic and genes that were once believed to be associated with hearing loss, such as *MYO1A* and *TSPEAR* are now disputed [21]. Efforts, such as ClinGen [22], make use of expert panels to review published data and have established criteria to determine if a gene is truly associated with hearing loss or not [4].

Criteria to determine whether a variant within a specific gene is pathogenic include previous identification in other affected individuals, relatively low prevalence of the variant in a population, significant impact on gene function through established laboratory assays or impact on gene function in animal models. A great deal of research effort is ongoing to determine whether variants are pathogenic or benign [10, 23]. Databases such as ClinVar (https://www.ncbi.nlm.nih.gov/clinvar/), ClinGen (https://clinicalgenome.org/), and the Deafness Variation Database (http://deafnessvariationdatabase.org/) maintain curated lists of benign, likely benign, unknown significance, pathogenic, and likely pathogenic hearing loss variants. Variant interpretation guidelines have been published specifically for hearing loss associated variant interpretation [24].

Dominant Pathogenic Variants Associated with Hearing Loss

Dominant inheritance implies that loss of one functional copy of a gene is sufficient to cause a condition. Genes associated with Autosomal Dominant Hearing loss at the time of this writing can be found at https://search.clinicalgenome.org listed in Fig. 8.2. Autosomal-dominant hearing loss is typically post-lingual and can occur in childhood to adulthood, but there are a few exceptions. While most dominant hearing loss affects the higher frequencies, there is one notable exception. The hearing loss associated with *WFS1* is typically low frequency, but this finding may vary according to specific variants [25].

X-Linked Pathogenic Variants Associated with Hearing Loss

X-linked hearing loss implies that the gene associated with hearing loss resides on the X-chromosome. For genetic males who have one X-chromosome, hearing loss will be

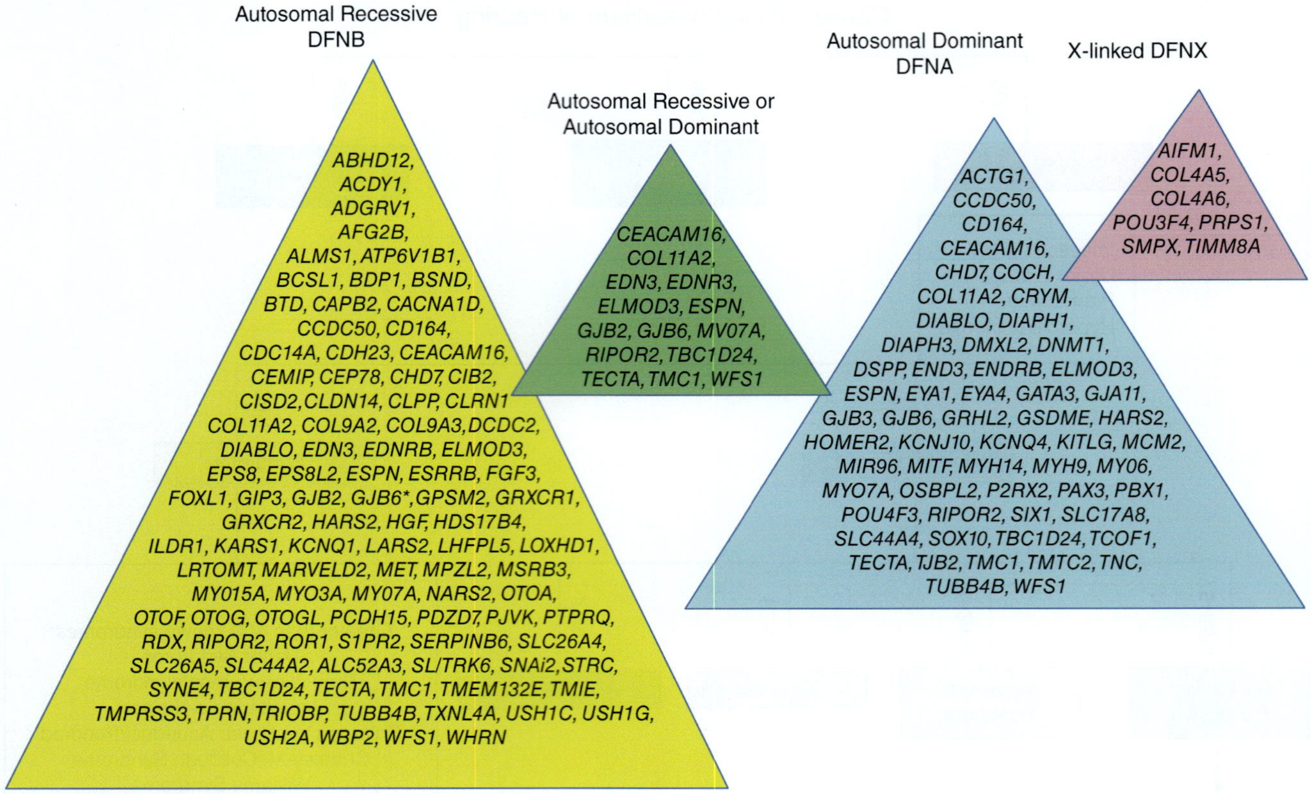

Fig. 8.2 List as of August 2024 of known non-syndromic hearing loss genes. Autosomal Recessive genes are listed in the yellow triangle. Autosomal-dominant genes are listed in the blue triangle. Genes that have variant specific Autosomal-Dominant or Autosomal-Recessive inheritance are listed in green. X-linked are listed in pink. **GJB6* can be found as a di-genic cause of hearing loss in trans with a pathogenic variant in *GJB2*. All genes are limited or greater evidence. Disputed and Refuted genes are not included in the listing. (Source: https://search.clinicalgenome.org/kb/gene-validity?page=1&size=All&search=hearing. Accession date August 6, 2024. Adapted from *Neurogenetics for the Practitioner*. Ed. Pastores GM. Elsevier. 2024)

fully penetrant and will typically be more severe and present earlier in life than in a female. Of note, the Y chromosome, which harbors genes associated with male sex determination, does not have any known hearing loss genes.

Genetic females have two X chromosomes and might escape the consequences of a pathogenic variant on the X chromosome. However, females can be affected by X-linked conditions, and for hearing genes, tend to have later onset or milder hearing loss. Much of the penetrance of X-linked hearing loss in females is related to X-inactivation. For females, to maintain normal dosage of X-linked genes, one X in every cell is inactivated. This is referred to as Lyonization, after Mary Lyon, who discovered this phenomenon [26]. If the majority of active X chromosomes in a female harbor an X-linked pathogenic allele, the individual is more likely to be affected by the condition; thus, the degree of X-inactivation modifies the phenotype of an X-linked condition in females.

While the terms X-linked dominant and X-linked recessive have been used in the past, they have been largely abandoned as there were more clinical exceptions to limit their usefulness in practice.

Mitochondria and Hearing Loss

All cells harbor hundreds of mitochondria with the role of generating energy and meeting other cellular metabolic needs. Unique among other organelles, mitochondria have multiple copies of their own genome. Each mitochondrial genome encodes proteins, transfer RNAs and ribosomal RNAs [27]. Mitochondria also rely upon the cell's nuclear genome to complete the full set of proteins needed to function properly. Mitochondria are inherited through the maternal line only and not through males. Normal mitochondrial function is essential to hearing.

The first reports of mitochondrial abnormalities as a cause of hearing loss date back to the early 1990s with observations of familial deafness that were only inherited through the maternal lineage [28, 29]. It was also observed that this deafness was associated with exposure to aminoglycoside antibiotics but could also occur at an older age and with variable penetrance without aminoglycoside exposure [29–32]. Furthermore, it was observed that deafness associated with aminoglycoside exposure did not result from elevated peak or trough levels but could occur within a short period of time after a single exposure [33, 34].

Mitochondrial deafness can occur as a non-syndromic condition or as part of a syndrome and is associated with the genes for the mitochondrial 12S ribosomal RNA1 *MT-RNR1* or the mitochondrial transfer RNA for serine, *MT-TS1*. Pathogenic variants in the gene for mitochondrial, *MT-RNR1*, specifically m.1555A > G and m.1494C > T, are the most described variants and are associated with aminoglycoside sensitivity [34]. Hearing loss is described as bilateral profound sensorineural hearing loss and occurs within days of aminoglycoside administration [35]. Hearing loss associated with the m.1555A > G variant has been reported in the absence of aminoglycoside exposure and can vary based on the degree of heteroplasmy of mitochondrial mutations [36]. Mutations in the MT-TS1, specifically m.7445 > C/T/G, are associated with non-syndromic hearing loss, but not associated with aminoglycoside sensitivity.

In addition to conditions where only deafness is observed in an apparent non-syndromic manner, nearly all maternally inherited mitochondrial syndromes present with deafness as one of the first signs of disease. Syndromic mitochondrial conditions characterized by hearing loss include Mitochondrial Encephalopathy, Lactic Acidosis, and Stroke (MELAS) [37], Mitochondrial Deafness and Diabetes (MIDD) [38], Mitochondrial Encephalopathy and Ragged Red Fibers (MERRF) [39], and Kearns-Sayre Syndrome [40]. It should be noted that in patients with symptoms of mitochondrial disease in addition to deafness, one should suspect a possible mitochondrial diagnosis. These symptoms include, but are not limited to, Type 2 diabetes, hypothyroidism, renal dysfunction, early onset stroke, myopathy, neuropathy, and cardiomyopathy [34].

The prevalence of mitochondrial pathogenic variants as a cause of non-syndromic hearing loss in the North American population may account for up to 3.5% in a large deaf cohort of 2434 probands from the National Hereditary Deafness DNA repository obtained between 1997 and 2009 [35]. It should be noted that this study was performed prior to the widespread use of targeted testing, thus it is unknown if the patients in this study had other causes of hearing loss [33].

Deaf/Hard of Hearing Genetics

The significant locus heterogeneity of hearing genes makes genetic testing and variant classification complex. To organize both hearing loss genotypes and phenotypes, a system was developed to communicate each deafness-associated gene according to its inheritance pattern and then numbered successively in the order of historical discovery based on genetic linkage studies in the 1990s and early 2000s. This system consists of the first three letters, *DFN* for deafness followed by *A* for dominant, *B* for recessive, and *X* for X-linked. Thus, the first locus identified on chromosome 13 that was associated with autosomal recessive hearing loss was *DFNB1,* known to be associated with pathogenic variants in *GJB2* and *GJB6.* While this system is used in much of the literature, as genes are being discovered by other means such as next-generation sequencing rather than linkage, this nomenclature is being used less often and the conditions more often recognized by association with a specific gene name.

Hearing Loss Associated with Pathogenic Variants in *GJB2* and *GJB6*

The most common genes associated with human hearing loss worldwide are *GJB2* and *GJB6*, and account for up 25% of deafness/hard of hearing in North American populations [41–43] with up to 50% prevalence among deaf/hard of hearing individuals in Europe, the Mediterranean basin, and East Asia [44–47]. The carrier frequency of pathogenic alleles is quite high in European and Asian populations.

Specific variants, such as c.35delG, which is a deletion of a G nucleotide at position 35 from the start codon in the cDNA transcript is the most common in Europe and North America and can be identified in 4% of hearing individuals who carry a single pathogenic variant [44, 48]. The variant c.235delC can be found in the carrier state in up to 2% of individuals of East Asian heritage [49]. The variant c.167delT can be found in up to 3% of individuals of Ashkenazi heritage [50]. The variant p.V37I is highly prevalent in East Asia, in up to 10% of individuals [51]. The variants that result from a nucleotide deletion are called frameshift variants. Frameshift variants result in premature stop codons and loss of the connexin 26 protein. The high carrier frequency of these known ethnic specific pathogenic variants is the reason why *GJB2*-related hearing loss is commonly encountered.

In addition to single nucleotide variants in *GJB2*, large deletions in *GJB6* are commonly encountered in European and Middle Eastern populations [52–55]. This deletion results in both loss of *GJB2* and *GJB6* expression from the chromosome bearing this deletion [56].

GJB2 and the adjacent gene on human chromosome 13, *GJB6*, encode the proteins named Connexin 26 and Connexin 30, respectively. These gap junction proteins are expressed throughout the cochlea in supporting cells surrounding hair cells, the stria vascularis, as well as other cells in the cochlear but *not* the hair cells themselves [57]. The mechanism by which loss of function variants in *GJB2* and *GJB6* cause hearing loss is a topic of intense study but current evidence supports a critical role in early development by facilitating the functional maturation of hair cells through gap junction mediated regulation of calcium transport in supporting cells and other surrounding cells of the cochlea [58].

The phenotype of hearing loss associated with autosomal-recessive *GJB2*-related hearing loss is congenital bilateral sensorineural hearing loss. Significant genotype–phenotype correlation has been observed. A large international consortium demonstrated that individuals harboring variants in *GJB2* that resulted in a premature stop codon, either a nonsense or frameshift variant in both copies of the gene, results in a severe to profound sensorineural hearing loss. Thus, an individual who has a c.35delG on both copies of *GJB2* would be expected to have severe to profound sensorineural hearing loss; however, variability has been observed. An individual who has two missense variants would be expected to have mild-moderate hearing loss. An individual who has one missense variant and one frameshift or early stop codon variant could have hearing loss somewhere in the mild-severe range depending upon the variant. Individuals who have a frameshift variant in *GJB2* and a deletion in *GJB6* are profoundly deaf [59].

It was initially believed that *GJB2*-related hearing loss was non-progressive. Two longitudinal studies have demonstrated mild progression of hearing loss over time [60, 61].

Individuals with autosomal-recessive pathogenic variants in *GJB2* have no other health issues as this is a non-syndromic form of hearing loss. Temporal bone anomalies are rare [61, 62].

There are a small number of individuals who have autosomal-dominant variants in *GJB2*. Hearing loss associated with autosomal-dominant *GJB2* pathogenic variants is typically bilateral, sensorineural hearing loss that ranges from mild to profound. Autosomal- dominant *GJB2* pathogenic variants are typically found in syndromic form with hyperkeratotic skin conditions such as Vohwinkle Syndrome, Bart-Pumphery, KID syndrome, Hystrix-like ichthyosis and deafness, and Palmoplantar Keratoderma and Deafness and Clouston Syndrome [63]. In contrast to the recessive variants that confer loss of function of the Connexin 26 protein, the autosomal-dominant variants confer a gain of function [64].

Hearing Loss Associated with *SLC26A4*

SLC26A4, a gene encoding protein that functions as a chloride, bicarbonate, and iodine transporter, is expressed in supporting cells of the cochlea, thyroid, and kidney. *SLC26A4* autosomal-recessive pathogenic variants are associated with non-syndromic hearing loss with enlargement of the vestibular aqueduct as well as Pendred Syndrome [65, 66]. Pendred Syndrome describes a condition characterized by bilateral sensorineural hearing loss with the development of thyroid goiter [67].

Variants in *SLC26A4* are the second-most commonly identified genetic cause found in patients who are deaf or hard of hearing [8, 68, 69]. In patients who have undergone temporal bone imaging and are identified to have enlarged vestibular aqueduct, bi-allelic pathogenic variants in *SLC26A4*, can be identified in up to 40% of individuals [68]. Furthermore, individuals with unilateral hearing loss and unilateral enlargement of the vestibular aqueduct, pathogenic variants in *SLC26A4* are frequently identified [70].

Patients with bi-allelic *SLC26A4* variants have a broad range of sensorineural hearing loss severity from mild to profound. Progression of hearing loss is typical, particularly rapid progression. Even within families, there is a range of hearing severity and progression with little genotype/phenotype correlation. Discovery of hearing loss can be at birth or shortly thereafter [71, 72].

The penetrance of thyroid phenotypes is quite variable with some family members developing thyroid goiter and others not [72, 73]. While it has been believed that thyroid goiter and thyroid insufficiency in Pendred syndrome occurred during or after the second decade, it has now become apparent that thyroid insufficiency can occur at birth and affected infants can present with congenital hypothyroidism [74].

Hearing Loss Associated with Variants in *MYO7A*, *CDH23*, and Other Genes Associated with Stereocilia Apparatus

The organ of Corti contains hair cells; specialized mechanosensors that respond to sound. The apical surface of each hair cell supports a size-organized cluster of actin fibril packed stereocilia [75]. Stereocilia, ordered from shortest to tallest, are tethered in succession through tip-links composed of PCDH15 and CDH23 [76–78]. Each tip link forms an attachment to the adjacent tallest stereocilia through an upper tip link density composed of MYO7A, Harmonin (USH1C), and Sans (USH1G) [79, 80].

Pathogenic variants in all genes encoding this group of proteins known to be expressed in stereocilia tip link [81], apart from *USH1G*, can be associated with either non-syndromic hearing loss or with Usher Syndrome. Autosomal-recessive pathogenic variants in *MYO7A*, *CDH23*, *PCDH15*, *USH1C*, and *USH1G* are associated with Usher Syndrome Type 1 as each are expressed in the retina as well the inner ear cite: [157]. *MYO7A* is associated with both recessive and dominant non-syndromic hearing loss, *DFNB2, DFNA11*; CDH23 is associated with recessive non-syndromic hearing loss *DFNB12*; PCDH15 is associated with *DFNB23;* and USH1C is associated with recessive non-syndromic hearing loss *DFNB18A* (OMIM).

One of the greatest challenges for patients who harbor pathogenic variants in genes that can cause either Usher Syndrome or non-syndromic hearing loss is to predict which patients will have non-syndromic hearing loss versus those that will go on to develop retinitis pigmentosa and fall under the category of Usher Syndrome Type 1. For *MYO7A, CDH23, or PCDH15 pathogenic variants identified* in deaf or hard of hearing infants, there remain ambiguities, but some correlations exist to reasonably predict whether a child has non-syndromic hearing loss or Usher Syndrome Type 1. For *CDH23*, genotype–phenotype correlations have emerged where missense variants that retain some functions are associated with non-syndromic hearing loss (*DFNB12*) while variants that result in absent or severely impaired proteins result in Usher Syndrome [82]. For individuals who harbor bi-allelic variants where at least one of the variants retains protein function, that individual is more likely to have only hearing loss and not develop vision loss. For *MYO7A*, similar predictions are made where variant proteins with residual function are more likely to result in hearing loss only (*DFNB2*) whereas those with loss of function are more likely to result in Usher Syndrome Type 1 [83]. For *PCDH15*, missense variants that retain protein function are more likely to be associated with *DFNB23* and variants causing loss of protein function associated with Usher Syndrome Type 1 [84].

Hearing Loss Associated with *TMC1* and Other Genes Associated with the Mechanoelectrical Transduction Channel

Despite two decades of research into the composition and function of the mechanotransduction channel, the complete set of proteins composing this channel remains unknown [85, 86]. Nonetheless, evidence points to a group of proteins encoded by the genes *TMC1, LHFPL5*, and *TMIE* that compose part of the mechanoelectrical transduction channel. Autosomal-recessive or autosomal-dominant pathogenic variants in *TMC1* are associated with sensorineural hearing loss [81]. *LHFPL5*, and *TMIE* are only associated with autosomal- recessive bilateral congenital sensorineural hearing loss. The phenotype associated with this group of genes is progressive bilateral sensorineural [87–89].

Syndromic Hearing Loss

Usher Syndrome

Usher Syndrome is an autosomal-recessive condition characterized by early onset sensorineural hearing loss with or without balance issues followed by the development of retinitis pigmentosa. Usher Syndrome is characterized into three types. Usher Syndrome Type 1 is characterized by profound congenital bilateral sensorineural hearing loss, balance dysfunction, and retinitis pigmentosa. Retinitis pigmentosa is typically absent in infancy and early childhood but symptoms can begin in the first decade of life. Early signs of retinitis pigmentosa can include difficulty with night vision with young children reporting being afraid of the dark. The retinopathy progresses to loss of peripheral vision with the remaining vision being a small area of central vision. Balance abnormalities may become evident in infancy and early childhood presenting as motor delays in the acquisition of sitting independently and walking prior to 16 months of age. The genes associated with Usher Syndrome Type 1 are *MYO7A, CDH23, PCDH15, USH1C*, and *USH1G* [90]. Prior to onset of retinal disease, Usher Syndrome Type 1 is clinically indistinguishable from non-syndromic profound sensorineural hearing loss. Hence, genetic testing is needed to identify this condition early and to help make habilitation decisions in an infant or young child who may have significant vision limitations in teenage years.

Usher Syndrome Type 2 is characterized by mild-moderate congenital sensorineural hearing loss that does not progress. Vision loss begins in the second decade and will present as difficulty with tasks requiring peripheral vision such as passing the vision screening to obtain a state-issued driver's license. The genes associated with Usher Syndrome Type 2 are *USH2A, ADGRV1*, and *WHRN* [91]. Like Usher Syndrome Type 1, this condition is clinically indistinguishable from non-syndromic hearing loss until the onset of retinitis pigmentosa during teenage years.

Usher Syndrome Type 3 is the most variable with later onset hearing loss with or without balance issues followed by the development of retinitis pigmentosa [92]. Until recently, Clarin (*CLR*) was the only gene associated with Usher Syndrome Type 3. There is much excitement and hope surrounding a small molecule-based therapy that will undergo clinical trials to treat Clarin associated Usher Syndrome Type 3 [93].

Jervell and Lange-Nielsen Syndrome

Jervell and Lange-Nielsen Syndrome describes a condition characterized by profound congenital bilateral sensorineural hearing loss and prolonged corrected QT interval (QTc) by electrocardiogram [94]. Affected individuals are at risk for life-threatening tachy-arrythmias and may require pharmacologic as well as electrophysiologic management to prevent life threatening events. Jervell and Lange-Nielsen is an autosomal-recessive condition caused by bi-allelic variants in *KCNQ1* or *KCNE1*. Parents of affected children will not have hearing loss, but will have prolonged QTc, known as Romano-Ward Syndrome [95].

The prevalence of Jervell and Lange-Nielsen Syndrome is a subject of debate. A study in California screening 707 children under 6 years of age with unilateral or bilateral severe to profound sensorineural or mixed hearing loss uncovered no cases of Jervell and Lange-Nielsen, however, they did uncover three cases of children with long-QT due to other genetic causes [96]. In specific populations, particularly those in Scandinavia and in the Middle East, the prevalence of Jervell and Lange-Nielsen is higher due to founder pathogenic variants as well as consanguinity [97, 98]. Recent studies using molecular testing suggest that the prevalence of Jervell and Lange-Nielsen Syndrome worldwide may be lower than expected, however, the prevalence of long QTc among the deaf population is higher than in the general population, suggesting that other genes may be responsible for this phenotype [99]. Currently, screening EKGs for deaf children are still recommended [100].

Alport Syndrome

Alport Syndrome describes a condition characterized by proteinuria and hematuria, corneal defects, and bilateral late childhood onset progressive sensorineural hearing loss due to defective basement membranes in the affected organs. Improper basement membrane function in the glomerulus, cornea, and organ of Corti is due to abnormalities in collagen 4 subunits encoded by *COL4A5*, *COL4A3,* and *COL4A4* [101].

While the X-linked form of Alport Syndrome, caused by pathogenic variants in *COL4A5*, has been the most prevalent, accounting for up to 80% of affected cases, the prevalence of the autosomal forms, both dominant and recessive due to pathogenic variants in *COL4A3* and *COL4A4*, are being detected more frequently due to the advent of unbiased next-generation sequencing of patients with glomerulonephritis [102].

Patients with Alport Syndrome will present first with kidney disease and later with hearing loss. The X-linked form is the most severe in males, although females are affected. End-stage kidney disease occurs more rapidly in the X-linked form and the prevalence of hearing loss is also greater [101].

Waardenburg Syndrome

Waardenburg syndrome describes a condition associated with congenital unilateral or bilateral non-progressive severe to profound sensorineural hearing loss and pigment abnormalities. It is divided into four types. Type I describes an individual with dystopia canthorum (widely spaced eyes) and pigmentary abnormalities that can include a lightly pigmented area of hair (white forelock) or skin, different colored eyes (heterochromia). Type II is the same as Type I but without the dystopia canthorum [103]. Type III, also known as Klein-Waardenburg Syndrome, has facial findings like Type I and is associated with limb contractures and hypoplasia of the hypothenar eminence [104]. Type IV is associated with Hirschsprung disease, a condition characterized by incomplete gut innervation resulting in functional bowel obstruction and severe constipation where unrecognized significant abdominal symptoms can lead to perforation and sepsis [103].

In all subtypes of Waardenburg Syndrome, penetrance of hearing loss is incomplete. Up to 60% of affected individuals within families of Type1 Waardenburg Syndrome will have hearing loss [103]. Temporal bone malformations are observed and can include enlargement of the vestibular aqueduct, hypoplasia of the modiolus and the internal auditory canal [105]. The hearing loss when it occurs in Waardenburg syndrome is typically severe/profound [105].

Autosomal-dominant variants in *PAX3* are associated with Type I and III, although autosomal- recessive variants have been associated with Type III [106–108]. Autosomal-dominant variants in *MITF* are associated with Type II and typically have a higher penetrance of hearing loss than patients with variants in Type III [103]. Autosomal-dominant variants in *EDNRB* [109], *EDN3* [110], *SNAI2* [111], and *SOX10* are associated with Type IV [112]. Variants in SOX10 can be associated with hypoplasia or absence of the eighth cranial nerve [113]. This is important to resolve by magnetic resonance imaging, as this will have implications for cochlear implantation.

POU3F4 and Endolymphatic Gusher

Pathogenic variants in *POU3F4* are the most common cause of X-linked hearing loss. This condition is associated with a mixed hearing loss and congenital fixation of the stapes (DFNX2). Temporal bone imaging reveals bilateral dilatation of the internal auditory canal that is considered classic for this condition, although cases have been reported to have normally interpreted imaging [114]. While males with this condition have pre-lingual hearing loss, females are also affected, but are typically milder and later onset [115]. Surgical intervention may result in endolymphatic gusher and acute loss of hearing although anticipation of this condition can allow planning for alternative surgical strategies to prevent complications [116].

Auditory Neuropathy

Auditory neuropathy refers to a form of deafness/hard of hearing that affects the eighth nerve while maintaining cochlear function [117]. Auditory neuropathy may appear non-syndromic but can be identified in conditions such as Friedreich's Ataxia or Charcot-Marie-Tooth. To date, four genes have been identified to be associated with non-syndromic auditory neuropathy: *OTOF, PJVK, DIAPH3, and GJB2* [118]. Early in 2024, multiple centers reported successful gene therapy in patients with OTOF-related auditory neuropathy [119–121]

Testing Strategies

Up until the last 15 years, genetic testing for hearing loss consisted of sequencing one single gene at a time using genomic DNA isolated from peripheral blood leukocytes. For most patients, testing was limited to sequencing *GJB2* and testing for deletions that encompassed the *GJB6* locus [42]. As this testing was diagnostic in only 25% of deaf/hard of hearing patients in North America, it became apparent that as many other non-syndromic (Fig. 8.1) and syndromic genes were discovered, it was important to provide patients with a more comprehensive diagnostic tool to determine the reason for hearing loss.

To meet this need, next-generation targeted sequencing panels were developed to interrogate the sequencing of a broad range of hearing loss genes with the first such targeted panel coming from the group at the University of Iowa [122]. Using "next-generation sequencing" techniques to simultaneously sequence between 80 and 200 known hearing loss genes, many groups have demonstrated benefits to patients in the form of more rapid diagnosis [123–126]. Next-generation targeted panels are helpful for patients to determine if they are at risk for progressive loss or an association with other health issues, particularly for patients with Usher Syndrome Type 1, who are profoundly deaf and may not be able to effectively use American Sign Language in their adult years as they lose their vision. Several studies have demonstrated the diagnostic advantage of offering targeted next-generation sequencing panels, but additional benefits may include an economic advantage as knowing the cause of hearing loss limits the number of other diagnostic tests and reduces cost [127].

Interpretation of Results

While genetic testing has several advantages, the interpretation of results is an evolving field and requires effort on the part of the laboratory providing results as well as the provider [10]. For most genetic testing, there are three types of results: a positive result, a negative result, and an ambiguous or indeterminate result.

A positive result: A positive result means that for an autosomal-recessive form of hearing loss, there are two confirmed pathogenic variants, in a specific gene. For example, in a 2-year-old patient who has bilateral congenital progressive sensorineural hearing loss with enlarged vestibular aqueduct, who has two pathogenic variants in *SLC26A4*, each variant confirmed to be inherited from each parent, would be considered a positive result. Another example would be a 9-month-old with congenital profound sensorineural hearing loss who is not yet sitting up and has two pathogenic variants in *MYO7A* inherited from each parent, may have Usher Syndrome or possibly non-syndromic hearing loss. There are important points in this interpretation. The first is that phenotype plays an important role in variant interpretation. The second is that each variant in a recessive condition must come from each parent (see next section on setting phase). For a dominant form of hearing loss, a positive result would be finding a pathogenic variant in one copy of the gene. For large families, many family members may need to be tested to determine if that variant segregates with the hearing phenotype or is a new or "*de novo*" genetic change in a child with two hearing parents.

A negative result: When a result is called "negative," no variants were identified in the patient's genomic DNA in any of the genes that are part of the targeted next-generation sequencing panel. This is not to be confused with hearing loss not being genetic. As all possible genes cannot be included on targeted panels, it is possible that the patient's genetic cause is not represented on the panel. Panels are designed to sequence coding regions of genes and have limited representation of genomic regions that are important for gene expression and other genetic regulation. Sequencing of the entire genome might be considered in this scenario, particularly if a patient has a phenotype that suggests a rare syndromic condition.

An ambiguous or indeterminate result: An ambiguous or indeterminate result can occur in several situations. One example of an indeterminate result is a single pathogenic variant in a known recessive gene. In this situation, it is difficult to disambiguate whether the patient is only a carrier of a recessive variant or if there is another variant that was not detected by the panel design. Another example would be the presence of variants of unknown significance in a specific gene that lack sufficient evidence of pathogenicity to be considered causative or benign. Additional testing and follow up might be considered in this situation.

Importance of Setting Phase

For a recessive condition, a patient must have two pathogenic variants in a specific gene, each variant must occur in each individual copy of the gene. Thus, each variant must come from each parent. If both variants are on the same copy of the gene, yet the patient has another copy with a normal sequence, then this is not the same as a recessive condition.

For most sequencing strategies, the technology that is used for sequencing cannot determine whether variants come from one parent or both parents, unless the variants are very close together in the DNA sequence, within tens of base-pairs. Thus, for many genetic testing results, the laboratory may request parental testing before providing a conclusive result. Other laboratories will provide a result but suggest that "segregation analysis," which is a synonym for "setting phase" is performed. In situations where only one parent is available, demonstrating that one variant comes from that parent is sufficient. If neither variant nor both variants come from the same parent, then the variants in each gene can be ruled out as causative. For example, a patient with bilateral moderate sensorineural hearing loss was found to have two variants in *MYO15A*. Testing both parents for the variants identified both variants coming from the father. The mother had neither variant. Thus, the variants in *MYO15A* could be ruled out as the cause of the child's hearing loss.

Variants of Unknown Significance

It is common to receive a genetic testing report from a targeted hearing loss exome panel that only identified several "variants of unknown significance" commonly referred to as a "VUS" or a "VOUS" [10, 128]. In this situation, the variant in DNA sequence cannot be interpreted to be pathogenic or benign and further effort or time is needed to disambiguate the interpretation. In a clinical setting, variant interpretation may include testing other affected family members if available and if the testing is covered or paid for by the laboratory. If a variant of unknown significance segregates with the affected individuals only, then the likelihood of the variant being pathogenic is more likely.

Other evaluations typically include the frequency of a given variant in known databases of apparently "normal" individuals gnomAD [129]. If a variant is found commonly in a population, then the likelihood of the variant being pathogenic is low. However, there are certain recessive variants, such as those in *GJB2*, that have high population frequencies. Other analysis may include impact on protein function or mRNA splicing using programs such as SIFT [130], Polyphen [131], Mutation Taster [132] SpliceAI (https://spliceailookup.broadinstitute.org/), and REVEL [158] to name a few of the more commonly used software packages. While these programs may provide conflicting results, they can be helpful in determining pathogenicity. Evaluations for the evolutionary conservation of a missense variant or the tolerance of a given gene to variation are also helpful adjuncts [10]. Curated lists of variants such as ClinVar [2] or the Deafness Variation Database [4] can also be used to identify whether a variant is pathogenic or not. A clinical report will frequently cite the bioinformatics tools used in the process of variant interpretation. On a research basis, efforts to interpret variants can include protein modeling [133] or functional modeling in a cell or animal model [134]. Keeping in mind the high frequency of some hearing loss variants in the population, the ClinGen working group has set specific parameters for variant interpretation [24, 135, 136].

Genetic Counseling and the Dynamic Nature of Our Understanding of Genomic Results

Genetic counseling is an integral part of genetic testing for hearing loss. Ideally, genetic counseling should consist of both pre-test and post-test counseling. Pre-test counseling should include the types of results that a patient could reasonably expect from genetic testing (positive, negative, ambiguous, or indeterminate) and that a negative test does not rule out a genetic cause. Post-test counseling is tailored to the type of result obtained. For example, if a recessive form of hearing loss is identified, then the parents should be made aware that they have a 1-in-4 chance with each pregnancy of having an affected child in the future [137]. Patients with negative or ambiguous results should also be informed that they should undergo genetic evaluation in the future as result interpretation may change or newer testing becomes available.

Neurofibromatosis Type 2-related Schwannomatosis

Neurofibromatosis Type 2-related schwannomatosis (NF2) is a genetically distinct condition separate from Neurofibromatosis Type 1. Originally described in the nineteenth century, early twentieth-century clinicians reported both Neurofibromatosis Type 1 and Type 2 to be the same condition. This confusion was not resolved until the middle of the 1980s, when it became clear that both conditions were distinct [138] with establishment of unique clinical criteria for each condition in the late 1980s [139], linkage of NF2 to chromosome 22 and the discovery of the *NF2* gene encoding the protein Merlin in the early 1990s [140].

Individuals with NF2 may present with unilateral or bilateral hearing loss, tinnitus, ear fullness, and balance difficulty followed by identification of enhancing lesions of the eighth nerve identified by MRI. Additional findings can include cranial meningioma, schwannomas of other cranial nerves, spinal meningioma, spinal cord ependymoma, peripheral nerve tumor, spinal schwannoma, subcutaneous tumors, skin plaques, and eye findings consisting of cortical wedge cataracts, thickened optic nerves, retinal hamartomas, and epiretinal membrane [141]. Neurofibromas are rarely reported as well as malignancy, yet malignant peripheral nerve sheath tumors have been reported [142].

In studies from the United Kingdom, the current prevalence is estimated to be 1 in 25,000 individuals [143]. Age of onset can be anywhere from birth through old age with 60 years as the median age of onset with nearly 100% penetrance [138].

The Revised International 2022 Criteria derived from the previous Manchester diagnostic criteria for NF2 consists of any one of the following [139, 141, 144, 145]:

1. Bilateral vestibular schwannomas.
2. An identical *NF2* pathogenic variant in at least two anatomically distinct NF2-related meningiomas and/or ependymomas.
3. Either two Major or one Major and two Minor criteria as follows:

Major criteria:

- Unilateral Vestibular Schwannoma (VS)
- First-degree relative other than sibling with *NF2*-related schwannomatosis
- Two or more meningiomas (note: single meningioma qualifies as minor criteria)
- *NF2* pathogenic variant in an unaffected tissue such as blood (Note: if the variants allele frequency (in blood) is significantly less than 50%, the diagnosis is mosaic *NF2*-related schwannomatosis).

Minor criteria:
Can count more than one of a type (e.g., two distinct schwannomas would count as two minor criteria)

- Ependymoma, Meningioma (Note: multiple meningiomas qualify as a major criteria), Schwannoma (Note: if the major criterion is unilateral VS, at least one schwannoma must be dermal in location).
- Juvenile subcapsular or cortical cataract; Retinal hamartoma; Epiretinal membrane aged less than 40 years, meningioma.

Genetic testing for NF2 consists of sequencing the *NF2* gene as well as deletion/duplication analysis as patients meeting diagnostic criteria can have either missense pathogenic variants or deletions/duplications of all or part of the gene (copy number variant). In patients with developmental disabilities, consideration of chromosome testing to detect ring 22q should also be considered [146]. In children and young adults, Manchester criteria should be relaxed; a child presenting with any schwannoma should be offered genetic testing. However, in clinical practice, testing for variants in *NF2* is accompanied by testing for variants in *LZTR1* and *SMARCB1* as a panel.

Phenotypic overlap of NF2 and Schwannomatosis has become only recently apparent [147]. In a recent study of 155 isolated schwannoma patients presenting under age 25, 30 (15%) had germline pathogenic variants in *NF2*, 7 (6%) had germline pathogenic variants in *SMARCB1,* and 10 (6%) had pathogenic variants in *LZTR1*. These data support evaluation of all three genes in young patients presenting with isolated schwannomas.

While it is true that schwannomatosis is a condition distinct both clinically and genetically from NF2, there is considerable phenotypic overlap. It was originally thought that patients with schwannomatosis and variants in *SMARCB1* or *LZTR1* did not have vestibular schwannomas [148], however very recent evidence has demonstrated that vestibular schwannomas can occur in patients with *SMARCB1* or *LZTR1* pathogenic variants [147, 149]. Thus, for patients with schwannomas who present under age 30 and have tested negative for *NF2* pathogenic variants, consideration should be given of additional testing for pathogenic variants in *SMARCB1* and *LZTR1* [147] or testing as a panel.

Twenty-five to fifty percent of individuals with NF2 will have mosaic pathogenic variants rather than germline pathogenic variants. For these individuals, a genetic variant occurred post-conception and the variant is only present in a sub-set of cells. In these individuals, blood studies are often negative, yet testing the tumor will identify two *NF2* variants, typically a deletion on one copy of chromosome 22 and a pathogenic variant within the *NF2* coding region on the other. Thus, simultaneous testing of both blood and tumor can help provide a diagnosis of mosaicism [147]. Ideally, if possible, testing of two tumors, to identify the mosaic germline variant is best practice if blood studies are negative. Testing should be performed in a laboratory where depth of read on next-generation sequencing is in the thousands to be able to identify mosaicism. Standard next-generation sequencing depth of read is typically 30x and will miss low-level mosaicism.

Paraganglioma-Pheochromocytoma Syndrome

Paraganglioma-Pheochromocytoma Syndrome describes a hereditary tumor predisposition condition where tumors arise from neural crest-derived paravertebral neuroendocrine tissues. Tumors may arise anywhere from the skull base to pelvis and are called paraganglioma. Tumors that arise within the adrenal medulla are pheochromocytomas. Skull base and neck tumors are of parasympathetic origin and typically do not secrete catecholamines. In contrast to those of the adrenal gland, thoracic, lumbar, and sacral paraspinal neuroendocrine tissue are typically sympathetic and secrete catecholamines [150]. While most tumors are benign, malignant degeneration has been reported in a genotype-specific manner.

The genetic basis of Paraganglioma-Pheochromocytoma was originally limited to pathogenic variants in genes comprising subunits of succinate dehydrogenase complex. The first gene identified to be associated with paraganglioma-pheochromocytoma syndrome was *SDHD* [151]. Subsequently, other subunits of the mitochondrial succinic dehydrogenase complex were identified, *SDHA, SDHAF2,*

SDHB, and *SDHC* and known collectively as *SDHx*. Paragangliomas-pheochromocytomas have the highest degree of heritability of any human tumor condition with over 40% having an identifiable germline driver predisposing pathogenic variant [152]. A recent consensus statement from the NGS in PPGL study group and published in 2017 Nature Reviews Endocrinology [153] lists 27 known genes associated with this condition and recommended panel testing that includes in addition to the *SDHx* group and includes *FH, MAX, NF1, RET, TMEM127, VHL, EGLN1/PHD2, EPAS1, KIF1B, MET, ATRX, BRAF, CDKN2A, EGLN2/PHD1, FGFR1, H3F3A, HRAS, IDH2, KMT2D, MDH2, MERTK, and TP53*.

While nearly all the genes listed to be associated with Paraganglioma-Pheochromocytoma Syndrome are inherited as an autosomal dominant, there are some important caveats to keep in mind. For patients with pathogenic variants in *SDHD*, it has been observed that there is a parent of origin effect where if the pathogenic variant is inherited from a father, then the offspring would be affected. However, if the pathogenic variant is inherited from a mother, then offspring would carry the pathogenic variant but not manifest paraganglioma-pheochromocytoma syndrome [151]. This observation has been called into question [154]. For patients with pathogenic variants in *SDHB*, there is a much higher chance of malignancy. Even small paragangliomas in an individual with an *SDHB* pathogenic variant should be resected due to the increased risk of malignancy and metastasis [155, 156]. Mosaicism has been reported and for patients with negative studies from genomic DNA from peripheral blood lymphocytes, testing of tumor derived DNA is encouraged [153].

Conclusions

Genetic testing can inform medical management in patients with hearing loss and head and neck tumors. Genetic testing has become increasingly complex as conditions thought to be caused by only a few genes are now known to be highly heterogeneous. While we have the technology to sequence many genes at once through next-generation sequencing, we are still limited by our ability to interpret sequence variants and establish their pathogenicity. Collaboration between clinical geneticists, genetic counselors, otologists, and neurotologists can help facilitate genetic testing and interpretation while informing medical management and decision-making.

References

1. Morton CC, Nance WE. Newborn hearing screening--a silent revolution. N Engl J Med. 2006;354(20):2151–64. https://doi.org/10.1056/NEJMra050700.
2. ClinVar. https://www.ncbi.nlm.nih.gov/clinvar/.
3. Online Mendelian Inheritance in Man. www.omim.org.
4. Van Camp G, Smith R. Hereditary hearing loss homepage. http://hereditaryhearingloss.org/.
5. Boudewyns A, van den Ende J, Peeters N, et al. Targeted next-generation sequencing in children with bilateral sensorineural hearing loss: diagnostic yield and predictors of a genetic cause. Otol Neurotol. 2023;44(4):360–6. https://doi.org/10.1097/MAO.0000000000003841.
6. Abou Tayoun AN, Al Turki SH, Oza AM, et al. Improving hearing loss gene testing: a systematic review of gene evidence toward more efficient next-generation sequencing-based diagnostic testing and interpretation. Genet Med. 2016;18(6):545–53. https://doi.org/10.1038/gim.2015.141.
7. Sloan-Heggen CM, Bierer AO, Shearer AE, et al. Comprehensive genetic testing in the clinical evaluation of 1119 patients with hearing loss. Hum Genet. 2016;135(4):441–50. https://doi.org/10.1007/s00439-016-1648-8.
8. Yan D, Tekin D, Bademci G, et al. Spectrum of DNA variants for non-syndromic deafness in a large cohort from multiple continents. Hum Genet. 2016;135(8):953–61. https://doi.org/10.1007/s00439-016-1697-z.
9. Zazo Seco C, Wesdorp M, Feenstra I, et al. The diagnostic yield of whole-exome sequencing targeting a gene panel for hearing impairment in The Netherlands. Eur J Hum Genet. 2017;25(3):308–14. https://doi.org/10.1038/ejhg.2016.182.
10. Richards S, Aziz N, Bale S, et al. Standards and guidelines for the interpretation of sequence variants: a joint consensus recommendation of the American College of Medical Genetics and Genomics and the Association for Molecular Pathology. Genet Med. 2015;17(5):405–24. https://doi.org/10.1038/gim.2015.30.
11. Moser T, Vogl C. New insights into cochlear sound encoding. F1000Res. 2016;5:F1000 Faculty Rev-2081. https://doi.org/10.12688/f1000research.8924.1.
12. Zhao B, Muller U. The elusive mechanotransduction machinery of hair cells. Curr Opin Neurobiol. 2015;34:172–9. https://doi.org/10.1016/j.conb.2015.08.006.
13. Alberts B, Johnson A, Lewis J, et al. Molecular biology of the cell. 6th ed. Garland Science; 2008.
14. Toriello HV, Smith SD. Hereditary hearing loss and its syndromes. Oxford: Oxford University Press; 2013.
15. Kimberling WJ, Hildebrand MS, Shearer AE, et al. Frequency of Usher syndrome in two pediatric populations: implications for genetic screening of deaf and hard of hearing children. Genet Med. 2010;12(8):512–6. https://doi.org/10.1097/GIM.0b013e3181e5afb8.
16. Fraser FC, Sproule JR, Halal F. Frequency of the branchio-oto-renal (BOR) syndrome in children with profound hearing loss. Am J Med Genet. 1980;7(3):341–9. https://doi.org/10.1002/ajmg.1320070316.
17. Ito T, Muskett J, Chattaraj P, et al. SLC26A4 mutation testing for hearing loss associated with enlargement of the vestibular aqueduct. World J Otorhinolaryngol. 2013;3(2):26–34. https://doi.org/10.5319/wjo.v3.i2.26.
18. ClinGen. 2024. https://www.clinicalgenome.org/affiliation/40007/.
19. Miyagawa M, Nishio SY, Usami S. A comprehensive study on the etiology of patients receiving cochlear implantation with special emphasis on genetic epidemiology. Otol Neurotol. 2016;37(2):e126–34. https://doi.org/10.1097/MAO.0000000000000936.
20. Park JH, Kim NK, Kim AR, et al. Exploration of molecular genetic etiology for Korean cochlear implantees with severe to profound hearing loss and its implication. Orphanet J Rare Dis. 2014;9:167. https://doi.org/10.1186/s13023-014-0167-8.

21. Panel CE. ClinGen Clinical Genomics Resource. https://www.clinicalgenome.org/.
22. DiStefano MT, Hemphill SE, Oza AM, et al. ClinGen expert clinical validity curation of 164 hearing loss gene-disease pairs. Genet Med. 2019;21(10):2239–47. https://doi.org/10.1038/s41436-019-0487-0.
23. Nussbaum RL, Rehm HL, ClinGen. ClinGen and genetic testing. N Engl J Med. 2015;373(14):1379. https://www.ncbi.nlm.nih.gov/pubmed/26430707.
24. Abou Tayoun AN, Pesaran T, DiStefano MT, et al. Recommendations for interpreting the loss of function PVS1 ACMG/AMP variant criterion. Hum Mutat. 2018;39(11):1517–24. https://doi.org/10.1002/humu.23626.
25. Chaussenot A, Rouzier C, Quere M, et al. Mutation update and uncommon phenotypes in a French cohort of 96 patients with WFS1-related disorders. Clin Genet. 2015;87(5):430–9. https://doi.org/10.1111/cge.12437.
26. Lyon MF. Gene action in the X-chromosome of the mouse (Mus musculus L.). Nature. 1961;190:372–3. https://www.ncbi.nlm.nih.gov/pubmed/13764598
27. Anderson S, Bankier AT, Barrell BG, et al. Sequence and organization of the human mitochondrial genome. Nature. 1981;290(5806):457–65. https://www.ncbi.nlm.nih.gov/pubmed/7219534.
28. Jaber L, Shohat M, Bu X, et al. Sensorineural deafness inherited as a tissue specific mitochondrial disorder. J Med Genet. 1992;29(2):86–90. https://doi.org/10.1136/jmg.29.2.86.
29. Prezant TR, Agapian JV, Bohlman MC, et al. Mitochondrial ribosomal RNA mutation associated with both antibiotic-induced and non-syndromic deafness. Nat Genet. 1993;4(3):289–94. https://doi.org/10.1038/ng0793-289.
30. Estivill X, Govea N, Barcelo E, et al. Familial progressive sensorineural deafness is mainly due to the mtDNA A1555G mutation and is enhanced by treatment of aminoglycosides. Am J Hum Genet. 1998;62(1):27–35. https://doi.org/10.1086/301676.
31. Fischel-Ghodsian N, Prezant TR, Bu X, Oztas S. Mitochondrial ribosomal RNA gene mutation in a patient with sporadic aminoglycoside ototoxicity. Am J Otolaryngol. 1993;14(6):399–403. https://doi.org/10.1016/0196-0709(93)90113-l.
32. Pandya A, Xia X, Radnaabazar J, et al. Mutation in the mitochondrial 12S rRNA gene in two families from Mongolia with matrilineal aminoglycoside ototoxicity. J Med Genet. 1997;34(2):169–72. https://doi.org/10.1136/jmg.34.2.169.
33. Dean L. Gentamycin therapy and MT-RNR1 genotype. Bethesda (MD): National Center for Biotechnology Information (US); 2012.
34. Usami S, Nishio S. Nonsyndromic hearing loss and deafness, mitochondrial. In: Adam MP, Ardinger HH, Pagon RA, et al., editors. GeneReviews((R)). Seattle (WA): University of Washington; 1993.
35. Yelverton JC, Arnos K, Xia XJ, Nance WE, Pandya A, Dodson KM. The clinical and audiologic features of hearing loss due to mitochondrial mutations. Otolaryngol Head Neck Surg. 2013;148(6):1017–22. https://doi.org/10.1177/0194599813482705.
36. Zhu Y, Huang S, Kang D, et al. Analysis of the heteroplasmy level and transmitted features in hearing-loss pedigrees with mitochondrial 12S rRNA A1555G mutation. BMC Genet. 2014;15:26. https://doi.org/10.1186/1471-2156-15-26.
37. Hougaard DD, Hestoy DH, Hojland AT, Gailhede M, Petersen MB. Audiological and vestibular findings in subjects with MELAS syndrome. J Int Adv Otol. 2019;15(2):296–303. https://doi.org/10.5152/iao.2019.5913.
38. Hendrickx JJ, Mudde AH, t Hart LM, Huygen PL, Cremers CW. Progressive sensorineural hearing impairment in maternally inherited diabetes mellitus and deafness (MIDD). Otol Neurotol. 2006;27(6):802–8. https://doi.org/10.1097/01.mao.0000224091.02506.a0.
39. DiMauro S, Hirano M. Merrf. In: Adam MP, Ardinger HH, Pagon RA, et al., editors. GeneReviews((R)). Seattle (WA): University of Washington; 1993.
40. Kornblum C, Broicher R, Walther E, et al. Sensorineural hearing loss in patients with chronic progressive external ophthalmoplegia or Kearns-Sayre syndrome. J Neurol. 2005;252(9):1101–7. https://doi.org/10.1007/s00415-005-0827-7.
41. Pandya A, Arnos KS, Xia XJ, et al. Frequency and distribution of GJB2 (connexin 26) and GJB6 (connexin 30) mutations in a large North American repository of deaf probands. Genet Med. 2003;5(4):295–303. https://doi.org/10.1097/01.GIM.0000078026.01140.68.
42. Putcha GV, Bejjani BA, Bleoo S, et al. A multicenter study of the frequency and distribution of GJB2 and GJB6 mutations in a large North American cohort. Genet Med. 2007;9(7):413–26. https://doi.org/10.1097/gim.0b013e3180a03276.
43. Schimmenti LA, Martinez A, Telatar M, et al. Infant hearing loss and connexin testing in a diverse population. Genet Med. 2008;10(7):517–24. https://doi.org/10.1097/gim.0b013e31817708fa.
44. Denoyelle F, Weil D, Maw MA, et al. Prelingual deafness: high prevalence of a 30delG mutation in the connexin 26 gene. Hum Mol Genet. 1997;6(12):2173–7. https://www.ncbi.nlm.nih.gov/pubmed/9336442.
45. Lee KY, Choi SY, Bae JW, et al. Molecular analysis of the GJB2, GJB6 and SLC26A4 genes in Korean deafness patients. Int J Pediatr Otorhinolaryngol. 2008;72(9):1301–9. https://doi.org/10.1016/j.ijporl.2008.05.007.
46. Prasad S, Cucci RA, Green GE, Smith RJ. Genetic testing for hereditary hearing loss: connexin 26 (GJB2) allele variants and two novel deafness-causing mutations (R32C and 645-648delTAGA). Hum Mutat. 2000;16(6):502–8. https://doi.org/10.1002/1098-1004(200012)16:6%3c502::AID-HUMU7%3e3.0.CO;2-4.
47. Tsukada K, Nishio S, Usami S, Deafness Gene Study C. A large cohort study of GJB2 mutations in Japanese hearing loss patients. Clin Genet. 2010;78(5):464–70. https://doi.org/10.1111/j.1399-0004.2010.01407.x.
48. Green GE, Scott DA, JM MD, Woodworth GG, Sheffield VC, Smith RJ. Carrier rates in the midwestern United States for GJB2 mutations causing inherited deafness. JAMA. 1999;281(23):2211–6. https://www.ncbi.nlm.nih.gov/pubmed/10376574.
49. Abe S, Usami S, Shinkawa H, Kelley PM, Kimberling WJ. Prevalent connexin 26 gene (GJB2) mutations in Japanese. J Med Genet. 2000;37(1):41–3. https://www.ncbi.nlm.nih.gov/pubmed/10633133.
50. Sobe T, Erlich P, Berry A, et al. High frequency of the deafness-associated 167delT mutation in the connexin 26 (GJB2) gene in Israeli Ashkenazim. Am J Med Genet. 1999;86(5):499–500. https://www.ncbi.nlm.nih.gov/pubmed/10508996.
51. Wattanasirichaigoon D, Limwongse C, Jariengprasert C, et al. High prevalence of V37I genetic variant in the connexin-26 (GJB2) gene among non-syndromic hearing-impaired and control Thai individuals. Clin Genet. 2004;66(5):452–60. https://doi.org/10.1111/j.1399-0004.2004.00325.x.
52. Del Castillo I, Moreno-Pelayo MA, Del Castillo FJ, et al. Prevalence and evolutionary origins of the del(GJB6-D13S1830) mutation in the DFNB1 locus in hearing-impaired subjects: a multicenter study. Am J Hum Genet. 2003;73(6):1452–8. https://doi.org/10.1086/380205.
53. del Castillo I, Villamar M, Moreno-Pelayo MA, et al. A deletion involving the connexin 30 gene in nonsyndromic hearing impairment. N Engl J Med. 2002;346(4):243–9. https://doi.org/10.1056/NEJMoa012052.

54. Lerer I, Sagi M, Ben-Neriah Z, Wang T, Levi H, Abeliovich D. A deletion mutation in GJB6 cooperating with a GJB2 mutation in trans in non-syndromic deafness: a novel founder mutation in Ashkenazi Jews. Hum Mutat. 2001;18(5):460. https://doi.org/10.1002/humu.1222.
55. Pandya A, O'Brien A, Kovasala M, Bademci G, Tekin M, Arnos KS. Analyses of del(GJB6-D13S1830) and del(GJB6-D13S1834) deletions in a large cohort with hearing loss: caveats to interpretation of molecular test results in multiplex families. Mol Genet Genomic Med. 2020;8(4):e1171. https://doi.org/10.1002/mgg3.1171.
56. Rodriguez-Paris J, Schrijver I. The digenic hypothesis unraveled: the GJB6 del(GJB6-D13S1830) mutation causes allele-specific loss of GJB2 expression in cis. Biochem Biophys Res Commun. 2009;389(2):354–9. https://doi.org/10.1016/j.bbrc.2009.08.152.
57. gEAR portal. 2024. http://umgear.org/.
58. Johnson SL, Ceriani F, Houston O, et al. Connexin-mediated signaling in nonsensory cells is crucial for the development of sensory inner hair cells in the mouse cochlea. J Neurosci. 2017;37(2):258–68. https://doi.org/10.1523/JNEUROSCI.2251-16.2017.
59. Snoeckx RL, Huygen PL, Feldmann D, et al. GJB2 mutations and degree of hearing loss: a multicenter study. Am J Hum Genet. 2005;77(6):945–57. https://doi.org/10.1086/497996.
60. Chan DK, Schrijver I, Chang KW. Connexin-26-associated deafness: phenotypic variability and progression of hearing loss. Genet Med. 2010;12(3):174–81. https://doi.org/10.1097/GIM.0b013e3181d0d42b.
61. Kenna MA, Feldman HA, Neault MW, et al. Audiologic phenotype and progression in GJB2 (Connexin 26) hearing loss. Arch Otolaryngol Head Neck Surg. 2010;136(1):81–7. https://doi.org/10.1001/archoto.2009.202.
62. Kenna MA, Rehm HL, Frangulov A, Feldman HA, Robson CD. Temporal bone abnormalities in children with GJB2 mutations. Laryngoscope. 2011;121(3):630–5. https://doi.org/10.1002/lary.21414.
63. Lee JR, White TW. Connexin-26 mutations in deafness and skin disease. Expert Rev Mol Med. 2009;11:e35. https://doi.org/10.1017/S1462399409001276.
64. Garcia IE, Bosen F, Mujica P, et al. From hyperactive connexin26 hemichannels to impairments in epidermal calcium gradient and permeability barrier in the keratitis-ichthyosis-deafness syndrome. J Invest Dermatol. 2016;136(3):574–83. https://doi.org/10.1016/j.jid.2015.11.017.
65. Everett LA, Glaser B, Beck JC, et al. Pendred syndrome is caused by mutations in a putative sulphate transporter gene (PDS). Nat Genet. 1997;17(4):411–22. https://doi.org/10.1038/ng1297-411.
66. Li XC, Everett LA, Lalwani AK, et al. A mutation in PDS causes non-syndromic recessive deafness. Nat Genet. 1998;18(3):215–7. https://doi.org/10.1038/ng0398-215.
67. Pendred V. Deaf-mutism and goitre. Lancet. 1896;148(3808):532.
68. Albert S, Blons H, Jonard L, et al. SLC26A4 gene is frequently involved in nonsyndromic hearing impairment with enlarged vestibular aqueduct in Caucasian populations. Eur J Hum Genet. 2006;14(6):773–9. https://doi.org/10.1038/sj.ejhg.5201611.
69. Park HJ, Shaukat S, Liu XZ, et al. Origins and frequencies of SLC26A4 (PDS) mutations in east and south Asians: global implications for the epidemiology of deafness. J Med Genet. 2003;40(4):242–8. https://www.ncbi.nlm.nih.gov/pubmed/12676893.
70. Chattaraj P, Reimold FR, Muskett JA, et al. Use of SLC26A4 mutation testing for unilateral enlargement of the vestibular aqueduct. JAMA Otolaryngol Head Neck Surg. 2013;139(9):907–13. https://doi.org/10.1001/jamaoto.2013.4185.
71. Kim BG, Roh KJ, Park AY, et al. Early deterioration of residual hearing in patients with SLC26A4 mutations. Laryngoscope. 2016;126(8):E286–91. https://doi.org/10.1002/lary.25786.
72. Suzuki H, Oshima A, Tsukamoto K, et al. Clinical characteristics and genotype-phenotype correlation of hearing loss patients with SLC26A4 mutations. Acta Otolaryngol. 2007;127(12):1292–7. https://doi.org/10.1080/00016480701258739.
73. Blons H, Feldmann D, Duval V, et al. Screening of SLC26A4 (PDS) gene in Pendred's syndrome: a large spectrum of mutations in France and phenotypic heterogeneity. Clin Genet. 2004;66(4):333–40. https://doi.org/10.1111/j.1399-0004.2004.00296.x.
74. Kuhnen P, Turan S, Frohler S, et al. Identification of PENDRIN (SLC26A4) mutations in patients with congenital hypothyroidism and "apparent" thyroid dysgenesis. J Clin Endocrinol Metab. 2014;99(1):E169–76. https://doi.org/10.1210/jc.2013-2619.
75. Flock A, Cheung HC. Actin filaments in sensory hairs of inner ear receptor cells. J Cell Biol. 1977;75(2 Pt 1):339–43. https://www.ncbi.nlm.nih.gov/pubmed/318131.
76. Kazmierczak P, Sakaguchi H, Tokita J, et al. Cadherin 23 and protocadherin 15 interact to form tip-link filaments in sensory hair cells. Nature. 2007;449(7158):87–91. https://doi.org/10.1038/nature06091.
77. Pepermans E, Petit C. The tip-link molecular complex of the auditory mechano-electrical transduction machinery. Hear Res. 2015;330(Pt A):10–7. https://doi.org/10.1016/j.heares.2015.05.005.
78. Siemens J, Lillo C, Dumont RA, et al. Cadherin 23 is a component of the tip link in hair-cell stereocilia. Nature. 2004;428(6986):950–5. https://doi.org/10.1038/nature02483.
79. Grati M, Kachar B. Myosin VIIa and sans localization at stereocilia upper tip-link density implicates these Usher syndrome proteins in mechanotransduction. Proc Natl Acad Sci USA. 2011;108(28):11476–81. https://doi.org/10.1073/pnas.1104161108.
80. Grillet N, Xiong W, Reynolds A, et al. Harmonin mutations cause mechanotransduction defects in cochlear hair cells. Neuron. 2009;62(3):375–87. https://doi.org/10.1016/j.neuron.2009.04.006.
81. Beurg M, Schimmenti LA, Koleilat A, et al. New Tmc1 deafness mutations impact mechanotransduction in auditory hair cells. J Neurosci. 2021;41(20):4378–91. https://doi.org/10.1523/JNEUROSCI.2537-20.2021.
82. Schultz JM, Bhatti R, Madeo AC, et al. Allelic hierarchy of CDH23 mutations causing non-syndromic deafness DFNB12 or Usher syndrome USH1D in compound heterozygotes. J Med Genet. 2011;48(11):767–75. https://doi.org/10.1136/jmedgenet-2011-100262.
83. Riazuddin S, Nazli S, Ahmed ZM, et al. Mutation spectrum of MYO7A and evaluation of a novel nonsyndromic deafness DFNB2 allele with residual function. Hum Mutat. 2008;29(4):502–11. https://doi.org/10.1002/humu.20677.
84. Ahmed ZM, Riazuddin S, Ahmad J, et al. PCDH15 is expressed in the neurosensory epithelium of the eye and ear and mutant alleles are responsible for both USH1F and DFNB23. Hum Mol Genet. 2003;12(24):3215–23. https://doi.org/10.1093/hmg/ddg358.
85. Wu Z, Grillet N, Zhao B, et al. Mechanosensory hair cells express two molecularly distinct mechanotransduction channels. Nat Neurosci. 2017;20(1):24–33. https://doi.org/10.1038/nn.4449.
86. Wu Z, Muller U. Molecular identity of the mechanotransduction channel in hair cells: not quiet there yet. J Neurosci. 2016;36(43):10927–34. https://doi.org/10.1523/JNEUROSCI.1149-16.2016.
87. Kalay E, Li Y, Uzumcu A, et al. Mutations in the lipoma HMGIC fusion partner-like 5 (LHFPL5) gene cause autosomal reces-

sive nonsyndromic hearing loss. Hum Mutat. 2006;27(7):633–9. https://doi.org/10.1002/humu.20368.
88. Kurima K, Peters LM, Yang Y, et al. Dominant and recessive deafness caused by mutations of a novel gene, TMC1, required for cochlear hair-cell function. Nat Genet. 2002;30(3):277–84. https://doi.org/10.1038/ng842.
89. Naz S, Giguere CM, Kohrman DC, et al. Mutations in a novel gene, TMIE, are associated with hearing loss linked to the DFNB6 locus. Am J Hum Genet. 2002;71(3):632–6. https://doi.org/10.1086/342193.
90. Lentz J, Keats BJB. Usher Syndrome Type I. In: Pagon RA, Adam MP, Ardinger HH, et al., editors. GeneReviews(R). Seattle (WA): University of Washington; 1993.
91. Lentz J, Keats B. Usher Syndrome Type II. In: Pagon RA, Adam MP, Ardinger HH, et al., editors. GeneReviews(R). Seattle (WA): University of Washington; 1993.
92. Adato A, Vreugde S, Joensuu T, et al. USH3A transcripts encode clarin-1, a four-transmembrane-domain protein with a possible role in sensory synapses. Eur J Hum Genet. 2002;10(6):339–50. https://doi.org/10.1038/sj.ejhg.5200831.
93. Alagramam KN, Gopal SR, Geng R, et al. A small molecule mitigates hearing loss in a mouse model of Usher syndrome III. Nat Chem Biol. 2016;12(6):444–51. https://doi.org/10.1038/nchembio.2069.
94. Jervell A, Lange-Nielsen F. Congenital deaf-mutism, functional heart disease with prolongation of the Q-T interval and sudden death. Am Heart J. 1957;54(1):59–68. https://www.ncbi.nlm.nih.gov/pubmed/13435203.
95. Tranebjaerg L, Samson RA, Green GE. Jervell and Lange-Nielsen syndrome. In: Pagon RA, Adam MP, Ardinger HH, et al., editors. GeneReviews(R). Seattle (WA): University of Washington; 1993.
96. Chang RK, Lan YT, Silka MJ, et al. Genetic variants for long QT syndrome among infants and children from a statewide newborn hearing screening program cohort. J Pediatr. 2014;164(3):590–5 e1–3. https://doi.org/10.1016/j.jpeds.2013.11.011.
97. Ocal B, Imamoglu A, Atalay S, Ercan TH. Prevalence of idiopathic long QT syndrome in children with congenital deafness. Pediatr Cardiol. 1997;18(6):401–5. https://doi.org/10.1007/s002469900215.
98. Tranebjaerg L, Bathen J, Tyson J, Bitner-Glindzicz M. Jervell and Lange-Nielsen syndrome: a Norwegian perspective. Am J Med Genet. 1999;89(3):137–46. https://www.ncbi.nlm.nih.gov/pubmed/10704188.
99. Sanecka A, Biernacka EK, Szperl M, et al. QTc prolongation in patients with hearing loss: electrocardiographic and genetic study. Cardiol J. 2016;23(1):34–41. https://doi.org/10.5603/CJ.a2015.0062.
100. Alford RL, Arnos KS, Fox M, et al. American College of Medical Genetics and Genomics guideline for the clinical evaluation and etiologic diagnosis of hearing loss. Genet Med. 2014;16(4):347–55. https://doi.org/10.1038/gim.2014.2.
101. Kashtan C. Alport syndrome: facts and opinions. F1000Res. 2017;6:50. https://doi.org/10.12688/f1000research.9636.1.
102. Fallerini C, Dosa L, Tita R, et al. Unbiased next generation sequencing analysis confirms the existence of autosomal dominant Alport syndrome in a relevant fraction of cases. Clin Genet. 2014;86(3):252–7. https://doi.org/10.1111/cge.12258.
103. Milunsky JM. Waardenburg Syndrome Type I. In: Pagon RA, Adam MP, Ardinger HH, et al., editors. GeneReviews(R). Seattle (WA): University of Washington; 1993.
104. Hoth CF, Milunsky A, Lipsky N, Sheffer R, Clarren SK, Baldwin CT. Mutations in the paired domain of the human PAX3 gene cause Klein-Waardenburg syndrome (WS-III) as well as Waardenburg syndrome type I (WS-I). Am J Hum Genet. 1993;52(3):455–62. https://www.ncbi.nlm.nih.gov/pubmed/8447316.
105. Madden C, Halsted MJ, Hopkin RJ, Choo DI, Benton C, Greinwald JH Jr. Temporal bone abnormalities associated with hearing loss in Waardenburg syndrome. Laryngoscope. 2003;113(11):2035–41. https://www.ncbi.nlm.nih.gov/pubmed/14603070.
106. Tassabehji M, Read AP, Newton VE, et al. Waardenburg's syndrome patients have mutations in the human homologue of the Pax-3 paired box gene. Nature. 1992;355(6361):635–6. https://doi.org/10.1038/355635a0.
107. Wollnik B, Tukel T, Uyguner O, et al. Homozygous and heterozygous inheritance of PAX3 mutations causes different types of Waardenburg syndrome. Am J Med Genet A. 2003;122A(1):42–5. https://doi.org/10.1002/ajmg.a.20260.
108. Zlotogora J, Lerer I, Bar-David S, Ergaz Z, Abeliovich D. Homozygosity for Waardenburg syndrome. Am J Hum Genet. 1995;56(5):1173–8. https://www.ncbi.nlm.nih.gov/pubmed/7726174.
109. Hofstra RM, Osinga J, Tan-Sindhunata G, et al. A homozygous mutation in the endothelin-3 gene associated with a combined Waardenburg type 2 and Hirschsprung phenotype (Shah-Waardenburg syndrome). Nat Genet. 1996;12(4):445–7. https://doi.org/10.1038/ng0496-445.
110. Edery P, Attie T, Amiel J, et al. Mutation of the endothelin-3 gene in the Waardenburg-Hirschsprung disease (Shah-Waardenburg syndrome). Nat Genet. 1996;12(4):442–4. https://doi.org/10.1038/ng0496-442.
111. Sanchez-Martin M, Rodriguez-Garcia A, Perez-Losada J, Sagrera A, Read AP, Sanchez-Garcia I. SLUG (SNAI2) deletions in patients with Waardenburg disease. Hum Mol Genet. 2002;11(25):3231–6. https://www.ncbi.nlm.nih.gov/pubmed/12444107.
112. Pingault V, Bondurand N, Kuhlbrodt K, et al. SOX10 mutations in patients with Waardenburg-Hirschsprung disease. Nat Genet. 1998;18(2):171–3. https://doi.org/10.1038/ng0298-171.
113. Pingault V, Faubert E, Baral V, et al. SOX10 mutations mimic isolated hearing loss. Clin Genet. 2015;88(4):352–9. https://doi.org/10.1111/cge.12506.
114. Krouchi L, Callonnec F, Bouchetemble P, Tollard E, Dehesdin D, Marie JP. Preoperative computed tomography scan may fail to predict perilymphatic gusher. Ann Otol Rhinol Laryngol. 2013;122(6):374–7. https://doi.org/10.1177/000348941312200605.
115. Marlin S, Moizard MP, David A, et al. Phenotype and genotype in females with POU3F4 mutations. Clin Genet. 2009;76(6):558–63. https://doi.org/10.1111/j.1399-0004.2009.01215.x.
116. Stanton SG, Griffin A, Stockley TL, et al. X-linked hearing loss: two gene mutation examples provide generalizable implications for clinical care. Am J Audiol. 2014;23(2):190–200. https://doi.org/10.1044/2014_AJA-13-0040.
117. Starr A, Picton TW, Sininger Y, Hood LJ, Berlin CI. Auditory neuropathy. Brain. 1996;119(Pt 3):741–53. https://www.ncbi.nlm.nih.gov/pubmed/8673487.
118. Carvalho GM, Ramos PZ, Castilho AM, Guimaraes AC, Sartorato EL. Molecular study of patients with auditory neuropathy. Mol Med Rep. 2016;14(1):481–90. https://doi.org/10.3892/mmr.2016.5226.
119. Lv J, Wang H, Cheng X, et al. AAV1-hOTOF gene therapy for autosomal recessive deafness 9: a single-arm trial. Lancet. 2024;403(10441):2317–25. https://doi.org/10.1016/S0140-6736(23)02874-X.
120. Qi J, Tan F, Zhang L, et al. AAV-mediated gene therapy restores hearing in patients with DFNB9 deafness. Adv Sci (Weinh). 2024;11(11):e2306788. https://doi.org/10.1002/advs.202306788.
121. Wang H, Chen Y, Lv J, et al. Bilateral gene therapy in children with autosomal recessive deafness 9: single-arm trial results.

Nat Med. 2024;30(7):1898–904. https://doi.org/10.1038/s41591-024-03023-5.
122. Shearer AE, DeLuca AP, Hildebrand MS, et al. Comprehensive genetic testing for hereditary hearing loss using massively parallel sequencing. Proc Natl Acad Sci USA. 2010;107(49):21104–9. https://doi.org/10.1073/pnas.1012989107.
123. Atik T, Onay H, Aykut A, et al. Comprehensive analysis of deafness genes in families with autosomal recessive nonsyndromic hearing loss. PLoS One. 2015;10(11):e0142154. https://doi.org/10.1371/journal.pone.0142154.
124. Brownstein Z, Friedman LM, Shahin H, et al. Targeted genomic capture and massively parallel sequencing to identify genes for hereditary hearing loss in Middle Eastern families. Genome Biol. 2011;12(9):R89. https://doi.org/10.1186/gb-2011-12-9-r89.
125. Sivakumaran TA, Husami A, Kissell D, et al. Performance evaluation of the next-generation sequencing approach for molecular diagnosis of hereditary hearing loss. Otolaryngol Head Neck Surg. 2013;148(6):1007–16. https://doi.org/10.1177/0194599813482294.
126. Vozzi D, Morgan A, Vuckovic D, et al. Hereditary hearing loss: a 96 gene targeted sequencing protocol reveals novel alleles in a series of Italian and Qatari patients. Gene. 2014;542(2):209–16. https://doi.org/10.1016/j.gene.2014.03.033.
127. Sabatini LM, Mathews C, Ptak D, et al. Genomic sequencing procedure microcosting analysis and health economic cost-impact analysis: a report of the Association for Molecular Pathology. J Mol Diagn. 2016;18(3):319–28. https://doi.org/10.1016/j.jmoldx.2015.11.010.
128. Cooper GM. Parlez-vous VUS? Genome Res. 2015;25(10):1423–6. https://doi.org/10.1101/gr.190116.115.
129. gnomAD browser | genome Aggregation Database v.4.1.0. http://gnomad.broadinstitute.org/.
130. Kumar P, Henikoff S, Ng PC. Predicting the effects of coding non-synonymous variants on protein function using the SIFT algorithm. Nat Protoc. 2009;4(7):1073–81. https://doi.org/10.1038/nprot.2009.86.
131. Adzhubei IA, Schmidt S, Peshkin L, et al. A method and server for predicting damaging missense mutations. Nat Methods. 2010;7(4):248–9. https://doi.org/10.1038/nmeth0410-248.
132. Schwarz JM, Cooper DN, Schuelke M, Seelow D. MutationTaster2: mutation prediction for the deep-sequencing age. Nat Methods. 2014;11(4):361–2. https://doi.org/10.1038/nmeth.2890.
133. Oliver GR, Zimmermann MT, Klee EW, Urrutia RA. "The molecule's the thing:" the promise of molecular modeling and dynamic simulations in aiding the prioritization and interpretation of genomic testing results. F1000Res. 2016;5:766. https://doi.org/10.12688/f1000research.8600.3.
134. Wang J, Al-Ouran R, Hu Y, et al. MARRVEL: integration of human and model organism genetic resources to facilitate functional annotation of the human genome. Am J Hum Genet. 2017;100(6):843–53. https://doi.org/10.1016/j.ajhg.2017.04.010.
135. Oza AM, DiStefano MT, Hemphill SE, et al. Expert specification of the ACMG/AMP variant interpretation guidelines for genetic hearing loss. Hum Mutat. 2018;39(11):1593–613. https://doi.org/10.1002/humu.23630.
136. Patel MJ, DiStefano MT, Oza AM, et al. Disease-specific ACMG/AMP guidelines improve sequence variant interpretation for hearing loss. Genet Med. 2021;23(11):2208–12. https://doi.org/10.1038/s41436-021-01254-2.
137. Schimmenti LA, Bower M, Steyermark J. Genetic testing for deaf and hard of hearing individuals: genetic counseling. Curr Genet Med Rep. 2016;4:27–34.
138. Evans DG. Neurofibromatosis type 2 (NF2): a clinical and molecular review. Orphanet J Rare Dis. 2009;4:16. https://doi.org/10.1186/1750-1172-4-16.
139. Baser ME, De Rienzo A, Altomare D, et al. Neurofibromatosis 2 and malignant mesothelioma. Neurology. 2002;59(2):290–1. https://www.ncbi.nlm.nih.gov/pubmed/12136076.
140. Trofatter JA, MacCollin MM, Rutter JL, et al. A novel moesin-, ezrin-, radixin-like gene is a candidate for the neurofibromatosis 2 tumor suppressor. Cell. 1993;72(5):791–800. https://www.ncbi.nlm.nih.gov/pubmed/8453669.
141. Evans DG. NF2-related schwannomatosis. In: Adam MP, Mirzaa GM, Pagon RA, et al., editors. GeneReviews((R)). Seattle (WA): University of Washington; 1993.
142. Asthagiri AR, Parry DM, Butman JA, et al. Neurofibromatosis type 2. Lancet. 2009;373(9679):1974–86. https://doi.org/10.1016/S0140-6736(09)60259-2.
143. Evans DG, Moran A, King A, Saeed S, Gurusinghe N, Ramsden R. Incidence of vestibular schwannoma and neurofibromatosis 2 in the North West of England over a 10-year period: higher incidence than previously thought. Otol Neurotol. 2005;26(1):93–7. https://www.ncbi.nlm.nih.gov/pubmed/15699726.
144. Halliday D, Emmanouil B, Evans DGR. Updated protocol for genetic testing, screening and clinical management of individuals at risk of NF2-related schwannomatosis. Clin Genet. 2023;103(5):540–52. https://doi.org/10.1111/cge.14310.
145. Plotkin SR, Messiaen L, Legius E, et al. Updated diagnostic criteria and nomenclature for neurofibromatosis type 2 and schwannomatosis: an international consensus recommendation. Genet Med. 2022;24(9):1967–77. https://doi.org/10.1016/j.gim.2022.05.007.
146. Evans DG. Neurofibromatosis 2. In: Pagon RA, Adam MP, Ardinger HH, et al., editors. GeneReviews(R). Seattle (WA): University of Washington; 1993.
147. Evans DGR, Salvador H, Chang VY, et al. Cancer and central nervous system tumor surveillance in pediatric neurofibromatosis 2 and related disorders. Clin Cancer Res. 2017;23(12):e54–61. https://doi.org/10.1158/1078-0432.CCR-17-0590.
148. Plotkin SR, Blakeley JO, Evans DG, et al. Update from the 2011 International Schwannomatosis Workshop: from genetics to diagnostic criteria. Am J Med Genet A. 2013;161A(3):405–16. https://doi.org/10.1002/ajmg.a.35760.
149. Smith MJ, Bowers NL, Bulman M, et al. Revisiting neurofibromatosis type 2 diagnostic criteria to exclude LZTR1-related schwannomatosis. Neurology. 2017;88(1):87–92. https://doi.org/10.1212/WNL.0000000000003418.
150. Kirmani S, Young WF. Hereditary paraganglioma-pheochromocytoma syndromes. In: Pagon RA, Adam MP, Ardinger HH, et al., editors. GeneReviews(R). Seattle (WA): University of Washington; 1993.
151. Baysal BE, Ferrell RE, Willett-Brozick JE, et al. Mutations in SDHD, a mitochondrial complex II gene, in hereditary paraganglioma. Science. 2000;287(5454):848–51. https://www.ncbi.nlm.nih.gov/pubmed/10657297.
152. Dahia PL. Pheochromocytomas and paragangliomas, genetically diverse and minimalist, all at once! Cancer Cell. 2017;31(2):159–61. https://doi.org/10.1016/j.ccell.2017.01.009.
153. Group NGSiPS, Toledo RA, Burnichon N, et al. Consensus Statement on next-generation-sequencing-based diagnostic testing of hereditary phaeochromocytomas and paragangliomas. Nat Rev Endocrinol. 2017;13(4):233–47. https://doi.org/10.1038/nrendo.2016.185.
154. Pigny P, Vincent A, Cardot Bauters C, et al. Paraganglioma after maternal transmission of a succinate dehydrogenase gene mutation. J Clin Endocrinol Metab. 2008;93(5):1609–15. https://doi.org/10.1210/jc.2007-1989.
155. Taieb D, Nolting S, Perrier ND, et al. Management of phaeochromocytoma and paraganglioma in patients with germline SDHB pathogenic variants: an international expert Consensus statement.

Nat Rev Endocrinol. 2024;20(3):168–84. https://doi.org/10.1038/s41574-023-00926-0.
156. Gimenez-Roqueplo AP, Favier J, Rustin P, et al. Mutations in the SDHB gene are associated with extra-adrenal and/or malignant phaeochromocytomas. Cancer Res. 2003;63(17):5615–21. https://www.ncbi.nlm.nih.gov/pubmed/14500403.
157. Cosgrove D, Zallocchi M. Usher protein functions in hair cells and photoreceptors. Int J Biochem Cell Biol. 2014;46:80–9. https://doi.org/10.1016/j.biocel.2013.11.001 Epub 2013 Nov 12.
158. Ioannidis NM, Rothstein JH, Pejaver V, Middha S, McDonnell SK, Baheti S, Musolf A, Li Q, Holzinger E, Karyadi D, Cannon-Albright LA, Teerlink CC, Stanford JL, Isaacs WB, Xu J, Cooney KA, Lange EM, Schleutker J, Carpten JD, Powell IJ, Cussenot O, Cancel-Tassin G, Giles GG, MacInnis RJ, Maier C, Hsieh CL, Wiklund F, Catalona WJ, Foulkes WD, Mandal D, Eeles RA, Kote-Jarai Z, Bustamante CD, Schaid DJ, Hastie T, Ostrander EA, Bailey-Wilson JE, Radivojac P, Thibodeau SN, Whittemore AS, Sieh W. REVEL: An Ensemble Method for Predicting the Pathogenicity of Rare Missense Variants. Am J Hum Genet. 2016;99(4):877–885. https://doi.org/10.1016/j.ajhg.2016.08.016. Epub 2016 Sep 22.

9 Local Drug Delivery to the Inner Ear

Athanasia Warnecke, Thomas Muhleman, and Hinrich Staecker

Introduction

Local delivery of medications to the inner ear by injection into the middle ear space has been used for over 30 years for the treatment of Ménière's disease. Our increased understanding of inner ear physiology and rapid advancements in biotechnology have significantly expanded the disorders that are being addressed by local therapy and resulting in the development of novel delivery systems. When considering inner ear pharmacotherapy, the anatomy and physiology, mode of application, as well as pharmacokinetics need thorough consideration. The inner ear connects to the middle ear space via the round window and oval window and to the cerebrospinal fluid (CSF) space via the cochlear aqueduct. The blood supply to the inner ear is derived from branches of the anterior inferior cerebellar artery (AICA). However, the blood-labyrinth barrier impedes the transfer of therapeutic molecules from systemic circulation to inner ear targets. Direct access to the middle and inner ear is, therefore, required to allow for effective transtympanic or intrascalar/intralabyrinthine drug delivery.

Transtympanic Drug Delivery: Why and How

Delivery of medication to the inner ear can broadly be thought of in two categories: systemic delivery and local therapy. The inner ear is separated from the systemic circulation by a blood-labyrinth barrier that limits penetration of certain molecules from the systemic circulation to the inner ear [1–3]. Since the human inner ear has a perilymph volume of approximately 160 μL, distribution of orally or intravenous administered drug is also inefficient since it must equilibrate through the volume of the human body (approximately 40 L) to deliver a therapeutic effect in the ear, raising the possibility of unwanted systemic side effects. The fact that the middle ear can be used as a reservoir for drugs that can then diffuse through the round window has been recognized for many years [4]. Direct access and delivery into the inner ear via an intrascalar or transcanal route allow the accumulation of higher concentrations of drugs within the inner ear without systemic side effects. This approach has become the most common focus of delivery efforts to date.

Medication can be delivered via a myringotomy or simple puncture of the tympanic membrane (TM) with a needle. It is important that the patient be in supine position to allow the drug to settle on the round window niche (see Fig. 9.1a, b). In this position, the Eustachian tube is oriented toward the ceiling, thus maintaining medication in the middle ear. If the medication has low viscosity or is water-like, it will flow toward the Eustachian tube as soon as the patient sits up. An important factor in performing the procedure is local anesthesia. Initially, injections of lidocaine into the ear canal were used, but this is painful and not tolerated by many patients. Anesthesia of the tympanic membrane can be induced with concentrated tetracaine or EMLA (lidocaine/prilocaine 2.5%) cream [5, 6]. This can be applied to a small region of the TM with a small cerumen loop or cotton piece. After 10 min, the drum can then be punctured. Alternately, application of phenol to the drum anesthetizes and cauterizes a small area. Single-use phenol applicators (Apdyne Medical Company, Denver CO, USA) are available and decrease the risk of storing and handling a large amount of phenol. Puncture myringotomies with topical anesthesia generally stay open for 3–4 days, whereas phenol cautery of the drum followed by puncture stays open for 2–3 weeks (Fig. 9.1c). Refinements of this procedure include the use of iontophore-

A. Warnecke
Department of Otorhinolaryngology, Hannover Medical School, Hannover, Germany

T. Muhleman
Ascentis Healthcare, Kansas City, KS, USA

H. Staecker (✉)
Department of Otolaryngology—Head and Neck Surgery, University of Kansas Health System, Kansas City, KS, USA
e-mail: hstaecker@kumc.edu

A. D. Sweeney et al. (eds.), *Haynes-Glasscock-Shambaugh Surgery of the Ear*, https://doi.org/10.1007/978-3-032-18264-7_9

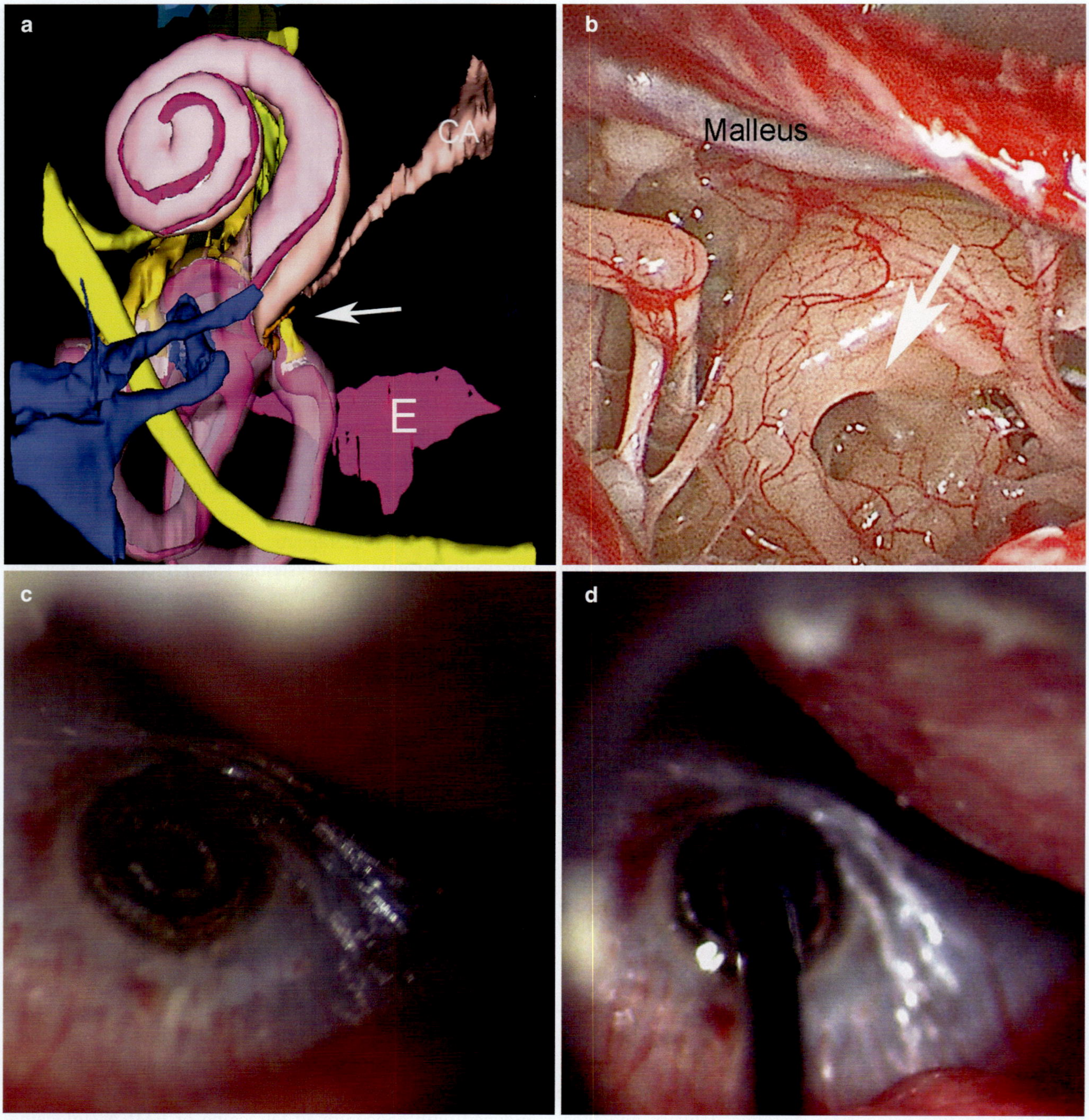

Fig. 9.1 Anatomic basis of middle ear drug delivery. Reconstruction of the middle and inner ear demonstrates the orientation of the ear when in the supine position (**a**). Medication needs to be applied in a large-enough volume to contact the round window (white arrow). The endolymphatic sac (E) can be directly accessed through the mastoid to allow delivery into the scala media. The cochlear aqueduct (CA) opens into the posterior fossa; substances injected into the inner ear can reach the CSF space through this route. The structures of the middle ear are seen in (**b**). The round window niche (white arrow) is often separated from the middle ear by a thin pseudomembrane. When injecting the middle ear space, filling the space to the level of the malleus results in both the round and oval window niches being covered with the drug. When performing serial injections, use of phenol to cauterize and anesthetize the TM results in a stable opening into the middle ear space (**c**). A 25# spinal needle can be used to fill the middle ear space (**d**)

sis to induce anesthesia or use of a laser-based myringotomy. This however requires additional equipment [7]. In clinical practice, a 25-gauge spinal needle can be used to perform the injections since these are long enough to reach through a speculum to the drum and can be bent at an angle to allow the surgeon an unobstructed view (Fig. 9.1d). The medication should then be slowly filled to about the level of the malleus (usually about 0.5 cc) to ensure that the round window niche and oval window niche are filled (Fig. 9.1b). The injection should be performed over 15–20 s to allow air bubbles to escape the middle ear. The patient is then instructed to lie supine for 20–45 min depending on the protocol to allow the drug to diffuse into the inner ear. As with all myringotomies, there is a theoretical risk of creating a permanent perforation, and this complication should be discussed as part of the consent process. Dry ear precautions postinjection are also needed to prevent post-procedure infections. When multiple injections are planned, some practitioners suggest placing a tube instead of performing repeat injections.

Anatomic Consideration for Delivery

Entry into the Inner Ear

In humans, medications can diffuse into the inner ear via either the round window or the oval window/stapediovestibular ligament. The round window membrane (RWM) is a three-layered membrane that separates the scala tympani from the middle ear space. It is integral to impedance matching of sound energy entering the middle ear, and its ability to transport medicines to the inner ear is a side effect of its physiologic function. The round window has an outer epithelium that faces the middle ear, a central core of connective tissue, and an inner epithelium. The outer epithelium consists of a single layer of cells with sparse microvilli. The connective tissue layer consists of fibroblasts, collagen myelinated and unmyelinated nerve fibers, blood vessels, and lymphatics. The inner epithelium is a squamous epithelium with lateral extensions that overlap. There are extensive extracellular spaces that allow the sequestration and transport of substances [8]. Factors impacting permeability include size, molecular weight, electrical charge of the substance being transported, and thickness of the round window. Additionally, adhesions causing obstruction of the round window have been shown to impede local drug delivery, making an argument for endoscopic inspection of the middle ear space prior to delivery [9, 10]. Electron microscopic studies have also demonstrated that there are different transport pathways for different types of substances suggesting that certain types of molecules may be more suited to local delivery than others [11]. When evaluating delivery in humans, one has to consider that the orientation of the round window is such that in normal sitting or standing position drugs are carried away from contact with the round window (Fig. 9.1a). Although the size of the round window is constant, there is significant variability between patients in the depth and orientation of the round window niche which may further alter delivery characteristics in patients. In addition, a false membrane covering the round window may further impair the entry of drugs to the inner ear. However, human cochlear pharmacokinetic studies showed the two active agents present in the investigational drug in FX-322 consistently entered the human cochlea regardless of anatomical variations such as false membranes or prominent bony round window overhangs [12]. To improve delivery of medications, drugs have to be modified to increase time of contact with the round window or directly injected into the inner ear [13–15]. Modeling of a potential drug's permeability and distribution within the cochlea can be used to design the optimal delivery route. Looking at an "egg plot" of medications that compares the hydrophobicity to the number of polar groups across the molecule surface can help predict the optimal formulation of a drug for distribution in the inner ear [16, 17]. Alternately, medications may also be delivered in conjunction with substances that increase the permeability of the RWM. Recent studies on liposome and polymersome delivery of fluorescent markers demonstrated effective delivery to the spiral ganglion and to a lesser degree the organ of Corti [13, 18]. Microparticle-based formulations have also been used to try to control the degree of release of an agent into the cochlea. Nanoparticles have also been shown to enhance cochlear entry and distribution [19].

Distribution in Perilymph

Animal studies suggest that there is also absorption directly through the otic capsule [20]. This may not occur in humans because of the thickness of the bone surrounding the cochlea but needs to be considered when translating animal studies to potential human trials [21]. Recently, there has also been documentation of absorption of drugs through the stapediovestibular ligament (the ligament that anchors the stapes bone in the oval window) allowing distribution to the scala vestibuli [22]. This implies that the oval window niche may also be used as a reservoir for drug delivery [23]. Interestingly, this anatomic feature of the middle ear may allow better retention of drugs in humans (Fig. 9.1b). The distribution of a molecule through the cochlea is dependent on the size of the cochlea and the diffusion coefficient of the substance being delivered. Using quantitative sampling methods developed in the Salt Lab (Washington University, USA, oto.wustl.edu/cochlea/), it has been determined that distribution of drugs within the scala tympani is passive. Therefore, once placed on the RWM and distributed to the inner ear by diffusion, drug concentration will be highest in the basal turn or the high-frequency region of the inner ear [24–26]. High molecular weight substances will tend to collect at the basal turn and will not reach the apical turn or low-frequency region of the cochlea. Similar techniques have also demonstrated that there is no significant flow within the cochlear fluids. The elimination of the drug from the cochlea is dependent on metabolism or elimination to blood. Improvements in delivery via the middle ear can therefore only be achieved by permeabilization of the RWM or formulation of drugs so that they have contact with the RWM for longer time periods (Fig. 9.2). Devices such as the Silverstein wick have also been proposed to prolong drug contact with the round window [27].

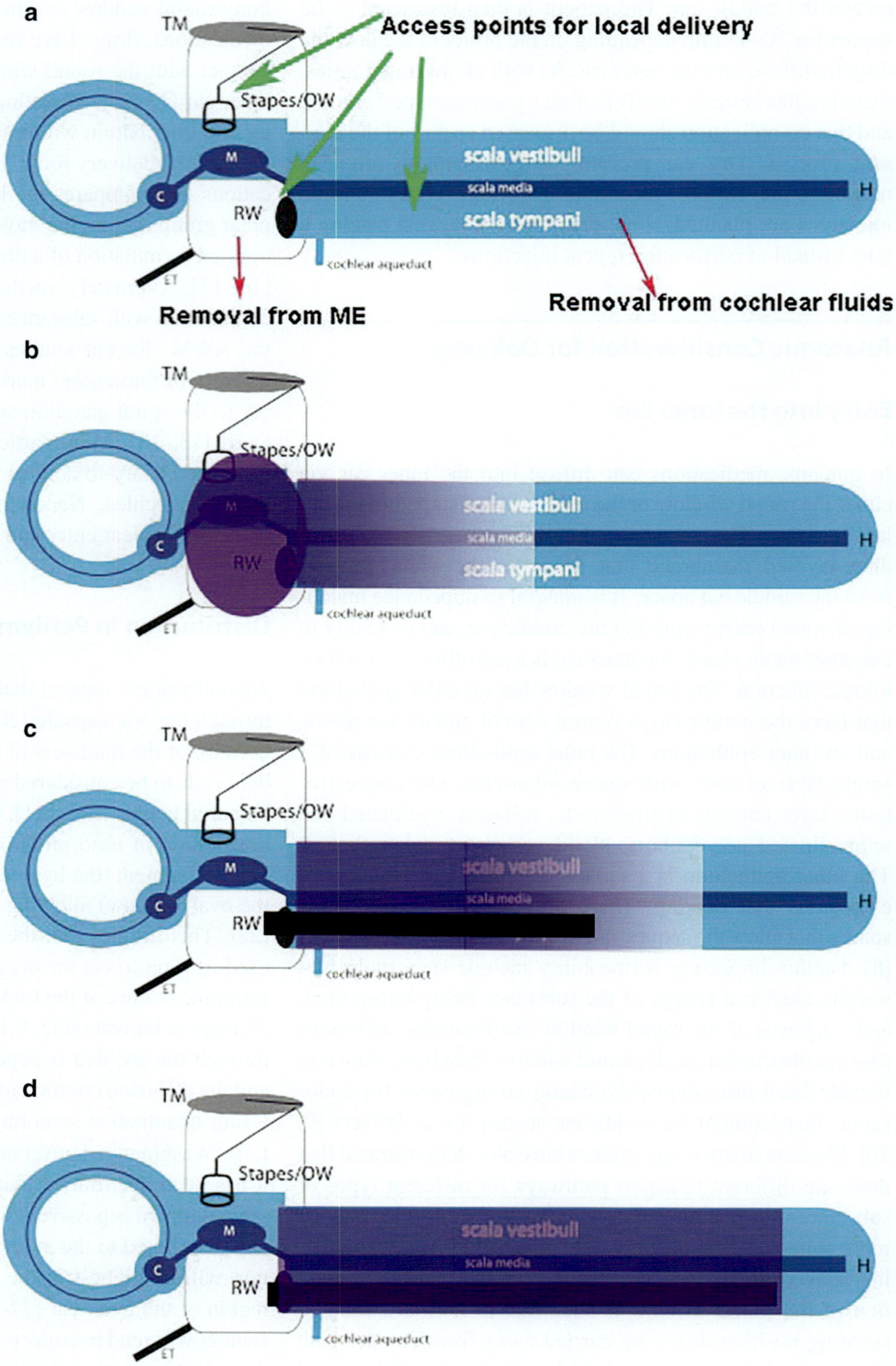

Fig. 9.2 Modeling distribution of medication in the inner ear. Routes of entry are shown in green (**a**). Drugs can be applied to or injected via the stapes footplate or the round window. Drugs can also be applied via a device in the perilymph space. Drugs are removed from the middle ear via absorption from the middle ear mucosa or by running down the Eustachian tube. When distributed in the perilymph, drugs diffuse into surrounding tissue and are removed by the cochlear blood supply. Application of a drug into the middle ear space (**b**) results in diffusion of the drug into the perilymph. Distribution is dependent on contact time in the middle ear, the physical properties of the drug, and the rate of removal. Modeling suggests that in humans most medications are unlikely to reach beyond the basal areas of the inner ear. Single-shot delivery of a drug into the inner ear can yield a more complete distribution of medications (**c**); however, medications are rapidly removed after delivery. Newer devices such as drug-eluting cochlear implants can produce more complete coverage of the entire inner ear (**d**)

Intrascalar Therapy

To overcome the limitations of diffusion-based therapy, active injection of drugs into the inner ear has been proposed [28]. Examples of direct delivery of pharmacologic agents via osmotic pumps without damage to residual inner ear function are present throughout the hearing research literature [29–31]. Recent advances in hearing preservation cochlear implantation demonstrate that instrumentation and displacement of perilymph within the human inner ear are possible without loss of residual function [32, 33]. Therefore, microinjection of drug into the scala tympani via the RWM or into the scala vestibuli via a stapedotomy could be performed without damage to residual inner ear function

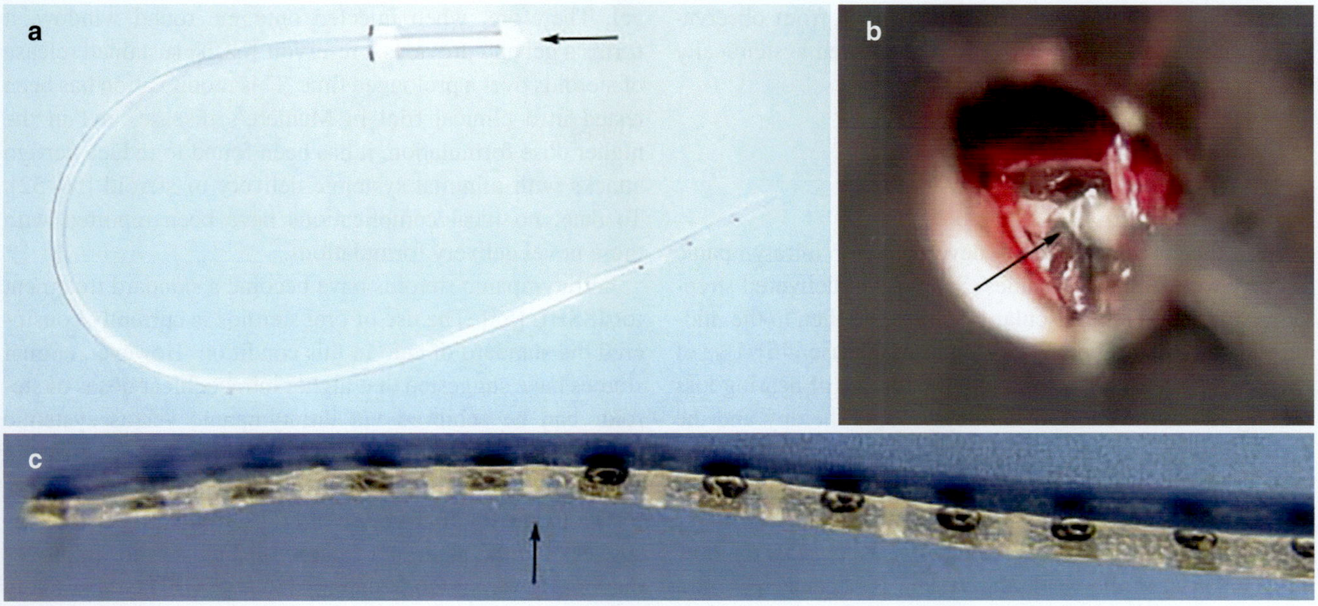

Fig. 9.3 Novel drug delivery devices for use in the ear. The Med-El cochlear catheter is a flexible catheter that can be inserted up to 20 mm into the scala tympani via the round window. It is presently CE marked in Europe and has been used in clinical studies (**a**). In the first-in-human inner ear gene therapy study, the study drug was infused through the stapes footplate via a 200-µm-wide metal catheter (arrow) (**b**). Most recently, medications have been incorporated in bands fused onto a cochlear implant to provide more long-term delivery

(Fig. 9.3). This would require the development of new equipment and injection devices that are not available in current neurotologic practice.

The endolymphatic sac has also been proposed as a potential space to deliver drugs. This organ connects to the scala media (Fig. 9.1a) and is thought to be involved in the reabsorption of endolymph. In an animal study, steroids were injected into the endolymphatic sac and shown to modulate aquaporin 3 expression [34, 35]. A recent study has also demonstrated that gadolinium injected into the endolymphatic sac of human patients undergoing a surgery for Ménière's disease is distributed all the way to the apical portion of the scala media. This occurred without any damage to residual hearing [36]. The endolymphatic sac is easily accessible in humans and could thus be used as a reservoir for drug delivery. Cochlear implant candidates may provide a population in which intrascalar drug delivery can be tested [37]. These patients already have a significant hearing loss, reducing the risk of drug-related hearing loss, and undergo an invasive procedure to improve their hearing. Drugs could be tested acutely via injection into the inner ear during placement of the electrode. Alternatively, several different electrode designs have been proposed in which a drug delivery channel is incorporated into the cochlear implant electrode [38, 39]. This could then be used to deliver drugs via a pump that is connected to the implant [37]. Catheter-based designs have been tested in humans. Single-shot intrascalar application of drugs via a catheter inserted in the cochlea does not require pumps or similar reservoirs and has been shown to be safe and effective in humans during cochlear implantation. Dose-dependent effects were also observed by using a catheter to deliver different steroid concentrations to more apical regions of the cochlea [40, 41]. However, the effects achieved with the catheter are transient and require depot formulation of drugs for longer efficacy periods (Figs. 9.2 and 9.3). Another approach to circumvent the lack of distribution of drugs within the cochlea after delivery via the RWM is the use of a reciprocating pump [42, 43]. The system works by picking up perilymph from the inner ear, which is then combined with the drug to be delivered and subsequently reinjected into the perilymph at controllable cycles. Studies in animals have shown effective delivery into the scala tympani with rapid equilibration of drug. Delivery from this type of system will probably be required to treat ear disease that evolves over long periods of time, such as presbycusis. Prior to implementation of long-term delivery in humans, researchers will have to address potential risks such as the transmission of infection into the cochlea from an externally refillable drug reservoir.

Medications Currently Being Applied Using Local Delivery

Local drug delivery is widely used to treat a number of acute inner ear diseases [44, 45]. Experience gained from these studies has led to increasing use of intratympanic medications. At present, medications being used in day-to-day practice are ones that have been developed from observations of the effects of these medications when systemically delivered.

Gentamicin

Among the first medications developed for intratympanic delivery were aminoglycosides. Schuknecht delivered streptomycin first by intramuscular injection and then to the middle ear space of patients with Ménière's disease [46]. Use of streptomycin was associated with a high rate of hearing loss leading to modification of aminoglycoside therapy and the use of gentamicin which has a lower incidence of hearing loss. A number of different delivery protocols have been proposed to ablate the vestibular system without auditory injury [47]. Interestingly, there is no consensus on exactly how much ablation of the vestibular system is needed to control Ménière's disease or the optimal delivery dose. Gentamicin treatment has evolved from a completely ablative treatment given through a series of consecutive injections over a 1-to-2-week period to mini-dose protocols. Most widely used in practice is the application of a single treatment of intratympanic gentamicin sulfate at a concentration of 40 mg/mL. When considering this treatment, it is important to determine that the contralateral ear has normal vestibular function.

Steroids

The most widely used medications for intratympanic delivery are steroids. Steroids have been used for the treatment of Ménière's disease, idiopathic sudden sensorineural hearing loss (ISSHL), and autoimmune inner ear disease (AIED). The use of steroids for Ménière's disease was first described in 1991 and evaluated in a randomized trial in 2005. Prospective studies show a 91% success rate in controlling vertigo using intratympanic dexamethasone; however, follow-up trials did not show any difference in improving hearing or tinnitus. Since distribution studies suggest limited distribution of dexamethasone to the cochlear apex when middle ear delivery is used, several attempts have been made to improve the availability of the drug at the RWM. These included the use of a microcatheter that pumps drug against the RWM as well as the use of a wick system that allows patients to self-administer drug into the ear canal which is then drawn up to the round window via a porous carrier [47–49]. Modification of steroids has also been attempted to improve contact time with the round window. A temperature-sensitive polymer in combination with steroids has been developed. This polymer exists in a liquid form at room temperature and when heated to body temperature becomes a gel. Therefore, when injected onto the round window, it forms a gel and provides a reservoir for the sustained release of steroids over a prolonged time. This modification has been tested in a clinical trial in Ménière's disease, and in the higher dose formulation, it has been found to reduce vertigo attacks with minimal systemic delivery of steroid [50–52]. To date, no local complications have been reported with these novel delivery formulations.

Intratympanic steroids have become a standard treatment for ISSHL [53]. The use of oral steroids is currently considered the standard of care in this condition. However, animal studies have suggested that higher intracochlear doses of steroids can be achieved via intratympanic versus systemic delivery. Early trials applied different doses, repetitions, and formulations of steroids injected through the eardrum as a rescue treatment after failure of oral steroids. Recent studies suggest that the addition of intratympanic steroids improves outcomes over systemic therapy alone [54]. The most likely explanation for this is that higher concentrations of steroids can be achieved in the inner ear when intratympanic delivery is used. A recent randomized prospective clinical trial also demonstrated that intratympanic steroids were equivalent in efficacy when compared directly with oral steroids [55]. Since intratympanic steroids would be expected to have a lower side effect profile, this may be the optimal way to treat these patients. In most studies that have performed meta-analysis or reviews of steroid delivery, the outcomes have been difficult to judge because of the variance in administration protocols and types of steroids used [56, 57].

Steroids may also be used to improve outcomes in cochlear implantation [58, 59]. Cochlear implants are now being inserted into patients with significant residual hearing and poor speech discrimination. Animal models suggest that intracochlear administration of steroids improves hearing preservation after manipulation of the inner ear. In one human trial, application of steroids to the RWM prior to cochlear implantation prevented postoperative dizziness, implying that the steroids protect inner ear function. The impact of preoperative steroids applied to the inner ear has also been prospectively studied in patients undergoing hearing preservation cochlear implantation. This study showed that steroid treatment improved hearing outcomes [23, 60]. A recent development in this field has been the incorporation of steroids into the matrix of cochlear implants. Diffusion of steroids out of the electrode would then give a cochlear protective effect that can be customized by the type and amount of steroids incorporated into the electrode [61–63]. Potential risks of this approach are increasing the risk of infection or decreasing healing at the cochleostomy site. What has not been defined is the optimal schedule of steroid treatment. For example, should steroids be delivered 24 h before surgery, and should they be maintained for a certain postoperative time?

NMDA Inhibitors

Cochlear N-methyl-D-aspartate (NMDA) receptors have been implicated in the initial generation of tinnitus after excitotoxicity [31, 64]. An intriguing study demonstrated that application of an NMDA inhibitor in animals undergoing acute sound trauma prevented the development of chronic tinnitus [65]. This has led to the development of NMDA inhibitors that can be used in humans and the launch of European and US clinical trials that evaluated these compounds for clinical use [66, 67]. These products were formulated in viscous hyaluronic acid gel to enhance the retention of the drug in the middle ear after injection.

Drugs Modulating Apoptosis

Modulation of apoptosis has been a focus of research aiming to attenuate ototoxicity and noise-induced hearing loss. The last 10 years have seen maturation of the understanding of the molecular biology underlying auditory hair cell apoptosis. The c-Jun and Jnk signaling cascades can be modulated via a variety of peptides that can abort apoptotic signaling [68]. The activation of Jnk signaling has been demonstrated in sound trauma, and delivery of Jnk blocking peptide has been shown to protect against impulse noise. A small study of patients presenting after acute sound from a firecracker explosion demonstrated the local RWM administration of Jnk inhibitor AM 111 (D isomer of Jnk-binding peptide) appears to protect from sound trauma [69, 70].

Antioxidants

Oxidative stress has been implicated in the pathophysiology of ototoxicity and noise trauma. A wide variety of different antioxidants have been tested both systemically and with local delivery after insults to the inner ear. D-Methionine has been proposed as a protective agent against cisplatin.

Development in the delivery of medications include both devices and novel therapeutic strategies for inner ear disease ototoxicity and noise trauma [44, 71]. Local delivery of these medications may have advantages of systemic delivery in terms of potency and lack of interference with chemotherapeutic agents such as cisplatin when locally delivered. Potential disadvantages are the requirement for repeated dosing to maintain inner ear drug levels. For drugs that have the potential for systemic toxicity, such as cisplatin, local delivery of a protectant molecule will of course only protect the inner ear and not offer any protection of other organs such as the kidneys.

The Future of Drug Delivery to the Inner Ear

Increasing data from human trials and cochlear implantation have demonstrated the ability to instrument the inner ear without loss of function. This opens the possibility of developing a range of novel therapeutics for inner ear disease. Delivery of large molecules, viral vectors, and cells requires direct delivery into the inner ear.

Gene Therapy

The same characteristics that make the inner ear an ideal target for local drug delivery also make it an ideal target for gene therapy. Gene delivery has the potential to address some of the concerns raised with treatment of chronic progressive inner ear disease, namely, that the presence of a catheter or pump predisposes the inner ear to infection. Gene therapy research in the inner ear has focused on regeneration of sensory cells and on chronic delivery of neurotrophins to the inner ear (refer to section "Neurotrophin Delivery to the Inner Ear"). Gene therapy also has the potential to address a number of genetic and degenerative disorders of the inner ear, and recently significant progress has been achieved in this domain in animal models [72–74]. The effort to determine the molecular basis for hair cell generation has led to examination of factors controlling hair cell differentiation [75]. One of the genes involved in the development of hair cells is the mammalian homolog of the atonal gene (*math1/atoh1*). Further investigation of this pathway has demonstrated that a complex regulatory pathway specifies the differentiation of hair cells and supporting cells and that suppression of atonal effects is what specifies a cell as a supporting cell. Transfer of atoh1 using an adenoviral vector was demonstrated to restore damaged auditory vestibular neuroepithelium [76, 77]. Translation to human clinical trials required intracochlear administration of the vector since diffusion through the round window for large biomolecules such as viruses is very inefficient [78]. For the human clinical trial NCT02133120, viral vector was infused though a stapedotomy (Fig. 9.3b). Currently, clinical trials for a variety of congenital genetic hearing loss are being planned with intrascalar injection approaches.

Neurotrophin Delivery to the Inner Ear

In animal models, the loss of neurotrophic support after destruction of the organ of Corti results in progressive degeneration of the spiral ganglion population which can potentially impact cochlear implant outcomes. The additional delivery of various growth factors to the cochlea has resulted in increased preservation of neurons after deafness, regrowth of peripheral processes, and reduction of the threshold of electrical stimulation, suggesting potential benefits for cochlear implant function. Functional recovery of ABR wave I was found in mice in whom neurotrophin-3 was administered to the round window niche 24 h after noise exposure [79, 80]. Feasible methodologies for short-term delivery of these agents include single-shot injection of particles, delivery from a pump or from a reservoir within the body of the electrode array, polymer-based delivery, or delivery from cells coating the electrode array [81, 82]. Longer-term delivery might be obtained using, for example, encapsulated cells or local cell manipulation through gene therapy-based approaches [83, 84]. Several animal cochlear implant models have shown effective support of spiral ganglion survival and function with neurotrophin gene therapy [85, 86]. Currently cochlear implants are being developed to deliver nonviral vectors expressing the neurotrophin BDNF using electroporation [87, 88].

Nanoparticles

Nanoparticles have been utilized to provide reservoirs for drugs on the RWM as well as materials to improve delivery to individual cells within the inner ear. As described above, a variety of different materials have been used to improve contact between a drug and the RWM. Most of these are various types of biodegradable polymers that prevent escape of a liquid drug formulation via the Eustachian tube, as well as a thermosensitive hydrogel-based delivery system, similar to that described for steroid administration above. Use of more sophisticated nanomaterials is currently improving delivery to the inner ear without the use of virus-derived vectors. Magnetic nanoparticles injected into the inner ear can potentially be driven to their target using a magnetic field [89].

Cell Therapy

Cell transplantation to the inner ear has been investigated in animal models for different purposes. Initial attempts aimed to replace lost sensory of neural cells by transplanting stem or progenitor cells to the cochlea [90]. Survival and integration of transplanted cells to the inner ear are limited and usually improved in sound-damaged cochleae or when co-transplanted with embryonic cells [91, 92]. Indeed, transplantation of cells into embryonic stages of the inner ear has been successfully performed to treat connexin 30 deficiency in mice suggesting that in the future cell therapy could be used in a range of different inner ear pathologies [93]. Factors impacting the integration of cells include the acuity of damage and the underlying matrix they are integrating into [94, 95].

Autologous cell transplantation may offer several advantages over allogeneic cell transplantation by reducing the risk of transmission of infectious diseases and of rejection reactions. When cells are transplanted as a source of protective and anti-inflammatory factors, the potency of the transplanted cells to release such factors needs to be considered. For example, mesenchymal stromal cells are well known for their protective and immunemodulative secretome and may present clinically feasible and effective methods for the delivery of human neuroprotective factors into the spatially constricted inner ear. Autologous mononuclear cells derived from the human bone marrow were investigated not only as suitable sources for regulating inflammation and mediating neuroprotective and immunomodulatory effects but also as sources of a balanced composition of various naturally occurring neuroprotective factors [96]. To overcome the disadvantages associated with cell therapies, extracellular vesicles (EVs) can be used since they are considered as a next-generation cell therapy. They allow the delivery of the therapeutic secretome of the cells without the need to transplant the cells themselves. As such, EVs can be delivered directly to the inner ear via a catheter as has been shown recently in a first-in-man application. They can be manufactured under GMP conditions and provide an opportunity to modulate a wide range of pathologic and physiologic pathways [97, 98].

Conclusion

Local drug delivery to the inner ear grew out of an attempt to avoid the side effects of systemically administered medications. Our increased understanding of inner ear drug distribution has shown that increased efficacy of drug delivery will require improvement of local delivery in terms of substances that maintain a drug in the middle ear and direct delivery of medication to the inner ear. Development of novel instrumentation to aid delivery also has to be considered. The first area of development will likely be micro-endoscopes to evaluate the middle ear prior to delivery of a drug to the middle ear. Further development of micromanipulators and microinjectors will be needed as more potential intracochlear interventions are developed. Currently, application of steroids and aminoglycosides is commonly used in middle ear-based delivery. Steroids have also been applied to the inner ear. As our diagnosis of inner ear disorders begins to reflect the molecular processes going on in the ear, local delivery of medication will play an increasing role in the treatment of inner ear disorders.

References

1. Nyberg S, Joan Abbott N, Shi X, Steyger PS, Dabdoub A. Delivery of therapeutics to the inner ear: the challenge of the blood-labyrinth barrier. Sci Transl Med. 2019;11(482). https://doi.org/10.1126/scitranslmed.aao0935.

2. Hirose K, Li SZ. The role of monocytes and macrophages in the dynamic permeability of the blood-perilymph barrier. Hear Res. 2019;374:49–57. https://doi.org/10.1016/j.heares.2019.01.006.
3. Shi X. Pathophysiology of the cochlear intrastrial fluid-blood barrier (review). Hear Res. 2016;338:52–63. https://doi.org/10.1016/j.heares.2016.01.010.
4. Kohonen A, Tarkkanen J. Cochlear damage from ototoxic antibiotics by intratympanic application. Acta Otolaryngol. 1969;68(1–6):90–7. https://doi.org/10.3109/00016486909121547.
5. Silverstein H, Call DL. Tetracaine base: an effective surface anesthetic for the tympanic membrane. Arch Otolaryngol. 1969;90(2):150–1. https://doi.org/10.1001/archotol.1969.00770030152010.
6. Jyväkorpi M. A comparison of topical Emla cream with Bonain's solution for anesthesia of the tympanic membrane during tympanocentesis. Eur Arch Oto-Rhino-Laryngol. 1996;253(4–5):234–6. https://doi.org/10.1007/bf00171133.
7. Comeau M, Brummett R. Anesthesia of the human tympanic membrane by iontophoresis of a local anesthetic. Laryngoscope. 1978;88(2):277–85. https://doi.org/10.1288/00005537-197802000-00010.
8. Goycoolea MV, Lundman L. Round window membrane. Structure function and permeability: a review. Microsc Res Tech. 1997;36(3):201–11. https://doi.org/10.1002/(SICI)1097-0029(19970201)36:3<201::AID-JEMT8>3.0.CO;2-R.
9. Plontke SK-R, Plinkert PK, Plinkert B, Koitschev A, Zenner H-P, Löwenheim H. Transtympanic endoscopy for drug delivery to the inner ear using a new microendoscope. In: Rational pharmacotherapy of the inner ear, vol. 59. Basel: KARGER; 2002. p. 149–55. https://doi.org/10.1159/000059253.
10. Marchioni D, Alicandri-Ciufelli M, Pothier DD, Rubini A, Presutti L. The round window region and contiguous areas: endoscopic anatomy and surgical implications. Eur Arch Otorrinolaringol. 2015;272(5):1103–12. https://doi.org/10.1007/s00405-014-2923-8.
11. Hentzer E. Ultrastructure of the human tympanic membrane. Acta Otolaryngol. 1969;68(1–6):376–90. https://doi.org/10.3109/00016486909121576.
12. McLean WJ, Hinton AS, Herby JTJ, et al. Improved speech intelligibility in subjects with stable sensorineural hearing loss following intratympanic dosing of FX-322 in a phase 1b study. Otol Neurotol. 2021; Publish Ah; https://doi.org/10.1097/MAO.0000000000003120.
13. Pritz CO, Dudás J, Rask-Andersen H, Schrott-Fischer A, Glueckert R. Nanomedicine strategies for drug delivery to the ear. Nanomedicine. 2013;8(7):1155–72. https://doi.org/10.2217/nnm.13.104.
14. Sakamoto T, Nakagawa T, Horie RT, et al. Inner ear drug delivery system from the clinical point of view. Acta Otolaryngol. 2010;130(SUPPL. 563):101–4. https://doi.org/10.3109/00016489.2010.486801.
15. Camarero G, Varela-Nieto I, Rivera T, Sanz L. Drug delivery to the inner ear: strategies and their therapeutic implications for sensorineural hearing loss IGF1R and chronic lung diseases view project genetic and molecular bases of age-related hearing loss view project drug delivery to the inner ear: strategies and their therapeutic implications for sensorineural hearing loss. Drug Deliv. 2012; https://doi.org/10.2174/156720112800389098.
16. Salt A, Plontke S. Pharmacokinetic principles in the inner ear: influence of drug properties on intratympanic applications. Hear Res. 2018; https://www.sciencedirect.com/science/article/pii/S0378595517306202?casa_token=YPoOxGJzSTsAAAAA:vFCxfsCkK2FRMSqL-cVj3Fj4vrCk__uGCYvy_avcOP6X6BetMyC8CF7KnubEs7Ow-yfv5T3V. Accessed 9 May 2020
17. Daina A, Zoete V. A boiled-egg to predict gastrointestinal absorption and brain penetration of small molecules. ChemMedChem. 2016:1117–21. https://doi.org/10.1002/cmdc.201600182.
18. Mäder K, Lehner E, Liebau A, Plontke SK. Controlled drug release to the inner ear: concepts, materials, mechanisms, and performance. Hear Res. 2018;368:49–66. https://doi.org/10.1016/j.heares.2018.03.006.
19. Dormer NH, Nelson-Brantley J, Staecker H, Berkland CJ. Evaluation of a transtympanic delivery system in Mus musculus for extended release steroids. Eur J Pharm Sci. 2018; https://doi.org/10.1016/j.ejps.2018.01.020.
20. Mikulec A, Plontke S, Hartsock J. Entry of substances into perilymph through the bone of the otic capsule following intratympanic applications in Guinea pigs: implications for local drug delivery. Otol Neurotol. 2009; https://www.ncbi.nlm.nih.gov/pmc/articles/PMC2729139/. Accessed 9 May 2020
21. Glueckert R, Chacko LJ, Rask-andersen H, Liu W, Handschuh S, Schrott-fischer A. Anatomical basis of drug delivery to the inner ear. Hear Res. 2018:1–18. https://doi.org/10.1016/j.heares.2018.06.017.
22. Salt AN, King EB, Hartsock JJ. Marker entry into vestibular perilymph via the stapes following applications to the round window niche of Guinea pigs. Hear Res. 2012;283:14. https://doi.org/10.1016/j.heares.2011.11.012.
23. Rajan GP, Kuthubutheen J, Hedne N, Krishnaswamy J. The role of preoperative, intratympanic glucocorticoids for hearing preservation in cochlear implantation: a prospective clinical study. Laryngoscope. 2012;122(1):190–5. https://doi.org/10.1002/lary.22142.
24. Salt A, Plontke SK. Local inner-ear drug delivery and pharmacokinetics. Drug Discov Today. 2005; https://www.sciencedirect.com/science/article/pii/S1359644605035749?casa_token=HG7sBDIRdqkAAAAA:4GMymmNmHgGiyHgs9uD5H0VYJAQUkRBlKnFDY1a_4Xifm6I-50O5gDpd1f1W2xuqJmRtg1nr. Accessed 9 May 2020.
25. Salt AN, Plontke SK. Pharmacokinetic principles in the inner ear: influence of drug properties on intratympanic applications. Hear Res. 2018;368:28–40. https://doi.org/10.1016/j.heares.2018.03.002.
26. Salt AN, Hartsock JJ, Gill RM. Perilymph pharmacokinetics of markers and dexamethasone applied and sampled at the lateral semi-circular canal. J Assoc Res Otolaryngol. 2012;13:771. https://doi.org/10.1007/s10162-012-0347-y.
27. Silverstein H. Use of a new device, the MicroWick™, to deliver medication to the inner ear. Ear Nose Throat J. 1999;78(8):595–600. https://doi.org/10.1177/014556139907800816.
28. Plontke SK, Hartsock JJ, Gill RM. Intracochlear drug injections through the round window membrane: measures to improve drug retention. Audiol Neurootol. 2016;21:72. https://doi.org/10.1159/000442514.
29. Davies E, Gladstone HB, Williams H, Hradek G, Shah SB, Schindler RA. A model for long-term intracochlear administration of pharmacologic agents. Am J Otol. 1994;15(6):757–61. http://www.ncbi.nlm.nih.gov/pubmed/8572088
30. Miller JM, Miller AL, Yamagata T, Bredberg G, Altschuler RA. Protection and regrowth of the auditory nerve after deafness: neurotrophins, antioxidants and depolarization are effective in vivo. Audiol Neurootol. 2002;7(3):175–9. https://doi.org/10.1159/000058306.
31. d'Aldin CG, Ruel J, Assie R, Pujol R, Puel JL. Implication of NMDA type glutamate receptors in neural regeneration and neoformation of synapses after excitotoxic injury in the Guinea pig cochlea. Int J Dev Neurosci. 1997;15(4–5):619–29. http://www.ncbi.nlm.nih.gov/pubmed/9263038
32. Pillsbury HC, Dillon MT, Buchman CA, et al. Multicenter US clinical trial with an electric-acoustic stimulation (EAS) system in adults: final outcomes. Otol Neurotol. 2018;39(3):299. https://doi.org/10.1097/MAO.0000000000001691.

33. Rodgers B, Prentiss S, Staecker H. Expanding cochlear implantation to patients with residual mid and high frequency hearing. Otorinolaringol. 2012;62(4):183.
34. Kitahara T, Fukushima M, Uno Y, Mishiro Y, Kubo T. Up-regulation of cochlear aquaporin-3 mRNA expression after intra-endolymphatic sac application of dexamethasone. Neurol Res. 2003;25(8):865–70. https://doi.org/10.1179/016164103771953989.
35. Kitahara T, Kubo T, Okumura SI, Kitahara M. Effects of endolymphatic sac drainage with steroids for intractable Ménière's disease: a long-term follow-up and randomized controlled study. Laryngoscope. 2008;118(5):854–61. https://doi.org/10.1097/MLG.0b013e3181651c4a.
36. Colletti V, Mandalà M, Carner M, et al. Evidence of gadolinium distribution from the endolymphatic sac to the endolymphatic compartments of the human inner ear. Audiol Neurootol. 2010;15(6):353–63. https://doi.org/10.1159/000292929.
37. Plontke SK, Götze G, Rahne T, Liebau A. Intracochlear drug delivery in combination with cochlear implants. HNO. 2017;65(S1):19–28. https://doi.org/10.1007/s00106-016-0285-9.
38. Jolly C, Garnham C, Mirzadeh H. Electrode features for hearing preservation and drug delivery strategies. In: Adv Otorhinolaryngol, vol. 67; 2010.
39. Shepherd RK, Xu J. A multichannel scala tympani electrode array incorporating a drug delivery system for chronic intracochlear infusion. Hear Res. 2002;172:92. https://doi.org/10.1016/S0378-5955(02)00517-8.
40. Prenzler NK, Salcher R, Timm M, Gaertner L, Lenarz T, Warnecke A. Intracochlear administration of steroids with a catheter during human cochlear implantation: a safety and feasibility study. Drug Deliv Transl Res. 2018;8(5):1191–9. https://doi.org/10.1007/s13346-018-0539-z.
41. Prenzler NK, Salcher R, Lenarz T, Gaertner L, Warnecke A. Dose-dependent transient decrease of impedances by deep Intracochlear injection of triamcinolone with a cochlear catheter prior to cochlear implantation–1 year data. Front Neurol. 2020;11:258. https://doi.org/10.3389/fneur.2020.00258.
42. Tandon V, Kang WS, Spencer AJ, et al. Microfabricated infuse-withdraw micropump component for an integrated inner-ear drug-delivery platform. Biomed Microdevices. 2015;17(2):37. https://doi.org/10.1007/s10544-014-9923-8.
43. Kim ES, Gustenhoven E, Mescher MJ, et al. A microfluidic reciprocating intracochlear drug delivery system with reservoir and active dose control. Lab Chip. 2014;14(4):710–21. https://doi.org/10.1039/c3lc51105g.
44. Rybak LP, Dhukhwa A, Mukherjea D, Ramkumar V. Local drug delivery for prevention of hearing loss. Front Cell Neurosci. 2019;13:300. https://doi.org/10.3389/fncel.2019.00300.
45. Piu F, Bishop K. Local drug delivery for the treatment of neurotology disorders. Front Cell Neurosci. 2019; https://www.frontiersin.org/articles/10.3389/fncel.2019.00238/abstract. Accessed 9 May 2020
46. Silverstein H. Streptomycin treatment for Meniere's disease. Ann Otol Rhinol Laryngol. 1984;93(4 II SUPPL. 112):44–8. https://doi.org/10.1177/00034894840930s408.
47. Miller MW, Agrawal Y. Intratympanic therapies for Menière's disease. Curr Otorhinolaryngol Rep. 2014;2(3):137–43. https://doi.org/10.1007/s40136-014-0055-8.
48. Devantier L, Djurhuus B, Hougaard D. Intratympanic steroid for Menière's disease: a systematic review. Otology. 2019; https://journals.lww.com/otology-neurotology/Fulltext/2019/07000/Intratympanic_Steroid_for_Meni_re_s_Disease__A.26.aspx?casa_token=fbugQNLQf_gAAAAA:wivGVtLOG0cI-JaMkdgvrR1TohKtT2qxITMpuHocfVVOlADvYQOpl4Xt09MX9Zm90JAnimO3kwV6DgYGlDPwa_dywabYjA7FTzkEnEAVang. Accessed 9 May 2020
49. Barrs DM, Keyser JS, Stallworth C, McElveen JT. Intratympanic steroid injections for intractable Ménière's disease. Laryngoscope. 2001;111(12):2100–4. https://doi.org/10.1097/00005537-200112000-00003.
50. Carey J, Mikulec A, LeBel C. Intratympanic sustained-exposure dexamethasone thermosensitive gel for symptoms of Meniere's disease: randomized phase 2b safety and efficacy trial. Otol Neurotol. 2016; https://www.ncbi.nlm.nih.gov/pmc/articles/PMC5414596/. Accessed 9 May 2020
51. Wang X, Dellamary L, Fernandez R, Ye Q, Lebel C, Piu F. Principles of inner ear sustained release following intratympanic administration. Laryngoscope. 2011;121(2):385–91. https://doi.org/10.1002/lary.21370.
52. Lustig L, Fletcher M, Bear M, LeBel C. Placebo-controlled clinical study to assess safety and clinical activity of OTO-104 given as a single intratympanic injection in patients with unilateral Ménière's .... Otology. 2012. https://journals.lww.com/otology-neurotology/Fulltext/2012/09000/A_Randomized,_Double_Blind,_Placebo_Controlled.25.aspx?casa_token=4GmyeYZ94HkAAAAA:FHKYeXk-J9VoTdCaQJqx8zIxrFWJDeulxQ_rhe8ll_aeBkMII1zkM9rFQ_4c85lIMBzTLoBSOA8Jxi67n0V-pGXNvyQFU1ZydGqezcp-5Q. Accessed 9 May 2020.
53. Vanwijck F, Rogister F, Pierre Barriat S, Camby S, Lefebvre P. Intratympanic steroid therapy for refractory sudden sensory hearing loss: a 12-year experience with the Silverstein catheter. Acta Otolaryngol. 2019;139(2):111–6. https://doi.org/10.1080/00016489.2018.1532107.
54. Taha A, Shlamkovitch N, AbuEta R. High dose of intratympanic steroids for sudden sensorineural hearing loss salvage. Otology. 2019; https://journals.lww.com/otology-neurotology/Fulltext/2019/10000/High_Dose_of_Intratympanic_Steroids_for_Sudden.7.aspx?casa_token=wTp58EbOfeQAAAAA:oityAdfxlR17jOsAR151ZdVAzH1wZ2-mFrS5ButEFptLqkvJErH5w50Zj_cqZDH7oKjcgsJzHrK1hrvde1lydJxroxYts3M9Pjd_jY0Yjg. Accessed 9 May 2020
55. Ermutlu G, Süslü N, Yılmaz T, Saraç S. Sudden hearing loss: an effectivity comparison of intratympanic and systemic steroid treatments. Eur Arch Oto-Rhino-Laryngol. 2017;274(10):3585–91. https://doi.org/10.1007/s00405-017-4691-8.
56. Witsell DL, Mulder H, Rauch S, Schulz KA, Tucci DL. Steroid use for sudden sensorineural hearing loss: a CHEER network study. Otolaryngol - Head Neck Surg (United States). 2018;159(5):895–9. https://doi.org/10.1177/0194599818785142.
57. Liebau A, Pogorzelski O, Salt A. Hearing changes after intratympanic steroids for secondary (salvage) therapy of sudden hearing loss: a meta-analysis using mathematical simulations of drug. Otol Neurotol. 2018; https://www.ncbi.nlm.nih.gov/pmc/articles/PMC6481671/. Accessed 9 May 2020
58. Kuthubutheen J, Joglekar S, Smith L, et al. The role of preoperative steroids for hearing preservation cochlear implantation: results of a randomized controlled trial. Audiol Neurootol. 2017;22(4–5):292–302. https://doi.org/10.1159/000485310.
59. OLeary S, Bester C, Tari S, Hearing ARJ of. Results of a double-blinded placebo controlled trial on the efficacy of high-dose systemic steroids for hearing preservation in cochlear implantation. J Hear. 2018; http://search.ebscohost.com/login.aspx?direct=true&profile=ehost&scope=site&authtype=crawl

er&jrnl=2083389X&AN=131274595&h=XSU4e9IDjubUSGkcIcZ8WGPMiLSn%2FJISNTFn6eo9CF8YB9w0BpUnAEvDIu0MqExffJV5G0VVGnnWk1vc%2BisaPA%3D%3D&crl=c. Accessed 21 October 2018
60. Lyu AR, Kim DH, Lee SH, Shin DS, Shin SA, Park YH. Effects of dexamethasone on intracochlear inflammation and residual hearing after cochleostomy: a comparison of administration routes. PLoS One. 2018;13(3):e0195230. https://doi.org/10.1371/journal.pone.0195230.
61. Liu Y, Jolly C, Braun S. Effects of a dexamethasone-releasing implant on cochleae: a functional, morphological and pharmacokinetic study. Hear Res. 2015;327:89. https://doi.org/10.1016/j.heares.2015.04.019.
62. Ghavi FF, Mirzadeh H, Imani M, Jolly C, Farhadi M. Corticosteroid-releasing cochlear implant: a novel hybrid of biomaterial and drug delivery system. J Biomed Mater Res - Part B Appl Biomater. 2010;94(2):388–98. https://doi.org/10.1002/jbm.b.31666.
63. Farhadi M, Jalessi M, Salehian P, et al. Dexamethasone eluting cochlear implant: histological study in animal model. Cochlear Implants Int. 2013;14(1):45–50. https://doi.org/10.1179/1754762811Y.0000000024.
64. Puel JL, Saffiedine S, Gervais d'Aldin C, Eybalin M, Pujol R. Synaptic regeneration and functional recovery after excitotoxic injury in the Guinea pig cochlea. CR Acad Sci III. 1995;318(1):67–75. http://www.ncbi.nlm.nih.gov/pubmed/7538893
65. Bing D, Lee SC, Campanelli D, et al. Cochlear NMDA receptors as a therapeutic target of noise-induced tinnitus. Cell Physiol Biochem. 2015;35(5):1905–23. https://doi.org/10.1159/000374000.
66. Staecker H, Maxwell KS, Morris JR, et al. Selecting appropriate dose regimens for AM-101 in the intratympanic treatment of acute inner ear tinnitus. Audiol Neurotol. 2015;20(3):172. https://doi.org/10.1159/000369608.
67. Van de Heyning P, Muehlmeier G, Cox T. Efficacy and safety of AM-101 in the treatment of acute inner ear tinnitus—a double-blind, randomized, placebo-controlled phase II study. Otology. 2014; https://www.ncbi.nlm.nih.gov/pmc/articles/PMC3966923/. Accessed 9 May 2020
68. Eshraghi AA, He J, Mou CH. D-JNKI-1 treatment prevents the progression of hearing loss in a model of cochlear implantation trauma. Otol Neurotol. 2006;27:504.
69. Suckfuell M, Canis M, Strieth S. Intratympanic treatment of acute acoustic trauma with a cell-permeable JNK ligand: a prospective randomized phase I/II study. Acta Otolaryngol. 2007;127:938. https://doi.org/10.1080/00016480601110212.
70. Suckfuell M, Lisowska G, Domka W. Efficacy and safety of AM-111 in the treatment of acute sensorineural hearing loss: a double-blind, randomized, placebo-controlled phase II study. Otol Neurotol. 2014;35:1317. https://doi.org/10.1097/MAO.0000000000000466.
71. Gabaizadeh R, Staecker H, Liu W, et al. Protection of both auditory hair cells and auditory neurons from cisplatin induced damage. Acta Otolaryngol. 1997;117(2):232.
72. Lustig LR, Akil O. Cochlear gene therapy. Curr Opin Neurol. 2012;25(1):57–60. https://doi.org/10.1097/WCO.0b013e32834f038c.
73. Ahmed H, Shubina-Oleinik O, Holt JR. Emerging gene therapies for genetic hearing loss. J Assoc Res Otolaryngol. 2017;18(5):649–70. https://doi.org/10.1007/s10162-017-0634-8.
74. Büning H, Schambach A, Morgan M, et al. Challenges and advances in translating gene therapy for hearing disorders. Expert Rev Precis Med Drug Dev. 2020;5(1):23–34. https://doi.org/10.1080/23808993.2020.1707077.
75. Hildebrand MS, Newton SS, Gubbels SP, et al. Advances in molecular and cellular therapies for hearing loss. Mol Ther. 2008;16(2):224–36. https://doi.org/10.1038/sj.mt.6300351.
76. Izumikawa M, Minoda R, Kawamoto K, Abrashkin K. Auditory hair cell replacement and hearing improvement by Atoh1 gene therapy in deaf mammals. Nat Med. 2005; http://www.nature.com/nm/journal/v11/n3/abs/nm1193.html. Accessed 7 June 2017
77. Schlecker C, Praetorius M, Brough DE, et al. Selective atonal gene delivery improves balance function in a mouse model of vestibular disease. Gene Ther. 2011;18(9):884. https://doi.org/10.1038/gt.2011.33.
78. Jero J, Mhatre AN, Tseng CJ, et al. Cochlear gene delivery through an intact round window membrane in mouse. Hum Gene Ther. 2001;12(5):539–48. https://doi.org/10.1089/104303401300042465.
79. Wan G, Gómez-Casati ME, Gigliello AR, Charles Liberman M, Corfas G. Neurotrophin-3 regulates ribbon synapse density in the cochlea and induces synapse regeneration after acoustic trauma. elife. 2014;2014:1–35. https://doi.org/10.7554/eLife.03564.
80. Suzuki J, Corfas G, Liberman MC. Round-window delivery of neurotrophin 3 regenerates cochlear synapses after acoustic overexposure. Sci Rep. 2016;6(1):24907. https://doi.org/10.1038/srep24907.
81. Radeloff A, Unkelbach MH, Mack MG, et al. A coated electrode carrier for cochlear implantation reduces insertion forces. Laryngoscope. 2009;119(5):959–63. https://doi.org/10.1002/lary.20206.
82. Richardson RT, Wise AK, Thompson BC. Polypyrrole-coated electrodes for the delivery of charge and neurotrophins to cochlear neurons. Biomaterials. 2009;30:2614. https://doi.org/10.1016/j.biomaterials.2009.01.015.
83. Scheper V, Hoffmann A, Gepp MM, et al. Stem cell based drug delivery for protection of auditory neurons in a Guinea pig model of cochlear implantation. Front Cell Neurosci. 2019;13:177. https://doi.org/10.3389/fncel.2019.00177.
84. Schwieger J, Hamm A, Gepp M. Alginate-encapsulated brain-derived neurotrophic factor–overexpressing mesenchymal stem cells are a promising drug delivery system for protection of auditory. J Tissue. 2020;11. https://doi.org/10.1177/2041731420911313.
85. Leake PA, Rebscher SJ, Dore C, Akil O. AAV-mediated neurotrophin gene therapy promotes improved survival of cochlear spiral ganglion neurons in neonatally deafened cats: comparison of AAV2-hBDNF and AAV5-hGDNF. J Assoc Res Otolaryngol. 2019:1–21. https://doi.org/10.1007/s10162-019-00723-5.
86. Pfingst BE, Colesa DJ, Swiderski DL, et al. Neurotrophin gene therapy in deafened ears with cochlear implants: long-term effects on nerve survival and functional measures. J Assoc Res Otolaryngol. 2017;18(6):731–50. https://doi.org/10.1007/s10162-017-0633-9.
87. Pinyon JL, von Jonquieres G, Crawford EN, et al. Neurotrophin gene augmentation by electrotransfer to improve cochlear implant hearing outcomes. Hear Res. 2019; https://doi.org/10.1016/J.HEARES.2019.06.002.
88. Pinyon JL, Tadros SF, Froud KE, et al. Close-field electroporation gene delivery using the cochlear implant electrode array enhances the bionic ear. Sci Transl Med. 2014; www.ScienceTranslationalMedicine.org. Accessed 9 May 2020
89. Frisina RD, Budzevich M, Zhu X, Martinez GV, Walton JP, Borkholder DA. Animal model studies yield translational solu-

tions for cochlear drug delivery. Hear Res. 2018; https://doi.org/10.1016/J.HEARES.2018.05.002.
90. Warnecke A, Mellott AJ, Römer A, Lenarz T, Staecker H. Advances in translational inner ear stem cell research. Hear Res. 2017; https://doi.org/10.1016/j.heares.2017.05.011.
91. Coleman B, Hardman J, Coco A, et al. Fate of embryonic stem cells transplanted into the deafened mammalian cochlea. Cell Transplant. 2006;15(5):369–80. https://doi.org/10.3727/000000006783981819.
92. Hildebrand MS, Dahl HHM, Hardman J, Coleman B, Shepherd RK, De Silva MG. Survival of partially differentiated mouse embryonic stem cells in the scala media of the Guinea pig cochlea. J Assoc Res Otolaryngol. 2005;6(4):341–54. https://doi.org/10.1007/s10162-005-0012-9.
93. Takeda H, Dondzillo A, Randall JA, Gubbels SP. Challenges in cell-based therapies for the treatment of hearing loss. Trends Neurosci. 2018;41(11):823–37. https://doi.org/10.1016/j.tins.2018.06.008.
94. Lang H, Ebihara Y, Schmiedt R, et al. Contribution of bone marrow hematopoietic stem cells to adult mouse inner ear: mesenchymal cells and fibrocytes. J Comp Neurol. 2006;496(2):187–201. https://doi.org/10.1002/cne.20929.
95. Schulze J, Sasse S, Prenzler N, et al. Microenvironmental support for cell delivery to the inner ear. Hear Res. 2018;368:109–22. https://doi.org/10.1016/j.heares.2018.06.015.
96. Roemer A, Köhl U, Majdani O, et al. Biohybrid cochlear implants in human neurosensory restoration. Stem Cell Res Ther. 2016;7(1):148. https://doi.org/10.1186/s13287-016-0408-y.
97. Warnecke A, Prenzler N, Harre J, et al. First-in-human intracochlear application of human stromal cell-derived extracellular vesicles. J Extracell Vesicles. 2021;10(8):e12094. https://doi.org/10.1002/JEV2.12094.
98. Warnecke A, Harre J, Staecker H, et al. Extracellular vesicles from human multipotent stromal cells protect against hearing loss after noise trauma in vivo. Clin Transl Med. 2020;10(8):e262. https://doi.org/10.1002/ctm2.262.

Tumor Biology of Vestibular Schwannomas

10

Archana Podury, Nicole T. Jiam, and D. Bradley Welling

Introduction

Recent advances in molecular biology have led to a better understanding of the etiology of many cranial base tumors. The ultimate goal of understanding the cellular mechanisms of tumorigenesis is to develop new treatment options that improve patient outcomes. Indeed, trials of several therapeutic agents targeting known pathways are underway.

As an example of the recent advances in cranial base tumors, vestibular schwannomas (VS) will be highlighted. VS generally arise as sporadic unilateral tumors in the internal auditory canal (IAC) and the cerebellopontine angle (CPA); however, they are also found bilaterally as the hallmark of the inherited genetic disorder *NF2*-related schwannomatosis, formerly known as neurofibromatosis type 2 (NF2) [Online Mendelian Inheritance in Man (OMIM) #101000]. NF2 syndrome is an autosomal-dominant disorder caused by the pathogenic biallelic variants on chromosome 22, which gives rise to VS, as well as meningiomas, ependymomas, epiretinal membranes, hamartomas, and presenile cataracts.

Fundamental understanding of the underlying molecular events leading to tumor formation began when the neurofibromatosis type 2 tumor suppressor gene (*NF2* gene) was identified, and pathogenic variants were confirmed in the VS or the germ line [1–3]. The clinical characteristics of VS and NF2 syndromes have both been related to alterations in the *NF2* gene. The clinical manifestations of NF2 have been described in association with various pathogenic variants, and signaling pathways affected by merlin (the product of the *NF2* gene) are becoming better understood.

For purposes of this chapter and elsewhere in the literature, abbreviations are as follows: "NF2" is used to indicate the human disease of neurofibromatosis type 2; the italicized "*NF2*" represents the human neurofibromatosis type 2 gene; and "*Nf2*" indicates the homolog or similar gene expressed in rodents. The mouse *Nf2* gene and the human *NF2* gene share greater than 98% amino acid homology, thus making the mouse a relevant model for study. Interestingly, chickens have 94% and drosophila have 50% human amino acid homology as well [4].

The nomenclature $nf^{+/+}$ is wild-type or normal nf gene. $nf^{-/-}$ refers to the absence of both alleles (homozygosity), and $nf^{+/-}$ refers to heterozygosity or one allele only being nonfunctional.

Vestibular schwannomas can be grouped into unilateral sporadic solid VS or bilateral NF2-associated schwannomas [5]. VS with true cysts or cystic schwannomas present with a unique and aggressive phenotype, which may distinguish it from the more benign solid unilateral sporadic schwannoma. Pathogenic variants in the *NF2* gene have been identified in all three tumor types, but at the molecular level, the tumors are only beginning to be distinguished from each other [6, 7].

Schwannomas most commonly present as solitary tumors and constitute 95% of all VS. Sporadic unilateral VS occur in approximately 10–20 persons per million per year [8, 9]. However, the true incidence may be higher. Anderson et al. [10] reported an incidence of 7 unsuspected schwannomas per 10,000 brain MRI studies (0.07%) or 70 per million. Sporadic tumors usually occur in the fourth and fifth decades with a mean presentation at about 50 years of age. Although histologically benign, schwannomas can compress the brain

A. Podury
Department of Otolaryngology—Head and Neck Surgery, University of California, San Diego, San Diego, CA, USA
e-mail: apodury@health.ucsd.edu

N. T. Jiam
Department of Otolaryngology—Head and Neck Surgery, University of California San Francisco School of Medicine, San Francisco, CA, USA
e-mail: Nicole.Jiam@ucsf.edu

D. B. Welling (✉)
Department of Otolaryngology—Head and Neck Surgery, Massachusetts Eye and Ear and Massachusetts General Hospital, Boston, MA, USA

Department of Otolaryngology—Head and Neck Surgery, Harvard Medical School, Boston, MA, USA
e-mail: Brad_Welling@meei.harvard.edu

A. D. Sweeney et al. (eds.), *Haynes-Glasscock-Shambaugh Surgery of the Ear*, https://doi.org/10.1007/978-3-032-18264-7_10

stem, leading to hydrocephalus, herniation, and death. Most commonly, they are associated with hearing loss, tinnitus, imbalance, facial paralysis, and facial paresthesias.

NF2 [OMIM #101000] is clinically an autosomal-dominant disease that is highly penetrant [11]. NF2-associated tumors account for about 5% of all VS. Patients who inherit an abnormal copy of the *NF2* tumor suppressor gene have a 95% chance of developing bilateral VS. However, about one-half of patients have no family history of NF2 in Caucasian populations. In a study by Teranishi et al., the number of familial NF2 cases in Japan was found to be around 7% [12]. As founders, patients without family history of NF2 represent new germ line mutations that were not inherited. Other disease features of NF2 include intracranial meningiomas, ependymomas, spinal schwannomas, epiretinal membranes, hamartomas, and presenile lens opacities [13–16]. The onset of symptoms is usually between 11 and 30 years of age, but for some patients, the symptoms may present in their fifth or sixth decade. The incidence is estimated at between 1 in 33,000 and 1 in 40,000 [17, 18]. NF2 is not to be confused with neurofibromatosis type 1 (NF1), historically referred to as von Recklinghausen's syndrome [OMIM #162200]. NF1 is associated with multiple peripheral neurofibromas and is caused by a pathogenic variant in the *NF1* tumor suppressor gene on chromosome 17.

The spectrum of phenotypic expression in NF2 varies widely. In the past, the more severe clinical presentations were termed the Wishart type [19]. In addition to bilateral VS, patients often suffered from associated spinal tumors with a typical onset of symptoms in the late teens or early 20s. The less severe phenotypes have been termed the Gardner type with a later onset of bilateral schwannomas and fewer associated intracranial or spinal tumors [20]. A third subtype known as segmental or mosaic NF2 has been described, where only a portion of cells carries the NF2 pathogenic variant due to a postzygotic mutation [21]. In truth, the spectrum of disease does not always allow a clear distinction but rather follows a continuum.

Mosaic NF2 may vary in its clinical presentation compared to familial cases of NF2 [22]. The cause of segmental NF2 may be due to somatic mosaicism where a pathogenic variant occurs later in embryogenesis rather than in the germ line DNA; therefore, only a portion of the patient's cells carry the pathogenic variant, and the disease is manifested in limited areas of the body [23, 24]. In contrast, patients with familial NF2 inherit one pathogenic variant from a parent at conception, and all cells carry one mutant allele. Kluwe et al. [22] estimated that mosaicism may account for 25% of the NF2 cases of any subtype among patients whose parents did not display the disease. Patients with somatic mosaicism could display bilateral VS if the postzygotic mutation occurred early in embryogenesis. However, they may also display an atypical presentation or segmental NF2, in which the patient has a unilateral vestibular schwannoma and an ipsilateral, additional intracranial tumor, such as a meningioma, if the postzygotic mutation occurred later in development [25]. Unlike the traditional forms of NF2, the risk of passing NF2 caused by mosaicism to future offspring is low.

Cystic Schwannomas

Cystic VS are a particularly aggressive group of unilateral, sporadic schwannomas, which invade the surrounding cranial nerves, splaying them throughout the tumors. Cystic VS are associated with either intratumoral or extratumoral cysts, which develop within Antoni B regions, a histologic term to describe loosely organized tissue within peripheral nerve sheath tumors. In addition, a higher degree of nuclear atypia is seen in cystic tumors [26, 27]. Careful distinction must be drawn between the truly cystic schwannomas and the very common heterogeneous schwannomas, which are not as aggressive in their clinical behavior. On magnetic resonance imaging (MRI), truly cystic regions of the tumors are hyperintense on T2-weighted images, and the cysts do not enhance with gadolinium administration. The noncystic component of cystic tumors enhances with gadolinium in a manner similar to the unilateral and NF2-associated schwannomas. Cystic tumors may grow rapidly and are difficult to manage due to the high rate of hearing loss, facial nerve paralysis, and recurrence that occurs after surgical removal [28]. When compared to solid tumors of a similar size, the rate of complete facial nerve paralysis (House-Brackmann grade VI) with surgical removal of cystic tumors was 41%, as compared to 27% for that of solid unilateral schwannomas [29]. Cystic tumors are also more likely to have continued growth and facial nerve paralysis when treated with stereotactic radiation therapy than either the unilateral spontaneous or NF2-associated schwannomas [30].

Although the effectiveness of treatment with current surgical and radiation treatments for VS is generally good, treatment-related morbidity continues to be problematic.

A brief review of recent discoveries and advances in the molecular biology of VS will follow.

The *NF2* Gene

The *NF2* gene was localized to chromosome 22 band q12 through genetic and physical mapping (Fig. 10.1) [31, 32]. Positional cloning studies led to the discovery of the *NF2* gene in 1993 by two independent groups, Rouleau et al. [2] and Trofatter et al. [1] The gene was found to be frequently mutated in NF2-related VS. Since that time, pathogenic variants in the *NF2* gene have been found not only in NF2-associated tumors but also in sporadic unilateral schwannomas and cystic schwannomas [3, 33–40]. Additionally, patho-

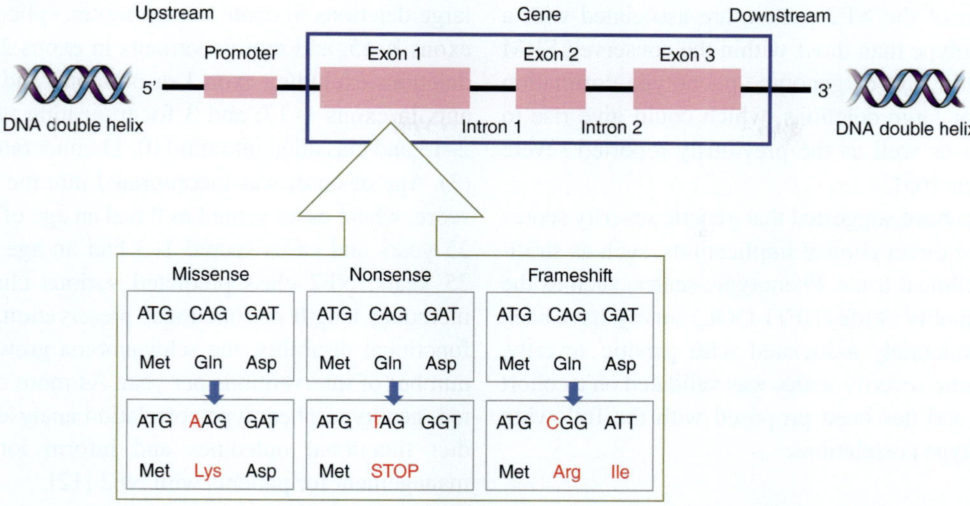

Fig. 10.1 Summary of genetic principles. Pathogenic variants can occur upstream of the gene itself in the promoter or regulatory regions or at the boundaries between introns and exons (splice sites). Pathogenic variants in the promoter or regulatory region may lead to over- or underexpression of the gene, while mutations in the intron/exon boundary may lead to aberrant splicing. Aberrant splicing might delete part of the resulting protein, add a new section of amino acids, or result in a frameshift. Single-nucleotide pathogenic variants within the exon may be classified as missense (single amino acid change), nonsense (premature stop codon), or frameshift (altered reading frame with multiple changes in downstream amino acids). Frameshift and nonsense pathogenic variants can be particularly disruptive to protein function. (Adapted from Surgery of the Ear. 6th Ed. Eds. PMPH. 2010)

genic variants within the *NF2* gene have been frequently identified in meningiomas and occasionally identified in other tumor types such as mesotheliomas [36–38, 41–45].

Human *NF2* Pathogenic Variants and Their Clinical Correlation

Specific *NF2* pathogenic variants in VS have been characterized in sporadic unilateral schwannomas and NF2-associated schwannomas [32–36, 38, 46–61]. The frequency, type, and distribution of *NF2* pathogenic variants were shown to be different between the sporadic and familial NF2 tumors [3]. Point mutations accounted for the majority of pathogenic variants identified in NF2 patients, whereas small deletions accounted for the majority of pathogenic variants found in sporadic unilateral tumors [47, 48, 56].

Two groups have recently published large databases of NF2 pathogenic variants. Ahronowitz et al. [62] presented a meta-analysis of 1070 small genetic changes detected primarily by exon scanning including 42 intragenic changes of 1 whole exon or larger and 29 whole gene deletions and gross chromosomal rearrangements. Overall, somatic events detected by tumor analysis showed a significantly different genetic profile than constitutional events detected in the patients' leukocytes. Over half of the pathogenic variants detected in tumors were frameshift pathogenic variants. The deletion of a single nucleotide from a gene can have particularly disrupting effects because all the codons downstream from the mutation are changed. In comparison, constitutional or system-wide inherited changes were primarily nonsense and splice site pathogenic variants (Fig. 10.1) [63]. Somatic events also differed markedly in meningiomas where most pathogenic variants were within the 5-prime protein 4.1 (ezrin, radixin, and moesin) (FERM) domain of the transcript with a complete absence of pathogenic variants in exons 14 and 15. Less than 10% of small alterations were nontruncating or lesions, which would not completely destroy the protein. These changes were clustered in exons 2 and 3, suggesting that this region may be especially crucial to tumor suppressor activity in the protein. We and others have shown a frequent pattern of mutation changing arginine codons (CGA) to the thymine stop codon (TGA). This type of "stop" codon not only terminates the transcription of mRNA but often results in degradation of the mRNA already transcribed in both VS and meningiomas, causing a truncating lesion [3, 64]. The chemical bonds associated with the configuration of these nucleotides make them less stable and more likely to undergo spontaneous mutation not only in NF2 but many other tumors as well. No pathogenic variants have been reported in exons 16 and 17, and few were noted in exon 9.

Studies to determine if genotype could be a predictor of disease severity showed that deletions that caused truncation of the NF2 protein have a more severe phenotype in NF2 pedigrees [47, 48, 56], while missense mutations (Fig. 10.1) or small in-frame insertions in the *NF2*-coding region have been reported to associate with a mild phenotype [3, 36, 37, 55, 57, 58]. However, exceptions are common as some missense mutations have been associated with severe phenotypes. The location of the mutation within the gene may influence phenotype as missense mutations within the α-helical domain of the NF2 protein are associated with a less severe phenotype than those within the conserved ERM domain [62]. This lack of genotype-phenotype correlation was also seen for large deletions, which could give rise to mild phenotypes as well as the previously reported severe disease expression [65].

Recent studies have suggested that genetic severity scores of NF2 may have direct clinical implications, such as stratification during clinical trials. Phenotypic scales, such as the NF2 impact on quality of life (NFTI-QOL) survey, have been shown to be moderately associated with genetic severity. One of such genetic severity scales was validated on a cohort of 142 patients and has been proposed with the following genotype-phenotype correlations:

- Type 1 cases present with a mild phenotype and include mosaic cases where the pathogenic variants are seen only in the tumor and not in the blood.
- Type 2a cases present with a mild phenotype and include missense mutations, truncating mutations in exons 1 and 13/14, splicing variants in exons 7–15, and mosaic variants in the blood (excluding those in exons 2–13).
- Type 2b cases present with a moderately severe phenotype and include large deletions, splicing variants in exons 1–6, and mosaics for truncating variants (exons 2–13) in the blood.
- Type 3 cases present with a severe phenotype and are frequently childhood onset with an expected mortality before the age of 60 years. These cases involve truncating mutations in exons 2–13.

The genetic severity score has been found to correlate with various hearing outcomes, including pure tone average (PTA) deterioration, hearing classification, and optimum discrimination scores (ODS). A weak correlation has also been reported between quality of life outcomes and the number of interventions. Genetic severity scores for NF2 have been used to counsel patients and may be implemented in clinical trial design, such as confining early phase trials to type 2b and 3 cases [66, 67].

This classification system has been supplemented with additional genotypic and phenotypic data. A cohort of 57 NF2 patients was sequenced and found to have a variety of germ line NF2 mutations, including truncating mutations, large deletions, splice site variants, and missense mutations, as well as mosaic NF2 mutations. Patients were assessed for progression of functional disability in hearing, swallowing, and gait function. The length of functional preservation differed significantly by mutation type, with longer functional preservation in mosaic variants and shortest preservation in truncating mutations. The authors used their findings and the previously described genetic severity score to generate a revised scale. Cases were scored by genotype: 0 for mosaic and variants in exons 1, 14, and 15; 1 for missense mutations, large deletions in exon 1 or promoter, splice site variants in exons 8–15, and mosaic variants in exons 2–13; 2 for large deletions excluding exon 1 or promoter and splice site variants in exons 1–17; and 3 for truncating variants in exons 2–15 and classified into mild (0, 1), moderate (2), and severe (3). Age of onset was incorporated into the genetic severity score, where cases scored as 0 had an age of onset at or after 25 years and cases scored 1–3 had an age of onset before 25 years. NF2 class predicted various clinical outcomes, including length of functional preservation, progression of functional disability, the schwannoma growth rate, and the number of interventions per year. As more cohorts are studied, genotype-phenotype correlation analyses may help predict functional outcomes and inform long-term disease management for patients with NF2 [12].

Clinical studies indicate that the phenotypic expression is more closely related within families than between families, but even within families, variability exists [68]. When statistically analyzed, the age of onset of NF2, the age at onset of hearing loss, and the number of intracranial meningiomas were all found to have a significant intrafamilial correlation [69]. It is not known whether this variability occurs by chance, by epigenetic phenomena, or by modifying genes at other loci [70]. Epigenetic phenomena are not caused by a change in the coding sequence of the DNA but rather alter the gene expression during gene development or cell proliferation. An example would be the methylation of segments of the promoter region of the *NF2* gene, which suppresses the expression of the gene. The *NF2*-coding region encompasses 17 exons spanning 90 kilobase pairs (kBp) of DNA on chromosome 22 [1, 2, 71]. By extensive screening of the entire *NF2* gene, Zucman-Rocci et al. [69] reported an 84% mutation detection rate in VS. Thus, additional mechanisms of inactivation of the *NF2* gene in some patients may exist. Mutation or methylation in the regulatory region of the *NF2* gene has been suggested (Fig. 10.1) as a possible mechanism of gene inactivation [72–74]. Posttranscriptional alternative splicing and differential polyadenylation may also be considered as possible means of inactivating the *NF2* gene [71]. Polyadenylation refers to the variable number of adenines that are attached at the 3′ end of the mRNA which may play a role in the way a gene is regulated. Alternative splicing refers to different patterns of splicing exons, in this case, the NF2 gene, resulting in differing isoforms of the gene. The two most common isoforms of NF2 have either exon 16 or exon 17 spliced out.

The NF2 Protein: Structure and Function

The *NF2* gene product is named merlin, for moesin-ezrin-radixin-like protein, or *schwannomin*, a name derived from schwannoma [1, 2]. For simplicity, the NF2 protein is referred to as "merlin" in this chapter. The *NF2* gene is transcribed into multiple RNA species by alternative splicing. Isoforms I and II are the two major RNA isoforms expressed in the cell. Isoform I encodes a 595-amino-acid protein and has exon 16 spliced out. Isoform II, containing all 17 exons, differs from Isoform I only at the C-terminus. Insertion of exon 16 into the mRNA provides a new stop codon, resulting in a 590-amino-acid protein that is identical to isoform I over the first 579 residues. Intriguingly, only isoform I possesses growth suppression activity [75].

Merlin shares a high degree of homology to the erythrocyte protein 4.1-related superfamily of proteins, which act to link the actin cytoskeleton to the plasma membrane [1, 2]. In particular, three proteins, ezrin, radixin, and moesin, referred to as the ERM family, share a great deal of structural similarity with merlin [76, 77]. The proteins belonging to this family have a similar N-terminal globular domain, also known as the FERM domain, followed by an α-helical stretch, and finally a charged carboxyl terminus [75, 78, 79]. The key functional domains of merlin may lie within the highly conserved FERM domains and the unique C-terminus of the protein. The ERM proteins have been shown to be involved in cellular remodeling involving the actin cytoskeleton [80]. These proteins bind actin filaments in the cytoskeleton via a conserved C-terminal domain and possibly via a second actin-binding site in the N-terminal half of the protein [81, 82].

Like the ERM proteins, merlin is expressed in a variety of cell types where it localizes to the areas of membrane remodeling, particularly membrane ruffles, although its precise distribution may differ from the ERM proteins expressed in the same cell [83]. Membrane ruffling is related to the interaction between the cytoskeleton with the cell body and the cell membrane. Schwannoma cells from NF2 tumors show dramatic alterations in the actin cytoskeleton and display abnormalities in cell spreading as well [84]. These results suggest that merlin may play an important role in regulating both the actin cytoskeleton-mediated processes and cell proliferation [85]. However, it should be noted that merlin has a growth suppression role, while other ERM family members seem to facilitate cell growth.

Merlin Acts as a Tumor Suppressor

Overexpression of the *NF2* gene in mouse fibroblasts or rat schwannoma cells limits cell growth [61, 86] and suppresses cell transformation by the ras oncogene [87]. Without the *NF2* gene overexpressed, transformation occurs when a cancer-causing protein, ras, allows the cellular proliferation machinery to become activated without proper regulatory mechanisms in place, causing malignant tumor growth. The growth control of certain Schwann cells and meningeal cells is lost in the absence of *NF2* function, suggesting that *NF2* mutations and merlin deficiency disrupt some aspect of intracellular signaling that leads to cellular transformation. Together, these findings demonstrate merlin's ability to act as a growth suppressor.

Nf2 knockout mouse models, which are either heterozygous or homozygous for the *Nf2* gene in the germ line, have been created [88, 89]. Heterozygous *Nf2* knockout mice go on to develop osteosarcomas and, less often, fibrosarcomas or hepatocellular carcinomas [86]. Metastatic disease is common in this model. Genetic analysis shows that nearly all these malignant tumors are missing both *Nf2* alleles. Tumor growth in the absence of both *Nf2* alleles indicates that the *Nf2* gene possesses a classical tumor suppressor function. However, none of the heterozygous *Nf2* mice develop tumors or clinical manifestations associated with human NF2. The *Nf2* gene also plays an important role during early embryogenesis. Homozygous *Nf2* mutant mice, which are missing both *Nf2* alleles, died at approximately 7 days of gestation from a gastrulation defect or failure of inward migration of cells. Merlin is important in cell migration during embryogenesis [90].

By engineering mice whose Schwann cells have exon 2 excised from both *Nf2* alleles, conditional homozygous *Nf2* knockout mice have been produced, which display some characteristics of NF2 including schwannomas, Schwann cell hyperplasia, cataracts, and osseous metaplasia [91]. A conditional knockout model is engineered by inserting a regulatory mechanism into the gene, allowing the investigator to choose the time at which the desired gene (in this case *Nf2*) will be knocked out. Although these results are in favor of the argument that loss of merlin is sufficient for schwannoma formation in vivo, none of the tumors observed in these conditional knockout mice were found on the vestibular nerve. This contrasts with those VS commonly found in patients with NF2.

Biallelic *NF2* inactivation is also frequently found in sporadic and in NF2-associated meningiomas. By engineering mice whose arachnoidal cells have exon 2 excised from both *Nf2* alleles, homozygous *Nf2*$^{-/-}$ mice show a range of meningioma subtypes histologically similar to human tumors [92]. Taken together, these results demonstrate a tumor suppressor function for merlin in both Schwann cells and arachnoidal cells, from which meningiomas commonly originate.

Merlin Signaling and Regulation

Merlin overexpression (Fig. 10.2), unlike other members of the ERM protein family, causes growth suppression. In addition to the actin cytoskeleton, merlin has been shown to associate with cell membrane domains, which are highly enriched in signaling molecules that regulate cellular responses to proliferative and antiproliferative stimuli [93]. Vestibular schwannoma cells with NF2 inactivation have dramatic alterations in cell spreading. To date, several proteins that are likely to interact with merlin have been identified including the ERM proteins [94, 95], CD44 [96, 97], F-actin [98], paxillin [99], microtubules [100], BII-spectrin [101], B1-integrin

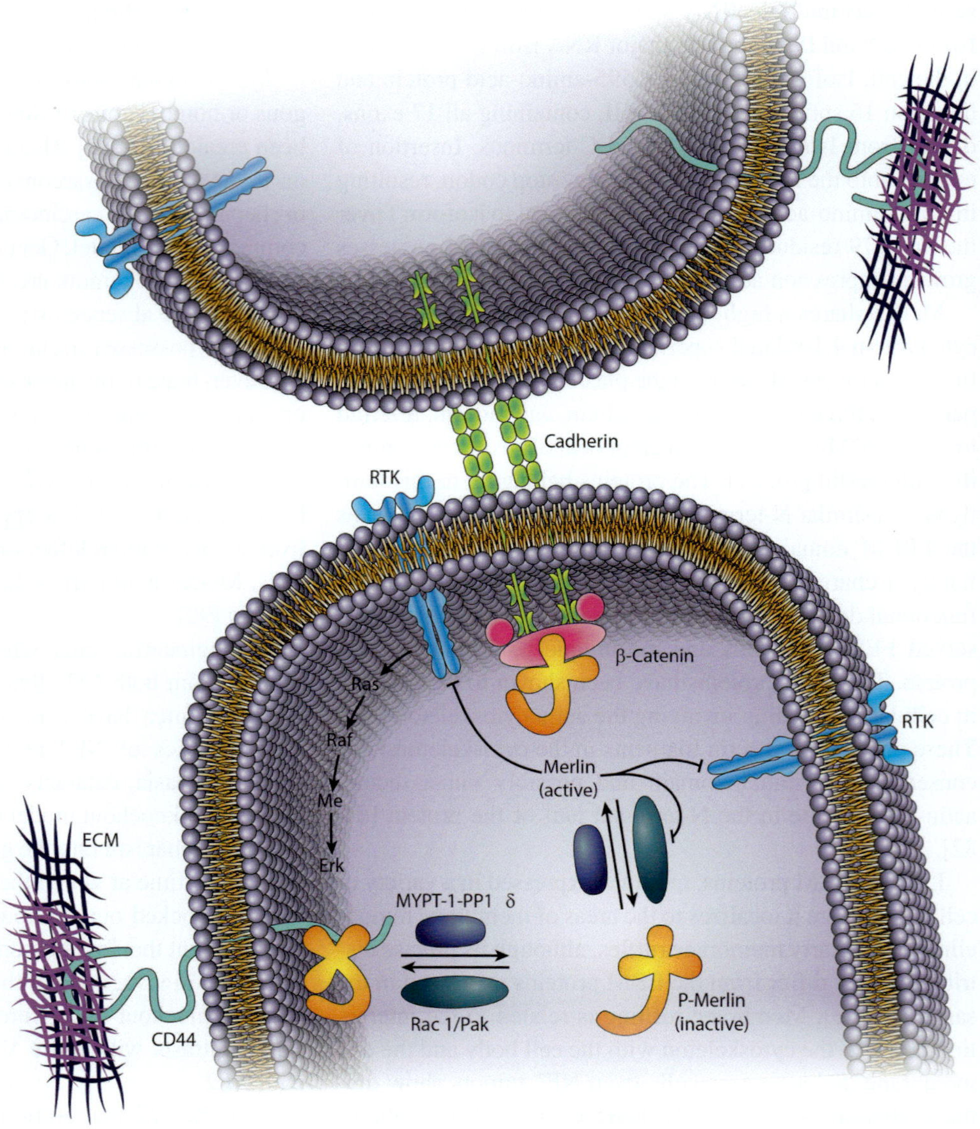

Fig. 10.2 Schematic diagram of merlin action. This diagram shows how Rac1 and Pak help convert the merlin protein from a closed conformation to an open conformation by phosphorylation of the protein. Consequently, merlin, in its open conformation, can interact with CD44 and facilitate linking the actin cytoskeleton to the cell membrane. p21-activated kinase 2 (Pak2) has been shown to phosphorylate merlin at serine 518 and thereby inactivating its function. Merlin is activated by dephosphorylation by myosin phosphatase (MYPT-1-PP1δ). (Adapted from Surgery of the Ear. 6th Ed. Eds. PMPH. 2010)

[102], B-fodrin [99], the regulatory cofactor of Na+-H+ exchanger (NHE-RF) [103, 104], SCHIP-1 [105], hepatocyte growth factor-regulated tyrosine kinase substrate (HRS) [106, 107], p21-activated kinase 1 and 2 (Pak1 and Pak2), Rac1, the RIB subunit of protein kinase A [108, 109], components of cadherin-mediated cell junctions [110], PIKE-L [phosphatidylinositol-3-kinase (PI3K) enhancer] [111, 112], erbin (erbB2-interacting protein) [113, 114], Hippo [115, 116], and NF-kB [84, 117, 118]. Major protein interactions are summarized in Table 10.1.

Presently, how these protein-protein interactions relate to the tumor suppressor activity of merlin is not well understood. Merlin is located in the cell membrane and binds to transmembrane proteins and actin with its N-terminal FERM domain. Merlin's ability to function as a growth regulator is also related to its ability to form such intramolecular associations [119]. Two such interactions have been identified. The first interaction is between residues that fold the N-terminal end of the protein onto itself, while the second interaction folds the entire protein so that there is no contact between N- and C-terminal ends of the protein [84, 105, 117]. In a fashion similar to the ERM proteins, merlin may cycle between the "open" and "closed" conformations that differentially determine whether it binds with the ERM proteins or other molecules to transduce merlin's growth inhibition signal [120]. Merlin's function is regulated by phosphorylation [108, 109]. Phosphorylation of the C-terminus disrupts N-terminal and C-terminal binding, which favors the "open" configuration of merlin. In this state, proliferation is favored. In the "closed" configuration, where the N-terminal FERM and C-terminal domains are bound to each other, merlin mediates contact-dependent growth inhibition.

The association of merlin with CD44 and B1-integrin raises the possibility that merlin might function as a molecular switch in the signaling pathways. CD44 is a transmem-

Table 10.1 Major protein-protein interactions that modulate merlin's growth regulatory function

Signal	Function	Regulation	Mechanism
Hippo	Growth-promoting kinase	Proliferation	Merlin activates Hippo by recruiting adaptor proteins Hippo activates downstream proteins, such as YAP1 and LATS1/2, which favors proliferation
B1-integrin	Integrin-dependent cell adhesion	Growth arrest	Effector of cell-cell adhesion modulated by kinases (YAP1, LATS1/2) that interact with merlin N-terminus and C-terminus, respectively Merlin phosphorylation reduces interactions with YAP1 and LATS1/2, which inhibits B1-integrin function and favors proliferation
Rac1 Cdc24	RhoGTPase	Proliferation	Activates p21-activated kinase (PAK) family proteins to phosphorylate merlin and favors proliferation
Pak1	Growth-promoting kinase	Proliferation	Inhibited by merlin. Loss of merlin expression inappropriately activates Pak1 and favors proliferation
Pak2	Growth-promoting kinase	Proliferation	Phosphorylates C-terminus of merlin, which favors "open" configuration and proliferation
Erbin	ErbB2-interacting protein	Growth arrest	Erbin/merlin complexes inactivate Pak2 Erbin knockout drives Pak2-mediated inhibition of merlin
PIKE-L	Phosphatidylinositol-3-kinase (PI3K) modulator	Growth arrest	Binds PI3K and stimulates lipid kinase activity. Merlin binds PIKE-L and inhibits PI3K activity PIKE-L knockout impairs merlin's tumor suppressor function and favors proliferation
PI3K/AKT	Growth-promoting kinase	Proliferation	Drives cell proliferation and survival Loss of merlin expression activates the PI3K/AKT pathway
CD44	Transmembrane hyaluronic acid receptor	Growth arrest	Activates CD44-dependent phosphatases to hypophosphorylate merlin and favor growth arrest Directly complexes with merlin, ezrin, and moesin in hypophosphorylated "closed" configuration
MYPT-1-PP1δ	Merlin phosphatase	Growth arrest	Hypophosphorylates merlin to favor growth arrest
CPI-17	Merlin phosphatase inhibitor	Proliferation	Inhibits MYPT-1-PP1δ, which drives merlin C-terminus phosphorylation into the "open" configuration and favors proliferation
HRS	Hepatocyte growth factor (HGF)-regulated tyrosine kinase substrate	Growth arrest	Reduced proliferation and contact-dependent cell growth Binds to merlin C-terminus in "open" configuration Overexpression mimics merlin overexpression phenotype
Cadherins	Contact inhibition via adherens junctions	Growth arrest	Mature cadherins form adherens junctions between cells and mediate contact inhibition Merlin drives maturation of cadherins. Loss of merlin expression impairs cadherin maturation and favors proliferation
NF-kB	Growth-promoting transcription factor	Proliferation	NF-kB promotes proliferation and protects against apoptosis Merlin's N-terminus inhibits NF-kB activation. Suppression of merlin favors proliferation

brane hyaluronic acid receptor implicated in cell-cell adhesion, cell-matrix adhesion, cell motility, and metastasis [92, 103]. Merlin mediates contact inhibition of cell growth through signals from the extracellular matrix. At high cell density, merlin becomes hypophosphorylated and inhibits cell growth in response to hyaluronate, a mucopolysaccharide that surrounds cells [121]. At low cell density, merlin is phosphorylated, growth permissive, and exists in a complex with ezrin, moesin, and CD44. CD44 is also thought to associate with anti-mitogenic signals, such as CD44-dependent MYPT1 phosphatase, which hypophosphorylate merlin at the C-terminus and maintain the closed configuration to inhibit cell growth. In this manner, CD44 may amplify the function of hyaluronate, which also maintains merlin in a hypophosphorylated state and signals growth arrest. These data indicate that merlin and CD44 form a molecular switch that specifies growth arrest or proliferation.

Various pro-mitogenic signals act via activating kinases that phosphorylate merlin, disrupt the binding between the N-terminal FERM and C-terminal domains, and allow for a growth-permissive configuration. For instance, Rac1, a member of the RhoGTPase family, has been demonstrated to promote the phosphorylation of merlin, thereby inactivating its growth suppressor mechanism [109, 110]. Among the effects of Rac1 and Cdc42 GTPases, members of the p21-activated kinase (PAK) family have demonstrated interactions with merlin. Specifically, Pak2 has been shown to phosphorylate merlin at serine 518 and inactivate its function [91, 105, 122, 123]. Other pro-mitogenic signals act by directly degrading merlin. The cyclic AMP-protein kinase A (PKA) pathway and AKT signaling pathways both modulate merlin phosphorylation and ubiquitination. Activating these pathways drives merlin into its open, growth-permissive configuration and tags merlin for proteasome-mediated degradation, both of which disrupt its tumor suppressor function [124].

Kissil et al. [121] also reported an interaction between merlin and Pak1, and merlin could inhibit the activation dynamic of Pak1. Loss of merlin expression leads to the inappropriate activation of Pak1, while overexpression of merlin results in the inhibition of Pak1 activity. Conversely, merlin is activated by dephosphorylation at serine 518, which occurs on serum withdrawal or on cell-cell or cell-matrix contact [119]. Although the members of the PAK family have been implicated in various cellular processes, such as cytoskeletal reorganization and apoptotic signaling, their exact roles and functions have not been clearly defined. Jin et al. [125] identified the myosin phosphatase (MYPT-1-PP1δ) as a merlin phosphatase. Interestingly, the cellular MYPT-1-PP1δ-specific inhibitor, CPI-17, could cause decreased merlin activity by merlin phosphorylation, Ras activation, and transformation. These results implicate MYPT-1-PP1δ and CPI-17 as important regulatory components in the merlin tumor suppressor pathway.

Merlin's Growth Regulatory Function Is Related to Its Conformation and Protein-Protein Interactions

The activities of the ERM proteins are controlled by self-association of the proteins' N-terminal and C-terminal regions [126, 127]. The ERM proteins can exist in the "closed" conformation, where the N- and C- terminal regions undergo an intramolecular interaction, thus folding the protein to mask the conserved actin-binding site (Fig. 10.3). The molecule can be converted to the "open" conformation in which the intramolecular interaction is disrupted by signals such as phosphorylation or treatment with phosphoinositides [107, 121, 128].

The association between merlin and HRS, a substrate implicated in the signaling pathway initiated by hepatocyte growth factor (HGF) binding to the c-met receptor [120], appears to be regulated by protein folding [105]. These results suggest that the ability of merlin to cycle between the "open" and "closed" conformations may integrate CD44 and HGF signaling pathways. All these findings are relevant to growth regulation. Also, merlin can exert its activity by inhibiting phosphatidylinositol 3-kinase (PI3-kinase) through binding to PIKE-L, a brain-specific GTPase that binds to PI3-kinase and stimulates its lipid kinase activity [109]. This finding suggests that PIKE-L is an important mediator of merlin growth suppression. Along this notion, we have found that the PI3-kinase/Akt pathway is activated in VS [129, 130].

The configuration of merlin also modulates the function of downstream proteins, such as B1-integrin. B1-integrin is involved in cell-cell adhesion and is a key protein that drives contact-dependent growth arrest. The N-terminal FERM domain of merlin interacts with the transcription factor Yes-associated protein 1 (YAP1) and with large tumor suppressor genes 1 and 2 (LATS1/2). LATS1/2 is thought to drive hypo-

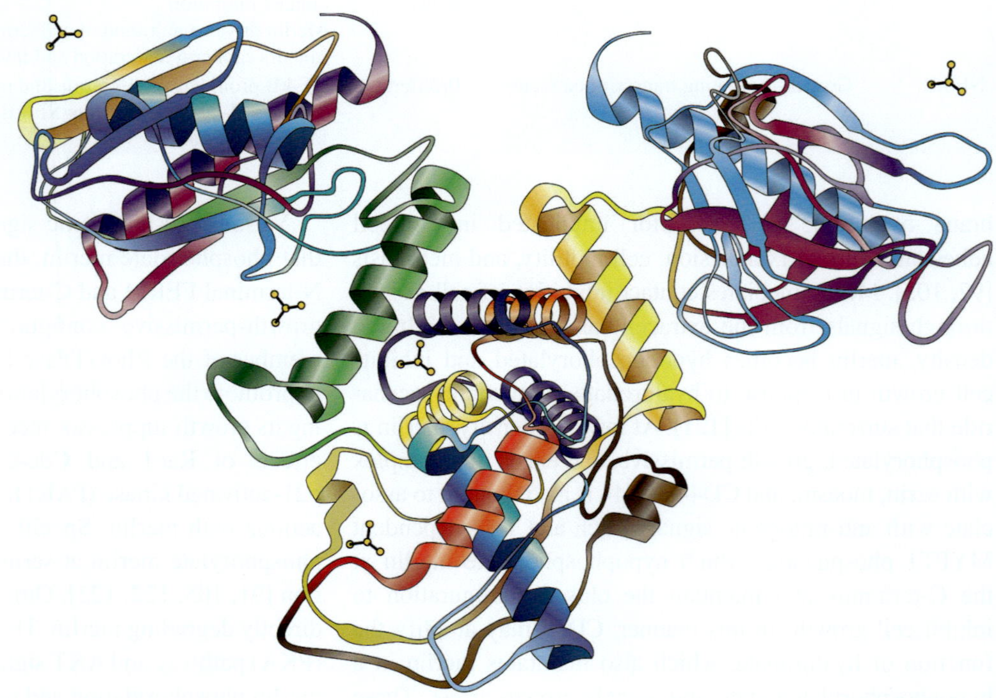

Fig. 10.3 The NF2 protein is divided into three general sections. The FERM domain is followed by an alpha-helical domain and a hydrophilic tail. Merlin can dimerize with itself and heterodimerize with other ERM family proteins. (Adapted from [79] and Adapted from Surgery of the Ear. 6th Ed. Eds. PMPH. 2010)

phosphorylation of YAP1, allowing for YAP1 relocation to the nucleus and inhibition of B1-integrin-dependent cell adhesion. When merlin is phosphorylated, by pro-mitotic kinases such as Pak2, FERM, and C-terminal domain interactions with YAP1 and LATS1/2 are reduced, resulting in YAP1 dephosphorylation and suppression of B1-integrin-mediated growth arrest. Thus, merlin phosphorylation is both mediated by upstream proteins and can regulate the function of downstream effectors involved in growth arrest and proliferation [131].

In addition, Lallemand et al. [108] showed that in *Nf2*$^{-/-}$ mouse embryo fibroblasts, *Nf2* deficiency led to piling up of cells, hyperproliferation, and defective cadherin-mediated cell-cell interactions. When functioning normally, these interactions terminate proliferation by contact inhibition through adherens junctions. Furthermore, merlin colocalizes and interacts with and causes maturation of adherens junction components in confluent wild-type cells. Stated simply, when normal Schwann cells contact each other, special signaling through these junctions stops further growth. In the absence of merlin, the adherens junctions are immature and do not stop the schwannoma cells from terminating their growth when they contact each other. These results indicate that merlin functions as a tumor suppressor at least in part by controlling cadherin-mediated cell-cell contact [132].

The *NF2* Gene Promoter

Characterization of the *NF2* regulatory regions is important for screening for mutations in both spontaneous and familial tumors in which no mutation was found in the *NF2*-coding region. We have shown that transcription of the *NF2* gene is initiated at multiple start sites, and multiple regions in the *NF2* promoter are required for full *NF2* promoter activity [71, 133]. Both positive and negative regulatory elements required for transcription of the *NF2* gene have been found in the 5′ flanking region of the promoter (Fig. 10.1). In particular, a sequence rich in guanine and cytosine nucleotide bases located in the proximal regulatory region, which can be bound by the Sp1 transcription factor, serves as a positive regulatory element [71]. This region is the area of the gene adjacent to the 5′ of the coding region which regulates, either positively or negatively, the translation of the DNA into messenger RNA as we have described. Both the 5′ and the 3′ flanking regions of the human *NF2* locus are G/C rich and could serve as a target for gene methylation and inactivation as a form of therapy [70, 71].

We have also shown that a 2.4-kb human *NF2* promoter could direct where the *NF2* gene expression would occur as early as embryonic day 5.5 [88]. During early embryonic development, strong *NF2* promoter activity was detected in the developing brain and in sites containing migrating cells including the neural tube closure and branchial arches. Interestingly a transient change of *NF2* promoter activity during neural crest cell migration was noted. While little promoter activity was detected in premigratory neural crest cells at the dorsal ridge region of the neural fold, significant activity was seen in the neural crest cells already migrating away from the dorsal neural tube. In addition, we detected considerable *NF2* promoter activity in various *NF2*-affected tissues such as the acoustic and trigeminal ganglia, spinal ganglia, optic chiasm, the ependymal cell-containing tela choroidea, and the pigmented epithelium of the retina. The *NF2* promoter expression pattern during embryogenesis suggests a specific regulation of the *NF2* gene during neural crest cell migration and further supports the role of merlin in cell adhesion, motility, and proliferation during development [88].

Alternatively Spliced *NF2* mRNA Isoforms in Vestibular Schwannomas and Other Cell Types

The *NF2* gene undergoes alternative splicing in the coding exons [42, 51, 71, 134–139]. Multiple alternatively spliced *NF2* transcripts have been identified in various human cells. The most common isoforms in these cells were isoforms II (containing all 17 exons) and isoform I (without exon 16). Presently, the role of alternative splicing of *NF2* mRNA is not well understood. It is possible that the functional contribution of the *NF2* tumor suppressor may require a balanced expression of various isoform proteins in Schwann cells and/or other cell lineages [71, 140]. Alternative splicing may be another mechanism for Schwann cells to inactivate merlin function and/or to generate isoforms that have additional properties conducive to tumor formation.

Immunohistochemical Markers of Growth in Vestibular Schwannomas: Clinical Correlation

Attempts to correlate clinical parameters with immunohistologic evaluation of protein expression in VS have been performed. An increase in Ki-67, a protein, which is an index of nuclear proliferation, was shown to correlate with the growth of solid schwannomas on MRI [130, 131]. Higher rates of tumor recurrence have also been suggested in tumors with an increased rate of nuclear proliferation and mitotic indices, although the supporting data for this claim was not conclusive [141]. Positron emission tomography (PET) scanning has been conducted to assess the metabolic activity of VS preoperatively and to assess the metabolic activity within the proliferation index, Ki-67. However, no correlation was found. Additionally, there was no correlation between 18-fluorodeoxyglucose (FDG) uptake (indicator of metabolic activity in tissues) and Ki-67 expression measured by immunostaining [142]. This is most likely because VS are slow-growing tumors with less than 5% of tumor cells being in S-phase or active division [143].

Another possible marker for tumor growth is the transforming growth factor β1 (TGF-β1). Immunostaining for TGF-β1 was positive in 96% of blood vessels within schwannomas and in 84% of schwannoma tissue samples; however, no direct correlation with tumor growth was found [144]. Immunohistochemical association of β1-integrin with merlin has been demonstrated but has not been related directly to tumor phenotypes [97]. Cystic schwannomas are associated with a 36-fold decrease in nuclear proliferation as measured with Ki-67 staining when compared to solid tumors, suggesting that the rapid clinical growth seen in cystic schwannomas is related to the accumulation of cyst formation but not by an actual increase in the growth rate of tumor cells [145, 146]. Also, NF2-associated schwannomas have been shown to have an increased proliferation index by Ki-67 and proliferating cell nuclear antigen (PCNA) immunostaining, when compared to unilateral solid schwannomas [147, 148]. PCNA is a proliferation index marker and is important in cell division.

Recently, we detected higher levels of cyclin D_3 expression, which is associated with G_1 cell cycle progression, in five of ten VS, compared to Schwann cells in adjacent normal vestibular nerve [46]. In contrast, expression of the cyclin D_1 protein, which controls Schwann cell differentiation, was not detected in any of the schwannomas examined [149]. Another study of 180 patients with previously untreated VS, including sporadic cases, who underwent surgical resection found that cyclin D_3 was overexpressed in 44% of tumors and cyclin D_1 in 68% of tumors [150]. These results suggest a possible role for cyclin D_3, and potentially cyclin D_1, in the growth of some VS cells.

Taken together, these studies demonstrate relatively little correlation between clinical growth as assessed by MRI scans, historical data, and nuclear growth indexes in solid unilateral and *NF2*-associated schwannomas. Cyclic tumor growth appears to occur via a different mechanism. Although the defective *NF2* gene is the underlying common denominator in tumor formation of all three tumor types, other differences at the molecular level likely account for the variable clinical presentations of these tumors.

Identifying Deregulated Genes in Vestibular Schwannomas

To further elucidate the growth pathways in VS, the gene expression profiles have been studied. The study of large-scale gene expression profiles utilizing the cDNA microarrays allows examination of the transcriptome of tissue and gives a means of exploring a broad view of the basic biology of tumors [151]. We studied gene regulation in VS using cDNA microarray analysis and found 42 genes, which were significantly upregulated including osteonectin, endoglin, and Rho B, when compared to normal vestibular nerve tissues [5, 152]. Additionally, multiple genes were found to be significantly downregulated in the majority of VS examined. Of these genes, a putative tumor suppressor gene LUCA-15 was downregulated in seven of eight schwannomas studied.

More recently, next-generation sequencing of sporadic VS has provided additional information about genetic alterations underlying tumorigenesis. In an analysis of fresh frozen tumor samples from 23 patients with sporadic VS, 31 unique variants in the *NF2* gene were identified, of which 10 were splice site, 2 were missense, 7 were premature stop, and 11 were frameshift mutations. Several major chromosomal anomalies were also observed, including loss of a chromosome 15, 18p, 16q, or an X or Y chromosome, which were noted only in tumors with an aggressive phenotype [153]. A second study of 46 sporadic vestibular schwannomas found mutations in a number of genes, including 25 patients who expressed mutations in axonal guidance pathways, 5 patients with CDC27 mutations, 2 patients with USP8 mutations, and 35 patients with at least one NF2 mutation. Of the tumors analyzed, none showed microsatellite instability [154].

Osteonectin is a secreted glycoprotein that interacts with extracellular matrix proteins to decrease adhesion of cells from the matrix, thereby inducing a biological state conducive to cell migration. Endoglin, a TGF-β receptor-binding protein, was found to be significantly upregulated in all the solid tumors but not in any of the cystic tumors examined. It is likely that increased endoglin expression may induce downstream signaling proteins, somehow leading to an aggressive cystic phenotype [5]. An example of a deregulated signaling pathway suggested by the microarray data is the retinoblastoma protein (pRB)-cyclin-dependent kinase (CDK) pathway [155]. Among genes involved in G_1-S phase progression, CDK2 was found to be downregulated in seven of eight tumors. In addition, upregulation of transforming factor RhoB was found in all the schwannomas examined. Further examination of these deregulated genes as potential downstream targets of the *NF2* tumor suppressor should provide us with targets for pharmacotherapeutic interventions.

Environmental Exposures

There is evidence that radiation may be associated with the induction of vestibular schwannoma growth. While other sites and tumors also show a propensity for growth in response to environmental exposure, the vestibular nerve appears to contain an increased sensitivity for tumor growth as compared to other regions within the central nervous system or elsewhere.

Evans and colleagues note an 18.8-fold increased relative risk of schwannoma induction and a 9.5-fold increased relative rate of meningioma induction following radiation doses of 2.5 Gy from the treatment of tinea capitis, adeno-tonsillar disease, and capillary hemangiomas [156]. The radiobiologic effect was dose dependent similar to the tissue effect and tumor growth response observed in post-WWII Japan. Preston and colleagues [157] showed that VS were the most abundant intracranial tumors encountered, with a high propensity for Schwann cell mutation in response to radiation damage.

Overall, the risk of tumors induced by therapeutic radiation appears to be approximately 0.1–3% after 30 years [146, 158]. In light of the 33–40% lifetime risk of malignancy in the general population, Evans [146] argues that the benefits of single-dose radiation treatment for VS may be justified for those with documented tumor growth that refuse surgery or for the elderly or infirm. However, patients with NF2 are disproportionate recipients of radiation-induced malignant tumors. Although only 7% of patients with VS have NF2, 50% of malignant changes induced by stereotactic irradiation of VS occur in NF2 patients. We strongly caution against the use of radiation treatment for benign tumors in childhood and in tumor-prone conditions such as neurofibromatosis.

Cellular Telephone Risk

Several studies addressed the risk of cellular telephone use and the formation of VS presumably secondary to electromagnetic radiation over a long exposure period. Hardell et al. [159] reviewed 13 case-controlled studies and found 9 case-control studies to have reported patients with over 10 years of cellular telephone use. They concluded that the odds ratio for ipsilateral cellphone use and the development of VS was 2.4 (95% confidence interval 1.1–5.3). Additional case-control studies suggest increased risk for vestibular schwannoma and glioma with risk elevation greatest for high-grade gliomas associated with unilateral long-term exposure [155, 160]. However, other studies have found no difference in VS size or incidence with long-term exposure and instead suggest that cell phone use may be correlated with earlier diagnosis of VS [161, 162].

Genetic Screening for NF2

A patient with NF2 has a 50% chance of passing the affected *NF2* allele along to their offspring if (1) their spouse does not have NF2 and if (2) they do not have a mosaic form of NF2. (Mosaicism occurs when a mutation in the *NF2* gene occurs after an embryo has undergone several sets of cell division. Therefore, only a portion of the child's cells carry a mutation in the *NF2* gene.) A child who inherits an abnormal copy of the *NF2* tumor suppressor gene has a 95% chance of developing bilateral VS.

Because early intervention is very important for clinical outcomes, genetic and clinical screening for at-risk patients is strongly advocated for those at risk to develop NF2. This includes anyone with a first-degree relative with NF2, patients under 30 years old with a unilateral VS, or any patient with multiple intracranial, spinal, or peripheral skin tumors that are associated with NF2. Any offspring of patients with NF2 should have annual ophthalmology examinations starting soon after birth since cataracts can begin at a very early age. Annual neurology examinations should be started at 7 years of age or earlier if neurologic deficits are noted. We recommend biannual audiograms and annual MRI evaluations beginning at age 7. Others have recommended starting a similar screening process at 10 years of age with an MRI every other year and annually once a tumor is found [163].

Mutation screening for the first-degree relatives of NF2 patients is recommended when the probands' mutation has been identified either from a schwannoma or from leukocyte screening [157, 164]. Other family members at risk can be identified and screened for developing NF2 or receive appropriate genetic counseling. Patients who are first-degree relatives of NF2 patients where the mutation in the *NF2* gene has not been identified may have more ambiguity regarding the screening of their *NF2* gene for mutations if no mutation is localized. Appropriate audiometric testing and neural imaging methods need to be carried out as false negatives in mutation screening can occur in up to 25% of patients. Annual MRI screening and biannual audiometric testing would still be recommended for children older than 7 years of age who had a negative test. Additionally, if a mutation was detected during DNA sequencing, we recommend annual MRIs and biannual audiometric testing in order to detect the development of VS at the earliest possible stage. Early detection in NF2 does make a significant difference in the ability to successfully preserve hearing and facial nerve function.

When an *NF2* mutation has already been identified in an affected family member, screening additional first-degree family members for the same mutation is considerably less costly and is recommended. The sensitivity of genetic testing in this circumstance is extremely high since the DNA being screened can be directly compared to the known mutation in the affected family member. In this case, knowing with near certainty that a child does not carry an *NF2* mutation can avoid the frequent MRI examinations that would otherwise be required [48, 158]. Therefore, if a family has multiple members diagnosed with NF2 and mutation testing has not been performed, it is worthwhile to identify the mutation in at least one family member so that future family members can be screened. This is most effectively done when tumor tissues are available for mutation screening. However, biopsy for genetic diagnosis alone is not suggested if tumor removal is otherwise not indicated as clinical screening protocols are also effective.

Potential Drug Treatments

As the understanding of merlin and its interacting partners is better, new means of targeting these pathways for intervention in schwannoma cells is occurring. Some treatments are aimed at restoring the wild-type merlin protein to the mutant cells, while other strategies attempt to block the proliferation of schwannoma cells by blocking its growth pathways or by increasing programmed cell death or apoptosis. For example, Messerli et al. [165] showed an effective reduction of schwannoma growth in both a transgenic and a xenograft mouse model by injecting wild-type merlin packaged in an oncolytic recombinant herpes simplex virus vector in the tumor. The vehicle for delivery was a replication competent herpes simplex virus, which has tumoricidal properties. There were no apparent toxicities with the injection of the oncolytic vector. A paradigm for the use of oncolytic vectors to reduce the volume of benign tumors when surgical resection may cause nerve damage is suggested. Likewise, reintroducing the *NF2* gene by direct injection resulted in tumor regression and reversion toward normal histology [166].

Hansen et al. [167] and Doherty et al. [168] demonstrated cell surface human epidermal growth factor, also known as erythroblastic leukemia viral oncogene homolog 2 or ErbB2, receptors as possible targets for VS cell growth inhibition. Blocking the ligand or interacting proteins, which activates this receptor by treatment with blocking antineuregulin antibodies, also inhibited schwannoma cell proliferation. ErbB2 is a tyrosine kinase receptor, a common cellular switch, on the VS cell surface, which triggers the MAPK kinase cascade, a process that leads sequentially to nuclear activation of cell division. One of its ligands, neuregulin-1, is a growth factor produced by schwannoma cells, thus creating an autocrine feedback loop; the schwannoma cells cause further stimulation of schwannoma growth.

Plotkin et al. showed that epidermal growth factor receptor (EGFR) blockage with erlotinib HCl was tolerated and showed radiographic and audiometric response to treatment in a patient with NF2 in short follow-up. Karajannis et al. demonstrated effectiveness of lapatinib, an Erb2 inhibitor for control of the growth of the majority of NF2-associated vestibular schwannomas although only 4 of 17 showed reduction in volume by greater than 15% [170].

Several investigators demonstrated that intervention at the intracellular proliferation pathways, specifically the MAPK pathway and the PI3K pathway, respectively, may also result in schwannoma growth suppression. Nakai et al. [169] showed that merlin is involved in suppression of Rac signaling, and cultured schwannoma cells contain elevated, GTP-bound, active Rac. Application of a Rac-specific inhibitor, the chemical compound NSC23766, to schwannoma cells restored neuronal interaction. The data support the significance of regulated Rac signaling in mediating Schwann cell-axon interaction and suggest controlling Rac activity as a possible therapy for schwannomas.

Jacob et al. [170] demonstrated the activation of the PI3K/AKT pathway in human schwannomas. It has been shown that merlin can inhibit PI3K through its binding to the PI3-kinase enhancer-L (PIKE-L), a GTPase which binds to and stimulates PI3K (Fig. 10.4). The suppression of PI3K activity results from merlin disrupting the binding of PIKE-L to PI3K. Our recent studies using cultured schwannoma cells further suggest that both an AKT pathway inhibitor and a histone deacetylase inhibitor could suppress schwannoma cell growth by blocking the PI3K pathway. Utilizing a quantifiable xenograft model for VS, we are currently testing the efficacy of these novel compounds. Recently, Zhao et al. performed a screening of 157 inhibitors targeting the PI3K/AKT pathway in an in vitro NF2 model and identified over a dozen inhibitors which suppressed schwannoma growth. Of these inhibitors, AZD8005 and PQR309, which are orally available, were found to inhibit growth both in vitro and in vivo. These findings highlight potential therapeutic benefit to targeting proteins within the PI3K/AKT pathway [171].

Transduction of growth factor stimulation of the mammalian target of rapamycin (mTOR) signaling pathway ultimately results in stimulation of protein synthesis and entry into the G_1 phase of the cell cycle. Decreased phosphatase and tensin homolog gene (PTEN), a human gene that acts as a tumor suppressor gene, manifests as AKT and mTOR activation stimulating growth. Additionally, hypoxia-inducible factors HIF-1 alpha and HIF-2 alpha show increased expression and account for enhanced angiogenesis with mTOR activation. This may lead to the necessary blood vessel supply to schwannomas. AKT and mTOR activation have been noted in VS. The immunosuppressant, rapamycin, inhibits mTOR and induces G_1 arrest and apoptosis. Newer mTOR inhibitors, such as temsirolimus, have shown good effect in the treatment of renal cell carcinoma alone and in combination with other agents (Fig. 10.5). Everolimus (or Rad001) is an orally administered mTORC1 inhibitor. Goutagny et al. in a prospective trial of everolimus for progressive VS in NF2 patients showed five of ten patients with decrease in growth rates and resumption of growth after termination of drug [172].

Karajannis et al. reported the results of a separate trial using everolimus in ten patients with NF2 and progressive vestibular schwannomas. No objective improvement in hearing or imaging response was reported [173]. Subsequently, in a phase 0 presurgical clinical trial, blood levels of everolimus were found to be in a high therapeutic range. Tumor tissue drug concentration was determined. Only partial inhibition of phospho-S6 was found in the treated tumors, indicating incomplete target inhibition compared with control tissues from untreated patients. Everolimus led to incomplete inhibition of mTORC1 and downstream signaling. The authors concluded that their data may explain the "limited antitumor effect of everolimus observed in clinical studies

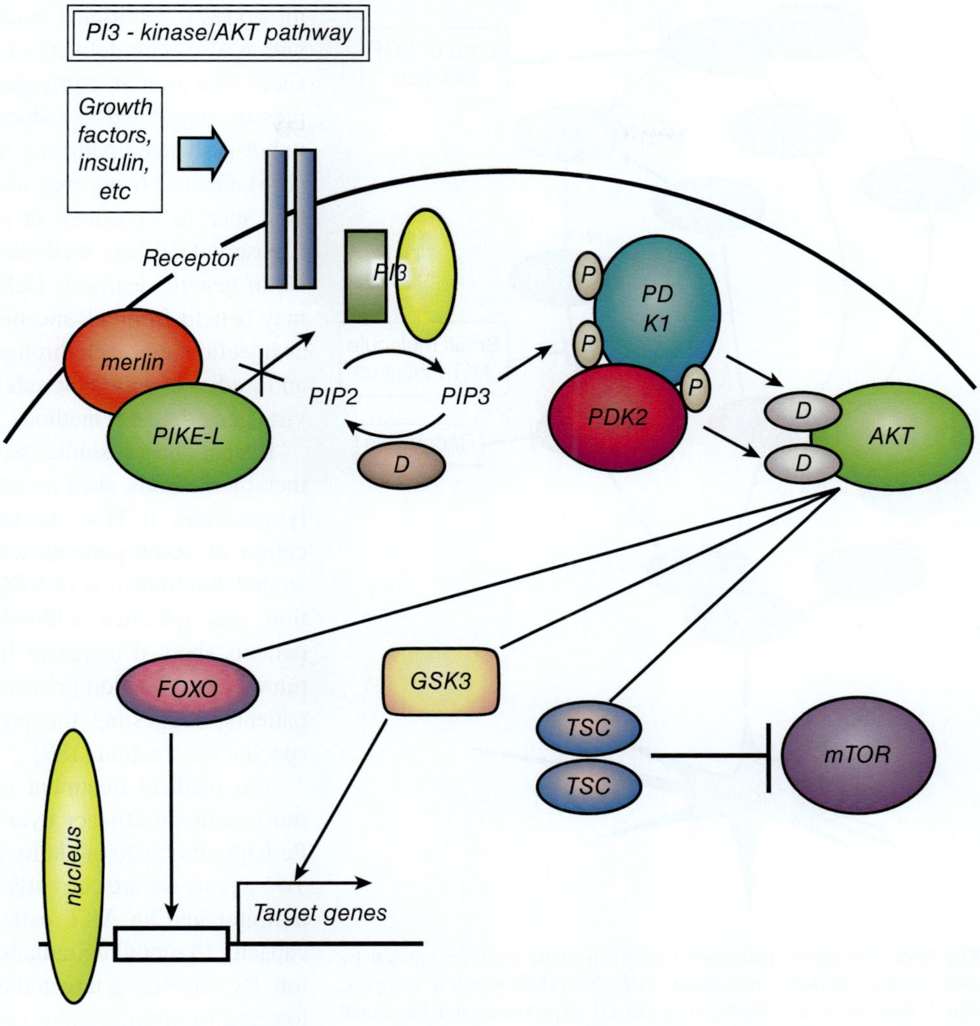

Fig. 10.4 PI3K/AKT signaling. Insulin and other growth factors activate cell surface tyrosine kinase receptors that stimulate PI3K activity. PI3K converts PIP2 to PIP3. PTEN is a negative regulator of the AKT pathway that catalyzes the conversion of PIP3 back to PIP2. PDK1 and PDK2 maximally activate AKT. Phosphorylation of downstream effectors of the AKT pathway inhibits these proteins. Existing as a complex, TSC1 and TSC2 normally inhibit mTOR activity. However, when TSC2 is phosphorylated by AKT, it dissociates from TSC1, and mTOR becomes active. Active GSK and FOXO function within the nucleus as transcriptional regulators that activate genes promoting apoptosis. Merlin, the NF2 gene product, can bind PIKE-L and inactivate PI3K. A small-molecule PDK1 inhibitor can inhibit phosphorylation of AKT at the 308 site. (PNAS 2004). (Adapted from Surgery of the Ear. 6th Ed. Eds. PMPH. 2010)

for patients with NF2" and that such preclinical surgical studies may influence future preclinical and clinical studies [174]. Side effects of everolimus include mouth ulcers early in the treatment course, anemia, decreased neutrophil and lymphocyte counts, peripheral edema, hyperglycemia, and pericardial effusion [175].

Angiogenesis inhibitors such as bevacizumab (Avastin) have been used alone or in combination for treatment of colorectal, lung, and prostate carcinomas [176–179]. It acts by inhibiting vascular endothelial growth factor (VEGF) and is used in several combination treatment protocols. Bevacizumab has shown temporary suppression of VS growth. Its temporary effect on tumor growth reduction, the potential side effects of leukopenia, and bleeding limit its use in surgical patients, and it is currently considered a temporizing agent.

Plotkin et al. reported a cohort of ten NF2 patients with poor candidacy for surgery or radiation therapy who received intravenous bevacizumab over 18 months. A volume reduction of 20% or more was observed in 41% of tumors, primarily within the first 12 months of treatment, with relapse and regrowth following discontinuation of bevacizumab treatment [180]. Significantly favorable effects were observed in patients above 25 years of age, while younger patients with faster-growing tumors showed a weaker response to bevacizumab. A second retrospective analysis of 31 VS patients receiving bevacizumab found a decrease in tumor volume of 20% or more in 55% of the sample and an increase in word recognition score in 57% of the sample. At 1 year, 88% of patients had stable or decreased tumor size [5]. Reduction in tumor volume and improvement in hearing response with bevacizumab have been reported in several other cohort studies, demonstrating that bevacizumab may have a significant therapeutic effect in VS in about one-third of patients [181–183]. Adverse effects including hypertension, proteinuria, hemorrhage, and tumor growth with interruption or discontinuation of therapy are all known side effects to be managed [184, 185].

Advancements in Nonpharmacological Methods

Gene delivery methods have shown promise in the treatment of various genetic conditions, such as heritable hearing loss and spinal muscular atrophy. Such methods may provide

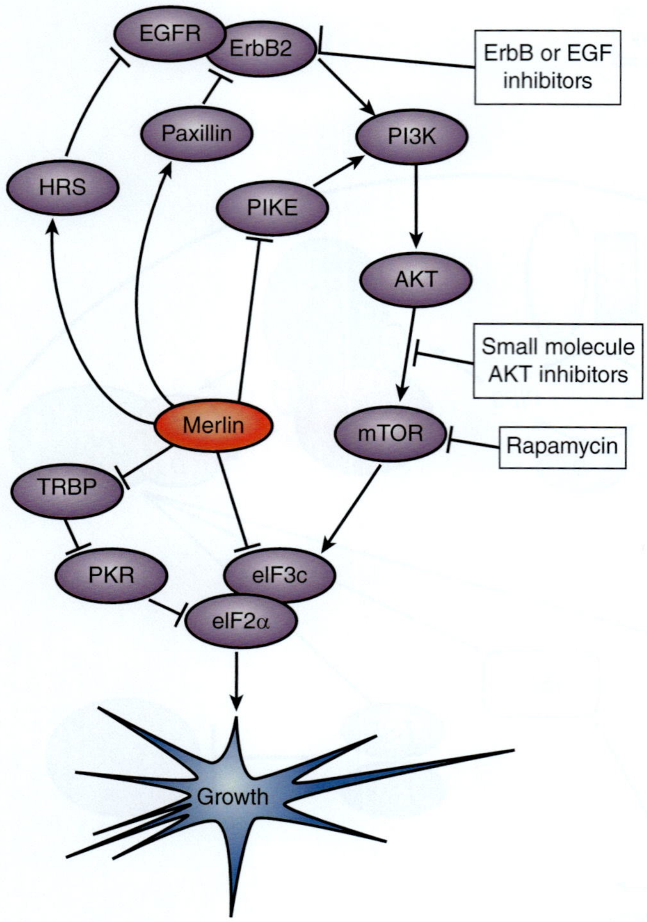

Fig. 10.5 Alternative pathways. In this schematic in a recent review by Dan Scoles, merlin's interaction with the ErbB2-paxillin complex, PIKE, and elF3c, its effects on cyclin D1 expression, and functional consequences of merlin loss suggest that signaling in the ErbB2-PI3K-mTOR-elF3c-cyclin D1 pathway may contribute to NF2 pathogenesis. PIKE-L enhances PI3K, which leads to phosphorylation and activation of PDK1 and PDK2, which in turn activates mitotic machinery. Drugs targeting this pathway therefore may be useful for inhibition of NF2 tumors with overactive mTOR signaling, including trastuzumab (Herceptin, LY294002, AKT inhibitors, UCN-01, Rad-001, CCI-779, and AP23573), small-molecule AKT pathway, and histone deacetylase inhibitors, and HSP90 inhibitor 17-allylamino-17-demethoxygeldanamycin (17AAG) may affect Akt and C-Raf, as well as Cdk4 and Cyclin D-1 (NexGenix). (Adapted from Surgery of the Ear. 6th Ed. Eds. PMPH. 2010)

benefits in NF2 cases with clear molecular targets. One approach involves the direct intratumoral injection of viral vectors carrying tumor-lytic agents such as caspases. In a mouse model with subcutaneously implanted immortalized human NF2 schwannoma cells, intratumoral injection of a herpes simplex virus-1 (HSV-1) vector encoding caspase-1 (ICE) under a Schwann cell-specific promoter (P0) led to reduction in tumor size [186]. A follow-up study demonstrated tumor regression with intratumoral injection of an adeno-associated viral (AAV) vector expressing ICE under P0 in schwannoma cells implanted into the sciatic nerve of mice [187]. Additional studies have demonstrated efficacy with AAV vector delivery of other molecular targets, such as speck-like protein, a pro-apoptotic schwannoma tumor suppressor, which led to reduced tumor growth and improved tumor-associated pain in a human xenograft model of NF2 [188]. Gene delivery may also involve nonviral vector methods, such as liposomal or peptide-based delivery systems. Liposomal delivery methods have been used in mouse models of genetic deafness. Delivery methods are evolving and may benefit from advancements in surgical technique, such as injection approach through the round window membrane, and studies to assess the safety and efficacy of viral and nonviral gene delivery methods.

Recent clinical studies have explored the use of immunotherapy methods, such as selective activation of cytotoxic T lymphocytes (CTLs), to target NF2 schwannomas. In a cohort of seven patients with NF2, Tamura et al. demonstrated that induction of VEGFR-specific CTLs via vaccination was tolerated without severe adverse effects. Two patients showed increases in word recognition scores, and tumor size reduction greater than 20% was observed in two patients, suggesting the preliminary efficacy of VEGFR-specific vaccination [189].

The medical treatment of slow-growing benign tumors must maintain efficacy over decades of potential treatment. Perhaps combined modality treatments might be considered. Two agents we are currently studying (a histone deacetylase inhibitor and an AKT pathway inhibitor) have shown the capacity to modulate radiation response in an additive fashion. By sensitizing targeted tissues, radiation doses could be lowered to optimistically promote a killing effect of tumor cells, reduce adverse effects on surrounding structures, preserve physiologic function, and decrease the risk of tumor promotion or malignant transformation.

Schwannomatosis (OMIM #162091), a distinct form of neurofibromatosis, is characterized by multiple schwannomas, but this condition most often lacks any VS. Patients with schwannomatosis frequently present with intractable pain rather than cranial nerve deficits. They seldom develop other intracranial tumors or malignancies. MacCollin et al. [190] noted that about one-third of patients with schwannomatosis had tumors in an anatomically limited distribution, such as a single limb, several contiguous segments of the spine, or one-half of the body. Sporadic cases of schwannomatosis are as common as NF2, but few cases of familial schwannomatosis have been identified in contradistinction to NF1 and NF2, which are autosomal dominant and highly penetrant. The underlying molecular disruption in schwannomatosis is a pattern of somatic *NF2* gene inactivation incompatible with NF1 or NF2, associated with alterations in the SMARCB1 or LZTR1 tumor suppressor genes in familial disease [191, 192].

Genetics of Paragangliomas

Paragangliomas of the head and neck are rare, mostly benign tumors. The hereditary paraganglioma syndromes are autosomal-dominant conditions with increased risk for multifocal tumors of the sympathetic and parasympathetic neuroendocrine systems. Approximately 30% of paraganglioma patients harbor a germ line mutation, which is carried by all the cells of the body (as opposed to a somatic mutation, which is only found in the tumor tissues). In more than a third of these patients, there is no prior family history, thus representing newer mutations.

About 10–15% of paragangliomas are caused by mutations in the succinate dehydrogenase (SDH) gene or its anchoring subunits B (SDHB), C (SDHC), or D (SDHD) [193]. They may be hormone secreting. Malignant paragangliomas have been partially associated with mutations in SDHB but have also been reported in SDHD [194]. The SDH genes provide a protein that is a small part of the cytochrome *b* complex in the mitochondrial complex H, one of the five protein assemblies or complexes that form the electron transport chain. By production of reactive oxygen molecules, this pathway is considered important in the signaling and detection of oxygen tension. The gene encoding SDHD consists of 4 exons and yields 159 amino acid polypeptides [195].

Other mutations found to be associated with paragangliomas include the prolyl hydroxylase domain (PDH) proteins, which play a major role in regulating HIF, which induces expression of genes involved in angiogenesis, erythropoiesis, and cell metabolism, proliferation, and survival. Mutations in the prolyl hydroxylase domain 2 gene (PHD2) have recently been described in a patient with erythrocytosis and recurrent paragangliomas [196].

Summary

Our understanding of the molecular mechanisms underlying VS formation is advancing. Elucidating merlin's function and its interactions with other proteins and signaling pathways and regulation of the *NF2* gene will accelerate the development of novel treatments for VS, such as drug therapies designed to stop schwannoma progression. This may offer alternatives to the current options of untreated observation of tumor growth, stereotactic radiation, or surgical removal.

References

1. Trofatter JA, MacCollin MM, Rutter JL, et al. A novel moesin-, ezrin-, radixin-like gene is a candidate for the neurofibromatosis 2 tumor-suppressor. Cell. 1993;72:791–800.
2. Rouleau GA, Merel P, Lutchman M, et al. Alteration in a new gene encoding a putative membrane-organizing protein causes neurofibromatosis type 2. Nature. 1993;363:515–21.
3. Welling DB, Guida M, Goll F, et al. Mutational spectrums in the neurofibromatosis type 2 gene in sporadic and familial schwannomas. Hum Genet. 1996;98:189–93.
4. Chen Y, Gutmann DH, Haipek CA, et al. Characterization of chicken Nf2/merlin indicates regulatory roles in cell proliferation and migration. Dev Dyn. 2004;229:541–54.
5. Plotkin SR, Messiaen L, Legius E, et al. Updated diagnostic criteria and nomenclature for neurofibromatosis type 2 and schwannomatosis: an international consensus recommendation. Genet Med. 2022;24(9):1967–97.
6. Welling DB, Lasak JM, Akhmametyeva E, et al. cDNA microarray analysis of vestibular schwannomas. Otol Neurotol. 2002;23(5):736–48.
7. Chang LS, Jacob A, Lorenz M, et al. Growth of benign and malignant schwannoma xenografts in severe combined immunodeficiency mice. Laryngoscope. 2006;116(11):2018–26.
8. Tos M, Thomsen J, Charabi S. Incidence of acoustic neuromas. Ear Nose Throat J. 1992;71:391–3.
9. Howitz MF, Johansen C, Tos M, et al. Incidence of vestibular schwannoma in Denmark. 1997–95. Am J Otol. 2000;21:690–4.
10. Anderson TD, Loevner LA, Bigelow DC, Mirza N. Prevalence of unsuspected acoustic neuroma found by magnetic resonance imaging. Otolaryngol Head Neck Surg. 2000;122:643–6.
11. World Health Organization. Prevention and control of neurofibromatosis: memorandum from a joint WHO/NNFF meeting. Bull World Health Organ. 1992;70:173–82.
12. Teranishi Y, Miyawaki S, Nakatomi H, et al. Early prediction of functional prognosis in neurofibromatosis type 2 patients based on genotype-phenotype correlation with targeted deep sequencing. Sci Rep. 2022;12:9543.
13. Fontaine B, Rouleau GA, Seizinger BR, et al. Molecular genetics of neurofibromatosis 2 and related tumors (acoustic neuroma and meningioma). Ann N Y Acad Sci. 1991;615:338–43.
14. Kaiser-Kupfer M, Freidlin V, Datiles MB, et al. The association of posterior capsular lens opacities with bilateral acoustic neuromas in patients with neurofibromatosis type 2. Arch Ophthalmol. 1989;107:541–4.
15. Kanter WR, Eldridge R, Fabricant R, et al. Central neurofibromatosis with bilateral acoustic neuroma: genetic, clinical and biochemical distinctions from peripheral neurofibromatosis. Neurology. 1980;30:851–9.
16. Martuza RL, Eldridge R. Neurofibromatosis 2 (bilateral acoustic neurofibromatosis). N Engl J Med. 1988;318:684–8.
17. Evans DGR, Huson SM, Donnai D, et al. A clinical study of type 2 neurofibromatosis. Q J Med. 1992;84:603–18.
18. Evans DGR, Huson SM, Donnai D, et al. A genetic study of type 2 neurofibromatosis in the United Kingdom. I: prevalence, mutation rate, fitness, and confirmation of maternal transmission effect on severity. J Med Genet. 1992;29:841–6.
19. Wishart JH. Case of tumors in skull, dura mater, and brain. Edinb Med Surg J. 1882;18:393–7.
20. Gardner WJ, Frazier CH. Bilateral acoustic neurofibromatosis: a clinical study and field survey of a family of five generations with bilateral deafness in thirty-eight members. Arch Neurol Psychiatr. 1930;23:266–302.
21. Celis-Aquilar E, Lassaletta L, Torres-Martin M, Rodrigues FY, Nistal M, Castresana JS, Gavilan J, Rey JA. The molecular biology of vestibular schwannomas and its association with hearing loss: a review. Genet Res Int. 2012;2012:856157.
22. Evans DGR, Wallace AJ, Wu CL, et al. Somatic mosaicism: a common cause of classic disease in tumor-prone syndromes: lessons from type 2 neurofibromatosis. Am J Hum Genet. 1998;63:727–36.

23. Ruggieri M, Huson SM. The clinical and diagnostic implications of mosaicism in neurofibromatosis. Neurology. 2001;56:1433–43.
24. Kluwe L, Mautner VF, Heinrich B, et al. Molecular study of frequency of mosaicism in neurofibromatosis 2 patients with bilateral vestibular schwannomas. J Med Genet. 2003;40:109–14.
25. Moyhuddin A, Baser ME, Watson C, et al. Somatic mosaicism in neurofibromatosis 2: Prevalence and risk of disease transmission to offspring. J Med Genet. 2003;40:459–63.
26. Kameyama S, Tanaka R, Kawaguchi T, et al. Cystic acoustic neurinomas: studies of 14 cases. Acta Neurochir. 1996;138:695–9.
27. Charabi S, Tos M, Thomsen J, et al. Cystic vestibular schwannoma-clinical and experimental studies. Acta Otolaryngol Suppl. 2000;542:11–3.
28. Charabi S, Tos M, Bordesen SE, Thomsen J. Cystic acoustic neuromas. Results of translabyrinthine surgery. Arch Otolaryngol Head Neck Surg. 1994;120:1333–8.
29. Fundova P, Charabi S, Tos M, Thomsen J. Cystic vestibular schwannoma: surgical outcome. J Laryngol Otol. 2000;114:935–9.
30. Pendl G, Ganz JC, Kitz K, Eustacchio S. Acoustic neuromas with macrocysts treated with gamma knife radiosurgery. Stereotact Funct Neurosurg. 1995;66(Suppl 1):103–11.
31. Shirato H, Sakamoto T, Takeichi N, et al. Fractionated stereotactic radiotherapy for vestibular schwannoma (VS): comparison between cystic-type and solid-type VS. Int J Radiat Oncol Biol Phys. 2000;48:1395–401.
32. Rouleau GA, Wertelecki W, Haines JL, et al. Genetic linkage of bilateral acoustic neurofibromatosis to a DNA marker on chromosome 22. Nature. 1987;329:246–8.
33. Wertelecki W, Routeau GA, Superneau DW, et al. Neurofibromatosis type 2: clinical and DNA linkage studies of a large kindred. N Engl J Med. 1988. 319(5): 278–283.
34. Welling DB. Clinical manifestations of mutations in the neurofibromatosis type 2 gene in vestibular schwannomas (acoustic neuromas). Laryngoscope. 1998;108:178–89.
35. Jacoby LB, MacCollin MM, Barone R, et al. Frequency and distribution of NF2 mutations in schwannomas. Genes Chromosomes Cancer. 1996;17:45–55.
36. Irving RM, Harada T, Moffat DA, et al. Somatic neurofibromatosis type 2 gene mutations and growth characteristics in vestibular schwannoma. Amer J Otol. 1997;18:754–60.
37. Lekanne Depres RH, Bianchi AB, Groen NA, et al. Frequent NF2 gene transcript mutations in sporadic meningiomas and vestibular schwannomas. Am J Hum Genet. 1994;54:1022–9.
38. Merel P, Hoang-Xuan K, Sanson M, et al. Predominant occurrence of somatic mutations of the NF2 gene in meningiomas and schwannomas. Genes Chromosomes Cancer. 1995;13:1211–6.
39. Merel P, Khe HX, Sanson M, et al. Screening for germ-line mutations in the NF2 gene. Genes Chromosomes Cancer. 1995;12:117–27.
40. Lasota J, Fetsch JF, Wozniak A, et al. The neurofibromatosis type 2 gene is mutated in perineurial cell tumors: a molecular genetic study of eight cases. Am J Pathol. 2001;158:1223–9.
41. Bianchi AB, Hara T, Ramesh V, et al. Mutations in transcript isoforms of the neurofibromatosis 2 gene in multiple human tumour types. Nat Genet. 1994;6:185–92.
42. Bianchi AB, Mitsunnaga SI, Cheng JQ, et al. High frequency of inactivating mutations in the neurofibromatosis type 2 gene (NF2) in primary malignant mesotheliomas. Proc Natl Acad Sci USA. 1995;92:10854–8.
43. Ruttledge MH, Sarrazin J, Rangaratnam S, et al. Evidence for the complete inactivation of the NF2 gene in the majority of sporadic meningiomas. Nat Genet. 1994;6:180–4.
44. Sekido Y, Pass HI, Bader S, et al. Neurofibromatosis type 2 (NF2) gene is somatically mutated in mesothelioma but not in lung cancer. Cancer Res. 1995;55:1227–31.
45. Deguen B, Goutebroze L, Giovannini M, et al. Heterogeneity of mesothelioma cell lines are defined by altered genomic structure and expression of the NF2 gene. Int J Cancer. 1998;77:554–60.
46. Sanson M, Marineau C, Desmaze C, et al. Germline detection in a neurofibromatosis type 2 kindred inactivates the NF2 gene and a candidate meningioma locus. Hum Mol Genet. 1993;2:1215–20.
47. MacCollin M, Mohney T, Trofatter JA, et al. DNA diagnosis of neurofibromatosis 2: altered coding sequence of the merlin tumor suppressor in an extended pedigree. JAMA. 1993;270:2316–20.
48. MacCollin MM, Ramesh V, Jacoby LB, et al. Mutational analysis of patients with neurofibromatosis 2. Am J Hum Genet. 1994;55:314–20.
49. Irving RM, Moffat DA, Hardy DG, et al. Somatic NF2 gene mutations in familial and non-familial vestibular schwannoma. Hum Mol Genet. 1994;3:347–50.
50. Jacoby LB, MacCollin MM, Louis DN, et al. Exon scanning for mutation of the NF2 gene in schwannomas. Hum Mol Genet. 1994;3:413–9.
51. Jacoby LB, Jones D, Davis K, et al. Molecular analysis of the NF2 tumor-suppressor gene in schwannomatosis. Am J Hum Genet. 1997;61:1293–302.
52. Sainz J, Figueroa K, Baser ME, et al. High frequency of nonsense mutations in the NF2 gene caused by C to T transitions in five CGA codons. Hum Genet. 1995;4:137–9.
53. Sainz J, Figueroa K, Baser ME, et al. Identification of three neurofibromatosis type 2 (NF2) gene mutations in vestibular schwannomas. Hum Mol Genet. 1996;97:121–3.
54. Sainz J, Huynh DP, Figueroa K, et al. Mutations of the neurofibromatosis type 2 gene and lack of the gene product in vestibular schwannomas. Hum Mol Genet. 1994;3:885–91.
55. Twist EC, Ruttledge MH, Rousseau M, et al. The neurofibromatosis type 2 gene is inactivated in schwannomas. Hum Mol Genet. 1994;3:147–51.
56. Bourn D, Carter SA, Mason S, et al. Germline mutations in the neurofibromatosis type 2 tumor suppressor gene. Hum Mol Genet. 1994;3:813–6.
57. Bourn D, Evans DGR, Mason S, et al. Eleven novel mutations in the NF2 tumor suppressor gene. Hum Genet. 1995;95:572–4.
58. Parry DM, MacCollin MM, Kaiser-Kupfer M, et al. Germ-line mutations in the neurofibromatosis 2 gene: Correlation with disease severity and retinal abnormalities. Am J Hum Genet. 1996;59:331–45.
59. Ruttledge MH, Andermann AA, Phelan CM, et al. Type of mutation in the neurofibromatosis type 2 gene (NF2) frequently determines severity of disease. Am J Hum Genet. 1996;59:331–42.
60. Gutmann DH, Geist RT, Xu HM, et al. Defects in neurofibromatosis 2 protein function can arise at multiple levels. Hum Mol Genet. 1998;7:335–45.
61. Stokowski RP, Cox D. Functional analysis of the neurofibromatosis type 2 protein by means of disease-causing point mutations. Am J Hum Genet. 2000;66:873–91.
62. Ahronowitz I, Xin W, Kiely R, et al. Mutational spectrum of the NF2 gene: a meta-analysis of 12 years of research and diagnostic laboratory findings. Hum Mutat. 2007;28:1–12.
63. Baser ME, Contributors to the International NF2 Mutation Database. The distribution of constitutional and somatic mutations in the neurofibromatosis 2 gene. Hum Mutat. 2006;27:297–306.
64. Gutmann DH, Hirbe AC, Haipek CA. Functional analysis of neurofibromatosis 2 (NF2) missense mutations. Hum Mol Genet. 2001;10:1519–29.
65. Bruder CE, Hirvela C, Tapia-Paez I, et al. High resolution deletion analysis of constitutional DNA from neurofibromatosis type 2 (NF2) patients using microarray-CGH. Hum Mol Genet. 2001;10:271–82.

66. Ferner RE, Shaw A, Evans DG, et al. Longitudinal evaluation of quality of life in 288 patients with neurofibromatosis 2. J Neurol. 2014;261(5):963–9.
67. Bettegowda C, Upadhayaya M, Evans DG, et al. Genotype-phenotype correlations in neurofibromatosis and their potential clinical use. Neurology. 2021;97(7 Suppl 1):S91–8.
68. Mautner VF, Baser ME, Kluwe L. Phenotypic variability in two families with novel splice-site and frameshift NF2 mutations. Hum Genet. 1996;98:203–6.
69. Zhao Y, Kumar RA, Bader S, et al. Intrafamilial correlation of clinical manifestations in neurofibromatosis 2 (NF2). Genet Epidemiol. 2002;23:245–59.
70. Bruder CE, Ichimura K, Blennow E, et al. Severe phenotype of neurofibromatosis type 2 in a patient with a 7.4-MC constitutional deletion on chromosome 22: possible localization of a neurofibromatosis type 2 modifier gene? Genes Chromosomes Cancer. 1999;25:184–90.
71. Zucman-Rossi J, Legoix P, Der Sarkissian H, et al. NF2 gene in neurofibromatosis type 2 patients. Hum Mol Genet. 1999;7:2095–101.
72. Kino T, Takeshima H, Nakao M, et al. Identification of the cis-acting region in the NF2 gene promoter as a potential target for mutation and methylation-dependent silencing in schwannoma. Genes Cells. 2001;6:441–54.
73. Chang LS, Akhmametyeva EM, Wu Y, et al. Multiple transcription initiation sites, alternative splicing, and differential polyadenylation contribute to the complexity of human neurofibromatosis 2 transcripts. Genomics. 2002;79(1):63–76.
74. Gonzalez-Gomez P, Bello MJ, Alonso ME, et al. CpG Island methylation in sporadic and neurofibromatosis type 2-associated schwannomas. Clin Cancer Red. 2003;9:5601–6.
75. Gutmann DH, Sherman L, Seftor L, et al. Increased expression of the NF2 tumor suppressor gene product, merlin, impairs cell motility, adhesion, and spreading. Hum Mol Genet. 1999;8:267–75.
76. Algrain M, Aprin M, Louvard D. Wizardry at the cell cortex. Curr Biol. 1993;3:451–4.
77. Golovnina K, Blinov A, Akhmametyeva EM, et al. Evolution and origin of merlin, the product of the *neurofibromatosis type 2* (NF2) tumor-suppressor gene. BMC Evol Biol. 2005;5:69–86.
78. Chisthti AH, Kim AC, Marfatia SM, et al. The FERM domain: a unique module involved in the linkage of the cytoplastic proteins to the membrane. TIBS. 1998;23:281–2.
79. Shimizu T, Seto A, Maita N, et al. Structural basis for neurofibromatosis type 2 crystal structure of the merlin FERM domain. J Biol Chem. 2002;277:10332–6.
80. Bretscher A, Chambers D, Nguyen R, et al. ERM-merlin and EBP50 protein families in plasma membrane organization and function. Ann Rev Cell Dev Biol. 2000;16:113–43.
81. Turunen O, Wahlstrom T, Vaheri A. Ezrin has a COOH-terminal actin-binding site that is conserved in the ezrin protein family. J Cell Biol. 1994;126:1445–53.
82. Gonzalez-Agosti C, Xu L, Pinney D, et al. The merlin tumor suppressor localizes preferentially in membrane ruffles. Oncogene. 1996;13:1239–47.
83. Pelton PD, Sherman LS, Rizvi TA, et al. Ruffling membrane, stress fiber, cell spreading and proliferation abnormalities in human schwannoma cells. Oncogene. 1998;17:2195–209.
84. Deguen B, Merel P, Goutebroze L, et al. Impaired interaction of naturally occurring mutant NF2 protein with actin-based cytoskeleton and membrane. Hum Mol Genet. 1998;7:217–26.
85. Lutchman M, Rouleau GA. The neurofibromatosis type 2 gene product, schwannomin, suppresses growth of NIH 3T3 cells. Cancer Res. 1995;55:2270–4.
86. Sherman L, Xu HM, Geist RT, et al. Interdomain binding mediates tumor growth suppression by the NF2 gene product. Oncogene. 1997;15:2505–9.
87. Tikoo A, Varga M, Ramesh V, et al. An anti-ras function of neurofibromatosis type 2 gene product (NF2/merlin). J Biol Chem. 1994;269:23387–90.
88. McClatchey AI, Saotome I, Mercer K, et al. Mice heterozygous for a mutation at the NF2 tumor suppressor locus develop a range of highly metastatic tumors. Genes Dev. 1998;12:1121–33.
89. McClatchey AI, Saotome I, Ramesh V, et al. The NF2 tumor suppressor gene product is essential for extraembryonic development immediately prior to gastrulation. Genes Dev. 1997;11:1253–65.
90. Akhmametyeva EM, Mihaylova MM, Luo H, et al. Regulation of the neurofibromatosis 2 gene promoter expression during embryonic development. Dev Dyn. 2006;235(10):2771–85.
91. Giovannini M, Robanus-Maandag E, van der Walk M, et al. Conditional biallelic *Nf2* mutation in the mouse promotes manifestations of human neurofibromatosis type 2. Genes Dev. 2000;14:1617–30.
92. Kalamarides M, Miwa-Kawakita M, Leblois H, et al. *Nf2* gene inactivation in arachnoidal cells is rate-limiting for meningioma development in the mouse. Genes Dev. 2002;16:1060–5.
93. Shaw RJ, Paez JG, Curto M, et al. The NF2 tumor suppressor, merlin, functions in rac-dependent signaling. Dev Cell. 2001;1:63–72.
94. Sherman L, Sleeman J, Herrlich P, et al. Hyaluronate receptors: key players in growth, differentiation, migration, and tumor progression. Curr Opin Cell Biol. 1994;6:726–33.
95. Takeshima H, Izawa I, Lee PS, et al. Detection of cellular proteins that interact with the NF2 tumor suppressor gene product. Oncogene. 1994;9:2135–44.
96. Sainio M, Zhao F, Heiska L, et al. Neurofibromatosis 2 tumor suppressor protein colocalizes with ezrin and CD44 and associates with actin-containing cytoskeleton. J Cell Sci. 1997;110:2249–60.
97. Herrlich P, Morrison H, Sleeman J, et al. CD44 acts as both a growth and invasiveness-promoting molecule and as a tumor-suppressing cofactor. Ann N Y Acad Sci. 2000;910:106–18.
98. Huang L, Ichimaru E, Pestonjamasp K, et al. Merlin differs from moesin in binding to F-actin and in its intra- and intermolecular interactions. Biochem Biophys Res Commun. 1998;248:548–53.
99. Fernandex-Valle C, Tang Y, Ricard J, et al. Paxillin binds schwannomin and regulates its density-dependent localization and effect on cell morphology. Nat Genet. 2000;31:354–62.
100. Xu HM, Gutmann DH. Merlin differentially associates with the microtubule and actin cytoskeleton. J Neurosci Res. 1998;51:403–15.
101. Scoles DR, Huynh DP, Morcos PA, et al. Neurofibromatosis 2 tumor suppressor schwannomin interacts with bII-spectrin. Nat Genet. 1998;18:354–9.
102. Obremski VJ, Hall AM, Fernandez-Valle C. Merlin, the neurofibromatosis type 2 gene product, and b1 integrin associate in isolated and differentiating schwann cells. J Neurobiol. 1998;37:487–501.
103. Gonzalez-Agosti C, Wiederhold T, Herndon ME, et al. Interdomain interaction of merlin isoforms and its influence on intermolecular binding to NHE-RF. J Biol Chem. 1999;274:34438–42.
104. Murthy A, Gonzalez-Agosti C, Cordero E, et al. NHE-RF, a regulatory cofactor for Na(+)-H+ exchange, is a common interactor for merlin and ERM (MERM) proteins. J Biol Chem. 1998;273:1273–6.
105. Goutebroze L, Brault E, Muchardt C, et al. Cloning and characterization of SCHIP-1, a novel protein in interacting specifically with spliced isoforms and naturally occurring mutant NF2 proteins. Mol Cell Biol. 2000;20:1699–712.

106. Scoles DR, Huynh DP, Chen MS, et al. The neurofibromatosis 2 tumor suppressor protein interacts with hepatocyte growth factor-regulated tyrosine kinase substrate. Hum Mol Genet. 2000;9:1567–74.
107. Guttman DH, Haipek CA, Burke SP, et al. The NF2 interactor, hepatocyte growth factor-regulated tyrosine kinase substrate (HRS), interacts with merlin in the "open" conformation and suppresses cell growth and motility. Hum Mol Genet. 2001;10(8):825–34.
108. Gronholm M, Vossebein L, Carlson CR, et al. Merlin links to the cAMP neuronal signaling pathway by anchoring the R1 beta subunit of protein kinase A. J Biol Chem. 2003;278:41167–72.
109. Kissil JL, Wilker EW, Johnson KC, et al. Merlin, the product of the NF2 tumor suppressor gene, is an inhibitor of the p21-activated kinase, PAK1. Mol Cell. 2003;12:841–9.
110. Lallemand D, Curto M, Santome I, et al. NF2 deficiency promotes tumorigenesis and metastasis by destabilizing adherens junctions. Genes Dev. 2003;17:1090–100.
111. Rong R, Tang X, Gutmann DH, et al. Neurofibromatosis 2 (NF2) tumor suppressor merlin inhibits phosphatidylinositol 3-kinase through binding to PIKE-L. Proc Natl Acad Sci USA. 2004;101:18200–5.
112. Petrill AM, Fuse MA, Donnan MS, et al. A chemical biology approach identified PI3K as a potential therapeutic target for neurofibromatosis type 2. Am J Transl Res. 2014;6(5):471–93.
113. Rangwala R, Banine F, Borg IF, Sherman LS. Erbin regulates mitogen-activated protein (MAP) kinase activation and MAP kinase-dependent interactions between merlin and adherens junction protein complexes in schwann cells. J Biol Chem. 1005;280:11790–7.
114. Wilkes MC, Repellin CE, Hong M, et al. Erbin and the NF2 tumor suppressor Merlin cooperatively regulate cell-type-specific activation of PAK2 by TGF-beta. Dev Cell. 2009;16(3):433–44.
115. Han Y. Analysis of the role of the Hippo pathway in cancer. J Transl Med. 2019;17:116.
116. Su T, Ludwig MZ, Xu J, Fehon RG. Kibra and Merlin activate the Hippo pathway spatially distinct from and independent of expanded. Dev Cell. 2017;40(5):478–90.
117. Kim JY, Kim H, Jeun S, et al. Inhibition of NF-kappaB activation by merlin. Biochem Biophys Res Commun. 2002;296(5):1295–302.
118. Ren Y, Chari DA, Vasilijic S, et al. New developments in neurofibromatosis type 2 and vestibular schwannoma. Neurooncol Adv. 2021;3(2):vdaa153.
119. Gutmann DH, Haipek CA, Hoang LK. Neurofibromatosis 2 tumor suppressor protein, merlin, forms two functionally-important intramolecular associations. J Neurosci Res. 1999;58:706–16.
120. Pearson MA, Reczek D, Bretscher A, et al. Structure of the ERM protein moesin reveals the FERM domain fold masked by an extended actin binding tail domain. Cell. 2000;101:259–70.
121. Morrison H, Sherman LS, Legg J, et al. The NF2 tumor suppressor gene product, merlin, mediates contact inhibition of growth through interactions with CD44. Genes Dev. 2001;15:968–80.
122. Xiao GH, Beeser A, Chernoff J, et al. P21-activated kinase links Rac/Cdc42 signaling to merlin. J Biol Chem. 2002;277:883–6.
123. Kissil JL, Johnson KC, Eckman MS, et al. Merlin phosphorylation by p21-activated kinase 2 and effects of phosphorylation on merlin localization. J Biol Chem. 2002;277:10394–9.
124. Mota M, Shevde LA. Merlin regulates signaling events at the nexus of development and cancer. Cell Commun Signal. 2020;18:63.
125. Jin H, Sperka T, Herrlich P, Morrison H. Tumorigenic transformation by CPI-17 through inhibition of a merlin phosphatase. Nature. 2006;442:576–9.
126. Bretscher A, Reczek D, Berryman M. Ezrin: a protein requiring conformational activation to link microfilaments to the plasma membrane in the assembly of cell surface structures. J Cell Sci. 1997;110:3011–8.
127. Tsukita S, Yonemura S, Tsukita S. ERM proteins: head-to-tail regulation of actin-plasma membrane interaction. TIBS. 1997;22:53–8.
128. Hirao M, Sato N, Kondo T, et al. Regulation mechanism of ERM (ezrin/radixin/moesin) protein/plasma membrane association: possible involvement of phosphatidylinositol turnover and rho-dependent signaling pathway. J Cell Biol. 1996;135:37–51.
129. Jacob A, Lee TX, Neff B, et al. Phosphatidylinositol 3 kinase/AKT pathway activation in human vestibular schwannoma. Otol Neurotol. 2003;29:58–68.
130. Rong R, Tang X, Gutmann DH, Ye K. Neurofibromatosis 2 (NF2) tumor suppressor merlin inhibits phosphatidylinositol 3-kinase through binding to PIKE-L. PNAS. 2004;101(52):18200–5.
131. Sabra H, Brunner M, Mandati V, et al. B1 integrin-dependent Rac/group I PAK signaling mediates YAP activation of Yes-associated protein 1 (YAP1) via NF2/merlin. J Biol Chem. 2017;292(47):19179–97.
132. Flaiz C, Utermark T, Parkinson DB, et al. Impaired intercellular adhesion and immature adherens junctions in merlin-deficient human primary schwannoma cells. Glia. 2008;56:506–15.
133. Welling DB, Akhmemetyava EM, Daniels RL, et al. Analysis of the human neurofibromatosis type 2 gene promoter and its expression. Otolaryngol Head Neck Surg. 2000;123(4):413–8.
134. Arakawa H, Hayashi N, Nagase H, et al. Alternative splicing of the NF2 gene and its mutation analysis of breast and colorectal cancers. Hum Mol Genet. 1994;3:565–8.
135. Hitotsumatsu T, Kitamoto T, Iwaki T, et al. An exon 8-spliced out transcript of neurofibromatosis 2 gene is constitutively expressed in various human tissues. J Biochem. 1994;116:1205–7.
136. Koga H, Araki N, Takeshima H, et al. Impairment of cell adhesion by expression of the mutant neurofibromatosis type 2 (NF2) gene which lacks exons in the ERM-homology domain. Oncogene. 1998;17:801–10.
137. Nishi T, Takeshima H, Hamada K, et al. Neurofibromatosis 2 gene has novel alternative splicing which controls intracellular protein binding. Int J Oncol. 1997;10:1025–9.
138. Pykett MJ, Murphy M, Harnish PR, et al. The neurofibromatosis type 2 tumor suppressor gene encodes multiple alternatively spliced transcripts. Hum Mol Genet. 1994;3:559–64.
139. Schmucker B, Tang Y, Kressel M. Novel alternatively spliced isoforms of the neurofibromatosis type 2 tumor suppressor are targeted to the nucleus and cytoplasmic granules. Hum Mol Genet. 1999;8:1561–70.
140. Giovannini M, Robanus-Maandag E, Niwa-Kawakita M, et al. Schwann cell hyperplasia and tumors in transgenic mice expressing a naturally occurring mutant NF2 protein. Genes Dev. 1999;13:978–86.
141. Light JP, Roland JT Jr, Fishman A, et al. Atypical and low-grade malignant vestibular schwannomas: clinical implications of proliferative activity. Otol Neurotol. 2001;22:922–7.
142. Chen JM, Houle S, Ang LC, et al. A study of vestibular schwannomas using positron emission tomography and monoclonal antibody ki-67. Am J Otol. 1998;19:840–5.
143. Kesterson L, Shelton C, Dressler L, et al. Clinical behavior of acoustic tumors. A flow cytometric analysis. Arch Otolaryngol Head Neck Surg. 1993;119:269–71.
144. Cardillo MR, Filipo R, Monini S, et al. Transforming growth factor-b1 expression in human acoustic neuroma. Am J Otol. 1999;20:65–8.
145. Charabi S, Manotni M, Tos M, et al. Cyclic vestibular schwannomas: neuroimaging and growth rate. J Laryngol Otol. 1994;108:375–9.
146. Charabi S, Klinken L, Tos M, Thomsen J. Histopathology and growth pattern of cystic acoustic neuromas. Laryngoscope. 1994;104:1348–52.
147. Antinheimo J, Haapasalo H, Seppala M, et al. Proliferative potential of sporadic and neurofibromatosis 2-associated schwannomas

as studied by MIB-I (ki-67) and PCNA labeling. J Neuropathol Exp Neurol. 1995;54:776–82.
148. Aguiar PH, Tatagiba M, Samii M, et al. The comparison between the growth fraction of bilateral vestibular schwannomas in neurofibromatosis 2 (NF2) and unilateral vestibular schwannomas using the monoclonal antibody MIB1. Acta Neurochir. 1995;134:40–5.
149. Neff BA, Oberstein E, Lorenz M, et al. Cyclin D(1) and D(3) expression in vestibular schwannomas. Laryngoscope. 2006;116(3):423–6.
150. Jabbour J, Earls P, Biggs N, et al. Role of cyclins D1 and D3 in vestibular schwannoma. J Laryngol Otol. 2016;130(Suppl 1):S2–10.
151. Bassett DEJ, Eisen MB, Boguski MS. Gene expression informatics—it's all in your mind. Nat Genet. 1999;21:51–5.
152. Lockhart DJ, Winzeler EA. Genomics, gene expression, and DNA arrays. Nature. 2000;405:827–36.
153. Carlson ML, Smadbeck JB, Link MJ, et al. Next generation sequencing of sporadic vestibular schwannoma: necessity of biallelic NF2 inactivation and implications of accessory non-HF2 variants. Otol Neurotol. 2018;39(9):e860–71.
154. Havik AL, Bruland O, Myrseth E, et al. Genetic landscape of sporadic vestibular schwannoma. J Neurosurg. 2018;128(3):911–22.
155. Lasak JM, Welling DB, Akhmametyeva EM, et al. Retinoblastoma-cyclin-dependent kinase pathway deregulation in vestibular schwannomas. Laryngoscope. 2002;112(9):1555–61.
156. Evans DGR, Birch JM, Ramsden RT, et al. Malignant transformation and new primary tumours after therapeutic radiation for benign disease: substantial risks in certain tumour prone syndromes. J Med Genet. 2006;43:289–94.
157. Preston DL, Ron E, Yonehara S, et al. Tumors of the nervous system and pituitary gland associated with atomic bomb radiation exposure. J Natl Cancer Inst. 2002;94:1555–63.
158. Schneider AB, Ron E, Lubin J, et al. Acoustic neuromas following childhood radiation treatment for benign conditions of the head and neck. Neuro-Oncology. 2008;10:73–8.
159. Hardell L, Carlberg M, Soderquist F, Mild KH. Meta-analysis of long-term mobile phone use and the association with brain tumors. Int J Oncol. 2008;32:1097–103.
160. Hardell L, Carlberg M, Söderquist F, et al. Long-term use of cellular phones and brain tumors: increased risk associated with use for > or = 10 years. Occup Environ Med. 2007;64:626–32.
161. Shuz J, Steding-Jessen M, Hansen S, et al. Long-term mobile phone use and the risk of vestibular schwannoma: a Danish Nationwide cohort study. Am J Epidemiol. 2011;174(4):416–22.
162. Hepsibah A, Pandey SK, Rupa V, et al. Changes in pattern of presentation of patients with unilateral vestibular schwannoma over two decades: influence of cell phone use in early diagnosis. J Clin Neuro. 2021;94:102–6.
163. Evans DGR, Sainio M, Me B. Neurofibromatosis type 2. J Med Genet. 2000;37:897–904.
164. Neff BA, Welling DB. Current concepts in the evaluation and treatment of neurofibromatosis type II. Otolaryngol Clin N Am. 2005;38(4):671–684, ix.
165. Messerli SM, Prabhakar S, Tang Y, et al. Treatment of schwannomas with an oncolytic recombinant herpes simplex virus in murine models of neurofibromatosis type 2. Hum Gene Ther. 2006;17:20–30.
166. Prabhakar S, Beauchamp RL, Cheah PS, et al. Gene replacement therapy in a schwannoma mouse model of neurofibromatosis type 2. Mol Ther Methods Clin Dev. 2002;22(26):169–80.
167. Hansen MR, Roehm PC, Chatterjee P, Green SH. Constitutive neuregulin-1/ErbB signaling contributes to human vestibular schwannoma proliferation. Glia. 2006;53:593–600.
168. Doherty JK, Ongekeko W, Crawley B, et al. ErbB and nrg potential targets for vestibular schwannoma pharmacotherapy. Otol Neurotol. 2008;29:50–7.
169. Nakai Y, Zheng Y, MacCollin MM, Ratner N. Temporal control of rac in schwann cell-axon interaction is disrupted in NF2-mutant schwannoma cells. J Neurosci. 2006;26:3390–5.
170. Jacob A, Lee TX, Neff BA, et al. Phosphatidylinositol 3 kinase/AKT pathway activation in human vestibular schwannoma. Otol Neurotol. 2008;29:58–68.
171. Zhao F, Chen Y, Li S, et al. Novel patient-derived xenograft and cell line models for therapeutic screening in NF2-associated schwannoma. J Pathol. 2022;257(5):620–34.
172. Goutagny S, Raymond E, Esposito-Farese M, et al. Phase II study of mTORC1 inhibition by everolimus in neurofibromatosis type 2 patients with growing vestibular schwannomas. J Neuro-Oncol. 2015;122(2):313–20.
173. Karajannis MA, Legault G, Hagiwara M. Phase II study of everolimus in children and adults with neurofibromatosis type 2 and progressive vestibular schwannomas. Neuro-Oncology. 2014;16(2):292–7.
174. Karajannis MA, Mauguen A, Maloku E, et al. Phase 0 clinical trial of everolimus in patients with vestibular schwannoma or meningioma. Mol Cancer Ther. 2021;20(9):1584–91.
175. Davies M, Saxena A, Kingswood JC. Management of everolimus-associated adverse events in patients with tuberous sclerosis complex: a practical guide. Orphanet J Rare Dis. 2017;12:35.
176. Pirker R, Filipits M. Targeted therapies in lung cancer. Curr Pharm Des. 2009;15:188–206.
177. Aragon-Ching JB, Dahut WL. The role of angiogenesis inhibitors in prostate cancer. Cancer J. 2008;14:20–5.
178. Ranieri G, Patruno R, Ruggieri E, et al. Vascular endothelial growth factor (VEGF) as a target of bevacizumab in cancer: from the biology to the clinic. Curr Med Chem. 2006;13:1745–57.
179. Chase JL. Clinical use of anti-vascular endothelial growth factor monoclonal antibodies in metastatic colorectal cancer. Pharmacotherapy. 2008;28:235–305.
180. Fujii M, Ichikawa M, Iwatate K, et al. Bevacizumab therapy of neurofibromatosis type 2 associated vestibular schwannoma in Japanese patients. Neurol Med Chir (Tokyo). 2020;60(2):75–82.
181. Goutagny S, Kalamarides M. Medical treatment in neurofibromatosis type 2. Review of the literature and presentation of clinical reports. Neurochirurgie. 2018;64(5):370–4.
182. Sverak P, Adams ME, Haines SJ, et al. Bevacizumab for hearing preservation in neurofibromatosis type 2: emphasis on patient-reported outcomes and toxicities. Otolaryngol Head Neck Surg. 2019;160(3):526–32.
183. Blakeley JO, Ye X, Duda DG, et al. Efficacy and biomarker study of Bevacizumab for hearing loss resulting from neurofibromatosis type 2-associated vestibular schwannomas. J Clin Oncol. 2016;34(14):1669–75.
184. Slusarz KM, Merker VL, Muzikansky A, et al. Long-term toxicity of bevacizumab therapy in neurofibromatosis 2 patients. Cancer Chemother Pharmacol. 2014;73(6):1197–204.
185. Alanin MC, Klausen C, Caye-Thomasen P, et al. The effect of bevacizumab on vestibular schwannoma tumor size and hearing in patients with neurofibromatosis type 2. Eur Arch Otorhinolaryngol. 2015;272(12):3627–33.
186. Prabhakar S, Brenner GJ, Sung B, et al. Imaging and therapy of experimental schwannomas using HSV amplicon vector-encoding apoptotic protein under Schwann cell promoter. Cancer Gene Ther. 2010;17(4):266–74.
187. Prabhakar S, Taherian M, Gianni D, et al. Regression of schwannomas induced by adeno-associated virus-mediated delivery of caspase-1. Hum Gene Ther. 2013;24(2):152–62.
188. Ahmed SG, Abdelnabi A, Maguire CA, et al. Gene therapy with apoptosis-associated speck-like protein, a newly described schwannoma tumor suppressor, inhibits schwannoma growth in vivo. Neuro-Oncology. 2019;21(7):854–66.

189. Tamura R, Fujioka M, Morimoto Y, et al. A VEGF receptor vaccine demonstrates preliminary efficacy in neurofibromatosis type 2. Nat Commun. 2019;10:5758.
190. MacCollin MM, Chiocca EA, Evans DGR. Diagnostic criteria for schwannomatosis. Neurology. 2005;18:38–45.
191. Boyd C, Smith MJ, Kluwe L, et al. Alterations in the SMARCB1 (IM11) tumor suppressor gene in familiar schwannomatosis. Clin Genet. 2008;74:358–66.
192. Sestini R, Bacci C, Provenzano A, et al. Evidence of a four-hit mechanism involving SMARCB1 and NF2 in schwannomatosis-associated schwannomas. Hum Mutat. 2008;29:227–31.
193. Papaspyrou K, Rossman H, Fottner C, et al. Malignant paraganglioma caused by a novel germline mutation of the succinate dehydrogenase D-gene: a case report. Head Neck. 2008;30:964–9.
194. Marvin ML, Bradford CR, Sisson JC, Gruber SB. Diagnosis and management of hereditary paraganglioma syndrome due to the F933>X67 SDHD mutation. Head Neck. 2009;31:689–94.
195. Mhatre AN, Lalwani AK. Molecular genetics in neurotology. In: Jackler RK, Brackmann DE, editors. Neurotology. Philadelphia: Elsevier Mosby; 2005.
196. Lasroue C, Carcenac R, Leporrier M, et al. PHD2 mutation and congenital erythrocytosis with paraganglioma. N Engl J Med. 2008;359:2685–92.

Part II

Clinical Evaluation

11 Clinical Diagnosis of the Otologic and Neurotologic Patient (History and Examination)

Daniel E. Killeen and Brandon Isaacson

Introduction

As with all medical conditions, the diagnosis of otologic and neurotologic disorders begins with a thorough history and physical examination, which is then augmented by ancillary audiologic, vestibular, and radiologic testing. While these ancillary tests are often important in establishing a definitive diagnosis to counsel the patients, complete and accurate history and physical exam are critical to narrowing down the differential diagnosis, thereby enabling directed and efficient use of additional testing. This chapter will discuss the important elements of the otologic history and physical exam with discussion about how these key points will help to narrow down the differential diagnosis.

History

The most crucial element in the evaluation of the otologic patient is a thorough and accurate history, which starts with the basic chief complaint. Eliciting the chief complaint related to the ear (i.e., hearing loss, dizziness, ear drainage, tinnitus, or otalgia) can then enable further categorization and enable more directed questions pertinent to the problem at hand. It is important to consider other systemic symptoms in addition to the otologic-focused historical questions as systemic diseases such as granulomatosis with polyangiitis, tuberculosis, diabetes, and multiple sclerosis can all impact the otologic system (Table 11.1 [1]). Furthermore, complete past medical and surgical history as well as a complete list of current medications is of utmost importance, as certain medications can be ototoxic and can account for various otologic complaints.

Table 11.1 Systemic diseases affecting the otologic system

Granulomatous and infectious diseases
Langerhans cell histiocytosis
Tuberculosis
Wegener granulomatosis
Sarcoidosis
Syphilis
Lyme disease
Mycotic diseases
Cytomegalic inclusion disease
Neoplastic diseases
Multiple myeloma
Leukemia
Lymphoma
Metastatic neoplasms
Diseases of the bone
Paget disease (osteitis deformans)
Osteogenesis imperfecta
Fibrous dysplasia
Osteopetroses
Osteitis fibrosa cystica
Storage and metabolic diseases
Mucopolysaccharidoses
Gout
Ochronosis
Collagen vascular and autoimmune diseases
Multiple sclerosis
Susac disease
Immunodeficiency disorders
Primary or congenital
Humoral immunodeficiency disorders
Cellular immunodeficiency disorders
Disorders of phagocyte function
Complement system defects
Acquired
Acquired immunodeficiency syndrome
Other
Genetically determined defects

Adapted from [1]

D. E. Killeen · B. Isaacson (✉)
Department of Otolaryngology—Head and Neck Surgery, University of Texas Southwestern Medical Center, Dallas, TX, USA
e-mail: Brandon.Isaacson@utsouthwestern.edu

A. D. Sweeney et al. (eds.), *Haynes-Glasscock-Shambaugh Surgery of the Ear*, https://doi.org/10.1007/978-3-032-18264-7_11

Direct interview of the patient is the standard for historical data gathering but can also be obtained with patient completed questionnaires or templates of questions, either generic or tailored to specific chief complaints. More recently, the institution of the electronic medical record has presented several other options for data gathering, including physician- or staff-completed templates, patient-completed templates or questionnaires prior to the visit, and interactive computerized interviews [2]. The advent of software to allow patient-entered data through directed lines of subsequent queries based on patient responses to initial questions holds the promise of a more efficient data-gathering system. Of course, physician review and refinement of additional questioning are likely warranted, but overall, an efficient and thorough history will make subsequent diagnosis and confirmatory testing more accurate and cost-effective. Directed questioning either by the physician or a computerized directed interview with self-reporting should address these bullet points based on chief complaints outlined in the following sections.

Hearing Loss

When approaching the chief complaint of hearing loss, the clinician should ask pertinent questions including but not limited to:

- Laterality—unilateral or bilateral?
  - Unilateral or asymmetric hearing loss often indicates localized ear pathology such as vascular insult, inflammatory disease, trauma, hydrops, or retrocochlear pathology. While the latter is often considered as a possible diagnosis, vestibular schwannomas have been only found in 1.5% of patients with asymmetric hearing loss [3].
  - Bilateral hearing loss suggests possible (1) degenerative etiology such as aging, noise damage, or ototoxicity or (2) systemic illness such as an autoimmune disease process.
- Duration—sudden (<3 weeks) or chronic?
  - Most hearing loss is chronic, and it is difficult to pinpoint the exact time of onset, but acute onset hearing loss raises concern for sudden sensorineural hearing loss, which must be treated promptly with corticosteroids, either intratympanic, oral, or a combination thereof [4].
- Stability—fluctuating or not?
  - Fluctuating hearing loss commonly occurs with endolymphatic hydrops, perilymph fistula, labyrinthitis, sarcoidosis, tuberculosis, and multiple sclerosis [5].
  - Autoimmune causes of hearing loss may have symptoms and characteristics similar to endolymphatic hydrops early in the disease course [5].
- Associated symptoms (otalgia, tinnitus, vertigo, otorrhea)
  - The presence of hearing loss with otalgia or otorrhea could be concerning for infections such as acute or chronic otitis media as well as cholesteatoma [5].
  - Fluctuating tinnitus, aural fullness, and vertigo with hearing loss can be concerning for endolymphatic hydrops [5].
- Past history of hearing problems, ear infections, head trauma, tympanostomy tubes, otologic surgery
- Family history of hearing loss
  - Approximately 60% of patients with otosclerosis will report family history of hearing loss [6].
  - Hereditary and familial hearing problems should prompt additional questions for syndromic conditions.
- Noise exposure (firearms, occupational, recreational, etc.)
- Ototoxic medications
  - Loop diuretics, aminoglycoside antibiotics, salicylates, chemotherapeutic agents (Table 11.2) [7–11].

Table 11.2 Agents and medications that can cause vestibular and auditory ototoxicity

Antibiotics
Aminoglycoside antibiotics
Primarily cochleotoxic
Neomycin
Kanamycin
Tobramycin
Dihydrostreptomycin
Amikacin
Primarily vestibulotoxic
Gentamicin
Streptomycin
Other
Erythromycin
Vancomycin
Antineoplastic agents
Cisplatin
Carboplatin
Nitrogen mustard
Vincristine
Vinblastine
Diuretics
Furosemide
Ethacrynic acid
Bumetanide
Anti-inflammatory agents
Salicylates
Quinine
Chloroquine
Chelating agents
Deferoxamine
Chemicals
Mercury
Gold
Lead
Arsenic
Aniline dyes

Adapted from [7–11]

Dizziness

History is especially important in the diagnosis of the dizzy patient. Approximately 61.4% of patients with dizziness were correctly diagnosed by history alone [12]. When approaching the chief complaint of dizziness, the clinician should ask pertinent questions including but not limited to:

- Character (lightheadedness, drop attacks, disequilibrium, room-spinning vertigo, syncope)
  - Vertigo is the sensation that either the patient is moving, either linearly or rotating while stationary, or the sensation that the room or objects are moving [13]. Vertigo is more concerning for vestibular dysfunction, either centrally or peripherally [13].
  - Generalized imbalance is more concerning for a central neurologic cause. One example is mal de debarquement, which typically occurs in patients after boat or air travel and is characterized by a back and forth rocking sensation [14].
- Hearing loss
  - Presence of hearing loss with vertigo is concerning for endolymphatic hydrops or labyrinthitis [12].
  - Absence of hearing loss is concerning for vestibular neuritis, vestibular migraine, or benign positional paroxysmal vertigo [12].
- Episodic or constant vertigo
  - Episodic vertigo is more concerning for endolymphatic hydrops or benign positional paroxysmal vertigo [12].
  - Constant vertigo is suggestive of labyrinthitis or vestibular neuritis [12]. The combination of this question and the presence or absence of hearing loss correctly diagnosed 61.4% of patients [12].
- Time course (lasting seconds, minutes, or hours)
  - Labyrinthitis and vestibular neuritis have a sudden onset with constant vertigo for a few days with gradually improving disequilibrium for days to weeks after the initial event [15].
  - Benign paroxysmal positional vertigo has frequent episodes of vertigo which last less than a minute [15].
  - Endolymphatic hydrops is characterized by more infrequent attacks that last hours but typically less than 24 h [15].
  - Vestibular migraine has a similar time course to endolymphatic hydrops—tends to last hours, but unlike endolymphatic hydrops, vestibular migraine can last more than 24 h and is usually not associated with hearing loss [15].
  - Persistent postural perceptual dizziness, mal de debarquement, uncompensated peripheral vestibulopathy, and presbystasis are all chronic vestibular conditions which can last from days to years [15].
- Associated symptoms (tinnitus, aural fullness, pulsatile tinnitus, headache, visual changes, nausea/vomiting)
  - Endolymphatic hydrops presents with roaring tinnitus, aural fullness, hearing loss, and severe vertiginous attacks [5].
  - Vestibular migraine typically occurs with other migraine symptoms, including visual auras, photophobia, phonophobia, and headache [16].
  - Presence of dysarthria, numbness of the face, hemiparesis, headache, diplopia, visual field defects, blindness, dysphagia, and ataxia raise concern for vertebrobasilar insufficiency, which causes vertigo lasting minutes that may be elicited by head turning [15].
- Exacerbating factors (positional, noise induced)
  - Dizziness triggered by standing or leaning forward and characterized by lightheadedness or the sensation that one is about to lose consciousness is concerning for presyncope [13]. Presyncope may be related to neural factors as in the case of vasovagal syncope or may be related to cardiovascular system, but usually, presyncope is not otologic in origin [13].
  - Vertigo triggered by turning the head to the side or looking up is concerning for benign paroxysmal vertigo [15]. Noise or pressure-induced vertigo is concerning for superior semicircular canal dehiscence or perilymph fistula, though it can also be associated with endolymphatic hydrops and congenital or acquired syphilis [5].
- History of trauma to the head and neck
  - Head trauma may predispose patients for perilymph fistula, benign positional paroxysmal vertigo, labyrinthine concussion, temporal bone fractures involving otic capsule, or endolymphatic hydrops [15].
  - Trauma can also cause cervical vertigo, which results from strain of the cervical muscles and is characterized by constant disequilibrium and restricted neck movement [15]. Palpation of the cervical muscles can occasionally replicate this sensation in cervical vertigo [15].
- History of chronic ear infections or cholesteatoma
  - Patients with cholesteatoma or chronic ear infection may develop labyrinthine fistulas. In a recent retrospective review, 6% of patients who underwent tympanoplasty for cholesteatoma had a lateral semicircular canal fistula [17].

Ear Drainage

When approaching the chief complaint of ear drainage, the clinician should ask pertinent questions including but not limited to:

- Type of fluid (clear, bloody, purulent)
  - Clear otorrhea is concerning for possible CSF leak.
  - Bloody or purulent otorrhea is more concerning for chronic ear infection, cholesteatoma, or otitis externa. Bloody drainage may also raise suspicion for an external auditory canal malignancy.
- Presence of associated symptoms (hearing loss, vertigo, otalgia)
  - Purulent otorrhea in combination with otalgia is concerning for possible otitis externa or acute otitis media with perforation of the tympanic membrane [5]. Severe otalgia with bloody otorrhea and hearing loss may be concerning for bullous myringitis [5]. Severe otalgia and bloody otorrhea with facial nerve paralysis may suggest Ramsay Hunt syndrome or necrotizing otitis externa [5].
  - Hearing loss with chronic purulent otorrhea without significant otalgia is concerning for possible cholesteatoma [5].
  - The presence of retro-orbital pain and diplopia with otorrhea is suggestive of Gradenigo syndrome and petrous apicitis [18]. However, only 36%, 55%, and 16% of patients with petrous apicitis had purulent otorrhea, retro-orbital pain, and abducens nerve palsy, respectively [18].
- Duration (acute vs. chronic)
  - Acute otorrhea is more concerning for acute bacterial infections such as otitis externa. Chronic otorrhea is more concerning for chronic suppurative otitis media with or without cholesteatoma.
- Predisposing factors (swimming, trauma)
  - Swimming and trauma to the ear canal with instrumentation such as Q-tips predispose patients to otitis externa [5].
  - Prior ear surgery or placement of tympanostomy tubes may suggest chronic otitis media with or without cholesteatoma.

Tinnitus

When approaching the chief complaint of tinnitus, the clinician should ask pertinent questions including but not limited to:

- Pulsatile or nonpulsatile
  - Nonpulsatile tinnitus is a common finding with sensorineural hearing loss but may also be associated with endolymphatic hydrops, superior semicircular canal dehiscence, vestibular schwannoma, and temporomandibular joint dysfunction [19].
  - Pulsatile tinnitus is more concerning for possible middle ear masses such as middle ear or jugular foramen paragangliomas. Sigmoid diverticulum and arteriovenous malformations are rare causes of venous and arterial pulsatile tinnitus, respectively [19]. Pulsatile tinnitus may also be related to benign idiopathic intracranial hypertension, carotid stenosis or hypertension, superior semicircular canal dehiscence, or patulous Eustachian tube [19].
- Presence of autophony with or without audible breathing
  - The presence of autophony with pulsatile tinnitus is suggestive of superior semicircular canal dehiscence or patulous Eustachian tube [20]. Audible breathing can be used to distinguish these two disorders. Audible breathing is associated with patulous Eustachian tube but not superior semicircular canal dehiscence [20].
- Associated comorbidities (obesity, smoking, heart disease)
  - Presence of obesity with pulsatile tinnitus could be concerning for benign idiopathic intracranial hypertension [20].
  - Cardiovascular risk factors may make cerebrovascular occlusive disease a more likely etiology [19].
- Associated symptoms (aural fullness, hearing loss, vertigo, otalgia with chewing)
  - Endolymphatic hydrops may present with aural fullness, tinnitus, hearing loss, and vertigo [5].
  - Jaw pain or otalgia may be indicative of temporomandibular joint dysfunction, necrotizing otitis externa, referred pain, or otitis media [19].

Otalgia

When approaching the chief complaint of otalgia, the clinician should ask pertinent questions including but not limited to:

- Unilateral or bilateral
  - Unilateral otalgia is more likely to have an otologic origin, usually infectious compared to bilateral, though bilateral otalgia can be related to infection.
- Associated symptoms (otorrhea, hearing loss, ear canal swelling/rash)
  - Otorrhea, periauricular swelling, and erythema can be concerning for otitis externa or cellulitis [5]. Otalgia associated with otorrhea and hearing loss is more concerning for acute otitis media with perforation or bullous myringitis [5]. Facial weakness may be concerning for Ramsay Hunt syndrome or necrotizing otitis externa [21]. Throat pain or difficulty swallowing may be concerning for referred throat pain from malignancy or acute infectious process of the throat such as peritonsillar abscess [21].

- Duration
  - Otalgia lasting less than 30 days is more concerning for an acute infection, while more chronic otalgia should be concerning for cholesteatoma, chronic otitis media or effusion, temporomandibular joint dysfunction, or malignancy.
- Dental issues or pain with eating
  - Bilateral otalgia associated with eating or a history of dental issues may be concerning for temporomandibular joint dysfunction [21].
- History of smoking, throat pain, and recent weight loss
  - Ear pain can be a presenting symptom for malignancies of the upper aerodigestive tract such as tonsil or base of tongue squamous cell carcinoma [21].
- History of cholesteatoma, otologic surgery, and tympanostomy tubes

Physical Exam

Following an accurate and thorough history with focused questions as demonstrated above, the next step in the clinical evaluation of the otologic patient is a focused physical examination.

Auricle

The otologic exam begins with examination of the auricle. Specifically, the auricle should be inspected for erythema, induration, fluctuance, which could be concerning for acute bacterial perichondritis [7]. Particular attention should be paid to the mastoid region. Erythema, induration, tenderness, and fluctuance of this region with proptosis of the auricle should be concerning for acute mastoiditis, which could be related to acute otitis media [7]. Additionally, the postauricular regions should be inspected for scars or evidence of prior otologic surgery. The preauricular area, particularly immediately superior to the tragus, should be inspected for auricular pits, which are developmental abnormalities that occur due to failure of fusion of the hillocks of His [7]. These pits and sinus tracts can be sources of recurrent infection [7].

External Auditory Canal

Attention is next directed to the external auditory canal (EAC), which is examined with either an otoscope or a microscope. Cerumen and debris first must be cleared to allow for adequate exam of proximal structures. Inspection of the canal skin for erythema, swelling, induration, or discharge can reveal the presence of otitis externa [22]. Careful attention should be paid to the bony cartilaginous junction of the external auditory canal; granulation in this location, especially in patients who are immunocompromised, is pathognomonic for necrotizing otitis externa, which can subsequently develop into skull base osteomyelitis [22]. The external auditory canal can also contain whitish or blackish spore like debris, concerning for possible otomycosis [22]. Additionally, the canal should be inspected for irregularities in the bony canal, such as bony outgrowths. A solitary pedunculated osseous mass is consistent with an osteoma, which is often attached to the tympanosquamous or tympanomastoid suture lines [23]. Bilateral, symmetric broad-based osseous elevations are more consistent with exostoses [23]. Significant squamous debris with bony erosion is concerning for canal cholesteatoma, malignancy, or keratosis obturans. Keratosis obturans is characterized by significant recurrent circumferential keratin debris with circumferential widening of the osseous canal [24]. Canal cholesteatoma, on the other hand, is often unilateral and is characterized by squamous debris and focal posterior-inferior bone erosion [24].

Tympanic Membrane

Careful inspection of the tympanic membrane (TM) and the scutum is crucial to the clinical evaluation of the otologic patient, especially regarding complaints of hearing loss, otalgia, and otorrhea. The operating microscope is well suited for identifying problems along the scutum and pars flaccida; however, the addition of endoscopes allows for inspection of areas out of the line of sight unlike the microscope. The endoscope also enables an expanded field of view of the tympanic membrane, which is especially useful for visualization of the anterior TM and EAC in the presence of a prominent anterior canal wall overhang. If a tympanic membrane perforation is present, the size and location of the perforation should be estimated. The middle ear mucosa should be assessed for the presence of edema, inflammation, and squamous debris in the setting of a TM perforation. A large subtotal perforation is demonstrated in Fig. 11.1 with healthy-appearing middle ear mucosa. Perforations extending to the osseous external canal are marginal and are the result of destruction of a portion of the TM annulus; these are thought to be associated with an increased risk of middle ear cholesteatoma formation [25]. Erosion of the scutum associated with an attic retraction pocket, which is demonstrated in Fig. 11.2, raises concern for the development of an epitympanic cholesteatoma [26].

The color and appearance of the tympanic membrane can also provide clues to abnormalities and disease processes affecting the middle ear. Additionally, pneumatic otoscopy is used to assess Eustachian tube function and/or the presence of middle ear fluid [27]. Either a bulging TM or a retracted TM can be associated with middle ear effusion; erythema

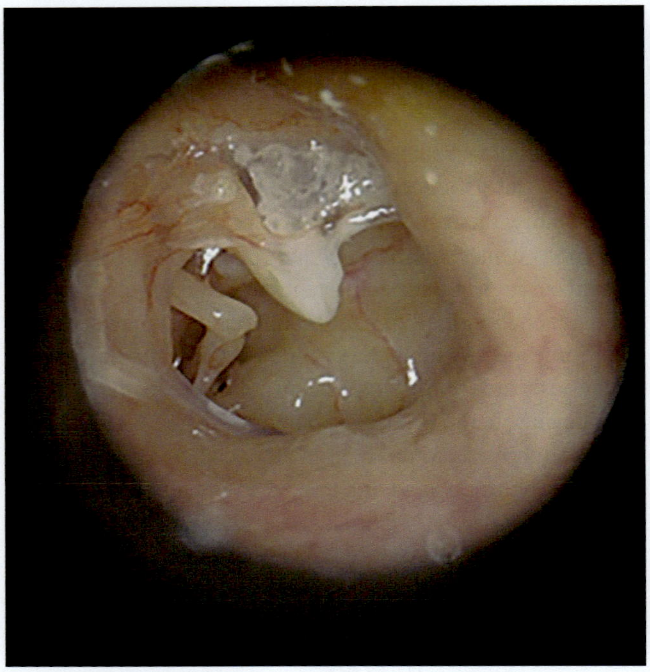

Fig. 11.1 A large subtotal perforation on otoscopic examination. The umbo of the malleus, long process of the incus, and incudostapedial joint are clearly seen through the perforation. The middle ear mucosa is normal and healthy appearing

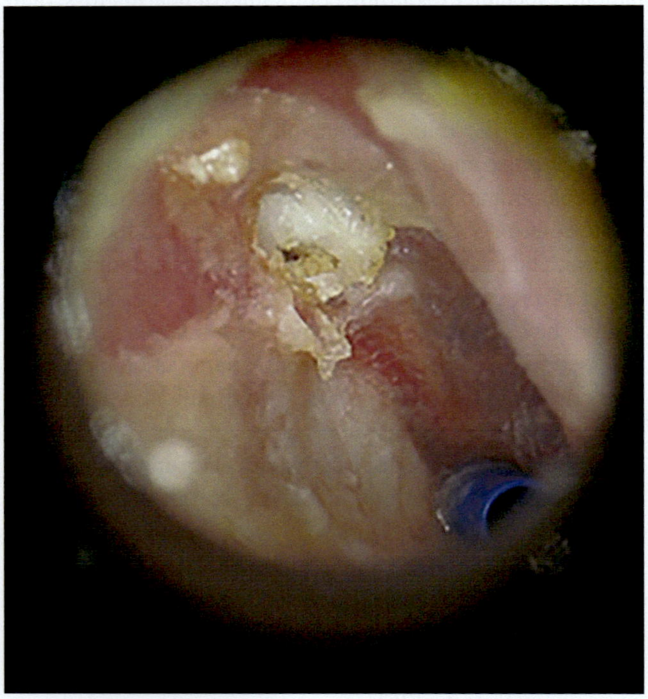

Fig. 11.2 An otoscopic image consistent with an attic cholesteatoma. There is a superior retraction pocket with erosion of the scutum and squamous debris coming from the retraction pocket, concerning for a cholesteatoma. Additionally, there is a tympanostomy tube placed in the inferior portion of the tympanic membrane, demonstrating likely previous retraction and Eustachian tube dysfunction

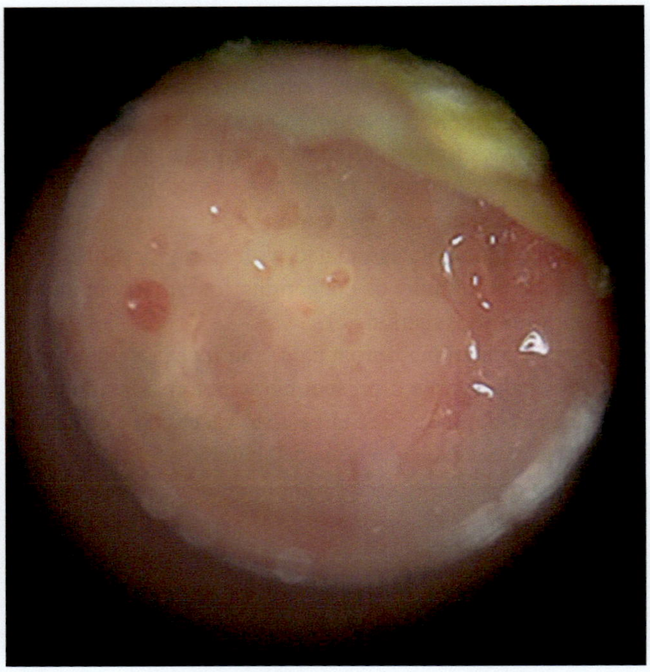

Fig. 11.3 An otoscopic examination concerning for granular myringitis. The tympanic membrane develops a mucosal appearance due to the granulation tissue throughout the tympanic membrane

suggests acute infection, and opacity suggests suppuration, while an amber or brown color suggests a serous or mucoid condition [27]. Erythematous granulation tissue on a thickened TM is concerning for granular myringitis, which is demonstrated in Fig. 11.3 [28]. Bullae or vesicles may also be apparent with bullous myringitis [5]. Marked retraction or atelectasis, signs of Eustachian tube dysfunction, may be flaccid and mobile with pneumatic otoscopy or static, the latter which may suggest either middle ear fluid or adhesions with possible myringoincudostapediopexy. Opacities in patches or circumferentially involving the TM are indicative of myringosclerosis which may develop after multiple infections but is also commonly seen after placement of a ventilation tube. Isolated erythema or injection of the posterior superior TM, corresponding to inflammation of the chorda tympani nerve, is seen in approximately 30–50% of cases of Bell's palsy and Ramsay Hunt syndrome suggesting a viral neuropathy [29, 30]. Additionally, middle ear paraganglioma, seen in Fig. 11.4, or jugular paragangliomas, seen in Fig. 11.4b, can be visualized as a red, pulsatile, retrotympanic mass. Blanching of a red, retrotympanic mass adjacent to the tympanic membrane with pneumatic otoscopy (Brown's sign) confirms the presence of a vascular tumor [31]. In a recent review, all middle ear paragangliomas were visible on physical exam, and 55% had Brown's sign [32]. In cases of conductive hearing loss, a reddish blush seen on the TM over the promontory anterior to the round window,

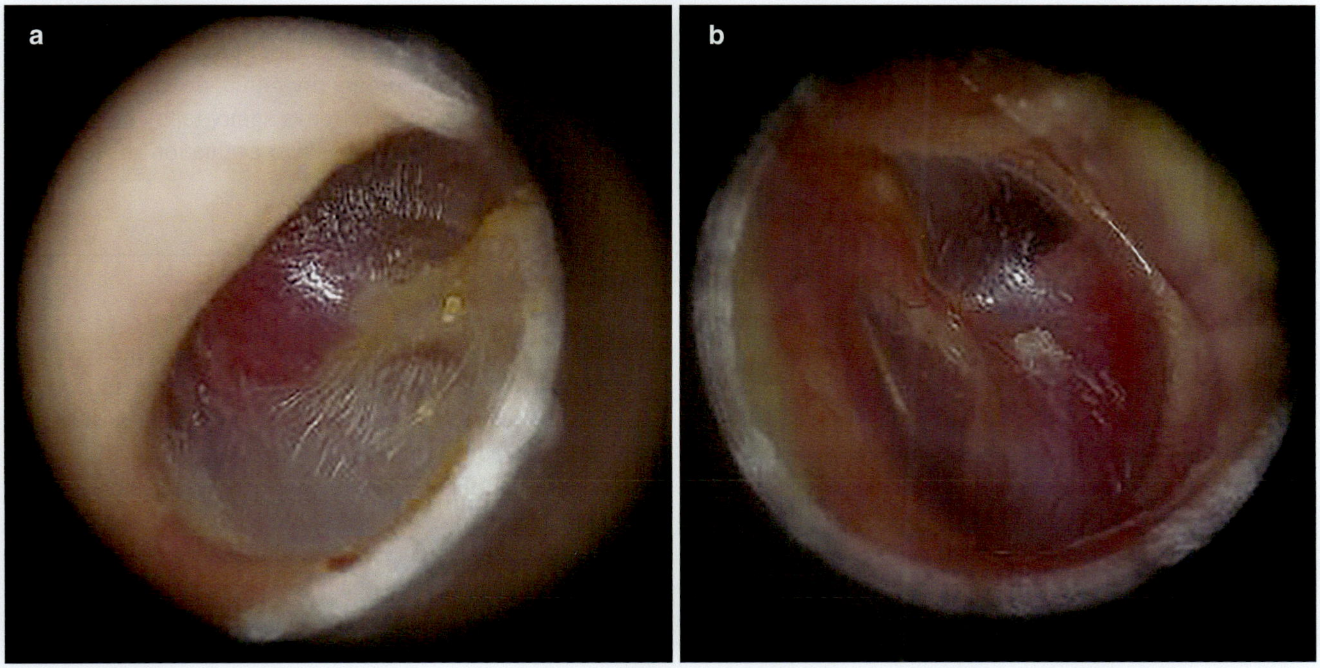

Fig. 11.4 (**a** and **b**) These figures demonstrate the typical appearance of retrotympanic red mass consistent with middle ear paraganglioma (**a**) or jugular paraganglioma (**b**). The red mass is typically pulsatile in nature, inferiorly based, and blanches with pneumatic pressure (Brown's sign)

termed the Schwartze's sign, can be indicative of active otosclerosis [33].

Tuning Fork

The tuning fork exam is a simple and effective means for the assessment of hearing loss. Although a more accurate hearing assessment can be obtained with audiometry, the tuning fork exam is still considered a reliable means to confirm surgical candidacy in patients with conductive or mixed hearing loss. The first test using the tuning forks is the Weber test, which assesses laterality with bone conduction. This test is performed by placing the vibrating tuning fork on the glabella or the central incisor and asking the patient to localize the sound. The normal response is midline. Lateralization to one side indicates possible conductive hearing loss in the ipsilateral ear or sensorineural hearing loss in the contralateral ear. The examiner then proceeds to test each ear with the Rinne test, which is performed by first placing the vibrating tuning fork on the mastoid process and then within 1 cm of the external auditory canal, with the patient queried to identify the location which is loudest. The normal response is to hear the tuning fork immediately next to the ear louder than when it is against the mastoid, indicating that air conduction is louder than bone conduction. If bone conduction is greater than air conduction, then there is likely a conductive hearing loss in that ear. The difference between air conduction and bone conduction at which bone conduction becomes louder than air conduction varies by the frequency of the tuning fork (Table 11.3). Bone conduction greater than air conduction with the most commonly used 512 Hz tuning fork indicates an air bone gap of at least 30–45 dB [34].

Table 11.3 Estimation of hearing loss by Rinne exam

Rinne test results	Estimated conductive loss
256 Hz: BC > AC 512 Hz: AC > BC 1024 Hz: AC > BC	20–30 dB
256 Hz: BC > AC 512 Hz: BC > AC 1024 Hz: AC > BC	30–45 dB
256 Hz: BC > AC 512 Hz: BC > AC 1024 Hz: BC > AC	45–60 dB

Adapted from [34]
AC denotes air conduction, *BC* denotes bone conduction

Head and Neck

Otalgia, hearing loss, and tinnitus may all be symptoms of underlying pathology elsewhere in the head and neck; as such, a thorough head and neck examination is often indicated. Unilateral middle ear effusion with associated conductive or mixed hearing loss in an adult may be a presenting condition for a nasopharyngeal mass [26], and nasopharyngoscopy or MRI is indicated. Even bilateral middle ear effusions may be likewise associated with nasopharyngeal masses, and investigation is warranted for persistent or recurrent problems with no obvious inflammatory etiology. Otalgia in the absence of any ear findings can also be a referred symptom of pharyngeal or laryngeal malignancy and should be further evaluated with thorough head and neck examination and possible flexible nasopharyngoscopy [5]. Pulsatile or objective tinnitus requires head and neck examination as well, with attention to the cranial nerves. In patients with pulsatile tinnitus, auscultation of the neck can reveal bruits and raise suspicion for carotid artery stenosis [20]. Additionally, improvement in the tinnitus with compression of the neck is more suggestive of a venous cause [20].

Vestibular Examination

Evaluation of the vestibular system is reliant upon assessing eye movements. The theoretical basis for the use of eye movements in the evaluation of the vestibular system is as follows:

- If there is a unilateral weakness, then the contralateral vestibular system sends signal while the ipsilateral vestibular system is silent, which is then interpreted as head movement to the contralateral side [7].
- The eyes then drift toward the side of the weakness in order to keep fixation and counter the aberrant signal indicating head movement to the contralateral side [7].
- The central processing system compensates for this drift by exerting a series of fast saccades toward the contralateral side to correct the eye drift and keep the eyes focused on the subject, resulting in nystagmus [7].

Evaluation of nystagmus involves identifying:

- Spontaneous or evoked by maneuvers (i.e., Dix-Hallpike maneuver)
- Direction
  - Direction is also denoted by the fast phase of the nystagmus. Nystagmus can be described as horizontal, vertical, or torsional geotropic (beating toward ground) or apogeotropic (beating away from the ground) [7].
- Intensity
  - Nystagmus is graded as first, second, or third degree. First degree occurs when the nystagmus occurs at end gaze in the direction of the fast phase of the nystagmus. Second degree describes nystagmus at mid-gaze and gaze in the direction of the fast phase. Third degree describes nystagmus occurring in all horizontal directions including toward the slow-phase side [7].
- Direction fixed or direction changing

Frenzel lenses are magnifying lenses that prevent fixation which can make the nystagmus more pronounced and aid in diagnosis without recording in clinic or at the bedside. Recording tests such as electronystagmography or videonystagmography provide an objective evaluation of vestibular function.

Fistula Test

The fistula test describes applying pressure to the tympanic membrane and observing for subjective vertigo (subjectively positive fistula test) or eye deviation (objective positive fistula test). A positive fistula test is associated with oval or round window fistula, post-stapedectomy perilymph leaks, semicircular canal fistula, endolymphatic hydrops, labyrinthitis, or syphilis [35, 36]. In addition to a positive fistula test, superior semicircular canal dehiscence can also demonstrate nystagmus with pressure applied to the tragus [37, 38].

Dix-Hallpike Maneuver

The Dix-Hallpike maneuver is the classic maneuver utilized to detect benign positional paroxysmal vertigo, specifically involving the posterior semicircular canals, which is the most common variant of benign positional paroxysmal vertigo [39]. The maneuver is performed by turning the patient's head 45° in the direction of the side being tested with patient started in a seated position [39]. The patient is then rapidly laid supine while the head is kept turned [39]. The neck is then slightly extended [39]. Subjective vertigo is considered subjectively positive [39]. Torsional nystagmus in the direction of the affected ear is considered an objective positive result [39].

Lateral canal benign positional paroxysmal vertigo can be assessed with a supine roll test [40]. The patient is laid supine, and the head is then rotated to right ear down and left ear down positions (the test ear is whichever ear is closest to the ground) [40]. Geotropic nystagmus is considered a positive result concerning for lateral canal benign positional paroxysmal vertigo of the lateral canal of the test ear [40].

Head Thrust Test

The head thrust test evaluates for unilateral vestibular weakness. The test is performed by rapidly rotating the head to the left or right with the chin inclined 30° downward. Normal response is no nystagmus or 1–2 beats of catch-up saccades [41]. A notable contralateral catch-up saccade will appear immediately following the rapid head turn in the direction of the weak ear, which would be concerning for a unilateral vestibular weakness [41].

Cranial Nerve Exam

A thorough cranial nerve examination is indicated in all otologic patients. Cranial nerves 1 and 9 are not routinely tested except with evaluation for a gag reflex in the latter. Examination begins with assessment of visual fields for cranial nerve 2. Cranial nerves 3, 4, and 6 are then assessed with gaze testing to evaluate extraocular motion. Cranial nerve 5 is then assessed by light touch or pinprick of the skin along the forehead, cheek, chin, and preauricular areas corresponding to V1, V2, and V3, respectively. Comparing contraction of the masseter and temporalis muscles bilaterally provides an assessment of the motor division of cranial nerve 5.

Cranial nerve 7 is assessed by evaluating facial function in all distal branch muscle groups (frontalis, zygomaticus major, nasalis, depressor labii, mentalis, orbicularis oculi and oris). Facial nerve deficits are commonly graded with the House-Brackmann scale (Table 11.4) [42]. Cranial nerve 8 has already been examined with the tuning fork exam as described above. Cranial nerve 10 can be assessed by palate elevation or by flexible laryngoscopy and examination for vocal cord mobility. Cranial nerve 11 is examined by abduction of arms above head, shoulder shrug, and head turn. Cranial nerve 12 is assessed by asking the patient to protrude their tongue out of the mouth and move it from side to side. Hypoglossal deficits show deviation of the mobile tongue toward the side of the deficit with protrusion and inability to lateralize the tongue toward the contralateral side.

Table 11.4 House-Brackmann facial nerve grading scale

Grade	Description
I	Normal facial function in all areas
II	*Gross:* slight weakness noticeable on close inspection; may have very slight synkinesis *At rest:* normal symmetry and tone *Motion* *Forehead:* moderate to good function *Eye:* complete closure with minimum effort *Mouth:* slight asymmetry
III	*Gross:* obvious but not disfiguring difference between two sides; noticeable but not severe synkinesis. Contracture and/or hemifacial spasm *At rest:* normal symmetry and tone *Motion* *Forehead:* slight to moderate movement *Eye:* complete closure with effort *Mouth:* slightly weak with maximum effort
IV	*Gross:* obvious weakness and/or disfiguring asymmetry *At rest:* normal symmetry and tone *Motion* *Forehead:* none *Eye:* incomplete closure *Mouth:* asymmetric with maximum effort
V	*Gross:* only barely perceptible motion *At rest:* asymmetry *Motion* *Forehead:* none *Eye:* incomplete closure *Mouth:* slight movement
VI	No movement

Adapted from [42]

Cerebellar Testing

Cerebellar testing is recommended in evaluation of patients with vertigo or disequilibrium to better assess for central causes of dizziness. Examination usually involves finger-nose-finger, heel-to-toe testing, rapid alternating movements, and tandem gait. Poor coordination on these exercises may point to cerebellar dysfunction [7]. Consistently falling to one side on gait testing can also be a sign of an uncompensated vestibular lesion [7]. The Romberg test consists of having a patient stand still with eyes closed. Falling to one side can be caused by cerebellar disease or by uncompensated unilateral vestibular loss [7]. The Fukuda test consists of marching in place with eyes closed and arms extended anteriorly. If there is a vestibular lesion, the arms may deviate toward the side of the lesion [7].

Conclusion

A thorough and focused history and physical examination can significantly narrow the differential diagnosis when evaluating a patient's chief complaint. With a preliminary or presumptive diagnosis, the clinician can then pursue appropriate confirmatory studies, including audiological, vestibular, radiological, and laboratory tests which are dealt with in depth in later chapters. A more focused and efficacious use of ancillary testing can thereby allow one to work through a differential diagnosis in both a time-efficient and a cost-effective manner.

References

1. Nadol JB, Merchant SN. Otologic manifestations of systemic disease. In: Flint PW, Haughey BH, Lund VJ, et al., editors. Cummings otolaryngology - head & neck surgery. 6th ed. Philadelphia, PA: Saunders; 2015. p. 2301–18.
2. Bachman J. Improving care with an automated patient history. Fam Pract Manag. 2007;14(7):39–43.
3. Wong BY, Capper R. Incidence of vestibular schwannoma and incidental findings on the magnetic resonance imaging and computed tomography scans of patients from a direct referral audiology clinic. J Laryngol Otol. 2012;126(7):658–62.
4. Stachler RJ, Chandrasekhar SS, Archer SM, et al. Clinical Practice Guideline. Otolaryngol Head Neck Surg. 2012;146(3_suppl):S1–S35.
5. Bauer CA, Jenkins HA. Otologic symptoms and syndromes. In: Flint PW, Haughey BH, Lund VJ, et al., editors. Cummings oto-

laryngology - head & neck surgery. 6th ed. Philadelphia, PA: Saunders; 2015. p. 2401–10.
6. Rudic M, Keogh I, Wagner R, et al. The pathophysiology of otosclerosis: review of current research. Hear Res. 2015;330(Pt A):51–6.
7. O'Malley MR, Haynes DS. Clinical Diagnosis. In: Gulya AJ, Minor LB, Poe D, editors. Glasscock-Shambaugh Surgery of the Ear. 6th ed. Shelton, CT: PMPH-USA; 2010. p. 171–88.
8. van der Hulst RJ, Dreschler WA, Urbanus NA. High frequency audiometry in prospective clinical research of ototoxicity due to platinum derivatives. Ann Otol Rhinol Laryngol. 1988;97(2 Pt 1):133–7.
9. Rybak LP. Ototoxicity of loop diuretics. Otolaryngol Clin N Am. 1993;26(5):829–44.
10. Jung TT, Rhee CK, Lee CS, Park YS, Choi DC. Ototoxicity of salicylate, nonsteroidal antiinflammatory drugs, and quinine. Otolaryngol Clin N Am. 1993;26(5):791–810.
11. Rybak LP, Brenner MJ. Vestibular and auditory ototoxicity. In: Flint PW, Haughey BH, Lund VJ, et al., editors. Cummings otolaryngology - head & neck surgery. 6th ed. Philadelphia, PA: Saunders; 2015. p. 2369–82.
12. Kentala E, Rauch SD. A practical assessment algorithm for diagnosis of dizziness. Otolaryngol Head Neck Surg. 2003;128(1):54–9.
13. Hullar TE, Zee DS, Minor LB. Evaluation of the patient with dizziness. In: Flint PW, Haughey BH, Lund VJ, et al., editors. Cummings otolaryngology - head & neck surgery. 6th ed. Philadelphia, PA: Saunders; 2015. p. 2301–18.
14. DeFlorio PT, Silbergleit R. Mal de debarquement presenting in the Emergency Department. J Emerg Med. 2006;31(4):377–9.
15. Kutz JW Jr. The dizzy patient. Med Clin North Am. 2010;94(5):989–1002.
16. O'Connell Ferster AP, Priesol AJ, Isildak H. The clinical manifestations of vestibular migraine: a review. Auris Nasus Larynx. 2017;44(3):249–52.
17. Meyer A, Bouchetemble P, Costentin B, Dehesdin D, Lerosey Y, Marie JP. Lateral semicircular canal fistula in cholesteatoma: diagnosis and management. Eur Arch Otorrinolaringol. 2016;273(8):2055–63.
18. Gadre AK, Chole RA. The changing face of petrous apicitis-a 40-year experience. Laryngoscope. 2017.
19. Hertzano R, Teplitzky TB, Eisenman DJ. Clinical evaluation of tinnitus. Neuroimaging Clin N Am. 2016;26(2):197–205.
20. Mattox DE, Hudgins P. Algorithm for evaluation of pulsatile tinnitus. Acta Otolaryngol. 2008;128(4):427–31.
21. Siddiq MA, Samra MJ. Otalgia. BMJ. 2008;336(7638):276–7.
22. Brant JA, Ruckenstein MJ. Infections of the external ear. In: Flint PW, Haughey BH, Lund VJ, et al., editors. Cummings otolaryngology - head & neck surgery. 6th ed. Philadelphia, PA: Saunders; 2015. p. 2115–22.
23. Kemink JL, Graham MD. Osteomas and exostoses of the external auditory canal - medical and surgical management. J Otolaryngol. 1982;11(2):101–6.
24. Persaud RA, Hajioff D, Thevasagayam MS, Wareing MJ, Wright A. Keratosis obturans and external ear canal cholesteatoma: how and why we should distinguish between these conditions. Clin Otolaryngol Allied Sci. 2004;29(6):577–81.
25. Ruggles RL, Koconis CA. Tympanic perforations: safe or not? Laryngoscope. 1967;77(3):337–40.
26. Chole RA. Chronic otitis media, mastoiditis, and petrositis. In: Flint PW, Haughey BH, Lund VJ, et al., editors. Cummings otolaryngology - head & neck surgery. 6th ed. Philadelphia, PA: Saunders; 2015. p. 2139–55.
27. Schilder AG, Chonmaitree T, Cripps AW, et al. Otitis media. Nat Rev Dis Primers. 2016;2:16063.
28. Neilson LJ, Hussain SS. Management of granular myringitis: a systematic review. J Laryngol Otol. 2008;122(1):3–10.
29. May M. Red chorda tympani nerve and Bell's palsy. Laryngoscope. 1974;84(9):1507–13.
30. May M. Red chorda tympani nerve in Herpes Zoster oticus. Laryngoscope. 1976;86(10):1572.
31. Sweeney AD, Carlson ML, Wanna GB, Bennett ML. Glomus tympanicum tumors. Otolaryngol Clin N Am. 2015;48(2):293–304.
32. Carlson ML, Sweeney AD, Pelosi S, Wanna GB, Glasscock ME 3rd, Haynes DS. Glomus tympanicum: a review of 115 cases over 4 decades. Otolaryngol Head Neck Surg. 2015;152(1):136–42.
33. House JW, Cunningham CD. Otosclerosis. In: Flint PW, Haughey BH, Lund VJ, et al., editors. Cummings otolaryngology - head & neck surgery. 6th ed. Philadelphia, PA: Saunders; 2015. p. 2211–9.
34. Teasley RA, Backous DB. Clinical assessment and surgical treatment of conductive hearing loss. In: Flint PW, Haughey BH, Lund VJ, et al., editors. Cummings otolaryngology - head & neck surgery. 6th ed. Philadelphia, PA: Saunders; 2015. p. 2200–10.
35. Hennebert C. A new syndrome in hereditary syphilis of the labyrinth. Presse Med Belg Brux. 1911;63:467.
36. Nadol JB Jr. Positive Hennebert's sign in Meniere's disease. Arch Otolaryngol. 1977;103(9):524–30.
37. Minor LB, Solomon D, Zinreich JS, Zee DS. Sound- and/or pressure-induced vertigo due to bone dehiscence of the superior semicircular canal. Arch Otolaryngol Head Neck Surg. 1998;124(3):249–58.
38. Minor LB. Superior canal dehiscence syndrome. Am J Otol. 2000;21(1):9–19.
39. Dix MR, Hallpike CS. The pathology symptomatology and diagnosis of certain common disorders of the vestibular system. Proc R Soc Med. 1952;45(6):341–54.
40. Imai T, Takeda N, Ikezono T, et al. Classification, diagnostic criteria and management of benign paroxysmal positional vertigo. Auris Nasus Larynx. 2017;44(1):1–6.
41. Hain TC, Fetter M, Zee DS. Head-shaking nystagmus in patients with unilateral peripheral vestibular lesions. Am J Otolaryngol. 1987;8(1):36–47.
42. House JW, Brackmann DE. Facial nerve grading system. Otolaryngol Head Neck Surg. 1985;93(2):146–7.

The Audiological Evaluation of Otologic and Neurotologic Disease

12

Christopher Ian Newberry and Richard K. Gurgel

Hearing Disorders

Hearing disorders can be classified as organic or nonorganic based on their underlying cause. Functional hearing loss is the term used for a nonorganic basis of the disorder. Organic hearing loss can be due to either hearing sensitivity loss or suprathreshold abnormalities. Hearing sensitivity loss necessitates that sounds be of higher intensity before they are perceived. Suprathreshold abnormalities are eclectic and include speech recognition deficits, abnormal loudness growth, atypical adaptation, hearing difficulty with competition, and problems processing temporal or spatial domain [1].

Nonorganic Hearing Loss

Functional hearing loss (FHL) is the exaggeration or complete feigning of hearing loss. The term is used interchangeably with nonorganic hearing loss and pseudohypacusis. Accurate diagnosis of FHL has serious treatment and medicolegal ramifications. For example, children with sudden hearing loss may have organic processes such as idiopathic sudden sensorineural hearing loss, enlarged vestibular aqueduct syndrome, or viral inner ear infection; however, the most frequent etiology of sudden hearing loss in children is FHL [2].

The hallmark of functional hearing loss is lack of consistent audiometric results. On pure-tone audiometry, there is often high test-retest variability, a lack of shadow curves with unmasked stimuli, and bone conduction thresholds may be higher than air. Speech audiometry can show an exaggerated disparity (>10 dB) between the speech recognition threshold and pure-tone average, as well as discrepancies between word recognition score and alleged audiometric thresholds [3].

Although clinical use of behavioral tests is declining, two commonly utilized measures are the Stenger and Lombard tests [4]. The Lombard test is a quick, inexpensive measure best used in the case of suspected bilateral FHL. It is based on the commonly observed principle that a person will regulate their vocal effort based on the level of ambient noise. Therefore, if a patient has FHL, they will have a compensatory increase in voice intensity with background noise [5]. The Stenger test is a valuable test in the workup of unilateral or significantly asymmetrical FHL (>30–40 dB interaural difference). A positive test result can confirm pseudohypacusis, while a negative test result provides reassurance that the patient's condition is not pseudohypacusis [6]. The test is based on the principle that the same frequency tone simultaneously presented to both ears will localize to the side in which the tone is perceived to be louder. Thus, if a difference exists between the ears, equal tones presented will become one fused tone that will localize to the ear that is better able to detect it. Whereas, if no difference in ear function exists, a fused tone will be perceived only in the ear in which a louder tone is presented.

Organic Hearing Loss Overview

Hearing sensitivity loss is the most common cause of organic hearing loss. Hearing sensitivity loss is caused by various conditions that lead to an abnormal reduction of sound signal being delivered to the brain. Typical hearing sensitive loss categories include conductive, sensorineural, and mixed hearing loss.

C. I. Newberry
Department of Otolaryngology—Head and Neck Surgery, University of Utah School of Medicine, Salt Lake City, UT, USA

Rhode Island ENT Physicians, Inc., Brown University, Providence, RI, USA
e-mail: richard.gurgel@hsc.utah.edu

R. K. Gurgel (✉)
Department of Otolaryngology—Head and Neck Surgery, University of Utah School of Medicine, Salt Lake City, UT, USA
e-mail: richard.gurgel@hsc.utah.edu

A. D. Sweeney et al. (eds.), *Haynes-Glasscock-Shambaugh Surgery of the Ear*, https://doi.org/10.1007/978-3-032-18264-7_12

Conductive hearing loss (CHL) is caused by an abnormal attenuation of sound as it travels from the outer ear through the middle ear. The conductive component can be quantified on audiogram as an air-bone gap, which is formed due to differences (>10 dB) in air and bone conductive thresholds. These abnormalities reduce the effective intensity of the air-conducted signal reaching the cochlea, but it does not affect the bone-conducted signal. Immittance testing will usually display abnormal tympanograms, and otoacoustic emissions are commonly absent [7]. However, as CHL acts principally as an attenuator of sound, it has minimal to no impact on suprathreshold hearing, and speech discrimination will be normal if sound is above the minimal threshold.

Sensorineural hearing loss (SNHL) is caused by irregularities in the conversion of sound energy into auditory nerve impulses by the cochlea and in the conduction of these signals along the cochlear nerve. SNHL causes can be divided into cochlear and retrocochlear processes. On an audiogram, both air and bone conduction thresholds will be elevated without a significant air-bone gap. The audiometric configuration of cochlear SNHL will vary depending on the location of disease along the basilar membrane—the base of the membrane is narrow and stiff and resonates with high-frequency waves, whereas the apical membrane is thin and flimsy and resonates with low-frequency waves [8]. If no conductive process is present, immittance testing will display normal tympanograms. Otoacoustic emissions (OAEs) will usually be absent in a cochlear disorder, whereas retrocochlear diseases often retain OAEs.

The Basic Audiological Test Battery

In addition to the essential history and physical exam, audiological testing helps to quantify hearing dysfunction. Audiologic test results should always be interpreted in the context of a battery of tests because no single test can provide a clear picture of a specific patient. The basic audiological test battery includes pure-tone audiometry, speech audiometry, and immittance measures.

Pure-Tone Audiometry

Pure-tone audiometry is the most commonly performed test for evaluating auditory sensitivity. Pure-tone signals are delivered at octave frequencies important for human communication, typically 0.25–8 kHz for air conduction (0.25–4 kHz for bone). Thresholds, defined as the lowest intensity that can be detected 50% of the time, are charted on a graphic plot called an audiogram. Audiograms chart sound intensity on a biologic scale in decibels hearing level (dB HL). The intensity scale is based on an audiometric 0 dB HL, which is the average intensity level for normal hearing young adults. Thus, an audiogram represents a subject's ability to hear compared with the hearing sensitivity of a group of normal-hearing young adults. Although hearing loss classification varies by source, a commonly used scale is depicted in Table 12.1 [9].

Table 12.1 Classification of hearing status

Classification	Hearing threshold	Interpretation
Normal hearing	0–25[a] dB HL	No difficulty with any speech
Mild hearing loss	25–40 dB HL	Difficulty with whispered speech
Moderate hearing loss	41–55 dB HL	Difficulty with conversational speech
Moderately severe hearing loss	56–70 dB HL	Difficulty even with loud speech
Severe hearing loss	71–90 dB HL	Can understand only shouted speech
Profound hearing loss	91+ dB HL	Cannot understand shouted speech

[a]In children >20 dB should be considered abnormal

Pure-tone audiograms are easily obtained in cooperative older children and adults. With standard audiometry, supra-aural or insert earphones deliver signals, and patients respond by raising their hand or pressing a button. Insert headphones are now the transducer of choice for routine testing as they reduce ear canal collapse and maximize interaural attenuation. When an infant is less than 6 months old, behavioral observation audiometry (BOA) is often used to estimate hearing thresholds by providing sound via speaker and observing responses (eye widening, startle, head turn) [10]. Although BOA estimates gross hearing thresholds, BOA inevitably estimates the better hearing ear. In children aged 6 months to 2–3 years, visual reinforcement audiometry (VRA) is used. VRA introduces sound via speakers or headphones, and the child is trained to turn toward auditory signals with visual reinforcement (toy, lights). Again, if sound field is used, VRA will solely estimate gross hearing and will not be ear specific. In children aged 2–3 to 5 years old, conditioned play audiometry (CPA) can be used in which the child performs a "fun" conditioned task (pegs in hole, balls in basket) in response to an auditory stimulus [11].

Audiograms compare thresholds obtained via air conduction (AC) and bone conduction (BC). AC thresholds measure the function of the total hearing system and therefore provide the overall hearing loss severity; however, since AC thresholds measure the entire system, when performed alone, they provide little information regarding the etiology of hearing loss. To determine both the type and severity of hearing loss, AC and BC testing are obtained. Because the skull vibrates as a whole, BC stimuli are presented via a bone oscillator placed on the mastoid to stimulate the cochlea's basilar

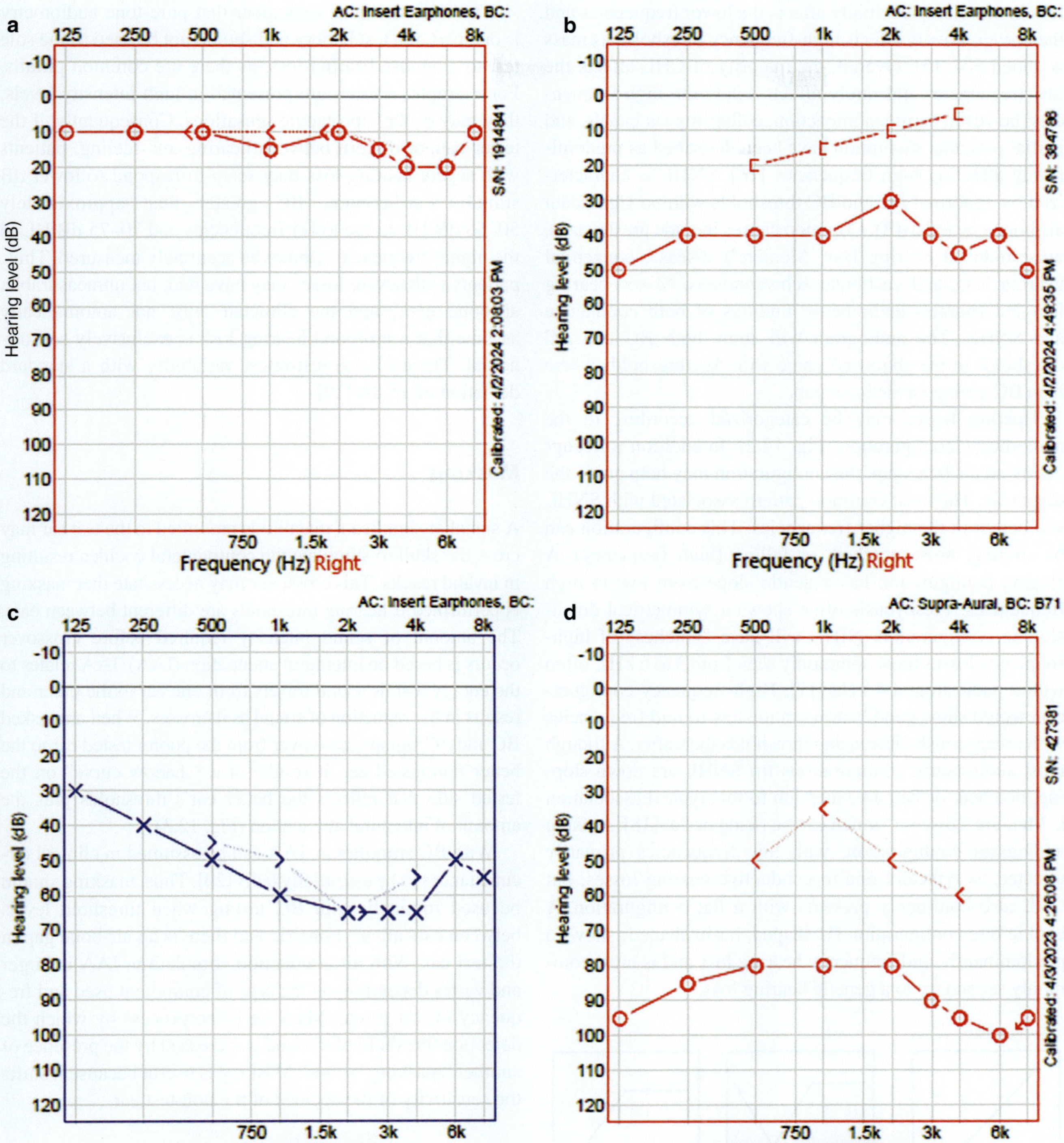

Fig. 12.1 Audiograms. (**a**) Normal hearing audiogram with thresholds below 25 dB hearing level (HL) and no air-bone gap. (**b**) Conductive hearing loss with air-bone gap, air thresholds >25 dB HL, and bone thresholds <25 dB HL. (**c**) Sensorineural hearing loss with no air-bone gap and both air and bone thresholds >25 dB HL. (**d**) Mixed hearing loss with air-bone gap present and both air and bone thresholds >25 dB HL. (Courtesy of Alex D. Sweeney, MD)

membrane directly to provide a measure of inner ear function [12]. The comparison of AC thresholds and BC thresholds provides an initial differentiation between conductive, mixed, and sensorineural involvement (Fig. 12.1).

On audiogram, a CHL is characterized by an air-bone gap (>10 dB) [13]. Generally, pathologies that add mass to the system limit higher frequencies, while pathologies that add stiffness limit lower frequencies [14]. For example, hearing loss in otosclerosis initially affects the lower frequencies and then progressively affects high-frequency thresholds as mass is added [14, 15]. Overall, the majority of CHL affects the low frequencies and rarely affects solely the high frequencies; however, cerumen impaction, collapsing ear canals, and partial ossicular disruption have been described as predominately affecting high frequencies [16]. SNHL is characterized by abnormal AC and BC thresholds with no significant air-bone gap (<10 dB). Common causes include presbycusis, noise-induced hearing loss, Ménière's disease, congenital hearing loss, and vestibular schwannomas. Mixed hearing loss incorporates audiometric findings of both conductive and SNHL. The audiogram will show both BC and AC thresholds in the abnormal range with AC thresholds worse than BC giving an air-bone gap.

Hearing losses may be categorized according to the audiometric configuration (Fig. 12.2). In addition to recognizing an air-bone gap, the configuration may help guide the diagnosis. The most common pattern associated with SNHL is a deficit in the higher frequencies. This configuration can be sloping, noise notched, or falling (high frequency). A sloping configuration has a gentle slope from low to high frequencies. Presbycusis often shows a symmetrical down-sloping configuration. NIHL will have "notches" of high-frequency losses most commonly seen from 3 to 6 kHz, often with a nadir around 4 kHz [17]. High-frequency configuration would show good hearing in the low to mid frequencies with precipitously decreasing thresholds thereafter. Although most audiometric configurations for SNHL are down sloping, notched, or flat, an exception to this typical association is Ménière's disease, which can be rising or flat [18]. A rising audiogram configuration, with low frequencies primarily affected, is typically due to conductive hearing losses, but CHL also commonly presents with a flat configuration. A cookie bite configuration (U shaped, basin shaped) shows a predominantly mid-frequency hearing loss and is most commonly secondary to a genetic hearing loss.

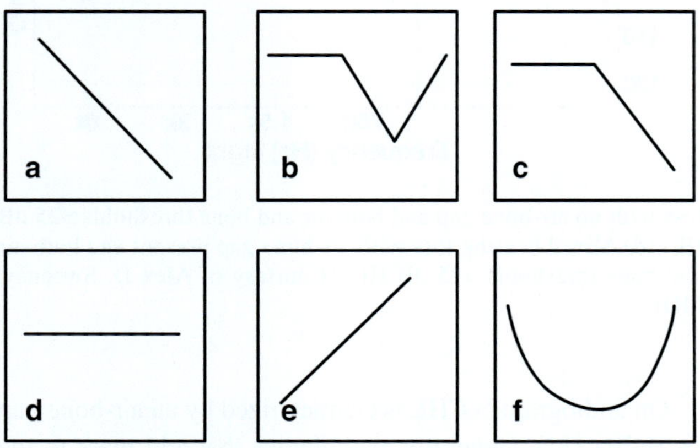

Fig. 12.2 Audiogram configurations. (**a**) Sloping, (**b**) notched, (**c**) falling, (**d**) flat, (**e**) rising, (**f**) cookie bite

The clinician must remember that pure-tone audiometry is one part of a test battery and should not be used as the sole test to diagnose hearing loss, as there are common pitfalls. For example, if tones are presented at high intensity levels, they may evoke vibrotactile sensations. Consequently, if the tester cannot discern between hearing and feeling, patients with severe hearing loss may seem to respond to lower dB stimuli. Furthermore, BC greater than approximately 50–60 dB HL in the lower frequencies and 70–75 dB HL in the higher frequencies cannot be accurately measured. Thus, patients with severe losses may have real, but unmeasurable, air-bone gaps, and the clinician must not automatically assume that a profound hearing loss is exclusively sensorineural. There is also test-retest variability with a standard deviation of ±5 dB [19].

Masking

A signal of significant magnitude presented to the test ear may cross the skull to stimulate the contralateral cochlea resulting in invalid results. This crossover may necessitate that masking is performed if hearing thresholds are different between ears. The amount of sound intensity required before crossover occurs is based on interaural attenuation (IAA). IAA relates to the energy lost as sound travels from one ear to the other and results in the reduction of sound as it crosses. When unmasked BC and AC signals cross over from the poorer tested ear to the better non-tested ear, it results in a "shadow curve" on the tested side that reflects the better ear's thresholds plus the amount of interaural attenuation (Fig. 12.3).

With BC stimulation, IAA can be assumed in clinical circumstances to be essentially 0 dB [20]. Thus, masking should be used routinely with BC testing when threshold levels between ears are asymmetric and there is an air-bone gap in the test ear. With air conduction stimulation, IAA is larger and varies depending on the type of equipment used and frequency of test signal. Masking is the process by which the detection threshold of a sound is increased by the presence of another "masking" sound. Masking is useful because it shifts the sensitivity of the cochlea of the non-test ear.

Speech Audiometry

Speech audiometry can be used to corroborate pure-tone thresholds, measure thresholds for speech, quantify ability to understand speech, and further assist in differential diagnosis. Speech detection threshold (SDT) is the softest level at which speech is sensed 50% of the time, whereas speech recognition threshold (SRT) is the level at which one can reliably repeat 50% of the spondee words presented. The main purpose of obtaining a SRT is for comparison with the

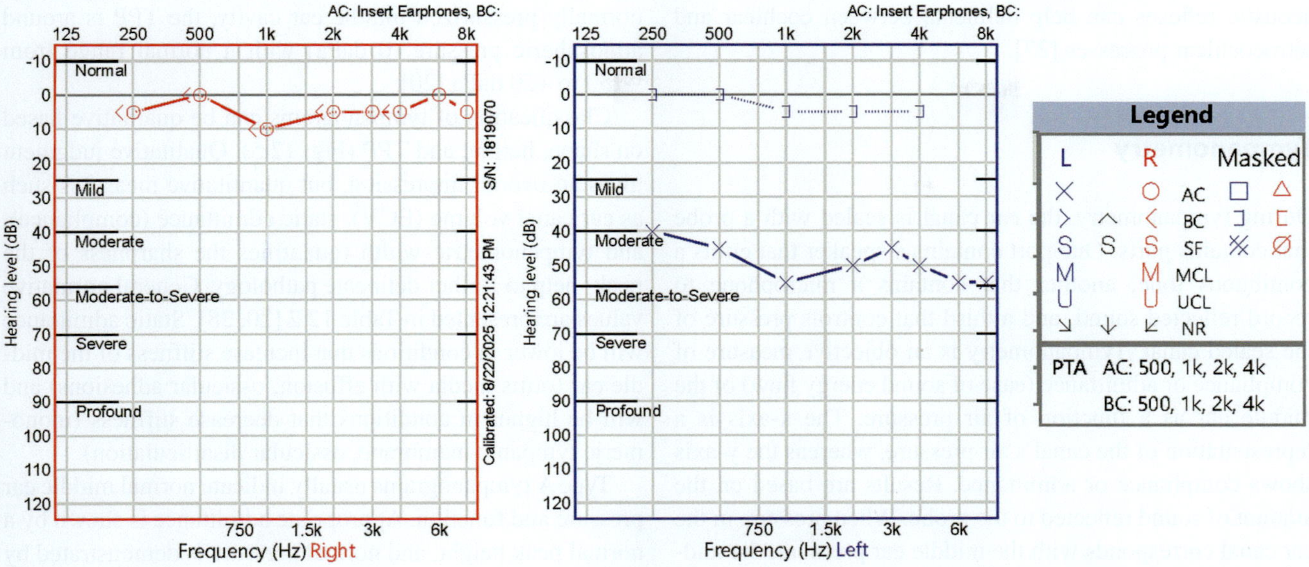

Fig. 12.3 Unmasked audiogram showing a shadow curve in a patient with left conductive hearing loss. The left bone conduction thresholds approximate the right because interaural attenuation is roughly zero. The right air conduction thresholds approximate the right thresholds plus the interaural attenuation amount (roughly 40 dB here)

pure-tone average (PTA), which is the average of 500, 1000, 2000 Hz thresholds and should also include 3000 Hz, as required by most hearing outcome reporting guidelines [21]. PTA and SRT should differ by no more than ±6 dB. Differences of 10 dB or more should raise suspicion of pseudohypacusis or inaccurate PTA results but can be seen when hearing loss differs drastically at various frequencies.

Most listening is actually done at suprathreshold levels. Word recognition score (WRS) quantitatively measures the ability to understand a list of phonetically balanced, single-syllable words presented at some suprathreshold level. WRS is expressed as a percentage of correct identification of presented words, with ≥90% being accepted as normal. WRS can be presented as a performance-intensity (PI) function (Fig. 12.4). A maximum WRS (WRSmax) is normally reached at approximately 30–40 dB SL and then remains persistent with increasing intensities [22]. For CHL, WRSmax will usually be normal (just achieved at higher presentation levels), and the PI function pattern will be similar to normal hearing but shifted right. For cochlear SNHL, the WRSmax can be 100%, but is often decreased, and will be predictable based on the degree of hearing loss [23, 24]. The PI function of a cochlear SNHL will usually show a "plateau effect" at a WRSmax less than 100% with no significant improvement in the score despite rising intensity. With retrocochlear SNHL, the WRS is frequently worse than predicted, and the PI function often shows a WRSmax of <100% with a significant decline (rollover) in percent correct scores at presentation levels above PB max. To define significant decline, the rollover index (RI) can be calculated using (WRSmax—WRSmin)/WRSmax and compared to norms [25, 26].

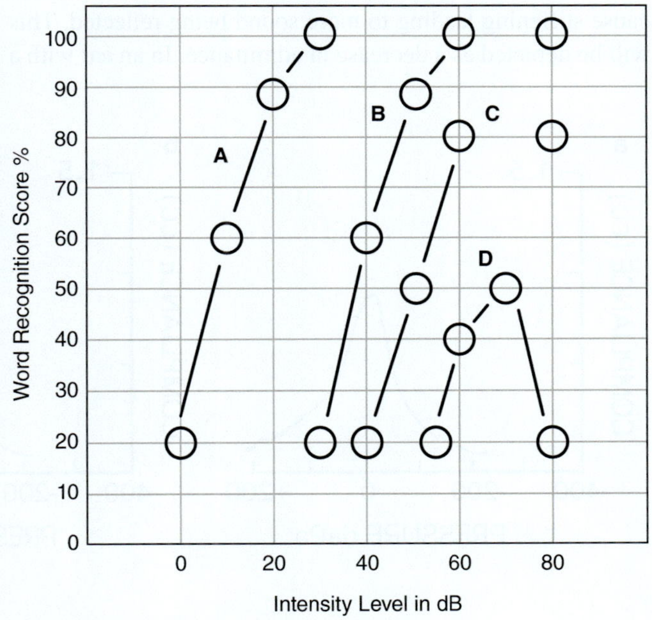

Fig. 12.4 Performance-intensity functions of various hearing categories: (A) Normal hearing, (B) conductive hearing loss, (C) cochlear hearing loss, and (D) retrocochlear hearing loss

Immittance Testing

Acoustic immittance is an important portion of the test battery. Generally, if the tympanogram and static immittance are normal, the hearing loss is often due to an SNHL, and acoustic reflexes can help delineate between cochlear and retrocochlear processes [27].

Tympanometry

During tympanometry, the ear canal is sealed with a probe that contains ports. One port contains a speaker that emits a continuous tone, another that contains a microphone to record reflected sound, and a third that controls pressure of the sealed canal. Tympanometry is an objective measure of compliance or admittance (ease of sound energy flow) of the middle ear as a function of air pressure. The x-axis is a representation of the canal's air pressure, whereas the y-axis shows compliance or admittance. Results are based on the amount of sound reflected to the probe. When pressure in the ear canal corresponds with the middle ear pressure, the middle ear is at its most compliant point and thus absorbs most sound. The pressure where the most sound is absorbed is known as the tympanometric peak pressure (TPP). Increases or decreases in canal pressure relative to the middle ear will cause stiffening leading to more sound being reflected. This will be depicted as a decrease in admittance. In an ear with a normally pressurized middle ear cavity, the TPP is around atmospheric pressure (0 daPa) with a normal range from −150 to +50 daPa [20].

Classification of tympanograms can be qualitative based on shape, height, and TPP (Fig. 12.5). Qualitative judgment gives an overall impression, but quantitative measures such as ear canal volume (ECV), static admittance (compliance), and tympanometric width (quantifies the sharpness of the peak) help to further delineate pathology. General normative values are presented in Table 12.2 [20, 28]. Static admittance will be lower in conditions that increase stiffness of the middle ear (otitis media with effusion, ossicular adhesions) and will be higher in conditions that decrease stiffness (monomeric tympanic membrane, ossicular disarticulation).

Type A tympanograms usually indicate normal middle ear pressure and function. Appropriate admittance is shown by a normal peak height, and normal pressure is demonstrated by TPP within the normal range. Two variations of type A are type As (shallow) and type Ad (deep). Both subtypes will have normal middle ear pressure, and thus admittance will be maximal within the normal range. The primary difference will be peak admittance height. Type As will have a stiffened middle ear system with reduced admittance (<0.3 mL) but

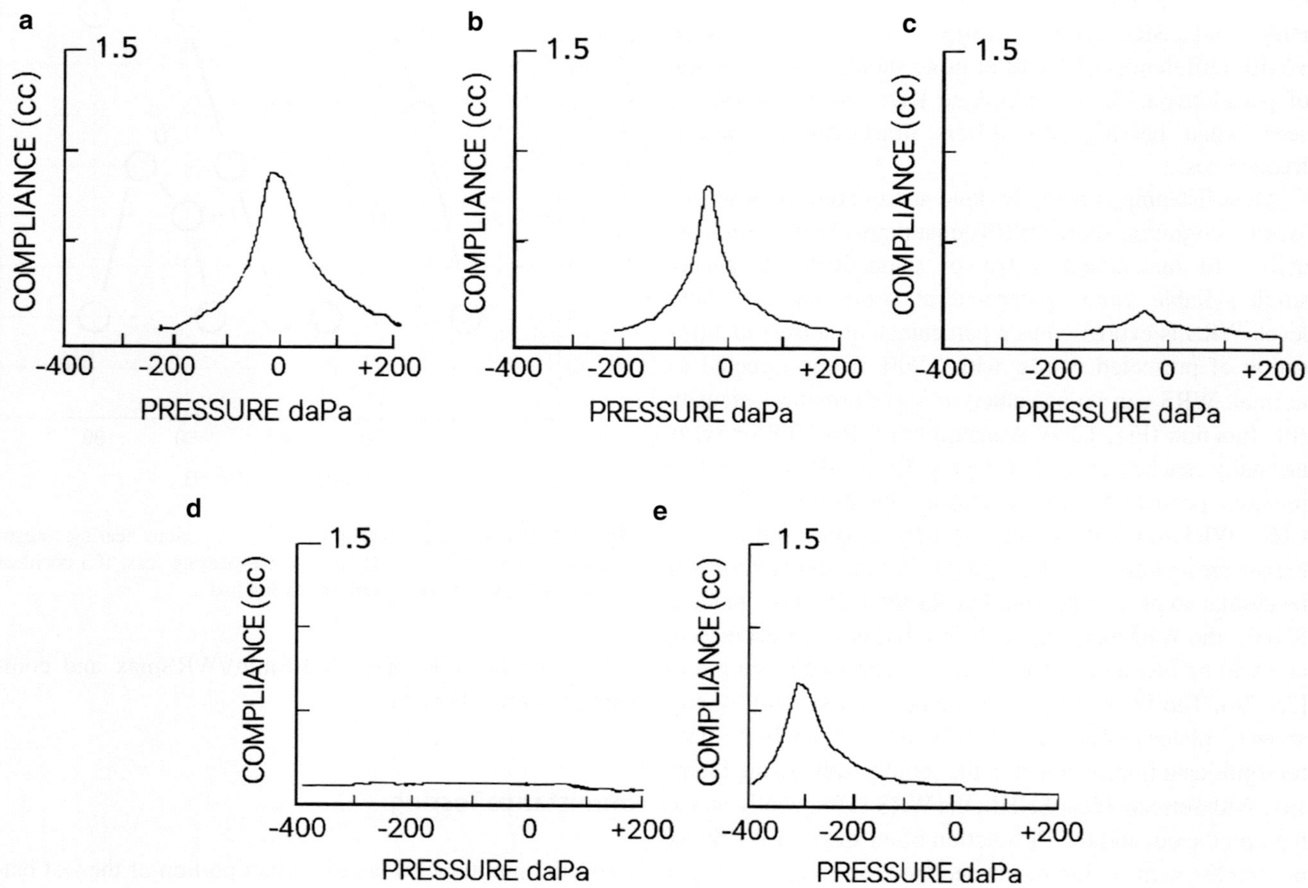

Fig. 12.5 Tympanograms. (**a**) Type A, (**b**) type As, (**c**) type Ad, (**d**) type B, (**e**) type C

Table 12.2 Normal ranges of equivalent ear canal volume (ECV), static acoustic admittance, and tympanometric width (TW)

Classification	ECV (mL)	TW (daPa)	Static admittance (mL)
Children	0.3–1.0	80–160	0.2–1.05
Adolescents and adults	0.6–2.0	40–125	0.3–1.6

will remain in the −150 to +50 daPa. This is seen in tympanosclerosis, otosclerosis, or fixation of the malleus. Type Ad will have increased compliance, and peak admittance will be >1.6 mL. This hypercompliant middle ear system is often due to a monomeric tympanic membrane (TM) or disarticulation of the ossicles.

Type B tympanograms will have low admittance that does not change drastically with variations in pressure. The tympanogram can be flat or very wide with a high TW. One of the primary differentiators will be the ECV. A type B tympanogram with normal ECV is due to added mass to the middle ear system, most commonly due to otitis media with effusion, but also sometimes in space-occupying lesions of the tympanic cavity, such as cholesteatoma. A decreased ECV indicates that the probe is blocked, commonly by cerumen, or that the probe tip is against the canal wall. Lastly, an increased ECV indicates a TM perforation or patent pressure equalization (PE) tube. It should also be noted that a type B with normal ECV could also be secondary to a perforation with an underlying middle ear mass occupying space.

A type C tympanogram will have a normal admittance peak, but the TPP will be less than −150 daPa. This is due to negative middle ear pressure often secondary to Eustachian tube dysfunction or initial/resolving stages of otitis media (OM).

Acoustic Stapedial Reflex

Another portion of the immittance battery is acoustic stapedial reflex (ASR) measurements. These are based on the stapedial reflex that occurs with exposure to high intensity sound. The ASR is a bilateral response [29]. Once sound reaches the cochlea, afferent signals are transmitted along the cochlear nerve to the ipsilateral ventral cochlear nucleus (VCN). The ipsilateral reflex is elicited as signals are conducted from the VCN directly to the ipsilateral motor nucleus of the facial nerve (MN7) and the ipsilateral medial superior olivary complex (MSO) which then conducts to MN7. From MN7, afferent signals are transmitted along the facial nerve to the stapedius muscle. The contralateral reflex is elicited when signals are transmitted from the ipsilateral VCN to both the ipsilateral and contralateral MSO. Both the ipsilateral and contralateral MSO then transmit to the contralateral MN7, which then signals the stapedius muscle.

Threshold is the most common measure of the ASR and is defined as the lowest intensity level that a middle ear admittance change can be detected in response to stimulus. Normally, reflex thresholds for pure tones will be reached at levels ranging from 70 to 100 dB HL (or dB SL) with an average threshold level of approximately 85 dB [30].

ASR measurements can help to delineate the type of impairment as well as the probable location. In an impaired middle ear, admittance is already abnormally altered, and further changes due to stapedius contraction are often undetectable, and CHL can reduce sound transmitted. Typically, thresholds measured on the side of the middle ear impairment will be absent, and contralateral thresholds stimulated from the side of impairment can be elevated or absent. For example, a right OME and a 15-dB air-bone gap could have right ipsilateral and left contralateral reflexes absent with right contralateral elevated/absent and left ipsilateral normal. In cochlear hearing loss, the ASR thresholds can be normal, elevated, or absent depending on the amount of hearing loss, and thresholds generally occur at reduced sensation levels due to cochlear recruitment [31]. For example, a patient with a 30-dB cochlear SNHL could have normal thresholds at 85 dB HL or at 55 dB SL. When the cochlear SNHL is 50 dB or less, reflex thresholds are often in the normal dB HL range [32]. Above this level, reflex thresholds are generally elevated in proportion to the degree of HL. Once hearing thresholds exceed 70–80 dB HL, the absence of a reflex is an equivocal finding because it can be attributed to either the degree of peripheral hearing loss or a retrocochlear disorder. Typically, in relation to the side with a significant cochlear SNHL, ipsilateral and contralateral reflexes will be absent or elevated. Accordingly, a left-sided cochlear SNHL will affect left ipsilateral and left contralateral reflexes, and right reflexes will be normal. ASR thresholds in ears with vestibular schwannomas are likely to be elevated or absent, even with a minimal SNHL, and thresholds are at elevated sensation levels. Thus, suspicion for a retrocochlear lesion is raised when the reflex threshold exceeds the normal range for the degree of hearing or is absent. For instance, the reflex threshold can be significantly elevated or absent with only a 5–10 dB HL [33]. The thresholds will be altered like that of a cochlear HL with thresholds of the stimulated ear (ipsilateral and contralateral) abnormal and reflexes present in the opposite normal ear. Intra-axial (within brain stem) and extra-axial brain stem pathologies can result in a variety of ART patterns depending on the size and location of the lesion. A textbook example for a small intra-axial lesion is solely contralateral reflexes affected. Facial nerve (if proximal to nerve to stapedius branch) or stapedius muscle injury can lead to reflexes on the side of injury being affected. Therefore, a right Bell's palsy can cause right ipsilateral and left contralateral reflexes to be absent, but unlike a right CHL the right contralateral reflex would not be affected.

Acoustic reflex decay (ARD) can help discern retrocochlear involvement from cochlear or conductive HL. ARD measures the ability of the stapedius muscle to maintain sustained contraction and not undergo the rapid adaptation that is seen in retrocochlear disease. During this test, a signal is presented 10 dB above the acoustic reflex threshold for 10 s [20]. A response is considered abnormal with positive decay if the response amplitude decreases to one half or less of its original amplitude within 5 s. This is considered suggestive of VIIIth nerve disorders.

Specialized Testing

The basic immittance battery is a good starting point for patients with suspected hearing loss. However, further testing may be required if the basic battery is abnormal or if other tests are more sensitive or feasible, such as in children or functional hearing loss.

Otoacoustic Emissions (OAEs)

OAEs are sounds that arise in the ear canal when the TM receives vibrations transmitted backwards through the middle ear from the cochlea. These vibrations occur as a nonlinear by-product of the cochlear amplification mechanism that is generated by outer hair cells (OHCs) [34]. The OHCs restore the traveling wave's energy that is lost as it progresses along the basilar membrane, but at the same time this amplification system transfers energy in the "reverse" direction along the basilar membrane that causes differential oscillating fluid pressure on the oval and round windows causing vibration of the ossicles and TM to produce measurable sounds in the ear canal [35].

There are two major categories of OAEs: spontaneous and evoked. Spontaneous OAEs are limited in their clinical significance [36]. Evoked OAEs (EOAEs) are elicited by a sound stimulus and are recorded by a sensitive microphone. The two most clinically useful EOAEs are transient otoacoustic emissions (TEOAEs) and distortion product otoacoustic emissions (DPOAEs).

With TEOAEs, a transient click or tone burst is presented to the ear, and a subsequent response occurs following a brief time delay. TEOAEs are broadband emissions that reflect the spectrum of the evoking stimuli. Click stimuli generally evoke broadband responses, while tone bursts are more frequency specific [37]. While TEOAEs are not frequency specific, they give information about frequency bands between 1 kHz and 4–5 kHz [38]. Averaged emission responses are alternately stored in two separate memory locations so that two responses are obtained and can be correlated as wave reproducibility. As the wave reproducibility increases, one can be more confident that an emission is present. If wave reproducibility is >50% and the signal-to-noise ratio (SNR) is at least 3 dB (often 6 dB), the TEOAE response is usually accepted as present [20, 39]. If TEOAEs are present, this demonstrates that hearing, up to the cochlea's OHCs, is normal or has no more than approximately a 30–40 dB SNHL in that frequency band [22].

DPOAEs are relatively frequency-specific OAEs that occur in response to two simultaneous brief pure tones of different frequencies (F1, F2). When the two stimuli are reasonably close in frequency, interaction on the basilar membrane results in the production of energy at other discrete frequencies, which are arithmetically related to the frequencies of the primaries (f2–f1, 2f1–f2, 2f2–f1) [20, 40]. DPOAEs occur simultaneously, as the two pure tones are evoking the responses. The 2f1–f2 DPOAE usually has the greatest amplitude and is most commonly measured to screen for an emission [41]. The actual cochlear frequency region assessed is closest to the F2 tone [15]. DPOAEs are generally used to estimate cochlear function in the 1–8 kHz range, and numerous points per octave can be evaluated. Multivariate analysis is used to detect DPOAEs taking into account DPOAE amplitude and SNR. If the DPOAE amplitude is sufficient and exceeds the background noise, often with DPOAE amplitude 6 dB or more above mean noise level, the DPOAE is often considered to be present. DPOAEs are generally not absent until hearing loss is worse than 40–50 dB [42].

Auditory Brain Stem Response

The ABR is the most clinically useful transient evoked response as it can be used for estimating hearing thresholds, neonatal hearing screening, furthering the differential diagnosis, and intraoperative monitoring. The ABR waveform contains 5–7 peaks that occur within 10 ms after stimulus onset presented at suprathreshold levels (Fig. 12.6). This waveform is a representation of the synchronized neuronal discharges from the auditory nerve through brain stem structures. The first five waves have received the most attention clinically, and extensive research has been conducted to delineate generator sites [43]. Wave I arises from the distal auditory nerve, whereas wave II arises from the proximal eighth nerve. Wave III is primarily generated by the cochlear nuclei and wave IV

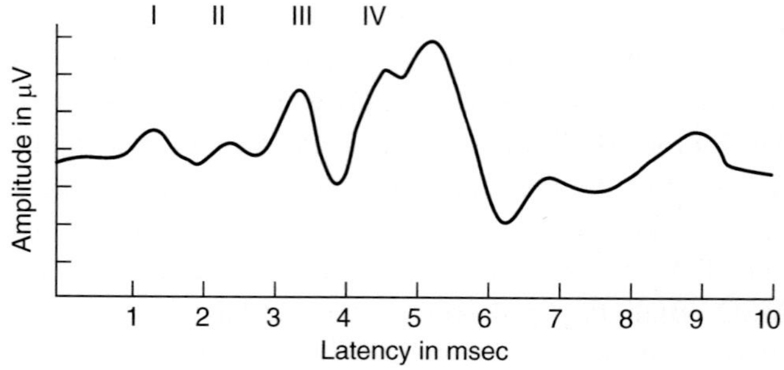

Fig. 12.6 Normal auditory brain stem response waveforms

by the superior olivary complex. Wave V (most prominent peak) appears to originate from the lateral lemniscus as it approaches the inferior colliculus (IC), whereas the trough following wave V may originate from the IC [43, 44].

ABR results are affected by several variables including core temperature, stimuli intensity, gender, and age. Very early in life, only waves I, III, and V are apparent, with wave I having greater amplitude than V. Their absolute latencies as well as interwave latencies are prolonged relative to adults [20]. In general, females show shorter absolute and interwave latency values and larger amplitudes [45]. ABR results are also altered by muscular activity, but results are not affected by sleep, sedation, or most general anesthetics.

During ABR testing, AC or BC stimuli are introduced to the ear of interest, and far-field recordings of electrical discharges are obtained. Both clicks (broadband) and narrow-spectrum stimuli (tone burst or tone pips) are used to elicit the ABR. The ABR is not a test of hearing itself but rather of the physiological function of the auditory nerve and brain stem in which results can be extrapolated. Clicks of high intensity levels are the commonly used stimuli in neurodiagnostic ABR because their abrupt rise time and broad spectrum enhance neural synchrony giving robust responses; however, these results are dominated by the high-frequency region, and lower-frequency tone pips have been used to circumvent effects of high-frequency cochlear hearing loss. During neurodiagnostic testing, latencies and amplitudes of waves are analyzed. Absolute values differ, but normal adult maximum absolute latencies include wave I, 2.0–2.1 ms; wave III, 4.15–4.25 ms; and wave V, 6.1–6.2 ms [46–48]. The upper limits for the interwave latencies (IWL) are I–III, 2.40–2.50 ms; III–V, 2.20–2.40 ms; and I–V, 4.40–4.60 ms. An interaural latency difference (ILD) of wave V of more than 0.3–0.4 ms is considered abnormal.

CHL reduces the effective stimulus intensity level activating the cochlea. Therefore, absolute latency values at a given air conduction stimulus intensity level are prolonged consistent with latencies expected for the intensity level actually reaching the cochlea. Most notably, the ABR will often show a clear, reliable wave I that is significantly delayed and will usually still be recordable even with a maximal CHL. The ABR will show good morphology that is just shifted to the right. This is because all absolute latencies will be delayed; however, IWL will be normal. There will be an elevation in ABR thresholds (lowest dB where wave V is initially observed), and ABR for bone conduction click stimulation will be normal.

With sensory (cochlear) hearing loss, findings are more variable. If available, ABR should be assessed in relation to audiological evaluation, as minimal loss or low-frequency sensory hearing loss should not drastically skew ABR results. Since click-evoked ABR response is more dependent on high-frequency hearing, low-frequency SNHL tends to affect waveform indices minimally. With high-frequency sensory HL, wave I latency may be normal, occasionally slightly earlier, but most commonly it is slightly delayed and smaller in amplitude, yet as hearing loss worsens, wave I can become undetectable [20]. If wave I is detectable, I–V and I–III IWL can be calculated and commonly fall within normal limits. If wave I is not identifiable, the differentiation between cochlear and retrocochlear dysfunction becomes more difficult as both can result in abnormal wave V latencies and abnormal ILD, especially in cases of asymmetrical hearing losses. If severe-to-profound high-frequency sensory HL is present, the absence of a response is equivocal as this can be explained by either degree of sensory HL or retrocochlear process, but if loss is only mild, some degree of a response is expected with cochlear dysfunction [44]. However, an absent wave V in the presence of a replicated wave I or III is suggestive of retrocochlear involvement.

Neural (retrocochlear) auditory dysfunction is associated with poor ABR morphology. If wave I is present, it often has a normal absolute latency, yet absolute latencies for later waves are usually delayed. Interwave latencies are typically delayed [49]. Although not an exact science, I–III IWL prolongation can imply eighth nerve or CN abnormality, and III–V IWL prolongation can imply the brain stem. While being mindful that drastic asymmetrical sensory HL could be contributing, a wave V ILD of greater than 0.3–0.4 ms is suggestive of retrocochlear involvement, especially if measured at equivalent sensation levels. Complete absence of an ABR response can be due to neural or significant sensory dysfunction. However, if there is minimal deficit, and no detectable ABR, this is suggestive of neural pathology.

Summary

The audiological evaluation for otologic and neurotologic disease is critical to determining the underlying pathology, quantifying the significance of dysfunction, and in assessing management success. It is important to remember that the basic audiological test battery and further specialized testing should be accessed in light of each other as no one test is usually definitive.

References

1. Central auditory processing disorders. American Speech-Language-Hearing Association; 2005.
2. Monsell EM, Herzon FS. Functional hearing loss presenting as sudden hearing loss: a case report. Am J Otol. 1984;5(5):407–10.
3. Schlauch RS, et al. Identification of pseudohypacusis using speech recognition thresholds. Ear Hear. 1996;17(3):229–36.
4. Lin J, Staecker H. Nonorganic hearing loss. Semin Neurol. 2006;26(3):321–30.
5. Durrant JD, Kesterson RK, Kamerer DB. Evaluation of the nonorganic hearing loss suspect. Am J Otol. 1997;18(3):361–7.
6. Durmaz A, et al. Efficiency of Stenger test in confirming profound, unilateral pseudohypacusis. J Laryngol Otol. 2009;123(8):840–4.
7. Margolis R, Trine MB. Influence of middle-ear disease on otoacoustic emissions. In: Otoacoustic emissions: clinical applications. New York: Thieme; 1997.

8. Kolb B, Whishaw IQ. Fundamentals of human neuropsychology. 6th ed. New York: Worth Publishers; 2009.
9. Clark JG. Uses and abuses of hearing loss classification. ASHA. 1981;23(7):493–500.
10. Schneider BA, et al. Auditory sensitivity in preschool children. J Acoust Soc Am. 1986;79(2):447–52.
11. Cunningham M, et al. Hearing assessment in infants and children: recommendations beyond neonatal screening. Pediatrics. 2003;111(2):436–40.
12. Dauman R. Bone conduction: an explanation for this phenomenon comprising complex mechanisms. Eur Ann Otorhinolaryngol Head Neck Dis. 2013;130(4):209–13.
13. Alshuaib WB, Al-Kandari JM, Hasan SM. Classification of hearing loss. InTech; 2015.
14. Kim J, Koo M. Mass and stiffness impact on the middle ear and the cochlear partition. J Audiol Otol. 2015;19(1):1–6.
15. Rosen CA, Bailey BJ, Johnson JT. Bailey's Head and Neck Surgery - Otolaryngology. 5th ed. Wolters Kluwer Health/ Lippincott Williams & Wilkins; 2014. 1 online resource (2 volumes (3484 pages)).
16. Mahoney CF, Luxon LM. Misdiagnosis of hearing loss due to ear canal collapse: a report of two cases. J Laryngol Otol. 1996;110(6):561–6.
17. Jansen E, et al. Noise induced hearing loss and other hearing complaints among musicians of symphony orchestras. Int Arch Occup Environ Health. 2009;82(2):153–64.
18. Hoa M, et al. Prognostic implications of and audiometric evidence for hearing fluctuation in Meniere's disease. Laryngoscope. 2015;125(Suppl 12):S1–12.
19. Henry JA, et al. Reliability of hearing thresholds: computer-automated testing with ER-4B Canal Phone earphones. J Rehabil Res Dev. 2001;38(5):567–81.
20. Katz J, et al. Handbook of clinical audiology. 7th ed. Philadelphia: Wolters Kluwer Health; 2015. xvi, 927 pages.
21. Gurgel RK, et al. A new standardized format for reporting hearing outcomes in clinical trials. Otolaryngol Head Neck Surg. 2012;147(5):803–7.
22. Kramer SJ. Audiology: science to practice. 2E ed. San Diego: Plural Publishing; 2014. xv, 425 p.
23. Yellin MW, Jerger J, Fifer RC. Norms for disproportionate loss in speech intelligibility. Ear Hear. 1989;10(4):231–4.
24. Dubno JR, et al. Confidence limits for maximum word-recognition scores. J Speech Hear Res. 1995;38(2):490–502.
25. Jerger J, Jerger S. Diagnostic significance of PB word functions. Arch Otolaryngol. 1971;93(6):573–80.
26. Lawson G, Peterson M. Speech audiometry. In: Core clinical concepts in audiology. San Diego: Plural Pub; 2011. 1 online resource (viii, 166 pages).
27. Jerger J, Jerger S, Mauldin L. Studies in impedance audiometry. I. Normal and sensorineural ears. Arch Otolaryngol. 1972;96(6):513–23.
28. Margolis RH, Heller JW. Screening tympanometry: criteria for medical referral. Audiology. 1987;26(4):197–208.
29. Silman S. The acoustic reflex: basic principles and clinical applications. Elsevier Science; 2012.
30. Moller AR. The sensitivity of contraction of the tympanic muscles in man. Ann Otol Rhinol Laryngol. 1962;71:86–95.
31. Jerger J, Hayes D, Anthony L. Effect of age on prediction of sensorineural hearing level from the acoustic reflex. Arch Otolaryngol. 1978;104(7):393–4.
32. Gelfand SA, Schwander T, Silman S. Acoustic reflex thresholds in normal and cochlear-impaired ears: effects of no-response rates on 90th percentiles in a large sample. J Speech Hear Disord. 1990;55(2):198–205.
33. Jerger J, et al. The acoustic reflex in eighth nerve disorders. Arch Otolaryngol. 1974;99(6):409–13.
34. Ashmore JF. A fast motile response in Guinea-pig outer hair cells: the cellular basis of the cochlear amplifier. J Physiol. 1987;388:323–47.
35. Kemp DT. Otoacoustic emissions, their origin in cochlear function, and use. Br Med Bull. 2002;63:223–41.
36. Penner MJ, Zhang T. Prevalence of spontaneous otoacoustic emissions in adults revisited. Hear Res. 1997;103(1–2):28–34.
37. Probst R, et al. Spontaneous, click-, and toneburst-evoked otoacoustic emissions from normal ears. Hear Res. 1986;21(3):261–75.
38. Ramos JA, Kristensen SGB, Beck DL. An overview of OAEs and normative data for DPOAEs. Hear Rev. 2013;20(11):30–3.
39. Uribe-Escamilla R, et al. Transient evoked otoacoustic emissions and cochlear dysfunction. Egypt J Ear Nose Throat Allied Sci. 2013;14(3):195–200.
40. Harris FP, et al. Acoustic distortion products in humans: systematic changes in amplitudes as a function of f2/f1 ratio. J Acoust Soc Am. 1989;85(1):220–9.
41. Gaskill SA, Brown AM. The behavior of the acoustic distortion product, 2f1-f2, from the human ear and its relation to auditory sensitivity. J Acoust Soc Am. 1990;88(2):821–39.
42. Lonsbury-Martin BL, Martin GK. The clinical utility of distortion-product otoacoustic emissions. Ear Hear. 1990;11(2):144–54.
43. Moller AR. Auditory neurophysiology. J Clin Neurophysiol. 1994;11(3):284–308.
44. Jacobson JT. The auditory brainstem response. San Diego: College-Hill Press; 1985. 444 p.
45. Wharton JA, Church GT. Influence of menopause on the auditory brainstem response. Audiology. 1990;29(4):196–201.
46. Jiang ZD, et al. Brainstem auditory evoked responses from birth to adulthood: normative data of latency and interval. Hear Res. 1991;54(1):67–74.
47. Hall JW. In: Education P, editor. New handbook for auditory evoked responses. Boston: Pearson; 2006.
48. Lima JP, et al. Polarity stimulation effects on brainstem auditory evoked potentials. Braz J Otorhinolaryngol. 2008;74(5):725–30.
49. Burkard RF, Don M, Eggermont JJ. Auditory evoked potentials: basic principles and clinical application. Baltimore: Lippincott Williams & Wilkins; 2007.

Vestibular Testing

13

Christopher A. Schutt, Caleb J. Fan, Wanda Fussell, and Dennis I. Bojrab

Introduction

Current technologies available for assessing the vestibular system include electronystagmography (ENG), the video head impulse test (vHIT), rotation testing, computerized dynamic posturography (CDP), and vestibular-evoked myogenic potential (VEMP) testing. The first three modalities evaluate the vestibular system by testing vestibulo-ocular interactions or the vestibulo-ocular reflex (VOR). Dynamic posturography is a test of postural stability and reveals information about the vestibulospinal reflex (VSR). VEMP testing evaluates inner ear vestibular function through the VSR or vestibulo-ocular pathway using auditory stimulation. We discuss how each of these tests is performed and what information each test provides and offer guidelines for their use in various clinical situations.

Electronystagmography

Electronystagmography is the most commonly employed method of laboratory evaluation of the vestibular system and consists of a battery of tests. The vestibular and ocular systems are connected through the VOR; thus, patients with peripheral and/or central vestibular disorders often exhibit abnormal eye movements that can be measured and recorded (Fig. 13.1). Electronystagmography assesses whether labyrinthine dysfunction is present and the degree of dysfunction and provides specific information about each ear separately allowing for the lateralization of dysfunction.

A variety of methods are available for recording eye movement and include electric potentials (ENG or electro-oculography), magnetic potentials (search coils), video cameras (video ENG or VNG), and infrared technology.

Corneoretinal Potential

Electrooculography is based on the steady direct current (DC) potential between the cornea and the retina, termed the corneoretinal potential. The retina possesses a negative charge relative to the cornea, due to its high metabolic requirements. This creates an electric field at the front of the head that rotates as the eyes rotate. The electrical potential can be measured by means of skin surface electrodes. When the eyes are looking straight ahead (primary gaze), the average potential measured at the cornea is about 1 mV. The potential changes as the eyes move relative to the skin electrodes. Rotation of this electric field produces a roughly linear change in the voltage between electrodes attached to the skin on either side of the eyes (Fig. 13.2a, b). Of note, it is difficult to detect torsional nystagmus with traditional electrooculography because rotation of the eye about the axis of the pupil does not effect a change in the corneoretinal potential. The best methods for recording torsional eye movements are search coils or video/infrared methods.

Video-Oculography and Other Methods

Other techniques have been developed to record eye motion but are not available in all ENG laboratories. These alternative methods of evaluating eye movement include videonystagmography (VNG), magnetic scleral search coil devices, and infrared recording devices.

Many vestibular laboratories have started to use VNG, which is computer based (Fig. 13.2c). Using this technique allows a computer to determine eye position by locating the pupil and tracking its center. Then, eye movement is tracked, measured, and analyzed similar to traditional ENG. An addi-

C. A. Schutt
Department of Neurotology, Michigan Ear Institute, Henry Ford Health System, Novi, MI, USA

C. J. Fan · W. Fussell · D. I. Bojrab (✉)
Department of Neurotology, Michigan Ear Institute, St. John Providence Hospital and Medical Centers, Novi, MI, USA

A. D. Sweeney et al. (eds.), *Haynes-Glasscock-Shambaugh Surgery of the Ear*, https://doi.org/10.1007/978-3-032-18264-7_13

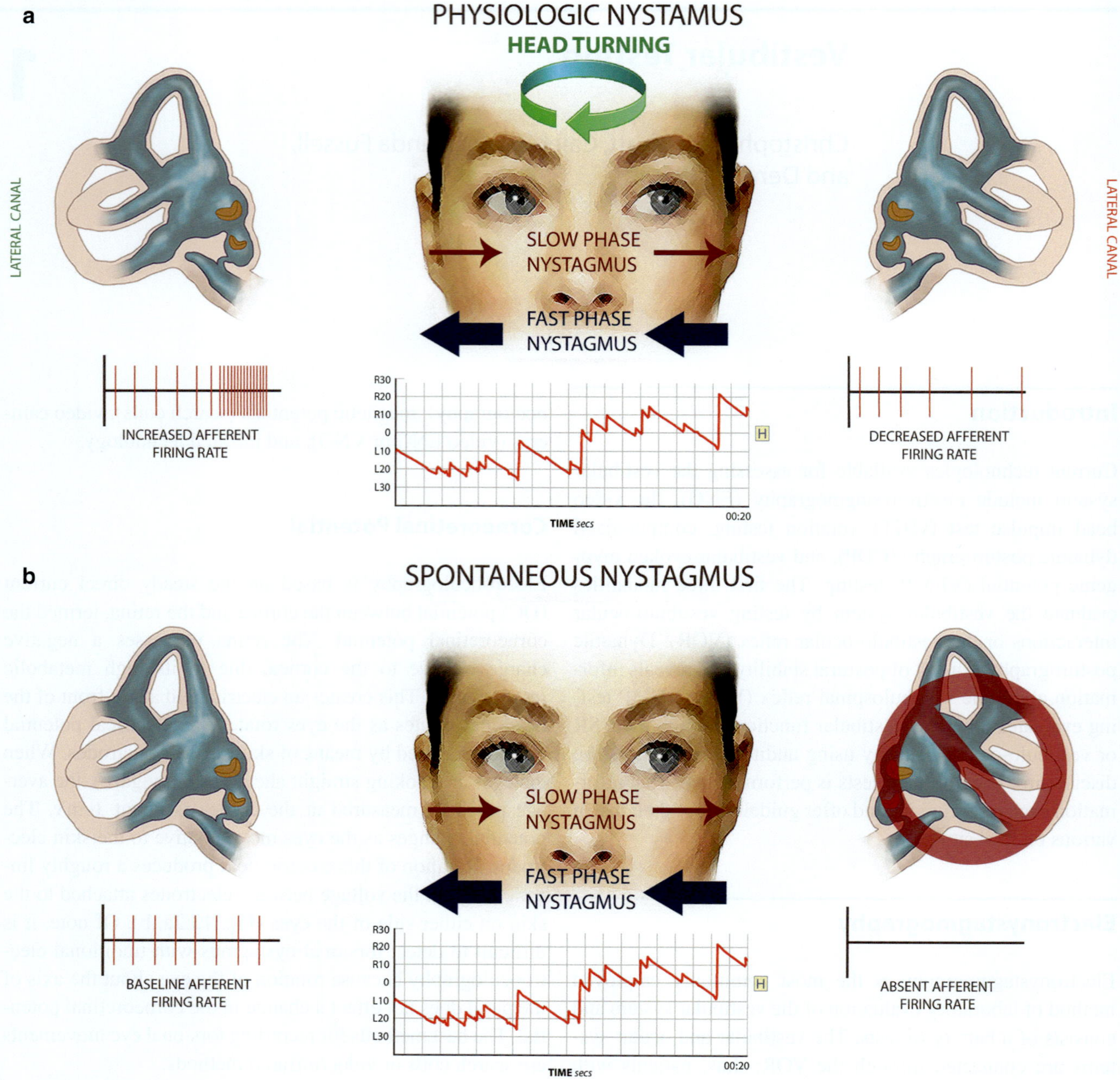

Fig. 13.1 Physiologic and spontaneous nystagmus are products of the vestibulo-ocular reflex. They are observed in clinical examination and recorded during vestibular testing. (Illustration courtesy of Wanda Fussell, MD)

tional benefit of the technique is the ability to record eye images, which can facilitate educational efforts and recall. VNG advocates would also suggest that tracings are clean with no drift, which improves accuracy. Without the need for traditional electrodes and frequent calibration, ease of use is also augmented. However, negatives of VNG use include the expense of the necessary equipment, intolerance of the equipment by patients with claustrophobia, and difficulty testing patients with eye and periocular abnormalities such as ptosis [1].

The magnetic search coil technique involves the patient sitting in a low-strength, alternating magnetic field. The patient wears a soft contact lens in which a wire coil is embedded. Motion of the coil in the alternating magnetic field induces a very small current in the wire, and this signal can be used to obtain a measurement of eye position. There are two major advantages of this method: it provides very precise determination of eye position in three dimensions, and it allows eye position to be sampled and recorded very rapidly (500–1000 times per second). These features are responsible for the search coil technique providing the most accurate measurement of eye movements. The major disadvantage of the search coil technique is that it requires a sophisticated laboratory and highly experienced personnel.

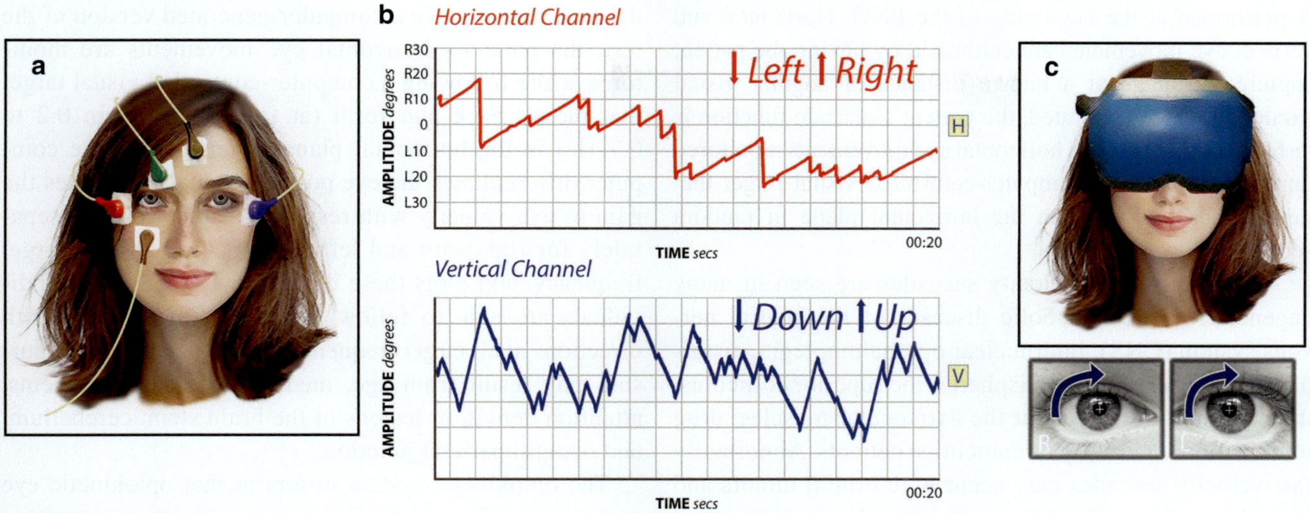

Fig. 13.2 Electrooculography (EOG) and videonystagmography (VNG). (**a**) EOG. The cornea is relatively positively charged in comparison to the retina; thus, an electric potential exists between the two. Electrodes are placed around the eyes, and rotation of the eye brings the cornea closer to one electrode and the negatively charged retina closer to the other. The relative voltage difference provides the basis for EOG. (**b**) Results are charted digitally with time plotted on the horizontal axis and eye movements recorded on the vertical axis. By convention, rightward eye movement is recorded as an upward deflection, and leftward eye motion is shown as a downward deflection. (**c**) VNG. VNG goggles contain video cameras that allow the patient's eye movements to be recorded for later viewing and analysis. Direct visualization of the eyes allows for superior documentation of torsional nystagmus, when compared with traditional EOG-based systems. (Adapted from Diagnosis and Treatment of Vestibular Disorders. Eds. Babu, Schutt, Bojrab. Springer. 2019)

For these reasons, the search coil technique is usually limited to research endeavors.

Infrared oculography is based on the differing reflectance properties of the iris compared to the sclera and the fact that the photocells of the eye remain stationary while the edge of the iris moves with the eye. As a result, the light sensed by the photocells differs according to eye position. The advantage of this technique is that a direct estimate of the eye position as a function of time can be calculated. The disadvantages of this technique include the physical bulk of the equipment, which limits visual stimulation, and the interference with eyelid motion, which makes vertical recording difficult at times [1].

Routine Components of Electronystagmography

The ENG test battery consists of three groups of tests, performed in a systematic fashion to assess the oculomotor and vestibular systems and their corresponding interaction. Test procedures are designed to test each function and to detect the presence of pathologic (spontaneous, gaze, positional, and positioning) nystagmus.

The first group of tests investigates visual-oculomotor function and evaluates non-vestibular eye movements. The saccade test detects disorders of the saccadic control system. The tracking test and the optokinetic test both detect disorders of the pursuit control system.

The second group of tests looks for the presence of abnormal eye movements and whether they change with altered head position. The gaze test evaluates limitations of gaze stability, spontaneous nystagmus, and latent nystagmus. The positional test determines whether various head positions cause or modify nystagmus. The Dix-Hallpike maneuver looks for positioning nystagmus.

The third group assesses vestibulo-oculomotor function. The bithermal caloric test, involving four irrigations, is the most indispensable test of the ENG battery and primarily detects dysfunction of the labyrinth or vestibular nerve.

Tests of Visual-Oculomotor Function

A variety of oculomotor testing paradigms are used to test the central oculomotor control system. The three types of eye movements assessed as part of the ENG are saccades, smooth pursuit, and optokinetic eye movements. As noted above, the saccade test assesses disorders of the saccade control system, and the tracking test and the optokinetic test assess disorders of the pursuit control system.

Saccade (Calibration) Test

The saccade control system is responsible for fast eye movements, voluntary and involuntary. Thus, this system facilitates rapid capture of—and focus on—visual targets in the periphery of the visual field. Due to the need to calibrate the vestibular test to a patient's eye movements, saccade testing is performed at the beginning of the ENG. Horizontal and vertical eye movements are calibrated by having the patient capture an image at a known distance of angular visual excursion. Once calibrated, the patient's saccade function is tested with the patient's horizontal eye movements monitored during fixation on a computer-controlled visual target that jumps back and forth in the horizontal plane in random sequence (Fig. 13.3).

Abnormally slow-velocity saccades are seen in many degenerative and metabolic diseases of the central nervous system (CNS): internuclear ophthalmoplegia, disturbances in the cerebral hemispheres, the superior colliculus, the oculomotor nucleus, or the extraocular muscles; drug intoxication; or drowsy or inattentive patients. Abnormally fast-velocity saccades may occur with orbital tumors and myasthenia gravis [2]. The cerebellum plays an important role in determining the accuracy of saccadic movements. Inaccurate saccades, or ocular dysmetria, are classified as hypermetria (overshooting the target) or hypometria (undershooting) and may be seen with cerebellar disease or brain stem disorders. Saccadic latency abnormalities may be seen in patients with abnormal vision, Parkinson's disease, Huntington's chorea, Alzheimer's disease, and focal hemispheric lesions [3].

Pursuit and Optokinetic Tests

The smooth pursuit system allows continuous tracking of slow-speed moving objects and maintains images on the fovea when a target is moving and the head is still. Two tests of pursuit, the tracking test and the optokinetic test, are performed as part of the ENG.

The pursuit tracking test can be performed simply with a pendulum swinging back and forth, producing a sinusoidal moving target. In a computer-generated version of the test, the patient's horizontal eye movements are monitored while following a computer-controlled visual target that moves back and forth (at frequencies from 0.2 to 0.7 Hz) in the horizontal plane. After testing, the computer differentiates the eye position signal, calculates the gain of eye velocity with respect to target velocity separately for rightward and leftward tracking at each target frequency, and plots these data (Fig. 13.4). Normal individuals are able to follow the target smoothly in both directions at all target frequencies. Deficits in smooth pursuit may result from age, medication, visual problems, attention deficit, or lesions of the brain stem, cerebellum, and occipitoparietal junction.

The optokinetic system differs in that optokinetic eye movements follow a moving object until the eye position becomes relatively eccentric. Optokinetic nystagmus consists of an involuntary pursuit of a repetitive image (slow phase) that is followed by a quick saccade that recenters the eyes (fast component). The specific methods and stimuli used in the optokinetic test vary according to testing laboratory. In one version, the patient's horizontal eye movements are monitored while following a series of visual targets that move to the right and then to the left. This stimulus evokes a nystagmus with the slow phase in the direction of target motion, periodically interrupted by fast phases in the opposite direction. The optokinetic test, like the tracking test, is a test of eye pursuit pathways, and the results of the tracking and optokinetic tests show concordance with tasks of similar difficulty. In normal individuals, the slow-phase eye velocities approximately match target velocities for both rightward- and leftward-moving targets.

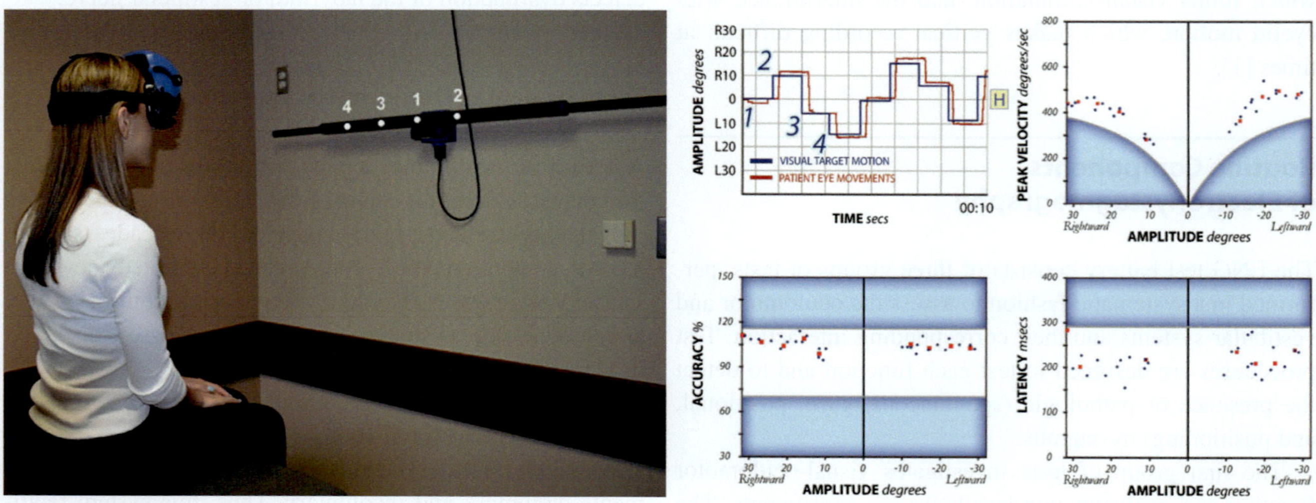

Fig. 13.3 The complete sequence of saccade testing often consists of 80 target jumps (40 to the right and 40 to the left), with amplitudes ranging from 5° to 25°. After testing, the computer calculates three values for each saccade: peak velocity, accuracy, and latency. (Adapted from Diagnosis and Treatment of Vestibular Disorders. Eds. Babu, Schutt, Bojrab. Springer. 2019)

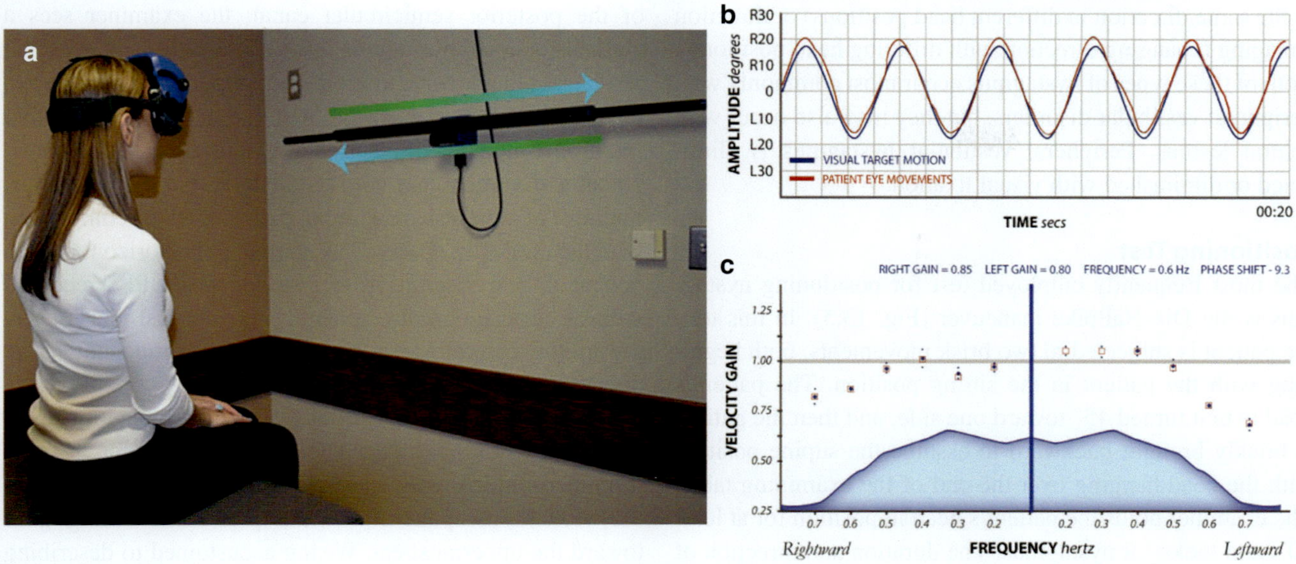

Fig. 13.4 (**a**) Tracking test performed by computer-generated sinusoidal moving target with patients. (**b**) Amplitude tracing. (**c**) Left and right gain plotted. (Adapted from Diagnosis and Treatment of Vestibular Disorders. Eds. Babu, Schutt, Bojrab. Springer. 2019)

Abnormal Eye Movements

Gaze Test

The gaze test is valuable in the detection of nystagmus that occurs without active vestibular stimulation. It may reveal disorders of peripheral vestibular origin, CNS origin, or congenital nystagmus. The test differentiates spontaneous, gaze-evoked, dysconjugate, and rebound nystagmus.

The gaze test is performed by recording eye movements first in the primary position and then while fixating on a target 30° to the right, left, above, and below the center position. Each position should be held for at least 30 s. Young, normal individuals rarely have nystagmus while fixating at any of these gaze positions, but many elderly individuals demonstrate end-gaze nystagmus. This nystagmus is usually subtle, with a centripetal slow phase, and generally is of equal intensity on right and left gaze.

Spontaneous vestibular nystagmus occurs when there is an imbalance in the tonic input from the labyrinth. It is typically seen with unilateral vestibular lesions, and the fast phase of the nystagmus beats away from the side of vestibular hypofunction. The intensity of the nystagmus may increase when visual fixation is denied or with a change in the direction of the gaze, being stronger when looking away from the side of vestibular hypofunction (Alexander's law). Spontaneous nystagmus that is not diminished or increases with visual fixation often suggests the presence of a central lesion. Upbeat nystagmus usually is a result of medullary lesions that involve the vertical vestibular pathways. Other types of central nystagmus seen in the gaze test are described by Leigh and Zee [4], and ENG tracings of many of these are illustrated by Barber and Stockwell [5].

Gaze-evoked nystagmus may be a side effect of a variety of medications, including anticonvulsants, sedatives, and alcohol. It can also occur in such diverse conditions as myasthenia gravis, multiple sclerosis, and cerebellar atrophy. Dysconjugate gaze nystagmus is commonly present with medial longitudinal fasciculus lesions, such as internuclear ophthalmoplegia [4].

Positional Test

The positional test helps to determine if different head positions inspire or modulate nystagmus. Nystagmus induced by positional testing is referred to as positional nystagmus or static positional nystagmus, to differentiate it from the positioning nystagmus of the Dix-Hallpike maneuver. During the positional tests, the patient's eye movements are monitored while the head is in at least four positions: sitting, supine, head right, and head left. If nystagmus appears or is modified in either of the latter two positions, the patient is tested again while lying on that side to determine if the effect is caused by neck rotation. Eye movements are monitored in each position for 20 s, both with and without visual fixation. When persistent nystagmus is seen, it is important to extend the observation period to at least 2 min in order to evaluate for signs of a CNS lesion. Specifically, certain types of direction-changing nystagmus, such as periodic alternating nystagmus, reverse direction in this timeframe [4].

Positional nystagmus may be intermittent or persistent, unlike positioning nystagmus, which fatigues over time. Persistent positional nystagmus is sustained as long as the head position is maintained and may reflect changing otolithic influences on the central processes involved in control of the VOR. The nystagmus may be direction fixed (beating to the same direction in different head positions) or direction changing (changing direction with differing head positions). Both of these types of nystagmus occur most commonly with peripheral vestibular disorders, but they may also occur with central lesions. Peripheral vestibular nystagmus is eliminated or diminished with visual fixation.

Positioning Test

The most frequently employed test for positioning nystagmus is the Dix-Hallpike maneuver (Fig. 13.5). In this test, the patient is subjected to two brisk movements, both beginning with the patient in the sitting position. The patient's head is first turned 45° toward one side, and then the patient is briskly brought backward to assume the supine position with the head hanging over the end of the examining table. The examiner holds the patient's head in position for at least 20 s and looks for nystagmus. The duration and direction of any nystagmus are noted. Next the patient is returned to the sitting position and again observed for the presence of nystagmus. The maneuver is then repeated with the patient's head turned 45° to the opposite side.

Patients with BPPV display a burst of intense nystagmus after a latency of 10–20 s dissipating after 15–45 s. In BPPV of the posterior semicircular canal, the examiner sees a vertical-torsional nystagmus that is upbeating with torsional fast phases that involve motion of the superior pole of the eye toward the downward ear. It should be noted, however, that traditional methods of electrooculography record only horizontal and vertical and not torsional eye movements. Thus, findings of this test may seem paradoxical in comparison with the clinically observed nystagmus. The horizontal component of the nystagmus from posterior canal BPPV recorded with electrooculography generally has the fast phase away toward the undermost ear, and the vertical component has an upbeating fast phase [6].

On exam, BPPV shows changes in direction with respect to the patient's gaze [7]. The rotary component is more prominent during gaze toward the undermost ear, whereas the vertical component is more prominent during gaze toward the uppermost ear. We are accustomed to describing eye movements with respect to an eye-fixed frame of reference, which explains why the direction of nystagmus appears to change with eye position. When described with respect to the canal planes, the nystagmus maintains the same alignment with the plane of the posterior canal regardless of eye position.

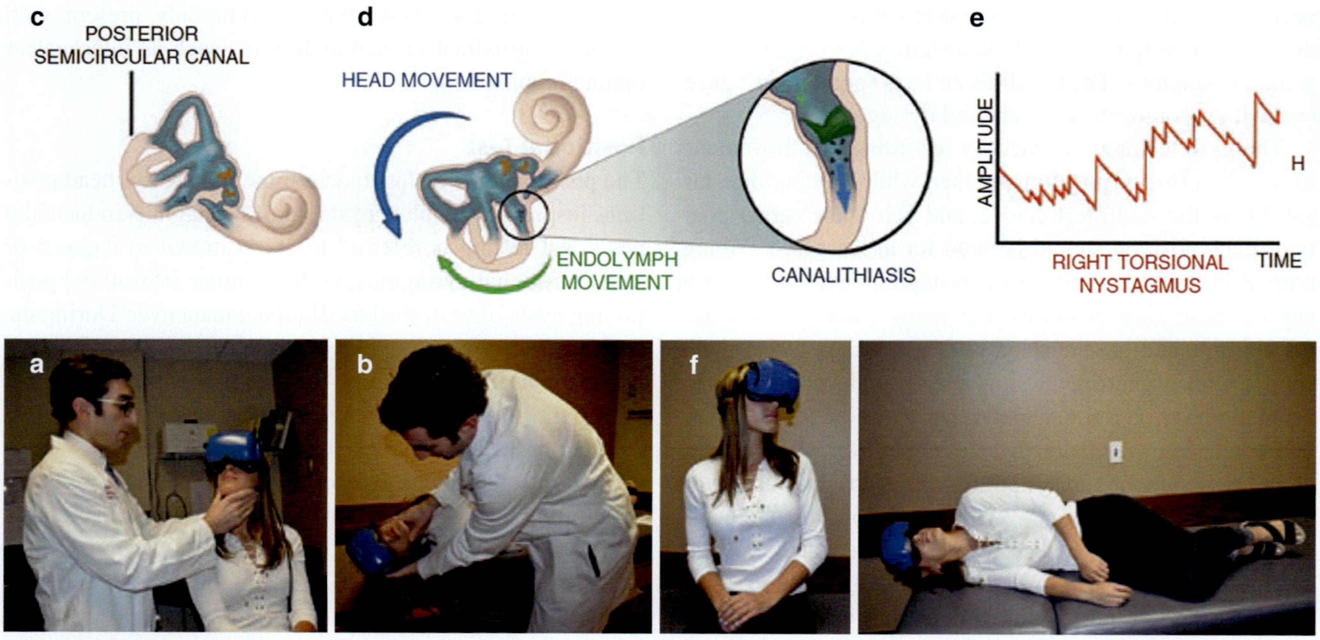

Fig. 13.5 Positioning testing. (**a**, **b**) Dix-Hallpike positioning maneuver demonstrated. The patient's head is first turned to the right. The patient is then rapidly brought into the head-hanging position. Patients with benign paroxysmal positional vertigo typically demonstrate a geotropic, torsional nystagmus with the affected ear down. (**c**) Corresponding labyrinth position which results in ampullofugal endolymphatic flow in the right posterior canal. (**d**) Stimulatory cupula deflection by right posterior canalithiasis. (**e**) VNG tracing representing right lateral canal electrode showing right-beating nystagmus which is seen with right posterior canal BPPV. (**f**) The Bojrab maneuver demonstrated as an alternative method for positional testing of the right posterior canal. The head is turned 45° to the left so that the pinna is perpendicular to the table surface. The examiner holds the head in that position as the patient is briskly lowered onto his/her shoulder with the head resting on the table. This position is held for at least 20 s, while eye movements are monitored. The patient is then returned to the sitting position. If nystagmus was elicited, the examiner repeats the same maneuver to determine if the nystagmus is fatigable. (Reused from Diagnosis and Treatment of Vestibular Disorders. Eds. Babu, Schutt, Bojrab. Springer. 2019)

One limitation of the Dix-Hallpike maneuver is that it cannot be performed on patients with cervical spine disease that limits neck extension or back disorders that prohibit rapid positioning of the patient into the head-hanging position. In those patients, a side-lying Bojrab-Calvert maneuver may be employed. This maneuver allows the same positioning of the posterior semicircular canal as with the Dix-Hallpike maneuver, without the head hanging (Fig. 13.5).

Lateral semicircular canal BPPV can often be detected with the Dix-Hallpike maneuver; however, a more effective maneuver involves placing the patient in the supine position, turning the head quickly to the right-ear-down position, and holding it there for at least 30 s (or, if nystagmus is provoked, for up to several minutes). The patient's head is then returned slowly to the supine position; lastly, the head is turned quickly into the left-ear-down position and held there for at least 30 s (or, if nystagmus is provoked, for up to several minutes). In patients with lateral canal BPPV, this maneuver provokes horizontal nystagmus, as described by Baloh and colleagues [8]. The nystagmus of lateral canal BPPV is (1) geotropic (right beating in the right-ear-down position and left beating in the left-ear-down position) and often followed by an ageotropic secondary nystagmus; (2) stronger when the ear presumed to be diseased is undermost; (3) transient (although more persistent than the response of posterior canal BPPV); (4) accompanied by vertigo, usually intense, which follows the same time course as the response; and (5) not delayed in onset.

Tests of Vestibulo-Oculomotor Function

Bithermal Caloric Test

The bithermal caloric test has proven to be both highly sensitive and laterality specific to unilateral lesions of the peripheral vestibular system because it allows the examiner to stimulate each ear separately. Other vestibular test procedures, such as rotation testing and posturography, stimulate both labyrinths simultaneously, thereby permitting the masking of abnormal responses from one labyrinth by normal responses from the opposite ear.

Caloric tests are designed to evaluate the integrity of the lateral semicircular canals and their afferent pathways through thermal induction of endolymphatic fluid flow. The patient is placed in the supine position with the head elevated 30°, thereby placing the lateral semicircular canal in the vertical plane (Fig. 13.6). Each ear is irrigated twice: once with air (or water) at 7° above body temperature and then with air (or water) at 7° below body temperature. In a healthy patient, irrigation with a warm stimulus provokes nystagmus with the fast phase directed toward the stimulated ear; irrigation with

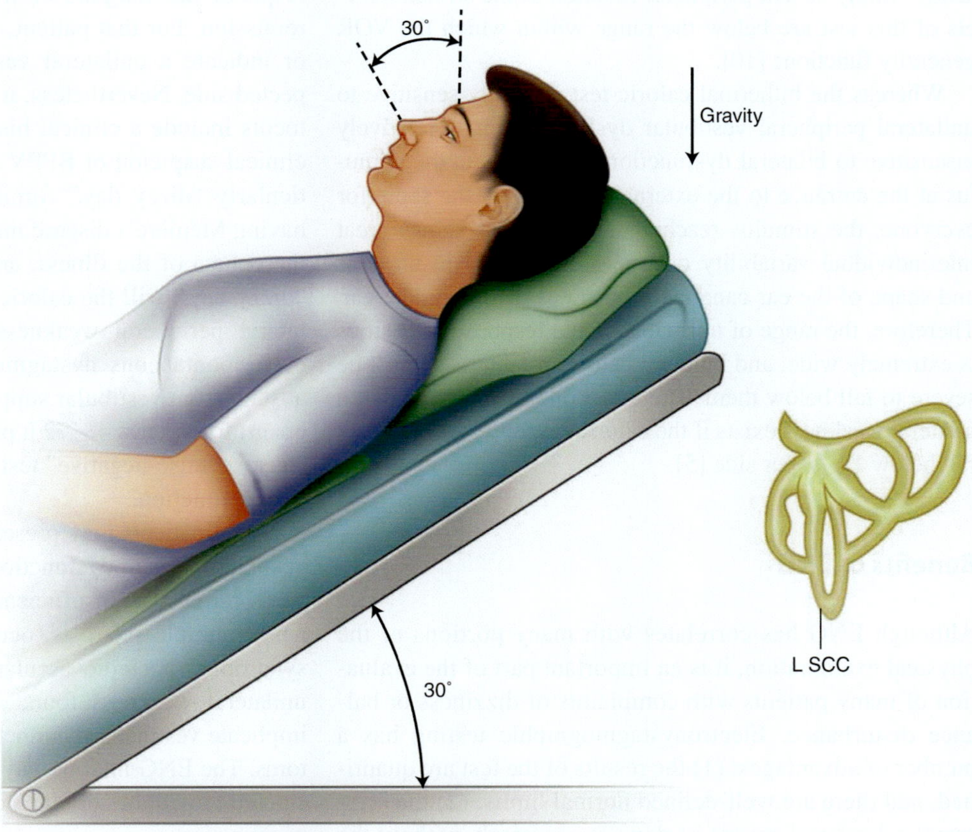

Fig. 13.6 Caloric testing may be performed with air or water. The correct position places the patient in the reclined position, 30° elevated from the table, which places the horizontal canal in the vertical plane. (Adapted from Surgery of the Ear. sixth Ed. Eds. Gulya, Minor, Poe. PMPH. 2010)

a cool stimulus evokes nystagmus with the fast phase directed away from the stimulated ear.

The caloric data are analyzed, and five characteristics of the nystagmus are calculated: duration, latency, amplitude, frequency, and velocity. Of these parameters, the most important variable is the peak slow-phase eye velocity. In normal individuals, the slow-phase eye velocity should be equally strong in both directions. Comparing the peak slow-phase eye velocity of the cool and warm caloric responses of the right ear with those of the left ear, using the following formula, allows the examiner to determine whether a unilateral vestibular weakness exists.

$$\frac{(\mathrm{RW}+\mathrm{RC})-(\mathrm{LW}+\mathrm{LC})}{\mathrm{RW}+\mathrm{RC}+\mathrm{LW}+\mathrm{LC}}\times 100\% = \mathrm{UW}$$

where RW, RC, LW, and LC are peak slow-phase eye velocities of the responses to right warm, right cool, left warm, and left cool responses, respectively, and UW is unilateral weakness. In general, a unilateral caloric weakness (CW) of greater than 20% indicates peripheral vestibular dysfunction on the side of the weaker response [9].

Patients with labyrinthine hypofunction may demonstrate reduced or absent caloric responses to the initial bithermal stimuli. In this case, the test is repeated with ice water (approximately 0 °C) irrigations. However, it should be kept in mind that the absence of a caloric response does not always imply absent peripheral function as the stimulus levels of this test are below the range within which the VOR generally functions [10].

Whereas the bithermal caloric test is highly sensitive to unilateral peripheral vestibular dysfunction, it is relatively insensitive to bilateral dysfunction. Even though the stimulus at the entrance to the external ear canal is the same for everyone, the stimulus reaching the inner ear shows great interindividual variability owing to differences in the size and shape of the ear canal and the status of the middle ear. Therefore, the range of normal absolute response intensities is extremely wide, and bilateral caloric weaknesses must be severe to fall below them. The usual rule of thumb is that a bilateral weakness exists if the caloric responses of both ears fall below 12°/s, per side [5].

Benefits of ENG

Although ENG has correlates with many portions of the physical examination, it is an important part of the evaluation of many patients with complaints of dizziness or balance disturbance. Electronystagmographic testing has a number of advantages: (1) the results of the test are quantified, and there are well-defined normal limits; (2) the bithermal caloric test cannot be done as accurately without the precise stimulus control and response quantification provided by ENG; (3) because ENG provides accurate documentation of results, it can be used to follow the patient with known vestibular disease; (4) standardized documentation is helpful in medical-legal and workers' compensation cases; and (5) it is the only test that assesses each ear separately and can give side-of-lesion localizing information.

Limitations of ENG

It is important to recognize that caloric stimulation tests only the lateral semicircular canal and provides little information about the status of the posterior or superior semicircular canals, utricle, or saccule. Traditional ENG testing using electrooculography is also relatively insensitive to torsional nystagmus because rotational movement of the eye about the axis of the pupil does not move the cornea with respect to any of the skin electrodes. However, this limitation is easily overcome using VNG.

The results of ENG testing may fluctuate in concordance with the patient's disease process. Two of the more common illnesses seen in vestibular clinics are BPPV and Ménière's disease. Both illnesses can be associated with a normal ENG despite "classic" symptomatology. For example, patients with BPPV may present for testing when the response has fatigued or when the disease has gone into remission. For that patient, the test results may be normal or indicate a unilateral vestibular weakness on the suspected side. Nevertheless, it is encouraged that testing protocols include a clinical history so that providers can use clinical suspicion of BPPV to facilitate retesting on a particularly "dizzy day." Similarly, the patient suspected of having Ménière's disease may have a normal ENG early in the course of the illness, and only later, on a particularly "dizzy day," will the caloric evaluation demonstrate a unilateral peripheral weakness, gaze-evoked nystagmus, or even spontaneous nystagmus. It is best to have patients abstain from vestibular suppressant medications (e.g. diazepam) for at least 48–72 h prior to ENG testing as they can cause a "false-negative" test or show abnormal central vestibular function.

Some patients may present with dizziness not related to vestibular system dysfunction (e.g., syncope or presyncope, vertebral-basilar insufficiency, migraine-associated dizziness, multiple sclerosis, ocular dizziness, motion sickness syndrome, or cardiovascular disease). In these patients, a unilateral weakness found on ENG does not necessarily implicate vestibular dysfunction as the cause of their symptoms. The ENG finding may be incidental and must be considered in light of the clinical history and physical examination.

Summary

Electronystagmography testing is an important tool in the management of the patient with dizziness. It is by no means a substitute for a thorough neurotologic history and physical examination, and the results should be interpreted in light of the clinical evaluation. Those who use ENG testing should have a thorough understanding of how the test is performed, what its components are, and the significance of the results. When used properly, ENG is the single most valuable test currently available in the vestibular laboratory.

The Video Head Impulse Test

The vHIT is a relatively newer test that can measure the function of each of the six semicircular canals individually. Essentially, it is a more sophisticated version of the head impulse test using technology that can track eye movements (similar to VNG) and head velocity transducers. The vHIT measures the VOR in response to abrupt head rotation (acceleration and deceleration) in the plane of each semicircular canal. Patients with a vestibular loss will exhibit a catch-up saccade either during or after the head impulse, and the gain of head movement in comparison to eye movement will not be equivalent [11]. The head impulse test and the vHIT are most useful in situations such as an acute unilateral vestibular loss where saccades are readily obvious or "overt," giving information about the VOR in response to stimuli in the high-frequency range. However, the vHIT is unique in its ability to also detect "covert" saccades [12]. Covert saccades can be present while a patient is compensating from a vestibular loss, e.g., a few weeks after vestibular neuritis, or even while a patient is taking a vestibular suppressant. On the other hand, the vHIT is not useful for central disorders such as strokes, brain tumors aside from vestibulocochlear tumors, or cerebellar pathology. Overall, the vHIT is an additional tool in the neurotologist's arsenal but does not replace the other vestibular tests.

Rotational Tests

Rotational tests provide another method of testing for vestibular disorders that affect the VOR. Rotational tests can be classified as either passive rotational tests, in which the patient's body is rotated without any movement between the head and body, or as active rotational tests, in which the patient rotates his or her own head back and forth while the body remains stationary.

Rotary Chair Test

The rotary chair test (RCT) is a passive rotational test in which the patient is seated in a chair so that the axis of rotation is vertical and passes through the center of the head, thus stimulating only the lateral semicircular canals [13, 14]. The base of the chair is bolted to a computer-controlled servomotor that determines the frequency of chair rotation. The patient's head is positioned so that the lateral semicircular canals are in the plane of rotation and is firmly restrained so that it exactly follows body and chair motion. Horizontal eye movements are monitored using electrooculography as in ENG testing.

Testing Paradigms

Rotary chair testing can be performed using various testing paradigms, but the one typically employed is slow harmonic acceleration. In this paradigm, the patient is oscillated in a sinusoidal fashion about a vertical axis at various test frequencies (ranging from 0.01 to 1.28 Hz). The exact test protocol varies somewhat among laboratories, but oscillation frequencies of 0.01, 0.02, 0.04, 0.08, 0.16, 0.32, and 0.64 Hz, with peak angular velocities of 50°/s at each frequency, are usually used. The stimulus level delivered by the rotary chair is much greater than that delivered in caloric testing, which delivers a stimulus equivalent of only 0.002 and 0.004 Hz.

Components of Rotary Chair Testing

Rotary chair testing stimulation generates right-beating nystagmus when the patient is moving rightward and left-beating nystagmus when moving to the left. After testing, the computer differentiates the eye position signal and removes the fast phase of nystagmus, yielding the slow-phase eye velocity (Fig. 13.7). The computer then compares the head velocity and slow-phase eye velocity and calculates three measurements, gain, phase and symmetry, for each of the test frequencies.

Gain

Gain is defined as slow-phase eye velocity divided by the head velocity. It is used as an indicator of overall responsiveness of the system. Clinically, a reduction in gain is used to help determine the overall level of decreased function in patients with bilateral vestibular disease.

Phase

The phase measures the temporal relationship between eye and head velocities and is measured in degrees. Of the three parameters, phase angle often has the greatest clinical significance. In normal individuals, through function of the vestibulo-ocular reflex, movement of the head to the right results in deviation of the eyes to the left. If the patient is

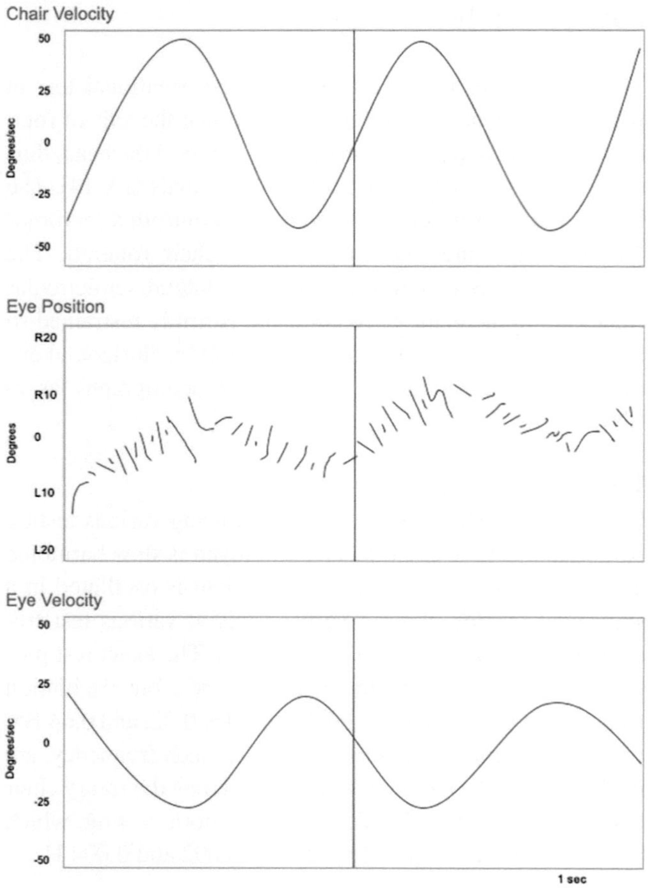

Fig. 13.7 Rotary chair test data from a normal individual. The oscillation frequency in this example was 0.16 Hz, near the middle of the test frequency range. Eye movements are 180° out of phase with head movement. The patient had nystagmus with leftward slow phases when their head was moving rightward and nystagmus with rightward slow phases when their head was moving leftward. (Adapted from Surgery of the Ear. 6th Ed. Eds. Gulya, Minor, Poe. PMPH. 2010)

rotated at a low frequency for a prolonged period of time, eye movement actually precedes the head movement. Increased phase lead implies peripheral vestibular system dysfunction, whereas decreased phase lead may suggest a cerebellar lesion.

Symmetry

Symmetry is the ratio of rightward to leftward slow-phase eye velocity. This parameter gives information as to whether any bias is present in the system, favoring one direction over the other. Asymmetry may result from a peripheral vestibular weakness on the side of the larger slow-phase component or an excitatory lesion of the contralateral labyrinth.

Importantly, phase and gain vary at high and low oscillation frequencies. When a normal individual is oscillated at low frequencies, slow-phase eye velocities exhibit progressively lower gains and are no longer exactly opposite in phase [15]. Instead, they display progressively larger phase leads, and changes in slow-phase eye velocity occur in advance of head velocity (Fig. 13.8). During rotary testing, abnormalities are often seen at the lowest and highest oscillation frequencies. Low-frequency oscillations reveal abnormal phase leads and gain reductions. High-frequency oscillations reveal asymmetries.

Abnormalities seen on RCT can be classified into four categories: (1) vestibular habituation and asymmetry, (2) vestibular habituation, (3) vestibular deficit, and (4) vestibular asymmetry.

Vestibular Habituation and Asymmetry

Abnormal low-frequency phase leads and high-frequency asymmetry are most often seen in patients with acute unilateral peripheral dysfunction (Fig. 13.9). At the lower oscillation frequencies, patients display progressively greater-than-normal phase leads, which are thought to be caused by a loss of velocity storage normally provided by the central vestibular system to enhance the low-frequency response of the vestibulo-ocular system [16, 17]. Loss of velocity storage seems to represent habituation to the strong tonic asymmetry produced by the unilateral peripheral vestibular lesion [17]. Loss of velocity storage is not an exclusive feature of unilateral peripheral vestibular lesions as it is also seen in a variety of vestibular disorders, both peripheral and central, and it has also been observed in normal individuals who have undergone prolonged rotation [18].

At low oscillation frequencies, asymmetry is essentially equal to the slow-phase velocities of the patient's spontaneous nystagmus, but at higher frequencies, the asymmetry is greater than can be accounted for by this bias. This additional asymmetry is thought to be attributable to either saturation of inhibitory responses of the intact labyrinth during rotation toward the side of the lesion or an asymmetric loss of velocity storage [19].

Vestibular Habituation (Abnormal Low-Frequency Phase Leads)

This finding is, by far, the most common abnormality seen in the slow sinusoidal rotation test. This abnormality is often seen in patients with a chronic, unilateral peripheral vestibular loss (Fig. 13.10). Stockwell reported abnormal low-frequency phase leads as the sole abnormality on the slow harmonic acceleration test in 109 of 305 patients with dizziness [20]. Twenty-seven of these patients (eight with a diagnosis of unilateral Ménière's disease and the rest with a variety of diagnoses) showed no abnormality on ENG. Moreover, 55 of the 305 patients showed evidence of a chronic unilateral peripheral vestibular lesion (i.e., a significant unilateral caloric weakness without significant spontaneous nystagmus), and most were diagnosed as having either Ménière's disease or a vestibular schwannoma. The reduc-

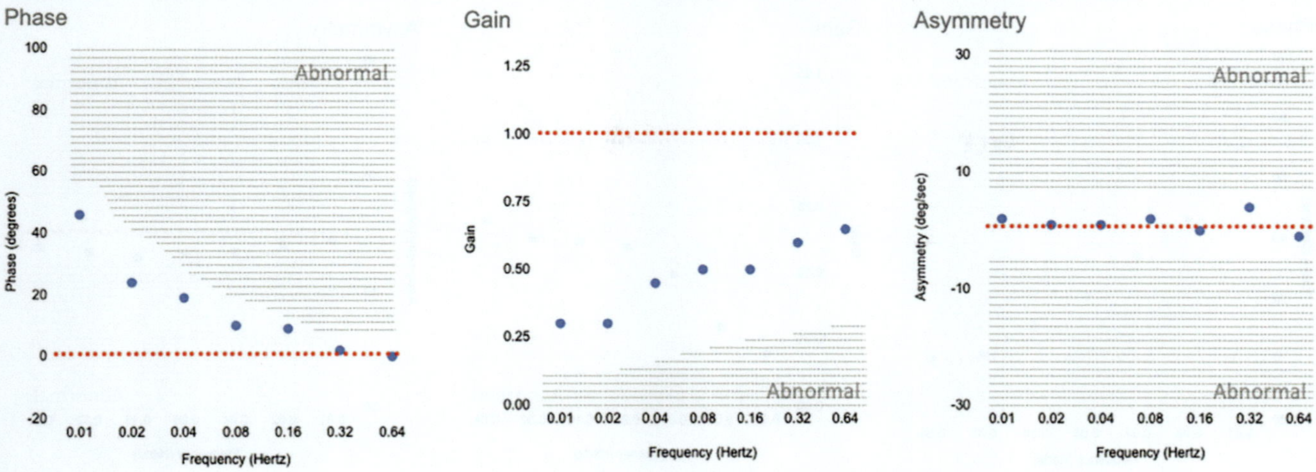

Fig. 13.8 Phase, gain, and asymmetry values in relation to oscillation frequency from a normal individual. Note that eye velocity signal is inverted during the analysis so that a phase angle of 180° is expressed as a phase angle of 0°. Phase leads become progressively larger and gains become progressively lower as oscillation frequency decreases. Symmetry values are approximately zero at all frequencies. (Adapted from Surgery of the Ear. 6th Ed. Eds. Gulya, Minor, Poe. PMPH. 2010)

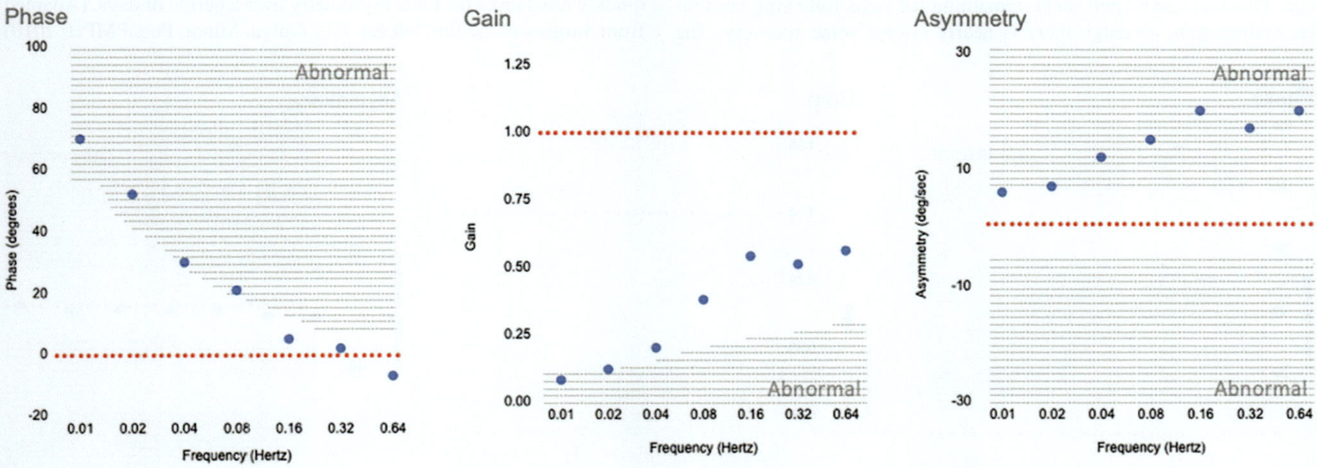

Fig. 13.9 Phase, gain, and asymmetry values in relation to oscillation frequency for a patient with an acute right peripheral vestibular lesion. At lower oscillation frequencies, this patient shows progressively greater-than-normal phase leads. The patient also has a rightward asymmetry. This response pattern—abnormal low-frequency phase leads and high-frequency asymmetry—is routinely observed in patients with acute unilateral vestibular loss. The asymmetry is always toward the side of the loss. (Adapted from Surgery of the Ear. 6th Ed. Eds. Gulya, Minor, Poe. PMPH. 2010)

tion in vestibular caloric response in these patients was nearly always greater than 50%. Patients with a unilateral caloric weakness of less than 50% generally did not have abnormal phase leads. The remaining 27 patients showed a variety of abnormalities on ENG, mostly consistent with either CNS dysfunction or a combination of abnormalities.

Vestibular Deficit (No Definite Nystagmus Response at Any Oscillation Frequency or Abnormal Low-Frequency Gain and Phase)

RCT has particular significance in cases of bilateral reduced or absent caloric responses. If rotatory chair responses are also diminished in these patients, then the findings provide a strong indication of bilateral vestibular hypofunction (Fig. 13.11). Some patients with bilaterally absent caloric responses, even to ice water, show absent or reduced response gains at the lower oscillation frequencies but normal gains at the highest frequencies [21]. An example is shown in Fig. 13.12 of a patient who developed unsteadiness following a course of gentamicin therapy and showed a bilateral absence of caloric response. In these cases, the results of caloric and rotation tests are not contradictory because the caloric response is instigated by a low-frequency stimulus and therefore should be similar to responses to low-frequency rotational stimuli. However, in other cases, RCT shows normal response gains at all frequencies, despite absent caloric responses, indicating a false-positive caloric test result [22]. This RCT is the procedure of choice in evaluating patients

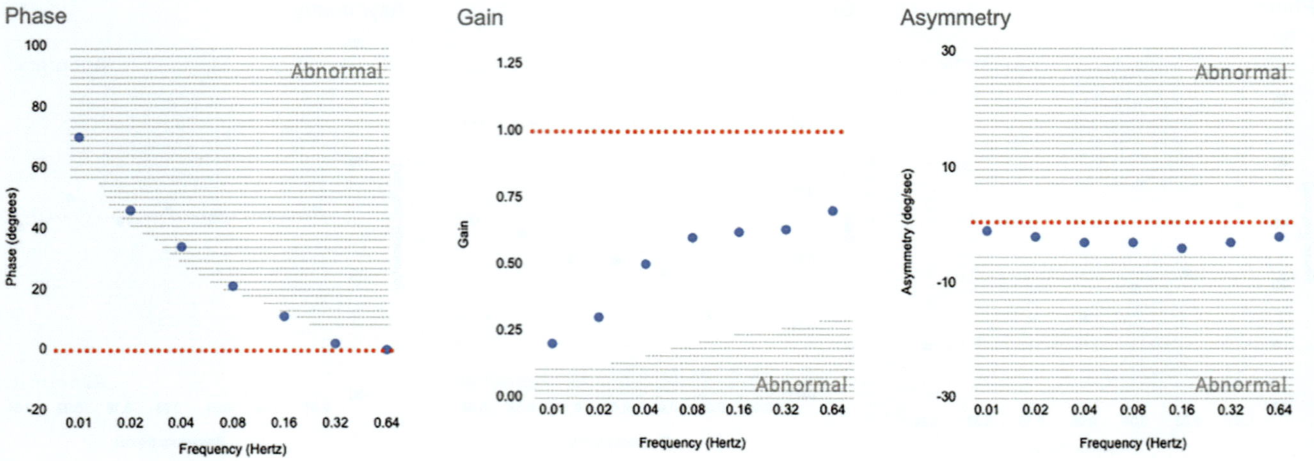

Fig. 13.10 Phase, gain, and asymmetry values in relation to oscillation frequency for a patient with a chronic left peripheral vestibular lesion (vestibular schwannoma). Electronystagmography showed a severe left caloric weakness. The rotational chair test shows greater-than-normal phase leads at lower test frequencies, reflecting a loss of velocity storage. This loss can be persistent, remaining for years following vestibular malfunction, although there is nearly always some recovery. The absence of tonic asymmetry in this individual illustrates the effect of vestibular compensation. If a peripheral vestibular lesion develops slowly, compensation is able to gradually rebalance the asymmetric input, preventing the vertigo and spontaneous nystagmus that would otherwise occur. Even when lesions develop suddenly, compensation quickly rebalances the tonic asymmetry over a period of days. (Adapted from Surgery of the Ear. 6th Ed. Eds. Gulya, Minor, Poe. PMPH. 2010)

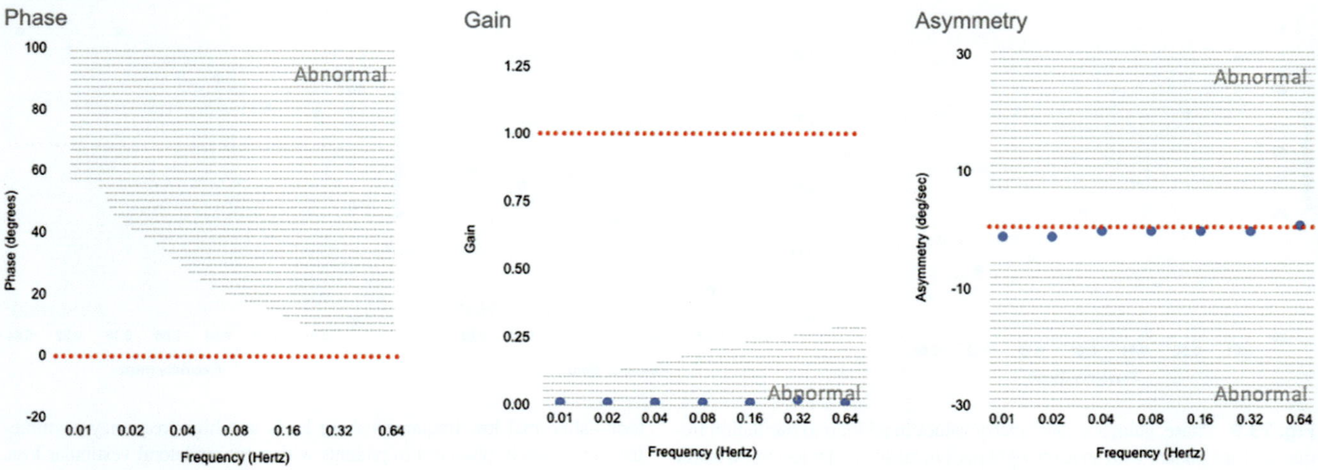

Fig. 13.11 Phase, gain, and asymmetry values in relation to oscillation frequency for a patient with bilateral absence of caloric responses, showing absent responses at all oscillation frequencies. Phase values were not plotted owing to low response gains. (Adapted from Surgery of the Ear. 6th Ed. Eds. Gulya, Minor, Poe. PMPH. 2010)

suspected of having bilateral loss of vestibular function because caloric testing, even with ice water, does not define the extent of the loss and sometimes yields false-positive results.

Vestibular Asymmetry (Asymmetry at High Frequencies)

This finding is similar to the high-frequency asymmetry seen in patients with acute unilateral peripheral lesions, which is attributed to low firing rates of central vestibular neurons. However, these patients have chronic complaints and do not show the spontaneous nystagmus and low-frequency phase leads of patients with acute peripheral lesions. We suspect that vestibular asymmetry reflects a central vestibular disorder because several patients have shown clear concomitant evidence of CNS dysfunction, but we do not have enough numbers to justify making a firm statement regarding the clinical significance of this finding.

Clinical Indications for Rotational Chair Testing

Rotational chair testing may be helpful when: (1) The ENG is normal and oculomotor results are either normal, or observed abnormalities would not invalidate rotational chair results. In this case, RCT is used to expand the assessment of peripheral

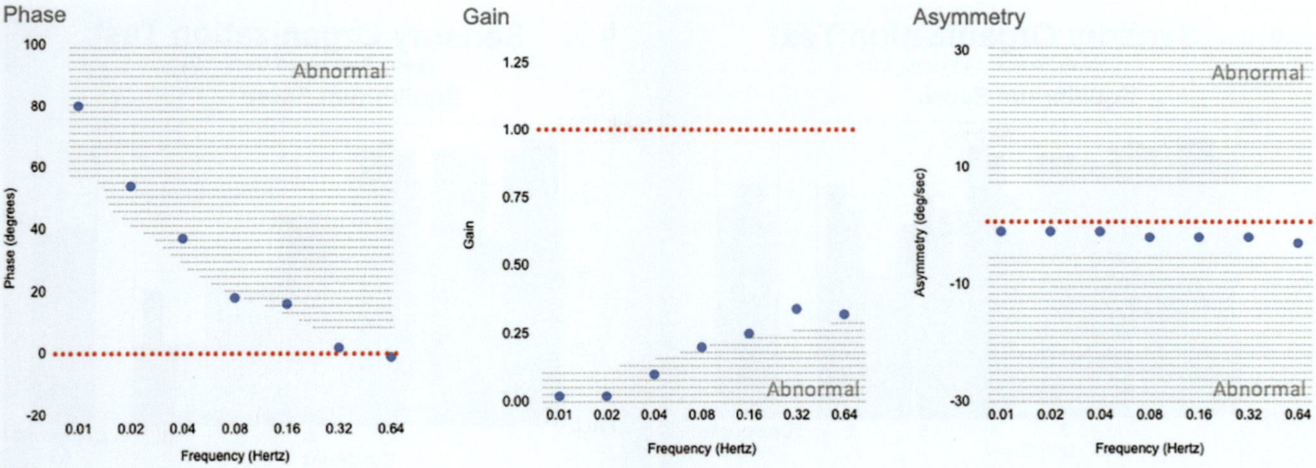

Fig. 13.12 Phase, gain, and asymmetry values in relation to oscillation frequencies for a patient with bilateral absence of caloric responses, showing normal response gains at the higher frequencies. (Adapted from Surgery of the Ear. 6th Ed. Eds. Gulya, Minor, Poe. PMPH. 2010)

system dysfunction (2). The ENG suggests a well-compensated state, despite the presence of a clinically significant unilateral caloric weakness and active symptomatology. In this case, RCT is used to investigate dysfunction and compensation. (3) The caloric irrigations are below 12°/s bilaterally, when caloric irrigations cannot be performed, or when results in the two ears may not be compared reliably because of anatomic variability. In this case, RCT is used to verify the presence, and define the extent, of a bilateral weakness (4). When it is necessary to establish a baseline measure to follow the natural history of the patient's disorder [23].

Vestibular Autorotational Testing

Vestibular autorotational testing is an active rotation test in which the patient actively shakes his/her head from side to side with increasing frequency. An angular sensor is fixed to a headband that is worn by the patient, and the eyes are evaluated with electro-oculography.

Advantages of vestibular autorotational testing over the other tests include portability of testing equipment, relatively brief duration of the test (18 s), and ability to test high-frequency (2–6 Hz) oscillations (when the VOR is active).

Posturography

Posturography is a quantitative balance test that assesses standing balance function under a variety of conditions. It is often performed on a computerized testing device, called the Equitest™ (manufactured by Neurocom International, Inc., Portland, Oregon). This device consists of a platform that is capable of moving back and forth and tilting in the pitch plane about an axis collinear with the patient's ankle joints. During the test, the patient stands independently on the platform, wearing a harness for safety and facing a visual screen that is capable of tilting about the same axis as the platform. As the patient sways on the platform, a built-in force plate measures the changes in the position of the patient's center of gravity. These data are transmitted to the computer, which calculates the angle of the body sway in the pitch plane.

Computerized dynamic posturography with the Equitest™ consists of two tests: the sensory organization test and the movement coordination test. Of the two, the sensory organization test is the more useful in the evaluation of patients with dizziness because it is designed primarily to test vestibular function. In the sensory organization test, the patient's postural stability is evaluated under six conditions in which either visual or proprioceptive cues (or both) are denied. Normally, individuals maintain their balance by integrating visual and somatosensory cues. The visual cues can be disrupted in one of two ways: visual input can be denied (by blindfolding), or visual cues can be disrupted by sway referencing the surroundings. Normal subjects ignore inaccurate sway-referenced visual input, relying on other information to maintain balance [24, 25].

The six test conditions in the sensory organization test are as follows:

1. Support fixed, eyes open, visual fixed
2. Support fixed, eyes closed, visual fixed
3. Support fixed, eyes open, visual sway referenced
4. Support swayed, eyes open, visual fixed
5. Support swayed, eyes closed, visual fixed
6. Support swayed, eyes open, visual sway referenced

The patient is subjected to each test condition three times, and an equilibrium score is calculated for each condition. The equilibrium score compares the patient's sway in the

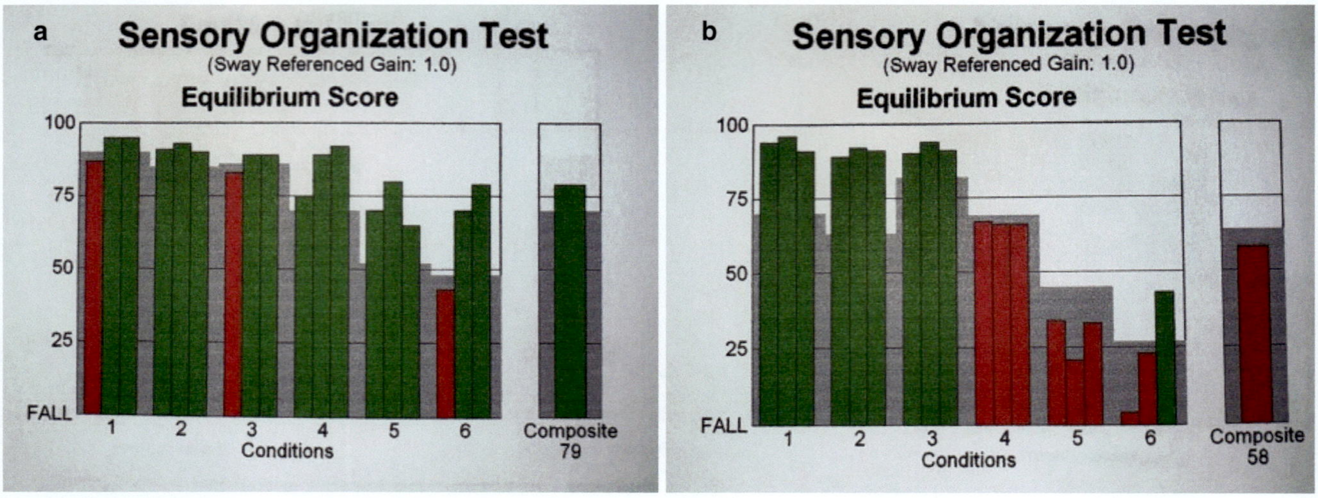

Fig. 13.13 Posturography tests demonstrating essentially normal results (**a**) versus instability (**b**). Note that the first test in a specific testing condition can be associated with a poorer outcome, though as shown in (**a**), subsequent trials can normalize. (Figure courtesy of Shireen Azeemuddin, DPT)

anteroposterior direction, compared to the theoretical limits of anteroposterior sway. A score of 100% implies little sway, and lower scores correspond to greater amounts of sway. The differences in scores for the six conditions are then analyzed to determine the specific nature of the patient's balance disorder. Of particular interest is the vestibular ratio, which compares conditions 1 and 5 and delineates the reduction in stability when visual and somatosensory inputs are disrupted. Although healthy subjects sway a little in condition 5, those with vestibular disease score poorer than average.

Posturography may be helpful in evaluating patients with balance disorders in whom the history and physical examination do not suggest any apparent etiology. In this regard, it is occasionally ordered for patients with vague symptoms of dizziness and unsteadiness, without vertigo. It can also be used to detect malingerers, who will tend to exaggerate their symptoms, thus producing results that are inconsistent with those seen in patients with true vestibular dysfunction. More than a diagnostic tool, it can also be used to evaluate how patients with known balance problems are progressing in terms of compensation and return to health. Examples of posturography testing are shown in Fig. 13.13.

Vestibular Evoked Myogenic Potential Testing

Vestibular evoked myogenic potentials (VEMP) are useful in evaluating portions of the inner ear not directly or individually assessed with other testing modalities. In particular, the cervical VEMP (cVEMP) is used to assess saccular and inferior vestibular nerve function, while the ocular VEMP (oVEMP) is used to evaluate the utricle and superior vestibular nerve. In addition, both oVEMP and cVEMP may show abnormalities in certain conditions including third window phenomenon.

cVEMP testing uses an intense sound to stimulate the saccule, which evokes a response via the inferior vestibular nerve. A vestibulospinal response with relaxation in the ipsilateral sternocleidomastoid muscle is measured as a change in activity recorded on the electromyogram (EMG). The VEMP response provides information by comparing the left side to the right side or by a change in certain parameters of the response including latency and stimulus threshold (Fig. 13.14).

The presence of the VEMP recording is dependent on the contraction of the muscle being monitored, so the test is performed by having the patient contract the muscle first, and then a loud (90–100 dB) repeating click or tone burst is delivered for 30 s to the ear being tested. In our laboratory in the supine position, lying flat, patients are instructed to lift the head 2 inches off the examination table thereby activating the SCM muscles bilaterally. If a patient is unable to perform a head lift maneuver, a head turn protocol is used. In this case, the patient is seated and instructed to turn the head sharply to the one side thereby activating the SCM muscle on the opposite side to the direction of the head turn.

After the sound is presented, the EMG tracing shows a sharp biphasic deflection in its baseline tracing. The first peak created by this wave is labeled P_1 (positive deflection), and the next peak is called N_1 (negative deflection). The peaks occur at predictable latencies in the normal patient: P_1 at 12–16 ms and N_1 at 22–24 ms. The amplitude of the wave (P_1 to N_1) generated by left ear stimulation is compared to the amplitude generated by right ear stimulation

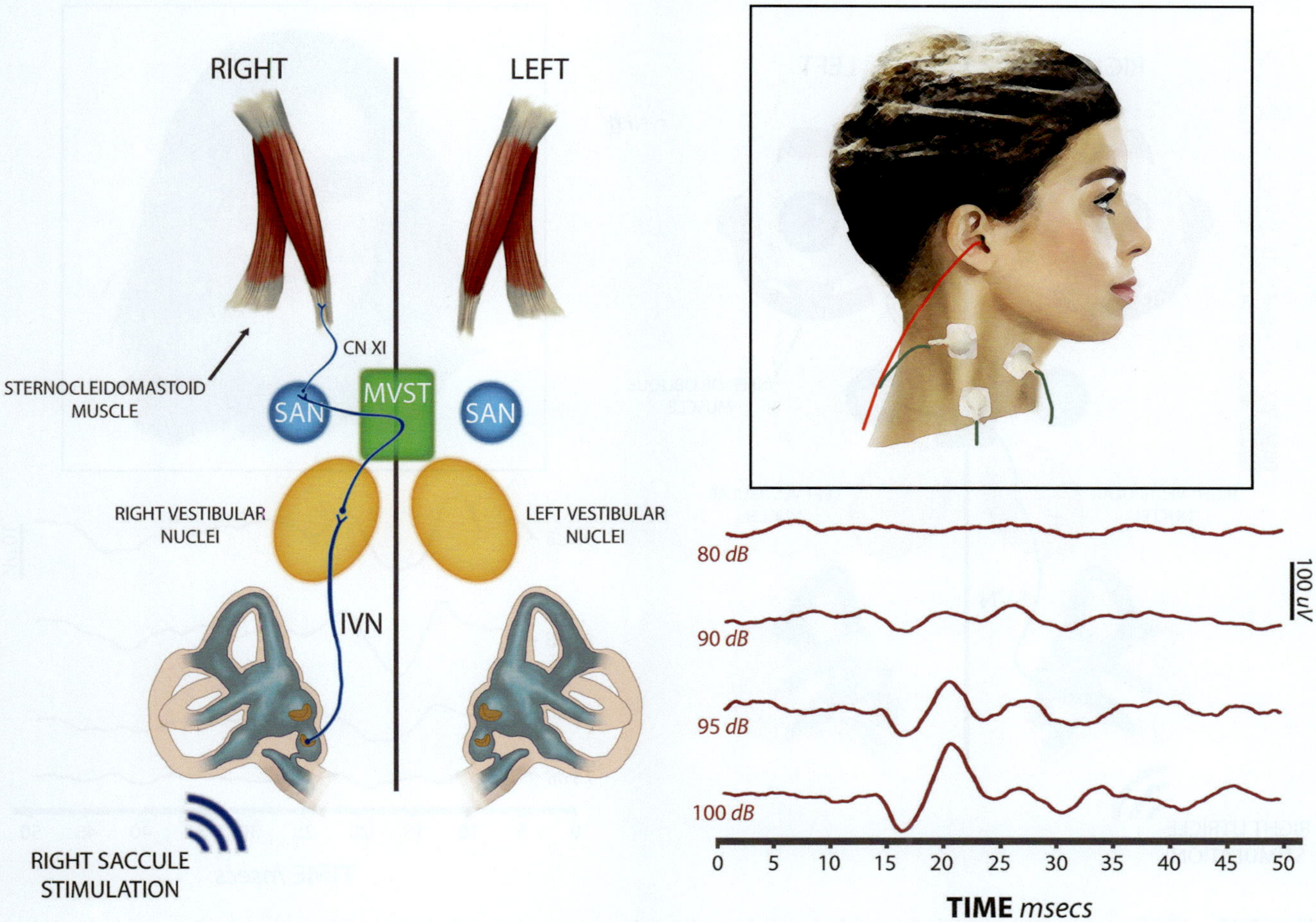

Fig. 13.14 cVEMP testing results in activation of the vestibulospinal response with relaxation in the ipsilateral sternocleidomastoid muscle after sound stimulation. (Illustration courtesy of Wanda Fussell, MD)

because the absolute amplitude varies significantly between individuals, but within-subject asymmetry is minimal in the normal condition. An interaural asymmetry ratio (AR) is calculated and determines whether one side is abnormally weak. The ratio is calculated by dividing the difference of the averages of each side by the sum of the averages from both sides: $AR = (A_L - A_R)/(A_L + A_R) \times 100$. This formula is analogous to Jongkee's formula, which is used to calculate unilateral weakness in ENG caloric testing. Since there is no standard AR that establishes abnormal, laboratories should establish normative data and consider using two standard deviations above and below as abnormal. In our laboratory, we consider a 30% difference significant.

A significantly decreased amplitude on one side (AR > Amplitude ±2SD) has been correlated with peripheral vestibular dysfunction from paretic lesions such as vestibular neuronitis, Ménière's disease, vestibular schwannoma, and intratympanic gentamicin therapy [26]. An increased amplitude is seen in peripheral vestibular dysfunction from irritative lesions such as Ménière's disease (recovery phase) and superior canal dehiscence syndrome (SCDS) [27]. The VEMP test is particularly useful in the diagnosis of SCDS. Patients with SCDS typically have a lower-than-normal VEMP threshold and elevated amplitude of VEMP responses in the affected ear. Increased latency of P_1 and N_1 has been associated with central vestibular dysfunction. In our laboratory, we consider a latency of P_1 greater than 17 ms abnormal.

oVEMPs are similar in nature to cVEMPs; however, they test the superior vestibular nerve and utricular function through monitoring inferior oblique muscle potential. Electrodes are placed under both eyes, the cheeks, and the forehead. The patient's head is then tilted forward 30° and instructed to look up and fixate on an object while repeating clicks or tone bursts are delivered (Fig. 13.15). In the evaluation of efficacy of cVEMPs and oVEMPs in diagnosing SCDS, oVEMPs show superiority with improved sensitivity and specificity [28].

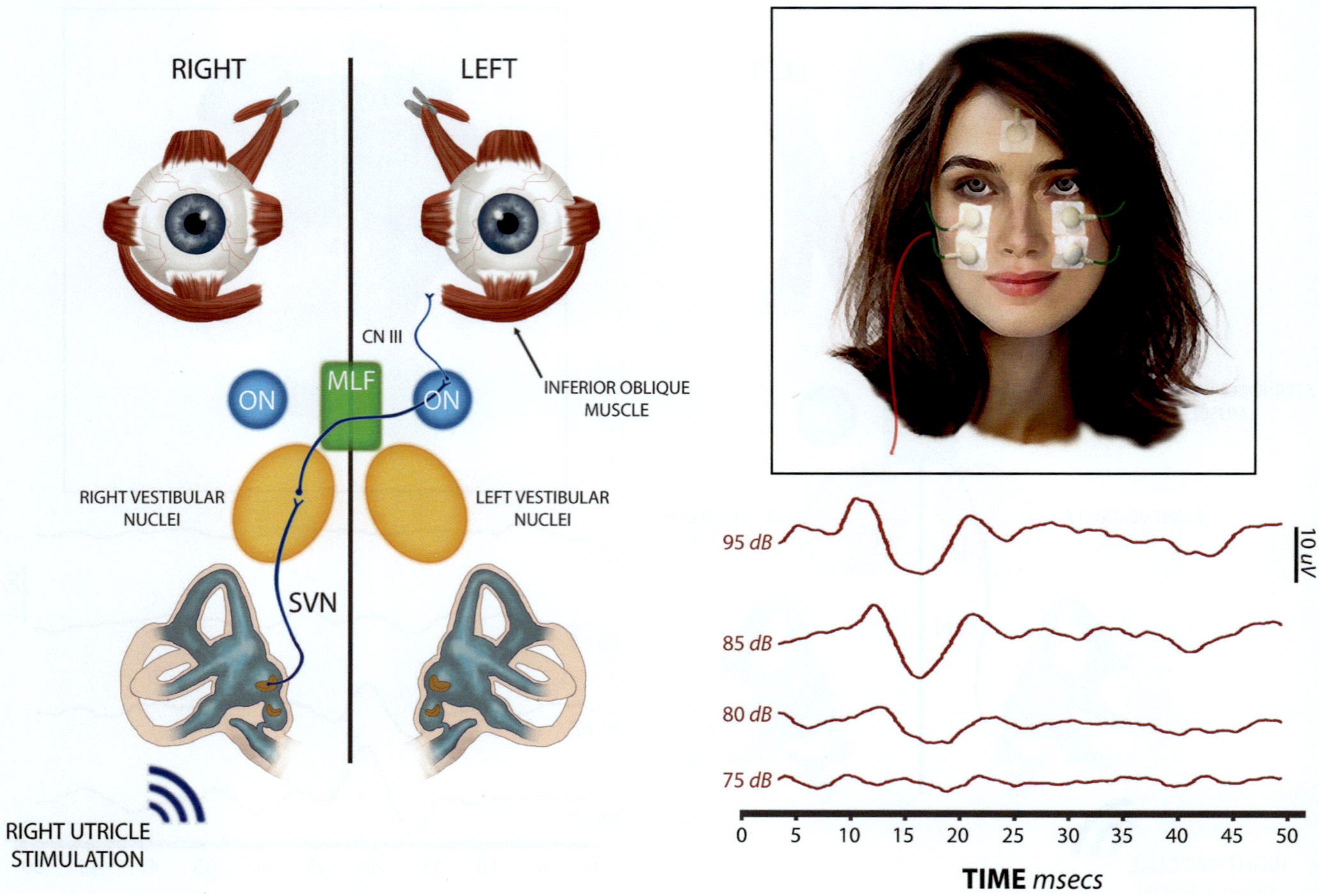

Fig. 13.15 oVEMP testing results in activation of the vestibulo-ocular pathway relaxation of the inferior oblique muscle after sound stimulation. (Illustration courtesy of Wanda Fussell, MD)

Conclusions

Objective vestibular tests are important diagnostic tools for any doctor who sees dizzy patients. While dizziness can arise from multiple etiologies, the vestibular system can cause debilitating symptoms and can also be affected by systemic and neurologic conditions in a measurable fashion. It is important for providers to understand indications and results from these tests in order to distinguish potentially treatable vestibular symptoms from those arising from other conditions.

References

1. Stockwell CW. Vestibular testing: past, present, future. Br J Audiol. 1997;31:387–98.
2. Bhansali SA, Honrubia V. Current status of electronystagmography testing. Otolaryngol Head Neck Surg. 1999;120:419–26.
3. Baloh RW, Honrubia V. Clinical neurophysiology of the vestibular system. Philadelphia: FA Davis; 1990.
4. Leigh RJ, Zee DS. The neurology of eye movements. Philadelphia: FA Davis; 1991.
5. Barber HO, Stockwell CW. Manual of electronystagmography. 2nd ed. St. Louis: CV Mosby; 1980.
6. Baloh RW, Honrubia V, Jacobson K. Benign positional vertigo: clinical and oculographic features in 240 cases. Neurology. 1987;37:371–8.
7. Baloh RW, Yue O, Jacobson KM, Honrubia V. Persistent direction-changing positional nystagmus: another variant of benign positional nystagmus? Neurology. 1995;45:1297–301.
8. Baloh RW, Jacobson K, Honrubia V. Horizontal semicircular canal variant of benign positional vertigo. Neurology. 1993;43:2542–9.
9. Jacobson GP, Newman CW, Peterson EL. Interpretation and usefulness of caloric testing. In: Jacobson GP, Newman CW, Kartush JM, editors. Handbook of balance function testing. San Diego: Singular; 1997. p. 193–234.
10. Bojrab DI, Bhansali SA, Battista RA. Peripheral vestibular disorders. In: Jackler RK, Brackman DE, editors. Neurotology. St. Louis: Mosby-Year Book; 1994. p. 629–50.
11. Alhabib SF, Saliba I. Video head impulse test: a review of the literature. Eur Arch Otorhinolaryngol. 2017;274(3):1215–22. https://doi.org/10.1007/s00405-016-4157-4. Epub 2016 Jun 21.
12. Blödow A, Pannasch S, Walther LE. Detection of isolated covert saccades with the video head impulse test in peripheral vestibular disorders. Auris Nasus Larynx. 2013;40(4):348–51. https://doi.org/10.1016/j.anl.2012.11.002. Epub 2012 Dec 11.
13. Bhansali SA, Stockwell CW, Bojrab DI. Oscillopsia in patients with loss of vestibular function. Otolaryngol Head Neck Surg. 1993;109:120–5.

14. Stockwell CW, Bojrab DI. Background and technique of rotational testing. In: Jacobson GP, Newman CW, Kartush JM, editors. Handbook of balance function testing. St. Louis: Mosby-Year Book; 1993. p. 237–48.
15. Stockwell CW, Bojrab DI. Interpretation and usefulness of rotational testing. In: Jacobson GP, Newman CW, Kartush JM, editors. Handbook of balance function testing. St. Louis: Mosby-Year Book; 1993. p. 249–58.
16. Raphan T, Matsuo V, Cohen B. Velocity storage in the vestibuloocular reflex arc (VOR). Exp Brain Res. 1979;35:229–48.
17. Honrubia V, Jenkins HA, Baloh RW, et al. Vestibulo-ocular reflexes in peripheral labyrinthine lesions: I. Unilateral dysfunction. Am J Otolaryngol. 1984;5:15–26.
18. Baloh RW, Henn V, Jager J. Habituation of the human vestibulo-ocular reflex by low frequency harmonic acceleration. Am J Otolaryngol. 1982;3:235–41.
19. Honrubia V, Jenkins HA, Baloh RW, et al. Evaluation of rotatory vestibular tests in peripheral labyrinthine lesions. In: Honrubia V, Brazier MAB, editors. Nystagmus and vertigo. Clinical approaches to the patient with dizziness. New York: Academic; 1982. p. 57–78.
20. Stockwell CW. Vestibular function testing: 4-year update. In: Cummings CW, Harker, Kralee, et al., editors. Otolaryngology-head and neck surgery: update II. St. Louis: Mosby-Year Book; 1989. p. 39–53.
21. Baloh RW, Honrubia V, Yee RD, et al. Changes in the human vestibulo-ocular reflex after loss of peripheral sensitivity. Ann Neurol. 1984;16:222–8.
22. Baloh RW, Sills AW, Honrubia V. Impulsive and sinusoidal rotatory testing: a comparison with results of caloric testing. Laryngoscope. 1979;89:646–54.
23. Shepard NT. Rotational chair testing. In: Goebel JA, editor. Practical management of the dizzy patient. Philadelphia: Lippincott Williams & Wilkins; 2001. p. 129–41.
24. Nashner LM. Computerized dynamic posturography. In: Goebel JA, editor. Practical management of the dizzy patient. Philadelphia: Lippincott Williams & Wilkins; 2001. p. 143–70.
25. Stockwell CW. Posturography. Otolaryngol Head Neck Surg. 1981;89:333–5.
26. Welgampola MS, Colebatch JG. Characteristics and clinical applications of vestibular-evoked myogenic potentials. Neurology. 2005;64:1682–8.
27. Minor LB, Solomon D, Zinreich JS, Zee DS. Sound- and/or pressure-induced vertigo due to bone dehiscence of the superior semicircular canal. Arch Otolaryngol Head Neck Surg. 1998;124:249–58.
28. Zuniga MG, Janky KL, Nguyen KD, Welgampola MS, Carey JP. Ocular versus cervical VEMPs in the diagnosis of superior semicircular canal dehiscence syndrome. Otol Neurotol. 2013;34(1):121–6.

Electrophysiological Testing of the Facial Nerve

14

Daniel Q. Sun and Marlan R. Hansen

Introduction

To understand the clinical role of various electrophysiologic tests, it is crucial to understand both the natural history of the disease process that caused facial palsy (e.g., Bell's palsy) and the process of neural injury that underlies paresis/paralysis. A detailed discussion of these topics is beyond the scope of this chapter. Idiopathic facial palsy (Bell's palsy) is the most common cause of facial paralysis. It generally has a favorable prognosis; 70–80% of patients recover function fully, while approximately 17% have poor function (House-Brackmann III or worse) [1]. The risk of poor recovery is higher in those that progress to complete paralysis. The rates of recovery to full function in patients with paresis versus paralysis are estimated to be 94% and 61%, respectively [1]. It is, therefore, in the latter group with complete paralysis that electrophysiologic testing is most useful as a tool to risk stratify patients at increased likelihood of poor outcome.

The clinicopathologic correlate of nerve injury has been provided by Seddon [2] and Sunderland [3] (Fig. 14.1). Compression-associated neuropraxia (Sunderland first degree) causes cessation of axoplasmic flow but still allows a stimulus applied distal to the site of blockage (e.g., electrical stimulation) to conduct normally and evoke a response at the muscle. Injuries of the second degree or higher, however, lead to Wallerian degeneration distal to the injury; consequently, external stimulation will not conduct and evoke a response once degeneration has progressed. The severity of injury and likelihood of good functional recovery are associated with the extent of endoneural, perineural, and epineural disruption. If the axon alone degenerates but the endoneural tubule remains intact (axonotmesis, Sunderland second degree), the axon can be expected to regenerate without synkinesis, whereas disruption of the endoneurium (neurotmesis, Sunderland third degree) leads to synkinesis during regeneration. Disruption of the perineurium (neurotmesis, Sunderland fourth degree) or epineurium (neurotmesis, Sunderland fifth degree) portends a poor prognosis for spontaneous recovery. While this framework helps conceptualize the pathology of neural injury, it has only limited applicability clinically. Different degrees of injury may coexist within the same clinical lesion (e.g., Bell's palsy). Furthermore, electrophysiologic testing is rooted in the presence or absence of Wallerian degeneration and cannot distinguish between all pathologic degrees of injury.

D. Q. Sun (✉)
Department of Otolaryngology—Head and Neck Surgery, University of Cincinnati, Cincinnati, OH, USA
e-mail: daniel.sun@uc.edu

M. R. Hansen
Department of Otolaryngology—Head and Neck Surgery, University of Iowa Hospitals and Clinics, Iowa City, IA, USA
e-mail: marlan-hansen@uiowa.edu

A. D. Sweeney et al. (eds.), *Haynes-Glasscock-Shambaugh Surgery of the Ear*, https://doi.org/10.1007/978-3-032-18264-7_14

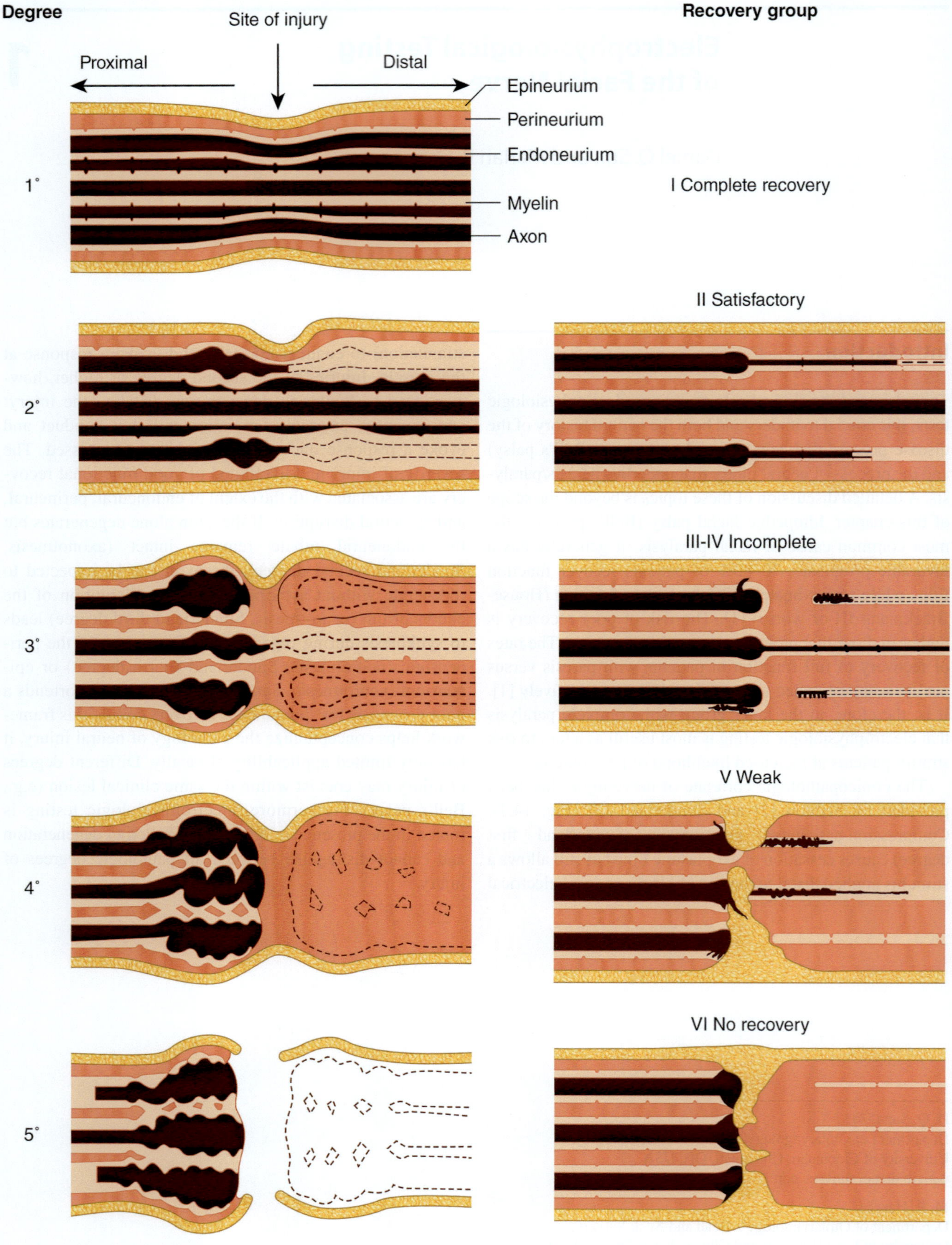

Fig. 14.1 Sunderland classification of neural injury. The potential for neural regeneration across the site of injury is related to the status of endoneural connective tissue elements. Endoneural disruption increases the risk of synkinesis. (Used with permission and adapted from May [4])

History

In 1862, Duchenne famously performed electrical stimulation of the facial nerve in awake humans to elicit various facial expressions [5]. He proceeded to stimulate the facial nerve of those with "rheumatismal" facial palsy and noted absence of muscular contractility in some and diminished contractility in others. Since then, many investigators have sought to use electrodiagnostic methods to diagnose and prognosticate facial palsies, which are hindered by the inaccessibility of the facial nerve in its long and tortuous course through the temporal bone. Others have sought to use the distinct efferent and afferent functions of the facial nerve and their discrete anatomical branch points to better localize lesions. Termed *topognostic* testing, these include tests of stapedial reflex, salivary secretion, and lacrimation (Schirmer test). However, they have been shown based on intraoperative studies to have little value in the diagnosis of facial nerve palsies such as Bell's [6], although they may continue to be useful in assessing end-organ function, such as dry eyes due to decreased lacrimation. The introduction of volitional electromyography (EMG) and stimulatory nerve excitability tests such as the minimal nerve excitability (NET) and maximal nerve stimulation tests (MST) allowed for electrophysiological assessments of the severity of facial nerve dysfunction and prognostication of facial palsies [7–11]. Since the development of electroneurography (ENoG) by Esslen [12], however, the NET and MST have largely been supplanted in the clinical assessment of facial nerve neurophysiology due to ENoG's ability to quantify the extent of Wallerian degeneration with both prognostic and treatment implications [13].

Electroneurography

In ENoG, suprathreshold electrical stimulation is delivered transcutaneously at the stylomastoid foramen to elicit a maximal muscle response, which is measured in the form of compound muscle action potentials (CMAP). Therefore, ENoG may be more aptly termed *evoked electromyography*. The test is performed using standard EMG equipment but requires the use of special surface stimulating and recording electrodes [6]. As originally described by Esslen [12], the recording electrodes are in a handheld carrier and are manipulated in the nasolabial fold. The recording electrodes are not taped to the skin, as has been described by others [14]. Manual manipulation of the surface recording electrode allows the technician to adjust the electrode location and orientation such that the maximum CMAP is recorded to allow comparison to the contralateral side and to minimize trigeminal artifact. Although frequently practiced, taping or using subdermal recording electrodes may result in recording non-maximum CMAP amplitudes and, as a result, inaccurate relative percent degeneration [15, 16]. The CMAP amplitude from the paralyzed side is compared with that of the normal side, and the result is reported as a percentage. In contrast to other forms of electrophysiological testing, ENoG is therefore able to provide a quantitative measurement of neural function across the entire muscle. Although CMAP latency has also been studied, its prognostic value has been unreliable [17]. Concerns regarding test-retest reliability can be overcome by performing multiple stimulations in each session and averaging the CMAP recordings [15]. In fact, increasing the number of stimulations also increases synchronization within the nerve, which improves ENoG accuracy [6, 18]. Some authors recommend stimulating 10–20 times before making an amplitude measurement [19], although other studies indicate as few as 5 times may be sufficient [20].

The amplitude of the biphasic CMAP has been found to correlate with the number of conducting nerve fibers [6]. As the percentage of degenerated fibers within the nerve increases, the amplitude of the CMAP decreases compared with the normal side of the face. Therefore, ENoG is only useful as a measure of distal Wallerian degeneration. That is, in neuropraxic injuries where a conduction block exists without distal Wallerian degeneration, ENoG would be normal. ENoG is also unable to distinguish between different pathologic classes of neural injury, such as axonotmesis versus neurotmesis, only whether Wallerian degeneration is present. Despite these pathophysiological limitations, ENoG carries tremendous prognostic value when used in the appropriate clinical context [19, 21–23]. Fisch and Esslen [24] determined that if 95% or more of the fibers within the facial nerve degenerate within the first 14 days of an acute paralysis, the chances of poor outcome in facial function were approximately 50%. A more recent study found that the ENoG threshold for increased likelihood of poor outcome in Bell's palsy may be lower, at approximately 85% degeneration [25]. ENoG is unable to perfectly prognosticate the extent of recovery even in the setting of severe degeneration because it cannot distinguish between axonotmesis and neurotmesis. Those with higher proportion of fibers that undergo neurotmesis and its associated endoneural disruption are more likely to recover with synkinesis and, therefore, poor function. Patients who do not reach the 90% degeneration level by 3 weeks have a very good prognosis and are likely to regain normal facial motion without synkinesis.

The time course of degeneration is also an important feature of electrophysiological testing; the more severe the injury, the more rapid the degeneration [26]. Following complete transection of the facial nerve, Wallerian degeneration of the distal axons reaches 100% over a course of 3–5 days. In contrast, a severe compression injury leading to delayed paralysis is associated with 100% Wallerian degeneration over a course of 14–21 days [19]. Patients with delayed paralysis typically return to normal facial function, suggesting that axonotmesis is the primary mode of injury. Thus, serial ENoG testing informs the clinician of the trajectory of degeneration, therefore the likely proportion of axonotmesis versus neurotmesis, and consequently the likelihood for good versus poor recovery (Fig. 14.2). A patient showing greater than 90% degeneration at 5 days would have a worse prognosis than a patient with 90% degeneration at 14 days.

By understanding the neurophysiological basis of ENoG testing, its clinical usage in acute facial paralysis becomes clear. Because ENoG is a measurement of neural degeneration, it is only useful when performed at least 3 days after the onset of complete paralysis, when Wallerian degeneration has occurred. Serial ENoGs performed every 2–3 days then reveal the trajectory of degeneration. If the percent degeneration decreases on serial ENoG, testing is stopped as the patient will have high likelihood of good functional recovery [19]. If degeneration reaches 90% within 14 days of complete paralysis and persistent paralysis is confirmed on EMG, treatment decisions will need to be made as the patient has a higher likelihood of poor functional recovery. The key decision is whether or not to offer surgical decompression of the labyrinthine and perigeniculate segments of the facial nerve in patients with >90% degeneration within 14 days of the onset of complete paralysis [13]. Case-control studies suggest improved recovery following surgical decompression in carefully selected patients, with ENoG providing the key prognostic information on which to base the clinical decision. If degeneration increases but does not reach 90% within 14 days, testing may also be stopped as the slow trajectory of degeneration portends a favorable prognosis.

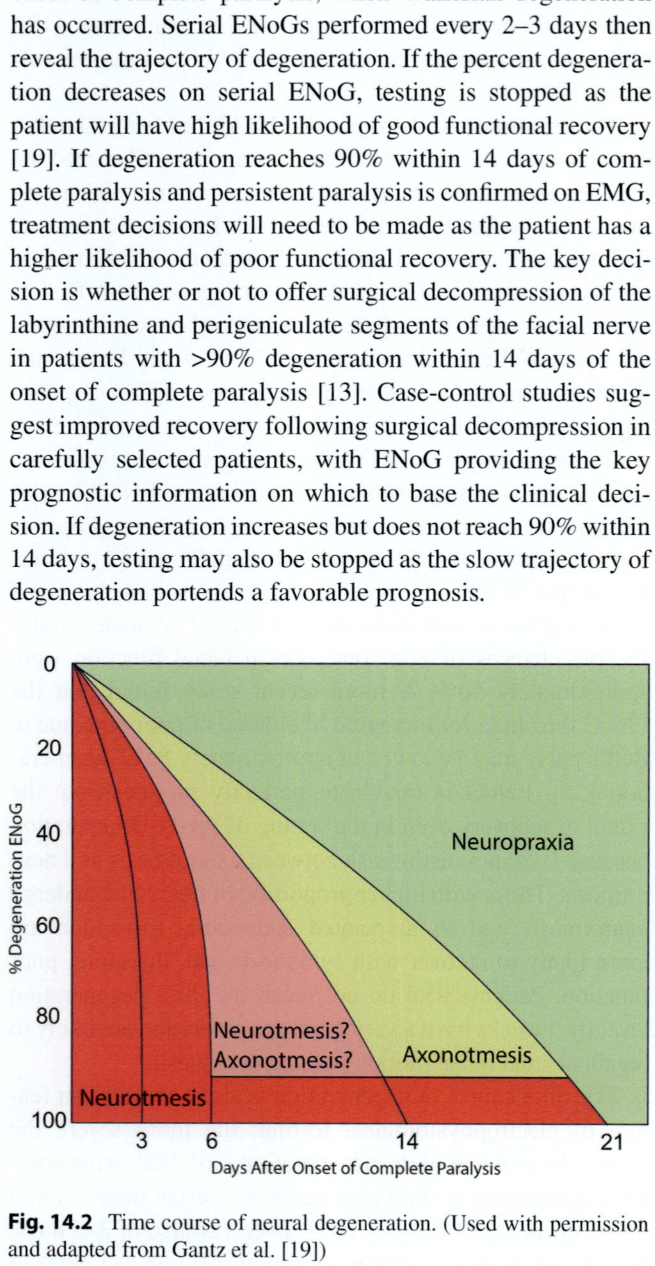

Fig. 14.2 Time course of neural degeneration. (Used with permission and adapted from Gantz et al. [19])

Since ENoG relies on the measurement of muscle action potentials, it is not useful in chronic paralysis where there is deterioration of the neuromuscular junction and muscle atrophy. Furthermore, since CMAP recording relies on synchronous firing of the stimulated nerve, ENoG is also inaccurate in chronic conditions such as facial nerve neuromas where individual nerve fibers undergo simultaneous degeneration and regeneration, which leads to dyssynchrony in neural response [19]. Since regenerating fibers do not fire synchronously, it is not uncommon to see voluntary facial movement, while ENoG recordings still reveal 100% neural degeneration. Termed *deblocking*, this phenomenon is frequently present in patients recovering from Bell's palsy [18, 22]. It is for this reason that all patients with severe degeneration on ENoG who are potential candidates for surgical decompression must undergo volitional EMG testing. Although rare, early deblocking occurring within 14 days of paralysis may result in the presence of voluntary motion that can be captured as muscle motor unit potentials on EMG, while ENoG recordings still yield severe degeneration due to dyssynchrony. Patients with early deblocking have a favorable prognosis for good recovery and therefore are not appropriate for surgical decompression. ENoG has not been shown to be prognostic in other etiologies of facial palsy that do not have discrete lesions, such as Ramsay Hunt syndrome or autoimmune vasculitides [27], and remains most useful in Bell's palsy and trauma.

Electromyography

EMG uses needle electrodes to record spontaneous and/or voluntary motor unit potentials (MUPs)—typically from *orbicularis oculi* and *oris* for facial palsies. In contrast to ENoG, no stimulation current is provided, and recordings are able to capture the activity of individual muscle fibers. Insertional activity can be measured upon needle placement and subsequently moving it within the muscle. Once the needle is at rest, spontaneous activity is measured. Normal muscle is electrically silent at rest; however, spontaneous firing of individual muscle fibers occurs when the muscle fibers are functionally denervated. Termed *fibrillation potentials*, they are indicative of Wallerian degeneration, decoupling of the motor endplate from its nerve terminal, and consequent spontaneous discharge of the denervated muscle membranes. Even after nerve transection, motor unit fibrillation potentials are not present until at least 10–14 days later even though clinical paresis/paralysis may be evident. Therefore, EMG is typically only clinically useful 2–3 weeks after onset of complete paralysis. In the acute phase of paralysis, EMG is used to rule out early deblocking when ENoG shows severe degeneration, as discussed previously. In this setting, since EMG is able to measure the activity of individual muscle fibers and does not rely on synchronous firing of the nerve, it is able to capture MUPs when the patient is asked to make voluntary movements that are indicative of regeneration despite minimal or absent CMAP amplitude.

EMG plays an important role in the evaluation of chronic paralysis. Polyphasic potentials are indicative of reestablishment of nerve terminals to motor endplates and, therefore, reinnervation; such potentials arise prior to evidence of motion on clinical exam. Thus, the presence of polyphasic potentials following nerve injury and/or repair reassures the clinician that at least partial neural regeneration has occurred and more time may be needed for its full clinical manifestation. If regeneration does not occur and chronic paralysis persists, muscle atrophy typically occurs after 12 months. On EMG, fibrillation potentials will diminish to electrical silence. Therefore, EMG can be used to guide facial reanimation decisions. Electrical silence in the setting of chronic paralysis indicates muscle atrophy, and therefore nerve grafts alone will be inadequate for reanimation. Grafting of the entire neuromuscular unit, such as gracilis free tissue transfer, will then be necessary.

Nerve Excitability and Maximum Stimulation Tests

NET and MSTs are tests of facial function that have been largely supplanted by ENoG in today's clinical practice. First introduced by Laumans and Jongkees in 1963 [10], NET uses a stimulating bipolar electrode to deliver successively higher current levels at the stylomastoid foramen until the technician notes a facial twitch. This is done for both the normal and lesioned sides, and the minimum current threshold required to elicit facial motion is compared between the two sides. A difference of 2–3.5 mA has been proposed as a sign of severe degeneration and predicts complete versus incomplete recovery with 80% accuracy [10].

MST also uses a stimulating current delivered at the stylomastoid foramen to elicit facial movement, but in contrast to NET, suprathreshold, maximal current levels are used. On the unaffected side, the current level is increased incrementally until no further increase in the magnitude of facial movement is seen. This current level is then used to stimulate the affected side, and the relative difference in the magnitude of facial movement is then noted and scored using a standardized rubric [28]. MST has also been found to have prognostic value in Bell's palsy; patients with marked reduction of facial movement on MST had 86% chance of incomplete recovery [29].

One weakness of both NET and MST is that subjective visual detection of facial movement is required. In contrast, ENoG records quantitative CMAP amplitudes as a marker of nerve function. Correlation between ENoG and NET has also been shown by some authors [15]. For these reasons, NET and MST are seldom used today for clinical decision-making in acute facial palsy.

Conclusions

Electrophysiological testing of the facial nerve provides significant diagnostic and prognostic information, with important treatment implications. Understanding the differential clinical role of various test modalities requires an understanding of the neuromuscular physiology on which they rely. In acute facial paralysis, ENoG is most useful in providing prognostic information on the severity and trajectory of neural degeneration. EMG is then used as a confirmatory test for those with severe-enough degeneration (≥90%) to warrant consideration for surgical decompression. In the chronic phase of paralysis, EMG provides valuable information on presence or absence of regeneration and helps select the most suitable option for facial reanimation. Their complementary roles are used in concert to optimize the diagnosis and management of patients with facial palsy.

References

1. Peitersen E. Bell's palsy: the spontaneous course of 2,500 peripheral facial nerve palsies of different etiologies. Acta Otolaryngol Suppl. 2002;122:4–30.
2. Seddon HJ, Medawar PB, Smith H. Rate of regeneration of peripheral nerves in man. J Physiol. 1943;102:191–215.
3. Sunderland S, Cossar DF. The structure of the facial nerve. Anat Rec. 1953;116:147–65.
4. May S. The facial nerve. 2nd ed. Thieme Publishers; 2000.
5. Duchenne GB. Mécanisme de la physionomie humaine, ou analyse électro-physiologique de ses différents modes de l'expression. Paris: Ve Jules Renouard, libraire; 1862.
6. Gantz BJ, Gmuer AA, Holliday M, et al. Electroneurographic evaluation of the facial nerve. Method and technical problems. Ann Otol Rhinol Laryngol. 1984;93:394–8.
7. Weddell G, Feinstein B, Pattle RE. The electrical activity of voluntary muscle in man under normal and pathological conditions. Brain. 1944;67:178.
8. Taverner D. Bell's palsy: a clinical and electromyographic study. Brain. 1955;78:209–28.
9. Campbell ED, Hickey RP, Nixon KH, et al. Value of nerve-excitability measurements in prognosis of facial palsy. Br Med J. 1962;2:7–10.
10. Laumans EP, Jongkees LB. On the prognosis of peripheral facial paralysis of endotemporal origin. Ann Otol Rhinol Laryngol. 1963;72:621–36.
11. Laumans EP, Jongkees LB. On the prognosis of peripheral facial paralysis of endotemporal origin. III. Ann Otol Rhinol Laryngol. 1963;72:894–9.
12. Esslen E. Electromyography and electroneurography. In: Fisch U, editor. Facial Nerve Surgery. Birmingham: Aesculapius; 1977. p. 93–100.

13. Schularick NM, Mowry SE, Soken H, et al. Is electroneurography beneficial in the management of Bell's palsy? Laryngoscope. 2013;123:1066–7.
14. Blumenthal F, May M. Electrodiagnosis. In: May M, editor. The facial nerve. New York: Thieme; 1986.
15. Coker NJ. Facial electroneurography: analysis of techniques and correlation with degenerating motoneurons. Laryngoscope. 1992;102:747–59.
16. Hughes GB, Josey AF, Glasscock ME, et al. Clinical electroneurography: statistical analysis of controlled measures in twenty-two normal subjects. Laryngoscope. 1981;91:1834–46.
17. Esslen E. The acute facial palsies: investigations on the localization and pathogenesis of meato-labyrinthine facial palsies. Berlin: Springer-Verlag; 1976.
18. Fisch U. Maximal nerve excitability testing vs electroneuronography. Arch Otolaryngol. 1980;106:352–7.
19. Gantz BJ, Rubinstein JT, Gidley P, et al. Surgical management of Bell's palsy. Laryngoscope. 1999;109:1177–88.
20. Gavilan J, Gavilan C, Sarria MJ. Facial electroneurography: results on normal humans. J Laryngol Otol. 1985;99:1085–8.
21. Thomander L, Stalberg E. Electroneurography in the prognostication of Bell's palsy. Acta Otolaryngol. 1981;92:221–37.
22. Sillman JS, Niparko JK, Lee SS, et al. Prognostic value of evoked and standard electromyography in acute facial paralysis. Otolaryngol Head Neck Surg. 1992;107:377–81.
23. Kartush JM, Lilly DJ, Kemink JL. Facial electroneurography: clinical and experimental investigations. Otolaryngol Head Neck Surg. 1985;93:516–23.
24. Fisch U, Esslen E. Total intratemporal exposure of the facial nerve. Pathologic findings in Bell's palsy. Arch Otolaryngol. 1972;95:335–41.
25. Byun H, Cho YS, Jang JY, et al. Value of electroneurography as a prognostic indicator for recovery in acute severe inflammatory facial paralysis: a prospective study of Bell's palsy and Ramsay Hunt syndrome. Laryngoscope. 2013;123:2526–32.
26. Fisch U. Prognostic value of electrical tests in acute facial paralysis. Am J Otol. 1984;5:494–8.
27. Honda N, Yanagihara N, Hato N, et al. Swelling of the intratemporal facial nerve in Ramsay Hunt syndrome. Acta Otolaryngol. 2002;122:348–52.
28. May M, Blumenthal F, Klein SR. Acute Bell's palsy: prognostic value of evoked electromyography, maximal stimulation, and other electrical tests. Am J Otol. 1983;5:1–7.
29. May M, Hardin WB, Sullivan J, et al. Natural history of Bell's palsy: the salivary flow test and other prognostic indicators. Laryngoscope. 1976;86:704–12.

Temporal Bone Imaging

15

Geoffrey C. Casazza, H. Ric Harnsberger, and Richard K. Gurgel

Introduction

The temporal bone is a complex anatomical region of the skull base harboring a diverse range of pathologic processes. Advances in diagnostic equipment and technique have enhanced the role of imaging in the assessment of temporal bone pathology. While computed tomography (CT) and magnetic resonance imaging (MRI) are the most frequently used modalities to assess the temporal bone and central auditory-vestibular pathways, other modalities, including angiography and nuclear imaging, have a role in evaluating temporal bone pathology. This chapter will address common temporal bone pathology and the role imaging plays in the diagnosis, treatment, and surveillance of these conditions.

Computed Tomography

CT is a radiographic technique that uses ionizing radiation to image patients. A well-collimated beam of ionizing radiation is passed through the area of interest. The beam is partially absorbed or scattered as it passes through the patient with tissues of varying thickness and density attenuating the beam to variable degrees. A bank of detectors arranged circumferentially around the patient measures the non-absorbed portion of the radiation and outputs a digital signal by measuring the amount of ionizing radiation absorbed by each pixel, or volumetric imaging unit (voxel), of tissue. Each voxel is assigned a numeric unit, also called a Hounsfield unit (HU), and displayed in a gray scale matrix resulting in a cross-sectional anatomic image. Various algorithms can then be applied to better evaluate different tissue types, and images can be reformatted for viewing the axial, coronal, sagittal, and oblique planes. Modern helical or spiral CT allows for continuous image acquisition as the beam and detectors continuously rotate around the patient, improving spatial resolution and allowing for large tissue volumes to be imaged with a reduced scan time. Using this technique, the entirety of the temporal bone can be imaged in ultrathin sections (≤1 mm) in less than 1 min.

CT provides excellent bony detail of the temporal bone, and it is the imaging modality of choice when evaluating patients with conductive hearing loss or those who sustained a traumatic injury. CT can also demonstrate variations in soft tissue density within the external auditory canal, middle ear, and air spaces of the mastoid; however, its application is limited to identification of a substance producing an abnormal density. Measuring the HUs of an unknown density can aid in its identification (water is assigned a HU value of 0). An intravenous infusion or bolus of contrast, which increases the density or enhancement of certain anatomic or pathologic processes, is used in CT to highlight specific structures. Contrast is commonly used in the evaluation of vascular anomalies, tumors, or infection.

MRI

MRI is a technologically advanced and complex imaging modality that uses the response of hydrogen atoms in biologic tissue to an applied and changing magnetic field to generate images. Most clinical MRI units use a field strength of 1.5 or 3 tesla (T). In general, the higher the field strength, the better the image quality. When the patient is placed into a strong magnetic field, protons within the soft tissue align

G. C. Casazza · R. K. Gurgel (✉)
Department of Otolaryngology—Head and Neck Surgery, University of Utah School of Medicine, Salt Lake City, UT, USA
e-mail: richard.gurgel@hsc.utah.edu

H. R. Harnsberger
Department of Radiology, University of Utah, Salt Lake City, UT, USA

A. D. Sweeney et al. (eds.), *Haynes-Glasscock-Shambaugh Surgery of the Ear*, https://doi.org/10.1007/978-3-032-18264-7_15

along with the polarity of the field. A radiofrequency pulse is applied to the patient, displacing protons from alignment. When the pulse is terminated, the displaced protons realign with the magnetic field, and a radiofrequency signal is released that can be detected by an array of receiving coils. The strength of the released radiofrequency signal is dependent on the concentration of hydrogen atoms within the area of interest and two tissue-specific magnet relaxation times, T1 and T2, respectively.

T1-weighted (T1W) sequences provide excellent soft tissue contrast with high signal-to-noise ratio. Fat is high signal intensity (bright), while air, bone, rapid blood flow, and other fluid-filled structures including CSF are low signal intensity (dark) on T1W imaging. The high contrast of fat relative to adjacent structures provides contrast to define planes between muscle, blood vessels, nerves, and mass lesions that abut tissue fat. Most head and neck lesions will have a comparable signal to muscle on T1W imaging. The combination of T1W and T2-weighted (T2W) imaging is useful for characterizing fluid-containing structures, solid masses, and hemorrhage within the head and neck. In T2W imaging, CSF, inflammatory processes, and mucosal surfaces are high signal intensity (bright) relative to the low or intermediate intensity (dark) of muscle and fat. Most head and neck masses are higher in signal intensity when compared to their low or intermediate signal on T1W imaging. Gadolinium contrast enhancement is often used in combination with T1W imaging to improve identification of pathologic processes relative to the lower signal intensity of surrounding muscle. Because fat is also hyperintense on T1W imaging and can obscure the contrast-enhanced lesion, gadolinium is commonly used with specific fat suppression techniques that turn fat dark. Gadolinium also enhances normal structures, including nasal and pharyngeal mucosa, lymphoid tissue, extraocular muscles, and slow-flowing blood. Gadolinium contrast should be used with caution in patients with decreased glomerular filtration rates (less than 30 mL/min/body surface area) as it can induce fatal nephrogenic systemic fibrosis.

MRI has the distinct advantage over CT in evaluation of fine soft tissue details without exposing the patient to ionizing radiation; however, longer imaging time, patient discomfort, and significant cost can limit its application. MRI is the imaging modality of choice with evaluating patients with sensorineural hearing loss or facial nerve symptoms. Most temporal bone MRI protocols use a combination of thin-cut pre-contrast T1W and T2W imaging to demonstrate the anatomy and evaluate for high-signal lesions. Contrast-enhanced T1W imaging with fat suppression can be used to evaluate for meningiomas or schwannomas along the course of the seventh and eighth cranial nerves. High-resolution T2W imaging is useful in examining the cranial nerves as they exit the brain stem and extend through the cistern and into the skull base. Other MRI sequences, including diffusion-weighted imaging (DWI) and apparent diffusion coefficient (ADC), can be helpful in identifying various soft tissue lesions of the temporal bone.

Angiography

Although not usually required for diagnosis of vascular tumors or anomalies, angiography can be helpful in defining feeding vessels for vascular tumors of the temporal bone. Contrast injection is usually performed through the common carotid to visualize both the internal and external carotid flow. Subtraction techniques can be used to remove the dense surrounding bone from the vascular tumor. Similar techniques can be used in the diagnosis of small, dural arteriovenous malformation not evident on conventional radiography. Development of magnetic resonance angiography (MRA) and CT angiography (CTA) can be used to evaluate vascular structures in three dimensions after electronic removal of bone and soft tissue. MRA can be useful in the demonstration of small dural arteriovenous malformation not evident on conventional MRI or vaso-occlusive pathology, including dural venous thrombosis.

Nuclear Imaging

In contrast to the other previously discussed imaging modalities, nuclear imaging provides important physiologic and biochemical information regarding tissue function. In evaluating temporal bone pathology, the main applications include positron emission tomography (PET) and skeletal (bone) scintigraphy. Both techniques rely on the use of radiotracers to demonstrate tissue metabolic activity. Generated data can be combined with CT to provide anatomical localization of increased uptake. The indium-tagged white blood cell scan uses the patient's own white blood cells, removed and tagged with indium 24 h prior to imaging, to evaluate areas of active infection. These techniques are helpful in the diagnosis and management of highly metabolic lesions, specifically metastatic disease, perineural invasion, and osteogenic infections of the temporal bone and skull base.

Anatomic Variations

The temporal bone is a heterogeneous structure. Anatomic variations in the size and position of normal structures are commonly encountered and should not be mistaken for a pathologic process. An understanding of these common anatomical variations will aid in diagnosis and treatment.

Mastoid

Mastoid development is variable, and extensive pneumatization, involving the petrous apex, mastoid tip, and squamosal temporal bone and even extending into the adjacent zygoma and occipital bone, may be seen in some patients, whereas in others, pneumatization may be limited to a single antral cell (Fig. 15.1). The non-pneumatized portions of the temporal bone may be made up of solid or diploic bone or filled with fatty marrow. Adult bone marrow is hyperintense on T1W imaging but hypointense on the T2W sequence; this pattern should be distinguished from fluid or from a pathologic process, which will often have a high signal intensity on T2W imaging.

Tegmen

The tegmen is the roof of the mastoid and the attic of the middle ear. It is usually oriented in the horizontal plane at a level just below the arcuate eminence. A low hanging tegmen, represented by the floor of the middle fossa deepening to form a groove lateral to the attic and labyrinth, is not an uncommon finding. In patients with congenital aural atresia, a stenotic external auditory canal may medialize a low hanging tegmen, causing it to dip laterally into the mesotympanum (Fig. 15.2).

Petrous Apex

Similar to the mastoid, variable petrous apex pneumatization is common. Asymmetric pneumatization, marrow replacement, and trapped fluid are identifiable based on characteristic imaging qualities. Whenever possible, fat-suppressed T1W MRI or CT should be used to distinguish these lesions from pathologic processes. These lesions are considered "leave me alone" lesions and generally are not managed surgically, though the surgeon may use clinical judgment if the patient is symptomatic.

Jugular Fossa

The jugular fossa is a depression on the inferior surface of the petrous temporal bone posterior to the inferior opening of the carotid canal. The size and contour of the jugular fossa can vary. A normal jugular fossa may only make a slight indentation into the petrous temporal bone or may extend superiorly up to the petrous ridge. The right jugular bulb is dominant in most patients. Often the jugular bulb can be lateralized or enlarged and extend into the hypotympanum or mesotympanum. There may be a bony cover over the vein, or it can be exposed within the middle ear and contact the tympanic membrane (Fig. 15.3). This may lead to misdiagnosis as a jugular paraganglioma on otoscopy or manifest as intractable bleeding during tympanostomy tube placement. A dehiscent jugular bulb may also extend superiorly to the superior petrosal ridge or laterally into the middle ear space. This can be a cause of pulsatile tinnitus in some patients. Slow or turbulent flow through the jugular bulb can create flow voids that can be misinterpreted as a glomus tumor on MRI. In contrast to the multiple small dots of signal voids in glomus tumors, linear streaks paralleling the walls of the jugular bulb are seen in a pathologically normal high-riding jugular bulb.

Carotid Artery

The intratemporal course of the carotid artery can be variable with little or no clinical significance. Occasionally the carotid artery may be displaced laterally, following an ectopic course through the middle ear. This aberrant internal carotid artery

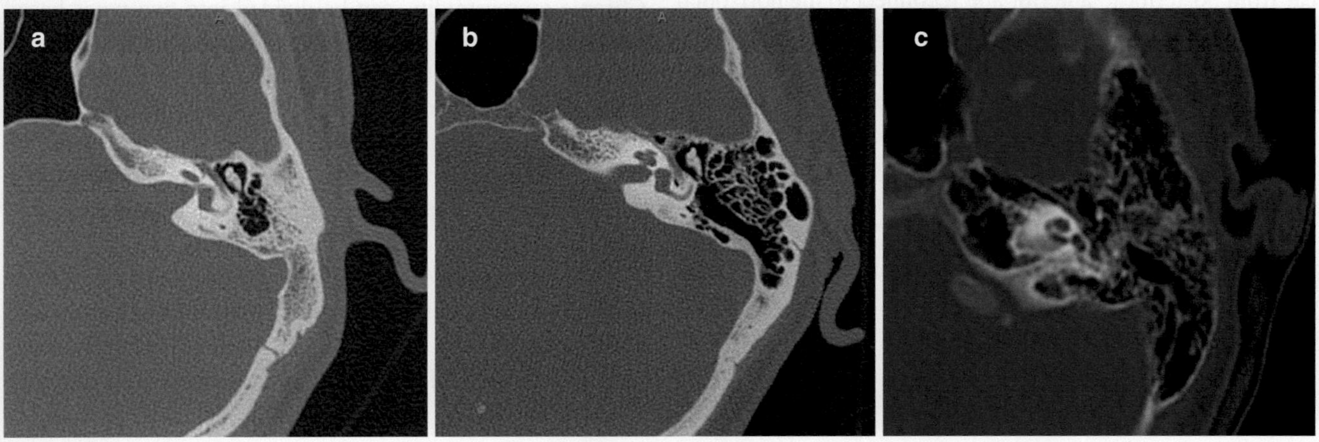

Fig. 15.1 Axial left bone CT's demonstrating variable mastoid pneumatization in otherwise healthy patients; (**a**) contracted, (**b**) normal, (**c**) extensive

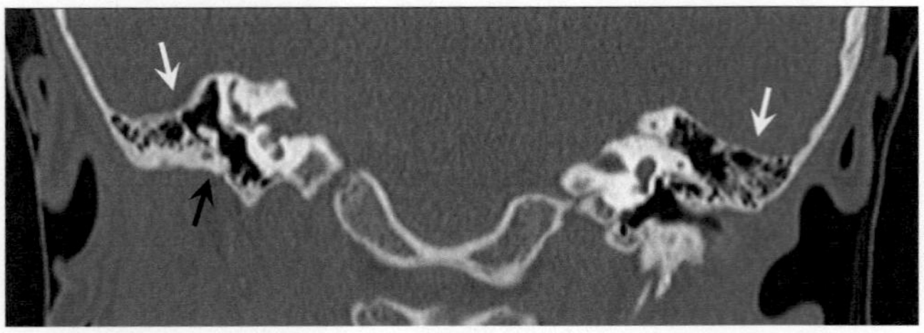

Fig. 15.2 Coronal temporal bone CT demonstrates down-sloping lateral tegmen seen in a child with congenital aural atresia (white arrow). There is normal middle ear anatomy (black arrow)

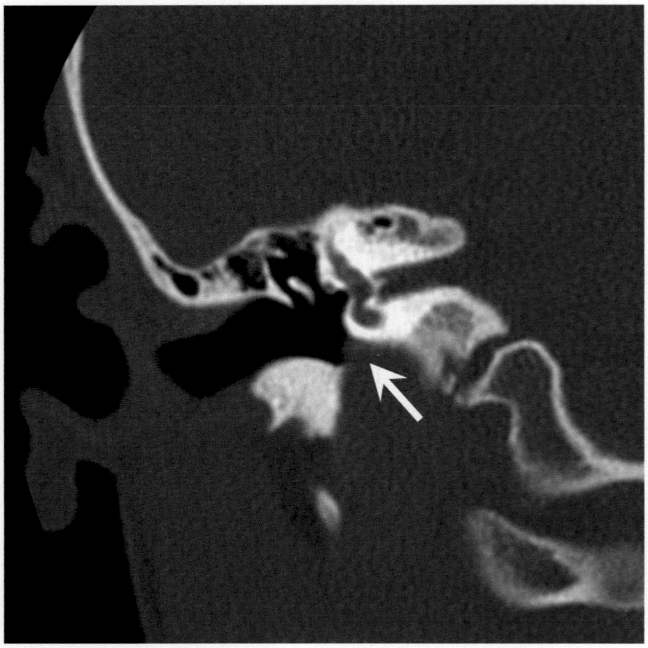

Fig. 15.3 Coronal right temporal bone CT demonstrating a high-riding jugular bulb with a dehiscent sigmoid plate resulting in protrusion of the jugular bulb (white arrow) into the mesotympanum

will enter the middle ear via an enlarged inferior tympanic canaliculus or through an opening in the floor of the hypotympanum. The artery will course the entirety of the middle ear from posterior to anterior and reconnect to the horizontal petrous ICA along its posterolateral margin (Fig. 15.4). The position of the artery coursing over the cochlear promontory can be easily mistaken as a glomus tympanicum, especially on the coronal CT view. The tubular shape, as represented on three-dimensional imaging, is the key observation distinguishing an aberrant carotid artery from a glomus tumor. Patients with an aberrant carotid artery will often be asymptomatic, and this will be discovered on routine physical exam, during middle ear surgery, or as an incidental imaging finding. Some patients may report some degree of pulsatile tinnitus or conductive hearing loss.

Arachnoid Granulations

Arachnoid granulations are projections of arachnoid membrane (villi) into the dural sinuses that allow for arachnoid space CSF to enter into the venous system. On CT, granulations are typically of CSF density and will appear as a filling defect within a dural sinus. MRI signal characteristics are similar to CSF. Occasionally, arachnoid granulations may contact the intracranial surface of the middle ear or posterior portion of the temporal bone. Over time, small pulsations within the granulations can lead to small areas of bony erosion. Although typically asymptomatic, these can become clinically significant when erosion opens a channel into adjacent air spaces (i.e., the epitympanum or mastoid air cells), which leads to spontaneous CSF otorrhea or serious intracranial complications, including meningitis or brain abscess, if the mastoid or middle ear cavity becomes infected.

Pathologic Conditions

Inflammatory and Infectious

Acute Otomastoiditis

Acute otitis media with mastoiditis is a clinical diagnosis. Initially, otomastoiditis is characterized by nonspecific opacification of the middle ear and mastoid air cells on CT. If the infection progresses, necrotic changes will lead to trabecular coalescence and abscess formation (Fig. 15.5). Erosion of the mastoid cortex can lead to subperiosteal abscess. If the infection erodes through the tegmen or sigmoid plate, intracranial complications including meningitis, epidural and intraparenchymal abscess (Fig. 15.6), and sigmoid sinus thrombosis can develop. While imaging is not required for the initial diagnosis, whenever an intracranial complication is suspected, MRI with contrast should be performed.

Chronic Otomastoiditis

Chronic otomastoiditis can be divided into two types based on the presence or absence of cholesteatoma. The role of imaging has been debated among those who treat chronic otomastoiditis, with some clinicians advocating for the routine use of CT in all operative cases [1], while others feel that imaging should be reserved for those undergoing surgery in an only hearing ear or in those patients with a suspected complication of chronic otitis media (i.e., lateral canal fistula).

Chronic otomastoiditis without cholesteatoma is usually the result of an infection of a low-virulence organism or of an acute infection with incomplete resolution. Changes associated with chronic infection are best evaluated on CT and may

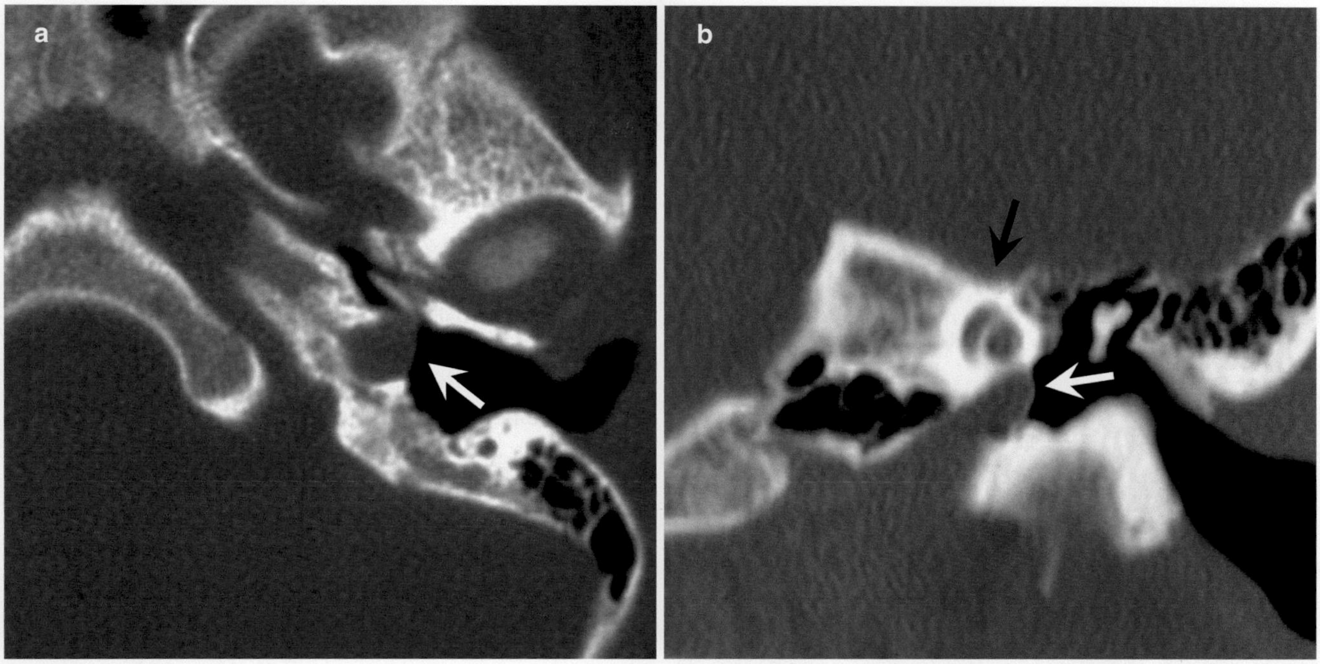

Fig. 15.4 Axial left ear temporal bone CT (**a**) shows a distal cervical ICA with no bony covering along its lateral margin (white arrow). The artery is protruding into the anteroinferior middle ear cavity. On a coronal bone CT (**b**), the left ICA extends more laterally into the middle ear and then the cochlea (black arrow)

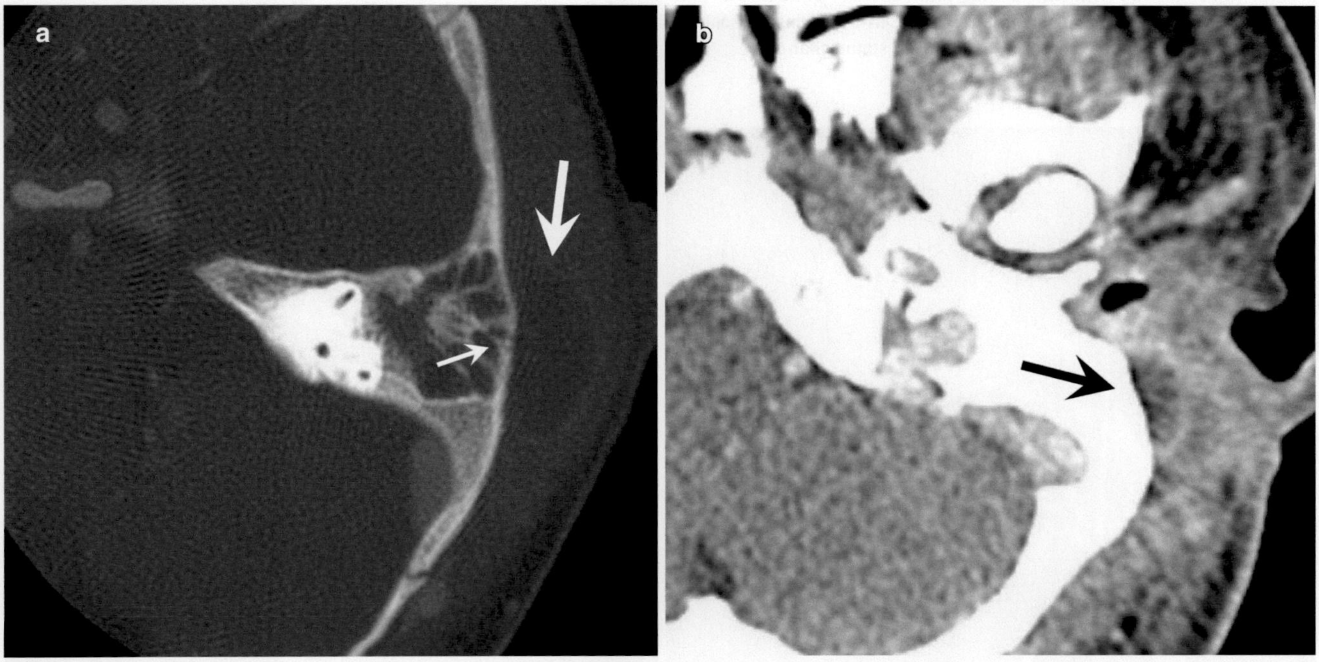

Fig. 15.5 Axial left temporal bone CT (**a**) showing an opacified mastoid with erosion of the mastoid cortex (small white arrow) and a rim enhancing fluid collection (large white arrow). In a different patient a soft tissue CT (**b**) demonstrates a rim-enhancing fluid (black arrow), consistent with a subperiosteal abscess. There is edema of the surrounding soft tissues

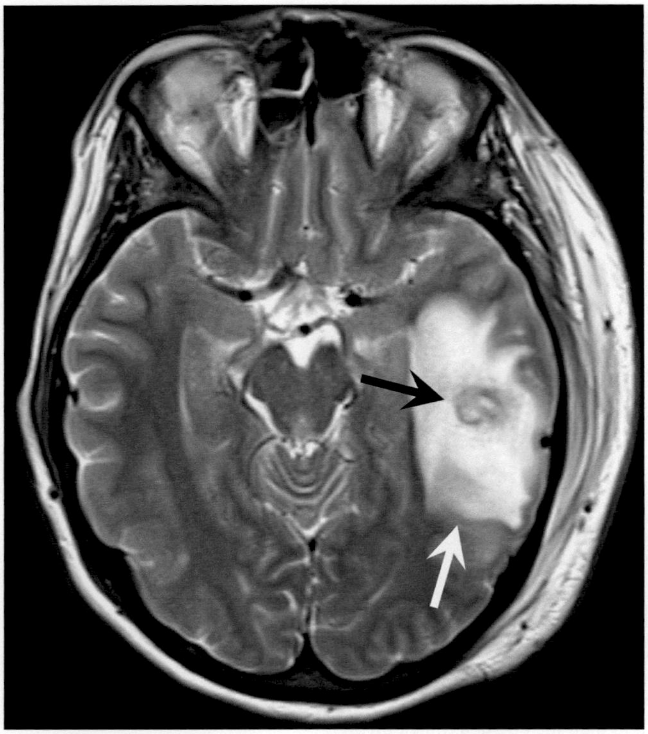

Fig. 15.6 Axial T2W axial MRI demonstrates an intraparenchymal abscess (black arrow) with surrounding brain edema (white arrow) and extensive overlying edema and inflammation in a patient presenting with acute otomastoiditis, seizures, and mental status changes

demonstrate thickening of the mastoid trabeculae, inhomogeneous air cell opacification, and, if no perforation is present, opacification of the middle ear. Over time, the involved air cells will be evident on temporal bone CT as a contracted mastoid with concomitant obliteration. Fluid or soft tissue density may fill the residual air cells, antrum, and middle ear. Ossicular erosion may be evident.

Chronic otomastoiditis with cholesteatoma is characterized by the presence of a cholesteatoma, which is an expansile and erosive lesion usually appearing as a soft tissue mass in the mesotympanum or hypotympanum. CT demonstrates an expansile soft tissue mass with surrounding erosive bony changes. Erosion of the lenticular process of the incus and stapes superstructure as well as enlargement of the attic, aditus, and mastoid antrum are common. Extension into the mastoid air cells leads to erosion of the bony trabeculae and similar findings of chronic otomastoiditis without cholesteatoma, including mastoid contraction and obliteration (Fig. 15.7). A labyrinthine fistula can result from involvement of the medial wall (Fig. 15.8). The ampullated limb of the lateral semicircular canal is the most common site of fistula formation. Axial and coronal oblique sections through the middle ear will demonstrate thinning or absence of the bone covering the lateral canal and flattening of the medial wall of the epitympanic recess due to erosion of the normal protuberance of the lateral

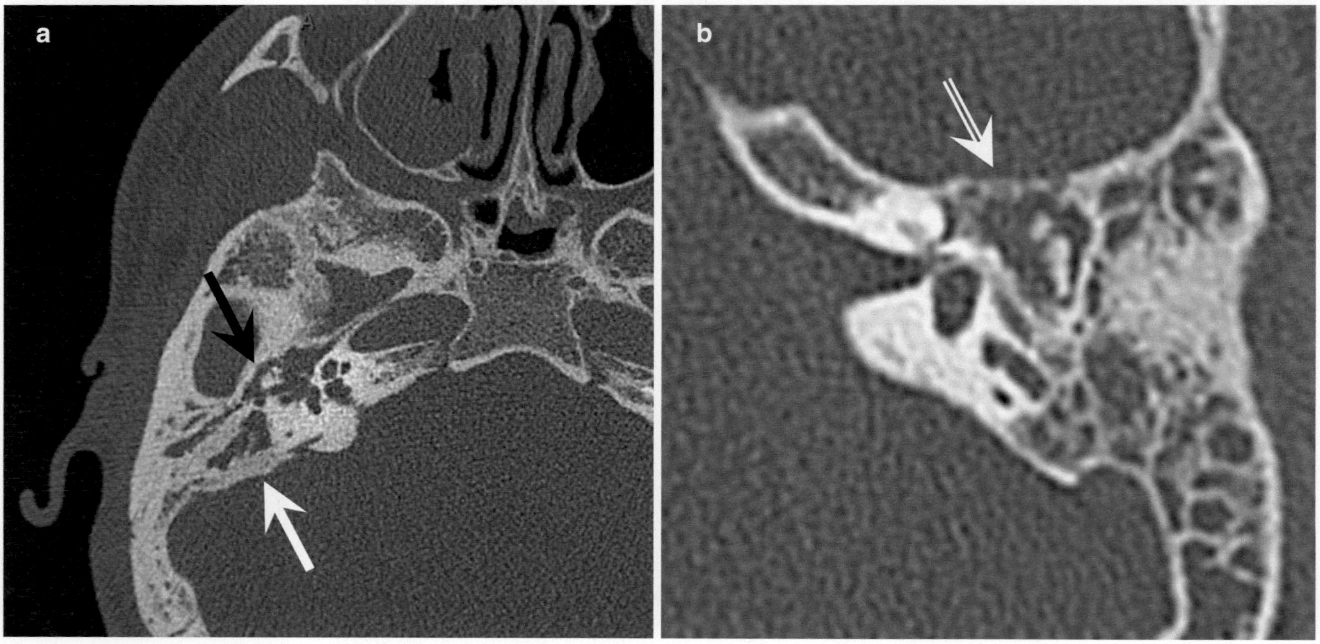

Fig. 15.7 Axial bone CT (**a**) through the right temporal bone demonstrating a contracted right mastoid with evidence of bony remodeling and thickening (single white arrow). There is a fluid density extending from the middle ear and into the mastoid with ossicular erosion (black arrow). In a different patient, an axial CT (**b**) demonstrates lateral displacement of the left ossicular chain (double white arrow) consistent with epitympanic cholesteatoma

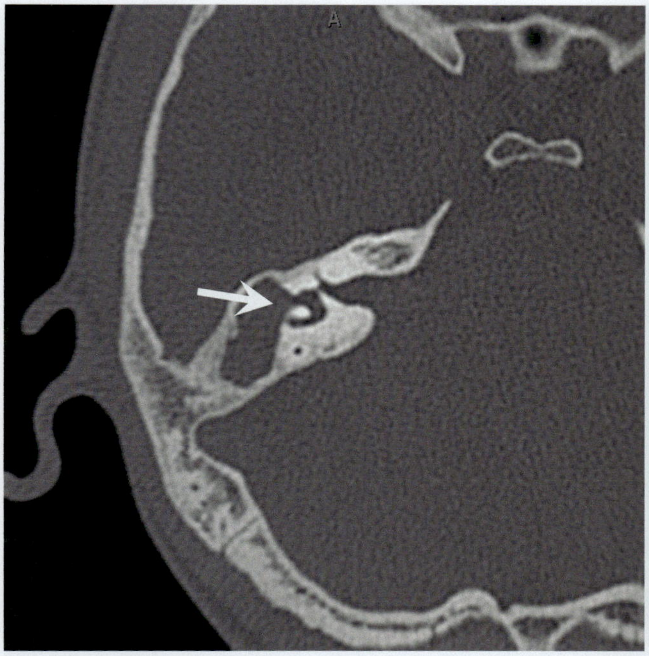

Fig. 15.8 Axial right temporal bone CT demonstrates a soft tissue mass filling the middle ear. Erosion of the entire ossicular chain and dehiscence of lateral semicircular canal have occurred (white arrow). Diagnosis of cholesteatoma was confirmed, and the patient underwent a canal wall down mastoidectomy

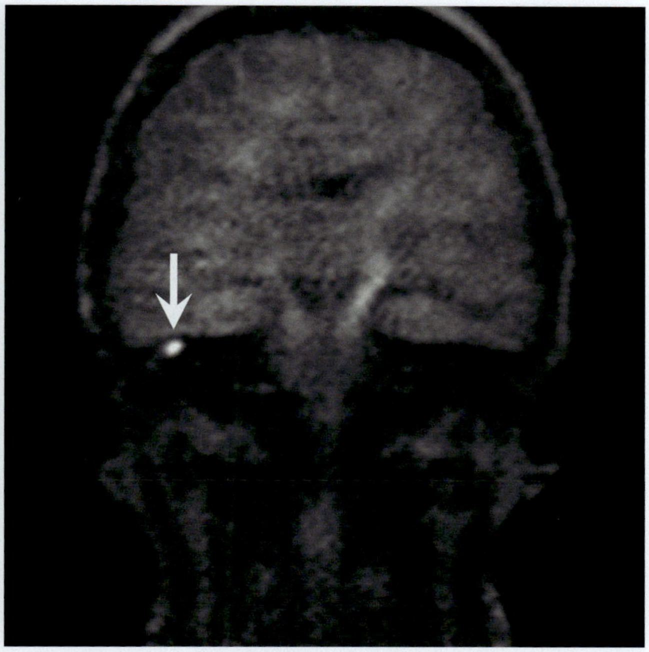

Fig. 15.9 Coronal MRI diffusion-weighted sequence (DWI) demonstrates marked hyperintensity (white arrow), consistent with cholesteatoma

canal. When fluid or inflammatory tissue fills the middle ear, the contour of the cholesteatoma can be obscured, limiting the use of CT. In these patients, MRI may be beneficial if clinical suspicion remains high.

Some clinicians have advocated for routine imaging instead of performing "second-look" procedures for residual or recurrent cholesteatoma [2], especially after canal wall up surgeries. Until recently, traditional CT and MRI were unreliable to monitor for cholesteatoma given the inability to differentiate between cholesteatoma and the normal mucosal lining. Improved techniques, including non-echo-planar diffusion-weighted MRI (DWI), are highly sensitive to identify cholesteatoma down to 3 mm in size (Fig. 15.9). While some cholesteatoma recurrence can be clinically evident, MRI can be particularly useful in the setting of an equivocal exam, such as a case when cartilage tympanoplasty has been previously performed and obscures examination of the middle ear and middle ear structures.

Skull Base Osteomyelitis

Skull base osteomyelitis, or necrotizing otitis externa, is a rare but often fatal infection of the temporal bone. The disease most commonly develops in diabetic or immunocompromised patients and is typically caused by *Pseudomonas aeruginosa*. The condition leads to severe otalgia and granulation tissue at the bony-cartilaginous junction of the external auditory canal. Eventually the infection will break through the floor of the external auditory canal at the bony-cartilaginous junction and spread along the floor of the temporal bone to involve the facial nerve at the stylomastoid foramen and lower cranial nerves at the jugular foramen.

Early in the clinical course, CT and MRI may be normal or show nonspecific deep nasopharyngeal and skull base enhancement (Fig. 15.10). If the clinical suspicion for skull base osteomyelitis is high, a technetium-99 m (Tc99m) bone scintigraphy will establish the diagnosis. Enhancement on Tc99m will lag behind clinical resolution of the infection, so serial gallium scintigraphy (Fig. 15.11) or indium-tagged white blood cell scans (Fig. 15.12) are used to follow patient recovery and are obtained until radiographic resolution of the infection. Positron emission tomography (PET) scan with co-registered CT scan has been reported for use in evaluating skull base osteomyelitis. Post-contrasted T1W MRI, while not preferred, is useful to determine the extent of comorbid soft tissue involvement, while pre-contrasted T1W MRI can also be useful in determining if the infection has involved the marrow spaces of the clivus and skull base.

Temporal Bone Trauma

Imaging studies of the temporal bone are necessary for evaluation of cerebrospinal rhinorrhea, hearing loss, or facial paralysis after trauma [3]. CT, including axial, coronal, and oblique sagittal sections, should be performed to define the location, severity of the injury, and any associated injuries

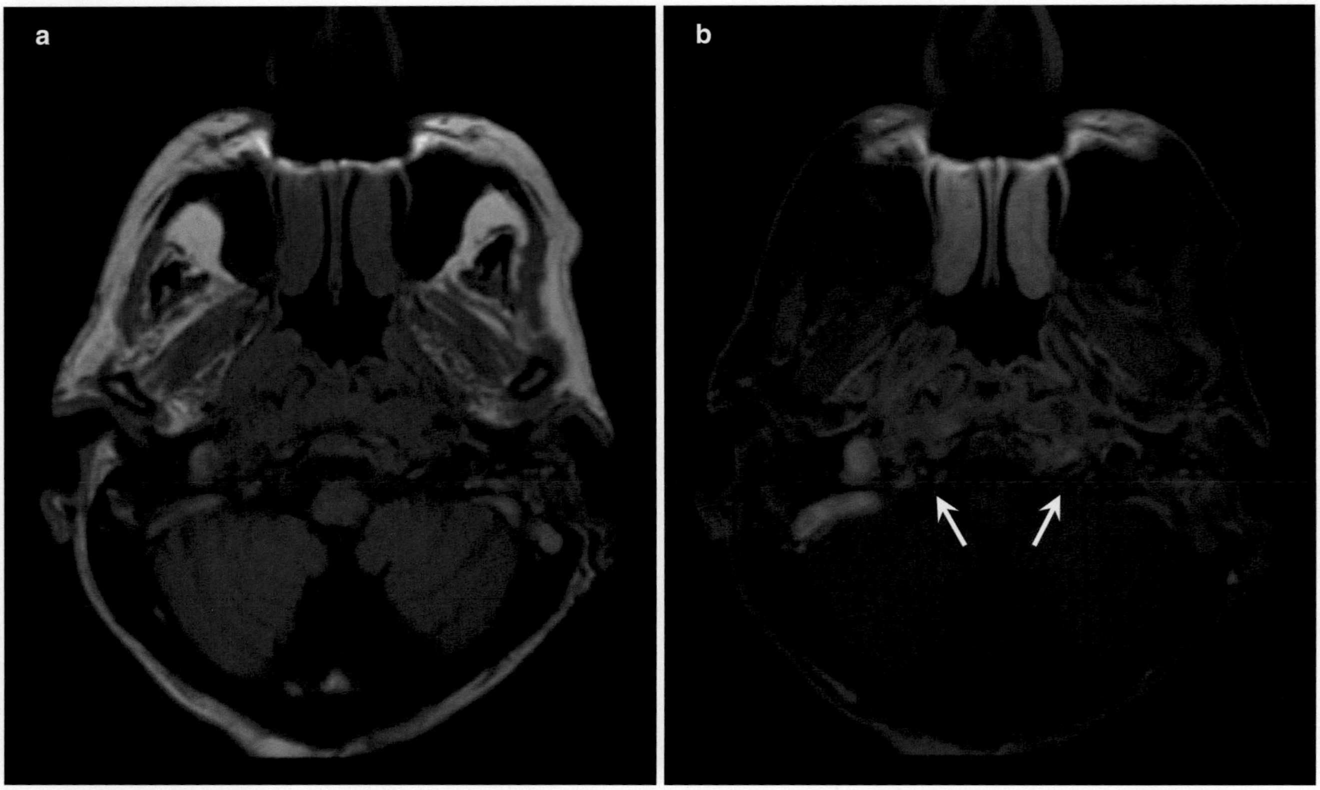

Fig. 15.10 Axial T1W (**a**) and C+ (**b**) MRI demonstrating nonspecific enhancement of the skull base (white arrow) in a patient with skull base osteomyelitis. The diagnosis was biopsy confirmed

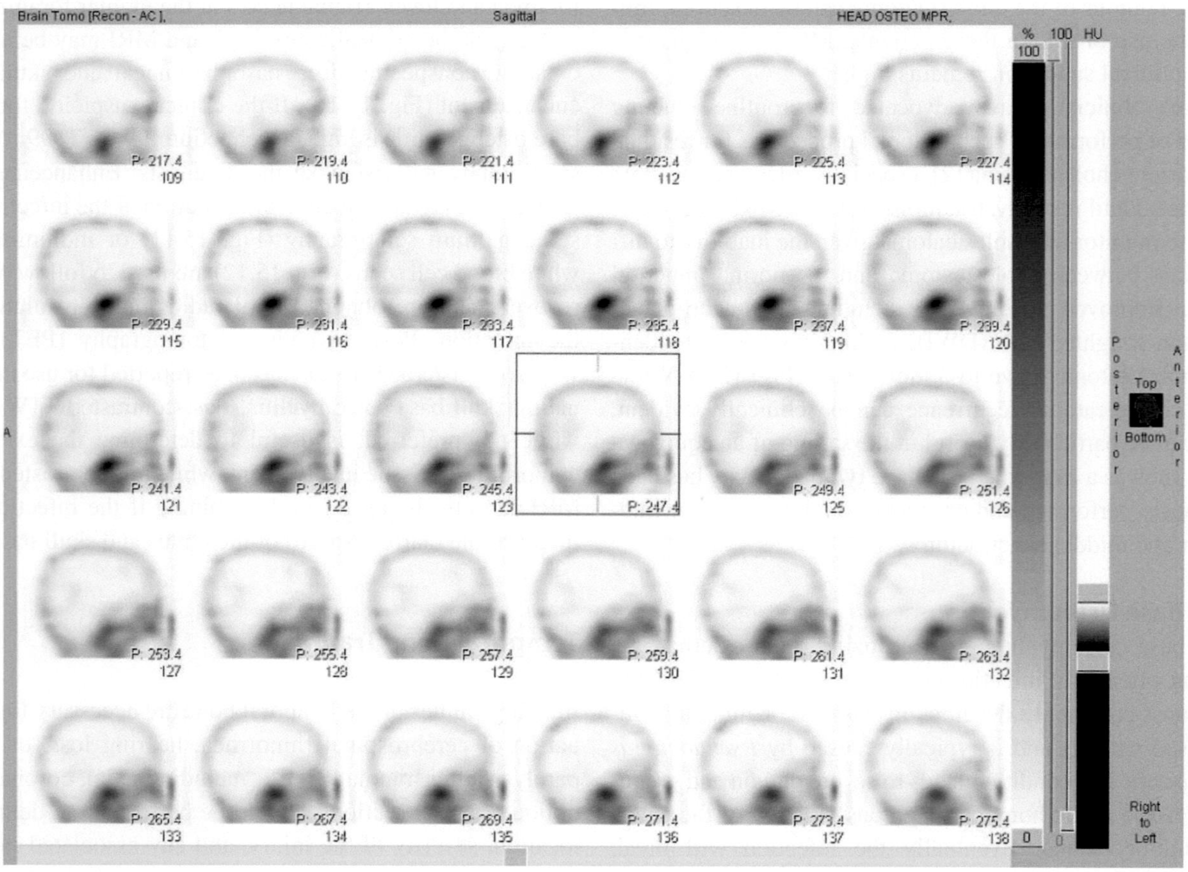

Fig. 15.11 Nuclear medicine gallium scan demonstrating increased uptake in the central skull base in a patient with skull base osteomyelitis

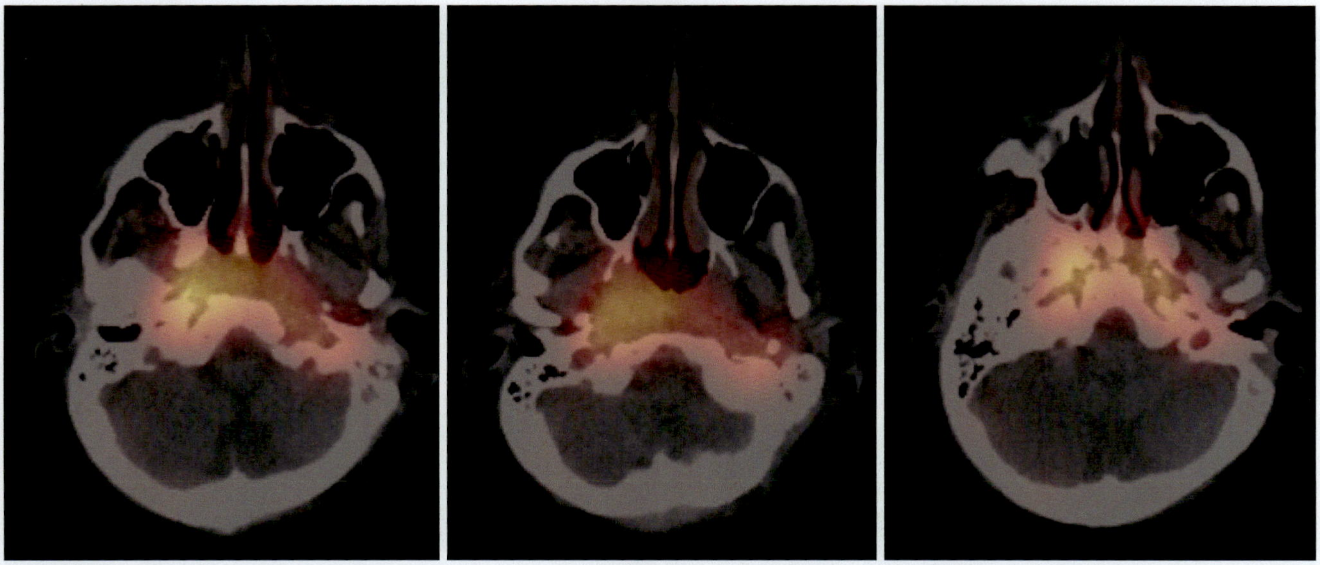

Fig. 15.12 Nuclear medicine indium-tagged white blood cell scan demonstrating increased uptake through multiple slices of the central skull base in a patient with skull base osteomyelitis

including involvement of the facial nerve, labyrinth, ossicles, or vascular structures. Traditionally, temporal bone fractures have been classified as longitudinal (parallel to the long axis of the temporal bone), transverse (perpendicular to the long axis of the temporal bone), or mixed (Fig. 15.13). Longitudinal fractures occur more frequently and are more likely to result in disruption of the ossicular chain, whereas transverse fractures are more likely to cross the course of the facial nerve. Disruption of the ossicular chain is difficult to assess on imaging. The malleus is rarely dislocated due to firm attachments to the tympanic membrane and malleal ligament. Dislocation of the incus is easily recognizable as widening of the incudomalleolar joint (Fig. 15.14), while fractures or dislocations of the stapes superstructure or footplate are seldom recognizable though air can occasionally be visible within the vestibule in this setting. A more current classification is to describe the integrity of the otic capsule [4] (i.e., otic capsule sparing versus involved, rather than fracture orientation). Fractures involving the immediate area surrounding the geniculate ganglion are more likely to lead to facial nerve injury. If the fracture extends toward the petrous portion of the carotid artery, or an injury is suspected, a dedicated CTA is indicated.

Bleeding within the membranous inner ear structures can occur after trauma. If the fracture traverses the otic capsule, then the detection of blood is irrelevant since the patient has an irreversible total deafness and/or vestibular injury; however, if bleeding occurs without fracture, MRI may be indicated to confirm the diagnosis. The study should be performed at least 2 days after the injury to allow for the transformation of deoxyhemoglobin into methemoglobin which has a bright signal on both T1W and T2W MRI.

Meningoceles and meningoencephaloceles are usually post-traumatic following a fracture of the tegmen but also may be iatrogenic after mastoid surgery. The brain and meninges will herniate through the defect and into the middle ear or mastoid antrum. CT can demonstrate a tegmen dehiscence and an adjacent soft tissue mass. The constant pulsation of CSF is transmitted through the walls of the meningocele causing gradual bony erosion and resorption. An MRI can be performed whenever the nature of the mass is unclear. On MRI, a meningocele will have similar signals to CSF, while the signal of an encephalocele will have a similar signal to the surrounding brain.

Congenital Hearing Loss

Congenital hearing loss is one of the most common birth defects in developed countries, occurring in 2–3 per 1000 live births and affecting nearly 28 million Americans [5]. For patients presenting with congenital hearing loss, both a conductive and sensorineural cause should be suspected. Imaging plays a critical role in the diagnosis of congenital hearing loss, and reviews have suggested that temporal bone imaging is cost-effective for evaluation of pediatric hearing loss [6].

Sensorineural

Anomalies of inner ear morphology, including the cochlea, vestibule and semicircular canals, and cochlear nerve, are the primary concern for patients with congenital sensorineural hearing loss (SNHL). A non-contrasted CT provides excellent resolution of the otic capsule and internal auditory canal

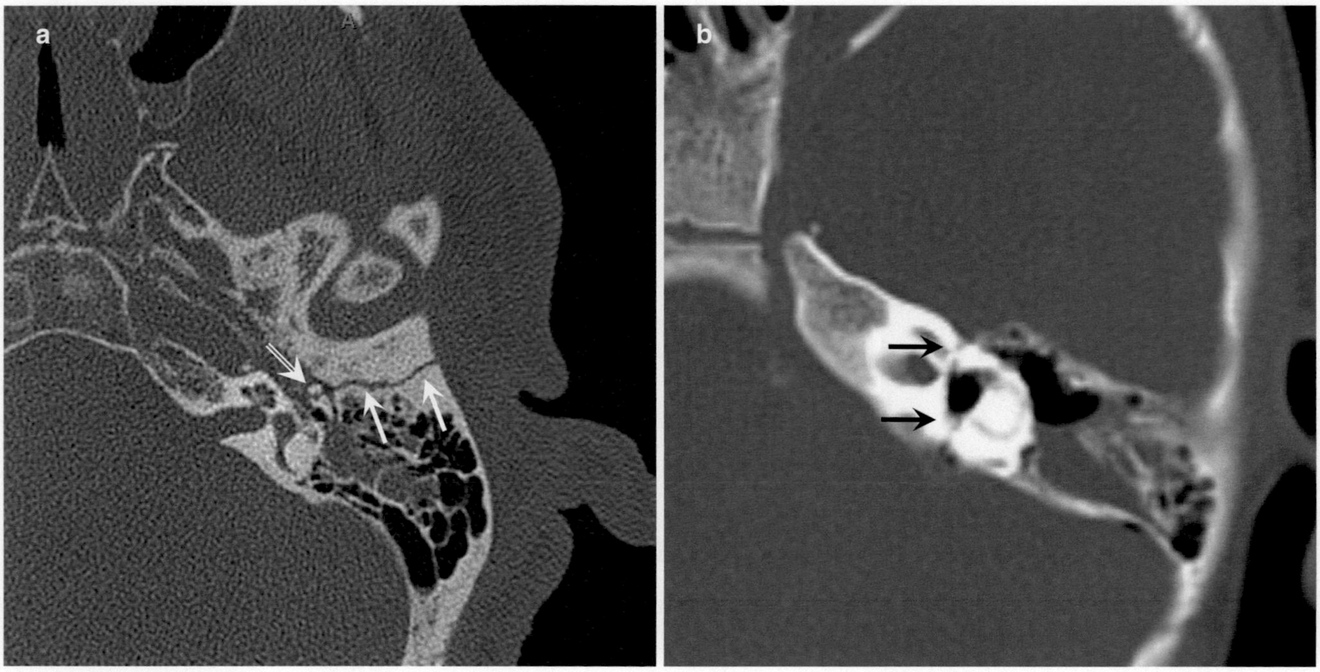

Fig. 15.13 Left axial bone CT (**a**) demonstrates a nondepressed longitudinal temporal bone fracture (single white arrow). The fracture extends through the malleoincudal joint (double white arrow) and spares the otic capsule. In contrast, a left axial bone CT (**b**) demonstrates a nondepressed transverse temporal bone fracture (black arrow) with involvement of the otic capsule and evidence of pneumocochlea

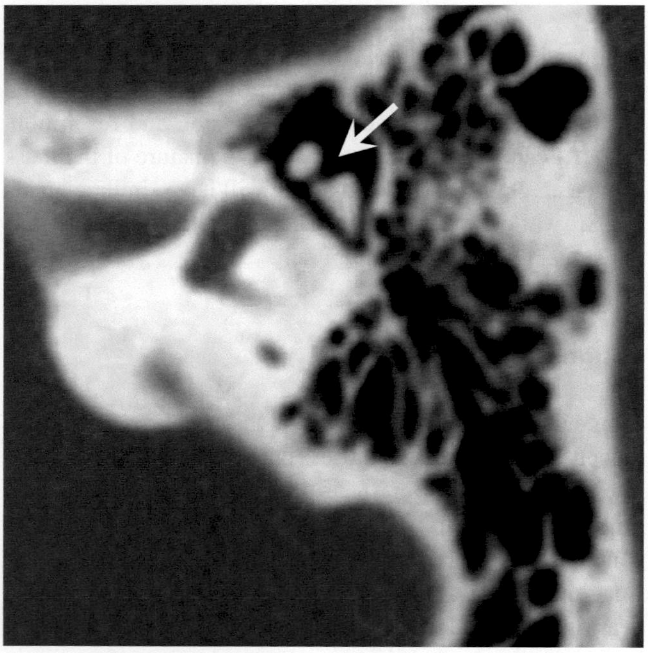

Fig. 15.14 Axial left temporal bone CT showing an abnormal widening of the malleoincudal joint (white arrow) representing a traumatic dislocation between the malleus and incus

and can evaluate for an enlarged vestibular aqueduct. T2W fast-spin echo MRI can detect defects of the membranous labyrinth.

Imaging studies can provide information that alters therapy for those with progressive SNHL. The detection of a large vestibular aqueduct may lead to restrictions of physical activity or any activity that could predispose to head trauma (Fig. 15.15), while in the older child, a retrocochlear lesion may be detected, particularly a vestibular schwannoma possibly associated with neurofibromatosis type II (Fig. 15.16). If there is suspicion of a vestibular schwannoma, a gadolinium-enhanced MRI is indicated. In these patients, multiple cranial nerve tumors may also be evident.

For patients meeting criteria for cochlear implant, preimplant imaging can provide important presurgical planning information, including patency of the cochlea, presence of cochlear malformations, any associated facial nerve anomalies, and the presence of a cochlear nerve. Both CT and MRI should be obtained during preoperative imaging [7]. CT may underestimate cochlear lumen occlusion, particularly if there is a history of meningitis making it possible that labyrinthine ossificans is present. In such a case, high-resolution T2W MRI is recommended to evaluate for the presence or absence

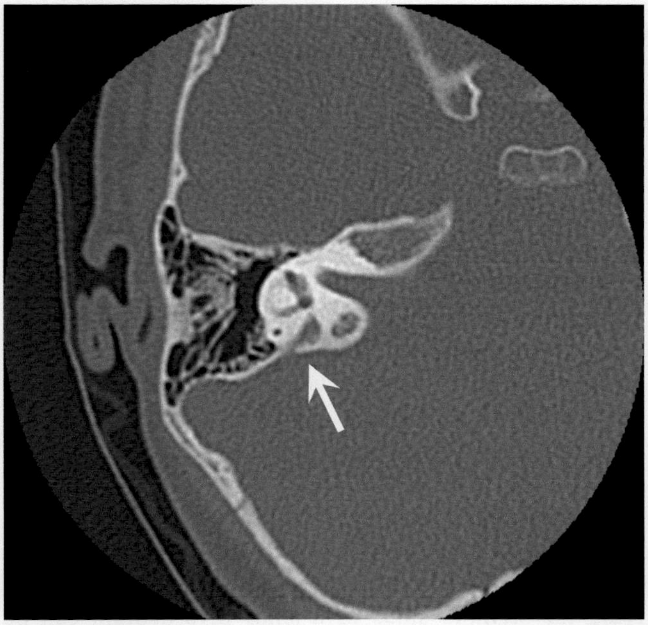

Fig. 15.15 Axial right temporal bone CT demonstrating an enlarged vestibular aqueduct (white arrow) in a 7-year-old patient who presented for evaluation of bilateral severe to profound sensorineural hearing loss

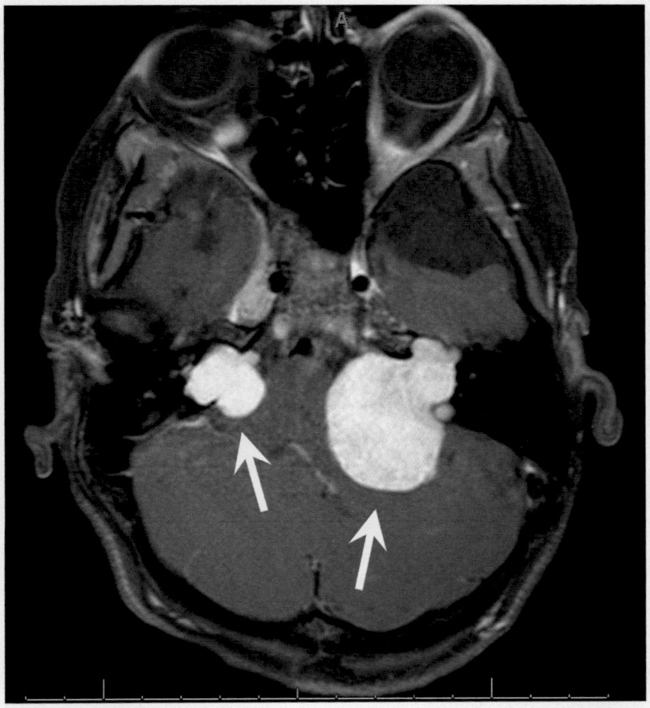

Fig. 15.16 Bilateral vestibular schwannomas seen in a patient with neurofibromatosis type II. Axial T1W C+ MRI reveals large bilateral enhancing vestibular lesions (white arrow)

of fluid within the cochlea. High-resolution T2W MRI with oblique sagittal views of the internal auditory canal (IAC) provides anatomical pictures of the nerves within the IAC to verify the presence of a cochlear nerve. Use of MRI in the pre-cochlear implant screening of children with profound congenital SNHL has the additional benefits of identifying other central nervous system (CNS) abnormalities while avoiding CT-associated radiation; however, contrast enhancement in young children should be avoided, as recent evidence has suggested that gadolinium can accumulate in the brain of patients with intact blood-brain barriers [8]. Long-term sequelae of this accumulation is unknown.

Conductive

Conductive hearing loss (CHL) is a result of abnormalities of the external or middle ear. Imaging can provide insight into any external canal, middle ear, or ossicular chain malformations. Normal imaging may suggest congenital stapes fixation. High-resolution CT scanning is usually recommended for evaluating a young child and prior to surgery for any congenital conductive hearing loss. Abnormalities, including oval window atresia, an anomalous facial nerve over the oval window, and an enlarged vestibular aqueduct (which can also cause a conductive loss), are reasons to consider nonsurgical management of a patient with congenital conductive hearing loss.

Imaging is critical in the evaluation of patients with congenital aural atresia. Jahrsdoerfer and others have shown that hearing results after atresia repair are correlated with the development and presence of specific anatomical features, including the presence of a stapes, a malleus/incus complex, incus to stapes connections, round and oval windows, middle ear space aeration, mastoid pneumatization, and a facial nerve in a favorable location [9, 10]. Imaging, specifically CT, can help identify these structures and is also critical in determining the feasibility of reconstruction, the presence of a coexisting congenital cholesteatoma, and any anatomic information that may facilitate surgery. Imaging should be delayed until the child is old enough to cooperate with the study and not require sedation. For many children, this will be at age 5–6 years, which is the age most surgeons will begin to offer reconstructive surgery.

Pulsatile Tinnitus and Vascular Tumors

For patients presenting with unilateral pulsatile tinnitus, the utility of imaging is dependent on clinical findings and suspicion [11]. MRI and MRA can be used to image intratemporal vascular structures; however, the juxtaposition between low-signal bone, low-contrast air, and flowing blood makes fine detail identification difficult. CT should be used as the initial imaging modality for those presenting with an obvious vascular middle ear mass. If an aberrant carotid artery, dehiscent or high-riding jugular bulb, or paraganglioma (glomus tumor) is identified on initial imaging, no further imaging is required. In cases of paraganglioma with suspected jugular bulb involvement or intracranial extension, a contrast-enhanced MRI will define the tumor margins, while CT can define precise bony surgical landmarks. Large glomus tumors may exhibit a characteristic "salt and pepper" appearance on unenhanced T1W MRI (Fig. 15.17). Subacute hemorrhage within the tumor represents the "salt," while flow voids through the tumor represent the "pepper." Angiography is useful for management of glomus jugulare tumors; however, it is primarily utilized in preoperative embolization rather than diagnostic imaging. Both angiography and CTA can also provide identification of feeding vessels and flow within the jugular vein. Some clinicians have also argued that CT angiography is superior at differentiating between glomus tumors and jugular foramen schwannomas [12].

For patients without a clinically evident middle ear mass but a strong clinical suspicion for a vascular pathology (i.e., pulse-synchronous tinnitus or objective pulsatile tinnitus), CTA and MRA are important imaging modalities, which can detect paragangliomas not visible on clinical exam, demonstrate a dural arteriovenous malformation, or find evidence of internal carotid stenosis. MRA can detect small dural arteriovenous malformations but may miss very small or inconspicuous lesions. If there is sufficient concern for a small dural arteriovenous malformation, the patient should undergo a diagnostic angiography with possible concomitant intervention if an arteriovenous malformation is found. A sigmoid sinus diverticulum or dehiscence (SSDD) can also be a cause of objective, pulse-synchronous tinnitus [13] (Fig. 15.18). Loss of bone overlying the sigmoid sinus or a sinus diverticulum can be identified on CT and can be diagnostic on SSDD if sufficient clinical concern exists [14].

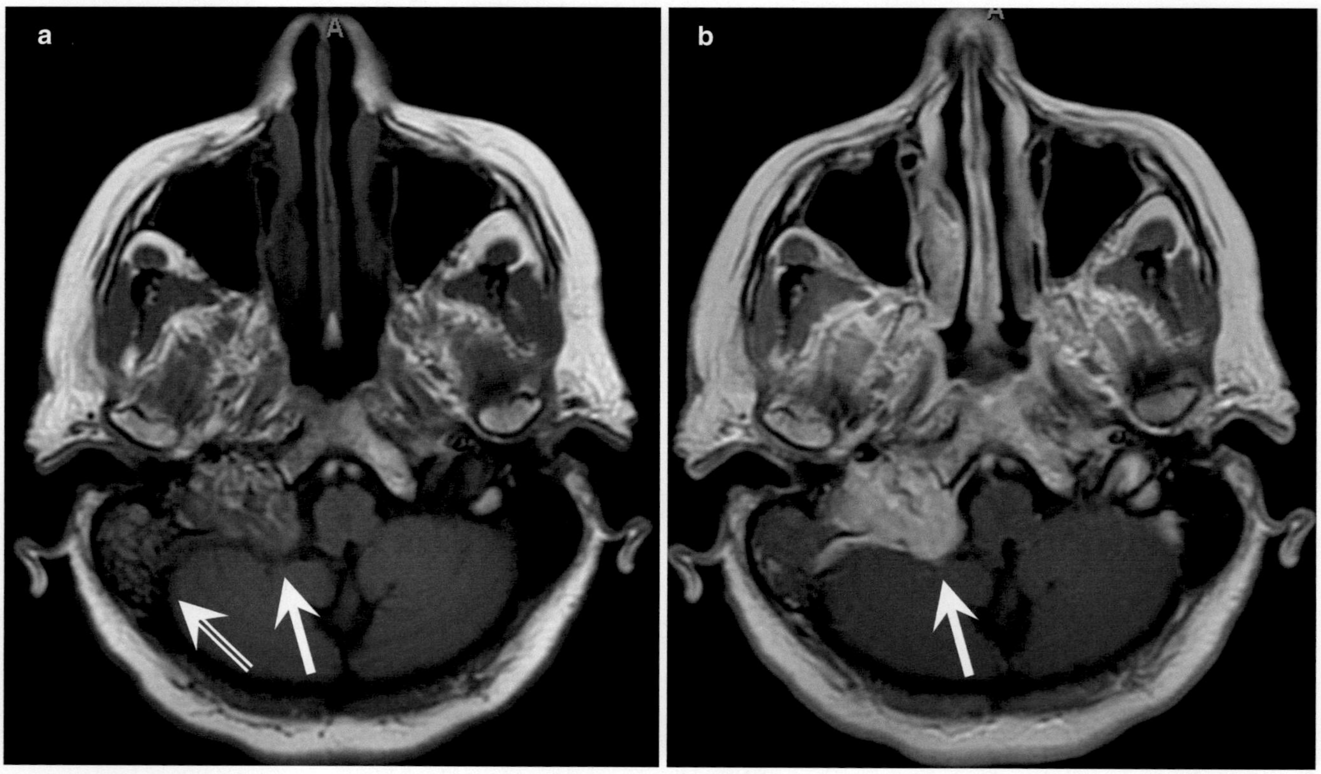

Fig. 15.17 Axial T1W MRI (**a**) demonstrates a large jugular foramen mass (single white arrow) with multiple areas of salt and pepper. The "salt" represents blood products or slow flow, while the "pepper" represents high-velocity arterial flow voids. Axial T1W C+ (**b**) in the same patient shows the classic intense enhancement of vascular glomus tumors (white arrow). There is an associated mastoid effusion due to Eustachian tube dysfunction (double white arrow)

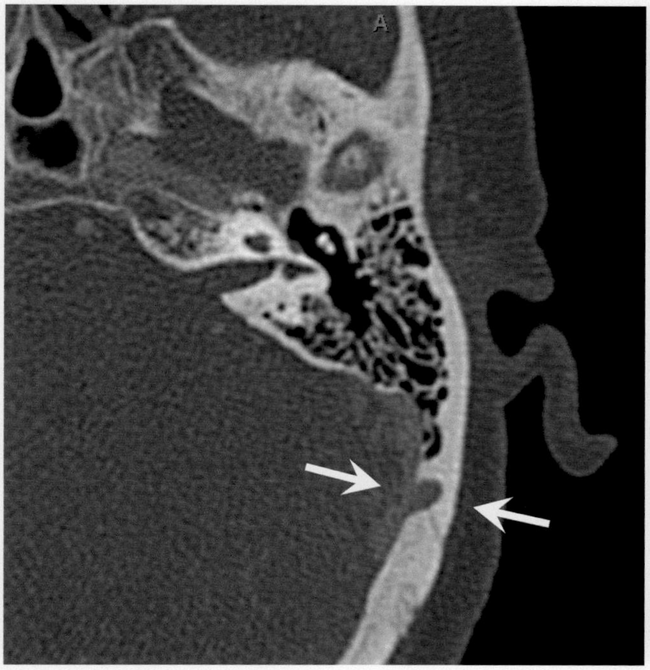

Fig. 15.18 Left axial bone CT reveals a sigmoid sinus diverticulum (white arrow). The patient had a history of pulsatile tinnitus that could be heard by the clinician with a Toynbee stethoscope

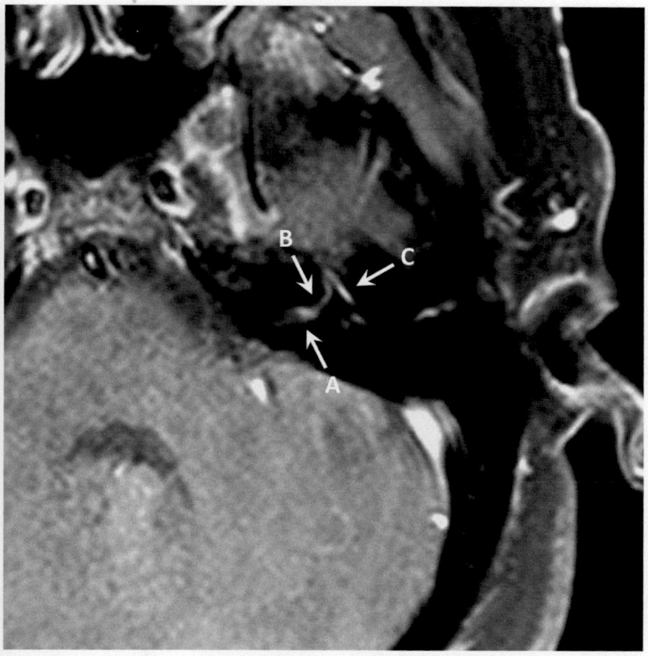

Fig. 15.19 Axial T1W C+ MRI showing classic findings of Bell's palsy including the internal auditory canal (IAC) fundal tuft sign (**a**), labyrinthine (**b**), and tympanic (**c**) facial nerve segment enhancement (white arrow)

Facial Nerve Lesions

Bell's palsy is the most common cause of acute unilateral facial paralysis. Most clinicians will agree that patients with the acute onset of facial paralysis and absence of other symptoms (i.e., parotid mass, voice changes, weight loss, trauma, etc.) do not require immediate imaging. An atypical presentation, including (1) recurrent ipsilateral paralysis, (2) slowly progressive paralysis, (3) no recovery at 6 months, or (4) palsy associated with ipsilateral facial twitching, requires imaging. High-resolution contrast-enhanced MRI from the brain stem through the parotid is the imaging modality of choice when evaluating facial nerve palsy. It is important to differentiate between facial nerve tumors and viral inflammation of the facial nerve (Fig. 15.19) (as seen in Bell's palsy and herpes zoster oticus). Specifically, facial nerve schwannomas significantly enlarge the facial nerve canal, while facial nerve inflammation does not.

Facial Nerve Schwannoma

Facial nerve schwannomas are the most common primary tumors of the facial nerve and may present with symptoms of hearing loss and facial hypesthesia. Symptoms of facial paralysis and contracture typically arise when lesions become large. Facial nerve schwannomas are isointense on T1W imaging and hyperintense on T2W imaging and will enhance homogeneously and intensely on T1W contrast-enhanced MRI (Fig. 15.20). Smooth, tubular enlargement of the affected area of the fallopian canal can be seen in CT. Multiple segments of the facial nerve are commonly involved, and skip lesions with a "bead on a string" appearance can be seen on MRI.

Facial nerve schwannomas can develop or extend into the CPA, only being distinguished from vestibular schwannomas by MRI enhancement along the course of the labyrinthine segment of the facial nerve. Other findings suggesting a facial nerve origin include erosion of the superior margin of the IAC, fallopian canal expansion, erosion of the region surrounding the geniculate fossa, and eccentricity of the CPA portion of the tumor relative to the porus of the IAC.

Facial Nerve Hemangioma

Facial nerve hemangiomas are vascular malformations most commonly arising in the geniculate ganglion. These tumors are slow-growing lesions that cause facial nerve paralysis out of proportion to their size. Unlike schwannomas, facial nerve hemangiomas have irregular bony margins with intratumoral bone spicules and calcifications. Erosion can extend into the cochlea leading to sudden hearing loss. MRI will demonstrate a T1W enhancing lesion with punctate areas of nonenhancement corresponding to ossified foci (Fig. 15.21).

Perineural Tumor Spread

Malignant tumors of the parotid gland, such as adenoid cystic and mucoepidermoid carcinoma, may spread retrograde to involve the intratemporal portion of the facial nerve

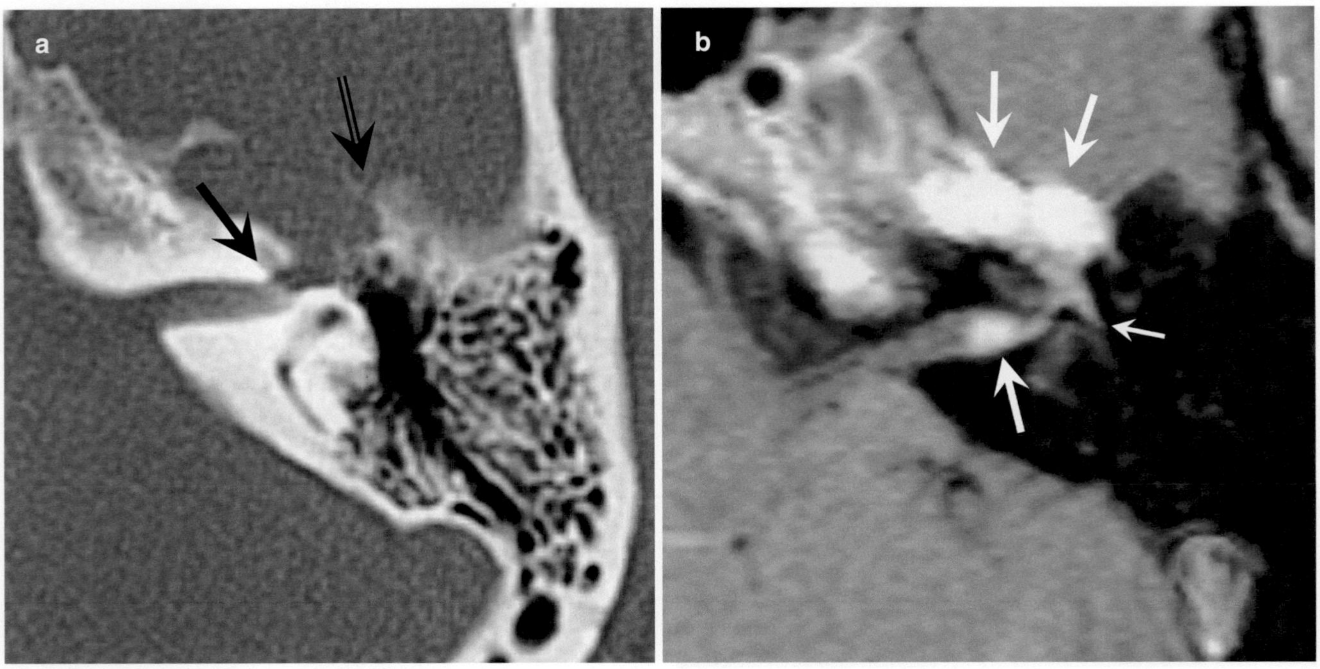

Fig. 15.20 Axial CT temporal bone (**a**) in a patient who presented with complete facial paresis demonstrating widening of the fallopian canal (single black arrow) and an expansile, nonerosive lesion of the petrous portion of the temporal bone (double black arrow). In the same patient, an axial T1W C+ MRI demonstrates (**b**) a homogeneously enhancing lesion arising from the geniculate ganglion with enhancement of the intracanalicular, labyrinthine, and tympanic segments of the facial nerve (large white arrow). The tympanic segment of the facial nerve extends from the lesion (small white arrow). Extension through the fallopian canal and presence of skip lesions giving a bead on a string appearance help differentiate facial nerve schwannomas from vestibular schwannomas

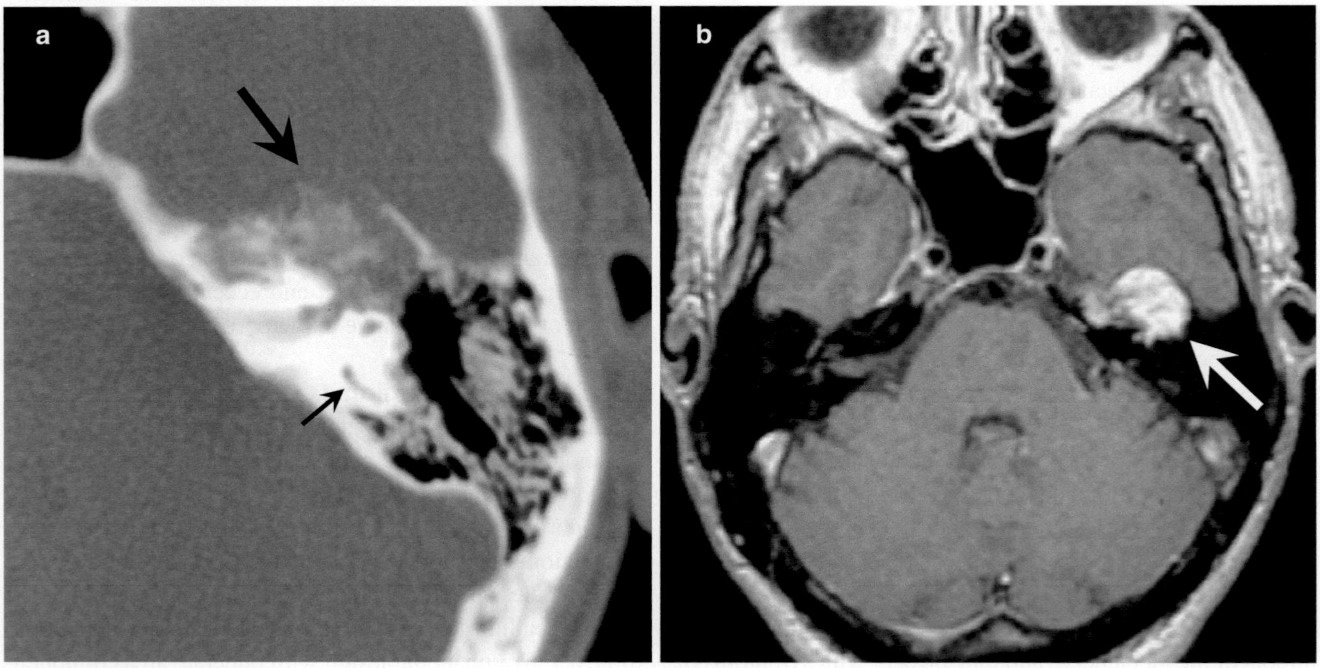

Fig. 15.21 Axial temporal bone CT (**a**) in a patient with left facial nerve palsy and left facial nerve hemangioma shows a petrous temporal bone lesion with irregular bony margins and intratumoral calcifications (large black arrow). There is no erosion of the cochlea (small black arrow). An axial T1W C+ MRI (**b**) in the same patient demonstrates an enhancing lesion with punctate areas of non-enhancement corresponding to areas of ossified foci (white arrow)

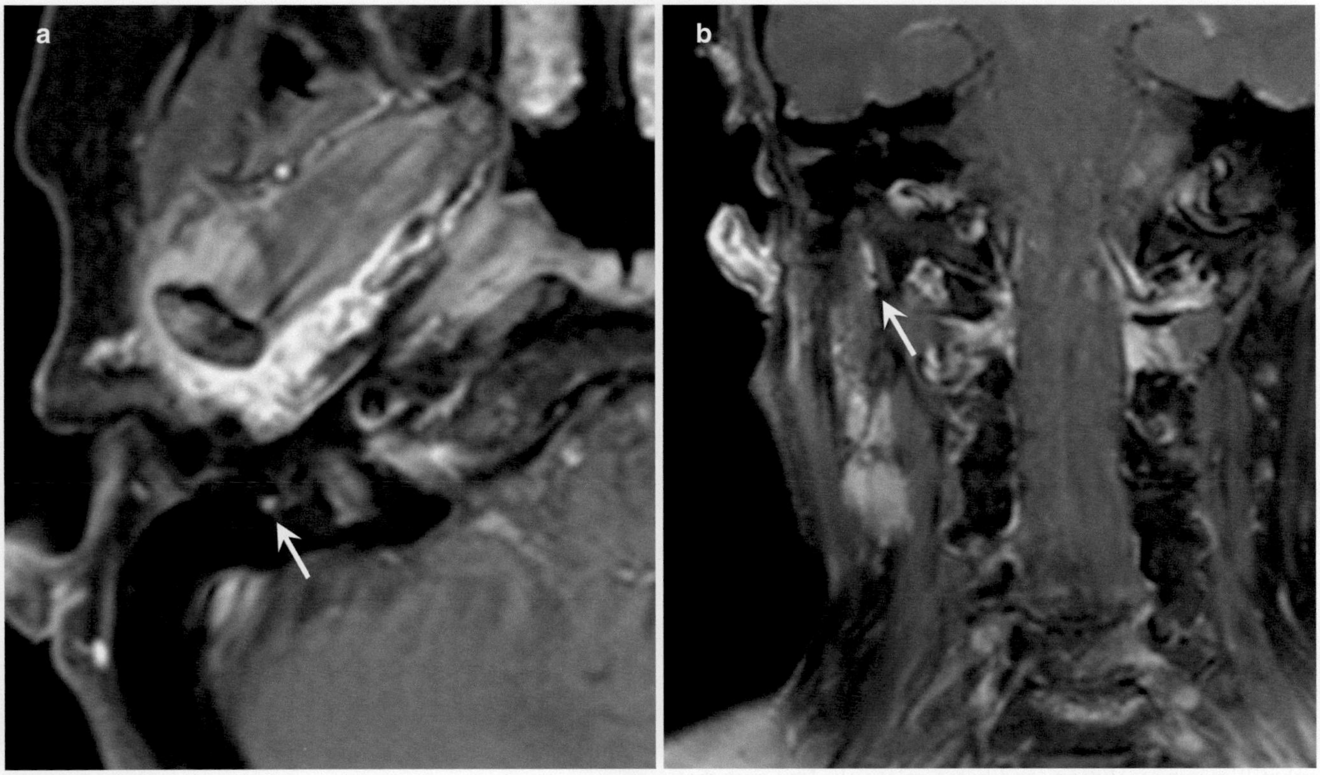

Fig. 15.22 Axial right T1W C+ MRI (**a**) demonstrating enhancement of the descending segment of the facial nerve within the mastoid bone (white arrow) in a patient with a large mucoepidermoid carcinoma of the parotid gland. In the same patient, a coronal T1W C+ MRI (**b**) demonstrates enhancement extending through the stylomastoid foramen and into the mastoid bone

(Fig. 15.22). For this reason, the entire course of the facial nerve should be included in the initial imaging in patients with an unresolved or progressive facial nerve palsy/paresis. Contrast-enhanced T1W MRI with fat suppression is used to increase the identification of the enhancing tumor by suppressing the enhancement of the surrounding fat. These images can be correlated with PET/CT to facilitate perineural tumor spread diagnosis.

Hemifacial Spasm

Radiologic investigation of patients with hemifacial spasm attempts to answer two principal questions: (1) Is there a lesion other than a vascular loop causing this problem? (2) Can an offending redundant vascular loop be identified? MRI and MRA are often used for evaluating patients with hemifacial spasm because of the ability both to visualize the relationships between the structures within the CPA cistern and to evaluate the complete course of the facial nerve (from pons to parotid gland). High-resolution T2W MRI images (constructive interference into steady state [CISS] or fast imaging employing steady-state acquisition [FIESTA] sequences) also show excellent neurovascular definition and can identify potential relationships between vascular loops and cranial nerves.

Retrocochlear Lesions

A common indication for temporal bone imaging is evaluation for a suspected retrocochlear lesion. Patients may present with a variety of unilateral auditory and vestibular symptoms, including progressive or sudden SNHL, tinnitus, and/or dizziness. Contrast-enhanced MRI is the gold standard for evaluation of these patients due to their high sensitivity. Both non-contrasted and contrasted CT scans have a relatively poor sensitivity for lesions within the IAC and CPA. The pertinent anatomic information regarding an IAC-CPA mass includes whether the lesion is intra-axial or extra-axial and where the lesion is centered relative to the IAC. Lesions of the cerebellopontine angle (CPA) have characteristic findings on contrast-enhanced MRI (Table 15.1).

Vestibular Schwannoma

Vestibular schwannoma (acoustic neuroma) is the most common extra-axial mass within the CPA. The majority of these lesions will arise from the vestibular nerve. Fine-cut MRI with contrast enhancement is the imaging modality of choice for evaluation of the CPA. These lesions are characteristically isointense to the brain on pre-contrast T1W MRI and mildly hyperintense on T2W MRI. Enhanced, post-contrast

Table 15.1 Retrocochlear lesions: MRI imaging characteristics

Lesion	T1	T2	Enhancement
Vestibular schwannoma*	Isointense	Hyperintense	Yes
Meningioma*	Isointense	Hyperintense	Yes
Epidermoid	Hypointense	Hyperintense	No, or rim enhancement
Lipoma	Hyperintense	Isointense	No (dark on fat saturation)
Arachnoid cyst	Isointense	Hyperintense	No

*For vestibular schwannoma and meningioma, comparisons are relative to the brain; for the remainder, comparisons are relative to CSF

T1W MRI features that define a vestibular schwannoma include a uniformly enhancing mass centered in the CPA over the porus acusticus (Fig. 15.23). The IAC component can often have an "ice cream cone" appearance, or the lesion can be entirely contained within the IAC. Care should also be taken to evaluate the inner ear on a post-contrasted MRI for an isolated intralabyrinthine or intracochlear schwannoma [15] (Fig. 15.24).

Fast spin-echo (FSE) MRI can be used for screening vestibular schwannoma growth after initial diagnosis. This technique does avoid contrast administration, can provide submillimeter resolution, and has a relatively low cost that approaches that of an ABR. It will also provide detailed anatomy of the IAC and CPA but is less sensitive to the variable intra-axial or intratemporal pathology. If the patient has had previous surgery for removal of a vestibular schwannoma, fat-suppressed images should always be obtained after contrast infusion to avoid enhancement of any residual or recurrent mass from being obscured by the surrounding fat graft.

A CT should be performed only if MRI is not available or is contraindicated in a patient because of an implanted medical device. CT scanning provides detailed assessment of the internal auditory canals. Although dimensions of the IAC are variable between patients, within one patient, both sides should be compared for symmetry. Enlargement of 2 mm or more or shortening of the posterior canal wall by at least 3 mm in comparison to the contralateral IAC is indicative of a space-occupying lesion within the IAC. Contrast infusion can aid in detection of extracanalicular lesions as small as 5 mm in size. If the CT findings are equivocal and clinical suspicion remains elevated, a CT cisternogram can be performed by injecting 3 cc of air into the subarachnoid space through a lumbar puncture. If a tumor is present, the gas will outline the medial contour of the mass and complete or partial block of the IAC. With this technique, intracanalicular tumors as small as 2–3 mm can be identified. However, this modality is rare in contemporary practice due to the high sensitivity of MRI and the relative risks associated with lumbar puncture.

Meningioma

Meningiomas are the second most common tumor of the CPA. Meningiomas can mimic vestibular schwannomas and will also enhance on post-contrasted MRI (Fig. 15.25). Location and shape are the most important criteria for diagnosing a CPA meningioma. Meningiomas are characteristically extra-axial and in a dural-based location off center from the IAC. A characteristic "dural tail" is considered highly suggestive of—although not specific for—meningiomas. Unlike vestibular schwannomas, meningiomas typically have a sessile growth pattern and will form an obtuse angle with the temporal bone due to hyperostosis or erosion of the bony canal. However they rarely extend into the IAC. When present, intralesional calcifications can suggest the diagnosis. Rarely, a meningioma may arise from the dura of the internal auditory canal; these will present as an intracanalicular mass with associated findings of meningioma. MRI will typically show contrast enhancement, T1 isointensity, and T2 hyperintensity.

Epidermoid Cysts

Epidermoid cysts are the third most common CPA lesions. They arise from epithelial rests of tissue during neural tube closure, and over time, keratin and cholesterol accumulation will lead to slow growth around and encasing the neurovascular structures of the CPA rather than displacing them. Epidermoid cysts rarely extend into the IAC. On CT, epidermoid cysts are hypoattenuating with characteristic lobular and irregular margins. MRI will show low signal on T1W and a high signal on T2W, similar to CSF, with non-enhancement after contrast administration (Fig. 15.26).

Although arachnoid cysts will have similar imaging characteristics, including lack of contrast enhancement and similar signal intensity to CSF across all sequences, they can be differentiated from epidermoid cysts using FLAIR or DWI (Fig. 15.26). Epidermoid cysts will show incomplete attenuation on FLAIR and evidence of diffusion restriction (bright) on DWI, whereas arachnoid cysts or surrounding CSF will not diffusion restrict (will be dark).

Lipomas

Lipomas occur less frequently in the CPA cistern than epidermoid and arachnoid cysts. Rarely they may be found within the IAC or the membranous labyrinth or vestibule. On MRI these lesions will appear bright on T1W but will lose signal on T2W MRI or fat-suppressed sequences (Fig. 15.27). Lipomas will typically surround the neurovascular structures of the IAC.

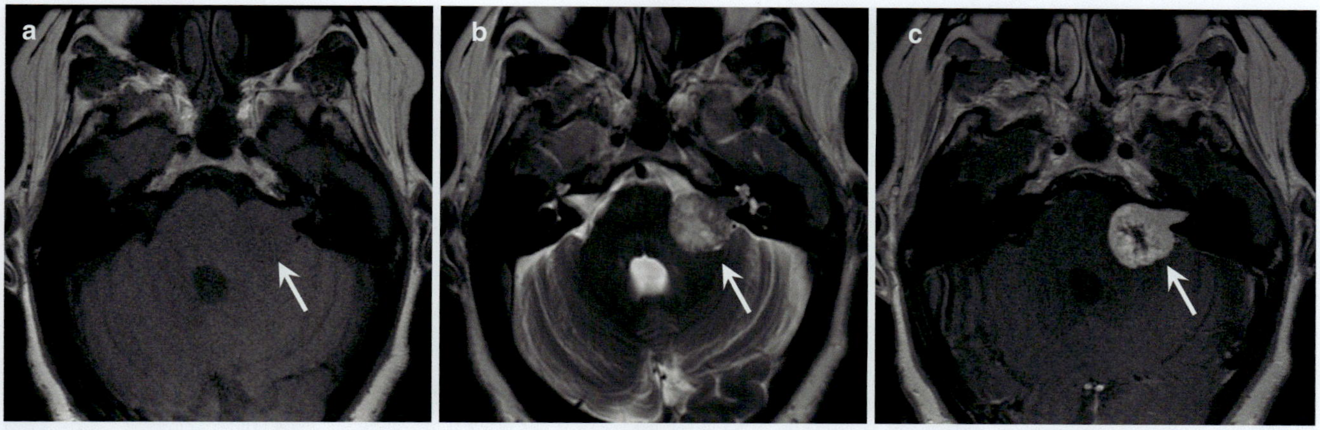

Fig. 15.23 A left vestibular schwannoma (white arrow) is seen in a patient who presented with left asymmetric hearing loss and tinnitus. Axial MRI demonstrates an isointense cerebellopontine angle (CPA) lesion on T1W MRI (**a**) that is hyperintense on T2W MRI (**b**) and enhances on T1W C+ MRI (**c**). The characteristic "ice cream cone" appearance is seen as a portion of the lesion extends into the internal auditory canal (IAC)

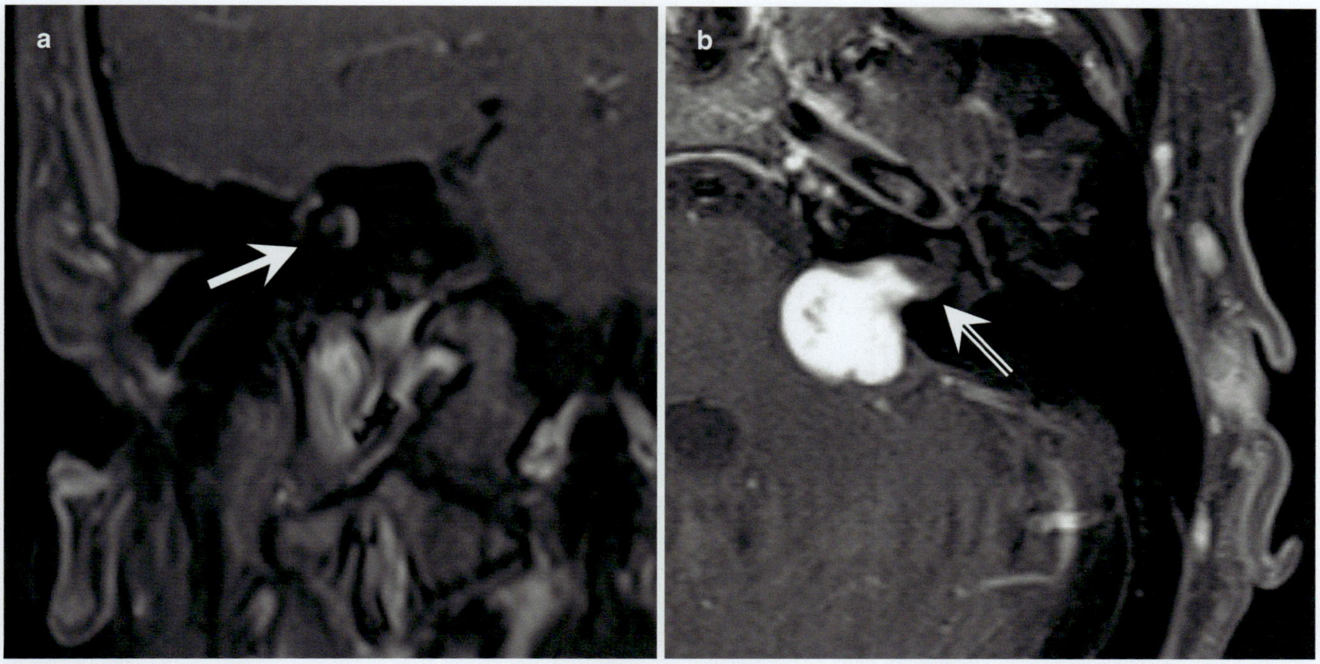

Fig. 15.24 Contrasting spectrum of vestibular schwannomas. Right coronal T1W MRI C+ (**a**) demonstrating an intracochlear vestibular schwannoma following the basal turn of the cochlea (single white arrow). This patient presented with profound sensorineural hearing loss. In contrast, a left axial T1W C+ MRI (**b**) demonstrates a large left vestibular schwannoma extending into the CPA with a "fundal cap" (double white arrow). This patient underwent a retrosigmoid approach for removal of the lesion

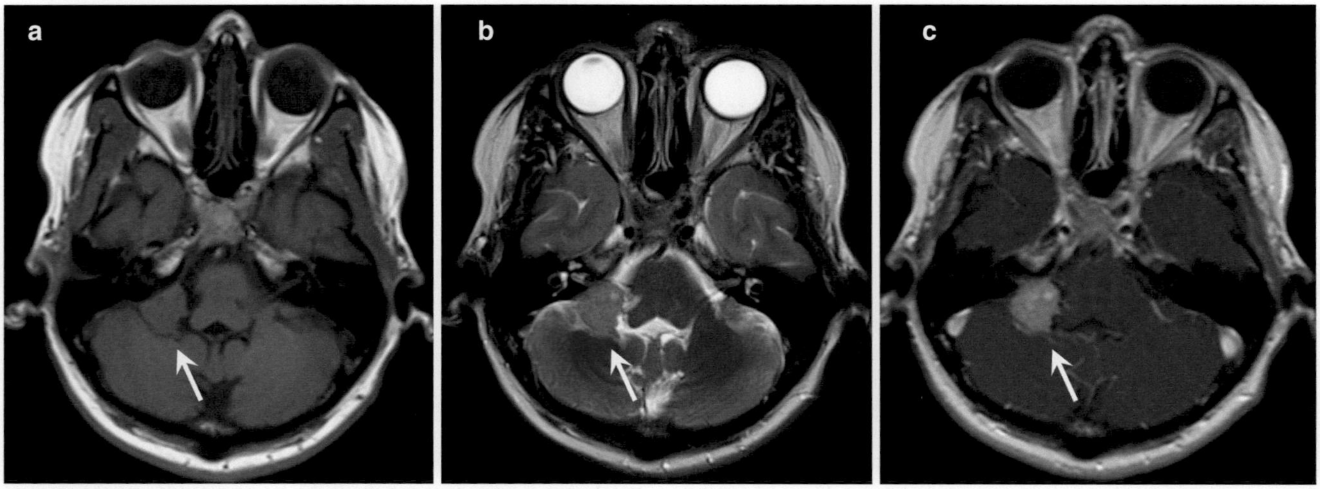

Fig. 15.25 A right cerebellopontine angle (CPA) meningioma (white arrow) is seen in a patient who presented with right asymmetric hearing loss. Axial MRI demonstrates an isointense cerebellopontine angle (CPA) lesion on T1W MRI (**a**) that is slightly hyperintense on T2W MRI (**b**) and enhances on T1W C+ MRI (**c**). A small "dural tail" can be seen extending into the internal auditory canal (IAC)

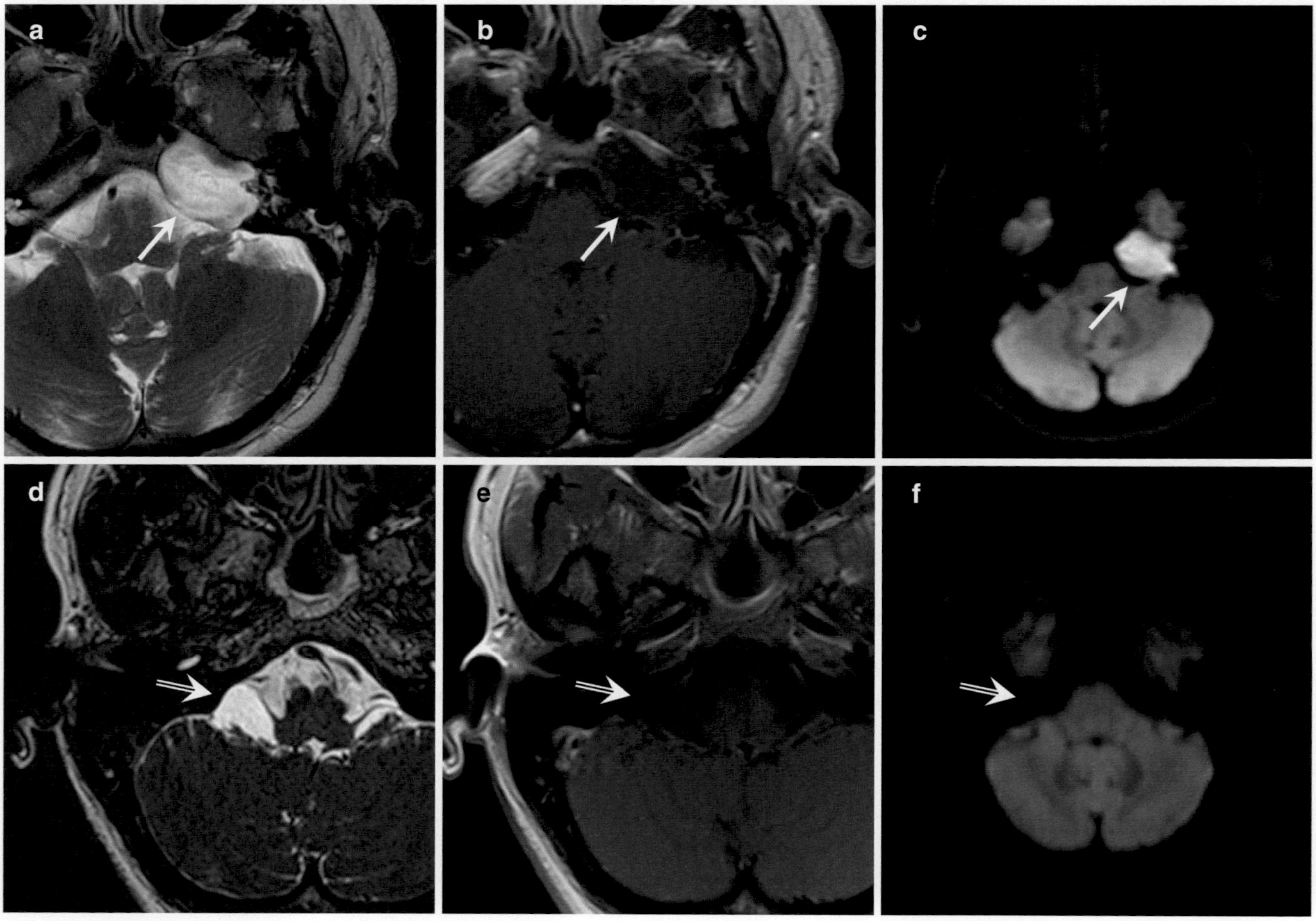

Fig. 15.26 Contrasting image series of an epidermoid cyst (single white arrow) and an arachnoid cyst (double white arrow). Axial T2W MRI (**a**) shows a high signal lesion within the left CPA cistern (white arrow). The lesion does not enhance on axial T1W C+ MRI (**b**). Axial DWI MRI (**c**) in the same patient demonstrates the characteristic restricted diffusion of the epidermoid cyst in the left CPA cistern. Without DWI information, the lesion could have been missed altogether. In comparison, an arachnoid cyst demonstrates similar patterns to an epidermoid cyst, high signal intensity on T2W MRI (**d**), and non-enhancement on T1W C+ (**e**); however, axial DWI MRI (**f**) (in the same patient) reveals that the arachnoid cyst has no associated signal (no restricted diffusion). DWI is the best way to differentiate an arachnoid cyst from an epidermoid cyst

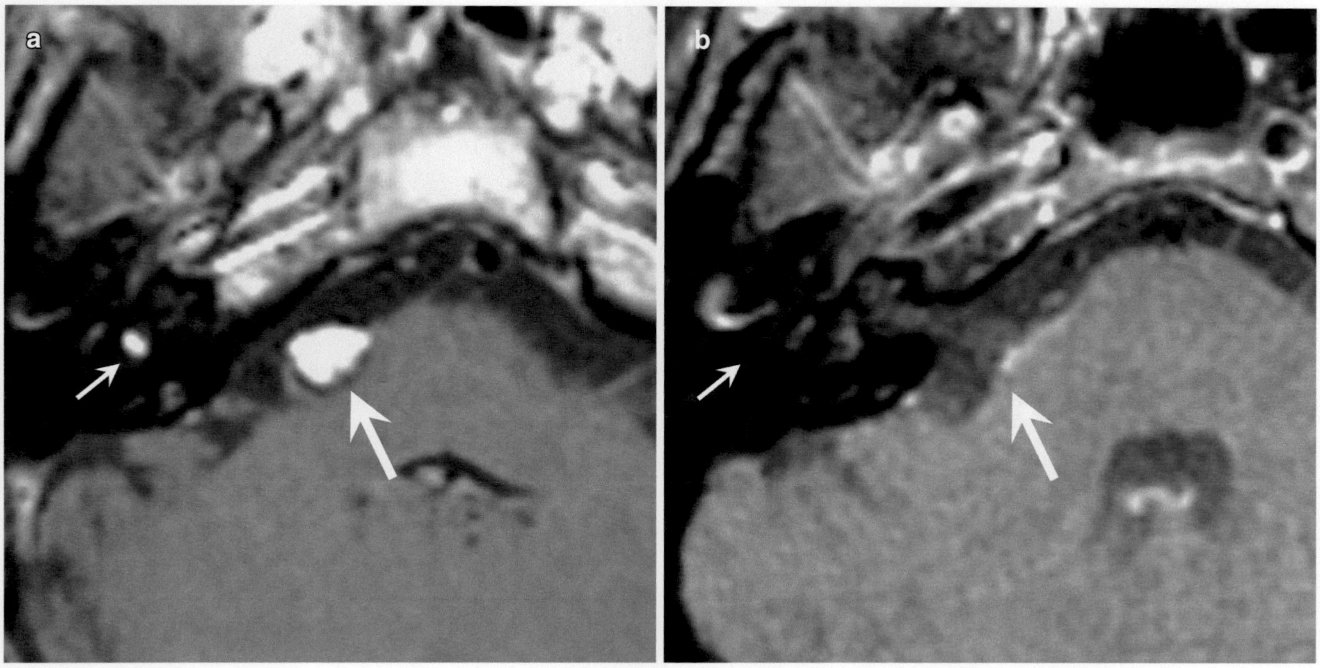

Fig. 15.27 Axial T1W MRI C+ (**a**) demonstrates a hyperintense CPA lipoma (large white arrow) abutting the lateral pons. A second (small white arrow) focus of hyperintensity represents a small intravestibular lipoma. Such intralabyrinthine lipomas are rare and may exist with or without CPA lipoma. The lesions become isointense to the surrounding tissue with fat suppression (**b**) confirming the diagnosis of a lipoma

Superficial Siderosis

Chronic bleeding into the subarachnoid space can cause superficial siderosis. The bleeding can be associated with arteriovenous or cavernous malformations, intracranial tumors, history of trauma, aneurysms, or past CNS surgery, though often, the source of bleeding is unknown. Superficial siderosis is a rare cause of progressive bilateral SNHL. On T2W MRI, hemosiderosis will appear as a dark lining of the arachnoid membranes on the surface of the brain stem and cerebellum [16] (Fig. 15.28).

Petrous Apex Lesions

The petrous apex is the pyramidal-shaped portion of the temporal bone anteromedial to the inner ear. It is pneumatized in approximately 33% of individuals. The petrous portion of the temporal bone lies within a complex anatomic region containing a number of critical neurologic and vascular structures often involved in the various pathologies developing in the region. The differential diagnosis of petrous apex lesions includes cholesterol granuloma, congenital cholesteatoma, and mucocele. The signal characteristics of these lesions are detailed in Table 15.2.

Cholesterol Granuloma

Cholesterol granuloma is the most common surgically managed lesion of the petrous apex. CT will demonstrate a soft tissue density in the petrous apex with loss of bony septations and smooth, pushing margins. Cholesterol granulomas have characteristic findings on MRI and are hyperintense on both T1W and T2W sequences, with signal remaining high on fat suppression imaging. Cholesterol granulomas will not usually enhance post-contrast (Fig. 15.29). The opposite petrous apex may be well pneumatized.

Petrous Apex Cholesteatoma

Patients with petrous apex cholesteatoma may present with chronic otomastoiditis; however, the etiology for many of these lesions is usually congenital. An expansile mass with bony destruction and irregular margins, different from cholesterol granuloma, can be seen on CT. Additionally, CT can be useful to evaluate the ossicles, otic capsule, and facial nerve in patients presenting with hearing loss or facial paralysis. MRI can be key to differentiating cholesteatoma from cholesterol granuloma. Cholesteatomas are isointense or hypointense to surrounding CSF on T1W imaging and hyperintense on T2W imaging. These lesions do not enhance on contrasted T1W imaging. Diffusion-weighted imaging is diagnostic of this lesion as it is hyperintense from diffusion restriction (Fig. 15.30).

Mucoceles

Petrous apex mucoceles are extremely rare. These lesions demonstrate similar findings on MRI (T1W hypointense and T2W hyperintense) to trapped fluid. However, petrous apex

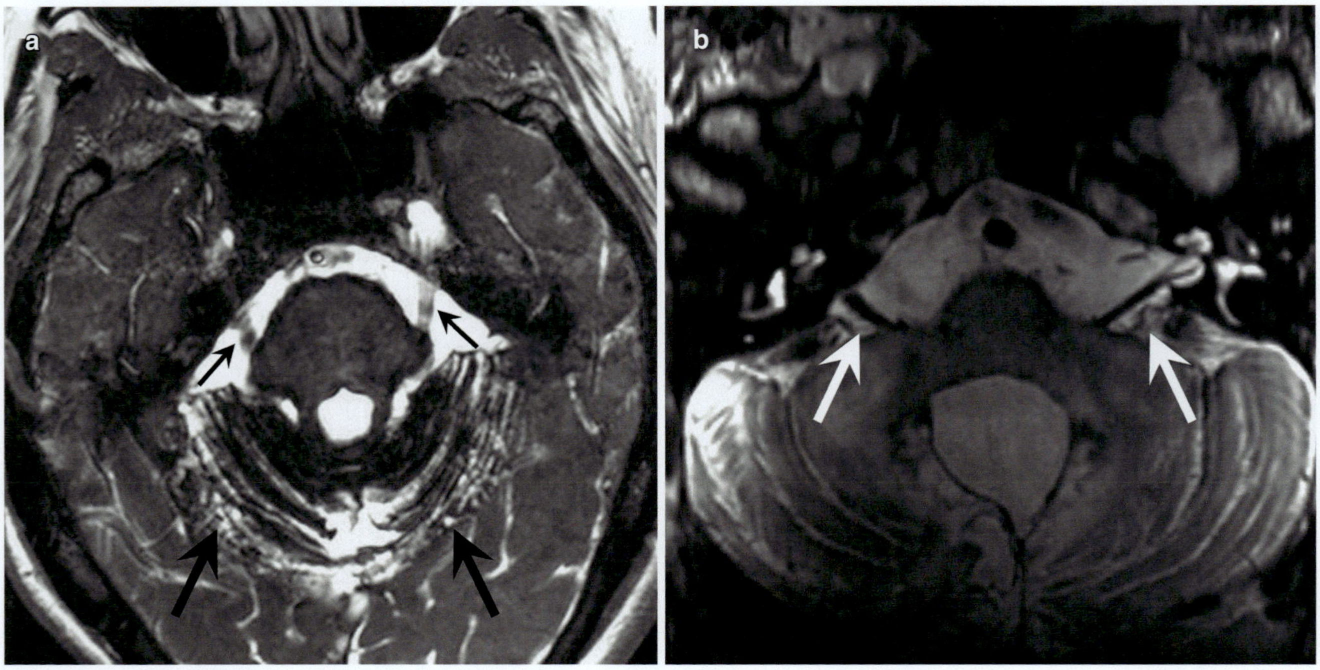

Fig. 15.28 Axial T2W MRI (**a**) revealing superficial siderosis in the posterior fossa (large black arrow) as represented as very low-signal lines within the posterior fossa. CNV is seen as very low-signal lines in the cerebellopontine cistern (small black arrow). In a different patient, an axial T2W MRI (**b**) demonstrates low signal outlining the bilateral IAC (white arrow)

Table 15.2 Petrous apex lesions: imaging characteristics

		MRI		
Lesion	CT	T_1	T_2	Enhancement
Cholesterol granuloma	Sharply marginated Expansile Trabecular breakdown	Hyperintense	Hyperintense	No
Cholesteatoma	Erosive changes Expansile Trabecular breakdown	Hypointense	Hyperintense	No
Trapped fluid	Trabecular preservation Nonexpansile	Hypointense, isointense, or hyperintense	Hyperintense	No
Mucocele	Sharply marginated Pushing borders Expansile Trabecular breakdown	Hypointense	Hyperintense	Rim enhancement

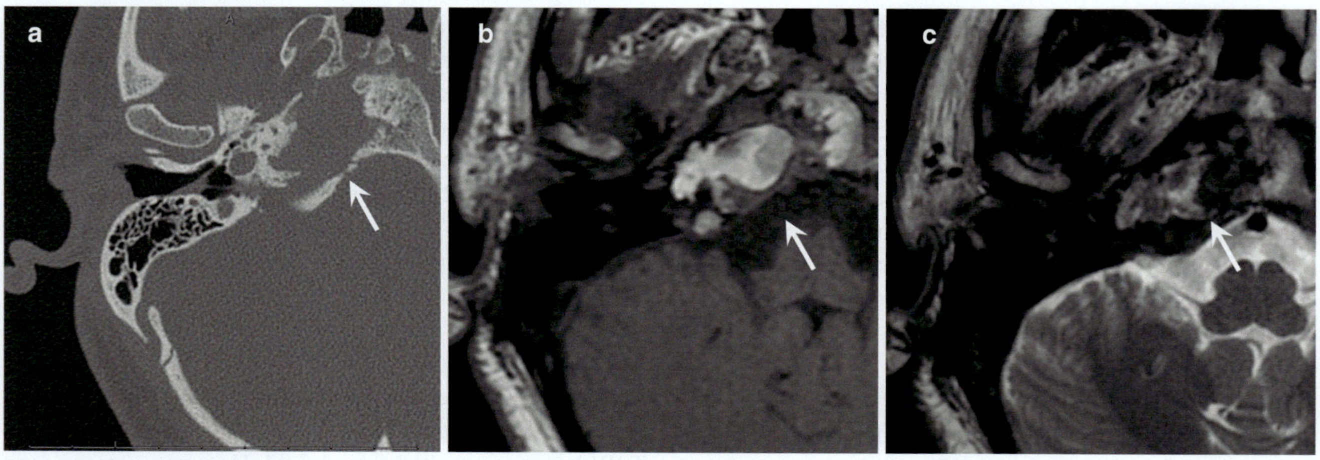

Fig. 15.29 Axial bone CT (**a**) reveals an expansile cholesterol granuloma in the right petrous apex (white arrow) with surrounding bone dehiscence. Axial T1W unenhanced MRI (**b**) in the same patient shows characteristic high signal (white arrow) of a cholesterol granuloma, while axial T2W MRI (**c**) demonstrates an inhomogeneous high signal (white arrow). Cholesterol granuloma contains "old blood." The T1 signal is therefore high (methemoglobin) and the T2 signal inhomogeneous (methemoglobin and hemosiderin)

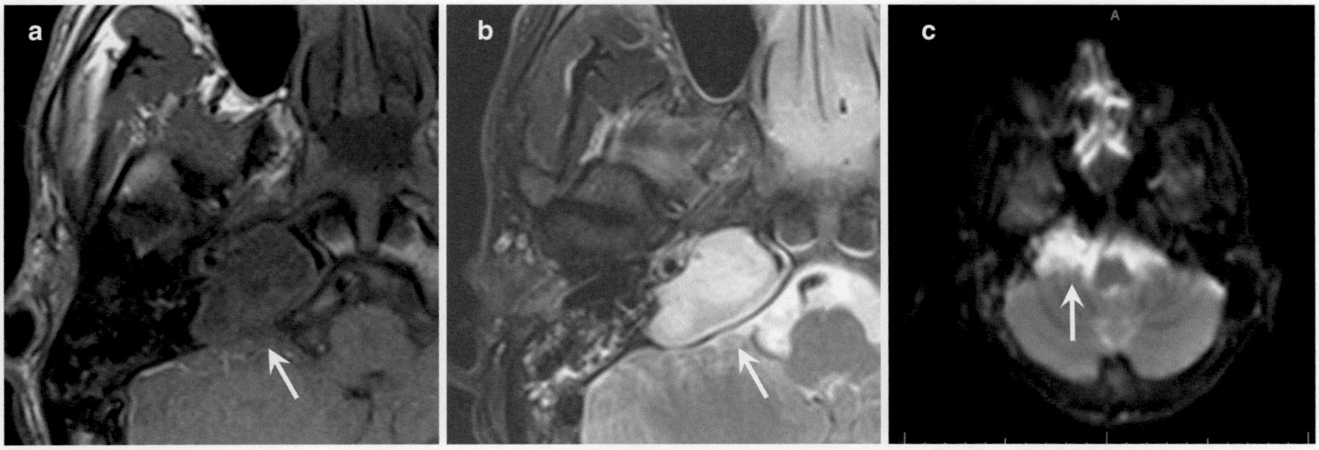

Fig. 15.30 Axial T1W MRI (**a**) demonstrates an ovoid, expansile inhomogeneous mixed low-intermediate signal petrous apex cholesteatoma (white arrow). In the same patient, axial T2W MRI (**b**) reveals the high-signal petrous apex cholesteatoma. DWI MRI (**c**) demonstrates the high signal (restricted diffusion) consistent with a petrous apex cholesteatoma (white solid arrow). DWI imaging helps differentiate cholesteatoma (restricted diffusion) from cholesterol granuloma (no restricted diffusion)

mucoceles are expansile and have smooth borders and fluid density (hypodensity) on CT. Diffusion-weighted imaging will not show any diffusion restrictions in the lesion.

Otosclerosis

The diagnosis of otosclerosis is made by clinical exam and audiogram. However, when the presentation is atypical, CT imaging can be helpful. Thin slice, non-contrasted CT of the temporal bone can adequately demonstrate subtle foci in the bony labyrinth. CT findings depend on the phase of the disease. During the active phase, demineralization of bone anterior to the oval window at the fissula ante fenestram suggests otosclerosis (Fig. 15.31). During remission, this region can become sclerotic, and in severe cases, the oval window can be completely filled with dense bone.

Retrofenestral or cochlear otosclerosis involves the otic capsule, and findings can be detected on CT using a bone algorithm. Often findings may appear as an "extra turn" of the cochlea as the dense bone of the otic capsule is demineralized. Advanced or cochlear otosclerosis develops when abnormal otospongiotic bone involves the otic capsule. This may create a "halo" signal around the cochlea (Fig. 15.32). A CT grading system was proposed in 2005 [17] (Table 15.3) and has been validated to yield excellent interobserver and intraobserver agreement [18]. MRI has little role in imaging for otosclerosis, though contrast enhancement can be seen in active disease [19].

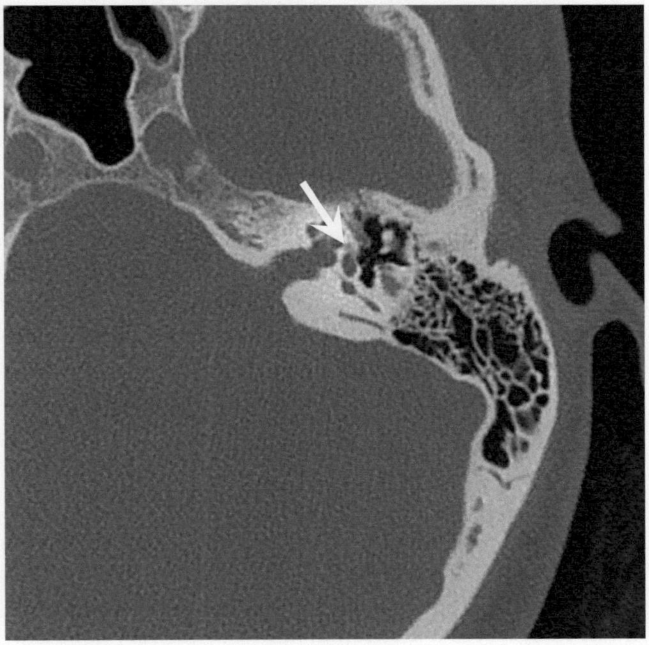

Fig. 15.31 Axial left temporal bone CT demonstrates fenestral otosclerosis blurring the margins of the oval window (white arrow)

Superior Semicircular Canal Dehiscence

Superior semicircular canal dehiscence (SSCD) occurs when a bone is missing over the superior semicircular canal, exposing the membranous labyrinth and creating a "third window" phenomenon. SSCD is otherwise known as the "great otologic mimicker" because it can cause many otologic-related symptoms, including sensorineural and conductive hearing loss, aural fullness, tinnitus, and vertigo. More specific symptoms include autophony to voice and bodily movement and sound- or pressure-induced vertigo [20, 21]. Given the possibility of an ambiguous presentation, imaging of the temporal bone is a mainstay of diagnosis. Temporal bone CT will demonstrate a defect in the arcuate eminence consistent with dehiscence over the superior canal (Fig. 15.33). This finding is best viewed on a reformatted sagittal oblique image that will show the entire course of the superior canal

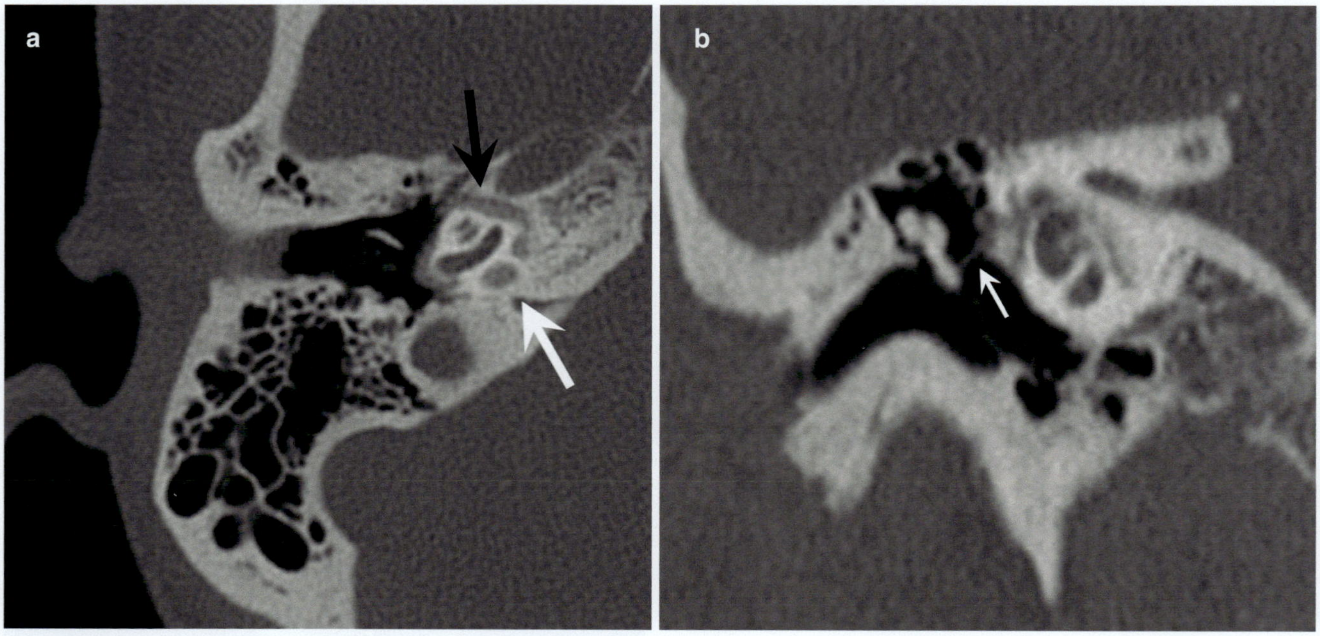

Fig. 15.32 Axial right temporal bone CT (**a**) demonstrating an osteolytic foci of cochlear otosclerosis as surrounding the cochlea (black arrow). Coronal right temporal bone CT (**b**) in a patient with mixed hearing loss reveals a "halo" of radiolucency surrounding the cochlea (large white arrow) representing cochlear otosclerosis. Concurrent fenestral otosclerosis is also seen as bony lucency along cochlear promontory extending from fissula ante fenestram (small white arrow). A stapes prosthesis is seen extending into the oval window

Table 15.3 CT grading of otosclerosis [18]

Grade	Description
1	Solely fenestral
2	Patchy localized cochlear disease (with or without fenestral involvement) with involvement of:
2a	Basal turn of the cochlea
2b	Middle or apical turns
2c	Diffuse confluent cochlear involvement of the otic capsule[a]
3	Diffuse confluent cochlear involvement of the otic capsule (with or without fenestral involvement)

[a]Grade 3 is differentiated from grade 2C by the diffuse involvement in grade 3 of the entire cochlea, whereas grade 2C has patchy focal involvement of the entire cochlea

in one image. It is not uncommon to also identify contralateral SSCD or a tegmen dehiscence [22]. MRI is not usually necessary for this diagnosis, as CT is far superior in defining the bony anatomy. However, MRI may be more sensitive to diagnose SSCD and have a higher negative predictive value when compared to CT [23]. MRI can also be used to follow patients after repair.

Distant Metastasis

Metastatic spread to the temporal bone should be suspected whenever a destructive lesion with atypical features is identified. Metastatic lesions to the temporal bone have been observed in carcinomas of the breast, kidney, prostate, lung, and thyroid and melanoma. Aggressive features with destructive and indistinct borders, internal calcifications, and extension into adjacent structures can be identified on CT. MRI characteristics are variable; however, hyperintensity on T2W imaging or low apparent diffusion coefficient (ADC) values correlates with the highly cellular lesions, suggesting a metastatic lesion (Fig. 15.34). PET/CT can be used to determine the location of the primary lesion.

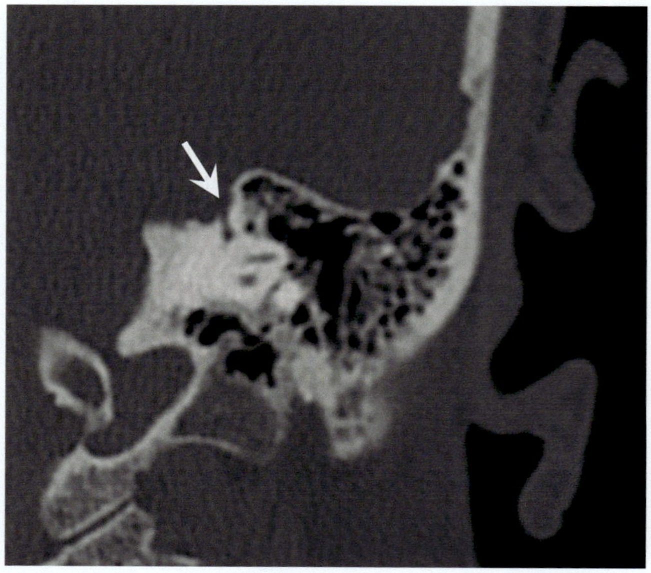

Fig. 15.33 Coronal bone CT demonstrating left superior semicircular canal dehiscence (white arrow). The patient presented for evaluation of vertigo. The dehiscence should be visible on two contiguous 1-mm cuts or three contiguous 0.5-mm cuts

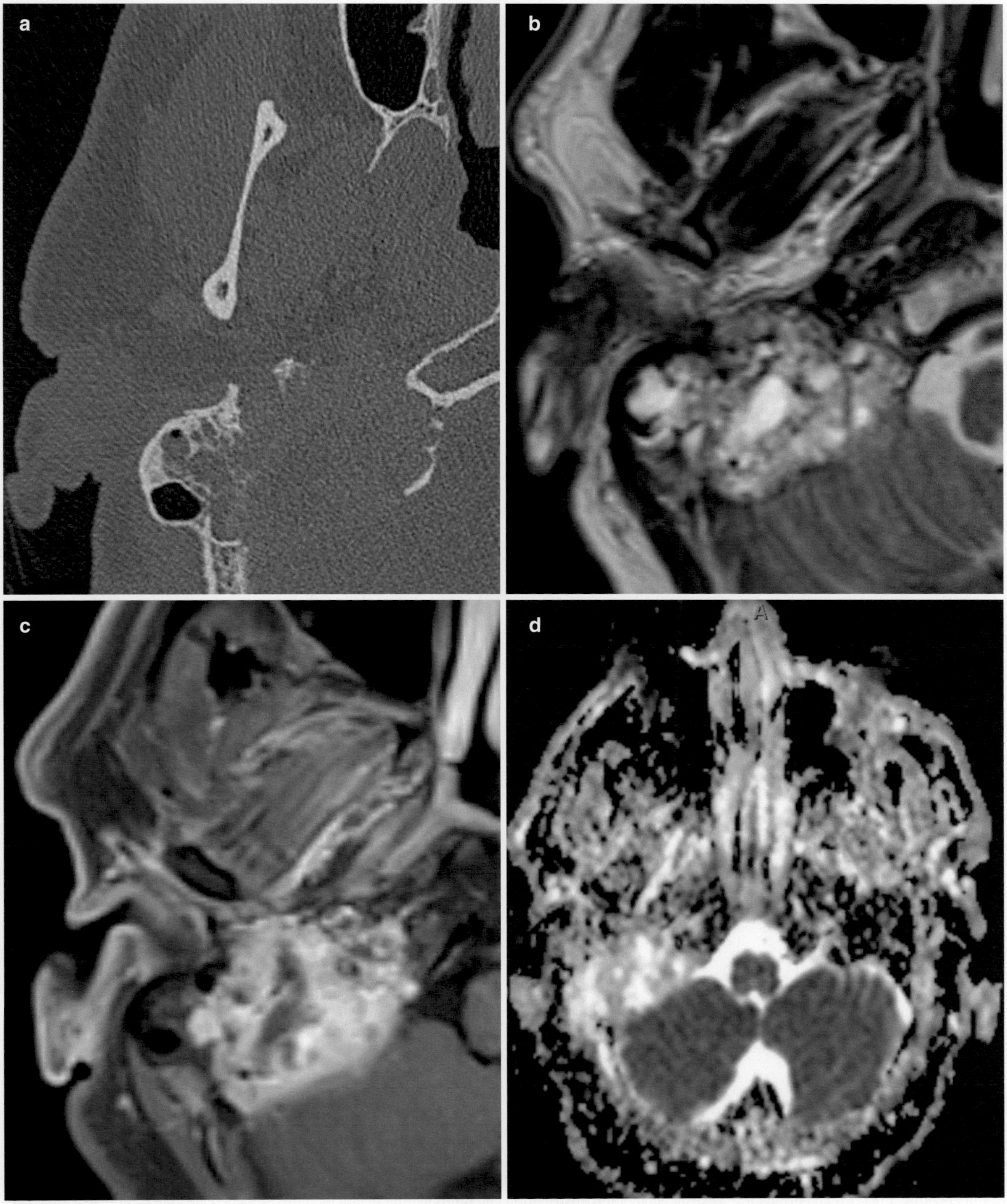

Fig. 15.34 This patient presented with a destructive right temporal bone lesion extending toward the jugular foramen (**a**). The lesion was hyperintense on T2W MRI (**b**) and enhanced after T1W C+ MRI (**c**). MRI ADC sequence (**d**) revealed a hyperintense lesion correlating with a highly cellular lesion. Biopsy demonstrated a metastatic renal cell carcinoma

Conclusions

Temporal bone imaging has become interwoven into the diagnostic paradigms of most otologic diseases. CT and/or MRI is commonly performed in the setting of temporal bone pathology to aid in creating and narrowing a differential diagnosis and for postoperative surveillance. In the contemporary practice of otology, it is imperative that surgeons have access to high-resolution and high-quality imaging modalities and interpretations.

References

1. Gul A, et al. Radiologic and surgical findings in chronic suppurative otitis media. J Craniofac Surg. 2014;25(6):2027–9.
2. Li PM, et al. Evaluating the utility of non-echo-planar diffusion-weighted imaging in the preoperative evaluation of cholesteatoma: a meta-analysis. Laryngoscope. 2013;123(5):1247–50.
3. Dempewolf R, Gubbels S, Hansen MR. Acute radiographic workup of blunt temporal bone trauma: maxillofacial versus temporal bone CT. Laryngoscope. 2009;119(3):442–8.
4. Little SC, Kesser BW. Radiographic classification of temporal bone fractures: clinical predictability using a new system. Arch Otolaryngol Head Neck Surg. 2006;132(12):1300–4.
5. Alford RL, et al. American College of Medical Genetics and Genomics guideline for the clinical evaluation and etiologic diagnosis of hearing loss. Genet Med. 2014;16(4):347–55.
6. Lin JW, et al. Comprehensive diagnostic battery for evaluating sensorineural hearing loss in children. Otol Neurotol. 2011;32(2):259–64.
7. Digge P, et al. Imaging modality of choice for pre-operative cochlear imaging: HRCT vs. MRI temporal bone. J Clin Diagn Res. 2016;10(10):TC01–4.
8. Ramalho J, et al. Gadolinium-based contrast agent accumulation and toxicity: an update. AJNR Am J Neuroradiol. 2016;37(7):1192–8.
9. Jahrsdoerfer RA, et al. Grading system for the selection of patients with congenital aural atresia. Am J Otol. 1992;13(1):6–12.
10. Frenzel H, et al. Grading system for the selection of patients with congenital aural atresia for active middle ear implants. Neuroradiology. 2013;55(7):895–911.
11. Mattox DE, Hudgins P. Algorithm for evaluation of pulsatile tinnitus. Acta Otolaryngol. 2008;128(4):427–31.
12. Christie A, Teasdale E. A comparative review of multidetector CT angiography and MRI in the diagnosis of jugular foramen lesions. Clin Radiol. 2010;65(3):213–7.
13. Grewal AK, et al. Clinical presentation and imaging findings in patients with pulsatile tinnitus and sigmoid sinus diverticulum/dehiscence. Otol Neurotol. 2014;35(1):16–21.
14. Dong C, et al. Association between the extent of sigmoid sinus dehiscence and an occurrence of pulsatile tinnitus: a retrospective imaging study. Clin Radiol. 2016;71(9):883–8.
15. Salzman KL, et al. Intralabyrinthine schwannomas: imaging diagnosis and classification. AJNR Am J Neuroradiol. 2012;33(1):104–9.
16. Kumar N. Superficial siderosis: associations and therapeutic implications. Arch Neurol. 2007;64(4):491–6.
17. Marshall AH, et al. Cochlear implantation in cochlear otosclerosis. Laryngoscope. 2005;115(10):1728–33.
18. Lee TC, et al. CT grading of otosclerosis. AJNR Am J Neuroradiol. 2009;30(7):1435–9.
19. de Oliveira Vicente A, et al. Magnetic resonance imaging in the evaluation of clinical treatment of otospongiosis: a pilot study. Otolaryngol Head Neck Surg. 2015;152(6):1119–26.
20. Minor LB. Clinical manifestations of superior semicircular canal dehiscence. Laryngoscope. 2005;115(10):1717–27.
21. Minor LB, et al. Sound- and/or pressure-induced vertigo due to bone dehiscence of the superior semicircular canal. Arch Otolaryngol Head Neck Surg. 1998;124(3):249–58.
22. Nadaraja GS, et al. Radiographic evaluation of the tegmen in patients with superior semicircular canal dehiscence. Otol Neurotol. 2012;33(7):1245–50.
23. Browaeys P, et al. Can MRI replace CT in evaluating semicircular canal dehiscence? AJNR Am J Neuroradiol. 2013;34(7):1421–7.

Part III

Rehabilitation of Otologic and Neurotologic Diseases

Hearing Aids and Assistive Listening Systems

16

Lara E. Strotheide and Esther X. Vivas

Introduction

For the otolaryngologist, a basic understanding of the various hearing aid styles, components, processing, and technological features is essential to ensuring comprehensive care strategies. While the selection, fitting, and programming of these devices do not fall directly under their purview, otolaryngologists consistently engage with patients with diverse hearing challenges and work alongside audiologists to effectively support patients in their journey to better hearing and communication. With the rapid advancement of technology, it becomes essential to remain up-to-date with the latest developments in hearing aid technology, features, and accessories, as well as assistive listening devices, all of which can significantly enhance quality of life [1–3]. This chapter offers an overview of hearing devices, patient candidacy, medical clearance, and fitting without delving into the nuances of hearing aid programming, verification, or follow-up.

Digital Hearing Aids

Hearing aid technology has come a long way since ear horns, body-worn devices, and analog hearing instruments. The signal processing technology built into current digital hearing aids is highly complex and does much more than amplify sound. Hearing technology is continually evolving, with new product releases from each manufacturer approximately every 1–3 years. As a result, it is essential to review current hearing aid technology and recommendations routinely to counsel patients with up-to-date and accurate information.

L. E. Strotheide · E. X. Vivas (✉)
Department of Otolaryngology—Head and Neck Surgery, Emory University Medical Center, Atlanta, GA, USA
e-mail: evivas@emory.edu

Hearing Aid Styles

Hearing aid options differ significantly depending on the style (Fig. 16.1) and the manufacturer. Table 16.1 lists the most common hearing aid styles, associated advantages, and disadvantages.

Nontraditional Hearing Aids

- *Contralateral Routing of Signal/Binaural Contralateral Routing of Signal (CROS/BiCROS)* hearing aids are indicated for use on unilateral or asymmetrical hearing losses when the worse ear cannot benefit from a traditional hearing aid. The user wears a microphone, resembling a hearing aid, on the unaidable ear. This microphone wirelessly transmits sound to the hearing aid on the better ear, allowing the auditory pathway of the best ear to process sounds from the opposite side more directly. The term "CROS" is used when transferring sound to a normal-hearing ear without amplification. "BiCROS" denotes that the better ear also needs amplification due to asymmetrical hearing loss. Studies indicate these systems do not improve localization in the horizontal plane but can improve speech-in-noise ability [4, 5]. Manufacturers offer CROS/BiCROS hearing aids in Behind-the-Ear (BTE), Receiver-in-the-Canal (RIC), and In-the-Ear (ITE) styles.
- *Extended-wear hearing aids* are concealed within the ear canal, do not need battery changes, and are worn 24/7 for weeks to months, making them attractive options for some patients. The deep placement of these devices has also been associated with improvements in personal image relative to more traditional hearing aids [6]. Extended-wear hearing aids use analog technology with minimal digital programming flexibility, can be more costly than traditional hearing aids, and have more strict candidacy guidelines [6, 7]. They require a subscription for purchase, and they require office visits every few months for replacement.

A. D. Sweeney et al. (eds.), *Haynes-Glasscock-Shambaugh Surgery of the Ear*, https://doi.org/10.1007/978-3-032-18264-7_16

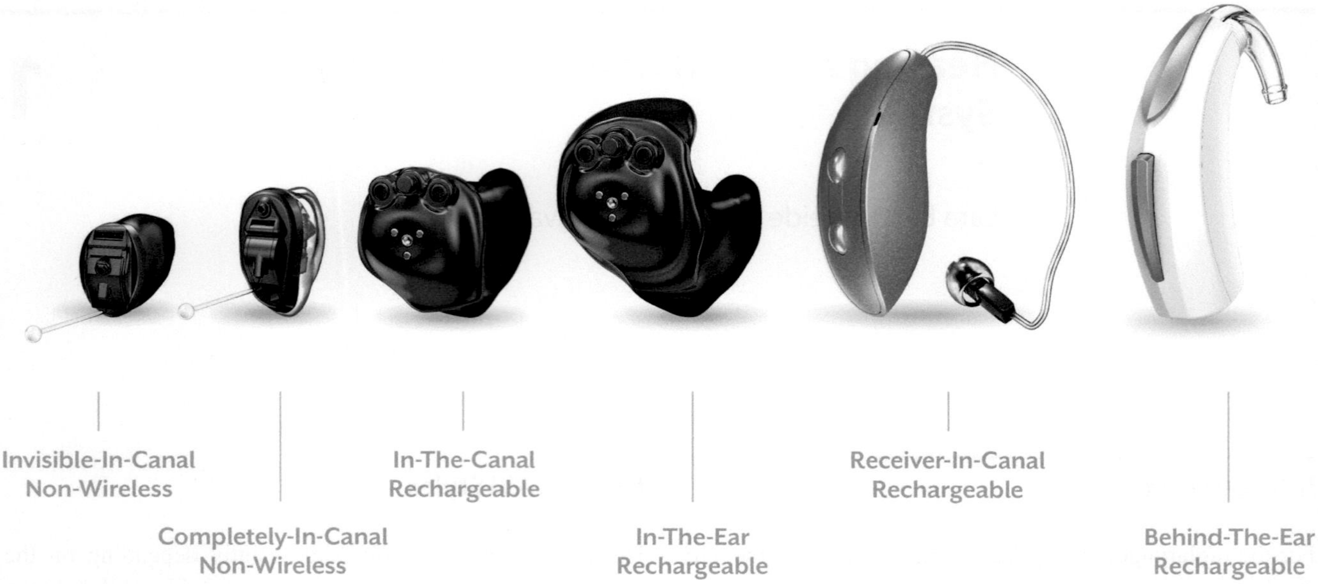

Fig. 16.1 Common hearing aid styles. This figure presents examples of six common hearing aid styles, illustrating their unique designs for quick visual reference. (Courtesy of Starkey)

- *Light-driven hearing aids* use a RIC-style external device to pick up sound and transfer it via ultraviolet (UV) light to a vibrating mechanical lens placed on the tympanic membrane. The UV light signal allows for detailed processing and usable/beneficial amplification at a much wider frequency range, with a very minimal chance of feedback [8–10]. Light-driven hearing aids can be more costly than traditional ones, do not have ITE or invisible options, are not widely available, and have relatively strict candidacy guidelines [9]. They also require a trained otologist or otolaryngologist to place the extended-wear lens on the tympanic membrane [9].

Electrical Components

Digital hearing aids are available in numerous brands, styles, technology levels, and fitting ranges. However, six essential electrical components fundamentally construct acoustic digital hearing aids.

- *Single or dual microphones* pick up external sound. Dual microphones allow for the detection of spatial cues from the environment and improve speech separation in noise compared to a single microphone.
- *Preamplifiers* increase the amplitude of the incoming analog signal to ensure it is loud enough for adequate conversion into a digital signal.
- *Analog-to-digital (A/D) converters* collect the incoming analog signal at regular intervals and translate it to binary code (a series of 0s and 1s) for digital processing.
  - *Sampling rate* is the number of analog sound samples captured per second. Hearing aids commonly sample at *~20 kHz*, allowing a usable bandwidth of up to *~9 kHz* [11–13].
  - *Bit depth* is the number of bits used to encode each sound sample. Higher bit depth improves signal clarity and dynamic range. Hearing aids typically use *12–24-bit precision*; *16-bit* provides a dynamic range of ~96 dB [11–13].
- *Digital signal processors* are computer chips that perform advanced processing of the binary codes to modify the incoming auditory signals. Digital processing allows for the most ideal amplified signal in each unique listening environment. Advanced digital processing commonly includes frequency-dependent gain adjustments, maximum power output limits, compression, speech enhancement and noise reduction processing, sound classifiers, and acoustic feedback systems [12, 14].
- *Receivers* collect the digitally processed signal and convert it back into acoustic sound waves, which they then send into the ear canal. Note: The digital-to-analog (D/A) converter is often a built-in part of the receiver; however, it can be a separate circuit between the processor and the receiver [12, 14].
- *Batteries* are the power source for digital hearing aids. Disposable zinc-air batteries last 4–30 days, while rechargeable lithium-ion batteries typically need to be charged nightly, depending on the battery type/size and power requirements of the hearing aids.

Table 16.1 Styles of hearing aids

Style	Description	Uses/advantages	Limitations/disadvantages
Behind-the-ear (BTE)	All electronics are positioned behind the pinna and are coupled by an ear hook and thick tubing to a custom earmold or, alternatively, by slim tubing to either a custom earmold or a non-custom dome situated in the ear canal	– Suitable for severe to profound hearing loss owing to versatile speaker size options – Optimal for individuals with conductive/mixed hearing loss – Offers a broad spectrum of acoustic coupling options – Provides a substantial fitting range – Integrates dual microphone technology – Ensures long-lasting battery performance – Available with rechargeable battery options – Allows for easy insertion and battery replacement – Encased in moisture/dust-resistant housing – Minimal feedback occurrence – Preferred choice for conditions with excessive moisture and cerumen – Has a prolonged lifespan with minimal repairs needed	– Lacks aesthetic appeal – Sound must travel through tubing, potentially reducing gain at certain frequencies, especially with slim tube coupling – Requires tubing changes every 4–6 months, typically necessitating an office visit – Speakers are not interchangeable – May present challenges for those wearing glasses, oxygen cannulas, and face masks
Receiver-In-The-Canal/ear (RIC/RITE)	Most electronics are housed behind the pinna, connected via a wire to the speaker/receiver, which is enclosed in either a custom earmold or a non-custom dome, positioned in the ear canal	– Suitable for individuals with "normal" low-frequency thresholds due to available open-fit options – Offers a wide variety of acoustic coupling options – Presents a substantial fitting range – Integrates dual microphone technology – Available with rechargeable battery options – Encased in a moisture/dust-resistant housing – Home-based routine maintenance is generally straightforward – Typically features the most advanced and inclusive technology – Minimal feedback occurrence – Location of the receiver in the ear enhances acoustical experience – Features interchangeable speakers	– Casing behind the ear may be noticeable – May present challenges for wearers of glasses, oxygen cannulas, and face masks – Prone to complications from moisture and wax buildup
In-the-ear (ITE) and In-The-Canal (ITC)	This is a custom-designed hearing aid constructed using an impression of the patient's ear. It represents the largest style among custom aids, occupying the helix and a portion or all of the concha	– Custom-fitted for individual ear anatomy – Allows for easy insertion – Integrates dual microphone technology – Features long-lasting battery life, compared to other custom styles – Available with rechargeable battery options – Home-based routine maintenance is generally straightforward – Ideal for individuals who wear glasses, oxygen cannulas, and facemasks	– Lacks aesthetic appeal – Does not offer an open-fit option – Is less suitable for individuals with "normal" low-frequency thresholds due to occlusion effects – Unable to demonstrate in the office – Speakers are not interchangeable – May pose challenges for patients with middle ear complications or those who have undergone ear surgeries – Less suitable for severe/profound losses due to an increased risk of feedback – Prone to complications from moisture and wax buildup

(continued)

Table 16.1 (continued)

Style	Description	Uses/advantages	Limitations/disadvantages
Completely in the canal (CIC)	This is a custom-designed hearing aid constructed using an impression of the patient's ear. It stands as the second smallest among the custom aids, filling the ear's canal portion. While it may be visible from the side, it is designed to remain inconspicuous from the front view	– Custom-fitted for individual ear anatomy – Provides a moderately aesthetic appearance – Allows for fairly easy insertion – Home-based routine maintenance is generally straightforward – Suitable for individuals who wear glasses, oxygen cannulas, and facemasks	– Does not offer an open-fit option – Is less suitable for individuals with "normal" low-frequency thresholds due to occlusion effects – Unable to demonstrate in the office – Handling and maintenance can be challenging due to the small size – Speakers are not interchangeable – May pose challenges for patients with middle ear complications or those who have undergone ear surgeries – Necessitates frequent battery replacements, typically every 4–7 days – Size constraints may limit available features and technology – Prone to complications from moisture and wax buildup – Generally, not suitable for severe/profound losses due to limitations in speaker size and a heightened risk of feedback
Invisible in the canal (IIC)	This is a custom-designed hearing aid constructed using an impression of the patient's ear. It represents the smallest variant among the custom aids. Its diminutive and deep design ensures it stays concealed within the ear canal, unobservable even from a side view	– Custom-fitted for individual ear anatomy – Completely concealed within the ear, offering utmost discretion – Experiences less occlusion compared to other custom styles due to deep insertion to the bony portion of the canal – Home-based routine maintenance is generally straightforward – Suitable for those who wear glasses, oxygen cannulas, and facemasks	– Does not offer an open-fit option – Is less suitable for individuals with "normal" low-frequency thresholds due to occlusion effects – Unable to demonstrate in the office – Handling and maintenance can be challenging due to the small size – Speakers are not interchangeable – May pose challenges for patients with middle ear complications or those who have undergone ear surgeries – Necessitates frequent battery replacements, typically every 4–7 days – Size constraints may limit available features and technology – Not suitable for severe/profound losses due to speaker size and increased chance of feedback – Candidacy depends on ear canal shape and size – Prone to complications from moisture and wax buildup

Acoustic Coupling and Venting

Various coupling and venting options exist within hearing aids, each playing a crucial role in determining the user's acoustic experience.

Tubing:

- *Traditional thick BTE tubing* connects a behind-the-ear hearing aid to a custom earmold. This tubing is available in different sizes and thicknesses to accommodate various degrees of hearing loss.
- *Slim tubing* is a less conspicuous BTE-style tubing that connects a behind-the-ear hearing aid to a custom earmold or dome; however, its narrow design can diminish high-frequency gain [15].
- *Thin wire* coupling digitally transfers sound from the body of the RIC hearing aid behind the patient's ear to the receiver placed in the patient's ear canal. A dome or a custom earmold attaches to the receiver for comfort and acoustic purposes.

Earmolds/Domes:

- *Custom earmolds* are manufactured using an impression of the patient's ear taken by an audiologist. These earmolds are compatible with traditional, slim tubing or RIC configurations.

- *Domes* are non-custom tips available in various shapes, sizes, and venting options. Domes can couple to RIC or slim tube BTE configurations.

Venting Considerations:
Hearing aid venting is most modifiable in BTE and RIC style fittings, ranging from fully open to complete occlusion. Venting also plays a crucial role in ITE, in the canal (ITC), completely in the canal (CIC), and invisible in the canal (IIC) hearing aids; however, the venting options are more limited due to all components being in the ear.

- *Open fittings* are characterized by large venting above 4–5 mm, offer a more natural sound quality, and are suited for individuals with essentially normal low-frequency thresholds and mid-high frequencies below 70 dB [16].
- *Occluded fittings* feature minimal to no venting, suitable for more severe losses, but elevate the risk of the "occlusion effect"—a phenomenon inducing a hollow sound sensation from trapped low frequencies [15, 16].

Understanding the different coupling options, tubing variations, earmold/dome compatibilities, and venting considerations is pivotal for ensuring adequate gain and optimal acoustic experiences in hearing aid users.

Digital Processing

Many different fitting algorithms and processing strategies are used in digital hearing aids. Digital processing attempts to provide the best signal possible for each environment the patient encounters. Advanced digital processing in hearing aids typically includes:

- *Frequency-dependent gain adjustments* amplify sections of the frequency range independently based on the patient's audiogram thresholds. The more frequency bands/channels available in the hearing aid, the more precisely it can be tuned. Most hearing aids have about 6–20 bands/channels.
- *MPO (Maximum Power Output) limits* the maximum hearing aid output for comfort and safety. MPO is a band/channel-specific limit, which varies for each hearing aid. The hearing aid MPO limits are contingent upon the device's fitting range and the individual's specific amplification requirements [17].
- *Compression* is a complex processing technique that modifies hearing aid gain across individual frequency bands/channels. Sensorineural hearing loss creates a limited dynamic range, characterized by an inability to hear soft sounds as well as increased sensitivity to loud sounds. Hearing aid compression aims to best fit the full range of environmental sounds into the patient's limited dynamic range. Wide dynamic range compression (WDRC) is a common compression strategy used in hearing aids to improve speech audibility in hearing aids by ensuring soft sounds are audible and loud sounds are available, but not uncomfortable, across all frequencies [17].
- *Speech enhancement and noise reduction processing* aim to amplify and clean up speech signals while separating them from background noise. Hearing aids with only a single microphone are limited to fewer and more basic processing strategies, like spectral subtraction, which decreases gain on bands/channels with excessive noise. Dual microphone hearing aids compare the signals received from the front vs. the back microphone for more complex processing strategies like adaptive polar plots and beamforming technology, which allow the hearing aid to change the direction and width of focus to amplify and enhance the primary speech signal over background noise [18]. Many hearing aids now use wireless communication between bilateral hearing aids to analyze input from all microphones to preserve binaural cues and further improve localization and speech perception in noise [19].
- *Sound classifiers* sample the patient's surroundings to determine different environment types, such as quiet, noise, speech with noise, or music [12]. These classifications automatically enable the hearing aid to adjust its processing strategies for distinct listening scenarios. Furthermore, the hearing aid can record a log of hearing aid wear time and duration spent in each environment type.
- *Acoustic feedback systems* notably reduce the risk of feedback or whistling due to improved digital adaptive feedback reduction and cancellation methods like gain reduction, notch filtering, and phase cancellation.

Additional Features

Hearing aid technology has many additional features, with availability based on the manufacturer and style.

Some of the possible features include:

- *Direct or hands-free streaming* of phone calls and media from smartphones to hearing aids without additional devices.
- *Tinnitus management* is available in many hearing aids via sound generators to help relieve tinnitus for patients with hearing loss and tinnitus [20, 21]. The sound generators allow patients to turn on low-level noise (e.g., white, pink, shaped) or sounds (e.g., ocean or tones) to help mask/suppress bothersome tinnitus.
- *Frequency-lowering technology* may be used for patients with severe/profound high-frequency hearing loss to pro-

vide them access to soft high-frequency consonants (i.e., "s," "sh," "f," "t," "th"). This technology allows high-frequency sounds to be shifted to lower frequencies where the hearing loss is less severe, and the hearing aid can provide sufficient gain [22].

- Artificial intelligence and deep neural network (DNN) learning are now used in some hearing aids to better classify environments and sounds for improved automatic adjustments of the hearing aids and improved hearing in background noise.
- *Rechargeable* hearing aids are now widely available due to improvements in battery technology and lower power consumption needs.
- *Compatible smart device apps* reduce the need to purchase/carry remotes or worry about pressing the small buttons on the hearing aids to access volume control and manual programs. Most apps also have specialized features within them, including, but not limited to, "Find my hearing aid" tracking, real-time adjustments using patient preferences, bass/treble balancing, background noise reduction, wear time and program use data logging, health fitness tracking, fall detection, instructional videos, and telehealth access for appointments and programming adjustments.
- Improved connectivity with services like Bluetooth or Auracast™ that allow public venues to stream audio directly to hearing aids without dedicated receivers. This type of broadcast is available in some airports, lecture halls, entertainment venues, and religious congregations.

Hearing Aid Candidacy

Patients rely on otolaryngologists and audiologists to interpret audiograms in an easily comprehensible manner and to provide them with guidance on the best amplification for their specific hearing needs. It is imperative to be well-versed in the indications for hearing aids and assistive listening devices to guide patients toward better hearing.

Multiple factors must be considered when determining hearing aid candidacy and appropriate recommendations. Hearing aids can help individuals with all three types of hearing loss (conductive, sensorineural, and mixed) and over a wide range of severity; however, not all individuals with hearing loss are ideal hearing aid candidates. The following considerations help to determine hearing aid candidacy.

Type of Hearing Loss

As described below, there are 3 different types of hearing loss: sensorineural, conductive, and mixed [23]. Hearing aids are typically an option for each of these categories of hearing loss, but some patients may benefit more from medical treatments or surgical options, including implantable devices [24]. Other chapters in this book discuss those options.

- *Sensorineural hearing loss* is the most common type of hearing loss, and hearing aids are typically the recommended treatment option. However, patients with sound distortion or poor speech recognition may not receive optimal benefit from hearing aids.
- *Conductive hearing loss* can often be appropriately managed with hearing aids. However, factors such as physical structures, surgical options, and the severity of the conductive component might make other devices, such as a bone-anchored implant, a more suitable choice. It is also important to note that extra acoustic power is required to overcome air-bone gaps, making moderate-to-large conductive hearing losses less ideal for hearing aid use due to limitations in power output and a heightened risk of feedback and distortion [24, 25].
- *Mixed hearing loss* is a combination of sensorineural and conductive hearing loss, and this type of loss is often challenging for traditional hearing aid fitting.

Degree of Hearing Loss

The degree of hearing loss (HL) is categorized from mild to profound and provides a general idea of how much difficulty a patient is experiencing with communication.

- *Mild hearing loss (26–40 dB HL)* may cause difficulty hearing soft speech and understanding speech in background noise. Compensation can often be manageable without amplification, making mild hearing loss challenging to determine hearing aid candidacy.
- *Moderate (41–55 dB HL)* to *moderately severe (55–70 dB HL) hearing loss* typically results in difficulty understanding soft and moderate speech. This more appreciable communication deficit often increases the patients' perceived necessity of hearing aids and allows for more noticeable benefits. Patients with this degree of loss are typically ideal candidates for hearing aids.
- *Severe (71–90 dB HL)* to *profound (91+ dB HL) hearing loss* usually *results* in an inability to hear soft and moderate speech and difficulty understanding loud speech. Most of these patients are ideal candidates for hearing aids; however, for some, a significant limitation to success with amplification is poor speech intelligibility. Patients who do not perceive enough clarity/benefit from well-fit hearing aids should be considered for cochlear implantation [26].

All hearing aids have recommended fitting ranges to ensure the hearing aid output is appropriate for the degree of loss. Fitting ranges help decide which hearing aids are ideal for the patient, but not whether the patient is ideal for hearing aids.

Audiometric Challenges

Reverse slope and steeply sloping high-frequency audiogram configurations are arguably two of the most challenging threshold configurations to fit successfully.

- *Reverse-slope (low-frequency) hearing loss* is characterized by hearing impairment up to 2000 Hz, coupled with normal high-frequency hearing thresholds. This loss is difficult to fit for several reasons. The ear canal must be sealed well to amplify the low frequencies effectively, but in turn, it can lead to an occlusion effect, which is generally bothersome to patients [27]. Amplifying low frequencies with hearing aids can also lead to poor sound quality by introducing more background noise and masking crucial mid- and high-frequency speech sounds, thereby reducing speech clarity [27].
- *Steeply sloping high-frequency hearing loss* is difficult to fit due to frequency range limitations of the hearing aid technology and venting needs. Many current hearing aids have increased bandwidths to 8–12 kHz; however, the amount of usable gain and whether it is truly beneficial at these high frequencies is debatable [28–30]. Hearing aids with non-occluding fittings, even with a broad frequency bandwidth, cannot provide useful amplification for frequencies above 4.4–6 kHz [31]. It may be necessary to occlude the ear to better meet the high-frequency gain requirements; however, this can increase the occlusion effect and decrease the natural sound quality of the hearing aids [32].

Current digital hearing aids have improved features, including detailed gain adjustments, own-voice algorithm adjustments, front-end processing, and frequency lowering, to help these difficult-to-fit patients maximize their benefits.

Other Candidacy Considerations

Although important, the type, degree, and configuration of hearing loss do not act as sole determining factors in hearing aid candidacy. Conducting an individualized, needs-based assessment is integral to the identification of suitable hearing aid candidates [12, 33]. While the specifics of assessment will vary from practice to practice, it remains essential to complete a detailed evaluation of each patient's individual hearing needs and lifestyle to determine candidacy and provide tailored hearing aid selection recommendations.

Patient Perception/Motivation

The patient's perception of their hearing deficit and their level of motivation are significant in determining hearing aid candidacy, especially for borderline candidates. Patients who struggle with communication will likely be more motivated to wear amplification consistently. Conversely, patients who report no hearing difficulties or who hold a negative stigma towards hearing aids are less likely to perceive significant benefits from amplification and may have poor usage compliance [34].

Patients who note a deficit in their ability to communicate with others have a gauge to measure the improvements in their everyday lives post-fitting with amplification. Patients who complain of difficulty hearing in background noise, decreased speech clarity, or the need for frequent repetition likely warrant a trial of amplification, even if their thresholds are borderline abnormal [35].

Lifestyle

A significant component of the needs-based assessment for hearing aid selection and fitting revolves around understanding the patient's lifestyle. To provide optimal benefits, assessing the environments the patient frequently interacts with is vital, ensuring the hearing aid features align with the patient's specific needs and expectations.

Lifestyle factors such as activity level, overall health, and the requirement for additional support also play pivotal roles in determining a suitable hearing aid recommendation. Some patients might not perceive themselves as active, social, or healthy enough to justify the acquisition of traditional hearing aids. While hearing aids are usually the best option, other assistive listening devices can also significantly benefit patients with hearing difficulty. Some patients may also need additional physical support from family members or caregivers to be successful hearing aid users. Maintenance, insertion/removal of the devices, or changing batteries can prove difficult for some patients, especially if they are frail, have reduced hand motor skills, or have visual difficulties.

Dementia and Cognitive Decline

The link between hearing impairment and cognitive function was formally reported as early as the 1980s. Since that time, untreated hearing loss has been reported as a strong predictor of early cognitive decline [36, 37]. Based on longitudinal studies of older adults, hearing loss has been implicated with not only accelerated cognitive decline but also an increased risk of all-cause dementia [38–42]. The degree of hearing loss is also important, as those with greater amounts of hearing loss have been shown to have a higher risk of developing dementia compared to those with less hearing loss [36].

Several theories have been proposed to describe this functional relationship, citing the following influencing changes in response to untreated hearing loss: increased cognitive load, brain function and structure changes, and reduced social engagement [39].

In 2023, a landmark study on hearing and cognition was published in the Lancet journal. The ACHIEVE study is a multicenter, parallel-group, unmasked, randomized control trial of adults 70–84 years old with untreated hearing loss. The ACHIEVE study findings suggest that a hearing intervention might reduce cognitive change over 3 years in populations of older adults at increased risk for cognitive decline [43]. This study aligns with the Lancet Commission on Dementia, which identified hearing loss as the largest modifiable dementia risk factor worldwide [55]. It is, therefore, important to emphasize the role of hearing rehabilitation, including hearing aids, in this at-risk population.

Cost

If cost is a barrier, patients can be provided with information about national and local financial assistance programs, low-cost hearing aids, over-the-counter (OTC) hearing aids, personal sound amplification products (PSAP), and other assistive listening devices.

In 2022, the U.S. Food and Drug Administration established an over-the-counter (OTC) hearing aid category for adults with perceived mild to moderate hearing loss, allowing these devices to be purchased without a prescription, medical evaluation, or professional fitting. Since their introduction, the OTC hearing aid market has expanded rapidly and continues to evolve, encompassing a wide range of device designs, technological features, and self-fitting approaches. Although a detailed review of OTC devices is beyond the scope of this chapter, they should be considered for select patients, particularly those with financial limitations, reduced access to hearing health professionals, or an anticipated short-term need for amplification, such as individuals awaiting otologic or reconstructive surgery. Clinicians should recognize that OTC hearing aids vary substantially in quality, electroacoustic performance, and suitability for individual hearing profiles, reinforcing the importance of careful patient counseling, appropriate medical screening, and individualized recommendations when considering OTC devices as part of a comprehensive hearing rehabilitation strategy (Table 16.2).

Table 16.2 Categories of hearing aids, per the United States Food and Drug Administration

	Over-the-counter (OTC) hearing aids	Prescription hearing aids*	Personal sound amplifiers
Type of product	Medical device and electronic product	Medical device and electronic product	Electronic product
Intended users	– People 18 years and older – People with perceived mild-to-moderate hearing loss	– People of any age – People with any degree of hearing loss	People of any age with normal hearing seeking to amplify sounds in certain environments
Conditions for sale	– Purchaser must be 18 years of age or older – No medical exam – No prescription – No fitting by audiologist – No need for licensed seller	– Prescription needed – Must purchase from licensed seller in some states	No applicable FDA requirements

Adapted from the FDA, as published in "Hearing Aids," 5/3/2023. Accessible at https://www.fda.gov/medical-devices/consumer-products/hearing-aids

[a]Any hearing aid that does not meet OTC requirements

Medical Clearance

Patients with possible ear disease should be medically evaluated, treated, and cleared by a physician, preferably an otolaryngologist or otologist, prior to referral to an audiologist for hearing aids [54].

Medical Considerations and Relative Contraindications

From our clinical experience, we have noted that the following ear conditions often need extra attention when evaluating for amplification purposes.

- *Actively draining* ears and those prone to chronic otitis can lead to clogged hearing aid receivers and tubing. The blockage results in no measurable output from the hearing aid and moisture damage to the electrical components. BTE-style hearing aids with a large fitting range and acoustically optimized venting are typically necessary for these patients. Implantable devices are often a favorable alternative for these patients [25, 44].

- *Tympanic membrane perforations* can lead to excess moisture in the ear canal when a hearing aid occludes it. Excessive moisture buildup may lead to chronic otorrhea and damage to the hearing aid components. Appropriate venting is essential, and if the ear is not dry, a BTE-style hearing aid with traditional or slim tubing may be warranted.
- *Excessive cerumen* can clog hearing aid receivers and tubing. Depending on the amount and consistency of the cerumen, it may be necessary to use a BTE-style hearing aid with traditional or slim tubing.
- *Atresia, stenosis, or surgical closure of the ear canal* are often contraindications for hearing aids due to the physical limitations of fitting the devices. In these cases, implantable devices or a CROS/BiCROS should be considered.
- *Mastoid cavities* can be more susceptible to recurrent infection when excess moisture is present in the surgical cavity. Large cavities require extra power from the hearing aid, which can be challenging to obtain with appropriate venting. Here, BTE-style hearing aids with custom earmolds are often a good option. Implantable devices may also be considered, especially if there is concern for recurrent infection.
- *Ménière's disease* can cause fluctuating hearing loss and sound distortion. The fluctuations in hearing may warrant a wide fitting range and patient access to multiple programs or volume control. If the hearing aids do not provide enough clarity due to distortion, they may benefit from a CROS/BiCROS system or an implantable device.
- *Sudden sensorineural hearing loss* is typically unilateral and can cause significant distortion. It is imperative that the hearing loss is stable and unlikely to recover before recommending amplification. Some patients may report hearing aids do not provide enough clarity due to distortion, and they may be a better candidate for a CROS/BiCROS or an implantable device.

Hearing Aid Fitting

Otolaryngologists and audiologists must stay up-to-date with hearing aid fitting advancements to provide patients with consistent and appropriate fitting recommendations. After determining a patient's suitability for hearing aids by evaluating the factors discussed in the previous section, the audiologist will outline fitting recommendations and set expectations.

Fitting Recommendations

Bilateral Amplification

Bilateral amplification is advised when fitting patients with bilateral hearing loss unless there are medical or audiological contraindications. The advantages of bilateral cues are numerous and include, but are not limited to:

- *Loudness summation*: a natural phenomenon where the loudness of a sound is increased by an average of 3–6 dB when presented bilaterally vs. unilaterally [45, 46].
- *Masking level*: uses bilateral differences in time and intensity to help separate a desired signal (i.e., speech) from background noise [47].
- *Localization:* uses bilateral differences in intensity and phase to locate where sounds are in the environment.
- *Head shadow effect:* the decrease in the amplitude of sounds, especially high frequencies, as they travel from one side of the head to the other.

Bilateral amplification will allow patients to use the above binaural cues to their advantage for better processing of the auditory information surrounding them. Many digital hearing aids can also connect to each other wirelessly to provide improved processing of speech with the use of bilateral cues, especially in complex environments.

Appropriate Fitting Expectations

The audiologist uses manufacturer-specific fitting software to program the hearing aid based on the patient's audiogram at the fitting appointment. Standard practice for fitting hearing aids typically includes evaluating the physical fit, analyzing potential feedback issues, programming gain and maximum output of the hearing aid based on research or proprietary algorithms, activating beneficial features, and adding programs tailored for various environments. Additionally, the process involves counseling the patient on device use and maintenance and may also entail linking the devices to the patient's phone and downloading and discussing relevant apps.

Verification

Current hearing aid fitting best-practice guidelines include using verification measurements for checking aided thresholds, aided speech understanding, or gain/output of the hearing aid(s) [33, 48, 49]. The gold standard of hearing aid verification is called Real Ear Measurements, which involves placing a probe microphone into the patient's ear canal to measure the actual gain and maximum output at the level of the eardrum. These measurements verify that the hearing aid is meeting the prescribed targets across all frequencies and are used to adjust hearing aid gain, as needed, for the best fitting.

Acclimatization

Providing guidance on the expectation of full-time hearing aid use is imperative. Increased exposure to sound by wearing hearing aids, even in quiet environments, is always preferable and will increase success in more difficult listening situations. Acclimatization improves auditory processing performance by separating speech from noise and suppressing environmental sounds that may be initially perceived as bothersome. Initial acclimatization to hearing aids takes about 2–4 weeks, but it may take up to 6 months of consistent use to receive optimal benefit from hearing aids [50, 51]. Some digital processing features, such as frequency lowering, have shown many benefits for speech, focusing on sound detection and consonants; however, it is important to note they can further increase the length of the acclimatization [52, 53].

Following the initial fitting session, the audiologist schedules subsequent follow-up appointments to ensure the patient's optimal experience with the hearing aid. During these sessions, the audiologist provides counseling, evaluates the device's performance and outcomes, reviews maintenance procedures, inspects the physical fit, cleans the device, and assesses whether any programming adjustments are necessary to enhance the user's listening experience.

Accessories and Assistive Listening Devices

While hearing aids generally offer the most significant benefit for individuals with hearing loss, hearing aid accessories and other listening devices are available to assist those experiencing hearing challenges. Table 16.3 lists examples of hearing aid accessories that potentially enhance the effectiveness of hearing aids in challenging listening environments. However, it is important to note that some hearing aids are incompatible with certain accessories. Figure 16.2 and Table 16.4 present examples of assistive listening devices that providers can recommend to improve the overall quality of life for individuals with hearing loss in various settings. It's important to remember that neither personal sound amplification products (PSAPs) nor assistive listening devices (ALDs) are considered medical devices.

Table 16.3 Common accessories for hearing aids

Devices	Description	Best use case/advantages	Limitations/disadvantages
Bluetooth (BT) clip/pendant/neck loop	Intermediate wireless accessory that connects hearing aids to Bluetooth-enabled devices (phones, tablets, computers)	– Enables hands-free phone calls and media streaming for hearing aids without native Bluetooth compatibility – Improves signal-to-noise ratio compared with acoustic phone use	– Typically sold separately – Compatible with select hearing aids only – Requires carrying/wearing the device – Setup and usage can be complex and confusing – Increasingly less necessary with newer direct-streaming hearing aids
TV streamer/ TV connector	Device that connects directly to a television and streams audio wirelessly to hearing aids	– Provides superior sound quality – Amplifies volume considering patient's hearing loss – Maintains signal quality irrespective of distance, room acoustics, or ambient noise – Offers signal enhancement with noise reduction	– Typically sold separately – Compatible with select hearing aids only – May necessitate a Bluetooth phone clip/necklace/device for pairing with TV – Setup and usage can be complex and confusing
Microphone clip-on/table/partner mic	Wearable or tabletop microphone that streams a speaker's voice(s) directly to hearing aids	– Ensures unaffected signal by distance, room acoustics, or ambient noise – Provides speech enhancement with noise reduction – Particularly useful for unilateral or poor speech-in-noise performers	– Typically sold separately – Compatible with select hearing aids only – Requires carrying/wearing the device – Setup and usage can be complex and confusing
Remote control	A remote permitting manual alteration to hearing aid settings, such as program settings and volume	– Facilitates control without interacting with small hearing aid buttons – Suitable for patients with limited dexterity – Adds control of hearing aids lacking onboard buttons	– Typically sold separately – Compatible with select hearing aids only – Requires carrying the device – Largely replaced by smartphone apps

(continued)

Table 16.3 (continued)

Devices	Description	Best use case/advantages	Limitations/disadvantages
FM device/ digital wireless classroom systems	Systems using dedicated digital or FM transmission to deliver speech directly to hearing aids	– Delivers speech enhancement, with some devices offering noise reduction – Ideal for classrooms and meetings	– Typically sold separately – Compatible with select hearing aids only – Often requires connecting and wearing extra devices – May require complex and costly setup for organizations
Streaming home/cell phone	A specialized phone or adapter enabling direct signal transfer to both hearing aids from cordless or cell phones	– Enhances speech intelligibility during phone calls – Offers binaural advantage for bilateral hearing aid users – User-friendly and compatible with non-Bluetooth devices – Allows unaltered phone use for other family members	– Typically sold separately – Compatible with select hearing aids only – Exclusively functions with the designated phone
Tele-coil(T-coil)/loop receiver	A copper coil, potentially integrated, transforming sounds from magnetic signals sent via various sources, enabling enhanced sound reception	– Compatible with certain phones to amplify phone frequencies – Facilitates speech enhancement with noise reduction when used in "looped" locations like religious congregations, theaters, and bank drive-throughs – Can be used to link hearing aids to Bluetooth or other accessories	– Integrated into select hearing aids only – Enlarges the hearing aid's size – Availability of "looped" environments is limited in the US, more prevalent in Europe – Declining use with growth of Bluetooth audio
Auracast™ broadcast audio	Next-generation Bluetooth public broadcast system allowing direct audio streaming to hearing aids in public venues	– Provides direct, clear audio in airports, theaters, and lecture halls without additional receivers – Scalable and privacy-controlled	– Requires Bluetooth LE audio–enabled hearing aids and venue infrastructure. Still emerging; availability varies by region

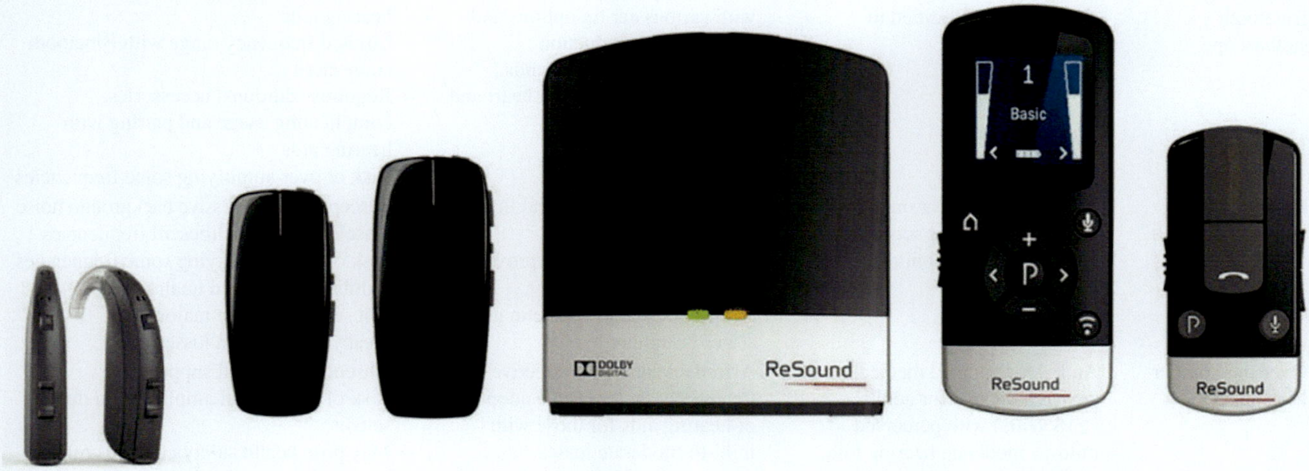

Fig. 16.2 Common accessories for hearing aids. This figure displays five common accessory variations from one manufacturer that patients can use in conjunction with their hearing aids, providing insights into the variety available in the market. (Courtesy of Resound)

Table 16.4 Assistive listening devices and smartphone-based assistive technologies

Devices	Description	Uses/advantages	Limitations/disadvantages
Amplified microphone headset	A microphone, integrated with an amplifier, connected to a headset for the patient	– Ideal in physicians' offices and hospitals for patients without hearing aids – Inexpensive solution for patients with severe losses waiting for hearing aids – Suitable for patients who will not tolerate or wear hearing aids – Appropriate for patients with limited lifespan or significant health concerns	– The individual speaking must be close due to wired microphone-headphone connection – Produces poor sound quality – Unselectively amplifies all frequencies – Prone to excessive background noise interference – Risk of over-amplifying some frequencies
Captioned home phone	Telephone that provides real-time speech-to-text captions in addition to amplified audio	– Improves telephone communication for patients with poor speech recognition – Often available at low or no cost under ADA-supported programs – Large, readable text	– May require a recommendation from an audiologist or physician – Necessitates adequate vision and reading capabilities – Internet connection is mandatory
Amplified home phone	A home phone equipped with additional amplification	– Enhances volume of phone receiver, improving user's communication	– Unselectively amplifies all frequencies – Risk of over-amplifying some frequencies – Restricted to this specific phone
Wireless TV headset	A headset that receives TV audio via infrared, Bluetooth, or radio frequency	– Unaffected by distance, acoustics, or background sounds – Allows individualized TV volume without disturbing others	– Unselectively amplifies all frequencies – Necessitates an individual unit for each TV – The device is bulky – May be incompatible when using hearing aids – Risk of over-amplifying some frequencies
Induction loop system	A device, either a headset or neck loop, suitable for looped environments, using T-coil technology	– Provides improved signal-to-noise ratio in looped venues (theaters, places of worship, government buildings), without needing a hearing aid	– Unselectively amplifies all frequencies – Availability of looped environments is limited in the US, more common in Europe – Risk of over-amplifying some frequencies – Declining use with expansion of Bluetooth LE audio
Amplified or Bluetooth stethoscope	A stethoscope that is electronically modified to amplify sounds	– Provides up to 24% louder sound with various ear tip options and ambient noise reduction – Can record and save sounds, offering choice between heart and lung frequencies	– Ear tips may be incompatible with certain hearing aids – Limited frequency range with Bluetooth connectivity – Requires additional accessories, complicating usage and pairing with hearing aids – Risk of over-amplifying some frequencies
Personal sound amplifier (PSAP)	A device worn in or on the ear to amplify sounds for activities like watching TV or monitoring others	– Designed to resemble and fit like hearing aids – Amplifies sounds for improved hearing – Affordable and available in general stores or online	– Susceptible to excessive background noise – Unselectively amplifies all frequencies – Risk of over-amplifying some frequencies – Exhibits poor sound quality – Not suitable for the majority of presbycusis-shaped losses
Over-the-counter hearing Aid	An FDA-regulated medical device indicated for adults (≥18 years) with perceived mild-to-moderate hearing loss, available without prescription or professional fitting through retail and online outlets	– Affordable and cost-effective option – Potentially increases the adoption of hearing aids for those with mild-to-moderate losses – Offers convenience and accessibility in purchasing – May contribute to reducing the stigma associated with hearing aids	– Absence of clinical support – Risk of suboptimal amplification due to self-fit – May pose health safety concerns related to underlying medical conditions – Lacks on-ear verification – Distinguishing between FDA-approved OTC hearing aids and amplifiers can be challenging for consumers
Speech-to-text Mobile Device and applications	A mobile device or mobile app, or a cell phone or tablet, capable of transcribing spoken words	– Faster than writing or typing – Useful in physicians' offices for patients without adequate amplification, speech understanding, or knowledge of sign language – Some applications allow communication in different languages	– Mandates carrying an electronic device – Slows the pace of communication – Requires adequate vision and reading capabilities – May be prone to transcription errors

(continued)

Table 16.4 (continued)

Devices	Description	Uses/advantages	Limitations/disadvantages
Alerting and safety devices	Visual, vibratory, or amplified alerts for alarms, doorbells, phones, and baby monitors	– Enhances safety and independence, especially when hearing aids are not worn (e.g., during sleep)	– Potential to be excessively loud and disruptive for individuals without hearing loss – Often requires multiple devices for full home coverage – Setup can be complex
Smartphone sound amplification/ accessibility modes	Built-in phone features that amplify sound through earbuds or headphones	– Readily available, no additional cost. Helpful for situational listening (lectures, one-on-one conversation)	– Not frequency-specific or audiogram-based – Risk of inappropriate amplification – Not intended to treat hearing loss
Consumer headphones	Earbuds or headphones with hearing aid-focused capabilities	– Lower-cost solution for people with mild-to-moderate hearing loss – Some models use audiograms for personalized frequency-dependent gain adjustments – Intelligent features can amplify conversations and calls while controlling noise – Familiar look may help overcome the stigma of traditional hearing aids – More suitable for music than other HA types	– Limited battery life may not last an entire day – Some might not find them comfortable for long-term wear – Often very visible – May be more suitable for situational use than all-day hearing assistance

Summary

A myriad of tailored solutions is available to manage hearing loss, from digital hearing aids to accessories and assistive listening systems. Given the diversity in solutions, it is crucial to reflect on all factors discussed in this chapter when guiding patients toward better hearing. Since the best solution varies significantly among individuals, clinicians must deeply empathize, recognizing the unique challenges hearing loss presents to patients and their families.

With the anticipated advancements and the increasing significance of amplification in the aging population, continuous adaptation of hearing healthcare recommendations is essential. Often being the initial consultants, otolaryngologists must remain abreast of current practices and ensure proper referrals and recommendations. The decision-making process for choosing the most suitable option is highly individualized and dynamic, requiring adaptation to the evolving landscape of amplification and the unique needs of each patient, many of whom will remain active well into their eighth and ninth decades of life.

References

1. Ferguson MA, et al. Hearing aids for mild to moderate hearing loss in adults. Cochrane Database Syst Rev. 2017;9(9):CD012023.
2. Holmes AE, Saxon JP, Kaplan HS. Assistive listening devices and systems: amplification technology for consumers with hearing loss. J Rehabil. 2000;66(3):56–9.
3. Mulrow CD, et al. Quality-of-life changes and hearing impairment. *A randomized trial*. Ann Intern Med. 1990;113(3):188–94.
4. Choi JE, et al. A comparison between wireless CROS/BiCROS and soft-band BAHA for patients with unilateral hearing loss. PLoS One. 2019;14(2):e0212503.
5. Snapp HA, et al. Comparison of speech-in-noise and localization benefits in unilateral hearing loss subjects using contralateral routing of signal hearing aids or bone-anchored implants. Otol Neurotol. 2017;38(1):11–8.
6. Gazia F, et al. Extended wear hearing aids: a comparative, pilot study. Eur Arch Otorhinolarygol. 2022;279(11):5415–22.
7. Phonak, "Phonak Lyric". https://www.phonakpro.com/content/dam/phonakpro/gc_us/en/products_solutions/hearing_aid/lyric/documents/028-6485-03_Keys_to_Success_for_Lyric_Fitters.pdf. Accessed 26 Jan 2026.
8. Arbogast TL, et al. Achieved gain and subjective outcomes for a wide-bandwidth contact hearing aid fitted using CAM2. Ear Hear. 2019;40(3):741–56.
9. Dundas D, Levy SC. A 10-year review of the Earlens system, part 3: what's the big deal about audibility and broader audible bandwidth? Hear Rev. 2022;29(2):24–7.
10. Perkins R, et al. The EarLens system: new sound transduction methods. Hear Res. 2010;263(1–2):104–13.
11. Dillon H., Hearing aids. Sydney: Boomerang Press. 2001.
12. Ricketts TA, Bentler R, Mueller HG. Essentials of modern hearing aids: selection, fitting, and verification. Plural Publishing, Inc.; 2019.
13. Launer S, Zakis J, Moore B. Hearing aid signal processing. In: Popelka GR, BCJ M, Fay RR, Popper AN, editors. Hearing aids; Springer handbook of auditory research. New York: Springer International Publishing; 2016. p. 93–130.
14. Sandlin, R. Digital hearing aids: hype, hoax or hope. https://www.audiologyonline.com/articles/digital-hearing-aids-hype-hoax-1221. Audiology Online. 2001.
15. Kuk F., Baekgaard M. Hearing aid selection and BTEs: choosing among various "open-ear" and "receiver-in-canal" options. Hear Rev. 2008.

16. Winkler A, Latzel M, Holube I. Open versus closed hearing aid fittings: a literature review of both fitting approaches. Trends Hear. 2016;20:1–13.
17. Starkey Hearing Technologies. The compression handbook. 4th ed. Eden Prairie: Starkey Laboratories; 2017.
18. Kuk F, et al. Performance of a fully adaptive directional microphone to signals presented from various azimuths. J Am Acad Audiol. 2005;16(6):333–47.
19. Geetha C, Tanniru K, Rajan RR. Efficacy of directional microphones in hearing aids equipped with wireless synchronization technology. J Int Adv Otol. 2017;13(1):113–7.
20. Ganesan P, et al. Combined amplification and sound therapy for individuals with tinnitus and coexisting hearing loss: a retrospective cohort study. J Int Adv Otol. 2021;17(6):514–9.
21. Tutaj L, Hoare DJ, Sereda M. Combined amplification and sound generation for tinnitus: a scoping review. Ear Hear. 2018;39(3):412–22.
22. Glista D, Scollie S. The use of frequency lowering technology in the treatment of severe-to-profound hearing loss: a review of the literature and candidacy considerations for clinical application. Semin Hear. 2018;39(4):377–89.
23. ASHA. Sensorineural hearing loss. https://www.asha.org/public/hearing/Sensorineural-Hearing-Loss/. Accessed 26 Jan 2026.
24. de Wolf MJ, et al. Better performance with bone-anchored hearing aid than acoustic devices in patients with severe air-bone gap. Laryngoscope. 2011;121(3):613–6.
25. Lerner S. Limitations of conventional hearing aids: examining common complaints and issues that can and cannot be remedied. Otolaryngol Clin N Am. 2019;52(2):211–20.
26. Zwolan TA, Schvartz-Leyzac KC, Pleasant T. Development of a 60/60 guideline for referring adults for a traditional cochlear implant candidacy evaluation. Otol Neurotol. 2020;41(7):895–900.
27. Kuk F., Keenan D, Ludvigsen C. Changing with the times: managing low-frequency hearing loss. Hear Rev. 2003.
28. Hornsby BW, Johnson EE, Picou E. Effects of degree and configuration of hearing loss on the contribution of high- and low-frequency speech information to bilateral speech understanding. Ear Hear. 2011;32(5):543–55.
29. Levy SC, et al. Extended high-frequency bandwidth improves speech reception in the presence of spatially separated masking speech. Ear Hear. 2015;36(5):e214–24.
30. Plyler PN, Fleck EL. The effects of high-frequency amplification on the objective and subjective performance of hearing instrument users with varying degrees of high-frequency hearing loss. J Speech Lang Hear Res. 2006;49(3):616–27.
31. Struck CJ, Prusick L. Comparison of real-world bandwidth in hearing aids vs Earlens light-driven hearing aid system. Hear Rev. 2017; 24(3):24–29.
32. Dillon H., Hearing aids. 2nd Ed. Sydney: Boomerang Press. 2012.
33. APSO, S2.1. Hearing Aid Fitting for Adult & Geriatric Patients https://www.audiologystandards.org/standards/display.php?id=102. Standard S2.1[2021] Adopted May 2, 2021. Accessed 26 Jan 2026.
34. Wilson C, Stephens D. Reasons for referral and attitudes toward hearing aids: do they affect outcome? Clin Otolaryngol Allied Sci. 2003;28:81–4.
35. Humes LE. What is normal hearing for older adults and can "normal-hearing older adults" benefit from hearing care intervention? Hear Rev. 2020;27(7):12–8.
36. Uhlmann RF, et al. Relationship of hearing impairment to dementia and cognitive dysfunction in older adults. JAMA. 1989;261(13):1916–9.
37. Deal JA, et al. Hearing impairment and cognitive decline: a pilot study conducted within the atherosclerosis risk in communities neurocognitive study. Am J Epidemiol. 2015;181(9):680–90.
38. Gallacher J, et al. Auditory threshold, phonologic demand, and incident dementia. Neurology. 2012;79(15):1583–90.
39. Lin FR, Albert M. Hearing loss and dementia – who is listening? Aging Ment Health. 2014;18(6):671–3.
40. Lin FR, et al. Hearing loss and cognition in the Baltimore longitudinal study of aging. Neuropsychology. 2011;25(6):763–70.
41. Lin FR, et al. Hearing loss and incident dementia. Arch Neurol. 2011;68(2):214–20.
42. Lin FR, et al. Hearing loss and cognitive decline in older adults. JAMA Intern Med. 2013;173(4):293–9.
43. Lin FR, et al. Hearing intervention versus health education control to reduce cognitive decline in older adults with hearing loss in the USA (ACHIEVE): a multicentre, randomised controlled trial. Lancet. 2023;402(10404):786–97.
44. Orji FT, Onyero OE, Agbo CE. The clinical implications of ear canal debris in hearing aid users. Pak J Med Sci. 2014;30(3):483–7.
45. Haggard MP, Hall JW. Forms of binaural summation and the implications of individual variability for binaural hearing aids. Scand Audiol Suppl. 1982;15:47–63.
46. Reynolds G, Stevens S. Binaural summation of loudness. J Acoust Soc Am. 1960;32:1337–44.
47. Kock W. Binaural localization and masking. J Acoust Soc Am. 1950;22:810–4.
48. Valente M., et al. Guidelines for the audiologic management of adult hearing impairment. American Academy of Audiology Task Force (US). https://www.audiology.org/practice-guideline/guidelines-for-the-audiologic-management-of-adult-hearing-impairment/.
49. Valente M, et al. Guidelines for hearing aid fitting for adults. Am J Aud. 1998;7:5–13.
50. Gatehouse S. The time course and magnitude of perceptual acclimatization to frequency responses: evidence from monaural fitting of hearing aids. J Acoust Soc Am. 1992;92(3):1258–68.
51. Karawani H, Jenkins K, Anderson S. Neural plasticity induced by hearing aid use. Front Aging Neurosci. 2022;14:884917.
52. Giroud N, et al. The impact of hearing aids and age-related hearing loss on auditory plasticity across three months – an electrical neuroimaging study. Hear Res. 2017;353:162–75.
53. Glista D, et al. Evaluation of nonlinear frequency compression: clinical outcomes. Int J Audiol. 2009;48(9):632–44.
54. American Academy of Otolaryngology – Head and Neck Surgery. Position Statement. Red flags – Warning of ear disease. Available from: https://www.entnet.org/resource/position-statement-red-flags-warning-of-ear-disease/. Revised April 21, 2021. Accessed 26 Jan 2026.
55. Livingston G, Huntley J, Liu KY, et al. Dementia prevention, intervention, and care: 2024 report of the Lancet standing Commission. Lancet. 2024;404(10452):572–628. https://doi.org/10.1016/S0140-6736(24)01296-0.

Active Middle Ear Implants

17

Susan D. Emmett, Anna Bareiss, and Debara L. Tucci

Introduction

An estimated 38 million adults in the United States live with hearing loss. Yet, of that number, less than 20% report regular use of hearing aids [1, 2]. Performance limitations, including distortion, acoustic feedback, and occlusion, as well as social stigma and self-image, contribute to dissatisfaction with conventional amplification [3]. Some candidates are unable to use hearing aids for medical reasons such as chronic otitis externa, eczema, otorrhea, and open mastoid cavities in which earmolds are impractical. Given the tremendous public health implications of hearing loss, including economic underachievement, social isolation, accelerated physical and cognitive decline, and increased likelihood of dementia, a range of hearing rehabilitation options are needed [4–9]. Active middle ear implants have evolved to address some of the inherent limitations of conventional amplification, providing an alternative for patients who do not derive benefit from hearing aids.

Addressing Limitations of Conventional Hearing Aids

Understanding hearing aid limitations is essential for distinguishing the role of surgical implants in hearing rehabilitation and weighing the benefits and risks in discussions with patients. First, individuals with moderately severe or severe losses often experience poor performance with conventional amplification due to insufficient gain, defined as the amount of amplification a hearing aid must generate for an individual to perceive quiet sounds at a normal threshold of 0 dB. Acoustic feedback often limits the potential gain in a conventional device because the speaker and microphone are located in close proximity. Distortion is another challenge with conventional hearing aids that results from selective amplification of the speech frequencies, often giving sound an artificial character. The occlusive seal formed by many conventional aids to minimize feedback can be uncomfortable, causes autophony, and produces a sense of aural fullness. It also blocks the natural sound entrance to the ear and increases risk of otitis externa due to moisture retention. While open-fit hearing aids mitigate occlusive effects, they perform less well when amplification at low and midrange frequencies is required. Lastly, there is inherent transduction inefficiency when using a microphone to transmit acoustic energy, which can worsen distortion. Active middle ear implants are coupled directly to the ossicular chain, which bypasses the transduction inefficiency observed in conventional hearing aids, boosting gain, minimizing feedback, and reducing distortion. Occlusive effects are also minimized if a processor in the ear canal is not required.

S. D. Emmett (✉)
Department of Otolaryngology—Head and Neck Surgery, College of Medicine; Department of Epidemiology, Fay W. Boozman College of Public Health; and Center for Hearing Health Access, University of Arkansas for Medical Sciences, Little Rock, AR, USA
e-mail: sdemmett@uams.edu

A. Bareiss
Department of Otolaryngology—Head and Neck Surgery, College of Medicine, University of Arkansas for Medical Sciences, Little Rock, AR, USA

D. L. Tucci
National Institute of Deafness and other Communication Disorders, National Institutes of Health, Bethesda, MD, USA

A. D. Sweeney et al. (eds.), *Haynes-Glasscock-Shambaugh Surgery of the Ear*, https://doi.org/10.1007/978-3-032-18264-7_17

Basic Design Features

In contrast to conventional hearing aids, which function by receiving acoustic energy through a microphone, processing and amplifying the signal, and transmitting the signal through a speaker near the tympanic membrane, active middle ear implants impart sound vibration directly to the ossicular chain. Two basic types of transducers have been incorporated into middle ear implantable hearing devices: electromagnetic and piezoelectric. Electromagnetic transducers generate a magnetic field that induces motion of a nearby magnet that moves the ossicles. Piezoelectric devices move ossicles using a piezoelectric crystal that bends or lengthens with changes in a signal voltage applied across it. Piezoelectric ossicular actuators generally yield greater power and less distortion than electromagnetic devices, but they are typically larger and require precise placement to ensure proper compressive force between the actuator (integrated into a housing rigidly connected to the temporal bone) and the ossicle it contacts. Both electromagnetic and piezoelectric designs can be adapted to contact the incus, stapes capitulum, stapes footplate, or round window membrane.

Active middle ear implants may be either partially or totally implanted. Partially implanted devices consist of an external processor comprising a microphone, speech processor, battery, and a transmitter coil that transcutaneously conveys signals and power to the internal device. This approach facilitates replacement of batteries, service and upgrade of processors, and minimization of the size of the internal device. However, it comes with the drawback of an external processor. In contrast, fully implantable systems house all of the components within the implanted portion of the device, including the battery pack and a microphone. This frees the patient from wearing a visible external processor, but it increases the size and complexity of the implanted components, mandates surgical procedures for battery replacement approximately every 5 years, and complicates design and placement of the microphone.

Challenges and Opportunities

In April 2021, the American Academy of Otolaryngology-Head and Neck Surgery endorsed the use of active middle ear implants for FDA-approved indications. The field of active middle ear implants is rapidly evolving. The technology has the potential to overcome many disadvantages of traditional hearing aids, but with it comes additional surgical risk and substantial cost. Out of pocket costs often include both the device and surgical costs, as none of the FDA-approved implants are routinely covered by private insurance at the time of this writing. Additionally, surgeons may be less likely to consider active middle ear implants, as there are no established reimbursement codes for device placement. Unlike cochlear implants, active middle ear implants are unlikely to be usable for the duration of a patient's lifetime, given likely deterioration of hearing and change in amplification requirements over time. Yet even with these cost and longevity disadvantages, active middle ear implants have still been found to be cost-effective in the Netherlands, Sweden, and Norway [10, 11].

An additional hurdle in the evolution of active middle ear implants is the expense of research and development and obtaining regulatory approval. Currently the subset of patients with hearing loss who are considered good candidates for middle ear implants is small, and several companies in the field have experienced financial collapse, resulting in temporary and sometimes permanent withdrawal of an implant from the market. This instability can be challenging for patients, surgeons, and audiologists, who can be left without needed technical support. Evaluation of the effectiveness of active middle ear implants is also challenging given the low level of evidence available. Aside from clinical trials, the majority of studies on active middle ear implants are retrospective case series, and to date there are no randomized controlled trials.

The following sections review the active middle ear implants that are currently approved by the FDA (Table 17.1). Excellent reviews are available that describe the history and evolution of middle ear implant technology, including devices not currently FDA approved [12–14].

Table 17.1 Distinctions between the FDA-approved active middle ear implants

	MED-EL Vibrant Soundbridge	Ototronix MAXUM[a]	Envoy Esteem
Transducer type	Electromagnetic	Electromagnetic	Piezoelectric
Semi- vs. fully implantable	Semi-implantable	Semi-implantable	Fully implantable
FDA-approved indication	Moderate to severe SNHL in adults[b]	Moderate to moderately severe SNHL in adults with normal bone conduction and at least 60% speech discrimination	Mild to severe SNHL in adults with speech discrimination of greater than 40%
Compatible with altered anatomy and/or chronic otitis media	Yes	No	No
Reversible	Yes	Yes	No[c]
MRI compatible	Conditional[d]	No[e]	No
Average battery lifespan	1 week	Unknown	5–9 years[f]

[a]Formerly SOUNDTEC direct system
[b]This device is not commercially available at the time of this writing. SNHL, sensorineural hearing loss
[c]Requires disarticulation of the ossicular chain
[d]Vibrant Soundbridge 503, released in 2014, was marketed as MR conditional for scans up to 1.5 Tesla. The prior version (502) was not MRI compatible
[e]The official manufacturer recommendation is avoidance of MRI; however, the SOUNDTEC device showed no complications with 0.3 Tesla scans
[f]Minor surgical procedure required for battery replacement

FDA-Approved Implants

MED-EL Vibrant Soundbridge

The Vibrant Soundbridge was the first active middle ear implant to receive FDA approval. It was first available in Europe beginning in 1998 and in the United States in 2000. However, it is no longer marketed for use anywhere in the world. This semi-implantable device was first marketed by Symphonix, but bankruptcy led to purchase of the technology by MED-EL in 2003 [12]. The implant consisted of an external processor and a vibrating ossicular prosthesis (VORP). The VORP served as an electromagnetic transducer, which was typically attached to the long process of the incus and connected via a thin signal wire to an implanted receiver/amplifier. A signal current driven through the coil induced vibration of the magnet, which in turn shook the long process of the incus to which it was attached. There were variations in coupling for the transducer, including round window, oval window, and stapes superstructure applications in addition to the originally described incus coupling. The external processor contained a microphone, telemetry coil, and standard zinc replaceable battery. It was positioned in the postauricular hairline through magnetic attraction with the underlying implanted receiver. The battery needed to be changed approximately once weekly [12].

Indications

The FDA-approved indication for the Vibrant Soundbridge is moderate to severe sensorineural hearing loss in adults. In 2006 Colletti and colleagues published on round window coupling for treatment of mixed and conductive losses [15]. This opened the potential for wider application of the implant, and European CE marking (regulatory approval) was obtained for conductive and mixed losses in adults and children in 2008 and 2009, respectively [12]. The flexibility of multiple coupling mechanisms allowed treatment of a broad array of etiologies of hearing loss. The Vibrant Soundbridge was used with ossicular chain defects, chronic otitis media, otosclerosis, and aural atresia [16–21]. It was reportedly safe and effective in obliterated mastoid cavities and subtotal petrosectomy, making it a feasible rehabilitative option for patients with severe middle ear disease [22–24].

Surgery

Though the device is not currently available, technical aspects of the implant procedure are presented here as an example of one form of active middle ear implant surgery. The internal device was typically implanted using a standard transmastoid, facial recess approach to the middle ear. The internal receiver was placed in a bony trough in the retrosigmoid bone several centimeters behind the ear, similar to placement of a cochlear implant processor. The VORP was crimped onto the long process of the incus. As in stapedectomy, crimping force during attachment of the prosthesis on the incus long process needed to reflect a balance between maximal vibration coupling and avoidance of incus ischemia and necrosis [25]. Additional coupling options to the round window, oval window, and stapes superstructure yielded flexibility in adapting the implant to an individual patient's anatomy for treatment of mixed hearing loss.

Objective Outcomes

Several important elements must be considered when evaluating audiometric results of an active middle ear implant. A primary concern is risk of hearing loss during device coupling. Across studies, there was no difference between pre- and postoperative air and bone conduction with the Vibrant Soundbridge [26, 27]. In a two-year follow-up study, Schmuziger and colleagues found a significant deterioration in pure-tone thresholds in the operated ear, which were an average of 8 dB worse than the preoperative assessment compared to 2.6 dB in the non-operated ear [28]. Another factor that is important when considering the benefits of active middle ear implants is the functional gain obtained postoperatively. Compared to preoperative unaided conditions, all studies demonstrate improvement [26]. However, a more useful comparison is with best-aided preoperative conditions. Results for this are mixed, with three studies showing equivalent gain between conventional hearing aids and the Vibrant Soundbridge and three others, including the phase III clinical trial, demonstrating significantly improved gain over aided conditions [29–34]. Finally, speech discrimination is an essential consideration. The Vibrant Soundbridge improved speech discrimination in quiet compared to unaided conditions in all studies [26]. Only two studies found a significant improvement in speech discrimination in quiet over conventional hearing aids, and Snik and Cremers found a significant decline [35–37]. One study found a significant improvement in speech discrimination in noise with the Vibrant Soundbridge compared to best-aided conditions [33]. Ernst and colleagues performed a systematic review of the Vibrant Soundbridge used in the treatment of conductive and mixed hearing loss and found overall benefit from the device in air conduction thresholds, functional gain, and speech recognition [38].

Patient-Reported Outcomes

One of the motivating factors behind development of active middle ear implants is to address the limitations of conventional hearing aids, including feedback, limits in gain, occlusion effect, and cosmesis. Patient-reported data provide insights into the ability of currently available active middle ear implants to overcome these limitations. Several instruments have been used to study patient reported outcomes with active middle ear implants, including the Abbreviated Profile of Hearing Aid Benefit (APHAB). Patients consistently rated the Vibrant Soundbridge as significantly decreasing feedback, improving sound quality, decreasing aversion to sound, improving ease of communication, and improving hearing in noise [31, 32, 39, 40]. In patients with external otitis, Zwartenkot and colleagues found that long-term patient satisfaction and quality of life were significantly improved with the Vibrant Soundbridge compared to hearing aids [41]. However, as has been true in quality of life studies of both hearing aids and active middle ear implants, the improvements trend down over time, possibly due to worsening of hearing loss with age, habituation to improvement with the device, or some unmeasured factor [41]. Seebacher and colleagues studied quality of life in patients with bilateral active middle ear implants compared to unilateral implant. This study found improvement in hearing specific and general quality of life measures, which also strongly correlated with improved speech discrimination scores with a second implant [42].

Complications

Device failure requiring explantation occurred in 6 of 92 patients (7%) in a retrospective cohort study with a mean follow-up of 4.4 years [43]. Explantation occurred in another eight patients (9%) in this study for incus erosion, pain, and wire extrusion into the external auditory canal. Of note, wire extrusions occurred in all patients in which a transcanal approach was used. Ten patients (11%) required revision surgery, and an additional three patients (3%) required two revisions [43]. Revision surgery was required to improve functional performance of the implant for 13 of 83 patients (15.6%) in series by Schraven and colleagues (2016) [25]. Revisions were most common with round window placement without the use of a coupler and coupling to the long process of the incus. Six patients (7%) demonstrated incus erosion at the time of revision surgery [25]. Spiegel and colleagues compared different coupling sites noting the round window patients had the highest rates of revision and explanation at 20% [27]. One delayed facial nerve paresis has been reported, which resolved completely within 6 weeks [32]. Other complications described included skin irritation and pain [26]. The systematic review by Ernst and colleagues regarding Vibrant Soundbridge implant for mixed and conductive hearing loss reported on adverse events. Interestingly, these rates were below the range for conventional tympanoplasty and bone conduction hearing implants, which are generally the alternative treatments for this type of hearing loss [38].

MRI Compatibility

The Vibrant Soundbridge was labeled MRI incompatible until 2014. Patients who underwent scans before this time have reported pain, noise, demagnetization, and movement of the VORP requiring revision surgery [44, 45]. No acoustic trauma has been reported [44, 45]. With the introduction of the 503 Vibrant Soundbridge in 2014, the implant has been labeled MR conditional for scans of 1.5 Tesla or less [46]. An MRI safety study with the 503 implant was published in temporal bones in 2016 [47].

Ototronix MAXUM (Formerly SOUNDTEC Direct System)

The second active middle ear implant to obtain FDA approval was the SOUNDTEC Direct Hearing System, approved in 2001 (Fig. 17.1). This semi-implantable device was developed based on experiments from the Hough Ear Institute and underwent a phase I clinical trial in 1998, followed by a multicenter phase II clinical trial that showed positive results [48, 49]. The device was voluntarily removed from the market in 2004, however, due to an audible rattle that occurred if the sound processor was not in place. Ototronix purchased the SOUNDTEC technology in 2009. After making some improvements, the device became commercially available as the MAXUM Hearing Implant. [12] The most significant upgrade is a self-crimping attachment wire that no longer requires separation of the incudostapedial (IS) joint.

Ototronix MAXUM uses electromagnetic energy to amplify sound from an in-the-canal external processor and coil to a surgically implanted internal magnet. This differs from the SOUNDTEC system, which relied on a behind-the-ear processor. The internal component is identical between systems and consists of a magnet attached to the IS joint [50].

Indications

The MAXUM system is FDA approved for adults (18 years of age and older) with stable moderate to severe sensorineural hearing loss. Unaided air conduction threshold upper limits should be 60, 70, 85, and 100 dB at 250, 500, 1000, and 2000–6000 Hz, respectively, with word recognition of 60% or better. Normal middle ear anatomy, without evidence of chronic otitis media, is required. A few studies have shown that a positive speech perception gap (defined as the difference in speech discrimination scores between unaided earphone and hearing aid testing) is correlated with active middle ear implant benefit [51–54]. While there is overlap with cochlear implant indications (especially for hybrid CI), the MAXUM system preserves the patient's native hearing function. In a study by Chang and colleagues, 7 of 9 patients implanted with MAXUM would have also met cochlear implant criteria. Patients' postoperative average speech discrimination with MAXUM was 67.4%. This was an average improvement of 52.6% over their hearing aids; thus, with the active middle ear implantable hearing aid, they no longer met cochlear implant criteria [52].

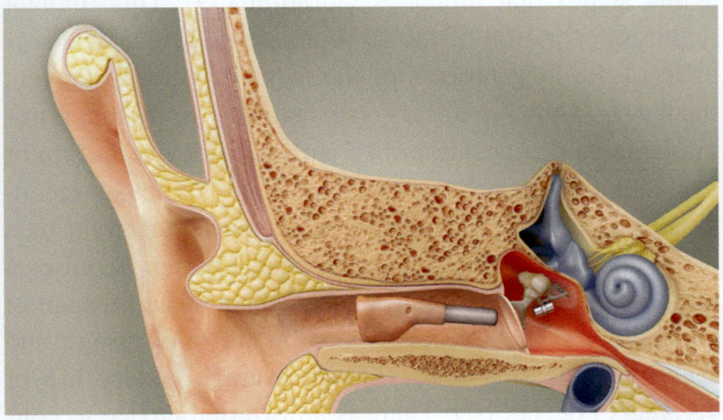

Fig. 17.1 The MAXUM hearing implant. (Used with permission from de Souza et al. Implantable Hearing Devices. Plural Publishing. 2017)

Preoperative Planning

Before surgery, the size and shape of the ear canal should be determined to ensure compatibility with the device. This is accomplished by a deep ear impression. A mold can be made from this process and used by the patient prior to surgery to help post operative acclimation of the device. For the in-the-canal external portion to fit properly, the canal must be a minimum of 20 mm in length from aperture to medial canal, 4 mm in width at the aperture, and 3 mm in diameter from the second bend to the medial canal [50].

Surgery

The MAXUM system is implanted under local anesthesia using a transcanal approach similar to a stapedotomy. Special nonmagnetic MAXUM instruments are available for handling the implant, which should not be touched directly by the surgeon. The nitinol attachment wire is placed around the IS joint and crimped using a low-temperature heating device such as the SMart Piston Heating Device [50]. Manual crimping is not recommended. Positioning affects performance of the MAXUM implant. In particular, the magnet on the IS joint should be positioned parallel to the electromagnetic coil in the ear canal mold to maximize vibration and therefore achieve the greatest functional gain. There is a 30 degree angle between the cylinder of the magnet and the attachment ring to aid in optimal placement. When the magnet is in the correct position, the surgeon sees only the end of the cylinder of the magnet and not the sides. The distance between the electromagnetic coil in the ear canal and the internal magnet also affects performance. The attachment wire is designed to be at the base of the magnet in order to position the magnet as close as possible to the tympanic membrane. If the magnet touches the tympanic membrane, however, a cartilage graft should be placed to prevent extrusion. Lastly, vibration of the magnet will be impeded if it comes into contact with the promontory. The magnet cylinder can be rotated into any of three positions in order avoid contact [50].

Objective Outcomes

The published audiometric results currently available were completed with the SOUNDTEC technology that required IS joint separation. In the phase II clinical trial, the average threshold change postoperatively was −4.2 dB for air conduction and − 1.1 dB for bone conduction [49]. Another series of 42 patients reported by Silverstein and colleagues observed an average decrease of 7 dB and 3 dB in air and bone conduction, respectively [55]. Neither study evaluated the statistical significance of these changes. In the phase II trial, there was a greater than 15 dB threshold shift in 2 of 95 participants (2%) at 20 weeks after surgery [49]. Silverstein and colleagues reported 21 of 47 patients (45%) experienced a threshold shift greater than 10 dB at 4 weeks [55]. Functional gain with the implant was compared to best fit hearing aids in two studies. Hough and colleagues demonstrated an average 7.9 dB gain over hearing aid in the speech frequencies, and Roland and colleagues observed 9.95 dB gain over best-aided conditions at the same frequencies [49, 56]. Again, neither study documented statistical significance of these findings. Findings on speech discrimination were mixed. Hough reported a 5.3% statistically significant increase in speech discrimination, while Silverstein reported an average 6% drop in speech discrimination (significance not measured), and Roland found no difference between SOUNDTEC and conventional hearing aids [49, 55, 56]. Chang and colleagues implanted 11 patients with MAXUM, showing an average 17.1 dB improvement in high frequencies over hearing aids, which was statistically significant. Additionally, there was an average 41.6% improvement in speech discrimination scores (23.1–64.7%), which was also statistically significant [52]. Hunter and colleagues reported on MAXUM implantation in 6 ears with high-frequency sensorineural hearing loss, namely, potential cochlear implant ears. Statistically significant results showed a median high-frequency pure tone average functional gain of 47.2 dB and median speech discrimination scores with 42% improvement over optimally fit hearing aids [57].

Patient-Reported Outcomes

Patients reported satisfaction with the SOUNDTEC device and improvement in sound quality in all studies [49, 55, 56]. Decreased feedback and reduced occlusive effects were also noted [49, 56]. On the APHAB, Hough found a statistically significant improvement in hearing in background noise and reverberant backgrounds compared to best-aided conditions [49]. Chang and colleagues found improvement in the ease of communication and background noise subscales, but this was not statistically significant [52].

Complications

Hematomas were reported after deep ear impressions in 5 of 6 patients (83%) surveyed by Roland for complications and 7 of 103 patients (7%) in the phase II clinical trial. [49, 56] Tympanic membrane perforations occurred in 3 of 103 patients (3%) in the phase II trial and 1 of 6 (17%) surveyed by Roland. [49, 56] Three of 64 patients (5%) in the Silverstein series required revision for magnet stabilization and four (6%) were explanted due to dissatisfaction [55]. Other complications reported included dizziness, tinnitus, otitis, and pain [49].

MRI Compatibility

Due to potential displacement of the ossicular chain, magnet heating, and demagnetization, the official manufacturer recommendation is to avoid MRI or close proximity to magnetic fields with an Ototronix MAXUM implant in place [50]. The issue of MRI compatibility was explored with the SOUNDTEC device, with no device-related complications in a series of 11 patients who underwent low-strength (0.3 T) MRIs [58]. Implant artifact can be reduced using a fast spin echo sequence [50].

Envoy Esteem

The Envoy Esteem is the only fully implantable device that is FDA approved and the only commercially available device that utilizes piezoelectric technology. Another fully implantable device, the Cochlear Carina system, had European CE marking but was discontinued in May 2020 [14]. The Envoy Esteem was developed by St. Croix Medical, which is now Envoy Medical Corporation, with a phase I clinical trial published in 2004 and two phase II trials from 2004 to 2009. CE marking was granted for the Esteem in 2006 and FDA approval in 2010.

The Esteem device does not use a traditional microphone or speaker, instead relying on the tympanic membrane and malleus to serve as a natural microphone [12]. The implant is comprised of a hermetically sealed sound processor, non-rechargeable lithium battery, and two piezoelectric transducers. One piezoelectric transducer, called the "sensor," is placed on the incus to detect motion in the tympanic membrane, which it converts into an electric signal sent to the processor. The signal is then transmitted to the "driver," the piezoelectric transducer attached to the stapes that produces vibration [59]. This implant requires separation of the IS joint and resection of a segment of the long process of the incus in order to prevent feedback. Thus, it differs substantially from the semi-implantable devices described earlier, as device failure or explantation for any reason necessitates ossicular reconstruction and may result in a permanent worsening of a patient's hearing. The non-rechargeable battery requires a minor surgical procedure for replacement. The lifespan of the battery is 5–9 years depending on daily usage and severity of hearing loss, with an average battery life of 4.9 years [12, 60, 61]. There is an external device to control volume and programming.

Indications

The Envoy Esteem is FDA approved for adults over the age of 18 years with stable, moderate to severe sensorineural hearing loss and a speech discrimination score of greater than or equal to 40%. Normal middle ear anatomy and function are required. A CT scan is typically obtained preoperatively to confirm sufficient space for the implant. The minimum space required is 22 mm from the stapes capitulum to the sigmoid and 2.5 mm from the tegmen to the incus body [62].

Surgery

Placement occurs through a standard postauricular transmastoid approach. The epitympanum is opened until the incus body and head of the malleus are visible and an extended facial recess is performed. Ossicular mobility is confirmed using Doppler vibrometry, with at least 100 nm of movement required of both the incus and stapes for the device to function correctly [62]. A well is drilled for the sound processor in similar fashion to placement of a cochlear implant receiver-stimulator. The distal 3–4 mm of the incus are removed with a laser to avoid the feedback inherent in having both the sensor and the driver on the ossicular chain [12]. The sensor is attached to the body of the incus using glass-ionomer cement, and the driver is similarly cemented to the stapes capitulum. Care should be taken to ensure that the tip of the driver does not contact soft tissue or bone, as this can create feedback between the sensor and driver [63]. Intraoperative testing using laser Doppler vibrometry is performed to confirm functioning of the implant.

Objective Outcomes

The first outcome consideration of active middle ear implants, assessing threshold shifts secondary to surgery, notably differs for the Envoy Esteem because resecting a portion of the incus creates a conductive hearing loss. Changes in cochlear function have been assessed with the device turned off; however, and no significant changes from preoperative bone conduction thresholds were identified [60, 63–66]. Pure-tone average with the Esteem was generally found to be equivalent to best-aided conditions [64, 67, 68]. Speech reception thresholds were found to have statistically significant improvement with the Esteem compared to best-aided conditions [60, 61, 64–66]. Speech testing delivered mixed results, with the phase I and II trials, as well as trial follow-up studies finding a significant improvement in speech discrimination in quiet with the Esteem compared to best-aided conditions, while two other studies found no difference [60, 64–68]. Shohet and colleagues suggested that patients with speech discrimination scores showing a speech perception gap (e.g., scores that are worse with a hearing aid than unaided with inserts) may have improved performance with active middle ear implantation [51].

Patient-Reported Outcomes

The Envoy Esteem has performed well with regard to patient-reported outcomes. Across studies, participants reported improvement in ease of communication and hearing in background noise and reverberant backgrounds [26]. In the phase II trial and 5-year follow-up study, patients found significantly decreased aversion to sound and preferred their implant over a hearing aid [65, 66]. In the phase I trial by Chen, positive results were reported in all the above listed measures, but statistical significance was not evaluated given the small sample size [64]. An unanticipated finding by Shohet et al. was resolution of tinnitus in 56.1% of subjects, although this finding is also seen with conventional hearing aids [60].

Complications

In the phase I clinical trial, four of seven devices (57%) malfunctioned and required explantation due to failure of the hermetic seal [64]. Two other studies reported explantations for device malfunction, including 3 of 13 devices (23%) in the series by Gerard and 3 of 57 devices (5%) in the phase II clinical trial [63, 66]. Wound infections requiring explantation occurred in 1 of 7 patients (14%) in the phase I trial, 1 of 57 patients (2%) in the phase II trial, and 2 of 13 patients (15%) in the series by Gerard and colleagues.[63 64 66] Walsh et al. reported explantation in 6 of 116 patients (13.8%) due to device exposure or infection. This case series also reported lower complication rates with increasing surgeon experience [69]. Facial paresis occurred in several studies, including permanent paralysis reported in 2 of 57 patients (4%) in the phase II trial and 1 of 10 patients (10%) in a study by Memari [66, 67]. However, in the 5-year follow-up study for the phase II trial, the previous reported permanent facial paralysis had resolved [65]. Temporary paresis has been reported in 1 of 13 patients (8%) by Gerard, 2 of 57 (4%) in the phase II trial, 1 of 10 (10%) by Memari, and in 3 of 34 (9%) and 5 of 41 (12%) patients in two studies by Barbara and colleagues [61, 63, 66, 67, 70]. Possible contributors to the higher likelihood of delayed facial paresis in Esteem surgery have included thermal damage from the drill during the extended facial recess approach, required resection of the chorda tympani nerve, postoperative swelling of the nerve secondary to the laser, or sustained elevated temperature from cement curing [70]. Other complications reported included pain, tinnitus, taste disturbance, and wound complications not requiring explantation [60, 63, 64, 66, 67]. A recent publication by Shohet and colleagues reports exclusively on revision procedures for the Envoy Esteem. Included are 60 revisions, with 27% due to wound issues, although most patients were noted to have risk factors predisposing them to their complication. Another 73% were due to device issues, notably device dysfunction and adverse body reactions to the device (i.e., middle ear adhesions) [71].

MRI Compatibility

As of 2018, the Envoy Esteem is MRI conditional for 1.5 T and 3.0 T scanning environments per the FDA.

Summary

The field of active middle ear implants is rapidly evolving, and these devices represent an important hearing rehabilitation option for patients who do not benefit from conventional hearing aids. There is tremendous potential to overcome the limitations of conventional amplification, and patient-reported outcomes are positive. Nonetheless, the lack of insurance coverage for these devices poses a significant barrier to widespread adoption of their use in hearing rehabilitation. With time, introduction of technological and surgical advances have the potential to decrease costs and make these devices more cost-effective and widely available.

References

1. Goman AM, Lin FR. Prevalence of hearing loss by severity in the United States. Am J Public Health. 2016;106(10):1820–2. https://doi.org/10.2105/AJPH.2016.303299. [published Online First: 20160823]. PMID: 27552261 PMC5024365
2. Reed NS, Garcia-Morales E, Willink A. Trends in hearing aid ownership among older adults in the United States from 2011 to 2018. JAMA Intern Med. 2021;181(3):383–5.
3. Kochkin S. MarkeTrak V:"why my hearing aids are in the drawer": the consumers' perspective. Hear J. 2000;53(2):34–6.
4. Emmett SD, Francis HW. The socioeconomic impact of hearing loss in U.S. adults. Otol Neurotol. 2015;36(3):545–50. https://doi.org/10.1097/mao.0000000000000562. [published Online First: 2014/08/28]. PMID: 25158616 PMC4466103
5. Jung D, Bhattacharyya N. Association of hearing loss with decreased employment and income among adults in the United States. Ann Otol Rhinol Laryngol. 2012;121(12):771–5. https://doi.org/10.1177/000348941212101201. [published Online First: 2013/01/25]. PMID: 23342548
6. Mick P, Kawachi I, Lin FR. The association between hearing loss and social isolation in older adults. Otolaryngol Head Neck Surg. 2014;150(3):378–84. https://doi.org/10.1177/0194599813518021. [published Online First: 20140102]. PMID: 24384545
7. Chen DS, Betz J, Yaffe K, et al. Association of hearing impairment with declines in physical functioning and the risk of disability in older adults. J Gerontol A Biol Sci Med Sci. 2015;70(5):654–61. https://doi.org/10.1093/gerona/glu207. [published Online First: 20141203]. PMID: 25477427. PMC4400396
8. Lin FR, Yaffe K, Xia J, et al. Hearing loss and cognitive decline in older adults. JAMA Intern Med. 2013;173(4):293–9. https://doi.org/10.1001/jamainternmed.2013.1868. PMID: 23337978. PMC3869227
9. Lin FR, Metter EJ, O'Brien RJ, Resnick SM, Zonderman AB, Ferrucci L. Hearing loss and incident dementia. Arch Neurol. 2011;68(2):214–20. https://doi.org/10.1001/archneurol.2010.362. PMID: 21320988. PMC3277836
10. Snik AF, van Duijnhoven NT, Mylanus EA, Cremers CW. Estimated cost-effectiveness of active middle-ear implantation in hearing-impaired patients with severe external otitis. Arch Otolaryngol Head Neck Surg. 2006;132(11):1210–5. https://doi.org/10.1001/archotol.132.11.1210. PMID: 17116816
11. Edfeldt L, Stromback K, Grendin J, et al. Evaluation of cost-utility in middle ear implantation in the 'Nordic School': a multicenter study in Sweden and Norway. Acta Otolaryngol. 2014;134(1):19–25. https://doi.org/10.3109/00016489.2013.834459. [published Online First: 20131121]. PMID: 24256038.
12. Carlson ML, Pelosi S, Haynes DS. Historical development of active middle ear implants. Otolaryngol Clin N Am. 2014;47(6):893–914. https://doi.org/10.1016/j.otc.2014.08.004. [published Online First: 20141001]. PMID: 25282038
13. Haynes DS, Young JA, Wanna GB, Glasscock ME 3rd. Middle ear implantable hearing devices: an overview. Trends Amplif. 2009;13(3):206–14. https://doi.org/10.1177/1084713809346262. PMID: 19762429. PMC4111438
14. Banakis Hartl RM, Jenkins HA. Implantable hearing aids: where are we in 2020? Laryngoscope Investig Otolaryngol. 2020;5(6):1184–91. https://doi.org/10.1002/lio2.495. [published Online First: 20201106]. PMID: 33364411. PMC7752069
15. Colletti V, Soli SD, Carner M, Colletti L. Treatment of mixed hearing losses via implantation of a vibratory transducer on the round window. Int J Audiol. 2006;45(10):600–8. https://doi.org/10.1080/14992020600840903. PMID: 17062502
16. Colletti L, Mandala M, Colletti V. Long-term outcome of round window Vibrant SoundBridge implantation in extensive ossicular chain defects. Otolaryngol Head Neck Surg. 2013;149(1):134–41. https://doi.org/10.1177/0194599813486255. [published Online First: 20130412]. PMID: 23585147
17. Luers JC, Huttenbrink KB. Vibrant Soundbridge rehabilitation of conductive and mixed hearing loss. Otolaryngol Clin N Am. 2014;47(6):915–26. https://doi.org/10.1016/j.otc.2014.08.002. [published Online First: 20141003]. PMID: 25282039
18. Streitberger C, Perotti M, Beltrame MA, Giarbini N. Vibrant Soundbridge for hearing restoration after chronic ear surgery. Rev Laryngol Otol Rhinol (Bord). 2009;130(2):83–8. PMID: 19813469
19. Coordes A, Jahreiss L, Schonfeld U, Lenarz M. Active middle ear implant coupled bilaterally to the round window despite bilateral implanted stapes prostheses. Laryngoscope. 2017;127(2):500–3. https://doi.org/10.1002/lary.26087. [published Online First: 20160627]. PMID: 27346704
20. Claros P, Pujol MC. Active middle ear implants: Vibroplasty in children and adolescents with acquired or congenital middle ear disorders. Acta Otolaryngol. 2013;133(6):612–9. https://doi.org/10.3109/00016489.2013.765969. PMID: 23675812
21. Cremers CW, O'Connor AF, Helms J, et al. International consensus on Vibrant Soundbridge(R) implantation in children and adolescents. Int J Pediatr Otorhinolaryngol. 2010;74(11):1267–9. https://doi.org/10.1016/j.ijporl.2010.07.028. [published Online First: 20100915]. PMID: 20828837.
22. Ihler F, Kohler S, Meyer AC, et al. Mastoid cavity obliteration and Vibrant Soundbridge implantation for patients with mixed hearing loss. Laryngoscope. 2014;124(2):531–7. https://doi.org/10.1002/lary.24180. [published Online First: 20130805]. PMID: 23918587
23. Linder T, Schlegel C, DeMin N, van der Westhuizen S. Active middle ear implants in patients undergoing subtotal petrosectomy: new application for the Vibrant Soundbridge device and its implication for lateral cranium base surgery. Otol Neurotol. 2009;30(1):41–7. https://doi.org/10.1097/MAO.0b013e31818be812. PMID: 18849883
24. Henseler MA, Polanski JF, Schlegel C, Linder T. Active middle ear implants in patients undergoing subtotal petrosectomy: long-term follow-up. Otol Neurotol. 2014;35(3):437–41. https://doi.org/10.1097/MAO.0b013e31829e8391. PMID: 24492140
25. Schraven SP, Gromann W, Rak K, Shehata-Dieler W, Hagen R, Mlynski R. Long-term stability of the active middle-ear implant

with floating-mass transducer technology: a single-center study. Otol Neurotol. 2016;37(3):252–66. https://doi.org/10.1097/MAO.0000000000000943. PMID: 26796211
26. Kahue CN, Carlson ML, Daugherty JA, Haynes DS, Glasscock ME 3rd. Middle ear implants for rehabilitation of sensorineural hearing loss: a systematic review of FDA approved devices. Otol Neurotol. 2014;35(7):1228–37. https://doi.org/10.1097/MAO.0000000000000341. PMID: 24643033
27. Spiegel JL, Kutsch L, Jakob M, Weiss BG, Canis M, Ihler F. Long-term stability and functional outcome of an active middle ear implant regarding different coupling sites. Otol Neurotol. 2020;41(1):60–7. https://doi.org/10.1097/MAO.0000000000002418. PMID: 31746816
28. Schmuziger N, Schimmann F, aWengen D, Patscheke J, Probst R. Long-term assessment after implantation of the Vibrant Soundbridge device. Otol Neurotol. 2006;27(2):183–8. https://doi.org/10.1097/01.mao.0000199754.51815.70. PMID: 16436987
29. Sziklai I, Szilvássy J. Functional gain and speech understanding obtained by Vibrant Soundbridge or by open-fit hearing aid. Acta Otolaryngol. 2011;131(4):428–33.
30. Todt I, Seidl RO, Gross M, Ernst A. Comparison of different vibrant soundbridge audioprocessors with conventional hearing AIDS. Otol Neurotol. 2002;23(5):669–73. https://doi.org/10.1097/00129492-200209000-00012. PMID: 12218618
31. Uziel A, Mondain M, Hagen P, Dejean F, Doucet G. Rehabilitation for high-frequency sensorineural hearing impairment in adults with the symphonix vibrant soundbridge: a comparative study. Otol Neurotol. 2003;24(5):775–83. https://doi.org/10.1097/00129492-200309000-00015. PMID: 14501456
32. Fraysse B, Lavieille JP, Schmerber S, et al. A multicenter study of the Vibrant Soundbridge middle ear implant: early clinical results and experience. Otol Neurotol. 2001;22(6):952–61. https://doi.org/10.1097/00129492-200111000-00041. PMID: 11698825.
33. Truy E, Philibert B, Vesson JF, Labassi S, Collet L. Vibrant soundbridge versus conventional hearing aid in sensorineural high-frequency hearing loss: a prospective study. Otol Neurotol. 2008;29(5):684–7. https://doi.org/10.1097/MAO.0b013e31817156df. PMID: 18434928
34. Luetje CM, Brackman D, Balkany TJ, et al. Phase III clinical trial results with the Vibrant Soundbridge implantable middle ear hearing device: a prospective controlled multicenter study. Otolaryngol Head Neck Surg. 2002;126(2):97–107. https://doi.org/10.1067/mhn.2002.122182. PMID: 11870337
35. Boeheim K, Pok SM, Schloegel M, Filzmoser P. Active middle ear implant compared with open-fit hearing aid in sloping high-frequency sensorineural hearing loss. Otol Neurotol. 2010;31(3):424–9. https://doi.org/10.1097/MAO.0b013e3181cabd42. PMID: 20042907.
36. Pok SM, Schlogel M, Boheim K. Clinical experience with the active middle ear implant Vibrant Soundbridge in sensorineural hearing loss. Adv Otorhinolaryngol. 2010;69:51–8. https://doi.org/10.1159/000318522. [published Online First: 20100705]. PMID: 20610914
37. Snik AF, Cremers CW. Vibrant semi-implantable hearing device with digital sound processing: effective gain and speech perception. Arch Otolaryngol Head Neck Surg. 2001;127(12):1433–7. https://doi.org/10.1001/archotol.127.12.1433. PMID: 11735810
38. Ernst A, Todt I, Wagner J. Safety and effectiveness of the Vibrant Soundbridge in treating conductive and mixed hearing loss: a systematic review. Laryngoscope. 2016;126(6):1451–7. https://doi.org/10.1002/lary.25670. [published Online First: 20151015]. PMID: 26468033
39. Monini S, Bianchi A, Talamonti R, Atturo F, Filippi C, Barbara M. Patient satisfaction after auditory implant surgery: ten-year experience from a single implanting unit center. Acta Otolaryngol. 2017;137(4):389–97. https://doi.org/10.1080/00016489.2016.1258733. [published Online First: 20161205]. PMID: 27918233
40. Bruchhage KL, Leichtle A, Schonweiler R, et al. Systematic review to evaluate the safety, efficacy and economical outcomes of the Vibrant Soundbridge for the treatment of sensorineural hearing loss. Eur Arch Otorhinolaryngol. 2017;274(4):1797–806. https://doi.org/10.1007/s00405-016-4361-2. [published Online First: 20161031]. PMID: 27796557
41. Zwartenkot JW, Hashemi J, Cremers CW, Mulder JJ, Snik AF. Active middle ear implantation for patients with sensorineural hearing loss and external otitis: long-term outcome in patient satisfaction. Otol Neurotol. 2013;34(5):855–61. https://doi.org/10.1097/MAO.0b013e31828f47c2. PMID: 23739560
42. Seebacher J, Weichbold V, Schorg P, et al. Subjective hearing impression and quality of life in patients with bilateral active middle ear implants. Otol Neurotol. 2020;41(6):e641–e47. https://doi.org/10.1097/MAO.0000000000002630. PMID: 32569243
43. Zwartenkot JW, Mulder JJ, Snik AF, Cremers CW, Mylanus EA. Active middle ear implantation: long-term medical and technical follow-up, implant survival, and complications. Otol Neurotol. 2016;37(5):513–9. https://doi.org/10.1097/MAO.0000000000001015. PMID: 27023016
44. Wagner JH, Ernst A, Todt I. Magnet resonance imaging safety of the Vibrant Soundbridge system: a review. Otol Neurotol. 2011;32(7):1040–6. https://doi.org/10.1097/MAO.0b013e31822a9816. PMID: 21844783
45. Renninger D, Ernst A, Todt I. MRI scanning in patients implanted with a round window or stapes coupled floating mass transducer of the Vibrant Soundbridge. Acta Otolaryngol. 2016;136(3):241–4. https://doi.org/10.3109/00016489.2015.1115552. [published Online First: 20151201]. PMID: 26624271
46. MED-EL. Secondary Magnetic Resonance Imaging with the SOUNDBRIDGE VORP 503. https://s3.medel.com/pdf/VSB_relaunch/29079EN_r1_0_VSBmriFS%20%28AUS%29.pdf. Accessed 6/2026.
47. Schnabl J, Wolf-Magele A, Pok SM, Hirtler L, Heinz G, Sprinzl GM. Magnetic resonance imaging compatibility of a new generation of active middle ear implant: a clinically relevant temporal bone laboratory study. Otol Neurotol. 2016;37(7):e222–7. https://doi.org/10.1097/MAO.0000000000001097. PMID: 27273396
48. Hough JV, Dyer RK Jr, Matthews P, Wood MW. Semi-implantable electromagnetic middle ear hearing device for moderate to severe sensorineural hearing loss. Otolaryngol Clin N Am. 2001;34(2):401–16. https://doi.org/10.1016/s0030-6665(05)70339-x. PMID: 11382578
49. Hough JV, Matthews P, Wood MW, Dyer RK Jr. Middle ear electromagnetic semi-implantable hearing device: results of the phase II SOUNDTEC direct system clinical trial. Otol Neurotol. 2002;23(6):895–903. https://doi.org/10.1097/00129492-200211000-00015. PMID: 12438853
50. Pelosi S, Carlson ML, Glasscock ME 3rd. Implantable hearing devices: the Ototronix MAXUM system. Otolaryngol Clin N Am. 2014;47(6):953–65. https://doi.org/10.1016/j.otc.2014.08.003. [published Online First: 20141005]. PMID: 25293787
51. Shohet JA, Gende DM, Bibee J, Patzkowski G, Tanita C. Speech perception gap is predictive of an active middle ear implant advantage. Otol Neurotol. 2020;41(5):663–8. https://doi.org/10.1097/MAO.0000000000002589. PMID: 32412724
52. Chang CYJ, Spearman M, Spearman B, McCraney A, Glasscock ME 3rd. Comparison of an electromagnetic middle ear implant and hearing aid word recognition performance to word recognition performance obtained under earphones. Otol Neurotol. 2017;38(9):1308–14. https://doi.org/10.1097/MAO.0000000000001554. PMID: 28885481.

53. Dyer RK, Spearman M, Spearman B, McCraney A. Evaluating speech perception of the MAXUM middle ear implant versus speech perception under inserts. Laryngoscope. 2018;128(2):456–60. https://doi.org/10.1002/lary.26605. [published Online First: 20170605]. PMID: 28581120
54. McRackan TR, Clinkscales WB, Ahlstrom JB, Nguyen SA, Dubno JR. Factors associated with benefit of active middle ear implants compared to conventional hearing aids. Laryngoscope. 2018;128(9):2133–8. https://doi.org/10.1002/lary.27109. [published Online First: 20180226]. PMID: 29481695. PMC6109627
55. Silverstein H, Atkins J, Thompson JH Jr, Gilman N. Experience with the SOUNDTEC implantable hearing aid. Otol Neurotol. 2005;26(2):211–7. https://doi.org/10.1097/00129492-200503000-00014. PMID: 15793407
56. Roland PS, Shoup AG, Shea MC, Richey HS, Jones DB. Verification of improved patient outcomes with a partially implantable hearing aid, The SOUNDTEC direct hearing system. Laryngoscope. 2001;111(10):1682–6. https://doi.org/10.1097/00005537-200110000-00002. PMID: 11801925
57. Hunter JB, Carlson ML, Glasscock ME 3rd. The ototronix MAXUM middle ear implant for severe high-frequency sensorineural hearing loss: preliminary results. Laryngoscope. 2016;126(9):2124–7. https://doi.org/10.1002/lary.25872. [published Online First: 20160312]. PMID: 26972428
58. Dyer RK Jr, Nakmali D, Dormer KJ. Magnetic resonance imaging compatibility and safety of the SOUNDTEC direct system. Laryngoscope. 2006;116(8):1321–33. https://doi.org/10.1097/01.mlg.0000230479.39551.4a. PMID: 16885731
59. Klein K, Nardelli A, Stafinski T. A systematic review of the safety and effectiveness of fully implantable middle ear hearing devices: the carina and esteem systems. Otol Neurotol. 2012;33(6):916–21. https://doi.org/10.1097/MAO.0b013e31825f230d. PMID: 22772013
60. Shohet JA, Gende DM, Tanita CS. Totally implantable active middle ear implant: hearing and safety results in a large series. Laryngoscope. 2018;128(12):2872–8. https://doi.org/10.1002/lary.27246. [published Online First: 20180908]. PMID: 30194720
61. Barbara M, Filippi C, Covelli E, Volpini L, Monini S. Ten years of active middle ear implantation for sensorineural hearing loss. Acta Otolaryngol. 2018;138(9):807–14. https://doi.org/10.1080/00016489.2018.1472807. [published Online First: 20180531]. PMID: 29852816
62. Marzo SJ. The envoy esteem implantable hearing aid system. In: de Souza CRP, Tucci DL, editors. Implantable hearing devices. San Diego: Plural Publishing; 2017.
63. Gerard JM, Thill MP, Chantrain G, Gersdorff M, Deggouj N. Esteem 2 middle ear implant: our experience. Audiol Neurootol. 2012;17(4):267–74. https://doi.org/10.1159/000338689. [published Online First: 20120522]. PMID: 22627489
64. Chen DA, Backous DD, Arriaga MA, et al. Phase 1 clinical trial results of the envoy system: a totally implantable middle ear device for sensorineural hearing loss. Otolaryngol Head Neck Surg. 2004;131(6):904–16. https://doi.org/10.1016/j.otohns.2004.05.027. PMID: 15577788
65. Shohet JA, Kraus EM, Catalano PJ, Toh E. Totally implantable hearing system: five-year hearing results. Laryngoscope. 2018;128(1):210–6. https://doi.org/10.1002/lary.26602. [published Online First: 20170413]. PMID: 28407310
66. Kraus EM, Shohet JA, Catalano PJ. Envoy esteem totally implantable hearing system: phase 2 trial, 1-year hearing results. Otolaryngol Head Neck Surg. 2011;145(1):100–9. https://doi.org/10.1177/0194599811401709. PMID: 21493292
67. Memari F, Asghari A, Daneshi A, Jalali A. Safety and patient selection of totally implantable hearing aid surgery: envoy system. Esteem Eur Arch Otorhinolaryngol. 2011;268(10):1421–5. https://doi.org/10.1007/s00405-011-1507-0. [published Online First: 20110217]. PMID: 21328002
68. Monini S, Biagini M, Atturo F, Barbara M. Esteem® middle ear device versus conventional hearing aids for rehabilitation of bilateral sensorineural hearing loss. Eur Arch Otorhinolaryngol. 2013;270(7):2027–33. https://doi.org/10.1007/s00405-012-2252-8. [published Online First: 20121110]. PMID: 23143506
69. McCarty Walsh E, Morrison DR, McFeely WJ. Totally implantable active middle-ear implants: a large, single-surgeon cohort. J Laryngol Otol. 2021;135(4):304–9. https://doi.org/10.1017/S0022215121000335. [published Online First: 20210322]. PMID: 33745469
70. Barbara M, Volpini L, Monini S. Delayed facial nerve palsy after surgery for the Esteem((R)) fully implantable middle ear hearing device. Acta Otolaryngol. 2014;134(4):429–32. https://doi.org/10.3109/00016489.2013.868602. [published Online First: 20140117]. PMID: 24433055
71. Shohet J, Bibee J, Gende D. Totally implantable hearing implant revision surgery indications and outcomes. Otol Neurotol. 2023;44(4):367–72. https://doi.org/10.1097/MAO.0000000000003820. [published Online First: 20230210]. PMID: 36764704

Bone-Anchored Hearing Implants

18

Alexander Chern, Francis X. Creighton Jr,
Lawrence R. Lustig, and Charles C. Della Santina

Introduction

Conventional hearing aids are the principal means of auditory rehabilitation for individuals with sensorineural hearing loss (SNHL) or conductive hearing loss (CHL) not amenable to medical or surgical treatment. Though continued technological advances, such as improved signal processing and decreased size, have increased hearing aid acceptance among patients, fewer than 20% of adults with hearing loss obtain hearing aids due to lack of perceived benefit, out-of-pocket expense, cosmetic concerns, and the social stigma associated with their use [1]. Conditions such as a chronically draining ear or extreme discomfort from the sound levels required from a conventional hearing aid can also complicate—or even prevent—successful use. Some patients are also unable to wear hearing aids due to anatomic abnormalities. Conventional hearing aids also have inherent limitations (e.g., insufficient gain, acoustic feedback) that can cause them to fall short in meeting patients' expectations.

Limitations of conventional hearing aids have resulted in the development of bone conducting devices (BCDs) and implants (BCIs). These devices convert ambient acoustic energy into vibration of the basilar membrane. In this chapter, we use the terms BCI to describe surgical implants and BCD to describe nonsurgical devices. Over the last 20 years, these devices have become a familiar solution in the treatment of patients with conductive or mixed hearing loss who are either poor surgical candidates or unable to tolerate a conventional hearing aid. These devices offer several potential advantages over conventional hearing aids, such as increased gain and dynamic range, improved cosmetic appearance, decreased feedback, reduced maintenance requirement, and insurance coverage.

This chapter provides an overview of bone conducting devices and implants, including background and history, mechanism and design, preoperative evaluation and candidacy, operative technique, and outcomes. Given that specific labeling and indications for individual devices are constantly changing, this information is not explicitly listed in this chapter, and our recommendation is to refer to the manufacturer and FDA labeling of any given device before use.

Background and History

The recognition of bone conduction as a hearing rehabilitation mechanism has been understood since antiquity. In the first century, Pliny the Elder described the potential of sound conduction through solid bodies; by placing one's ear to the end of a long beam of wood, a tap on the other side could be distinctly heard and help one assess the character of the wood [2]. During renaissance times, Girolamo Cardano, an Italian physician, philosopher, and mathematician, demonstrated that sound could be transmitted to the ear using a rod or the shaft of a spear held between one's teeth, allowing that person to "hear distant sounds, voice and words that he could not hear under normal circumstances." [3, 4].

Development of Non-implanted Bone-Conduction Devices and Their Limitations

In the second half of the nineteenth century, the first bone-conduction devices (BCDs) were developed. Instruments such as the Fonifero, Audiphone, and Dentaphone enabled bone conduction through teeth. The development of the carbon microphone and magnetic receiver (or earphone) at the beginning of the twentieth century facilitated the development of BCDs that relied on bone stimulators pressed against the skin over the mastoid that were held up by eyeglasses.

A. Chern · F. X. Creighton Jr · C. C. Della Santina
Department of Otolaryngology—Head and Neck Surgery, Johns Hopkins University School of Medicine, Baltimore, MD, USA

L. R. Lustig (✉)
Department of Otolaryngology—Head and Neck Surgery, Columbia University Irving Medical Center, New York, NY, USA
e-mail: lrl2125@cumc.columbia.edu

A. D. Sweeney et al. (eds.), *Haynes-Glasscock-Shambaugh Surgery of the Ear*, https://doi.org/10.1007/978-3-032-18264-7_18

These external BCDs began to lose popularity with the rapid advancement of air conduction hearing aid technology [3]. Moreover, external BCDs had several inherent problems, including variable fixation of the vibrator and consequences of chronically applied firm pressure on the skin and subcutaneous soft tissues. Other limitations included an unsatisfactory cosmetic appearance and poor sound quality due to soft tissue attenuation [3]. To this day, BCDs still have distinct indications. These include adult patients who are unfavorable surgical candidates and infants with ear canal atresia whose temporal bones are not thick enough to accommodate an osseointegrated device. Contemporary examples of BCDs include the MED-EL (Innsbruck, Austria) ADHEAR and Cochlear™ (Lane Cove, Australia) Baha® SoundArc™, Baha® Softband.

Osseointegrated Implants

In the 1960s, Per-Ingvar Brånemark, a Swedish physician, discovered that titanium had a unique ability to firmly anchor in the bone and be subjected to considerable forces without long-term changes in stability. Additionally, adverse reactions with respect to surrounding bone/soft tissue and epithelial proliferation/invasion were minimal. With these permanent fixtures, Brånemark predicted the ability of these titanium implants to support human prostheses and coined the term "osseointegration." Although first applied in dentistry, Brånemark hypothesized such implants could be extended to skin-penetrating (or percutaneous) implants. In 1977, Brånemark and his colleagues, including Albrektsson, Jacobsson, and Tjellström, implemented a clinical program with percutaneous titanium implants [5, 6]. Brånemark and Tjellström reported in 1982 that these implants could pierce the skin of the upper arm and be anchored for long periods without any inflammatory or adverse soft tissue reaction provided that the free movements of the skin around the implant were restricted [7]. In 1987, Brånemark and his colleagues reported their case series of 389 percutaneous titanium implants that provided an anchor for various facial prostheses, including those for a missing pinna, eye, or nose (due to congenital malformations, reconstruction after head and neck cancer surgery, or facial trauma) and for bone-anchored hearing implants [6]. From this foundational work, a number of percutaneous bone conduction devices have emerged, and currently, two percutaneous osseointegrated devices are labeled for use: the Baha® (Cochlear™, Fig. 18.1) and the Ponto (Oticon Medical, Askim, Sweden). Surgical and outcomes details for these devices are discussed later in this chapter.

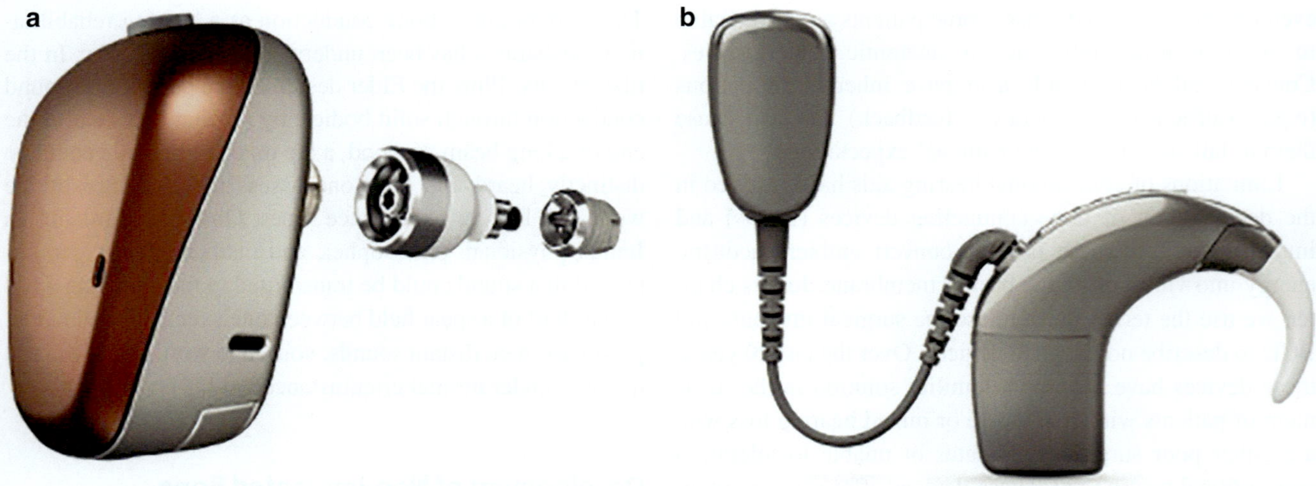

Fig. 18.1 Example of an Osseointegrated Baha® Connect and associated processor. (**a**) The Baha® 5 Connect system is depicted with its attachment to the abutment and titanium implant. (**b**) The Baha® 5 SuperPower processor offers increased amplification for patients with a more severe sensorineural component in their hearing loss. (© Cochlear™ North America. Do not reproduce)

Transcutaneous Bone-Conduction Implants

Though percutaneous BCIs have proven to be useful options for management of CHL and SSD, several new technologies have been developed to address some of the limitations of these devices. These most notably include skin breakdown, need for daily cleaning/maintenance, and poor cosmetic appearance. Transcutaneous bone-conduction implant systems are increasingly popular and feasible alternatives because they can operate through intact skin. These devices can be divided into passive (skin-drive) and active (direct-drive) devices [8].

Passive transcutaneous BCIs have an external transducer that vibrates the bone through the skin, which is attached to a magnet implanted into the skull. Examples include the Baha® Attract (Cochlear™) and the Alpha 2 (Sophono Inc., Boulder, CO). Outcomes of the Baha® Attract and Alpha 2 are similar; patients experience improved hearing (compared to the unaided condition) for conductive, mixed, and unilateral SNHL, but the degree of amplification is often less than that of percutaneous devices (e.g., the traditional Baha® or Ponto) due to increased soft tissue attenuation. However, compared to percutaneous devices, patients noted minimal skin complications and better cosmetic appearance [9–11].

Active transcutaneous BCIs have an implanted transducer permanently placed in the temporal bone and an external processor that transmits the sound signal through the intact skin. These devices combine the advantage of direct bone conduction stimulation (similar to a percutaneous BCI) with the additional benefit of maintaining intact skin. Examples include the BONEBRIDGE (MED-EL), the Sentio™ (Oticon Medical) and the Osia® (Cochlear™, Fig. 18.2). The BONEBRIDGE system was the first active transcutaneous BCI, introduced globally in 2012 and cleared by the FDA in July of 2018; the second-generation device (BCI 602) received FDA clearance in 2019. This active system uses an electromagnetic transducer implanted underneath the skin that vibrates the skull in response to a magnetically coupled external sound processor. While the device does osseointegrate, osseointegration is not required prior to activation of the processor, providing an advantage for fitting external components without waiting for osseointegration to occur. The Osia® system is considered an active osseointegrated steady-state implant. It employs an implanted piezoelectric transducer to directly vibrate the skull in response to an external sound processor. The benefit of a piezoelectric design is that there is no movement between the internal parts, which potentially provides long-term performance and durability. Following a 1-year multicenter clinical investigation and limited release of a first-generation device, the second-generation Osia® 2 system recently gained FDA approval in December of 2019. The Sentio™ received FDA clearance in 2024, and involves the use of a Sentio Ti implant that magnetically attaches to an external processor.

Osseointegration: Mechanism and Design

Osseointegration is critical to successful surgical BCI use, percutaneous or transcutaneous. Osseointegration has been described as the optimal coexistence among the implant, bone, and soft tissue. Successful osseointegration occurs if the load-bearing implant is rigidly fixed into living bone with no reaction at the implant-bone interface [12, 13]. Living bone and the implant must have *direct* contact at the histological level, without interposed connective or soft tissue [14]. Moreover, there should not be any inflammation at the implantation site, such as an infiltrate surrounding the implant or evidence of osteolysis. There are several key determinants of successful osseointegration of an implant, which are discussed below.

Implant Material

Chemical composition of the implant is an important factor for osseointegration. The ideal implant material is tissue-tolerant, corrosion-resistant, and capable of withstanding heavy loads at the implantation site [14]. In the 1970s, many attempts were made to implant different metals (e.g., stainless steel, vitallium, tantalum, and titanium) into various bones of the body [15]. Due to complications such as adverse tissue reactions, most of these did not allow for direct contact between the implant and bone, which is required for long-term osseointegration [5]. In comparison, titanium's extraordinary biocompatibility and characteristics that enable seamless integration into living bone have been well-documented over the past 50 years. Titanium is available commercially in two forms—as 99.75% "pure" titanium and as a titanium alloy, which contains 90% titanium, 6% aluminum, and 4% vanadium. Similar to other metals, titanium forms several types of oxides when exposed to oxygen (e.g., TiO, Ti_2O_3, and TiO_2). It is important to note that metals and their respective oxides can have completely different characteristics. Since the oxide coating of the implant is in contact with host tissue, the biocompatibility of the oxide layer ultimately determines the implant's interaction with host tissue [13]. Unlike many other metals, titanium forms a tightly bonded and highly corrosion-resistant oxide layer on its surface, making it mostly inert at the implant-bone interface. It is also important to account for the toxicity of the oxide coating, since the implant may be worn for several decades; tita-

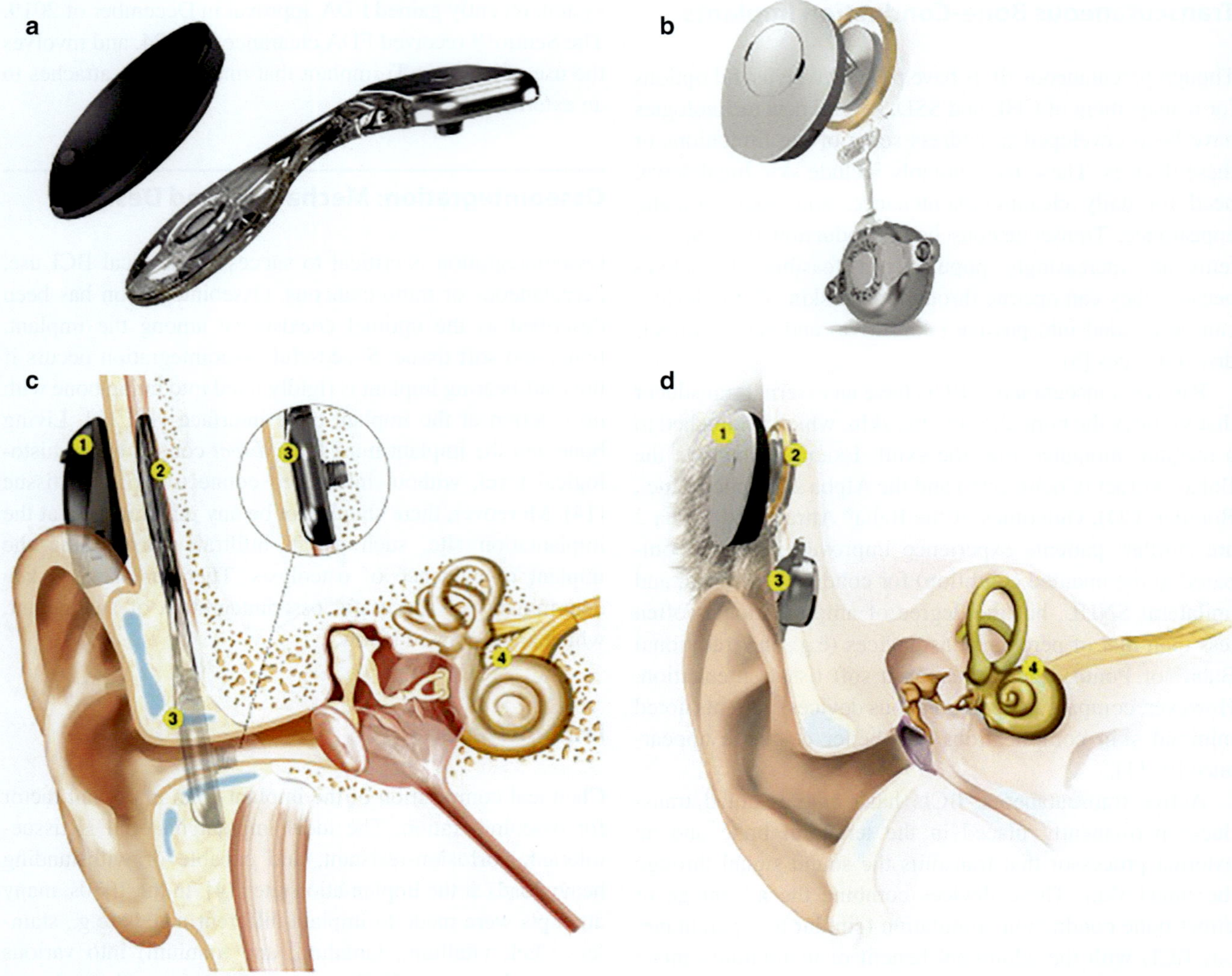

Fig. 18.2 Two of the transcutaneous active bone-conduction devices. (**a**) Osia® 2. (**b**) BONEBRIDGE BCI 602. (**c**) Osia® Mechanism. (**d**) BONEBRIDGE Mechanism. (1) External sound processor captures and analyzes sound signal. (2) Processed signal is sent transcutaneously to the implant. (3) Piezoelectric (**c**) or electromagnetic (**d**) transducer directly vibrates bone. (4) Vibrations travel to the inner ear and are converted to electrical impulses to be sent to the brain. ((**a** and **c**) © Cochlear™ North America. Do not reproduce. (**b** and **d**) © MED-EL GmbH. Do not reproduce)

nium is less toxic compared to many other implant materials (e.g., steel, vitallium) [14]. Though not as strong as steel, titanium still has approximately 10 times the strength of the bone, more than adequate for implant purposes [13]. These characteristics make titanium an ideal and highly biocompatible implant material that represents a standard by which all other biomaterials are measured.

Implant Design: Microstructure and Macrostructure

Implant micro- and macrostructure are also determinants of successful osseointegration. Though a rough porous surface may be advantageous from a load distribution perspective, this considerable increase in surface area would also confer an increased risk of corrosion or an adverse reaction to the implant, even with a relatively corrosion-free material like titanium. According to Eriksson and Brånemark, the microarchitecture of the implant surface should ideally have a topography with micropits that fit the dimensions of the cell membrane and large biomolecules [13]. This enables direct bonding of the implant's oxide layer with bone tissue. The macrostructure of the implant also heavily influences establishment and maintenance of osseointegration, as well as effective distribution of load. Studies have demonstrated that osseointegration is more easily achieved with threaded, screw-shaped implants, which provide maximal contact between bone and implant, and distribute stress more effectively than smooth implants. Threaded implants are also more effective at maintaining stability during initial stages of healing. If the implant is not absolutely stable after placement, fibrous connective tissue may form instead of bone at the contact surface, preventing effective osseointegration [13, 14].

Other Considerations

Healthy living bone is essential for osseointegration. Conditions such as osteoporosis and previous exposure to ionizing radiation may yield suboptimal healing conditions; dental and craniofacial implants in previously irradiated bone in patients with head and neck cancer have been shown to have increased failure and complication rates [16–18]. The comparatively small number of studies on BCIs in patients with previous history of radiation to the temporal bone have demonstrated mixed results with respect to implant failure and complication rates [19, 20]. The rate and severity of complications from BCI placement may be minimized by implanting the device prior to irradiation, ideally at the time of primary oncologic surgery [19]. A stable healing environment is also required for osseointegration. If the implant is not stable during the first few months of healing, connective tissue rather than the bone may form at the implant surface. Even micromovements of the implant during this healing phase have been found to inhibit osteogenesis [14].

Operative Technique: Percutaneous BCI

Proper operative technique is another key determinant for successful osseointegration, and perhaps the one factor over which the surgeon has greatest control. Insertion of an osseointegrated implant for a BCI typically takes place as a single-stage procedure for adults and children over the age of 5. The surgery is typically an outpatient procedure performed in the operating room using local anesthesia with intravenous sedation or general anesthesia. However, some surgeons prefer performing the procedure in an outpatient clinic setting because it may be more cost-effective for the patient and the surgeon [21].

The surgery was originally based on the same principles seen in nature, after trial and error ensured successful osseointegration. While many aspects of the original surgery are not typically used today, occasionally, these same principles must be reemployed, and thus, they are described here. The goal of this form of surgery was to create a thin, immobile, dry, hairless, ~1 cm rim of skin adjacent to the planned implant site, with a gradual increase in soft tissue thickness back to undisturbed tissues ~3 cm from the implant. This skin-implant interface is analogous to biological principles found elsewhere in humans and other species—teeth, nails, tusks, and claws all interface with a thin, firmly attached cutaneous or mucosal border with little or no hair. This arrangement increases stability of the area and minimizes tissue mobility, reducing the risk of inflammation or infection [22, 23].

The implant site is typically chosen 50–60 mm posterior to the ear canal, preferably on—or just inferior to—the linea temporalis. The linea temporalis is well suited for screw placement because it has relatively thick bone, avoids the mastoid air cells, and avoids the thinner squamous temporal bone superiorly. The ideal location is in a region of thin, relatively immobile skin, sufficiently posterior so that subsequent attachment of the Baha® processor will not cause it to touch the pinna. Traditionally, it has been believed that two conditions should be met to create a reaction-free cutaneous-implant interface. First, the skin to be penetrated by the implant must be hairless so the implant site is easily kept clean. Second, subcutaneous tissue should be aggressively thinned to minimize skin mobility against the implant, which allows the dermal layer to heal directly over the mastoid periosteum. This creates a solid, fixed foundation for the implant [24]. Some authors previously advocated for removal of the skin and replacement with a full-thickness skin graft, but this measure was found to be associated with a high rate of skin graft loss [25]. To achieve these conditions, hair is shaved from the site and an adhesive drape is applied after skin preparation. A ~0.6-mm-thick, ~2.5 × 2.5 cm skin flap is elevated using either a dermatome or scalpel. Of note, a dermatome has been designed specifically for use with the Baha® and has been found to reduce the incidence of skin necrosis [26]. All soft tissue deep to this dissection, including hair follicles, is excised down to (but not including) periosteum. An additional ring of subcutaneous tissue is then excised for ~2.5 cm in all directions around the skin wound edges. The final skin flap should be less than 1 mm thick at the site of the implant and surrounding area. The edges of the surrounding skin flaps are then sutured down to the mastoid periosteum to reduce tension on the flap.

The "Punch" Technique Variation

An alternative cutaneous technique that has grown in popularity in recent years is the performance of a 4 or 5 mm skin punch to the level of the periosteum at the designated site. This is followed by removal of the resulting skin plug and obtainment of hemostasis if necessary. This technique is much quicker, though it will require a longer abutment depending on skin thickness. A method used by one of the manufacturers (Oticon Medical), termed "MIPS" (Minimally Invasive Ponto Surgery), employs a cannula inserted into the cutaneous punch site that protects soft tissue during drilling.

Bone Drilling

After cutaneous work is performed, attention turns toward drilling. A 3-mm-deep pilot hole is drilled at the planned implant site with or without the use of a cannula; if the floor of the hole is solid, the hole is extended to a 4 mm depth. The pilot hole is used to align a countersink burr, which widens the pilot hole and creates a shallow countersink in the adjacent bone surface. The titanium implant with the attached abutment (the percutaneous post to which a processor will be secured 2–3 months postoperatively) is then advanced at a slow revolution rate and constant torque until secured. The implant insertion must be performed with meticulous attention to technique because minimizing surrounding tissue damage is essential for osseointegration. Insertion of the implant should be performed precisely and as delicately as possible to minimize thermal injury to the surrounding bone. Employing a high-torque drill at slow speeds (1500–3000 rpm) with sharp drill bits can help the surgeon achieve this goal. Using new, disposable drill bits can help prevent the possibility of worn cutting surfaces damaging the implant bed. Drilling and implant insertion should occur along the same axis to prevent premature thread locking of the screw. Copious irrigation should be used to keep bone clean and cool while drilling. Studies have shown that heating tissue to temperatures as little as 47 °C for 1 minute can cause osteocyte death and hinder proper osseointegration. High-speed drilling typically used in otologic surgery without adequate irrigation can also cause temperature elevations as high as 89 °C [27]. That being said, it is generally recommended that irrigation not be used during the actual implant insertion until the threads of the implant are engaged within the bone of the countersink hole.

After the implant is secured, a hole is then punched into the flap directly over the implant site, allowing it to slip around the abutment down to the bone. This step is not required for the skin punch technique, as a hole in the skin already exists. The abutment is screwed into the implant if it is not already pre-attached. A plastic healing cap is snapped onto the abutment, and a gently compressive antibiotic-soaked dressing is applied to prevent hematoma formation. After 5–7 days, the compressive dressing is removed. After waiting 12 (for adults) or 16 weeks (for children >5 years old) for osseointegration, the processor can be placed onto the abutment.

Variations in operative technique continue to evolve—most are centered on methods to minimize soft tissue complications. These include use of stellate and linear incisions, use of full-thickness skin flaps, choice of dermatome or knife for flap elevation, various dressings, and early postoperative loading of the hearing device [28–30].

Operative Technique: Active Transcutaneous Devices

Active transcutaneous implants, such as the Cochlear™ Osia®, the Oticon Medical Sentio™ and the MED-EL BONEBRIDGE, have become increasingly popular over time. As noted below, performance with these devices appears to be relatively good, and the transcutaneous nature of the device mitigates some of the soft tissue risks associated with a percutaneous implant. However, to accommodate the larger size of the implant, a larger incision generally needs to be made.

Cochlear™ Osia®

Prior to making an incision, it is recommended that a template be used to ensure that the device position is designed to accommodate the actuator of the implant as close as possible to the ear canal and in vertical alignment with the ear canal, if possible. A superior placement is also permitted. Care should be taken to ensure that the placement of the processor will not come into contact with the external ear.

Different incisions have been utilized for the Osia® device. The manufacturer recommends using a standard postauricular incision with superior or inferior extension vs. a "C-shape" incision posterior to the device placement. Keeping 1.5 cm of distance between the incision and the edge of the implant is recommended, though some centers have advocated for an incision immediately over the mid portion of the Osia® or over the site of the implant and screw [31]. A subperiosteal pocket is generally developed for the placement of the entire Osia® device.

Inserting the implant onto which the Osia® will be placed, which is the same style of implant used in Baha® Connect surgery, proceeds as described above in terms of drilling and insertion. After the implant ® has been placed, care is taken to ensure that the surface of the surrounding bone will not interfere with the Osia®. If concerns of this sort exist, a conventional Otologic drill can be used to lower the bone height. Thereafter, the Osia® is placed into the tight pocket and secured into place on the implant. The surgical site is then irrigated and closed in a multilayer fashion.

MED-EL BONEBRIDGE

Similar to the Osia®, prior to making an incision, it is recommended that a template be used to ensure that the device position is designed to accommodate the implant and avoid the external ear. Also similar to the Osia®, different incisions and techniques have been described over time [32].

Following exposure of the bone into which the Bone Conduction-Floating Mass Transducer (BC-FMT) will be placed, a subperiosteal pocket is created to allow for placement of the remainder of the implant. A template for the BC-FMT is provided by the manufacturer to allow for a size match between the device and the countersink hole. The latter can be created with a conventional otologic drill and irrigation. Both dura and venous sinus compression may be necessary for placement of the device, depending on the location of the hole. It is important that the countersink hole has edges that are perpendicular to the floor of the hole so that the BC-FMT will fit. In cases where the BC-FMT cannot be fully seated into the depth of the hole, 1 mm "lifts" are provided to allow the device to function without being completely recessed. Specifically, the lifts can be placed under the screw ports on the side of the implant to "lift" the implant off the bone slightly. The BC-FMT is secured with self-tapping screws, which are provided by the manufacturer. Once the device has been secured in place, the surgical site is irrigated and closed in multiple layers.

Oticon Medical Sentio™

As a newer device, less literature exists for the Sentio™ regarding variations on the manufacturer's surgical technique. Similar to the BONEBRIDGE and Osia®, however, template use for surgical planning is important to ensure that the device avoids the auricle. Distinct from the other devices, the Sentio™ is secured in place using a fixation band, which is packaged with the implant. Once the appropriate location for the implant has been determined, the procedure begins with an incision that is large enough to accommodate the implant as well as the fixation band. It is important to consider that the latter is wider than the actual footprint of the implant. Once the incision is made, it is carried down to bone. Next, a subperiosteal pocket is dissected to house the receiver coil of the implant. The site of the transducer is planned using a template, and additionally, dissection is used to free the periosteum from around the planned site of the transducer in order to create room for the fixation band. A drill is then used to create a recess in the planned location of the transducer. It is important that the recess not exceed 3 mm in depth because a deeper recess may prevent device fixation. A gentle slope can be drilled in the planned location of the implant neck. Once the transducer site is prepared, the surgical site, including the subperiosteal pocket, should be irrigated. The device is then placed into the recess (transducer) and pocket (receiver coil). The implant can be bent up to 30 degrees to accommodate the curvature of the skull. Horizontal bending of up to 30 degrees is also permitted twice. The fixation band is then placed over the center of the transducer and secured into place with 2.7mm screws. The surgical site is then irrigated and closed in multiple layers.

Osseointegrated Implants in Young Children

BCIs are generally not recommended for children under the age of 5 because their temporal bones are thin and may not be well developed enough to support successful osseointegration. For children under 5 years who may benefit from bone conduction hearing, a headband with mounted BCD (e.g., Baha® Softband) is recommended. This device functions by securing a standard BCD to the head using a soft headband and has been shown to allow for bone-conduction hearing nearly equivalent to the osseointegrated device [33]. However, some groups have reported a high rate of success with a traditional osseointegrated implant in this younger population [34, 35]. To maximize the chance of successful osseointegration, the surgery is typically performed as a two-stage procedure for this population, especially in patients with temporal bone that is under 2.5 mm in thickness. In the first stage, the implant is placed into the bone, with or without the abutment, over which the skin is closed directly [34, 35]. The second stage can take place up to 6 months later if the temporal bone is particularly thin; at this point, the skin flap is re-elevated, the abutment is attached to the implant, and the rest of the surgery is completed similarly to the single-stage procedure. During the second stage, it is recommended that a scalpel be used, rather than the dermatome, when the skin is tented upward by the protruding implant screw. Alternatively, the flap can be infiltrated with local anesthetic to cause the site to balloon prior to using the dermatome [34]. Using the two-stage approach in children under 5 years has been shown to yield comparable hearing outcomes to those achieved in older children who undergo the traditional one-stage approach [35].

Complications of Osseointegration

Skin and soft tissue reactions at the percutaneous implant site are the most common complications associated with osseointegrated implants. Studies have reported a wide range of complication rates [24, 36–38]. A meta-analysis of 20 studies (2310 total implants) reported skin reactions from Holgers Grade 2 to 4 occurred in anywhere from 2.4% to 38.1% of patients. Observations from these studies indicate that soft tissue reactions around percutaneous implants are best prevented by thinning skin around the abutment, removing underlying soft tissue, and suturing dermis to underlying bone to minimize skin mobility. Patient compliance with routine cleaning of the abutment site and close monitoring of adjacent skin is also essential for avoiding soft tissue reactions [39].

Other complications are relatively rare. The second most common complication associated with insertion of an osseointegrated implant is osseointegration failure. Risk factors include a thin temporal bone, young age, syndromic status, and prior radiation. A two-stage procedure is often recommended in patients with a high risk of osseointegration failure. Some data supports use of hyperbaric oxygen therapy to reduce the risk of implant failure or osteoradionecrosis in irradiated patients [17, 40]. Osseointegration failure rates have been found to range anywhere from 0% to 18% [24, 38, 39]. One meta-analysis found revision surgery rates ranged from 1.7% to 34.5% in adult and mixed populations and 0.0% to 44.4% in pediatric populations, while the overall rate of implant loss ranged from 1.6% to 17.4% in adult and mixed populations and from 0.0% to 25% in pediatric populations [39]. Additional complications cited for implant removal include poor cochlear function, unexplained pain, and uncooperative patients exhibiting poor compliance [38]. Another rarely described complication is intracerebral abscess [39].

Newer minimally invasive and soft tissue preservation techniques have been developed to decrease the complications associated with percutaneous osseointegrated implants (Fig. 18.3). These include using a small linear incision (without skin thinning) and using a single skin punch to access the skull (using a longer abutment). Studies comparing these new techniques to traditional cutaneous techniques have found comparable or even lower rates of skin complications [41–44]. These techniques are becoming increasingly popular because they are associated with significantly reduced operative time, decreased healing time, and increased cost-effectiveness [30, 41, 42, 45, 46]. Despite the relatively low complications rate associated with osseointegrated implants, the costs of these complications should be taken into account when considering treatment options for patients with hearing loss [47].

One disadvantage of any metallic implant is interference with subsequent radiologic studies. Although the Baha® abutment causes some scatter artifact on CT, the implant is typically located out of the plane of axial and coronal slices through key temporal bone structures. Fortunately, pure titanium produces relatively little degradation of images on MRI, and the presence of a Baha® Connect implant without its external processor is not a contraindication for MRI [48]. However, transcutaneous devices that contain an implanted magnet can be problematic for patients needing an MRI, and manufacturer guidelines should be consulted when this situation is encountered. Consideration should also be given when using such a device in a patient who may need future MRIs, particularly in the setting of cholesteatoma [49].

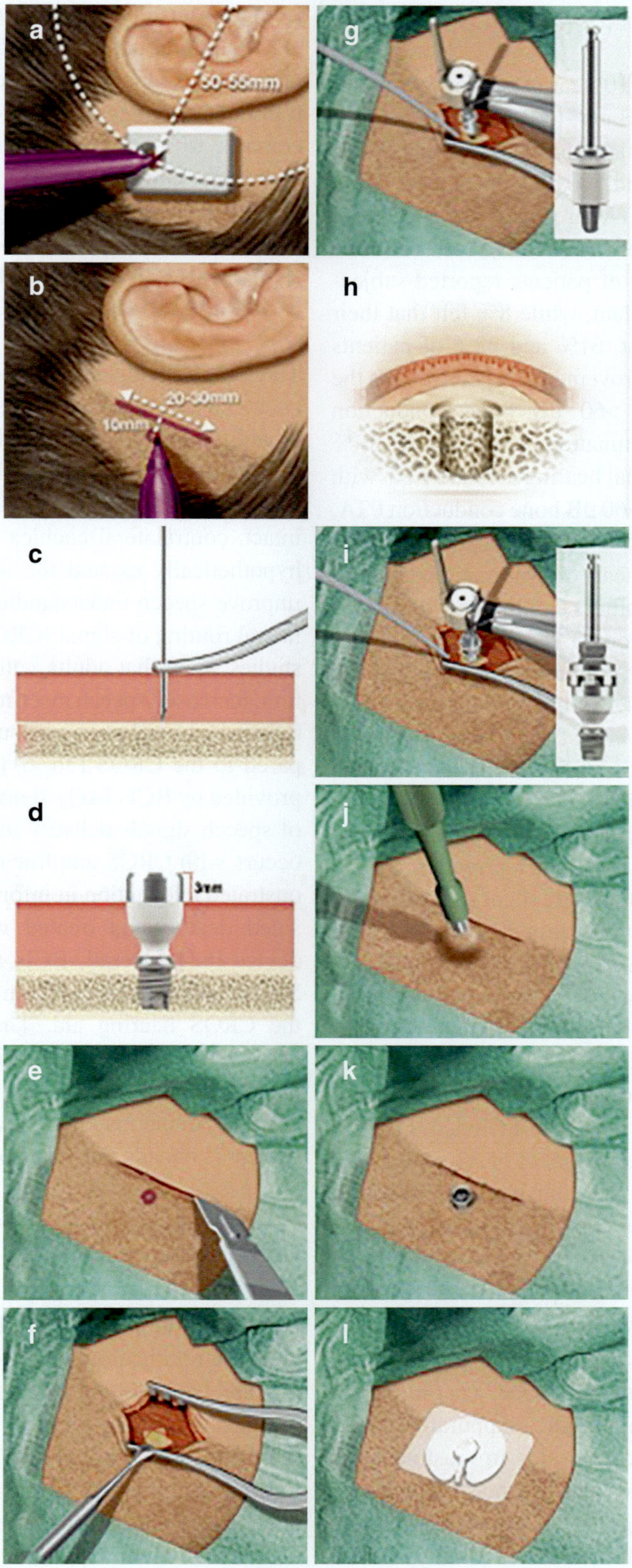

Fig. 18.3 Minimally invasive operative technique for placement of Baha® Connect. (**a**) Implant site is chosen 50–55 mm posterior to the ear canal aligned to the top of the pinna. (**b**) A 20–30 mm incision is planned 10 mm anterior to the abutment site. (**c**) Soft tissue thickness is measured with a needle. (**d**) Appropriate abutment size is chosen. (**e**) Incision to periosteum is made. (**f**) Implant placement 10 mm posterior to incision is identified with a cross-shaped incision made in the periosteum and elevated off bone. (**g**) A 3–4 mm hole is drilled into the bone. (**h**) Countersink creates recessed surface for implant placement. (**i**) Titanium implant with abutment is drilled into the bone. (**j**) Hole punch is made to create an opening for the abutment 10 mm posterior to the incision (sutured). (**k**) Flap is slipped around the abutment down to the bone. (**l**) Healing cap is placed. (©Cochlear™ North America. Do not reproduce)

Outcomes

Håkansson et al. reported their 10-year experience with 147 adult patients who received the Baha® [50]. Dividing patients into three groups [bone conduction pure tone average (PTA) between 0–45 dB, 46–60 dB, and >60 dB], the authors noted a strong relationship between PTA thresholds and successful outcome. In the group with the best cochlear reserve (bone conduction PTA <45 db), 89% of patients reported subjective improvement with the implant, while 8% felt that their hearing was worse. By contrast, 61% and 22% of patients reported subjective hearing improvement, respectively, in the groups with 46–60 dB and >60 dB bone conduction PTA. Average speech discrimination scores were 14% unaided, 67% with a conventional hearing aid, and 81% with the Baha®. Excluding subjects >60 dB bone conduction PTA, mean discrimination improved to 85%; excluding 46 to 60 dB PTA, subjects raised mean discrimination to 89%. Based upon these results, the authors recommended a candidacy criterion of bone conduction PTA <45 dB for the standard Baha® system. However, improvements in hearing should still be expected for a PTA of up to 60 dB, especially with development of more powerful Baha® processors. The Baha® has also been used successfully in children; studies have demonstrated increased aided PTAs, improved quality of life, and high level of patient compliance in the pediatric population [51–53]. Overall, the Baha® provides a high degree of hearing rehabilitation and excellent satisfaction to patients with a bone conduction PTA less than 45 dB.

In the first review of the US experience with the Baha®, the most common indications for implantation included chronic otitis media and/or draining ears and external auditory canal stenosis or aural atresia [38]. Patients who had undergone prior skull base surgery and had complete closure of the external auditory canal were also included. Overall, each patient had an average improvement of 32 dB ±19 dB with use of the Baha®. Closure of the air-bone gap to within 10 dB of the preoperative bone conduction thresholds was observed in 80% of patients, while closure to within 5 dB occurred in 60%. Nearly one-third of patients demonstrated "overclosure" of the preoperative bone conduction threshold of the better hearing ear.

BCIs have also been shown to be cost-effective. Implantation in patients with chronic suppurative otitis media who previously used hearing aids in mastoid bowl resulted in fewer treatments and visits for mastoid debridement as well as a net cost savings [54]. A cost-benefit analysis of management options for external auditory canal atresia favored the osseointegrated implant over atresia repair [55].

The introduction of active transcutaneous BCIs has added new considerations for surgeons and patients. Evidence is emerging that these devices, though generally more involved from a surgical perspective, are able to offer significant benefit to eligible patients [56–60]. Though passive percutaneous devices continue to be offered and utilized, active transcutaneous devices are promising systems that will likely continue to increase in popularity and become more common in the United States [8].

Bone-Anchored Hearing Implants for Single-Sided Deafness

Though originally designed for patients with CHL, the bone-anchored hearing implant system has proven valuable in the rehabilitation of single-sided deafness (SSD), or severe-to-profound unilateral SNHL. Placing the device on the side with hearing loss can capture sound and convey it to the intact, contralateral cochlea via cranial vibration. This can hypothetically expand the sound field for the patient and improve speech understanding in noise, similar to a contralateral routing of signal (CROS) hearing aid. Indeed, several studies show that adults with SSD have increased satisfaction, increased speech discrimination (notably in background noise), and similarly poor sound localization with BCIs compared to the CROS [36, 61]. Improved speech recognition provided by BCIs likely stems from averting the interference of speech signals delivery to the better ear, which typically occurs with CROS amplification [61]. One study also demonstrated a reduction in informational masking when single-sided deafness is treated with a bone-anchored hearing device [62]. Overall, BCIs are useful for rehabilitation of SSD and seem to outperform the only other available option: the CROS hearing aid. The main benefit appears to be improved speech perception in noise, with little to no benefit in sound localization. For contemporary SSD patients, cochlear implantation may also be an option, though this subject is outside the scope of this chapter.

Conclusion

BCIs have the potential to deliver improved sound quality, greater amplification, less distortion, better directional hearing, and better cosmetic appearance than conventional hearing aids. However, these potential desirable benefits come with trade-offs including increased cost to the patient and insurer, surgical risks, postoperative complications, and dependence on the sometimes-uncertain long-term viability of manufacturers supporting these devices. While conventional hearing aids continue to improve and cochlear implantation criteria continue to expand, implantable BCIs will continue to develop and ultimately play a critical role in the care of patients whose hearing loss is not adequately addressed by those competing technologies.

References

1. Chien W, Lin FR. Prevalence of hearing aid use among older adults in the United States. Arch Intern Med. 2012;172(3):292–3.
2. Pliny the Elder. The Natural History. Translated by Bostock J, Riley H (London: Bohn, 1855), Perseus Digital Library. http://www.perseus.tufts.edu/hopper/text?doc=urn:cts:latinLit:phi0978.phi001.perseus-eng1:16.73. Accessed April 26, 2020.
3. Mudry A, Tjellström A. Historical background of bone conduction hearing devices and bone conduction hearing aids. Adv Otorhinolaryngol. 2011;71:1–9.
4. Cardano G. De subtilitate libri XXI. Parisiis [Paris]: Michaelis Fezendat et Roberti Granjon. 1550., liber XIII. p. 234.
5. Tjellström A, Lindström J, Hallén O, Albrektsson T, Brånemark PI. Osseointegrated titanium implants in the temporal bone. A clinical study on bone-anchored hearing aids. Am J Otol. 1981;2(4):304–10.
6. Albrektsson T, Brånemark PI, Jacobsson M, Tjellström A. Present clinical applications of osseointegrated percutaneous implants. Plast Reconstr Surg. 1987;79(5):721–31.
7. Brånemark PI, Albrektsson T. Titanium implants permanently penetrating human skin. Scand J Plast Reconstr Surg. 1982;16(1):17–21.
8. Reinfeldt S, Håkansson B, Taghavi H, Eeg-Olofsson M. New developments in bone-conduction hearing implants: a review. Med Devices (Auckl). 2015;8:79–93.
9. Hol MK, Nelissen RC, Agterberg MJ, Cremers CW, Snik AF. Comparison between a new implantable transcutaneous bone conductor and percutaneous bone-conduction hearing implant. Otol Neurotol. 2013;34(6):1071–5.
10. Briggs R, Van Hasselt A, Luntz M, et al. Clinical performance of a new magnetic bone conduction hearing implant system: results from a prospective, multicenter, clinical investigation. Otol Neurotol. 2015;36(5):834–41.
11. Iseri M, Orhan KS, Tuncer U, et al. Transcutaneous bone-anchored hearing aids versus percutaneous ones: multicenter comparative clinical study. Otol Neurotol. 2015;36(5):849–53.
12. Brånemark PLJ, Ericson L, Thomsen P, Brånemark R, Skalak R. Anatomy of osseointegration and the transfer of load. In: Reconstructive preprosthetic oral and maxillofacial surgery; 1995. p. 165–224.
13. Eriksson E, Brånemark PI. Osseointegration from the perspective of the plastic surgeon. Plast Reconstr Surg. 1994;93(3):626–37.
14. Albrektsson T, Brånemark PI, Hansson HA, Lindström J. Osseointegrated titanium implants. Requirements for ensuring a long-lasting, direct bone-to-implant anchorage in man. Acta Orthop Scand. 1981;52(2):155–70.
15. Pazzaglia UE, Bernini F, Zatti G, Di Nucci A. Histology of the metal-bone interface: interpretation of plastic embedded slides. Biomaterials. 1994;15(4):273–7.
16. Ihde S, Kopp S, Gundlach K, Konstantinović VS. Effects of radiation therapy on craniofacial and dental implants: a review of the literature. Oral Surg Oral Med Oral Pathol Oral Radiol Endod. 2009;107(1):56–65.
17. Granström G, Bergström K, Tjellström A, Brånemark P-I. A detailed analysis of titanium implants lost in irradiated tissues. Implant Dent. 1995;4(3):204.
18. Granström G, Tjellström A, Brånemark PI, Fornander J. Bone-anchored reconstruction of the irradiated head and neck cancer patient. Otolaryngol Head Neck Surg. 1993;108(4):334–43.
19. Nader ME, Beadle BM, Roberts DB, Gidley PW. Outcomes and complications of osseointegrated hearing aids in irradiated temporal bones. Laryngoscope. 2016;126(5):1187–92.
20. Soo G, Tong MC, Tsang WS, et al. The BAHA hearing system for hearing-impaired postirradiated nasopharyngeal cancer patients: a new indication. Otol Neurotol. 2009;30(4):496–501.
21. Catalano PJ, Choi E, Cohen N. Office versus operating room insertion of the bone-anchored hearing aid: a comparative analysis. Otol Neurotol. 2005;26(6):1182–5.
22. Adell R, Lekholm U, Rockler B, et al. Marginal tissue reactions at osseointegrated titanium fixtures (I). A 3-year longitudinal prospective study. Int J Oral Maxillofac Surg. 1986;15(1):39–52.
23. Lekholm U, Adell R, Lindhe J, et al. Marginal tissue reactions at osseointegrated titanium fixtures. (II) A cross-sectional retrospective study. Int J Oral Maxillofac Surg. 1986;15(1):53–61.
24. Tjellström A, Håkansson B. The bone-anchored hearing aid. Design principles, indications, and long-term clinical results. Otolaryngol Clin N Am. 1995;28(1):53–72.
25. Snyder MC, Moore GF, Johnson PJ. The use of full-thickness skin grafts for the skin-abutment interface around bone-anchored hearing aids. Otol Neurotol. 2003;24(2):255–8.
26. Tjellström A, Granström G. How we do it: frequency of skin necrosis after BAHA surgery. Clin Otolaryngol. 2006;31(3):216–20.
27. Eriksson RA, Albrektsson T, Magnusson B. Assessment of bone viability after heat trauma. A histological, histochemical and vital microscopic study in the rabbit. Scand J Plast Reconstr Surg. 1984;18(3):261–8.
28. Strijbos RM, Salameh S, Bezdjian A, Daniel SJ, Thomeer HG. The minimally invasive star-shaped incision technique and the linear incision technique with tissue preservation for percutaneous bone conduction devices: a retrospective cohort study. Front Surg. 2022;9:863997.
29. Stalfors J, Tjellström A. Skin reactions after BAHA surgery: a comparison between the U-graft technique and the BAHA dermatome. Otol Neurotol. 2008;29(8):1109–14.
30. de Wolf MJ, Hol MK, Huygen PL, Mylanus EA, Cremers CW. Clinical outcome of the simplified surgical technique for BAHA implantation. Otol Neurotol. 2008;29(8):1100–8.
31. Deep NL, Johnson BJ, Kay-Rivest E, et al. Modifications to implanting the OSIA® 2 bone conduction hearing implant: how I do it. Laryngoscope. 2022;132(9):1850–4.
32. You P, Siegel LH, Kassam Z, et al. The middle fossa approach with self-drilling screws: a novel technique for BONEBRIDGE implantation. J Otolaryngol Head Neck Surg. 2019;48(1):35.
33. Verhagen CV, Hol MK, Coppens-Schellekens W, Snik AF, Cremers CW. The Baha Softband. A new treatment for young children with bilateral congenital aural atresia. Int J Pediatr Otorhinolaryngol. 2008;72(10):1455–9.
34. Yellon RF. Bone anchored hearing aid in children--prevention of complications. Int J Pediatr Otorhinolaryngol. 2007;71(5):823–6.
35. Davids T, Gordon KA, Clutton D, Papsin BC. Bone-anchored hearing aids in infants and children younger than 5 years. Arch Otolaryngol Head Neck Surg. 2007;133(1):51–5.
36. Niparko JK, Cox KM, Lustig LR. Comparison of the bone anchored hearing aid implantable hearing device with contralateral routing of offside signal amplification in the rehabilitation of unilateral deafness. Otol Neurotol. 2003;24(1):73–8.
37. House JW, Kutz JW Jr. Bone-anchored hearing aids: incidence and management of postoperative complications. Otol Neurotol. 2007;28(2):213–7.
38. Lustig LR, Arts HA, Brackmann DE, et al. Hearing rehabilitation using the BAHA bone-anchored hearing aid: results in 40 patients. Otol Neurotol. 2001;22(3):328–34.
39. Kiringoda R, Lustig LR. A meta-analysis of the complications associated with osseointegrated hearing aids. Otol Neurotol. 2013;34(5):790–4.
40. Granström G, Tjellström A, Brånemark PI. Osseointegrated implants in irradiated bone: a case-controlled study using adjunctive hyperbaric oxygen therapy. J Oral Maxillofac Surg. 1999;57(5):493–9.
41. Dumon T, Medina M, Sperling NM. Punch and drill: implantation of bone anchored hearing device through a minimal skin punch

incision versus implantation with dermatome and soft tissue reduction. Ann Otol Rhinol Laryngol. 2016;125(3):199–206.
42. Gordon SA, Coelho DH. Minimally invasive surgery for osseointegrated auditory implants: a comparison of linear versus punch techniques. Otolaryngol Head Neck Surg. 2015;152(6):1089–93.
43. Høgsbro M, Agger A, Johansen LV. Bone-anchored hearing implant surgery: randomized trial of dermatome versus linear incision without soft tissue reduction--clinical measures. Otol Neurotol. 2015;36(5):805–11.
44. Mohamad S, Khan I, Hey SY, Hussain SS. A systematic review on skin complications of bone-anchored hearing aids in relation to surgical techniques. Eur Arch Otorhinolaryngol. 2016;273(3):559–65.
45. Husseman J, Szudek J, Monksfield P, Power D, O'Leary S, Briggs R. Simplified bone-anchored hearing aid insertion using a linear incision without soft tissue reduction. J Laryngol Otol. 2013;127(Suppl 2):S33–8.
46. Verheij E, Bezdjian A, Grolman W, Thomeer HG. A systematic review on complications of tissue preservation surgical techniques in percutaneous bone conduction hearing devices. Otol Neurotol. 2016;37(7):829–37.
47. Pross SE, Layton A, Tong K, Lustig LR. Cost of placement and complications associated with osseointegrated bone-conducting hearing prostheses: a retrospective analysis of medicare billing data. Otol Neurotol. 2014;35(3):476–81.
48. Fritsch MH, Naumann IC, Mosier KM. BAHA devices and magnetic resonance imaging scanners. Otol Neurotol. 2008;29(8):1095–9.
49. Nassiri AM, Messina SA, Benson JC, et al. Magnetic resonance imaging artifact associated with transcutaneous bone conduction implants: cholesteatoma and vestibular schwannoma surveillance. Otolaryngol Head Neck Surg. 2024;170(1):187–94.
50. Håkansson B, Lidén G, Tjellström A, et al. Ten years of experience with the Swedish bone-anchored hearing system. Ann Otol Rhinol Laryngol Suppl. 1990;151:1–16.
51. Stevenson DS, Proops DW, Wake MJ, Deadman MJ, Worrollo SJ, Hobson JA. Osseointegrated implants in the management of childhood ear abnormalities: the initial Birmingham experience. J Laryngol Otol. 1993;107(6):502–9.
52. McDermott AL, Williams J, Kuo M, Reid A, Proops D. The Birmingham pediatric bone-anchored hearing aid program: a 15-year experience. Otol Neurotol. 2009;30(2):178–83.
53. McDermott AL, Williams J, Kuo M, Reid A, Proops D. Quality of life in children fitted with a bone-anchored hearing aid. Otol Neurotol. 2009;30(3):344–9.
54. Watson GJ, Silva S, Lawless T, Harling JL, Sheehan PZ. Bone anchored hearing aids: a preliminary assessment of the impact on outpatients and cost when rehabilitating hearing in chronic suppurative otitis media. Clin Otolaryngol. 2008;33(4):338–42.
55. Evans AK, Kazahaya K. Canal atresia: "surgery or implantable hearing devices? The expert's question is revisited". Int J Pediatr Otorhinolaryngol. 2007;71(3):367–74.
56. Harris MK, Kaul VF, Bergman M, Dodson EE, Ren Y, Adunka OF. Outcomes after transcutaneous bone-conduction implantation in adults and children. Otol Neurotol. 2023;44(4):317–23.
57. Miller ME. Osseointegrated auditory devices: Bonebridge. Otolaryngol Clin N Am. 2019;52(2):265–72.
58. Gerdes T, Salcher RB, Schwab B, Lenarz T, Maier H. Comparison of audiological results between a transcutaneous and a percutaneous bone conduction instrument in conductive hearing loss. Otol Neurotol. 2016;37(6):685–91.
59. Lau K, Scotta G, Wright K, et al. First United Kingdom experience of the novel Osia active transcutaneous piezoelectric bone conduction implant. Eur Arch Otorhinolaryngol. 2020;277(11):2995–3002.
60. Goycoolea M, Ribalta G, Tocornal F, et al. Clinical performance of the Osia™ system, a new active osseointegrated implant system. Results from a prospective clinical investigation. Acta Otolaryngol. 2020;140(3):212–9.
61. Lin LM, Bowditch S, Anderson MJ, May B, Cox KM, Niparko JK. Amplification in the rehabilitation of unilateral deafness: speech in noise and directional hearing effects with bone-anchored hearing and contralateral routing of signal amplification. Otol Neurotol. 2006;27(2):172–82.
62. May BJ, Bowditch S, Liu Y, Eisen M, Niparko JK. Mitigation of informational masking in individuals with single-sided deafness by integrated bone conduction hearing aids. Ear Hear. 2014;35(1):41–8.

Pediatric Cochlear Implantation

19

Jacob B. Hunter, J. Walter Kutz Jr., and Kenneth H. Lee

Introduction

Despite the general acceptance that cochlear implantation (CI) benefits bilateral severe to profound sensorineural hearing loss (SNHL) in children, pediatric utilization rates demonstrate regional differences. It is estimated that only 50% of children in the United States who qualify for a cochlear implant actually receive one, which is notably less than the 90+% found in European countries [1]. In this chapter, we will discuss patient evaluation, candidacy criteria, the surgical procedure, and current outcomes in pediatric CI.

Preoperative Evaluation

Patients with severe-to-profound SNHL should be assessed to determine their candidacy from a medical, surgical, and audiological perspective. The medical evaluation requires a complete history and physical, including discussion of the patient's birth, immunization, family, and otologic history, which can assist in potentially identifying the hearing loss etiology. Prenatal exposure to teratogens, select infections, prematurity, low birth weight or APGAR scores, anoxia, intubation, aminoglycoside and/or furosemide administration, meningitis, mumps, sepsis, neonatal intensive care unit stay, and hyperbilirubinemia, such as drug abuse, alcohol, thalidomide, and methyl mercury, as well as (TORCH) infections (toxoplasmosis, other (varicella and syphilis), rubella, cytomegalovirus (CMV), and herpes), have all been associated with congenital SNHL. With CMV being the most common nongenetic cause of pediatric SNHL, universal targeted CMV screening with timely diagnostic evaluations for hearing loss in children may yield substantial benefits [2].

It is recommended to obtain an immunization history given the high rates of meningitis in children with hearing loss, as well as in children with cochlear implants [3–5]. In 2003, Reefhuis et al. reported a 30-fold increased risk of pneumococcal meningitis following CI, which was more pronounced in those individuals where an electrode positioner was used [6]. This was the result of the posterior fossa communicating with the inner ear through the basal turn of the cochlea via the cochlear aqueduct and/or via microscopic canaliculi into the internal auditory canal. Not surprisingly, cochleovestibular malformations lead to an increased risk of meningitis, as one study reported 32% of patients with inner ear malformations had cerebrospinal fluid (CSF) leaks noted at the time of CI (Fig. 19.1) [7].

As a result, the Centers for Disease Control and Prevention (CDC) Advisory Committee on Immunization Practices recommends that pediatric cochlear implant patients under 2 years of age who are unvaccinated or have received less than three pneumococcal conjugate vaccine (PCV) doses receive two doses of PCV15 or PCV20. If the patient has not received a dose of PCV20, and they are not immunocompromised, they should receive one dose of PCV20 or the pneumococcal polysaccharide vaccine (PPSV23) [8]. Though the vaccines work via different mechanisms, there is a synergistic effect through carrier priming. To achieve optimal results based on their mechanisms, there are guidelines on when each vaccine can be administered [9]. For patients who are immunocompromised and have not received PPSV23 should receive one dose of PCV20 or PPSV23. When PCV20 is used, their pneumococcal vaccinations are complete, but when PPSV23 is used, they need another pneumococcal vaccine at least five years later. [8]. As for the *Haemophilus influenzae* type B (Hib) vaccine, only children under 5 years of age should receive the Hib series, since immunity is presumed in all older children [8]. While the CDC recommends that all immunizations are completed at least 2 weeks prior to surgery, the Medicines and Healthcare

J. B. Hunter (✉)
Department of Otolaryngology—Head and Neck Surgery, Thomas Jefferson University School of Medicine, Philadelphia, PA, USA

J. W. Kutz Jr · K. H. Lee
Department of Otolaryngology—Head and Neck Surgery, University of Texas Southwestern Medical Center, Dallas, TX, USA

A. D. Sweeney et al. (eds.), *Haynes-Glasscock-Shambaugh Surgery of the Ear*, https://doi.org/10.1007/978-3-032-18264-7_19

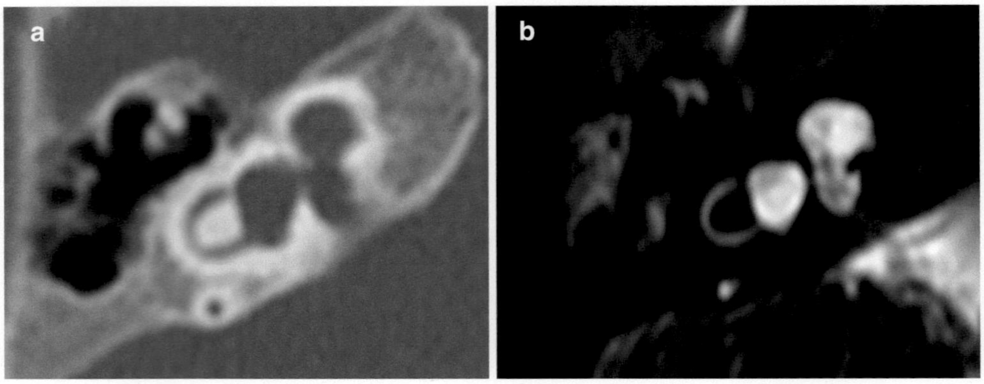

Fig. 19.1 Cochleovestibular anomaly. Axial CT image on the left (**a**) and an axial T2 MR image on the right (**b**), demonstrating an incomplete partition type II with a dilated vestibule and incomplete interscalar septum within the cochlea

Products Regulatory Agency of Great Britain states that CI should not be delayed secondary to immunizations [9, 10]. Furthermore, there are no human studies correlating meningitis in cochlear implant patients and pneumococcal vaccination status.

Approximately 50% of pediatric SNHL is genetic; therefore directed questions regarding early-onset and congenital SNHL is a key element of the preoperative evaluation. Genetic hearing loss is associated with either syndromic or non-syndromic causes, with the latter being far more common. Specifically, the most common genetic cause of non-syndromic severe-to-profound autosomal recessive hearing loss is a gap junction protein B2 mutation (connexin 26) [11–15]. These patients are excellent CI candidates, demonstrating significantly better outcomes as compared to those patients with acquired deafness via environmental etiologies [16, 17]. Syndromic SNHL etiologies that are associated with successful CI include Pendred, Waardenburg, Usher, branchio-oto-renal (BOR), and Jervell and Lange-Nielsen syndromes. Patients with CHARGE (coloboma of the eye, congenital heart defects, choanal atresia, mental and/or growth retardation, genital hypoplasia, and ear anomalies and or deafness) association have variable outcomes due to associated developmental delays [18]. Usher syndrome and Refsum disease can lead to retinitis pigmentosa and progressive blindness. Thus, CI should be completed in these patients prior to severe vision loss [19]. Since Jervell and Lange-Nielsen syndrome is associated with a prolonged QT interval, cardiac arrhythmias, and syncope, it is generally recommended that all patients with congenital SNHL undergo an electrocardiogram when no other etiology is identified. If confirmed, a cardiology consultation and complete family testing should be completed before CI, as many consider a defibrillator or pacemaker before surgery, along with perioperative beta-blockade [20]. Regardless of the family history, children should undergo a speech and language evaluation prior to CI to determine if other factors contribute to their auditory development [21].

Developmental disabilities are an important factor to consider and affect approximately 30% of children with hearing loss [22]. Corrales and Oghalai highlight that many centers are resistant to implanting patients who may never develop speech and language [23]. While Boons and colleagues found that the presence of an additional learning disability led to lower receptive language scores 1, 2, and 3 years following CI, studies have shown that CI increases acquisition of language skills, speech intelligibility, social interaction, environmental awareness, and development of adaptive behavior in patients with disabilities [24–28]. Palmieri and colleagues utilized the Deafness and Additional Disabilities Questionnaire (DADQ) in 50 children who were CI candidates with additional disabilities and demonstrated quality of life improvements in physical, neuropsychological, and social domains following CI [29]. Gerard and colleagues used the Acceptance, Perception, Comprehension, Expression, Intelligibility (APCEI) scale in 89 children with cochlear implants, and while an associated disability was linked with slower progress in APCEI scores after CI, children still derived substantial improvement [30]. In conclusion, while parents with children with additional disabilities should be counseled that development of oral communication skills may not occur, they can expect increased sound awareness, improved family activity, social and personal interactions, environmental connectivity, and improvement in quality of life [23].

Imaging Evaluation

Imaging is obtained to evaluate for cochleovestibular anomalies, presence of a cochlear nerve, and retrocochlear pathology. Anomalies (some of which may preclude CI) can occur in 35–40% of pediatric cochlear implant candidates and are bilateral in 65% of patients [21, 31]. Imaging studies also enable the surgeon to identify anatomical variations that may complicate surgery, including facial nerve anomalies or luminal obstruction. It is estimated that 15% of pediatric patients with cochleovestibular anomalies have anomalous facial nerve anatomy, which may impede a traditional facial recess approach [32, 33]. Vascular anatomy can also be assessed: in one study, an anteriorly positioned sigmoid sinus prevented adequate facial recess exposure in 1.6% of patients [34]. In addition, a high-riding jugular bulb or a diverticulum can make access to the round window difficult, while, an aberrant or dehiscent carotid artery may complicate drill-out procedures. Imaging also identifies patients with incomplete partition type III or enlarged vestibular or cochlear aqueducts, all of which may lead to an increased risk of a CSF gusher [35, 36]. While cochleovestibular anomalies will be discussed in another chapter, most pediatric patients with anomalies may successfully undergo CI, with the exception of those patients with complete cochlear and labyrinthine aplasia. Even some patients with radiographically absent eighth nerves have obtained open set speech recognition following CI [21].

Preoperative imaging can also direct the surgeon to select the best side when a unilateral implant is planned or to confirm the feasibility of bilateral CI. Such pathology includes cochlear luminal obstruction, which most commonly occurs from post-meningitis labyrinthitis ossificans but can also be seen after suppurative labyrinthitis secondary to cholesteatoma, otitis media, viral infections, septicemia, rubella, and mumps. Labyrinthitis ossificans is most commonly bilateral, but the severity can be asymmetric. This pathology can be identified on imaging, and though variable, the cochlear obstruction typically begins in the basal turn and progresses toward the apex [31]. It is important to keep in mind that the onset is unpredictable, with ossification occurring anytime from weeks to years after the insult [37]. Fibrosis occurs first, prior to mineralization, and both are visualized as a loss of normal T2-hyperintensity on magnetic resonance (MR) imaging. Computed tomography (CT) imaging can provide additional value as it may help differentiate between fibrosis or mineralization [31]. Other causes of luminal obstruction include osseous dysplasias (e.g., Paget disease) or sequelae from temporal bone fracture [21]. While MRI is more sensitive in identifying labyrinthitis ossificans and inner ear soft tissue anomalies as compared to CT, no benefit has been shown demonstrating a difference in imaging studies in predicting abnormal inner ear anatomy [38].

Lastly, MRI can determine the presence of a cochlear nerve. Considered to be one of the more common etiologies for pediatric SNHL, one study found that an absent or deficient cochlear nerve was present in 18% of patients with SNHL (Fig. 19.2) [39]. However, there are reports of patients with absent cochlear nerves who benefited from CI, presumably due to cochlear nerve fibers traveling with vestibular nerve fibers [40–43]. Kutz and colleagues reported on seven patients with imaging suggestive of cochlear nerve absence,

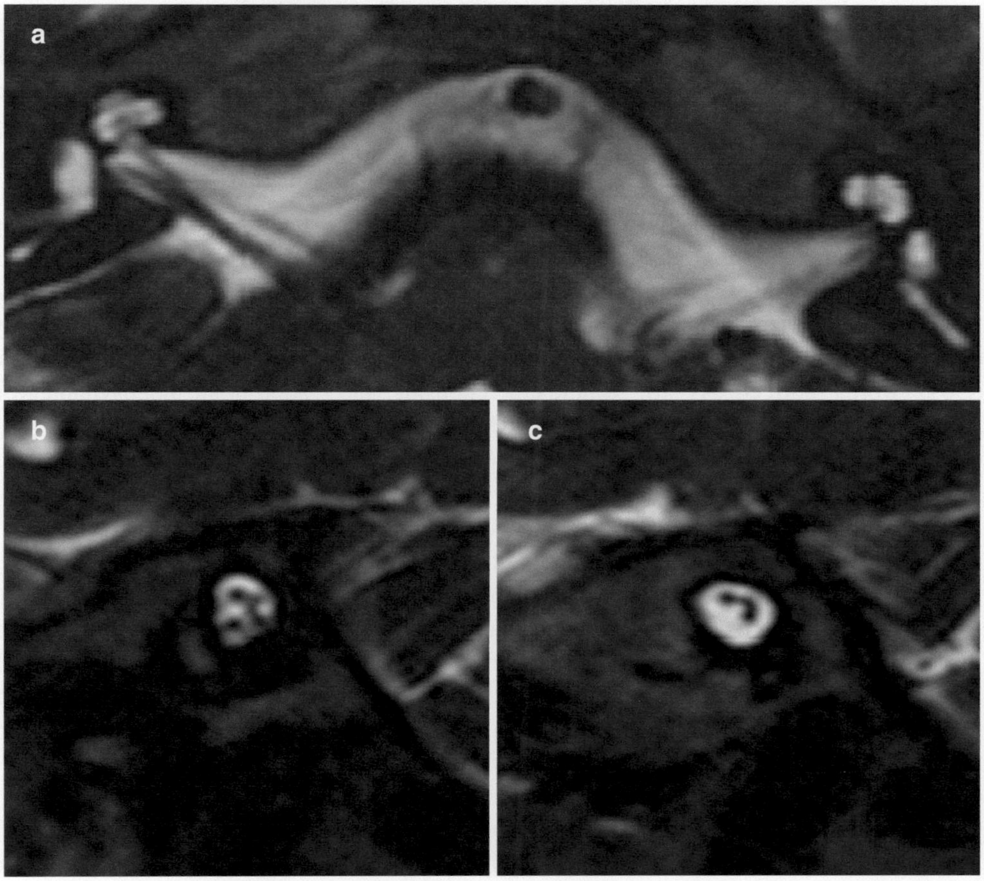

Fig. 19.2 Cochlear nerve aplasia. Axial T2 MRI (**a**), with parasagittal images demonstrating absence of the cochlear nerve in the left ear (**b**), with presence of the cochlear nerve in the right ear (**c**) (arrow)

all of whom underwent CI [41]. Six children developed speech detection or pattern reception, while one developed closed-set speech recognition [41]. With two patients demonstrating deficient cochlear nerves on imaging, both of which were implanted and both of which developed closed-set word recognition, the authors concluded that patients with at least a deficient cochlear nerve may develop some speech recognition, but not to the level of those children with normal cochlear nerves [41]. In another study, Birman and colleagues identified 50 pediatric CI recipients, 27 of which had a developmental delay, who had either an absent or dysplastic/hypoplastic cochlear nerve, the latter of which was defined as when the cochlear nerve is smaller than the facial nerve in the midportion of the internal auditory canal [28]. Utilizing Categories of Auditory Performance (CAP), 89% of dysplastic cochlear nerves and 47% of aplastic nerves achieved CAP scores of 5–7, representing some verbal understanding [28].

Candidacy Guidelines

With respect to bilateral SNHL, CI was first approved in children in 1990 as young as 24 months of age. This approval was lowered to 9 months of age in 2020, when the FDA labeled the Nucleus Cochlear Implant System (Cochlear Americas, Sydney, Australia), and then 7 months of age in 2025, when the FDA approved the SYNCHRONY Cochlear Implant System (MED-EL, Innsbruck, Austria) of January 1, 2026, FDA-approved device labeling for pediatric CI is manufacturer-dependent. For Advanced Bionics and the HiResolution Ultra 3D implant, children should have a profound bilateral hearing loss greater than 90 dB HL. For Cochlear Americas and their Cochlear Nucleus Cochlear Implant System, children older than two years of age must demonstrate bilateral severe to profound SNHL, with profound bilateral loss for children 9-24 months of age. Cochlear Americas' labeling for aided word recognition is limited to ≤30% words correct. As for candidates choosing the MED-EL (Innsbruck, Austria) SYNCHRONY cochlear implant system, their device insert defines pediatric candidacy in children aged 7 months and older with bilateral, severe to profound SNHL in the low frequencies, while children 12 months to 5 years and 11 months of age can have bilateral, mild to profound SNHL in the low frequencies.

However, despite recent changes to pediatric CI candidacy, many believe the criteria are still too strict. Park et al. note that recently lowering the age requirement does not adhere to Joint Committee on Infant Hearing (JCIH) standards, additionally highlighting that the adult audiometric criteria for CI are not as restrictive as in children [44].

In assessing a group of children with better audiometric and speech recognition performance than delineated by relatively recent FDA criteria, Carlson et al. conducted a retrospective review of pediatric patients who underwent CI surgery between 2 and 17 years of age and had better than 70 dB HL pure-tone average (PTA) in the ipsilateral ear. This study also included children under 24 months in age with 90 dB HL PTA, and in both groups, age-appropriate sentence and/or word recognition scores greater than 30% in the best-aided condition [45]. Identifying 51 patients, at a mean follow-up of 17.1 months, speech recognition scores improved an average of 62.8 percentage points in the implanted ear and 39.9 percentage points in the bimodal condition, both of which were statistically significant improvements [45]. Furthermore, in patients who could not participate in speech perception testing before CI, language development questionnaires were used to demonstrate an average of a 26.5 percentage point improvement after CI, which also was statistically significant [45]. Based on these findings, the authors concluded that pediatric CI criteria should be reassessed [45].

In a different approach, Lovett and colleagues sought to determine the PTA associated with odds of 4:1 that patients with bilateral cochlear implants would have a better outcome than those patients with bilateral digital hearing aids. They found that children with an unaided pure-tone average of 80 dB HL or poorer in both ears should be considered bilateral CI candidates [46].

Regardless of the device selected, one exception to the age criteria above is in children with deafness secondary to meningitis with imaging demonstrating cochlear ossification. In such cases, it is recommended to implant these children as soon as it is medically safe and logistically possible.

Most recently, the FDA has approved both Med-El SYNCHRONY 2 and Cochlear Nucleus Implants for the treatment of unilateral hearing loss (UHL)/single-sided deafness (SSD) in patients 5 years and older. SSD is defined as profound SNHL in one ear with normal or mild SNHL in the contralateral ear. Additionally, candidates must demonstrate aided speech perception test scores ≤5% on developmentally appropriate monosyllabic word lists in the ear to be implanted alone.

Age of Implantation

CI in children younger than 12 months of age has been associated with earlier acquisition of receptive language skills and mastery of auditory skills earlier when compared to older recipients [47, 48]. Some data suggest speech production and vocabulary development are superior in children implanted before 12 months of age compared to older children [49, 50]. Nonetheless, surgical and anesthetic issues that are unique to infants add additional risks, which complicate surgery. Anatomical studies have demonstrated a more lateral location of the facial nerve, along with thinner calvaria. Additionally, there are increased risks of bradycardia and hypoxia in children with an underdeveloped sympathetic response undergoing general anesthesia [51–53]. O'Connell and colleagues performed a retrospective review of institutional and national databases to determine the safety of CI in infants younger than 12 months of age [54]. Comparing infants younger than 12 months of age to those aged between 12 and 18 months of age, they found that there was no difference in the incidence of 30-day postoperative surgical complications, and there was no significant difference in long-term surgical complications [54]. A separate study explored the development of auditory skills in children activated before 9 months of age, indicating that earlier access to sound with earlier CI activations achieved greater number of auditory skills than those with later CI activations [55].

Various studies have also looked at those children who had delayed CI. Dunn and colleagues determined the effect of age on CI in 83 children with prelingual hearing loss implanted prior to 4 years of age. They found that long-term language and reading performance did not differ between children who were implanted before 2 years of age and those implanted between 2 and 4 years of age. The authors attributed this finding to additional factors besides age of implantation, such as the amount of time children used the cochlear implant, as well as the richness of the linguistic input. Specifically, the quality of maternal language input was critical to the outcome measures in these patients [56]. They also found the effect of age at CI diminishes over time. While the best results are obtained with CI in younger children, analysis of speech perception demonstrates the effect of age did not differ between patients implanted at 7, 11, or 13 years of age [56]. In adolescents who were prelingually deaf and were implanted at 12 years of age, one review found them able to obtain open-set speech understanding [57]. In another study, pure-tone thresholds have been reported as low as 40 dB HL in prelingually deafened patients implanted during adolescence [58]. In summary, factors affecting CI outcomes in prelingually deafened patients implanted during adolescence include degree of hearing loss, hearing loss etiology, education, speech therapy, device, and therapeutic strategy [59].

Bilateral Implantation

It has been established that binaural hearing provides better sound localization, speech understanding in noise, reduced listening effort, and an improved quality of life [60–64]. Specifically in children, bilateral CI improves sound localization and speech understanding in quiet and noise compared to unilateral CI alone or with the use of a hearing aid [65–68]. As a result, many studies have compared simultaneous versus sequential bilateral CI in children. One early study showed poorer outcomes in children who underwent sequential CI, possibly due to increased time to receive the second implant [69]. However, other studies have shown no differences in outcomes [61, 65].

The risks and complications of bilateral CI are theoretically higher than unilateral CI. However, Ramsden and colleagues looked at simultaneous bilateral CI, compared with unilateral CI, and found no difference in complication rates, immediate postoperative-pain, or length of stay [70]. Nonetheless, in another study, the authors found that 26% of families declined simultaneous CI, most commonly citing a lack of acceptance of their child's deafness for pursuing sequential CI [71]. Other reasons for pursuing unilateral CI include waiting for future technologies, concerns about postoperative appearance, and a child's inability to give up a hearing aid [71]. However, studies have shown when combining the operative time between two sequential implants, the total operative time was significantly shorter in 50 patients with simultaneous bilateral CI compared with sequential CI [70].

As a result, several studies have sought to determine if simultaneous or sequential CI have better outcomes. Chadha et al. compared patients with bilateral early onset deafness who underwent sequential CI more than 2 years apart with patients who were implanted simultaneously [72]. They found that when background noise and target speech were spatially separated, also known as spatial unmasking, the patients with simultaneous implants scored significantly better than those implanted sequentially, and the former group of children were comparable to those with normal hearing [72].

In a larger sample size, with a longer listening period, Kocdor et al. retrospectively reviewed 290 pediatric patients under 18 years of age who received bilateral cochlear implants with at least 12 months of listening experience [73]. With an average interdevice interval of 3.4 years, they created a ratio of the best Phonetically Balanced Kindergarten (PBK) scores of the second side with the first side, plotting it against the interdevice interval [73]. Performing multivariate regression, they found that gender, age, laterality, intellectual disability, labyrinthine malformations, medical comorbidities, hearing loss onset, hearing loss etiology, ANSD, and hearing loss stability all led to little variation in the plot [73]. However, they found that there was a worse speech perception score with the second implant, as compared to the first, with prolonged interdevice intervals. This was noted to be more pronounced in those individuals with stable severe to profound SNHL [73]. They concluded that the second device should be implanted within 3–4 years of the first device [73].

Gordon and Papsin reviewed 58 pediatric patients with early-onset deafness and found that patients who were frequent cochlear implant users had better speech perception scores when the time difference between bilateral implants was less than 12 months as opposed to more than 2 years [61]. Nonetheless, patients still benefit from sequential CI up to 10 years after initial implantation [60, 63, 74, 75].

One study analyzed those patients with a significant delay between sequential CI surgery. Friedmann et al. identified 25 individuals who underwent sequential CI, first during childhood, with the second between 10 and 17 years of age and an average time interval of 8.2 years between implants [76]. Though there are concerns that delayed sequential CI would lead to central auditory system reorganization and poorer outcomes, they found that age at CI or the time interval between implants did not predict performance outcomes [76].

Accordingly, the European Bilateral Pediatric Cochlear Implant Forum released a consensus statement in 2010 that an "infant or child with unambiguous cochlear implant candidacy should receive bilateral cochlear implants simultaneously as soon as possible after definitive diagnosis of deafness" [77]. They mention that bilateral CI was not initially offered given concerns of chorda tympani nerve injuries, vestibular failure, and loss of an intact cochlea to benefit from future therapies. Because the first two reasons are not substantiated by the literature, simultaneous bilateral CI should be the ideal approach [77]. Similarly, Santa Maria and Oghalai reviewed the literature and concluded that the best practice was to implant bilateral candidates simultaneously, considering the surgeon experience, as well as the patient's family and social situation [64].

Cost-Effectiveness

Bilateral CI raises debate regarding cost-effectiveness. A second implant has been demonstrated to be of substantial added benefit in children [78, 79]. In addition, Emmett and colleagues found that CI and deaf education are also cost-effective in six lower-middle and upper-middle income sub-Saharan African countries [4, 80]. Furthermore, Summerfield and colleagues estimated the additional quality-adjusted life years (QALYs) gained by deaf children implanted bilaterally versus unilaterally and found that bilateral CI is probably cost-effective use in the United Kingdom [81].

Single-Sided Deafness

Unilateral hearing loss has long been known to have detrimental effects on the development of children [82]. Studies have shown that unilateral hearing impairment in children can negatively affect social interactions, language development, and academic performance [83–85]. Sangen and colleagues assessed 21 children with SSD between 5 and 15 years of age, matching them each with two normal hearing children [86]. They found that children with SSD had lower scores in assessing language syntax, morphology, and vocabulary compared to normal controls [86]. Using resting state functional connectivity MRI, Tibbetts et al. noted differences in brain network interconnections between normal hearing and SSD children [87]. Recognizing there are differences between normal hearing and SSD pediatric patients, several studies provided the framework for the FDA to approve CI in UHL/SSD children as young as 5 years of age in 2019.

Arndt and colleagues reviewed 50 children who presented with SSD, 32 of which qualified for CI surgery and 20 of which had been implanted at the time of publication [88]. They reported that the two most frequent causes of SSD in children were cochlear nerve hypoplasia or aplasia, followed by congenital CMV infections [88]. With few patients having completed a 12-month follow-up, and separating patients based on congenital, perilingual, and postlingual SSD, they found that patients obtained varying improvements in the ability to localize sound and speech comprehension in noise, with a trend toward improved outcomes in those children with an acquired, shorter duration hearing loss compared to congenitally deafened children [88].

In another study, Rahne and colleagues reported the CI outcomes of four children with SSD, all of whom had at least pure-tone thresholds above 90 dB HL in the implanted ear and no worse than 35 dB HL air-conduction thresholds in the contralateral ear [89]. Three children had borderline indications (hypoplastic cochlear nerve, unknown etiology and duration, and a "common vestibulo-cochlear nerve with questionable patency"), but each reported deficits in everyday life. Sound localization and speech perception in noise was significantly improved in all three patients [89].

Brown et al. recently conducted a prospective clinical trial in 20 children with at least moderate to profound SNHL and speech perception scores <30% in one ear, with normal hearing in the contralateral ear [90]. Using BKB-SIN to assess speech perception in noise, by 12 months, there were significant improvements in all three noise configurations (head shadow, summation, and squelch). Furthermore, localization improved by 26° at 9 months, and Speech, Spatial, and Qualities (SSQ) demonstrated significant improvement in all three domains, as well as listening effort. The authors concluded that children with UHL significantly benefited from CI. In a meta-analysis that pre-dated Brown et al., including 12 observational studies with 119 children, almost 80% of children demonstrated clinically meaningful improvement in speech perception in noise, while long duration of deafness, older than 4 years in congenital SSD, was the most commonly proposed reason for lack of improvement [91].

The handicap to children with SSD is well documented. Therefore the potential for benefit is substantial. But while

Brown et al. included patients as young as 3.5 years of age, FDA approval for CI in UHL/SSD patients includes patients only as young as 5 years of age [90]. Therefore, further research is needed to demonstrate benefit sufficient to justify insurance and government agencies to expanding coverage of surgery for this indication as a standard of care.

Auditory Neuropathy

Patients with auditory neuropathy spectrum disorder (ANSD) demonstrate speech reception testing scores that are disproportionately poor relative to what would be expected based on their pure-tone thresholds. Given the discrepancy between the PTA and speech perception testing, CI was initially limited in patients with ANSD. However, more recent studies have shown that CI improves hearing performance in ANSD patients [92, 93]. In particular, when the etiology of AN is due to an Otoferlin (*OTOF*) mutation, the CI outcomes are relatively superior to other causes of AN [94]. This is likely due to the fact that Otoferlin is a protein involved with synaptic transmission of the signal from the hair cell to the auditory nerve. A cochlear implant bypasses the causative defect and directly stimulates the auditory nerve. Pelosi and colleagues compared the auditory performances of hearing aids versus CIs in patients with ANSD [95]. Twenty-six patients with ANSD, as defined by having absent ABR waveforms with measurable otoacoustic emissions, underwent a hearing aid trial, and 16 of these patients eventually received a cochlear implant [95]. With a median duration of device use of 48 months, 4 of 8 hearing aid patients and 6 of 16 cochlear implant recipients achieved higher than 60% on open-set speech perception scores [95]. Carvalho et al. reviewed 10 pediatric patients with ANSD who received a cochlear implant. All patients demonstrated significant improvement in hearing levels after CI, and all of them reported increased satisfaction using a Likert scale 1 year following the surgery [96].

Surgical Procedure

Preoperative Consideration

Currently most high volume CI centers perform pediatric CI in the United States on an outpatient basis. Alyono and Oghalai reviewed the literature to determine whether pediatric otologic surgery, specifically CI, is safe as an outpatient procedure [97]. Admitting that most studies only included patients older than 2 years of age, they found that postoperative nausea and vomiting were the most common reason to admit patients overnight, with Liu and colleagues finding that it was the result of anesthetic recovery, not surgery [98]. Two studies have assessed parental opinions via questionnaires and found that 19% and 33% of parents would have preferred overnight observation [98, 99].

As for device selection, which is highly dependent on the CI center, most centers leave the device selection to the patient and/or their family. In hopes of assessing how cochlear implant devices were chosen by CI candidates, Migirov and colleagues mailed a questionnaire to 429 patients, with 112 pediatric patients responding. They found that children, and their surrogates, were more significantly influenced by the experience of other CI users, medical staff, and religious considerations, compared to adult cochlear implant patients [100].

Prophylactic Antibiotics

Though no double-blinded studies have assessed the role of perioperative antibiotics in otologic surgery, most cochlear implant surgeons administer at least one intravenous dose, typically an antistaphylococcal agent, 20 min before the incision is made. Not surprisingly, the literature is inconclusive as to the role of perioperative antibiotics in CI. Basavaraj et al. retrospectively reviewed 292 adult and pediatric patients who underwent CI with 3 different surgical incisions and 3 different antibiotic prophylaxis regimens [101]. They not only found a statistical difference between the infection rate and incision type, with large c-shaped and extended endaural incisions having more infections than postauricular incisions; they also found that 5- and 7-day antibiotic regimes, most commonly involving a second-generation cephalosporin or amoxicillin with clavulanic acid, had statistically higher infection rates than a single antibiotic dose [101]. More recently, Anne and colleagues performed a systematic review on the effects of perioperative antibiotics in CI and concluded there was insufficient evidence to make definitive conclusions regarding perioperative antibiotics [102].

Incision and Skin Flap

Over the years a number of different incisions have been used for CI. It is generally thought that the skin incision should not cross the receiver-stimulator. Early cochlear implant surgeons employed an inverted U-shaped incision thinking that the predominant blood supply to the postauricular skin originated inferiorly. Other surgeons utilized large C-shaped incisions; however, rare cases of flap necrosis occurred in patients with previous mastoidectomy incisions. With increased experience, the U-shaped incision was converted to an inverted "L" or inverted 'J" incision. And while some implant surgeons still employ the inverted "L" or "J" incisions, most high volume CI centers now implement a

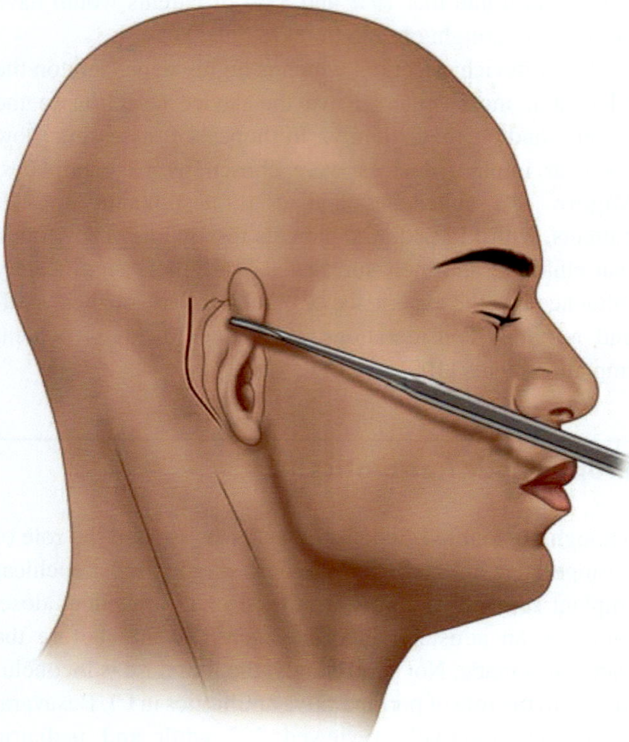

Fig. 19.3 Right cochlear implant incision. (Adapted from Glasscock and Shambaugh's Surgery of the Ear. 6th edition. Eds. Gulya, Minor, Poe. PMPH. 2010)

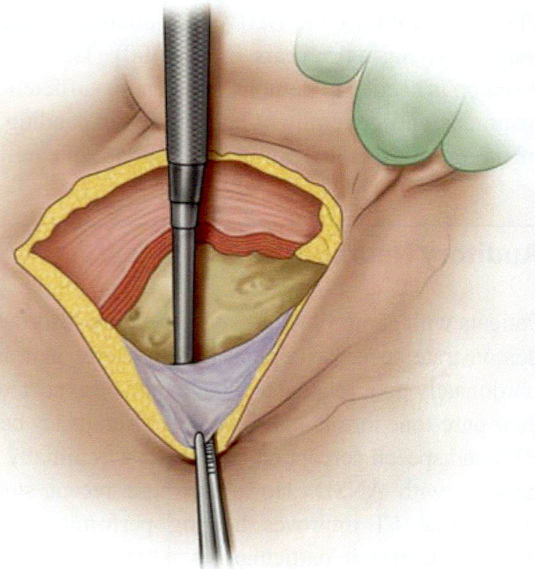

Fig. 19.4 Creation of a tight subperiosteal pocket with a Freer elevator. (Adapted from Glasscock and Shambaugh's Surgery of the Ear. 6th edition. Eds. Gulya, Minor, Poe. PMPH. 2010)

3–4 cm postauricular incision, approximately 0.5 cm posterior to the sulcus (Fig. 19.3).

After the skin incision, a single- or double-layer flap, the latter of which consists of an anteriorly based Palva flap, is elevated. For a single-layer flap, many surgeons carry the incision down through the periosteum to the bone, elevating the periosteum with the overlying soft tissue anteriorly. For a double-layer flap, the superficial layer should be elevated first, leaving at minimum the mastoid periosteum intact. Once the superficial layer is elevated anteriorly, the mastoid periosteum and any overlying tissue can be elevated as an anteriorly based Palva flap. At the conclusion of the case, the periosteum can be sutured into its original position to protect the electrode array in the mastoid cavity. The Palva flap should also be designed to cover at least the take off point of the cochlear implant electrodes.

Receiver-Stimulator Pocket Versus Well

With an ear-level processor, it is generally thought the receiver-stimulator should be placed 2.5 cm posterior to the posterior border of the bony external auditory canal in order to prevent interference with the processor. Historically, many surgeons would drill a depression in the skull, also known as a "well," to accommodate the protrusion on the deep surface of the receiver-stimulator, to stabilize the receiver-stimulator position, and to prevent displacement. However, in young children with thin calvarium, sometimes only 2–3 mm in thickness, drilling the well would result in the implant resting on exposed dura. In addition to the well, a channel to the mastoid cavity would be required for the electrode array, avoiding sharp edges.

Currently, many cochlear implant surgeons are omitting the well entirely. One modification is that some surgeons drill a slight depression, leading to a bony ridge. Another option is creating a tight subperiosteal pocket and avoiding direct fixation (Fig. 19.4). This shortens operative times and still firmly secures the receiver-stimulator. Sweeney et al. reviewed 193 adult and pediatric patients who received 228 cochlear implants with creation of a tight postauricular subperiosteal pocket for the receiver-stimulator without drilling or fixation [103]. Called the direct subperiosteal pocket technique (DSPT), an approximately 4 cm postauricular incision is made, carried directly to the mastoid periosteum, with use of a curved 7 mm square tip Lempert elevator to create a posterior-superior subperiosteal receiver-stimulator pocket, designed to be slightly larger than the receiver-stimulator [103]. Not only did the DSPT lead to a mean 18.9% reduction in operative time, receiver-stimulator migration was not observed, with a mean follow-up time of 18.1 months (range, 6.1–45.3 months) [103].

Recognizing the concerns of drilling a well in the calvarium in children 12 months or younger, Cohen and colleagues reported on six children younger than 12 months of age who had the receiver-stimulator placed within a subperiosteal pocket [104]. Emphasizing that the pocket was not much larger than the receiver-stimulator, no postoperative wound complications or observed device migration were noted [104].

However, some argue that device migration still occurs with a subperiosteal pocket. Orhan and colleagues identified 8 out of 280 pediatric cochlear implant patients who required revision surgery because of device migration after using a subperiosteal technique. Revision surgery was performed an average of 9 months following the primary surgery (5–54 months). Nonetheless, several groups have reported the presence of spontaneous bone formation around the bed of the receiver-stimulator when revision surgery, regardless of the indication, has been warranted [105–108]. Thus surgeons performing revision cochlear implant surgeries should be prepared to use a drill when needed.

As an adjunct to the subperiosteal technique, Papsin et al. describe the addition of a linear, silastic pedestal to the medial surface of the receiver-stimulator, which, per their report, significantly increases the force required to displace the implant [109]. Utilizing the same pedestal, Parkes and colleagues described drilling a 2.5-mm-wide linear groove into the calvarium for the silastic pedestal, allowing deliberate device placement [110].

The receiver-stimulator can also be secured with tie-down sutures secured to drilled holes or to small plating screws placed in the calvarium. Many surgeons will drill two holes angled into the mastoid cavity on either side of where the electrode takes off the receiver-stimulator, with a single suture placed across the device through both drill holes. Another option is to place 3 mm self-tapping, self-drilling screws on each side of the receiver stimulator and securing a suture to each screw. The suture is then tied over the top of the receiver stimulator. Other surgeons have employed a strip of material, such as a miniplate, Gortex, or AlloDerm, to secure the device. In patients with a thin calvarium, surgeons must be cautious in avoiding an intracranial and/or subdural injury, such as a CSF leak and or postoperative intracranial hemorrhage.

Mastoidectomy

In regard to the mastoidectomy, the mastoid cavity does not need to be large, and it is encouraged to avoid unnecessary saucerization to help retain the electrode array within the mastoid cavity (Fig. 19.5). Once the lateral semicircular canal and incus are identified, the facial recess is widely opened to expose the round window overhang and niche. In certain cases, the bone medial to the facial recess, as well as the bone in the inferior portion of the recess, will need to be removed to provide adequate exposure.

While it is generally recognized that the facial nerve can be located in a more lateral position in pediatric patients as compared to adults, there is not thought to be a difference in the size of the facial recess between children and adults. Bielamowicz et al. analyzed the facial recess width in children younger than 1 year of age, comparing it to those patients between 2 and 3 years old, as well as adults, and found that there does not appear to be a difference in the facial recess width [111]. However, in assessing more than just the facial recess, McRackan et al. compared 46 pediatric ears with 40 adult ears utilizing a model-based segmentation algorithm and high-resolution CT temporal bone studies and found there were statistically significant differences in the orientations between the facial recess, round window, external auditory canal, and the long axis of the basal turn of the cochlea [112].

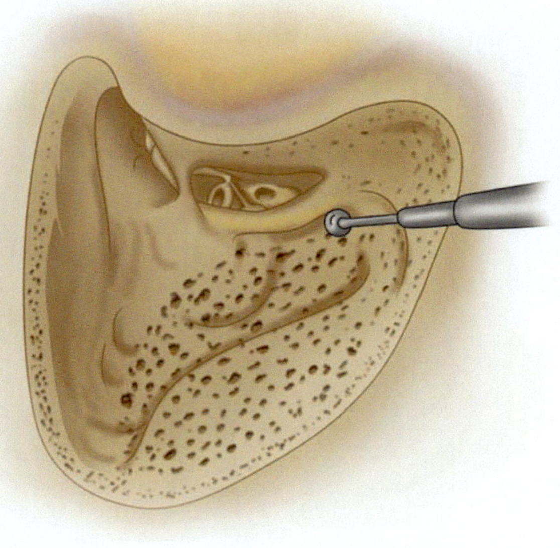

Fig. 19.5 A mastoidectomy with facial recess has been performed to access the cochlea. (Adapted from Glasscock and Shambaugh's Surgery of the Ear. 6th edition. Eds. Gulya, Minor, Poe. PMPH. 2010)

Almost all anomalous facial nerves are displaced anteriorly and medially. Just distal to the oval window, they turn directly into the hypotympanum and run just inferior to or directly over the round window area. Consequently, when the facial nerve is absent from its usual position, it does not form the typical posterior boundary of the facial recess. As the facial recess is opened, if it seems that the recess is unusually large, a facial nerve anomaly should be suspected.

Approaches: Round Window, Extended Round Window, or Cochleostomy

After the facial recess has been widely opened, the round window niche is identified. Frequently the bony overhang needs to be removed with a 1 mm diamond burr to visualize

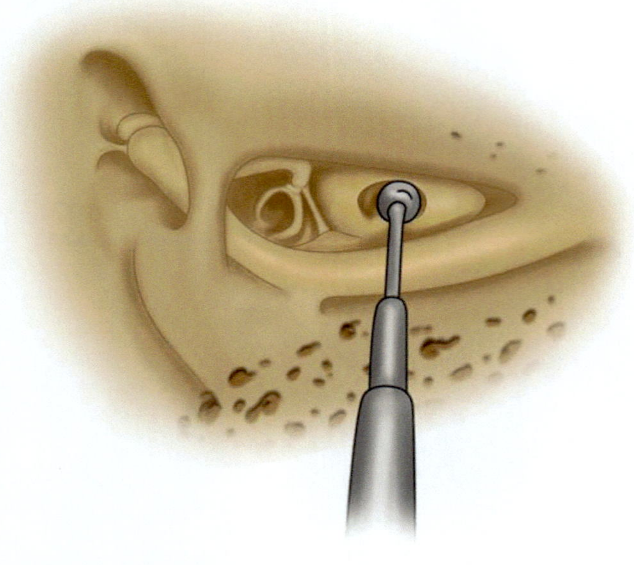

Fig. 19.6 The cochleostomy is performed through the facial recess. A drill is employed to perform an extended round window or cochleostomy, the latter, anterior and inferior to the actual round window. (Adapted from Glasscock and Shambaugh's Surgery of the Ear. 6th edition. Eds. Gulya, Minor, Poe. PMPH. 2010)

the round window membrane. Once the round membrane is visualized, there are three different approaches to accessing the scala tympani. Many surgeons favor the round window approach, which requires use of a sharp, fine instrument (Fig. 19.6). Other surgeons utilize a cochleostomy, drilling anterior and inferior to the round window membrane to create a complete 0.8–1.2 mm separate opening to the scala tympani. If the patient's facial recess precludes adequate visualization of the round window, an extended round window approach can also be utilized, drilling the anterior-inferior portion of the bony round window to enlarge the opening into the scala tympani. Some surgeons will also employ the extended round window approach if the round window has an unfavorable angle.

Insertion of the Electrode Array

Monopolar cautery has the risk of damaging the electronic components of the cochlear implant and is avoided when the implant is in the operative field. While many surgeons insert the electrode only after the receiver-stimulator has been placed and/or secured, some surgeons believe they have more flexibility, leading to a more atraumatic insertion, if the receiver-stimulator has not been placed and secured.

Some surgeons use lubricants to help facilitate placement, i.e. hyaluronic acid, also theorizing that the lubricants encourage bone dust and other debris to either "float out" of the scala tympani or prevent the ingress of such debris, hopefully minimizing postoperative osteoneogenesis. Some older electrodes also require special tools and techniques, with appropriate orientation of the electrode to optimize its electrode contacts. Generally the tip of the electrode should be directed inferiorly along the lateral wall of the basal turn, with some implant surgeons employing their right hand to insert the electrode in left ears and their left hand to insert the electrode in right ears, to optimize the insertion angle.

The electrode should be inserted slowly to minimize trauma. If resistance is encountered, slow gentle pressure often allows for continued insertion of the electrode array. Incomplete insertions are uncommon, except in cases with cochleovestibular anomalies. Also, in hearing preservation cases, when resistance is encountered, it is advised to settle for incomplete insertion to avoid trauma and loss of residual hearing. Once placed, surgeons use fascia and/or muscle over the round window or in the facial recess to secure the positioning of the electrode and provide another barrier between the scala tympani and the middle ear.

Intraoperative fluoroscopy has been used as an adjunct in those pediatric patients undergoing CI as it allows real-time assessment. With most fluoroscopy units producing less than 10 rad per minute, radiation exposure to the patient should be less than 200 rads, with the average exposure time during CI being less than 3 minutes in total [21]. Fishman and colleagues used live intraoperative fluoroscopy in nine patients, some of whom had severe malformations or ossification, and achieved insertion in all cases with no electrode damage [113]. In addition, Coelho and colleagues compared surgical outcomes in patients with common cavity deformities, with and without the assistance of fluoroscopy, and found that half of the patients who had electrode placement without image guidance had suboptimal placement of the arrays, higher incidence of complications, more extra cochlear electrodes, and fewer active electrodes at follow-up [114].

Closure

Regardless of the surgical approach, the incision needs to be closed in layers. Some surgeons will place dissolvable packing lateral to the electrode array, covering the mastoid cavity, to reduce the chances a suture catches the electrode array. Ideally the Palva flap should cover not only the mastoid cavity, but also where the electrode exits the receiver-stimulator. Buried, interrupted sutures are used to re-approximate the dermis, while tissue adhesive, absorbable and non-absorbable sutures, and staples have been used to close the skin. Many surgeons will then apply a pressure dressing that can be removed after 24 hours.

Alternative Approaches

Other surgical approaches include the middle fossa and suprameatal approaches, as well as a subtotal petrosectomy. The suprameatal approach, designed to avoid a mastoidectomy, introduces the electrode into the middle ear by a suprameatal route via a retroauricular tympanotomy. More specifically, a tunnel is drilled in a posterosuperior to anteroinferior orientation, beginning just superior to the spine of Henle [115]. Kronenberg et al. reported the outcomes in 126 pediatric patients who underwent the procedure, as young as 11 months of age, and with an average follow-up of 22 months [115]. Reporting outcomes for 188 children and adults, there appeared to be no significant differences in speech perception results compared with a traditional cohort, but four patients had tympanic membrane perforations [115]. In a similar study, Postelmans et al. reported on the outcomes of 104 patients undergoing the same surgical technique, albeit with a smaller post-auricular incision, as well as opening the attic through the suprameatal tunnel as opposed to transmeatally. They reported a major complication rate of 3.7%, including two electrode extrusions due to wound infection, one device failure, and one electrode that was placed incorrectly [116].

Jackler has highlighted the many difficulties with the suprameatal procedure, including the blind dissection, electrode insertion not along the axis of the basal turn, placement of electrodes in an external auditory canal groove, and utilizing skills and techniques not normally practiced by otologists, thus cautioning against the implementation of this technique [115]. However, in cases where a facial recess or retrofacial approach to the round window is not possible, following a mastoidectomy, a tympanomeatal flap can be elevated to facilitate placement of an electrode through the aditus ad antrum, avoiding the need for a suprameatal tunnel.

In cases with a radical cavity, history of chronic middle ear infections, or cerebrospinal fluid (CSF) leakage in patients with cochleovestibular anomalies, a subtotal petrosectomy with blind sac closure of the external auditory canal, packing of the Eustachian tube, and obliterating the mastoid cavity with abdominal fat may be performed [117]. In overclosing the canal, all mucosa from the middle ear and mastoid must be removed, and the cavity should be isolated from the nasopharynx by plugging the Eustachian tube. While some surgeons stage the CI, overclosing the canal prevents electrode extrusions and extractions in an open cavity [118]. Other cochlear implant surgeons have bypassed the middle ear altogether. Coletti and colleagues have described approaching the cochlea from the floor of the middle fossa [119].

Ossified Cochlea

Roughly 5% of pediatric patients with meningitis present with profound SNHL [120]. Because meningitis can result in rapid cochlear ossification (Fig. 19.7), earlier CI is associ-

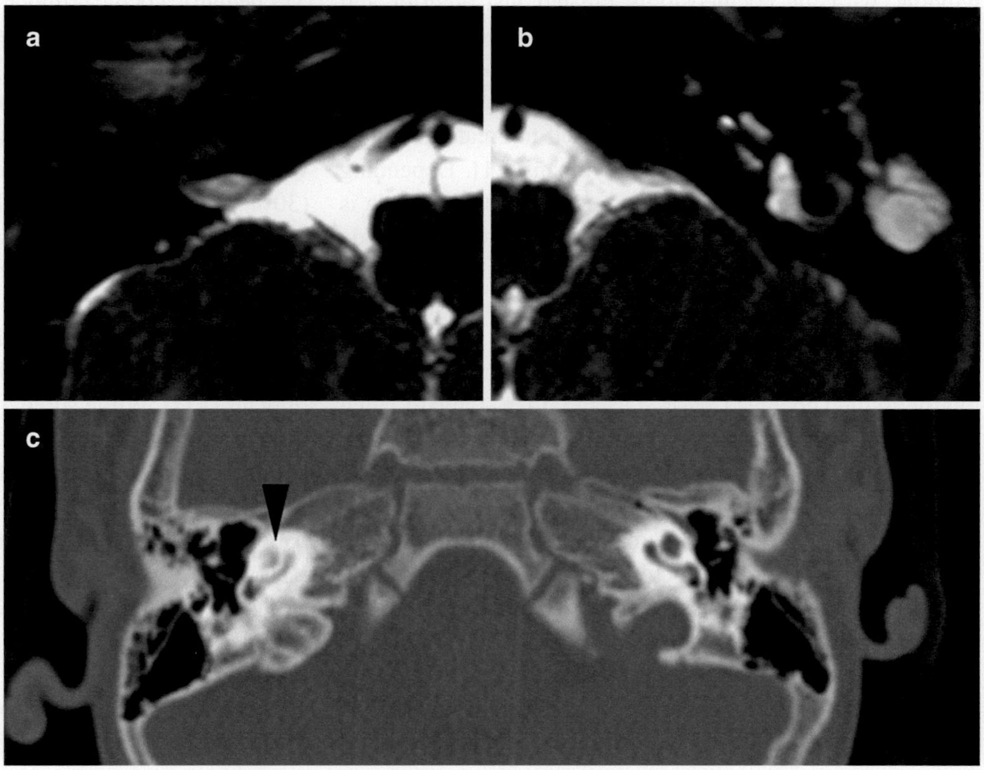

Fig. 19.7 Ossified right cochlea. Axial T2 MR imaging (**a**, **b**) demonstrates a hypointense right basal turn of the right cochlea with the left cochlea having normal intensity. Corresponding CT temporal bone imaging (**c**) shows partial ossification of the right cochlea (black arrowhead)

ated with improved speech intelligibility and sound localization [121]. Ossification may result in incomplete insertion; however, studies have shown that patients have developed open-set speech recognition with at least 10 electrodes [122]. Liu and colleagues reviewed 39 patients who received cochlear implants for hearing loss secondary to bacterial meningitis, 19 (48.7%) of whom had intraoperative evidence of labyrinthitis ossificans [123]. Comparing the speech perception performances between groups, there was a trend ($p = 0.17$) toward better postimplantation speech perception scores in patients without labyrinthitis ossificans, though each group demonstrated significant speech perception improvements following CI [123].

However, different surgical approaches are required depending on which segments of the cochlea are ossified. When the round window is obliterated, a drill-out should be initiated about 1.5 mm inferior to the pyramidal process or stapes, allowing exposure of the scala tympani [21, 124]. When the basal turn is ossified, drilling out the round window niche and extending into the basal cochlea may be needed for 8–10 mm [21]. But one must recognize the carotid artery just anterior to the basal turn, and thus a pick or laser may be needed to tunnel out the remaining fibrous tissue obliterating the basal turn.

When the upper portions of the cochlea are ossified, while a partial insertion can be accomplished through a drilled basal turn, a middle turn cochleostomy can also be completed to accommodate a double-array electrode [21]. The incus and stapes are removed to improve access to the oval window, with the cochleostomy created just anterior and adjacent to the stapes annular ligament. In such cases, the cochleariform process is used as the superior limit of dissection [21]. If no lumen is identified in the upper cochlea, a rasp or small diamond burr can be used to create an apical tunnel directed toward the tensor tympani [21]. Depending on the manufacturer and surgical anatomy, the electrode is placed, preferably anterograde with cochlear and retrograde with MED-EL [21]. If both the scala tympani and the scala vestibuli are ossified beyond the basal turn, a perimodiolar trough can be drilled out [125].

Balkany et al. described a surgical technique for the totally ossified cochlea [124]. Starting with a standard facial recess approach, using a 1.5-mm diamond drill, an approximately 8-mm-long tunnel is drilled through an anterior-inferior cochleostomy. Then, after elevating a tympanomeatal flap, removing the malleus, flattening the promontory, and removing the cochleariform process and tensor tympani, a 1-mm drill is used to unroof the previously drilled tunnel approximately 4 mm from the round window. Abnormal bone is then followed around the ascending bend of the basilar turn, which is followed posteriorly toward the anterior edge of the oval window and then inferiorly, completing a course approximating the spiral ganglion and modiolus. The electrode can then be placed through the tunnel and into the trough, fixed with bone wedges at various points [124]. The authors reported on four pediatric patients implanted with this technique, with two English-speaking children developing open-set PBK word scores of 24% and 16%, with the other two children, who spoke Portuguese, developing limited open-set word recognition [124].

Postoperative Complications

While complications can be characterized as early and late based on their time course relative to the procedure, most literature dichotomizes complications between minor and major. In most cases, the former are managed with conservative measures, which may include minimal surgery, and the latter most often require surgical revision or hospital admission. Early complications include infection, wound dehiscence, device failure, CSF leak, balance disturbance, facial palsy, and meningitis. Late complications include pain, displacement, device failure, otitis media, and meningitis.

While the chorda tympani nerve is injured in 20% of cases, and device failure occurs in about 2% of all cases, it is understood that inner ear malformations are associated with increased risk of complications [126–130]. Nonetheless, the most common immediate complications tend to be related to dizziness and or nausea and vomiting. Sivam et al. reviewed 579 pediatric cochlear implants, 1–17 years of age, with nausea/vomiting (50%) and dizziness (32%) being the most common complications [131]. While patients between 1 and 3 years of age did not demonstrate greater complications compared to older patients, those who received bilateral CI were significantly more likely to develop a complication (30%) compared to those who were unilaterally implanted (19%) [131]. Surprisingly, patients 13–15 years of age had the highest rate of complications when comparing age groups (36%) [131].

In another single institutional experience, Farinetti and colleagues reviewed 235 children who received a cochlear implant [132]. While some question defining otitis media as a complication, they found that 10.2% experienced minor complications, with acute otitis media being the most frequent minor complication (58.3%, 14/24), while 4.7% of patients had major complications, the most frequent being mastoiditis (36.4%, 4/11) [132]. They also reviewed 168 adults who received a cochlear implant, observing that the global complication rate was significantly higher in the adult population (26.8% versus 14.9%; $P = 0.002$), though no significant difference was found in the major complication rate between adults and children [132].

With the increased incidence of otitis media in the pediatric population, several studies have looked at the role of tympanostomy tubes in patients with a cochlear implant. Javia and colleagues studied 557 pediatric cochlear implant patients, with 24.2% having a ventilation tube at some point with their cochlear implant, and found there was no difference in complication rates between those with and without a ventilation tube [133]. Similarly, Googe and Carron reviewed a single institutional experience of 248 cochlear implants, with major and minor complication rates of 5.2% and 11.3%, respectively [134]. They reported that a history of tympanostomy tubes did not affect the complication rate, with the most common major complication rate being device failure (2.4%) [134].

However, patients with otitis media can go on to develop mastoiditis. Raveh et al. reviewed 490 pediatric CI surgeries, with 3.5% developing acute mastoiditis. [135] All patients were treated with a myringotomy and intravenous broad-spectrum antibiotics, though surgical drainage was required in 8/13 patients for subperiosteal abscesses or lack of symptomatic improvement, seven of which required a tympanostomy tube [135]. However, there was no need for a wider surgical approach, with no intracranial complications or middle ear pathology with a mean follow-up of 3.8 years [135].

For management of postoperative otitis media and/or meningitis, the American Academy of Pediatrics recommends intravenous antibiotics if acute otitis media or meningitis develops within 60 days following CI. Specifically, intravenous vancomycin and Gram-negative bacilli coverage, such as meropenem, is recommended for meningitis, while ceftriaxone or cefotaxime is recommended for acute otitis media [136]. Beyond 60 days, oral antibiotics are an acceptable treatment option for uncomplicated acute otitis media, while a standard bacterial meningitis regimen is recommended for meningitis (e.g., ceftriaxone plus vancomycin) [136]. Currently it is thought that if meningitis develops between 30 days and 2 years postoperatively, it is most likely the result of acute otitis media [9].

Additional complications include CSF leaks, which can occur as the result of dural tears, either the result of drilling a bony well in young children, placement of drill holes for tie-down sutures, or CSF gushers in the presence of a modiolar defect and cochleovestibular anomalies. For the latter, these can generally be managed by head of bed elevation, passive suctioning, and, once slowed, occluding the opening. However, occasionally oversewing the external auditory canal and filling the middle ear and mastoid with fat is needed.

Rarely one may encounter an exposed electrode array. Walgama and colleagues described their experience with seven patients who had exposed electrodes, five of which were children [137]. While two children required revision surgery, both of which demonstrated destructive otologic comorbidities, the three remaining children were managed conservatively with a combination of oral and topical antibiotics and careful observation.

Occasionally the magnet may become displaced secondary to trauma or MR imaging (Fig. 19.8). Young and colleagues evaluated their experience with 11 pediatric patients who underwent MRI studies with the cochlear implant magnet in place [138]. With a total of 13 MRI studies, with all but one patient receiving a compression head wrap, as well as sedation or general anesthesia, complications occurred in 30.8% of studies: the magnet polarity was reversed in three cases, while the magnet strength was reduced and the magnet displaced in one case each. Some of these complications occurred even when the imaging directed at body regions inferior to the head [138]. Only one of these complications required surgery, but they concluded that complications do arise. However, obtaining the imaging study with the magnet in situ avoids multiple surgeries to remove and replace the implant, as well as the associated costs [138]. In cases when the magnet becomes displaced, depending on its position, it

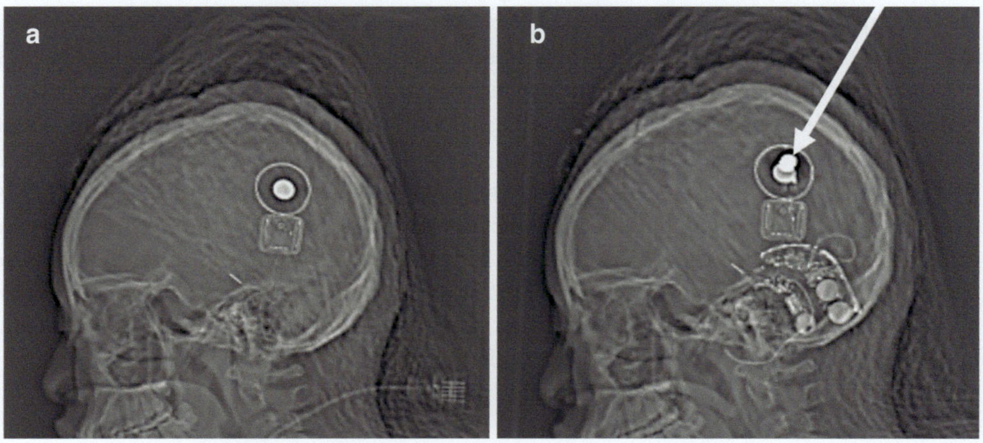

Fig. 19.8 Displaced cochlear implant magnet. Scout head x-ray on the left (**a**) demonstrates a cochlear implant magnet in place. Follow-up head x-ray on the right (**b**) demonstrates a dislodged cochlear implant magnet (arrow)

can rarely be repositioned at the bedside manually; however, usually this situation requires surgery with a C-shaped incision posterior-superior to the receiver-stimulator, identification of a fibrous capsule, and replacement of the magnet. If future MRI studies are needed, a non-magnet plug can be placed in lieu of the magnet to facilitate placement of a magnet at a later date.

Results

Within this chapter, audiometric outcomes for various pathologies have been described in each appropriate section. Nonetheless, this section will briefly describe pediatric cochlear implant recipients compared to their normal hearing peers. Waltzmann and colleagues evaluated 36 prelingually deafened children, implanted earlier than 5 years of age, all of whom developed significant open-set speech recognition [139]. Robbins et al. assessed 23 pediatric patients who had received a cochlear implant and found that they developed language at the same rate as normal-hearing children [140]. Similarly, Geers and colleagues assessed 181 children implanted before 5 years of age and noted that more than half of the patients produced and understood English at the same level as their normal-hearing peers [141]. In a more recent study, Fitzpatrick and colleagues compared pediatric patients with hearing aids and cochlear implants [142]. They found that the groups did not differ in open-set speech recognition abilities or speech production abilities. However, children with moderately severe to severe hearing loss using hearing aids obtained better scores in receptive vocabulary, language, phonological memory, and reading comprehension than their cochlear implant peers. While briefly mentioned earlier when discussing delayed implantation, the younger the patient at CI, the better the performance. Tobey and colleagues found that later ages of implantation are associated with higher probabilities of continued language delays, specifically in grammar and pragmatic domains [143].

The mode of communication also has a significant impact on audiometric outcomes. Hodges and colleagues showed that cochlear implant patients using only oral communication had better outcomes than those children using total communication [144]. In support of this finding, Geers et al. found that children in oral communication environments received more benefit from their cochlear implants [141]. Nonetheless, in the Robbins et al. cohort mentioned previously, they found no difference in outcomes between those patients who utilized oral or total communication [140].

Beyond hearing and language acquisition, other studies have shown long-term differences between pediatric cochlear implant patients and their normal-hearing peers. The Hannover cochlear implant program recently sent a questionnaire to all pediatric patients who had a cochlear implant placed between 1986 and 2000, with an average follow-up time of 17.8 years [145]. While they found that age of implantation was significantly associated with auditory performance, education, vocational, and occupational levels in these patients were significantly poorer compared to the normal German population [145].

In summary, cochlear implants allow children to acquire speech and language skills that enable them to participate in society. While the gap between their chronological and language age progressively increases in unimplanted children, it remains constant after surgery in children who undergo CI.

Hearing Preservation

The adult literature contains more data and outcomes on patients with serviceable low-frequency hearing receiving cochlear implants. And while there is a desire to expand the pediatric candidacy criteria, there are relatively few pediatric patients with the classic "ski slope" hearing loss pattern ideal for hearing preservation cochlear implant surgery. Thus, there remains a relative paucity of pediatric patients with low-frequency hearing that have been implanted. Brown et al. reviewed 31 pediatric patients 19 years and younger with a preoperative unaided audiogram that demonstrated a 90 dB HL or better threshold at 250, 500, or 1000 Hz [146]. The surgical protocol included a perioperative dose of 0.25 mg/kg intravenous dexamethasone, a cochleostomy approach, injection of sodium hyaluronate into the scala tympani, and a standard length electrode array. Complete hearing preservation, defined as a change in low-frequency PTA of less than 10 dB, was achieved in 45.2% of patients at a mean audiometric follow-up of 10.7 months (range, 1–30 months) [146]. In this cohort, 9/18 (50%) of patients maintained functional hearing defined as having a 75 dB HL or better threshold at 250, 500, or 1000 Hz, following implantation [146].

Skarzynski and colleagues describe the case of a 16-year-old boy who had preoperative pure-tone audiometry thresholds ranging from 10–30 dB HL up to 1500 Hz, with a profound hearing loss from 2000 to 8000 Hz, who was subsequently implanted with a 24 mm electrode through a round window approach to a depth of 18 mm [147]. This patient was given intravenous dexamethasone, 0.1 mg/kg/day, for 3–4 days, as well as dexamethasone solution placed into the middle ear prior to opening the round window [147]. Utilizing the hearing classification system proposed by

Skarzynski et al., they found that the patient had complete hearing preservation (82.5%) 5 years postoperatively, which progressed to partial hearing preservation (74.6%) at 7 years. Based on this, they have suggested that CI criteria for adolescents should be expanded [147].

Bruce and colleagues reviewed their experience in implanting 14 adolescent patients who were candidates for hearing preservation surgery between 10 and 18 years of age [148]. Criteria included recordable thresholds at 125, 250, and 500 Hz. These patients received implants ranging from 20 to 31.5 mm in length, 12/14 had arrays placed via a cochleostomy, and in all cases, insertion was stopped at first resistance [148]. With a mean follow-up of 34 months, half of the patients lost less than 10 dB HL at 125, 250, and 500 Hz at less than 6 weeks postimplantation. In addition, 7 of 10 patients with at least 2 years follow-up had less than a 10 dB decrease in thresholds. Based on this, the authors of this study concluded that residual hearing can be consistently preserved and maintained in adolescents [148].

Assessing the role of the Nucleus Hybrid implant, Gantz and colleagues implanted 10 children between 12 and 16 months of age with a Nucleus Freedom implant in one ear and the Nucleus Hybrid S12 in the contralateral side [149]. Since the S12 is a 10-mm electrode array, the authors hypothesized that by using a shorter electrode, the apical end of the cochlea would not be damaged following insertion and be available for possible future therapies. At the same time, the electrode would stimulate the basal end of the cochlea to allow for adequate speech perception [149]. Preliminary results showed these patients had similar results to age-matched children implanted with standard electrode arrays. They concluded that shorter-length cochlear implants in one ear may provide a viable "option for bilateral CI in children." [149]

Lastly, Carlson and colleagues reviewed their experience in 35 pediatric patients with 43 ears who underwent CI with a preoperative low-frequency PTA (250–500 Hz average) less than or equal to 75 dB HL in the implanted ear [150]. In summary, while 65% maintained functional low-frequency hearing, they conclude that favorable rates of hearing preservation provide further evidence that pediatric cochlear implant candidacy should be expanded [150].

Conclusion

Pediatric CI has been proven to be beneficial by significantly improving speech perception and language acquisition in children with severe to profound SNHL. It is understood that the younger patients are implanted, the shorter the auditory deprivation period, and thus, the better the outcomes. While the FDA approves CI as early as 9 months of age, several studies have demonstrated the safety of the procedure in children younger than 9 months. Therefore, it may warrant investigation in pushing the age qualification of CI to children of younger age. In addition, several studies have demonstrated the benefits of bilateral CI. While no consensus exists as to the best time interval between surgeries, it is generally encouraged to sequentially implant patients within 2 years. Nonetheless, as some studies have demonstrated benefits to children with longer interdevice intervals, a sequential implant should be considered in any patient that may potentially benefit from a second implant. And lastly, if medically and logistically possible, a simultaneous bilateral implant should be considered the default ideal approach for children.

Cochlear implant candidacy criteria are being challenged as implanting patients with serviceable low-frequency hearing and SSD is actively being investigated. The approach and surgical techniques however remain relatively the same, with only slight variations in incision planning, scala tympani approaches, and receiver-stimulator fixation. Currently, it is popular among surgeons to enter the scala tympani with a round window approach and to utilize a tight subperiosteal pocket to secure the receiver-stimulator. Complications remain minimal, demonstrating that it is a safe procedure that can generally be performed on an outpatient basis.

References

1. Sorkin DL, Buchman CA. Cochlear implant access in six developed countries. Otol Neurotol. 2016;37(2):e161–4.
2. Diener ML, et al. Outcomes from a hearing-targeted cytomegalovirus screening program. Pediatrics. 2017;139(2)
3. Biernath KR, et al. Bacterial meningitis among children with cochlear implants beyond 24 months after implantation. Pediatrics. 2006;117(2):284–9.
4. Parner ET, et al. Hearing loss diagnosis followed by meningitis in Danish children, 1995-2004. Otolaryngol Head Neck Surg. 2007;136(3):428–33.
5. Cohen NL, Hirsch BE. Current status of bacterial meningitis after cochlear implantation. Otol Neurotol. 2010;31(8):1325–8.
6. Reefhuis J, et al. Risk of bacterial meningitis in children with cochlear implants. N Engl J Med. 2003;349(5):435–45.
7. Pakdaman MN, et al. Cochlear implantation in children with anomalous cochleovestibular anatomy: a systematic review. Otolaryngol Head Neck Surg. 2012;146(2):180–90.
8. Centers for Disease Control and Prevention (CDC). Available from: www.cdc.gov/vaccines/vpd/mening/hcp/dis-cochlear-gen.html.
9. Kahue CN, et al. Vaccination recommendations and risk of meningitis following cochlear implantation. Curr Opin Otolaryngol Head Neck Surg. 2014;22(5):359–66.
10. Medicines and Healthcare products Regulatory Agency. Available from: https://www.gov.uk/drug-device-alerts/medical-

device-alert-all-cochlear-implants-update-on-immunisation-recommendations.
11. Riga M, et al. Etiological diagnosis of bilateral, sensorineural hearing impairment in a pediatric Greek population. Int J Pediatr Otorhinolaryngol. 2005;69(4):449–55.
12. Siem G, et al. Causes of hearing impairment in the Norwegian paediatric cochlear implant program. Int J Audiol. 2010;49(8):596–605.
13. Kenneson A, Van Naarden Braun K, Boyle C. GJB2 (connexin 26) variants and nonsyndromic sensorineural hearing loss: a HuGE review. Genet Med. 2002;4(4):258–74.
14. Dahl HH, et al. Prevalence and nature of connexin 26 mutations in children with non-syndromic deafness. Med J Aust. 2001;175(4):191–4.
15. Snoeckx RL, et al. GJB2 (connexin 26) mutations are not a major cause of hearing loss in the Indonesian population. Am J Med Genet A. 2005;135(2):126–9.
16. Rayess HM, et al. Predictive factors and outcomes of cochlear implantation in patients with connexin 26 mutation: a comparative study. Am J Otolaryngol. 2015;36(1):7–12.
17. Abdurehim Y, Lehmann A, Zeitouni AG. Predictive value of GJB2 mutation status for hearing outcomes of pediatric Cochlear implantation. Otolaryngol Head Neck Surg. 2017;157(1):16–24.
18. Lanson BG, et al. Cochlear implantation in children with CHARGE syndrome: therapeutic decisions and outcomes. Laryngoscope. 2007;117(7):1260–6.
19. Loundon N, et al. Usher syndrome and cochlear implantation. Otol Neurotol. 2003;24(2):216–21.
20. Yanmei F, et al. Cochlear implantation in patients with Jervell and Lange-Nielsen syndrome, and a review of literature. Int J Pediatr Otorhinolaryngol. 2008;72(11):1723–9.
21. Heman-Ackah SE, et al. Pediatric cochlear implantation: candidacy evaluation, medical and surgical considerations, and expanding criteria. Otolaryngol Clin N Am. 2012;45(1):41–67.
22. Meinzen-Derr J, et al. Children with cochlear implants and developmental disabilities: a language skills study with developmentally matched hearing peers. Res Dev Disabil. 2011;32(2):757–67.
23. Corrales CE, Oghalai JS. Cochlear implant considerations in children with additional disabilities. Curr Otorhinolaryngol Rep. 2013;1(2):61–8.
24. Oghalai JS, et al. Cognitive outcomes and familial stress after cochlear implantation in deaf children with and without developmental delays. Otol Neurotol. 2012;33(6):947–56.
25. Wiley S, et al. Longitudinal functional performance among children with cochlear implants and disabilities: a prospective study using the Pediatric Evaluation of Disability Inventory. Int J Pediatr Otorhinolaryngol. 2012;76(5):693–7.
26. Boons T, et al. Predictors of spoken language development following pediatric cochlear implantation. Ear Hear. 2012;33(5):617–39.
27. Pierson SK, et al. Cognition in children with sensorineural hearing loss: etiologic considerations. Laryngoscope. 2007;117(9):1661–5.
28. Birman CS, Elliott EJ, Gibson WP. Pediatric cochlear implants: additional disabilities prevalence, risk factors, and effect on language outcomes. Otol Neurotol. 2012;33(8):1347–52.
29. Palmieri M, et al. Evaluating benefits of cochlear implantation in deaf children with additional disabilities. Ear Hear. 2012;33(6):721–30.
30. Gerard JM, et al. Evolution of communication abilities after cochlear implantation in prelingually deaf children. Int J Pediatr Otorhinolaryngol. 2010;74(6):642–8.
31. Young JY, Ryan ME, Young NM. Preoperative imaging of sensorineural hearing loss in pediatric candidates for cochlear implantation. Radiographics. 2014;34(5):E133–49.
32. Papsin BC. Cochlear implantation in children with anomalous cochleovestibular anatomy. Laryngoscope. 2005;115(1 Pt 2 Suppl 106):1–26.
33. Sennaroglu L, Sarac S, Ergin T. Surgical results of cochlear implantation in malformed cochlea. Otol Neurotol. 2006;27(5):615–23.
34. Tomura N, et al. Normal variations of the temporal bone on high-resolution CT: their incidence and clinical significance. Clin Radiol. 1995;50(3):144–8.
35. Chadha NK, et al. Bilateral cochlear implantation in children with anomalous cochleovestibular anatomy. Arch Otolaryngol Head Neck Surg. 2009;135(9):903–9.
36. Kim LS, et al. Cochlear implantation in children with inner ear malformations. Ann Otol Rhinol Laryngol. 2006;115(3):205–14.
37. Sugiura S, Paparella MM. The pathology of labyrinthine ossification. Laryngoscope. 1967;77(11):1974–89.
38. Gleeson TG, et al. High resolution computed tomography and magnetic resonance imaging in the pre-operative assessment of cochlear implant patients. J Laryngol Otol. 2003;117(9):692–5.
39. McClay JE, et al. Evaluation of pediatric sensorineural hearing loss with magnetic resonance imaging. Arch Otolaryngol Head Neck Surg. 2008;134(9):945–52.
40. Zanetti D, et al. Favorable outcome of cochlear implant in VIIIth nerve deficiency. Otol Neurotol. 2006;27(6):815–23.
41. Kutz JW Jr, et al. Cochlear implantation in children with cochlear nerve absence or deficiency. Otol Neurotol. 2011;32(6):956–61.
42. Govaerts PJ, et al. Cochlear implants in aplasia and hypoplasia of the cochleovestibular nerve. Otol Neurotol. 2003;24(6):887–91.
43. Ozdogmus O, et al. Connections between the facial, vestibular and cochlear nerve bundles within the internal auditory canal. J Anat. 2004;205(1):65–75.
44. Park LR, Gagnon EB, Brown KD. The limitations of FDA criteria: inconsistencies with clinical practice, findings, and adult criteria as a barrier to pediatric implantation. Semin Hear. 2021;42(4):373–80.
45. Carlson ML, et al. Evidence for the expansion of pediatric cochlear implant candidacy. Otol Neurotol. 2015;36(1):43–50.
46. Lovett RE, Vickers DA, Summerfield AQ. Bilateral cochlear implantation for hearing-impaired children: criterion of candidacy derived from an observational study. Ear Hear. 2015;36(1):14–23.
47. Colletti L. Long-term follow-up of infants (4-11 months) fitted with cochlear implants. Acta Otolaryngol. 2009;129(4):361–6.
48. Colletti L, et al. Infants versus older children fitted with cochlear implants: performance over 10 years. Int J Pediatr Otorhinolaryngol. 2011;75(4):504–9.
49. Leigh J, et al. Communication development in children who receive a cochlear implant by 12 months of age. Otol Neurotol. 2013;34(3):443–50.
50. Houston DM, Miyamoto RT. Effects of early auditory experience on word learning and speech perception in deaf children with cochlear implants: implications for sensitive periods of language development. Otol Neurotol. 2010;31(8):1248–53.
51. Keenan RL, et al. Bradycardia during anesthesia in infants. An epidemiologic study. Anesthesiology. 1994;80(5):976–82.
52. Holman MA, et al. Cochlear implantation in children 12 months of age and younger. Otol Neurotol. 2013;34(2):251–8.
53. Roland JT Jr, et al. Cochlear implantation in the very young child: long-term safety and efficacy. Laryngoscope. 2009;119(11):2205–10.
54. O'Connell BP, et al. Safety of cochlear implantation before 12 months of age: Medical University of South Carolina and Pediatric American College of Surgeons-National Surgical Quality improvement program outcomes. Laryngoscope. 2016;126(3):707–12.

55. Culbertson SR, et al. Younger age at cochlear implant activation results in improved auditory skill development for children with congenital deafness. J Speech Lang Hear Res. 2022;65(9):3539–47.
56. Dunn CC, et al. Longitudinal speech perception and language performance in pediatric cochlear implant users: the effect of age at implantation. Ear Hear. 2014;35(2):148–60.
57. Waltzman SB, Roland JT Jr, Cohen NL. Delayed implantation in congenitally deaf children and adults. Otol Neurotol. 2002;23(3):333–40.
58. Kos MI, et al. What can be expected from a late cochlear implantation? Int J Pediatr Otorhinolaryngol. 2009;73(2):189–93.
59. Arisi E, et al. Cochlear implantation in adolescents with prelinguistic deafness. Otolaryngol Head Neck Surg. 2010;142(6):804–8.
60. Litovsky RY, et al. Bilateral cochlear implants in children: localization acuity measured with minimum audible angle. Ear Hear. 2006;27(1):43–59.
61. Gordon KA, Papsin BC. Benefits of short interimplant delays in children receiving bilateral cochlear implants. Otol Neurotol. 2009;30(3):319–31.
62. Mok M, et al. Spatial unmasking and binaural advantage for children with normal hearing, a cochlear implant and a hearing aid, and bilateral implants. Audiol Neurootol. 2007;12(5):295–306.
63. Scherf FW, et al. Functional outcome of sequential bilateral cochlear implantation in young children: 36 months postoperative results. Int J Pediatr Otorhinolaryngol. 2009;73(5):723–30.
64. Santa Maria PL, Oghalai JS. When is the best timing for the second implant in pediatric bilateral cochlear implantation? Laryngoscope. 2014;124(7):1511–2.
65. Zeitler DM, et al. Speech perception benefits of sequential bilateral cochlear implantation in children and adults: a retrospective analysis. Otol Neurotol. 2008;29(3):314–25.
66. Dunn CC, et al. Comparison of speech recognition and localization performance in bilateral and unilateral cochlear implant users matched on duration of deafness and age at implantation. Ear Hear. 2008;29(3):352–9.
67. Dunn CC, et al. Bilateral and unilateral cochlear implant users compared on speech perception in noise. Ear Hear. 2010;31(2):296–8.
68. Eapen RJ, et al. Hearing-in-noise benefits after bilateral simultaneous cochlear implantation continue to improve 4 years after implantation. Otol Neurotol. 2009;30(2):153–9.
69. Illg A, et al. Speech comprehension in children and adolescents after sequential bilateral cochlear implantation with long interimplant interval. Otol Neurotol. 2013;34(4):682–9.
70. Ramsden JD, et al. Bilateral simultaneous cochlear implantation in children: our first 50 cases. Laryngoscope. 2009;119(12):2444–8.
71. Ramsden JD, et al. Parental and program's decision making in paediatric simultaneous bilateral cochlear implantation: who says no and why? Int J Pediatr Otorhinolaryngol. 2009;73(10):1325–8.
72. Chadha NK, et al. Speech detection in noise and spatial unmasking in children with simultaneous versus sequential bilateral cochlear implants. Otol Neurotol. 2011;32(7):1057–64.
73. Kocdor P, et al. The effect of interdevice interval on speech perception performance among bilateral, pediatric cochlear implant recipients. Laryngoscope. 2016;126(10):2389–94.
74. Sparreboom M, Snik AF, Mylanus EA. Sequential bilateral cochlear implantation in children: development of the primary auditory abilities of bilateral stimulation. Audiol Neurootol. 2011;16(4):203–13.
75. Wolfe J, et al. 1-year postactivation results for sequentially implanted bilateral cochlear implant users. Otol Neurotol. 2007;28(5):589–96.
76. Friedmann DR, et al. Sequential bilateral cochlear implantation in the adolescent population. Laryngoscope. 2015;125(8):1952–8.
77. Ramsden JD, et al. European bilateral pediatric cochlear implant forum consensus statement. Otol Neurotol. 2012;33(4):561–5.
78. Schulze-Gattermann H, et al. Cost-benefit analysis of pediatric cochlear implantation: German experience. Otol Neurotol. 2002;23(5):674–81.
79. Barton GR, et al. Hearing-impaired children in the United Kingdom, IV: cost-effectiveness of pediatric cochlear implantation. Ear Hear. 2006;27(5):575–88.
80. Emmett SD, et al. GDP matters: cost effectiveness of cochlear implantation and deaf education in Sub-Saharan Africa. Otol Neurotol. 2015;36(8):1357–65.
81. Summerfield AQ, et al. Estimates of the cost-effectiveness of pediatric bilateral cochlear implantation. Ear Hear. 2010;31(5):611–24.
82. Bess FH, Tharpe AM. Unilateral hearing impairment in children. Pediatrics. 1984;74(2):206–16.
83. Friedmann DR, et al. Single-sided deafness cochlear implantation: candidacy, evaluation, and outcomes in children and adults. Otol Neurotol. 2016;37(2):e154–60.
84. Lieu JE, Tye-Murray N, Fu Q. Longitudinal study of children with unilateral hearing loss. Laryngoscope. 2012;122(9):2088–95.
85. Bess FH, Tharpe AM. Performance and management of children with unilateral sensorineural hearing loss. Scand Audiol Suppl. 1988;30:75–9.
86. Sangen A, et al. Single-sided deafness affects language and auditory development - a case-control study. Clin Otolaryngol. 2017;42:979.
87. Tibbetts K, et al. Interregional brain interactions in children with unilateral hearing loss. Otolaryngol Head Neck Surg. 2011;144(4):602–11.
88. Arndt S, et al. Cochlear implantation in children with single-sided deafness: does aetiology and duration of deafness matter? Audiol Neurootol. 2015;20(Suppl 1):21–30.
89. Rahne T, Plontke SK. Functional result after cochlear implantation in children and adults with single-sided deafness. Otol Neurotol. 2016;37(9):e332–40.
90. Brown KD, Dillon MT, Park LR. Benefits of cochlear implantation in childhood unilateral hearing loss (CUHL trial). Laryngoscope. 2022;132(Suppl 6):S1–S18.
91. Benchetrit L, et al. Cochlear implantation in children with single-sided deafness: a systematic review and meta-analysis. JAMA Otolaryngol Head Neck Surg. 2021;147(1):58–69.
92. Peterson A, et al. Outcomes of cochlear implantation in children with auditory neuropathy. J Am Acad Audiol. 2003;14(4):188–201.
93. Breneman AI, Gifford RH, Dejong MD. Cochlear implantation in children with auditory neuropathy spectrum disorder: long-term outcomes. J Am Acad Audiol. 2012;23(1):5–17.
94. Zheng D, Liu X. Cochlear implantation outcomes in patients with OTOF mutations. Front Neurosci. 2020;14:447.
95. Pelosi S, et al. Cochlear implantation versus hearing amplification in patients with auditory neuropathy spectrum disorder. Otolaryngol Head Neck Surg. 2013;148(5):815–21.
96. de Carvalho GM, et al. Performance of cochlear implants in pediatric patients with auditory neuropathy spectrum disorder. J Int Adv Otol. 2016;12(1):8–15.
97. Alyono JC, Oghalai JS. Should pediatric tympanomastoidectomy and cochlear implantation routinely be performed as outpatient surgery? Laryngoscope. 2015;125(5):1041–2.
98. Liu JH, Roland PS, Waller MA. Outpatient cochlear implantation in the pediatric population. Otolaryngol Head Neck Surg. 2000;122(1):19–22.
99. Stephens J, Cruise A, Shaida A. Cochlear implants as a paediatric day surgery service. Cochlear Implants Int. 2010;11(Suppl 1):221–4.

100. Migirov L, et al. Factors affecting choice of device by cochlear implant candidates. Otol Neurotol. 2009;30(6):743–6.
101. Basavaraj S, et al. Short-term versus long-term antibiotic prophylaxis in cochlear implant surgery. Otol Neurotol. 2004;25(5):720–2.
102. Anne S, Ishman SL, Schwartz S. A systematic review of perioperative versus prophylactic antibiotics for cochlear implantation. Ann Otol Rhinol Laryngol. 2016;125(11):893–9.
103. Sweeney AD, et al. 228 cases of cochlear implant receiver-stimulator placement in a tight subperiosteal pocket without fixation. Otolaryngol Head Neck Surg. 2015;152(4):712–7.
104. Cohen MS, et al. Surgical outcomes with subperiosteal pocket technique for cochlear implantation in very young children. Int J Pediatr Otorhinolaryngol. 2014;78(9):1545–7.
105. Orhan KS, et al. Spontaneous bone bed formation in cochlear implantation using the subperiosteal pocket technique. Otol Neurotol. 2014;35(10):1752–4.
106. Balkany TJ, et al. The temporalis pocket technique for cochlear implantation: an anatomic and clinical study. Otol Neurotol. 2009;30(7):903–7.
107. Guldiken Y, et al. Subperiosteal temporal pocket versus standard technique in cochlear implantation: a comparative clinical study. Otol Neurotol. 2011;32(6):987–91.
108. Jethanamest D, et al. Cochlear implant fixation using a subperiosteal tight pocket without either suture or bone-recess technique. Laryngoscope. 2014;124(7):1674–7.
109. Papsin BC, et al. Characterization of retentive capacity of the subpericranial pocket in cochlear implants with and without a pedestal. Laryngoscope. 2016;126(5):1175–9.
110. Parkes WJ, et al. Preliminary experience using a cochlear implant with a novel linear pedestal design. Int J Pediatr Otorhinolaryngol. 2017;93:42–6.
111. Bielamowicz SA, et al. Surgical dimensions of the facial recess in adults and children. Arch Otolaryngol Head Neck Surg. 1988;114(5):534–7.
112. McRackan TR, et al. Comparison of cochlear implant relevant anatomy in children versus adults. Otol Neurotol. 2012;33(3):328–34.
113. Fishman AJ, et al. Fluoroscopically assisted cochlear implantation. Otol Neurotol. 2003;24(6):882–6.
114. Coelho DH, Waltzman SB, Roland JT Jr. Implanting common cavity malformations using intraoperative fluoroscopy. Otol Neurotol. 2008;29(7):914–9.
115. Kronenberg J, et al. The suprameatal approach: an alternative surgical approach to cochlear implantation. Otol Neurotol. 2004;25(1):41–4; discussion 44–5.
116. Postelmans JT, et al. The suprameatal approach: a safe alternative surgical technique for cochlear implantation. Otol Neurotol. 2010;31(2):196–203.
117. Free RH, et al. The role of subtotal petrosectomy in cochlear implant surgery--a report of 32 cases and review on indications. Otol Neurotol. 2013;34(6):1033–40.
118. Hunter JB, O'Connell BP, Wanna GB. Systematic review and meta-analysis of surgical complications following cochlear implantation in canal wall down mastoid cavities. Otolaryngol Head Neck Surg. 2016;115(4):555–63.
119. Colletti V, et al. New approach for cochlear implantation: cochleostomy through the middle fossa. Otolaryngol Head Neck Surg. 2000;123(4):467–74.
120. Baraff LJ, Lee SI, Schriger DL. Outcomes of bacterial meningitis in children: a meta-analysis. Pediatr Infect Dis J. 1993;12(5):389–94.
121. Tsuji RK, et al. Neural response thresholds in the Nucleus Contour cochlear implant before and after stylet removal. Acta Otolaryngol. 2009;129(11):1330–6.
122. Cohen NL, Waltzman SB. Partial insertion of the nucleus multichannel cochlear implant: technique and results. Am J Otol. 1993;14(4):357–61.
123. Liu CC, et al. The impact of postmeningitic labyrinthitis ossificans on speech performance after pediatric cochlear implantation. Otol Neurotol. 2015;36(10):1633–7.
124. Balkany T, et al. Surgical technique for implantation of the totally ossified cochlea. Laryngoscope. 1998;108(7):988–92.
125. Gantz BJ, McCabe BF, Tyler RS. Use of multichannel cochlear implants in obstructed and obliterated cochleas. Otolaryngol Head Neck Surg. 1988;98(1):72–81.
126. Bhatia K, et al. Surgical complications and their management in a series of 300 consecutive pediatric cochlear implantations. Otol Neurotol. 2004;25(5):730–9.
127. Loundon N, et al. Medical and surgical complications in pediatric cochlear implantation. Arch Otolaryngol Head Neck Surg. 2010;136(1):12–5.
128. Francis HW, et al. Surgical factors in pediatric cochlear implantation and their early effects on electrode activation and functional outcomes. Otol Neurotol. 2008;29(4):502–8.
129. McJunkin J, Jeyakumar A. Complications in pediatric cochlear implants. Am J Otolaryngol. 2010;31(2):110–3.
130. Hou JH, et al. Postoperative complications in patients with cochlear implants and impacts of nursing intervention. Acta Otolaryngol. 2010;130(6):687–95.
131. Sivam SK, et al. Consideration for routine outpatient pediatric cochlear implantation: a retrospective chart review of immediate post-operative complications. Int J Pediatr Otorhinolaryngol. 2017;94:95–9.
132. Farinetti A, et al. Cochlear implant complications in 403 patients: comparative study of adults and children and review of the literature. Eur Ann Otorhinolaryngol Head Neck Dis. 2014;131(3):177–82.
133. Javia L, et al. Infectious complications and ventilation tubes in pediatric cochlear implant recipients. Laryngoscope. 2016;126(7):1671–6.
134. Googe BJ, Carron JD. Analyzing complications of minimally invasive pediatric cochlear implantation: a review of 248 implantations. Am J Otolaryngol. 2016;37(1):44–50.
135. Raveh E, et al. Acute mastoiditis in children with a cochlear implant. Int J Pediatr Otorhinolaryngol. 2016;81:80–3.
136. Rubin LG, et al. Cochlear implants in children: surgical site infections and prevention and treatment of acute otitis media and meningitis. Pediatrics. 2010;126(2):381–91.
137. Walgama ES, et al. Management of electrode exposure after cochlear implantation. Otol Neurotol. 2012;33(7):1197–200.
138. Young NM, et al. Magnetic resonance imaging of cochlear implant recipients. Otol Neurotol. 2016;37(6):665–71.
139. Waltzman SB, et al. Open-set speech perception in congenitally deaf children using cochlear implants. Am J Otol. 1997;18(3):342–9.
140. Robbins AM, Svirsky M, Kirk KI. Children with implants can speak, but can they communicate? Otolaryngol Head Neck Surg. 1997;117(3 Pt 1):155–60.
141. Geers AE, et al. Effects of communication mode on skills of long-term cochlear implant users. Ann Otol Rhinol Laryngol Suppl. 2000;185:89–92.
142. Fitzpatrick EM, et al. Comparison of outcomes in children with hearing aids and cochlear implants. Cochlear Implants Int. 2012;13(1):5–15.
143. Tobey EA, et al. Influence of implantation age on school-age language performance in pediatric cochlear implant users. Int J Audiol. 2013;52(4):219–29.

144. Hodges AV, et al. Speech perception results in children with cochlear implants: contributing factors. Otolaryngol Head Neck Surg. 1999;121(1):31–4.
145. Illg A, Haack M, Lesinski-Schiedat A, et al. Long-term outcomes, education, and occupational level in cochlear implant recipients who were implanted in childhood. Ear Hear. 2017;38(5):577–87.
146. Brown RF, et al. Residual hearing preservation after pediatric cochlear implantation. Otol Neurotol. 2010;31(8):1221–6.
147. Skarzynski H, et al. Expanding pediatric cochlear implant candidacy: a case study of electro-natural stimulation (ENS) in partial deafness treatment. Int J Pediatr Otorhinolaryngol. 2015;79(11):1896–900.
148. Bruce IA, et al. Hearing preservation cochlear implantation in adolescents. Otol Neurotol. 2014;35(9):1552–9.
149. Gantz BJ, et al. Bilateral cochlear implants in infants: a new approach--Nucleus Hybrid S12 project. Otol Neurotol. 2010;31(8):1300–9.
150. Carlson ML, Patel NS, Tombers NM, et al. Hearing preservation in pediatric cochlear implantation. Otol Neurotol. 2017;38(6):e128–e133.

20 Cochlear Implants in Adults

Nathan R. Lindquist and David S. Haynes

Introduction

Cochlear implants (CIs) are the most successful neural prostheses developed to date, a designation based on both the sheer number of implant recipients and the degree of functional restoration of speech understanding and hearing for patients with sensorineural hearing loss (SNHL). [1, 2] The first cochlear prosthesis was implanted by William F. House and John Doyle in 1961, with innumerable contributors and improvements over the subsequent decades [3–5]. The first multichannel CI was approved by the US Food and Drug Administration (FDA) in 1985. Despite early concerns regarding the safety and efficacy of stimulation of the residual neural elements of the cochlea, CIs continue to demonstrate other positive effects beyond their primary aim of treating advanced hearing loss. Increasingly, cochlear implantation is associated with improved quality of life, psychosocial health, and cognition [6–8].

As of 2015, an estimated 170,000 adults and children with 240,000 total devices had undergone implantation in the United States alone. In that year, approximately 1.34 million people in the United States met the traditional audiometric criteria of severe-to-profound hearing loss in the better-hearing ear, putting device utilization at approximately 12.7% of the population meeting that criterion [9].

Recently the criteria for CI have expanded to include patients with better residual hearing [10–13], single-sided deafness (SSD) [14–16], asymmetric hearing loss (AHL) [17, 18], and increasingly younger pediatric patients [19–22]. Estimates accounting for these additional potential adult and pediatric candidates put CI device utilization at approximately 2.1% overall. While device utilization rates for children are approximately 50% in the United States and 90% in parts of Europe, adult rates remain much lower [23]. Despite improved characterization of patient benefits as well as expanded criteria for cochlear implantation, CI provision remains a major challenge. Moving forward, we must work to improve patient awareness, the knowledge of healthcare professionals, and streamline referral pathways and uncover financial and cost-effectiveness data to improve the penetrance of these important devices.

Indications

In the United States, the FDA regulates three manufacturers with approved CI devices: Advanced Bionics Corporation (Valencia, CA), Cochlear Corporation (Sydney, Australia), and MED-EL Corporation (Innsbruck, Austria). While CI device technology, programming strategies, and patient outcomes continued to improve into the twenty-first century, a relative stagnation of FDA indications followed the approval of the Cochlear Nucleus system for adults scoring ≤50% on open set sentence recognition in the ear to be implanted and ≤ 60% in the best-aided listening condition in the year 2000. Carlson and coauthors highlighted this trend in a 2017 survey of the American Neurotology Society wherein 78% of surgeons performed implantations for off-label or non-traditional indications within the preceding 2 years [24]. Fortunately, the past decade has seen a significant expansion of FDA criteria to include millions of new potential implant candidates (Table 20.1).

FDA approval of the Cochlear Nucleus Hybrid CI device (2014) and the MED-EL EAS device (2016) made it possible for patients with serviceable low-frequency thresholds to

N. R. Lindquist
Bobby R. Alford Department of Otolaryngology—Head and Neck Surgery, Baylor College of Medicine, Houston, TX, USA
e-mail: nathan.lindquist@bcm.edu

D. S. Haynes (✉)
Department of Otolaryngology—Head and Neck Surgery, Vanderbilt University Medical Center, Nashville, TN, USA
e-mail: david.haynes@vumc.org

A. D. Sweeney et al. (eds.), *Haynes-Glasscock-Shambaugh Surgery of the Ear*, https://doi.org/10.1007/978-3-032-18264-7_20

Table 20.1 FDA indications for cochlear implants in adults in the United States

Manufacturer and device	Pure tone audiometric indications	Speech recognition indications
Advanced Bionics HiRes™ Ultra/ Ultra 3D	Severe-to-profound bilateral SNHL (PTA ≥70 dB HL)	≤50% on open-set sentence recognition test (originally HINT sentences)
Cochlear Nucleus Profile™, Profile™ Plus, and Nexa™ Series	Moderate-to-profound SNHL below 500 Hz (≥40 dB HL) and profound SNHL above 1000 Hz (≥90 dB HL) in both ears	≤50% sentence recognition in the ear to be implanted and ≤ 60% in the opposite ear or binaurally (best-aided condition)
Cochlear Nucleus Profile™, Profile™ Plus, and Nexa™ Series for UHL/SSD	Severe-to-profound SNHL (PTA >80 dB HL) in ear to be implanted with normal or near-normal hearing (PTA ≤30 dB HL) in contralateral ear	≤5% CNC word score for ear to be implanted
Cochlear Nucleus® Hybrid™ L24	Normal-to-moderate hearing loss in the low frequencies (≤60 dB HL up to and including 500 Hz) with severe-to-profound mid- to high-frequency SNHL (≥75 dB HL for average of 2000 Hz, 3000 Hz, 4000 Hz)	CNC word recognition score between 10% and 60% in the ear to be implanted, with contralateral ear CNC score <80% and better than ear to be implanted
MED-EL SYNCHRONY™ and SYNCHRONY 2™	Severe-to-profound bilateral SNHL (≥70 dB HL for average of 500 Hz, 1000 Hz, 2000 Hz)	≤40% on open-set sentence recognition test (originally HINT sentences)
MED-EL SYNCHRONY™ and SYNCHRONY 2™ - EAS	Normal-to-moderate hearing loss in the low frequencies (<65 dB HL up to and including 500 Hz) with severe-to-profound mid- to high-frequency SNHL (≥70 dB HL for 2000 Hz and above)	CNC word recognition score ≤ 60% in the best-aided condition, in the ear to be implanted and the contralateral ear
MED-EL SYNCHRONY™ and SYNCHRONY 2™ for SSD	Profound SNHL (PTA ≥90 dB HL) in ear to be implanted with normal-to-mild SNHL (PTA ≤30 dB HL) in contralateral ear	≤5% CNC word score for ear to be implanted
MED-EL SYNCHRONY™ and SYNCHRONY 2™for AHL	Profound SNHL (PTA ≥90 dB HL) in ear to be implanted with mild-to-moderately severe SNHL (PTA 31–55 dB HL) in contralateral ear, with a difference > 15 dB HL in PTA between ears	≤5% CNC word score for ear to be implanted

AHL indicates asymmetric hearing loss; CNC indicates consonant-nucleus-consonant; FDA indicates US Food and Drug Administration; HINT indicates hearing in noise test; PTA indicates pure tone average (defined for most of these indications as the average of 500 Hz, 1000 Hz, 2000 Hz, and 4000 Hz frequencies); SNHL indicates sensorineural hearing loss, SSD indicates single-sided deafness; UHL indicates unilateral hearing loss. Data current as of March 2026.

receive a CI. Importantly, the criteria for these devices was based on open-set word scores in the ear to be implanted and not open-set sentence scores in the best-aided (often bilateral) condition [25]. Further approvals for SSD and AHL with the MED-EL device (2019) and the Cochlear device (2022) stressed the importance of the individual ear in consideration of candidacy.

Preoperative Evaluation

Medical Evaluation

Strictly speaking, the only two absolute contraindications to cochlear implantation are the complete absence of the cochlea and/or the absence of the cochlear nerve. Relative contraindications to implantation may include fibrosis or ossification of the cochlea, inner ear malformations including cochlear nerve hypoplasia/deficiency, active infection, prelingually deafened adults, other medical conditions stemming from inability to tolerate anesthesia, or neuropsychiatric comorbidities that would preclude the successful usage of the device. A complete history should focus on uncovering other potential contraindications or conditions that would make the surgery or auditory rehabilitation process either more difficult or less likely to succeed. The assessment of factors such as etiology, progression, and duration of hearing loss as well as psychosocial well-being is vital. The clinician is wise to investigate a history of meningitis, post-traumatic SNHL, prior infections, surgeries, family history, and associated otologic/neurotologic symptoms and conditions.

A thorough physical examination of the head and neck serves to identify any craniofacial abnormalities or prior surgical sites. Examination includes otomicroscopy with pneumatic otoscopy to assess for any pathology of the external auditory canal, tympanic membrane, and middle ear. Straightforward tuning fork assessment and documentation of the cranial nerves, including facial nerve function, is performed. Clinical and laboratory vestibular testing may be utilized at the discretion of the clinician for associated otologic symptoms, elderly patients more likely to have preoperative vestibular hypofunction, or bilateral implant recipients.

Patients on antiplatelet and/or anticoagulation therapy may be maintained on these regimens throughout the perioperative period, especially for those at risk of major complications (deep venous thrombosis, myocardial infarction, pulmonary embolism, or stroke) with the cessation of these medications [26]. These patients should be cautioned as to possible sequelae such as bruising or hematoma, but the overall risk of complications is low if these therapies are continued in the perioperative period.

Audiologic Evaluation

While complete ear-specific audiometric testing remains at the core of CI candidacy evaluation, considerable variability still exists among audiologists regarding their choice of testing materials, testing environment, and definition of the "best-aided" listening condition [27]. In a 2018 survey of adult CI audiologists, most respondents utilized at least some components from the Minimum Speech Test Battery (MSTB) to identify adult CI candidates [28]. The most recent iteration of the MSTB (Version 3, 2024) refines the definition of "best-aided" condition to refer to an individual ear with properly fit hearing aid and streamlines the test to start with testing with CNC monosyllabic words [29] prior to testing with AzBio sentences +10 signal-to-noise ratio (SNR) [30]. The battery aims to streamline clinical testing, encourages usage of patient reported outcome measures (PROMS), recommends when to consider CI evaluation, and provides test batteries for patients with asymmetric hearing loss or single-sided deafness (https://www.cochlearimplanttraining.com/minimum-speech-test-battery).

In terms of CI candidacy, the most important aspect of a patient's audiometric profile is speech understanding with properly fitted hearing aids (HAs), as patients undergoing CI placement should obtain limited benefit from these devices. A challenging clinical scenario exists when patients are borderline CI candidates based on audiometric criteria but still struggle with properly fitted HAs. In these situations, a multidisciplinary, patient-centered discussion regarding options, outcomes, and expectations of both rehabilitation strategies should occur. For patients with less-than-ideally fitted HAs, a retrial after proper fitting may better elucidate the benefit of these assistive devices versus CI for that individual patient.

In addition to audiometric criteria, other considerations influencing CI candidacy may be multifaceted and nuanced. Clinicians must consider criteria such as CI manufacturer-specific FDA labeling, especially considering the recent expansion in CI indications. However, such FDA indications are meant as guidelines and should not supersede clinical judgment [31]. Off-label implantation is often performed in the setting of well-informed clinical judgment, solid medical evidence and rationale, ample patient counseling, and proper documentation [24]. The surgeon and audiologist must be mindful of insurance criteria and coverage, as this may differ starkly among third-party payors. Other factors such as cognitive function, patient expectations, and quality of life measures are important; however, routine assessment of these concerns is not yet ubiquitous [27].

Radiographic Evaluation

In general, high-resolution computed tomography (CT) and magnetic resonance imaging (MRI) of the temporal bones/internal auditory canals (IACs) are the two main radiographic studies utilized in the work-up for prospective CI candidates. Imaging should aim to complete the work-up for the patient's hearing loss, enable improved surgical planning, and inform any necessary anticipatory guidance for expectations and outcomes. Unlike children, most adult candidates present with postlingual hearing loss, making etiologies such as inner ear malformations or cochlear nerve aplasia less probable. Pediatric patients with sensorineural hearing loss, discussed in Chap. 19, may be reasonable to undergo MRI IAC protocol without contrast CT temporal bone if indicated as part of the CI evaluation. Centers may choose to utilize one or both studies for adult CI candidates depending on clinician preference, insurance coverage, and institution protocol.

While all three FDA-approved manufacturers currently market MRI-conditional devices, CI magnet-related artifact is a major concern for head and brain imaging [32]. MRI studies are advisable prior to CI placement if necessary for the work-up of hearing loss, neurologic processes, or evaluation of intracranial pathology. Careful consideration of the device/magnet placement, specific manufacturer guidelines, and imaging techniques to reduce artifact are prudent depending on the need for surveillance of intracranial pathology after cochlear implantation [33].

CT and MRI provide different information with regard to the anatomy of the temporal bone (Table 20.2). High-resolution CT provides superior evaluation of bone including the otic capsule structures such as the cochlea and its aperture, semicircular canals, and vestibular aqueduct. CT also enables assessment of the location/dehiscence of the fallopian canal as well as the overall aeration/pneumatization of the middle ear and mastoid. MRI, given its improved characterization of soft tissue and neurologic structures, is useful for assessing the T2 fluid signal of the inner ear in cases of meningitis, labyrinthitis, or cochlear fibrosis [34]. MRI also allows for superior assessment of the vestibulocochlear nerve and identification of potential retrocochlear pathologies. As a result, the CT and MRI modalities should be viewed as complementary in the work-up for adults undergoing cochlear implantation candidacy evaluation.

Table 20.2 CT and MRI evaluation of the temporal bone

	CT	MRI
Morphology of cochlea and semicircular canals	+++	++
Patency of cochlear duct	+	+++
Status of cochlear nerve	–	+++
Anatomy of facial nerve and fallopian canal	+++	+
Defect of the modiolus	++	++
Defect of the cribriform area	+++	++
Enlarged vestibular aqueduct	+++	+++
Enlarged cochlear aqueduct	+++	+
Presence of round or oval window	+++	–
CNS abnormalities	+	+++

Deciding Which Ear to Implant

For patients undergoing candidacy evaluation for their first CI, several conditions enable decision-making regarding the ear to undergo surgery. These criteria broadly consist of audiologic criteria and anatomic factors, although other considerations may prove valuable as well. The potential impact of patient-related factors such as handedness, subjective hearing, and personal preference should not be ignored.

From an audiologic perspective the degree of hearing loss, objective speech recognition scores, ability to utilize a hearing aid, and the duration of deafness for each ear should all be considered. The etiology of hearing loss and any history of vestibular dysfunction should be evaluated as well.

From an anatomic perspective, investigation into the status of the cochlea and the mastoid are paramount and may affect which side undergoes implantation. While congenital malformations of the cochlea are more common in the pediatric population, acquired etiologies for cochlear duct fibrosis or labyrinthitis ossificans in the adult population may include a history of temporal bone/otic capsule trauma, meningitis, otosclerosis, or labyrinthitis. The most common approach to cochlear implantation involves a mastoidectomy and facial recess drill-out; adequate pneumatization and accessibility of these regions are requisite. A history of prior neurotologic surgery, chronic/active ear disease, or the presence of a canal-wall-down mastoid cavity may also influence laterality of device placement or necessitate a staged approach to implant placement.

With all other factors being equal, we recommend implantation of the poorer-hearing ear. This aligns with the otologic principle of preventing damage to the hearing and balance organ with better residual function. Several decades of studies demonstrate that speech recognition outcomes are no different based on implantation of the better or worse ear [35–37]. Even for patients with different durations of hearing deprivation between ears, outcomes are more reflective of the overall health of the central auditory pathways than the individual ears [38–40]. Furthermore, implantation of the poorer ear allows for bimodal stimulation (cochlear implant in one ear with hearing aid in the contralateral ear) with improvements in sound localization, speech recognition, and patient-reported outcomes measures [17, 41, 42].

Immunization

Patients with cochlear implants are thought to have an increased risk for some types of bacterial meningitis. This evidence is based primarily on a 2002 study of pediatric CI recipients experiencing episodes of postimplantation bacterial meningitis. In this analysis, risk factors included the use of a silastic intracochlear surgical positioner, inner ear malformations, cerebrospinal fluid leak or gusher, prior episodes of meningitis, presence of ventriculoperitoneal shunt, or recurrent/acute otitis media. Nonetheless, the US Centers for Disease Control and Prevention (CDC) issues a clear recommendation for all cochlear implant recipients to undergo vaccination. These guidelines include recently approved pneumococcal conjugate vaccines (PCV15, PCV20, and PCV21) as well as a 23-valent pneumococcal polysaccharide vaccine (PPSV23). Adults undergoing CI placement, if they have not previously received pneumococcal vaccines, should receive PCV15, PCV20, or PCV21. If PCV15 is used, it should be followed with 1 dose of PPSV23 at least 8 weeks later [43]. The patient's chosen vaccination regimen should be completed at least 2 weeks prior to surgery, if possible.

Device/Electrode Selection

Broadly, CI electrode arrays are divided into two main designs: straight, lateral wall (LW), and pre-curved, perimodiolar (PM) types. LW electrodes are designed to skirt the outer wall of the cochlea within the scala tympani. PM electrodes are intended to be placed more medially within the scala tympani abutting the cochlear modiolus and spiral ganglion cells, theoretically providing improved frequency resolution and decreased power consumption due to the proximity of stimulation. However, PM electrodes are at higher risk of scalar translocation and tip fold-over events which may negatively impact speech recognition performance and the degree of residual hearing in hearing preservation CI surgery [44–46]. Interestingly, a PM electrode array with external introducer sheath, rather than traditional stylet, resulted in just a single scalar translocation event for 24 patients undergoing CI with this device [47].

With LW arrays, longer electrodes portend greater angular insertion depths and are associated with better speech recognition performance [48–53]. This relationship is theorized to arise from (1) broader cochlear "coverage" with improved acoustic and electrical pitch-matching between the tonotopic map of the cochlea and the stimulating bands of the electrode array and (2) improved spectral resolution given the greater distance between the stimulating bands of the electrode array [49, 50]. Moving forward, patient-specific measurements of cochlear duct length may inform clinician decision-making regarding specific electrode length and type.

Hearing Preservation

With the continued expansion of CI criteria, an increasing percentage of patients present with some degree of usable residual low-frequency hearing. Preservation of this low-frequency hearing allows for combined electro-acoustic stimulation (EAS), which yields improved speech understanding, performance in complex listening environments, and binaural timing cues [54–57]. Advances in electrode design and atraumatic surgical technique have greatly improved hearing preservation rates [57, 58]. It is our opinion that a "soft" surgical technique to minimize trauma to the cochlear structures during electrode placement should apply to all patients, regardless of preoperative hearing status.

In general, the best hearing preservation results are attained for electrodes placed entirely within the scala tympani; LW electrodes placed through a round window (RW) or extended round window (ERW) approach appear to maximize the likelihood of such positioning [59]. At our center, we emphasize a low drill speed while removing the bony niche to expose the RW. At that point, we employ a large, atraumatic opening of the RW membrane to allow ample egress of perilymph as the electrode is inserted slowly and smoothly into the cochlea. Introduction with excessive force or against resistance is avoided. Care is taken to not suction the perilymph within the cochlea, and blood or bone dust is not permitted to enter the open labyrinth. In addition to soft surgical technique, other methods such as perioperative steroids [60–62], topical middle ear steroids [63], topical hyaluronic acid [64], and robotic insertion techniques [65, 66] have all been proposed to improve hearing preservation rates.

While opinions vary across centers, it is the authors' preference to utilize a full-length rather than a shortened/hybrid electrode array for patients with residual low-frequency thresholds. With an appropriately selected full-length array and meticulous soft surgical technique, these patients demonstrate excellent hearing preservation rates [67, 68]. Furthermore, the apical electrical stimulation available from longer electrode arrays may prevent revision surgery for patients undergoing low-frequency threshold shifts immediately after surgery or further progression of their hearing loss years down the road.

Surgery

Preoperative

CI surgery is almost universally performed on an outpatient basis, unless observation is indicated by the patient's health condition(s), post-anesthetic concerns, or another complicating factor. In the preoperative area, the surgeon verifies any changes to the history and physical examination and marks the ear to be implanted. In considering the placement of the CI, the surgeon should consider the position of a contralateral implant, if present, and discuss any occupational or recreational head-covering utilized by the patient.

Antibiotics

Robust data regarding the utility of perioperative and postoperative antibiotics for CI surgery is lacking [69]. The available data do not support the notion that prophylactic antibiotics decrease infection rates, which are approximately 1% [70, 71]. There is limited evidence that more than 2 days of antibiotic treatment after surgery may be beneficial.

In a large cohort study of 1180 patients of all ages, those receiving less than 48 hours of antibiotics were nearly three times more likely to have surgical site infection than those with more than 48 hours of antibiotics, although there were only 12 patients (1%) with this complication [72]. In this cohort, children were much more likely to have postoperative infections than adults.

Despite a paucity of high-level evidence, the authors favor prophylactic antibiotics for CI surgery to cover skin flora pathogens. Typically, this involves cefazolin for patients without risk factors for methicillin-resistant *S. aureus* (MRSA) colonization and consideration of vancomycin for those at risk of MRSA infection or with colonization. Patients with a history of chronic ear disease or recent infection may warrant prophylactic and postoperative coverage of respiratory tract pathogens with ceftriaxone or amoxicillin-clavulanic acid. We typically utilize antibiotic irrigation during the surgery and may send a short course of postoperative antibiotics. Arguments against routine postoperative antibiotic usage arise due to concerns of bacterial resistance, possible side effects/allergic reactions, and cost. [73]

Incision, Soft Tissue, and Device Positioning

Standard surgical technique involves a transmastoid, facial recess approach to the round window and scala tympani. General anesthesia with continuous facial nerve monitoring is utilized, so paralysis for induction occurs either with a short-acting agent or with a longer-acting agent that has been adequately reversed. Prophylactic antibiotics are administered, device position is marked, and a time-out is performed.

Over time, most surgeons have adopted a simple, routine postauricular incision for this procedure (Fig. 20.1). Designs such as the large C-shaped, inferiorly based inverted U-shaped, or S-shaped incisions are mainly historical relics. In practice, it is difficult to completely avoid the incision line crossing some portion of the CI electrode; more important is positioning the receiver-stimulator (RS) and fantail at least 1 cm from the skin incision. After skin incision, the ear is raised forward under the temporoparietal fascia in an avascular plane. The Palva musculoperiosteal flap is elevated ante-

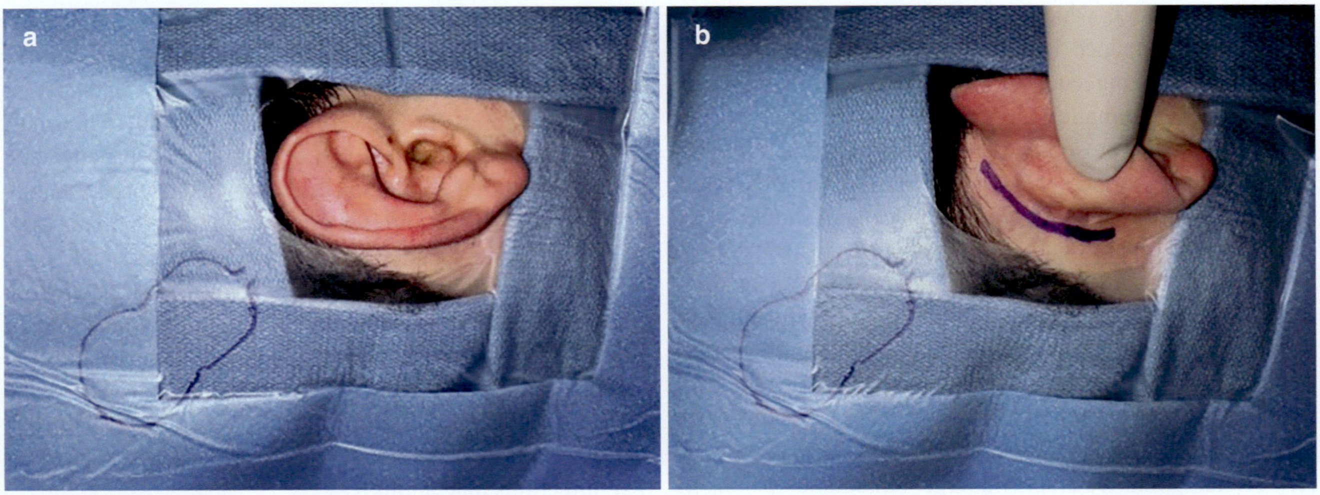

Fig. 20.1 (**a**) Planned device position is outlined and (**b**) a simple postauricular incision is designed 5–10 mm behind the ear crease

riorly to the spine of Henle to fully expose the mastoid cortex, and the posterior-superior elevation of a tight subperiosteal pocket is performed. Adequate elevation of the pocket is confirmed with a device-specific template, as the RS must be adequately positioned away from the incision line and as to not interfere with a behind-the-ear processor device. Given the low rate of clinically apparent device migration and decreased operative time for the tight subperiosteal pocket technique, we do not routinely advocate the use of a bony well, tie-down sutures, or other hardware to secure the device [74–76]. We assert that avoidance of a bony well lowers the risk of intracranial or fixation hardware complications [77].

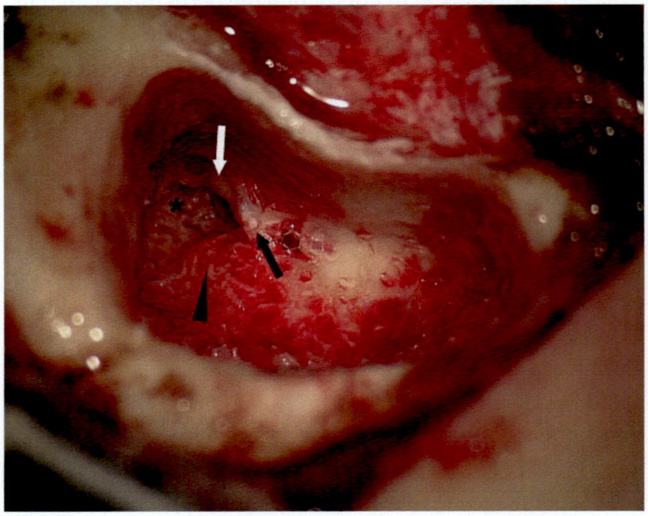

Fig. 20.2 Cortical mastoidectomy demonstrates an appropriately thin ear canal with identification of the antrum (asterisk), lateral semicircular canal (black arrowhead), and incus (white arrow). The posterior ligament of the incus is demarcated by the black arrow

Mastoidectomy

Once the RS pocket has been confirmed, a standard mastoidectomy is performed with progressively smaller cutting burrs and suction-irrigators to identify the tegmen, sigmoid sinus, lateral semicircular canal, and incus (Fig. 20.2). Some surgeons advocate against wide saucerization of the mastoid cortex to allow retention of the electrode leads within the mastoid cavity; it is important that such a philosophy does not preclude adequate visualization of vital structures, especially for trainees. Adequate thinning of the bony ear canal without compromising its integrity is essential to allow proper visualization of the round window after the facial recess (posterior tympanotomy) has been opened. Violation of the bony ear canal should be avoided to minimize the risk of exposed hardware postoperatively.

Facial Recess

After the cortical mastoidectomy is completed, the facial recess is opened with diamond drill bits under continuous irrigation (Fig. 20.3). This may be completed by carefully skeletonizing and thus discretely identifying the facial nerve and chorda tympani in the mastoid bone, although such an approach may create a greater risk of inadvertent injury or thermal damage to these structures. Alternatively, identification of the posterior ligament of the short process of the incus (the "white dot") as it attaches to the incus buttress is a reli-

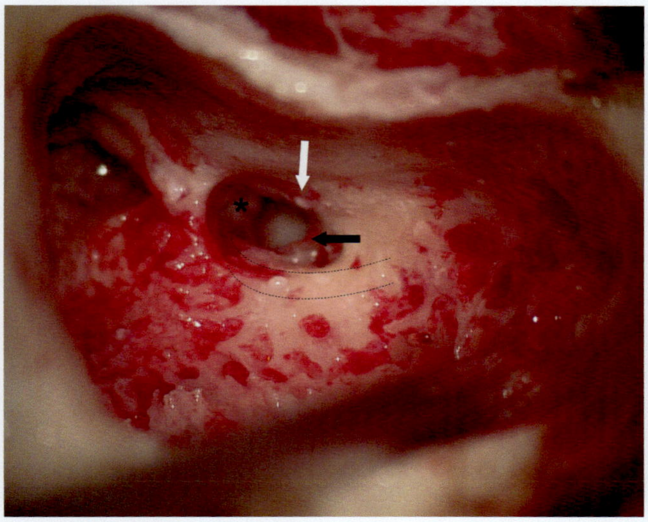

Fig. 20.3 The facial recess has been opened immediately inferior to the posterior ligament of the incus. The chorda tympani nerve is identified anteriorly (white arrow). The path of the facial nerve is demarcated by the dashed lines. Through the facial recess, the stapes is identified (asterisk). The ridge of bone marked by the black arrow is medial to the facial nerve and will be drilled away to reveal the round window niche

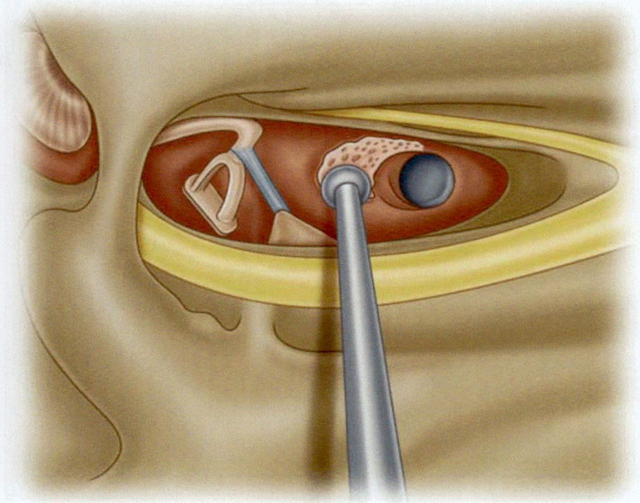

Fig. 20.4 The round window niche is removed with a small diamond bit to expose the obliquely oriented round window membrane. (Adapted from Glasscock and Shambaugh's Surgery of the Ear, 6th Ed. Eds. Gulya, Minor, Poe. PMPH. 2010)

able surgical landmark for both novice and advanced CI surgeons [78]. Identification of this "white dot" allows the surgeon to open the facial recess directly at its widest point just inferior to the incus buttress. Methodical and judicious enlargement of the facial recess is performed anterior and parallel to the anticipated path of the facial nerve. Rarely does the path of the chorda tympani nerve preclude visualization of the round window requiring sacrifice of this structure via an extended facial recess approach. Removal of bone medial to the facial nerve is performed with progressively smaller burrs. Careful attention must be taken to avoid resting the drill shaft on the facial nerve during this maneuver. It is prudent to avoid rotating the burr while moving the tip of the drill through the facial recess corridor to access the middle ear space and bone medial to the facial nerve to avoid inadvertent contact with the facial and chorda tympani nerves. Identification of the stapes and the stapedius tendon is useful in identifying the location of the round window (RW) as this structure is reliably 2 mm inferior and posterior to the oval window [79].

Electrode Placement

We favor a RW approach to electrode insertion in order to minimize intracochlear trauma, aid in positioning the electrode closer to cochlear neural elements, maximize hearing preservation results, and improve speech perception outcomes (Fig. 20.4) [44, 80–82]. The RW approach entails

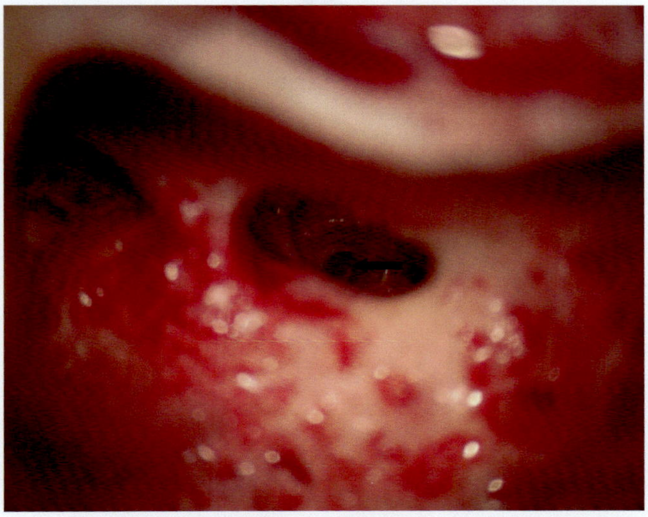

Fig. 20.5 The round window niche has been drilled to allow visualization of the round window membrane (black arrow)

removal of the oblique bony overhang of the round window to allow visualization of the full membrane (Fig. 20.5). Alternative approaches may be dictated by electrode choice or obstructive pathologies at the round window. The extended-RW approach entails enlargement at the anterior-inferior edge of the RW, while a formal cochleostomy is a fenestration separate from the RW at an anterior-inferior location.

After completing the bony exposure of the cochlear fenestration, ample irrigation with antibiotic-soaked solution removes any residual bone dust or blood from the working area. The tight subperiosteal pocket is irrigated and the

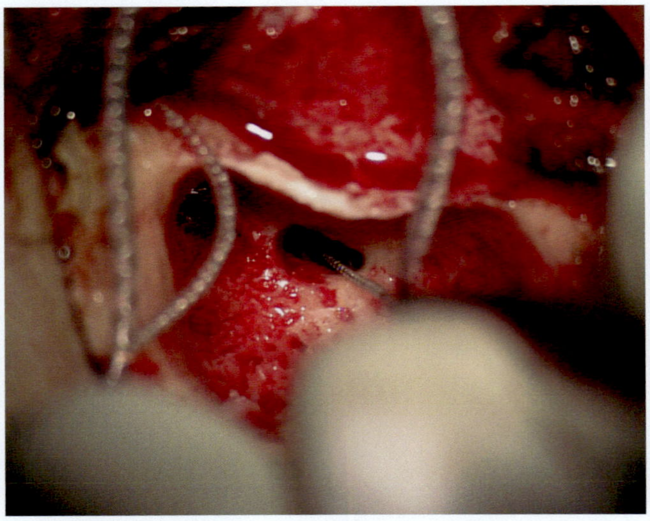

Fig. 20.6 The grounding electrode, if present, is placed under the temporalis muscle. Placement of the electrode array within the scala tympani proceeds via soft technique through the round window cochleostomy

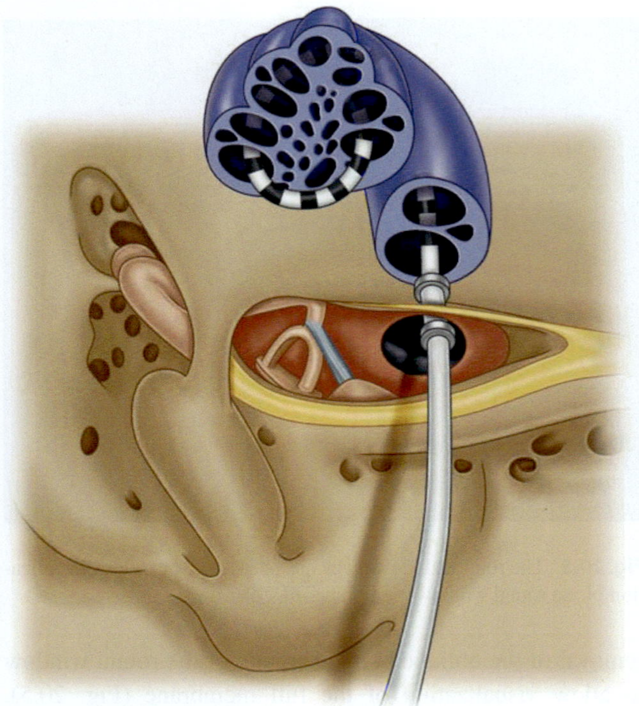

Fig. 20.7 A cross-sectional illustration after electrode insertion demonstrates a scala tympani location. (Adapted from Glasscock and Shambaugh's Surgery of the Ear, 6th Ed. Eds. Gulya, Minor, Poe. PMPH. 2010)

device brought onto the field and placed in the pocket. If the device has a separate grounding electrode, this is usually placed in a subperiosteal pocket over the squamous portion of the temporal bone. The round window membrane or cochleostomy is then opened widely, and the electrode is inserted into the scala tympani in an atraumatic manner (Figs. 20.6 and 20.7). This is discussed further in the section on hearing preservation techniques. The device is then coiled within the mastoid cavity (Fig. 20.8). Muscle or periosteum is packed inferiorly and then superiorly around the cochleostomy and facial recess to maintain optimal electrode position and prevent egress of perilymph [83].

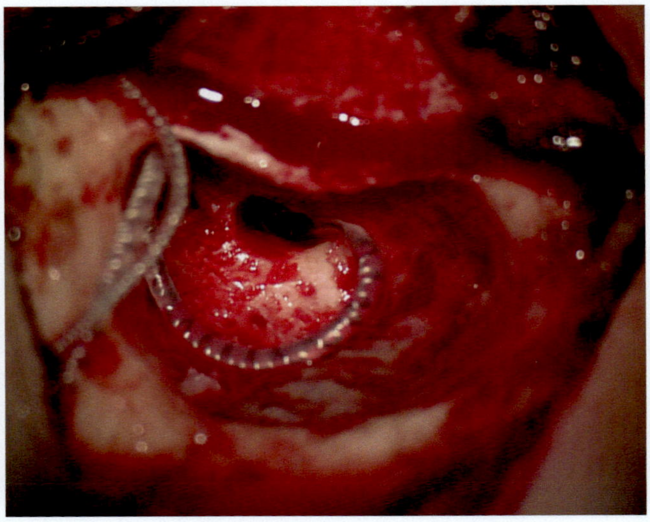

Fig. 20.8 The device is coiled within the mastoid cavity in preparation for soft tissue packing of the facial recess

A large piece of absorbable gelatin foam is placed over the RS fantail and electrode within the mastoid to prevent device migration during closure. A multilayered closure with absorbable sutures returns the musculoperiosteal flap and subcutaneous tissues to their anatomic positions. Confirmation of electrode placement may be accomplished with a plain-film radiograph or computed tomography (CT) scan (Fig. 20.9) [84, 85]. We routinely perform intraoperative monitoring to assess device integrity and the cochlea's neural responses while the incision is being closed. This testing involves impedance testing and neural response testing but may also include spread-of-excitation testing to rule out electrode fold-over events.

Postoperative Considerations: Activation, MRI, and Monopolar Electrocautery

Generally, patients are seen for their first postoperative visit 2 to 3 weeks after surgery. With routine healing, patients may be activated and fit with their sound processors at this time. Earlier activation is certainly feasible, although careful attention should be paid to postoperative healing and flap thickness. The surgeon and audiologist should anticipate variable magnet strength and retention. With early activation at 5–7 days, predictable changes in impedance and electrical stimulation levels are expected

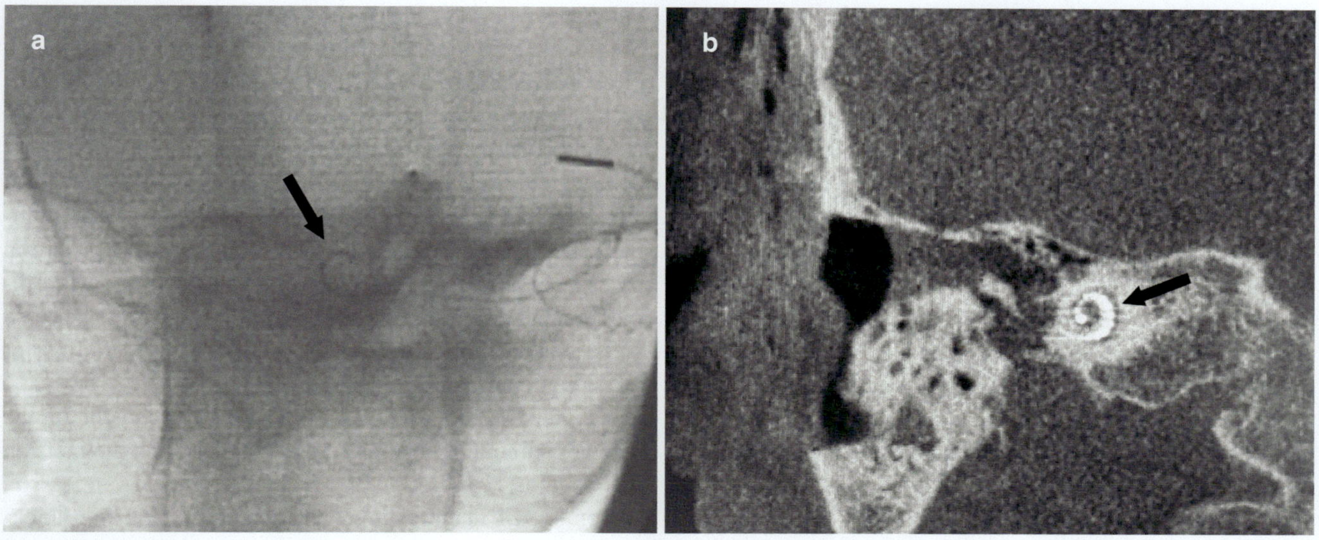

Fig. 20.9 Intraoperative placement of the electrode array is confirmed either with (**a**) fluoroscopy (left ear, black arrow) or (**b**) intraoperative CT scan (right ear, black arrow). Images courtesy of Matthew R. O'Malley, MD and Noah Whittenbarger

and may necessitate reprogramming within the first month [86].

With the introduction of diametric and rotating magnets, the latest generation of internal devices from all three manufacturers are MRI-conditional without removal of the implant magnet. Previously, some CI devices with axial magnets were able to undergo MRI with placement of a headwrap splint kit to keep the magnet from "flipping" in the magnetic field. In 2015, Carlson et al. demonstrated that tight headwrap placement allows successful 1.5 Tesla MRI obtainment for most patients without CI magnet removal, although patients should be counseled regarding the risk of internal magnet movement [87]. The radiologist, surgeon, and audiologist should refer to current manufacturer guidelines for MRI as some CI models may require surgical removal of the magnet or the device may be completely contraindicated for MRI. For patients with known pathology of the temporal bone or IAC, a more posterior and horizontally positioned RS may allow better characterization of these structures on postoperative MRI, especially at 3 T (Fig. 20.10) [88].

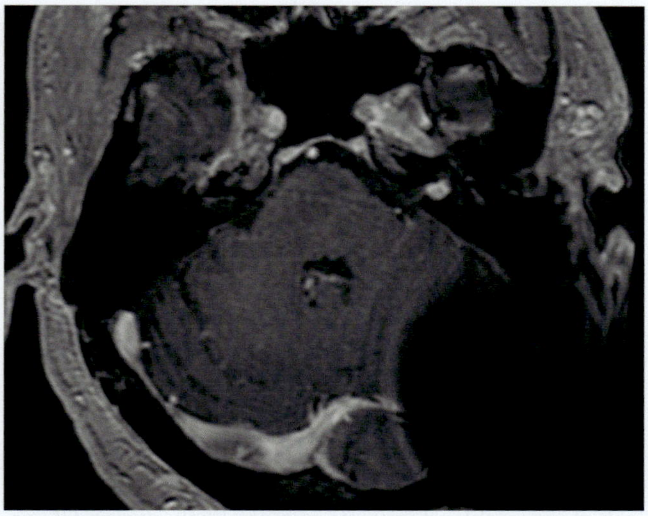

Fig. 20.10 Post-gadolinium T1-weighted MRI sequence for a patient with known, stable left intracanalicular tumor. The artifact from left cochlear implant allows adequate surveillance of the likely vestibular schwannoma

Current practice is to avoid monopolar electrocautery (MES) in certain situations after placement of CIs, as there is a theoretical risk of diversion of the electrical current to the device. Of the three FDA-approved CI manufacturers, two device labels prohibit MES in the head and neck after CI placement (with no specific recommendation as to the rest of the body), while the other company discourages MES with a CI in the opposite ear, although it is unclear whether this relates only to contralateral otologic surgery. Despite these recommendations, reports of unintentional MES exposure have failed to demonstrate any damage to the internal devices, even for surgeries of the head and neck [89–92]. Further clarification and guidance from the manufacturers will be paramount as CI surgery and other surgeries requiring MES continue to become more common; surgeons will likely be asked to assess the relative risks and benefits for patients with CIs undergoing surgical procedures with or without MES.

Complications

The risks associated with CI surgery are similar to chronic ear surgery but with the additional complexity of placing an implantable device within the inner ear. We routinely discuss the risks of bleeding, infection, pain, scar, facial paralysis/

stimulation, taste changes, hearing loss, tinnitus, vertigo, cerebrospinal fluid (CSF) leakage, meningitis, as well as extrusion, migration, and/or failure of the internal device. While CI surgery is generally considered to be safe and reliable, even the most experienced otologic surgeon should anticipate a small rate of short- and long-term complications. Complications arising during the perioperative and acute postoperative phase are rare but may include damage to surrounding structures such as the facial nerve or chorda tympani or soft tissue complications such as infection, hematoma, and flap necrosis. The rates of these complications may be minimized by meticulous surgical technique and diligent postoperative regimens [93]. As a result, we advocate attention to sterile technique, observing Halsted's principles for tissue handling, and the intraoperative identification and avoidance of critical structures.

While exceedingly rare, permanent facial nerve injury from cochlear implantation is certainly a devastating complication. Even transient facial weakness is considered a rare sequela of CI surgery, with an incidence much less than 1%. In the absence of an obvious intraoperative injury to the nerve, patients with postoperative facial weakness are more likely to have an inadvertent thermal injury and less likely dysfunction due to infiltration of local anesthetic, as this is usually limited to the postauricular region. More common after CI surgery is taste disturbance due to irritation or injury to the chorda tympani nerve during the posterior tympanotomy or facial recess drill-out. Fortunately, these issues tend to resolve for the vast majority of patients within the weeks to months following surgery, and permanent taste dysfunction is unusual [94]. The intentional sacrifice of the chorda tympani should be avoided, if possible, especially for patients potentially undergoing bilateral otologic surgery thus placing them at risk for bilateral, permanent taste dysfunction.

Intraoperative identification of a perilymph fistula or CSF leak at the cochleostomy site is more likely during CI surgery for congenitally malformed inner ears. For adult patients, enlargement of the cochlear aqueduct or vestibular aqueduct may lead to both progressive sensorineural hearing loss and intraoperative perilymph fistula [95]. Control of profuse CSF outflow should be managed by first allowing ample egress of fluid to slow the gusher. After electrode insertion, packing of the cochleostomy with muscle or fascia with or without fibrin glue ensures a tight seal to prevent further leakage. The risk of perioperative or postoperative meningitis is diminished by control of the cerebrospinal leak and adequate vaccination.

Soft tissue complications such as hematoma or seroma are uncommon, but may be treated either conservatively or through needle aspiration/drainage depending on the size and quality of the fluid collection [96]. Such issues should be monitored carefully in the setting of ongoing anticoagulation. The utility of pressure dressings in these situations is unknown, but such headwraps remain relatively low risk. Surgical site infections such as cellulitis, acute otitis media, or chondritis are best treated with broad-spectrum oral antibiotics. Rarely does infection progress to a drainable fluid collection requiring further intervention. Simple incisional dehiscence is usually treated conservatively with local wound care; adequate intraoperative closure of the musculoperiosteal layer is paramount to prevent device exposure in cases of superficial dehiscence. We tend to have a low threshold to start postoperative antibiotics for known or suspected soft tissue complications such as hematoma, cellulitis, or incisional dehiscence.

As mentioned previously, thoughtful placement of the receiver stimulator ensures ample distance from the incision and avoids conflict with a behind-the-ear processor. Generally, CI manufacturers recommend a skin flap thickness of less than 7 mm. Greater thickness of the soft tissue envelope may adversely affect signal transmission, battery life, and processor retention [97]. Conversely, thin skin flaps or improperly strong magnets may lead to headaches, skin irritation, or pressure necrosis [98]. Fortunately, complications from this including skin flap necrosis, wound dehiscence, and cochlear implant extrusion are rare (Fig. 20.11) [99, 100]. Healing issues and flap breakdown may be managed by the increasingly aggressive options of local wound care, antibiotics, locoregional reconstruction, explantation, or even microvascular free tissue transfer [100–102].

Migration of the internal electrode during either the surgical closure or postoperative period may result in increased impedances for the basal electrodes and decreased auditory performance [103]. Prevention of electrode migration is

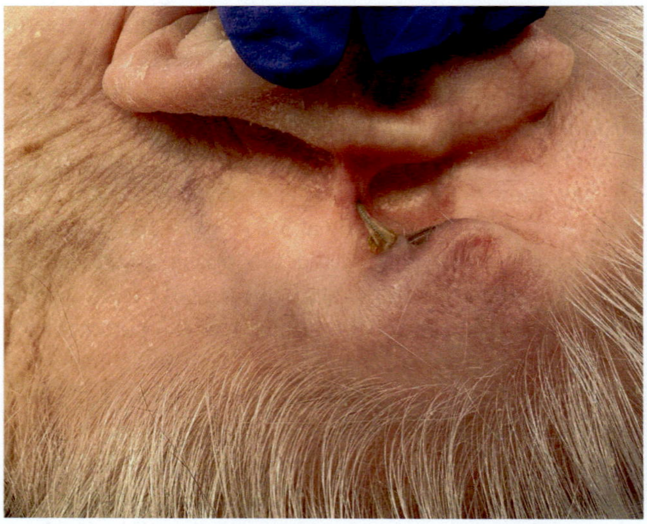

Fig. 20.11 Extrusion of the receiver-stimulator fantail. In this case, the fantail lies directly over the mastoid cavity, and the RS is positioned adjacent to the postauricular incision. Retraction of this patient's already thin soft tissue envelope into the prior mastoid cavity was thought to expedite extrusion

attempted by careful tissue packing of the electrode array at the round window and facial recess. In cases of suspected migration, CT imaging is often sufficient for diagnosis.

Unfortunately, CIs are not immune from device failure, with reported rates varying from 0.5% to 14.7%, with an average of 6% [104–106]. Hard failures are due specifically to malfunction of the internal CI device resulting in the absence of useful auditory stimuli and are diagnosed on integrity testing [107]. Hard failures should be suspected in cases of decreased auditory performance, alterations in sound quality, or decreased impedances and should be verified with integrity testing [104]. On the other hand, soft failures are due to suspected device malfunction that does not appear abnormal on imaging or with current methods of in vivo integrity testing. Symptoms related to soft failure may include abnormal auditory or nonauditory symptoms or decreased audiometric performance; this type of failure is confirmed after revision surgery ameliorates the issue [107, 108].

On average, approximately 9% of CI recipients may report some degree of transient, short-term vertigo or vestibular disturbance after surgery, with increasing age the main risk factor for unilateral vestibular loss [109, 110]. However, the rate of new disability due to vestibular hypofunction at 1 year is rare (~1%) due to compensatory mechanisms of central nervous system [111–113]. A recent meta-analysis demonstrated no significant change in postoperative Dizziness Handicap Inventory after CI surgery, suggesting a minimal clinical effect on the vestibular system [114]. Nonetheless, vestibular evaluation and patient counseling are important considerations for the CI surgeon, especially for elderly patients, patients undergoing bilateral implantation, or CI surgery on an "only-balancing" ear.

Postoperative facial stimulation after CI may be immediate or delayed and is more common for patients with a history of otosclerosis, inner ear malformation, otosyphilis, meningitis, or temporal bone fracture [115, 116]. Such stimulation is best managed by deactivation of the offending electrodes, although this may result in decreased speech recognition scores [117].

Outcomes

In the nearly four decades since FDA approval in the United States, CI outcomes continue to improve as the result of improved hardware, software/programming, and the expansion of implant criteria to include patients with better preoperative and residual hearing [118]. The 1995 National Institutes of Health consensus statement set expectations for postoperative sentence scores of at least 80% [119]. While speech recognition testing through open-set word and sentence lists remain the gold standard for measuring objective benefit from the device, increasingly quality of life questionnaires are emerging as essential, complementary tools to assess the patient condition both prior to and after CI surgery [120, 121].

A flurry of recent research has focused on analyzing and affecting the factors that determine hearing outcomes for the individual patient undergoing CI surgery. However, there remains a considerable degree of variability among postoperative speech performance, even among high-volume CI centers. A recent, large multicenter report estimated mean word recognition score testing at 1 year between 42.1% and 51.2% [122]. These differences may be the result of institutional practices, referral patterns, primary spoken language, timing of postoperative assessment, programming methodologies, and patient population, among other factors. In terms of predicting outcomes for the individual postlingually deafened adult patient, factors such as age at implantation, duration of deafness, sex, etiology of the hearing loss, and preoperative speech recognition scores are statistically significant but are associated with a low effect size [122, 123]. Other factors known to affect individual outcomes include spiral ganglion cell count [124], top-down processing, neural health [125, 126], electrode position and depth [44, 45, 49, 59, 127], utilization of residual low-frequency acoustic hearing [128, 129], aural rehabilitation [130, 131], and daily device usage "datalogging" [132, 133].

In certain situations, patients may benefit from cochlear implantation even when objective speech outcomes may be lower than average. As a result, careful preoperative counseling and a multidisciplinary approach to decision-making should be considered for patients with auditory neuropathy spectrum disorder (ANSD) [134, 135], traumatic brain injury [136, 137], neurofibromatosis type II [138, 139], as well as stable observed or treated sporadic vestibular schwannomas [140, 141]. Outcomes for patients receiving CI for post-meningitis hearing loss are dictated by time-to-intervention, intraoperative findings, and other neurological sequelae [142].

Congenitally or prelingually deafened adults with bilateral auditory deprivation tend to have poor speech intelligibility after CI with variable detection of speech sounds or environmental cues and will likely require continued lipreading and/or sign language postimplantation [143, 144]. However, modest improvements in health-related quality of life metrics after CI suggest that even improvement in sound perception may be a meaningful result for these patients [145, 146]. As a result, careful counseling is required to assess motivations and define expectations for this group of patients. In contrast, adults with a single long-deafened ear in the presence of aided contralateral hearing tend to have similar outcomes regardless of the ear that is implanted, supporting the notion that central auditory processing persists despite monaural auditory deprivation.

Special Considerations

Several scenarios deserve special mention with regard to clinical decision-making and CIs. We are currently in a period of rapid expansion for CI indications, which implies a much broader and diverse population of potential CI candidates. As clinician and public awareness improves, patients that were not previously considered to be candidates may be referred for CI evaluation. CI surgeons and audiologists must evaluate their own outcomes to provide the best recommendations for patients that may still benefit more from regular amplification, have different or unrealistic expectations, or be at risk of becoming a nonuser.

Bilateral Implantation

For patients who are CI candidates for both ears, it is well-established that bilateral CI placement provides additional benefits as compared to a single, unilateral device. While a unilateral CI generally provides good speech recognition in quiet environments, restoration of useful binaural hearing through bilateral implantation is advantageous for hearing comprehension in noise, sound localization, and overcoming the head shadow effect [147, 148]. In practice, we generally advise adults to first undergo implantation in the poorer-hearing ear. With adequate follow-up and device usage, it is not uncommon to see patients exceed the speech recognition performance of their contralateral, previously better-hearing ear. For bimodal patients (utilizing one CI with a hearing aid on the non-implanted side), the clinical decision-making with regard to second-side implantation is not always straightforward. Standard audiometric setups with a single loudspeaker are not sensitive enough to distinguish performance between bimodal and the bilateral CI conditions. Interestingly, the patient's response to the question "Do you think you need a second CI?" provides a high sensitivity for identifying patients that would benefit from a second CI and a moderately high specificity in determining patients that would perform better in their existing bimodal configuration [149]. As a result, we tend to offer a second CI to adults once they express a desire to undergo bilateral implantation.

Single-Sided Deafness (SSD) and Asymmetric Hearing Loss (AHL)

Traditionally, evaluation of CI candidacy was based on the best-aided or bilateral condition rather than consideration of each individual ear. As a result, patients with SSD or AHL were not considered candidates for CI given that their bilateral performance was above FDA labeling thresholds. While the recent FDA approvals for SSD and AHL have focused on speech performance for the ear to be implanted, they remain relatively conservative in their criteria ($\leq$5% CNC word score for the ear to be implanted). Recent studies examining outcomes for patients with bimodal rehabilitation of AHL suggest that CI candidacy should be based solely on the ear to be implanted, rather than the bilateral condition or the status of the better-hearing ear [17, 150, 151].

Electroacoustic Stimulation (EAS)

Early investigations regarding hearing preservation CI surgery and EAS were focused on the utilization of shorter electrode arrays in an effort to avoid acoustic trauma at the lower frequencies. We now know that a combination of soft surgical technique with newer, full-length electrode designs allows hearing preservation in a majority of cases [152]. Patients utilizing combined EAS demonstrate improved speech perception in noise of approximately 10–15% on speech testing or 2–3 dB improvement in the signal-to-noise ratio (SNR) [31]. The presence of low-frequency acoustic cues allows improved sound localization and music appreciation as compared to the electric-only stimulation of traditional CIs [153]. EAS continues to be underutilized in the adult CI population [154].

Tinnitus

The modulation and/or suppression of tinnitus is a well-known sequelae of CI surgery. In fact, some of the earliest studies regarding CI for patients with SSD were focused on methods to improve incapacitating, unilateral tinnitus [155]. Recent meta-analyses suggest that approximately 88% of patients with SSD experience some improvement or resolution of their tinnitus symptoms after CI [156, 157]. While not an approved indication for these devices, CI surgery may actually be one of the more successful treatment options for incapacitating unilateral tinnitus for patients with SSD. In contrast, effects on tinnitus remain much more variable for patients with bilateral SNHL after CI. For this group, tinnitus questionnaire scores generally tend to improve after CI surgery, but a non-trivial group of patients experience either worsening or new-onset tinnitus symptoms. [158, 159] As a result, CI candidates with bilateral SNHL and bothersome tinnitus should be counseled thoroughly regarding the wide range of possible effects on tinnitus before undergoing surgery.

Labyrinthitis Ossificans

Labyrinthitis may occur as the result of infection, inflammation, temporal bone trauma, hemorrhage, or tumor. Pathologic ossification of the membranous labyrinth or endosteum as a sequela of labyrinthitis is referred to as labyrinthitis ossificans. Clinicians should monitor patients with temporal bone trauma, especially those with otic-capsule involving fractures, for progressive sensorineural hearing loss and radiographic signs of ossification. With a properly timed intervention, outcomes for CI among temporal bone trauma patients are excellent [160]. A separate scenario involves patients with profound hearing loss after bacterial meningitis, as up to a third of this group subsequently develop labyrinthitis ossificans [161]. Early intervention and counseling is essential for patients at risk of developing labyrinthitis ossificans, as progressive ossification may preclude successful CI device placement in these scenarios.

Imaging is particularly useful in cases of temporal bone fracture or post-meningitis SNHL to evaluate the inner ear for labyrinthitis ossificans and guide the timing of potential intervention. In the acute phase of labyrinthitis, contrast enhancement of the labyrinth on MRI is common (Fig. 20.12). In the months after initial insult, T2-weighted sequences may be useful for detecting the presence of intracochlear fibrosis and assessing the patency of the membranous labyrinth. CT has a role in the diagnosis of temporal bone fractures and the assessing the degree of intracochlear ossification (Fig. 20.13). In general, we advise early implantation for patients meeting CI candidacy who are at risk of developing labyrinthitis ossificans.

Intraoperative management of labyrinthitis ossificans is dependent on the degree of fibrous tissue or bony obstruction. For cases of isolated basal turn ossification, the surgeon should utilize a standard cochleostomy to drill out and remove the new bony tissue until encountering the patent scala tympani, if present. For cases of more extensive ossification, the surgeon may opt for partial electrode insertion, middle turn cochleostomy [162], split-array electrodes [163], scala vestibuli insertion [164], or complete cochlear drill-out [165].

Chronic Ear Disease

CI is an excellent, albeit usually more difficult, management strategy for patients with sensorineural hearing loss and chronic ear disease [166]. For patients with stable disease and favorable facial recess approach, standard placement may be performed. The strategy of subtotal petrosectomy with blind sac closure of the external auditory canal (EAC) with or without abdominal fat graft and eustachian tube obliteration may be useful for patients with difficult anatomy, chronic inflammation, cerebrospinal fluid leak, or recurrent meningitis [167]. CI surgery in a prior canal wall down (CWD) cavity may be performed via EAC overclosure or while maintaining an open mastoid cavity [168]. While maintenance of the open CWD cavity for patients undergoing CI may be necessary for patients with unusually large prior meatoplasties, EAC overclosure is associated with significantly fewer global complications [169]. These patients undergoing subtotal petrosectomy and EAC closure in a

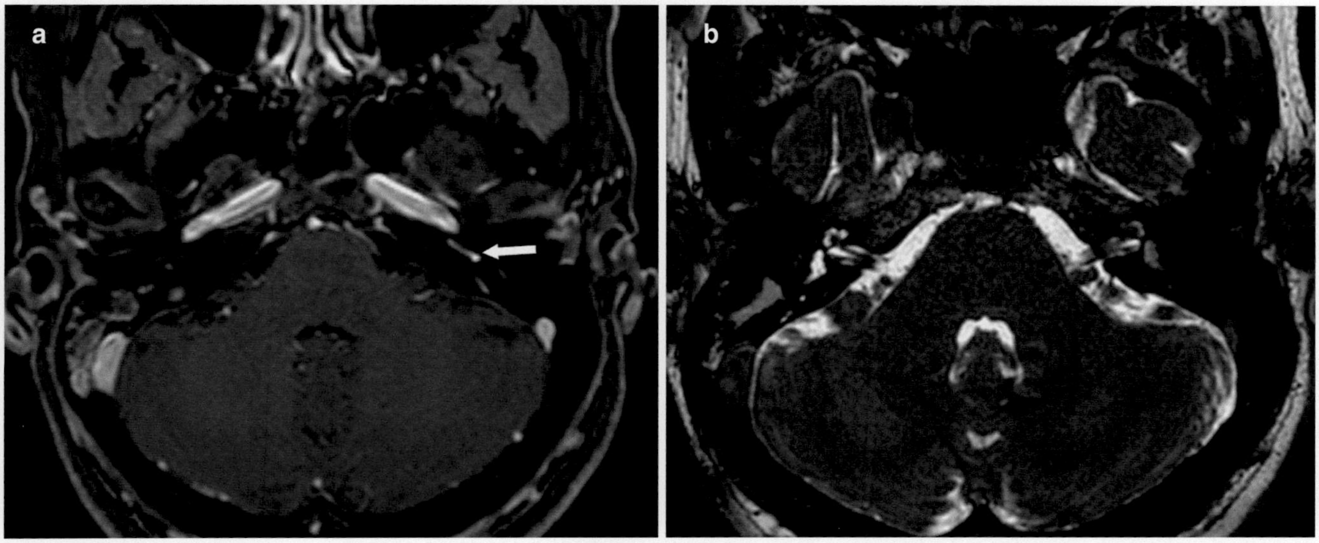

Fig. 20.12 MRI for a patient with profound bilateral SNHL after meningitis demonstrates (**a**) enhancement of the left inner ear on post-contrast T1-weighted sequences including the basal turn of the cochlea (white arrow), semicircular canals, and vestibule as well as (**b**) decreased fluid signal within the left labyrinthine on T2-weighted sequences. CT scan performed the same day demonstrated no abnormalities aside from scatter right-sided opacification of the mastoid. This patient ultimately underwent bilateral simultaneous CI placement, with intraoperative findings notable for fibrosis of the membranous labyrinth

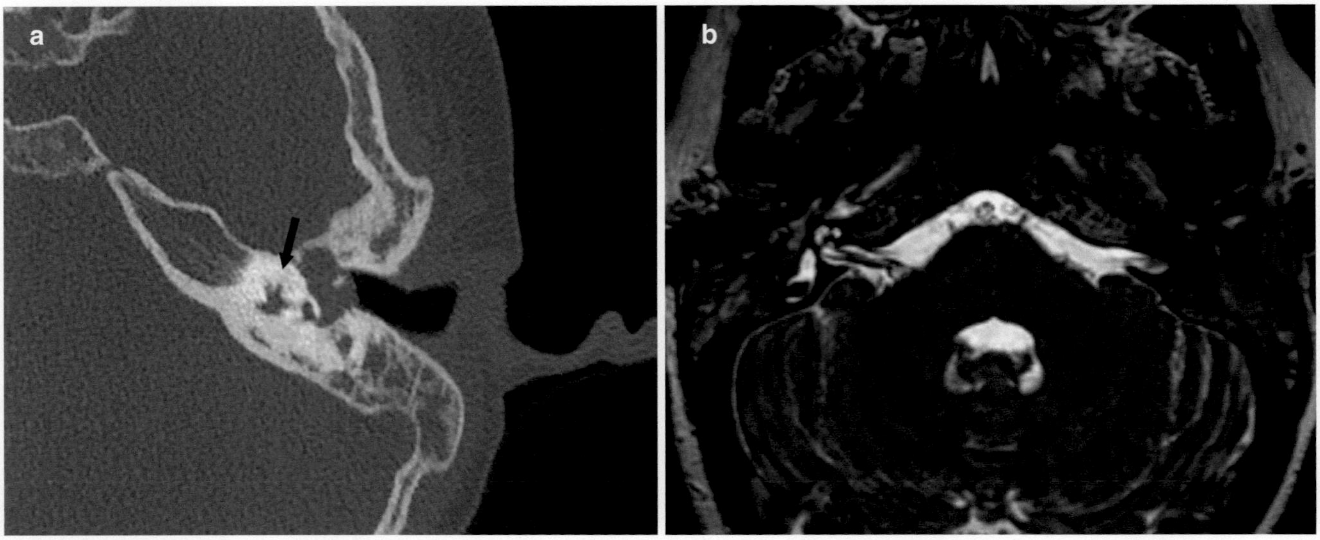

Fig. 20.13 A patient presented with single-sided deafness from recurrent left otitis media. (**a**) bone-window CT scan of the left temporal bone demonstrates labyrinthine ossification of the left cochlea, semicircular canals, and vestibule. (**b**) The MRI of the temporal bones with a thin-cut T2-weighted protocol demonstrates normal fluid signal on the right and absent fluid signal in the left labyrinth

CWD cavity may undergo concomitant or staged CI placement [170]. With either strategy, patients should be monitored for breakdown of the blind sac closure and recidivistic cholesteatoma. Inherently, a staged procedure for CI placement in these patients allows a functional second-look procedure as well. Either way, these patients often require long-term surveillance, which is now possible with the latest generation of MRI-conditional implants in the form of non–echo-planar diffusion-weighted sequences on MRI though magnet artifact is a concern as well.

Revision Surgery

Like most implantable devices, CIs come with a low but inherent rate of revision surgery. Reasons for replacement include hard device failure, soft or inconclusive failure, upgrade of a legacy device, as well as medical/surgical issues such as infection or extrusion [105]. Fortunately, revision surgery will often yield restoration of original speech recognition outcomes [104, 171].

Put simply, revision CI surgery is defined by removal of the original device, placement of the new device, and correct positioning of the electrode array within the cochlea. In practice, the CI surgeon must avoid certain pitfalls to ensure completion of these tasks. Removal of the original device should be performed in such a manner to avoid prematurely withdrawing the electrode array from the inner ear. Thus, we recommend severing the electrode just lateral to the facial recess prior to removing the RS. This maneuver allows 1) the device to be delivered to pathology and the manufacturer in just two pieces and 2) keeps the fibrous tract surrounding the electrode patent until the moment the surgeon is ready to reinsert the new device. The soft tissue of the facial recess is dissected free to allow clear visualization of the electrode entering the RW/cochleostomy. Occasionally, drilling of the cortical mastoid, ear canal, or facial recess is needed to improve visualization. The RS pocket is irrigated, and the new device is placed. Removal of the cut electrode array is performed immediately prior to insertion of the new electrode to avoid collapse of the fibrous sheath surrounding the device; loss of visualization of this tract may make reinsertion difficult. Closure and intraoperative testing proceed as in a primary CI surgery.

Conclusion

Cochlear implantation has become an integral part of otologic surgery. Though the majority of these surgeries are straightforward, the potential for—and implications of—complexity necessitate a robust knowledge of ear anatomy and physiology.

References

1. Wilson BS, Dorman MF, Woldorff MG, Tucci DL. Cochlear implants: matching the prosthesis to the brain and facilitating desired plastic changes in brain function. Prog Brain Res. 2011;194:117–29. https://doi.org/10.1016/B978-0-444-53815-4.00012-1.
2. Carlson ML. Cochlear implantation in adults. N Engl J Med. 2020;382:1531–42. https://doi.org/10.1056/NEJMra1904407.
3. Hainarosie M, Zainea V, Hainarosie R. The evolution of cochlear implant technology and its clinical relevance. J Med Life. 2014;7:1–4.

4. Mudry A, Mills M. The early history of the Cochlear implant: a retrospective. JAMA Otolaryngol. 2013;139:446–53. https://doi.org/10.1001/jamaoto.2013.293.
5. Eisenberg LS. The contributions of William F. House to the field of implantable auditory devices. Hear Res. 2015;322:52–6. https://doi.org/10.1016/j.heares.2014.08.003.
6. Völter C, Götze L, Haubitz I, et al. Benefits of cochlear implantation in middle-aged and older adults. Clin Interv Aging. 2020;15:1555–68. https://doi.org/10.2147/CIA.S255363.
7. Andries E, Gilles A, Topsakal V, et al. Systematic review of quality of life assessments after cochlear implantation in older adults. Audiol Neurootol. 2021;26:61–75. https://doi.org/10.1159/000508433.
8. Mertens G, Andries E, Claes AJ, et al. Cognitive improvement after cochlear implantation in older adults with severe or profound hearing impairment: a prospective, longitudinal, controlled, multicenter study. Ear Hear. 2021;42:606–14. https://doi.org/10.1097/AUD.0000000000000962.
9. Nassiri AM, Sorkin DL, Carlson ML. Current estimates of cochlear implant utilization in the United States. Otol Neurotol. 2022;43:e558. https://doi.org/10.1097/MAO.0000000000003513.
10. Arnoldner C, Lin VYW. Expanded selection criteria in adult cochlear implantation. Cochlear Implants Int. 2013;14(Suppl 4):S10–3. https://doi.org/10.1179/1467010013Z.000000000123.
11. Varadarajan VV, Sydlowski SA, Li MM, et al. Evolving criteria for adult and pediatric cochlear implantation. Ear Nose Throat J. 2021;100:31–7. https://doi.org/10.1177/0145561320947258.
12. Buchman CA, Gifford RH, Haynes DS, et al. Unilateral cochlear implants for severe, profound, or moderate sloping to profound bilateral sensorineural hearing loss: a systematic review and consensus statements. JAMA Otolaryngol Head Neck Surg. 2020;146:942–53. https://doi.org/10.1001/jamaoto.2020.0998.
13. Roland JT, Gantz BJ, Waltzman SB, et al. United States multicenter clinical trial of the cochlear nucleus hybrid implant system. Laryngoscope. 2016;126:175–81. https://doi.org/10.1002/lary.25451.
14. Friedmann DR, Ahmed OH, McMenomey SO, et al. Single-sided deafness cochlear implantation: candidacy, evaluation, and outcomes in children and adults. Otol Neurotol. 2016;37:e154–60. https://doi.org/10.1097/MAO.0000000000000951.
15. Deep NL, Spitzer ER, Shapiro WH, et al. Cochlear implantation in adults with single-sided deafness: outcomes and device use. Otol Neurotol. 2021;42:414–23. https://doi.org/10.1097/MAO.0000000000002955.
16. Lindquist NR, Holder JT, Patro A, et al. Cochlear implants for single-sided deafness: quality of life, daily usage, and duration of deafness. Laryngoscope. 2022; https://doi.org/10.1002/lary.30452.
17. Patro A, Lindquist NR, Holder JT, et al. Further evidence for individual ear consideration in cochlear implant candidacy evaluation. Otol Neurotol. 2022;43:1033–40. https://doi.org/10.1097/MAO.0000000000003677.
18. Dillon MT, Buss E, Rooth MA, et al. Cochlear implantation in cases of asymmetric hearing loss: subjective benefit, word recognition, and spatial hearing. Trends Hear. 2020;24:2331216520945524. https://doi.org/10.1177/2331216520945524.
19. Chweya CM, Smith AJ, May MM, et al. Prevalence of surgical, anesthetic, and device-related complications among infants implanted before 9 and 12 months of age versus older children: evidence for the continued expansion of pediatric cochlear implant candidacy criteria. Otol Neurotol. 2021;42:e666–74. https://doi.org/10.1097/MAO.0000000000003060.
20. Chweya CM, May MM, DeJong MD, et al. Language and audiological outcomes among infants implanted before 9 and 12 months of age versus older children: a continuum of benefit associated with cochlear implantation at successively younger ages. Otol Neurotol. 2021;42:686–93. https://doi.org/10.1097/MAO.0000000000003011.
21. Brown C, Gifford RH. Expansion of audiologic criteria for pediatric cochlear implantation. Otolaryngol Clin N Am. 2021;54:1181–91. https://doi.org/10.1016/j.otc.2021.08.002.
22. Carlson ML, Sladen DP, Haynes DS, et al. Evidence for the expansion of pediatric cochlear implant candidacy. Otol Neurotol. 2015;36:43–50. https://doi.org/10.1097/MAO.0000000000000607.
23. Sorkin DL. Cochlear implantation in the world's largest medical device market: utilization and awareness of cochlear implants in the United States. Cochlear Implants Int. 2013;14:S4–S12. https://doi.org/10.1179/1467010013Z.00000000076.
24. Carlson ML, Sladen DP, Gurgel RK, et al. Survey of the American Neurotology Society on Cochlear implantation: part 1, candidacy assessment and expanding indications. Otol Neurotol. 2018;39:e12. https://doi.org/10.1097/MAO.0000000000001632.
25. Zwolan TA, Basura G. Determining cochlear implant candidacy in adults: limitations, expansions, and opportunities for improvement. Semin Hear. 2021;42:331–41. https://doi.org/10.1055/s-0041-1739283.
26. Hunter JB, Carlson ML, Sweeney AD, et al. Cochlear implantation in the setting of perioperative anticoagulation and antiplatelet therapy. Otolaryngol Head Neck Surg. 2016;154:513–7. https://doi.org/10.1177/0194599815621738.
27. Prentiss S, Snapp H, Zwolan T. Audiology practices in the preoperative evaluation and Management of Adult Cochlear Implant Candidates. JAMA Otolaryngol Head Neck Surg. 2020;146:136–42. https://doi.org/10.1001/jamaoto.2019.3760.
28. Auditory Potential, LLC. Minimum Speech Test Battery (MSTB) For Adult Cochlear Implant Users 2011. Accessed at https://www.auditorypotential.com/MSTBfiles/MSTBManual2011-06-20%20.pdf. Accessed 6/2026.
29. Peterson GE, Lehiste I. Revised CNC lists for auditory tests. J Speech Hear Disord. 1962;27:62–70. https://doi.org/10.1044/jshd.2701.62.
30. Spahr AJ, Dorman MF, Litvak LM, et al. Development and validation of the AzBio sentence lists. Ear Hear. 2012;33:112–7. https://doi.org/10.1097/AUD.0b013e31822c2549.
31. Haynes DS, Gifford RH, Wanna GB, Rivas AC. Cochlear implants: from principles to practice. 1st ed. Jaypee Brothers Medical Pub; 2020.
32. Cass ND, Totten DJ, Ross JD, O'Malley MR. Characterizing cochlear implant magnet-related MRI artifact. Ann Otol Rhinol Laryngol. 2022;00034894221089143 https://doi.org/10.1177/00034894221089143.
33. Edmonson HA, Carlson ML, Patton AC, Watson RE. MR imaging and cochlear implants with retained internal magnets: reducing artifacts near highly inhomogeneous magnetic fields. Radiographics. 2018;38:94–106. https://doi.org/10.1148/rg.2018170135.
34. Digge P, Solanki RN, Shah DC, et al. Imaging modality of choice for pre-operative cochlear imaging: HRCT vs. MRI temporal bone. J Clin Diagn Res. 2016;10:TC01–4. https://doi.org/10.7860/JCDR/2016/18033.8592.
35. Francis HW, Yeagle JD, Bowditch S, Niparko JK. Cochlear implant outcome is not influenced by the choice of ear. Ear Hear. 2005;26:7S–16S. https://doi.org/10.1097/00003446-200508001-00003.
36. Chen JM, Shipp D, Al-Abidi A, et al. Does choosing the "worse" ear for cochlear implantation affect outcome? Otol Neurotol. 2001;22:335–9. https://doi.org/10.1097/00129492-200105000-00011.
37. Lazard DS, Vincent C, Venail F, et al. Pre-, per- and postoperative factors affecting performance of postlinguistically deaf adults using cochlear implants: a new conceptual model over

time. PLoS One. 2012;7:e48739. https://doi.org/10.1371/journal.pone.0048739.
38. Friedland DR, Venick HS, Niparko JK. Choice of ear for cochlear implantation: the effect of history and residual hearing on predicted postoperative performance. Otol Neurotol. 2003;24:582–9.
39. Gantz BJ, Tyler RS, Rubinstein JT, et al. Binaural cochlear implants placed during the same operation. Otol Neurotol. 2002;23:169–80. https://doi.org/10.1097/00129492-200203000-00012.
40. Boisvert I, Lyxell B, Mäki-Torkko E, et al. Choice of ear for cochlear implantation in adults with monaural sound-deprivation and unilateral hearing aid. Otol Neurotol. 2012;33:572–9. https://doi.org/10.1097/MAO.0b013e3182544cdb.
41. Firszt JB, Reeder RM, Holden LK, Dwyer NY. Results in adult cochlear implant recipients with varied asymmetric hearing: a prospective longitudinal study of speech recognition, localization and participant report. Ear Hear. 2018;39:845–62. https://doi.org/10.1097/AUD.0000000000000548.
42. Kelsall D, Lupo J, Biever A. Longitudinal outcomes of cochlear implantation and bimodal hearing in a large group of adults: a multicenter clinical study. Am J Otolaryngol. 2021;42:102773. https://doi.org/10.1016/j.amjoto.2020.102773.
43. Cochlear implants and vaccination recommendations: information for public. CDC. 2022. https://www.cdc.gov/vaccines/vpd/mening/public/dis-cochlear-faq-gen.html. Accessed 11 Dec 2022.
44. Wanna GB, Noble JH, Carlson ML, et al. Impact of electrode design and surgical approach on scalar location and cochlear implant outcomes. Laryngoscope. 2014;124(Suppl 6):S1–7. https://doi.org/10.1002/lary.24728.
45. Holden LK, Finley CC, Firszt JB, et al. Factors affecting open-set word recognition in adults with cochlear implants. Ear Hear. 2013;34:342–60. https://doi.org/10.1097/AUD.0b013e3182741aa7.
46. Jwair S, Prins A, Wegner I, et al. Scalar translocation comparison between lateral wall and perimodiolar cochlear implant arrays - a meta-analysis. Laryngoscope. 2021;131:1358–68. https://doi.org/10.1002/lary.29224.
47. Nassiri AM, Yawn RJ, Holder JT, et al. Hearing preservation outcomes using a precurved electrode array inserted with an external sheath. Otol Neurotol. 2020;41:33–8. https://doi.org/10.1097/MAO.0000000000002426.
48. Buchman CA, Dillon MT, King ER, et al. Influence of cochlear implant insertion depth on performance: a prospective randomized trial. Otol Neurotol. 2014;35:1773–9. https://doi.org/10.1097/MAO.0000000000000541.
49. O'Connell BP, Hunter JB, Haynes DS, et al. Insertion depth impacts speech perception and hearing preservation for lateral wall electrodes. Laryngoscope. 2017;127:2352–7. https://doi.org/10.1002/lary.26467.
50. Canfarotta MW, Dillon MT, Brown KD, et al. Insertion depth and cochlear implant speech recognition outcomes: a comparative study of 28- and 31.5-mm lateral wall arrays. Otol Neurotol. 2022;43:183. https://doi.org/10.1097/MAO.0000000000003416.
51. Hochmair I, Arnold W, Nopp P, et al. Deep electrode insertion in cochlear implants: apical morphology, electrodes and speech perception results. Acta Otolaryngol. 2003;123:612–7.
52. Yukawa K, Cohen L, Blamey P, et al. Effects of insertion depth of cochlear implant electrodes upon speech perception. AUD. 2004;9:163–72. https://doi.org/10.1159/000077267.
53. Morrel WG, Holder JT, Dawant BM, et al. Effect of Scala tympani height on insertion depth of straight cochlear implant electrodes. Otolaryngol Head Neck Surg. 2020;162:718–24. https://doi.org/10.1177/0194599820904941.
54. Gifford RH, Dorman MF, Skarzynski H, et al. Cochlear implantation with hearing preservation yields significant benefit for speech recognition in complex listening environments. Ear Hear. 2013;34:413–25. https://doi.org/10.1097/AUD.0b013e31827e8163.
55. Gantz BJ, Dunn C, Oleson J, et al. Multicenter clinical trial of the Nucleus Hybrid S8 cochlear implant: final outcomes. Laryngoscope. 2016;126:962–73. https://doi.org/10.1002/lary.25572.
56. Lorens A, Polak M, Piotrowska A, Skarzynski H. Outcomes of treatment of partial deafness with cochlear implantation: a DUET study. Laryngoscope. 2008;118:288–94. https://doi.org/10.1097/MLG.0b013e3181598887.
57. Pillsbury HC, Dillon MT, Buchman CA, et al. Multicenter US clinical trial with an electric-acoustic stimulation (EAS) system in adults: final outcomes. Otol Neurotol. 2018;39:299–305. https://doi.org/10.1097/MAO.0000000000001691.
58. Helbig S, Adel Y, Rader T, et al. Long-term hearing preservation outcomes after cochlear implantation for electric-acoustic stimulation. Otol Neurotol. 2016;37:e353–9. https://doi.org/10.1097/MAO.0000000000001066.
59. O'Connell BP, Hunter JB, Wanna GB. The importance of electrode location in cochlear implantation. Laryngosc Investig Otolaryngol. 2016;1:169–74. https://doi.org/10.1002/lio2.42.
60. Sweeney AD, Carlson ML, Zuniga MG, et al. Impact of perioperative oral steroid use on low-frequency hearing preservation after cochlear implantation. Otol Neurotol. 2015;36:1480–5. https://doi.org/10.1097/MAO.0000000000000847.
61. Skarżyńska MB, Kołodziejak A, Gos E, et al. The clinical effect of steroids for hearing preservation in cochlear implantation: conclusions based on three cochlear implant systems and two administration regimes. Pharmaceuticals (Basel). 2022;15:1176. https://doi.org/10.3390/ph15101176.
62. Shaul C, Venkatagiri PK, Lo J, et al. Glucocorticoid for hearing preservation after cochlear implantation: a systemic review and meta-analysis of animal studies. Otol Neurotol. 2019;40:1178–85. https://doi.org/10.1097/MAO.0000000000002383.
63. Rajan GP, Kuthubutheen J, Hedne N, Krishnaswamy J. The role of preoperative, intratympanic glucocorticoids for hearing preservation in cochlear implantation: a prospective clinical study. Laryngoscope. 2012;122:190–5. https://doi.org/10.1002/lary.22142.
64. Laszig R, Ridder GJ, Fradis M. Intracochlear insertion of electrodes using hyaluronic acid in cochlear implant surgery. J Laryngol Otol. 2002;116:371–2. https://doi.org/10.1258/0022215021910816.
65. Torres R, Daoudi H, Lahlou G, et al. Restoration of high frequency auditory perception after robot-assisted or manual cochlear implantation in profoundly deaf adults improves speech recognition. Front Surg. 2021;10:8:729736.
66. Tarabichi O, Jensen M, Hansen MR. Advances in hearing preservation in cochlear implant surgery. Curr Opin Otolaryngol Head Neck Surg. 2021;29:385–90. https://doi.org/10.1097/MOO.0000000000000742.
67. Van de Heyning PH, Dazert S, Gavilan J, et al. Systematic literature review of hearing preservation rates in cochlear implantation associated with medium- and longer-length flexible lateral wall electrode arrays. Front Surg. 2022;9:893839. https://doi.org/10.3389/fsurg.2022.893839.
68. Bruce IA, Bates JEHM, Melling C, et al. Hearing preservation via a cochleostomy approach and deep insertion of a standard length cochlear implant electrode. Otol Neurotol. 2011;32:1444–7. https://doi.org/10.1097/MAO.0b013e3182355824.
69. Anne S, Ishman SL, Schwartz S. A systematic review of perioperative versus prophylactic antibiotics for cochlear implantation. Ann Otol Rhinol Laryngol. 2016;125:893–9. https://doi.org/10.1177/0003489416660113.
70. Košec A, Živko J, Marković S, et al. Impact of preoperative antibiotic use in preventing complications of cochlear implantation

surgery. Cochlear Implants Int. 2022;23:134–8. https://doi.org/10.1080/14670100.2021.2013586.

71. Hirsch BE, Blikas A, Whitaker M. Antibiotic prophylaxis in cochlear implant surgery. Laryngoscope. 2007;117:864–7. https://doi.org/10.1097/MLG.0b013e318033c2f9.
72. Sayed-Hassan A, Hermann R, Chidiac F, et al. Association of the duration of antibiotic therapy with major surgical site infection in cochlear implantation. JAMA Otolaryngol Head Neck Surg. 2019;145:14–20. https://doi.org/10.1001/jamaoto.2018.1998.
73. Almosnino G, Zeitler DM, Schwartz SR. Postoperative antibiotics following cochlear implantation: are they necessary? Ann Otol Rhinol Laryngol. 2018;127:266–9. https://doi.org/10.1177/0003489418758101.
74. Sweeney AD, Carlson ML, Valenzuela CV, et al. 228 cases of cochlear implant receiver-stimulator placement in a tight subperiosteal pocket without fixation. Otolaryngol Head Neck Surg. 2015;152:712–7. https://doi.org/10.1177/0194599814567111.
75. Jethanamest D, Channer GA, Moss WJ, et al. Cochlear implant fixation using a subperiosteal tight pocket without either suture or bone-recess technique. Laryngoscope. 2014;124:1674–7. https://doi.org/10.1002/lary.24426.
76. Maxwell AK, Cass SP. Cochlear implant receiver-stimulator migration using the subperiosteal pocket technique: objective measurements of early and late positioning. Otol Neurotol. 2019;40:328. https://doi.org/10.1097/MAO.0000000000002117.
77. Dodson KM, Maiberger PG, Sismanis A. Intracranial complications of cochlear implantation. Otol Neurotol. 2007;28:459. https://doi.org/10.1097/mao.0b013e31802fba94.
78. McMillan RA, Nassiri AM, Leonel LC, et al. The posterior ligament of the incus ("white dot"): a reliable surgical landmark for the facial recess. Am J Otolaryngol. 2022;43:103304. https://doi.org/10.1016/j.amjoto.2021.103304.
79. Jain S, Gaurkar S, Deshmukh PT, et al. Applied anatomy of round window and adjacent structures of tympanum related to cochlear implantation. Braz J Otorhinolaryngol. 2019;85:435–46. https://doi.org/10.1016/j.bjorl.2018.03.009.
80. Richard C, Fayad JN, Doherty J, Linthicum FH. Round window versus cochleostomy technique in cochlear implantation: histological findings. Otol Neurotol. 2012;33:1181–7. https://doi.org/10.1097/MAO.0b013e318263d56d.
81. Jiam NT, Jiradejvong P, Pearl MS, Limb CJ. The effect of round window vs cochleostomy surgical approaches on Cochlear implant electrode position: a flat-panel computed tomography study. JAMA Otolaryngol. 2016;142:873–80. https://doi.org/10.1001/jamaoto.2016.1512.
82. Avasarala VS, Jinka SK, Jeyakumar A. Complications of cochleostomy versus round window surgical approaches: a systematic review and meta-analysis. Cureus. 2022;14(5):e25451. https://doi.org/10.7759/cureus.25451.
83. Dedmon MM, O'Connell BP, Yawn RJ, Rivas A. Cochleostomy and facial recess packing alter cochlear implant electrode location in a human cochlea model. Am J Otolaryngol. 2018;39:489–92. https://doi.org/10.1016/j.amjoto.2018.05.008.
84. Gallant S, Friedmann DR, Hagiwara M, et al. Comparison of skull radiograph and computed tomography measurements of cochlear implant insertion angles. Otol Neurotol. 2019;40:e298–303. https://doi.org/10.1097/MAO.0000000000002121.
85. Cooper T, Hildrew D, McAfee JS, et al. Optimization of intraoperative imaging protocol to confirm placement of cochlear implant electrodes. Otol Neurotol. 2019;40:625–9. https://doi.org/10.1097/MAO.0000000000002200.
86. Hagr A, Garadat SN, Al-Momani M, et al. Feasibility of one-day activation in cochlear implant recipients. Int J Audiol. 2015;54:323–8. https://doi.org/10.3109/14992027.2014.996824.
87. Carlson ML, Neff BA, Link MJ, et al. Magnetic resonance imaging with cochlear implant magnet in place: safety and imaging quality. Otol Neurotol. 2015;36:965–71. https://doi.org/10.1097/MAO.0000000000000666.
88. Todt I, Rademacher G, Mittmann P, et al. MRI artifacts and cochlear implant positioning at 3 T in vivo. Otol Neurotol. 2015;36:972. https://doi.org/10.1097/MAO.0000000000000720.
89. Tien DA, Woodson EA, Anne S. Safety of monopolar electrocautery in patients with cochlear implants. Ann Otol Rhinol Laryngol. 2016;125:701–3. https://doi.org/10.1177/0003489416646792.
90. Poetker DM, Runge-Samuelson CL, Firszt JB, Wackym PA. Electrosurgery after cochlear implantation: eighth nerve electrophysiology. Laryngoscope. 2004;114:2252–4. https://doi.org/10.1097/01.mlg.0000149469.03575.91.
91. Page JC, Chapel AC, Silva RC, et al. Monopolar cautery use in pediatric cochlear implant users. Otolaryngol Head Neck Surg. 2022;1945998221108051 https://doi.org/10.1177/01945998221108051.
92. Cass ND, Lindquist NR, Bennett ML, Haynes DS. Monopolar electrosurgery with cochlear implants. Laryngoscope. 2023; 133(4):933–37. https://doi.org/10.1002/lary.30323.
93. Ikeya J, Kawano A, Nishiyama N, et al. Long-term complications after cochlear implantation. Auris Nasus Larynx. 2013;40:525–9. https://doi.org/10.1016/j.anl.2013.04.012.
94. Alzhrani F, Lenarz T, Teschner M. Taste sensation following cochlear implantation surgery. Cochlear Implants Int. 2013;14:200–6. https://doi.org/10.1179/1754762812Y.0000000018.
95. Bianchin G, Polizzi V, Formigoni P, et al. Cerebrospinal fluid leak in cochlear implantation: enlarged cochlear versus enlarged vestibular aqueduct (common cavity excluded). Int J Otolaryngol. 2016;2016:6591684. https://doi.org/10.1155/2016/6591684.
96. Filipo R, D'Elia C, Covelli E, et al. Haematoma after cochlear implantation: management of a minor complication. Acta Otolaryngol. 2010;130:108–13. https://doi.org/10.3109/00016480902939657.
97. Zaubitzer L, Schaefer E, Wallhaeuser-Franke E, et al. Methods for measuring pre-, intra-, and postoperative skin thickness for cochlear implants. J Otol. 2022;17:72–7. https://doi.org/10.1016/j.joto.2021.12.001.
98. Günther S, Baumann U, Stöver T. Early fitting in cochlear implantation: benefits and limits. Otol Neurotol. 2018;39:e250. https://doi.org/10.1097/MAO.0000000000001745.
99. Davids T, Ramsden JD, Gordon KA, et al. Soft tissue complications after small incision pediatric cochlear implantation. Laryngoscope. 2009;119:980–3. https://doi.org/10.1002/lary.20204.
100. Gawecki W, Karlik M, Borucki L, et al. Skin flap complications after cochlear implantations. Eur Arch Otorhinolaryngol. 2016;273:4175–83. https://doi.org/10.1007/s00405-016-4107-1.
101. Geraghty M, Fagan P, Moisidis E. Management of cochlear implant device extrusion: case series and literature review. J Laryngol Otol. 2014;128(Suppl):S55–8. https://doi.org/10.1017/S002221511300323X.
102. Lindquist NR, Vinh DB, Appelbaum EN, et al. Microvascular free tissue transfer and cochlear implants: a case series and literature review. Laryngoscope. 2020;130:1552–7. https://doi.org/10.1002/lary.28300.
103. Dietz A, Wennström M, Lehtimäki A, et al. Electrode migration after cochlear implant surgery: more common than expected? Eur Arch Otorhinolaryngol. 2016;273:1411–8. https://doi.org/10.1007/s00405-015-3716-4.
104. Lindquist NR, Cass ND, Patro A, et al. HiRes ultra series recall: failure rates and revision speech recognition outcomes.

Otol Neurotol. 2022;43:e738–45. https://doi.org/10.1097/MAO.0000000000003598.
105. Lane C, Zimmerman K, Agrawal S, Parnes L. Cochlear implant failures and reimplantation: a 30-year analysis and literature review. Laryngoscope. 2020;130:782–9. https://doi.org/10.1002/lary.28071.
106. Wang JT, Wang AY, Psarros C, et al. Rates of revision and device failure in cochlear implant surgery: A 30-year experience. Laryngoscope. 2014;124(10):2393–9. https://doi.org/10.1002/lary.24649.
107. Stevens SM, Dougherty H, Wenstrup L, et al. Is hard failure still a common indication for revision surgery in adult cochlear implant recipients? Otol Neurotol. 2019;40:321. https://doi.org/10.1097/MAO.0000000000002118.
108. Balkany TJ, Hodges AV, Buchman CA, et al. Cochlear implant soft failures consensus development conference statement. Otol Neurotol. 2005;26:815–8. https://doi.org/10.1097/01.mao.0000178150.44505.52.
109. Enticott JC, Tari S, Koh SM, et al. Cochlear implant and vestibular function. Otol Neurotol. 2006;27:824. https://doi.org/10.1097/01.mao.0000227903.47483.a6.
110. Hänsel T, Gauger U, Bernhard N, et al. Meta-analysis of subjective complaints of vertigo and vestibular tests after cochlear implantation. Laryngoscope. 2018;128:2110–23. https://doi.org/10.1002/lary.27071.
111. Melvin T-AN, Della Santina CC, Carey JP, Migliaccio AA. The effects of cochlear implantation on vestibular function. Otol Neurotol. 2009;30:87–94.
112. Buchman CA, Joy J, Hodges A, Telischi FF, Balkany TJ. Vestibular effects of cochlear implantation. Laryngoscope. 2004;114 https://doi.org/10.1097/00005537-200410001-00001.
113. Woodson EA, Aaron K, Nguyen-Huynh A, et al. Mythbusters! The truth about common misconceptions in cochlear implantation. Semin Hear. 2021;42:352–64. https://doi.org/10.1055/s-0041-1739368.
114. Ibrahim I, da Silva SD, Segal B, Zeitouni A. Effect of cochlear implant surgery on vestibular function: meta-analysis study. J Otolaryngol Head Neck Surg. 2017;46:44. https://doi.org/10.1186/s40463-017-0224-0.
115. Bigelow DC, Kay DJ, Rafter KO, et al. Facial nerve stimulation from cochlear implants. Am J Otol. 1998;19:163–9.
116. Espahbodi M, Sweeney AD, Lennon KJ, Wanna GB. Facial nerve stimulation associated with cochlear implant use following temporal bone fractures. Am J Otolaryngol. 2015;36:578–82. https://doi.org/10.1016/j.amjoto.2015.04.003.
117. Berrettini S, Vito A, Bruschini L, et al. Facial nerve stimulation after cochlear implantation: our experience. Acta Otorhinolaryngol Ital. 2011;31:11–6.
118. Hoppe U, Hocke T, Hast A, Iro H. Maximum preimplantation monosyllabic score as predictor of cochlear implant outcome. HNO. 2019;67:62–8. https://doi.org/10.1007/s00106-019-0648-0.
119. NIH consensus conference. Cochlear implants in adults and children. JAMA. 1995;274:1955–61.
120. McRackan TR, Hand BN, Cochlear Implant Quality of Life Development Consortium, et al. Cochlear implant quality of life (CIQOL): development of a profile instrument (CIQOL-35 profile) and a global measure (CIQOL-10 global). J Speech Lang Hear Res. 2019;62:3554–63. https://doi.org/10.1044/2019_JSLHR-H-19-0142.
121. McRackan TR, Hand BN, Velozo CA, et al. Development of the cochlear implant quality of life item bank. Ear Hear. 2019;40:1016–24. https://doi.org/10.1097/AUD.0000000000000684.
122. Goudey B, Plant K, Kiral I, et al. A multi-center analysis of factors associated with hearing outcome for 2,735 adults with cochlear implants. Trends Hear. 2021;25:23312165211037525. https://doi.org/10.1177/23312165211037525.
123. Zhao EE, Dornhoffer JR, Loftus C, et al. Association of patient-related factors with adult cochlear implant speech recognition outcomes: a meta-analysis. JAMA Otolaryngol. 2020;146:613–20. https://doi.org/10.1001/jamaoto.2020.0662.
124. Cheng Y-S, Svirsky MA. Meta-analysis—correlation between spiral ganglion cell counts and speech perception with a cochlear implant. Audiol Res. 2021;11:220–6. https://doi.org/10.3390/audiolres11020020.
125. Kramer S, Vasil KJ, Adunka OF, et al. Cognitive functions in adult Cochlear implant users, Cochlear implant candidates, and Normal-hearing listeners. Laryngosc Investig Otolaryngol. 2018;3:304–10. https://doi.org/10.1002/lio2.172.
126. Moberly AC. A surgeon-scientist's perspective and review of cognitive-linguistic contributions to adult cochlear implant outcomes. Laryngosc Investig Otolaryngol. 2020;5:1176–83. https://doi.org/10.1002/lio2.494.
127. Finley CC, Holden TA, Holden LK, et al. Role of electrode placement as a contributor to variability in cochlear implant outcomes. Otol Neurotol. 2008;29:920–8. https://doi.org/10.1097/MAO.0b013e318184f492.
128. Incerti PV, Ching TYC, Cowan R. A systematic review of electric-acoustic stimulation: device fitting ranges, outcomes, and clinical fitting practices. Trends Amplif. 2013;17:3–26. https://doi.org/10.1177/1084713813480857.
129. Gifford RH, Davis TJ, Sunderhaus LW, et al. Combined electric and acoustic stimulation with hearing preservation: effect of Cochlear implant low-frequency Cutoff on speech understanding and perceived listening difficulty. Ear Hear. 2017;38:539–53. https://doi.org/10.1097/AUD.0000000000000418.
130. Dornhoffer JR, Reddy P, Ma C, et al. Use of auditory training and its influence on early Cochlear implant outcomes in adults. Otol Neurotol. 2022;43:e165. https://doi.org/10.1097/MAO.0000000000003417.
131. Chow K, Kaul VF, Levine-Madoff J, et al. Does auditory environment predict speech perception outcomes in elderly Cochlear implant patients? Audiol Neurootol. 2021;26:378–86. https://doi.org/10.1159/000513637.
132. Holder JT, Gifford RH. Effect of increased daily Cochlear implant use on auditory perception in adults. J Speech Lang Hear Res. 2021;64:4044–55. https://doi.org/10.1044/2021_JSLHR-21-00066.
133. Holder JT, Dwyer NC, Gifford RH. Duration of processor use per day is significantly correlated with speech recognition abilities in adults with Cochlear implants. Otol Neurotol. 2020;41:e227–31. https://doi.org/10.1097/MAO.0000000000002477.
134. Shearer AE, Hansen MR. Auditory synaptopathy, auditory neuropathy, and cochlear implantation. Laryngosc Investig Otolaryngol. 2019;4:429–40. https://doi.org/10.1002/lio2.288.
135. De Siati RD, Rosenzweig F, Gersdorff G, et al. Auditory neuropathy spectrum disorders: from diagnosis to treatment: literature review and case reports. J Clin Med. 2020;9:1074. https://doi.org/10.3390/jcm9041074.
136. Lubner RJ, Knoll RM, Trakimas DR, et al. Long-term cochlear implantation outcomes in patients following head injury. Laryngosc Investig Otolaryngol. 2020;5:485–96. https://doi.org/10.1002/lio2.378.
137. Lindquist NR, Stapp M, Choi JS, et al. Cochlear implantation after traumatic brain injury without otic capsule fracture: a case report and literature review. Am J Otolaryngol. 2020;41:102512. https://doi.org/10.1016/j.amjoto.2020.102512.
138. Carlson ML, Breen JT, Driscoll CL, et al. Cochlear implantation in patients with neurofibromatosis type 2: variables affecting auditory performance. Otol Neurotol. 2012;33:853–62. https://doi.org/10.1097/MAO.0b013e318254fba5.

139. Lustig LR, Yeagle J, Driscoll CLW, et al. Cochlear implantation in patients with neurofibromatosis type 2 and bilateral vestibular schwannoma. Otol Neurotol. 2006;27:512. https://doi.org/10.1097/01.mao.0000217351.86925.51.
140. Patel NS, Carlson ML, Link MJ, et al. Cochlear implantation after radiosurgery for vestibular schwannoma. J Neurosurg. 2021;135:126–35. https://doi.org/10.3171/2020.4.JNS201069.
141. Longino ES, Manzoor NF, Cass ND, et al. Cochlear implantation outcomes in observed vestibular schwannoma: a preliminary report. Otolaryngol Head Neck Surg. 2022;167:149–54. https://doi.org/10.1177/01945998211045903.
142. Singhal K, Singhal J, Muzaffar J, et al. Outcomes of Cochlear implantation in patients with post-meningitis deafness: a systematic review and narrative synthesis. J Int Adv Otol. 2020;16:395–410. https://doi.org/10.5152/iao.2020.9040.
143. Teoh SW, Pisoni DB, Miyamoto RT. Cochlear implantation in adults with prelingual deafness. Part I clinical results. Laryngoscope. 2004;114:1536–40. https://doi.org/10.1097/00005537-200409000-00006.
144. Chao TN, Levi J, O'Reilly RC. How old is too old for cochlear implantation for congenital bilateral sensorineural hearing loss? Laryngoscope. 2018;128:2221–2. https://doi.org/10.1002/lary.27134.
145. Straatman LV, Huinck WJ, Langereis MC, et al. Cochlear implantation in late-implanted prelingually deafened adults: changes in quality of life. Otol Neurotol. 2014;35:253–9. https://doi.org/10.1097/MAO.0b013e3182a4758e.
146. Ovari A, Hühnlein L, Nguyen-Dalinger D, et al. Functional outcomes and quality of life after cochlear implantation in patients with long-term deafness. J Clin Med. 2022;11:5156. https://doi.org/10.3390/jcm11175156.
147. Brown KD, Balkany TJ. Benefits of bilateral cochlear implantation: a review. Curr Opin Otolaryngol Head Neck Surg. 2007;15:315–8. https://doi.org/10.1097/MOO.0b013e3282ef3d3e.
148. Wanna GB, Gifford RH, McRackan TR, et al. Bilateral cochlear implantation. Otolaryngol Clin N Am. 2012;45:81–9. https://doi.org/10.1016/j.otc.2011.08.018.
149. Gifford RH, Dorman MF. Bimodal hearing or bilateral cochlear implants? Ask the patient. Ear Hear. 2019;40:501. https://doi.org/10.1097/AUD.0000000000000657.
150. Misztal C, Peña S, Martinez D, et al. Comparison of speech test outcomes after Cochlear implantation in patients with and without asymmetric hearing loss. Otol Neurotol. 2022;43:559–66. https://doi.org/10.1097/MAO.0000000000003515.
151. Sydlowski SA, Farrokhian N, Carrozza M, et al. (Even off-label) cochlear implantation in single-sided deafness and asymmetric hearing loss results in measurable objective and subjective benefit. Otol Neurotol. 2022;43:e895–902. https://doi.org/10.1097/MAO.0000000000003623.
152. Spitzer ER, Waltzman SB, Landsberger DM, Friedmann DR. Acceptance and benefits of electro-acoustic stimulation for conventional-length electrode arrays. AUD. 2021;26:17–26. https://doi.org/10.1159/000507975.
153. Gifford RH, Grantham DW, Sheffield SW, et al. Localization and interaural time difference (ITD) thresholds for cochlear implant recipients with preserved acoustic hearing in the implanted ear. Hear Res. 2014;312:28–37. https://doi.org/10.1016/j.heares.2014.02.007.
154. Perkins E, Lee J, Manzoor N, et al. The reality of hearing preservation in cochlear implantation: who is utilizing EAS? Otol Neurotol. 2021;42:832–7. https://doi.org/10.1097/MAO.0000000000003074.
155. Van de Heyning P, Vermeire K, Diebl M, et al. Incapacitating unilateral tinnitus in single-sided deafness treated by cochlear implantation. Ann Otol Rhinol Laryngol. 2008;117:645–52. https://doi.org/10.1177/000348940811700903.
156. Peter N, Liyanage N, Pfiffner F, et al. The influence of cochlear implantation on tinnitus in patients with single-sided deafness: a systematic review. Otolaryngol Head Neck Surg. 2019;161:576–88. https://doi.org/10.1177/0194599819846084.
157. Levy DA, Lee JA, Nguyen SA, et al. Cochlear implantation for treatment of tinnitus in single-sided deafness: a systematic review and meta-analysis. Otol Neurotol. 2020;41:e1004–12. https://doi.org/10.1097/MAO.0000000000002711.
158. Ramakers GGJ, van Zon A, Stegeman I, Grolman W. The effect of cochlear implantation on tinnitus in patients with bilateral hearing loss: a systematic review. Laryngoscope. 2015;125:2584–92. https://doi.org/10.1002/lary.25370.
159. van Zon A, Smulders YE, Ramakers GGJ, et al. Effect of unilateral and simultaneous bilateral cochlear implantation on tinnitus: a prospective study. Laryngoscope. 2016;126:956–61. https://doi.org/10.1002/lary.25493.
160. Cowan B, Oska S, Arianpour K, et al. A systematic review of cochlear implantation in temporal bone fractures and the significance of otic capsule involvement. Otol Neurotol. 2020;41:1309. https://doi.org/10.1097/MAO.0000000000002779.
161. Caye-Thomasen P, Dam MS, Omland SH, Mantoni M. Cochlear ossification in patients with profound hearing loss following bacterial meningitis. Acta Otolaryngol. 2012;132:720–5. https://doi.org/10.3109/00016489.2012.656323.
162. Isaacson B, Roland PS, Wright CG. Anatomy of the middle-turn cochleostomy. Laryngoscope. 2008;118:2200–4. https://doi.org/10.1097/MLG.0b013e318182ee1c.
163. Millar DA, Hillman TA, Shelton C. Implantation of the ossified cochlear: management with the split electrode array. Laryngoscope. 2005;115:2155–60. https://doi.org/10.1097/01.MLG.0000181494.21654.5E.
164. Kiefer J, Weber A, Pfennigdorff T, von Ilberg C. Scala vestibuli insertion in cochlear implantation: a valuable alternative for cases with obstructed scalar tympani. ORL J Otorhinolaryngol Relat Spec. 2000;62:251–6. https://doi.org/10.1159/000027755.
165. Balkany T, Bird PA, Hodges AV, et al. Surgical technique for implantation of the totally ossified cochlear. Laryngoscope. 1998;108:988–92. https://doi.org/10.1097/00005537-199807000-00007.
166. El-Kashlan HK, Telian SA. Cochlear implantation in the chronically diseased ear. Curr Opin Otolaryngol Head Neck Surg. 2004;12:384–6. https://doi.org/10.1097/01.moo.0000134439.99357.c9.
167. Free RH, Falcioni M, Di Trapani G, et al. The role of subtotal petrosectomy in cochlear implant surgery–a report of 32 cases and review on indications. Otol Neurotol. 2013;34:1033. https://doi.org/10.1097/MAO.0b013e318289841b.
168. Hunter JB, Fernando SJ, Bennett ML, et al. Cochlear implantation in canal wall down mastoid cavities. Otolaryngol Head Neck Surg. 2016;155:312–6. https://doi.org/10.1177/0194599816641064.
169. Hunter JB, O'Connell BP, Wanna GB. Systematic review and meta-analysis of surgical complications following cochlear implantation in canal wall down mastoid cavities. Otolaryngol Head Neck Surg. 2016;155:555–63. https://doi.org/10.1177/0194599816651239.
170. Szymański M, Ataide A, Linder T. The use of subtotal petrosectomy in cochlear implant candidates with chronic otitis media. Eur Arch Otorhinolaryngol. 2016;273:363–70. https://doi.org/10.1007/s00405-015-3573-1.
171. Reis M, Boisvert I, Looi V, da Cruz M. Speech recognition outcomes after Cochlear reimplantation surgery. Trends Hear. 2017;21:2331216517706398. https://doi.org/10.1177/2331216517706398.

Inner Ear Pathology for the Cochlear Implant Surgeon

21

Ophir Handzel, Omar Ungar, and Alicia M. Quesnel

Introduction

Cochlear implantation (CI) is the treatment of choice for most patients with severe to profound sensorineural hearing loss and insufficient benefit from hearing aids. In 2022, it was estimated that one million people worldwide had received cochlear implants (CIs) [85]. Indications for implantation continue to expand. Current candidates include children as young as 9 months old, children and adults with single-sided deafness, some types of malformed cochleae, and those with residual low-frequency hearing. When residual hearing is preserved after CI, patients benefit from simultaneous acoustic and electric stimulation in the same ear and may have improved word understanding in noise and in quiet [71]. In most countries, the population is aging. Since the incidence of hearing loss increases dramatically after the age of 65 years, the portion of the general population expected to meet the audiometric criteria for CI continues to increase [14].

Although most patients benefit significantly from CI with improved speech understanding and communication capabilities, the results vary significantly between recipients. The factors determining CI performance are only partially known. Some of the variance in outcome may be attributed to the etiology of hearing loss, residual function of the cochlea, duration of deafness, age at implantation, and central factors such as neural plasticity and cognition [5, 61, 68, 78]. However, some variance in outcome is also likely attributable to the neural substrate of the cochlea [78] and the pathologic response in the cochlea to implantation, both of which may impact the quality of the electrode-neuron interface.

Human temporal bones (TBs) from patients who had been implanted during life and donated their temporal bones to scientific study are an invaluable source for understanding the consequences of CI and the pathophysiology of hearing loss in implanted patients. The histopathologic study of these specimens provides an essential perspective on the cochlear microanatomy in humans, immediate surgical trauma after CI, and long-term histopathologic effects of implantation. These studies may help inform surgical methods and guide CI electrode design. Human TB studies, for example, have aided the understanding of the intricate three-dimensional anatomy of the cochlea adjacent to the round window [42]. Understanding this level of anatomical detail is helpful for CI surgeons, especially for the round window insertion technique. In addition, human TB specimens enable investigation of the long-term effects of CI in humans, including inflammatory, immune, and foreign body responses to CI [59]. Insights from histopathology after CI may be useful in improving hearing preservation surgical methods and in developing personalized CI programming strategies [64], which are two current areas of research aimed at improving CI outcomes.

Successful processing of human temporal bones is labor- and time-intensive and requires experience and specialized equipment and skills. Large amounts of dense bone, particularly in the otic capsule, mandate histologic preparation procedures, which are unique compared to other tissues of the human body. Although new techniques are being developed, the traditional method, which yields excellent histologic morphology, requires approximately 6–9 months for decalcification and typically utilizes celloidin as the embedding material. Cutting the specimens with the electrode array left in situ is challenging and can lead to artifactual disruption of the tissue. Hence, in most cases, the electrode is gently removed after the embedment has been completed but before the bone is sectioned. In essentially all cases, a fibrous capsule develops around the electrode, and therefore, the location of the implant can be readily and accurately determined

O. Handzel
Department of Otolaryngology, University of Rochester, Rochester, NY, USA

O. Ungar
Department of Otolaryngology, Tel Aviv Sourasky Medical Center and Tel Aviv University, Tel Aviv, Israel

A. M. Quesnel (✉)
Department of Otolaryngology—Head and Neck Surgery, Harvard Medical School, Boston, MA, USA
e-mail: alicia_quesnel@meei.harvard.edu

A. D. Sweeney et al. (eds.), *Haynes-Glasscock-Shambaugh Surgery of the Ear*, https://doi.org/10.1007/978-3-032-18264-7_21

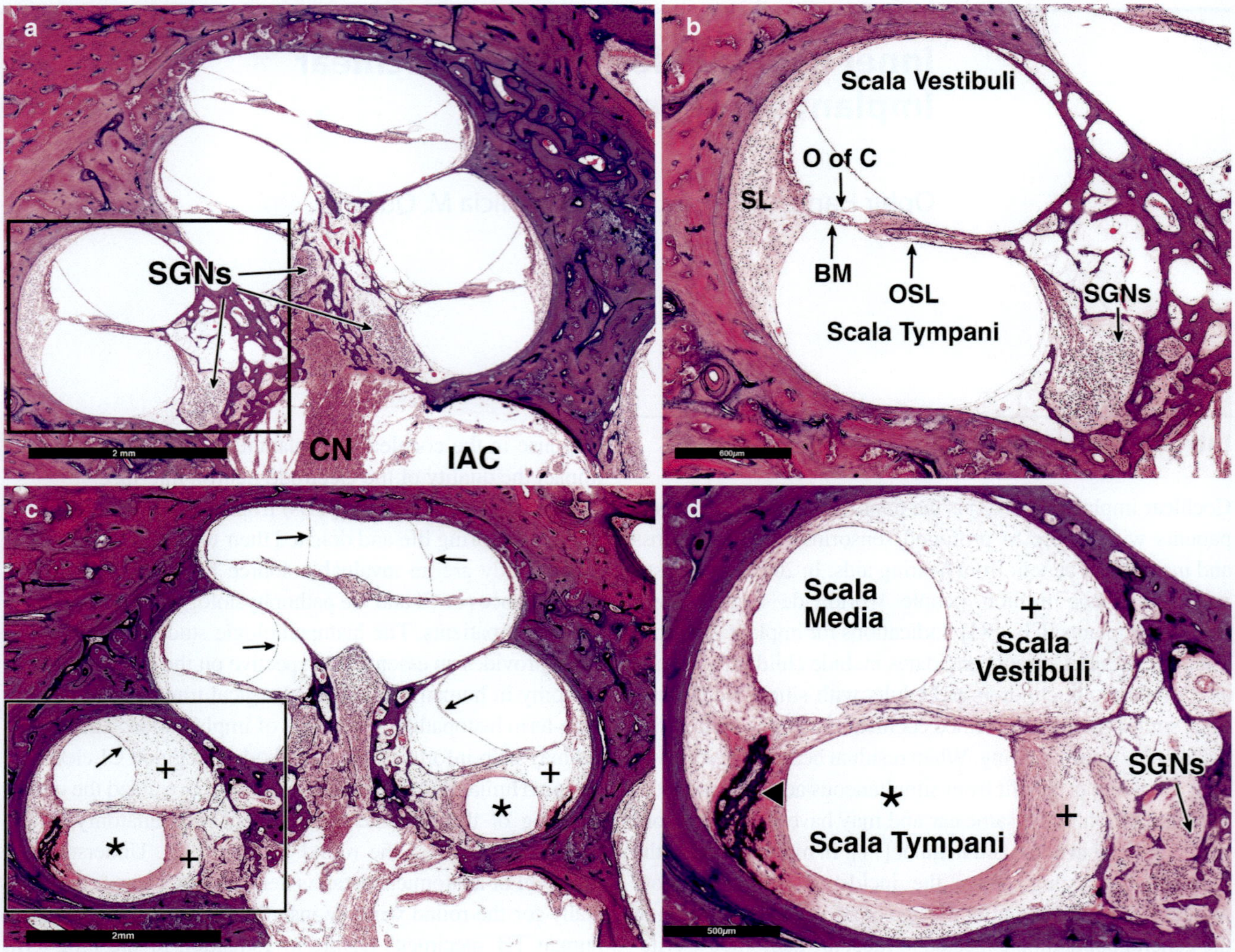

Fig. 21.1 Normal human cochlea (**a**, **b**) versus an implanted human cochlea (**c**, **d**). (**a**) Normal cochlea approximate mid-modiolar section, low magnification (scale bar = 2 mm). (**b**) Higher magnification of cross-section through basal turn of cochlea shown in boxed area of A (scale bar = 600 μm). (**c**) An implanted human cochlea (Advanced Bionics helix electrode) approximate mid-modiolar section, low magnification (scale bar = 2 mm). The electrode array was removed before the specimen was sectioned. The electrode array tract is apparent (*) due to the fibrous sheath. There is fibrous tissue (+) and new bone growth. Endolymphatic hydrops is present throughout the cochlea, indicated by the distorted position of the Reissner's membrane (arrows). (**d**) Higher magnification of cross section through basal turn of cochlea shown in boxed area of C (scale bar = 500 μm). The electrode array tract (*) with surrounding fibrous tissue (+) in the scala vestibuli and scala tympani is shown, along with new bone growth (arrowhead) at the lateral cochlear wall. SGNs spiral ganglion neuron cell bodies, CN cochlear nerve, IAC internal auditory canal, SL spiral ligament, OSL osseous spiral lamina containing the peripheral axons of the SGNs, BM basilar membrane, O of C organ of Corti. (Horizontal sections, H&E stain)

in the histologic sections (Fig. 21.1). For all its virtues, utilizing human TBs for investigation does reflect older cochlear implant models and surgical techniques. From the time of surgery to the death of the donor, years and decades may elapse. In the example presented in the figures of this chapter, we have made an effort to represent implant designs that are relevant to those currently in clinical use.

This chapter focuses on some of the most critical insights from studying implanted human temporal bone histopathology. We have selected findings with clinical and surgical implications, emphasizing data that cannot be collected with other techniques. The data presented regarding the anatomy of the human cochlea and the response to implantation has been used in debates, such as in favor of lateral wall versus perimodiolar electrodes and longer versus shorter electrode arrays, to name just two of the debates related to optimizing outcomes of CI. The readers are encouraged to evaluate the evidence presented in the chapter with these implications in mind.

Anatomy of the Inner Ear

Cochlear Size and Shape

Knowledge of the exact shape and dimensions of the cochlea and Rosenthal's canal is essential for cochlear implant electrode array design, its introduction to the cochlea, and optimal placement. As the basis for sound perception is the organ of Corti, the length and coiling of the cochlear duct (CD) are commonly used to represent the dimensions of the cochlea. The parasagittal length of the average human cochlea is about 9 mm [56, 84]. The CD coils for 2.5–2.9 turns (rarely for three complete turns). CD length averages 33 mm but can vary widely from 31 to 42 mm [60]. Another study found the CD length to vary from 35.4 mm to 43.57 mm, with no intergender difference [12]. A review article concluded that the average observed length of the male cochlea is about 34 mm, and the average observed length of the female cochlea is about 33 mm. Still, the observed sex difference in cochlear length is small compared to the observed variability of the lengths of normal cochleae [44]. The wide variability in CD length is one reason it can be advantageous to obtain a preimplantation CT scan and compute the length of the CD. The two cochleae of the same person tend to be of similar size and shape [12, 60]. This can influence electrode choice when implanting a second ear based on the outcome of the electrode array placed in the first ear.

Detailed imaging-derived measurement of a patient's CD length can dictate the length of an electrode array, which may optimize chances for hearing preservation and CI performance [75]. Of note, the radius of the lateral wall of the scala tympani can be almost twice as long as the radius of medial wall of the scala tympani. Therefore, depending on the medial to lateral position of the electrode within the scala tympani, the same length electrode may terminate at a much different angular insertion depth as measured from the round window [12]. For example, the tip of a 26 mm lateral wall electrode array will not necessarily be located deeper than an 18 mm modiolar hugging electrode array.

For optimal outcomes, the electrode array is placed in the scala tympani [52] and should remain in that compartment. Fujiwara et al. measured the cross-sectional area and height of the scala tympani from three-dimensional (3D) reconstruction of horizontal histological preparations of ten temporal bones [17]. The vertical height of the scala tympani at its lateral wall significantly decreased from 1.28 to 0.88 mm from 0 to 180°, and the perimodiolar height decreased from 1.20 to 0.85 mm. The cross-sectional area decreased from 2.29 mm^2 (standard deviation, 0.60) to 1.38 mm^2 (standard deviation, 0.13) from 0 to 180° ($p < 0.001$). After 360°, the scala tympani shape transitioned from an ovoid to a triangular shape, corresponding with a significantly decreased lateral height relative to perimodiolar height. These measurements influence the location of both perimodiolar and lateral cochlear wall electrode arrays along the scala tympani and in relation to the spiral ganglion neurons (SGN).

The spiral ganglion neurons, which are the primary auditory neurons and the target for CI electrical stimulation, are located in Rosenthal's canal. This bony canal is 13.7 mm long [72] on average, and it coils for 1.5–1.8 turns [3]. On average, Rosenthal's canal linear length is 34–46% of the total CD length. The 26% apical most CD is innervated by SGN located more basally [12].

The length of CD and the length of RC can be expressed by the angle from the round window as suggested by a consensus panel [82]. The round window is the reference point (assigned a 0°). Intracochlear structures and electrode array depth can be expressed in degrees of angular length. An example of the advantage of this measurement technique is allowing comparison of the depth of location of a lateral cochlear wall to perimodiolar electrodes.

Due to inconsistencies of the TB "cutting angle" (the angle between the sectioning plane and modiolar axes) two-dimensional Rosenthal's canal (RC) reconstruction might miss the distal, projecting portion of the RC toward the helicotrema [34]. Recent three-dimensional cochlear reconstructions have demonstrated that RC is projected apically in a trajectory that travels centrally with little radial extension, which is missed in a two-dimensional cochlear reconstruction. Hence, SGNs are present more apically along the cochlear duct than a two-dimensional reconstruction can perceive [41]. Recently, optimized three-dimensional reconstruction techniques using digitized human temporal bone histopathologic sections can utilize mathematical alignment algorithms and machine learning to faithfully translate RC and SGNs back to three-dimensional reconstructions [18, 19, 80].

Histology is currently the only method to count the number of spiral ganglion neurons, evaluate the dendrites connecting the inner hair cells to the neuron cell body, and look for morphological changes in the SGN cell bodies. The normal cochlea of a child has more than 30,000 spiral ganglion neurons residing in Rosenthal's canal [46]. However, even in normal-hearing patients, it can vary considerably, between 23,910 and 33,702 [10, 11]. In a review article, it was shown that the apical quadrant of RC or segment IV of the cochlea accounts for approximately 25–30% of the entire SGN population, regardless of the cochlear condition (normal vs. pathologic) [10, 11]. Aging, noise, genetics, infections [48], congenital anomalies [46], and multiple other known [10, 11] and unknown factors result in a decline in the number of primary auditory neurons.

The Round Window Region

Currently, cochlear implants are inserted using one of three approaches in most non-malformed inner ears. These approaches include directly through the round window (RW), through a drilled opening adjacent to and incorporating the RW (called extended round window approach) or through a separate drilled opening near the RW (called a cochleostomy approach). Therefore, the RW and its surrounding structures are the sites of penetration of the implant array, and detailed anatomical knowledge of this area may aid the surgeon. The anatomy of the RW comprises the bone framework of the otic capsule, the RW membrane (Fig. 21.2), the commonly present fibrous and soft tissue in the niche [1], and the intricate intracochlear bone and soft tissues.

From the surgeon's view through the mastoid and the facial recess, the RW membrane is most commonly partially or completely hidden from view and direct access by the operculum of the niche (mostly by the posterior pillar) (Fig. 21.3). RW pseudomembranes (false membranes) may be present (Fig. 21.2) or soft tissue may occupy the RW niche. In one study, 11% of the ears were found to have fibrous tissue or a fat plug, and 21% had an extraneous (false) round window membrane [1]. Adequate access to the RW requires the removal of the surrounding bone (Figs. 21.2 and 21.3). Medial to the RW and in close proximity to it are two additional important structures. The cochlear aqueduct, which connects the perilymphatic scala tympani space to the cerebrospinal fluid containing posterior fossa space and lies close to the RW, may be impacted by the post-CI inflammatory response (Figs. 21.3 and 21.4). The ductus reuniens is closely related to the posterior margin of the RW membrane (RWM), whereas the inferior cochlear vein and cochlear aqueduct are closely related to the inferior margin of the RWM [42]. To avoid the basilar membrane and osseous spiral lamina, the trajectory of the implant from a round window approach should be slanted inferiorly (Figs. 21.2 and 21.3). The scala tympani tapers toward the RW, while the distance to the spiral ligament, basilar membrane, and osseous spiral lamina quickly decreases. The center point of the RW is 0.5 mm away from the primary osseous spiral lamina and the basilar membrane [42]. They are located superior to the central point of the RW and can be avoided by a more inferior trajectory that introduces the electrode array parallel to these structures. RW insertion can avoid the ductus reuniens and the entrance to the adjacent cochlear vein.

The cochlear aqueduct originates from the scala tympani at the inferior aspect of the basal turn, in close proximity to the round window. At this location, the cochlear aqueduct is at risk of direct injury from implantation and the effect of subsequent new fibrous and bone formation. In a study of 101 TBs from donors of variable ages, the cochlear duct was narrowest near its cochlear end and widened progressively as it traversed the otic capsule in an inferior direction toward the subarachnoid space [21]. It was found to be occluded or obliterated by the bone in 7% of the human TBs studied.

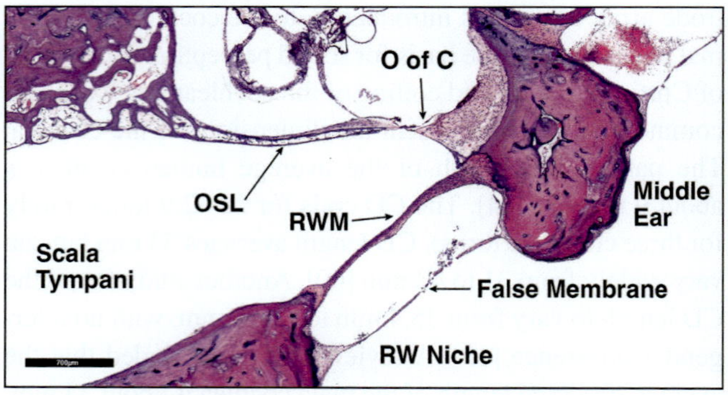

Fig. 21.2 The round window area shown in a histologic section in an approximate Stenver's plane. Notice the relationship and proximity of the round window membrane (RWM) to the adjacent osseous spiral lamina (OSL) and organ of Corti (O of C) in this specimen. While the organ of Corti is mostly degenerated in this specimen, the location is shown to indicate proximity to potential pathway of a cochlear implant electrode. A false membrane (arrow), also called pseudomembrane, is present in the round window niche. (Parasagittal section similar to Stenver's plane, H&E stain, scale bar = 700 μm)

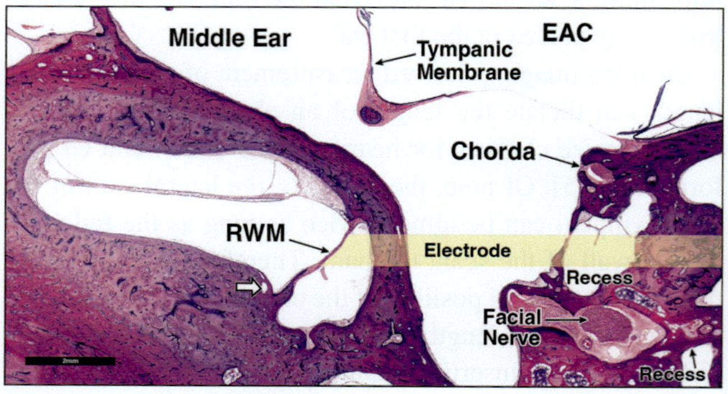

Fig. 21.3 The facial recess approach and round window area. The approximate pathway of a cochlear implant electrode is sketched in light gray. The round window niche (Niche), round window membrane (RWM), and anatomy just medial to the RWM are shown. The entrance to the cochlear aqueduct (black arrow) and accompanying vein (white arrow) can be seen near the RWM. The approach through the facial recess (Recess) can be appreciated, with the chorda tympani nerve (Chorda) laterally and the facial nerve medially. The cochlear vein (open arrow) is seen adjacent to the opening for the cochlear aqueduct just inside the scala tympani near the RWM (Horizontal section, H&E stain)

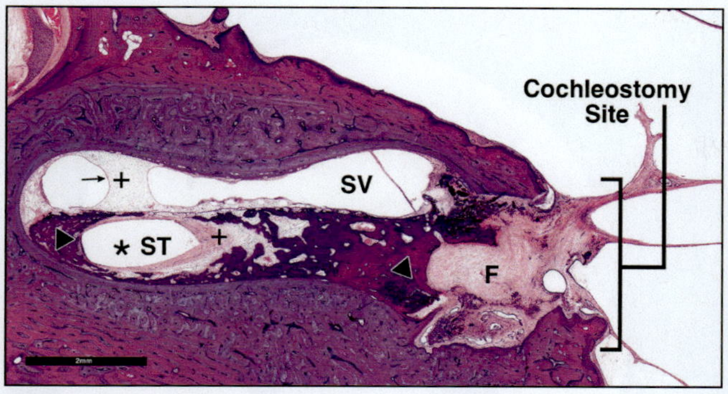

Fig. 21.4 Typical pathologic changes in the basal turn of the cochlea near the cochleostomy site from a donor who received a cochlear implant during life, with the electrode successfully introduced into the scala tympani. Abundant new bone formation (arrowheads), fibrous tissue deposition (+), hydrops (arrow indicates Reissner's membrane), electrode tract (*), and a fibrous plug (F) at the cochleostomy are apparent. ST scala tympani, SV scala vestibuli (horizontal section, H&E stain, scale bar = 2 mm)

Intracochlear Effect of Implantation and Response to the Electrode Array

Acute Injury Patterns Due to Insertion Trauma

CI involves opening the cochlea and the surgical introduction of the electrode array to the perilymphatic space, preferably the scala tympani. Acute injury refers to the mechanical trauma caused by the surgical opening of the cochlea and the passage of the array. This may include injury to the lateral cochlear wall, the osseous spiral lamina and adjacent structures or even the modiolus in rare circumstances. Injuries to the lateral cochlear wall include penetration of the spiral ligament (Fig. 21.5a, b), direct trauma to the cochlear endosteum on the bony lateral cochlea wall, and translocation through the spiral ligament from one scala to another. Injuries to the osseous spiral lamina (Fig. 21.5c, d) may be associated with trauma to the dendrites of the SGNs that pass through the osseous spiral lamina, the basilar membrane, and the organ of Corti structures such as the hair cells, supporting cells, and/or tectorial membrane. Electrodes may also translocate medially in the scala tympani by penetrating through the osseous spiral lamina and/or basilar membrane (Fig. 21.6). Some degree of intracochlear trauma seems inevitable, but it can be reduced or minimized.

In a study of 21 implanted human TBs, acute trauma patterns were segregated by electrode design (Fig. 21.7). The perimodiolar electrodes were more commonly associated with osseous spiral lamina fracture (at an average of ~120° angular insertion) and were less often associated with spiral ligament perforation at the lateral wall. In contrast, the straight electrodes were associated with spiral ligament perforation (most commonly at ~170° angular insertion), and no instances of osseous spiral lamina fracture were seen with straight electrodes [20].

Long-Term Sequelae

Cochlear implants are designed to be introduced and left in place for the recipient's life. CI is approved by the FDA for patients as young as 9 months old, and there is evidence that activation of implants at an age younger than 9 months old can result in better outcomes [9]. Accordingly, the effects of implantation and the host's response to its introduction and presence in the inner ear must be analyzed with respect to decades of implantation and use. TBs implanted premortem are an excellent model for studying these long-term effects.

Fibrous Tissue and New Bone Formation

The most striking histological observation in TBs after CI is new soft tissue and bone formation that develops within the cochlea and the fibrous tissue sheath surrounding the electrode array (Fig. 21.1c, d). These findings are seen in nearly every implanted human TB. The inflammatory response to both the trauma and the continued presence of the electrode array contribute to the formation of fibrous tissue and new bone (Fig. 21.8). In a study of 20 implanted TBs, which were three-dimensionally reconstructed, intracochlear new bone and fibrous tissue formation were seen in each case [19]. On average, 33% of the total cochlear volume was occupied by fibro-osseous tissue, with 26% occupied by fibrous tissue and 7% by new bone growth, indicating a significant biologic response occurs in nearly all implanted cases [19].

Damage to the lateral cochlear wall correlates with the three-dimensional volume of fibrosis and new bone growth [43]. The number of years after CI was a predictor of new bone formation but not fibrosis [13]. Similarly, there was no significant correlation between the fibrous tissue's thickness and the implantation duration [27].

A few studies investigated the impact of electrode length on new tissue formation. It can be difficult to separate the effect of the length of the electrode array from the possible effect of its translocation. Very short electrodes, used mainly in the initial efforts for hearing preservation (<10 mm), exhibit minimal tissue reaction; none translocated [29]. In a study of 15 human temporal bones, the depth of electrode insertion, as measured by distance and angle in relation to the round window, did not correlate with the extent of new bone formation [13].

Electric current emitted by the implant may play a role in tissue formation. Ishai et al. compared the fibrous tissue surrounding perimodiolar and lateral wall full banded electrodes. The latter was surrounded by uniform thickness

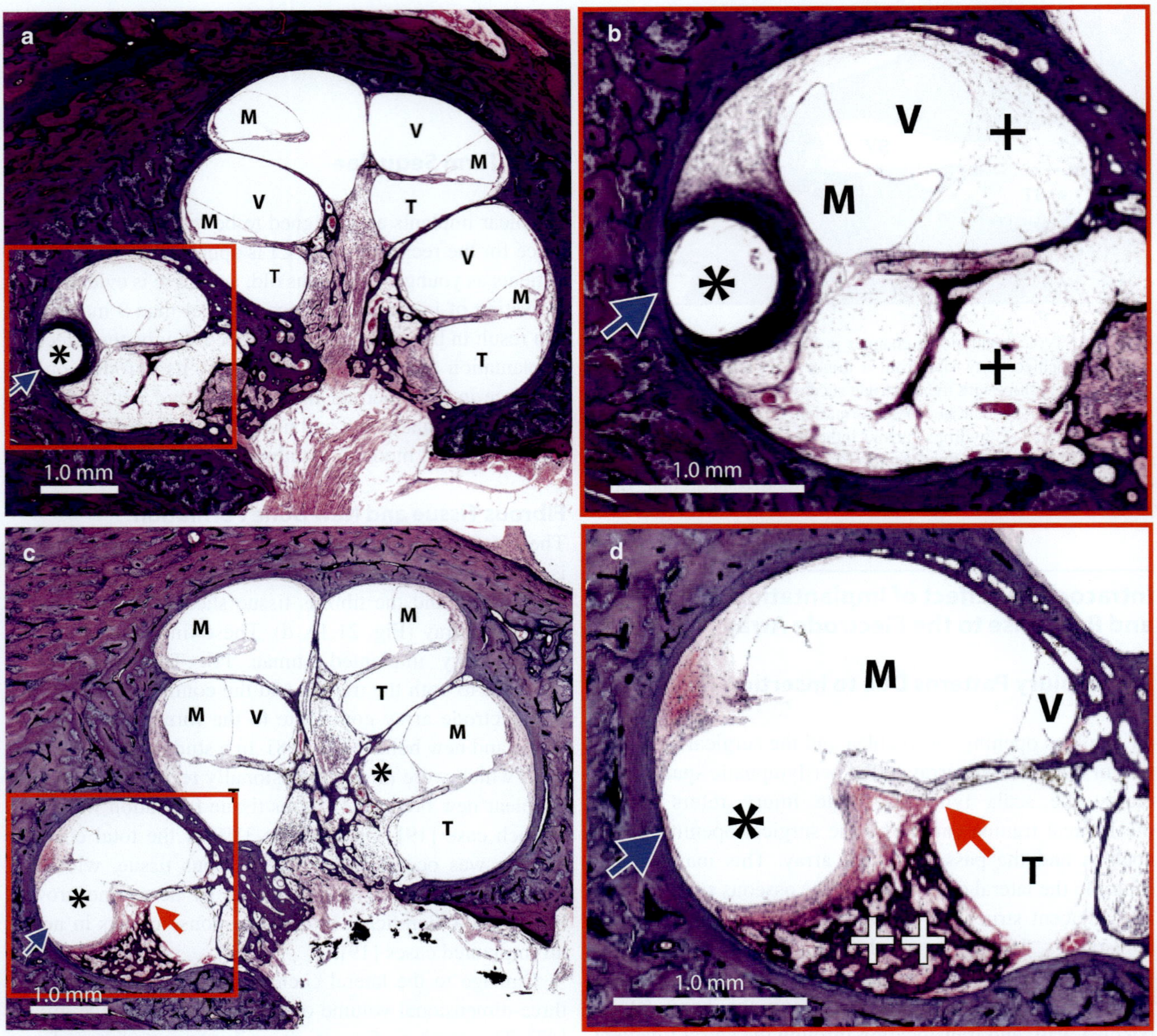

Fig. 21.5 Perforation of the spiral ligament (blue arrows) at the lateral wall of the cochlea shown in low (**a**) and high (**b**) magnification. Fracture of the osseous spiral lamina (red arrows) is shown in low (**c**) and high (**d**) magnification, and this example also has perforation of the spiral ligament. M scala media, V scala vestibuli, T scala tympani, + fibrous tissue, ++ new bone growth. (Reproduced with permission from Geerardyn et al. [20])

fibrous tissue, whereas in the former, it was asymmetric, thicker on the medial, stimulating side [27].

The insertional approach, i.e., RW vs. extended RW vs. cochleostomy, may impact patterns of fibrosis and bony osteoneogenesis in the cochlea. Based on a 3-dimensional reconstruction of 15 temporal bones, total tissue formation was measured and expressed as a percentage of cochlear volume. Median total tissue formation in cochleostomy vs. round window insertions was 25.98% and 10.34%, respectively [13]. In another human TB histology study, virtual resectioning was applied three-dimensionally reconstructed cochleae in order to assess fibrosis and osteoneogenesis patterns which may impact hearing preservation after CI, such as when soft tissue or bone directly abutted the RWM or the basilar membrane itself, potentially limiting acoustic movement [19]. In this study, which consisted of all ERW or cochleostomy cases, the reactive soft tissue fibrosis and bony osteoneogenesis completely covered/obliterated the RWM in 85% cases and abutted the basal portion of the basilar membrane in 100% of cases. In 89% cases, however, the basilar membrane *apical* to the 500 Hz frequency location in the cochlea remained free of impingement by fibro-osseous tis-

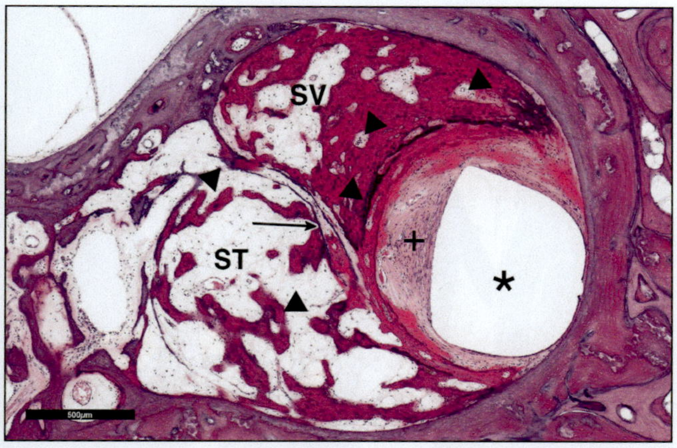

Fig. 21.6 Translocated electrode array which is shown in the scala vestibuli (SV) of the basal turn, after transgressing through the basilar membrane and fracturing the osseous spiral lamina (arrow). New bone growth is indicated by arrowheads throughout scala vestibuli (SV) and scala tympani (ST) (horizontal section, H&E stain, scale bar = 500um)

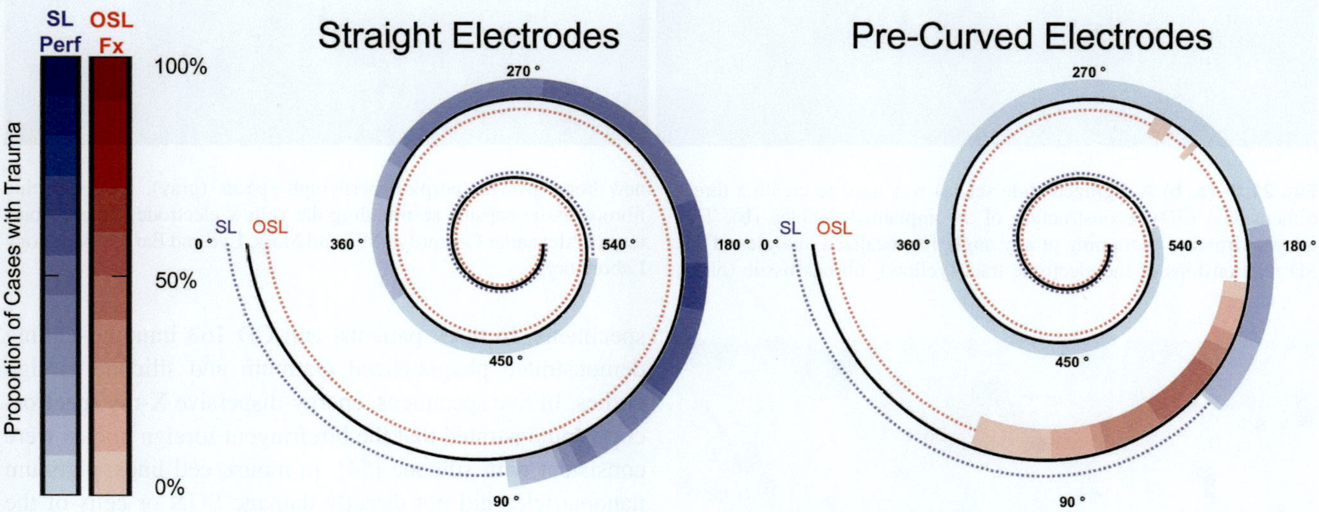

Fig. 21.7 Patterns of intracochlear trauma differ based on electrode style, as shown in a series of 21 human temporal bones. Straight electrodes were associated with spiral ligament (SL) perforation (SL Perf) and none had osseus spiral lamina (OSL) fracture (OSL Fx). Pre-curved electrodes were associated with OSL fracture and SL perforation. The location of the injury is shown in two-dimensional maps, which demonstrate the length of the site of injury varies. Darker color represents higher number of cases with injury at that location. (Reproduced with permission from: Geerardyn et al. [20])

sue. Hodges et al. compared new bone formation in otosclerotic cochleae implanted via cochleostomy or round window approaches. In cochleostomy cases, extensive osteoneogenesis and fibrosis, which was more prominent at the cochleostomy insertion site in the basal turn of the cochlea, often obliterating the scala tympani in the basal turn and, in some cases, extending to the scala media and scala vestibuli. This contrasted with the round window insertion, which exhibited minimal osteoneogenesis within the cochlear duct [25]. The percentage volume of new bone in the scala media/vestibuli was positively correlated with the degree of intracochlear insertional trauma, especially trauma to the basilar membrane [32]. Endolymphatic hydrops was prevalent in cochleae implanted via cochleostomy but not the round window approach [28].

Foreign Body Response

The electrode array interface with the host is made of biocompatible materials: a silicone carrier and metal electrode contacts, predominantly made of platinum. However, biocompatible does not equal bio-inert [50]. A foreign body response to biomaterials is almost universal [2]. Histologic evidence of a foreign body reaction has been described in approximately 75% [50] to 96% [67] of cases in patients who in life had undergone cochlear implantation. A cochlear implant generates a vigorous cellular immune response of B and T lymphocytes, foreign body giant cells, and macrophages (Fig. 21.9). The inflammatory response to the electrode array is greater at the basal turn of the cochlea close to the cochleostomy and lesser at the apex [67]. Insertional trauma may initiate a cascade of inflammatory effects that

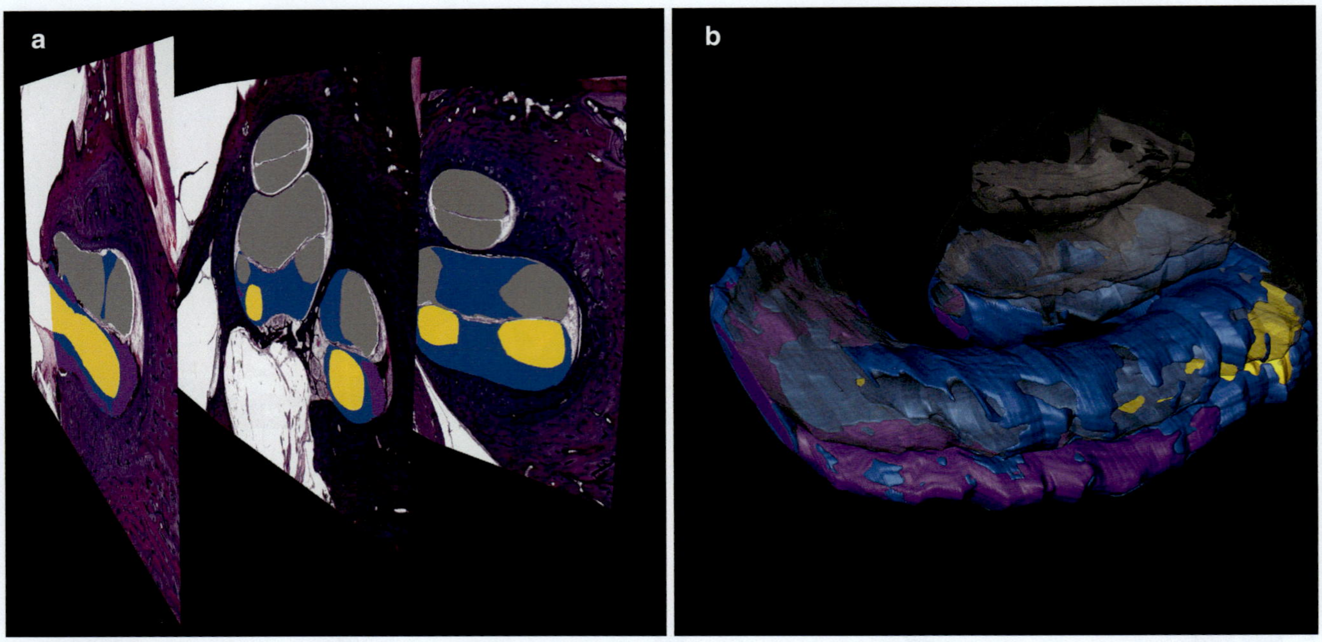

Fig. 21.8 (**a**, **b**) A digitized slide set (**a**) was used to create a three-dimensional (3D) reconstruction of an implanted cochlea (**b**). This allows virtual re-sectioning at any angle for localized analyses of the 3D relationships of the electrode tract (yellow), fibrous tissue (blue), new bone growth (purple), perilymph spaces (gray). Note the blue fibrous tissue capsule surrounding the yellow electrode. (Image courtesy of Alexander Geerardyn MD and Mass. Eye and Ear Otopathology Laboratory)

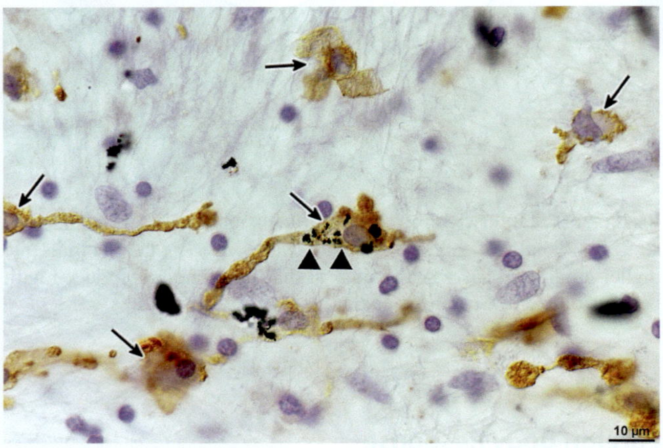

Fig. 21.9 Macrophages phagocytizing platinum particles from the electrode array contacts. The image was taken from the fibrous sheath abutting the electrode array. Macrophages (arrows) are labeled using an anti-Iba1 antibody. The platinum particles (arrow heads) are black in color. The slide is counterstained with hematoxylin to show nuclei in blue. (Image courtesy of Jennifer O'Malley, Mass. Eye and Ear Otopathology Laboratory)

organizes itself around the electrode array [16]. The observation that fibrous tissue tends to be most pronounced around the electrode array supports the electrode array as a source of the inflammatory response.

Platinum was identified as one of the materials likely responsible for this cellular response [50]. In a study of 44 temporal bone specimens from 36 patients, evidence for the presence of both platinum and silicone was found in all 44 specimens. In three patients, anti-CD 163 immunostaining demonstrated phagocytized platinum and silicone foreign bodies. In five specimens, energy-dispersive X-ray spectroscopy demonstrated that the birefringent foreign bodies were consistent with silicone [54]. In mouse cell lines, platinum nanoparticles did not directly damage SGN or cells of the organ of Corti [4].

Macrophages have a role in the immune response to CI (Fig. 21.9). Okayasu et al. found an increase in macrophages' densities in the vestibular end-organs of implanted inner ears compared to the contralateral non-implanted ears [53]. Based on their morphology, it was established that the macrophages were actively phagocytizing near the fibrous sheath with lymphocytic infiltration surrounding the electrode array [53]. Noonan et al. noted that the fibrous capsule surrounding the electrode arrays and areas of fibrosis, possibly due to translocation and/or cochleostomy trauma, was populated by both Iba1 and CD68 macrophages [51]. It is speculated that this foreign body response may result in migration or even extrusion of an implant device [50, 54]. However, in addition to the potential contribution to migration, the foreign body response can have a negative effect on CI performance by contributing to the formation of fibrous tissue and new bone formation.

Effects on Ganglion Cells

Insertion of a cochlear implant electrode has been associated with a reduced number of inner and outer hair cells along and apical to the electrode array and a reduced number of dendritic processes in the osseous spiral lamina along the electrode [33]. Translocation is associated with a reduced number of spiral ganglion cells at that segment and slower postimplantation improvement in speech recognition scores [38]. Interscalar translocation was found to trigger fibrosis and new bone formation, which is accentuated by damage to the lateral cochlear wall [29]. Electrode array tip fold-over in the basal turn resulted in atypical fibro-osseous changes and lower SGN counts [76].

Effects on the Vestibular System

Long-term effects on the vestibular system can be caused by tissue formation obstructing the ductus reuniens and the inflammatory response. Handzel et al. found that there was no difference in the densities of hair cells of the five vestibular sense organs or the number of Scarpa's ganglion neurons, concluding that CI does not cause deafferentation of the vestibular organs [23]. This observation is important because a number of publications measured reduced vestibular responses (such as to caloric stimulation and VEMP). Cochlear endolymphatic hydrops was common and seen in 60% of the implanted cochleae, apical to the location of the electrode array.

Intracochlear Factors Influencing Implantation Outcome

The outcome of cochlear implantation is generally satisfactory. However, there is significant variability in the outcomes between implantees [26]. Sources of the variation may include patient-related (i.e., duration of deafness), central processing, and intracochlear variables (i.e., the distance of the electrode from modiolus) [26].

Spiral Ganglion Neurons

CI results in electrical stimulation of the primary auditory neurons. Intuitively, having more neurons should allow for better speech recognition with a CI, but this has not been the case in older publications. In a study from 2005 of 15 temporal bones, no clear correlation between the number of neurons and post-implantation speech understanding as measured by the NU6 test was found [35]. A study from 2006 found a trend to a negative correlation between surviving spiral ganglion neurons and performance variability [16]. In 2014, analyzing 12 TB from 6 patients, differences in SGN counts were highly correlated with the differences in word recognition scores [67]. A recent meta-analysis did not find a significant correlation between SGN counts and word recognition scores in CI users. The authors concluded that the result is consistent with the possibility that a relatively small number of SGNs is sufficient to understand speech with a cochlear implant, and therefore the correlation does not exist for patients with SGN counts above that threshold. Alternatively, any influence of SGN count on speech perception by CI users is obscured by other factors that are more strongly associated with speech perception outcomes [8]. Newer histology techniques for the analysis of the SGNs in implanted cases include the application of machine learning [80] (Fig. 21.10), the use of three-dimensional reconstructions based on digitized slide sets, and improvements in immunohistochemistry. Application of these techniques may yield further clarification on the correlation between the SGN population and CI performance for an individual implantee.

A number of studies have demonstrated the positive effect of electrical stimulation with an implant on the number of spiral ganglion cells [35]. In one study comparing the implanted to the non-implanted side in patients with bilateral symmetric profound hearing loss, the segment of the spiral ganglion influenced by stimulation had more neurons on the implanted side [65]. The effect was seen only with bipolar but not mono-polar stimulation. In the same study, the apical segment of the spiral ganglion in the implanted bone had a smaller population of spiral ganglion neurons as compared to the non-implanted side, supporting a possible positive effect of implantation on the neurons adjacent to the electrode. In deafened cats, unilateral chronic electrical stimulation increased the number of SGN as compared to a contralateral ear and increased the cross-sectional soma area of the largest cells measured [39].

Future development may allow noninvasive imaging to provide an estimation of the number of primary auditory neurons. The cross-sectional area of the auditory nerve on parasagittal sections was found to be significantly different between postlingually deafened and normal-hearing adults [24] and has been shown to be positively associated with CI performance and adult implantees [36]. In pediatric implantees with prelingual deafness, no correlation was found between the diameter of the auditory nerve and 6 months postimplantation performance. The authors conclude the finding supports the theory of a low threshold for the number of SGN (and nerve diameter) required to reach adequate performance [30].

New Bone and Fibrous Tissue Formation

There is some evidence that new bone formation has a negative impact on the outcome of CI as measured by speech understanding scores. Postimplantation CNC word scores were negatively correlated with the volume of new bone within the scala tympani, scala media/vestibuli, and the cochlea but not the volume of fibrous tissue [32]. The thick-

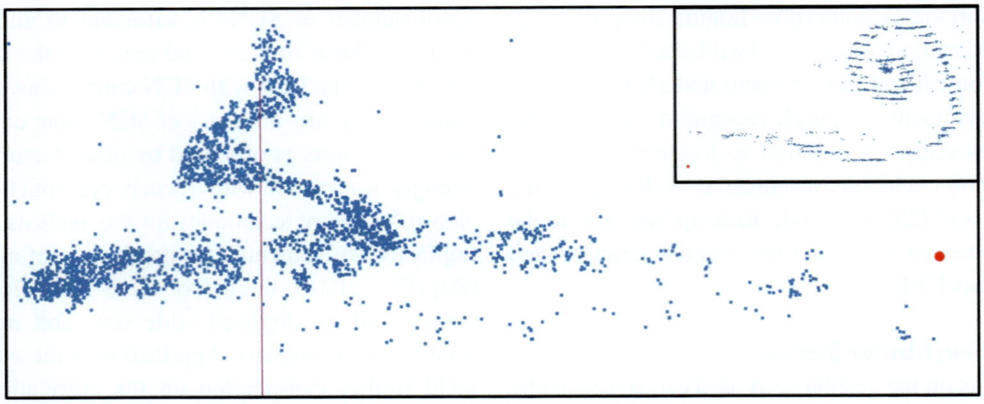

Fig. 21.10 Spiral ganglion neurons (SGNs) in an implanted cochlea plotted in 3D using a machine learning algorithm based on a digitized slide set, as described in Wu P, O'Malley J, Liberman MC 2023. Each blue dot represents a single SGN cell body in Rosenthal's canal. Red dot indicates round window location. Red line indicates mid-modiolar axis. The inset box in upper right shows the top-down view (rotated relative to the large image). Since every tenth 20-um-thick slide is stained with H&E, digitized, and used for identifying SGNs by the machine learning program, there are spaces between the H&E sections used for SGN analyses. (Image courtesy of Anbuselvan Dharmarajan MD, Mass. Eye and Otopathology Laboratory)

ness of the fibrous sheath surrounding the electrode array does not correlate with CI performance or duration of implantation but does correlate with intracochlear trauma [27]. The thickness and pattern of the fibrous sheath vary by electrode type and stimulation pattern [27]. New bone growth can be associated with elevated electrode impedance [27]. Labyrinthitis ossificans is associated with a reduced number of spiral ganglion neurons [49].

For older implant designs, patients with interscalar translocation of the array and damage to the lateral cochlear wall had inferior speech understanding as compared to patients only with translocation [29].

The Vestibular System

Studying the effects of cochlear implantation on vestibular function and structures is an ongoing effort. Factoring vestibular function in the process of CI is becoming more important. Implanting ears with residual hearing, bilateral implantation, implanting babies before they learn to stand and walk, and elderly recipients are examples of potentially sensitive recipients. Although several studies have demonstrated decreased vestibular function after implantation (vHIT, VEMP, ENG, etc.) [70], the decreased function does not necessarily correlate well with symptoms and results of targeted questionnaires. In a series of 107 patients with residual hearing undergoing CI, the preservation of vestibular function was correlated with the preservation of residual hearing [70].

In one of the few human temporal bone studies available, differences in Scarpa's ganglion cell counts and hair cell densities in the five vestibular sense organs between the implanted and nonimplanted sides were not statistically significant. In 59% of the implanted bones, the cochlea was hydropic, and in the majority of these bones, the saccule collapsed. The ductus reuniens was patent in most hydropic ears [23]. Ishiyama et al. hypothesize that cochleostomy involving the scala vestibuli incites fibrosis, compromising the ductus reuniens and causing hydrops [28]. This effect was seen in implantation via cochleostomy rather than a round window approach. Su-Velez et al. studied 17 human TBs implanted via cochleostomy with straight electrodes. They found cochlear hydrops and fibrosis, atrophy, or obstruction of the ductus reuniens [74]. Hydrops of the utricle was seen in close to half of the TB and was correlated with the presence of vestibular symptoms. The authors conclude these findings support round window (rather than cochleostomy) implantation.

One possible explanation for the commonly seen endolymphatic hydrops is damage to the lateral cochlear wall and the response to it. This theory is supported by clinical observation of a spike in electrode impedance following the implantation of straight electrodes (that touch the lateral cochlear wall) but not a perimodiolar one [69].

To summarize, CI does not damage the vestibular neuroepithelium or vestibular neurons but may result in endolymphatic hydrops. Round window approach, minimizing lateral cochlear wall damage and avoiding inter-scala translocation, may decrease the risk of hydrops. A yet-to-be-answered question is whether the observed hydrops implies that patients with Ménière's- like dizziness post-CI should be treated like those with Ménière's disease.

Special Pathologies

Implantation in Ears with Residual Hearing

Simultaneous electric and acoustic stimulation of ears with residual low-tone hearing requires the preservation of essential structures of the inner ear, particularly in the apical regions representing frequencies up to and including 750 Hz, as well as allowing energy passage from the footplate to the basilar membrane at the apex. Clinical protocols for hearing preservation CI include variable amounts, duration, and timing of administration of steroids. In an animal model, the addition of local dexamethasone to electrical stimulation increased the number of SGN (as compared to no local dexamethasone) [63].

Hearing initially preserved can deteriorate in the subsequent months and years. The histopathology correlate of delayed hearing loss in a patient implanted with a short 10 mm array was fibrosis and new bone formation in the basal turn of the cochlea and hydrops apical to the array [58]. The authors offer a number of possible pathogenesis of delayed hearing loss: new tissue increasing impedance of the round window membrane and cochlear partitioning, disturbance of the inter-scala pressure gradient, and damage to the cochlear aqueduct [58]. Hair cells and spiral ganglion neuron counts were comparable to the contralateral non-implanted ear when counted with a traditional histologic method [58]. Based on a study of 29 human temporal bones implanted with the intent of low-tone hearing preservation, it was hypothesized that a cochleostomy involving scala vestibuli incites fibrosis, compromising the ductus reuniens, causing hydrops which may cause the delayed loss of residual low frequency hearing in a cochlear implant [28].

The Ossified Cochlea

Implantation of the ossified cochlea poses intraoperative challenges and may negatively impact outcomes. Bacterial meningitis is commonly complicated by labyrinthitis ossificans. The source of bacterial spread to the meninges is often otogenic but can be hematogenic or from other sources. Nonbacterial infections do not usually result in labyrinthitis ossificans. Ossification can be seen in other etiologies. Cogan's syndrome is an example of an immune-mediated disease [31]. Other etiologies include genetic disorders such as Cockayne's syndrome, vascular infarcts, otitis media, trauma (Fig. 21.11), and rarely cholesteatoma [73].

The perilymphatic space is in a continuum with the CSF space. Bacteria present in the CSF can directly reach the inner ear (and vice versa). Bacterial labyrinthitis often results in fibrosis and variable ossification of the membranous labyrinth. The exact cause of the new bone formation has not been completely elucidated [6]. Although damage can initially be seen in the vestibular organs, fibrosis and ossification of the scala tympani and then scala vestibuli may follow. In a study of 32 TB of patients who had bacterial meningitis, 9 had fibrosis and 10 labyrinthitis ossificans [77]. Fibrosis was present as early as 1.5 weeks after meningitis. In all cases of ossification, the round window and the basal turn of the scala tympani were involved. The scala vestibuli was not necessarily spared but was involved in a patchy and more distal pattern. In an animal model, ossification appeared 3 weeks post pneumococcal meningitis [47]. Tympanogenic ossification involves the round window and the adjacent scala tympani [22]. The introduction of an electrode array to the ossified cochlea can be challenging. For this reason, hearing loss after bacterial meningitis requires prompt implantation.

Postmeningitic ossification is associated with a significantly reduced number of spiral ganglion cells. In a human temporal bone study, the population of spiral ganglion neurons averaged 45% less than age-matched normal controls [55]. There is an inverse relation between the number of postmeningitis years and the neuron population [48]. Drill-out of the ossified scala tympani can damage the modiolus and further deplete the population of auditory neurons [77]. The technical challenges of introducing the electrode array to a cochlear lumen and the reduced number of neurons are why outcomes of cochlear implantation in the setting of labyrinthitis ossificans tend to be inferior compared to other etiologies.

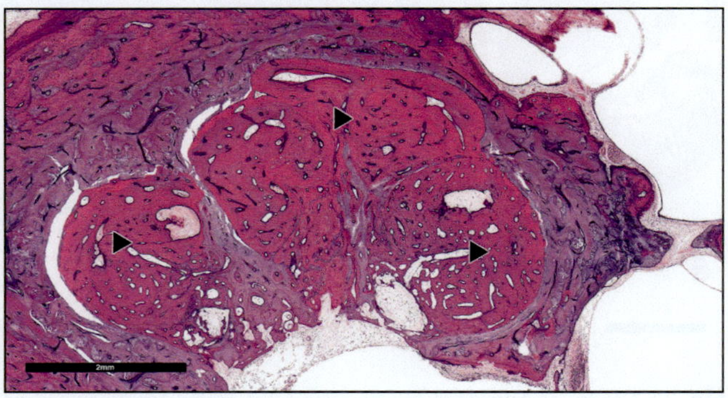

Fig. 21.11 Extensive labyrinthitis ossificans due to temporal bone fracture. The cochlea is filled with abnormal bone (arrow heads), making the introduction of an electrode array challenging. The number of SGNs in Rosenthal's canal (RC) is extremely reduced and looks almost empty at low magnification. (Horizontal section, H&E stain, scale bar = 2 mm)

Otosclerosis

In some patients with otosclerosis, hearing loss will reach a severity meeting the indication for cochlear implantation. There are a few unique considerations in implanting a cochlea with otosclerosis. Milder forms of otosclerosis tend to be confined to the otic capsule. Sensorineural hearing loss is seen with involvement of the lateral cochlear wall, presumably due to damage to the spiral ligament or stria vascularis. In advanced (previously referred to as "far advanced" or "malignant") otosclerosis, the abnormal growth of lamellar bone is present in the scala tympani (Fig. 21.12a–c). In most cases, new bone growth is limited to the basal turn and does not preclude implantation [15]; the RW niche is typically obliterated (Fig. 21.12b). In one study, cochlear otosclerosis adjacent to the round window caused significantly more damage to spiral ganglion cells and outer hair cells than cochlear otosclerosis adjacent to the oval window without loss of spiral ligament [62]. Hence, removing the abnormal bone is required for scala tympani insertion. Alternatively, the scala vestibuli can be inserted. These considerations are similar in labyrinthitis ossificans.

The otic capsule forms a partial barrier to the leak of electrical currents generated by the electrodes of the intracochlear array. Facial nerve stimulation by adjacent electrodes is more common in etiologies such as cochlear malformation, TB fractures, and otosclerosis. In these pathologies, the otic capsule's electrical isolation is compromised (Fig. 21.12c). A recent meta-analysis has computed the rate of facial nerve stimulation at 5.6% of all otosclerotic ears with CI [81]. In addition to otosclerosis, lateral wall electrodes had a higher rate of facial nerve stimulation as compared to pre-curved one arrays [81]. Facial nerve stimulation can be reduced or eliminated by switching off or reprogramming some electrodes. Still, it may become so significant as to require re-implantation [57]. The electrodes located at the apex of the basal cochlear turn are most likely to trigger unwanted facial stimulation. Histologic finding correlated with facial nerve stimulation is full-thickness replacement of the otic capsule with otosclerotic bone

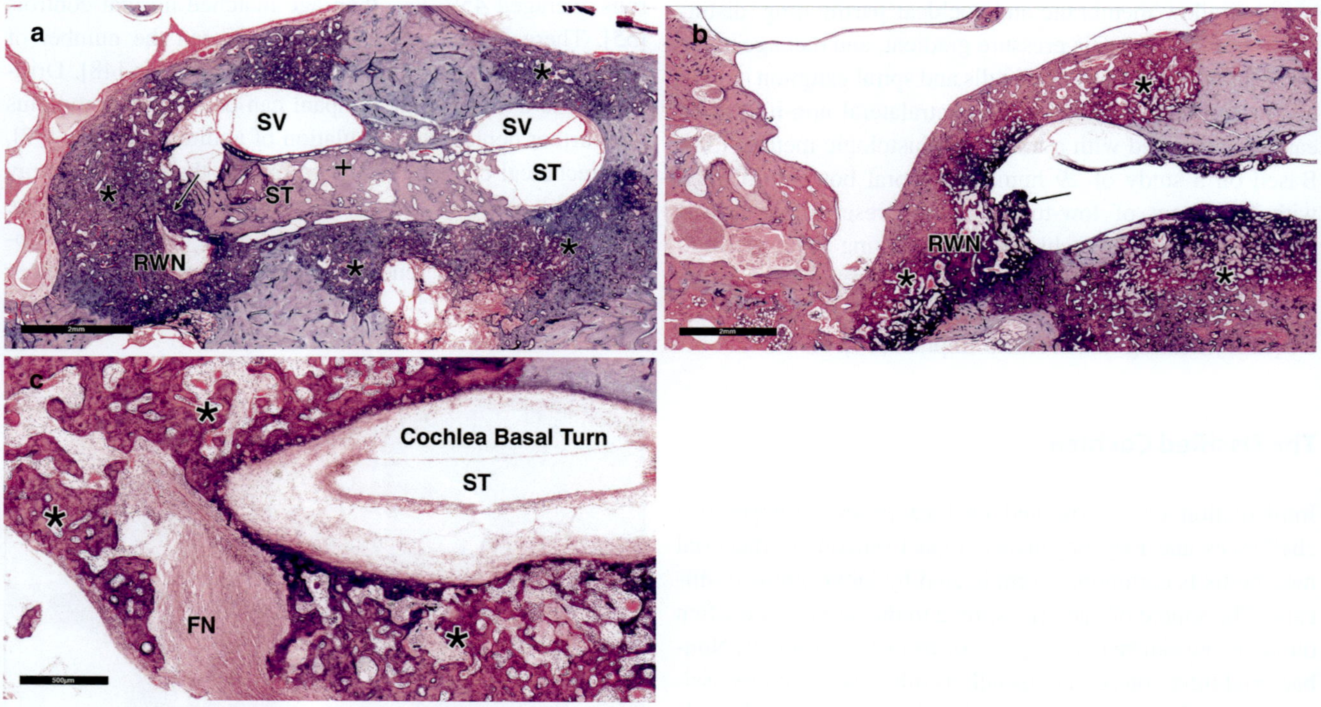

Fig. 21.12 (**a–c**) Advanced otosclerosis (also called far advanced or "malignant") poses specific challenges for cochlear implantation including direct intracochlear extension of otosclerotic bone and new bone growth (**a**), obliteration of the round window (**b**), and increased incidence of facial nerve stimulation (**c**). In A, note the extensive otosclerotic foci (*) involving the otic capsule and obliterating the round window niche (RWN). In this particularly advanced case, there is otosclerosis (*) and new bone growth (+) filling the basal end of the scala tympani (ST). SV, scala vestibuli. (**b**) Another advanced otosclerosis case, in which the RWN is filled with otosclerosis and the RW membrane would not be visible from the facial recess approach (or any approach) prior to surgical removal of the otosclerotic bone. In this case, there is a small amount of otosclerosis extending just into the scala tympani (arrow). (**c**) Otosclerotic foci (*) with large pseudovascular spaces between the labyrinthine facial nerve (FN) and the upper basal turn of the cochlea may potentially result in current leakage and unwanted stimulation of the facial nerve. ST scala tympani (horizontal sections, H&E stain, scale bars = 2 mm (**a**), 2 mm (**b**), 500 μm (**c**))

adjacent to the labyrinthine segment of the facial nerve [66]. The partitioning otic capsule at this point is often thinned down by otosclerosis. Facial nerve stimulation is more likely to happen with straight vs. modiolar hugging electrodes, even when the extent of otosclerosis is similar [66]. Cavitary otosclerosis is a rare presentation of otosclerosis that may create a diverticulum to the internal auditory canal resulting in a "third window phenomenon," conductive hearing loss, and risk of electrode misplacement at cochlear implantation [7]. This extensive type of otosclerosis is usually seen in older patients and can involve the anterior portion of the internal auditory canal. Compared to histological diagnosis, postmortem high-resolution CT scans had the sensitivity and specificity of detecting IAC diverticula of 77% and 63%, respectively [79].

Temporal Bone Fracture

Relevancy of TB fractures to cochlear implants arises in cases involving the otic capsule. Violation of the otic capsule almost always results in severe-profound hearing loss. When fractured, the middle layer of the otic capsule does not form a callus but heals by fibrosis (Fig. 21.11) [45]. One consequence is the possibility of aberrant facial nerve stimulation, similar to the phenomenon discussed in relation to otosclerosis. Cochlear implantation in fractured TB is feasible [83]. In a study of two implanted TB from patients with bilateral fractures, the implanted TB showed extensive intracochlear ossification, which was greater when the fracture involved the cochlea. In contrast, the nonimplanted cochleae were patent with small osseous deposits at the round window membrane. Interaural SGN counts were lower on the implanted side, and hearing results were moderate to poor [77].

On histopathology of the peripheral vestibular organs, structural changes such as atrophy of the semicircular cristae and reduced number of Scarpa's ganglion neurons are commonly present [37]. These likely result in hyporeflexia and should be considered in patients such as candidates for implantation of the contralateral side (risk of bilateral vestibular loss).

Cochlear Reimplantation

Although cochlear implants are reliable and robust devices, revision surgery is not rare. Reasons to replace an implant include errors in the design or manufacturing of the implants, infections, dehiscence of the overlying skin, and traumatic damage. In a study of four temporal bones, all revised implants were placed deeper than the original arrays [40]. The primary track of the initial implantation did not interfere with the insertion of a revision cochlear implant, and the trajectory of the revision electrode did not always follow the primary track [40].

Summary

CI is no longer a rare form of hearing rehabilitation, and its applications are likely to grow with the aging population. Despite the generally favorable response, there is a variance in outcomes, and more data is required to improve implant design and optimize surgery, to name just two gaps in our knowledge. The study of temporal bones of human CI recipients, accompanied by their clinical data, is a powerful tool for gaining insights into the interaction of this successful neural prosthesis with the human body. Future developments in TB analysis techniques and the evolution of indications and surgery for CI are expected to make histopathology an even more powerful research tool in the future.

Acknowledgments The images in this chapter are based on temporal bone cases from the Massachusetts Eye and Ear Otopathology Laboratory. We acknowledge the generosity of donors who enroll to donate an anatomic gift, surgeons and clinicians who raise awareness for the program, and the support of the National Institute on Deafness and Other Communication Disorders (U24 DC020849, U24 DC013983, R01 DC021606). We thank Dr. Joseph B Nadol Jr, Barbara Burgess, Diane Jones, Jennifer T. O'Malley, Meng Yu Zhu, and Anbuselvan Dharmarajan MD, who were instrumental in beginning the cochlear implant collection and/or doing the histologic processing for the cases included here. We thank Garyfallia Pagonis for assistance with figure labeling.

References

1. Alzamil KS, Linthicum FH Jr. Extraneous round window membranes and plugs: possible effect on intratympanic therapy. Ann Otol Rhinol Laryngol. 2000;109(1):30–2. https://doi.org/10.1177/000348940010900105.
2. Anderson JM, Rodriguez A, Chang DT. Foreign body reaction to biomaterials. Semin Immunol. 2008;20(2):86–100. https://doi.org/10.1016/j.smim.2007.11.004.
3. Avci E, Nauwelaers T, Lenarz T, Hamacher V, Kral A. Variations in microanatomy of the human cochlea. J Comp Neurol. 2014;522(14):3245–61.
4. Berger E, Brandes G, Reifenrath J, Lenarz T, Durisin M, Wissel K. In vitro impact of platinum nanoparticles on inner ear related cell culture models. PLoS One. 2023;18(4):e0284794. https://doi.org/10.1371/journal.pone.0284794.
5. Blamey P, Artieres F, Başkent D, Bergeron F, Beynon A, Burke E, Dillier N, Dowell R, Fraysse B, Gallégo S, Govaerts PJ, Green K, Huber AM, Kleine-Punte A, Maat B, Marx M, Mawman D, Mosnier I, O'Connor AF, O'Leary S, Rousset A, Schauwers K, Skarzynski H, Skarzynski PH, Sterkers O, Terranti A, Truy E, Van de Heyning P, Venail F, Vincent C, Lazard DS. Factors affecting auditory performance of postlinguistically deaf adults using cochlear implants: an update with 2251 patients. Audiol Neurootol. 2013;18(1):36–47. https://doi.org/10.1159/000343189.
6. Bloch SL, McKenna MJ, Adams J, Friis M. Labyrinthitis ossificans: on the mechanism of perilabyrinthine bone remodeling. Ann Otol Rhinol Laryngol. 2015;124(8):649–54. https://doi.org/10.1177/0003489415573960.

7. Bou-Assaly W, Mukherji S, Srinivasan A. Bilateral cavitary otosclerosis: a rare presentation of otosclerosis and cause of hearing loss. Clin Imaging. 2013;37(6):1116–8. https://doi.org/10.1016/j.clinimag.2013.07.007. Epub 2013 Sep 17. PMID: 24050941.
8. Cheng YS, Svirsky MA. Meta-analysis-correlation between spiral ganglion cell counts and speech perception with a cochlear implant. Audiol Res. 2021;11(2):220–6. https://doi.org/10.3390/audiolres11020020.
9. Culbertson SR, Dillon MT, Richter ME, Brown KD, Anderson MR, Hancock SL, Park LR. Younger age at cochlear implant activation results in improved auditory skill development for children with congenital deafness. J Speech Lang Hear Res. 2022;65(9):3539–47. https://doi.org/10.1044/2022_JSLHR-22-00039.
10. Dhanasingh A, Jolly NC, Rajan G, van de Heyning P. Literature review on the distribution of spiral ganglion cell bodies inside the human cochlear central modiolar trunk. J Int Adv Otol. 2020a;16(1):104–10. https://doi.org/10.5152/iao.2020.7510.
11. Dhanasingh AE, Rajan G, van de Heyning P. Presence of the spiral ganglion cell bodies beyond the basal turn of the human cochlea. Cochlear Implants Int. 2020b;21(3):145–52. https://doi.org/10.1080/14670100.2019.1694226.
12. Danielian A, Ishiyama G, Lopez IA, Ishiyama A. Morphometric linear and angular measurements of the human cochlea in implant patients using 3-dimensional reconstruction. Hear Res. 2020;386:107874. https://doi.org/10.1016/j.heares.2019.107874.
13. Danielian A, Ishiyama G, Lopez IA, Ishiyama A. Predictors of fibrotic and bone tissue formation with 3-D reconstructions of post-implantation human temporal bones. Otol Neurotol. 2021;42(7):e942–8. https://doi.org/10.1097/MAO.0000000000003106.
14. Fakurnejad S, Vail D, Song Y, Alyono J, Blevins NH. Trends in age of cochlear implant recipients, and the impact on perioperative complication rates. Otol Neurotol. 2020;41(4):438–43. https://doi.org/10.1097/MAO.0000000000002558.
15. Fayad J, Moloy P, Linthicum FH Jr. Cochlear otosclerosis: does bone formation affect cochlear implant surgery? Am J Otol. 1990;11(3):196–200. PMID: 2188511.
16. Fayad JN, Linthicum FH Jr. Multichannel cochlear implants: relation of histopathology to performance. Laryngoscope. 2006;116(8):1310–20. https://doi.org/10.1097/01.mlg.0000227176.09500.28.
17. Fujiwara RJT, Ishiyama G, Lopez IA, Ishiyama A. Morphometric analysis and linear measurements of the scala tympani and implications in cochlear implant electrodes. Otol Neurotol. 2023;44(5):e343–9. https://doi.org/10.1097/MAO.0000000000003848.
18. Geerardyn A, Zhu M, Klabbers T, Huinck W, Mylanus E, Nadol JB Jr, Verhaert N, Quesnel AM. Human histology after structure preservation cochlear implantation via round window insertion. Laryngoscope. 2023a; https://doi.org/10.1002/lary.30900.
19. Geerardyn A, Zhu M, Wu P, O'Malley J, Nadol JB Jr, Liberman MC, Nakajima HH, Verhaert N, Quesnel AM. Three-dimensional quantification of fibrosis and ossification after cochlear implantation via virtual re-sectioning: potential implications for residual hearing. Hear Res. 2023b;428:108681. https://doi.org/10.1016/j.heares.2022.108681.
20. Geerardyn A, Zhu M, Nadol JB Jr, Verhaert N, Quesnel AM. Intracochlear trauma and local ossification patterns differ between straight and pre-curved cochlear implant electrodes. Otol Neurotol. 2024;45(3):245–55. https://doi.org/10.1097/MAO.0000000000004102. Epub 2024 Jan 17.
21. Gopen Q, Rosowski JJ, Merchant SN. Anatomy of the normal human cochlear aqueduct with functional implications. Hear Res. 1997;107(1–2):9–22. https://doi.org/10.1016/s0378-5955(97)00017-8.
22. Green JD Jr, Marion MS, Hinojosa R. Labyrinthitis ossificans: histopathologic consideration for cochlear implantation. Otolaryngol Head Neck Surg. 1991;104(3):320–6. https://doi.org/10.1177/019459989110400306.
23. Handzel O, Burgess BJ, Nadol JB Jr. Histopathology of the peripheral vestibular system after cochlear implantation in the human. Otol Neurotol. 2006;27(1):57–64. https://doi.org/10.1097/01.mao.0000188658.36327.8f.
24. Herman B, Angeli S. Differences in cochlear nerve cross-sectional area between normal hearing and postlingually deafened patients on MRI. Otolaryngol Head Neck Surg. 2011;144(1):64–6. https://doi.org/10.1177/0194599810390884.
25. Hodge SE, Ishiyama G, Lopez IA, Ishiyama A. Histopathologic analysis of temporal bones with otosclerosis following cochlear implantation. Otol Neurotol. 2021;42(10):1492–8. https://doi.org/10.1097/MAO.0000000000003327.
26. Holden LK, Finley CC, Firszt JB, Holden TA, Brenner C, Potts LG, Gotter BD, Vanderhoof SS, Mispagel K, Heydebrand G, Skinner MW. Factors affecting open-set word recognition in adults with cochlear implants. Ear Hear. 2013;34(3):342–60. https://doi.org/10.1097/AUD.0b013e3182741aa7.
27. Ishai R, Herrmann BS, Nadol JB Jr, Quesnel AM. The pattern and degree of capsular fibrous sheaths surrounding cochlear electrode arrays. Hear Res. 2017;348:44–53. https://doi.org/10.1016/j.heares.2017.02.012.
28. Ishiyama A, Doherty J, Ishiyama G, Quesnel AM, Lopez I, Linthicum FH. Post hybrid cochlear implant hearing loss and endolymphatic hydrops. Otol Neurotol. 2016;37(10):1516–21. https://doi.org/10.1097/MAO.0000000000001199.
29. Ishiyama A, Ishiyama G, Lopez IA, Linthicum FH Jr. Temporal bone histopathology of first-generation cochlear implant electrode translocation. Otol Neurotol. 2019;40(6):e581–91. https://doi.org/10.1097/MAO.0000000000002247.
30. Jain S, Sharma V, Patro SK, Khera P, Yadav T, Tiwari S, Kaushal D, Soni K, Goyal A. Correlation of cochlear nerve cross-sectional area and auditory performance after cochlear implantation in prelingual children with bilateral profound hearing loss. Int J Pediatr Otorhinolaryngol. 2020;137:110173. https://doi.org/10.1016/j.ijporl.2020.110173.
31. Jung DH, Nadol JB Jr, Folkerth RD, Merola JF. Histopathology of the inner ear in a case with recent onset of Cogan's syndrome: evidence for vasculitis. Ann Otol Rhinol Laryngol. 2016;125(1):20–4. https://doi.org/10.1177/0003489415595426.
32. Kamakura T, Nadol JB Jr. Correlation between word recognition score and intracochlear new bone and fibrous tissue after cochlear implantation in the human. Hear Res. 2016;339:132–41. https://doi.org/10.1016/j.heares.2016.06.015.
33. Kamakura T, O'Malley JT, Nadol JB Jr. Preservation of cells of the organ of corti and innervating dendritic processes following cochlear implantation in the human: an immunohistochemical study. Otol Neurotol. 2018;39(3):284–93. https://doi.org/10.1097/MAO.0000000000001686.
34. Kawano A, Seldon HL, Clark GM. Computer-aided three-dimensional reconstruction in human cochlear maps: measurement of the lengths of organ of Corti, outer wall, inner wall, and Rosenthal's canal. Ann Otol Rhinol Laryngol. 1996;105(9):701–9.
35. Khan AM, Handzel O, Damian D, Eddington DK, Nadol JB Jr. Effect of cochlear implantation on residual spiral ganglion cell count as determined by comparison with the contralateral nonimplanted inner ear in humans. Ann Otol Rhinol Laryngol. 2005;114(5):381–5. https://doi.org/10.1177/000348940511400508.
36. Kim BG, Chung HJ, Park JJ, Park S, Kim SH, Choi JY. Correlation of cochlear nerve size and auditory performance after cochlear implantation in postlingually deaf patients. JAMA Otolaryngol

Head Neck Surg. 2013;139(6):604–9. https://doi.org/10.1001/jamaoto.2013.3195.
37. Knoll RM, Ishai R, Lubner RJ, Trakimas DR, Brodsky JR, Jung DH, Rauch SD, Nadol JB Jr, Remenschneider AK, Kozin ED. Peripheral vestibular organ degeneration after temporal bone fracture: a human otopathology study. Laryngoscope. 2020;130(3):752–60. https://doi.org/10.1002/lary.28010.
38. Knoll RM, Trakimas DR, Wu MJ, Lubner RJ, Nadol JB Jr, Ishiyama A, Santos F, Jung DH, Remenschneider AK, Kozin ED. Intracochlear new fibro-ossification and neuronal degeneration following cochlear implant electrode translocation: long-term histopathological findings in humans. Otol Neurotol. 2022;43(2):e153–64. https://doi.org/10.1097/MAO.0000000000003402.
39. Leake PA, Hradek GT, Snyder RL. Chronic electrical stimulation by a cochlear implant promotes the survival of spiral ganglion neurons after neonatal deafness. J Comp Neurol. 1999;412(4):543–62. https://doi.org/10.1002/(sici)1096-9861(19991004)412:4<543::aid-cne1>3.0.co;2-3.
40. Lee J, Eddington DK, Nadol JB. The histopathology of revision cochlear implantation. Audiol Neurootol. 2011;16(5):336–46. https://doi.org/10.1159/000322307.
41. Li H, Schart-Moren N, Rohani SA, Ladak HM, Rask-Andersen H, Agrawal S. Synchrotron radiation-based reconstruction of the human spiral ganglion: implications for cochlear implantation. Ear Hear. 2020;41(1):173–81.
42. Li PM, Wang H, Northrop C, Merchant SN, Nadol JB Jr. Anatomy of the round window and hook region of the cochlea with implications for cochlear implantation and other endocochlear surgical procedures. Otol Neurotol. 2007;28(5):641–8. https://doi.org/10.1097/mao.0b013e3180577949.
43. Li PM, Somdas MA, Eddington DK, Nadol JB Jr. Analysis of intracochlear new bone and fibrous tissue formation in human subjects with cochlear implants. Ann Otol Rhinol Laryngol. 2007a;116(10):731–8. https://doi.org/10.1177/000348940711601004.
44. Miller JD. Sex differences in the length of the organ of Corti in humans. J Acoust Soc Am. 2007;121(4):EL151–5. https://doi.org/10.1121/1.2710746.
45. Milroy CM, Michaels L. Pathology of the otic capsule. J Laryngol Otol. 1990;104(2):83–90. https://doi.org/10.1017/s0022215100111946.
46. Miura M, Sando I, Hirsch BE, Orita Y. Analysis of spiral ganglion cell populations in children with normal and pathological ears. Ann Otol Rhinol Laryngol. 2002;111(12 Pt 1):1059–65. https://doi.org/10.1177/000348940211101201.
47. Nabili V, Brodie HA, Neverov NI, Tinling SP. Chronology of labyrinthitis ossificans induced by Streptococcus pneumoniae meningitis. Laryngoscope. 1999;109(6):931–5. https://doi.org/10.1097/00005537-199906000-00017.
48. Nadol JB Jr, Hsu WC. Histopathologic correlation of spiral ganglion cell count and new bone formation in the cochlea following meningogenic labyrinthitis and deafness. Ann Otol Rhinol Laryngol. 1991;100(9 Pt 1):712–6. https://doi.org/10.1177/000348949110000904.
49. Nadol JB Jr. Patterns of neural degeneration in the human cochlea and auditory nerve: implications for cochlear implantation. Otolaryngol Head Neck Surg. 1997;117(3 Pt 1):220–8. https://doi.org/10.1016/s0194-5998(97)70178-5.
50. Nadol JB Jr, O'Malley JT, Burgess BJ, Galler D. Cellular immunologic responses to cochlear implantation in the human. Hear Res. 2014;318:11–7. https://doi.org/10.1016/j.heares.2014.09.007.
51. Noonan KY, Lopez IA, Ishiyama G, Ishiyama A. Immune response of macrophage population to cochlear implantation: cochlea immune cells. Otol Neurotol. 2020;41(9):1288–95. https://doi.org/10.1097/MAO.0000000000002764.
52. O'Connell BP, Hunter JB, Wanna GB. The importance of electrode location in cochlear implantation. Laryngoscope Investig Otolaryngol. 2016;1(6):169–74. https://doi.org/10.1002/lio2.42.
53. Okayasu T, O'Malley JT, Nadol JB Jr. Density of macrophages immunostained with anti-iba1 antibody in the vestibular endorgans after cochlear implantation in the human. Otol Neurotol. 2019;40(8):e774–81. https://doi.org/10.1097/MAO.0000000000002313.
54. O'Malley JT, Burgess BJ, Galler D, Nadol JB Jr. Foreign body response to silicone in cochlear implant electrodes in the human. Otol Neurotol. 2017;38(7):970–7. https://doi.org/10.1097/MAO.0000000000001454.
55. Pauna HF, Knoll RM, Lubner RJ, Brodsky JR, Cushing SL, Hyppolito MA, Nadol JB Jr, Remenschneider AK, Kozin ED. Histopathological changes to the peripheral vestibular system following meningitic labyrinthitis. Laryngoscope Investig Otolaryngol. 2020;5(2):256–66. https://doi.org/10.1002/lio2.349.
56. Pelliccia P, Venail F, Bonafé A, Bonafé A, Makeieff M, Iannetti G, Bartolomeo M, Mondain M. Cochlea size variability and implications in clinical practice. Acta Otorhinolaryngol Ital. 2014;34(01):42–9.
57. Polak M, Ulubil SA, Hodges AV, Balkany TJ. Revision cochlear implantation for facial nerve stimulation in otosclerosis. Arch Otolaryngol Head Neck Surg. 2006;132(4):398–404. https://doi.org/10.1001/archotol.132.4.398.
58. Quesnel AM, Nakajima HH, Rosowski JJ, Hansen MR, Gantz BJ, Nadol JB Jr. Delayed loss of hearing after hearing preservation cochlear implantation: human temporal bone pathology and implications for etiology. Hear Res. 2016;333:225–34. https://doi.org/10.1016/j.heares.2015.08.018. Epub 2015 Sep 1.
59. Rahman MT, Chari DA, Ishiyama G, Lopez I, Quesnel AM, Ishiyama A, Nadol JB, Hansen MR. Cochlear implants: causes, effects and mitigation strategies for the foreign body response and inflammation. Hear Res. 2022;422:108536.
60. Rask-Andersen H, Liu W, Erixon E, Kinnefors A, Pfaller K, Schrott-Fischer A, Glueckert R. Human cochlea: anatomical characteristics and their relevance for cochlear implantation. Anat Rec (Hoboken). 2012;295(11):1791–811. https://doi.org/10.1002/ar.22599.
61. Roditi RE, Poissant SF, Bero EM, Lee DJ. A predictive model of cochlear implant performance in postlingually deafened adults. Otol Neurotol. 2009;30(4):449–54. https://doi.org/10.1097/MAO.0b013e31819d3480.
62. Sato T, Morita N, Cureoglu S, Terao K, Joglekar SS, Deroee AF, Ishikawa K, Paparella MM. Cochlear otosclerosis adjacent to the round window and oval window: a histopathological temporal bone study. Otol Neurotol. 2010;31(4):574–9. https://doi.org/10.1097/MAO.0b013e3181d8d73b.
63. Scheper V, Hessler R, Hütten M, Wilk M, Jolly C, Lenarz T, Paasche G. Local inner ear application of dexamethasone in cochlear implant models is safe for auditory neurons and increases the neuroprotective effect of chronic electrical stimulation. PLoS One. 2017;12(8):e0183820. https://doi.org/10.1371/journal.pone.0183820.
64. Schurzig D, Repp F, Timm ME, Batsoulis C, Lenarz T, Kral A. Virtual cochlear implantation for personalized rehabilitation of profound hearing loss. Hear Res. 2023;429:108687.
65. Seyyedi M, Eddington DK, Nadol JB Jr. Effect of monopolar and bipolar electric stimulation on survival and size of human spiral ganglion cells as studied by postmortem histopathology. Hear Res. 2013a;302:9–16. https://doi.org/10.1016/j.heares.2013.04.007.
66. Seyyedi M, Herrmann BS, Eddington DK, Nadol JB Jr. The pathologic basis of facial nerve stimulation in otosclerosis and multichannel cochlear implantation. Otol Neurotol. 2013b;34(9):1603–9. https://doi.org/10.1097/MAO.0b013e3182979398.
67. Seyyedi M, Viana LM, Nadol JB Jr. Within-subject comparison of word recognition and spiral ganglion cell count in bilateral cochlear

implant recipients. Otol Neurotol. 2014;35(8):1446–50. https://doi.org/10.1097/MAO.0000000000000443. PMID: 25120196; PMCID: PMC4139064.
68. Shafieibavani E, Goudey B, Kiral I, Zhong P, Jimeno-Yepes A, Swan A, Gambhir M, Buechner A, Kludt E, Eikelboom RH, Sucher C, Gifford RH, Rottier R, Plant K, Anjomshoa H. Predictive models for cochlear implant outcomes: performance, generalizability, and the impact of cohort size. Trends Hear. 2021;25:23312165211066174. https://doi.org/10.1177/23312165211066174.
69. Shaul C, Bester CW, Weder S, Choi J, Eastwood H, Padmavathi KV, Collins A, O'Leary SJ. Electrical impedance as a biomarker for inner ear pathology following lateral wall and peri-modiolar cochlear implantation. Otol Neurotol. 2019;40(5):e518–26. https://doi.org/10.1097/MAO.0000000000002227.
70. Sosna-Duranowska M, Tacikowska G, Gos E, Krupa A, Skarzynski PH, Skarzynski H. Vestibular function after cochlear implantation in partial deafness treatment. Front Neurol. 2021;12:667055. https://doi.org/10.3389/fneur.2021.667055.
71. Spitzer ER, Waltzman SB, Landsberger DM, Friedmann DR. Acceptance and benefits of electro-acoustic stimulation for conventional-length electrode arrays. Audiol Neurootol. 2021;26(1):17–26. https://doi.org/10.1159/000507975.
72. Stakhovskaya O, Sridhar D, Bonham BH, Leake PA. Frequency map for the human cochlear spiral ganglion: implications for cochlear implants. J Assoc Res Otolaryngol. 2007;8(2):220–33. https://doi.org/10.1007/s10162-007-0076-9.
73. Suga F, Lindsay JR. Labyrinthitis ossificans due to chronic otitis media. Ann Otol Rhinol Laryngol. 1975;84(1 Pt 1):37–44. https://doi.org/10.1177/000348947508400106.
74. Su-Velez BM, Lopez IA, Ishiyama A, Ishiyama G. Human temporal bone study of vestibular histopathology in cochlear implant patients with cochlear hydrops. Otol Neurotol. 2020;41(5):e607–14. https://doi.org/10.1097/MAO.0000000000002609.
75. Timm ME, Majdani O, Weller T, Windeler M, Lenarz T, Büchner A, Salcher RB. Patient-specific selection of lateral wall cochlear implant electrodes based on anatomical indication ranges. PLoS One. 2018;13(10):e0206435. https://doi.org/10.1371/journal.pone.0206435.
76. Trakimas DR, Kozin ED, Ghanad I, Nadol JB Jr, Remenschneider AK. Human otopathologic findings in cases of folded cochlear implant electrodes. Otol Neurotol. 2018;39(8):970–8. https://doi.org/10.1097/MAO.0000000000001886.
77. Trakimas DR, Knoll RM, Castillo-Bustamante M, Kozin ED, Remenschneider AK. Otopathologic analysis of patterns of postmeningitis labyrinthitis ossificans. Otolaryngol Head Neck Surg. 2021;164(1):175–81. https://doi.org/10.1177/0194599820934748.
78. Walia A, Shew MA, Varghese J, Ioerger P, Lefler SM, Ortmann AJ, Herzog JA, Buchman CA. Improved cochlear implant performance estimation using tonotopic-based electrocochleography. JAMA Otolaryngol Head Neck Surg. 2023;149(12):1120–9. https://doi.org/10.1001/jamaoto.2023.2988.
79. Wells D, Knoll RM, Kozin E, Chen JX, Reinshagen KL, Staecker H, Curtin HD, McKenna MJ, Nadol JB Jr, Quesnel AM. Otopathologic and computed tomography correlation of internal auditory canal diverticula in otosclerosis. Otol Neurotol. 2022;43(9):e957–62. https://doi.org/10.1097/MAO.0000000000003665.
80. Wu PZ, O'Malley JT, Liberman MC. Neural degeneration in normal-aging human cochleas: machine-learning counts and 3D mapping in archival sections. J Assoc Res Otolaryngol. 2023;24(5):499–511. https://doi.org/10.1007/s10162-023-00909-y.
81. Van Horn A, Hayden C, Mahairas AD, Leader P, Bush ML. Factors influencing aberrant facial nerve stimulation following cochlear implantation: a systematic review and meta-analysis. Otol Neurotol. 2020;41(8):1050–9. https://doi.org/10.1097/mao.0000000000002693.
82. Verbist BM, Skinner MW, Cohen LT, Leake PA, James C, Boëx C, Holden TA, Finley CC, Roland PS, Roland JT Jr, Haller M, Patrick JF, Jolly CN, Faltys MA, Briaire JJ, Frijns JH. Consensus panel on a cochlear coordinate system applicable in histologic, physiologic, and radiologic studies of the human cochlea. Otol Neurotol. 2010;31(5):722–30. https://doi.org/10.1097/MAO.0b013e3181d279e0.
83. Yousef MF, Theyab R, Garadat SN, Hagr A. Bilateral cochlear implantations in temporal bone fracture: a viable treatment option. Laryngoscope. 2021;132(10):2050–5. https://doi.org/10.1002/lary.29994.
84. Zahara D, Dewi RD, Aboet A, Putranto FM, Lubis ND, Ashar T. Variations in cochlear size of cochlear implant candidates. Int Arch Otorhinolaryngol. 2019;23(2):184–90. https://doi.org/10.1055/s-0038-1661360.
85. Zeng FG. JASA Express Lett. 2022;2(077201). https://doi.org/10.1121/10.0012825.

Auditory Brainstem Implantation

22

Daniel S. Roberts, Steven R. Otto, Marc S. Schwartz, and Eric P. Wilkinson

Introduction

Frequently, loss of integrity of the auditory nerve after removal of vestibular schwannomas in neurofibromatosis type 2 (NF2) leaves patients completely deafened. Other communication methods such as signing and lipreading have provided some assistance, but obviously, these modalities cannot restore audiologic perception. The auditory brainstem implant (ABI) was developed to bypass the auditory nerve by directly stimulating the cochlear nucleus complex. Remarkably, useful auditory perception is possible [1, 2]. The multichannel version of the ABI (Nucleus®, Cochlear Corporation, Englewood, Colorado) successfully completed US Food and Drug Administration (FDA) clinical trials in July, 2000, and it received approval for commercial release shortly thereafter. Since then, ABIs have also been produced by other implant manufacturers, including MED-EL GmbH (Innsbruck, Austria), which are not approved for use in the United States. This chapter summarizes the history, surgical, and clinical aspects of ABI implantation and perceptual performance.

History of Development

In 1979, William House and William Hitselberger first implanted an electrode to stimulate the cochlear nucleus of a patient with NF2 facing deafness after removal of a vestibular schwannoma. The patient was persistent in her requests that an ABI be tried in the hope that it would allow her to continue to have some auditory perception. The electrode was a simple ball type, and electrical stimulation was supplied by a modified, body-worn hearing aid. Useful auditory perception was achieved, but the electrode proved somewhat unstable and was shortly removed. A two-electrode (later three) mesh-type array was subsequently developed by Huntington Medical Research Institute (HMRI, Pasadena, California) and was used successfully in 25 recipients. The speech processors were modified 3 M/House-type cochlear implant processors that provided patients with sound awareness, ability to discriminate some environmental sounds, and significantly improved understanding of speech in conjunction with lipreading. Experiments also suggested that multichannel stimulation was feasible and would be potentially beneficial with a multiple-electrode array. This led to the development and successful use of the current multichannel ABI.

Patient Selection

At least 90% of individuals with NF2 have bilateral vestibular schwannomas [3]. Treatment of these, and other tumors associated with NF2, has significantly prolonged the lifespan of such patients. Although audiologic performance with an ABI is typically less robust than with a cochlear implant, the auditory information provided can significantly enhance quality of life and the ability to function in occupational and social environments relative to anacusis.

Hearing preservation is a goal in management of NF2-related vestibular schwannomas, and early diagnosis and treatment can be helpful in this effort. However, when hearing preservation is not possible, the ABI provides an alternative auditory rehabilitative option.

The multichannel ABI is approved for use in individuals with NF2 who are at least 12 years of age. There are no preoperative audiologic criteria because the surgical procedure for tumor resection and electrode array placement generally

D. S. Roberts (✉)
Division of Otolaryngology—Head and Neck Surgery, University of Connecticut School of Medicine, Farmington, CT, USA

S. R. Otto
House Clinic and House Ear Institute, Los Angeles, CA, USA

M. S. Schwartz
Department of Neurological Surgery, University of California—San Diego, San Diego, CA, USA

E. P. Wilkinson
Idaho Ear Clinic, Meridian, ID, USA

A. D. Sweeney et al. (eds.), *Haynes-Glasscock-Shambaugh Surgery of the Ear*, https://doi.org/10.1007/978-3-032-18264-7_22

eliminate residual hearing. Implantation may occur during first- or second-side vestibular schwannoma removal or in patients with previously resected bilateral tumors. A small but significant number of patients (9% at House Clinic) fail to experience auditory responses from the implant, primarily because of anatomic difficulties. In this instance, a second opportunity for ABI placement can be realized if a vestibular schwannoma is sequentially removed from the contralateral side.

Realistically, an ABI may not be the best option for every patient with NF2. A number of non-implant-related factors including general health, vision, social activity, and anatomic factors (as seen on magnetic resonance imaging [MRI]) can influence ABI benefit. Age can also be an important consideration. For example, the House Ear institutional experience is that teenage implant recipients, in general, have been less successful than older recipients. Patients with limited vision also have shown relatively less benefit, since the ABI works best in conjunction with lipreading; however, a few blind ABI recipients have benefited from their ABIs. Candidates for ABIs should be apprised of the potential effects of these factors on their ability to benefit from the device.

Off-label applications of the ABI include bilateral temporal bone fractures that involve the cochlea and cause deafness in a manner that precludes cochlear implantation (such as ossification), cochlear ossification from meningitis, cochlear nerve avulsion, and cochlear agenesis. The ABI also may be beneficial in cases of demyelinating diseases affecting the eighth cranial nerve but sparing at least one cochlear nucleus. Congenitally deaf children who have been deemed not to be candidates for cochlear implantation (CI) or who have failed to progress with CI due to severe cochlear malformation or cochlear nerve aplasia have been implanted with success, which is an area of active investigation. A clinical trial at the House Ear Clinic recently studied these outcomes in children [4], and outcomes from other centers are described in the results section of this chapter [5–7].

Preoperative Evaluation and Counseling

Preoperative determination of informed consent regarding the ABI is extremely important to the success of an ABI program. Preoperative evaluation and counseling help prepare patients for the loss of hearing after tumor removal and lay the groundwork for acclimation to a new modality of hearing with the ABI. Prospective recipients and their families should have appropriate expectations regarding the potential benefits and limitations of the device. A frank and thorough explanation of what is involved in using an ABI is necessary. Inadequate preparation can significantly delay and complicate acceptance and use of the implant.

A major criterion for successful integration and use of the device is a high level of motivation and determination to make maximal use of whatever auditory sensations the ABI provides. Willingness to participate in the postoperative follow-ups is also very important in optimizing device function. Preoperative counseling provides an opportunity to explore motivation issues and to explain the need for judicious compliance with the follow-up audiologic and rehabilitative protocols. Special counseling may also be helpful in patients having difficulties coping with deafness and other disabilities related to NF2. Such difficulties can distract patients from learning to use an ABI in the postoperative period.

Patients should also be counseled preoperatively about the likelihood that they will experience mild nonauditory sensations such as tingling or dizziness on some electrodes, as well as the possibility that the ABI may not ultimately provide meaningful auditory sensations. The focus at House Ear has been to maintain a tone of hopeful and cautious optimism in preoperative counseling of relevant patients. This approach has worked well in eliminating unpleasant surprises and properly setting the stage for postoperative rehabilitation.

The participation of an experienced, skilled, and coordinated multidisciplinary team is necessary for the successful treatment and management of patients with NF2. Each team member is essential to the success of an ABI program. Chief among these is the surgeon's skill and experience in removing tumors, preserving necessary structures, and accurately placing the electrode array. Electrophysiologic monitoring expertise contributes to proper identification of the implant site. Postoperatively, implant audiology expertise is required to program the speech processor and optimize perceptual performance. Even under ideal circumstances, adapting to and learning to use an ABI is an ongoing process that typically extends over a longer period than in cochlear implantation. New recipients should be encouraged that performance almost always improves with experience.

Device

Hitselberger and colleagues originally used a cochlear implant ball-type electrode in their first ABI recipient [8]. Subsequently, patients received a 2 × 8-mm fabric mesh array with two or three platinum ribbon electrodes. In 1992, House Ear Institute (HEI) collaborated with Cochlear Corporation and Huntington Medical Research Institute (Pasadena, California) in the development of an eight-electrode multichannel ABI system. This was further upgraded to the 21-electrode Cochlear Nucleus 24 device. The preponderance of implanted patients in the United States have received this device. The production of the Cochlear Nucleus 24 device was discontinued in 2015, and the substitute Cochlear Device, ABI541, was not approved by the FDA until 2016. During this period, both Cochlear and the MED-EL Synchrony devices were implanted under the auspices of "Compassionate Use" approval by the FDA in the United States on an individual, case-by-case basis [9]. FDA approval was granted in June of 2016 for the ABI541. The MED-EL device has been used in the United States through an open clinical trial (ClinicalTrials.gov ID NCT01736267).

The ABI541 electrode array comprises a flexible perforated silicone and mesh substrate with 0.7-mm platinum disk electrodes. This design facilitates conformation of the array to the surface of the cochlear nucleus and promotes long-term stability. The MED-EL Synchrony device uses a smaller surface array profile with the goal of aiding placement. The device also has a four-channel test electrode that allows confirmation of electric auditory brainstem responses (EABRs) prior to ABI implantation. Two potential advantages of the test electrode array exist: if no EABR response is present, implantation may be deferred preventing implantation of a device that will not be functional, and the test electrode is slightly smaller with no Dacron backing, allowing for mobility and minimizing damage while conforming to the location of the cochlear nucleus.

The penetrating electrode ABI (PABI) system was used at the House Ear Institute in a research setting. The device includes two electrode arrays with a 10- (or 12-) electrode surface-type array, plus an array with 8 (or 10) penetrating needle-type microelectrodes. The PABI system used the same external sound processor equipment and strategies as the regular surface ABI. While this device resulted in increased selectivity and lowered charge requirements in the usable penetrating electrodes, improved speech discrimination was not demonstrated [10]. Currently, all commercially available devices do not utilize penetrating electrodes. Examples of electrodes are shown in Fig. 22.1.

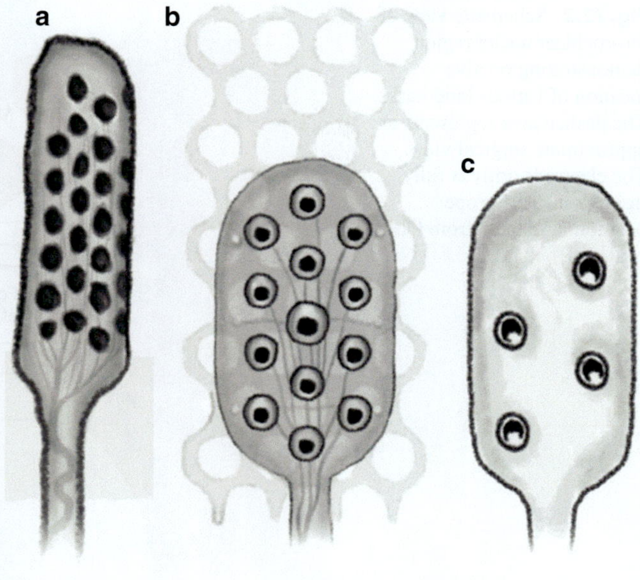

Fig. 22.1 Illustration of ABI electrode arrays. (**a**) Cochlear ABI541 21 electrode array, (**b**) MED-EL Synchrony ABI electrode array with a Dacron backing, (**c**) MED-EL Synchrony ABI four-channel ABI placing electrode without a Dacron backing. (Republished with permission from Roberts et al. [9])

Anatomic Considerations

The dorsal and ventral cochlear nuclei are the targets for placement of the ABI electrode array. Although the nuclei are hidden by the cerebellar peduncle, surface landmarks are useful in identifying this region. Frequently, however, these structures may be distorted by tumors. Figure 22.2 shows the major structures of the pontomedullary junction and the surgical field of view afforded by the translabyrinthine approach. Important landmarks include the terminus of the sleeve-like lateral recess forming the foramen of Luschka, the root of the glossopharyngeal (ninth) nerve, and the vestibulocochlear and facial nerve roots.

Normally, the intact choroid plexus marks the entrance to the lateral recess (foramen of Luschka), and the taenia obliquely traverses the roof of the lateral recess, marking the surface of the ventral cochlear nucleus. These structures may not be clearly identifiable when a large tumor distorts the lateral surface of the pons and medulla. In such cases, the stump of the eighth nerve may be traced to the opening of the lateral recess. The ninth cranial nerve can

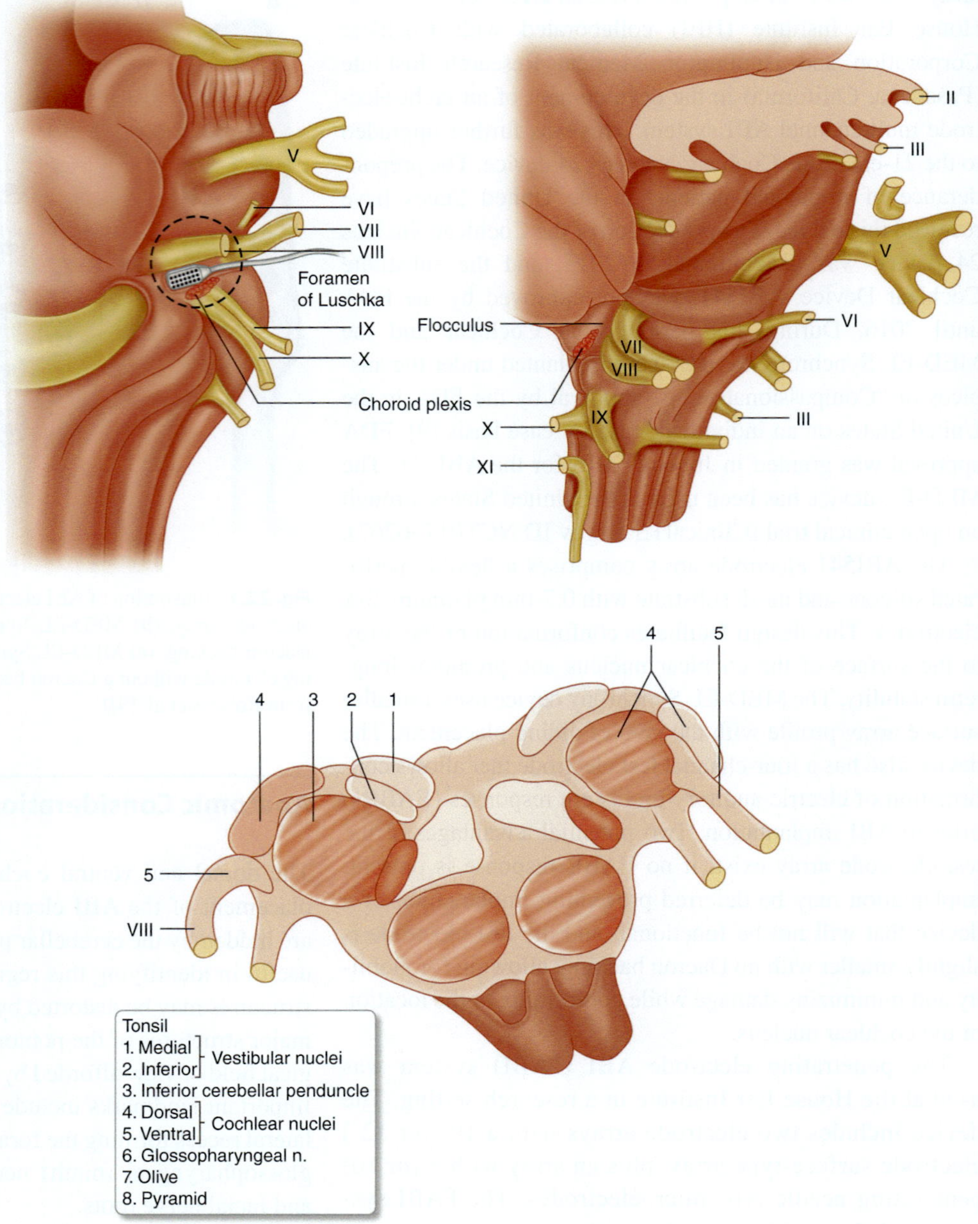

Fig. 22.2 Schematic view of the cochlear nuclei region demonstrating relative location of various landmarks. The dashed area represents an approximate surgical view. The electrode array is fully inserted into the proper position. (Adapted from Otto et al. [28])

also be used as a reference point for the lateral recess. A concavity sometimes visualized between the eighth and ninth nerves should not be confused with the introitus of the recess.

Within the lateral recess and on its superior aspect are found the dorsal and ventral cochlear nuclei. The electrode array is positioned well within the recess to provide positional stability. Electrical stimulation of the ventral cochlear nucleus, the main relay for eighth nerve input, and the major portion of the ascending auditory pathway is probably the primary source of auditory sensations, even though some part of the array also lies adjacent to the dorsal cochlear nucleus.

Surgical Considerations

At the House Clinic, the translabyrinthine craniotomy is preferred for tumor removal and exposure of the lateral recess of the fourth ventricle. However, other centers offer the retrosigmoid approach with success [7, 11]. The retrosigmoid approach is useful in cases where the sigmoid sinus is located anteriorly or in pediatric cases. A typical translabyrinthine tumor removal process is followed except that recording electrodes are placed for monitoring EABRs and any activity from cranial nerves VII and IX. Also, a standard postauricular incision is used and the device is placed into a pocket in the temporal area (Fig. 22.3). Intravenous antibiotics, such as

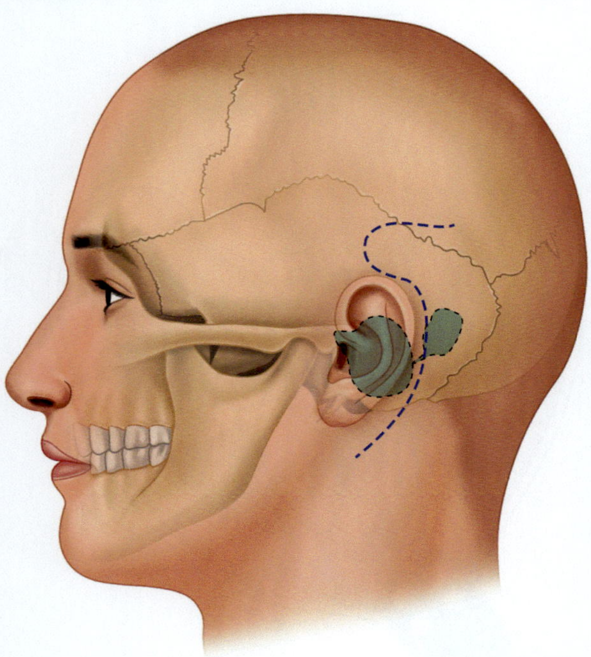

Fig. 22.3 Location of the incision with respect to the planned site of receiver/stimulator. The superior extension may not be necessary. The implant is then placed into a subcutaneous pocket. (Adapted from Gulya et al. [29])

cefuroxime (Zinacef®, GlaxoSmithKline), are administered prophylactically on induction of anesthesia in a weight-specific manner. Monitoring of the EABR assists with confirmation that the electrode array is properly positioned. Slight adjustments of the array may be necessary to minimize responses that suggest activation of nonauditory neural structures. For EABR monitoring, subdermal needle electrodes are inserted at the vertex of the head, over the seventh cervical vertebra, and at the hairline of the occiput. For electromyographic recording of nonauditory activation, the facial nerve is monitored in the standard fashion [12], and bipolar electrodes are inserted in the ipsilateral pharyngeal (soft palate) muscles to monitor activity from cranial nerve IX. After the receiver/stimulator has been secured and the array placed, a transmitter coil is placed over the receiver antenna. The EABR obtained with biphasic pulsatile stimulation of the cochlear nucleus differs from responses obtained using acoustic stimulation and from electrical stimulation using cochlear implants [13]. An experienced electrophysiologist interprets these waveforms intraoperatively and provides feedback to the neurosurgeon regarding device placement.

Implantation Procedure

Tumor dissection proceeds in the normal fashion via a translabyrinthine craniotomy. After complete tumor removal and adequate hemostasis, the site for the internal receiver posterosuperior to the mastoid cavity is determined, and temporalis muscle in this area is elevated off the parietal skull and excised. Using a replica of the receiver/stimulator as a guide, a well is fashioned from the bony cortex in this area using cutting burs, and a trench is created between the implant seat and the mastoid cavity for placement of the electrode wires (Fig. 22.4). Tunnel holes are then created on either side of the receiver/stimulator, and suture is placed through these holes prior to electrode array positioning so that manipulation of the leads does not alter electrode placement (Fig. 22.5). A tight periosteal pocket is also a viable alternative to a tie-down technique. Once the internal receiver has been implanted, only bipolar electrocautery should be used for hemostasis since current transmission through the implant to the brainstem is a potential hazard with monopolar electrocautery.

The location of the lateral recess may be confirmed by noting the egress of cerebrospinal fluid (CSF) as the anesthesiologist induces the Valsalva maneuver in the patient. This technique should be reserved as a final check after the opening to the recess has been located using standard landmarks since CSF will be drained quickly, and the advantage of this technique is lost with multiple Valsalva maneuvers.

After identifying the foramen of Luschka, the electrode array is mounted on a Rosen needle and inserted into the lateral recess with the electrodes oriented superiorly (Fig. 22.6). With experience, we have found that the implant functions better, with fewer nonauditory side effects, when the electrodes are placed fully within the lateral recess [4]. After placement, selected electrodes in the array are activated to confirm their position over the cochlear nucleus. They are tested for the presence of EABRs, stimulation of adjacent cranial nerves (VII and IX), and changes in vital signs. The position of the electrode array usually needs very slight adjustment to maximize auditory stimulation and minimize electromyographic responses from the other nerves. If nerve IX is activated, a small insulating pad of Teflon is interposed between the electrodes and the nerve. For the MED-EL Synchrony device, a four-channel ABI test electrode is first used to generate EABR responses from the cochlear nucleus. Measurements are repeated until adequate EABR tracings are obtained for all electrode combinations.

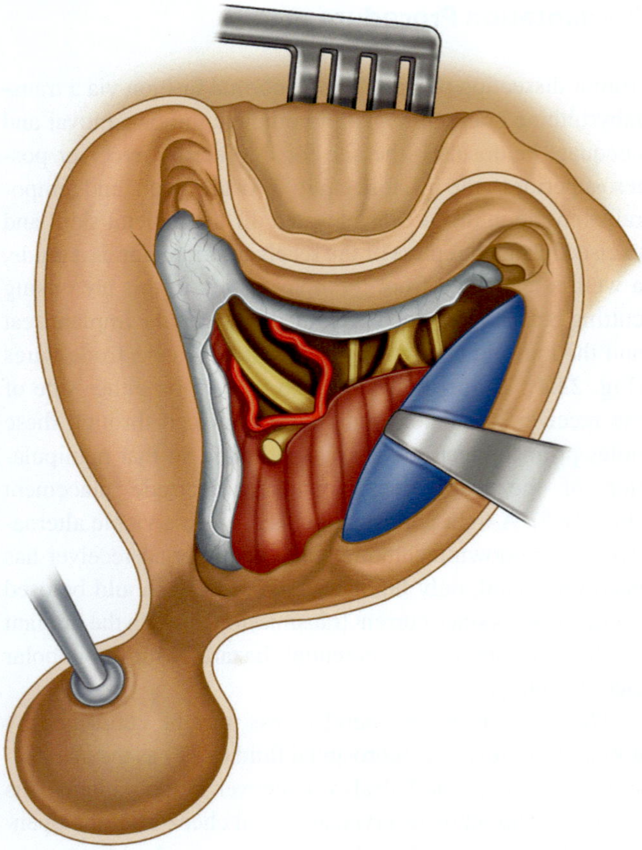

Fig. 22.4 Schematic surgical view of the completed translabyrinthine craniotomy, trench for receiver/stimulator wires, and receiver/stimulator seat being drilled. (Adapted from Gulya et al. [29])

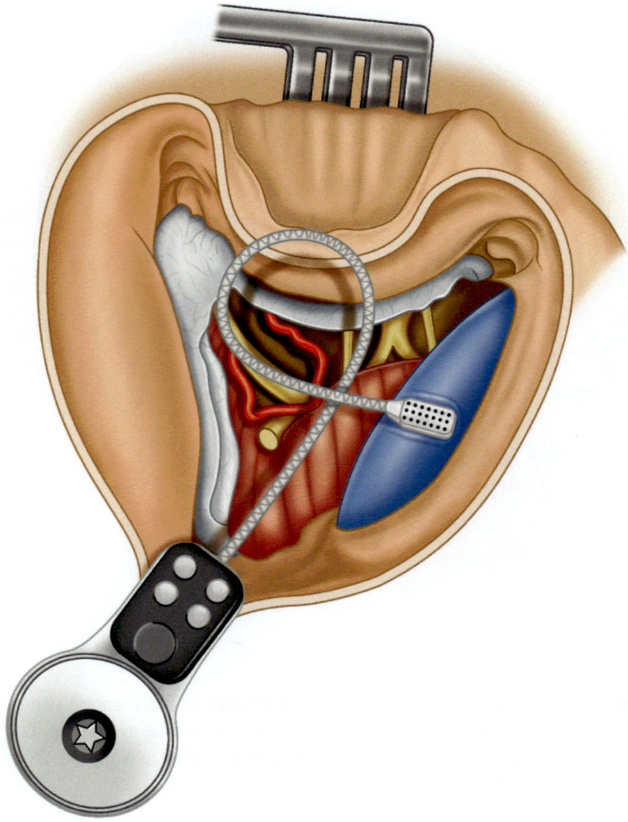

Fig. 22.5 The receiver/stimulator has now been placed into the bone seat. (Adapted from Gulya et al. [29])

The test electrode is then removed, and the active implant is then placed, again using EABR data to assist with positioning. A final EABR recording using the active electrode array is then performed to confirm correct placement.

The electrode array is secured using a small piece of Teflon packed into the meatus of the lateral recess. Subsequent ingrowth of fibrous tissue eventually stabilizes the array in position. The electrode wiring is positioned within the mastoid cavity and bony trench. The eustachian tube and middle ear are then packed with oxidized cellulose (Surgicel®) and muscle. Abdominal fat is used to obliterate the mastoid defect (Fig. 22.7).

At that time, the magnet in the receiver/stimulator can be removed to allow for future surveillance MRIs when using Cochlear ABI541 device. The MED-EL Synchrony ABI magnet can generally remain in place due to MRI conditionality. Since the magnet is typically removed from the receiver/stimulator at the time of implantation for the Cochlear ABI541, there may be difficulty in identifying the location of the receiver/stimulator at the time of initial stimulation. Improper positioning of the external transmitter coil in such cases may lead to the false impression of

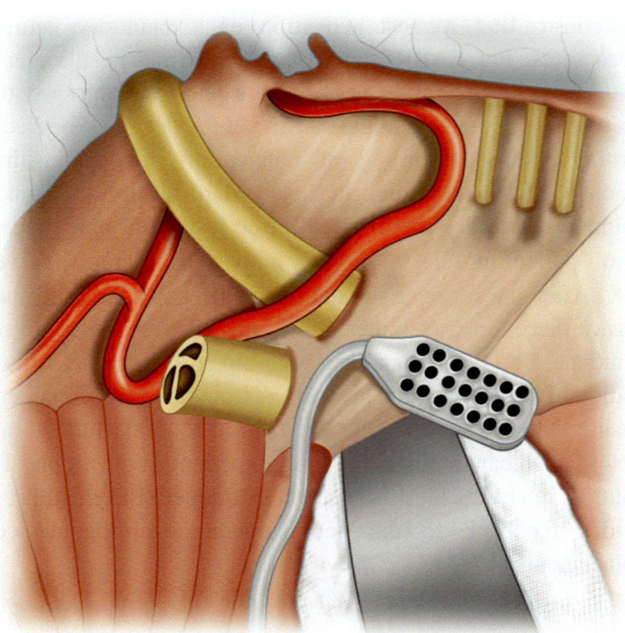

Fig. 22.6 The ABI electrode array being placed into the lateral recess. (Adapted from Gulya et al. [29])

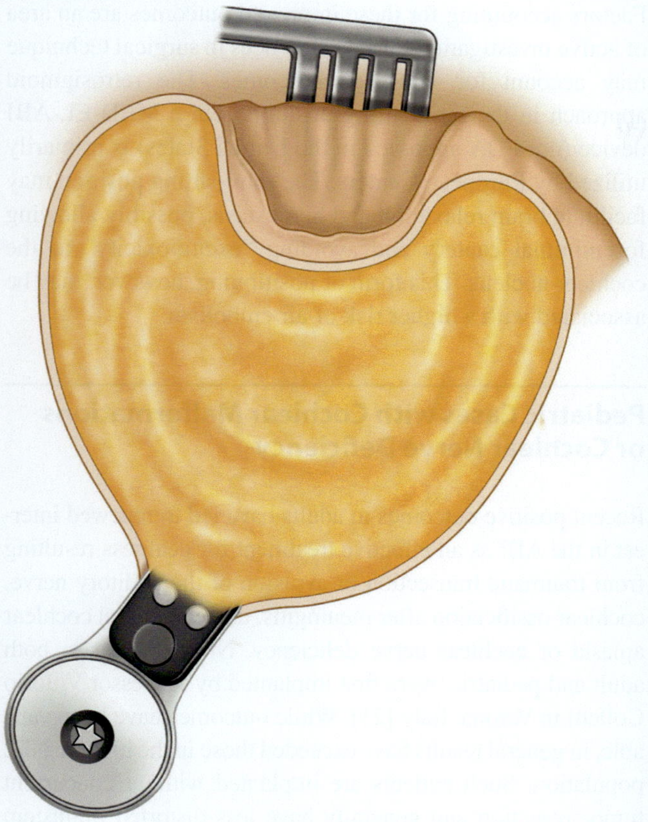

Fig. 22.7 Fat obliteration of the surgical cavity. (Adapted from Gulya et al. [29])

device failure or stimulation failure on the part of the patient. We now routinely tattoo the center location of the circular receiver/stimulator antenna at the time of surgery to facilitate its location postoperatively. The incision is then closed in layers.

Postoperative Care

Postoperative care after ABI is similar to that following routine craniotomies for tumor removal. A large mastoid-type dressing is left in place for 3 days. Careful attention to any moisture on the bandages allows prompt identification of CSF leak through the postauricular wound. The device is typically activated for the first time as many as 8 weeks after implantation, allowing for resolution of edema in the skin flap overlying the receiver/stimulator, which would otherwise prevent an adequate signal from reaching the implant. In actual use, implant patients may need to shave this area and apply a thin tape and metal disk ("retainer" disk) to which the magnetic transmitter coil adheres. The patient, or a companion, must be trained to ensure proper and consistent positioning of the transmitter coil over the implant receiver/stimulator. Many complaints about poor signal or deterioration in sound quality can be traced to improper positioning of the retainer disk.

Postoperative Complications

The most significant complication in the immediate postoperative period is CSF leak. Unlike routine translabyrinthine surgery, in which the fluid usually takes the nasal route via the eustachian tube, the ABI electrode and wires provide a pathway along which CSF can travel under the skin flap. Prevention of a leak begins with meticulous dural approximation. Although the dural opening cannot be closed in a watertight manner, it should be approximated as closely as possible and strips of abdominal fat are used to plug the residual dural defect.

Surgicel® and muscle are commonly employed for eustachian tube and middle ear closure, and autologous fat packs the mastoid cavity. Titanium mesh is placed over the fat to hold it in position. Finally, a multilayered closure of the wound reduces the risk of CSF leak through the incision.

Despite these precautions, patients with ABIs appear more prone to CSF leak than those undergoing translabyrinthine procedures without implantation. Leaks from the nose and wound usually respond to reapplication of a mastoid pressure dressing and bed rest. A lumbar-subarachnoid drain is inserted for persistent leaks. When these maneuvers fail to control a leak, we perform a blind sac closure of the ear canal with removal of the external auditory canal skin, tympanic membrane, malleus, and incus. The eustachian tube is then closed with Surgicel® packing and bone wax, and the middle ear is filled with muscle. This is a safer way to control CSF leaks than surgical exploration and repacking of the wound. Meningitis can occur either spontaneously or as a result of postoperative CSF leak. This unusual complication, when identified promptly, responds to antibiotics and control of the leak.

Results

Comprehensive performance results from the initial group of multichannel ABI recipients have been reported elsewhere [2]. With some notable exceptions, speech perception with the ABI typically does not reach the very high levels generally attained with modern cochlear implants. However, the auditory sensations in combination with lipreading can be highly beneficial in facilitating oral communication. With regular and continued use of the ABI, recipients typically show substantial improvements in performance over time. Regular use of the device greatly enhances performance, and patients should be counseled about this necessity preoperatively.

Over 310 patients with NF2 have been implanted with the Nucleus multichannel ABI system at House Clinic between 1992 and the present. Approximately 1300 patients have been implanted worldwide. With notable exceptions, ABI performance generally has not reached the high levels typically seen with CIs at our center. Eighty percent of ABI patients are device users, and 92% have received auditory sensations from their ABIs. The majority of patients recognize a high percentage of environmental sounds, and speech understanding ability is enhanced an average of 35% when ABI sound is combined with lipreading. This enhancement has reached as high as 75% in some individuals. Although improvements are generally greatest during the first year, many patients have continued to improve even after 10 years of use. All patients used the SPEAK (spectral maxima) speech processing strategy [14].

Approximately 25% of ABI users at our center have achieved some open-set speech discrimination (at least 20% correct without lipreading cues on the CUNY Sentence Test) [15, 16]. Several of these individuals were also able to communicate on the telephone to a limited extent. Ten patients at the House Clinic have scored 65% or better, and three patients have scored 82% or better on this test. Cumulative data from our center and others is presented in Table 22.1 (Adapted from Roberts et al., 2017) [17].

Recent reports notably illustrate the successful outcomes among NF2 patients with as high as 37% rate of open speech perception at 1 year and 41% at 2 years after activation [18, 19]. An inverse relationship between deafness duration and open speech perception was noted among these patients. Factors accounting for these improved outcomes are an area of active investigation [20]. Differences in surgical technique may account for improved outcomes. The retrosigmoid approach in the semi-sitting position with a MED-EL ABI device (not FDA approved in the United States) is primarily utilized by European Centers. The semi-sitting position may facilitate brain relaxation and hemostasis, possibly allowing for minimal cautery and avoiding "excitotoxicity" to the cochlear nucleus. This form of positioning, however, may be associated with a higher risk of air embolism.

Table 22.1 ABI outcomes in NF2

First author	Year	N	Daily users, N (%)	Open-set sentence recognition, N (%)	No auditory response, N (%)
Laszig	1995	9	4 (42%)	0 (0%)	1 (11%)
Lenarz	2002	13	13 (93%)	0 (0%)	1/13 (8%)
Vincent	2002	14	12 (85%)	3 (21%)	1 (7%)
Nevison	2002	26	23 (88%)	2 (8%)	1 (4%)
Otto	2002	61	55 (90%)	5%	6 (9%)
Kanowitz	2004	18	11 (61%)	0 (0%)	1 (6%)
Behr	2006	20	18 (90%)	8 (42%)	NR
Grayeli	2008	23	16 (70%)	8 (34%)	5 (22%)
Schwartz	2003	230	NR	5%	15%
Maini	2009	10	7 (70%)	5%	1 (10%)
Sanna	2012	24	19 (79%)	4 (17%)	4 (17%)
Matthies	2013	32	27 (84%)	37%	3 (9%)
Matthies	2014	18	16 (88%)	41%	2 (11%)
Thong	2016	8	3 (38%)	1 (13%)	2 (25%)
Ramsden	2016	49	29 (59%)	5 (10%)	4 (8%)
Average			74%	14%	12%

Adapted from Roberts et al. [17]

Pediatric Cases with Cochlear Malformations or Cochlear Nerve Deficiency

Recent positive outcomes in adults have led to renewed interest in the ABI as an effective treatment for deafness resulting from traumatic transection or avulsion of the auditory nerve, cochlear ossification after meningitis, and congenital cochlear aplasia or cochlear nerve deficiency. Non-NF2 cases, both adult and pediatric, were first implanted by Professor Vittorio Colletti in Verona, Italy [21]. While outcomes have been variable, in general results have exceeded those in the historic NF2 population. Such patients are implanted without concurrent tumor resection and generally have less distorted brainstem anatomy, which helps preserve neural function and facilitates the identification of important anatomical landmarks used in device implantation. This factor may be particularly important in maximizing ABI outcomes in pediatric cases.

ABIs are being trialed in Los Angeles by a multidisciplinary team including House Clinic surgeons under the auspices of the FDA and with funding from the National Institutes of Health for the treatment of deafness in pediatric cases with cochlear malformations or cochlear nerve deficiency [4]. Other centers are also performing ABIs in non-NF2 children in the research setting [22]. Results indicate that some children develop a substantial level of auditory function, including discrimination of environmental sounds. Long-term data from other centers suggests that open set recognition of speech, development of expressive speech and language skills, and, in some cases, attendance in a "normal-hearing" classroom with appropriate support services may be possible [5–7]. Pediatric cases without concurrent developmental delay tend to perform best. A retrosigmoid surgical approach has typically been used because the mastoid is less developed in pediatric cases, and the patients have generally been positioned in the lateral position. Early implantation seems to provide the best outcomes, and generally, diminishing returns are seen as duration of deafness increases. In all cases, benefits of ABI surgery must be weighed against the risk of craniotomy.

Auditory Midbrain Implant and Inferior Colliculus Implant

The inferior colliculus (IC) is a desirable target for an auditory prosthesis because the central nucleus of the inferior colliculus (ICC) is a locus of convergence for ascending auditory pathways and may have utility as a primary modality for auditory rehabilitation or when tumor location makes ABI unattainable [23, 24]. Two approaches, to include the use of a surface array and a penetrating array, have shown promise to safely produce auditory sensations [23, 25]. Two studies have examined the effect of bypassing the lower brainstem by stimulating the IC with either a surface electrode array (the auditory midbrain implant [AMI]) [25] or a penetrating array (the inferior colliculus implant [ICI]) [26]. The AMI was safe and provided auditory sensations, aided with lipreading, sound awareness, and some speech perception in a clinical trial from 2006 to 2008 of five patients [27]. However, AMI has not yet demonstrated the outcomes comparable to the highest ABI performers, with no patients achieving open-set sentence recognition. Despite these limitations, device and surgical modifications are an area of active investigation with further clinical trials planned [27].

Summary

The multichannel ABI is a viable means of providing useful hearing sensation to individuals deafened by NF2. The sound information provided by the device facilitates sound awareness, recognition, and spoken communication when used in conjunction with lipreading. A small percentage of ABI recipients also experience significant degrees of speech understanding even without lipreading. The recent performance increases have resulted in renewed interest in ABI. Current research seeks to understand the factors that may lead to better audiometric outcomes. Recent data also suggests significant benefits for non-NF2 patients and current research is investigating optimal outcomes in pediatric patients with cochlear malformations or cochlear nerve deficiency.

Acknowledgments The authors are grateful to the patients and staff of House Ear Institute for their time and effort on behalf of ABI research. We also thank the previous authors of this chapter (S. Otto, D. Brackmann, W. Hitselberger, E. Toh, R. Shannon, L. Friesen) who created the foundation for this contribution.

References

1. Eisenberg LS, Maltan AA, Portillo F, et al. Electrical stimulation of the auditory brainstem structure in deafened adults. J Rehabil Res Dev. 1987;24:9–22.
2. Otto SR, Brackmann DE, Hitselberger WE, et al. Multichannel auditory brainstem implant: update on performance in 61 patients. J Neurosurg. 2002;96:1063–71.
3. Riccardi VM. Neurofibromatosis. Neurol Clin. 1987;5:337–49.
4. Wilkinson EP, Eisenberg LS, Krieger MD, et al. Initial results of a safety and feasibility study of auditory brainstem implantation in congenitally deaf children. Otol Neurotol. 2017;38(2):212–20.
5. Colletti V, Carner M, Miorelli V, et al. Auditory brainstem implant (ABI): new frontiers in adults and children. Otolaryngol Head Neck Surg. 2005;133(1):126–38.
6. Colletti V, Shannon RV. Open set speech perception with auditory brainstem implant? Laryngoscope. 2005;115(11):1974–8.
7. Colletti V, Sacchetto L, Giarbini N, et al. Retrosigmoid approach for auditory brainstem implant. J Laryngol Otol Suppl. 2000;27:37–40.
8. Hitselberger WE, House WF, Edgerton BS, Whitaker S. Cochlear nucleus implant. Otolaryngol Head Neck Surg. 1984;92:52–4.
9. Roberts DS, Slattery WH, Chen BS, et al. Compassionate use protocol for auditory brainstem implantation in neurofibromatosis type 2: early House ear institute experience. Cochlear Implants Int. 2017;18:1–62. https://doi.org/10.1080/14670100.2016.1258203.
10. Otto SR, Shannon RV, Wilkinson EP, et al. Audiologic outcomes with the penetrating electrode auditory brainstem implant. Otol Neurotol. 2008;29(8):1147–54.
11. Puram SV, Herrmann B, Barker FG 2nd, et al. Retrosigmoid craniotomy for auditory brainstem implantation in adult patients with neurofibromatosis type 2. J Neurol Surg B Skull Base. 2015;76(6):440–50.
12. Niparko JK, Kileny PR, Kemink JL, et al. Neurophysiologic intraoperative monitoring: II. Facial nerve function. Am J Otol. 1989;10:55–61.
13. Waring MD. Refractory properties of auditory brain-stem responses evoked by electrical stimulation of human cochlear nucleus: evidence of neural generators. Electroencephalogr Clin Neurophysiol. 1998;108:331–4.
14. McDermott HJ, McKay CM, Vandali AE. A new portable sound processor for the University of Melbourne/nucleus multielectrode cochlear implant. J Acoust Soc Am. 1992;91:3367–71.
15. Brackmann DE, Hitselberger WE, Nelson RA, et al. Auditory brainstem implant: I. Issues in surgical implantation. Otolaryngol Head Neck Surg. 1993;108:624–33.
16. Shannon RV, Fayad J, Moore JK, et al. Auditory brain- stem implant: II. Postsurgical issues and performance. Otolaryngol Head Neck Surg. 1993;108:634–42.
17. Roberts D, Otto SR, Schwartz MS, Wilkinson EP. Auditory rehabilitation in neurofibromatosis type 2. In: Comprehensive management of vestibular schwannoma. New York: Thieme Publishers; 2017.
18. Matthies C, Brill S, Kaga K, et al. Auditory brainstem implantation improves speech recognition in neurofibromatosis type II patients. ORL J Otorhinolaryngol Relat Spec. 2013;75(5):282–95.
19. Matthies C, Brill S, Varallyay C, et al. Auditory brainstem implants in neurofibromatosis type 2: is open speech perception feasible? J Neurosurg. 2014;120(2):546–58.

20. Schwartz MS. Letters to the editor. Auditory brainstem implants in neurofibromatosis type 2. J Neurosurg. 2014;121(3):760–2.
21. Colletti V, Shannon R, Carner M, Veronese S, Colletti L. Outcomes in non-tumor adults fitted with the auditory brainstem implant: 10 years experience. Otol Neurotol. 2009;30(5):614–8.
22. Puram SV, Barber SR, Kozin ED, et al. Outcomes following pediatric auditory brainstem implant surgery: early experiences in a north American center. Otolaryngol Head Neck Surg. 2016;155(1):133–8.
23. Lim HH, Lenarz M, Lenarz T. Auditory midbrain implant: a review. Trends Amplif. 2009;13(3):149–80.
24. Casseday JH, Fremouw T, Covey E. The inferior colliculus: A hub for the central auditory system. In: Oertel D, Fay RR, Popper AN, editors. Springer handbook of auditory research: Integrative functions in the mammalian auditory pathway, vol. 15. New York: Springer-Verlag; 2002. p. 238–318.
25. Colletti V, Shannon R, Carner M, et al. The first successful case of hearing produced by electrical stimulation of the human midbrain. Otol Neurotol. 2007;28:39–43.
26. Lenarz T, Lim HH, Reuter G, et al. The auditory midbrain implant: a new auditory prosthesis for neural deafness—concept and device description. Otol Neurotol. 2006;27:838–43.
27. Lim HH, Lenarz T. Auditory midbrain implant: research and development towards a second clinical trial. Hear Res. 2015;322:212–23.
28. Otto SR, Hitselberger WE, Telischi FF, et al. Auditory brainstem implant. In: Brackmann DE, Shelton C, Arriaga MA, editors. Otologic surgery. 2nd ed. Philadelphia: WB Saunders; 2001. p. 594–603.
29. Gulya AJ, Minor LB, Poe D, editors. 6th Edition of Glasscock and Shambaugh's surgery of the ear. PMPH; 2010.

Vestibular Rehabilitation

23

Devin L. McCaslin, Neil T. Shepard, and Courtney D. Hall

Introduction

Current vestibular rehabilitation for peripheral vestibular hypofunction is an exercise-based approach that typically includes a combination of four different exercise elements: (1) gaze stabilization exercises; (2) habituation exercises as needed based on symptoms; (3) balance and gait training; and (4) endurance and strength exercises. There is considerable evidence that vestibular rehabilitation is effective in improving symptoms and function in patients with unilateral or bilateral peripheral vestibular dysfunction [1–3].

The Physiologic Basis for Vestibular Rehabilitation

Background on Physiology

The majority of insults that occur to the peripheral vestibular system are unilateral and can occur as the result of a number of disorders. The loss of function can be localized to either the hair cells in the labyrinth or the nerve fibers that connect those cells to the brain. If the damage is severe enough, this type of impairment will generate a neural asymmetry between the inputs to the central vestibular system from the two end-organs. This imbalance in neural firing rate is interpreted by the brain as rotation toward the intact side in the plane of the impaired semicircular canal (SCC). The extended asymmetry in neural firing is sensed by the brain as being aberrant and central vestibular system structures (i.e., cerebellum and brainstem) are recruited to restore the balance. This adjustment process is referred to as vestibular compensation and occurs naturally after most significant vestibular insults. In the majority of cases, this centrally mediated process will reliably relieve vestibular symptoms provided that the unilateral impairment is either stable or producing only gradual progressive deterioration. The underlying physiologic stages of this process are the foundations of vestibular rehabilitation.

At least four distinct stages of vestibular compensation are recognized: *static compensation*, which occurs regardless of movement, and three dynamic compensatory processes, *adaptation*, *habituation*, and *sensory substitution*, each of which is promoted by various exercise techniques targeted in vestibular rehabilitation.

Peripheral Vestibular Impairments and Static Compensation

Vertigo of acute onset due to unilateral vestibular deafferentation (uVD) is accompanied by nystagmus and a variety of autonomic signs and symptoms, such as nausea and pallor (Table 23.1). Unilateral VD refers to either a partial or complete loss of vestibular afferent input from one labyrinth [4].

Table 23.1 Characteristic clinical symptoms associated with unilateral vestibular deafferentation (uVD), including the typical pattern of sudden onset vertigo, early spontaneous episodes, and progression to head-motion– provoked symptoms during central compensation

Unilateral vestibular deafferentation (uVD) symptoms
Sudden memorable onset
Typically true vertigo at onset
Paroxysmal spontaneous events <24 hours
Head movement provoked symptoms <2 minutes
Vestibular crisis—Sudden onset vertigo slowly improving from continuous to head movement provoked symptoms in days
More likely to have auditory involvement

D. L. McCaslin (✉) · N. T. Shepard
Department of Otolaryngology—Head and Neck Surgery, Division of Audiology, University of Michigan, Ann Arbor, MI, USA
e-mail: mccaslin@med.umich.edu

C. D. Hall
James H. Quillen Veteran's Affairs Medical Center, Auditory and Vestibular Research Enhancement Award Program, Mountain Home, TN, USA

Department of Physical Therapy, East Tennessee State University, Johnson City, TN, USA

A. D. Sweeney et al. (eds.), *Haynes-Glasscock-Shambaugh Surgery of the Ear*, https://doi.org/10.1007/978-3-032-18264-7_23

The process of static compensation is invoked soon after a patient incurs uVD. Following a lesion to one end-organ, the central vestibular system (i.e., vestibular nuclei) receives a reduced tonic level of neural input from the impaired side. This asymmetrical tonic neural firing rate registered at the level of the brainstem is falsely interpreted as a head movement toward the intact side (Fig. 23.1). The vestibulo-ocular reflex (VOR) is triggered into action generating what is referred to as "spontaneous vestibular nystagmus." In the absence of head movement, the patient perceives a head rotation away from the impaired side (i.e. vertigo). The magnitude of the nystagmus is an indication the severity of the vestibular impairment. Acutely, the fast phase of the nystagmus beats away from the impaired ear.

Within hours following an uVD, a phenomenon referred as cerebellar clamping is initiated. During this stage, neural activity from the intact side is reduced at the vestibular nuclei in an effort to decrease the magnitude of the tonic neural asymmetry. Specifically, this central mechanism has the effect of reducing the amplitude of the spontaneous vestibular nystagmus thereby decreasing the severity of vertigo as well as the symptoms generated by the autonomic nervous system (e.g., nausea). In fact, this is the physiological equivalent of the vestibular suppressants that are prescribed during the acute phase of an attack. The process of cerebellar clamping is beyond the scope of this chapter, and a more detailed account of the process is provided by Curthoys and Halmagyi (1996) [5].

Once the activity to the intact vestibular nucleus (VN) has been "clamped," the next stage in the process of static compensation begins. In order to restore the static response properties of the VOR to its pre-insult level, two fundamental changes in the neural activity need to occur. First, the level of clamping must be reduced on the intact side [6]. The reduction in the clamping allows the intact side to assume its normal neural resting rate and operate as it did prior to the insult. Second, the tonic resting rate at the VN must be restored on the impaired side. This is thought to be accomplished by the ipsilesional side using the contralesional side (i.e., intact labyrinth/nerve) as a reference and is made possible by the commissural fibers that connect the two vestibular systems together. This direct communication between the two sides facilitates the process for the system to equilibrate the activity at both VN [7]. Reports have shown that as soon as 52 h

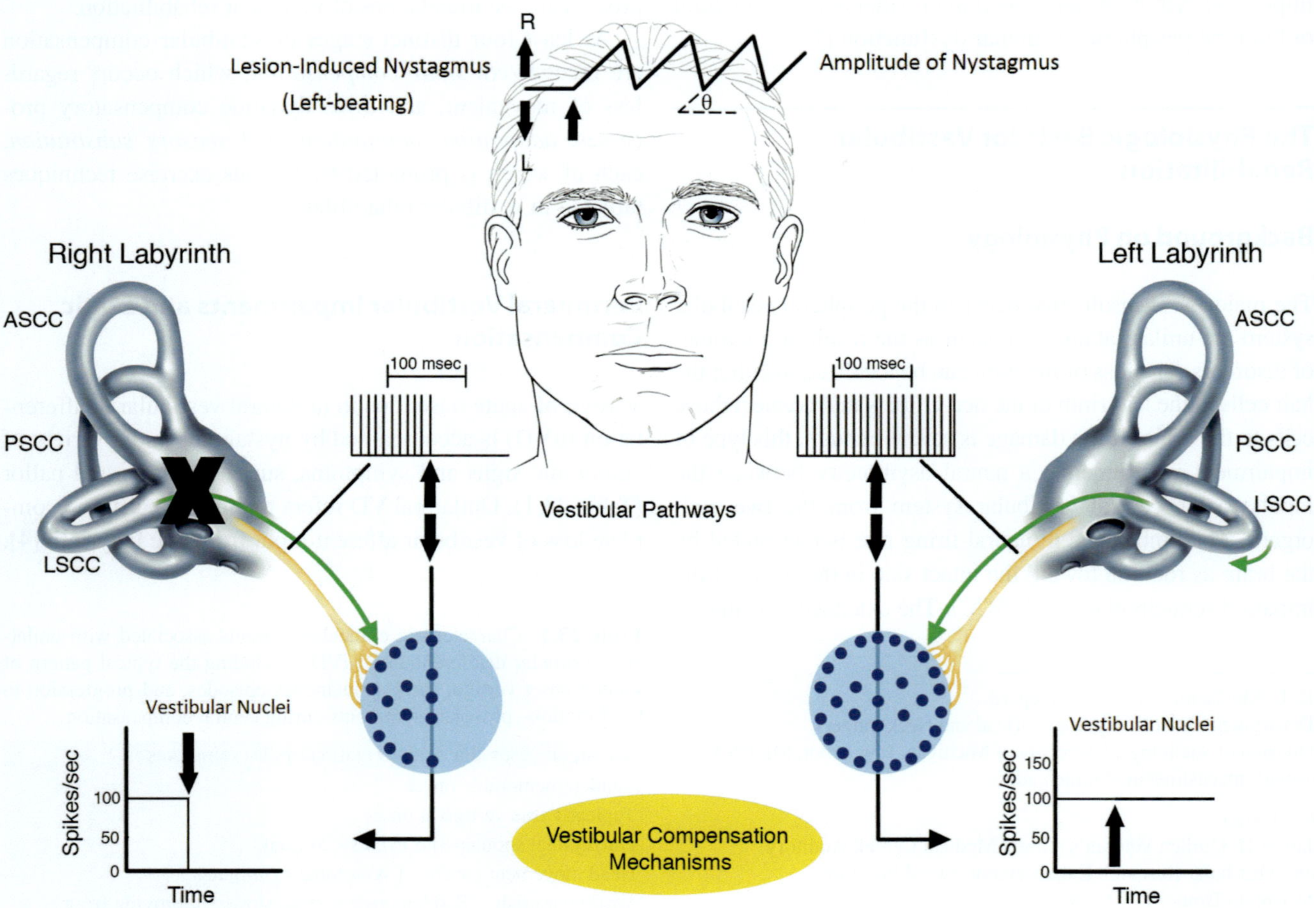

Fig. 23.1 Illustration of the change in primary afferent firing rate that occurs as a result of an acute loss of peripheral vestibular function on the right side and the accompanying left-beating nystagmus. (Adapted from McCaslin [78])

following uVD, the neural resting rate in the ipsilesional VN can be equivalent to rates that preceded the insult [4].

These neural changes minimize side-to-side differences between the tonic firing rates in the second-order neurons originating in the VN and occur without the need of head movement or vision [5]. Successful static compensation is only possible if the impairment is stable. This series of events will generally provide relief from the most intense symptoms of vertigo and nausea within 24–72 h. Complete static compensation, in theory, is a complete reduction in neural asymmetry and absence of spontaneous vestibular nystagmus [5].

Peripheral Vestibular Impairments: Dynamic Compensation

Following completion of static compensation, patients may no longer complain of vertigo when the head is at rest; however, they may continue to experience considerable dysequilibrium and head-motion provoked vertigo. This is because the dynamic response properties of the vestibular reflexes (i.e., VOR and vestibulospinal reflex, VSR) remain impaired. To eliminate persistent dysequilibrium and motion-provoked vertigo after a vestibular lesion, the system must predict and produce accurate responses to head movements. This process is referred to in the literature as *dynamic compensation*. The dynamic compensation phase is thought to be accomplished by reorganization of brainstem and cerebellar pathways, without modulation of the neural input to the vestibular nuclei from the peripheral system [6]. The two primary facilitators of dynamic compensation are visual input and the vestibulocerebellum [7]. This process requires more time than static compensation and is based largely on the severity of the impairment, level of activity of the patient, and the integrity of the central vestibular nervous system. Dynamic compensation consists of reprogramming of eye movements and postural control responses to head movements. The necessary reprogramming is accomplished by exposure to sensory stimuli that challenge both the gaze stabilization and postural control systems. Because of the brainstem commissural pathways linking the vestibular nuclei together, appropriate (but not always adequate) central vestibular responses can be produced from inputs arriving from one functioning labyrinth [4]. This feature of the compensation process is critical to recovery after extensive pathologic insults or ablative vestibular surgery (i.e., labyrinthectomy and vestibular nerve section). As discussed in the following section, there are three major mechanisms that facilitate dynamic compensation: adaptation, habituation, and sensory substitution.

Vestibular adaptation refers to the neural plasticity of the vestibular system that exists to compensate for disease and/or age. It is the neurologic mechanism that provides us with long-term physiological adjustments in both gait and gaze, that, if not present, would lead to debilitating effects on our ability to navigate our environment. For example, in the case of a complete unilateral vestibular loss, when the head is turned quickly in the direction of the impairment, the neural asymmetry between the intact side and the impaired side is reduced to half. Therefore, the head velocity is interpreted by the brain to be much less than it actually is. This aberrant difference between the velocity of the head and the velocity of the eye results in the fovea (located in the retina) coming off the target. Patients will report that their vision becomes blurry with quick head movements, and this is referred to in the literature as "oscillopsia." This velocity error signal between the head and the eyes is the stimulus that is used to reduce retinal slip. This process has been termed adaptation, but it remains unclear what the mechanism is for changing the functional performance of the VOR since it has not been shown to consistently change the gain of the VOR. There are two primary stimuli that facilitate this neural rewiring and promote the effect of improvement in the functional aspect of the use of the VOR. One is the ability to see (vision), and the other is movement of the head. This process of adaptation that is initiated by retinal slip is context-dependent. That is, specific physiological adjustments must be made to the VOR for movements of different frequency, directions of head movement, eye position in the orbit, and distances from the visual target [8]. The complex nature of the adaptation process explains why residual symptoms are almost unavoidable even in a fairly well-compensated patient in some conditions.

Vestibular habituation is the reduction in symptoms following exposure to repeated provocative stimuli that exacerbate patient's symptoms. This concept was first set forth by Cawthorne and Cooksey in the 1940s in an effort to develop a method to treat patients with dizziness and poor balance. The process of habituation is context-dependent and should be customized for the patient's specific symptoms. Habituation exercises are not limited to treating patients with peripheral vestibular asymmetries. Application of habituation has been shown to be successful in patients with central and peripheral nervous system impairments that have comorbid conditions such as anxiety disorders and migraines [9]. Recently, habituation exercises have shown great promise in treating people with chronic dizziness. In particular, patients diagnosed with persistent postural-perceptual dizziness (PPPD) present with sensitivities to visually complex environments, visually focused tasks, and visual motion. Habituation exercises have been reported to be successful in reducing symptoms in this patient population [10]. Although the reduction in symptoms produced by habituation exercises can be realized in the short term in patients with stable impairments, irritative disorders of the vestibular system are much more challenging. For this reason, patients with fluctuating vestibular lesions, such as

Ménière's disease or vestibular migraine, may derive less benefit than their counterparts.

Sensory substitution in the context of an impaired vestibular system refers to process of aiding the rehabilitation process by adopting alternate strategies for the use of vision and somatosensation to aid with recovery of balance. This form of rehabilitation is often applied to patients suffering from severe bilateral vestibular hypofunction. In these cases, the patients must rely on their visual and proprioceptive inputs in order to maintain postural stability and compensate for an inadequate VOR. It is current practice to develop these strategies in a therapeutic setting where it is safe for the patient to learn to rely on different sensory modalities in a way that is not natural. However, it is often the case that by the time they arrive for their first appointment, they have already learned a number of techniques that help with their balance. Although sensory substitution may be helpful in many instances, it may be maladaptive in some environmental settings. For example, a patient may be overly dependent on vision and therefore cannot use proprioceptive and residual vestibular inputs to successfully navigate in darkness.

Influential Factors on Vestibular Compensation

While it is now well-known that head movement is a prime driver of central vestibular compensation, there are also a number of factors that can inhibit or block this process. The site of the impairment can affect vestibular compensation. The efficiency of compensation has been shown to be inhibited by central vestibular dysfunction [11, 12]. Patients with a purely central or mixed vestibular lesion who are undergoing therapy may need to be counseled regarding realistic expectations about the time of recovery [13]. Patients that have cerebellar dysfunction or have suffered a head injury also demonstrate significantly decreased therapy outcomes when compared to their counterparts with only peripheral vestibular disease [14]. Interestingly, patients with mixed (peripheral and central) impairments have been shown to have poorer outcomes than those patients with purely central vestibular impairments [15]. This fact makes a strong case for performing vestibular tests prior to any destructive procedures targeted at reducing episodes of vertigo.

The level of activity that a patient adopts following a vestibular impairment, regardless of whether it is central or peripheral, is critical to the time it will take to recover. Research has shown that head movement and physical activity soon after a vestibular deficit promotes vestibular compensation, reduces head-motion provoked symptoms, and improves postural stability earlier [16].

The psychological well-being of patients is now recognized as an important consideration for patients with vestibular impairments. Generalized anxiety, depression, and numerous other psychiatric disorders can inhibit the compensation process and decrease therapy outcomes [17, 18].

Medications that typically are used for acute symptoms of vertigo, such as meclizine, scopolamine, and benzodiazepines all cause sedation and central nervous system depression. Although they may provide helpful symptomatic relief during the initial stages of an acute labyrinthine crisis, their effects are potentially counterproductive with respect to vestibular compensation, especially with use over extended periods [19]. Therefore, judicious use of medications is needed to allow early symptom reduction in order to promote natural and exercise-based head movements with reduction of medication over time. The clinical practice guidelines for vestibular rehabilitation in unilateral hypofunction states that the vestibular suppressive medication should not be automatically withdrawn for the acute patient; however, there is no evidence to support medication use in the chronic patient [3].

Although remarkably reliable, vestibular compensation seems to be a somewhat fragile, energy-dependent process. Even after it is apparently complete, periods of symptomatic relapse may occur because of decompensation. A period of inactivity, extreme fatigue, a change in medications, or an acute illness may trigger a relapse [20]. A relapse of vestibular symptoms in this situation does not imply ongoing, progressive, or new vestibular dysfunction.

To summarize, the underlying tenants of vestibular compensation are that the patient must be active (i.e., head movement in the pitch, roll, and yaw planes) and have an intact central vestibular system. The goal of the clinician should be to have the patient start a formal vestibular rehabilitation program as early as possible once uVD has been identified. In some cases, symptoms may persist for a longer period of time in patients that become sedentary and/or avoid head movements because of the deleterious effects of the uVD on everyday activities involving motion. Additionally, following the vestibular crisis, the patient may have been prescribed vestibular suppressants but continues to take them long after the event has occurred. This can essentially "blind" the central vestibular structures responsible for compensation to the fact that there is an ongoing asymmetry. Because the stimulus that drives central compensation is centered on repeated exposure to the sensory conflicts produced by head (i.e., retinal slip) and body movement (i.e. postural instability), medications prescribed to reduce the patient's vertigo should be discontinued as quickly as possible with consideration being given to the symptoms of the patient. For the majority of patients suffering from a significant uVD, recovery will occur quickly provided they are physically active. In cases of patients diagnosed with central vestibular pathologies, the design of the intervention is more challenging. The therapist should make clear to the patient what the expectations for recovery are and the time it may take to realize a significant decrease in symptoms. Some examples of factors that can influence compensation include medications being taken and physical well-being. Impairment of the central vestibular structures responsible for driving recovery can greatly reduce a patient's response to therapy. If the level of the central vestibular impairment can be determined (e.g., brainstem or cortex), then appropriate activities can be recommended.

Evaluating the State of Vestibular Compensation

History of the Dizzy Patient

Taking a thorough neurologic, psychiatric, and otologic history is the key component in beginning any evaluation of the dizzy patient. Balance function studies should always be interpreted in the context of the symptoms the patient presents with as well their past medical history [1]. With regard to the history, the interviewer should query the patient about, the qualities of the dizziness, the time course and aggravating factors, associated otologic symptoms, and neurologic symptoms. Additionally, any predisposing factors in the medical history such as exposure to ototoxic drugs, cardiovascular disease, head trauma, medications, or other management strategies should be considered. Factors that can inhibit a patient's compensation should be identified and documented. These include complications such as visual impairment, sensory neuropathies, and dependence on medications that can disrupt compensation. It is now well accepted that psychological comorbidities such as depression and anxiety can influence a patient's recovery; thus, the interview should also include inquiry into the stability of the patient's psychological well-being and the commitment of the family support system.

While the majority of patients compensate quickly, chronic symptoms following a peripheral vestibular insult suggest that vestibular compensation is incomplete. To elucidate the reason for delayed recovery, the history and presenting symptoms are used to determine whether these continuing sensations may be a result of an irritative or progressive labyrinthine disorder. In the case of the fluctuating lesions, inadequate compensation occurs because the central nervous system must continually rebalance the asymmetrical input originating from the peripheral system. When taking a history, an irritative lesion can be suspected when there are continued multiple events of vertigo that have a spontaneous onset (e.g., Ménière's disease). Vestibular compensation is most efficient when the impairment is stable. Patients with inadequate compensation that have a stable lesion will typically report that symptoms are exacerbated by head or eye movements. Individuals with stable lesions are the population most likely to derive maximum benefit from a vestibular rehabilitation program. A vestibular rehabilitation program for patients with unstable lesions as part of their management may derive some benefit between spells; however, this should be coupled with medical management in order to minimize the episodes as much as possible.

Role of Vestibular Testing

Over the last few decades, the standard assessment of the vestibular system has been greatly expanded. Traditionally, vestibular function tests have been used for three primary purposes. First, the tests are used for site-of-lesion localization, motor output function, and the evaluation of the vestibular neural pathways. Second, the tests are used to evaluate patients' ability to integrate sensory input for functional activities. This includes evaluating a patient's ability to maintain stance before and after induced sway and coordination of head and eye movements to maintain gaze stability with the head moving. Lastly, select vestibular studies can be used, in a limited manner, to describe a patient's degree of physiologic and functional compensation [21]. Until recently, vestibular function testing was limited to measuring one part of the vestibular system, the horizontal semicircular canal; it is now possible through the use of vestibular function tests to determine the function in all five vestibular end-organs. Otolith organ testing is becoming more widely used in vestibular clinics; yet, it is unclear how otolith organ dysfunction contributes to postural instability and the incidence of falls. Furthermore, results from these tests do not enable the clinician to predict the nature or magnitude of a patient's vestibular symptoms or the level of disability/handicap. For example, when findings from the vestibular test battery are compared with a patient's performance on activities of daily living, there is very little relationship between the two except in extreme cases (e.g., bilateral hypofunction) [22]. It is speculated that this disconnect is the result of our inability to fully characterize the status of the compensation process. For this reason, therapists should proceed with careful questioning to clearly characterize the patient's symptoms while at the same time taking into account findings from the quantitative vestibular assessment.

Information regarding where the patient is in the compensation process can be obtained using a number of tests including videonystagmography (VNG), video head impulse testing (vHIT), rotary chair, posturography, computerized dynamic visual acuity (DVA) and gaze stabilization tests, and vestibular evoked myogenic potentials (VEMP). Depending on the test, information obtained from these studies can relate to either the static or dynamic phase of compensation. Ocular motor subtests of the VNG (with and without vision) can be used to identify significant spontaneous nystagmus and positional nystagmus thereby providing a snapshot of whether the patient has statically compensated. The caloric examination can document whether or not a peripheral impairment exists and if there is a persistent asymmetry (bias) in vestibular tone due to incomplete compensation (i.e., directional preponderance). There are, however, a number of weaknesses associated with the caloric test. The test is poorly controlled, measures only the relative function of one ear compared to the other, and simulates a very low frequency rotation (0.003 Hz). Rotational chair testing addresses a number of the aforementioned issues encountered in caloric testing. The rotary chair test is well tolerated and independent of the anatomical features of the ear. Passive whole-body rotation using a sinusoidal harmonic acceleration stimulus evaluates the horizontal semicircular canals and their corresponding neural connections through the VOR over a broad range of frequencies (0.01 Hz–1 Hz). Rotational testing provides information about the VOR that is not obtained from the VNG. For instance, the test can describe the severity and frequency range of bilateral vestibular loss which can have critical prognostic implications for therapy. In acute cases, abnormalities in the timing (phase) or amplitude (gain) of eye responses generated by rotational testing can provide evidence of incomplete dynamic compensation of the VOR. As with the caloric response, asymmetrical nystagmus in response to rightward versus leftward rotation is indicative of a peripheral lesion that is physiologically uncompensated.

Recently, a quantitative evaluation of the semicircular canals known as the video head impulse test (vHIT) has emerged as a potential way to evaluate dynamic vestibular compensation. This test employs small amplitude (20 degree), high frequency head movements (2000–3000 deg./sec/sec) delivered in an unpredictable manner while a patient maintains gaze on an earth fixed target. In patients with intact vestibular function, the VOR generates a smooth compensatory eye movement that is equal and opposite of the head movement. The functional effect of this is that the eye is kept on the object of interest throughout the head movement and the observer can maintain clear vision. In patients with uVD, when the head is thrust in the direction of the impaired ear, a slower than normal movement of the eye is generated due to the lesion. This results in the eye coming off the target during the head turn. When the head stops, the subject is no longer looking at the point of interest, and a refixation saccade must be generated to reacquire the target. This has been termed an *overt* saccade and is a classic marker for vestibular impairment. A second saccade termed *covert* has been described and occurs during the head movement [23]. Covert saccades result in reduction of the provocative symptoms associated with head motion, as well as reduced gaze position error [24]. It has been suggested that covert saccades can reduce retinal slip (i.e., image moving across the retina due to a deficient VOR) in three ways. First, a high velocity eye movement (i.e., saccade) occurring during the head movement will reduce the visibility of the slip (i.e., the eye is effectively blind during an eye movement of this speed); second, visual perception is suppressed immediately before and after generation of a saccade. Finally, the covert saccade effectively moves the eye in a direction opposite of the head movement (i.e., compensating for a defective VOR response) thereby reducing the amount of error realized at the end of the head movement. This adaptation illustrates how the substitution of other eye movements can effectively reduce the amount of retinal slip and the associated symptoms that accompany head movements in patients with uVD. Long after compensation has occurred, the VOR gain will continue to be decreased. Therefore, vestibular rehabilitation of uVD patients should be targeted at facilitating new strategies for saccades to accommodate the vestibular loss rather than trying to restore function.

Over the last decade vestibular function testing has expanded to include assessment of the otolith organs. Vestibular evoked myogenic potentials (VEMP) are short latency sonomotor responses evoked by acoustical stimulation of the vestibular system [25]. These sonomotor responses can be recorded from a number of muscles including the sternocleidomastoid (SCM) and the inferior oblique muscles. The most effective stimuli to elicit VEMPs are low-frequency tone bursts (e.g., 500 Hz tone bursts) or unfiltered clicks that are presented at relatively high intensity levels 85–100 dB nHL [26, 27]. The cervical VEMP (cVEMP) response is generated by the saccule and reflects a stimulus-induced reduction in the electromyographic (EMG) activity in an activated SCM bilateral pathway. The ocular VEMP (oVEMP) is generated by the utricle and has a crossed and bilateral pathway. The ipsilateral response stimulates the superior rectus muscle, while the contralateral response stimulates the inferior oblique muscle. There is very little research that describes the effect of otolith impairment on rehabilitation outcomes. Murray and colleagues (2010) studied patients with impaired semicircular canal function only and participants with combined lesions of semicircular canal and otolith organs [28]. The research findings suggest that the additional otolith dysfunction does not negatively influence the response to rehabilitation of individuals with a peripheral vestibular disorder; however, individuals with isolated otolith organ dysfunction were not included in the study. Patients with isolated otolith impairments have been shown to have poorer performance on the sensory organization test and significantly more severe dizziness handicap when compared to their normal counterparts [29].

Computerized dynamic posturography (CDP) is a quantitative method for assessing upright and standing balance function under a variety of conditions that simulate the conditions encountered in daily life. The sensory organization test (SOT), subtest of CDP, is a test of a patient's functional ability to effectively use visual, vestibular, and somatosensory inputs to maintain upright stance. It does not provide information regarding site of lesion. Specifically, the test uses a clever process known as *sway-referencing* to disrupt somatosensory and/or visual information and then measures patients' ability to orient themselves in order to maintain balance. Sensory input is systematically altered across six conditions, the first three involving a stable support surface with eyes open (condition 1), eyes closed (condition 2), and sway-referenced visual surround (condition 3) and the last three involving a sway-referenced surface with eyes open (condition 4), eyes closed (condition 5), and sway-referenced visual surround (condition 6). A quantitative measure of functional compensation is obtained by analyzing estimating the amount of postural sway for each of the six sensory conditions. However, if a patient is not tested shortly after the vestibular crisis, findings on CDP will often be normal even though motion provoked symptoms persist. Alternatively, it may be the case that patients will show grossly abnormal performance on tests of postural control; whereas, vestibular function testing (e.g., ocular motor and rotational testing) would suggest that compensation is complete.

In 1984, Barber described a test that permitted quantification of dynamic visual acuity by measuring the degradation in acuity that occurs with oscillation (2 Hz) of the head when a patient reads a wall eye chart [30]. This test was termed the "oscillopsia test." Since the initial description of the test, there have been numerous variations, and it is now most commonly referred to as dynamic visual acuity (DVA) test. One of the key changes that have occurred over the years has involved using more appropriate eye charts. For example, the modified ETDRS (Early Treatment Diabetic Retinopathy Study) chart uses SLOAN letters (Lighthouse Distance Visual Acuity Tests, Long Island City, New York) and has been shown to be superior to the Snellen. Handheld Snellen cards are not appropriate due to the distance at which the test is performed, unequal decrease in letter size from line to line, and the letters are not adjusted for difficulty. Advances in technology have led to the development of commercially available computerized DVA systems that have been reported to enhance the sensitivity of the test to vestibular impairments [31]. In addition to identifying vestibular disorders, the computerized DVA has also shown clinical utility in predicting a patients' risk of falling. Specifically, when computerized DVA was used in the yaw plane, it was found to be a sensitive (92%) and accurate screening measure of falls when using a cutoff value of >0.25 logMAR [26]. DVA has also been reported to have predictive value with regard to therapy outcomes. Patients with more severe vestibular deficits have been reported to be less likely to return to normal DVA following a round of vestibular rehabilitation [32].

In an attempt to address visual acuity issues using different target sizes, Goebel and colleagues developed a modified test of dynamic visual acuity called the gaze stabilization test (GST) [33]. The GST is a computerized DVA test that registers the maximum head velocity an individual can achieve and still accurately report the orientation of the target optotype, which is 0.3 LogMAR (or 3 lines) above static acuity. Performance of the GST showed that the test was 93% specific and 64% sensitive and had a reliability index of 0.91 using a cut point of <91 deg./s for identifying unilateral vestibular dysfunction [33].

To summarize, vestibular function test results can provide important indications regarding both the physiological and functional status of both static and dynamic compensation. However, the findings must be taken in context with a patient's symptoms before a treatment plan is devised. As indicated below, functional tests of balance (e.g., posturography and DVA) can be useful in defending what specific exercises may go into a vestibular rehabilitation program but in a stand-alone manner cannot be used to select the patients for whom vestibular rehabilitation would be appropriate.

Choosing Appropriate Candidates for Therapy

Vestibular Rehabilitation to Treat Benign Paroxysmal Positional Vertigo

It is well accepted that vestibular rehabilitation for patients with benign paroxysmal positional vertigo (BPPV) is the frontline approach to treating this disorder [34]. Our understanding of the pathophysiological mechanism of BPPV has evolved since the original description of the disorder by Barany [35]. Up until the early 1990s, non-customized programs such as Brandt-Daroff exercises were employed to treat BPPV [36]. This is because these early treatments were based on the findings from Schuknecht suggesting that cupulolithiasis was the primary mechanism [37]. In 1980 John Epley postulated the canalithiasis theory of BPPV which represented a shift in treatment for this common disorder [38]. Patients presenting with BPPV generate nystagmus when the SCC with displaced otoconia from the otolith organs is placed into gravity-dependent positions, as in the Dix-Hallpike test (Fig. 23.2). When the impaired SCC is stimulated, an eye movement specific to the affected canal is generated that directs the clinician to choose the appropriate treatment (Figs. 23.3, 23.4 and 23.5). To date, there are three accepted treatment approaches each of which are based on the pathophysiologic theories of this disorder. The techniques include the canalith repositioning maneuver, the liberatory (Semont) maneuver, and Brandt-Daroff exercises. A full discussion regarding the non-medical management of

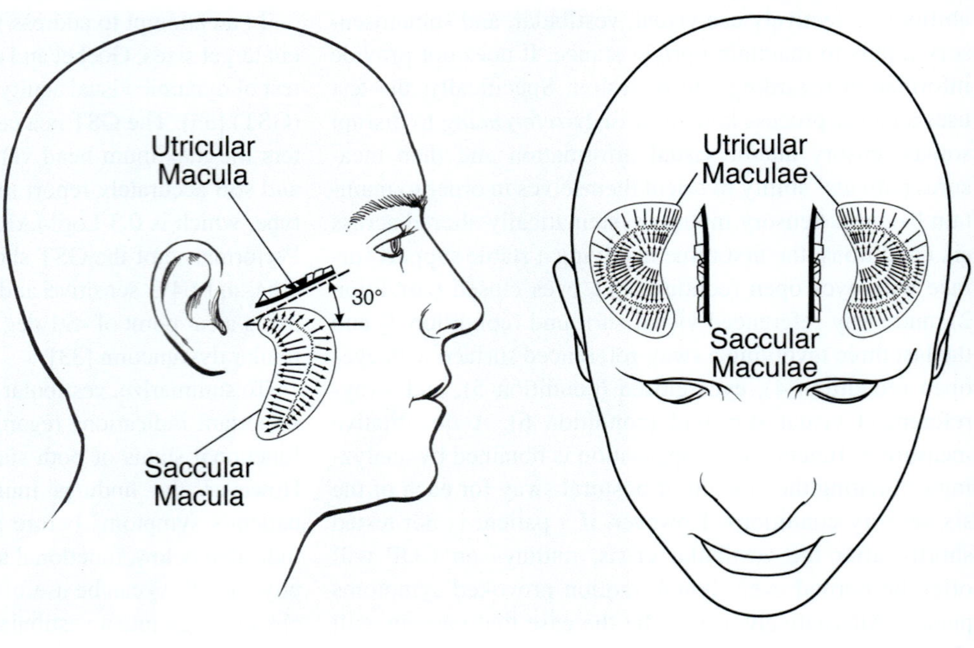

Fig. 23.2 Figure illustrating the otolith organs and their orientation in the head

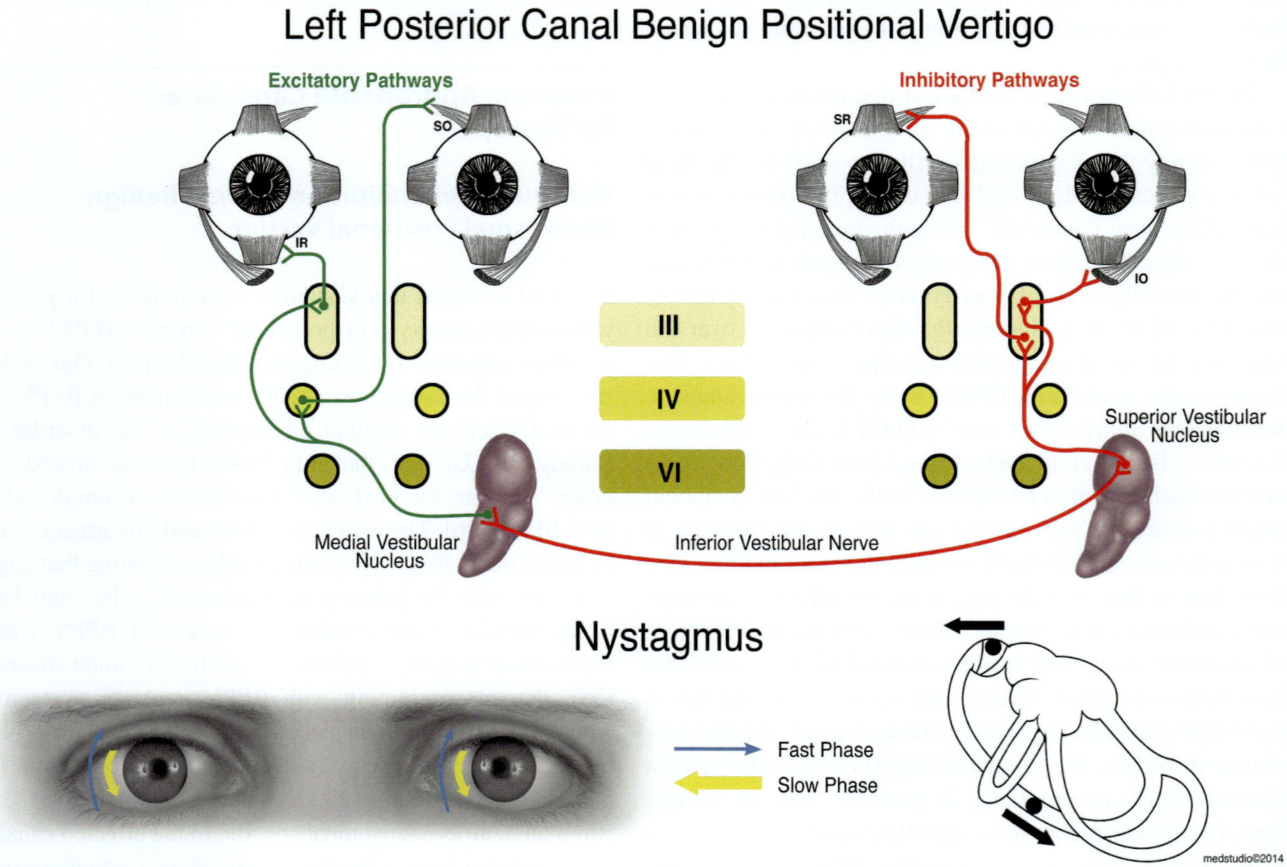

Fig. 23.3 Figure illustrating left ear posterior canal BPPV and the excitatory and inhibitory receptor connections to the extraocular muscles and the direction of nystagmus. Upbeating with a right torsional component to the left when the head is placed in the head-down left position

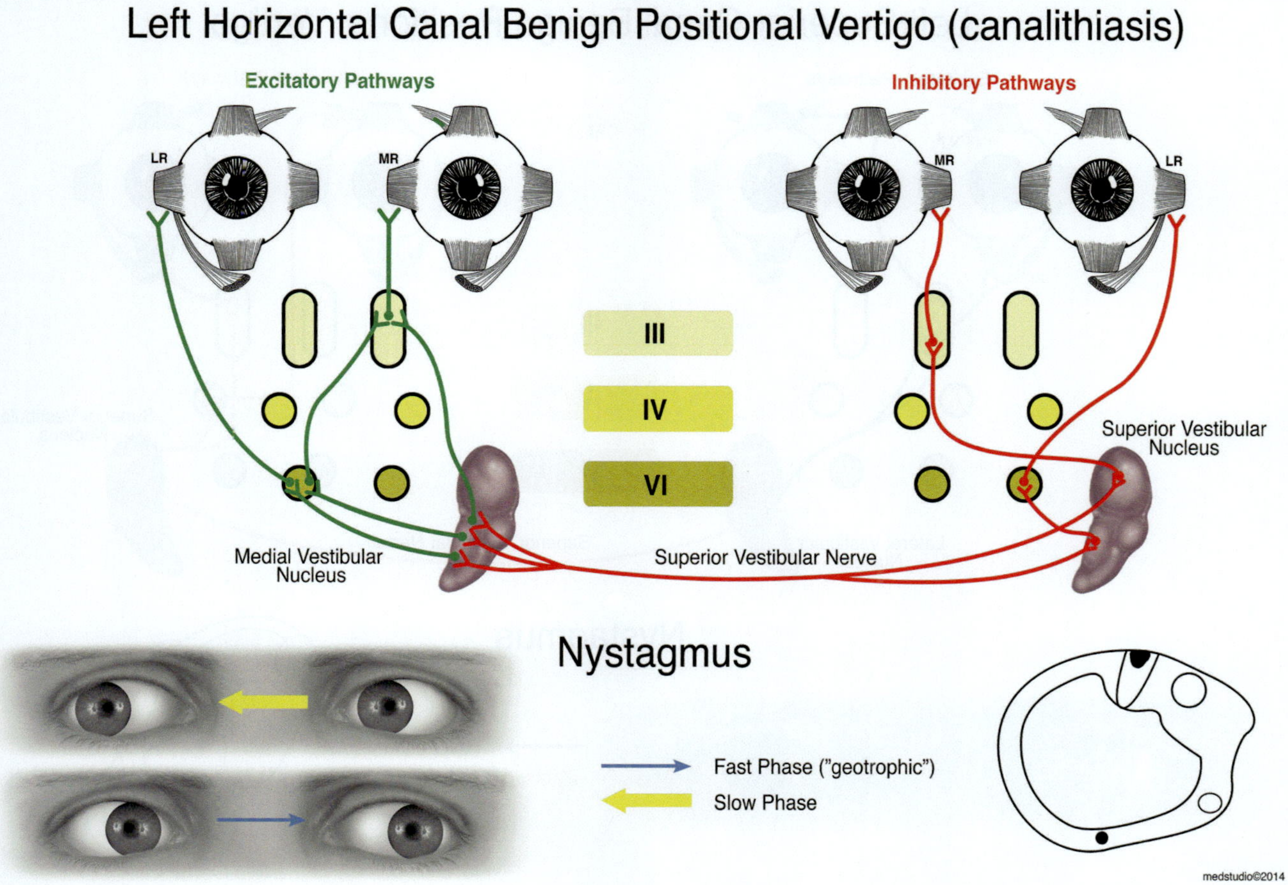

Fig. 23.4 Figure illustrating left ear horizontal canalithiasis BPPV and the excitatory and inhibitory receptor connections to the extraocular muscles and the direction of nystagmus. Horizontal nystagmus with a stronger response when the head is turned to the left and the left ear is down (geotropic)

BPPV is beyond the scope of this chapter. Readers should refer to Chap. 11 in Jacobson, Shepard, et al. (2021) for a complete review [39].

The canalith repositioning maneuver (CRM) is based on the idea that there are free-floating densities known as "canaliths" that create aberrant endolymphatic flow when the patient's head is moved into provocative positions. CRMs are designed to migrate the canaliths through the membranous labyrinth using a sequence of head position changes based on the anatomy of the labyrinth. Specifically, the goal is to move the debris out of the involved SCC and into the vestibule. If the treatment is successful, the BPPV nystagmus disappears, and patient's symptoms of positionally provoked vertigo should resolve shortly following the procedure.

Liberatory or Semont maneuvers were designed to treat BPPV based on the cupulolithiasis theory of BPPV [40]. These maneuvers utilize rapid clinician-guided movements of the patient to dislodge the canaliths that are assumed to be attached to the cupula. This form of treatment has been shown to be effective as an alternative treatment to the CRM for canalithiasis form of BPPV [41].

Brandt-Daroff exercises were devised to habituate the CNS to the provoking position [36]. However, these maneuvers may also have a secondary effect of dislodging the canaliths from the cupula and/or migrating them out of the canal. The maneuvers are typically suggested to be performed by the patient for 5–10 repetitions, three times a day until the patient has no symptoms for 2 consecutive days. Modifications to this protocol can be instituted based on the severity of the patients' symptoms (e.g., if the patient has severe vertigo or complaints of nausea).

Vestibular Rehabilitation to Treat Peripheral Vestibular Hypofunction

In cases of stable unilateral or bilateral peripheral vestibular hypofunction, the use of vestibular rehabilitation as the primary treatment approach is appropriate when the patient has not fully compensated. Determination of compensation is through careful documentation of the patient's symptoms, risk of falling, DVA, postural stability, and dynamic gait at the time of the visit with the therapist. A patient who reports

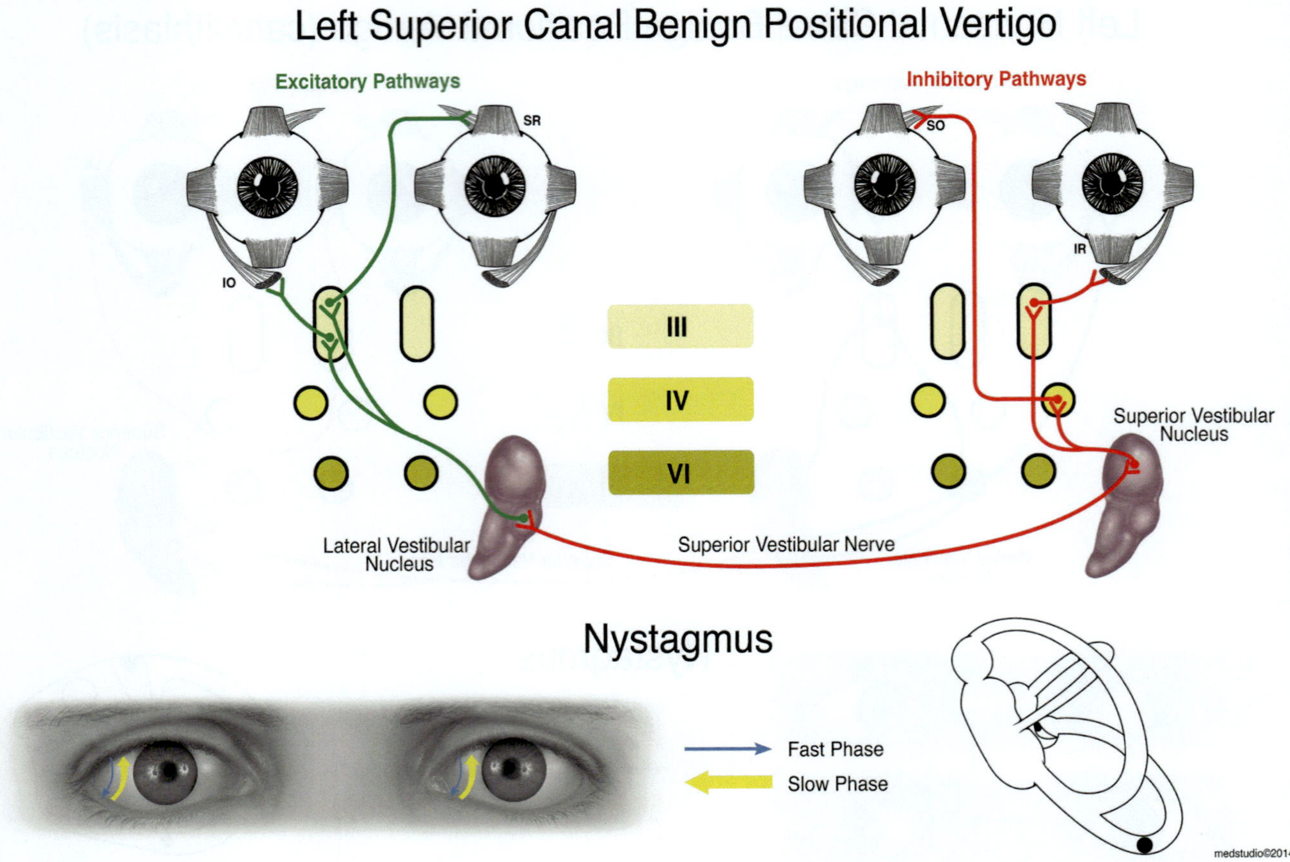

Fig. 23.5 Figure illustrating left ear superior canal BPPV and the excitatory and inhibitory receptor connections to the extraocular muscles and the direction of nystagmus. Downbeating with a left torsional component to the left when the head is placed in the head-down left position

ongoing symptoms of dizziness that occur spontaneously or fluctuating hearing in combination with spells of vertigo may suggest an irritative lesion. If, after a detailed interview with the patient, there is no evidence of symptoms that indicate a fluctuating or progressive vestibular disorder, and the patient reports that symptoms are exacerbated with head or visual motion, the patient is a candidate for vestibular rehabilitation. There is no question that leveraging the body's natural compensation mechanisms is preferable to extended used of vestibular suppressants (e.g., meclizine) [42]. In patients suffering from stable unilateral vestibular impairments, other than reducing symptoms in the acute phase of the crisis, there is no role for the long-term use of anti-vertigo medications. In select cases, this class of medication may be used to help reduce symptoms in order to help the patient begin a vestibular rehabilitation program [43]. In most instances, extended use of these types of medications following a vestibular insult inhibit the speed of recovery and may reduce the effectiveness of the therapy program.

Vestibular Rehabilitation and Medical Treatment

There are a number of instances where the use of vestibular rehabilitation should be provided as treatment modality for patients undergoing surgical or chemical treatment of the vestibular system. In cases where an ablative procedure (e.g., labyrinthectomy or vestibular schwannoma removal) is performed, there is clear evidence that vestibular rehabilitation optimizes outcomes when initiated acutely or subacute [43]. For example, Herdman and colleagues (1995) followed two groups of patients that had undergone vestibular schwannoma resection [44]. One group of patients received gaze stabilization exercises 3 days after their surgery, and these were continued until discharge. Another group was provided with a set of control exercises. The group that received the gaze stabilization exercises reported significantly less dysequilibrium than their control counterparts; furthermore, the gaze stabilization group had significantly more stable posture and gait than the control group. Patients that present with irritative vestibular disorders can realize a significant decrease in their episodic symptoms following an ablative procedure. However, while the patient may experience a decrease in the number of spontaneous events, they now face the challenge of compensating for a more severe (albeit stable) unilateral peripheral impairment. Following the destructive procedure, the patient may experience symptoms (i.e., vertigo, nausea, oscillopsia, dysequilibrium) similar to a spontaneous vestibular crisis; the intensity of which is dependent on the level of vestibular function prior to ablation. Provided the necessary central compensation mechanisms are intact, the natural process of vestibular compensation will begin within hours to reduce the patient's symptoms and disequilibrium.

In order to optimize the patient's outcomes, the therapist should design and implement a program during this acute/subacute phase to address four key issues: (1) decrease disequilibrium; (2) improve balance while ambulating (especially, with head movement); (3) improve the ability to see clearly during head movements; and (4) resumption of normal activities as soon as possible [43]. Factors that may contribute to prolonged recovery time include central nervous system disorders (e.g., Parkinson's disease), sedating medications, or poor motivation. It is noteworthy that prior to any destructive procedure, patients should be educated regarding the symptoms that they will encounter postoperatively and that movement is critical to central nervous system compensation.

Patients with Ménière's disease represent a challenging patient population due to the fluctuating nature of their symptoms. In addition to episodic attacks of true vertigo, they also may report positional vertigo (e.g., BPPV) and disequilibrium between episodes. These patients can benefit from vestibular rehabilitation between attacks for disequilibrium, head movement-induced dizziness, and deficits related to vestibular hypofunction. There is a clear role for therapy in patients receiving medical treatment for this disorder. Gottshall and colleagues (2005) reported that vestibular rehabilitation can improve symptoms in patients receiving nondestructive intraear medicines (e.g., steroid injections or diuretics) for Ménière's disease. Patients with a diagnosis of Ménière's disease were assessed prior to receiving and following diuretic therapy or transtympanic steroid injections. Following treatment, patients reporting no vertigo episodes for 3 months were enrolled in a vestibular rehabilitation program. Eighty-eight percent of the patients undergoing vestibular rehabilitation showed resolution of their dizziness and disequilibrium symptoms [45].

Patients who are unable to control their Ménière's disease-related episodes of vertigo with diet or medical therapy may elect to have a destructive procedure. These procedures are aimed at reducing or eliminating the episodes of vertigo (i.e., stabilizing the disease) by partially or completely deadening the vestibular system on the impaired side. One destructive method of treatment is intra- or transtympanic gentamicin. Following gentamicin injection therapy, patients may report vertigo and unsteadiness [46]. These patients can be treated using the same methods as individuals with a naturally incurred vestibular hypofunction. The goal should be to enroll the patient in a vestibular rehabilitation program soon after treatment to help facilitate the compensation process and reduce symptoms.

The most aggressive form of treatment employed to control episodes of Ménière's disease are ablative surgical procedures. These procedures are intended to completely destroy the vestibular system on the affected side. The symptoms the patient experiences following the surgery depends, to some degree, on the amount of residual function that the impaired ear has remaining. That is, if the ear is almost completely "burned out," then the symptoms of vertigo and disequilibrium that follow may be slight. However, if the impaired ear is functioning at near normal levels at the time of surgery, then the postsurgical symptoms can be extremely severe. Regardless of the severity of the symptoms, vestibular rehabilitation is a critical component to reducing the patient's symptoms and ensuring they will be able to function as soon as possible [47]. In cases where a complete ablation is the treatment of choice, it is recommended that the therapist consult with the patient prior to the surgical intervention. This allows the treating clinician to describe and explain the use of adaptation exercises in a situation where the patient can comfortably ask questions. A presurgical therapy appointment ensures that the patient will understand techniques, the reasons behind doing rehabilitation, and how they can reduce their symptoms as quickly as possible given their condition. When working with patients that have had success in minimizing their episodes either through diet or surgery, the prognosis of reducing their chronic symptoms and reducing their dizziness handicap is considerably improved when they are enrolled in a vestibular therapy program [48].

Vestibular rehabilitation should also be considered as a treatment option in patients with vestibular dysfunction as a result of traumatic brain injury (TBI) or concussion. TBI is defined as damage to the brain, resulting from an external force such as a blow to the head, blast waves, or penetration from a projectile object. The term concussion is used interchangeably with mild TBI (mTBI). Dizziness is a common and sometimes persistent symptom following a concussion or mTBI. The presence of dizziness at 6 months post-injury is an adverse prognostic indicator and may be the most persistent symptom adversely affecting quality of life [49, 50]. Patients suffering from mTBI may manifest impairments in dizziness and balance and may present with cognitive deficiencies on neurocognitive testing and central vestibular findings during the oculomotor subtest of the VNG. It is often the case that diagnostic imaging is normal in this cohort of patients. Depending on the type and severity of the head injury, patients may have a peripheral vestibular component that is identified using laboratory testing. Patients that present with temporal bone fractures have a high risk of incurring peripheral vestibular hypofunction. In cases of moderate to severe TBI, vestibular rehabilitation techniques are best used as a complementary rehabilitative approach that is integrated into a comprehensive, multidisciplinary head injury program. Lastly, patients that have been identified as having a visual impairment (e.g., vergence insufficiency and diplopia) following a TBI may benefit from a combination of vision therapy and vestibular rehabilitation [51].

Another group of patients that present with chronic dizziness and have been shown to respond well to vestibular rehabilitation are those that have an anxiety disorder and go on to develop what has been termed persistent postural-perceptual dizziness (PPPD). PPPD is a specific set of symptoms that reflects a conditioned response, often to a trigger event that causes dizziness (e.g., BPPV or concussion). Patients with a diagnosis of PPPD report sensitivities to self-motion, visual motion, visual complexity, and focused visual tasks (e.g., reading). The treatment regimen for PPPD involves a combination of medication (selective serotonin reuptake inhibitors) for the conditioned response and habituation exercises to reduce the developed sensitivities to both head movement and visual stimuli. Patients that respond positively to the treatment will typically begin to see significant improvement in 4–6 weeks and complete resolution in 3–4 months. A full discussion of the issue of PPPD and the use of therapy for a portion of the treatment are beyond the scope of this chapter, and the interested reader is referred to other published literature [52].

Vestibular Rehabilitation as a Therapeutic Trial

There are circumstances when it is unclear whether a patient's complaints of dizziness are in response to a poorly compensated stable unilateral impairment or an irritative labyrinthine disorder, such as a perilymphatic fistula or third window disorder (e.g., enlarged vestibular aqueduct or canal dehiscence). In these cases vestibular function testing in combination with vestibular rehabilitation is an appropriate recommendation for use as a therapeutic trial. The use of vestibular rehabilitation in this context is directed at assisting the physician in distinguishing between these two patient states. The concept is that if the patient's symptoms resolve following a therapy program, it could be assumed that the impairment is stable and the patient was incompletely compensated. No change or exacerbation of a patient's symptoms would be suggestive of an impairment that is unstable or even progressive. In this latter case, the physician may decide to proceed with appropriate surgical management based on the severity of the symptoms and the findings from vestibular function testing. In cases where exploratory surgery for a spontaneous perilymph fistula or a canal plugging for a superior canal near-dehiscence are being considered, this conservative treatment approach is recommended [53].

In this same vein, a patient with uVD as a result of a definitive procedure of the labyrinth that has shown a resolution of symptoms and is considered well compensated may have a relapse (i.e., decompensation). In situations such as this, vestibular compensation may be nullified, and the patient has a return of spontaneous vestibular nystagmus, the sensations of vertigo, and disequilibrium. The challenge for the clinician in these cases is to determine whether the return to the uVD syndrome is a result of central decompensation, a progression of the disease on the affected side, or a change in function on the side that was previously unaffected (i.e., the good ear) [54]. When a definitive destructive procedure has been performed (e.g., transmastoid labyrinthectomy), patients may report a return of symptoms. A key component in the differential diagnosis for this phenomenon is the time course. If a patient decompensates following the destructive procedure, a number of factors should be considered. Was the diagnosis correct, was the neuroepithelium completely removed at the time of surgery, or is this simply a manifestation of the patient not being completely compensated immediately following the procedure? Decompensation that occurs long after the procedure has been hypothesized to be due to "post-labyrinthectomy neuromas." [54] If central decompensation is suspected, rather than proceeding to additional surgery, a therapeutic trial of vestibular rehabilitation should be initiated, and the patient response to the therapy program carefully tracked.

Patients for Whom Vestibular Rehabilitation Is Inappropriate

Patients who suffer from irritative vestibular impairments such as Ménière's disease are less likely to have long-lasting improvement following a vestibular rehabilitation program. The reason is that vestibular rehabilitation will not treat the spontaneous episodes of vertigo. If a patient with a fluctuant vestibular disorder is evaluated for therapy and there are no complaints of head or body motion symptoms or disequilibrium, they are not a candidate for vestibular rehabilitation at that time. In these cases, the patient may have an underlying vestibular hypofunction but has compensated since the last episode. Regardless, all patients should be instructed to adopt an active and healthy lifestyle that is appropriate for their age and physical condition.

Quantitative tests of vestibular function such as VNG, VEMPs, and rotational chair are site of lesion tests and do not provide information that assists in determining who would be a successful candidate for a vestibular therapy program.

Where these tests of vestibular function are of value is when they can be used in conjunction with a patient's symptoms to determine if a specific form of exercise should be used to maximize therapy outcomes. For example, a patient may present with a severe bilateral vestibular impairment on rotational testing which would indicate a different treatment approach than a patient identified with a unilateral vestibular lesion. What is important for the therapist and physician to understand is that when provided with balance function study results, these tests should not be used as a metric against which to measure the success of a rehabilitation program. In cases where a patient is not meeting expected outcomes, or is undergoing medical treatment in conjunction with the rehabilitation program, repeating components of the VNG or rotational chair examination may be indicated to rule out a progressive or new additional vestibular impairment [55].

Functional Balance Outcome Measures and Vestibular Rehabilitation

Uncompensated vestibular hypofunction results in postural instability, visual blurring with head movement, subjective complaints of dizziness and/or imbalance, and disability. Successful rehabilitation requires the identification of patient-specific problems in order to design a customized exercise program. Appropriate evaluation of patients with vestibular deficits involves a test battery including assessment of self-report disability and symptoms, balance, gait, dynamic visual acuity, and fall risk [56]. Validated physical performance measures that assess balance and gait function include but are not limited to the Dynamic Gait Index (DGI), Functional Gait Assessment (FGA), Timed Up and Go (TUG), Physiological Profile Approach (PPA), and the Balance Evaluation Systems Test (BESTest) (Table 23.2).

Subjective Self-Report Outcome Measures

It is important to measure symptoms of dizziness and/or imbalance and their impact on dizziness-related quality of life (DRQoL), including perceived disability, for three primary reasons. First, and as has been discussed earlier in this chapter, it is well-known that vestibular function studies do not correlate significantly with measures of DRQoL unless a patient suffers from a severe vestibular impairment (e.g., complete bilateral vestibular loss) [22]. Second, it is important to document to payers that vestibular rehabilitation is efficacious. Demonstrating pre-versus posttherapy outcomes is critical in today's healthcare environment. Finally, DRQoL measures enable therapists to obtain information about a patient's disorder that can help design and guide treatment programs (i.e., patients with anxiety disorders). While an entire discussion regarding the assessment of DRQoL is beyond the scope of this chapter, readers can refer to Chap. 8 in Jacobson, Shepard, et al. (2021) [77]. Two self-report outcome measures that are validated and widely used include the Dizziness Handicap Inventory (DHI) and the Activities-specific Balance Confidence Scale (ABC). The DHI was developed in response to the need to have a standardized measure of self-report of participation restriction and activity limitation resulting from dizziness and unsteadiness [57]. The DHI is a 25-item measure of self-perceived disability-related to dizziness. The patient is asked to respond to each

Table 23.2 Commonly used functional balance and gait outcome measures in patients with vestibular and balance dysfunction, including descriptions of each assessment and clinically relevant scoring thresholds associated with fall risk

Assessment	Description	Scoring
Dynamic Gait Index (DGI) (Shumway-Cook et al. 1997) [69]	Index assesses dynamic postural stability and gait in patients with vestibular dysfunction The DGI is an eight-item test that uniquely challenges balance in part by incorporating deliberate head and body turns	Scores of ≤19/24 are correlated to falls in community living elderly adults
The Time up and Go (TUG) (Podsiadlo and Richardson 1991) [70]	Index assesses multiple functional skills including transitioning sit to stand, walking 3 m, and changing direction	Generally scores less than 10 seconds are considered normal, while scores greater than 12 s indicate an increased fall risk, and/or imply significant mobility limitations or functional deficits [71]
Balance evaluation systems test (Horak 2009) [72]	Targets six different balance control systems so that specific rehabilitation approaches can be designed for different types of balance deficits	Combines commonly used validated outcome measure scores such as the Dynamic Gait Index, Berg Balance Scale, Timed up and Go, including dual task cognitive challenges
Functional Gait Assessment (Wrisley et al. 2010) [73]	A modification of the Dynamic Gait that incorporates an obstacle course, double-task activities, stairs, ramps	A total score ≤ 22/30 indicates fall risk
Physiological Profile Approach (PPA) (Lord 1993) [74]	The PPA involves a series of simple tests of vision, cutaneous sensation on the feet, leg muscle force, reaction time, and postural sway in stance	Composite PPA scores below 0 indicate a low risk for falling, scores between 0 and 1 indicate a mild risk for falling, scores between 1 and 2 indicate a moderate risk for falling, and scores above 2 indicate a high risk for falling

question about the impact of dizziness on daily life by choosing "yes" (4 points), "sometimes" (2 points), or "no" (0 points). Higher total scores indicate greater perceived handicap due to dizziness. Total scores of 30 or less indicate mild self-perceived disability; scores of 31–60 indicate moderate disability; and scores greater than 60 indicate severe disability [58]. The DHI has been shown to have high test-retest reliability, and the standard error of measurement (SEM) has been calculated to be 6.23 pretreatment and posttreatment.

The ABC was developed by Powell and Myers in 1995 to measure balance-related confidence across a spectrum of activities in community-dwelling older adults. The measure is different from many other self-report instruments in that it evaluates self-efficacy or the belief in one's ability to perform daily activities without falling. Patients are asked to rate confidence in maintaining their balance on a scale of 0–100% (0% indicates no confidence and 100% indicates complete confidence) when performing specific activities, and an overall average score is calculated. The instrument has high internal consistency reliability and is moderately correlated ($r = -0.63$) to the total DHI score [59].

Vestibular Rehabilitation: Core Exercises

Depending on the degree and type of impairment a patient presents with, the vestibular rehabilitation therapist has a variety of treatment options that can be drawn on to develop a personalized program (Table 23.3). The intent of the following section is to provide the reader with a broad overview of the categories of vestibular rehabilitation exercises that are commonly used. A more in-depth discussion that details both the diagnostic and therapeutic options that are available to therapists can be found in the following texts [60].

Table 23.3 Common vestibular disorders and functional impairments with corresponding core vestibular rehabilitation strategies, including repositioning maneuvers, gaze stabilization exercises, balance training, and habituation exercises

Balance and vestibular deficit	Impairments or functional limitations	Rehabilitation approach
Benign paroxysmal positional vertigo	Positive Dix-Hallpike or roll test	Canalith repositioning maneuver; liberatory (Semont) maneuver; Brandt-Daroff exercise
VOR insufficiency due to unilateral or bilateral vestibular hypofunction	Symptoms with head motion; abnormal DVA or increased symptoms with DVA testing; gait unsteadiness with head turns	Gaze stabilization exercises (VORx1, VORx2, gaze shifting, and remembered target) as needed
VSR insufficiency (i.e., postural instability)	Abnormal static balance with altered sensory input (e.g., mCTSIB or SOT); abnormal dynamic balance, including reduced limits of stability, impaired reactive balance, and/or gait unsteadiness, especially with head turns (e.g., DGI or FGA)	Balance training under challenging sensory (altered visual and somatosensory input) and dynamic conditions (altered base of support, weight shifts). Gait training involving dynamic conditions and may include walking with head turns or performing a cognitive task while walking. General conditioning, such as walking for endurance or Aerobic exercise, is frequently prescribed because people with vestibular dysfunction often Limit physical activity to avoid symptom provocation
Motion sensitivity	Symptoms with self-motion (e.g., mSQ) or with visual motion or visually complex environments (e.g., VVAS) [75]	Habituation exercises based on the provocative situation (i.e., self-motion or visual motion)

Gaze Stabilization Exercises

Gaze stabilization exercises were developed based on the concept of VOR adaptation and substitution to increase the functional performance of the VOR. An appropriate set of activities for patient's demonstrating impaired DVA and head-motion provoked symptoms are gaze stabilization exercises. There are three primary types of gaze stability exercises that are prescribed to address a deficient VOR. First, exercises based on the assumption that they promote vestibular adaptation have been shown to be efficacious in patients with vestibular hypofunction. These exercises consist of having the patient turn the head (in the yaw or pitch planes) as fast as possible without losing focus of a target, which may be stationary (VORx1) or moving (VORx2) (Fig. 23.6). The second type of gaze stability exercise is based on the idea of substitution with the goal of promoting alternative eye movement strategies (e.g., compensatory saccades) to substitute for lost vestibular function. The gaze stability exercises can be made more and more difficult with progressions such as placing a visually active background behind the target or changing the distance of the patient from the target. Resolution of symptoms for patients with a confirmed unilateral vestibular hypofunction averages 6–8 weeks following the initiation of therapy. Finally, the use of optokinetic stimuli has been shown to increase the gain of the VOR [61]. While it is now known that head movement paired with a visual stimulus is optimal, optokinetic stimuli have been

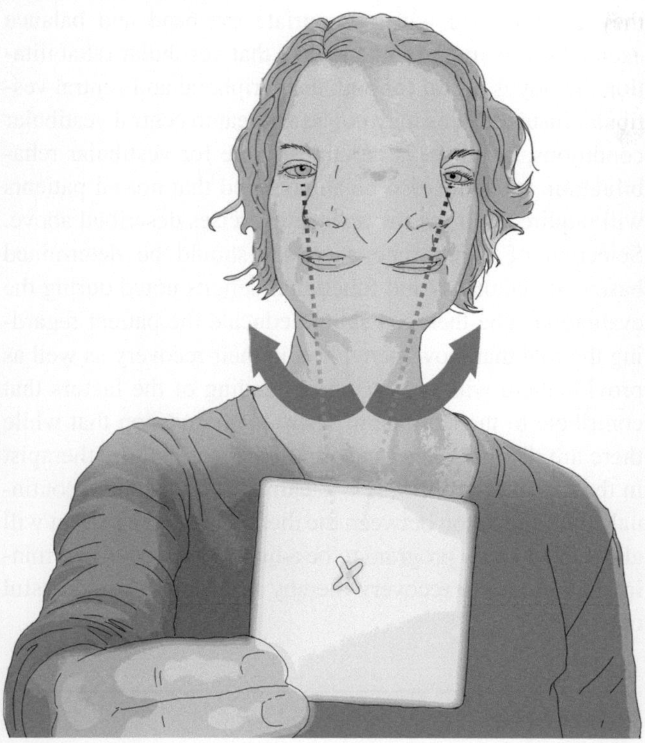

Fig. 23.6 Gaze stabilization exercises that show the "X1" exercise. During the X1 viewing paradigm, the visual target is stationary, and the patient directs her gaze on a target located on the card. The goal is for her to move her head back and forth in the yaw plane as fast as possible while still being able to clearly see the target. During the X2 exercise, the target and the head are moved simultaneously in opposite directions. (For additional illustrations and information, please see Hall et al. [79])

used successfully in treating patients with vestibular impairments [62]. The underlying physiological mechanisms of vestibular compensation are not completely understood; however, there is sufficient evidence that demonstrates that prescribed therapy programs produce significant changes in the functional abilities of an impaired VOR (Fig. 23.6) [63].

Vestibular Habituation Exercises

Habituation exercises are based on the principle that a patient's symptoms can be diminished or extinguished with brief, repeated exposure to the stimuli that are noxious. For example, in the case of motion provoked symptoms, the clinician should identify the specific movements that generate symptoms of dizziness and design a targeted and progressive program of exercises. A structured way to evaluate motion provoked symptoms is through use of the Motion Sensitivity Quotient (MSQ). The MSQ, developed by Michael Smith-Wheelock, is a series of prescribed movements for which the patient rates the severity (0–5) and duration of his/her symptoms [64]. Identification of provocative motions from the MSQ enables the therapist to design a habituation program and then track progress of rehabilitation by change in MSQ scores. A new reliable and validated shortened version of the MSQ test is now available by Heusel-Gillig, et al. (2022) [76]. The habituation approach typically consists of having the patient perform the exercises two to three times per day. The duration and frequency of the program are customized based on the intensity of the symptoms experienced when doing the exercise (e.g., dizziness and nausea). In order to motivate patients to perform the prescribed exercises, they should be educated that they may experience an increase in symptoms initially but that the symptoms will resolve over time. The majority of patients that are neurologically intact will report a reduction in their positional vertigo within 2–6 weeks [65]. The habituation approach has also been shown to be successful in treating patients that suffer from sensitivity to visual motion, visually complex environments, and visually focused tasks (e.g., persistent postural-perceptual dizziness (PPPD) [66]. It is noteworthy that habituation exercises show little clinical utility when used with patients with severe bilateral hypofunction [67].

Postural Control Exercises

Patients may continue to have deficiencies in postural control even after head motion-induced symptoms have resolved. This is not an uncommon occurrence as VOR function has been shown to be restored more quickly than postural stability [68]. It is important to note that recovery of postural control in patients with vestibular lesions can vary greatly based on their history and medical condition. A key principle for postural control exercises is to challenge the patient's balance system by altering the sensory input provided for balance. For example, a patient who is overly reliant on visual input despite having accurate somatosensory cues (i.e., standing on a firm surface) would be forced to utilize somatosensory cues by altering visual input. In this situation, the therapist would provide verbal cues to bring attention to the somatosensory input and alter visual input by providing a complex visual background and a visual task such as throwing or catching a ball or by having the patient close his/her eyes. Exercises such as this force patients to use different sensory systems and work toward appropriately weighting sensory input for a given task. Additional balance exercises are prescribed, as needed. For example, static balance training may include maintaining balance with progressively narrower base of support with vision and/or somatosensory cues altered. Dynamic balance exercises may include voluntary weight shifts and performance of ankle, hip, and step strategies.

Gait Exercises

Patients that have incurred an acute vestibular loss will often manifest ataxic gait for a period of time that is determined by a number of factors (e.g., health, medications, age). The goals of therapy for improving gait should be centered on improving postural stability when walking, especially with head turns, as well as increasing endurance to walking. Once a patient has shown that they can ambulate safely and confidently over a short distance, more challenging activities can be assigned. These include, but are not limited to, walking with head turns, walking and turning quickly, walking in different environments with varied surfaces, walking over/around obstacles, and walking in a crowded environment. Each of these activities is focused on improving a patient's ability to perform daily activities. However, precautions should be taken to ensure that the patient is able to perform these activities safely, especially in patients with bilateral hypofunction.

Conditioning and Maintenance Activities

It is not uncommon for patients to become less active following a vestibular crisis. This is due to the fact that head motion may exacerbate their symptoms. For this reason, general conditioning exercises, such as walking or aerobic activities, are frequently prescribed. It is important that the therapist counsel the patient that a sedentary lifestyle can both delay recovery and cause symptoms to persist. Once patients reach their maximum potential or a plateau, a maintenance program targeted at maintaining physical activity should be prescribed. Although there is little evidence to support prescribing specific vestibular exercises after discharge from rehabilitation, it is clear that an active lifestyle is important for health and maintaining balance into old age.

The therapist should consider recommending an exercise program that is appropriate for a patient's age and physical condition, but is also fun and aligns with their hobbies or interests. As the patient becomes more confident and has adequate balance function, sports such as tennis or golf may be undertaken. Of note, swimming can pose significant danger to patients with bilateral vestibular impairments due to their inability to sense direction when underwater.

Conclusion

There is strong evidence that exercise and customized vestibular rehabilitation can reduce symptoms, improve postural and gaze stability, and reduce fall risk [69]. It is well-established that patients who have suffered a vestibular insult can realize significant improvements in their condition if they are provided with appropriate eye/head and balance exercises. It is important to realize that vestibular rehabilitation therapy is useful for both the peripheral and central vestibular insults. Gains may not be as great in central vestibular conditions, but there is certainly a role for vestibular rehabilitation. It should also be emphasized that not all patients will require all of the therapeutic exercises described above. Selection of appropriate exercises should be determined based on symptoms and functional deficits noted during the evaluation. The therapist should educate the patient regarding the role that movement plays in their recovery as well as provide them with a clear understanding of the factors that contribute to their problem. There is no question that while there are distinct roles for both the patient and the therapist in the recovery process, it is a team effort. Open and continual communication between the therapist and the patient will allow the therapy program to be adjusted as needed and minimize the time to recovery thereby resulting in a successful outcome.

References

1. McDonnell MN, Hillier SL. Vestibular rehabilitation for unilateral peripheral vestibular dysfunction. Cochrane Database Syst Rev. 2015;1(1):CD005397.
2. Porciuncula F, Johnson CC, Glickman LB. The effect of vestibular rehabilitation on adults with bilateral vestibular hypofunction: a systematic review. J Vestib Res. 2012;22(5–6):283–98.
3. Hall CD, Herdman SJ, Whitney SL, et al. Vestibular rehabilitation for peripheral vestibular hypofunction: an updated clinical practice guideline from the academy of neurologic physical therapy of the American Physical Therapy Association. J Neurol Phys Ther. 2022;46(2):118–77. https://doi.org/10.1097/NPT.0000000000000382.
4. Baloh RW, Honrubia V. Clinical neurophysiology of the vestibular system. 2nd ed. Philadelphia: F.A. Davis; 1989.
5. Baloh and Halmagyi. Disorders of the vestibular system. 2nd ed. New York: Oxford University Press; 1996.
6. Beraneck M, Idoux E, Uno A, Vidal, Moore LE, Vibert N. Unilateral labyrinthectomy modifies the membrane properties of contralesional vestibular neurons. J Neurophysiol. 2004;92(3):1668–84.
7. Olabi B, Bergquist F, Dutia MB. Rebalancing the commissural system: mechanisms of vestibular compensation. J Vestib Res. 2009;19(5–6):201–7.
8. Zee DS. Vestibular adaptation. In: Herdman S, editor. Vestibular rehabilitation. 2nd ed. Philadelphia: F.A. Davis; 2000. p. 77.
9. Shepard NT, Asher A. Treatment of patients with nonvestibular dizziness and disequilibrium. In: Herdman S, editor. Vestibular Rehabilitation. 2nd ed. Philadelphia: F.A. Davis- USA; 2000.
10. Thompson KJ, Goetting JC, Staab JP, Shepard NT. Retrospective review and telephone follow-up to evaluate a physical therapy protocol for treating persistent postural-perceptual dizziness: a pilot study. J Vestib Res. 2015;25(2):97–10.
11. Igarashi M, Levy JK, Reschke MF, et al. Locomotor dysfunction after surgical lesions in the unilateral vestibular nuclei region in squirrel monkeys. Arch Otorhinolaryngol. 1978;221:89.
12. Beraneck M, McKee JL, Aleisa M, Cullen KE. Asymmetric recovery in cerebellar-deficient mice following unilateral labyrinthectomy. J Neurophysiol. 2008;100:945–58.

13. Telian SA, Shepard NT, Smith-Wheelock M, Kemink JL. Habituation therapy for chronic vestibular dysfunction: preliminary results. Otolaryngol Head Neck Surg. 1990;103:89–95.
14. Furman JM, Balaban CD, Pollack IF. Vestibular compensation in a patient with a cerebellar infarction. Neurology. 1997;48:916–20.
15. Shepard NT, Telian SA. Programmatic vestibular rehabilitation. Otolaryngol Head Neck Surg. 1995;112:173–82.
16. Igarashi M, Ishikawa M, Yamane H. Physical exercise and balance compensation after total ablation of vestibular organs. Prog Brain Res. 1988;76:405.
17. Staab J. Diagnosis and treatment of psychologic symptoms and psychiatric disorders in patients with dizziness and imbalance. In: Shepard NT, Solomon D, editors. Practical issues in the management of the dizzy and balance disorder patient, vol. 34. Otolaryngol Clin North Am; 2000. p. 617.
18. Yardley L. Overview of the psychologic effects of chronic dizziness and balance disorders. In: Shepard NT, Solomon D, editors. Practical Issues in the management of the dizzy and balance disorder patient, vol. 34. Otolaryngol Clin North Am; 2000. p. 603.
19. Peppard SB. Effect of drug therapy on compensation from vestibular injury. Laryngoscope. 1986;96:878.
20. Curthoys IS, Halmagyi MG. Vestibular compensation-recovery after unilateral vestibular loss. In: Herdman S, editor. Vestibular rehabilitation. 4th ed. Philadelphia: F.A. Davis; 2014.
21. Shepard NT. Management of the patient with chronic complaints of dizziness: an overview of laboratory studies. Clackamas, Ore: Neurocom International; 2007.
22. Jacobson GP, Calder JH. Self-perceived balance disability/handicap in the presence of bilateral peripheral vestibular system impairment. J Am Acad Audiol. 2000;11(2):76–83.
23. MacDougall HG, Weber KP, McGarvie LA, Halmagyi GM, Curthoys IS. The video head impulse test. Diagnostic accuracy in peripheral vestibulopathy. Neurol. 2000;73(14):1134–41.
24. Schubert MC, Hall CD, Das V, Tusa RJ, Herdman SJ. Oculomotor strategies and their effect on reducing gaze position error. Otol Neurotol. 2010;31(2):228–31.
25. Colebatch JG, Halmagyi GM. Vestibular evoked potentials in human neck muscle before and after unilateral vestibular deafferentation. Neurol. 1992;42(8):1635–6.
26. Todd NP, Cody FW, Banks JR. A saccular origin of frequency tuning in myogenic vestibular evoked potentials: implications for human response to loud sounds. Hear Res. 2000;141(1–2):180–8.
27. Makowiec K, McCaslin DL, Jacobson GP, Hatton K, Lee J. Effect of electrode montage and head position on air conducted ocular vestibular evoked myogenic potential (oVEMP). Am J Audiol. 2017;16:1–9.
28. Murray KJ, Hill PB, Waterson J. Does otolith organ dysfunction influence outcomes after a customized program of vestibular rehabilitation? J Neurol Phys Ther. 2010;34(2):70–5.
29. McCaslin DL, Jacobson GP, Grantham SL, Piker EG, Verghese S. The influence of unilateral saccular impairment on functional balance performance and self-report dizziness. J Am Acad Audiol. 2011 Sep;22(8):542–9.
30. Barber HO. Vestibular neurophysiology. Otolaryngol Head Neck Surg. 1984;92:151–7.
31. Herdman SJ, Tusa RJ, Blatt P, Suzuki A, Venuto PJ, Roberts D. Computerized dynamic visual acuity test in the assessment of vestibular deficits. Am J Otol. 1998;19:790–6.
32. Schubert MC, Migliaccio AA, Clendaniel RA, Allak A, Carey JP. Mechanism of dynamic visual acuity recovery with vestibular rehabilitation. Arch Phys Med Rehab. 2008;89(3):500–7.
33. Goebel JA, Tungsiripat N, Belinda S, Carmody J. Gaze stabilization test: a new clinical test of unilateral vestibular dysfunction. Otol Neurotol. 2006;28:68–73.
34. Herdman S, Tusa R. Assessment and treatment of patients with benign paroxysmal positional vertigo. In: Herdman S, editor. Vestibular rehabilitation. 4th ed. Philadelphia: F.A. Davis; 2014. p. 461.
35. Barany R. Physiologie und Pathologie des Bogengangapparates beim Menshen. Vienna: Deuticke; 1907.
36. Brandt T, Daroff RB. Physical therapy for benign paroxysmal positional vertigo. Arch Otolaryngol. 1980;106:494.
37. Schuknecht HF. Cupulolithiasis. Arch Otolaryngol. 1969;90(6):765–78.
38. Epley JM. The canalith repositioning procedure for treatment of benign paroxysmal positional vertigo. Otolaryngol Head Neck Surg. 1992;107:399–404.
39. Clendaniel RA. Positional testing and treatment. In: Jacobson GP, Shepard NT, Barin K, Burkard RF, Janky K, McCaslin DL, editors. Balance function and management. 3rd ed. San Diego: Plural Publishing; 2021. p. 225.
40. Semont A, Freyss G, Vitte E. Curing the BPPV with a liberatory maneuver. Adv Otorhinolaryngol. 1998;42:290.
41. Cohen HS, Kimball KT. Effectiveness of treatments for benign paroxysmal positional vertigo of the posterior canal. Otol Neurotol. 2005;26:1034–40.
42. Baloh RW. Dizziness, hearing loss, and tinnitus. Philadelphia, Davis; 1998.
43. Herdman SJ, Shepard NT. Vestibular rehabilitation and pre-Hab in sporadic acoustic neuroma. In: Carlson ML, link MJ, Driscoll CL, editors. Comprehensive Management of Acoustic Neuroma. New York: Thieme Publishers, 2019.
44. Herdman SJ, Clendaniel RA, Mattox DE, Holliday MJ, Niparko JK. Vestibular adaptation exercises and recovery: acute stage after acoustic neuroma resection. Otolaryngol Head Neck Surg. 1995;113(1):77–87.
45. Gottshall KR, Hoffer ME, Moore RJ, Balough BJ. The role of vestibular rehabilitation in the treatment of Meniere's disease. Otolaryngol Head Neck Surg. 2005;133:326–8.
46. Assimakopoulos D, Patrikakos G. Treatment of Meniere's disease by intratympanic gentamicin application. J Laryngol Otol. 2003;117:10–6.
47. Clendaniel RA, Tucci DL. Vestibular rehabilitation strategies in Meniere's disease. Otolaryngol Clin N Am. 1997;30:1145–59.
48. Mruzek M, Barin K, Nichols DS, Burnett CN, Welling DB. Effects of vestibular rehabilitation and social reinforcement on recovery following ablative vestibular surgery. Laryngoscope. 1995;105:686–92.
49. Chamelian L, Feinstein A. Outcome after mild to moderate traumatic brain injury: the role of dizziness. Arch Phys Med Rehabil. 2004;85:1662–6.
50. Yang C-C, Tu Y-K, Hua M-S, Huang S-J. The association between the postconcussion symptoms and clinical outcomes for patients with mild traumatic brain injury. J Trauma. 2007;62:657–63.
51. Zasler ND, Ross ZD, Arciniegas DB, Ross MR, Kreutzer JS. Brain injury medicine, 2nd Edition: Principles and practice. New York: Demos Medical; 2012.
52. Staab JP. Chronic subjective dizziness. Continuum. 2012;18:1118–41.
53. Shepard NT, Telian SA, Niparko JK, et al. Platform pressure test in identification of perilymphatic fistula. Am J Otol. 1992;13:49.
54. Monsell EM, Brackmann DE, Linthicum FH. Why do vestibular destructive procedures sometimes fail? Otolaryngol Head Neck Surg. 1988;99:482.
55. Wall C 3rd. The sinusoidal harmonic acceleration rotary chair test. Theoretical and clinical basis. Neurol Clin. 1990;8:269.
56. Clendaniel RA. Outcome measures for assessment of treatment of the dizzy and balance disorder patient. Otolaryngol Clin N Am. 2000;33:519–33.
57. Jacobson GP, Newman CW. The development of the dizziness handicap inventory. Arch Otolaryngol Head Neck Surg. 1990;116(4):424–7.

58. Whitney SL, Wrisley DM, Brown KE, Furman JM. Is perception of handicap related to functional performance in persons with vestibular dysfunction? Otol Neurotol. 2004;25(2):139–43.
59. Powell LE, Myers AM. The activities-specific balance confidence (ABC) scale. J Gerontol A Biol Sci Med Sci. 1995;50A(1):M28–34.
60. Whitney SL, Rossi MM. Efficacy of vestibular rehabilitation. In: Shepard NT, Solomon D, editors. Practical issues in the management of the dizzy and balance disorder patient, vol. 34. Otolaryngol Clin North Am; 2000. p. 659.
61. Herdman S, editor. Vestibular rehabilitation. 3rd ed. Philadelphia: F.A. Davis; 2007.
62. Shelhamer M, Robinson DA, Tan HS. Context-specific adaptation of the gain of the vestibulo-ocular reflex in humans. J Vestib Res. 1992;2:89.
63. Gonshor A, Melvill Jones G. Short-term adaptive changes in the human vestibulo-ocular reflex arc. J Physiol. 1976;256(2):361–79.
64. Smith-Wheelock M, Shepard NT, Telian SA. Physical therapy program for vestibular rehabilitation. Am J Otol. 1991;12:218–25.
65. Shepard NT, Telian SA, Smith-Wheelock M, et al. Vestibular and balance rehabilitation therapy. Ann Otol Rhinol Laryngol. 1993;102:198.
66. Yardley L. Overview of the psychologic effects of chronic dizziness and balance disorders. Otolaryngol Clin N Am. 2000;33:603.
67. Telian SA, Shepard NT, Smith-Wheelock M, et al. Bilateral vestibular paresis: diagnosis and treatment. Otolaryngol Head Neck Surg. 1991;104:67.
68. Horak FB, Nashner LM. Central programming of postural movements: adaptation to altered support surface configurations. J Neurophysiol. 1986;55:1379.
69. Shumway-Cook A, et al. Predicting the probability for falls in community-dwelling older adults. Phys Ther. 1997;77:812.
70. Podsiadlo D, Richardson S. The timed "Up & Go": a test of basic functional mobility for frail elderly persons. J Am Geriatr Soc. 1991 Feb;39(2):142–8.
71. Whitney SL, Marchetti GF, Schade A, Wrisley DM. The sensitivity and specificity of the Timed "Up & Go" and the Dynamic Gait Index for self-reported falls in persons with vestibular disorders. J Vestib Res. 2004;14(5):397–409.
72. Horak FB, Wrisley DM, Frank J. The balance evaluation systems test (BESTest) to differentiate balance deficits. Phys Ther. 2009;89(5):484–98.
73. Wrisley DM, Kumar NA. Functional gait assessment: concurrent, discriminative, and predictive validity in community-dwelling older adults. Phys Ther. 2010;90(5):761–73.
74. Lord SR, Menz HB, Tiedemann A. A physiological profile approach to falls risk assessment and prevention. Phys Ther. 2003;83(3):237–52.
75. Dannenbaum E, Chilingaryan G, Fung J. Visual vertigo analogue scale: an assessment questionnaire for visual vertigo. J Vestib Res. 2011;21(3):153–9.
76. Heusel-Gillig L, Santucci V, Hall CD. Development and validation of the modified motion sensitivity test. Otol Neurotol. 2022;43:944–9.
77. Piker EG, Jacobson GP, Newman CW. Assessing dizziness-related quality of life. In: Jacobson GP, Shepard NT, Barin K, Burkard RF, Janky K, McCaslin DL, editors. Balance function and management. 3rd ed. San Diego: Plural Publishing; 2021. p. 143.
78. McCaslin DL. Electronystagmography and videonystagmography. Plural; 2013.
79. Hall CD, et al. Treatment of vestibular disorders (inner ear balance problems): how does your physical therapist treat dizziness related to inner ear balance problems? J Neurol Phys Ther. 2022;46(2):178–9.

Rehabilitation of Facial Paralysis

24

Andrew T. Huang, David Wilde, Evan Jones,
and Michael Baddour

Introduction

Facial paresis or paralysis is a feared complication and, sometimes, inevitability, following neurotologic and otologic procedures. Whether inadvertent or necessary, iatrogenic injury to the facial nerve leads to significant functional impairments including oral incompetence, dysarthria, lack of ocular protection, and challenges with self-expression and identity [1]. The consequences of facial paralysis are extensive and can lead to the development of psychosocial sequelae including depression and anxiety [2]. In fact, survey studies demonstrate that those with facial paralysis are more likely to be deemed unattractive, unlikable, and less trustworthy [3].

Neurotologic procedures represent a minority of iatrogenic facial nerve injuries, despite proximity of the nerve to the lateral skull base and organs of hearing and balance, with injury rates estimated to be less than 2% [4, 5]. Unfortunately, surgeons will encounter this complication in practice, especially with increasing levels of case complexity and revision surgery. Reports on lateral skull base procedures for resection of vestibular schwannoma and glomus jugulare have demonstrated facial nerve alterations in 39% and 56%, respectively, making understanding and familiarity with management and reconstructive rehabilitation of this consequence significantly important [6, 7].

The pathophysiology of nerve injury and degeneration are beyond the scope of this chapter, but a relevant discussion is found elsewhere in this book. The current chapter is focused on the rehabilitation, through surgery and post-treatment physical therapy, of facial nerve injury and paralysis in the acute and chronic setting. Overall, identifying facial rehabilitation goals of the individual patient is critical to selecting the appropriate intervention. Setting expectations, both for the provider and patient, is a vital component of achieving success with facial rehabilitation, especially in the situation of complete nerve transection when complete recovery of function is not yet achievable. Balancing the risks of any procedural option with the pre-determined goals will help optimize the ultimate result for the patient.

A. T. Huang (✉) · D. Wilde · E. Jones
Bobby R. Alford Department of Otolaryngology—Head and Neck Surgery, Baylor College of Medicine, Houston, TX, USA
e-mail: andrew.huang@bcm.edu

M. Baddour
Department of Otolaryngology—Head and Neck Surgery, Emory University, Atlanta, GA, USA

Immediate Management

Immediately recognized facial nerve injuries during neurotologic procedures are generally only repairable when isolated at the vertical segment. When only partial thickness, these injuries can best be managed by thorough decompression to prevent pressure-related damage, microsurgical axonal coaptation, and wrapping the injury site with a nerve protecting graft, either venous or allograft. In this setting, complete recovery to House-Brackmann (HB) I can be possible if the disruption of nerve axons is minimized [8].

When complete transection of the nerve is detected or anticipated, immediate reconstruction should be planned and performed concurrently, with both static and dynamic options considered. Ideally, when possible, primary neurorrhaphy or autologous grafting should be performed, and these options have been shown to be superior to selective re-innervation techniques such as hypoglossal nerve to facial nerve anastomosis (XII-VII) [9]. Historically, the best functional outcome after immediate primary neurorrhaphy is HB III, but these results are being challenged and optimized through newer repair techniques and nerve connecting options, which will be discussed in the next section (Fig. 24.1) [8]. However, as the proximal stump of the facial nerve at the lateral skull base is usually inaccessible, immediate facial reanimation utilizing selective re-innervation, nerve substitution, or other dynamic techniques should be

A. D. Sweeney et al. (eds.), *Haynes-Glasscock-Shambaugh Surgery of the Ear*, https://doi.org/10.1007/978-3-032-18264-7_24

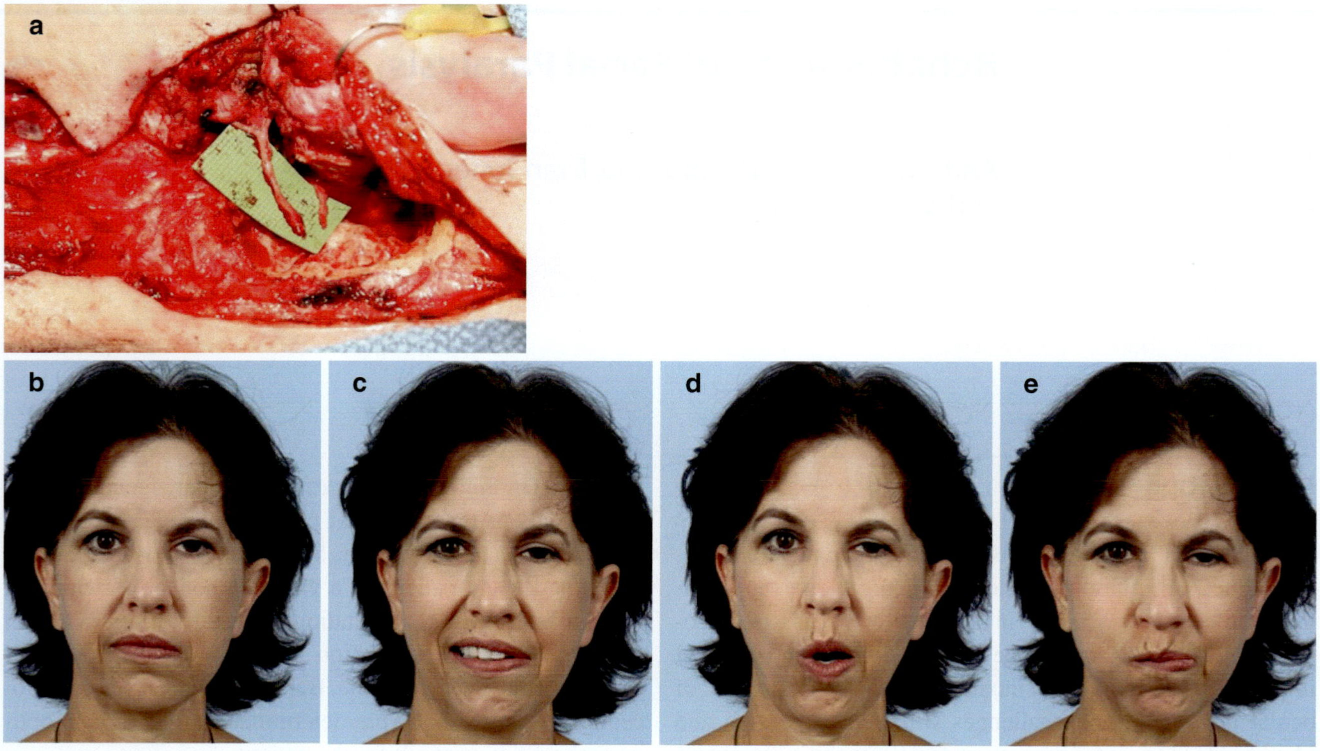

Fig. 24.1 Immediate primary repair of complete facial nerve transections (**a**) can result in HBIII or better facial nerve function (**b–e**) Photographs used with permission

employed, and these will be discussed in the following sections. In retrospective analyses, utilizing these techniques in the immediate setting, or even chronic setting following facial nerve injury, has been associated with excellent functional outcomes [10].

The use of static repair techniques to protect the eye, improve oral competence, and maintain facial symmetry in repose is well-established. In the immediate post-injury setting, the utility of these techniques in minimizing flaccid paralysis and improving the outcomes of dynamic reconstruction techniques through optimizing facial mimetic sarcomere length is important [11]. These static repair techniques are described in later sections.

Delayed Management

When a facial nerve injury did not involve complete transection during the index procedure, at least partial functional recovery may be achieved within 6 months postoperatively. Timing and extent of recovery are mostly age and comorbidity dependent, and specifically, patients over 60 years of age are generally considered poor candidates for functional return; however, through newer techniques and improved surgical and pharmacologic modalities, age limitations are now being challenged with facial dynamic restoration now being achievable in even those over 70 years of age [12]. In general, if no discernible facial function has returned within 6 months on clinical evaluation and electrodiagnostic testing, then the performance of static and dynamic reconstructive should be considered [13].

There are many options for objective testing of facial nerve function in the postoperative setting. It is prudent to document both pre- and postoperative function of the facial nerve using the House-Brackmann scale for all patients undergoing otologic surgery. In addition, neurophysiologic testing is important to quantify the degree of a facial nerve injury and assess candidacy for appropriate intervention in those with delayed diagnosis. Modalities include nerve excitability testing (NET), maximal stimulation testing (MST), and electroneuronography (ENoG).

Static Reconstruction Techniques

Static facial reconstructive procedures are defined as techniques that improve facial symmetry at rest or facilitate normal facial function without nerve intervention. While not expected to restore function to the motor units of the affected facial mimetic musculature, these procedures can positively affect a patient's postoperative outcome. Also, considering the additive effect of static procedures on quicker and more robust dynamic repair outcomes, static repair procedures are integral in the surgical rehabilitation of facial paralysis at any stage, immediate or long-standing.

Upper Face

The upper face consisting of the forehead, brow, and eyelids is important in non-verbal communication and, specifically considering the eyelids, serves functionally in the protection and maintenance of the eye. Static procedures to address these areas focus on achieving symmetry of brow position and facilitation of eyelid closure through reduction in eyelid retraction and weighted correction of the upper eyelid.

When planning static procedures for the upper face, the brow should always be evaluated and targeted first through a brow lift. Failure to correct brow ptosis prior to addressing the upper eyelid can result in inaccurate measurement of upper eyelid closure deficiency, generally resulting in inadequate correction of lagophthalmos. There are multiple approaches to accomplish a brow lift (e.g. coronal, pretrichial/trichophytic, direct, indirect, and endoscopic). Determining the correct approach requires careful facial analysis, including hairline position and rhytids. However, recognizing the nature and severity of the injury is a key to the success of any approach.

Commonly performed static procedures for the eyelids include gold or platinum weight placement and the lateral tarsal strip procedure for the upper and lower lid, respectively. With upper eyelid weight placement, a small weight is placed in either a pretarsal or prelevator aponeurotic plane and fixed to the tarsal plate as close to the lash line as possible to aid with gravity-assisted closure. The weight chosen must not be too heavy as to overpower the levator palpebrae superioris and lead to upper eyelid ptosis, but not too light as to fail to achieve complete eyelid closure in both upright and supine positioning. To identify the correct weight, sizing can be performed in the office setting using serially increasing weights taped to the inferior margin of the upper eyelid until full closure in both upright and supine positions without impairment of visual fields is achieved. The choice in use of a gold or platinum weight is based on patient sensitivity to gold (platinum being less reactive than gold) as well as weight requirement, taking into account the quality of upper eyelid skin and soft tissue and space available. As platinum is denser than gold, a platinum weight will be smaller and lower profile, decreasing the risk of pressure-related necrosis of the overlying upper eyelid soft tissue which may result in implant extrusion.

The lateral tarsal strip procedure is indicated when increased lower eyelid laxity results in clinically significant ectropion preventing contact with the upper eyelid despite full excursion. The procedure entails sectioning of the inferior division of the lateral canthal tendon and resuspension of the posterior lamella of the lid to Whitnall's tubercle. This procedure increases the height and tension of the lateral canthus, improving contact with the upper eyelid during closure and preventing ectropion.

Mid- and Lower Face

While the aesthetic impact of a drooping mid- and lower face cannot be trivialized, functionally, loss of facial tone will result in ipsilateral nasal obstruction from alar collapse and rotation of the nose contralaterally, as well as oral incompetence from orbicularis oris weakness. Fascial suspension grafts are, thus, an invaluable tool in the maintenance of facial symmetry at rest, static opening of the affected nasal ala to improve nasal breathing, and placement of tension on the atonic oral commissure to improve oral competence. Tensor fascia lata is commonly used for autograft and can be harvested from the upper lateral thigh either through an open or endoscopic approach. The grafts are prepared either as individual or conjoined strips, which should be secured under tension to the upper and lower orbicularis oris, modiolus, and alar part of the nasalis. They are then tunneled in a supra-superficial musculoaponeurotic system (SMAS) plane to be fixated to the root of the zygoma, which then creates the appropriate vector of support for the mid- and lower face structures (Fig. 24.2). High rates of patient satisfaction can be achieved with this procedure, and complication rates can be as low as 8% [14].

Contralateral Face

In order to improve facial symmetry non-invasively, chemodenervation of the contralateral face with botulinum neurotoxin serotype A (BoNT-A) can be considered. BoNT-A can target hyperkinesis of the non-paralyzed face in the clinic setting without major surgical intervention [15]. Duration of action for the most common formulations is 3–4 months. The forehead should be treated with relatively high doses, while the mid- and lower face should be treated conservatively to minimize the risk of developing oral incompetence on the treated side. This technique can be particularly useful in patients with the potential for functional recovery of the paralyzed face given the transient nature of BoNT-A. Studies suggest that treatment of the contralateral face may modulate the degree of re-innervation achieved after injury in the paralyzed side through biofeedback regulation [16, 17].

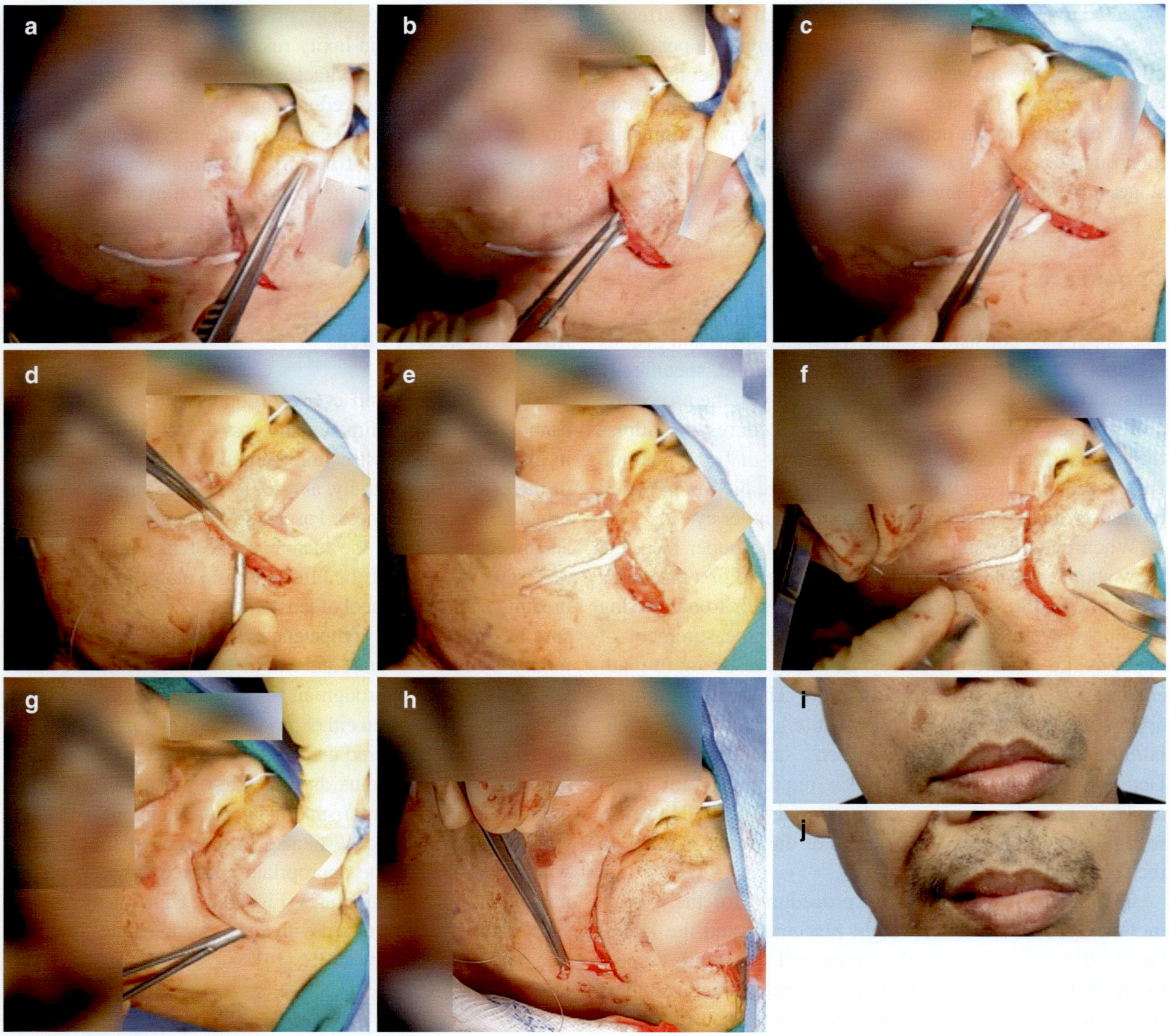

Fig. 24.2 Mid- and lower face static repair techniques. Tensor fascia lata grafts can be used to suspend the nasal ala, upper lip, oral commissure, and lower lip (**a**–**h**) to achieve facial symmetry at rest, improving nasal breathing and oral competence (**i**, **j**)

Dynamic Reconstruction Techniques

Dynamic facial reconstruction procedures restore active, volitional facial movement. As stated earlier in this chapter, in the situation of acute facial nerve injury, early intervention with primary nerve repair or selective re-innervation is associated with improved facial movement outcomes [10]. In some instances, such as with cerebellopontine angle tumor resections with preserved facial nerve continuity, the degree of facial nerve dysfunction cannot definitively be assessed until postoperatively when the patient is awake and alert enough to follow commands. While some cases involving postoperative facial weakness will resolve with conservative management, close follow-up is important so that intervention can be planned within the first 6 months, if necessary [13, 18, 19].

Principles of Nerve Repair

Nerve repair requires optimization of tissue handling from the perspective of both instrumentation and microsurgical technique. Jeweler forceps with tips of 0.1 to 0.3 mm allow for precise handling of the epineurium, avoiding crush injury of the peri- and endoneurium. Loupe or microscope-assisted visualization facilitates proper identification of nerve sheath layers and placement of coaptation sutures, usually sized 9–0 or smaller.

When repairing a nerve, preparation of the nerve ends, performance of a tension-free anastomosis, and avoidance of axonal bundling are imperative to prevent aberrant axonal regeneration. The cut ends of both the donor and recipient nerves, when not utilizing auto- or allografts, should be examined for healthy bleeding from the endoneurium. Freshening the nerve edges is preferentially performed with as sharp of an instrument as possible, such as a scalpel, to avoid crushing of the axonal bundles. Ensuring the vitality of the nerve mitigates the risk of degeneration at the anastomotic site, which can lead to neural tissue loss and failure of axonal regeneration. Similarly, tension-free anastomosis using a minimum amount of suture material and disrupting only the epineural layer may help prevent neural devascularization and optimize healing [20]. In addition to minimizing repair tension, care must be taken to ensure that the anastomotic site demonstrates no axonal interference or overlap, which can lead to aberrant axonal regeneration and failure of appropriate nerve propagation. As axonal regeneration between opposing nerve ends requires transduction of neural growth factors from the donor-to-recipient end, it is recommended that a gap of 1 millimeter or less be left at the repair site, with gaps of up to 5 millimeters demonstrated to still allow for appropriate nerve regrowth [21, 22]. Use of nerve connector-assisted coaptation aids and nerve autografts can be helpful when gaps between nerve endings preclude a tension-free primary anastomosis; however, attention must be paid to the donor nerve graft for epineural defects or nerve branches that will lead to aberrant axonal growth [23]. Failure to address these areas may lead to loss of nerve growth signaling before maximal potentiation through the desired repair site can occur.

Bridging long segment nerve deficits can be accomplished using an autograft or, more recently, an allograft (Fig. 24.3). Donor sites for autologous nerve graft include, but are not limited to, the greater auricular nerve, transverse cervical nerve, and the sural nerve. Use of nerve allografts has become more widespread due to the wider availability of suitable allograft options and due to the avoidance of a donor sensory or motor deficit from autograft harvesting. While there are no prospective results of facial nerve repair outcomes utilizing allograft, several large database reviews have been published on their benefits in peripheral nerve repair, with comparable sensory and motor outcomes demonstrated between autograft and allograft use [24].

Regardless of whether primary repair or grafting is used, newer techniques using biologic materials and topical pharmacologic agents to improve nerve repair outcomes have become more widespread. In general, biologic materials assist nerve coaptation by reducing suture tension and protecting donor and recipient nerves from wound bed inflammation and aberrant axonal propagation. Examples of biologic materials used for this purpose are decellularized porcine small intestinal submucosa, chitosan, and type I collagen. While several topical pharmacologic agents have been reported to improve nerve regeneration when placed at the time of nerve repair, calcium channel blockers are the most widely accepted. The mechanism of action is not completely understood, but animal studies have shown reduction in axonal resistance and scar tissue formation at the anastomotic site [25, 26].

Nerve Substitution and Selective Re-innervation

The premise of nerve substitution and selective re-innervation relies on the use of separate donor motor nerves of the head and neck, non-facial or contralateral facial, as a source of distal facial nerve branch stimulation. With these techniques, conscious activation of the donor nerve can stimulate targeted facial mimetic muscular groups and lead to adaptive spontaneous return of facial movement. In general, these techniques are most utilized when complete loss of the affected facial nerve is realized and primary grafting is not a good option. Most commonly, these techniques are used for restoring a spontaneous smile, but there are reports demonstrating their usefulness with spontaneous eyelid closure and forehead movement, as well [27]. Importantly, these techniques can be used either alone or in conjunction with primary facial nerve grafting or microvascular free tissue transfer in a "supercharging" fashion to augment spontaneous facial movement [28]. Currently, the most common sources of donor nerve for re-innervation include distal branches of the contralateral facial nerve, the hypoglossal nerve, and the masseteric nerve, with lesser reported nerves including the spinal accessory nerve [29].

Nerve substitution and selective re-innervation techniques were originally published in the early 1900s when the first hypoglossal-to-facial nerve re-innervation was reported [30]. Early attempts utilized end-to-end coaptation of the cut distal end of the facial nerve with the ipsilateral hypoglossal nerve. Unfortunately, while reasonable return of spontaneous smile could be achieved, loss of ipsilateral control of the tongue musculature resulted in dysphagia or dysarthria in nearly half of patients [31]. Refinements in the procedure were thus developed to reduce tongue morbidity through less aggressive manipulation of the hypoglossal nerve, including limited transection of the nerve (less than one-half) with end-to-side facial-to-hypoglossal coaptation, and more recently, selective hypoglossal axonal connection to distal facial nerve targets [32, 33]. In cases where the distal facial nerve branches are not able to be mobilized to safely reach the hypoglossal nerve, jump grafts may be used and have shown good results [32]. Large series have demonstrated achievement of HB III in greater than 90% of patients with minimal

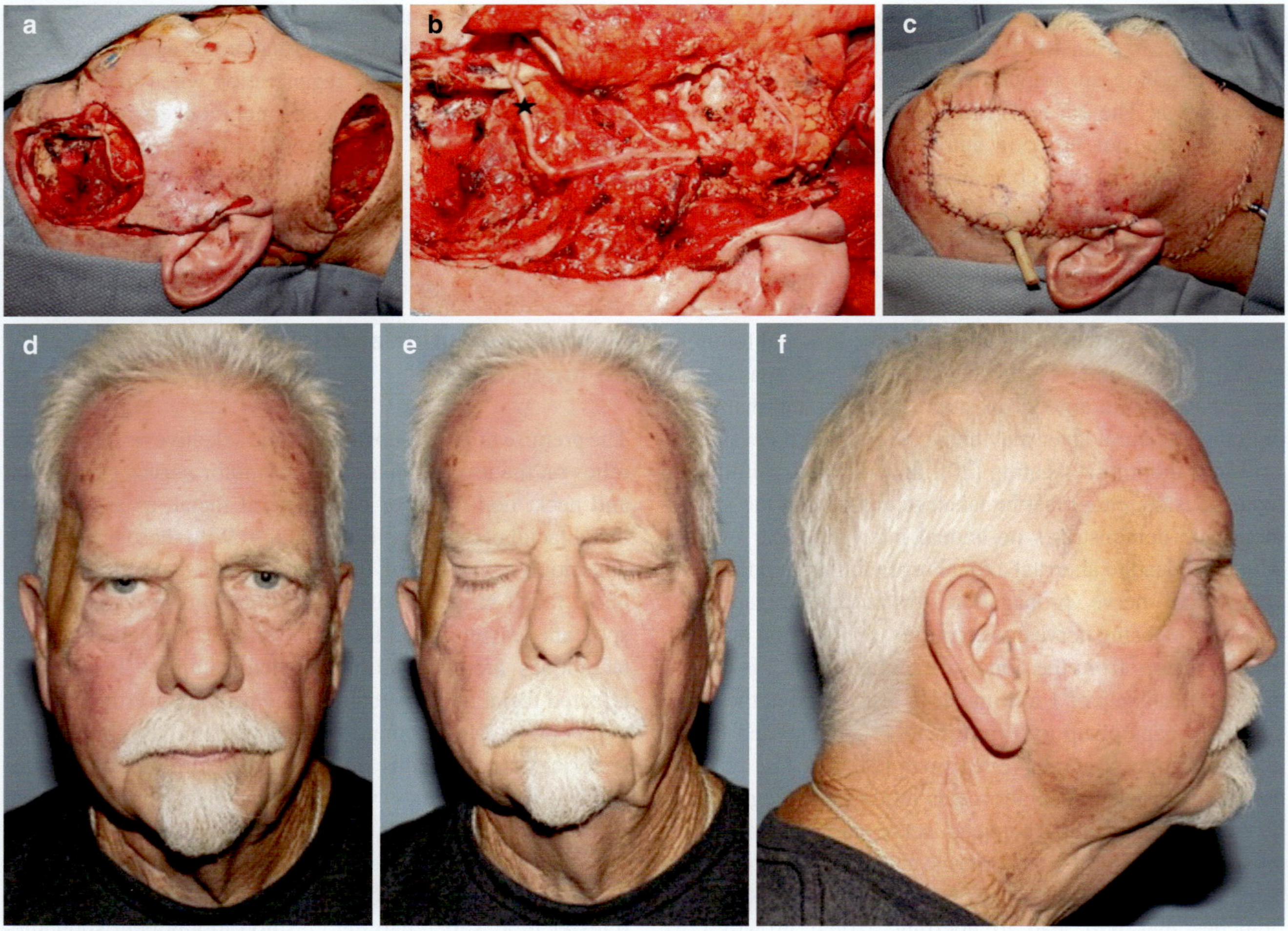

Fig. 24.3 Long segmental defect of the zygomatic branch of the facial nerve from sacrifice during resection of a locally extensive cutaneous squamous cell carcinoma of the temple (**a**). Repair of the zygomatic branch using a nerve allograft (**b**) and anterolateral thigh free flap (**c**). The patient's final outcome over 1 year out from adjuvant radiotherapy (**d**–**f**). Photographs used with permission

tongue atrophy [18]. Due to the large amount of experience and reliability with hypoglossal-to-facial selective re-innervation, this option remains commonly employed.

While the hypoglossal nerve has proven its reliability over time, the masseteric nerve has become a preferential donor nerve for many surgeons given its relatively close proximity to the buccal branch of the facial nerve and the synergistic nature of jaw clenching and smiling. The shorter distance of the donor masseteric nerve at the subzygomatic triangle to the distal buccal branches of the facial nerve and its high concentration of axons have demonstrated production of an earlier functional recovery than hypoglossal nerve transfer (Fig. 24.4) [13, 34, 35]. In a large meta-analysis comparing the two techniques, Sunnybrook Facial Nerve Grading Scale scores were higher in masseteric transfer; however, oral commissure symmetry at rest was better for hypoglossal transfer. Given these findings, concurrent selective re-innervation using the masseteric and hypoglossal nerves for smile reanimation has been recommended to optimize functional outcome.

Cross-face nerve grafting is another technique, which uniquely allows for synchronicity of facial expression; however, considering the long distance between the contralateral functional distal branches of the facial nerve and the paralyzed face, a major downside is the prolonged time period required for axon regeneration before re-innervation occurs. Long autologous nerve grafts such as the sural nerve must be utilized to span these long distances, resulting in sacrifice of a distant sensory distribution and increasing risk of graft-related failure due to aberrant axonal regeneration through microscopic defects that may occur in the epineurium during graft harvest. When performed meticulously in the right candidate, cross-face nerve grafting offers unparalleled rehabilitative potential due to its ability to give spontaneous and symmetric movement to the paralyzed face. Newer techniques, called "babysitter" procedures, also help mitigate the lack of facial mimetic stimulation and potential loss of motor end plates during cross-face nerve graft healing. These procedures combine selective re-innervation using the masseteric and/or hypoglossal nerves combined with cross-face

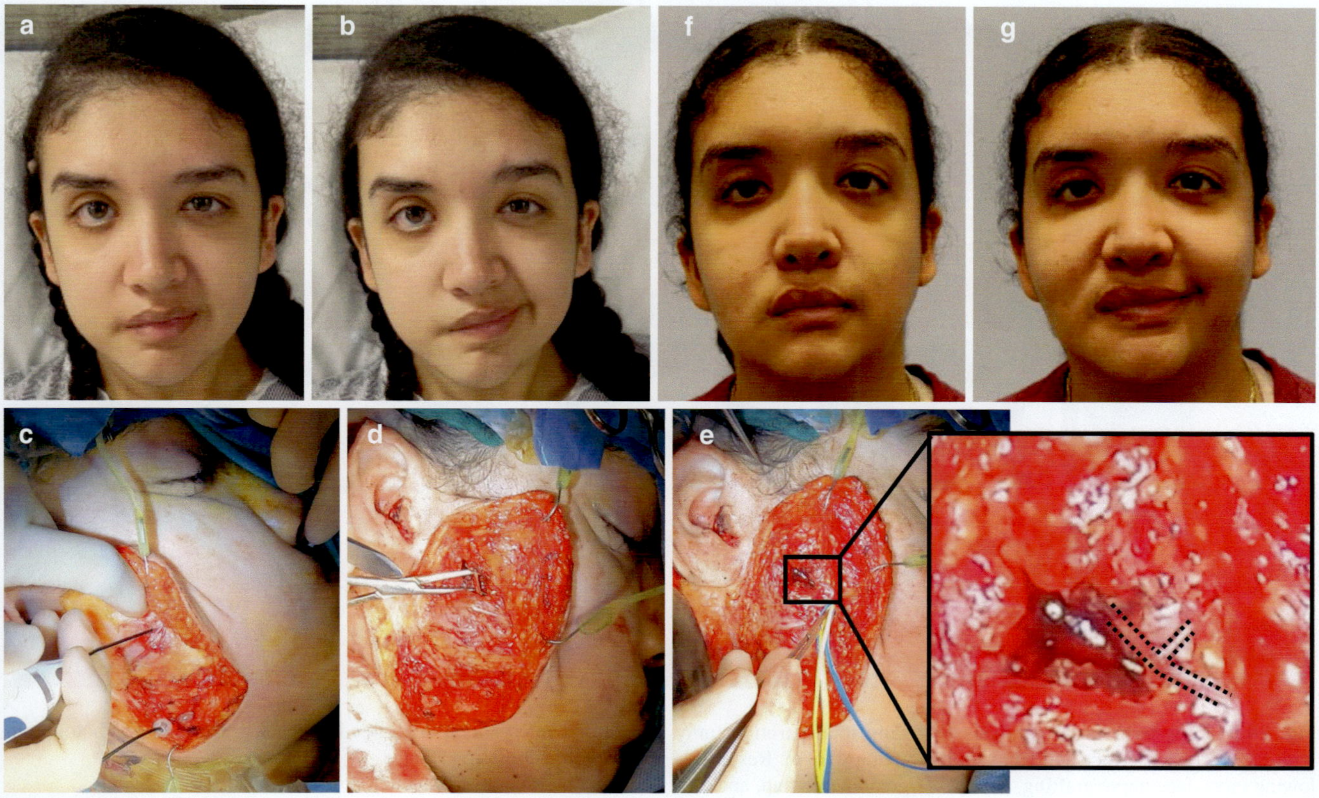

Fig. 24.4 Complete facial nerve paralysis from a facial nerve schwannoma requiring transcochlear resection and nerve sacrifice (**a**, **b**). Immediate repair using selective re-innervation of distal buccal branches of the facial nerve with the masseteric nerve (**c**–**e**) resulting in excellent functional return of spontaneous smile (**f**, **g**). Photographs used with permission

grafting in a single stage to provide earlier facial mimetic muscle stimulation, preventing potential motor end plate loss and muscle elongation that can limit recovery [28, 36, 37].

Microvascular Free Tissue Transfer

For patients with previously failed re-innervation, severe motor end plate degeneration and muscular atrophy (> 2 years), or loss of facial mimetic muscles, microvascular free tissue transfer (MVFTT) of functional muscle can recreate dynamic movement of the paralyzed face through ipsilateral or contralateral facial nerve, masseteric nerve, and/or hypoglossal nerve coaptation. Several options exist for donor functional muscle including the latissimus dorsi, the pectoralis minor, platysma, and, most commonly, the gracilis [38–41]. For free functional gracilis muscle transfers, innervation of the obturator nerve from the donor nerve allows restoration of smile movement. While variations exist on how to inset the gracilis muscle, how to select the thickness of the functional muscle units harvested, and how to determine the best points of the lower face to target, universally accepted practices to optimize smile appearance and excursion include orientation of the muscle from the upper lip and modiolus toward the root of the zygoma and maintenance of resting gracilis sarcomere length during planning and placement into the facial deformity [42]. This method can reliably restore both resting tone and oral commissure excursion (Fig. 24.5).

Temporalis Tendon Transfer

The temporalis muscle has been reported as a donor muscle for facial paralysis rehabilitation since the early 1900s [43, 44]. Similar to selective re-innervation and nerve substitution techniques using the masseteric nerve, temporalis muscle or temporalis tendon transfer (TTT) achieves function through learned collaboration of jaw clench and smile excursion. However, by utilizing neurotized functional muscle, TTT has the added benefit over selective re-innervation and cable grafting of immediate return of resting facial tone and movement.

Originally described as a method to reanimate the lip by harvesting the muscle and turning it over the zygoma, the procedure has been refined to preserve the muscle in situ, capitalizing on its placement in a natural vector with the oral commissure. Due to this relationship, TTT, compared to gracilis muscle free tissue transfer, has demonstrated achievement of superior angular symmetry of the oral commissure with the

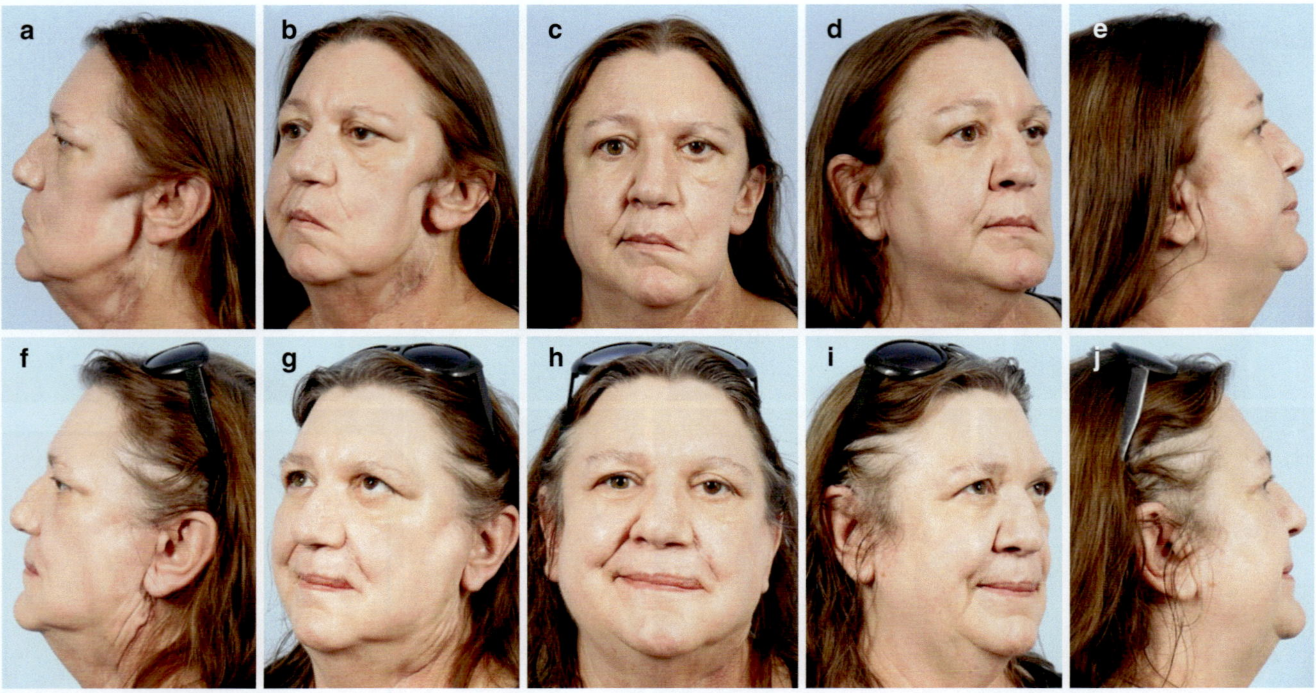

Fig. 24.5 Long-term facial paralysis following total parotidectomy with facial nerve sacrifice and adjuvant radiotherapy (**a–e**). Result following cross-face nerve grafting, neurotized gracilis free flap, and adipofascial anterolateral thigh free flap reconstruction (**f–j**). Photographs used with permission

non-paralyzed side [45]. Through evolution of the TTT procedure from an open procedure to now a minimally invasive transoral approach (the orthodromic temporalis tendon transfer procedure, or OTTT), its use as a dynamic facial rehabilitation option has been proven to be safe and highly reliable, especially for patients with significant comorbidities that preclude longer and more complex operations like MVFTT (Fig. 24.6) [46, 47]. However, while patient satisfaction rates following TTT are high, comparative studies examining smile excursion have demonstrated greater smile movement with gracilis MVFTT over TTT [45, 48, 49].

Management of Synkinesis

In addition to the above considerations, synkinesis is an important, long-term sequela of facial nerve injury and repair, and this development can be a significant burden for patients. Synkinesis is the involuntary activation of facial motor units when separate volitional facial muscles are activated. It is thought to result from aberrant re-innervation after nerve injury [50]. Chemodenervation with BoNT-A is highly effective to achieve temporary relief from synkinesis. In a double-blind trial, BoNT-A significantly improved patients' perception of social interaction and quality of life.

Surgical options also exist for the definitive management of synkinesis in the form of modified selective neurectomy or muscle transection, and these options are often employed following a successful trial of BoNT-A. In these techniques, distal facial nerve branches (or the mimetic muscle units themselves) that are contributing to the individual pattern of synkinetic activity are ligated [51]. Patient-reported quality of life outcomes as measured by the Synkinesis Assessment Questionnaire and Facial Clinimetric Evaluation scale have been shown to be improved in patients undergoing these procedures.

Facial Retraining

Facial retraining, or neuromuscular retraining, is an adjunctive rehabilitative modality performed by specially trained physical, occupational, or speech-language pathology therapists and is an integral part in the multidisciplinary management of facial paralysis. By combining techniques including biofeedback training, muscular strengthening, and tissue lengthening, facial retraining improves facial mimetic muscle recovery while also assisting in cortical adaptation to reduce aberrant muscular action such as synkinesis. When performed at the optimal time, generally when nerve regeneration is occurring and visible, facial function outcomes have been demonstrated to be improved both objectively and subjectively in post-viral or post-traumatic/iatrogenic etiologies of facial nerve injury regardless of age or chronicity of injury [52, 53]. As such, initiation of facial retraining therapy should not be overlooked even in the setting of prolonged facial paralysis. Length of facial retraining therapy may differ based on provider, but at least 12 months is recommended with prolonged therapy indicated depending on the degree of improvements achieved.

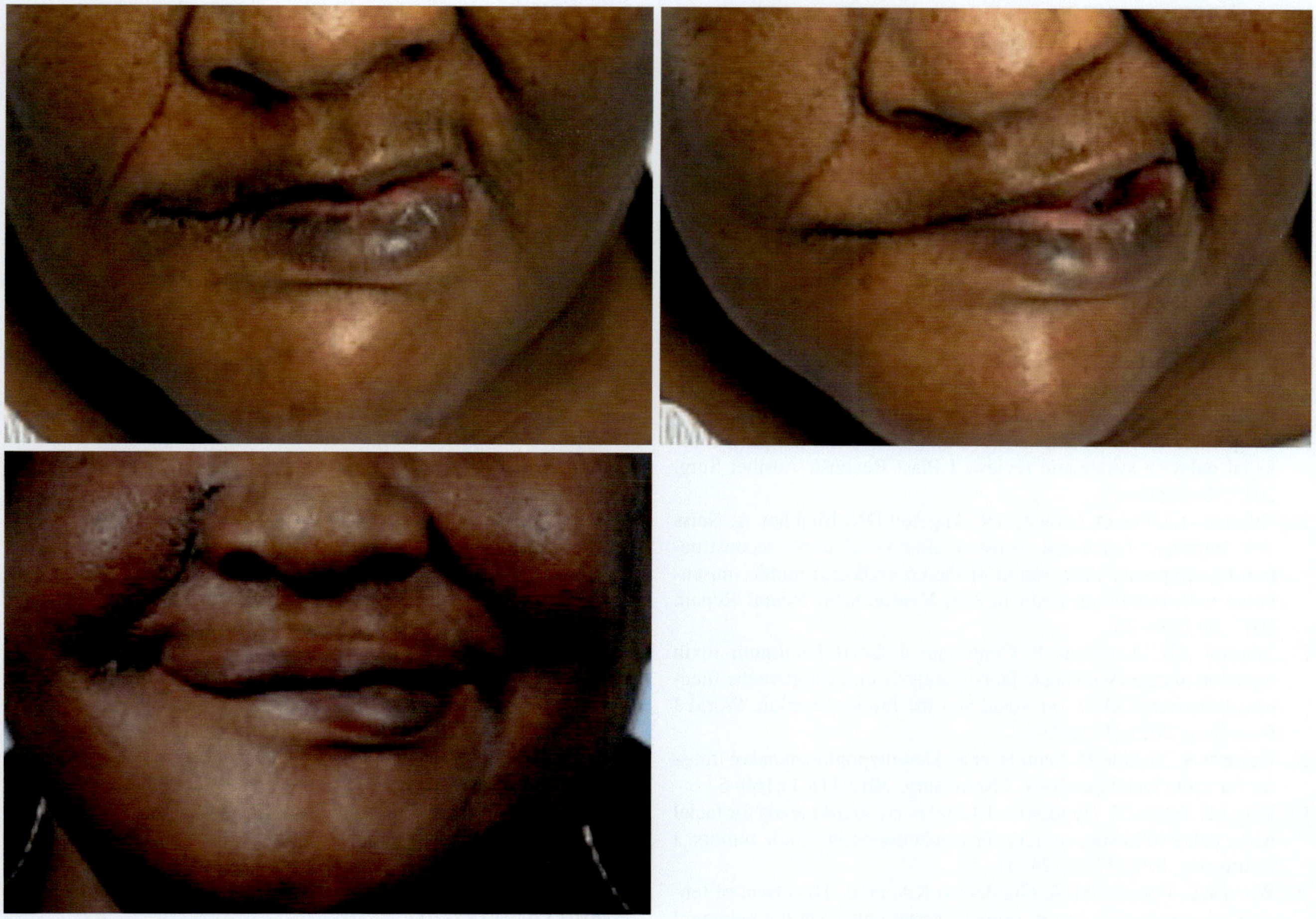

Fig. 24.6 Orthodromic temporalis tendon transfer. In patients that are beyond the window or not amenable to facial nerve re-innervation or substitution techniques, OTTT offers a reliable option in regaining spontaneous smile

Conclusions

Facial nerve injury remains an important risk of neurotologic surgery and can be a source of considerable physical and psychologic morbidity. In addition to sound surgical technique and intimate knowledge of facial nerve anatomy, familiarity with management of intraoperatively and\ postoperatively diagnosed facial nerve injury is a requisite for the neurotologic surgeon. Prevention of ophthalmologic complications is paramount, and a plethora of management options are available for the rehabilitation of facial nerve paralysis. Understanding patient goals and the benefits of each reconstructive technique optimizes functional and aesthetic outcomes.

References

1. Charters E, Low TH, Coulson S. Utility of an oral competence questionnaire for patients with facial nerve paralysis. J Plast Reconstr Aesthet Surg. 2023;77:201–8.
2. Hotton M, Huggons E, Hamlet C, et al. The psychosocial impact of facial palsy: a systematic review. Br J Health Psychol. 2020;25(3):695–727.
3. Parsa KM, Hancock M, Nguy PL, et al. Association of facial paralysis with perceptions of personality and physical traits. JAMA Netw Open. 2020;3(6):e205495.
4. Hohman MH, Bhama PK, Hadlock TA. Epidemiology of iatrogenic facial nerve injury: a decade of experience. Laryngoscope. 2014;124(1):260–5.
5. Nilssen EL, Wormald PJ. Facial nerve palsy in mastoid surgery. J Laryngol Otol. 1997;111(2):113–6.
6. Rinaldi V, Casale M, Bressi F, et al. Facial nerve outcome after vestibular schwannoma surgery: our experience. J Neurol Surg B. 2012;73:21–7.
7. El Shazly MA, Mokbel MAM, Elbadry AA, Badran HS. Management of the facial nerve in lateral skull base surgery analytic retrospective study. Clin Med Insights: Ear, Nose Throat. 2011;4:21–30.
8. Green JD, Shelton C, Brackmann DE. Surgical management of iatrogenic facial nerve injuries. Otolaryngol Head Neck Surg. 1994;111(5):606–10.
9. Wang Z, Zhang Z, Huang Q, Yang J, Wu H. Long-term facial nerve function following facial reanimation after translabyrinthine vestibular schwannoma surgery: a comparison between sural grafting and VII-XII anastomosis. Exp Ther Med. 2013;6(1):101–4.

10. Yawn RJ, Wright HV, Francis DO, Stephan S, Bennett ML. Facial nerve repair after operative injury: impact of timing on hypoglossal-facial nerve graft outcomes. Am J Otolaryngol. 2016;37(6):493–6.
11. Oyer SL. Static lower facial reconstruction in facial paralysis. Oper Tech Otolaryngol-Head Neck Surg. 2021;32(4):219–25.
12. Hembd A, Harrison B, Rocha CSM, et al. Facial reanimation in the seventh and eighth decades of life. Plast Reconstr Surg. 2018;141(5):1239–51.
13. Albathi M, Oyer S, Ishii LE, Byrne P, Ishii M, Boahene KO. Early nerve grafting for facial paralysis after cerebellopontine angle tumor resection with preserved facial nerve continuity. JAMA Facial Plast Surg. 2016;18(1):54–60.
14. Leckenby JI, Harrison DH, Grobbelaar AO. Static support in the facial palsy patient: a case series of 51 patients using tensor fascia lata slings as the sole treatment for correcting the position of the mouth. J Plast Reconstr Aesthet Surg. 2014;67(3):350–7.
15. Cooper L, Lui M, Nduka C. Botulinum toxin treatment for facial palsy: a systematic review. J Plast Reconstr Aesthet Surg. 2017;70(6):833–41.
16. Guntinas-Lichius O, Glowka TR, Angelov DN, Irintchev A, Neiss WF. Improved functional recovery after facial nerve reconstruction by temporary denervation of the contralateral mimic musculature with botulinum toxin in rats. Neurorehabil Neural Repair. 2011;25(1):15–23.
17. Jahromi AH, Konofaos P. Contralateral facial botulinum toxin injection in cases with acute facial paralysis may improve the functional recovery: where we stand and the future direction. World J Plast Surg. 2021;10(2):89–92.
18. Hayashi A, Nishida M, Seno H, et al. Hemihypoglossal nerve transfer for acute facial paralysis. J Neurosurg. 2013;118(1):160–6.
19. Pitty LF, Tator CH. Hypoglossal-facial nerve anastomosis for facial nerve palsy following surgery for cerebellopontine angle tumors. J Neurosurg. 1992;77(5):724–31.
20. Wood KL, Fonseca MIA, Gunderson KA, et al. The effect of tension on gene expression in primary nerve repair via the epineural suture technique. J Surg Res. 2022;277:211–23.
21. Ismayilzade M, Ince B, Zuhour M, Oltulu P, Aygul R. The effect of a gap concept on peripheral nerve recovery in modified epineurial neurorrhaphy: an experimental study in rats. Microsurgery. 2022;42(7):703–13.
22. Kornfeld T, Borger T, Radtke C. Reconstruction of critical nerve defects using allogenic nerve tissue: a review of current approaches. Int J Mol Sci. 2021;22(7):3515.
23. Ducic I, Safa B, DeVinney E. Refinements of nerve repair with connector-assisted coaptation. Microsurgery. 2017;37(3):256–63.
24. Lans J, Eberlin KR, Evans PJ, Mercer D, Greenberg JA, Styron JF. A systematic review and meta-analysis of nerve gap repair: comparative effectiveness of allografts, autografts, and conduits. Plast Reconstr Surg. 2023;151(5):814e–27e.
25. Xue JW, Jiao JB, Liu XF, et al. Inhibition of peripheral nerve scarring by calcium antagonists, also known as calcium channel blockers. Artif Organs. 2016;40(5):514–20.
26. Divac N, Aksic M, Rasulic L, Jakovcevski M, Basailovic M, Jakovcevski I. Pharmacology of repair after peripheral nerve injury. Int J Clin Pharmacol Ther. 2021;59(6):447–62.
27. Mohanty AJ, Perez JL, Hembd A, Thrikutam N, Bartley J, Rozen SM. Orbicularis oculi muscle reinnervation confers corneal protective advantages over static interventions alone in the subacute facial palsy patient. Plast Reconstr Surg. 2020;145(3):791–801.
28. Bianchi B, Bergonzani M, Stella E, et al. Supercharged masseteric-facial cross-graft for gracilis reinnervation in unilateral facial palsy treatment. Microsurgery. 2022;42(3):231–8.
29. Placheta E, Tinhofer I, Schmid M, et al. The spinal accessory nerve for functional muscle innervation in facial reanimation surgery: an anatomical and histomorphometric study. Ann Plast Surg. 2016;77(6):640–4.
30. Korte W, Bernhardt M. [A case of nerve transfer from the facial nerve to the hypoglossal nerve]. Dtsch Med Wochenschr. 1903;29:293–5.
31. Hammerschlag PE. Facial reanimation with jump interpositional graft hypoglossal facial anastomosis and hypoglossal facial anastomosis: evolution in management of facial paralysis. Laryngoscope. 1999;109(2 Pt 2 Suppl 90):1–23.
32. May M, Sobol SM, Mester SJ. Hypoglossal-facial nerve interpositional-jump graft for facial reanimation without tongue atrophy. Otolaryngol Head Neck Surg. 1991;104(6):818–25.
33. Cusimano MD, Sekhar L. Partial hypoglossal to facial nerve anastomosis for reinnervation of the paralyzed face in patients with lower cranial nerve palsies: technical note. Neurosurgery. 1994;35(3):532–4.
34. Collar RM, Byrne PJ, Boahene KDO. The subzygomatic triangle: rapid, minimally invasive identification of the masseteric nerve for facial reanimation. Plast Reconstr Surg. 2013;132(1):183–8.
35. Urban MJ, Eggerstedt M, Varelas E, et al. Hypoglossal and masseteric nerve transfer for facial reanimation: a systematic review and meta-analysis. Facial Plast Surg Aesthet Med. 2022;24(1):10–7.
36. Terzis JK, Tzafetta K. The "babysitter" procedure: minihypoglossal to facial nerve transfer and cross-facial nerve grafting. Plast Reconstr Surg. 2009;123(3):865–76.
37. Yoshioka N, Tominaga S. Masseteric nerve transfer for short-term facial paralysis following skull base surgery. J Plast Reconstr Aesthet Surg. 2015;68(6):764–70.
38. Park JH, Park SO, Chang H. Facial reanimation using free partial latissimus dorsi muscle transfer: single versus dual innervation method. J Craniomaxillofac Surg. 2022;S1010-5182(22):128–7.
39. Kejner AE, Rosenthal EL. Lower facial reanimation techniques following cancer resection and free flap reconstruction. Laryngoscope. 2016;126(9):1990–4.
40. Vincent AG, Bevans SE, Robitschek JM, Groom KL, Herr MW, Hohman MH. Sterno-omohyoid free flap for dual-vector dynamic facial reanimation. Ann Otol Rhinol Laryngol. 2020;129(2):195–200.
41. Bove A, Chiarini S, D'Andrea V, Di Matteo FM, Lanzi G, De Antoni E. Facial nerve palsy: which flap? Microsurgical, anatomical, and functional considerations. Microsurgery. 1998;18(4):286–9.
42. Boonipat T, Robertson CE, Meaike JD, Vyas KS, Asaad M, Mardini S. Dual innervation of free gracilis muscle for facial reanimation: what we know so far. J Plast Reconstr Aesthet Surg. 2020;73(12):2196–209.
43. Conley J, Gullane PJ. Facial rehabilitation with temporal muscle: new concepts. Arch Otolaryngol. 1978;104(8):423–6.
44. Brown JB. The utilization of the temporal muscle and fascia in facial paralysis. Ann Surg. 1939;109(6):1016–23.
45. Oyer SL, Nellis J, Ishii LE, Boahene KD, Byrne PJ. Comparison of objective outcomes in dynamic lower facial reanimation with temporalis tendon and gracilis free muscle transfer. JAMA Otolaryngol Head Neck Surg. 2018;144(12):1162–8.
46. Parker NP, Eisler LS, Dresner HS, Walsh WE. Orthodromic temporalis tendon transfer: anatomical considerations. Arch Facial Plast Surg. 2012;14(1):39–44.
47. Patel NN, Zebolsky AL, Park AM, Seth R, Knott PD. Smile outcomes of an externally scarless, intraoral orthodromic temporalis tendon transfer. Facial Plast Surg Aesthet Med. 2022;24(2):83–8.
48. Byrne PJ, Kim M, Boahene K, Millar J, Moe K. Temporalis tendon transfer as part of a comprehensive approach to facial reanimation. Arch Facial Plast Surg. 2007;9(4):234–41.
49. Sidle DM, Fishman AJ. Modification of the orthodromic temporalis tendon transfer technique for reanimation of the paralyzed face. Otolaryngol Head Neck Surg. 2011;145(1):18–23.
50. Cabin JA, Massry GG, Azizzadeh B. Botulinum toxin in the management of facial paralysis. Curr Opin Otolaryngol Head Neck Surg. 2015;23(4):272–80.

51. Azizzadeh B, Hjelm N. Modified selective neurectomy: a new paradigm in the management of facial palsy with synkinesis. Facial Plast Surg Clinic North Am. 2021;29(3):453–7.
52. Beurskens CH, Heymans PG. Positive effects of mime therapy on sequelae of facial paralysis: stiffness, lip mobility, and social and physical aspects of facial disability. Otol Neurotol. 2003;24:677–81.
53. Karp E, Waselchuk E, Landis C, et al. Facial rehabilitation as noninvasive treatment for chronic facial nerve paralysis. Otol Neurotol. 2019;40:241–5.

Rehabilitation of Non-facial Cranial Nerve Dysfunction Following Skull Base Surgery

25

Michael H. Freeman and James L. Netterville

Introduction

Cranial nerves IV through XII can be compromised by lateral skull base pathology and its treatment. These nerves are responsible for coordinating a number of important functions, including speech, mastication, swallow, and maintenance of airway patency. Hypofunction of cranial nerves in patients with lateral skull base pathology can be acute, such as that seen after surgery, or chronic and gradually progressive, as typically seen due to compression from a mass. Traditionally, patients are better able to compensate for cranial nerve weakness or sensation loss due to gradual compressive pathology than to a sudden decrease in lower cranial nerve function. Cranial nerves IX, X, and XII characteristically have the most significant impact on functional outcomes related to speech and swallowing (Fig. 25.1).

Some procedures, such as resection of jugular paragangliomas, very commonly result in significant lower cranial nerve weakness, whereas smaller tumors and those nearer to the internal auditory canal are far less likely to impair lower cranial nerve function. The rise of subtotal resection and radiosurgery for benign tumors has allowed for improved neural preservation rates over time, with reduced morbidity from skull base surgery [1]. Clinical history can give important clues as to the preoperative or baseline status of the lower cranial nerves, and physical examination in the office can help guide care to ensure that functional deficits after surgery are corrected in a timely fashion. This chapter will discuss each of the affected cranial nerves and how it is placed at risk in managing lateral skull base pathology, as well as the available options for rehabilitation. Due to the special relationship between the facial and vestibulocochlear nerves and ear and skull base surgery, these nerves will be the focus of other chapters and will not be addressed here.

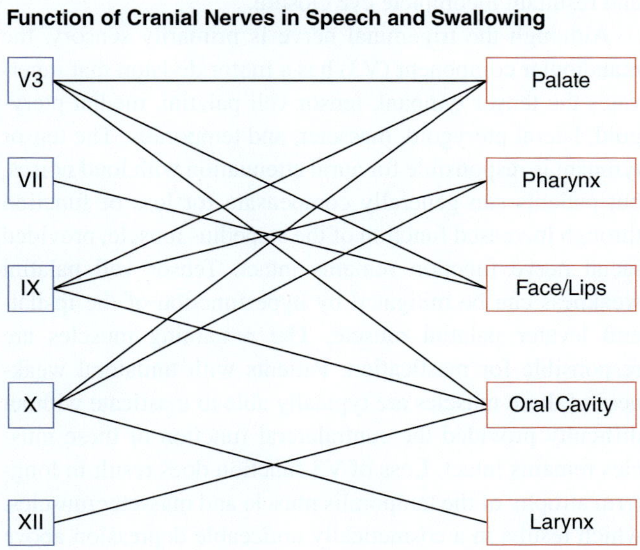

Fig. 25.1 The function of the upper aerodigestive tract is coordinated by the complex innervation of lower cranial nerves. (Adapted from Netterville and Civantos [15])

Trigeminal Nerve (Cranial Nerve V)

The trigeminal nerve passes from the root entry zone in the mid-pons through the prepontine cistern. Once there, it courses through a dural thickening at the medial face of the petrous temporal bone known as Meckel's cave and converges as the trigeminal (aka Gasserian) ganglion. The fibers of the nerve leave the ganglion as three divisions, namely, the ophthalmic (V1), maxillary (V2), and mandibular (V3). Due to its location in the prepontine cistern, the trigeminal nerve is placed at risk when working on the ventral surface of large cerebellopontine angle masses and also during approaches to the anterior petrous face and middle cranial fossa. The V3 branch of the nerve is placed at special risk during extended jugular foramen approaches due to the proximity of foramen ovale, where this nerve exits the skull base.

M. H. Freeman · J. L. Netterville (✉)
Department of Otolaryngology—Head and Neck Surgery, Vanderbilt University Medical Center, Nashville, TN, USA
e-mail: james.netterville@vumc.org

A. D. Sweeney et al. (eds.), *Haynes-Glasscock-Shambaugh Surgery of the Ear*, https://doi.org/10.1007/978-3-032-18264-7_25

The bulk of the trigeminal nerve is sensory. Loss of the meningeal and auriculotemporal branches of V3 can result in numbness of the scalp and face, increasing risk of burns with hair dryers and curling irons and making shaving the face more dangerous. Patients should be cautioned of this if there is a sensory deficit in these areas. Loss of the buccal, inferior alveolar, and lingual nerves can result in difficulty with swallowing due to loss of intraoral sensation. This is generally managed with swallowing therapy and rarely results in permanent swallowing dysfunction. The ophthalmic branch of the nerve (V1) provides corneal sensation. Loss of this function greatly increases risk of corneal abrasion and exposure keratitis, especially in patients with facial nerve weakness and resultant incomplete eye closure.

Although the trigeminal nerve is primarily sensory, the mandibular component (V3) has a motor division that innervates the tensor tympani, tensor veli palatini, medial pterygoid, lateral pterygoid, masseter, and temporalis. The tensor tympani is responsible for aural attenuation with loud noises, but patients can generally compensate for loss of function through increased function of the stapedius muscle, provided facial nerve function remains intact. Tensor veli palatini weakness can be mitigated by hyperfunction of the ipsilateral levator palatini muscle. The remaining muscles are responsible for mastication. Patients with unilateral weakness of these muscles are typically able to masticate without difficulty provided the contralateral function of these muscles remains intact. Loss of V3 function does result in long-term atrophy of the temporalis muscle and masseter muscles, which results in a cosmetically noticeable depression above the zygoma within a year of surgery. In patients for whom this is bothersome, cosmetic implants to fill this depression are an option.

Some lesions of the lateral skull base (e.g., vestibular schwannoma) can cause trigeminal neuropathy when lesions grow large. This neuropathy is common, affecting nearly half of patients with large vestibular schwannomas, and presents with hypesthesia of the ipsilateral face [2, 3]. True trigeminal neuralgia, which is described by patients as intense, stabbing pain, is less common in the setting of skull base masses. Surgery of the lateral skull base can often improve the symptoms of trigeminal neuralgia but is less likely to improve the trigeminal distribution numbness and paresthesia more often seen in these patients. Radiation to the lateral skull base can exacerbate or cause trigeminal neuralgia as well. First-line treatments include carbamazepine and oxcarbazepine, but a wide array of second-line therapies including baclofen, lamotrigine, and others have been used [4].

Nerves of Extraocular Movement (Cranial Nerves III, IV, VI)

The oculomotor nerve is fortunately rarely involved in lateral skull base surgery due to its position in the anterior cranial fossa. The trochlear (cranial nerve IV) and abducens nerve (cranial nerve VI) are commonly encountered during surgery of the lateral skull base and consequently merit discussion here.

Trochlear Nerve (Cranial Nerve IV)

The trochlear nerve is a motor nerve that supplies only the superior oblique muscle of the eye. After leaving the midbrain, it courses superior to the superior cerebellar artery and along the free edge of the tentorium. It can be encountered and endangered in dissection in lateral skull base tumors with significant anterior and superior extension, as well as in cases where the tentorium is divided for expanded access. The trochlear nerve is a thin structure and is highly susceptible to injury if manipulated but can fortunately be avoided in most skull base approaches. Weakness of the trochlear nerve manifests with vertical or torsional diplopia. Isolated trochlear nerve weakness is addressed much like abducens nerve weakness (see below).

Abducens Nerve (Cranial Nerve VI)

The abducens nerve is a motor nerve that exits the brainstem at the pontomedullary junction and crosses the prepontine cistern, where it can be encountered during approaches to the lateral skull base. It later courses through Dorello's canal to the cavernous sinus and past the carotid and then exits the skull base at the superior orbital fissure. Its long intracranial course and narrow diameter make it susceptible to traction injury in lateral skull base approaches. Its course through the cavernous sinus also places it at risk in anterior skull base approaches, especially when the cavernous sinus is packed to control hemorrhage.

The abducens nerve innervates only one muscle—the lateral rectus muscle of the eye. Injury results in a lateral gaze palsy and lateral diplopia. Most injuries can be managed conservatively, with Fresnel prisms placed in a patient's glasses. Botulinum toxin injection is sometimes performed to weaken the medial rectus muscle in the affected eye, which can accelerate recovery and minimize diplopia [5]. If the nerve has been transected or does not recover function with time, surgical options center around extraocular muscle transposition [6]. Evaluation of abducens nerve function is fairly straightforward and can be performed with standard extraocular muscle function testing in any clinical or bedside setting.

Glossopharyngeal Nerve (Cranial Nerve IX)

The glossopharyngeal nerve exits the medulla and crosses the flocculus to exit the skull base at the pars nervosa of the jugular foramen. Once there, it courses between the carotid artery and internal jugular vein. The glossopharyngeal nerve has more complex functions than the previously discussed nerves in that it encodes branchial motor, visceral motor, somatic sensory, and special sensory functions.

Branchial motor innervation is limited to the stylopharyngeus muscle and is not independently clinically significant, provided the deficit is (1) unilateral and (2) there are not significant accompanying sensory deficits. If there are also deficits of other palatal elevators such as the levator veli palatini (innervated by CN X), then significant velopharyngeal insufficiency and dysphagia can result. The visceral motor function provides for parasympathetic innervation of the parotid salivary gland. Damage to CN IX or the auriculotemporal branch of V3 (also part of the parasympathetic pathway to the parotid gland) can impair salivary flow and lead to parotitis.

The glossopharyngeal nerve carries somatic sensory information from the tonsillar pillars and base of tongue as well as the portions of the external ear, middle ear, and tympanic membrane. Even unilateral interruption in sensation to the base of tongue and tonsillar pillars can impair the oropharyngeal phase of swallowing and reduce bolus control. Patients can learn to safely swallow through swallow therapy focused on bolus positioning on the side of intact sensation. Isolated glossopharyngeal nerve impairment is rare in the setting of skull base surgery. Typically, injury to the glossopharyngeal nerve also carries implications for the function of the vagus nerve, which increases the difficulty of speech and swallow recovery for these patients (this will be addressed in more detail in the next section).

The final and most unique function of the glossopharyngeal nerve is that it carries signals from the carotid body and carotid sinus via one of its branches, the carotid sinus nerve. Unilateral impairment is rarely clinically significant, as the intact contralateral side allows for normal carotid baroreceptor reflexes. In fact, disruption of the affected carotid sinus (either through transection of the glossopharyngeal nerve or of the carotid sinus nerve more specifically) remains a means of treatment of carotid sinus syndrome. Bilateral interruption of the glossopharyngeal nerve or carotid sinus nerve, however, has more significant physiologic consequences. In the immediate postoperative period, this state is characterized by severe reactive hypertension requiring the help of an intensivist. Eventually, patients are able to be weaned to a maintenance regimen including beta blockers and/or nitrates to prevent significant hypertension, although orthostatic hypotension often remains a problem.

As the most significant functional roles of this nerve are sensory and visceral, there is not a clear established role for intraoperative glossopharyngeal nerve monitoring. Physical examination can isolate impaired glossopharyngeal nerve function via observation of palatal elevation and through palpation of the tonsillar pillars to assess sensation.

Vagus Nerve (Cranial Nerve X)

Of the lower cranial nerves at risk in skull base surgery, the vagus nerve has the widest-ranging and most significant symptomatic implications. It carries both general and visceral sensory functions as well as branchial and visceral motor components. Skull base surgery resulting in injury to the vagus nerve typically results in a "high" vagal injury, which impairs both motor and sensory function. This has cumulative effects on swallowing function and results in severe dysphagia and dysphonia [7].

The motor and sensory nuclei of the vagus nerve exit the medulla at the posterolateral sulcus and course through the basal cistern to enter the pars vascularis of the jugular foramen. Upon exiting the skull base, the nerve courses through the neck within the confines of the carotid sheath. Once in the neck, the nerve splits into its various motor and sensory subdivisions. The general sensory components of the vagus nerve provide for sensation of portions of the ear canal and tympanic membrane, lateral pharyngeal walls, and supraglottic larynx. Swallowing therapy is the mainstay of care for overcoming unilateral loss of sensation to the pharyngeal walls and supraglottic larynx. Visceral sensory innervation of the glottic and infraglottic larynx, trachea, and esophagus is encoded through smaller sensory fibers. The visceral motor/parasympathetic functions of the vagus nerve are wide-ranging, enabling function of the lower esophageal sphincter, esophageal contraction, gastric motility, and upper abdominal viscera function. Bilateral loss of vagal innervation can lead to a need for surgical modification of the lower esophageal sphincter and placement of a gastro-jejunal feeding tube to bypass a hypo-motile stomach. Longstanding impairment of the lower esophageal sphincter due to loss of vagal tone can result in a condition called secondary achalasia, or pseudoachalasia, which like primary achalasia can be managed with balloon dilation or targeted myotomy [8].

The branchial motor components of CN X course through three branches that leave the main trunk of the nerve in the neck:

1. The pharyngeal branch—responsible for pharyngeal constrictor and palatal muscle function (except for stylopharyngeus and tensor veli palatini; see above sections on trigeminal and glossopharyngeal nerves).
2. The superior laryngeal nerve—responsible for supraglottic sensation and cricothyroid muscle innervation.
3. The recurrent laryngeal nerve—responsible for infraglottic sensation as well as innervation of the remaining intrinsic muscles of the larynx.

Loss of the motor function of these three branches has significant functional implications. Loss of the palatal innervation of the vagus nerve results in incomplete closure of the velopharynx, known as velopharyngeal insufficiency (VPI). Nearly every sound in the English language is produced with a closed velopharynx, except for "m," "n," and "ng" sounds. Apart from speech deficits, VPI also manifests with nasopharyngeal regurgitation with swallows. Surgical management of velopharyngeal insufficiency is addressed in a subsection below. Loss of pharyngeal constrictor function results in significant delay in the pharyngeal phase of swallow. This delay places food in the supraglottis and hypopharynx for a prolonged period of time, greatly increasing aspiration risk. Aggressive swallowing therapy with compensatory maneuvers that force the paralyzed side closed (e.g., head turn/tilt) is the mainstay of treatment.

In cranial base surgery, isolated injury of the superior laryngeal or recurrent laryngeal nerves is uncommon. Typically, both branches will be affected if one is impaired. Therefore, concerns regarding pitch modulation seen with isolated superior laryngeal nerve injury are rare. Impairment of the recurrent laryngeal nerve's motor function manifests with unilateral paralysis of the vocal fold as well as impairment of the cricopharyngeus muscle's contraction and relaxation functions. This results in significant dysphonia as well as aspiration due to incomplete glottic closure and impaired upper esophageal sphincter function. Surgical management of the upper esophageal sphincter can be undertaken through cricopharyngeal myotomy or balloon dilation [9].

The use of a neural integrity monitoring (NIM) endotracheal tube allows for easy monitoring of the vagus nerve intraoperatively. This has benefits of allowing for surgeons to identify the nerve in patients with distorted intracranial anatomy as well as providing feedback during dissection to facilitate safe tumor resection. Although there is a high rate of false-positive signals through this system, in appropriately selected patients, this monitoring can be very helpful.

Role of Tracheostomy in Vagus Injuries

In the 1970s and 1980s, routine tracheostomy concurrent to approaches to the jugular foramen were performed. That approach is less common, provided patients have reasonable pulmonary reserve and preoperative swallowing function precluding tracheostomy [10]. Tracheostomy can impair postoperative swallowing compensation by mechanically preventing normal elevation and depression of the larynx during swallow function and therefore should be avoided if possible. The balloon of cuffed tracheostomy tubes can also compress the esophagus through the party wall of the trachea and esophagus, leading to impaired food bolus passage. Unfortunately, tracheostomy still may play a role in the patients with a high vagal injury if poor pulmonary hygiene is not able to be remedied.

Preoperative Evaluation

Patients undergoing cranial base surgery in which cranial nerve IX or X will be placed at risk should undergo preoperative flexible laryngoscopy to establish preoperative status of vocal fold motion, swallowing function, and supraglottic sensation. If there are concerns regarding preoperative swallowing function based on history or the fiberoptic laryngoscopy (e.g., pooled secretions, hypomobile vocal fold, insensate hemilarynx), a formal radiographic swallowing assessment like a modified barium swallow study can be performed. Engagement of a speech and language pathologist prior to surgery can also be useful to coach patients on compensatory swallowing techniques. Early involvement of a laryngologist to create a team-based approach can also help facilitate care.

Swallow therapy and multidisciplinary nonsurgical care are the first line in treatment for postoperative lower cranial nerve deficits, but interventions are often required for postoperative velopharyngeal insufficiency and vocal fold paralysis and can have significant benefit in appropriately selected patients. Nonsurgical therapy can take over a year to determine functional baseline due to the gradual pace of recovery of speech and swallowing deficits, especially if the integrity of the nerve is unclear following surgery.

Management of Postoperative Velopharyngeal Insufficiency

The nature and severity of velopharyngeal insufficiency should be assessed with flexible endoscopy and videofluoroscopic swallowing assessments prior to undertaking surgical attempts at velopharyngeal closure. Speech-language pathology has developed metrics for grading the severity of VPI, such as the Pittsburgh Weighted Speech Scale [11]. These metrics can help grade response to therapy and surgery. There are many surgical options for VPI management, many of which were designed in the setting of cleft palate repair. Recently, injection augmentation of the posterior pharyngeal wall to reduce the size of the adynamic velopharynx has been utilized as a temporizing option before more permanent surgical options are undertaken. Definitive surgery for VPI should not be undertaken until the care team is confident that a delayed vagal nerve recovery will not take place—at least several months from the time of initial insult. Prosthetic devices such as palatal lifts and pharyngeal bulbs can yield fair outcomes in patients who prefer to avoid surgery [12, 13].

Patients with high vagal injuries have a unique type of VPI, in that they have an adynamic lateral pharyngeal wall. This is in contrast to more common causes of VPI, such as cleft palate. The most popular surgical approaches to VPI overall are the pharyngeal flap surgery, palate lengthening procedures such as Furlow/double-opposing z-plasty, and dynamic sphincter pharyngoplasty [13]. Pharyngeal flap surgery relies on a superiorly based pharyngeal flap attached to the soft palate to create a small lateral velopharyngeal port to reduce insufficiency. In patients with dynamic pharyngeal walls, this port can be selectively closed during speech and swallow and opened otherwise, giving a highly functional result. Due to concurrent inability to contract the lateral pharyngeal constrictors on the side of injury, VPI from skull base surgery does not respond well to pharyngeal flap surgery. Similar issues arise with pharyngoplasties that rely on the dynamic function of the pharyngeal constrictors. High vagal injuries seen in skull base surgery result in a palatal paralysis that is also not improved with palate lengthening procedures commonly utilized in other populations with VPI.

Interestingly, a modification of the first surgery developed for VPI is the best option for patients with VPI following skull base surgery. This approach entails direct adhesion of the soft palate to the posterior pharyngeal wall, pioneered in 1862 by Passavant [14]. This procedure does not alter the size of the pharynx, and the lack of long mucosal flaps improves healing outcomes. After placement of a Dingman mouth gag, the posterior pharyngeal wall and the soft palate are infiltrated with local anesthetic and epinephrine. A transpalatal incision is placed in the soft palate on the side of paralysis (Fig. 25.2). The posterior pharyngeal wall is identified through this incision and is itself incised to the level of the prevertebral fascia, taking care to make this incision below the level of the adenoid pad. Roughly 1 centimeter of undermining is performed above and below the pharyngeal wall incision to optimize adhesion. Multiple mattress sutures using absorbable material are placed to approximate the pharyngeal surface of the soft palate to the posterior pharyngeal wall (Figs. 25.3 and 25.4). The oral mucosal surface of the soft palate is then reapproximated. From a surgical perspective, the patient is immediately cleared for a liquid diet, provided their other cranial nerve deficits do not preclude this.

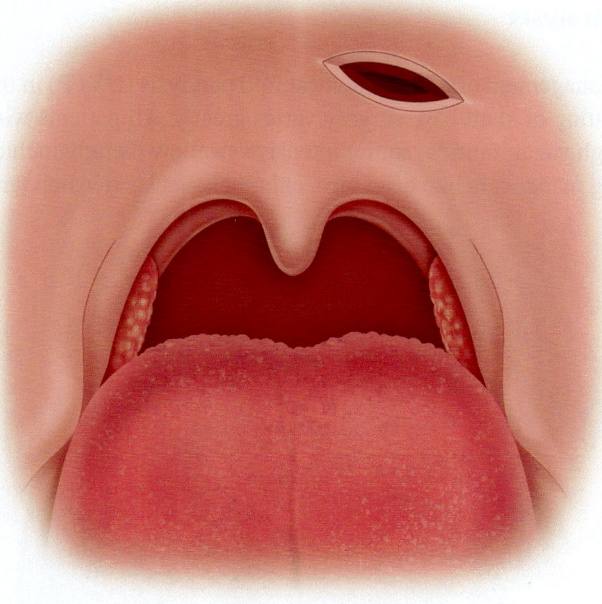

Fig. 25.2 The incision through the palate is outlined in the palatal crease unilaterally. (Adapted from Netterville and Civantos [15])

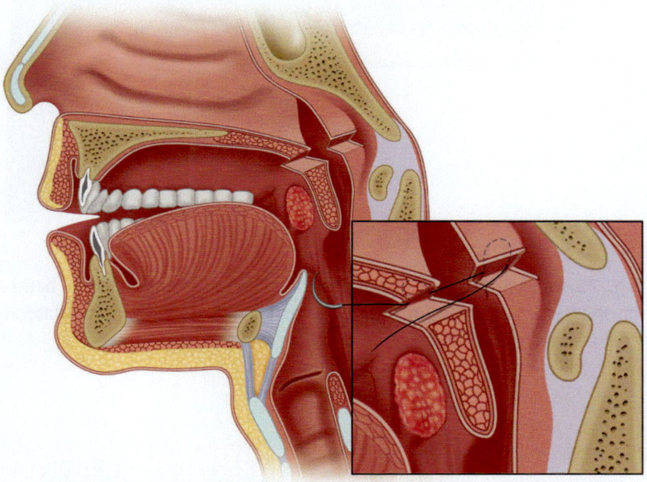

Fig. 25.3 A parallel incision is created down to the prevertebral fascia; the dorsal surface of the hemipalate is approximated to the nasopharyngeal surface with deep mattress sutures. (Adapted from Netterville and Civantos [15])

Transnasal endoscopy reveals closure of half of the velopharynx, with a very small adynamic lateral port (Fig. 25.5). The main complication is wound dehiscence, which can require revision surgery. A theoretical concern for these patients is the development of obstructive sleep apnea due to the narrowed velopharyngeal airway, although in practice this is uncommon [15]. Nearly all patients undergoing this procedure experience improvement in hypernasality of speech and nasal regurgitation with swallow [15–17].

Surgical Management of Unilateral Vocal Fold Paralysis

Management of unilateral vocal fold paralysis (UVFP) in the setting of skull base surgery varies greatly. All patients with high vagal injuries require intensive swallow therapy including maneuvers like head turn, chin tuck, neck extension, and supraglottic or supersupraglottic swallow. The role of voice therapy is less clear and is clouded by the fact that the patients who benefit most from voice therapy are those who experience neurologic recovery [18]. Nevertheless, many surgeons do recommend voice therapy for patients with UVFP in the setting of skull base surgery regardless of expectation of neural recovery. Postoperative baseline assessment of palatal function, vallecula and pyriform pooling, voice quality, and maximum phonation time (~12 s is considered lower limit of normal) can help determine the course of recovery.

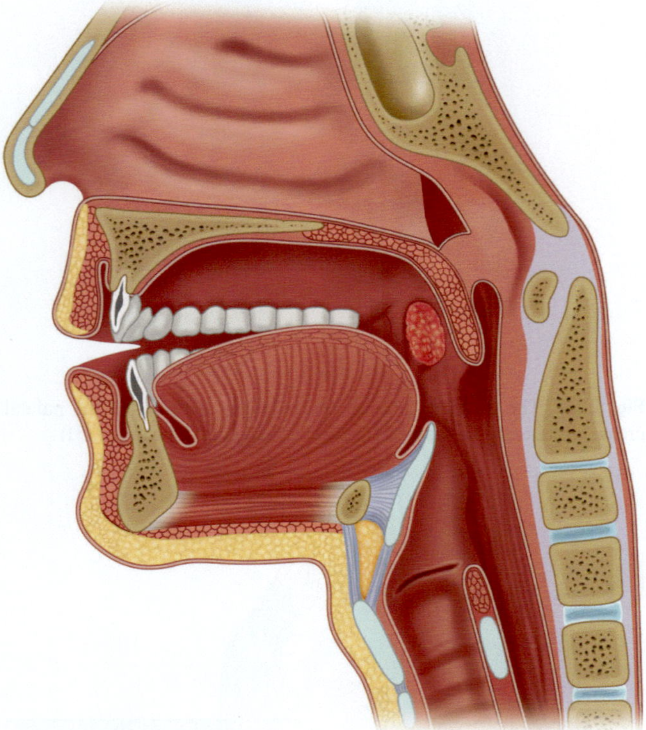

Fig. 25.4 The resultant adhesion obliterates the incompetent hemi-nasopharynx, allowing for normal palatal function on the contralateral side. (Adapted from Netterville and Civantos [15])

Medialization of the paretic vocal fold is the mainstay of surgical treatment. Some authors advocate for injection laryngoplasty of the affected side concurrent with skull base surgery. Others advocate for a delayed approach, in which the injection laryngoplasty is undertaken shortly after paralysis has occurred to allow for optimal medialization without inducing airway compromise. Early medialization (within the first 5 days after paralysis onset) is associated with reduced rates of pneumonia [19]. Injection materials are widely variable and are also subject to surgeon preference, but include hyaluronic acid, collagen, methylcellulose, hydroxyapatite, and autologous fat. Complications of injection laryngoplasty are rare and mostly revolve around under-injection and over-injection. Under-injection results in breathy voice and poor swallow, and over-injection can result in strained voice, airway narrowing, and stridor. Voice outcomes can be assessed through the GRBAS (Grade, Roughness, Asthenia, Breathiness, and Strain) scale and a number of voice handicap indices [20]. Maximum phonation time is also a good metric for improvement in glottic competency.

Some patients elect to undergo periodic injection medializations of the affected vocal fold indefinitely, but spontaneous recovery in these patients is poor, and most patients

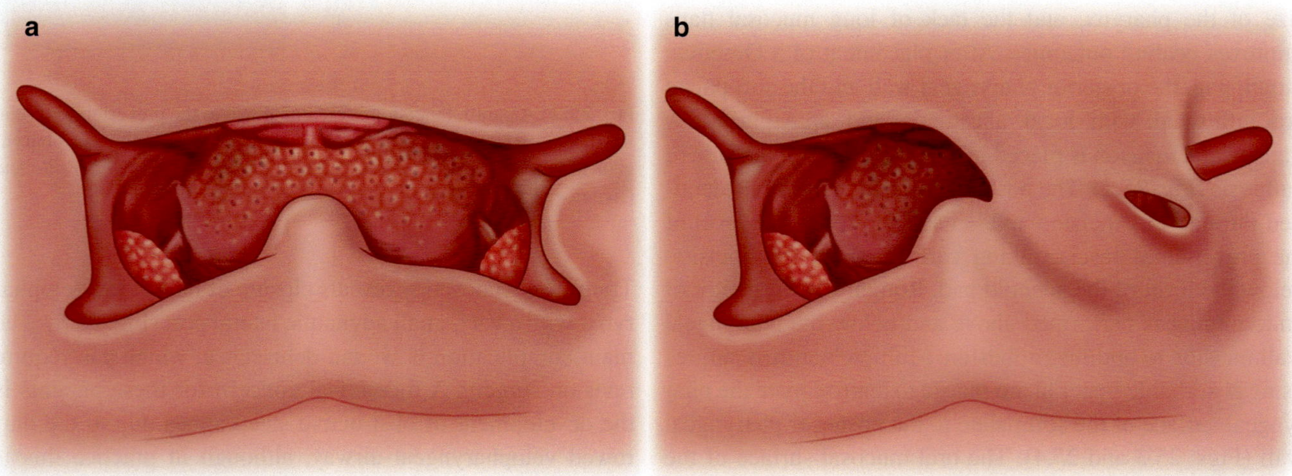

Fig. 25.5 Open nasopharynx before (**a**) and after (**b**) the unilateral adhesion. A small opening which is seen laterally through the fossa of Rosenmuller usually occludes nicely with speech. (Adapted from Netterville and Civantos [15])

eventually undergo definitive surgery such as type 1 thyroplasty with or without arytenoid adduction [21]. In cases of unclear nerve prognosis, electromyography can play a role in determining eventual outcome. Just as there are a variety of available injection materials, there exist a variety of materials for type 1 thyroplasty surgery including hydroxyapatite and Gore-Tex®, but a hand-carved Silastic™ block remains the most common implant for this type of surgery.

Type 1 Thyroplasty and Arytenoid Adduction

Type 1 thyroplasty is typically performed under local anesthesia to allow for intraoperative phonation while sizing the implant. A flexible laryngoscope is positioned in the pharynx for the duration of the case to allow for intraoperative assessment of vocal fold position. An incision is made horizontally overlying the midportion of the thyroid cartilage on the affected side. Subplatysmal flaps are elevated, the sternohyoid muscle is partially divided, and remaining strap muscle attachments are freed in a subperichondrial plane to reveal the surface of the thyroid cartilage (Figs. 25.6 and 25.7). Once cartilage is sufficiently exposed, a rectangular window is marked 13 mm in length and 5 mm in height (Fig. 25.8). This window should be located 3 mm superior to the inferior border of the thyroid ala, to avoid fracture when implant is inserted. The anterior limb of the rectangular window should be placed 7 mm from the midline in males and 5 mm from the midline in females (difference due to testosterone-related size differences in laryngeal size).

The cartilage window is carefully removed with either curettage or a drill, taking care not to violate inner perichondrium. Once the window has been cleared of cartilage, a blade is used to incise the perichondrial layer from the rectangular area, creating an anteriorly based perichondrial flap. The paraglottic space is elevated from the inner cortex

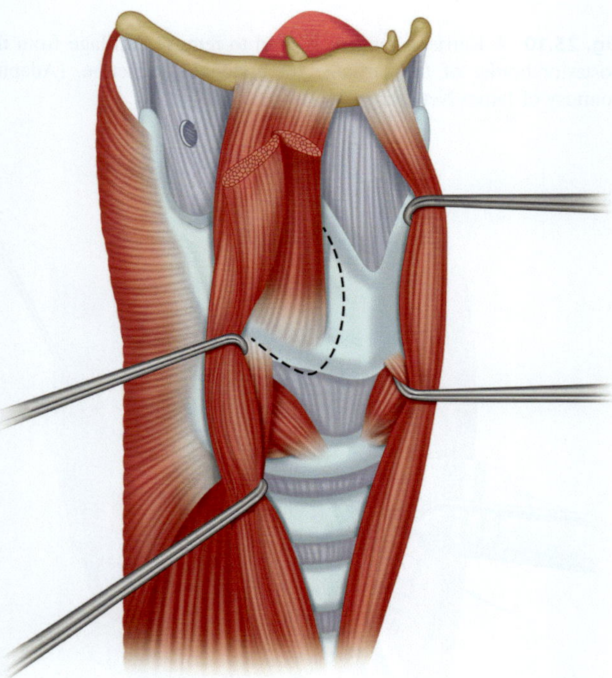

Fig. 25.6 Releasing strap muscles and perichondrium to reveal the thyroid cartilage. Dotted lines indicate the location of a scoring incision to allow for perichondrial and muscle removal. (Adapted courtesy of James Netterville, MD)

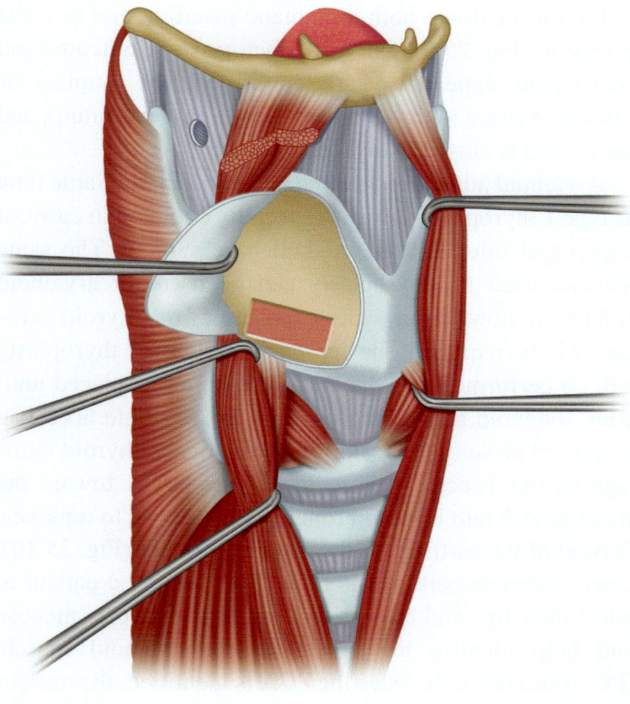

Fig. 25.7 Subperichondrial dissection has been performed, and a rectangle is measured for removal. (Adapted courtesy of James Netterville, MD)

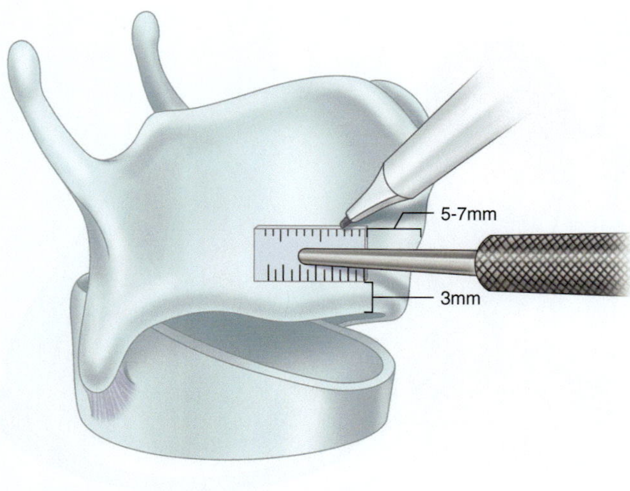

Fig. 25.8 A rectangular window is marked into the cartilage 13 mm in length, 5 mm in height, approximately 3 mm superior to the inferior border. (Adapted from Netterville and Civantos [15])

of cartilage in all directions except anteriorly, so as to permit atraumatic insertion of the Silastic™ block while preserving the vocal ligament. Excessively anterior placement of the implant can result in a strained voice. A depth gauge can be used to determine implant size required for optimal voice outcome and vocal fold position. The implant is then carved to size on the basis of the depth gauge assessment. The average final block is 13–18 mm long, with thickness of 2–3 mm anteriorly and 5–7 mm at maximum before tapering off posteriorly. The implant is carved in a beveled fashion to facilitate both atraumatic insertion and to resist extrusion (Fig. 25.9). Once satisfactory voice outcome and endoscopic appearance are confirmed, the implant is sutured in place to the cartilage using a Prolene suture, and the wound is closed in layered fashion.

Arytenoid adduction is often performed at the same time as type 1 thyroplasty. This is especially common in cases of high vagal injuries seen in skull base surgery. The same incision used for thyroplasty can be used for arytenoid adduction; however, a wider exposure of the thyroid cartilage will be required. The approach for a type 1 thyroplasty will be performed, but the implant will not be placed until after arytenoid adduction is completed. A single hook can be placed around the posterior border of the thyroid cartilage on the affected side to retract the larynx toward the surgeon. A 5 mm Kerrison rongeur can be used to remove a portion of the cartilage at the posterior border (Fig. 25.10). Once sufficient cartilage is removed, asking the patient to purse their lips and blow can expand the pyriform mucosa and help identify the posterior cricoarytenoid muscle (PCA) anterior to it. Once the PCA is identified, the muscular process of the arytenoid to which it attaches is palpated, and a double-armed Prolene suture is passed through it (Fig. 25.11). One needle of the double-armed suture is tunneled under the thyroid cartilage and passed through the cartilage anterior to the thyroplasty window. The other needle is tunneled under the thyroid cartilage and passed through the cricothyroid membrane. The ends of this suture can be gently pulled to rotate the arytenoid inferiorly and medially. If this is performed concurrent to type 1 thyroplasty, suture tension adjustment can be performed concurrent to implant sizing (Fig. 25.12). The arytenoid adduction suture can be adjusted and tied at the desired tension. The wound is then closed in layered fashion.

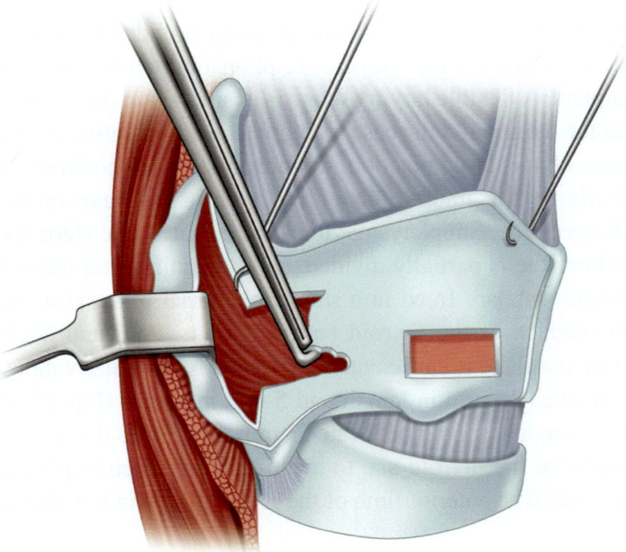

Fig. 25.10 A Kerrison rongeur is used to remove cartilage from the posterior border of the cartilage for arytenoid adduction. (Adapted courtesy of James Netterville, MD)

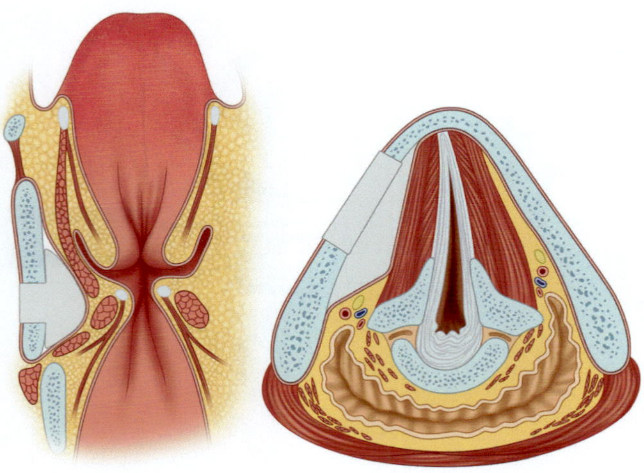

Fig. 25.9 Posterior perspective coronal (left) and axial (right) image of the beveled medialization implant in place. (Adapted from Netterville and Civantos [15])

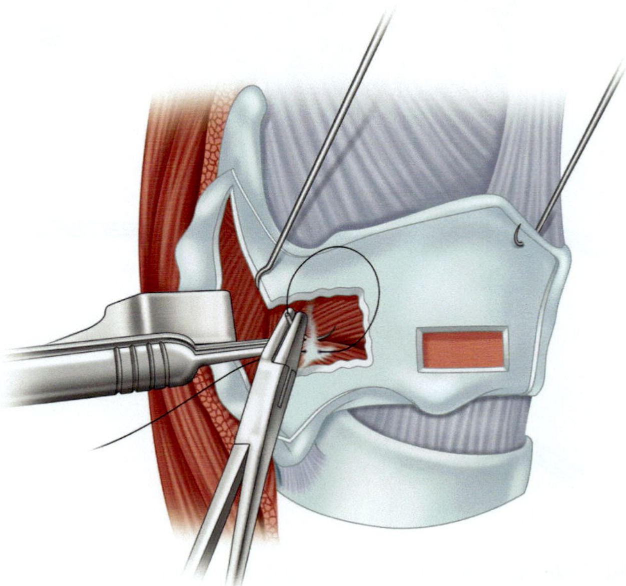

Fig. 25.11 A Prolene suture is used to manipulate the posterior cricoarytenoid muscle (PCA). (Adapted courtesy of James Netterville, MD)

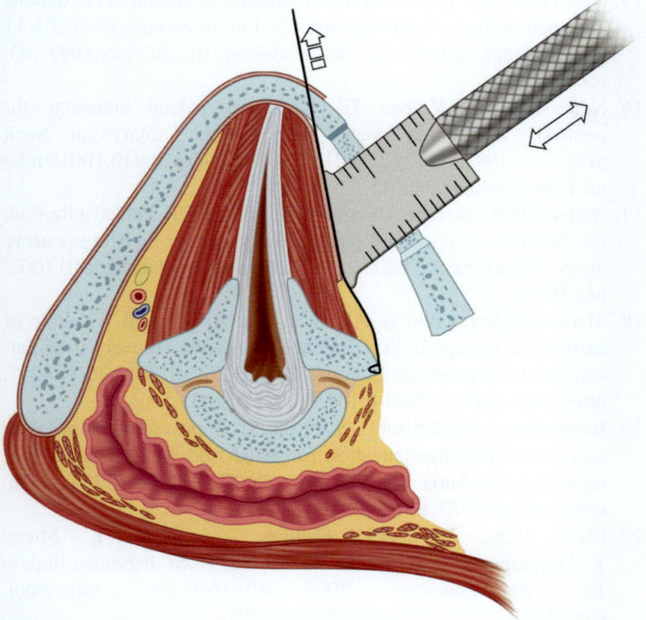

Fig. 25.12 A Prolene suture is used to regulate tension (dashed arrow) while sizing (solid, double ended arrow) a thyroplasty implant. (Adapted courtesy of James Netterville, MD)

The most common complication of these procedures is malposition of the implant, most commonly too superiorly or too medially, resulting in a weak or strained voice. Insufficient implant sizing typically results in a satisfactory voice outcome for about a week while postoperative swelling persists, but after swelling fades, the vocal fold will appear insufficiently medialized. To account for the role of intraoperative edema, the voice should be slightly strained and over-medialized at the time of closure. More serious complications such as fistula, infection, airway compromise, and implant extrusion are fortunately quite rare. A variety of laryngeal reinnervation procedures have been attempted in conjunction with and as an alternative to medialization procedures, especially in children. The most common of these procedures is the ansa cervicalis to recurrent laryngeal nerve anastomosis. The role for these procedures following skull base surgery has not been specifically studied, but outcomes generally appear better in younger patients, and swallowing function appears to improve more avidly than voice function [22–24].

Spinal Accessory Nerve (Cranial Nerve XI)

The spinal accessory nerve exits the lateral surface of the medulla oblongata inferior to the vagus nerve and courses superiorly to exit the skull base through the pars nervosa of the jugular foramen adjacent to the vagus nerve. The intracranial portion of the nerve can be at risk in posterior fossa surgery, and in approaches to the jugular foramen, the transition zone between the cranial portion of the nerve and the spinal portion of the nerve can be injured. The function of cranial nerve XI is motor innervation of the ipsilateral sternocleidomastoid and trapezius muscles. Function is evaluated through resisted head turn away from the side of interest or through resisted shrugging of the shoulders. Loss of function typically results in a shoulder droop and a winged scapula, which can be uncomfortable and limit use of the upper extremity. Shoulder pain is a common long-term issue in these patients. Intraoperative monitoring is possible through the use of needle electrodes inserted into the body of the sternocleidomastoid muscle, although monitoring of this nerve is less common than monitoring of the vagus or hypoglossal nerves, due to their role in speech and swallowing function. Rehabilitation is centered around physical therapy to strengthen surrounding neck muscles to compensate for loss of function of the sternocleidomastoid and trapezius.

Hypoglossal Nerve (Cranial Nerve XII)

The hypoglossal nerve exits the medulla as a cluster of rootlets that converge into the cisternal segment of the nerve. This bundle courses anteriorly to enter the hypoglossal canal, which sits between the jugular tubercle and the occipital condyle. The hypoglossal nerve provides motor innervation to all of the intrinsic and extrinsic muscles of the tongue with the exception of the palatoglossus. The nerve is placed at risk in the surgery of large posterior fossa masses with anteroinferior extension. Hypoglossal weakness is the most common deficit preoperatively with large jugular paragangliomas, but new postoperative deficits are uncommon if subtotal resection is attempted [1]. Intraoperative monitoring can be performed using bipolar needle electrodes inserted into the body of the tongue. Longstanding hypoglossal weakness tends to result in hemiatrophy of the tongue, but rarely results in significant dysphagia or dysarthria due to compensation by the contralateral tongue. Early in the course of hypoglossal weakness, patients tend to have difficulty with oral bolus coordination, but aspiration is rare. Swallow therapy can accelerate the process of recovery.

References

1. Manzoor NF, Yancey KL, Aulino JM, et al. Contemporary management of jugular paragangliomas with neural preservation. Otolaryngol Head Neck Surg. 2021;164(2):391–8. https://doi.org/10.1177/0194599820938660.
2. Matsuka Y, Fort ET, Merrill RL. Trigeminal neuralgia due to an acoustic neuroma in the cerebellopontine angle. J Orofac Pain. 2000;14(2):147–51.

3. Karkas A, Lamblin E, Meyer M, Gay E, Ternier J, Schmerber S. Trigeminal nerve deficit in large and compressive acoustic neuromas and its correlation with MRI findings. Otolaryngol Head Neck Surg. 2014;151(4):675–80. https://doi.org/10.1177/0194599814545440.
4. Al-Quliti KW. Update on neuropathic pain treatment for trigeminal neuralgia. Neurosciences. 2015;20(2):107–14. https://doi.org/10.17712/nsj.2015.2.20140501.
5. Rowe FJ, Noonan CP. Botulinum toxin for the treatment of strabismus. Cochrane Database Syst Rev. 2017;3(3):CD006499. https://doi.org/10.1002/14651858.CD006499.pub4.
6. Akbari MR, Masoomian B, Mirmohammadsadeghi A, Sadeghi M. A review of transposition techniques for treatment of complete Abducens nerve palsy. J Curr Ophthalmol. 2021;33(3):236–46. https://doi.org/10.4103/joco.joco_42_21.
7. Miles ER, Krishna PD, Inman JC, et al. Dysphagia Severity and Outcomes Following Iatrogenic High Vagal Nerve Injury. Ann Otol Rhinol Laryngol. 2022; 131(5): 493–98. https://doi.org/10.1177/00034894211026991.
8. Schizas D, Theochari NA, Katsaros I, et al. Pseudoachalasia: a systematic review of the literature. Esophagus Off J Jpn Esophageal Soc. 2020;17(3):216–22. https://doi.org/10.1007/s10388-020-00720-1.
9. Jung B, Choi I, Lee NJ, Jung KI, Yoo WK, Ohn SH. Videofluoroscopy-guided balloon dilatation for the opening dysfunction of upper esophageal sphincter by postoperative Vagus nerve injury: a report on two cases. Ann Rehabil Med. 2014;38(1):122–6. https://doi.org/10.5535/arm.2014.38.1.122.
10. Netterville JL, Jackson CG, Miller FR, Wanamaker JR, Glasscock ME. Vagal Paraganglioma: a review of 46 patients treated during a 20-year period. Arch Otolaryngol Neck Surg. 1998;124(10):1133–40. https://doi.org/10.1001/archotol.124.10.1133.
11. McWilliams BJ, Philips BJ. Velopharyngeal incompetence: audio seminars in speech pathology. W.B. Saunders; 1979.
12. Sell D, Mars M, Worrell E. Process and outcome study of multidisciplinary prosthetic treatment for velopharyngeal dysfunction. Int J Lang Commun Disord. 2006;41(5):495–511. https://doi.org/10.1080/13682820500515852.
13. Gart MS, Gosain AK. Surgical management of velopharyngeal insufficiency. Clin Plast Surg. 2014;41(2):253–70. https://doi.org/10.1016/j.cps.2013.12.010.
14. Passavant G. Uber die Operation der angeborenen Spalten des harten Gaumens und der damit complicirten Hasenscharten. Archiv fur Ohr- Nasen- und Kehlkopfheilkunde. 1862;3:193.
15. Netterville JL, Civantos FJ. Rehabilitation of cranial nerve deficits after neurotologic skull base surgery. Laryngoscope. 1993;103(11 Pt 2 Suppl 60):45–54. https://doi.org/10.1002/lary.1993.103.s60.45.
16. Netterville JL, Vrabec JT. Unilateral palatal adhesion for paralysis after high vagal injury. Arch Otolaryngol Neck Surg. 1994;120(2):218–21. https://doi.org/10.1001/archotol.1994.01880260088017.
17. Netterville JL, Fortune S, Stanziale S, Billante CR. Palatal adhesion: the treatment of unilateral palatal paralysis after high vagus nerve injury. Head Neck. 2002;24(8):721–30. https://doi.org/10.1002/hed.10134.
18. Mattioli F, Bergamini G, Alicandri-Ciufelli M, et al. The role of early voice therapy in the incidence of motility recovery in unilateral vocal fold paralysis. Logoped Phoniatr Vocol. 2011;36(1):40–7. https://doi.org/10.3109/14015439.2011.554433.
19. Bhattacharyya N, Batirel H, Swanson SJ. Improved outcomes with early vocal fold medialization for vocal fold paralysis after thoracic surgery. Auris Nasus Larynx. 2003;30(1):71–5. https://doi.org/10.1016/s0385-8146(02)00114-1.
20. Rosen CA, Lee AS, Osborne J, Zullo T, Murry T. Development and validation of the voice handicap index-10. Laryngoscope. 2004;114(9):1549–56. https://doi.org/10.1097/00005537-200409000-00009.
21. Oestreicher-Kedem Y, Agrawal S, Jackler RK, Damrose EJ. Surgical rehabilitation of voice and swallowing after jugular foramen surgery. Ann Otol Rhinol Laryngol. 2010;119(3):192–8. https://doi.org/10.1177/000348941011900308.
22. Paniello RC, Edgar JD, Kallogjeri D, Piccirillo JF. Medialization versus reinnervation for unilateral vocal fold paralysis: a multicenter randomized clinical trial. Laryngoscope. 2011;121(10):2172–9. https://doi.org/10.1002/lary.21754.
23. Buyukatalay ZC, Brisebois S, Sirin S, Merati AL. Does dysphagia improve following laryngeal reinnervation for treatment of hoarseness in unilateral vocal fold paralysis? J Voice Off J Voice Found. 2021;35(2):307–11. https://doi.org/10.1016/j.jvoice.2019.08.005.
24. Fadhil M, Havas T, Jacobson I. Timing of Ansa Cervicalis-to-recurrent Laryngeal Nerve Reinnervation: a systematic review. J Voice Off J Voice Found. Published online June 4, 2022:S0892-1997(22)00114-X. https://doi.org/10.1016/j.jvoice.2022.04.010.

Part IV

Fundamentals of Otologic and Neurotologic Surgery

Instrumentation in Otologic and Neurotologic Surgery

26

Kenny F. Lin and Justin S. Golub

Introduction

Otologic and neurotologic surgery is highly specialized and uniquely challenging because the critical portions are performed within the temporal bone and lateral skull base. Adequate exposure and visualization are the foremost considerations. To this end, many instruments have been specially created or adapted to facilitate exposure of the middle ear, temporal bone, and lateral skull base. The anatomy is highly compressed, usually requiring microscopic visualization of a small, deep surgical field. Rigorous hemostasis is critically important to the safety of each operation, as even a single drop of blood may obscure landmarks and cause inadvertent injury to surrounding structures.

This chapter begins with a guide to common instruments in otology and neurotology. Next, we review hemostatic agents and techniques. Finally, a brief overview of laser technology is provided.

Instrumentation

There is a vast array of highly specialized instrumentation used in otologic/neurotologic surgery. Below is a summary of the most commonly used instruments. For a more comprehensive discussion, the reader is referred to dedicated texts [1].

K. F. Lin
Department of Otolaryngology—Head and Neck Surgery, Houston Methodist Hospital, Houston, TX, USA

J. S. Golub (✉)
Department of Otolaryngology—Head and Neck Surgery, Columbia University Vagelos College of Physicians and Surgeons, New York, NY, USA

NewYork-Presbyterian/Columbia University Irving Medical Center, New York, NY, USA
e-mail: justin.golub@columbia.edu

Specula and Retractors

Aural specula and retractors are used to gain and maintain exposure. Unlike soft tissue surgery, most otologic surgery is performed within the depths of the temporal bone. Efforts to maximize exposure are often focused on removing rigid bone with a drill, rather than retracting compressible and fragile structures. Nonetheless, the lateral surgical field always includes soft tissue that must be retracted. This most commonly includes the cartilaginous external auditory canal and postauricular skin and muscle.

The *Lempert speculum* (Fig. 26.1) is a handheld speculum used to examine the external auditory canal and tympanic membrane. It looks similar to a nasal speculum but with a curved neck for improved ergonomics and flatter blades. When unavailable, a standard nasal speculum will usually suffice. It can be helpful when working on the lateral external auditory canal, such as trimming hairs or making endaural incisions. The standard *aural speculum* (Fig. 26.2) is widely used in otologic surgery for operating on the tympanic membrane or middle ear through a transcanal microscopic approach. Many sizes and style variations are available. Often the tip is beveled; when present, the longer part should be directed anteriorly to retract the obstructing anterior external auditory canal. It is an important pearl to use the *largest size possible* for maximal visualization. Speculum holders exist to aid with transcanal approaches. Transcanal endoscopic surgery does not employ a speculum.

Self-retaining retractors (Fig. 26.3) include variations of the widely used Weitlaner; subtypes include Perkins, Wullstein, and Carlson-Haynes retractors. In otologic surgery, these are most commonly used to retract soft tissue and maintain exposure of the mastoid cortex through the postauricular incision. This can allow access to the external auditory canal (by incising the skin of the external auditory canal) or to the mastoid in order to perform a mastoidectomy or translabyrinthine approach. Style variations have different angulations of the

A. D. Sweeney et al. (eds.), *Haynes-Glasscock-Shambaugh Surgery of the Ear*, https://doi.org/10.1007/978-3-032-18264-7_26

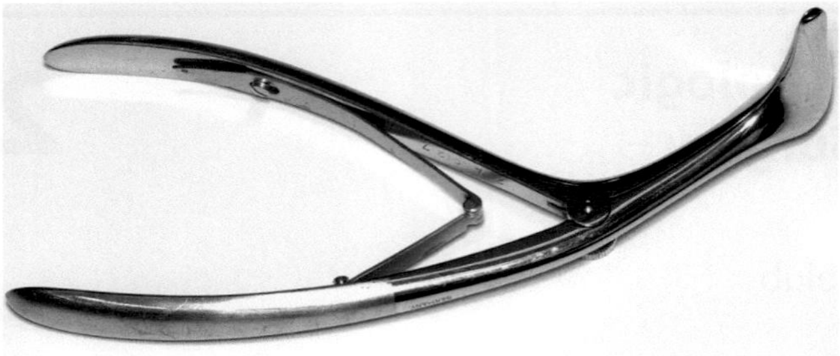

Fig. 26.1 Lempert speculum. (Golub and Schmitt [1]. Used with permission)

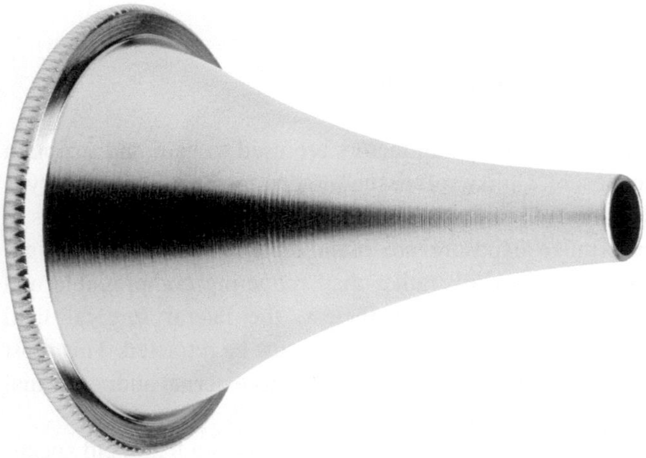

Fig. 26.2 Aural specula. (Image courtesy of MytaMed)

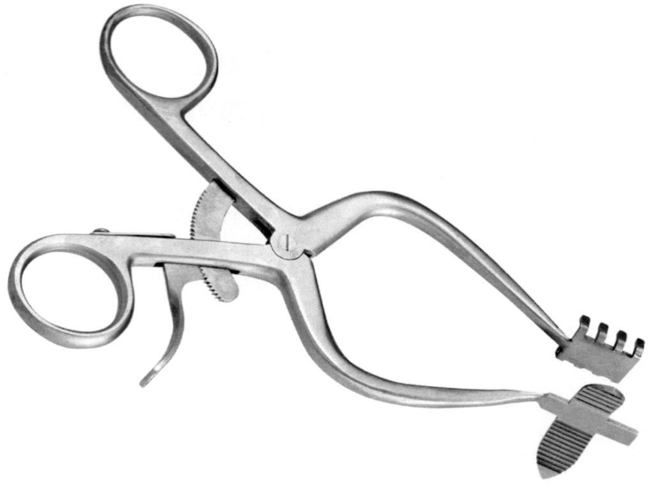

Fig. 26.3 Self-retaining retractor. The standard retractor is the Weitlaner; however, many variations better suited to postauricular surgery exist. Pictured here is the Carlson-Haynes Universal Otologic Retractor. (Image courtesy of Grace Medical)

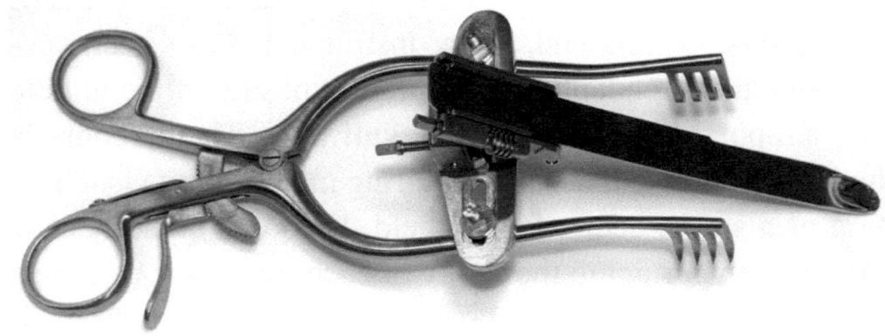

Fig. 26.4 House-Urban middle fossa retractor. The system includes a self-retaining retractor that resembles a Weitlaner with a hinged adapter. A long blade slides into the hinged adapter and displaces the temporal lobe superomedially. The hinged adapter has several screws and pins that allow fine-tuning of the exposure. These adjustments are made with a specialized wrench. (Golub and Schmitt [1]. Used with permission)

neck and different configurations of the blades/teeth. In mastoid surgery, two self-retaining retractors are often used at right angles to one another for improved exposure.

The *House-Urban Middle Fossa Retractor* (Fig. 26.4) is used to retract the temporal lobe dura during middle cranial fossa approaches. Several variations are available.

Suction and Irrigation

Suctions are used to clear the field of blood and irrigation during otologic surgery. Within the middle ear, they can be put to more delicate work, including placing grafts or maneuvering resorbable packing. The *Frazier suction* is generally larger than 7 French and has a square thumb plate. The *Baron suction* often comes in 3, 5, and 7 French and has a round thumb plate. Pressing on the hole contained in the thumb plate increases suction power.

Microsuctions (Fig. 26.5) are generally smaller than 3 French. Unfortunately, they are usually sized in gauge rather than French. In the gauge system, a larger number indicates a smaller diameter. 20, 22, and 24 gauge microsuctions are common. A 20 gauge is slightly smaller than a 3 French. Only microsuctions should be used around critical inner ear structures, such as the oval window.

When drilling a mastoidectomy, some otologists will use a combined suction-irrigator (Fig. 26.6). Others will use a dedicated suction, and the irrigation will be adapted onto the drill. This preferred configuration is based purely on surgeon preference.

Elevators

Periosteal elevators are used to elevate tissue, including periosteum, off bone. Larger elevators, such as the *Lempert* (Fig. 26.7) *and Joseph elevators*, are commonly used to remove muscle and periosteum off the mastoid cortex before mastoidectomy. Dissection must become gentler when near

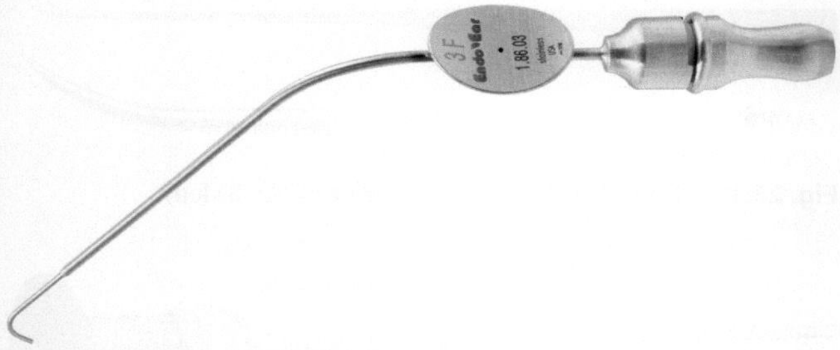

Fig. 26.5 Microsuction. This particular model, designed for endoscopic ear surgery, features a curved tip

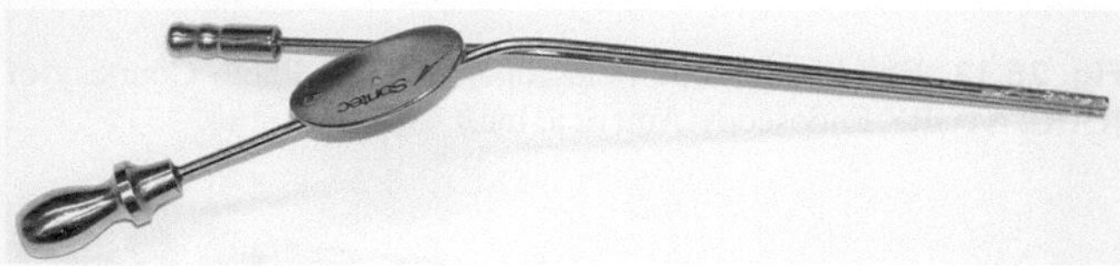

Fig. 26.6 Suction-irrigator

the external auditory canal to avoid tearing its delicate skin. Smaller elevators are used within the middle ear. The *round knife* (Fig. 26.8) is used both to incise the skin of the external auditory canal and then elevate the medial segment off the bone. This process is termed creation and raising of the tympanomeatal flap. Once the middle ear is reached and entered, the *Gimmick elevator* (also called an annulus elevator, Fig. 26.9) can be used to "unzip" the tympanic membrane's annulus from its bony sulcus by a side-to-side sweeping motion. The flattened tip with sharper sides allows safe elevation without cutting of deeper middle ear structures. To minimize middle ear damage, however, the elevator should not be placed deep inside the middle ear when elevating the annulus.

Pistol-Grip Instruments

While not technically a proper name for the category, the term "pistol-grip" is instructive. They are so-called because they are held in the hand similar to a pistol. The design allows opening and closing of small forceps or scissor jaws via a long, narrow shaft. Unlike standard forceps or scissors, the jaws do not open widely. These features allow working in narrow spaces. *Alligator forceps*, named for their long, ridged alligator-like jaws (Fig. 26.10) are used to grasp delicate soft tissue and other small objects such as myringotomy tubes. *Cup forceps* are often superior for grabbing smaller tissue and obtaining biopsies. *Bellucci scissors*, as the name implies, are microscissors.

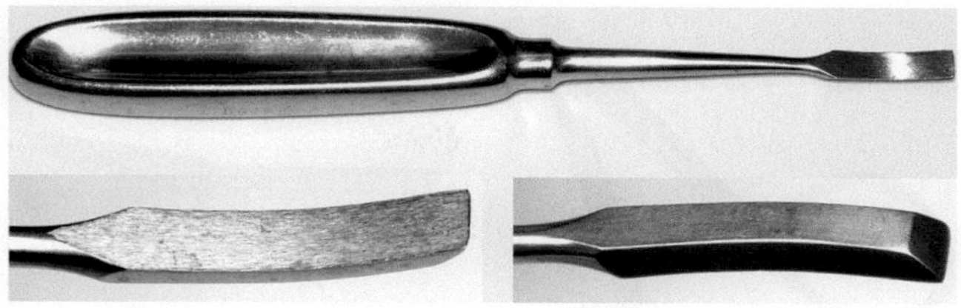

Fig. 26.7 Periosteal elevator. Tip enlargements appear at the bottom. (Golub and Schmitt [1])

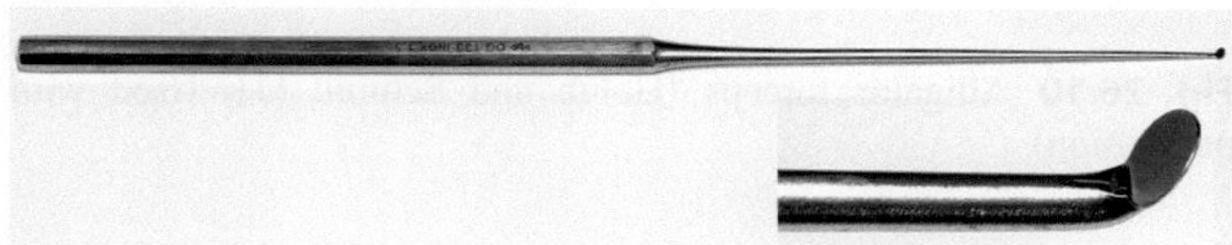

Fig. 26.8 Round knife

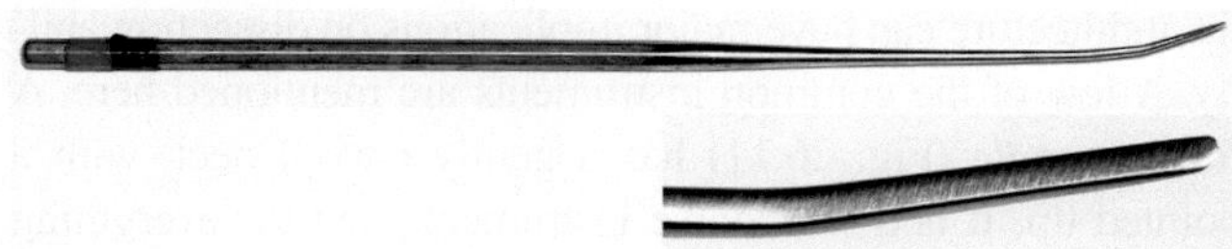

Fig. 26.9 Gimmick (annulus) elevator (Golub and Schmitt [1]. 2012. Used with permission)

Cochlear Implant Instruments

Jeweler's forceps are used to grasp delicate structures, such as the electrode array of a cochlear implant. Specialized forceps are also made by device manufacturers. The *electrode claw* has a tip containing a claw-like groove for manipulating the electrode array during insertion.

Curettes

Bone curettes are used for removing bone without the aid of a drill. They come in a variety of sizes. A small *double-ended curette* is helpful for removing bone in the lateral middle ear, such as removing the scutum to improve exposure. As the name implies, cerumen curettes (or loops) are used to remove cerumen.

Microsurgical Knives, Picks, and Rasps

A wide array of microsurgical knives, picks, and rasps are used for microsurgical dissection in the middle ear and skull base. These instruments often look the same upon gross inspection:

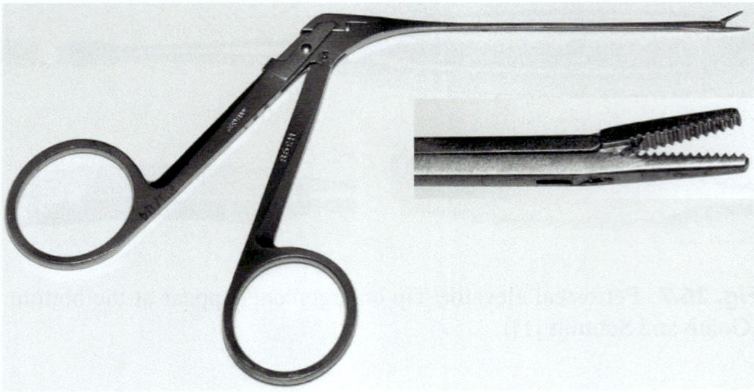

Fig. 26.10 Alligator forceps (Golub and Schmitt [1]. Used with permission)

a cylindrical handle with straight shaft ending in a near-point. Occasionally there is an angulation between the handle and the shaft. Under the microscope, however, subtle differences in the tip architecture can have major implications on dissection ability. A few of the common instruments are mentioned here. A *Rosen needle* (Fig. 26.11) has a gently curved neck with a pointed tip. It is a workhorse instrument used for everything from positioning a tympanostomy tube to assessing the ossicular chain for mobility. The *incudostapedial (I-S) joint knife* looks like a small round knife and is designed to disarticulate the incus from the stapes; however, its small right-angle shaped tip can be used in a variety of dissections. The *oval window (or stapes) rasp* can be used to enlarge a stapedotomy or cochleostomy. The tip is small and mushroom shaped. The *whirlybird* has an apparently whimsical tip with multiple bends. It can be used to remove tissue, particularly cholesteatoma, out of curved recesses. The *sickle knife*, containing a sickle-shaped tip, is another workhorse instrument that can be used for making small incisions, separating ossicles from surrounding scar, or middle ear dissection.

Telescopes (Endoscope) and Mirrors

A microscope requires a direct line of sight, making it difficult to visualize recesses and corners. Small mirrors can be used to see around corners, which is important to verify complete removal of pathology such as cholesteatoma. Endoscopes (or telescopes, such as the Hopkins rod; Fig. 26.12), particularly angled endoscopes, allow enhanced ability to see otherwise-hidden areas. In certain circumstances, endoscopes may be used to perform completely transcanal surgery that would otherwise require a postauricular incision with a microscope.

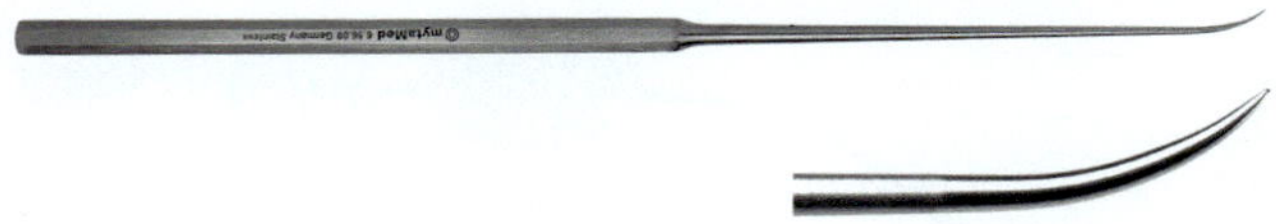

Fig. 26.11 Rosen needle. (Image courtesy of MytaMed)

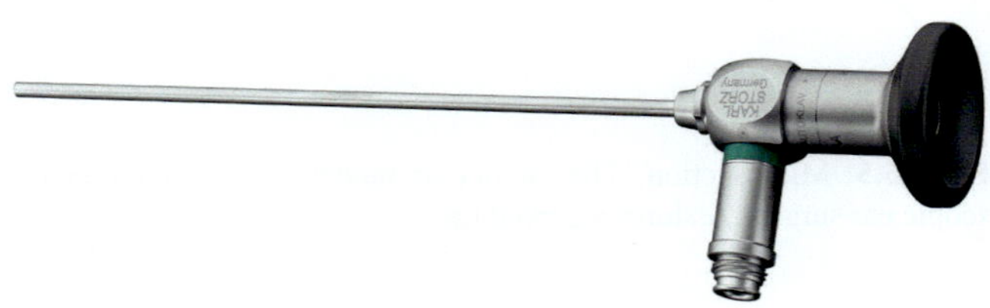

Fig. 26.12 Rigid endoscope (telescope). (©2017 Photo Courtesy of KARL STORZ Endoscopy-America, Inc.)

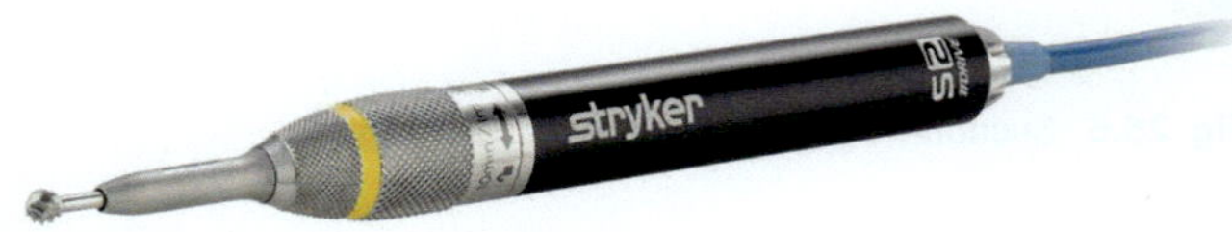

Fig. 26.13 Otologic drill. (Image courtesy of Stryker)

Drills

Drills are a mainstay in otologic surgery. Drills are used to remove non-vital bone to access deeper pathology or resect diseased tissue. Standard otologic drills (Fig. 26.13) are commonly used to perform a mastoidectomy. Most drills are electric, allowing them to be quieter and lighter than their pneumatic predecessors. A variety of burs are available, in terms of aggressiveness and size. Cutting burs are used to remove bone faster. Diamond burs are used in more delicate areas. As a general rule, always use the largest bur possible to avoid plunging a small bur into a critical structure. Smaller microdrills are useful in the middle ear and external auditory canal. Specifically, these drills are commonly used for footplate fenestration during stapes surgery.

Hemostatic Agents

While few procedures routinely pose a risk of significant blood loss in otology and neurotology, several anatomic features of the ear and lateral skull base make hemostasis a unique challenge and supreme safety requirement. First, the critical portions of otologic and neurotologic surgery are performed within the bone. Only the initial approach traverses the soft tissue, where conventional techniques such as electrocautery or ligature apply. Second, the anatomy is highly compressed, frequently requiring microscopic visualization and operating in a deep and narrow space. Third, critical sensorineural and vascular structures are densely located throughout the temporal bone and are frequently millimeters from the operative field. Fourth, transcanal endoscopic approaches have emerged in which hemostatic control is even more important because the non-dominant hand holds an endoscope rather than suction.

Especially in temporal bone approaches to the lateral skull base and petrous apex, neurotologists should be able to manage potentially catastrophic carotid or dural sinus injuries. In all cases, even a small amount of blood in the operative field reduces visualization and raises the risk of damaging neighboring structures and prolongs surgery. The consequences of inadvertent injury may be severe, ranging from deafness to facial paralysis to stroke.

There are many products available, often with non-intuitive naming, and the selection of one agent versus another is not usually standardized. The physical consistency and deliverability of topical compounds are often more important than their chemical composition. Topical agents are effective on the bone and are particularly relevant when operating in small, deep cavities adjacent to the bone or sensorineural structures. Agents with biologically active components that directly interact with the coagulation cascade may be most effective. This section will cover common hemostatic techniques with a focus on topicals. The category, composition, and usage of available agents are explained.

Hemostatic techniques for otology and neurotology can be divided into three broad categories: non-topical techniques, powered instruments, and topical agents (Table 26.1). Non-topical techniques include systemic measures such as administration of blood products as well as locoregional measures such as preoperative embolization of blood vessels or local injection of epinephrine. Powered instruments include a variety of thermal or electrosurgical devices that coagulate by applying energy to bleeding surfaces or vessels. Topical agents are similarly applied directly to a bleeding area, but act via physical compression or an active biological mechanism rather than energy.

Non-topical Hemostatic Techniques

Systemic techniques provide hemostasis through prevention of bleeding. One example is the administration of blood products in a patient with a coagulopathy (e.g., platelets for thrombocytopenia). A thorough review of correcting coagulopathy is presented elsewhere [2, 3]. Other examples are the type of anesthesia administered and the positioning of the patient. Several randomized studies in endoscopic sinus surgery have shown an advantage of total intravenous anesthesia (TIVA) compared to inhalation anesthesia [4, 5]. A randomized trial investigating systemic measures of blood loss in tympanoplasty, however, did not find any difference [6]. Head of bed elevation may decrease venous congestion and reduce bleeding. Similarly, appropriately decreasing blood pressure may limit bleeding. Surgical hypotension is emphasized more in sinus surgery [5]; however, non-controlled trials have anecdotally suggested efficacy in otologic surgery as well [7, 8].

Preoperative embolization of vascular tumors can have a dramatic effect on hemostasis. Embolic agents include metal coils and both solid and liquid materials. The prototypical lesions requiring embolization are paragangliomas (e.g., glomus jugulare). Blood loss reductions and decreased operative time have been demonstrated [9, 10]. Consultation with an interventional neuroradiologist to consider embolization is recommended before operating on a potentially vascular tumor. Risks, while rare, include ischemia, cranial neuropathy, and stroke.

Local injection of the surgical site with a vasoconstrictor, most commonly epinephrine mixed with a local anesthetic, is a commonly employed technique. A rare side effect when using local anesthetic in otologic surgery is transient facial paralysis. Injection of vasoconstrictors is particularly important in transcanal middle ear procedures wherein a single drop of blood can obscure visualization of the surgical field [11]. The concentration of epinephrine may be varied, commonly between 1:50,000–1:200,000. In this effort, it is important to avoid over-concentrated epinephrine, as skin necrosis, or even systemic toxicity, can result.

Powered Hemostatic Instruments

Powered hemostatic agents play a minor role in otology and neurotology. Within the soft tissue, bleeding vessels respond readily to conventional techniques such as cautery. However, once within the temporal bone, powered instruments become less useful for reasons including access and potential injury to adjacent structures. Indeed, monopolar cautery should be avoided once deep to the lateral boundary of the skull.

There are some scenarios that lend themselves to specific powered instruments. Skull base tumors may be treated with bipolar cautery, which also reduces their volume. When removing bone around the sigmoid sinus, such as during a translabyrinthine approach, bipolar cautery has the combined effect of hemostasis and tissue shrinkage, thus improving visualization. Bleeding dural edges are also readily controlled with bipolar.

Lasers have the unique ability to ablate and coagulate without mechanical manipulation. This is particularly advantageous in the middle ear, where mechanical forces on the ossicular chain can cause hearing loss. Several laser systems are available (discussed later in this chapter) with flexible fibers and handpieces allowing maneuverability and precision. Care must be taken when using the laser adjacent to the facial nerve or other critical neurovascular structures because

Table 26.1 Methods for hemostasis in otologic and neurotologic surgery

Method class	Examples	Mechanism	Ideal uses	Advantages	Disadvantages
Non-topical techniques					
Systemic	Surgical hypotension Head of bed elevation Total IV anesthesia Drugs (e.g., desmopressin) Administration of deficient blood products (e.g., platelets)	Various	Various	May affect entire surgical field, blood products may correct coagulopathy	Effect variable, drugs and blood products may have side effects
Embolization	Various materials and devices	Vessel occlusion	Vascular tumor	May affect entire surgical field	Risk of ischemia, cerebrovascular accident
Local injection	Epinephrine	Vessel constriction	Prevent incisional bleeding	Diffusely affects superficial field, prophylactic	Limited to superficial tissue, effect is temporary
Powered instruments					
Powered instruments	Monopolar electrocautery (Bovie) Bipolar electrocautery Drill with diamond bur Laser (argon, KTP, CO_2) Ultrasonic forceps Thermal knives, scissors Radiofrequency (Coblation*)	Energy (usually heat) induced sealing of vessels and adjacent tissue	Small- medium vessels	Combined cutting/ ablating/dissecting functionality, rapid	Less effective on diffuse oozing, challenging if poor exposure, ineffective for bone (except drill with diamond), may leave devitalized/coagulated tissue (impaired visualization, poorer healing), potential injury to adjacent structures
Topical agents					
Nonimplantable	Gauze/sponge/pledget/ patty (e.g., Cottonoid*) Hemostatic forceps Scalp clips (e.g., Raney*)	Physical occlusion of vessels	Small-large vessels, temporary for rapid hemorrhage	Immediate, temporizing measure	No long-term biocompatibility; must be removed at end of surgery
Passive Nonresorbable	Bone wax Ligature (e.g., suture, clips/staples) (Note: some ligature is resorbable)	Physical occlusion of vessels	Focal bleeding from vessel or bone	Immediate	Ligature is very challenging if poor exposure. Bone wax may impair bone healing
Passive Resorbable	Gelatin (Gelfoam®*, Surgifoam™*) Oxidized cellulose (Surgicel™*, Oxycel®*) Collagen (e.g., microfibrillar collagen/ Avitene™*) Synthetic bone wax (Ostene®*)	Physical occlusion of vessels >> biological activation of clotting cascade	Diffuse or focal oozing	Quick action	Foreign body reaction, infection
Active	Epinephrine Thrombin Fibrinogen/thrombin (Tisseel™*)	Vasoconstriction (epinephrine) Biological activation of clotting cascade (thrombin products)		Still effective if coagulopathy	Delay to take effect
Combination	Gelatin/thrombin matrix (Floseal®*, Surgiflo™*) Epinephrine-soaked gelatin Thrombin-soaked gelatin	Combined active + passive mechanisms	Diffuse or focal oozing	May have synergistic effect	Non-human products have small immunologic or infectious risk

thermal damage is possible. In addition, structures in the path of the beam but deep to the target may be inadvertently injured. Applications with hemostatic benefit include lysis of adhesions, stapes surgery, and tumor removal. The latter is particularly precedented in cholesteatoma or paragangliomas [12, 13].

Drilling on bleeding bone with a diamond bur under minimal irrigation produces heat (resulting in cautery) and packs bone dust into small pores (tamponade). Care must be taken when critical structures underlie thin bone to avoid thermal or direct mechanical injury.

While employed elsewhere in otolaryngology, ultrasonic forceps, thermal knives and scissors, and radiofrequency devices do not have widespread application in otology or neurotology.

Topical Hemostatic Agents

Topical agents can be divided into four subcategories based on their basic biologic properties: nonimplantable, passive nonresorbable, passive resorbable, and active. Nonimplantable agents (e.g., cotton sponges) are for transient use and do not possess long-term biocompatibility. If left within the body, they will cause infection. Implantable agents can be further divided into passive or active. Passive is defined as exerting a hemostatic influence by physical compression or occlusion of a vessel. This includes both nonresorbable agents (e.g., bone wax) and resorbable agents. Active is defined as biologically altering blood vessel function (e.g., vasoconstriction) or, more commonly, directly manipulating the coagulation cascade.

Some products combine more than one agent to work via multiple mechanisms. In addition, different topical agents may be applied in a specific sequence for a synergistic effect.

Nonimplantable Agents

Nonimplantable topical agents include a heterogenous group of tools. Hemostatic forceps are used for temporarily clamping vessels. This allows ligature (i.e., sutures, clips/staples) to be used. Such techniques have existed since the dawn of modern surgery. Scalp clips (e.g., Raney clips) are used to clamp bleeding skin edges for the duration of the surgery. Compared to electrocautery, this may result in less tissue injury and faster healing.

Surgical gauze (sponge) is made from nonresorbable woven fabric, such as cotton. The material contains numerous pores that allow absorption many times its weight in blood. Numerous sizes and consistencies are available, all with accompanying nicknames ("lap sponge," "4x4"). Gauze sponges in otology/neurotology can be practically divided into two sizes: "large" (e.g., 4x4 inch or greater) that is held in your hand and "small" (e.g., pledget, patty, neuropatty, cottonoid) that is handled with forceps and typically under microscopy. Disadvantages include the need for removal (with possible rebleeding) and the difficulty cutting to custom sizes (which can lead to unwanted retention or complicate safety counting protocols).

Passive Nonresorbable Agents

Bone wax dates to at least the late 1800s [14]. Bleeding bone can be occluded with wax, leading to tamponade. Care must be taken not to wax a widely open dural venous sinus, because intravenous dislocation could cause embolization. Wax application is most effectively followed by compression with a conformable material, such as a fingertip or small pledget. A sideways "smearing" motion is usually more effective than pushing or packing. The size and quality of the wax are also relevant. Undersized pieces will inadequately tamponade, while oversized pieces will interfere with effective compression into the bleeding bone. In our experience, a slightly sticky consistency is easier to use.

Ligature involves physically tying a vessel with suture or clamping with a small clip/staple. In otology/neurotology, this technique is primarily confined to initial soft tissue work. One exception is aneurysm clips, which can control catastrophic intracranial bleeding. Aneurysm clips should be available whenever brainstem vessels are exposed.

Passive Resorbable Agents

Passive resorbable agents exert their hemostatic effect primarily through local pressure. A secondary effect is that the materials act as a scaffold to encourage clotting. Unlike standard surgical gauze, resorbables can be cut and packed into small spaces. In addition, removal, which may lead to rebleeding, is not necessary. Passive resorbables are also generally inexpensive. Passive resorbable agents may continue to swell, thus should not be tightly packed next to neurovascular structures [15]. Rarely, foreign body reactions or infection may occur prior to resorption [16, 17]. Therefore, it is best to use the minimum amount needed.

Oxidized cellulose (e.g., Surgicel™, Oxycel®) is one of the most common topical agents. Standard surgical gauze is composed of cotton, which is 90% cellulose. Thus, these products can be thought of as specially treated resorbable gauze. The consistency of oxidized cellulose products varies widely, from woven sheets (Surgicel™) to cottonball-like tufts that can be shaped into cigars (Oxycel®). The malleability and diversity allow them to be packed into various bleeding corners and crevices. Resorption occurs over weeks.

Gelatin (e.g., Gelfoam®) is composed of mostly collagen, typically of porcine origin. The most common consistency (Gelfoam®) is sponge-like. It can be used dry, pressed, or soaked in active hemostatic agents (see below).

Collagen agents have a similar compositional makeup to gelatin. Various consistencies are available, including an ultrafine texture (microfibrillar collagen, Avitene™).

Lastly, a synthetic polymer that functions as a resorbable bone wax substitute (Ostene®) is available. This agent, which resorbs in 48 hours, may allow improved bone healing compared to wax [18, 19]. However, for regions where bone healing is not critical (e.g., mastoid cavity), this may not represent a meaningful advantage.

Active Agents

Epinephrine (adrenaline) is a potent vasoconstrictor. Within the temporal bone, it is administered via a carrier material (e.g., pledget or gelatin).

Thrombin is an enzyme that catalyzes the conversion of fibrinogen into fibrin in the last step of the coagulation cascade. For this reason, it remains effective in most clotting disorders. Like epinephrine, it is often administered via a carrier (see below).

Fibrin and thrombin preparations have been used since the early 1900s by purifying blood plasma or using nonhuman sources [20, 21]. More recently, off-the-shelf products have been FDA approved with essentially no immunologic/infectious risk. Fibrinogen/thrombin "sealant" preparations (e.g., Tisseel™) contain both thrombin and its substrate, fibrinogen [22]. Different formulations may contain additional ingredients. For example, Tisseel™ also contains aprotinin, a fibrinolysis inhibitor [23]. Thawing and preparation are required. Delivery via a double barrel syringe combines the thrombin and fibrinogen. The active mixture possesses a cured gel-like consistency. One disadvantage of this delivery is that the resulting gel sheet is not conveniently manipulated or suctioned. Thus, fibrinogen/thrombin sealant products are often administered just prior to closure as a final measure.

No randomized controlled trials comparing fibrinogen/thrombin sealant agents to other products were found in the otology/neurotology literature. In a randomized trial of several surgical specialties, hemostasis was more readily achieved with an autologous fibrin sealant (without thrombin) compared to oxidized cellulose (Surgicel™) (94% versus 65% at 5 minutes) [24]. Randomized trials in cardiac and spine surgery also showed superiority of fibrin sealant to conventional agents (e.g., gelatin, oxidized cellulose, microfibrillar collagen) [25, 26].

Combination Agents

Passive resorbable agents may be combined with biologically active agents for a synergistic effect. For example, gelatin (e.g., Gelfoam®) or gauze patties may be soaked in epinephrine or thrombin, resulting in an additional vasoconstrictive or pro-coagulation effect.

A prefabricated mixture (or "matrix") of gelatin and thrombin (Floseal®, Surgiflo™) combines a foam-like consistency with easy delivery. Brief preparation is required. The unique granular gelatin formulation provides the foamy texture that imparts a compressive effect. Advantages include high conformability to the bleeding region and easy suctioning so that it may be repeatedly applied as needed. Like all hemostatic agents, care must be taken not to inject intravascularly [27]. One disadvantage is cost; however, this may be outweighed by decreased operative time.

No randomized controlled trials comparing gelatin/thrombin matrix to other products were found in the otology/neurotology literature. In cardiac, vascular, and spine surgery randomized trials, hemostasis was more readily achieved with gelatin/thrombin matrix products compared to traditional gelatin (Gelfoam®) soaked in thrombin (88–99% versus 57–93% at 10 minutes) [28–30]. This illustrates that the formulation, consistency, and deliverability of topical hemostatic products are important, rather than only the chemical composition.

Sealants, Adhesives, and Glues

The use of the terms sealant, adhesive, and glue can cause confusion because these products may provide hemostatic, sealing, or combined effects. Furthermore, the term "sealant" can refer to both sealing blood vessels and sealing closed a cavity or incision. For example, fibrinogen/thrombin (Tisseel™; described above) is both a hemostatic and sealing agent, whereas polyethylene glycol and trilysine amine (DuraSeal®) is primarily a non-hemostatic sealing agent for obtaining watertight closure to prevent cerebrospinal fluid leak [31]. Products that possess overlapping hemostatic and sealing effects are previously described. Products that exert a sealing function only are beyond the scope of this chapter.

Conclusions

Conventional soft tissue hemostatic techniques are frequently not applicable when operating within the temporal bone. Topical agents that contain active components that directly promote the clotting cascade may be more effective in certain situations than agents that only exert physical compression. Comparing among hemostatic techniques is difficult because high-quality trials are limited.

Lasers

The advantage of laser surgery comes from reduced mechanical manipulation and trauma. This might result in a lower risk of iatrogenic sensorineural hearing loss when manipulating the ossicular chain. Lasers have also been used successfully to remove (via vaporization) glomus tumors, vestibular schwannomas, and small arteriovenous (AV) malformations. In chronic ear surgery, lasers have also been used to vaporize granulation tissue and cholesteatoma, particularly on a mobile stapes footplate. Prosthesis manufacturers have also developed nitinol implants that crimp onto ossicles simply by heating with laser energy.

Three lasers are commonly utilized in otologic surgery. These include argon (514 nm wavelength), potassium titanyl phosphate (KTP, 532 nm), and carbon dioxide (CO_2, 10,600 nm). Argon and KTP lasers are in the visible spectrum (visible laser dot without an aiming beam), whereas CO_2 is infrared (requiring an optional separate visible laser as an aiming beam). This section includes a brief overview of the principles of quantum mechanics that explain the basis of lasers in surgery as well as an introduction to the common lasers used in otology and neurotology.

Understanding Lasers

The term laser was originally an acronym for light amplification by stimulated emission of radiation. A laser generates a *monochromatic* (one wavelength), *coherent* (phase locked), and *collimated* (parallel waves) beam of electromagnetic (EM) energy. Depending on the wavelength, the laser beam may be in the infrared, visible, or ultraviolet spectrum. Each wavelength of EM energy is associated with a specific amount of energy, which is proportional to the frequency and inversely proportional to the wavelength. At the molecular level, the electrons orbiting each atom exist in quantized energy levels and are only able to move between these specific energy levels. When an electron moves to a lower energy level, the lost energy is emitted as a photon of EM energy. Conversely, each atom can only absorb photons that contain the precise amount of EM energy that will move an electron to a higher quantized energy level.

On the molecular level, energy may be described as vibrational kinetic energy, rotational kinetic energy, and translational kinetic energy. Long-wavelength lasers in the infrared spectrum contain less energy in each photon; absorption primarily occurs in the form of increased kinetic energy resulting in heat. As the target molecule is heated, a solid may turn to gas (vaporize) or liquid (coagulate).

The key, therefore, is that each atom can only absorb specific photons determined by its available energy states. By extension, knowledge of the composition of the target tissue allows one to design a selective laser by picking a specific wavelength. Those wavelengths that are best absorbed by the target tissue are the safest to use because there is less energy transmission and scatter through the tissue. For example, water molecules absorb energy from CO_2 lasers well, making CO_2 lasers a good choice for soft tissue dissection given the prevalence of water molecules in tissues.

Applications of Lasers

Early applications for otologic lasers were focused on otosclerosis because of the theoretical benefit of reducing mechanical trauma and iatrogenic sensorineural hearing loss when opening the oval window. Lasers had to be designed to have precise optics, efficient absorption by the bone and collagen, minimal heating of perilymph, and not damaging to inner ear structures from photons transmitted through the perilymph [32].

The earliest lasers developed for stapedectomy were argon and KTP [13, 33]. The development to meet the above listed requirements necessitated an understanding of the absorption profile of bone, collagen, and water. When a laser is applied to the bone, kinetic energy (heat) increases until water and collagen reach their boiling points and are vaporized. Therefore, the ideal laser wavelength to ablate bone and collagen should be readily absorbed by water and collagen. Moreover, such a laser would be safe for the inner ear because any laser energy directed into the footplate would be absorbed by water molecules in perilymph at the footplate without transmitting the energy directly to the inner ear structures. CO_2 is one laser that fits this profile well. KTP and argon will travel 70 m in water before half of its energy is absorbed, compared to 0.007 mm for CO_2 [34]. However, KTP and argon lasers are absorbed well by hemoglobin and melanin, allowing for precise dissection of soft tissue containing pigmented molecules such as hemoglobin and melanin with minimal thermal damage to surrounding tissues.

Otologic Surgical Lasers

The most commonly used otologic lasers in modern practice are the argon, KTP, and CO_2. They were initially designed as microscope-mounted micromanipulator systems, but have all been adapted with flexible fibers to allow use through handhold probes.

The predominant use of lasers in otologic surgery has been for stapes surgery and for lysis of adhesions or vaporizing small amounts of granulation tissue during middle ear surgery. There have been reported uses of lasers to vaporize cholesteatomas, acoustic neuromas, glomus tumors, and other skull base tumors [35–37]. However, the rate of tumor ablation with lasers is slow. Coupled with the risk of thermal injury to adjacent tissues and nerves or inadvertent misdirected laser beams, the use of lasers has been limited for these applications.

In transcanal endoscopic ear surgery (TEES), lasers have been used to dissect soft tissue lesions such as cholesteatoma and adhesions. In this application lasers are advantageous in their ability to maintain hemostasis while dissecting. This allows the surgeon to better operate with a one-handed technique, since the non-dominant hand holds the endoscope [38].

Reports of the use of argon lasers (514 nm wavelength) in middle ear and stapes surgery began in the 1980s [13, 33, 39, 40]. The argon laser was initially designed as a microscope-mounted micromanipulator system and later adapted into a handheld handpiece in the late 1980s [41]. Argon lasers are absorbed well by pigmented molecules and are well suited for soft tissue ablation. Indeed, argon lasers are also used for photocoagulation of pigmented lesions such as port-wine stains, hemangiomas, and telangiectasias [42]. However, as discussed above, argon lasers are poorly absorbed by water molecules, so should not be aimed directly into the vestibule because the laser energy will transmit through the perilymph and directly damage inner ear structures. KTP lasers (532 nm) were developed concurrently with argon lasers in the 1980s and share the same absorption profile due to the similar wavelengths. Compared to argon, the KTP laser features even better absorption by hemoglobin.

The development and use of the CO_2 laser (10,600 nm) was limited by the difficulty of transmitting the laser beam. In its earliest forms, CO_2 lasers were bulky attachments to a microscope and lacked the precision required for otologic surgery. In addition, being an infrared laser, CO_2 lasers required a separate laser (typically helium-neon, HeNe) in the visible spectrum as an aiming beam which must be tested for alignment before each use. A flexible fiber (OmniGuide®) with a diameter of 0.9 mm and spot size 0.25 mm was brought to market in 2007. In the handheld system, the HeNe aiming beam is replaced with a continuous jet of helium that gently displaces the target tissue. This can approximate an aiming mechanism and also clears the plume of smoke off the field [43].

References

1. Golub JS, Schmitt NC. Otolaryngology surgical instrument guide. San Diego, CA: Plural Publishing; 2012.
2. Johansson PI. Hemostatic strategies for minimizing mortality in surgery with major blood loss. Curr Opin Hematol [Internet] 2009;16(6):509–514. Available from: http://www.ncbi.nlm.nih.gov/pubmed/19701086.
3. Mahdy AM, Webster NR. Perioperative systemic haemostatic agents. Br J Anaesth. 2004;93(6):842–58.
4. Pavlin JD, Colley PS, Weymuller EA, Van Norman G, Gunn HC, Koerschgen ME. Propofol versus isoflurane for endoscopic sinus surgery. Am J Otolaryngol - Head Neck Med Surg. 1999;20(2):96–101.
5. Wormald PJ, van Renen G, Perks J, Jones JA, Langton-Hewer CD. The effect of the total intravenous anesthesia compared with inhalational anesthesia on the surgical field during endoscopic sinus surgery. Am J Rhinol [Internet]. 2005;19(5):514–20. Available from: http://www.ncbi.nlm.nih.gov/pubmed/23258603.
6. Özer E, Çeliker V, Aypar Ü, Başgül E. Influence of total intravenous and inhalational anaesthesia on haemostasis during tympanoplasty. Acta Anaesthesiol Scand. 2003;47(10):1242–7.
7. Deacock AR. Aspects of anaesthesia for middle ear surgery and blood loss during stapedectomy. Proc R Soc Med [Internet]. 1971;64(12):1226–8. Available from: http://www.pubmedcentral.nih.gov/articlerender.fcgi?artid=1813161&tool=pmcentrez&rendertype=abstract.
8. Kerr AR. Anaesthesia with profound hypotension for middle ear surgery. Br J Anaesth. 1977;49(5):447–52.
9. Murphy TP, Brackmann DE. Effects of preoperative embolization on glomus jugulare tumors. Laryngoscope [Internet]. 1989;99(12):1244–7. Available from: http://www.ncbi.nlm.nih.gov/pubmed/2557501.
10. Larouere MJ, Zappia JJ, Wilner HI, Graham MD, Lundy LB. Selective embolization of glomus jugulare tumors. Skull Base Surg [Internet]. 1994;4(1):21–5. Available from: http://www.pubmedcentral.nih.gov/articlerender.fcgi?artid=1656471&tool=pmcentrez&rendertype=abstract.
11. Smith C. Haemostasis in ear surgery. Proc R Soc Med [Internet]. 1971;64(12):1225–6. Available from: http://www.pubmedcentral.nih.gov/articlerender.fcgi?artid=1813201&tool=pmcentrez&rendertype=abstract.
12. Saeed SR, Jackler RK. Lasers in surgery for chronic ear disease. Otolaryngol Clin North Am. 1996;29(2):245–55.
13. Perkins RC. Laser stapedotomy for otosclerosis. Laryngoscope [Internet]. 1980;90(2):228–40. Available from: http://www.ncbi.nlm.nih.gov/pubmed/7354691.
14. Gupta G, Prestigiacomo CJ. From sealing wax to bone wax: predecessors to Horsley's development. Neurosurg Focus [Internet]. 2007;23(1):E16. Available from: http://www.ncbi.nlm.nih.gov/pubmed/17961057.
15. Dutton JJ, Tse DT, Anderson RL. Compressive optic neuropathy following use of intracranial oxidized cellulose hemostat. Ophthalmic Surg [Internet]. 1983;14(6):487–90. Available from: http://www.ncbi.nlm.nih.gov/pubmed/6348621.
16. Andrychowski J, Czernicki Z, Taraszewska A, Frontczak-Baniewicz M, Przytuła E, Zębala M. Granulomatous inflammation of dura mater—a rare side effect after application of hemostatic and insulation materials in case of two-stage operation of huge meningioma. Folia Neuropathol [Internet]. 2012;50(4):417–24. Available from: http://www.termedia.pl/doi/10.5114/fn.2012.32377.
17. Kothbauer KF, Jallo GI, Siffert J, Jimenez E, Allen JC, Epstein FJ. Foreign body reaction to hemostatic materials mimicking recurrent brain tumor. Report of three cases. J Neurosurg [Internet]. 2001;95(3):503–6. Available from: http://www.ncbi.nlm.nih.gov/pubmed/11565875.
18. Vestergaard R, Jensen H, Vind-Kezunovic S, Jakobsen T, Soballe K, Hasenkam J. Bone healing after median sternotomy: a comparison of two hemostatic devices. J Cardiothorac Surg. 2010;24(5):117.
19. Vestergaard R, Nielsen P, Terp K, Soballe K, Andersen G, Hasenkam J. Effect of hemostatic material on sternal healing after cardiac surgery. Ann Thorac Surg. 2014;97(1):153–60.
20. Bailey OT, Ingraham FD. Chemical, clinical, and immunological studies on the products of human plasma fractionation. XXI. The use of fibrin foam as a hemostatic agent in neurosurgery: clinical and pathological studies. J Clin Invest [Internet]. 1944;23(4):591–6. Available from: http://www.pubmedcentral.nih.gov/articlerender.fcgi?artid=435377&tool=pmcentrez&rendertype=abstract.

21. Senturia BH, Ogura JH, Walsh TE. The use of thrombin and absorbable sponge for hemostasis in otolaryngology. Laryngoscope [Internet]. 1949;59(10):1068–83. Available from: http://www.ncbi.nlm.nih.gov/pubmed/15392462.
22. Nissen AJ, Johnson AJ, Perkins RC, Welsh JE. Fibrin glue in otology and neurotology. Am J Otol [Internet]. 1993;14(2):147–50. Available from: http://www.ncbi.nlm.nih.gov/pubmed/8503488.
23. Dhillon S. Fibrin sealant: a review of its use as supportive treatment for haemostasis in surgery. Drugs. 2011;71(14):1893–915.
24. Hanks JB, Kjaergard HK, Hollingsbee DA. A comparison of the haemostatic effect of Vivostat patient-derived fibrin sealant with oxidised cellulose (Surgicel) in multiple surgical procedures. Eur Surg Res. 2003;35(5):439–44.
25. Rousou J, Levitsky S, Gonzalez-Lavin L, Cosgrove D, Magilligan D, Weldon C, et al. Randomized clinical trial of fibrin sealant in patients undergoing resternotomy or reoperation after cardiac operations. A multicenter study. J Thorac Cardiovasc Surg [Internet]. 1989;97(2):194–203. Available from: http://www.ncbi.nlm.nih.gov/pubmed/2464722.
26. Tredwell SJ, Sawatzky B. The use of fibrin sealant to reduce blood loss during Cotrel-Dubousset instrumentation for idiopathic scoliosis. Spine (Phila Pa 1976) [Internet]. 1990;15(9):913–5. Available from: http://www.ncbi.nlm.nih.gov/pubmed/2259980.
27. Singleton RH, Jankowitz BT, Wecht DA, Gardner P. Iatrogenic cerebral venous sinus occlusion with flowable topical hemostatic matrix. J Neurosurg [Internet]. 2011;115(3):576–83. Available from: http://www.ncbi.nlm.nih.gov/pubmed/21456896.
28. Oz MC, Cosgrove DM, Badduke BR, Hill JD, Flannery MR, Palumbo R, et al. Controlled clinical trial of a novel hemostatic agent in cardiac surgery. Ann Thorac Surg [Internet]. 2000;69(5):1376–82. Available from: http://linkinghub.elsevier.com/retrieve/pii/S0003497500011942.
29. Renkens KL, Payner TD, Leipzig TJ, Feuer H, Morone MA, Koers JM, et al. A multicenter, prospective, randomized trial evaluating a new hemostatic agent for spinal surgery. Spine (Phila Pa 1976) [Internet]. 2001;26(15):1645–50. Available from: http://www.ncbi.nlm.nih.gov/pubmed/11474348.
30. Weaver FA, Hood DB, Zatina M, Messina L, Badduke B. Gelatin-thrombin-based hemostatic sealant for intraoperative bleeding in vascular surgery. Ann Vasc Surg. 2002;16(3):286–93.
31. Osbun JW, Ellenbogen RG, Chesnut RM, Chin LS, Connolly PJ, Cosgrove GR, et al. A multicenter, single-blind, prospective randomized trial to evaluate the safety of a polyethylene glycol hydrogel (duraseal dural sealant system) as a dural sealant in cranial surgery. World Neurosurg [Internet]. 2012;78(5):498–504. https://doi.org/10.1016/j.wneu.2011.12.011.
32. Lesinski S, Palmer A. Lasers for otosclerosis: CO2 vs. Argon and KTP-532. Laryngoscope. 1989;99(6):1–8.
33. McGee T. The argon laser in surgery for chronic ear disease and otosclerosis. Laryngoscope. 1983;93:1177–82.
34. Wolfe W, Zissis G. The infrared handbook. Washington, DC: Office of Naval Research; 1978. p. 3–107.
35. Hamilton JW. Systematic preservation of the ossicular chain in cholesteatoma surgery using a fiber-guided laser. Otol Neurotol [Internet]. 2010;31(7):1104–8. Available from: http://www.ncbi.nlm.nih.gov/pubmed/20616760.
36. Nissen AJ, Sikand A, Welsh JE, Curto FS. Use of the KTP-532 laser in acoustic neuroma surgery. Laryngoscope [Internet]. 1997;107(1):118–21. Available from: http://www.ncbi.nlm.nih.gov/pubmed/9001275.
37. le Nobel GJ, James AL. Recommendations for potassium-titanyl-phosphate laser in the treatment of cholesteatoma. J Int Adv Otol [Internet]. 2016;12(3):332–6. Available from: http://www.advancedotology.org/eng/makale/973/93/Full-Text.
38. Yau AY, Mahboubi H, Maducdoc M, Ghavami Y, Djalilian HR. Curved adjustable fiberoptic laser for endoscopic cholesteatoma surgery. Otol Neurotol. 2015;36(1):61–4.
39. Glasscock ME III, Jackson CG, Whitaker SR. The argon laser in acoustic tumor surgery. Laryngoscope. 1981;91(9):1405–16.
40. DiBartolomeo J, Ellis M. The argon laser in otology. Laryngoscope. 1980;90(11):1786–96.
41. Horn KL, Gherini S, Griffin GM Jr. Argon laser stapedectomy using an endo-otoprobe system. Otolaryngol Head Neck Surg. 1990;102(2):193–8.
42. Garret CG, Ossoff RH, Reinisch L. Laser surgery: basic principles and safety considerations. In: Flint PW, Haughey BH, Lund VJ, Niparko JK, Richardson MA, Robbins KT, et al., editors. Cummings otolaryngology: head & neck surgery. 5th Ed. Mosby Elsevier; 2010. p. 25–37.
43. Landegger LD, Cohen MS. Use of the flexible fiber CO2 laser in pediatric transcanal endoscopic middle ear surgery. Int J Pediatr Otorhinolaryngol [Internet]. 2016;85:154–7. https://doi.org/10.1016/j.ijporl.2016.03.039.

Principles of Temporal Bone and Skull Base Surgery

27

Roberto A. Cueva

Preoperative Assessment

In a tertiary care setting, patients will often be referred for surgery with all the appropriate tests and workup completed. However, both tertiary care specialists and general otolaryngologists must ensure that the workup is complete before performing surgery. Preoperative assessment includes evaluation of the disease process requiring surgery and evaluation of the patient's suitability for surgery/anesthesia.

General Health

Integral to any specialist's consultation is both a thorough history of the presenting illness/disease process and detailed review of the patient's general health status. Depending on the findings of this inquiry, more extensive medical evaluation may be required before surgery may be safely undertaken, or the consideration of surgery may be abandoned entirely and other management options recommended. A patient's suitability to undergo surgery/anesthesia depends on numerous factors including type of anesthetic to be used, nature and duration of the surgical procedure, hemodynamic challenges of the operation (either from blood loss or fluid shifts), and anticipated morbidity of the surgery. Ever-increasing life expectancy, along with successful treatment of chronic illness, has resulted in greater numbers of older patients being considered for surgical management of temporal bone/skull base diseases. Proactive involvement of appropriate medical specialists in the perioperative management of a patient's chronic illness is necessary to reduce risks associated with surgery. Consultation with an anesthesiologist, in advance of the morning of surgery, may be required to assess suitability to undergo general anesthesia or to avoid anesthetic complications.

Healthy patients, taking no daily medication, typically do not require any preoperative blood tests. Patients with chronic medical illness or patients who are on daily medication may require blood tests as indicated by their circumstances. Otherwise, asymptomatic men over the age of 40 and women over the age of 50 should have an electrocardiogram. Patients with complex medical histories may require formal consultation with an internist or other specialist (e.g., cardiologist). Medications and/or dietary supplements that inhibit proper blood clotting (anticoagulants, aspirin, nonsteroidal anti-inflammatory drugs (NSAIDs), ginkgo biloba extract, vitamin E, fish oil, etc.) should be stopped approximately 10 days before the planned procedure. The emergence and popularity of glucagon-like peptide-1 (GLP-1) receptor agonist weight loss drugs must also be considered, and recent guidelines suggest that delayed gastric emptying associated with this class of drugs can increase perioperative risk [1].

Disease Specific Evaluation

In addition to a thorough head and neck examination, including cranial nerve testing, patients considered for temporal bone/skull base surgery require specific examinations and testing appropriate to their diagnosis.

Otologic Surgery

Patients considered for surgery of the middle ear, tympanic membrane, and/or mastoid should all undergo microscopic otoscopy. Such careful examination reduces the likelihood that the surgeon will be surprised in the operating room and have to extend the operation beyond what was planned. Particularly important is the careful removal of any crusts

R. A. Cueva (✉)
Southern California Permanente Medical Group, San Diego, CA, USA

University of California, San Diego, CA, USA
e-mail: Cueva@cox.net

A. D. Sweeney et al. (eds.), *Haynes-Glasscock-Shambaugh Surgery of the Ear*, https://doi.org/10.1007/978-3-032-18264-7_27

covering the pars flaccida region that may hide the neck of a cholesteatoma. Furthermore, in patients requiring revision surgery following a previous intact canal wall mastoidectomy, careful inspection of the postero-lateral ear canal is important as a canal-mastoid fistula may be present if the previous surgeon unnecessarily reduced the height of the posterior canal bone. The opening to such a fistula may be easily missed if attention is solely focused on the tympanic membrane.

Preoperative audiometry of both ears is mandatory. Operating on the only hearing ear should be approached with the utmost of caution as a potential complication is complete deafness. The preoperative audiogram not only serves as a baseline for postoperative comparison but also allows the surgeon to counsel the patient regarding the potential for hearing improvement related to the planned surgery. Electronystagmography (ENG) should be performed on all patients prior to surgery targeting the vestibular system. Although rare, a patient may have one ear symptomatic for hearing fluctuation, tinnitus, and aural pressure, while the opposite ear is the cause of vertigo. Performing surgery on the incorrect ear in this setting will not help patients and likely leave them worse.

The role of computed tomography (CT) scanning prior to middle-ear/mastoid surgery is dependent on the surgeon's judgment and disease process in question. An adult suspected of having otosclerosis with a normal microscopic otoscopy does not necessarily need a CT scan of the temporal bones. The opposite is true for a patient with two previous surgeries, recurrent cholesteatoma, and a history of transient facial weakness following the last surgery. Other indications for preoperative temporal-bone CT scanning include ear canal atresia/hypoplasia; suspected middle-ear/mastoid/jugular foramen tumor; suspected cerebrospinal fluid (CSF) otorrhea; suspected fracture; suspected X-linked conductive hearing loss; preoperative cochlear assessment prior to cochlear implantation; and sensorineural hearing loss/vertigo/facial weakness in the setting of chronic otitis media and/or cholesteatoma.

Neurotologic/Skull Base Surgery

Patients being prepared for neurotologic/skull base surgery not only require the evaluation process described above but also require a more extensive neurological examination. Skull base tumors often negatively impact the central nervous system in addition to regional cranial nerves. Sensory and motor function of the extremities, deep tendon reflexes, Hoffman's sign, pronator drift, cerebellar testing (Romberg—normal and tandem, heel to shin, finger to nose, rapid alternating movements), and gait should all be assessed. Consultation with a neurosurgeon is typically sought since such cases are managed in a team setting. In practice settings with sufficient patient volume, a highly efficient multidisciplinary clinic can be established in which the neurotologist and neurosurgeon see the patient simultaneously. Such a "skull base clinic" promotes greater exchange of information between specialties and facilitates discussion of management options and approach selection, as well as other aspects of perioperative planning. Consultation with a plastic/reconstructive surgeon is recommended when complex reconstruction is anticipated following tumor extirpation.

Patients with skull base lesions commonly require preoperative audiologic and neurophysiologic testing. The results of the audiogram will help in determining whether a hearing preservation type approach should be employed and help predict potential for hearing preservation or loss. Auditory brain stem response (ABR) testing, while not essential, may help prognosticate chances of hearing preservation in vestibular schwannoma cases. The absence of ABR waveforms does not preclude attempted hearing preservation as intraoperative direct eighth nerve monitoring (DENM) routinely detects cochlear nerve action potentials when ABR is absent [2, 3]. Postoperative testing of hearing demonstrates whether hearing was preserved and the quality of hearing, if still present. Electronystagmography (ENG) has historically been used to try and predict the nerve branch of origin for vestibular schwannomas, but is unreliable and therefore of limited utility. Vestibular evoked myogenic potentials (VEMP) should be tested in all patients suspected of superior semicircular canal dehiscence to corroborate with their CT findings.

Radiological studies are always required for patients undergoing neurotologic/skull base surgery. For most lesions magnetic resonance imaging (MRI), with and without gadolinium contrast, is the study of choice. Axial and coronal images help the surgeon form a three-dimensional picture of the tumor's relationship to the patient's anatomy. Lesions in the region of the sella turcica (i.e., pituitary macroadenomas, craniopharyngiomas, and chordomas) warrant contrast-enhanced sagittal views as well. For epidermoid cysts/tumors of the central nervous system, which can mimic arachnoid cysts, diffusion-weighted images are optimal for establishing the diagnosis and delineating extent of disease [4].

In cases where tumor embolization is not required, the use of magnetic resonance angiography (MRA) and magnetic resonance venography (MRV) may be used to assess a tumor's relationship to major vascular structures such as the internal carotid artery and jugular bulb/vein. When tumor embolization is anticipated, formal cerebral angiography, with its attendant risks, is necessary. Angiography with embolization is scheduled 24–48 hours prior to the planned tumor surgery to maximize tumor vessel occlusion without allowing excess time for dense fibrosis to occur within and/or around the tumor. Octreotide scanning can be useful for finding metachronous lesions in patients with neuroendocrine tumors such as paragangliomas, if cranial MRI does not include the neck down to the carotid bifurcation. CT scanning may be indicated to better define the bony anatomy of the skull base in lesions causing deformity, erosion, or destruction of the temporal bone or skull base.

Specific diseases require blood or urine testing for diagnosis and prevention of perioperative complications. Paragangliomas require 24-hour urine collection testing for vanillylmandelic acid (VMA) and metanephrines. Patients with glomus tumors that secrete epinephrine/norepinephrine should have preoperative alpha blockade to prevent potentially dangerous intraoperative hypertension. Such blockade should be in place at the time of angiography with embolization, as release of these vaso-active hormones can also occur related to embolization.

Preoperative Patient Preparation

Once the patient and the disease process have been appropriately evaluated and the decision made to proceed with surgery (after fully discussing the other management options), the patient must be prepared for the event.

Education

This preparation includes educating the patient about the disease process, the planned surgical procedure, type of anesthesia, associated risks/complications, expected outcome of surgery, anticipated recovery time, postoperative care, and follow-up plans. The discussion of the surgical procedure should include location and size of incisions, amount of hair to be clipped (if any), basic steps of the procedure, method of wound closure, and dressing(s). The description of the risks/complications and expected outcomes will occasionally overlap. The expected outcome in many temporal bone procedures involves improvement or preservation of function. However, in some procedures the expected outcome may involve a decline in function (hearing loss, cranial nerve dysfunction, altered cosmesis, etc.), which should not be considered as a complication. Complications are unplanned adverse events that may occur within a recognized statistical range. This difference should be made clear in settings when the expected outcome involves such an anticipated decrement of function. Whenever possible the quoted likelihood of success and/or risk of developing a complication should be based on the individual surgeon's practice experience. Surgeons early in their practice should rely on published statistical data.

Choice of anesthetic is dependent on the planned procedure, the temperament of the patient, and the surgeon's preference. Most transcanal middle-ear surgery is readily accomplished with local anesthetic and sedation. This allows intraoperative testing of hearing and more speedy recovery. Postauricular otologic procedures including tympanoplasty with or without mastoidectomy may also be done under local anesthesia with sedation, but proper patient selection is important. Additionally, the surgeon must reliably be able to complete the planned procedure within 2 to 3 hours. Of course, all otologic procedures may also be done under general anesthetic. Skull base procedures are done under general anesthesia.

Anticipated course of recovery and timing for return to work/activities should be discussed. If hospitalization is required, duration of hospital stay will vary and should be determined by the patient's postoperative functional status. At the Skull Base Surgery Center for Southern California Permanente Medical Group, patients are advised that they will be able to leave the hospital when they are maintaining oral alimentation, ambulating with little or no assistance, pain relief is provided by oral medications, and there are no signs of complications. This focuses the issue of hospital discharge on achieving appropriate functional level rather than a specific number of days. Using this simple algorithm over the past two decades, length of stay for vestibular schwannoma patients has averaged about 2.5 days. Reassuring the patient that he or she will not be discharged until they have achieved a suitable level of function relieves anxiety about readiness to go home. Identifying the functional goals required for discharge also motivates patients to achieve those goals. Creating the proper expectation regarding discharge criteria during the preoperative discussion is critical to optimizing duration of hospitalization. Hospitalization beyond what is medically or functionally indicated increases the risk of nosocomial infection, deep vein thrombosis, and other hospitalization-related complications.

The patient and family should be informed about proper postoperative care following discharge. Topics to address are proper wound care, symptoms or changes to watch for, eye care (if facial nerve weakness is present), medication schedule, activity level, and physician contact information should problems arise. Providing this information in written form is helpful as patients are often overwhelmed by the volume of information during this stressful time. Once home, patients are encouraged to pursue an appropriate level of activity to reduce the risk of deep venous thrombosis, as well as maintain mobility and stamina. Exertion requiring a Valsalva maneuver, particularly in patients at risk for CSF leak, is discouraged for 1 month following surgery. The number, timing, and purpose of postoperative visits should be well delineated. Neurotologic/skull base lesions commonly require long-term radiological monitoring. The type and timing of imaging to be done should be discussed in advance as well as postoperatively. Establishing a system for tracking patients needing scans at recommended intervals is necessary to avoid losing a patient to follow-up.

Medical Preparation

A brief discussion between a surgeon and anesthesiologist regarding the surgery can help optimize the patient's surgical experience and avoid complications. Review of the anesthetic choice, anticipated duration of surgery, use/nonuse of neurophysiological monitoring, concerns regarding intracranial pressure, intraoperative fluid management, hyperventilation to lower Pco_2, and patient-specific health issues are topics worthy of review. In centers where otologic/neurotologic surgery is common, the discussion may be more abbreviated as the anesthesia team will likely be familiar with the surgeon's preferences. The surgeon should visit the patient in the preoperative area and confirm the site for surgery, marking it personally.

The topic of intraoperative fluid management during skull base surgeries merits specific attention. From the perspective of the anesthesiologist, the patient arrives in the preoperative area in a dehydrated state having foregone oral hydration for at least 8 hours. The anesthesiologist will commonly want to "make up" the patient's fluid deficit using intravenous fluids. The author and his neurosurgical colleague have instructed their anesthesia team to resist this impulse. Our instructions regarding fluid balance are to match the volume of intravenous fluids given to the quantity of urine output and blood loss during the course of the surgery. This avoids overhydration and possible brain edema. We have experienced situations in which the anesthetic team did not follow this request, giving patients as much as 3 liters of fluids during the course of an uncomplicated 3-hour surgery, causing the patients to develop cerebellar edema a few hours later requiring emergent measures. Excessive dehydration is to be avoided as well since it increases the risk of venous thrombosis.

Anxiolysis is typically provided by the anesthesiologist in the preoperative area depending on patient need. To reduce nausea related to otologic procedures, 4 to 8 mg of dexamethasone (Decadron) and 4 mg of ondansetron (Zofran) given intravenously at the start of surgery are a useful combination. Perioperative antibiotics for clean otologic procedures (intact tympanic membrane or dry perforation) are not employed as the infection rate is in the range of 1% [5, 6]. Actively draining ears have a higher rate of postoperative infection compared to non-draining ears. The administration of a single dose of preoperative (within 1 hour of incision) cephalosporin, in draining ears, has been shown to reduce early (within the first week) postoperative infection rates threefold. However, this protective effect disappears in the second postoperative week [5]. As such, there is no compelling indication for the use of perioperative antibiotics for otologic surgery. Patients with diabetes have their blood glucose level checked and if necessary treated to prevent hyperglycemia, which has been associated with surgical site infection (SSI) [7]. Neurotologic and skull base procedures require medications aimed at brain protection and infection control. For the purpose of brain protection, preoperative intravenous mannitol 0.5 to 1 g/kg (usually 75 g) and dexamethasone 10 mg are given intravenously. In contrast to otological surgery, prophylactic antibiotics are routinely used for skull base procedures. The antibiotic of choice should be effective against *Staphylococcus aureus* as this is the most commonly cultured organism from neurosurgical SSIs. Either oxacillin 1 g, or a cefazolin 1 g, is given intravenously within 1 hour of incision. If the patient is allergic to both penicillin and cephalosporins, then vancomycin is employed in a dose appropriate to the patient's weight. If the procedure is lengthy, intraoperative doses of antibiotics should be given at appropriate intervals. Prophylactic intravenous antibiotics are discontinued 24 hours postoperatively [7–9].

Transition to the Operating Room

As the patient is brought into the operating room, the staff present should introduce themselves to the patient and identify their role. If music is playing, it should be soothing and at a low volume to avoid affecting conversation. The patient is then assisted in transferring onto the operating table. The patient's head should be at the end of the bed with the most space underneath to accommodate the surgeon's legs while seated. While the patient is still awake, identity is confirmed, and the planned procedure and site are reconfirmed with all staff participating in this "time out" check.

Once the patient is sedated or under general anesthetic, positioning for the planned surgery is undertaken. For all otologic and neurotologic surgeries, the anesthetist is at the patient's feet. In addition to providing appropriate sedation/anesthesia, the anesthetist is charged with managing the bed controls to adjust side-to-side tilt and height. Attention is paid to protecting the patient's airway when moving the head during patient positioning. Stabilization of the endotracheal tube, once the patient is positioned, should be done in such a way so that movement of the head during dressing placement at the conclusion of surgery does not inadvertently extubate the patient. The patient then is secured to the operating table with adjustable straps to prevent patient movement when the bed is tilted side to side. For trans-temporal bone procedures, the patient's head is placed on a "donut" pillow with the head turned to place the operative site "up." Additional elevation of the head may be needed in patients with large shoulders. Often slight neck flexion will help the surgeon gain access to the temporal bone in robustly proportioned patients. Pin fixation of the head is used in retrosigmoid craniotomy and most supratentorial craniotomy cases. Clipping of hair and skin cleansing with isopropyl alcohol is undertaken before incision marking is done. Injection of local anesthetic with epinephrine along the incision site is done for hemostasis. Electrophysiological monitoring setup is then undertaken as appropriate for the planned procedure.

The scrub technician/nurse (scrub) is positioned directly opposite the surgeon in most cases. In cases where the surgeon is positioned at the top of the patient's head, the scrub is positioned on the side of the surgeon's dominant hand to facilitate instrument transfers. A video monitor is positioned so the scrub can see it, follow the course of surgery, and anticipate instrument changes. Some surgeons prefer that the scrub operate the foot pedals of all devices such as bipolar cautery and drills. Other surgeons control such foot pedals themselves as there is an inherent delay in starting and stopping the devices, since the surgeon must vocalize a command, and the scrub then reacts to it. Figures 27.1, 27.2, 27.3, and 27.4 demonstrate idealized operating room organization of patient, equipment, and staff for different surgical site examples. Each surgeon's operating room size and configuration will dictate specifics of personnel and equipment positioning.

More important than the physical organization of the operating room are the personnel that make up the operative team. It is optimal to have a consistent crew of scrub technicians, circulating nurse, anesthesia team, and neurophysiologist working with the surgeon's team. By repetition and experience, this consistent team will increase the quality of care as well as improve safety for the patient and for each other. Familiarity with the types of procedures, disease processes, surgeon preferences, and routines will decrease inadvertent errors and foster excellence from all participants.

Surgical Site Preparation

Surgical site preparation is undertaken for the purpose of limiting colonization of the wound by normal skin flora. Adequate clipping of hair to accommodate the anticipated incision(s) and extent of surgery should be done. Shaving of hair with a razor has been associated with higher wound infection rates, and clipping with an electric clipper is now recommended [7]. Cleansing of the skin with isopropyl alcohol helps to further reduce the bacterial count as well as remove skin oils in preparation for incision marking,

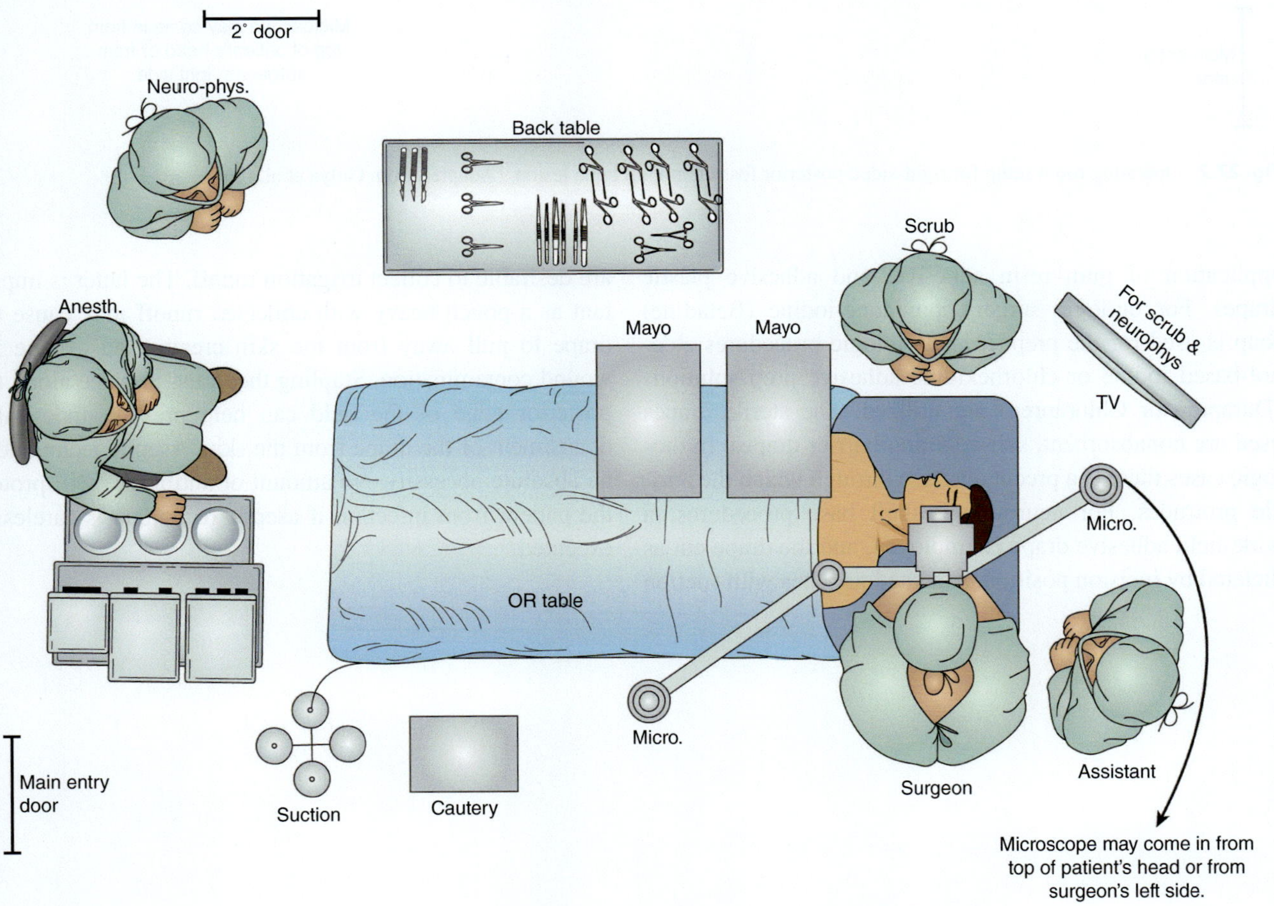

Fig. 27.1 Operating room setup for left-sided posterior fossa/temporal bone lesion. (Adapted from Gulya et al. [16])

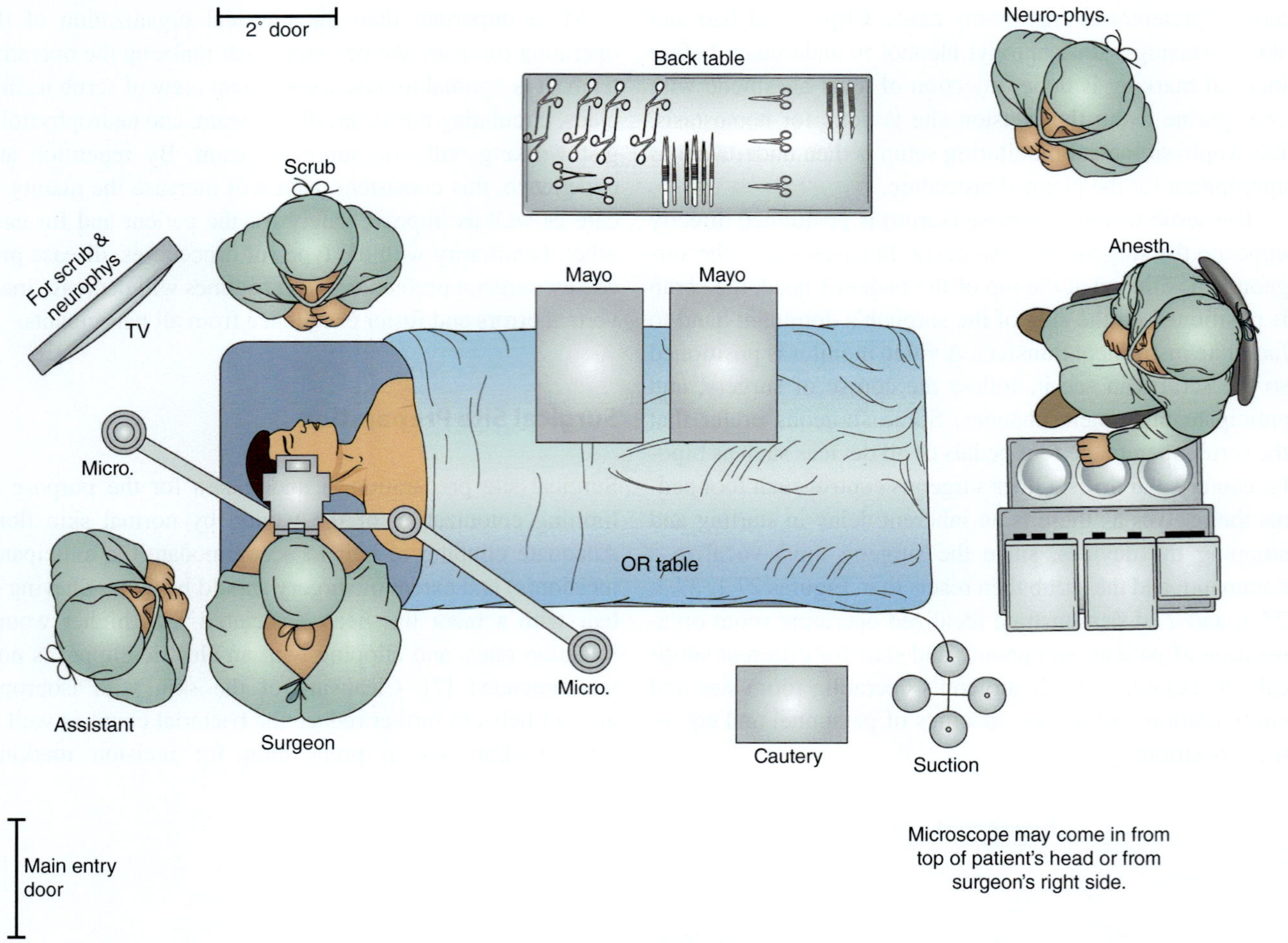

Fig. 27.2 Operating room setup for right-sided posterior fossa/temporal bone lesion. (Adapted from Gulya et al. [16])

application of gum resin adhesive, and adhesive plastic drapes. For otologic surgery, povidone-iodine (Betadine) soap is used for the prep. In neurotologic procedures alcohol-based iodine or chlorhexidine adhesive prep solutions (Duraprep or Chloraprep) are utilized. The sterile drapes used are nonabsorbent, self-adhering barrier drapes. In otologic cases there is a precut aperture through which the auricle protrudes. For neurotologic/skull base procedures, a wide-field adhesive drape is employed, and the drape cut as dictated by incision position. Attached pouches with suction are desirable to collect irrigation runoff. The latter is important as a pouch heavy with collected runoff may cause the drape to pull away from the skin creating an avenue for wound contamination. Stapling the drape in place along the posterior edge of the field can help prevent undesirable detachment of the drape from the skin. Aseptic technique is an absolute necessity. No amount of antibiotics will protect the patient from infection if aseptic technique is carelessly executed.

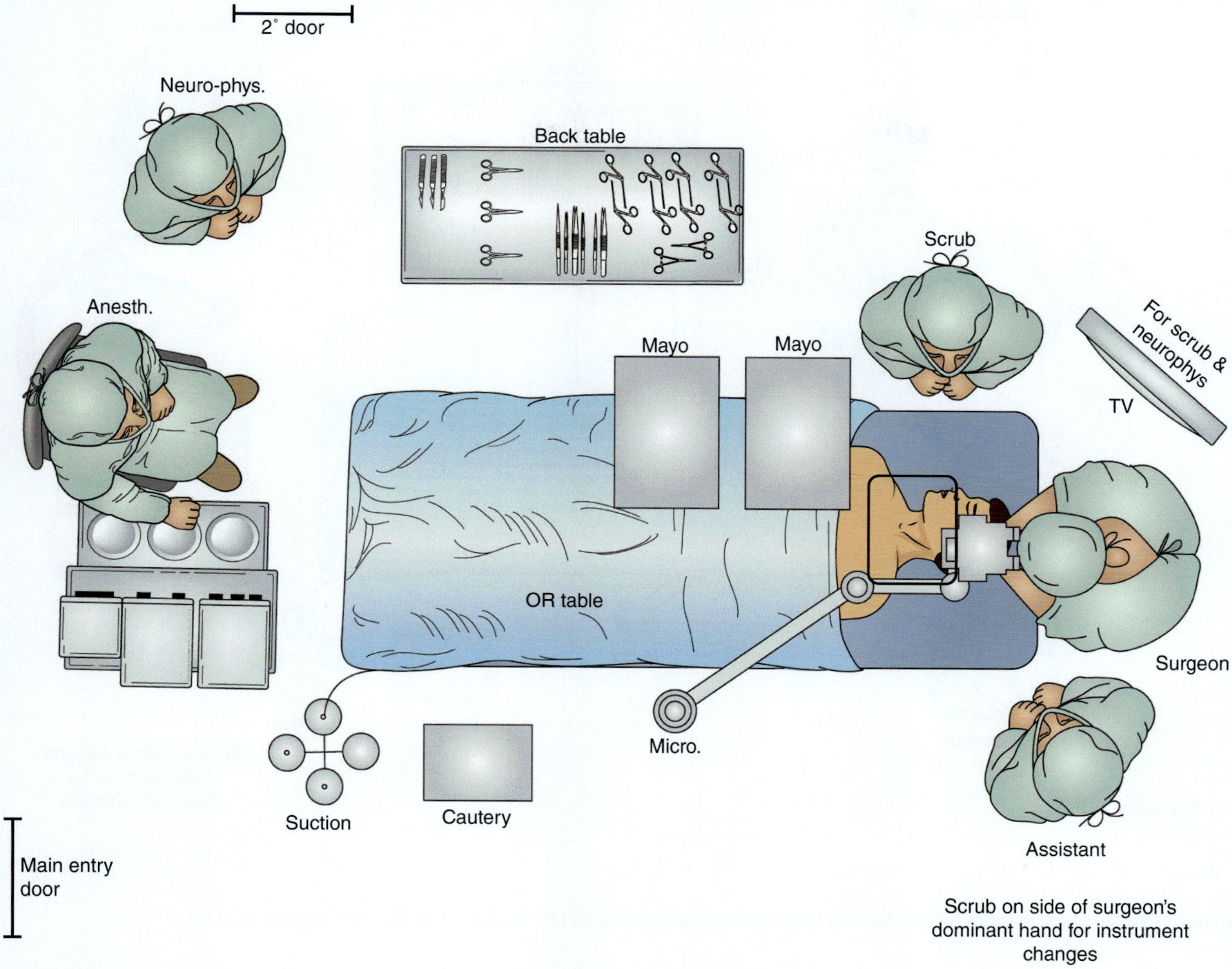

Fig. 27.3 Operating room setup for a right-handed surgeon seated at top of patient's head. (Adapted from Gulya et al. [16])

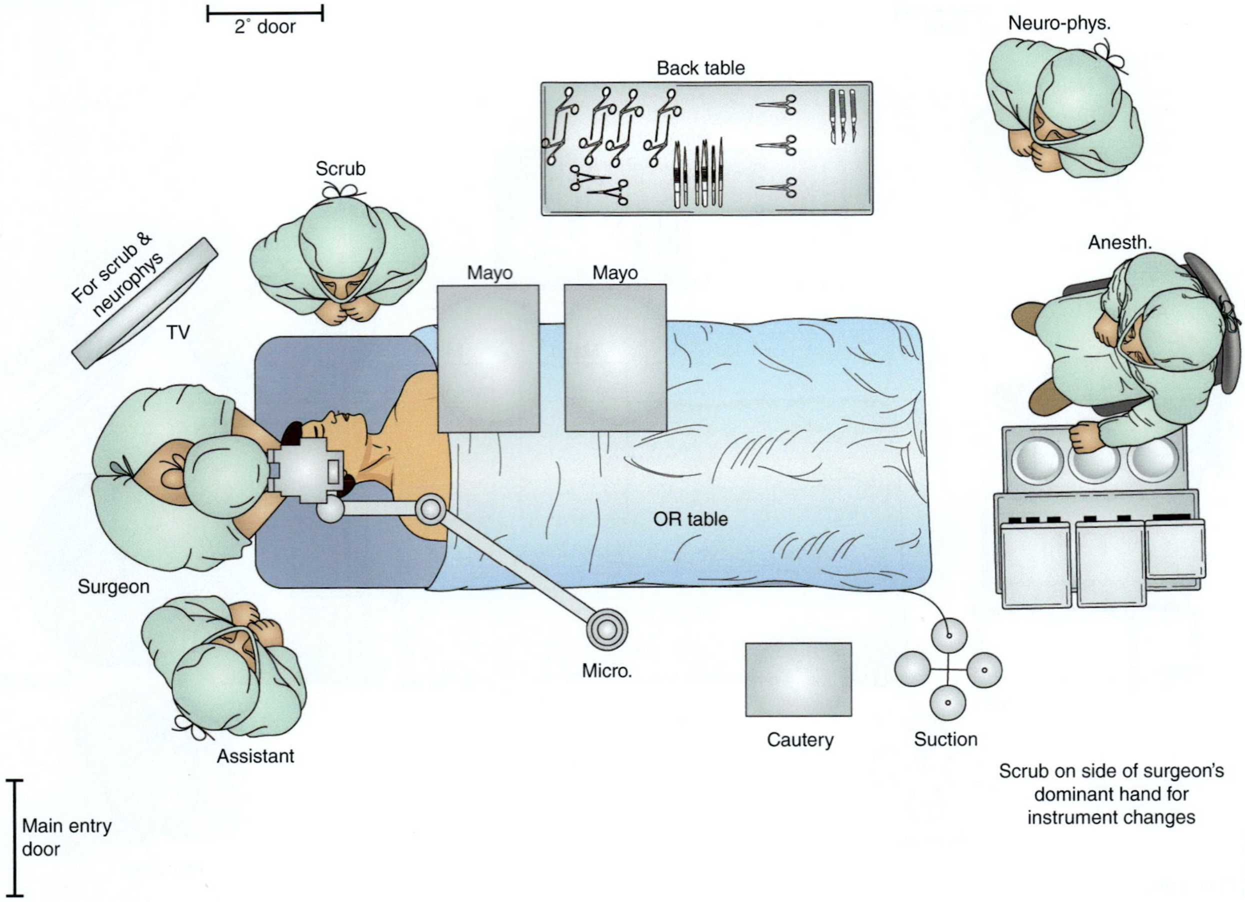

Fig. 27.4 Operating room setup for left-handed surgeon seated at top of patient's head. (Adapted from Gulya et al. [16])

Surgical Technique

This section will focus on basic principles. Specifics related to incisions, degree of bone removal, etc. for particular approaches/diseases will be covered in their respective chapters. Proper handling of tissues throughout the procedure will maximize tissue vitality and consequently proper healing. Tissue that is crushed, devascularized, or allowed to desiccate will not heal well and will be more susceptible to infection and necrosis. Maintaining hemostasis and optimal exposure is a critical element contributing to successful otologic/neurotologic surgery. Proper bone dissection technique is critical for maximizing speed and safety during this phase of temporal bone/skull base surgery. Identification of vital structures away from involvement by pathology makes for safer disease removal. Finally, meticulous multilayered wound closure will provide better cosmesis and lower risk of complications such as CSF leak.

Hemostasis

The demand for hemostasis in microsurgery surpasses that required during more typical procedures in the head and neck. To achieve the degree of hemostasis required for microsurgery, special tactics must be mastered. Injection of local anesthetic with epinephrine is the first step of both providing comfort for the patient and vasoconstriction of vessels in the surgical field. For otologic surgeries done under local anesthetic with sedation, the pattern of injections will differ based on the specific procedure. For transcanal procedures, injections of 2% xylocaine with 1:100,000 epinephrine (total volume usually 2–3 mL) are placed in the tragus (Fig. 27.5), the incisura (cleft between the tragus and root of helix; Fig. 27.6), and the floor and posterior aspect of the lateral portion of the canal (Figs. 27.7 and 27.8). Deeper canal injections can be made with 2% xylocaine with 1:50,000 epinephrine (usually less than 1 mL) starting in the vascular

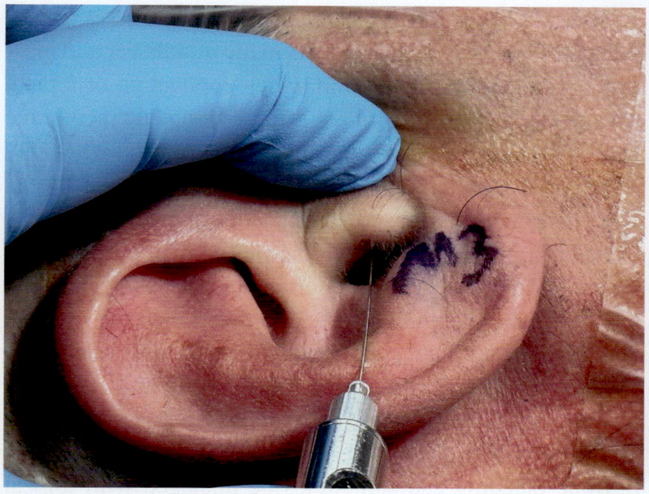

Fig. 27.5 Tragal injection of local anesthetic with epinephrine

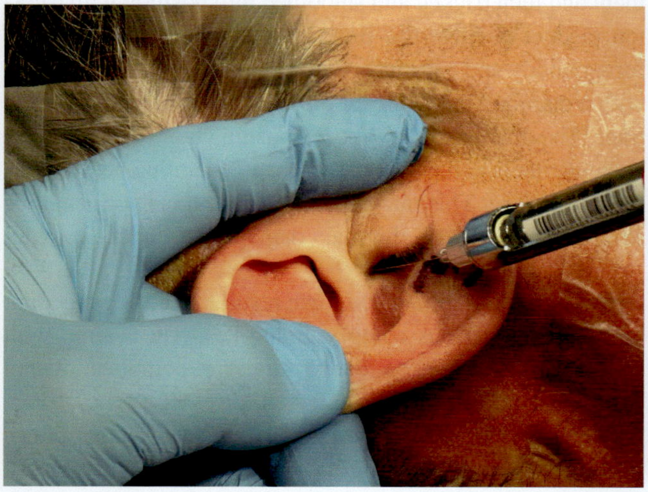

Fig. 27.6 Local anesthetic injection in incisura

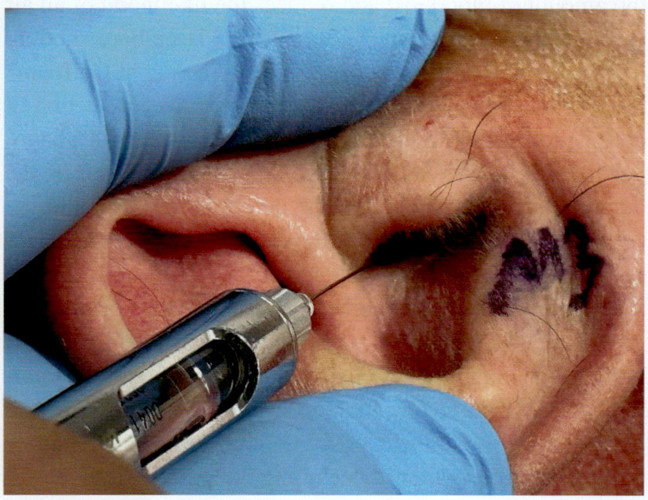

Fig. 27.7 Floor of lateral ear canal injection

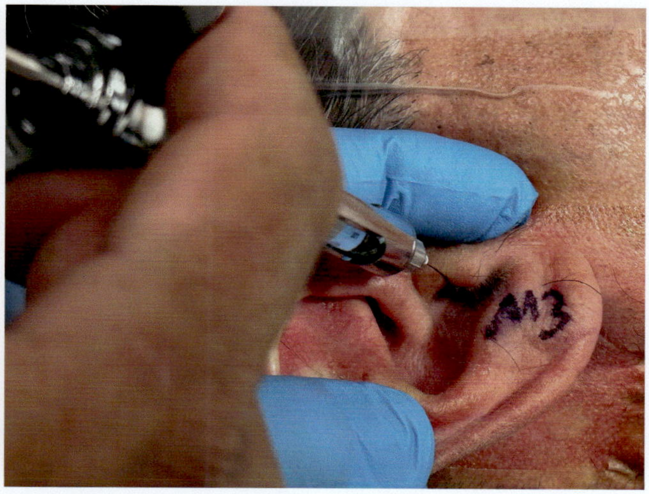

Fig. 27.8 Posterior ear canal injection

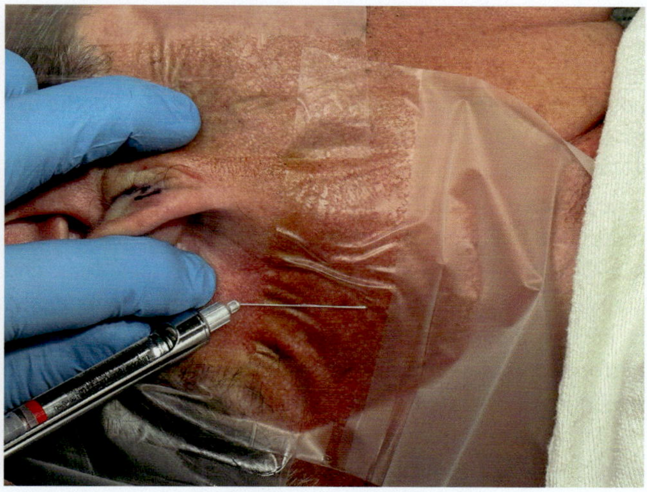

Fig. 27.9 Demonstration of entry point and subcutaneous course of needle for greater auricular nerve block

strip, then two anterior canal injections, and the last injection along the floor of the canal. These deeper injections start in the more mobile, hair bearing, portion of the canal skin with the needle tip contacting the bone of the medial-ear canal. Gentle injection pressure must be used to prevent a bleb in the deep canal skin.

For postauricular procedures under local anesthetic, the canal injections are the same, but are preceded first by placement of a greater auricular nerve block (Fig. 27.9). This is followed by injection of the postauricular tissues along the anticipated incision line (Fig. 27.10). The tissues from dermis to periosteum are injected with 2% xylocaine with 1:100,000 epinephrine. The areas of the zygomatic root, superior and posterior to the incision line, receive additional injection for a total volume of 5 to 6 mL. If mastoidectomy is anticipated, these latter areas are augmented with 0.5%

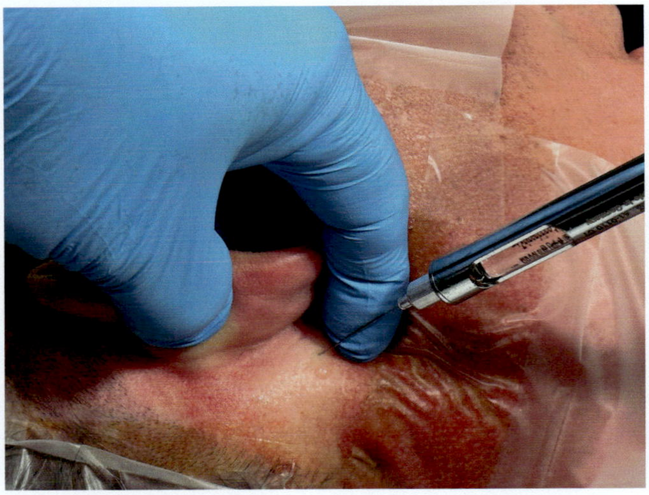

Fig. 27.10 Injection of postauricular tissues. The index finger palpates the mastoid tip

marcaine with 1:200,000 epinephrine (total of 3–5 mL). To better control the rate of injection, the author favors the use of dental syringes with commercially available carpules of xylocaine/marcaine and epinephrine in the concentrations noted above. Additionally, the carpules are labeled and reduce the likelihood of a medication error. The needle used is a 27-gauge, 1 ¼-inch-long dental needle. Total volume and concentration of the injected local anesthetic are announced to the anesthetist and nurse, to be recorded. For procedures performed under general anesthetic, the same pattern of injections is used (with the elimination of the greater auricular nerve block and marcaine injections) as a carrier for the epinephrine. The injections (apart from the deep canal injections) are administered prior to the surgeon scrubbing as this gives adequate time for optimal vasoconstriction to occur. Infiltration of the intended incision sites for neurotologic procedures with xylocaine/epinephrine is also undertaken for hemostasis.

Electrocautery is an indispensable tool for achieving hemostasis. Use of monopolar electrocautery is limited to the soft tissues of the skin and muscles. Bipolar cautery, specifically microbipolar cautery (usually irrigating), is most helpful once the microscope is being used. With bipolar cautery the strength of current required for hemostasis and the related current spread is reduced resulting in a lower risk of adjacent tissue damage. Bipolar cautery is most useful for achieving hemostasis on exposed dura, the exposed sigmoid sinus, adjacent to the facial nerve, middle-ear mucosa, ear canal skin flaps, and the internal auditory canal. The surgeon's experience and familiarity with their equipment will guide the current level suitable for specific sites, but if questions arise, the current level may be tested on exposed muscle or other soft tissue in the surgical field.

Topical application of concentrated epinephrine is a valuable tool for achieving hemostasis in the middle ear and mastoid. Specific circumstances in which application of topical epinephrine is most helpful are prior to tympanic membrane graft placement, prior to stapes manipulation, and when dissecting diseased middle-ear mucosa or granulation tissue. One can employ an absorbable gelatin sponge (Gelfoam®) soaked in 1:1000 epinephrine. The Gelfoam® is placed in the area requiring hemostasis and left in place for a few minutes. Work is undertaken elsewhere, and then when the surgeon removes the Gelfoam®, remarkably good hemostasis is usually encountered. It is rare to have even minimal change in heart rate or blood pressure with the topical use of epinephrine as described.

Bone bleeding can sometimes be managed with topical epinephrine, but commonly bone wax is needed to achieve hemostasis. A piece of bone wax is delivered on an instrument and then packed and smoothed into position with a cotton pledget or fingertip. Bone wax should be considered a foreign body and used judiciously in infected fields. Drilling with a diamond bur is useful for achieving hemostasis in the bone. The diamond bur works by pushing bone dust into vascular channels in the bone rather than generating heat to cauterize the bone. This maneuver should be done with copious irrigation to avoid thermal damage to adjacent vital structures.

Injury to the sigmoid sinus can result in startling bleeding and potential serious complications. Properly dealing with this event is necessary to reduce the risk of complication and to maximize the chance of maintaining vessel patency. Since the sigmoid sinuses are the main avenue for venous return from the brain, "packing it off" should remain a last resort. Should the sinus be violated, rather than place suction at the opening while getting ready to deal with the injury, the surgeon should occlude the defect with a fingertip. This limits the amount of blood lost and reduces the likelihood of an air embolus. Next the scrub should attach a large-bore suction/irrigation tip to the tubing, assemble a selection of Gelfoam® squares soaked in saline or thrombin, and have a selection of cotton pledgets ready. The surgeon then selects, with a bayonet forceps, a Gelfoam® square larger than the size of the defect. The finger occluding the defect is removed and the Gelfoam® square placed over the defect. Next a cotton pledget larger than the Gelfoam® square is picked up using the suction and placed over the Gelfoam®. Compression with the large-bore suction and bayonet forceps on this "Gelfoam® patch" is maintained with irrigation turned on and off intermittently. Within a few moments, the Gelfoam® will have become adherent to the exposed dura of the sinus effectively sealing the defect without occluding the vessel. Slight elevation of the patient's head done by placing the table in reverse Trendelenburg position will reduce venous pressure and can assist in achieving hemostasis. However, this maneuver must be used with caution to avoid an air embolus. Defects in the sinus, as large as 1 cm, may be "patched" with this technique. Should this technique fail, suture repair of the sinus may be employed. Small openings in the sinus may be "welded" shut using bipolar cautery if there is sufficient mobility of the sinus wall to pinch the hole closed with the bipolar forceps.

Should all other options fail, then packing the sinus becomes necessary. Proximal flow can often be managed by extraluminal packing. The dura of the sinus is dissected from its bony covering near the sinodural angle. Then absorbable oxidized regenerated cellulose (Surgicel™) is packed between the bone and dura to extraluminally compress the sinus. The same technique may be used with the distal portion of the sinus. Should intraluminal packing be needed, longer strips of Surgicel™ should be used with a tail left coming out of the defect in the sinus. This prevents embolization of the packing material into the central venous circulation. Panic is to be avoided, as the medial wall of the sinus may be breached and the intracranial contents compressed by overzealous packing.

Exposure

The key to all surgery, and in particular otologic/neurotologic surgery, is adequate exposure. One simply must see what one is doing in the anatomically complex temporal bone. Developing a sequential pattern of bone dissection for various temporal bone procedures will ensure that the optimal exposure is achieved for the task at hand. One must resist the temptation to reach the deeper structure of interest prior to achieving the desired degree of lateral exposure first. Creating a narrow, deep corridor can yield disorientation from a lack of anatomic landmarks and result in injury to vital structures. While the details of specific incisions and bone removal will be left to other chapters, the principle of adequate exposure must be emphasized. Incision and bone-removal planning should allow appropriate visualization and access (distal and proximal control) to the neurovascular structures traversing the intended surgical field. Furthermore, contingencies must be made should the exposure need extension to deal with intraoperative complications.

The authors recommend use of the operating microscope for all aspects of temporal bone and skull base surgery with the exception of initial soft tissue work. The microscope should possess the following characteristics: high-quality optics, variable magnification, objectives with appropriate focal distances, adjustable eye pieces, mounted camera for photo/video documentation, and finally a suitable stand, which may be finely balanced. The microscope must be prepared by the surgeon prior to draping. The surgeon should check the diopter settings and ensure that the observer and operating oculars are par focal. The microscope should be balanced to allow full range of motion with minimal effort. During surgery, the surgeon should be in an ergonomically sound sitting position using a chair which provides good back support during microscope use. This will reduce fatigue and avoid back and neck problems related to improper sitting position. Starting temporal bone drilling under microscopic magnification provides better illumination, a better view of the anatomy, and protection against bone dust and irrigation, which may carry potentially lethal viruses (hepatitis C, HIV, prions). By using the lowest magnification suitable for each step in the surgery maximizes field of view and depth of field.

An intimate knowledge of the three-dimensional anatomic relationships (and their variations) within the temporal bone, especially the course of the facial nerve, is mandatory for efficient and safe bone removal. The temporal bone lab is where a temporal bone surgeon should begin to explore the complex temporal-bone anatomy. Likewise, the lab is where a practicing surgeon can rehearse an uncommonly done procedure. Learning the anatomic "pointers" to the facial nerve, the digastric ridge, chorda tympani, the lateral and posterior semicircular canals, the incus/fossa incudus, the cochleariform process, the "cog," the pyramidal process, the oval window, Jacobson's nerve, greater and lesser superficial petrosal nerves, Bill's bar, and the eighth cranial nerve are crucial to becoming an accomplished temporal bone surgeon [10]. This knowledge provides the surgeon a number of options for finding the nerve in a location away from where it is affected by pathology. The facial nerve should then be traced into the area of pathology. As the facial nerve is dissected, should direct exposure of the sheath be required, the bone overlying the nerve is thinned to an "eggshell," and then this thin layer of bone is carefully dissected from the sheath. This sequence of dissection will reduce the likelihood of facial nerve injury. The facial nerve should be viewed as a welcome landmark, routinely sought out during all manner of temporal bone procedures. Use of electromyographic facial nerve monitoring is a useful tool for informing the surgeon during dissection directly on the sheath or nerve itself. However, such monitoring is no substitute for knowledge of anatomy or proper technique when seeking out the nerve during dissection.

Fearing the facial nerve and avoiding its identification make inadvertent injury more likely. The same is true of the internal carotid artery in complex skull base surgeries. Identifying this important vessel away from the area of disease involvement and achieving proximal and distal control are prerequisites for embarking on tumor dissection along its course. The potential for morbidity/mortality is greatest in those tumors that intimately involve the internal carotid artery. The modern skull base surgeon should be prepared to manage injury to this vessel themselves or by having appropriate team members assembled for such cases.

Bone Dissection

Next in importance is the use of drilling technique that allows for rapid bone removal while sequentially identifying and delineating anatomic landmarks, which then help lead the surgeon to subsequent structures. Modern high-speed, high-torque drills (both pneumatic and electric) should rightfully be called bone dissection tools. These tools allow for rapid bone removal with minimal force needed from the surgeon's hand. This combination of attributes allows a sense of feel with the drill similar to that of a scalpel on tissue. Just as a surgeon would not use a dull scalpel, brand new burs should be used with every case. Dull burs require more pressure to remove bone, reduce sense of feel, and escalate the risk of injury.

Just as it takes time and experience to develop the "feel" required for soft tissue surgery, the same is true of bone dissection. The novice temporal bone surgeon will commonly use a very light pressure stroke with rapid side-to-side motion of the drill, which results in very little bone removal and sets up a dangerous rhythm that may be difficult to stop when a vital structure is encountered. Additionally, the irrigation component of the suction irrigator is commonly poorly aimed and either kept too wet or too dry. The safest and most efficient technique of bone dissection is similar to that of a computer numerical control (CNC) milling machine. In a CNC machine, the computer has a shape three-dimensionally programmed as numerical coordinates. The computer then drives a milling tool to create the programmed shape out of a block of solid material. The temporal bone surgeon should have in mind the idealized temporal bone anatomy as that programmed three-dimensional shape. Different from a CNC machine, the surgeon is able to see the temporal bone structures as they are approached and modify the bone dissection to follow the contours of the structures encountered. In this way the anatomy of the neurovascular structures that traverse the temporal bone are "liberated" from their bony encasement.

When drilling with well-applied suction irrigation, the bone is kept moist and does not develop significant, opaque, white dusting. Wet bone remains translucent. If one cannot see an anatomic structure through the wet bone to be drilled, it is likely to be at least 2 to 3 mm thick. That much bone can be safely removed in a single, measured stroke with a cutting bur; the pressure exerted to remove the bone should be measured, not maximal. If maximal pressure is used, there is greater risk of loss of control and therefore injury. The hands should be supported against the patient's head for optimal stability. Using the side of the bur achieves the most effective bone removal. Use of the tip should be avoided. The largest bur suitable for the task should be used as it will expose structures in a broader fashion. Inappropriately small burs tend to penetrate structures and cause injury. Expose and delineate the lateral anatomy developing a sequence of anatomic landmarks that lead to deeper structures. Broad, saucerized-lateral exposure eliminates ledges or overhangs that may obscure structures, reduce illumination, and inadvertently catch the flute of a cutting bur causing it to jump. Keep the field clear of bone dust as it can hide vital structures making them susceptible to injury. Furthermore, bone dust is prone to osteoneogenesis and if left in the middle ear may contribute to conductive hearing loss.

The depth of bone removal should be predetermined by the surgeon and modified by feedback from one's senses. The senses of sight, touch, and hearing should be employed while drilling. The sound generated by drilling will change to a high-pitched tone when approaching areas of thin bone overlying the dura. The structures to be identified through thin bone will have different colors and characteristic locations through the temporal bone. Differences in bone density can be discerned by the degree of pressure required for bone removal while drilling. When the edge of a landmark is approached, pressure is reduced to avoid the drill flipping past the edge or injuring the structure. When the bone over a structure is thinned, it may be visible through 0.5 to 1 mm of wet bone. The different bur types are used for different purposes. The cutting burs are aggressively fluted and used for rapid bone removal. The diamond bur is used for finer, more gradual bone removal when approaching a vital structure. However, care must be taken to use adequate irrigation as the diamond bur can generate significant heat that can burn bone and cause thermal injury to vital structures such as the facial nerve.

Integral to all surgery is the closure. While important in otologic surgery, attention to detail during wound closure in skull base surgery is essential. CSF leakage remains one of the most commonly reported complications of skull base surgery [11]. Attention to approach design and meticulous, multilayer closure techniques can reduce the incidence to 1% or 2% [12, 13]. Complex closures, more frequently seen in revision surgeries, may require regional or free-flap reconstructions [14].

To close this section on operative technique, it must be emphasized that part of doing the best possible job for the patient includes knowing when one has reached their own (or the team's) limit of expertise, encountered a problem they are unprepared to manage, or have become disoriented in the surgical field. In such circumstances often the best service rendered to the patient means "backing out." By persisting under the aforementioned conditions, one greatly increases the risk of injuring the patient. Remember, *Primum non nocere*. Reassessment may allow reoperation in better circumstances or may prompt referral to a helpful colleague.

Postoperative Care

Patients following otologic/neurotologic surgery should be transferred from the operating room to a post-anesthesia care unit (PACU). The PACU staff should be trained to recognize facial nerve, cranial nerve, and other neurological dysfunction related to these surgeries. Patients are closely monitored until they are sufficiently recovered to go home or be transferred to their hospital room (intensive care unit, ICU, or medical/surgical unit). Patients undergoing otologic surgery are routinely discharged to home the day of surgery. Should severe nausea persist, then they are admitted overnight for hydration and control of nausea. This latter circumstance is most commonly seen in procedures that open the labyrinth.

Patients undergoing craniotomy are observed in the ICU. The following day, if they are in suitable condition, then they may be transferred to a medical/surgical unit for the remainder of their hospital stay. Prevention of perioperative deep venous thrombosis is important [15]. Routine use of sequential compression stockings is initiated in the operating room as part of the patient positioning. Subcutaneous heparin injections of 5000 units twice daily are started the morning following surgery. Rapid mobilization of the patient further reduces the risk of thrombus formation in the lower extremities. As permitted by the presence or absence of postoperative vertigo, patients are encouraged to be out of bed the day following surgery. Physical therapy consultation is obtained on the first postoperative day to assess and assist in ambulating patients.

Following surgery for tumors affecting the lower cranial nerves, patients may have significant problems with swallowing function and airway protection and are kept *nil* per os (NPO). Early consultation with speech/swallowing therapists is critical before starting oral intake to reduce the likelihood of aspiration pneumonia. Older patients have more difficulty compensating for these problems than do younger patients, and rehabilitation can be a lengthy process. Procedures for temporary vocal cord medialization are suitable for patients in whom recovery of nerve function is expected. Otherwise more permanent vocal cord medialization may be needed. Though uncommon, tracheotomy and gastrostomy may be necessary temporary measures for such patients. For patients without lower cranial nerve involvement, a clear liquid diet is ordered postoperatively with advance as tolerated. Rehabilitation of lower cranial nerve injury is discussed in Chap. 25.

As previously mentioned, prophylactic antibiotics following skull base surgery are continued for only 24 hours postoperatively. The use of postoperative dexamethasone (4 mg every 6 hours) for 48 hours after neurotologic cases is used to prevent/reduce brain or nerve edema. Patients with tumors causing significant preoperative brainstem/pontine compression are at risk for symptomatic re-expansion edema. Re-expansion edema can be so severe that it can cause cytotoxic changes in brain tissue resulting in permanent dysfunction. In such cases, low-dose mannitol (25 g every 6 hours for 2–3 days) may be prophylactically employed to mitigate the re-expansion edema and reduce the likelihood of cytotoxic damage. Urine and serum osmolality are monitored during the period of mannitol use. Care must be taken not to excessively dehydrate the patient as this increases the risk for venous thrombosis.

Patients with facial nerve weakness following surgery require special attention to maintaining corneal lubrication. These issues are discussed preoperatively with patients in whom the facial nerve is in peril. Use of lubricating eye drops at least hourly during the day is recommended. Moisturizing ophthalmologic ointment is used at night. A moisture chamber may also be used. Ongoing monitoring of corneal status by an ophthalmologist is recommended in patients with significant facial weakness and poor eye closure. Consultation with an oculoplastic surgeon may be necessary if more aggressive measures (gold weight, lateral tarsorrhaphy, etc.) are required to protect the cornea.

Skin staple removal occurs 10 to 14 days following skull base surgery. At this visit, the patient's recovery progress is assessed. Encouragement is given, and instructions are reinforced regarding activity level and, if appropriate, eye care. For patients experiencing vertigo following their surgery, Cawthorne exercises are given at this time. For patients not recovering well with Cawthorne exercises after 1 month, referral to physical therapy for balance rehabilitation is initiated. Most patients are able to return to work within 4 to 6 weeks following neurotologic surgery. If the patient is recovering well and there is no facial nerve dysfunction, then radiological follow-up is arranged with telephonic visits arranged to review results and plan future studies. If facial nerve or other neurological dysfunction is present, then follow-up visits every 3 to 6 months, to monitor pace of recovery, are planned.

Summary

Temporal bone and skull base surgery requires precision planning and execution to achieve the best results for patient and surgeon alike. The level of expectation for a favorable outcome is very high, and while we strive to achieve perfection, the disease process will often thwart our efforts. Proper patient education and preparation will help align expectations with the anticipated results. Every surgeon should constantly strive for excellence and routinely pursue self-critique to find opportunities for improvement in all aspects of care. Rigorous application of the principles discussed in this chapter will assist the temporal bone/skull base surgeon reach the highest levels of achievement possible.

References

1. Sen S, Potnuru PP, Hernandez N, et al. Glucagon-like peptide-1 receptor agonist use and residual gastric content before anesthesia. JAMA Surg. 2024;159:660–67.
2. Roberson JB Jr, Jackson LE, McAuley JR. Acoustic neuroma surgery: absent auditory brainstem response does not contraindicate attempted hearing preservation. Laryngoscope. 1999;109(6):904–10.
3. Danner C, Mastrodimos B, Cueva RA. A comparison of direct eighth nerve monitoring and auditory brainstem response in hearing preservation surgery for vestibular schwannoma. Otol Neurotol. 2004;25(5):826–32.
4. Doll A, Abu Eid M, Kehrli P, et al. [Aspects of FLAIR sequences, 3D-CISS and diffusion-weight MR imaging of intracranial epidermoid cysts]. J Neuroradiol. 2000;27(2):101–6.
5. Govaerts PJ, Raemaekers J, Verlinden A, Kalai M, Somers T, Offeciers FE. Use of antibiotic prophylaxis in ear surgery. Laryngoscope. 1998;108(1 Pt 1):107–10.
6. Jackson CG. Antimicrobial prophylaxis in ear surgery. Laryngoscope. 1988;98(10):1116–23.
7. Mangram AJ, Horan TC, Pearson ML, Silver LC, Jarvis WR. Guideline for prevention of surgical site infection, 1999. Hospital Infection Control Practices Advisory Committee. Infect Control Hosp Epidemiol. 1999;20(4):250–78. quiz 279-280
8. Korinek AM, Golmard JL, Elcheick A, et al. Risk factors for neurosurgical site infections after craniotomy: a critical reappraisal of antibiotic prophylaxis on 4,578 patients. Br J Neurosurg. 2005;19(2):155–62.
9. Barker FG 2nd. Efficacy of prophylactic antibiotics against meningitis after craniotomy: a meta-analysis. Neurosurgery. 2007;60(5):887–94. discussion 887-894
10. Sanna M, Khrais T, Mancini F, Russo A, Taibah A, editors. The facial nerve in temporal bone and lateral skull base microsurgery. New York: Thieme Medical Publishers; 2006.
11. Selesnick SH, Liu JC, Jen A, Newman J. The incidence of cerebrospinal fluid leak after vestibular schwannoma surgery. Otol Neurotol. 2004;25(3):387–93.
12. Cueva RA, Mastrodimos B. Approach design and closure techniques to minimize cerebrospinal fluid leak after cerebellopontine angle tumor surgery. Otol Neurotol. 2005;26(6):1176–81.
13. Sanna M, Taibah A, Russo A, Falcioni M, Agarwal M. Perioperative complications in acoustic neuroma (vestibular schwannoma) surgery. Otol Neurotol. 2004;25(3):379–86.
14. Jackson CG, Netterville JL, Glasscock ME 3rd, et al. Defect reconstruction and cerebrospinal fluid management in neurotologic skull base tumors with intracranial extension. Laryngoscope. 1992;102(11):1205–14.
15. Epstein NE. A review of the risks and benefits of differing prophylaxis regimens for the treatment of deep venous thrombosis and pulmonary embolism in neurosurgery. Surg Neurol. 2005;64(4):295–301; discussion 302.
16. Gulya AJ, Minor LB, Poe D, editors. Glasscock and Shambaugh's surgery of the ear. 6th ed. PMPH; 2010.

Neurophysiologic Monitoring in Otologic and Neurotologic Surgery

28

William J. Riggs, Michael S. Harris, and Oliver F. Adunka

Introduction

Intraoperative neurophysiologic monitoring is a valuable tool which allows for the assessment of neural elements of both the central and peripheral systems during surgery. As such, consistent and reliable monitoring typically serves as an important adjuvant to localization and protection of critical neural structures and helps to improve outcomes in complex procedures of the lateral skull base where both peripheral and central nervous system structures are at risk of injury. Specifically, surgeries involving the cerebellopontine angle (CPA) have utilized the latest advances in monitoring to aid with real-time intraoperative decision making. Otologic/neurotologic surgeons have been at the forefront of these developments and have been able to successfully utilize these monitoring techniques to minimize neurological deficits while providing adequate resections [1, 2, 3].

Facial Nerve Monitoring

The utility of neurophysiologic monitoring of the facial nerve during surgery of the internal auditory canal and CPA has been reflected in decreasing incidence in facial paralysis following surgery [4, 5]. Currently, facial nerve monitoring can involve two approaches: electromyography (EMG) or facial nerve motor evoked potentials (FNMEPs) using transcranial electrical stimulation. Both techniques measure compound motor evoked potentials at the peripheral muscle innervated by the facial nerve but differ in how these responses are elicited. EMG monitoring is most commonly utilized and often readily available, whereas FNMEPs require a more sophisticated setup including dedicated equipment and a highly trained technologist well versed in this modality. However, both facial nerve monitoring techniques have their advantages and disadvantages. When used together, these two approaches can provide the operating surgeon with significant advantages in evaluation of the integrity of the facial nerve.

W. J. Riggs · O. F. Adunka (✉)
Department of Otolaryngology—Head and Neck Surgery, The Ohio State University Wexner Medical Center, Columbus, OH, USA
e-mail: oliver.adunka@osumc.edu

M. S. Harris
Division of Otology and Neurotologic Skull Base Surgery, Department of Otolaryngology and Communication Sciences, Medical College of Wisconsin, Milwaukee, WI, USA

Electromyography (EMG)

Typically, there are three separate or simultaneous EMG acquisition formats: continuous or free-run EMG (FEMG), triggered EMG (TEMG), and stimulated EMG (SEMG). Free-run EMG is recorded in real time, typically employing sweep durations of 200 milliseconds to 5 seconds. Triggered EMG allows for the capture of spontaneous responses that exceed a preset voltage. Many commercial systems provide an audible warning when the EMG activity exceeds the preset voltage. Stimulated EMG records responses to a stimulus source such as a hand-held probe designed specifically for cranial nerve stimulation. Depending on the manufacturer, commercially available systems may employ one or a combination of the three acquisition formats. Figure 28.1 demonstrates free-run EMG in two different conditions of stimulus.

Generally, two configurations may be employed for monitoring EMG from the face and other cranial nerves: monopolar and bipolar. In a monopolar and bipolar electrode configuration, the amplifier records the difference in activity between two strategically placed electrodes. Monopolar recordings use active electrodes placed in the desired myotomes (e.g., orbicularis oculi muscle for the facial [VII] nerve or the masseter muscle for the trigeminal [V] nerve), and a reference electrode is neutrally placed (e.g., lateral forehead on the opposite side of the head from the active electrodes). Bipolar recordings are obtained by placing both the active and reference electrodes in

A. D. Sweeney et al. (eds.), *Haynes-Glasscock-Shambaugh Surgery of the Ear*, https://doi.org/10.1007/978-3-032-18264-7_28

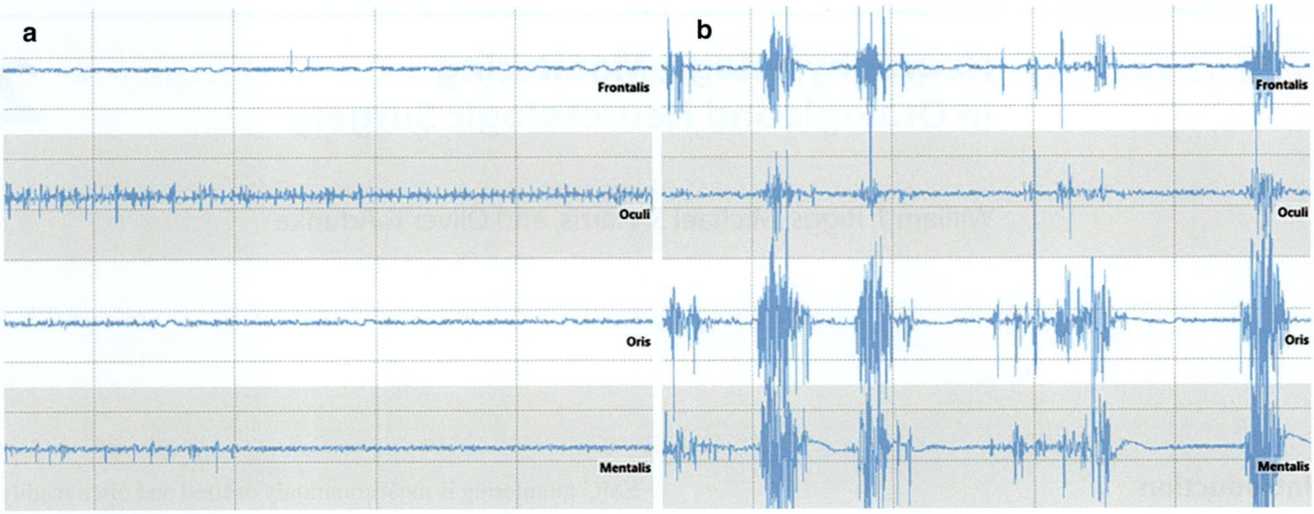

Fig. 28.1 Free-run electromyography (FEMG) and triggered EMG (TEMG) acquired during surgery. All of the muscles exhibit spontaneous activity secondary to inadvertent stimulation of the facial nerve during tumor manipulation. The first panel shows neurotonic discharges following manipulation of the facial nerve (**a**). Repetitive EMG burst activity is seen with manipulation of the nerve (**b**). (Figure courtesy of Scott Crosby, CNIM)

the muscle. Both methods are acceptable and use a differential amplifier common to most current recording systems. True referential recorders may be used only with amplifiers specifically designed to provide this type of recording methodology. A referential amplifier subtracts the activity of the reference electrode from the activity of the active electrode or electrodes. This results in greater specificity, reduced noise, and the convenience of using fewer electrodes.

EMG Response Type

The EMG response displayed on the recording device should be evaluated for its duration as well as its waveform morphology. A single motor unit potential EMG response is termed a "spike," whereas multiple quick spikes are termed a "burst." When the EMG activity is sustained over an extended period of time, >1 s, it is termed a "train" [6, 7]. Further, the morphology of the response can be described and has been correlated to outcomes. Romstock and colleagues [8] identified three main types of EMG train activity: A, B, and C (Fig. 28.2). An "A train" is characterized by rapid onset and offset sinusoidal, high-frequency activity ranging in magnitude of approximately 100–200 μV. "B-trains" can be either made of spikes or bursts and usually have a slow onset and last up to several minutes. "C-trains" are identified by a continuous irregular activity or spikes and trains ranging from less than 100 μV to several thousand microvolts. Outcomes of Romstock et al. [8] found that A-trains correlated highly with postoperative facial palsy in patients undergoing CPA tumor resection, whereas "B" and "C" trains failed to correlate with postoperative facial nerve dysfunction.

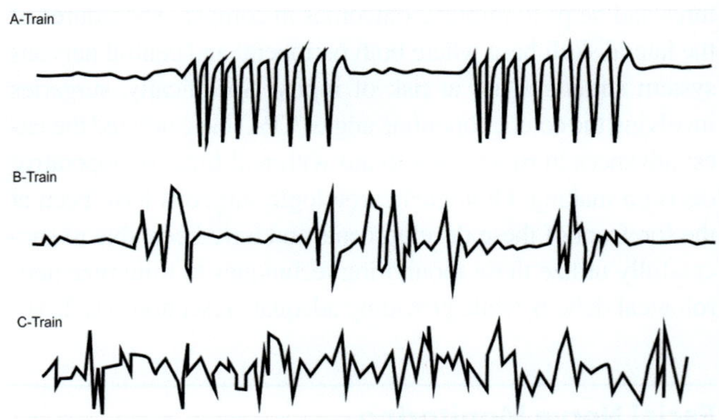

Fig. 28.2 Three types of electromyographic (EMG) train responses as described by Romstock and colleagues [8]: A-train, B-train, and C-train. Note the A-trains have a distinct pattern with abrupt on- and off-set morphology. The A-train pattern was shown to be associated with postoperative facial nerve deficits

Direct Nerve Stimulation

If the surgeon chooses to utilize stimulated EMG, the electrode setup will require a reference or return electrode, which is usually placed at the shoulder near the ground. In most surgical conditions, two channels of facial nerve EMG are adequate. However, in large tumors in which the seventh nerve may be splayed across the surface of the tumor, three or four channels of EMG representing additional branches of the facial nerve provide greater sensitivity. Figure 28.3 shows EMG activity recorded continuously from four facial muscles. EMG activity limited to the oris and mentalis muscles in response to stimulus is evident.

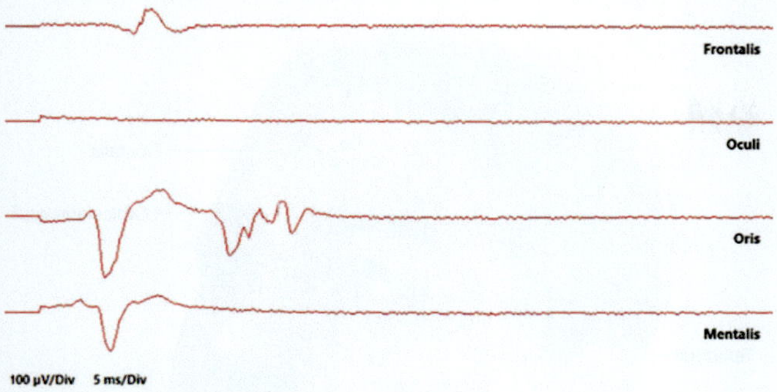

Fig. 28.3 Triggered electromyographic activity showing responses captured to a 0.5 mA trigger. (Figure courtesy of Scott Crosby, CNIM)

Stimulation of the nerve with electric current should be performed at the lowest possible current level possible. Pulse duration and the voltage or current determine the strength of the stimulus. Most commercial systems use a pulse width of 0.05 or 0.10 μs and provide intensity integrals of 0.05 or 0.10 mA. During initial stages of tumor resection, when the location of the seventh nerve may not be obvious, spontaneous EMG activity would suggest close proximity to the nerve. In this instance, a slightly higher pulse intensity (0.10–0.20 mA) is useful when searching for the nerve in a field in which anatomy is distorted (referred to as "search mode" by the authors). At the conclusion of surgery, the functional integrity of the facial nerve may be estimated by determining the lowest current level required for facial nerve stimulation. If robust amplitude motor responses are obtained from the facial nerve at its exit from the brain stem with stimulation at 0.05 to 0.10 mA, then good facial function is expected. Neff and colleagues [9] showed that upon completion of tumor resection a response of ≥240 mV at ≤0.05 mA portended a House-Brackmann Grade I or II outcome in 85% (56/66) at 12 months after surgery.

Facial nerve monitoring during otologic surgery may be helpful in reducing the risk of facial nerve injury during cases in which the facial nerve may be exposed by disease (cholesteatoma, granulation tissue) or congenital variation of anatomy. Because of the fibrous sheath surrounding the nerve in the temporal bone, higher current levels, in the 0.20 to 0.50 mA range, are required to stimulate EMG responses. If attempts to stimulate the nerve are being performed through a thin bony layer, higher current levels, 0.50–1.0 mA, are required.

Facial Nerve Motor Evoked Potentials (FNMEPs)

The use of FNMEPs is growing in popularity during vestibular schwannoma surgery and provides an alternative means of evaluating the integrity of the facial nerve beyond

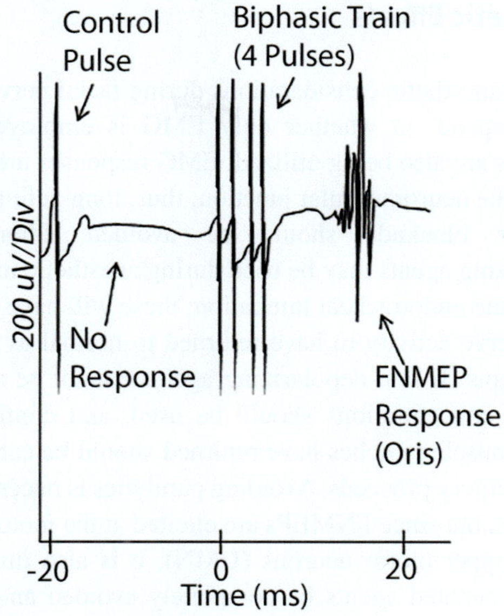

Fig. 28.4 Example of a facial nerve motor evoked response (FNMEP) recorded from the orbicularis oris muscle. No response can be seen following an initial control pulse, confirming no current spread across the scalp is occurring. A true FNMEP response is seen approximately 12 ms following a train of biphasic electrical pulses to the cortex

traditional EMG. FNMEPs involve electrical activation at the motor cortex which creates a descending volley down the supranuclear tract, ultimately out the internal auditory canal to the peripheral muscular junction [10, 11]. The technical aspects of monitoring FNMEPs are crucial to ensuring proper monitoring. Electrical stimulation utilizes a fast charge delivery paradigm (single or double train—1 or more trains of four to five pulses each) using anodal stimulation with short rapid pulse charges (pulse width of 0.5 ms) delivered to the area corresponding to the face of the contralateral motor cortex (C3-Cz [right FN stimulation] or C4-Cz [left FN stimulation]) [11]. It is imperative for meaningful interpretation of FNMEPs that direct current spread across the scalp to the extracranial muscles is avoided. To identify this, the authors urge using a single "control" pulse delivered prior to each train stimulation (Fig. 28.4). Current intensity decreases as a function of distance, and therefore it is more feasible to obtain a reliable response (not artifact due to current spread) from the orbicularis oris than oculi. Typically, the true FNMEP response will occur approximately 10–12 ms or later following stimulation of the cortex. Responses earlier than this are likely artifactual in nature and not representative of the evoked motor pathway originating at the cortex and traveling out to the periphery. Anytime FNMEPs are used, a proper bite block should be placed in the patient's mouth between the molars to prevent tongue lacerations. Outcomes in patients undergoing vestibular schwannoma resection have been reported to be an unfavorable prognosis when the FNMEP amplitude drops below 30% of its baseline amplitude [12].

Anesthetic Effects

Specific anesthetic considerations during facial nerve monitoring depend on whether only EMG is employed or if FNMEPs are also being utilized. EMG responses are dependent on the neuromuscular junction; thus, long-acting neuromuscular blockade should be avoided. Short-acting depolarizing agents may be used during anesthetic induction to facilitate endotracheal intubation; these will have allowed motor nerve activity to have returned to normal as the surgery begins. If non-depolarizing agents cannot be avoided, minimal concentrations should be used, and confirmation that all muscle twitches have returned should be carried out before surgery proceeds. Avoiding paralytics is necessary for FNMEPs, but since FNMEPs are elicited at the motor cortex via the upper motor neurons (UMN), it is also imperative that halogenated agents be completely avoided and a total intravenous anesthetic (TIVA) regimen used [13]. Inhalation agents cause a severe inhibition of the UMNs, which cannot be overcome to elicit the FNMEP needed to properly monitor the facial nerve. This is critical for obtaining optimal baselines because induction with a volatile agent and then switching to a TIVA protocol can cause inaccurate baseline measures rendering it difficult to determine a significant change in response.

Ephaptic Responses

The condition of hemifacial spasm (HFS) is thought to be caused by irritative arterial compression of the facial nerve near its root entry zone at the brainstem. Electrophysiological studies indicate that this vascular contact creates a physiologically active bridge between fibers, allowing crossover of antidromic impulses. These crossed impulses then travel distally through other branches to activate the facial muscles. The abnormal muscle response generated by nonsynaptic axonal activation (ephapse) may be recorded during EMG as the ephaptic response (ER) [14]. Monitoring the facial nerve for ER during microvascular decompression (MVD) for HFS may help the surgeon identify the offending vessel. Figure 28.5 demonstrates the stimulus and acquisition positions for EMG with ER. Stimulus electrodes are used to pass a stimulating current, and crossover motor activity is recorded on EMG.

If the surgeon is very familiar with a particular, dedicated, motor nerve monitoring device and is able to differentiate true motor responses from artifactual signals, then they may be comfortable interpreting the output of the monitoring equipment themselves. Otherwise, the use of personnel trained and qualified to perform neurophysiologic monitoring is strongly recommended. Using more sophisticated equipment and trained personnel has distinct advantages. As

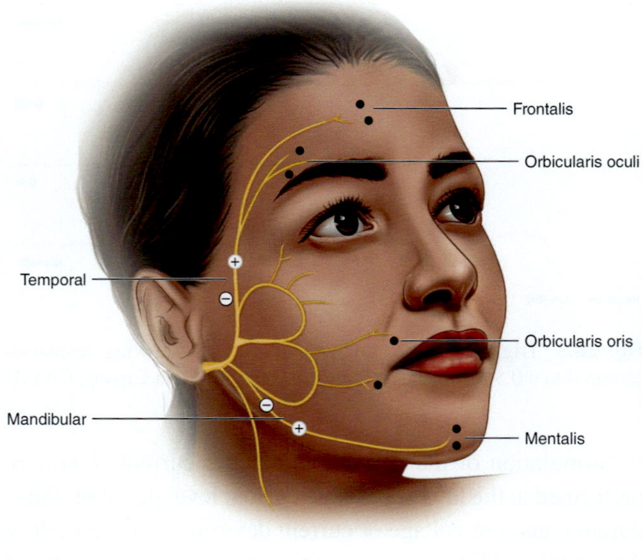

Fig. 28.5 The stimulus and acquisition sites are displayed. For stimulation of the temporal (T) and mandibular (M) branches of the seventh nerve, the anode is typically placed proximally to enhance the antidromic conduction of the action potential. A bipolar recording montage is recommended for each muscle: (**a**) frontalis, (**b**) orbicularis oculi, (**c**) orbicularis oris, and (**d**) mentalis. (Adapted from Gulya et al. [27])

noted above, multichannel monitoring equipment allows monitoring of other motor nerves and helps differentiate true facial nerve stimulation from artifact or other cranial nerve stimulation. Additionally, a diffuse increase in EMG activity in multiple muscle groups may indicate reduced depth of anesthesia, which can be disastrous during posterior cranial fossa surgery. Furthermore, use of monitoring personnel allows the surgeon to focus on dissecting rather than having to divert attention to interpret the EMG feedback. Finally, for monitoring to be successful, the surgeon must respond appropriately to the feedback provided and alter activities to reduce or eliminate facial nerve irritation.

There is no substitute for an intimate and thorough knowledge of facial nerve anatomy and its variations within the temporal bone. For the experienced surgeon, facial nerve monitoring may reduce the risk of facial nerve injury during dissection of cholesteatoma or granulation tissue from an exposed nerve. It should not serve as a crutch for finding the nerve during otherwise routine otologic surgery. Clearly, any patient who has had facial nerve symptoms related to cholesteatoma or ear infection or as a consequence of previous otologic surgery warrants facial nerve monitoring during surgery. These symptoms warn the surgeon of the high likelihood that the nerve is dehiscent and directly affected by the disease process, increasing surgical risk.

Routine facial nerve monitoring for otologic surgery remains somewhat controversial as there is disagreement regarding whether it provides significant, protective benefit to the nerve. Some authors express concern that routine use of facial nerve monitoring is no substitute for thorough knowledge of anatomy and may create a false sense of confidence for the inexperienced surgeon. For the experienced surgeon, medico-legal concerns may drive the decision regarding routine facial nerve monitoring during uncomplicated otologic cases. Therefore it is up to each surgeon to decide this issue for himself/herself.

Auditory Monitoring

Monitoring of the auditory system to achieve hearing preservation has a historical presence during vestibular schwannoma surgery and continues to be employed especially in cases which involve the CPA [15, 16]. Two techniques to carry this out are auditory brainstem response (ABR) monitoring or direct eighth nerve monitoring (DENM). Some authors not only use DENM but adapt this technique to record from the brainstem by placing a special electrode at the cochlear nucleus [17]. ABR has become the preferred and more commonly used technique; however, it is limited by the amount of time needed to obtain a reliable response. Whereas DENM is almost instantaneous, access to the recording location and electrode stability limit its use.

The best way to improve hearing preservation rates, apart from earlier diagnosis of smaller tumors, is to obtain the most rapid intraoperative feedback possible regarding the functional status of the cochlear nerve. DENM provides the closest approximation of real-time auditory function during CPA surgery and has been shown to be superior to ABR in facilitating hearing preservation [18, 19]. Reports on the use of DENM during resection of vestibular schwannomas 10 mm and smaller demonstrate hearing preservation rates in the range of 80–85% [20].A combination of both of these techniques is often utilized and provide for the optimal protocol for monitoring the integrity of the auditory pathway during lateral skull base surgery.

Auditory Brainstem Response (ABR)

The ABR is evoked by acoustic stimulation to the ear and consists of five vertex positive waves labeled I–V [21], each thought to be representing neural generators at the distal and proximal eighth nerve (waves I and II) to the level of cochlear nucleus/superior olivary complex (wave III) up to the lateral lemniscus and inferior colliculus (waves IV and V) [22, 23]. Waves I, III, and V are most reliable and, therefore, are used for continuous assessment during surgery. Amplitude (μV) and latency (ms) of the ABR can vary among subjects and are all affected by degree of hearing loss as well as neural compression to the auditory pathway caused by the tumor. Typically, the ABR waves are all captured within the first 10 ms of stimulus onset. In the normal ABR (Fig. 28.6), the poststimulus latency of wave I evoked by a suprathreshold (60–80 dB nHL [normal hearing level]) click occurs at or before 2 millisecond. Subsequent waves exhibit latencies at approximately 1 millisecond intervals. However, patients with larger tumors can show latencies past the first 10 ms if significant neural alteration exists. It is a necessary requirement to obtain a reliable ABR baseline after anesthetic induction but prior to surgical intervention. Each subject will then serve as his/her own control because all subsequent ABR recordings throughout the surgery will then be compared back to the baseline recording to determine significant changes in responses in which the surgeon needs to be alerted to.

Intraoperatively, scalp-recorded ABR is acquired by arranging sub-dermal needle electrodes around the head at opposing ends of the dipole or direction of the neuroelectric activity of the auditory neural pathway. In the operating room, it is recommended that a two-channel recording system be utilized and the waves be displayed in a vertex positive direction. The first channel setup requires the active electrode placed at midline/center of head and a reference placed at the ipsilateral mastoid or preauricular point. The second channel should utilize the aforementioned active midline electrode but should be referenced to an electrode placed at the contralateral mastoid or preauricular point. Benefits to the second channel are an enhancement of the IV-V wave complex as well as serving as a back-up in case the first channel becomes contaminated by electrical noise or an electrode becomes dislodged. Designating the midline electrode as the active allows for display of the ABR signal with vertex positive peaks.

Sound delivery is accomplished via insert ear phones placed into the ear canals and then sealing the canal off with bone wax or adhesive tape or surgical draping taking caution not to crimp any portion of the sound tube. This will ensure preparatory or other fluids do not enter the canal as well as secure the ear phone and sound tube connectors and earphones in place. For optimal ABR monitoring, the delivered stimulus typically consists of several hundred to several thousand click stimuli generated by a 100 μV square wave pulse which are then averaged by the monitoring system to display the small click-evoked responses (usually <1.0 μV) of the ABR waveform. This process is carried out every few minutes throughout the course of the procedure with the surgeon being alerted to significant changes from the baseline ABR (Fig. 28.6).

It is important to note that sensorineural hearing loss will affect the amplitude of the ABR waves, especially wave I, which is sometimes rendered absent when recording from the mastoid. However, enhancement of wave I of the ABR can be attained by placing an ear canal electrode (tiptrode). This allows for a more near-field recording at the level of the

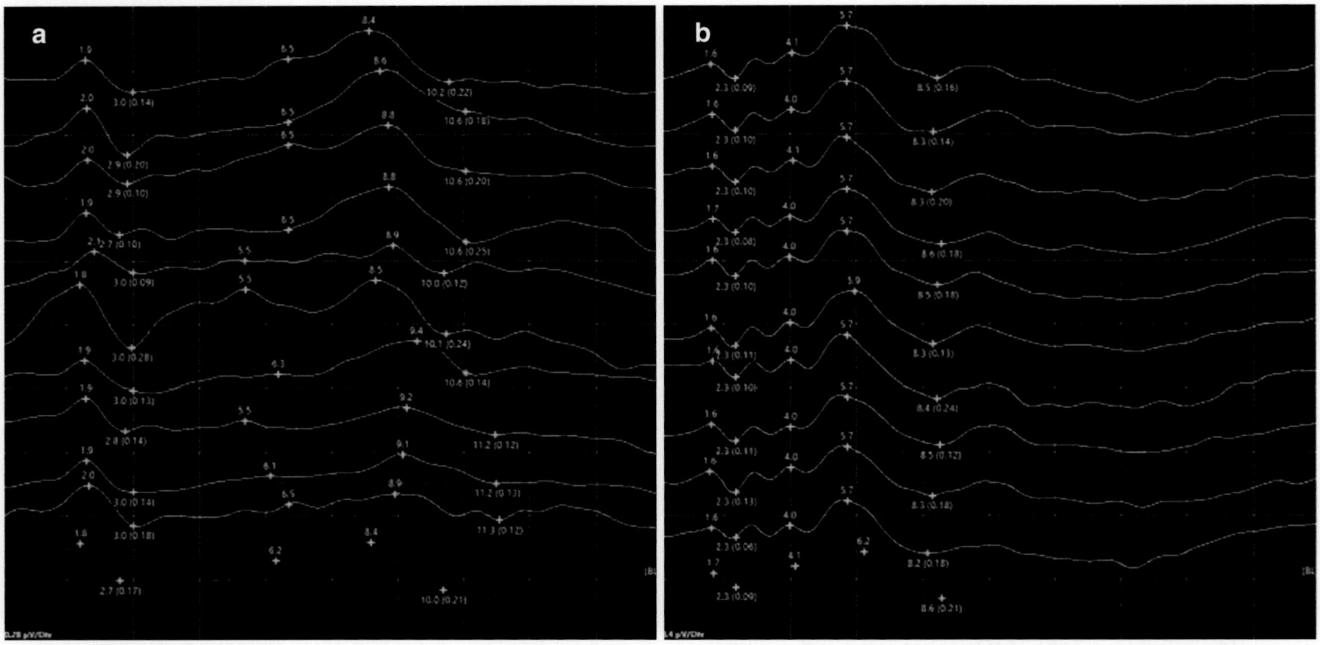

Fig. 28.6 Scalp-recorded auditory brainstem response (ABR) traces for the tumor (**a**) and non-tumor (**b**) ears of a patient with a unilateral vestibular schwannoma are shown. Serial recordings are captured in each ear. The top trace was acquired prior to tumor dissection and was used as a baseline trace by which all subsequent traces were compared. Note in the tumor ear that subsequent traces exhibit progressively greater morphologic and latency abnormalities. The non-tumor ear ABR exhibits normal morphology and normal absolute and interpeak latencies. (Figure courtesy of Scott Crosby, CNIM)

inner ear. Patients with eighth nerve or brainstem lesions rarely exhibit normal ABRs on the affected side and require interpretation by an experienced clinician or technologist.

Compound Nerve Action Potential (CNAP)

Direct eighth nerve monitoring is achieved by placing an electrode directly on cranial nerve VIII. The stimulation and acquisition parameters are similar to that of ABR monitoring, but the recorded response is the afferent compound nerve action potential (CNAP) of the vestibulocochlear nerve. The CNAP, first described by Moller and Jannetta [24], provides a robust response within a few seconds due to the near field recording directly from the nerve. Special electrodes (AD-Tech Medical Instrument Corporation; Racine, Wisconsin) are currently designed to be placed directly on the nerve proximal to the tumor and stay relatively stable and out of the surgeon's way so that continuous auditory monitoring can be carried out. A drawback to this technique is that to reach the proximal aspect of cranial nerve VIII some degree of tumor manipulation and dissection must take place prior to the electrode being placed. However, reliance on scalp ABR is typically sufficient for auditory monitoring until the electrode can be placed. The advantage of the CNAPs has previously been demonstrated by Roberson et al. [25], who reported their findings in a series of patients undergoing surgery for a vestibular schwannoma in whom the ABR was absent, yet all had a detectable CNAP.

Alarm Criteria

It is critical that the monitoring personnel continually follow the course of the procedure. This allows for correlating changes in the recorded ABR to events taking place in the field. This also helps identify non-significant changes due to other causes, such as artifact from instrumentation (bipolar, microscope, etc.) contaminating/distorting the ABR waveform. Alarm criteria for significant changes in the ABR are typically a shift (increase) in latency (ms) of wave V by 1 ms or a decrease in the amplitude (μV) of wave V by 50% or more from its baseline amplitude [26]. Other significant changes in ABR responses can include a change/increase in the interpeak latency of waves I–III, I–V, or III–V. The interpeak latency changes are thought to indicate a stretching of the vestibulocochlear nerve. Significant CNAP changes include the same criteria as the ABR alert: decrease by 50% from baseline amplitude and 1 ms increase in latency.

Other Cranial Nerve Monitoring

Electromyography is widely used to monitor other motor cranial nerves during neurotologic surgery. The motor branch of the trigeminal nerve, the vagus nerve, the spinal accessory nerve, and the hypoglossal nerve are commonly monitored using EMG [8]. These nerves have been monitored primarily in patients undergoing surgery for tumors affecting the CPA, jugular foramen, and Meckel's cave.

Monitoring of the other motor cranial nerves involves placing either needle or surface electrodes in or near the muscles innervated by the nerve of interest. In the case of the trigeminal nerve, the masseter or temporalis muscle may be used. Needle electrode placement into the trapezius and tongue muscles for monitoring the spinal accessory and hypoglossal nerves, respectively, is readily accomplished. Monitoring the vagus nerve is more challenging and requires either direct laryngoscopy for needle electrode placement into the vocalis muscles of the true vocal cords or use of a specially designed endotracheal tube that incorporates surface electrodes on its surface. As with facial nerve monitoring using EMG, neuromuscular paralysis must be avoided during the course of surgery.

Summary

Intraoperative neurophysiologic monitoring is a valuable tool available to the surgeon working with and around critical neural structures. It serves as a powerful adjuvant, but is not a substitute for a comprehensive knowledge of surgical anatomy and technical skill. In applications such as vestibular schwannoma resection in the internal auditory canal and CPA, intraoperative neurophysiologic monitoring has been shown to aid in the improvement of functional outcomes of patients and predict their postoperative functional status. Working with evolving techniques for neurophysiologic monitoring requires an understanding of the underlying principles, the expertise of trained personnel, and close communication between the surgeon, neural monitoring personnel, and the anesthesiologist.

References

1. Delgado TE, Buchheit WA, Rosenholtz HR, et al. Intraoperative monitoring of facial muscle evoked responses obtained by intracranial stimulation of the facial nerve: a more accurate technique for facial nerve dissection. Neurosurgery. 1979;4:418–21.
2. Møller AG, Jannetta PJ. Preservation of facial function during removal of acoustic neuromas. J Neurosurg. 1984;61:757–60.
3. Gantz BJ. Intraoperative facial nerve monitoring. Am J Otol. 1985;6(Suppl):58–61.
4. Hammerschlag PE, Cohen NL. Intraoperative monitoring of facial nerve function in cerebellopontine angle surgery. Otolaryngol Head Neck Surg. 1990;103(5):681–4.
5. Jellinek DA, Tan LC, Symon L. The impact of continuous electrophysiological monitoring on preservation of the facial nerve during acoustic tumour surgery. Br J Neurosurg. 1991;5:19–24.
6. Prass RL, Luders H. Acoustic (loudspeaker) facial electromyographic monitoring: part 1. Evoked electromyographic activity during acoustic neuroma resection. Neurosurgery. 1986;19:392–400.
7. Minahan RE, Mandir AS. Neurophysiologic intraoperative monitoring of trigeminal and facial nerves. J Clin Neurophysiol. 2011;28:551–65.
8. Romstock J, Strauss C, Fahlbusch R. Continuous electromyography monitoring of motor cranial nerves during cerebellopontine angle surgery. J Neurosurg. 2000;93:586–93.
9. Neff BA, Ting J, Dickinson SL, Welling DB. Facial nerve monitoring parameters as a predictor of postoperative facial nerve outcomes after vestibular schwannoma resection. Otol Neurotol. 2005;26(4):728–32.
10. Bozinov O, Grotzer M, Sarnthein J. Intraoperative monitoring of facial nerve motor-evoked potentials in children. World Neurosurg. 2015;84(3):786–94.
11. Tomáš R, Klener J, Šetlík M. Transcranial facial motor evoked potentials: a continuous monitoring of the facial motor function during vestibular schwannoma surgery. Clin Neurophysiol. 2014;125(5):e41.
12. Zhou HH, Zhu C. Comparison of isoflurane effects on motor evoked potential and F wave. Anesthesiology. 2000;93:32–8.
13. Bovo N, Momjian S, Gondar R, et al. Sensitivity and negative predictive value of motor evoked potentials of the facial nerve. J Neurol Surg A Cent Eur Neurosurg. 2021;82(4):317–24.
14. Nielsen VK. Pathophysiology of hemifacial spasm: I. Ephaptic transmission and ectopic excitation. Neurology. 1984;34:418–26.
15. Rausdzens PA, Shetter AG. Intraoperative monitoring of brainstem auditory evoked potentials. J Neurosurg. 1982;57:341–8.
16. Grundy BL, Jannetta PJ, Procoio PT, et al. Intraoperative monitoring of brain stem auditory evoked potentials. J Neurosurg. 1982;57:674–81.
17. Miyazaki H, Thomasen PC, Magnan J. Advanced intraoperative continuous Cochlear monitoring and Cochlear nerve mapping for CP angle surgery: dramatic improving the hearing preservation. J Neurosurg B. 2014:75–a206.
18. Danner C, Mastrodimos B, Cueva RA. A comparison of direct eighth nerve monitoring and auditory brainstem response in hearing preservation surgery for vestibular schwannoma. Otol Neurotol. 2004;25(5):826–32.
19. Jackson LE, Roberson JB. Acoustic neuroma surgery: use of cochlear nerve action potential monitoring for hearing preservation. Am J Otol. 2000;21:249–59.
20. Meyer TA, Canty PA, Wilkinson EP, Hansen MR, Rubinstein JT, Gantz BJ. Small acoustic neuromas: surgical outcomes versus observation or radiation. Otol Neurotol. 2006;27(3):380–92.
21. Jewett DL, Romano MN, Williston JS. Human auditory evoked potentials: possible brain stem components detected on the scalp. Science. 1970;167:1517–8.
22. Musiek FE, Baran JA. Neuroanatomy, neurophysiology, and central auditory assessment. Part 1: brainstem. Ear Hear. 1986;7:207–19.
23. Moller AR. Neural generators of auditory evoked potentials. In: Jacobson JT, editor. Principles and applications in auditory evoked potentials. Boston: Allyn and Bacon; 1994. p. 23–46.
24. Moller AG, Jannetta PJ. Compound action potentials recorded intracranially from the auditory nerve in man. Exp Neurol. 1981;74:862–74.
25. Roberson JB, Jackson LE, McAuley JR. Acoustic neuroma surgery: absent auditory brainstem response does not contraindicate attempted hearing preservation. Laryngoscope. 1999;109:904–10.
26. Kileny PR, Niparko JK, Shepard NT, Kemink JL. Neurophysiologic intraoperative monitoring: I. Auditory function. Am J Otol. 1988;Suppl:17–24.
27. Gulya AJ, Minor LB, Poe D. Glasscock and Shambaugh's surgery of the ear. 6th ed. PMPH; 2010.

Image-Guided Systems in Temporal Bone and Skull Base Surgery

29

Robert F. Labadie and J. Michael Fitzpatrick

Introduction

While many drivers take it for granted, the automobile global positioning system (GPS) is a relatively new innovation, which gained widespread adoption in the mid-1990s. Prior to GPS, navigation occurred with the driver referring to a paper map often unfolded on the passenger's seat. The driver would (a) try to locate their current position on the map, (b) identify a desired target, and then (c) mentally formulate the most desirable path between the two. GPS revolutionized the process by constantly tracking the position of the car in relation to a map overlaid on the terrain and then providing voice prompts guiding the driver to follow the optimal path. Taking this technology one step further, self-driving cars are becoming reality with many transportation experts predicting widespread adoption.

Intraoperative navigation, more appropriately called image-guided surgery (IGS), is following a similar trajectory albeit at a slower pace (e.g., maps have been around for millennia while radiographic images are just over 100 years old). While many ear surgeons have been exposed to IGS by either their neurosurgical or rhinology colleagues, who employ it regularly, it has not gained widespread usage despite some obviously beneficial applications such as draining petrous apex lesions or navigating within the middle cranial fossa. Analogous to the self-driving car, future endeavors such as robotic excavation of the lateral skull base—already demonstrated by at least two groups [1–4]—are likely to become clinical realities. Toward this end, a basic understanding of IGS will be required of ear surgeons, and that is the purpose of this chapter. The motivated reader is directed toward a more comprehensive textbook—*Image-Guided Surgery: Fundamentals and Clinical Applications in Otolaryngology* written by the authors of this chapter—should this brief treatise not satisfy their intellectual curiosity about IGS [5].

History

Shortly after the discovery of the radiograph by Röntgen in 1895, surgeons capitalized upon it to guide surgical dissection, with the first image-guided surgery credited to JH Clayton, who used an X-ray machine to identify and assist in removing a sewing needle from the hand of a victim of an industrial accident [6]. Further development and clinical adoption of IGS awaited the discovery and clinical deployment of computerized tomography (CT) machines in 1973 and MRI in 1978. These 3D imaging modalities allowed referencing to fiducial markers on the patient consisting first of the N-bar reference system employed in neurosurgery in the late 1970s and still used today. The cumbersome N-bar was soon replaced by individual fiducial markers placed on the patient prior to CT or MRI scanning with various mechanisms for identifying the fiducial markers in space first with mechanical linkages and then with infrared (IR) or electromagnetic (EM) tracking, both of which are still used today. Identification of these markers is crucial as they form the link between the patient and the imaging in an overlay process known as registration. The transformation that relates individual fiducial markers on the patient to their corresponding positions in the image is then used to transform any given anatomical point from physical space in the OR to the image space of the CT or MRI. If the alignment (aka registration) between the fiducials is accurate, the alignment between the rest of the anatomy and ongoing navigation should be accurate as well. But, if the alignment between fiducials is not

R. F. Labadie (✉)
Department of Otolaryngology—Head and Neck Surgery, Medical University of South Carolina (MUSC), Charleston, SC, USA
e-mail: labadie@musc.edu

J. M. Fitzpatrick
Professor Emeritus of Computer Science, Computer Engineering, Electrical Engineering, Radiology, and Neurosurgery, Vanderbilt University, Nashville, TN, USA
e-mail: j.michael.fitzpatrick@vanderbilt.edu

A. D. Sweeney et al. (eds.), *Haynes-Glasscock-Shambaugh Surgery of the Ear*, https://doi.org/10.1007/978-3-032-18264-7_29

accurate, the alignment between the rest of the anatomy and the ongoing navigation will not be accurate. There are a number of factors that determine how accurate the registration will be including (i) the truthfulness of the CT or MRI image, (ii) the accuracy of the tracking system (IR or EM), and (iii) the geometric relationship of the fiducial markers to the anatomical target of interest. Each of these factors will be discussed below in sufficient detail for clinical use of IGS systems, following which specific commercially available IGS systems available at the time of this writing and prognostications on robotic systems will be discussed.

Computerized Tomography (CT) and Magnetic Resonance Imaging (MRI)

Computerized tomography (CT) consists of an X-ray source rotating around the volume of interest with an X-ray detector located 180° opposite the source. X-rays absorbed by the tissue are prevented from reaching the detector. The tissue in the line of the X-ray can be divided into discrete volumes, referred to as voxels. After assigning a variable to each voxel denoting the absorption—or attenuation—of X-rays due to that voxel, an equation relating the amount of X-ray emitted, I_O, to the amount of X-ray recorded on the detector, I, based on the attenuation of each voxel is generated. By simultaneously solving a multitude of equations, the attenuation coefficients (measured in Hounsfield units in recognition of Sir Godfrey Hounsfield the Nobel Prize-winning pioneer of CT development) of each voxel can be calculated and represented on a gray scale (Fig. 29.1). Modern CT scanners typically utilize more advanced image acquisition techniques (e.g., helical scanners, cone beam scanners), but the underlying principle remains the same.

While clinicians are accustomed to very sharp CT images, such images are almost always modified from the raw data which assigned a single Hounsfield unit to each voxel (Fig. 29.2). The concept of a single Hounsfield unit assigned

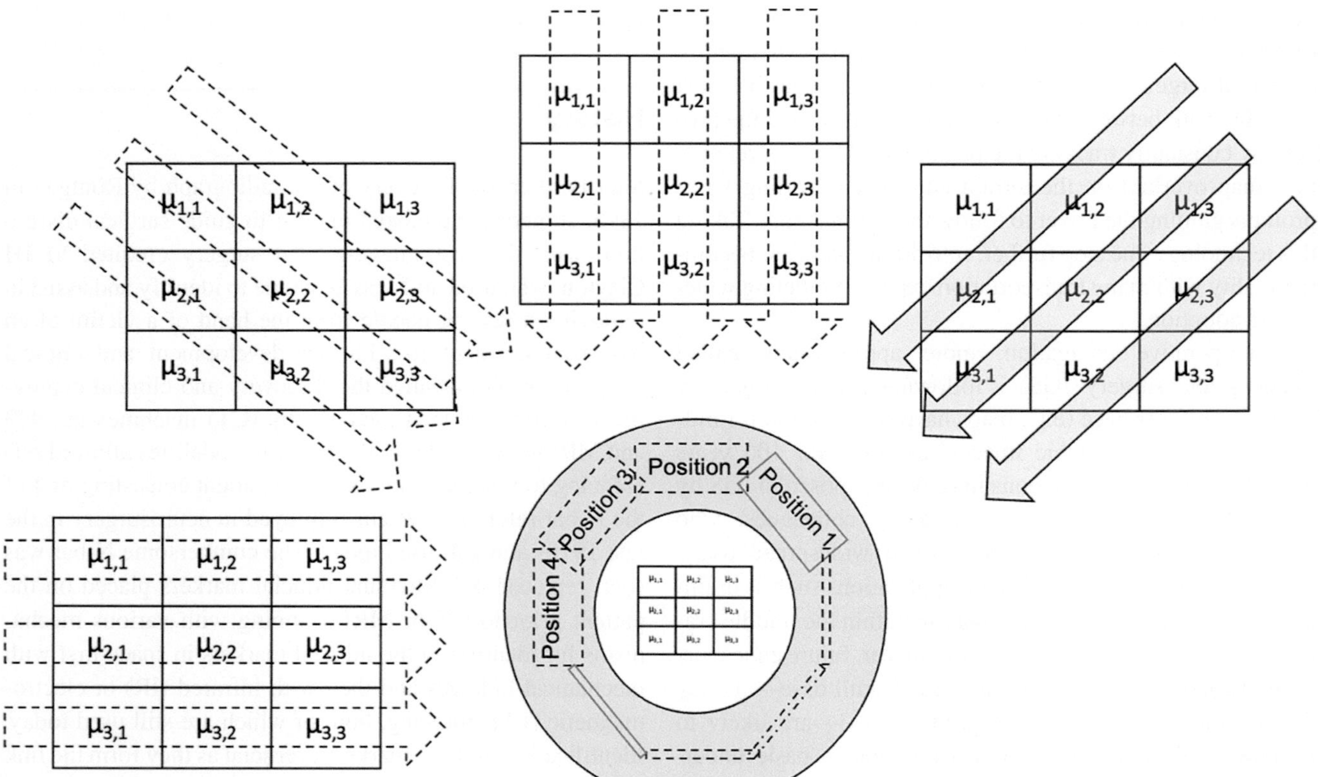

Fig. 29.1 As shown in the circular figure, CT scanning employs an X-ray emitter (large rectangles) and opposing detector (thin rectangles) rotating around an object in the bore of the scanner. At discrete orientations, in this simplified example, positions 1, 2, 3, and 4, the detector records the amount of radiation passing through the object for multiple rays (arrows), three in this example. At each orientation, for each ray, one equation relates the amount of radiation emitted, I_1, and detected, I_2, to the attenuation coefficients, $\mu_{m,n}$, of tiny pieces of tissue through which the ray passes, e.g., the equation for the middle ray of position 1 is $I_2 = I_1 e^{-(\mu 1,3 + \mu 2,2 + \mu 3,1)}$, where $e = 2.7183$. After scanning, these equations (12 of them in this example) can be solved simultaneously for the $\mu_{m,n}$, which are then used to create a pixelated image like that shown in the left panel of Fig. 29.2, where each pixel (or voxel in 3D) is assigned a gray-scale value (aka "Hounsfield number") based on its attenuation coefficient. (Adapted from Labadie and Fitzpatrick [25] © 2016. Plural Publishing. Inc. All rights reserved. Used with permission)

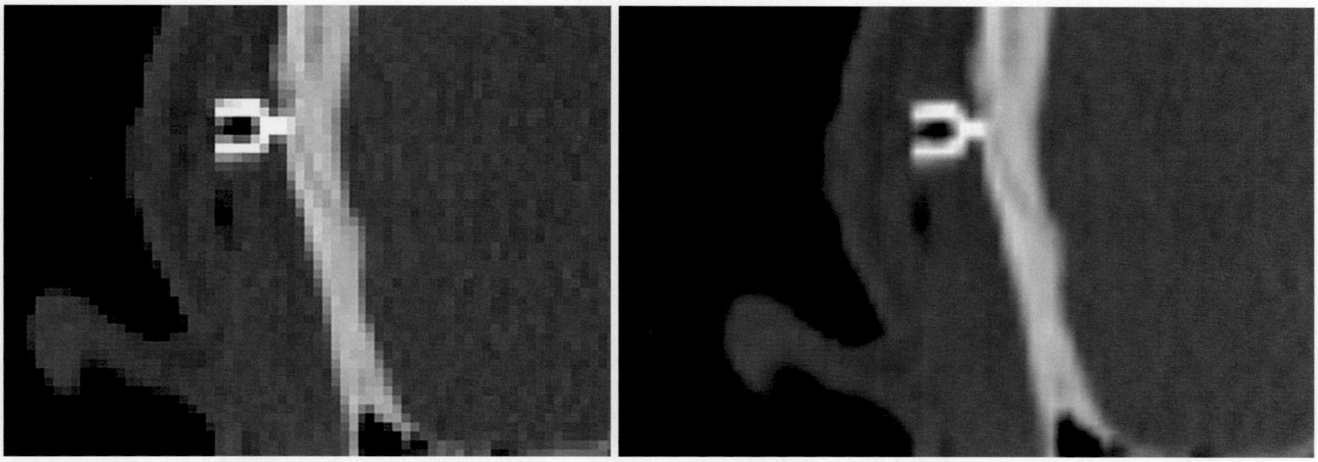

Fig. 29.2 Raw CT data with each voxel assigned a single Hounsfield unit on the left and a processed image on the right demonstrating the problems inherent in precisely localizing an object in a CT image resulting in fiducial localization error (FLE). (Adapted from Labadie and Fitzpatrick [25] © 2016. Plural Publishing. Inc. All rights reserved. Used with permission)

to a voxel is important to keep in mind when considering the accuracy afforded by CT scanners. While it would seem intuitive that the voxel size indicates the lower limit of accuracy for a CT scanner, because most meaningful measurements take place over a volume composed of multiple voxels, the accuracy can be less than a voxel. For most modern CT scanners which have voxel sizes of 0.8 mm or less, the error localizing an anatomical location within a volume about the size of a human head is approximately 0.25 mm.

Of note, portable CT scanners that acquire scans by incrementally acquiring a portion of a scan over a small volume and then inching forward using tank treads to propel themselves over the floor, following which the next portions are acquired, are not suitable for IGS in our opinion. Unfortunately, because floors are not perfectly planar, this design results in geometrically skewed images which are not geometrically true [7].

Magnetic resonance imaging is a completely different and more complex imaging modality than CT and far beyond the scope of this chapter. However, a couple of points are warranted to understand MRI scanning accuracy as it relates to IGS. MRI is accomplished by repeatedly applying spatially varying magnetic fields which excite hydrogen nuclei via nuclear magnetic resonance in a manner determined by the spatial variation. By analyzing the electromagnetic signal emitted by the nuclei, their spatial distribution can be inferred. Both CT and MRI produce a 3D matrix of gray-scale values that can be viewed after scanning with adjustable levels of brightness, contrast, and intensity windowing, but despite this post-scan adjustability, each CT image maps only tissue density, while an MRI image can map any one of multiple soft tissue properties via properly selected scanner settings. Unfortunately, MRI's advantage in versatility is offset by a significant level of geometrical distortion that makes it unreliable for surgical guidance. *As a general rule, CT should be used for image guidance with MRI "fused" to the CT when additional soft tissue information from MRI is necessary.*

Infrared (IR) and Electromagnetic (EM) Tracking Systems

To localize position in the operating room, the most commonly used tracking systems use light or electromagnetic (EM) radiation. Unlike EM, light travels in straight rays and so is amenable to "triangulation" methods. Light tracking can be affected by sending light from multiple sources toward reflective spherical fiducial markers affixed to the patient and then triangulating the reflected rays to determine the positions of the markers (Fig. 29.3). Because the OR is awash with intense visible light, most intraoperative trackers use infrared (IR) light. When within the optimal field of view, the root mean square (RMS) error is approximately 0.35 mm. We stress that this does not mean that the error of an IR tracking system is 0.35 mm. Rather it means that the RMS, which is calculated by summing the squares of deviations from true position, dividing by the number of measurements, and taking the square root, is 0.35 mm. RMS error is specified, instead of, say, mean error, because it can be used in mathematical calculations that are predictive of the tracking error of a system. Error in optical tracking and navigation is known empirically to follow a Maxwell distribution, which differs from a normal distribution in that it excludes all negative numbers and is asymmetrically skewed

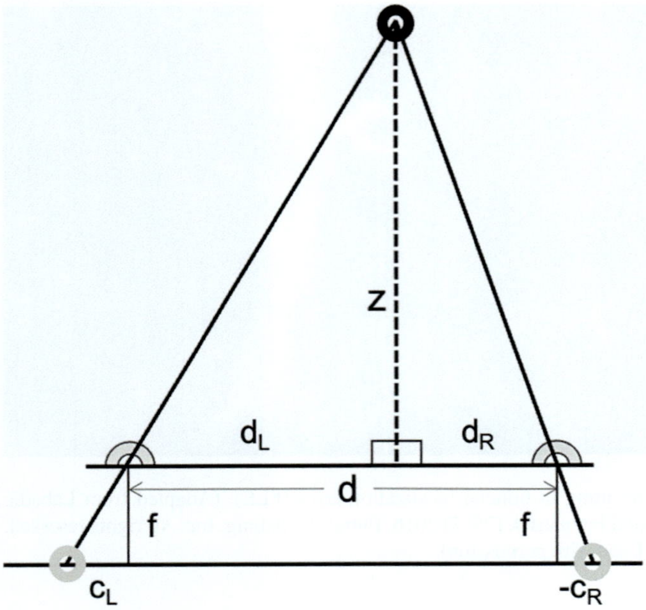

Fig. 29.3 Triangulation in two dimensions. Two cameras (lenses shown as gray half-donuts) with known focal lengths, *f*, and placed a fixed distance, *d*, apart from each other. Basic geometry is used to find *z*, the perpendicular distance from the line joining the cameras to the point of interest, in this case a black circle. *d* is bisected by *z* into d_R and d_L. The circle projects onto the left camera at c_L and on the right camera at $-c_R$. (Note: With perspective taken from the point of the circle, moving to the left is considered a positive direction and to the right considered negative.) Using similarities of triangle, $z/d_L = f/(c_L)$ and $z/d_R = f/-c_R$, and with substitution of $d = d_R + d_L$, we get $d = (c_L - c_R)z/f$ or $z = fd/(c_L - c_R)$. This same principle is also applied in the plane coming out of the page to allow specification of 3D location. (Adapted from Labadie and Fitzpatrick [25] © 2016. Plural Publishing. Inc. All rights reserved. Used with permission)

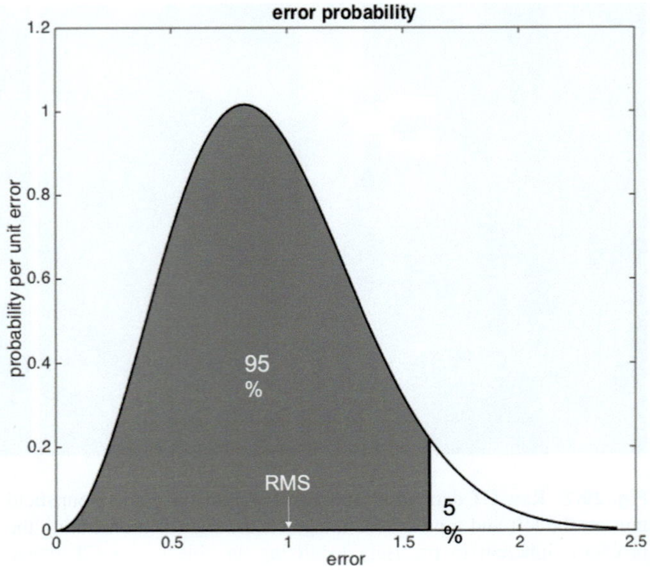

Fig. 29.4 Maxwell distribution of error associated with optical tracking. If a root mean square (RMS) error of 1 mm is specified, 95% of the time the error will be less than 1.61 mm, but at any given point, larger or smaller recordings are possible. While target registration error, TRE (aka accuracy of the IGS system) follows a slightly different distribution; the principle of statistical distribution is important to keep in mind when using IGS. Reiterating, when taking a measurement with an optical tracker or navigating with a surgical system that has a specified error, e.g., 1 mm, any specific recording will not be 1 mm but rather fall somewhere within the statistical distribution. (Adapted from Labadie and Fitzpatrick [25] © 2016. Plural Publishing. Inc. All rights reserved. Used with permission)

for the positive ones (Fig. 29.4). For a RMS of 0.35 mm, the Maxwell distribution has a mean ± standard deviation of 0.32 ± 0.15 mm and a 95% confidence interval of zero to 0.56 mm, indicating that 95% of measurements will be ≤0.56 mm (but 5% will be higher!).

Electromagnetic (EM) tracking is much more complicated than optical tracking. EM tracking involves generating a magnetic field of known geometric distribution and then embedding sensors within surgical instruments to make measurements of the magnetic field at a particular location and via the measurements determining three-dimensional location. While the upside is very clear—obviating the need for line of sight required by IR tracking—the downside is that magnetic fields can be distorted by many components commonly used in the OR including large metallic objects (e.g., the OR bed). In ideal settings, the RMS of an EM tracking system can be as low as 0.7 mm with a 95% confidence interval of 1.4 mm, but in real-world settings, the error is likely to be double these values.

Registration

If you take home anything from the prior two sections—imaging and tracking—we hope it is that an accurate mapping of a point in either CT or MRI to 3D space with either IR or EM has limits. This realization is very helpful in understanding the subsequent limits of a crucial step of IGS, registration, in which the image is overlaid on the patient in the OR allowing surgical navigation to take place (Fig. 29.5). If this step is done poorly, all the anatomical information that passively follows the transformation from the CT/MRI to the patient based on the localization of the fiducial markers in CT/MRI and in the operating room is done poorly as well. As a surgeon, there are steps you can take to make this registration as optimal as possible including choice of fiducials and their placement.

Fiducials that do not move or deform from imaging to the OR will result in the best registration, and the gold standard is bone-implanted markers (e.g., facial plating screws). When used with point-based registration (subsequently picking the location of at least three bone-implanted markers in the CT/MRI and matching them up as best as possible

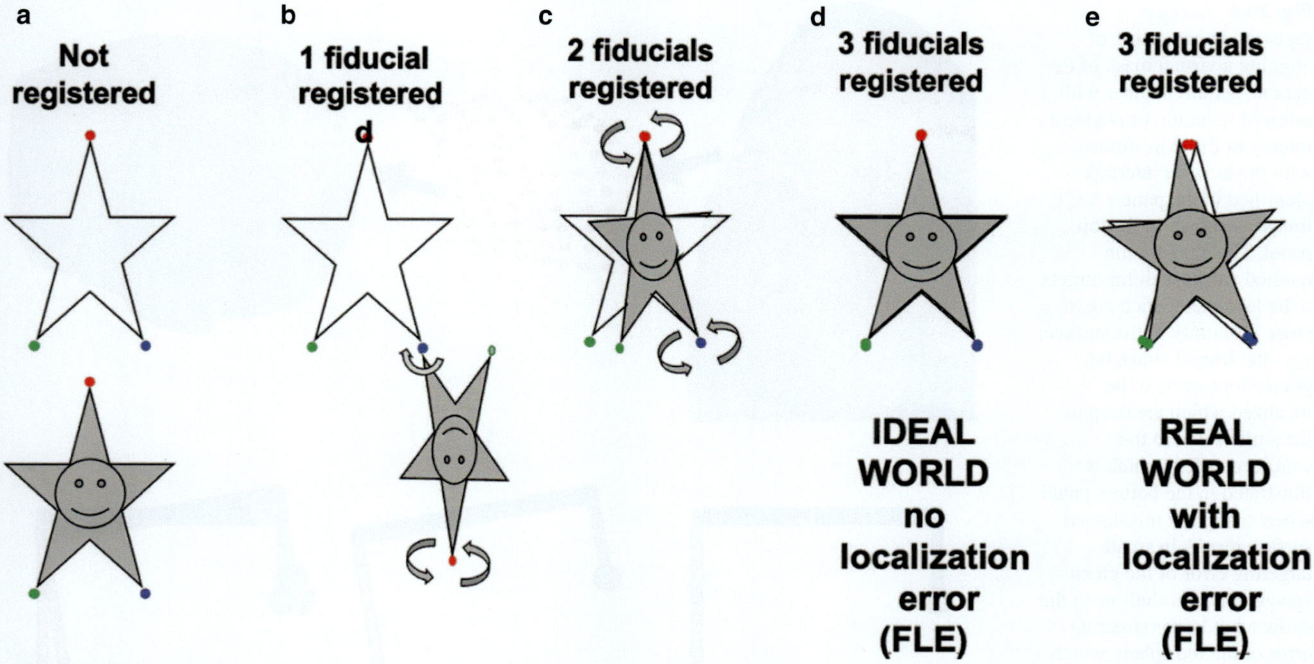

Fig. 29.5 Rigid point registration requires at least three points to align in 3D space. The gray star with the smiley face is to be registered to the white star. (**a**) No registration. (**b**) Registration with one fiducial (blue). (**c**) Registration with two fiducials (blue and red). (**d**) Perfect registration with three fiducials (blue, red, and green). (**e**) Real-world registration where the fiducial localization also has some error associated with it. (Adapted from Labadie and Fitzpatrick [25] © 2016. Plural Publishing. Inc. All rights reserved. Used with permission)

with the corresponding three points as identified in the operating room with the tracking system), submillimetric error (RMS error < 1 mm) is achievable. Next best is using surface registration in which a coordinate reference frame is either screwed into the skull or affixed to the patient with a Velcro headband, following which the surface of the face is scanned with an IR wand creating a virtual mask of the face. This mask is then aligned as best as possible with the surface from the CT scan identified by the drop-off of Hounsfield units from soft tissue to air (Fig. 29.6). "Aligned as best as possible" means that, after an iterative fitting process to get the two "masks" as close as possible to each other, the sum of squares of distances between corresponding locations (e.g., tip of nose in image and in OR) is minimized. As one can imagine, surface matching works pretty well if one is looking at anatomical locations shallow to the mask but starts to generate much more significant error when getting deep to the mask. This concept has been quantified by neurosurgeons, who reported that targeting error (the error in localizing anatomy) after surface-based registration resulted in error of 1.8 ± 0.8 mm of locations in the front part of the skull and 2.8 ± 2.1 mm in the temporal, parietal, occipital, and infratentorial locations. The values in the right and left external auditory canals were 3.3 ± 1.9 mm and 3.9 ± 2.2 mm, respectively [8].

Error associated with mapping a point from image to OR using an IGS system is formally known as the target registration error or TRE. Then targeting is based on fiducials, TRE results from the error in localizing the fiducials, which is formally known as fiducial localization error, FLE. There are two sources of fiducial localization error: localization in the CT/MRI image, FLE_{im}, and physical localization on the anatomy in the operating room using whatever tracking is employed, FLE_{OR}. These errors are invisible and not directly measurable, but their presence is revealed by the visible and directly measurable error in the alignment of the fiducials, which is formally known as fiducial registration error, FRE. While a deep dive into error analysis is beyond the scope of this chapter (the interested reader is directed to reference [9]), there are a number of practical steps that can be followed by surgeons to reduce error. First, as noted above, pick the most stable fiducial markers possible with bone implanted markers resulting in the best accuracies, which can be submillimetric. Second, choose fiducials such that the centroid of the configuration of the fiducials is near the target of interest. This can best be seen in the case of surface registration where locations closest to the surface have the least targeting error or TRE. Why this occurs is illustrated in Fig. 29.6. Third, space the fiducials as widely as possible. This method reduces error and increases the range of target points that qualify as being near the center of the fiducial configuration. This point is illustrated in Fig. 29.7 [10]. And, fourth, and perhaps the most important, use more fiducials even if the system tells you that dropping one improves FRE. This non-intuitive paradox—lower FRE but higher TRE—has been the source of great misunderstanding by clinicians resulting

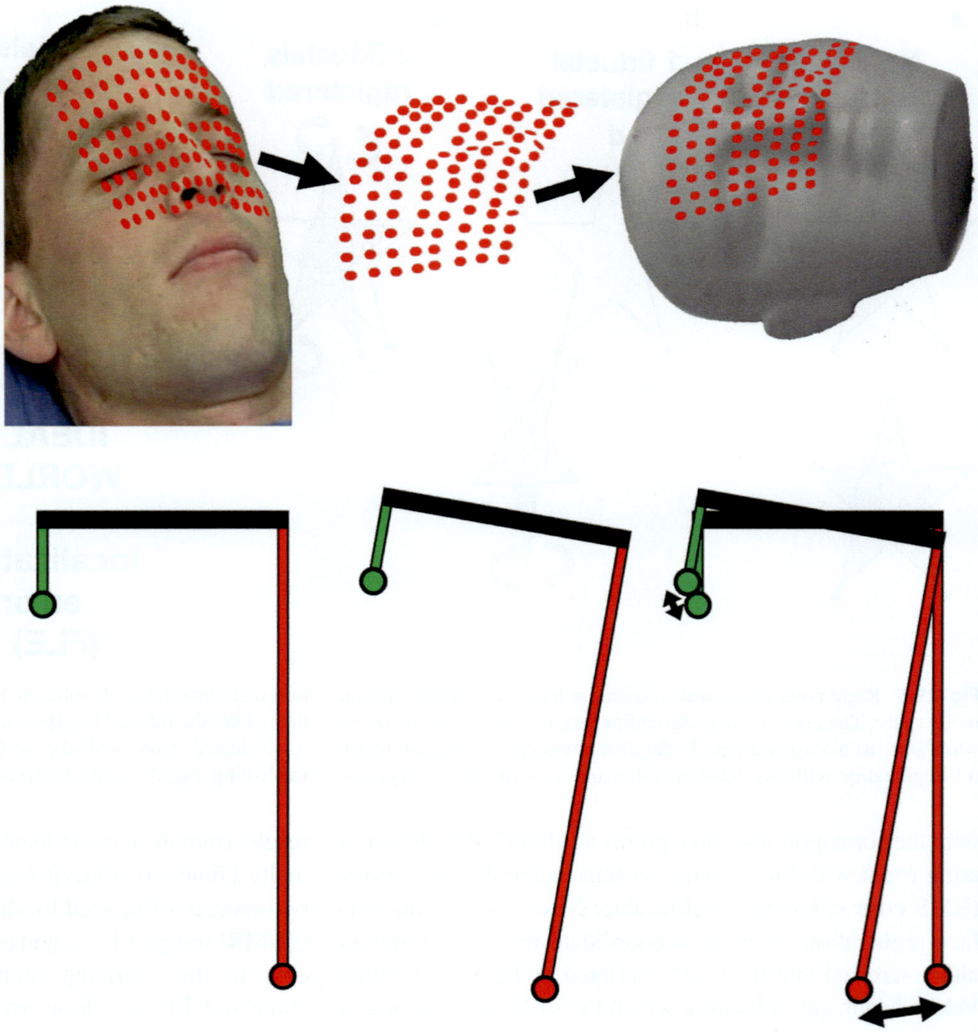

Fig. 29.6 Surface registration consisting of aligning a virtual mask of the patient, acquired either with infrared scanning or physical tracing of the skin surface, with the air-skin interface identified in the patient's CT image as shown in the top panel. This registration method works well for targets to be localized which are in close proximity to the surface, e.g., the frontal sinus, but poorly for targets to be localized which are deep to the surface due to the cantilever effect which is illustrated in the bottom panel where a slightly misaligned surface results in small targeting error of the green sphere which is shallow to the surface but larger targeting error of the red sphere which is deep to the surface. (Adapted from Labadie and Fitzpatrick [25] © 2016. Plural Publishing. Inc. All rights reserved. Used with permission. The top panel is also adapted from Germano [5])

unfortunately in at least one highly cited paper that recommends dropping a fiducial to decrease FRE [11]! An intuitive illustration of why this paper is wrong is provided by the example shown in Fig. 29.8. As fiducials beyond the three necessary for 3D registration are added, each additional fiducial results in a better alignment of the two spaces, but at the same time increases the FRE because FRE is defined as the square root of the sum of the squares of the differences between fiducials divided by the number of fiducials, and the effect of adding an extra squared term for the additional fiducial more than offsets the effect of increasing by one the number of fiducials in the division. Intuition is not sufficient to guess which of these two effects tends to be stronger—guesswork has no place here. A statistical analysis is required to render the right verdict, and that verdict is that dropping a fiducial just because it decreases FRE is a mistake. Dropping the fiducial with the worst alignment can also be problematic considering that detailed statistical simulations show that the fiducial with the worst alignment is probably the most important one to keep! Perhaps one final example will convince you not to drop fiducials to decrease FRE: If one aligns a surface alone, the cantilever seen in Fig. 29.6 occurs. But, if one adds to that surface just one point on the contralateral part of the skull, even if that point is not aligned so well and increases the FRE, it adds great value in bettering the registration. We do not recommend dropping fiducials during registration unless you have a good reason (e.g., a bone-implanted fiducial has come loose). *And, by all means, after registration is done, do a sanity check of known anatomy to make sure the IGS system's results seem reasonable to you—if they don't, reassess and re-register.*

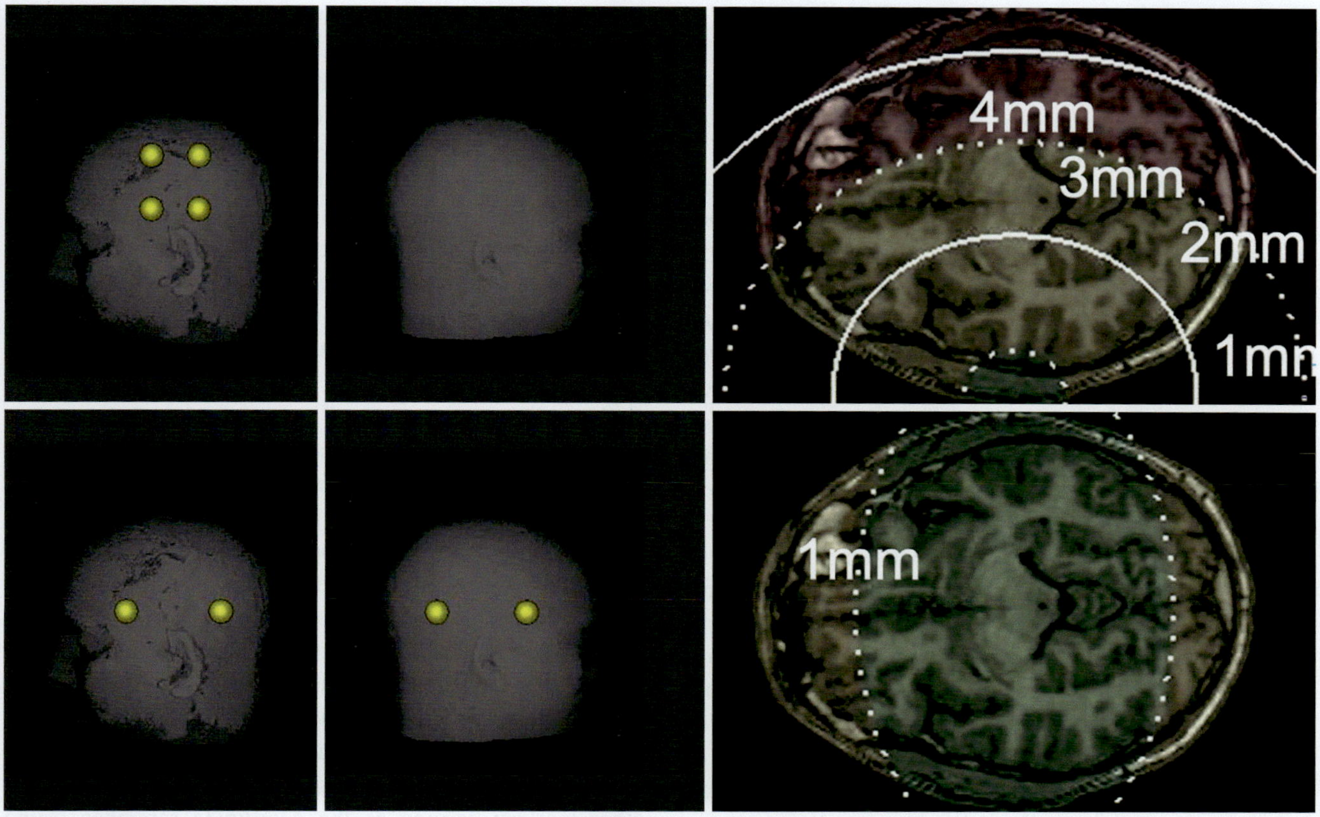

Fig. 29.7 Example of how placing fiducial markers as wide as feasible with markers shown as yellow spheres in the left panels and zones of predicted accuracy in the corresponding right panels. Using four markers on one side of the head produces depth of accuracy similar to the cantilever effect shown in the preceding figure. By moving two of the fiducials to the other side of the head, the 1 mm accuracy zone is enlarged to cover almost the entire head. (Used with permission from West et al. [10])

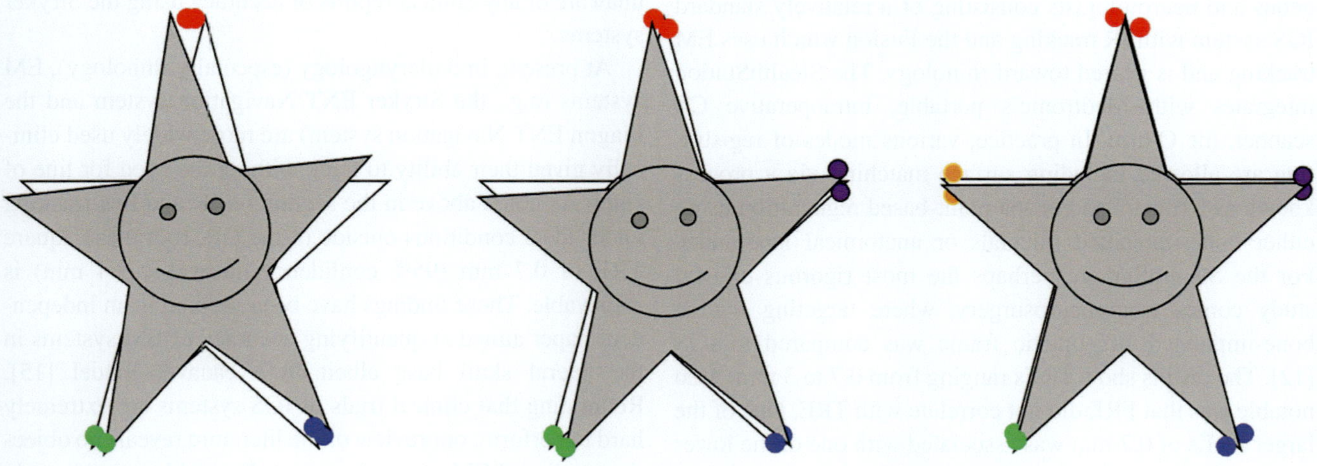

Fig. 29.8 Increasing the number of fiducials results in better registration as can be seen in this example using three (left), four (center), and then five (right) fiducial markers. However, the fiducial registration error, FRE, which is defined as the square root of the sum of the distances between individual fiducials squared divided by the number of fiducials. Because adding one term to this sum tends to have a larger effect than increasing the number in the division by one, FRE typically increases when more fiducials are used. Our recommendation is, if you do not have a good reason to drop a fiducial marker during registration (e.g., the marker became unstable and/or moved from between CT scan and the patient being registered in the OR), do not disregard any markers. You will get a better overall registration. (Adapted from Labadie and Fitzpatrick [25] Used with permission)

Commercial IGS Systems

After registration is complete, the surgeon is ready to navigate, but there is one additional constraint—either the patient or tracker has to be immobilized relative to each other (e.g., neurosurgical Mayfield head holder), or the patient needs to be continually tracked by using what is known as a coordinate reference frame (CRF). As with fiducials used for localization in CT or MRI and the OR, the CRF needs to be fixed as tightly as possible to the patient because any slippage will result in an erroneous transformation during navigation. Bone-affixed CRFs are best—and often achievable given that patients are already anesthetized—but pressure-affixed CRFs (e.g., a headband) tend to be used more predominantly by rhinologists. *We strongly recommend that for neurotology applications, bone-affixed CRFs be used.*

While the field continues to evolve at a rapid pace, much of the ENT market consists of equipment from Medtronic, Brainlab, and Stryker. While each offers unique features, the core components can be similar (e.g., Brainlab and Medtronic use Northern Digital IR tracking). Accuracy studies of commercial systems are extremely difficult to perform and inconsistent in setup from one report to the other. While we are certain that each company has very detailed accuracy data, it is not publicly available leaving us only incommensurate peer-reviewed studies from which to make generalizations.

Medtronic entered the IGS market in 1998. Medtronic offers both the StealthStation marketed toward neurosurgeons and neurotologists consisting of a relatively standard IGS system with IR tracking and the Fusion which uses EM tracking and is geared toward rhinology. The StealthStation integrates with Medtronic's portable, intraoperative CT scanner, the O-arm. In practice, various modes of registration are allowed including surface matching via a process known as "Tracer" and/or via point-based registration using either bone-implanted fiducials or anatomical landmarks. For the StealthStation, perhaps the most rigorous clinical study comes from neurosurgery, where targeting with a bone-implanted stereotactic frame was compared to IGS [12]. The results show TREs ranging from 0.7 to 3 mm. Also notable was that FRE did not correlate with TRE. One of the larger FREs of 0.7 mm was associated with one of the lower TREs of 1.6 mm. Keep in mind that each of these TRE values represents a statistical distribution of accuracy with values much higher and lower possible during any given data acquisition (see description of this under Tracking regarding Maxwell and normal distributions and Fig. 29.4) [10].

Brainlab offers the VectorVision for neurosurgical applications and the Curve for rhinology. As mentioned above, it utilizes the NDI IR tracking system as does the Medtronic StealthStation. Registration occurs via either surface (non-contacting laser scanning) or point-based registration. For the Brainlab system, perhaps the most rigorous study is preclinical and was done with cadaver heads but yields some insights regarding the best possible outcomes understanding that these are unlikely to be duplicated on a regular basis in the clinical world. With surface registration and using facial plating screws as targets, TREs varied from 0.77 ± 0.30 mm at the frontal sinus to 1.76 ± 0.45 mm in the petrous bone [13]. In clinical practice, on a regular basis target, registration error with a statistical distribution centered about 2 mm can likely be achieved in the region of the sinus cavities with laser surface scanning.

Stryker acquired Image Guided Technologies in 2000, a company that manufactured active IR tracking systems. Active systems emit a signal from the fiducial rather than passively reflecting IR light as described above. In practice, while passive systems suffer from user error (e.g., smearing a passive spherical marker by touching it with the ungloved hand inhibits its reflective properties), active and passive systems should have roughly equivalent localization error. Stryker does not currently offer an IR-based system for otolaryngology but does offer the Q guidance system for neurosurgery. This IGS system utilizes a battery-powered face mask which has integrated active IR markers. Using the mask, the guidance system can automatically register using some of the markers to determine facial surface features and other markers serving as the coordinate reference frame relating overall position of the patient to the tracking system. While a strong preclinical study exists showing TREs of 1.45 +/− 0.63 mm for point-based registration and 2.51 +/− 1.49 mm for surface-based registration [14], the authors are unaware of any clinical reports of accuracy using the Stryker systems.

At present, in otolaryngology (especially rhinology), EM systems (e.g., the Stryker ENT Navigation system and the Fiagon ENT Navigation system) are more widely used clinically given their ability to track without the need for line of sight. As noted above in the section on IR and EM tracking under ideal conditions outside of the OR, root mean square TRE of 0.7 mm (95% confidence interval < 1.4 mm) is achievable. These findings have been verified in an independent paper aimed at quantifying accuracy of EM systems in the lateral skull base albeit in a cadaver model [15]. Reiterating that clinical trials of IGS systems are extremely hard to perform, our review of the literature reveals no objective studies of EM system in neurotology, although the study just cited also included three demonstrative procedures (middle cranial fossa (MCF) approach, cochleostomy from MCF, and infralabyrinthine access to the petrous apex "without anatomical injury of important anatomical structures" [15]. Within the field of IGS, the 1997 report by Friedman et al. [16] on the InstaTrak system (no longer commercially available) is considered the best study to date and was recently republished as a "historical classic." While not directly applicable to skull base surgery—the registration method utilized a proprietary headframe, and the targets were skin-affixed fiducials—the TRE results (mean ± standard deviation) of 2.28 ± 0.91 mm with a maximum of 5.08 mm show that real-world results are worse than optimal results in phantom or cadaver models. *Out of concerns regarding accuracy, the authors urge caution using EM systems rather than IR systems with bone-implanted fiducials.*

Evidence-Based Medicine for IGS

So we have all these cool technological marvels. Should we use them? What value do they add to the surgical encounter? While it seems obvious that IGS would result in better surgical outcomes, the literature is surprisingly sparse. The overall perception among users of IGS is that their benefit is obvious and that studies proving their efficacy are unnecessary [17]. Evidence, however, is beginning to mount showing that IGS may hold tangible benefits including fewer complications. A meta-analysis published in 2013 compiling 13 articles showed incidence of major and minor complications were fewer in the 1119 patients who underwent IGS intervention (1.25% major and 3.9% minor) versus the 1282 who underwent non-IGS interventions (3.3% major and 6.3% minor) [18]. And, a retrospective chart review of 48,848 trans-sphenoidal pituitary resections published in 2015 showed fewer CSF leaks (1.1% when using CT-guided IGS and 1.9% when not using CT-guided IGS) but an increased rate of leaks (2.5%) when using MRI-guided IGS possibly attributed to the lower fidelity of MRI images as noted in the bolded sentence in the section above entitled Computerized Tomography and Magnetic Resonance Imaging [19].

In the field of otology and neurotology, IGS would seem to be a natural fit for complex cases (e.g., common-cavity cochlear-implant placement) and when surgical landmarks are not reliable (e.g., endolymphatic sac surgery, petrous apex lesions, MCF approaches). However, if IGS is used only in such cases, most surgeons would be unfamiliar with the technology and unlikely to rely upon it. A rational approach warrants otologists and neurotologists familiarizing themselves with IGS systems before a critical need arises. Because neurosurgeons and rhinologists have integrated these machines more widely into their routine surgical practices, we highly recommend "picking their brains" when doing combined cases and then starting to use IGS in routine otology and neurotology cases to become familiar with the pros and cons.

Robotic Surgery in Otology and Neurotology

Recent trends suggest that the next step in the evolution of surgical intervention will include robots. These trends include numbers of publications involving robotics within our field, number of new surgical robotics companies, and recent publications from professional organizations.

From an engineering standpoint, robots are classified as systems that mimic and refine human motions (e.g., the da Vinci surgical system) or surgical computer-assisted design (CAD) robots that autonomously perform interventions (e.g., RoboDoc). Within the field of otolaryngology, the only "robot"—placed in quotations because the FDA does not allow Intuitive, the manufacturer of the da Vinci surgical system, to market using the word "robot"—which has seen routine clinical use is the da Vinci surgical system as used for trans-oral resection of tongue base (aka trans-oral robotic surgery or TORS).

Looking to neurosurgery, which was an early adopter of IGS and is an early adopter of robots, we may be able to predict where surgical robots are headed in otology/neurotology. Robots have been used to place deep brain stimulators by mounting motorized micromanipulators on microstereotactic frames to guide electrodes to sites of stimulation (e.g., the subthalamic nucleus). Similar technology has been used to gain access to the cochlea for cochlear implant electrode insertion (Fig. 29.9) with the potential upside of simplifying and standardizing the surgical approach leading to wider availability especially in underserved societies [20, 21]. Perhaps the "lowest hanging fruit" for a robot would be cochlear implant electrode insertion. Several technologies have shown decreased insertion forces and better electrode positioning [22]. With electrode insertion at about

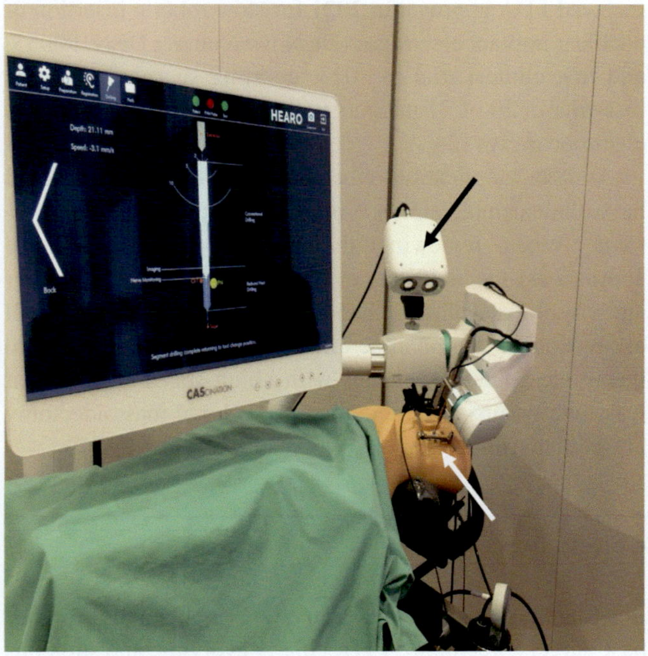

Fig. 29.9 Investigational robot used for cochlear access developed by investigators at the University of Bern, Switzerland [21]. The computer screen shows progress of a tracked drill bit as it bypasses the facial nerve (yellow circle on computer screen) and the multi-articulated arm robot holding a drill (silver with black cord) and guided by an IR camera (black arrow) which tracks both the drill and patient position (coordinate reference frame screwed into skull shown by white arrow). This system has CE mark approval and has been used in live cases

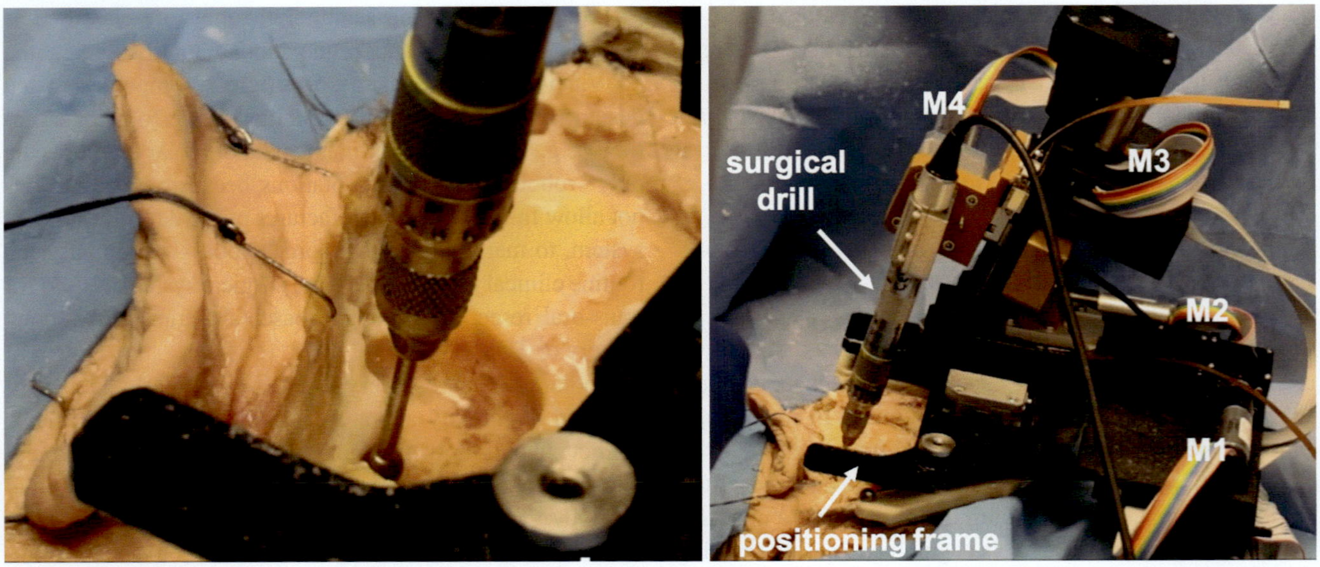

Fig. 29.10 Bone attached lateral skull base robot for translabyrinthine approaches to the internal auditory canal. Right panel—overview showing robot rigidly affixed to the skull via positioning frame (white arrow) which is screwed into the skull. The robot has 4° of freedom being able to move in the *x*, *y*, and *z* direction as well as rotate anteriorly and posteriorly as controlled by four motors each of which has a multi-colored ribbon control wire (M1, M2, M3, M4). Left panel—close-up of robot performing right translabyrinthine approach. This robot is intended to quickly and efficiently perform bulk bone removal leaving a 1–2 mm margin of bone over vital structures allowing the surgeon to spend their time and effort doing fine bone removal and soft tissue dissection [3]

the level of human motor and sense perception [23], such technology would potentially augment the abilities of human surgeons and lead to improved outcomes. IotaMotion received FDA approval in 2021 for slow robotic insertion of cochlear implant electrodes (De Novo Number DEN190055) and first clinical trial in 2023 reporting successful robotic insertion in 20 of 21 patients with straight (aka lateral wall) electrode arrays [24].

Another application where robotic technology would have clinical applicability is mastoidectomy and labyrinthectomy. When reviewing the history of these surgical approaches, the field has evolved from handheld hammer and chisel excavation to handheld high-speed surgical-drill excavation. In the manufacturing world, the next step would be robotic-guided excavation with a high-speed drill. And, at least two groups have demonstrated robotic mastoidectomy [1] and labyrinthectomy [3, 4] in cadavers (Fig. 29.10).

Conclusion

Image-guided surgery has numerous applications to skull base surgery. Technology is regularly evolving, and surgeons should stay apprised of new developments in order to maintain a cutting-edge practice.

References

1. Danilchenko A, et al. Robotic mastoidectomy. Otol Neurotol. 2011;32(1):11–6.
2. Dillon N, et al. A compact, bone-attached robot for mastoidectomy. J Med Device. 2015;9(3):0310031–7.
3. Dillon NP, et al. Cadaveric testing of robot-assisted access to the internal auditory canal for vestibular schwannoma removal. Otol Neurotol. 2017;38(3):441–7.
4. Couldwell WT, et al. Computer-aided design/computer-aided manufacturing skull base drill. Neurosurg Focus. 2017;42(5):E6.
5. Germano IM. Advanced techniques in image-guided brain and spine surgery. New York: Thieme; 2002.
6. Burrow EH. Pioneers and early years: a history of British radiology. Alderney: Colophon Press; 1986.
7. Balachandran R, Blachon G, Fitzpatrick JM. Geometric fidelity testing of CT scanners. IJCARS. 2015;7(2):315–21.
8. Raabe A, et al. Laser surface scanning for patient registration in intracranial image-guided surgery. Neurosurgery. 2002;50(4):797–801; discussion 802–3.
9. Fitzpatrick JM. The role of registration in accurate surgical guidance. Proc Inst Mech Eng H. 2010;224(5):607–22.
10. West JB, et al. Fiducial point placement and the accuracy of point-based, rigid body registration. Neurosurgery. 2001;48(4):810–6; discussion 816–7.
11. Snyderman C, Zimmer LA, Kassam A. Sources of registration error with image guidance systems during endoscopic anterior cranial base surgery. Otolaryngol Head Neck Surg. 2004;131(3):145–9.

12. Henderson JM. Frameless localization for functional neurosurgical procedures: a preliminary accuracy study. Stereotact Funct Neurosurg. 2004;82(4):135–41.
13. Ledderose GJ, et al. Surface laser registration in ENT-surgery: accuracy in the paranasal sinuses--a cadaveric study. Rhinology. 2007;45(4):281–5.
14. Paraskevopoulos D, et al. Comparative study of application accuracy of two frameless neuronavigation systems: experimental error assessment quantifying registration methods and clinically influencing factors. Neurosurg Rev. 2010;34(2):217–28.
15. Komune N, et al. The accuracy of an electromagnetic navigation system in lateral skull base approaches. Laryngoscope. 2017;127(2):450–9.
16. Fried MP, et al. Image-guided endoscopic surgery: results of accuracy and performance in a multicenter clinical study using an electromagnetic tracking system. Laryngoscope. 1997;107(5):594–601.
17. Smith TL, et al. Indications for image-guided sinus surgery: the current evidence. Am J Rhinol. 2007;21(1):80–3.
18. Dalgorf DM, et al. Image-guided surgery influences perioperative morbidity from endoscopic sinus surgery: a systematic review and meta-analysis. Otolaryngol Head Neck Surg. 2013;149(1):17–29.
19. Chung TK, Riley KO, Woodworth BA. The use of image-guidance during transsphenoidal pituitary surgery in the United States. Am J Rhinol Allergy. 2015;29(3):215–20.
20. Labadie RF, et al. Minimally invasive image-guided cochlear implantation surgery: first report of clinical implementation. Laryngoscope. 2014;124(8):1915–22.
21. Caversaccio M, et al. Robotic cochlear implantation: surgical procedure and first clinical experience. Acta Otolaryngol. 2017;137(4):447–54.
22. Majdani O, et al. Force measurement of insertion of cochlear implant electrode arrays in vitro: comparison of surgeon to automated insertion tool. Acta Otolaryngol. 2010;130(1):31–6.
23. Kratchman LB, et al. Force perception thresholds in cochlear implantation surgery. Audiol Neurootol. 2016;21(4):244–9.
24. Gantz JA, et al. A steadier hand: the first human clinical trial of a single-use robotic-assisted surgical device for cochlear implant electrode array insertion. Otol Neurotol. 2023;44(1):34–9.
25. Labadie RF, Fitzpatrick JM. Image-guided surgery: fundamentals and clinical applications in otolaryngology. Plural Publishing Inc.; 2016. p. 1–232.

30 Medicolegal Aspects of Otologic Clinical Practice

Douglas S. Ruhl and Philip D. Littlefield

Background

It has been estimated that approximately 80% of physicians in surgical subspecialties will be involved in a lawsuit by the time they are 45 years of age [1]. Patterns have changed, and there has been a decrease in the number of litigations and insurance claims over the last decade [2, 3]. However, a recent review of US malpractice claims demonstrated a continuous increase in payments over time, with statistically higher payouts for permanent and debilitating injuries [4]. Furthermore, insurance data indicate that otologic cases have the highest payouts in otolaryngology [5].

Most patients that suffer negligent injuries do not pursue litigation [6], but further analysis is difficult because malpractice databases can yield conflicting data. For example, a 2013 study of cases involving otolaryngologists showed that all otology-related verdicts were in favor of the defending surgeon [7]. However, an otology-specific review the same year (with larger numbers) found that only half of verdicts favored the surgeon [8]. Another study that reviewed otology claims using insurance data found that 84% resulted in payment to the patient [9].

Components of Negligence

In the US legal system, a bad outcome alone is not enough to demonstrate malpractice. The plaintiff must prove four elements to the jury [4, 10]. First, the physician had a duty to care for the patient. Second, the physician violated an accepted standard of care. Third, the patient experienced a compensable injury. Finally, the physician's substandard care caused the injury. It is generally not difficult to prove that the physician had a duty to treat the patient and an injury occurred. However, the breach of duty due to deviation from a standard of care is a more arduous fact to establish, and this is often the focus of courtroom discussion.

Standard of Care

Establishing a standard of care is of paramount importance in the courtroom [11]. This begins with the process of discovery. The medical record and available communication with the patient are obtained for review by both the defense and prosecution teams. Expert witnesses are used often,

D. S. Ruhl (✉)
Otology & Neurotology, Department of Otolaryngology—Head & Neck Surgery, Madigan Army Medical Center, Tacoma, WA, USA
e-mail: douglas.s.ruhl.mil@health.mil

P. D. Littlefield
Otology & Neurotology, Sharp Rees—Stealy Medical Group, San Diego, CA, USA
e-mail: philip.littlefield@sharp.com

A. D. Sweeney et al. (eds.), *Haynes-Glasscock-Shambaugh Surgery of the Ear*, https://doi.org/10.1007/978-3-032-18264-7_30

and they testify their opinions in order to help the jury decide what the reasonable standard of practice is. For the same reasons, medical literature is frequently cited as authoritative material.

Role of Guidelines

There is growing momentum for academic organizations to create Clinical Practice Guidelines (CPGs) for a multitude of medical situations. According to the Institute of Medicine, these are "statements that include recommendations intended to optimize patient care that is informed by a systematic review of evidence and an assessment of the benefits and harms of alternative care options." [12] It seems expected for lawyers to use CPGs as a means to establish a medicolegal standard of care. Indeed, guidelines may be admissible as learned treatise or authoritative text [13]. However, guidelines have historically been used conservatively in the courtroom [14] and often in conjunction with expert testimony rather than as independent authorities [11]. The American Academy of Otolaryngology—Head & Neck Surgery (AAO-HNS) has eleven CPGs that pertain to otology (Table 30.1), and we should be familiar with them. Although the quality of evidence varies for each guideline, physicians are in a more favorable position when they follow their recommendations [13]. An astute clinician may deviate from guidelines when a unique situation arises, but it is advisable to discuss this with the patient and document it (Table 30.2).

Table 30.1 List of AAO-HNS Clinical Practice Guidelines related to otology and year published and updated

Clinical practice guideline topic	Year published
Otitis media with effusion	2004; updated 2016
Acute otitis externa	2006; updated 2014
Cerumen impaction	2008; updated 2017
Benign positional paroxysmal vertigo	2008; updated 2017
Sudden hearing loss	2012; updated 2019
Bell's palsy	2013
Tympanostomy tubes in children	2013; updated 2022
Tinnitus	2014
Ménière's disease	2020
Opioid prescribing for analgesia after Common otolaryngology operations	2021
Age-related hearing loss	2024

Adapted from the American Academy of Otolaryngology—Head and Neck Surgery. Accessed on 10/1/2024 at http://www.entnet.org/content/clinical-practice-guidelines

Table 30.2 Statement on qualifications and guidelines for the physician expert witness

I. Qualifications for the physician expert witness
A. The physician expert witness must have a current, valid, and unrestricted license to practice medicine in the state in which he or she practices.
B. Members who act as physician experts in the courts will be familiar with the Academy's educational materials on expert witness testimony.
C. The physician expert witness should be fully trained in a specialty or a diplomate of a specialty board recognized by the American Board of Medical Specialties and qualified by experience and demonstrated competence in the subject of the case. The specialty of that physician should be appropriate to the subject matter in the case.
D. The physician expert witness should be familiar with the clinical practice of the specialty and the subject matter of the case and should be actively involved in the clinical practice of the specialty and the subject matter of the case, for three (3) of the previous 5 years at the time of the testimony.
II. Guidelines for behavior of the physician expert witness
A. Physicians have an obligation to testify in court as expert witnesses when appropriate to assist in the administration of justice and/or necessary to protect a patient's legal rights.
B. Physician expert witnesses should not adopt a position as an advocate or partisan in the legal proceedings.
C. The physician expert witness should review all the appropriate medical information in the case and testify to its content fairly, truthfully, and objectively.
D. Within a reasonable time prior to testifying, physician expert witnesses should review and be thoroughly familiar with the relevant standards of practice and medical literature prevailing at the time of the occurrence and limit their testimony to their areas of expertise, both in terms of the specialty and the subject matter of the case.
E. The physician expert witness should state the basis of the testimony presented and whether it is based on personal experience or specific clinical references or is a generally accepted opinion in the specialty field.
F. Compensation of the physician expert witness should be reasonable and commensurate with the time and effort given to preparing for deposition and court appearance. It is unethical for a physician expert witness to link compensation to the outcome of the case.
G. The physician expert witness should be aware that transcripts of their deposition and courtroom testimony are public records, subject to independent peer review.

From the American Academy of Otolaryngology—Head and Neck Surgery Code of Ethics. Adapted from the American Academy of Otolaryngology—Head and Neck Surgery. Revised 5/2016. Accessed 10/1/2024 at https://www.entnet.org/about-us/leadership-governance/ethics/expert-witness-qualifications-and-testimony/

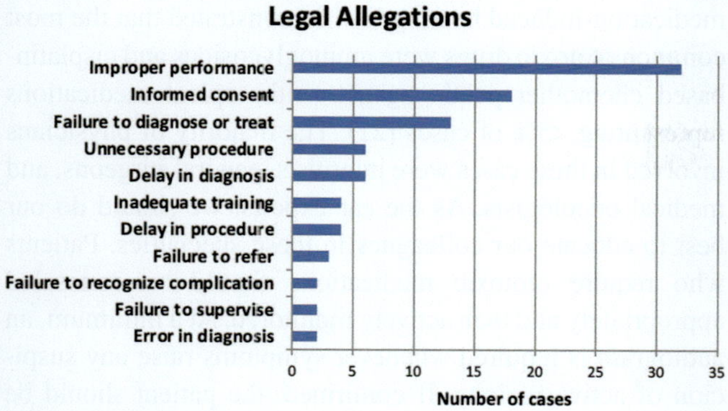

Fig. 30.1 Frequency of legal allegations in otology malpractice cases. (From: Ruhl et al. [8]. Used with permission)

Clinical Insights

Otologists spend a substantial amount of their time in clinic. Although we commonly attribute negligence and injury to events that occur in the operating room, the clinic also provides numerous opportunities for error and harm. Furthermore, the bulk of the informed consent process is carried out in the clinic. We reviewed otology malpractice cases from several prominent legal databases and identified that, aside from improper performance of surgery, issues with the informed consent were the second most common legal allegation against otologists (Fig. 30.1) [8].

Informed Consent

Many malpractice claims allege that there was a problem with the informed consent [10]. This may include the lack of a signed document, or the inability to prove that an appropriate discussion occurred between the patient and surgeon. It is essential to explain the procedure and, within reason, the potential risks and alternatives prior to any intervention [10, 15]. The absence of informed consent in the presence of negligence may be considered battery [10, 16]. However, there are exceptions, such as in extreme emergencies where taking the time to review a consent document would put the patient's life in further jeopardy [17].

Informed consent is more than just a piece of paper—it is a process. This ideally begins well before any procedure. In addition to the detailed, procedure-specific form, this process may include patient education materials, anatomical drawings, pre-/post-procedure instructions, and clinical discussions [16]. It is good practice to document that the patient understands the situation and elects to proceed with treatment. Every clinical encounter is an opportunity to cultivate rapport with the patient, and then they are truly informed [16].

Many hospitals standardize their consent forms. It is wise to ensure that these are thorough and consistent. Use terminology that a patient will understand, and do not use abbreviations on the actual consent. Although obvious, any handwritten document should be legible.

Clinical Documentation

Most clinicians are pressured for time, and we all deal with cumbersome checklists, forms, and medical record requirements. These cost us quality time with our patients, but nonetheless are important, and documentation needs to be thorough and complete. Notes should be written in a way that not only helps you provide continuing care but also informs providers in other specialties. It also is helpful to use odd abbreviations sparingly since they often are confusing and may need to be deciphered later.

Be cautious of any "copy and paste" feature in an electronic medical record. We have reviewed many cases where these perpetuated errors. They make it easy for a lawyer to create a narrative that you are thoughtless and lazy and then any of your documentation is suspect. Litigation can begin years after an incident. This depends on statutes of limitations, but you probably will be unable to recall many details accurately, and they will not be verifiable without prior documentation. It is easy for copied notes to leave out new details or to include outdated ones. This absence of evidence often does not work well for the defendant. However, thoughtful notes will make this a non-issue. Remember that your notes may be the only insight you and the jury have about your prior thought process and plan [8].

Clinic Staff and Protocol

Perception is crucial, and the patient's perception of the clinic visit usually begins and ends with ancillary staff. It is therefore important that you and your support staff are professional, insightful, and courteous. If you work in a teaching hospital, it is beneficial to make it clear that trainees may be a part of the patient's care but that you are directly in charge. Establishing rapport as a team can be presented in a positive way and help alleviate a patient's anxiety. It is also important to have a system that assures timeliness of follow-up. The time between the availability of a laboratory result and when the patient is notified may be crucial in a malpractice case. This is also true of correspondence, such as when calls/questions are returned. Evidence is not limited to the medical record, and an astute attorney may request e-mails, text messages, and call records from the physician and ancillary staff [18]. Do not assume that *any* type of information is protected. Trial records occasionally show otherwise, although we will avoid going into the specifics.

If you did not physically look at the images of a radiology scan, do not state so in your notes or tell a patient that you did. There have been cases where login records and the time a physician spent reviewing digital images were compared against the clinical notes. It is also inappropriate to state that you reviewed images with a particular radiologist unless the same radiologist is also named on the imaging report. Should there be a disagreement between your assessment and the imaging report, it is best to explain why or to review the case with the radiologist and request an addendum.

Patients May Record You?

We live in a digital age and recording devices are cheap and readily available. Surgeons should be aware that patients might be secretly recording them [19]. As alarming as this sounds, it does not automatically mean that there is suspicion or malicious intent. They may want to use the recording to recall the details later or to share the information with family and caregivers. However, the legality of these recordings depends on jurisdiction. Each state has different wiretapping laws. Some are "single-party" states where only one person on the recording (viz., the patient) needs to consent to be recorded [20]. If interested, you should check your regional wiretapping laws to see what rules may apply in your situation. Regardless, it is not unheard of to have recordings show up in the courtroom as evidence. Therefore, assume that you are being recorded, and it is obvious that you need to be honest, thorough, and polite. This is worthwhile since you never know what may surface later and because it is the right thing to do.

Ototoxicity

Otologists are familiar with the ototoxic effects of many drugs, including topical aminoglycosides, gentian violet, and chlorhexidine gluconate. After all, we use gentamicin for chemical labyrinthectomy in order to intentionally damage vestibular hair cells. Following this logic, there are few reasons to use an ototoxic agent topically with a non-intact tympanic membrane when far safer alternatives (i.e., fluoroquinolones) are readily available. It would certainly make for an awkward defense in court, unless the reasoning for the practice deviation was documented beforehand.

Our colleagues in other specialties may not be as attuned to these hazards. They are also more likely to use systemic drugs with ototoxic profiles, and this is reflected in the legal records. A review of malpractice cases associated with medication-induced hearing loss demonstrated that the most common ototoxic drugs were aminoglycosides and cisplatin-based chemotherapeutic agents, with topical medications representing <5% of cases [21]. The majority of physicians involved in these cases were internists, general surgeons, and medical oncologists. As the ear experts, we should do our best to educate our colleagues in these specialties. Patients who require ototoxic medications should be counseled appropriately and then actively monitored. At a minimum, an audiogram is required whenever symptoms raise any suspicion of active toxicity. If confirmed, the patient should be switched to a less ototoxic medication as soon as possible [21]. Drug interactions may enhance ototoxicity [22], so co-administration of medications should be performed judiciously, and providers must be aware of every medication that a patient is taking [23].

Clinic Procedures

Myringotomies and intratympanic injections are a routine part of any otology clinic, and we all know their risks. So it may come as a surprise that cerumen removal is the most common otology procedure leading to litigation (including operating room procedures!) and the most likely to yield a payment [24]. Otologists are infrequently blamed as 80% of these cases involved primary care providers [24]. However, mid-level providers perform cerumenectomy in many practices, including otology clinics, and adequate training and supervision are essential. It is good practice to perform a tuning fork exam before and after removing cerumen or middle ear fluid. The note should also state if the patient tolerated the procedure well and had an improvement in symptoms since this is sometimes debated during litigation.

Surgical Insights

Common Surgical Injuries in Otology Malpractice Cases

Although serious surgical injury is uncommon, otologists work in a high-risk field. Not unexpectedly, facial nerve injury and hearing loss are the most common alleged injuries in surgical otology (Fig. 30.2) [8, 9, 24, 25]. A review of otology court cases showed that mastoidectomies were the most common procedure (Fig. 30.3). When injury occurred, case outcomes for mastoidectomy overwhelmingly favored the patient, more so than for any other procedure [8]. It is worth discussing several aspects of these procedures and special considerations in malpractice cases.

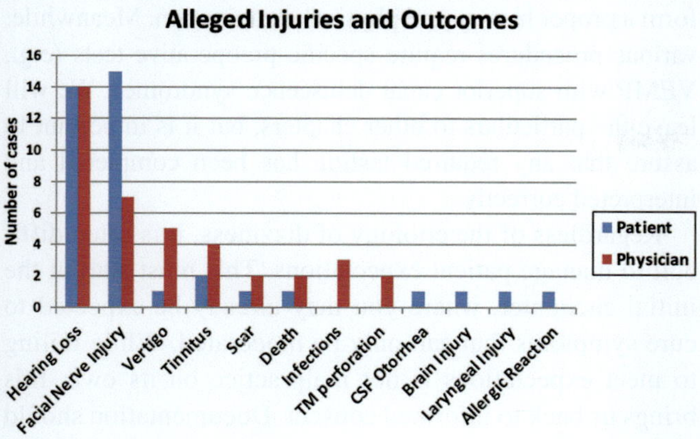

Fig. 30.2 Alleged injuries and outcomes from otology litigation. Cases resulting in either a settlement or a verdict in favor of the plaintiff were considered an outcome in favor of the patient. (From: Ruhl et al. [8]. Used with permission)

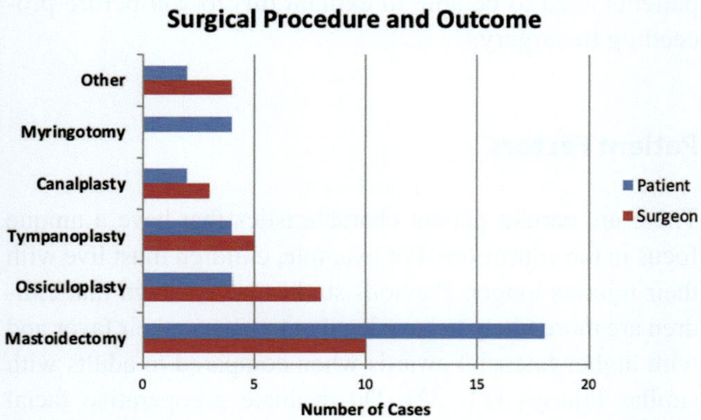

Fig. 30.3 Surgical procedures and verdict outcomes from otology litigation. Cases resulting in either a settlement or a verdict in favor of the plaintiff were considered an outcome in favor of the patient. (From: Ruhl et al. [8]. Used with permission)

Wrong Site Surgery

Wrong site surgery is arguably indefensible [26]. While many otolaryngology procedures are midline, the otologist never enjoys this luxury and must always be mindful of laterality [27]. All hospitals are required to have systems that confirm patient identity and surgical laterality, but errors occur despite this. Imaging (not just the reports, the actual images), notes, and audiograms should be reviewed to ensure consistency. Surgeons should have an adequate discussion with the patient in order to establish which ear to operate on—and cases with bilateral disease are particularly treacherous. The appropriate side should be marked prior to administering sedatives, and the patient *must* participate in this process. We also recommend having the most recent audiogram and imaging displayed in the operating room, and these should be reviewed with near-paranoia immediately before the procedure. Unfortunately, the surgeon is often the only member of the operative team that fully understands these tests, so there is little opportunity for cross-verification. Despite teamwork-based "universal protocols," the responsibility inevitably falls on the attending surgeon, so use all of the available information to verify the correct side of surgery.

Facial Nerve Injuries

Injuries of the facial nerve are arguably the most devastating complication in otologic surgery. Fortunately, they are not common, but they bear a high probability of litigation. A review of claims involving cranial nerve injuries found that the facial nerve was the most commonly litigated [28]. In our review of otology malpractice cases, 38% alleged facial nerve injury, and they were more than twice as likely to yield a verdict in favor of the patient [8]. Moreover, facial nerve injuries have the highest payout in otology [24].

Lawyers often scrutinize the details of operative notes—including any delay in dictation. There have been cases where a surgeon's operative note put poor anatomical knowledge and surgical technique on ignominious display in the courtroom [8]. Relevant landmarks and pathology should be described clearly. Some errors are harder to defend than others, such as causing a thermal injury due to inadequate irrigation or failing to follow the nerve from an area of normal anatomy into the disease [9]. Also, the function of the facial nerve must be thoroughly assessed and documented prior to surgery. It is easy to forget how important this is, but it would be awful to operate on someone with a pre-existing facial palsy only to become the object of blame.

Facial nerve monitoring (FNM) is becoming more popular. A recent survey of otologists found that 49% believe that FNM should be used in all chronic ear surgery. This is a marked increase from 32% a decade earlier [29]. It is our opinion that FNM should not replace a good understanding of anatomy, which is paramount in otologic surgery, and yet we use it in every chronic ear case, as well as stapedectomy and canalplasty. This is because it has surprised us several times, and then we were grateful that we were using it. We hope that we would have avoided injury anyway, but our point is that FNM provides an additional protection (when used appropriately), even if it is not the legal standard of care [8].

Hearing Loss

Hearing loss is one of the most alleged injuries in otology [8]. The degree of hearing loss correlates with higher monetary awards [30]. Therefore, it is important to know the actual degree and type of hearing loss prior to surgery. This is not only for prognosis and counseling, but also in order to accurately assess any change in hearing due to surgery. We recommend an updated audiogram shortly before surgery, and it should not be more than 6 months old.

If a patient has hearing loss, it is important to adequately discuss possible options for hearing rehabilitation. Children with hearing loss should be followed for progressive loss, and they need to be adequately rehabilitated in order to develop proper speech. In these cases, it is important to communicate with audiology, pediatricians, family, and school caregivers as a team.

Dizziness

A review of malpractice claims that alleged dizziness associated with otolaryngology care found that over half of the verdicts were in the patient's favor. Forty-seven percent of the cases were surgical (i.e., stapes surgery and tympanomastoidectomy), and most cited inadequate informed consent [31]. In other words, nearly half were from supposedly unsuspecting patients that were not dizzy until after a surgery, and the legal arguments in these cases generally hinged on informed consent. The remainder is a mixed group, but the actual malpractice errors follow a short list of storylines:

- Misdiagnosing a patient with a benign vestibular disease, but something more serious is causing the symptoms. Cases range from small vestibular schwannomas to intra-axial brain tumors and aneurysms. The plaintiff has a strong malpractice case if it can be established that early treatment is potentially less morbid or if the delay caused a complication.
- Performing a procedure on a presumed peripheral vestibulopathy, but the symptoms were actually caused by a non-vestibular condition (e.g., chemical labyrinthectomy for migraine-associated vertigo). One can argue that the symptoms were exacerbated by an unnecessary surgery.
- Treating a peripheral vestibular disease with an ablative procedure and causing worse symptoms. This is more of a problem when the clinician does not recognize an important second condition. For example, performing a vestibular neurectomy without recognizing a contralateral vestibulopathy will result in chronic oscillopsia and imbalance.

There are other possibilities, but staying out of trouble (as for all of medicine) is foremost a matter of making a correct and timely diagnosis and skillfully employing the appropriate treatments. As in nearly every textbook chapter, we have come to the place where the clinician is admonished to perform a proper history and physical examination. Meanwhile, various procedures require specific preoperative tests (e.g., VEMP with superior canal dehiscence syndrome). We will leave the particulars to other chapters, but it is important to assure that any required testing has been completed and interpreted correctly.

Regardless of the etiology of dizziness, it is often difficult to manage patient expectations. This must start at the initial encounter, where you may already be expected to cure symptoms that can only be moderated. While failing to meet expectations is not malpractice on its own, this brings us back to informed consent. Documentation should be particularly cautious with procedures that may trade one set of symptoms for a presumably less bothersome set of symptoms. Using a common example, labyrinthectomy will stop vertigo spells from Ménière's disease, at the cost of a lifetime of gaze slip with rapid head motion. Your patients need to be able to explain this to *you* before proceeding to surgery.

Patient Factors

There are certain patient characteristics that have a unique focus in the courtroom. For example, children must live with their injuries longer. Previous studies have shown that children are more likely to have legal outcomes in their favor and with higher financial awards when compared to adults with similar injuries [21, 32]. Do evaluate preoperative facial nerve function carefully because it is surprisingly easy to miss a congenital facial palsy in a small child. Elderly patients are also unique. Common factors are less resilient organ systems, a higher chance of operative complications, increased fall risk (even after simple interventions such as an Epley maneuver), and polypharmacy. Therefore, counseling should be patient specific, and the medication list should be thoroughly reviewed prior to any intervention. In particular, older patients may have reduced renal clearance and accumulate ototoxic medications [23].

What to Do After an Adverse Event

Should the unfortunate occur, and you inadvertently injure a patient, it is best to be open and honest [27]. This is often difficult for surgeons, since an apology is often feared to indicate an admission of guilt [33]. It is natural to want to distance oneself from complications, but these patients need to be kept close. Do this directly, but also place any consults required for ancillary care. Although it is neglectful to provide inadequate care to anyone, distancing yourself from this type of patient may elicit a feeling of abandonment and increase the risk of litigation.

When an injury is identified during a procedure, it is prudent to seek advice from a trusted colleague [8]. Do not be ashamed to request intraoperative consultation. We owe that to each other as professionals. If you are struggling, it is best to pause, step away from the table, and regain your composure and mental clarity. Many injuries must be dealt with immediately, but others are best approached at a second stage. For example, unless you have a lot of experience with facial nerve repair, it is best to close, regroup, and then return in a day or two with someone who does [34]. Whatever the situation may be, do not proceed while bewildered and make a bad situation worse.

Hospital policy is changing, and it is wise to understand the disclosure procedures wherever you work. It is best if your hospital's legal team hears your side of the story first, rather than from an unhappy patient.

Expert Witness

The primary purpose of a trial is to discover and clarify the truth [27]. Surgeons may find themselves on the other side of the courtroom as an expert witness—for either the plaintiff or the defense. This is not necessarily a bad thing as our experience and insight may help clarify a situation. However, it is imperative that an expert witness is impartial and provides fair and unbiased testimony [35, 36]. The AAO-HNS has previously published guidance for potential expert witnesses [37].

Should you be called upon to give testimony, it is wise to contact peers or mentors to seek advice and to ease any fears. Your hospital may have assistance available through the legal department as well. In the courtroom, it is best to bring a list of medical terms for the legal transcriptionist. This will minimize interruptions during this stressful process [27].

Conclusion

While the number of otology malpractice claims has been decreasing, cases appear to favor the patient more often than the surgeon. The payouts are high and continue to grow. Facial nerve injury and hearing loss are the most common injuries associated with otologic surgery litigation. Ultimately, the habits that minimize litigation are not new. The best approach is to stay up to date in your field, be surgically proficient, cultivate good doctor-patient relationships, and provide support should the unwanted occur.

Disclaimer The views expressed are those of the authors and do not reflect the official policy of the Department of the Army, the Department of War, or the US Government.

References

1. Jena AB, Seabury S, Lakdawalla D, Chandra A. Malpractice risk according to physician specialty. N Engl J Med. 2011;365(7):629–36.
2. Kreimer S. Managing risk: how to prevent patient injury and avoid lawsuits. Med Econ. 2013;90(23):46–9.
3. Mello MM, Studdert DM, Kachalia A. The medical liability climate and prospects for reform. JAMA. 2014;312(20):2146–55.
4. Orosco RK, Talamini J, Chang DC, Talamini MA. Surgical malpractice in the United States, 1990-2006. J Am Coll Surg. 2012;215(4):480–8.
5. Physician Insurers Association of America (PIAA). Risk management report – otolaryngology. Rockville: PIAA; 2010.
6. Studdert DM, Thomas EJ, Burstin HR, Zbar BI, Orav EJ, Brennan TA. Negligent care and malpractice claiming behavior in Utah and Colorado. Med Care. 2000;38(3):250–60.
7. Svider PF, Husain Q, Kovalerchik O, et al. Determining legal responsibility in otolaryngology: a review of 44 trials since 2008. Am J Otolaryngol. 2013;34(6):699–705.
8. Ruhl DS, Hong SS, Littlefield PD. Lessons learned in otologic surgery: 30 years of malpractice cases in the United States. Otol Neurotol. 2013;34(7):1173–9.
9. Mathew R, Asimacopoulos E, Valentine P. Toward safer practice in otology: a report on 15 years of clinical negligence claims. Laryngoscope. 2011;121(10):2214–9.
10. Nepps ME. The basics of medical malpractice: a primer on navigating the system. Chest. 2008;134(5):1051–5.
11. Recupero PR. Clinical practice guidelines as learned treatises: understanding their use as evidence in the courtroom. J Am Acad Psychiatry Law. 2008;36(3):290–301.
12. Institute of Medicine (US) Committee on Standards for Developing Trustworthy Clinical Practice Guidelines; Graham R, Mancher M, Miller Wolman D, et al., editors. Clinical practice guidelines we can trust. Washington (DC): National Academies Press (US); 2011.
13. Ruhl DS, Siegal G. Medical malpractice implications of clinical practice guidelines. Otolaryngol Head Neck Surg. 2017;157(2):175–77.
14. Mello M. Of swords and shields: the role of clinical practice guidelines in medical malpractice litigation. Univ Penn Law Review. 2001;149:645–710.
15. Saravanappa N, Balfour A, Bowdler D. Informed consent for middle ear operations: a United Kingdom survey. Clin Otolaryngol Allied Sci. 2003;28(2):91–9.
16. Baum N. Informed consent--more than a form. J Med Pract Manage. 2006;22(3):145–8.
17. Hartman K, Liang B. Exceptions to informed consent in emergency medicine. In: Perspective in Legal Medicine and Health Law; 1999. p. 53–9.
18. Huff D, Mackenzie D. Practice tips to reduce malpractice exposure. J Med Assoc Ga. 2014;103(2):24–6.
19. Jerrold L. Litigation and legislation. You secretly did what? Am J Orthod Dentofacial Orthop. 2015;147(1):143–5.
20. Rodriguez M, Morrow J, Seifi A. Ethical implications of patients and families secretly recording conversations with physicians. JAMA. 2015;313(16):1615–6.
21. Ruhl DS, Cable BB, Martell DW. Medication associated with hearing loss: 25 years of medical malpractice cases in the United States. Otolaryngol Head Neck Surg. 2014;151(3):431–7.
22. Das-Purkayastha P, Rutka J. How should awareness of ototoxicity change the way medicine is practiced? Semin Hear. 2011;32(3):236–47.
23. Cianfrone G, Pentangelo D, Cianfrone E, et al. Pharmacological drugs inducing ototoxicity, vestibular symptoms and tinnitus: a reasoned and updated guide. Eur Rev Med Pharmacol Sci. 2011;15(6):601–36.

24. Blake DM, Svider PF, Carniol ET, Mauro AC, Eloy JA, Jyung RW. Malpractice in otology. Otolaryngol Head Neck Surg. 2013;149(4):554–61.
25. Hong SS, Yheulon CG, Wirtz ED, Sniezek JC. Otolaryngology and medical malpractice: a review of the past decade, 2001-2011. Laryngoscope. 2014;124(4):896–901.
26. Liou TN, Nussenbaum B. Wrong site surgery in otolaryngology-head and neck surgery. Laryngoscope. 2014;124(1):104–9.
27. Ruhl DS, Littlefield PD. Updates in medical malpractice: an otology perspective. Curr Opin Otolaryngol Head Neck Surg. 2015;23(5):348–54.
28. Svider PF, Sunaryo PL, Keeley BR, Kovalerchik O, Mauro AC, Eloy JA. Characterizing liability for cranial nerve injuries: a detailed analysis of 209 malpractice trials. Laryngoscope. 2013;123(5):1156–62.
29. Hu J, Fleck TR, Xu J, Hsu JV, Xu HX. Contemporary changes with the use of facial nerve monitoring in chronic ear surgery. Otolaryngol Head Neck Surg. 2014;151(3):473–7.
30. Reilly BK, Horn GM, Sewell RK. Hearing loss resulting in malpractice litigation: what physicians need to know. Laryngoscope. 2013;123(1):112–7.
31. Tolisano AM, Song SA, Ruhl DS, Littlefield PD. Dizziness, malpractice, and the otolaryngologist. Am J Otolaryngol. 2017;38:401. Epub 2017 Mar 31.
32. Rose C, Svider PF, Sheyn A, et al. Protecting the most vulnerable: litigation from pediatric otolaryngologic procedures and conditions. Laryngoscope. 2014;124(9):2161–6.
33. Gustin A. The art and science of disclosing unanticipated outcomes to patients. ASA Refresher Courses Anesthesiol. 2013;41(1):53–8.
34. Wiet R, Harvey S, Littlefield P. Complications of surgery for otitis media. In: Brackmann D, Shelton C, Arriaga M, editors. Otologic surgery. 4th ed. New York: WB Saunders; 2015.
35. Ferreres AR. Ethical issues of expert witness testimony. World J Surg. 2014;38(7):1644–9.
36. Sanders J. Expert witness ethics. Fordham Law Rev. 2007;76(3):1539–84.
37. American Academy of Otolaryngology – Head and Neck Surgery: expert witness qualifications and testimony. Revised 5/2016. Accessed 10/1/2024 at https://www.entnet.org/about-us/leadership-governance/ethics/expert-witness-qualifications-and-testimony/.

Part V

Diseases of the External Ear

31 Diseases of the Auricle, External Auditory Canal, and Tympanic Membrane

Stephanie Moody Antonio, Mikayla Huestis, Peter Volsky, and Barry Strasnick

Developmental Considerations

The auditory and vestibular systems develop as distinct anatomic units. During the sixth week of gestation, auricular development begins with the formation of the six hillocks of His, mesenchymal proliferations originating from the first and second pharyngeal arches. The first arch contributes three hillocks, which eventually form the tragus and the root and superior portion of the helix. The second arch also contributes three hillocks, destined to become the antihelix, antitragus, and lobule. The definitive auricle develops from the fusion of the hillocks and is usually complete by the 12th week of gestation. The auricle will not reach its adult shape, however, until the 20th gestational week, and it continues to grow for the first 5 years of life. Given the complexity of this process, it is not surprising that developmental abnormalities of the auricle are common.

The ectoderm of the first branchial groove invaginates to form the primitive EAC. As the cells continue to grow inward, they eventually meet endodermal tissue of the developing tubotympanum, a derivative of the first pharyngeal pouch. Mesodermal anlages encroach on this area of apposition from ventral and dorsal sites. The resulting solid core of tissue is named the meatal plug or plate. By the 28th week of fetal development, the plate resorbs and the EAC recanalizes. Ectodermal elements from the meatal plate form the epithelial lining of the EAC and the lateral tympanic membrane, whereas mesodermal elements contribute to the development of the cartilaginous EAC, ossification centers of the tympanic ring, and the ossicular chain. Failure of EAC recanalization results in congenital aural atresia [1].

S. M. Antonio · M. Huestis · P. Volsky · B. Strasnick (✉)
Department of Otolaryngology—Head and Neck Surgery, Eastern Virginia Medical School, Norfolk, VA, USA
e-mail: moodysa@evms.edu; vhuestimj@evms.edu; volskypg@evms.edu; strasnb@evms.edu

Anatomy

The Auricle

Fibroelastic cartilage, perichondrium, and skin comprise the auricular framework. The cartilage of the auricle is continuous with that of the lateral EAC. The skin of the topographically complex lateral surface of the auricle is firmly attached to the perichondrium; however, the skin of the posterior surface is less adherent, due to a layer of loose areolar tissue between it and the perichondrium. The auricle is fixed to the temporal bone by its cartilaginous contribution to the external meatus, the three auricular ligaments—anterior, superior, and posterior—and by six poorly developed intrinsic muscles. Additionally, three distinctly better-developed extrinsic muscles exist, also named anterior, superior, and posterior. Voluntary contraction of the extrinsic musculature is responsible for the ability possessed by some to "wiggle" the auricle. These muscles are innervated by the facial nerve.

Sensory innervation of the auricle is characterized by a great deal of overlap between multiple nerves [2]. The auriculotemporal branch of the mandibular division of the trigeminal nerve supplies sensation to the tragus and the helix and its crus; it also supplies sensation to the anterior and superior portions of the EAC and corresponding areas of the lateral surface of the tympanic membrane. Fibers from cervical sensory nerves (C2, C3), contained in the great auricular nerve, innervate the posterior surface of the auricle, the posterior region of the helix, the antihelix, and the lobule. Fibers from the ninth and tenth cranial nerves supply the majority of the conchal concavity, with additional contribution from the seventh cranial nerve.

The external carotid artery supplies blood to the auricle and external meatus via the postauricular and superficial temporal branches. Venous drainage parallels the arterial supply. The superficial temporal vein joins the retromandibular vein and ultimately the internal jugular system, whereas the postauricular vein joins the external jugular

A. D. Sweeney et al. (eds.), *Haynes-Glasscock-Shambaugh Surgery of the Ear*, https://doi.org/10.1007/978-3-032-18264-7_31

system [3]. There also may be drainage to the sigmoid sinus via the mastoid emissary vein [4]. The lymphatics of the anterior auricle and meatus drain into the preauricular and periparotid nodes. Lymphatics of the posterior auricle, however, empty into the retroauricular (mastoid) and infra-auricular nodes [5].

The External Auditory Canal

The EAC is a tube measuring approximately 2.5 cm in length that extends from the concha to the tympanic membrane. The most lateral one-third of the canal is cartilaginous, whereas the medial two-thirds are osseous. The narrowest segment of the EAC, the isthmus, corresponds to the junction of the cartilaginous and bony portions. The canal's anteroinferior wall is slightly longer than the posterosuperior wall, creating an acute angle between the anterior canal wall and the tympanic membrane. The EAC is also slightly convex anteriorly, which can prevent complete examination of the tympanic membrane. Improved tympanic membrane visualization is achieved by retracting the auricle in a posterosuperior direction during otoscopy.

The skin and subcutaneous tissue surround the cartilage of the lateral EAC. Hair follicles and sebaceous and apocrine (ceruminous) glands exist within this subcutaneous tissue. These structures form an apopilosebaceous unit and produce a protective layer of cerumen. In contrast, the more medial, osseous EAC lacks glandular adnexae and consists only of the tympanic bone and a tightly adherent epidermis. The clinical significance of this difference lies in the fact that infected sebaceous cysts and furuncles occur only in the lateral EAC. The epidermis of the EAC is continuous with the squamous epithelial layer of the tympanic membrane. Infectious processes of the EAC may spread to the temporomandibular joint and periparotid soft tissue via inconstant dehiscences of the cartilaginous canal called the fissures of Santorini. An anterior gap of the tympanic bone, named Huschke's foramen, may similarly permit spread of infection to the preauricular tissue. This developmental dehiscence usually closes in late childhood but may persist into adulthood [6].

Sensory innervation of the EAC is variable, with suspected contributions from cranial nerves V, VII, IX, and X. Generally, the auriculotemporal branch of the mandibular division of the trigeminal nerve innervates the anterior and superior walls of the EAC. Fibers from the facial, glossopharyngeal, and vagus nerves, traveling with the auricular branch (Arnold's nerve) of the vagus nerve, enter the EAC through the tympanomastoid suture to supply the posterior and inferior aspects of the canal [2].

The blood supply of the EAC is the same as that of the auricle, with additional contributions from the deep auricular artery. This vessel, a branch of the internal maxillary artery, passes through the substance of the parotid gland and travels posterior to the temporomandibular joint capsule before penetrating the EAC in the region of the isthmus. Venous drainage is via the superficial temporal and posterior auricular veins, which join the internal and external jugular systems, respectively. Lymphatics of the inferior EAC drain to the infra-auricular nodes, those of the posterior canal drain to the retroauricular nodes, and the periparotid, superficial, and deep cervical nodes receive drainage from the anterior region of the canal.

Cerumen is a mixture of desquamated epidermal cells and secretions from sebaceous and ceruminous glands of the EAC, including fatty acids, alcohols, triglycerides, cholesterol, cholesterol precursors, and amino acids. The composition of wax may be in part hereditary. Cerumen that tends to be wet as opposed to dry wax tends to contain more lipid and pigment. Cerumen lubricates the EAC and keeps the canal clean by trapping dirt and repelling water. Whether cerumen has further antimicrobial benefits is not entirely clear [7].

The Tympanic Membrane

The tympanic membrane is a thin fibrous sheet interposed between the EAC and middle ear. Its diameter measures approximately 9 mm, and it is oriented obliquely at the lateral end of the external canal. Its appearance is one of a cone directed medially, the apex of which corresponds to its attachment to the umbo. Three cell layers form the tympanic membrane: a lateral epithelial lining that is continuous with the skin of the EAC, a middle fibrous layer composed of both radiating and circular fibers of connective tissue, and an internal mucosal layer. A coalescence of the fibrous layer at its rim, known as the fibrous annulus, helps anchor the tympanic membrane within the bony tympanic sulcus. The pars tensa refers to the majority of the membrane area, which is separated from the pars flaccida (Shrapnell's membrane) superiorly by the anterior and posterior alveolar folds. The lamina propria of the pars tensa is thin and strong, made up of abundant type II collagen. The medial layer of the pars flaccida contains thicker and more loosely arranged collagen fibrils, mainly type I collagen, and it is more elastic than the pars tensa [8]. The pars flaccida sits in a region of the tympanic ring deficient of bone, named the notch of Rivinus. Medial to the pars flaccida is Prussak's space, the most common site of primary cholesteatoma formation.

Sensory innervation to the lateral surface of the tympanic membrane mirrors that of the EAC. The auriculotemporal nerve supplies the posterior and inferior region of the tympanic membrane, and the auricular branch (Arnold's nerve) of the vagus nerve innervates its anterior and superior aspect, with additional fibers originating from the seventh cranial nerve. The tympanic branch (Jacobson's nerve) of the glossopharyngeal nerve provides sensation to the medial surface of the tympanic membrane.

The blood supply to the tympanic membrane is derived from vessels that supply the external canal and middle ear cavity. The deep auricular branch of the internal maxillary artery forms a peripheral ring from which arise branches destined for the tympanic membrane's lateral surface. The internal maxillary artery also supplies the internal surface of the tympanic membrane via its anterior tympanic branch [9]. The manubrial artery paralleling the malleus accounts for much of the blood supply of the central tympanic membrane. Venous drainage tends to parallel corresponding arterial anatomy.

Diseases of the Auricle

Frostbite

The auricle, with its high ratio of surface area to mass, is at increased risk for this type of injury. Blood vessels supplying this region lie superficially within the subcutaneous tissues, increasing their exposure to colder temperatures. Prolonged exposure blocks afferent sensory nerve transmission, reducing the patient's awareness of ongoing injury. The initial physiologic response is vasoconstriction. The frozen tissue appears yellow-white and waxy and is cold and hard to the touch. This appearance, combined with the loss of sensation, is diagnostic of frostbite. Extracellular ice formation during the freezing and thawing process results in cell dehydration and cell membrane rupture. The blood vessels are also damaged, resulting in extravasation of fluid and clotting. As tissues warm, extravasated fluid causes edema and bullae formation, which are painful.

Management consists of rapid tissue warming via circulating warm water or warmed moistened dressings. Use of radiant heat is contraindicated as it may worsen the injury, especially if warming and refreezing take place. The pinna should be dressed aseptically with 1% silver sulfadiazine cream, similar to management of a burn injury. Secondary infection is treated with antimicrobial agents directed against *Pseudomonas aeruginosa* and *Staphylococcus aureus*. In some cases, tissue initially appearing devitalized will recover after a period of observation and conservative management. Therefore, debridement of necrotic tissue should be delayed until a reliable line of demarcation develops [10]. Recently, tissue plasminogen activator has decreased the rate of digit amputation and has been incorporated into frostbite treatment protocols [11].

Hematoma

Blunt trauma to the auricle may result in hematoma. The trauma causes a shearing injury, resulting in separation of auricular cartilage from its associated perichondrium and bleeding into this newly created space. The cartilage is subsequently deprived of its perichondrium-dependent blood supply and may become ischemic. Hematoma may present immediately following an injury or in delayed fashion, as painful swelling, which causes effacement of the normal topography of the auricle.

Management consists of evacuation and compression. The former task may be accomplished by needle aspiration if the hematoma is acute and small in size. For larger collections, incision and drainage are required. The incision is placed along the helical fold, thereby minimizing the conspicuousness of the resultant scar, and the blood clot is expelled. Curettage may be used to completely remove all of the hematoma. In terms of compression, it is critical to place of a pressure dressing to prevent reaccumulation. One technique is to use dental rolls as bolsters, secured with through-and-through sutures on both the lateral and medial auricular surfaces. Close follow-up is necessary to address recurrences in a timely fashion. Failure to evacuate a hematoma leads to fibrosis and new cartilage formation. The resulting deformity is permanent and ranges from mild cartilaginous thickening to the severe "cauliflower" ear, seen most frequently in wrestlers and boxers [12].

Perichondritis

Infection of the auricular perichondrium and underlying cartilage is a possible complication of surgery, trauma, or external otitis. Perichondritis presents with erythema, edema, and exquisite tenderness of the involved pinna. Progression of the infectious process can lead to abscess formation and loss of cartilage. The most common offending organism is *Pseudomonas aeruginosa*. Diabetes and other causes of immunosuppression have been implicated as predisposing factors [13].

If diagnosed early, perichondritis may be managed on an outpatient basis with oral antibiotics, aural toilet and debridement, and close observation. Because of its excellent cartilaginous penetration and high activity against *Pseudomonas* species, ciprofloxacin is the drug of choice. In children with early perichondritis, outpatient management with antibiotics can be initiated. Fluoroquinolones in children may be used with caution and with appropriate monitoring for cartilage toxicity [14]. If significant clinical improvement is not observed within the first 24 to 36 hours of oral therapy, or if the patient presents initially with severe infection, parenteral antibiotic therapy is warranted. An auricular abscess requires prompt incision and drainage. Additionally, all necrotic cartilage and tissue should be debrided and cultures obtained. A drain under a conforming pressure dressing may help reduce permanent deformity.

Sebaceous Cyst

Sebaceous cysts form as a result of sebaceous gland obstruction. The lobule and retroauricular areas are common locations for these soft, mobile masses. Normally, asymptomatic sebaceous cysts do not require treatment unless cosmetic deformity exists. Occasionally, however, the cyst will become acutely infected and require antibiotic therapy. Formal excision should be delayed until the infection has resolved. When excision is performed, the entire cyst capsule must be removed, or recurrence is likely [15].

Preauricular Sinus

The incidence of preauricular pits or sinuses are estimated at less than 1 in 100 births in the United States [16]. Resulting from abnormalities in the fusion of the hillocks of His during auricular development, they present as pit-like depressions anterior to the root of the helix and superior to the level of the tragus. Preauricular sinuses are bilateral in 25–50% of cases. Genetic inheritance is more likely involved in the case of bilateral pits. These sinuses are prone to acute infection requiring antibiotic therapy. If infection does not respond to oral antibiotics, incision and drainage may be necessary. However, acute incision and drainage are ideally avoided since subsequent scarring and fibrosis will obliterate normal tissue planes and make future excision more difficult. When symptomatic or associated with recurrent infection, surgical resection of a preauricular sinus is indicated [17].

Other related lesions include preauricular skin tags and branchial cleft anomalies. Similar to preauricular sinuses, skin tags in this location represent duplication anomalies of the ectodermal hillocks of His. Although generally benign in their natural history, the skin tags may be excised for cosmetic purposes. First branchial cleft cysts, sinuses, and fistulas, on the other hand, result from duplication anomalies of the membranous EAC. A fistulous tract may exist between the skin of the neck and an intact EAC. The Work classification divides first branchial cleft sinuses into two types [18]. Type I anomalies contain only ectodermal derivatives, whereas type II anomalies possess tissues of both ectodermal and mesodermal origin. Management of first branchial cleft lesions consists of surgical resection. Caution is required when dealing with branchial cleft anomalies as their mesodermal origin results in an intimate association with the parotid gland, placing the facial nerve at risk during attempts at excision. Surgical approach should include superficial parotidectomy and consideration of continuous facial nerve monitoring.

Hearing loss may be associated with preauricular pits, branchial cleft anomalies, and other congenital external ear and EAC anomalies. For example, branchiootorenal syndrome, which is the second most common type of autosomal dominant syndromic hearing loss, manifests with conductive, sensorineural, or mixed hearing loss with branchial cleft cysts or fistulae, preauricular pits, and renal anomalies. CHARGE association, Townes-Brocks syndrome, branchiootorenal syndrome, Nager syndrome, Miller syndrome, and diabetic embryopathy also may include both auricular and renal anomalies. Patients who present with auricular anomalies should be examined for dysmorphic features such as facial asymmetry, colobomas, choanal atresia, branchial cysts or sinuses, or other abnormal features. Renal ultrasound may be indicated if syndromic features such as these are found. Isolated preauricular pits are infrequently associated with hearing loss and rarely associated with renal abnormalities [19]. Audiologic testing is warranted to rule out hearing loss, but follow-up audiologic testing is probably not indicated, unless there is a significant family history of hearing loss or other risk factors. Wang et al. suggest that a renal ultrasound should be performed in patients with preauricular pits, cup ears, or any other ear anomaly accompanied by other dysmorphic features or in the setting of other genetic risk factors such as family history of hearing loss or renal malformations [20].

Surgical Technique for Resection of Preauricular Pit and Sinuses

Pits and sinuses that have been subject to infection or discharge are appropriately considered for resection. It is best to avoid operating on an actively infected pit or sinus.

Surgical details: An elliptical incision is designed incorporating the pit. Some surgeons prefer a wide local excision with a supra-auricular approach, citing reduced recurrence [21]. Placement of a lacrimal probe into the tract aids in determining its extent. After making the incision and beginning the dissection of the tissues, the probe may be stabilized by clamping it to the surrounding soft tissues. The tract is followed while avoiding violation to the medial extent, usually at the helical cartilage. Care should be taken to avoid violating the sinus, and an adequate margin of tissue should be resected with the specimen. Preauricular sinuses tend to have multiple “fingers,” which can cause recurrences if left behind. At the medial extent, a section of the cartilage is removed with the specimen to prevent recurrence.

Pitfalls and Complications: The most significant challenge with resection of preauricular sinuses is recurrence. Meticulous dissection is needed to completely remove the sinus and cyst. Some surgeons inject methylene blue to help delineate the extent of the lesion. Attempting to perform resection during acute infection will increase the risk of recurrence. Also, if the cyst has been infected on multiple occasions, tissue planes will have been disrupted, and it will be more difficult to achieve a complete excision. Thus, once a lesion has been infected, surgical treatment should be strongly considered. In cases of postoperative recurrent sinus or cyst, a wider resection incorporating tissue between the superficial temporal vessels, temporalis fascia, and conchal cartilage will improve the likelihood of removing all the epithelial remnants [22]. A new technique pioneered by one institution termed "inside out" involves incising the tract and using magnification to follow all branches and remove them, similar to other methods. They report no recurrences with this technique [23].

Keloid

Keloids are benign, hypertrophic, fibrous lesions that generally develop following trauma or surgery. They are more common in darkly pigmented people and are frequently found on the lobule as a result of ear piercing. An excess of extracellular matrix, particularly glycoproteins, characterizes the histologic appearance of keloids [24]. Treatment generally requires a combination of medical and surgical therapy. For small lesions or developing keloids, intralesional injections of triamcinolone acetonide may be used as first-line therapy. Because of their poor absorption through hypertrophic tissue, topical corticosteroids play a very limited role in the management of keloids. For larger and more mature lesions, excision is required. Intralesional corticosteroid injection is performed at the time of surgery and repeated every 4 to 6 weeks thereafter for a minimum of three postoperative injections. Patient compliance with this postoperative regimen is required to minimize the risk of recurrence. Some advocate additional pre-excisional injections to ensure that patients understand and accept the need for multiple treatments and are likely to adhere to the prescribed postoperative regimen [25]. Despite combined excision and intralesional corticosteroid therapy, recurrence rates approach 50% [26]. Extremely gentle tissue management may reduce activation of the inflammatory response that can increase recurrence. Low-dose radiation therapy can be considered for cases resistant to conventional therapy, but the risk of radiation-induced malignancy in these predominantly young patients tempers our enthusiasm for this aggressive approach.

Tophi

Gout is a severe monoarticular inflammatory arthritis triggered by the presence of urate crystals in synovial joint fluid. Tophaceous deposition of urate crystals in and around joints is one of the hallmark physical findings associated with hyperuricemia. Frequently, patients will present with deposits in the helix, appearing as moderately painful, salmon-pink nodules. When compressed, tophi exude a whitish, chalky substance consisting of sodium biurate. Crystals appear negatively birefringent when examined under polarized light. Treatment of acute attacks of gouty arthritis focuses on pain relief and correction of the underlying abnormality in uric acid metabolism [27]. No specific surgical therapy directed at auricular tophi is necessary.

Chondrodermatitis Nodularis Chronica Helicis

Chondrodermatitis nodularis chronica helicis, or Winkler's nodule, is an intensely painful solitary nodule, usually found in the helix or antihelix of older men. They appear spontaneously and are thought to be caused by pressure or trauma-induced damage to underlying cartilage. The right side is more commonly involved, possibly due to favored sleeping position. The nodules are tender, round, well-defined and firm, and usually pale, grey, or slightly erythematous. The edge may be raised, and the center may be ulcerated or crusted. A shave biopsy should be performed to rule out malignancy. Conservative treatment options range from laser to pressure relief. Surgical treatment has lower recurrence rates and involves removal of involved cartilage [28].

Neoplasms

The external ear is a common site for benign and malignant processes of the skin, including actinic keratosis, papilloma, melanoma, basal cell carcinoma, and squamous cell carcinoma. The otologic surgeon should be aware of the differential diagnosis of skin lesions and apply appropriate management. Auricular cancers commonly originate in areas with maximal sun exposure, such as the helical rim or antihelix. Basal cell carcinoma may be less likely associated with sun exposure and is the more common type of tumor found on the posterior surface of the auricle. The thin skin of the pinna provides very little resistance to spread to the underlying perichondrium, but embryonic lines of fusion may limit disease to an anatomical subunit, at least temporarily [29]. Biopsy is required to make a diagnosis and should not be delayed. Management is varied and may include curettage, electrodissection, cryosurgery, topical 5-fluorouracil, local excision, or radiation therapy. The auricle is particularly amenable to surgical excision with Mohs technique. After surgical excision, reconstruction is geared toward covering defects and restoring cosmesis and function. The optimal reconstructive technique is greatly influenced by the deficit tissue and can be as simple as allowing healing by secondary intention or skin grafting to rotating tissue flaps onto reconstructed structural elements [30].

Congenital Deformities of the Pinna

Congenital deformities of the pinna, including protruding ear and lop ear, are frequently encountered in the otologic practice. The deformity may be unilateral or bilateral. Frequently, the auricular cartilage is of appropriate size but lacks a well-defined antihelical fold. An excessively high or spherical conchal cartilage contributes to the prominent ear. If identified at birth, splinting can be an option for possible correction. The entity has no significant otologic ramifications aside from cosmesis; therefore, its importance is determined by the psychological disturbance endured by the patient. By age 5, the auricle has essentially reached adult size, and children generally start school [31]. Teasing from peers may become severe at this time, and surgical correction may be sought at this time if it was not before.

Although differences in opinion regarding "normative values" for auricular position and protrusion exist, Tolleth provided some general guidelines on which surgical correction can be based [32]. With the head oriented vertically, the desired position of the auricle is approximately one ear length posterior to the lateral orbital rim. The level of the brow defines the preferred position of the top of the ear, whereas the base of the columella marks the appropriate inferior extent of the lobule. The axis of the auricle should not lie in the vertical plane; rather, it should be rotated 15 to 20 degrees in the posterior direction. A distance of 15 to 20 mm between the scalp and the outer edge of the helix provides an esthetically pleasing degree of auricular protrusion.

Surgical Technique for Correction of Protruding Ear

Preoperative Planning: The goals of otoplasty include correction of protrusion of the helix and lobe, creation of an antihelical fold, avoidance of overcorrection, and creation of auricles that are symmetric in appearance and position. A surgical plan will include a detailed analysis of the anatomy and, potentially, a combination of techniques to address each component of the deformity. Preoperative photographs will assist in planning and counseling. A wide variety of techniques can be used to reshape the auricular cartilages, including abrasion and scoring or suture fixation. We prefer a modification of the technique described by Mustarde, employing a combination of posterior auricular skin excision and mattress sutures [33]. The technique is relatively simple and provides predictable results.

Surgical Details (Fig. 31.1): The ear is again examined, and the plan is reviewed. Markings are applied with an ink marker to define the crest of the antihelix and with a needle to define the suture sites. The location for the Mustarde sutures may also be made by placing marking sutures through the anterior skin while folding the ear into position. An elliptical incision is made in the postauricular sulcus. Most surgeons will plan to resect an ellipse of skin, but others do not. In the latter case, a simple linear incision is made. The posterior auricular skin is elevated to the helical rim and triangular fossa, taking care to avoid nicking the cartilage. The tissues are also elevated from the conchal cartilage toward the periosteum of the mastoid. The intrinsic and extrinsic muscles will need to be divided. Several Mustarde sutures (a row of horizontal mattress sutures) are placed through cartilage and anterior perichondrium to roll and create a smooth antihelical fold and approximate the scaphoid fossa closer to the concha. A 5–0 or 6–0 non-absorbable suture with a taper needle is used. Once a suture is set, it is temporarily tightened with just enough pull to fold the antihelix, but not necessarily to fully approximate the gap. The tie is clamped, while the next sutures are thrown. Once three or four sutures are in good position, they can be individually tied. Repetitive reevaluation of the created fold is done to ensure a good result. The helix should be visible beyond the new antihelix. An excessively high concha is reduced by tacking the proximal conchal cartilage to the periosteum of the mastoid [34]. The appropriate position is first evaluated by holding the ear. A 4–0 or 5–0 suture should be used and more than one stitch used for support, as these sutures tend to bear more force. If needed, conchal cartilage can be thinned or excised. At this point, examine the upper pole of the ear and the lobule to ensure these areas do not appear excessively prominent. A prominent upper pole can be corrected with a stitch between the triangular fossa and the deep temporal fascia [35]. Redundant posterior auricular skin is excised in elliptical fashion, and the incision is then closed. The ear is dressed by packing the auricular contours with cotton, padding the posterior surface, and placing a mastoid dressing.

Postoperative care: The dressing should be removed at postoperative day 1 and examined for hematoma and signs of excessive pressure. It can then be replaced for a few days. The patient should be examined frequently in the postoperative period to check the ear position. Some surgeons ask the patient to wear a headband for 3 or 4 months.

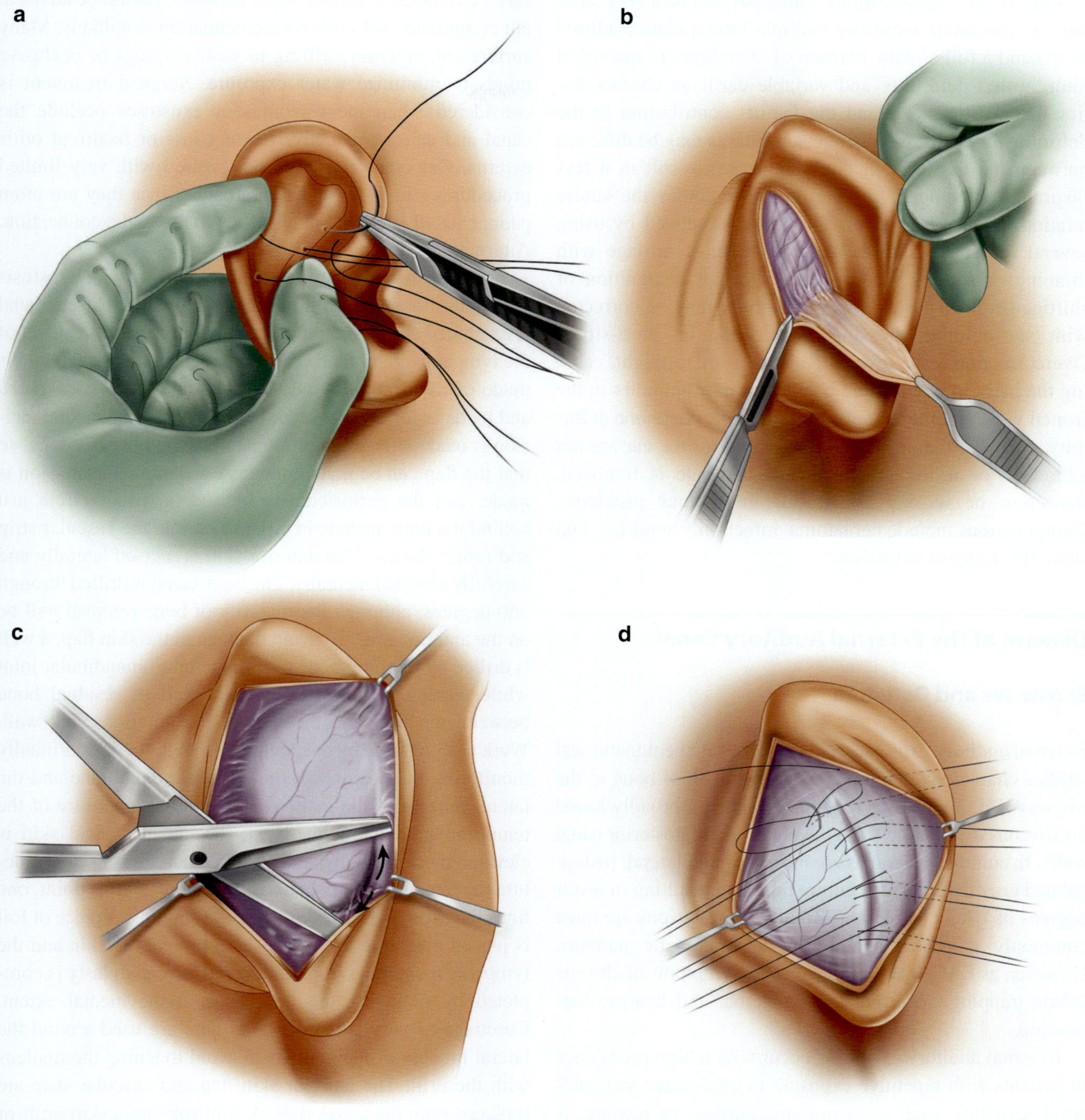

Fig. 31.1 Procedural steps for otoplasty. Adapted from Glasscock and Shambaugh's Surgery of the Ear. Eds. Gulya, Minor, Poe. PMPH. 2010. (**a**) Marking the suture sites by a through and through silk suture (after raising the skin from the posterior aspect of the pinna). (**b**) Postauricular elliptical skin incision. (**c**) Elevating the postauricular skin to the helical rim. (**d**) Placing multiple horizontal mattress sutures at the site of the marking sutures

Pitfalls and Complications: Otoplasty can be a very challenging procedure requiring multiple intraoperative adjustments and a full armamentarium of techniques to manage a multifaceted deformity and variable cartilage characteristics. Failure to understand the factors contributing to the deformity of each ear, which in some cases may be different between the two ears in one patient, can result in a less favorable outcome. If the cartilage overcomes the suture fixation, relapse can occur. This can be reduced by using several redundant sutures and by relaxing cartilage with thinning or scoring when needed. Prompt recognition of shifting or other postoperative deformity may be corrected with a molding dressing, headband, or steri-strips. Overcorrection results when the sutures are too tight, causing the helix to be invisible behind the new antihelix in the frontal view. Another undesirable outcome, telephone deformity, occurs if the upper and lower poles of the ear are not addressed or if too much conchal cartilage is removed. Resection or scoring can result in contour problems. Complications include hematoma, infection, chondritis, and suture bridging or extrusion.

Disease of the External Auditory Canal

Exostoses and Osteoma

External auditory exostoses and osteomas are benign clinical entities characterized by hyperplastic growth of bone in the osseous EAC. Exostoses tend to be bilateral, broadly based protrusions originating from the anterior and posterior canal walls. In contrast, osteomas are more often unilateral, pedunculated growths located at suture lines and resulting in lesser degrees of EAC obstruction. Both types of lesions are most commonly noted incidentally in asymptomatic patients. However, as EAC obstruction worsens, symptoms of chronic debris trapping, recurrent otitis externa, and hearing loss develop.

External auditory exostoses occur with a high prevalence in patients with repetitive exposure to cold-water and cold-wind activities, such as swimming, surfing, or boating. A causal relationship between cold water exposure and the development of exostoses was first proposed by van Gilse, who showed that irrigation of the EAC with water colder than 17 °C results in prolonged meatal erythema [36]. Exposure to cold temperature is thought to produce a periosteitis, which seems to cause new bone growth.

Surgical Technique for Removal of Exostosis and Osteoma

Indications and Preoperative Planning: Management of exostoses and osteomas consists of periodic cerumen disimpaction and debridement and treatment of infection as necessary. Avoidance of further water exposure should be advised, but compliance with this recommendation is unlikely. Many surfers are, however, willing to wear earplugs or occlusive hoods to minimize water exposure. Surgical treatment is considered when the osteomas or exostoses occlude the canal and cause conductive hearing loss or recurrent otitis externa. Osteomas can often be resected with very limited procedures and a transcanal approach. Since they are often pedunculated, a curette may suffice to break the connection. Alternatively, it may be drilled.

Surgical details for removal of exostosis: Exostosis removal is done with a postauricular approach. The ear canal is examined and injected with local anesthesia. If the level of the tympanic membrane can be appreciated, a mental note is made of its location. A posterior vascular strip is designed and made as long as possible. In some cases, the medial incision is made after some of the lateral canalplasty is done, so that the flap can be made longer. A postauricular incision is made, and the periosteum is incised in a half circle just behind the bony meatus in order to elevate the vascular strip and reflect the ear. The anterior skin is incised laterally and carefully elevated medially. The bony canal is drilled through 360 degrees, although the majority of bone removal will be on the anterior wall. To avoid damage to the skin flap, a well is drilled by thinning bone over the temporomandibular joint while leaving a thin "egg-shelled" wall of residual bone between the well and the skin of the anterior canal wall. Work can continue by deepening this well, while continually monitoring the position of the tympanic membrane and the lateral process of the malleus and avoiding exposure of the temporomandibular joint. Next, the anterior canal skin is elevated more medially, and finally, a curette is used to fracture the remaining egg-shelled bone. Often, at this point, one finds the exostosis extending over the annulus. A piece of foil is placed medial to the exostosis to protect the skin and the tympanic membrane from injury, and the canalplasty is completed by removing the final bone at the medial extent. Curettage or very small diamond burs are used around the lateral process of the malleus to avoid touching the malleus with the drill. The anterior skin flap and vascular strip are replaced onto the canal wall. A split-thickness skin graft or fascial graft may be necessary if significant areas of exposed bone remain. The canal is packed with gelfoam soaked in saline or antibiotic. The incision is closed.

Postoperative care: Antibiotic drops are applied to the packed ear canal twice daily. Water exposure is avoided. Packing material is removed during weekly or biweekly visits over 4–6 weeks.

Pitfalls and Complications: Risks of canalplasty for excision of exostoses include facial nerve injury, perforation of the tympanic membrane, infection, recurrence of exostoses, and sensorineural hearing loss. Facial nerve injury is avoided by using intraoperative facial nerve monitoring and by limiting posterior and inferior bone removal. Complete excision is safer with a postauricular approach and is therefore preferred over a transcanal approach which will limit exposure and understanding of the presumed location of the facial nerve. The anterior canal wall skin and tympanic membrane should be protected from injury by careful technique and by using a small disk made from foil suture packing material. Also, great care should be taken to identify and protect the lateral process of the malleus from drill trauma, which can induce sensorineural hearing loss.

Keratosis Obturans

Keratosis obturans is characterized by the accumulation of large keratin plugs in the osseous EAC, resulting in obstruction, acute pain, and hearing loss. The underlying epithelium is hyperplastic with an increased rate of desquamation and loss of normal migration. Additionally, it is often chronically inflamed. Interestingly, upward of 90% of patients suffering from keratosis obturans also have a past history of bronchiectasis or sinusitis [37, 38]. Clinically, keratosis obturans presents as occlusion of the external meatus by tightly compacted plugs of laminar desquamated keratin debris. Over time, the osseous external canal may become significantly widened, frequently to the point at which the tympanic membrane and annulus "stand out in relief." The tympanic membrane typically shows moderate degrees of thickening, and some cases report tympanic membrane perforation with associated cholesteatoma. Management consists of local debridement of the plug, occasionally requiring general anesthesia secondary to severe discomfort and appropriate ototopical therapy to address residual tissue inflammation or secondary infection. Routine cleaning with acetic acid solution or irrigation with hydrogen peroxide and warm water may reduce accumulation of debris. Infrequently, patients will suffer from repeated canal occlusion and pain despite vigilant home maintenance, office surveillance, and debridement. In these difficult situations, canalplasty with skin grafting can be an effective treatment option by replacing chronically diseased epithelium with the healthy epidermis of a skin graft [39]. Surgery is also indicated if there is concern for cholesteatoma. Given that the disease process starts from the tympanic membrane, disease is limited and more easily cleared compared to external auditory canal cholesteatoma [40].

External Auditory Canal Cholesteatoma

Cholesteatoma of the EAC is similar to keratosis obturans in that each is characterized by the presence of keratin debris within the canal. They are, however, distinct clinical entities. Patients with EAC cholesteatoma are generally older and often present with unilateral disease that can be characterized by otorrhea, dull pain, and hearing loss. This rare variety of cholesteatoma can be acquired secondary to trauma, surgery, stenosis, or chronic inflammation, or it can arise spontaneously [41]. The precise etiology of spontaneous EAC cholesteatoma is unclear, but pathologic studies consistently cite a localized periosteitis and bone sequestra formation [42].

Clinically, EAC cholesteatomas cause focal erosion of the bony canal wall, usually in an inferior and posterior location. The accumulated debris is loose and random as opposed to the laminated plug of keratosis obturans. The severity can range from limited, superficial erosion and minimal debris accumulation to extensive involvement of surrounding structures, such as the TMJ, facial nerve, or mastoid. Complete microscopic examination of the cholesteatoma is critical in determining its extent. For localized lesions, frequent office debridement of necrotic bone and debris may suffice. For cholesteatomas eroding into the canal wall and when office management is difficult or painful, a canalplasty may successfully exteriorize the defect. External auditory canal healing can be aided by obliterating large defects with cartilage or cartilage-perichondrial grafts and/or covering exposed bone with skin or fascial grafts. Disease involving the mastoid may warrant tympanomastoidectomy to remove involved bone and repair associated defects.

Foreign Body

Children are frequently referred to otolaryngologists for the management of ear canal foreign bodies. Primary care physicians often discover the foreign body when evaluating a child for possible otitis, or it may be found incidentally during a well-child visit. Inorganic objects are commonly present. A greater challenge to manage in the office, however, are organic objects, such as popcorn and peanut fragments, which tend to absorb moisture and swell to completely obstruct the meatus. Foreign bodies are removed under microscopic visualization with a cerumen loop, right-angle pick, or suction. For the uncooperative child, removal under general anesthesia is required, given the risk of tympanic membrane and ossicular chain injury that can result from the sudden movement of a distressed patient. Occasionally, an endaural incision is necessary to remove a severely impacted object. Postoperative antibiotic drops should be used when an incision is required or extensive trauma to the skin of the external canal is observed [43].

Furuncle

Also known as acute localized otitis externa, acute furunculosis is the result of obstruction of pilosebaceous glands present in the subcutaneous tissue of the cartilaginous EAC. Elevation of the tightly adherent skin of the external canal causes exquisite pain and discomfort. The pinna and preauricular soft tissue may display associated cellulitic changes. Treatment of acute furunculosis consists of antibiotics directed against *S. aureus* and warm compresses. If significant fluctuance develops, incision and drainage are required and generally provide pain relief. If possible, a small wick of packing material should be placed into the abscess cavity following drainage to prevent recurrence.

Aural Polyp

Aural polyps are well-circumscribed, soft, fleshy masses frequently found in the EACs of patients presenting with otorrhea and hearing loss. They are usually inflammatory and suggest active middle ear disease. An association between aural polyps and cholesteatoma, especially in children, is well established and may be as high as 45% [44, 45]. Polyps are frequently seen in pediatric patients, the result of a foreign body reaction to pressure equalization tubes. Polyps may arise from middle ear mucosa and protrude into the external meatus through a tympanic membrane perforation or tube. Additionally, polyps may be a manifestation of myringitis, malignant otitis externa, temporal bone malignancy, or other neoplastic or inflammatory lesion, such as inflammatory pseudotumor or giant cell granuloma. Histopathologic analysis is therefore required when the etiology of a polyp is unknown.

Gentle aural cleansing and the application of antibiotic-corticosteroid-containing drops can effectively reduce a polyp's size and allow adequate examination of the medial EAC and tympanic membrane. Cauterization with silver nitrate can also be a helpful adjunctive measure in initial therapy. Aggressive debridement or avulsion of an aural polyp should be avoided as it may have attachments to a dehiscent facial nerve, the stapes footplate, or cholesteatoma overlying a labyrinthine fistula. Biopsy and histologic analysis should be performed on polyps of uncertain origin, both to rule out malignancy and possibly to help in diagnosing an underlying cholesteatoma. Patients who fail to respond to medical management require surgery. Removal and biopsy of aural polyps with middle ear involvement should be performed in conjunction with middle ear exploration, tympanoplasty, and possibly mastoidectomy to appropriately address the primary disease [46].

Dermatologic Processes

The EAC is essentially a blind pouch lined with skin. Its epidermis is susceptible to the same dermatologic processes encountered elsewhere in the body. Because it encompasses a small space and its skin is so thin, dermatologic processes of the external meatus produce troubling symptoms. These conditions present with chronic itching, serous or mucoid drainage, fullness, and subjective hearing loss. During the acute phase, the skin of the EAC and concha may appear edematous, erythematous, and wet and may have vesicles, excoriations, and serous or mucoid otorrhea. Bacterial or fungal superinfections may occur, with associated purulent otorrhea and, potentially, microabcesses and cellulitis. In the chronic disease state, the skin becomes lichenified and often has the appearance of dryness with flaking and excoriations. The EAC may display purely local disease, such as contact dermatitis, asteatosis, or neurodermatitis (lichen simplex chronicus) which is a skin disorder caused by primary scratching and often associated with stress [47]. However, in some cases, EAC problems are a manifestation of a systemic condition, such as psoriasis, atopic dermatitis, seborrheic dermatitis, acne vulgaris, and sarcoidosis [48]. Generally, all of these conditions will respond to local care with topical steroid cream or ointment, antibiotic or antifungal preparations, and modification of exposure to moisture, dryness, or allergens.

Topical steroids should be used sparingly, as complications are more common with prolonged use and high potency formulations. Although systemic absorption from the ear canal has not been specifically described, the face in general has higher potential for absorption and even more so for thinner skin regions such as the eyelids. Though speculative, the ear canal may have a similarly elevated risk of absorption and consequent side effects. Complications include steroid atrophy, ulceration, exacerbation of underlying fungal infection, steroid acne or rosacea, and tachyphylaxis with chronic use. More serious complications include suppression of the hypothalamic pituitary axis, hyperglycemia, and increased intraocular pressure. Continuous courses longer than 2 weeks for moderated potency steroids should be avoided for these reasons. Examples of commonly used high potency formulations include betamethasone dipropionate ointment 0.05% and clobetasol propionate ointment 0.05% followed by fluocinonide ointment 0.05% (Lidex) and triamcinolone acetonide ointment 0.5% (Kenalog), with decreasing concentrations and cream variations as milder potency. Other commonly used creams such as 1% hydrocortisone cream are available over the counter and are the least potent [49].

Systemic steroids may be considered for severe inflammatory disease. Surgical therapy for dermatologic conditions is largely limited. However, deep cysts of the EAC may manifest secondary to generalized acne vulgaris. Uncomplicated acne can be managed with salicylic acid cleansers, topical tretinoin or antibiotic, or intralesional steroids [50]. Large cysts may easily become superinfected, then causing generalized pain, swelling, and inflammation of the EAC. Incision and drainage may be needed along with systemic antibiotics.

Bacterial and Fungal Otitis Externa

Cerumen plays an important protective role in EAC physiology. A relatively acidic pH and hydrophobic nature account for its bacteriostatic properties. [7] A warm, moist environment favors bacterial growth, accounting for the increased incidence of acute otitis externa during summer months and in regions with tropical climates. Overzealous removal of cerumen not only compromises the natural defenses of the EAC, it may also cause sufficient trauma to allow for bacterial inoculation. Patients with pruritic dermatologic conditions often suffer from recurrent bouts of infection as a result of frequent scratching and excoriation of the canal skin.

Acute diffuse otitis externa (swimmer's ear) refers to bacterial infection and inflammation of the skin and subcutaneous tissue of the cartilaginous EAC. Characteristic symptoms include itching, pain, and tenderness of the pinna with associated hearing loss and aural fullness. Examination typically reveals erythema and edema of the external canal skin, which may spread to involve the concha and lobule. Seropurulent otorrhea often results in crusting of the EAC and concha. Manipulation of the pinna and mastication generally elicit pain. In advanced cases, worsening edema significantly narrows the external canal lumen, preventing visualization of the tympanic membrane, and associated inflammatory changes may spread to involve preauricular soft tissue.

Otomycosis refers to an acute fungal infection of the EAC. *Candida* and *Aspergillus* are the most common fungal species implicated in otomycosis. The initial symptoms of fungal otitis externa mirror those of bacterial otitis externa, with the exception that associated pain is less severe. Intense pruritus is the most common complaint in otomycosis. Examination typically reveals canal skin erythema and the presence of abundant fungal debris, often embedded in a cheesy material thicker than that seen in bacterial otitis externa. Recognizing the white, gray, or black filamentous elements characteristic of fungal growth is critical to make the diagnosis of otomycosis. When unsure, a potassium hydroxide preparation can be helpful in demonstrating branching filaments or budding yeasts.

Treatment of acute otitis externa requires the thorough removal of all purulent or fungal material and desquamated debris to allow penetration of antimicrobial therapy. The frequency of aural cleansing is dictated by the amount of debris present in the canal. When significant, debridement may be required several times per week. This measure is essentially the only procedural component of otitis externa management. Ototopical preparations containing acidifying agents and antibiotics active against *P. aeruginosa* and *S. aureus* address the bacterial component of this process. When edema is severe, inserting a non-absorbable wick into the canal aids in the delivery of medication to its deeper portions. Wicks should be replaced every 2 to 3 days until canal patency is restored. Many otic preparations contain a corticosteroid, helpful in reducing inflammation and edema of the canal as well as associated pain. Oral antibiotics may be necessary when bacterial infection has extended to involve preauricular soft tissue. Pain control is another cornerstone in the treatment of otitis externa. Nonsteroidal anti-inflammatory medications or narcotic analgesics are required if over-the-counter analgesics fail to provide sufficient relief. Treatment of otomycosis requires appropriate topical antifungal medications. Many options are available, including M-cresyl-acetate (Cresylate™), 1% clotrimazole cream or solution, and vital dyes such as gentian violet. The majority of treatment failures are believed to result from inadequate skin penetration of the prescribed ototopical medication, further emphasizing the importance of adequate EAC debridement [51].

Efforts to prevent recurrent episodes of otitis externa focus on minimizing the moisture content within the EAC. Water precautions should be recommended. Occlusive ear plugs are effective in preventing water entry into the canal. Carefully directing a hair dryer at the EAC after water exposure followed by use of drying agents such as boric acid in ethyl alcohol can also be helpful if a perforation in the tympanic membrane is not present.

The potential for ototoxicity must be considered when treating patients with tympanic membrane perforations or pressure equalization tubes. Instillation of ototopical drops into the middle ear of chinchillas was shown to result in cochlear toxicity [52]. Nevertheless; this appears to be an exceedingly rare complication in humans. In his review, Roland documented only four cases in the English literature of sensorineural hearing loss potentially related to topical antibiotic use [53]. A possible explanation is provided by the work of Schachern and colleagues, who demonstrated that the thickness of the round window membrane increases while in the presence of inflammation or infection [54]. Use of potentially ototoxic medications in nondiseased middle ears should therefore be employed with caution as they lack this potentially protective characteristic.

Malignant Otitis Externa (Skull Base Osteomyelitis)

Malignant otitis externa was first described by Meltzer and Keleman in 1959 and was later named by Chandler in 1968 [55, 56]. The term skull base osteomyelitis more accurately describes the pathophysiology of this life-threatening infection of the EAC and skull base. Usually seen in diabetic patients and those with other forms of immunocompromised, infection spreads from the skin and subcutaneous tissue of the cartilaginous canal to involve the tympanic bone. Skull base osteomyelitis spreads via the Haversian system of compact bone, forming multiple abscesses and sequestra of necrotic bone. As infection progresses, periparotid and cervical soft tissues become involved. A facial nerve paralysis implies infection encasing the extratemporal portion of the nerve or involvement of the stylomastoid foramen. Palsies of cranial nerves IX, X, XI, and XII present as infection extends to involve the jugular foramen. Centrally invasive disease can involve the labyrinth, clivus, temporomandibular joint, and intratemporal carotid artery, putting the patient at risk for ischemic events (Fig. 31.2).

The cerumen of patients with diabetes has been shown to be of higher pH than that of nondiabetics, perhaps responsible for the increased incidence of external otitis in this population [57]. Impaired polymorphonuclear leukocyte function and microangiopathic disease typical of advanced diabetes contribute to the progression of otitis externa to skull base osteomyelitis in elderly diabetic patients [58].

Patients with osteomyelitis of the skull base often report a previous history of otitis externa. Intense otalgia exceeding that expected for routine otitis is common and can be associated with otorrhea. Granulation tissue seen protruding into the EAC from the bony-cartilaginous junction is a cardinal sign of skull base osteomyelitis, present in as many as 80% of patients in one series [59]. Biopsy is required both to rule out malignancy and for culture purposes. Sedimentation rate will be elevated, but osteomyelitis may occur in the absence of fever and elevated white blood cell count. Computed tomographic scans help to evaluate the extent of bony involvement. Magnetic resonance imaging provides more detail regarding soft tissue disease and, when combined with magnetic resonance angiography, can evaluate the patency of the dural sinuses. Technetium-99 and gallium-67 (Tc-99m and Ga-67, respectively) bone scans help in confirming the diagnosis of skull base osteomyelitis. Only the gallium scan, however, can be used to monitor response to therapy. Gallium scans image the activity of white blood cells and proteins at sites of active infection. This study will normalize as infection resolves, whereas the technetium scan may remain positive for many months. Similarly, patients will clinically improve before significant improvement is seen on CT or MRI [60]. More recently, PET has been used to monitor clinical improvement and patients with clear PET scans after treatment remain asymptomatic. It is unclear at this time if when inflammatory markers normalize despite continued PET activity if the disease is actually latent, as relapse has been reported in this situation [61].

Treatment of osteomyelitis of the skull base generally requires long-term administration of parenteral antibiotics in combination with daily aural debridement and vigilant management of diabetes and other compromising medical conditions. The vast majority of skull base osteomyelitis results from infection by *P. aeruginosa*. Central skull base osteomyelitis is more commonly secondary to *S. aureus*. Immunocompromised patients can also present with fungal or mycobacterial infections [62]. Underlying sinusitis and presentation with sinonasal pain and facial or periorbital swelling was more common in fungal etiologies as compared to bacterial [63]. Double coverage directed against *Pseudomonas* is empirically begun after cultures have been obtained. Fluoroquinolones offer potent activity against *Pseudomonas* via oral administration and may be effective as monotherapy. However, recent resistance to fluoroquinolones has emerged, suggesting that monotherapy may not be

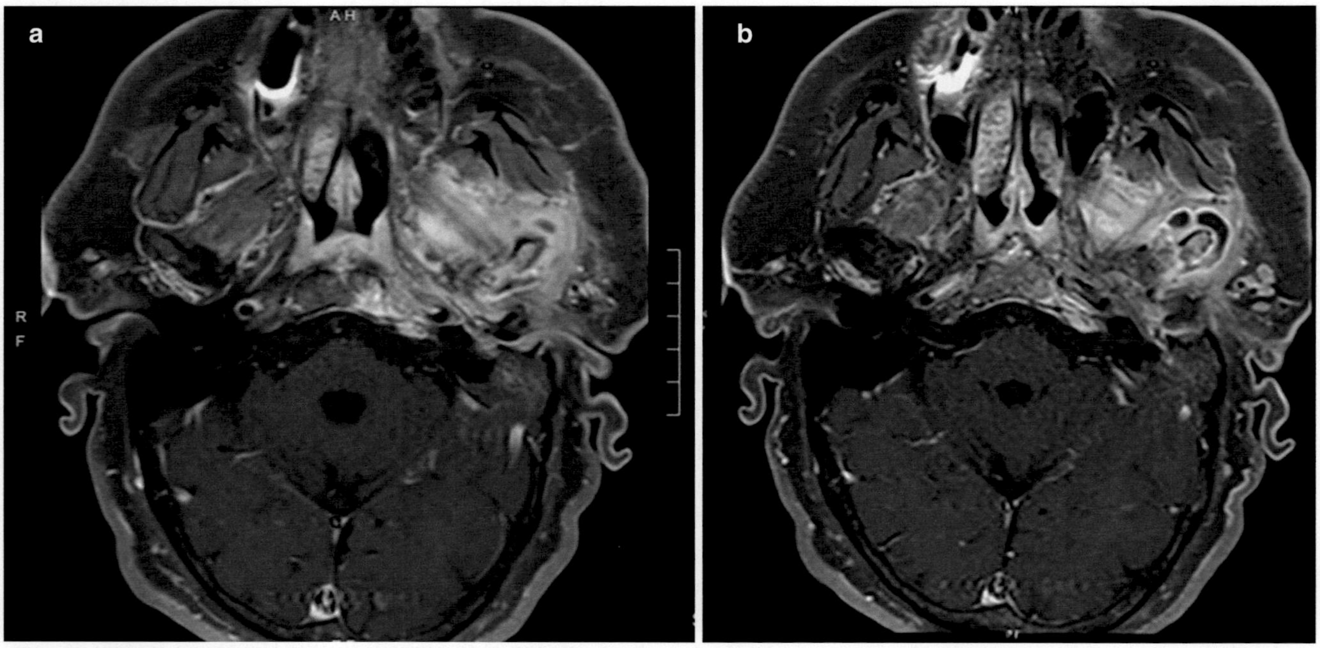

Fig. 31.2 Central osteomyelitis of the skull base as shown on a contrast-enhanced MRI, axial views. (**a**) Shows extension into the clivus and anterior skull base. (**b**) Shows extension into the glenoid fossa, where rim-enhancing hypointensities are seen. (*Images courtesy of MJH*)

adequate in some cases [64]. Strong consideration for parenteral antifungal treatment should be considered when patients do not respond to antibiotics as fungus can be an etiologic concern even in immunocompetent patients [63]. There is no standard antifungal regimen, though most often, an azole is used (i.e., posaconazole or voriconazole) if *Aspergillus* is speciated, with or without amphotericin B [65]. It is generally recommended that an infectious disease provider be consulted in the management of these patients. Surgical therapy is controversial, though it is usually pursued for new cultures, the debridement of necrotic bony sequestra, and/or the drainage of abscesses. Justification for the latter is rooted in the notion that antibiotic penetration into necrotic bone or an abscess cavity will be poor. Further discussion of this condition is provided in Chap. 30.

Atresia and Stenosis

Acquired stenosis and atresia of the EAC, also known as medial canal fibrosis, refers to a condition characterized by the cicatricial formation of fibroinflammatory tissue lateral to the tympanic membrane. A distinct clinical entity that must be differentiated from congenital aural atresia, acquired stenosis usually results from chronic infection and inflammation but may also represent a complication related to prior otologic surgery or EAC trauma [66]. As the developing stenosis progresses, affected patients suffer a worsening conductive hearing loss. Examination reveals edema and hypertrophy of the canal wall skin, and once fibrosis matures, the EAC becomes a foreshortened skin-lined pouch. The lateral aspect of the tympanic membrane frequently becomes incorporated into the scar tissue, obliterating any potential intervening space.

The best treatment of acquired stenosis of the EAC is prevention. Chronic otitis externa refers to a diffuse inflammatory process of the external canal of long duration, and while a distinct etiology of this condition remains unclear, it appears to be the most frequent cause of medial canal fibrosis [67]. Bilateral in 50% of cases and twice as common in women than men, this entity is probably related to a combination of infection, allergy, and dermatoses [68]. A paucity of literature analyzing treatment options for chronic otitis externa exists, but management is primarily medical until complete medial canal fibrosis develops. A regimen consisting of topical corticosteroid and antibiotic preparations in combination with periodic, atraumatic cleansing may prevent the need for surgical intervention. Cauterization of granulation tissue may also aid in drying and halting the inflammatory process.

Surgical Technique for Repair of Acquired Stenosis of EAC

Preoperative Planning: Surgical therapy of acquired stenosis is indicated for correction of conductive hearing loss (hearing aids tend to exacerbate underlying inflammation) and to prevent or remove cholesteatoma in cases related to trauma or prior surgery where an epithelialized tympanic membrane or canal may exist medial to the stenotic segment. Generally, canalplasty with a wide meatoplasty is the procedure of choice. This may be performed endaurally if adequate exposure can be obtained but usually requires a postauricular approach. Computed tomography may be helpful to determine the status of the middle ear and the presence of cholesteatoma medial to the stenosis and to define the pertinent anatomy.

Surgical Details (Fig. 31.3): A vascular strip is designed and made with the medial incision at the level of the stenosis or blind sac. The flap should be made as long as possible. It may be helpful to make the medial incision from behind after making the postauricular incision. Similar to the incision for exostosis, the periosteal incision may be made as a semicircle, corresponding to the bony meatus. The flap is elevated and the ear is retracted anteriorly. Next, the anterior canal skin is either incised medially and "window-shaded" by elevating it as a laterally based flap or incised laterally and removed to be replaced as a free graft. The scar can frequently be dissected free of the medial layer of the tympanic membrane, but, if not, the drum remnant is resected. A drill is used to perform a wide canalplasty. For reconstruction, a fascial graft is taken from the temporalis muscle and used to reconstruct any perforation of the tympanic membrane, with either a medial or lateral technique. The anterior canal skin is trimmed of disease and prepared for replacement. Usually, a split-thickness skin graft will be needed, and it can be harvested from the inner arm or thigh. Postauricular skin can be taken as a free graft, but in the author's experience, the full-thickness graft is too thick, suffers from inward curling of the graft edges, and shrinks, leaving less than desirable bony coverage. Fascia can also be used to cover bone where inadequate skin is available. The tympanic membrane may be covered with a disk of Gelfilm™. The postauricular incision is closed and the canal is packed with gelfoam. A stent or rosebud packing fashioned from silk or silicone strips filled with gelfoam is helpful in many cases to encourage adherence of the grafts and vascular strip.

Postauricular Care: Antibiotic drops are used twice daily and the packing is removed over 4–6 weeks during biweekly visits. The packing can be removed and replaced and allowed to support the canal for 10–14 days or longer. Granulation

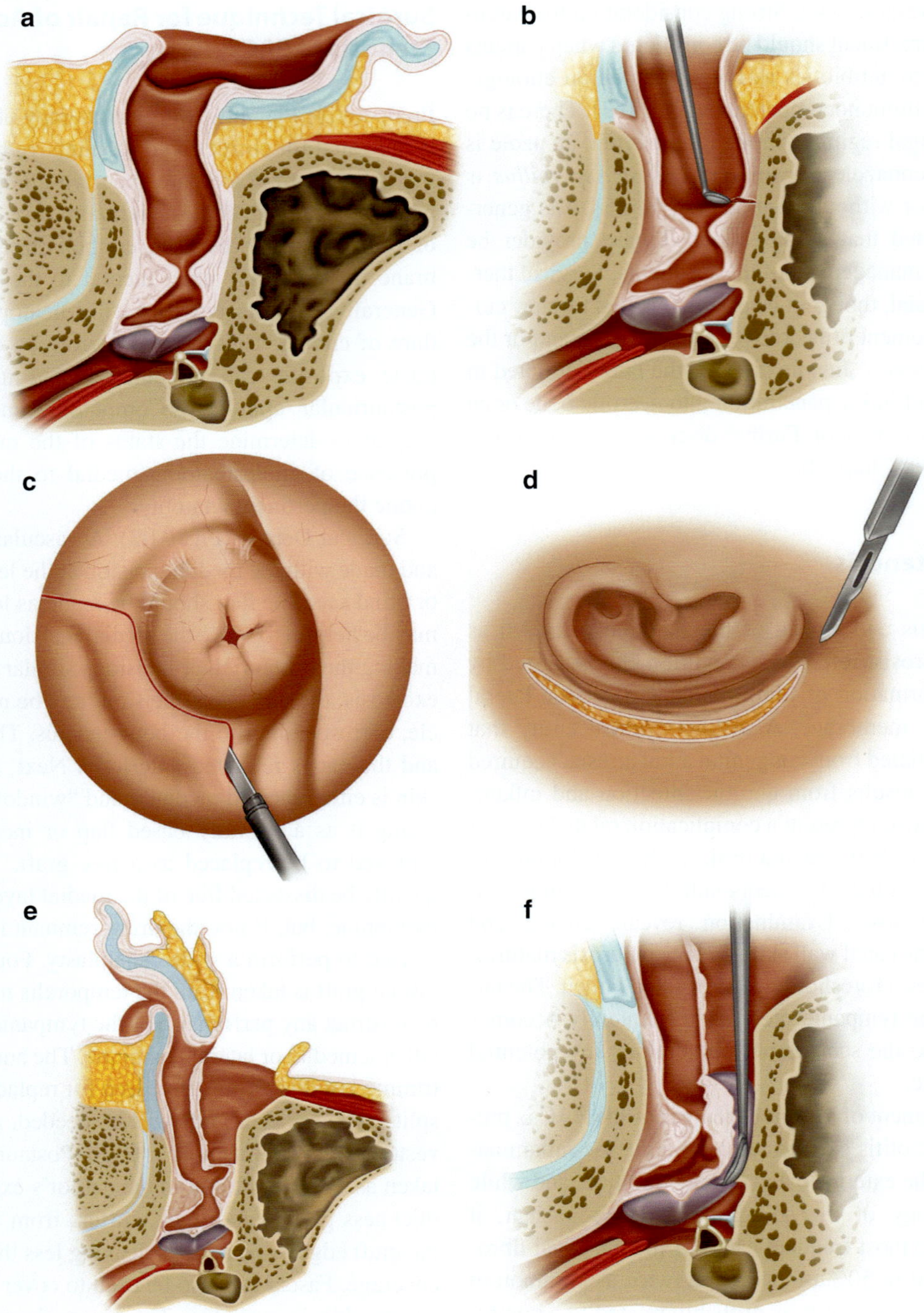

Fig. 31.3 Surgical treatment of acquired external canal stenosis. Adapted from Glasscock and Shambaugh's Surgery of the Ear. Eds. Gulya, Minor, Poe. PMPH. 2010. (**a**) Cicatricial fibrous stenosis at the level of the bony external auditory canal. (**b, c**) Vascular strip incisions are made as far medial as is safe and practicable. (**d**) A postauricular incision is made. (**e**) The vascular strip is elevated out of the external canal. (**f**) The mass of scar tissue is elevated from the posterior wall of the ear canal until the middle ear space is entered. (**g**) Posterior fibrous stenosis excised. (**h**) The stenotic scar tissue anteriorly is excised, leaving the anterior drum remnant if at all possible. The canal is enlarged with a drill until air cells can be seen through bone. (**i**) The drum and canal are grafted with fascia and the canal is filled with ointment

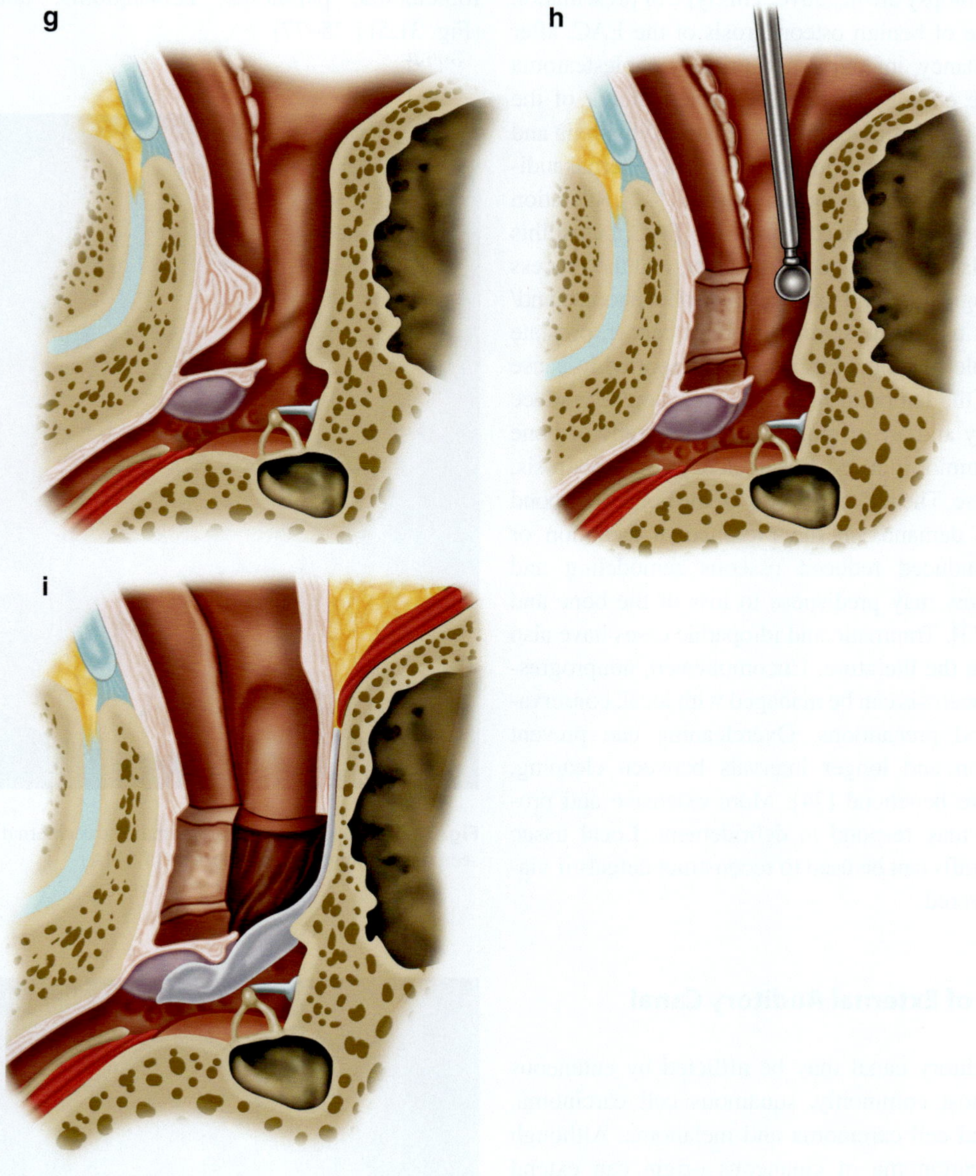

Fig. 31.3 (continued)

tissue is carefully monitored and treated with chemical cautery. Close monitoring is needed, as restenosis can occur very quickly. Postoperative infection should be managed aggressively as it will contribute to failure.

Pitfalls and Complications: Recurrence is a very distinct risk. All involved tissue must be removed and the bony canal enlarged to allow for some element of postoperative restenosis. Critical to the success of this procedure is resurfacing the osseous canal with epithelium. If the bone is left exposed, and the formation of granulation tissue and healing by secondary intention are allowed, the rate of recurrent stenosis is unacceptably high. Usually, a split-thickness skin graft is employed, but a variety of pedicled flaps, as well as full-thickness skin grafts, have been described [69–71]. Other risks include sensorineural hearing loss, conductive hearing loss, facial nerve injury, and tympanic membrane perforation. Intraoperative facial nerve monitoring may be used to reduce the risk of facial nerve injury.

Necrosis of the External Auditory Canal

Occasionally, one will encounter a benign-appearing, painless ulcer in the EAC, often near the bony-cartilaginous junction in the inferior or posterior canal. The edges of the ulcer may appear healthy without evidence of infection. The underlying bone is exposed, sometimes with sequestra, but does not appear infected. Over time, the lesion does not appear to progress. Culture and biopsy are negative. This type of presentation may be indicative of benign osteonecrosis of the EAC, after ruling out malignancy, infection, and primary cholesteatoma of the EAC. The etiology of primary cholesteatoma of the external auditory canal is thought to be related to hypoxia and is usually found along the inferior portion of the external auditory canal and rarely can erode into the mastoid [72]. Radiation may also predispose to osteonecrosis of the EAC, but in this case, there is a history of radiation treatment, and the process may be more progressive and extensive. Bisphosphonate and/or chemotherapy use in the setting of breast cancer, prostate cancer, or multiple myeloma has also been reported to cause osteonecrosis of the temporal bone. Bisphosphonates reduce osteoclast activity and are a frequently used therapy of bone metastases and tumor-induced hypercalcemia, osteoporosis, and Paget's disease. The reduced ability of the bone to respond to physiological demands in the presence of radiation or bisphosphonate-induced reduced osseous remodeling and reduced blood flow may predispose to loss of the bone and overlying skin [73]. Traumatic and idiopathic cases have also been presented in the literature. Uncomplicated, nonprogressive, focal EAC necrosis can be managed with local, conservative cleaning and precautions. Overcleaning can prevent re-epithelialization and longer intervals between cleaning, 4–5 months, were beneficial [74]. More extensive and progressive disease may respond to debridement. Local tissue grafts and skin grafts can be used to reconstruct defects if viable bone is uncovered.

Malignancies of External Auditory Canal

The external auditory canal may be afflicted by cutaneous malignancies, most commonly, squamous cell carcinoma, followed by basal cell carcinoma and melanoma. Although squamous cell carcinoma of cutaneous origin can extend from the auricle into the external auditory canal, it can also occur primarily within the canal (Fig. 31.4). Adenoid cystic carcinoma, ceruminal gland adenocarcinoma, as well as more rare tumors may also occur within the EAC. Malignancies of the EAC typically present as ulcerated or nodular skin lesions, which are associated with chronic bloody otorrhea. Temporal bone invasion is classically heralded by complaints of a deep-boring otalgia. Radiographic imaging helps define the extent of tumor invasion. Successful treatment usually requires wide excision by temporal bone resection, frequently combined with postoperative radiation therapy. Chemotherapy may also play a role. A thorough discussion of the management of this class of malignancy is beyond the scope of this chapter. However, it is important to keep benign and malignant processes in mind when forming a differential diagnosis for disorders of the EAC. Benign neoplasms to consider include folliculoma, papilloma, hemangioma, and ceruminoma (Fig. 31.5) [75–77].

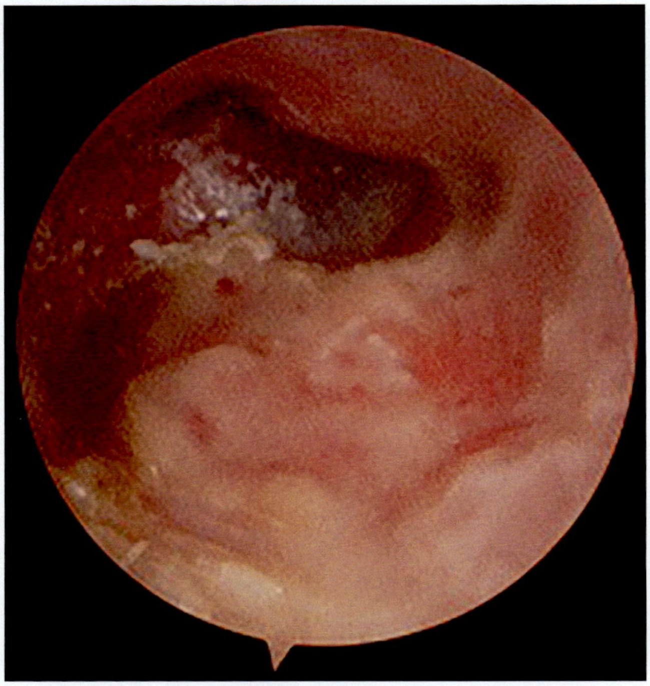

Fig. 31.4 Squamous cell carcinoma of the external auditory canal as seen on otoscopy. (Image courtesy of SMA)

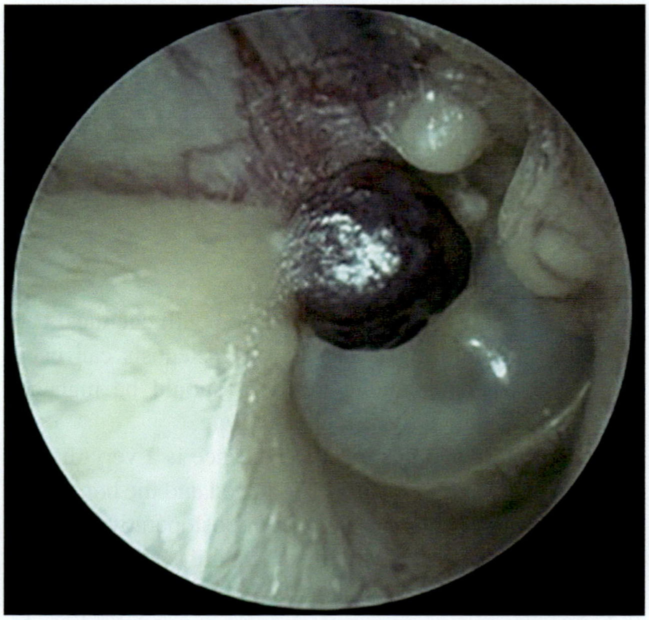

Fig. 31.5 A violaceous-appearing hemangioma of the right external auditory canal as seen on otoscopy. Small, white exostoses are also seen. (Image courtesy of SMA)

Diseases of the Tympanic Membrane

Bullous Myringitis

Bullous myringitis is a poorly understood condition characterized by inflammation of the tympanic membrane and the formation of serous or hemorrhagic bullae on its epithelial surface. Middle ear effusion may also be present. Most commonly, the disease is unilateral and results in severe otalgia, often disproportionate to findings seen on physical examination. Sensorineural hearing loss frequently accompanies bullous myringitis. In Hoffman and Shepsman's review of 15 patients with 21 affected ears, 67% showed evidence of sensorineural loss, either alone or as a component of a mixed loss [78]. Hearing loss associated with bullous myringitis is generally transient, and the majority of patients recover full auditory function [79].

The etiology of bullous myringitis remains unknown. It often follows a nonspecific upper respiratory illness, and early studies indeed suggested a causal relationship with influenza infection [80]. Later, Rifkin and colleagues induced bullous myringitis in nearly half of healthy subjects inoculated with *Mycoplasma pneumoniae* [81]. However, when examining the acute and postconvalescent sera of patients diagnosed with bullous myringitis, Merifield and Miller found no consistent changes in antibody titers to suggest an etiologic role for *M. pneumoniae* or a variety of common upper respiratory viruses [82]. It may be that the bullous lesions characteristic of this illness represent a nonspecific response to inflammation of the tympanic membrane and that bullous myringitis is not, in fact, a distinct entity.

Treatment of bullous myringitis has traditionally included decompression of the painful vesicles and oral analgesics. In cases complicated by sensorineural hearing loss, it is our practice to treat aggressively with antibiotics and systemic corticosteroids (prednisone 1 mg/kg/day for 7 days, then tapered) as if it represents a complication of otitis media. Myringotomy may be performed if a middle ear effusion accompanies bullae formation. Randomized trials comparing management options for bullous myringitis with associated sensorineural hearing loss do not exist.

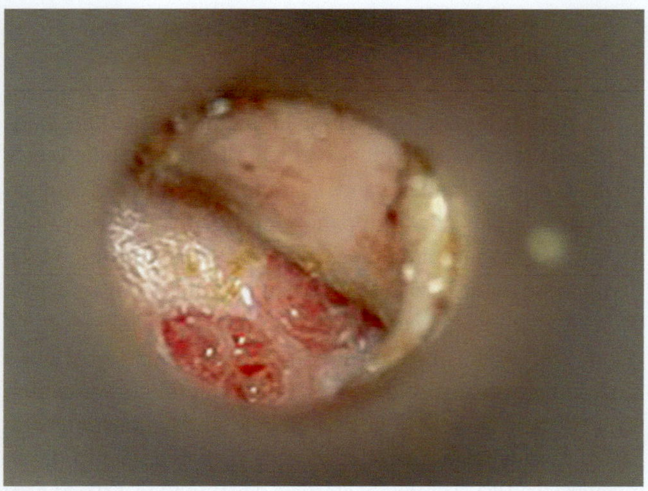

Fig. 31.6 Granular myringitis of tympanic membrane as seen on otoscopy. (Image courtesy of PGV)

Granular Myringitis

Another poorly understood condition, granular myringitis is characterized by chronic inflammation of the tympanic membrane leading to the replacement of its epithelial surface and, occasionally, adjacent deep meatal skin with proliferating granulation tissue (Fig. 31.6). The predominant presentation of granular myringitis is a unilateral scant constant or recurrent, often malodorous otorrhea. Symptoms of pruritus and aural fullness are also common, but the ear is usually painless. Otoscopy reveals a mucoid, serous, mucopurulent, or frankly purulent discharge bathing the tympanic membrane. Careful aural cleansing is required to visualize characteristic granulation tissue, which may involve the tympanic membrane in focal patches, segmental distributions, or diffusely, where most of the pars tensa surface is replaced. Perforations may occur in conjunction with myringitis [83]. A mild conductive hearing loss is frequently noted on audiometric evaluation.

The etiology of granular myringitis is unknown. Acute infection or mechanical trauma leading to loss of the squamous epithelial layer of the tympanic membrane appears to be a critical event in the development of granular myringitis, which disrupts normal epithelial migration responsible for the healing properties of the tympanic membrane [84]. In their review, Blevins and Karmody found that 60% of patients with granular myringitis had previously undergone an otologic procedure [85]. Once the epithelial layer has been compromised, infection by those organisms commonly responsible for otitis externa, especially *Pseudomonas* and *Staphylococcus*, further inhibits healing of the tympanic membrane. *Pseudomonas aeruginosa*, *Staphylococcus aureus*, *Proteus*, and *Staphylococcus epidermidis* have been linked to the process [86].

Management of granular myringitis often requires protracted therapy. Initially, external infection must be controlled. Antibiotic-steroid drops, diluted vinegar, gentian violet, antifungal agents, and oral quinolone antibiotics have also been used with some success. Once infection has been addressed, granulation tissue may be cauterized with silver nitrate, trichloroacetic acid, or phenol, if abundant, and is controlled with daily use of topical corticosteroid drops until resolution is observed. Frequent office visits are often required until the process is under good control. Unfortunately, recurrence is typical. Other options include laser therapy, which was recently shown to be initially more effective with similar recurrence rates at one year of approximately 15% as compared to trichloroacetic acid [87]. The role of surgery in the management of granular myringitis remains controversial. It is generally reserved for those refractory cases that fail prolonged topical therapy. The involved area of the tympanic membrane is excised and repaired with an underlay or overlay graft. Some authors have reported excellent success rates for surgical therapy of granular myringitis, but available data are sparse and limited by short follow-up periods [86].

Traumatic Perforation

Acute perforations of the tympanic membrane generally result from episodes of acute otitis media or trauma. The majority of infectious perforations heal as the inciting condition resolves. Traumatic tympanic membrane perforation may result from blunt or penetrating injuries as well as rapid changes in barometric pressure (barotrauma). Slap injuries to the head, frequently encountered in cases related to assault or aquatic sports accidents, create a column of compressed air within the EAC of sufficient pressure to implode the tympanic membrane. Blast injuries inflict similar implosive forces on the tympanic membrane. Penetrating injuries are most frequently self-inflicted during overzealous cerumen removal. Barometric trauma commonly occurs following rapid airplane descent or deep-water diving or during hyperbaric oxygen therapy. Rather than causing a perforation, barotrauma generally results in hemorrhage of tympanic membrane vasculature. Thermal injuries to the tympanic membrane, commonly seen in welders and those struck by lightning, result in a small percentage of perforations. However, because of associated tissue necrosis, burn-related perforations have a high rate of nonhealing [88].

Most studies suggest that upward of 90% of traumatic perforations heal spontaneously within 3 months of injury [88–90]. Epithelial migration patterns on the tympanic membrane and within the EAC responsible for the removal of desquamated cells and keratin debris form the basis for the tympanic membrane's impressive healing properties. Studies by Litton and Alberti used India ink to mark epithelial elements on the tympanic membrane and documented cell migration that originates from the region of the umbo and proceeds in a centripetal fashion [91, 92]. Following an acute injury, platelets gather to cause vasoconstriction and form a thrombus. An inflammatory response ensues, attracting neutrophils, macrophages, and bioactive cytokines to the wound. A matrix of proteoglycans and glycosaminoglycans is formed and allows for proliferation of the tympanic membrane's squamous epithelial layer across the perforation, forming a scaffold on which the mucosal and, later, the fibrous layers of the tympanic membrane can grow. The squamous elements responsible for bridging the perforation originate from "upstream" and must traverse the length of the defect. It is not surprising, therefore, that larger perforations are associated with delayed healing and higher rates of chronicity.

Patients who have suffered a traumatic tympanic membrane perforation often complain of mild hearing loss and aural fullness. Vertigo is uncommon and should prompt concern for stapes injury and a perilymphatic fistula. Audiometric assessment often shows conductive hearing loss of varying severity. Ritvik et al. suggest that the conductive hearing loss associated with a perforation is frequency-dependent and varies directly with the size of the perforation, inversely with the volume of the middle ear space, and is not related to the location [93]. Management of traumatic perforations ranges from observation along with dry ear precautions to early myringoplasty. Either approach will result in perforation closure in approximately 90% of cases. Those who practice expectant management of traumatic tympanic membrane perforations cite the high likelihood of spontaneous healing, whereas supporters of early intervention report quicker resolution of hyperacusis and prompt return of patients to their preferred lifestyles. Myringoplasty can be performed as an office-based procedure under local anesthesia. After injecting the external canal with 1% lidocaine, the margins of the tympanic membrane are everted and aligned with a pick. A patch of paper is then placed over the perforation. The patch helps prevent inversion of the tympanic membrane edges and promotes prompt healing. Use of ototopical medications in the setting of an uncomplicated traumatic tympanic membrane perforation is discouraged given theoretical risk of ototoxicity. Additionally, the wet environment resulting from medication application impairs fibroblast proliferation and may therefore hinder perforation healing.

Tympanosclerosis

Tympanosclerosis is characterized by hyaline degeneration of the fibrous layer of the tympanic membrane and the middle ear mucosa. Isolated involvement of the tympanic membrane is most common and is more appropriately named myringosclerosis, but tympanosclerotic plaques may also present within the middle ear cleft and mastoid (Fig. 31.7). Tympanosclerosis is irreversible and results from infection or inflammation of the middle ear space. The incidence of tympanosclerosis in patients with a previous history of otitis media ranges from 14 to 43% in different clinical series [94, 95]. In their review, Tos and Stangerup demonstrated an association between ventilation tube placement and tympanosclerosis [96]. Tympanosclerosis developed in 13% of ears with secretory otitis media treated with paracentesis compared with 59% treated with grommet tube insertion. Additionally, Kay and colleagues' recent meta-analysis of

134 studies regarding sequelae of tympanostomy tube insertion revealed a 32% incidence of postintubation tympanosclerosis compared with 10% of controls [97].

Rarely does isolated tympanic membrane tympanosclerosis result in a clinically significant hearing loss. Middle ear tympanosclerosis, on the other hand, can cause ossicular fixation and result in more severe degrees of conductive hearing loss.

Retraction Pockets of the Tympanic Membrane

Retraction of the tympanic membrane is a common finding in both children and adults. Middle ear negative pressure (atelectasis) results in retraction or retraction pockets that range in severity from shallow nonprogressive and self-cleaning pockets to deep, adherent, and problematic retractions into the attic and mastoid. Even shallow retractions into the posterior superior region of the pars tensa can cause progressive hearing loss from erosion of the ossicular chain. Deeper attic retractions can remain asymptomatic for years while collecting keratin debris, expanding by erosion of bone, and eventually developing into extensive cholesteatoma. Sade's grading system is clinically useful for staging retraction of the tympanic membrane. Grade I retractions are simple, shallow, and nonadherent. Grade II retractions touch the incus and/or stapes with or without erosion. Grade III pockets retract to the promontory without adhesion, and grade IV retractions are adherent to the promontory (Fig. 31.8) [98].

The primary cause of atelectasis is the loss of normal middle ear ventilation and the development of negative pressure in the middle ear as the middle ear mucosa absorbs nitrogen from the air. The inherent structure of the posterior superior portion of the pars tensa and the pars flaccida make these areas of the tympanic membrane more prone to retraction. The posterior superior pars tensa has thinner, more

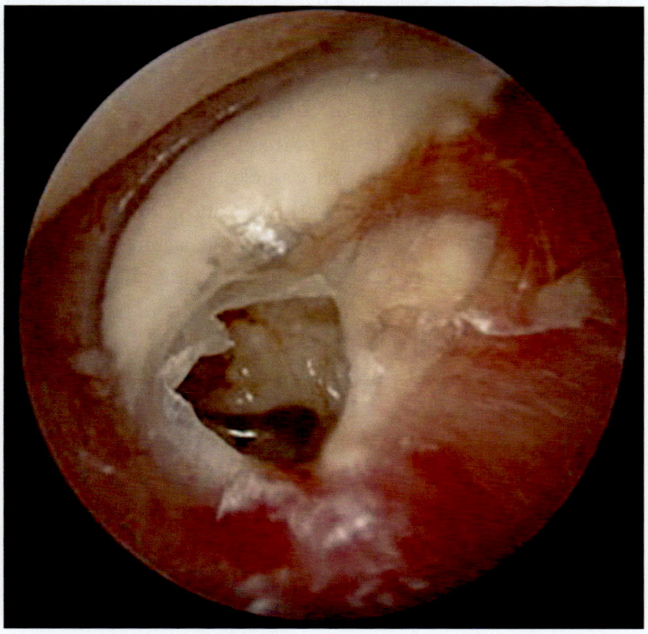

Fig. 31.7 Tympanosclerosis of a left tympanic membrane as seen on otoscopy. A perforation is also noted. (Images courtesy of PGV)

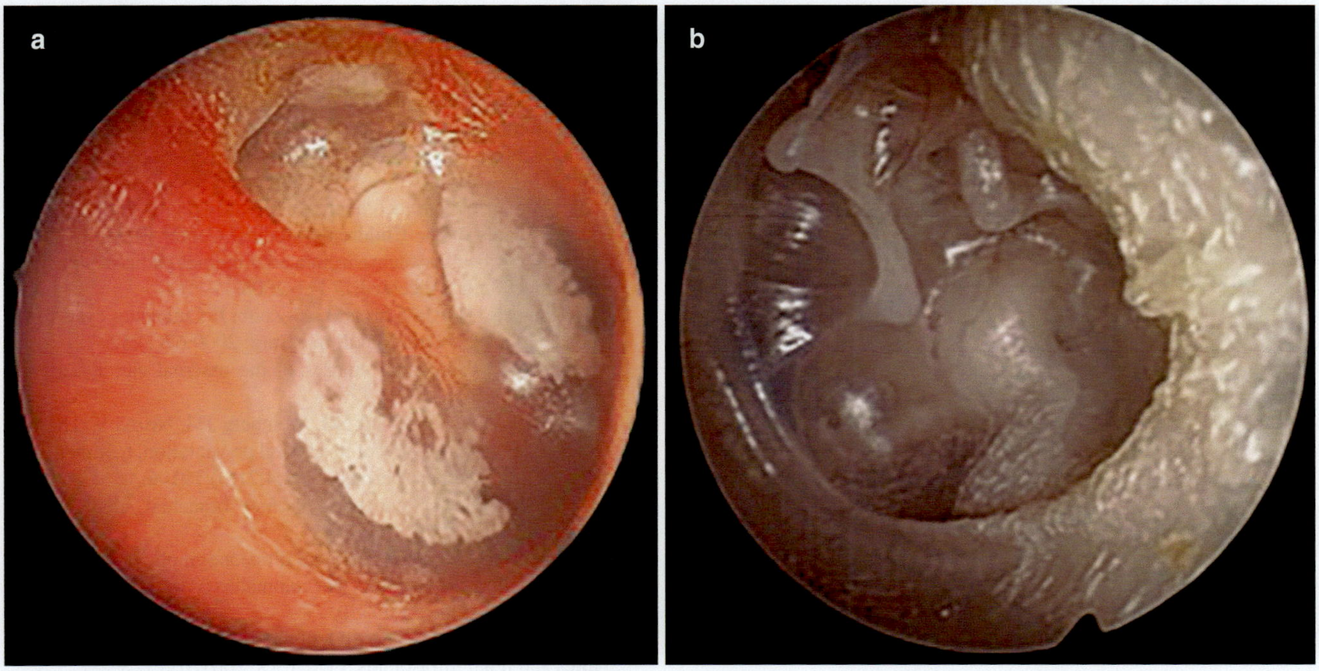

Fig. 31.8 (**a**) Atelectasis of a right-sided tympanic membrane in the pars flaccida as seen on otoscopy. Scattered sclerosis is also noted. (**b**) Retraction of the pars tensa with adherence of the tympanic membrane to the incus and stapes. (Images courtesy of PGV)

sparsely distributed collagen and increased vascular supply. The pars flaccida is actually thicker than the pars tensa, but has thinner, less organized collagen fibers loosely arranged in a vascular lamina propria. Inflammation and infection damage the inherent collagenous support, making the tympanic membrane weaker and more susceptible to increased and persistent negative middle ear pressure and eventual retraction [98–100]. The atelectatic tympanic membrane is characterized by hyperkeratosis, edema, and inflammation of the lamina propria and loss of collagen organization [101].

The dilemma at diagnosis is distinguishing stable from progressive disease. Problematic pockets will manifest with recurrent otorrhea, hearing loss, and cholesteatoma. Sometimes, a "trail sign" is evident as a line of keratin extending from the pocket onto and along the posterior wall of the EAC. This line of migrating keratin may represent cholesteatoma within the pocket. Other red flags include deep pockets where the medial extent cannot be appreciated, conductive hearing loss, recurrent otorrhea, polypoid tissue, or crusts or cerumen covering a pocket that is difficult to clean. Management options include observation, medical therapy, and surgery. Routine microscopic exams can over time identify stable disease. Shallow pockets should be cleaned of debris and cerumen. Acetic acid drops, mineral oil, or other cleansing and lubricating agents may reduce the accumulation of debris in the pockets. Eustachian tube function is supported by managing contributing factors, such as allergy, adenoid disease, and gastroesophageal reflux, and by encouraging autoinsufflation. Progressive or risky pockets can often be managed by placement of a tympanostomy tube. Some advocate simple excision of the damaged tympanic membrane, which can then heal similar to a perforation with thicker collagen and scar, less prone to retraction, either with or without placement of a tube. Ostrowski and Bojrab describe a novel technique of laser-assisted contraction myringoplasty to address the redundant and weakened atelectatic tympanic membrane [102]. Other surgical options for progressive or complicated disease include tympanoplasty, cartilage tympanoplasty, and tympanoplasty combined with mastoidectomy. Postoperative recurrence is not uncommon with any of these techniques.

Conclusions

Despite being a relatively small structure, the external auditory canal can be affected by a plethora of pathologic processes. A comprehensive otologic history and physical exam are critical when evaluating ear canal disease, given that many conditions are progressive and can even be rooted in embryologic development, and given that visual identification of disease can often distinguish between entities with similar symptom profiles (i.e., bacterial vs. fungal otitis externa). Surgical intervention for ear canal disease requires careful planning, meticulous microsurgical technique, and, often, radiographic and electrophysiologic adjuncts given the relative proximity of the facial nerve, ossicular chain, temporomandibular joint, and middle cranial fossa.

References

1. Mallo M. Formation of the outer and middle ear, molecular mechanisms. Curr Top Dev Biol. 2003;57:85–113.
2. Hollinshead WH. Anatomy for surgeons: the head and neck. 3rd ed. Philadelphia: Lippincott-Raven; 1982. p. 159–67.
3. Park C, Lineaweaver WC, Rumly TO, Buncke HJ. Arterial supply of the anterior ear. Plast Reconstr Surg. 1992;90(1):38–44.
4. Reis CV, Deshmukh V, Zabramski JM, et al. Anatomy of the mastoid emissary vein and venous system of the posterior neck region: neurosurgical implications. Neurosurgery. 2007;61(5 Suppl 2):193–201.
5. Pan WR, le Roux CM, Levy SM, Briggs CA. Lymphatic drainage of the external ear. Head Neck. 2011;33(1):60–4.
6. Donaldson JA, Duckert LG. Anson-Donaldson: surgical anatomy of the temporal bone. 4th ed. Lippincott Williams & Wilkins; 1992.
7. Lum CL, Jeyanthi S, Prepageran N, Vadivelu J, Raman R. Antibacterial and antifungal properties of human cerumen. J Laryngol Otol. 2009;123(4):375–8.
8. Stenfeldt K, Johansson C, Hellstrom S. The collagen structure of the tympanic membrane: collagen types I, II, and III in the healthy tympanic membrane, during healing of a perforation, and during infection. Arch Otolaryngol Head Neck Surg. 2006;132(3):293–8.
9. Schuknecht HF. Pathology of the ear. 2nd ed. Philadelphia: Lea & Febiger; 1993. p. 31–41.
10. McAdams TR, Swenson DR, Miller RA. Frostbite: an orthopaedic perspective. Am J Orthop. 2000;16(2):21–6.
11. Bruen KJ, Ballard JR, Morris SE, Cochran A, Edelman LS, Saffle JR. Reduction of the incidence of amputation in frostbite injury with thrombolytic therapy. Arch Surg. 2007;142:546–51.
12. Choung YH, Park K, Choung PH, Oh JH. Simple compressive method for treatment of auricular haematoma using dental silicone material. J Laryngol Otol. 2005;119(1):27–31.
13. Bassiouny A. Perichondritis of the auricle. Laryngoscope. 1981;91:422–31.
14. Buck ML. Ciprofloxin use in children: a review of recent findings. Pediatric pharmacotherapy, a monthly review for health care professionals of the Children's Medical Center. 1998;4(12):1–8. http://www.healthsystem.virginia.edu/internet/pediatrics/pharma-news/dec98.pdf. Accessed 17 Feb 2008.
15. Al-Khateeb TH, Al-Masri NM, Al-Zoubi F. Cutaneous cysts of the head and neck. J Oral Maxillofac Surg. 2009;67(1):52–7.
16. Ewing MR. Congenital sinuses of the external ear. J Laryngol Otol. 1946;61:18–23.
17. Scheinfeld NS, Silverberg NB, Weinberg JM, Nozad V. The preauricular sinus: a review of its clinical presentation, treatment, and associations. Pediatr Dermatol. 2004;21(3):191–6.
18. Work WP. Newer concepts of first branchial cleft defects. Laryngoscope. 1972;82:1581–93.
19. Deshpande SA, Watson H. Renal ultrasonography not required in babies with isolated minor ear anomalies. Arch Dis Child Fetal Neonatal Ed. 2006;91:29–30.
20. Wang RY, Earl DL, Ruder RO, Graham JM. Syndromic ear anomalies and renal ultrasounds. Pediatrics. 2001;108:1–8.

21. Prasad S, Grundfast K, Milmoe G. Management of congenital preauricular pit and sinus tract in children. Laryngoscope. 1990;100(3):320–1.
22. Bruijnzeel H, van den Aardweg MT, Grolman W, Stegeman I, van der Veen EL. A systematic review on the surgical outcome of preauricular sinus excision techniques. Laryngoscope. 2016;126(7):1535–44.
23. Baatenburg de Jong RJ. A new surgical technique for treatment of preauricular sinus. Surgery. 2005;137(5):567–70.
24. Kischer CW, Shetlar MR. Collagen and mucopolysaccharides in the hypertrophic scar. Connect Tissue Res. 1974;2:205–13.
25. Sherris DA, Larrabee WF, Murakami CS. Management of scar contractures, hypertrophic scars, and keloids. Otolaryngol Clin N Am. 1995;28:1057–67.
26. Farrior RT, Stambaugh KI. Keloids and hyperplastic scars. In: Thomas JF, Holt JR, editors. Facial scars, revisions, and camouflage. St. Louis: CV Mosby; 1989. p. 211–28.
27. Wortmann RL. Gout and other disorders of purine metabolism. In: Isselbacher KJ, editor. Harrison's principles of internal medicine. 13th ed. New York: McGraw-Hill; 1994. p. 2079–88.
28. Salah H, Urso B, Khachemoune A. Review of the etiopathogenesis and management options of chondrodermatitis nodularis chronica helicis. Cureus. 2018;10(3):e2367.
29. Mohs F, Larson P, Iriondo M. Micrographic surgery for the microscopically controlled excision of carcinoma of the external ear. J Am Acad Dermatol. 1988;19:729–37.
30. Ouyang YH. Skin cancer of the head and neck. Semin Plast Surg. 2010;24(2):117–26.
31. Nazarian R, Eshraghi AA. Otoplasty for the protruded ear. Semin Plast Surg. 2011;25(4):288–94.
32. Tolleth H. A hierarchy of values in the design and construction of the ear. Clin Plast Surg. 1990;17:193.
33. Mustarde JC. The treatment of prominent ears by buried mattress suture—a ten years' survey. Plast Reconstr Surg. 1967;39:382.
34. Furnas DW. Correction of prominent ears with multiple sutures. Clin Plast Surg. 1978;5(3):491–5.
35. Lin SJ, Furnas DW. Ear, prominent ear. Emedicine. 2007. http://www.emedicine.com/plastic/TOPIC454.HTM. Accessed 18 Feb 2008.
36. van Gilse PHG. Des observations ulterieures sur la genes des exostoses du conduit externe par l'irriations d'eau froide. Acta Otolaryngol (Stockh). 1938;26:343.
37. Corbridge RJ, Michaels L, Wright T. Epithelial migration in keratosis obturans. Am J Otolaryngol. 1996;17:411–4.
38. Morrison AW. Keratosis obturans. J Laryngol Otolaryngol. 1956;70:317–21.
39. Paparella MM, Goycoolea MV. Canalplasty for chronic intractable external otitis and keratosis obturans. Otolaryngology. 1981;89:440–3.
40. Shinnabe A, Hara M, Hasegawa M, et al. A comparison of patterns of disease extension in keratosis obturans and external auditory canal cholesteatoma. Otol Neurotol. 2013;34(1):91–4.
41. Vrabec JT, Chaljub G. External canal cholesteatoma. Am J Otol. 2000;21:608–14.
42. Piepergerdes JC, Kramer BM, Behnke EE. Keratosis obturans and external auditory canal cholesteatoma. Laryngoscope. 1980;90:383–90.
43. Prasad N, Harley E. The aural foreign body space: a review of pediatric ear foreign bodies and a management paradigm. Int J Pediatr Otorhinolaryngol. 2020;132:109871.
44. Veitch D, Brockbank M, Whittet H. Aural polyp and cholesteatoma. Clin Otolaryngol. 1988;13:395–7.
45. Gliklick RE, Cunningham MJ, Eavey RD. The cause of aural polyps in children. Arch Otolaryngol Head Neck Surg. 1993;119:669–71.
46. Tay HL, Hussain SS. The management of aural polyps. J Laryngol Otol. 1997;111(3):212–4.
47. Lotti T, Buggiani G, Prignano F. Prurigo nodularis and lichen simplex chronicus. Dermatol Ther. 2008;21(1):42–6.
48. Oztürkcan S, Oztürkcan S. Dermatologic diseases of the external ear. Clin Dermatol. 2014;32(1):141–52.
49. Hengge UR, Ruzicka T, Schwartz RA, Cork MJ. Adverse effects of topical glucocorticosteroids. J Am Acad Dermatol. 2006;54(1):1–18.
50. Strauss JS, Krowchuk DP, Leyden JJ, et al. Guidelines of care for acne vulgaris management. J Am Acad Dermatol. 2007;56(4):651–63.
51. Hannley MT, Dennery JC, Holzer SS. Consensus panel report: use of ototopical antibiotics in treating 3 common ear diseases. Otolaryngol Head Neck Surg. 2000;122:934–40.
52. Wright CG, Meyerhoff WL. Ototoxicity of otic drops applied to the middle ear in the chinchilla. Am J Otolaryngol. 1984;5:166–76.
53. Roland PS. Clinical ototoxicity of topical antibiotic drops. Otolaryngol Head Neck Surg. 1994;110:598–602.
54. Schachern PA, Paparella MM, Goycoolea MV. Thickness of the human round window membrane in different forms of otitis media. Arch Otolaryngol Head Neck Surg. 1987;110:630–4.
55. Meltzer P, Keleman G. Pyocyaneus osteomyelitis of the temporal bone, mandible and zygoma. Laryngoscope. 1959;69:1300–16.
56. Chandler JR. Malignant external otitis. Laryngoscope. 1968;78:1257–94.
57. Driscoll PV, Ramachandrula A, Drezner DA, et al. Characteristics of cerumen in diabetic patients: a key to understanding malignant external otitis? Otolaryngol Head Neck Surg. 1993;109:676.
58. Smitherman KO, Peacock JE. Infectious emergencies in patients with diabetes mellitus. Med Clin North Am. 1995;79:53–77.
59. Bhat V, Aziz A, Bhandary SK, Aroor R, Kamath PSD, Saldanha M. Malignant otitis externa - a retrospective study of 15 patients treated in a tertiary healthcare center. J Int Adv Otol. 2015;11(1):72–6. https://doi.org/10.5152/iao.2015.430.
60. Adams A, Offiah C. Central skull base osteomyelitis as a complication of necrotizing otitis externa: imaging findings, complications, and challenges of diagnosis. Clin Radiol. 2012;67(10):e7–e16.
61. Faizal B, Surendran B, Kumar M. Comparative study of reliability of inflammatory markers over 18-FDG-PET CT scan in monitoring skull base osteomyelitis. Braz J Otorhinolaryngol. 2022;88(5):691–700.
62. Johnson AK, Batra PS. Central skull base osteomyelitis: an emerging clinical entity. Laryngoscope. 2014;124(5):1083–7.
63. Blyth CC, Gomes L, Sorrell TC, Da Cruz M, Sud A, Chen SA. Skull-base osteomyelitis: fungal vs. bacterial infection. Clin Microbiol Infect. 2011;17(2):306–11.
64. Djalilian HR, Shamloo B, Thakkar KH, Najme-Rahim M. Treatment of culture-negative skull base osteomyelitis. Otol Neurotol. 2006;27(2):250–5.
65. Akhtar F, Iftikhar J, Azhar M, Raza A, Sultan F. Skull base osteomyelitis: a single-center experience. Cureus. 2021;13(12):e20162.
66. El-Sayed Y. Acquired medial canal fibrosis. J Laryngol Otol. 1998;112:145–9.
67. Selesnick S, Nguyen TP, Eisenman DJ. Surgical treatment of acquired external auditory canal atresia. Am J Otol. 1998;19:123–30.
68. Roland PS. Chronic external otitis. Ear Nose Throat J. 2001;80(Suppl 6):12–6.
69. Adkins WY, Ogusthorpe JD. Management of canal stenosis with a transposition flap. Laryngoscope. 1981;91:1267–9.
70. Heeneman H. Surgical correction of the stenosed ear canal. J Otolaryngol. 1979;8:461–2.

71. McCary WS, Kryzer TC, Lambert PR. Application of split-thickness skin grafts for acquired diseases of the external auditory canal. Am J Otol. 1995;16:801–5.
72. Naim R, Linthicum F, Shen T, Bran G, Hormann K. Classification of the external auditory canal cholesteatoma. Laryngoscope. 2005;115(3):455–60.
73. Thorsteinsson AL, Vestergaard P, Eiken P. External auditory canal and middle ear cholesteatoma and osteonecrosis in bisphosphonate-treated osteoporosis patients: a Danish national register-based cohort study and literature review. Osteoporos Int. 2014;25(7):1937–44.
74. Abelardo E, Jaramillo M. Give ears some respite from regular microsuctioning in bisphosphonate-induced osteonecrosis of the external ear canal. J Laryngol Otol. 2022;136(10):1002–4.
75. Saleem MI, Tham T, Ponder B, Georgolios A. Trichofolliculoma of the external auditory canal: a case report and review of the literature. J Surg Case Rep. 2022;2022(4):rjac147.
76. Chang NC, Chien CY, Wu CC, Chai CY. Squamous papilloma in the external auditory canal: a common lesion in an uncommon site. World J Clin Cases. 2013;1(2):92–5.
77. Psillas G, Krommydas A, Karayannopoulou G, Chatzopoulos K, Kanitakis J, Markou K. Ceruminous adenoma of the external auditory canal: a case report with imaging and pathologic findings. Case Rep Med. 2015;2015:359627.
78. Hoffman RA, Shepsman MA. Bullous myringitis and sensorineural hearing loss. Laryngoscope. 1983;93:1544–5.
79. Lashin N, Zaher S, Ragab A, et al. Hearing loss in bullous myringitis. Ear Nose Throat J. 1988;67:206–10.
80. Milligan W. Hemorrhagic types of ear disease occurring during epidemics of influenza. J Laryngol Otol. 1926;41:493–8.
81. Rifkind D, Chanock R, Kravetz H, et al. Ear involvement (myringitis) and primary atypical pneumonia following inoculation of volunteers with Eaton agent. Am Rev Respir Dis. 1962;85:479–89.
82. Merifield D, Miller G. The etiology and clinical course of bullous myringitis. Arch Otolaryngol. 1966;84:41–3.
83. DeWeese DD, Saunders WH, Schuller DE, Schleuning AJ. Infection and inflammation of the ear. In: DeWeese DD, Saunders WH, Schuller DE, Schleuning AJ, editors. Otolaryngology - head and neck surgery. 7th ed. St Louis: The C.V. Mosby Company; 1988. p. 395–425.
84. Makino K, Amatsu M, Kinishi M, et al. The clinical features and pathogenesis of granular myringitis. Arch Otorhinolaryngol. 1988;245:224–9.
85. Blevins NJ, Karmody CS. Chronic myringitis: prevalence, presentation, and natural history. Otol Neurotol. 2001;22:3–10.
86. El-Seifi A, Fouad B. Granular myringitis: is it a surgical problem? Am J Otol. 2000;21:462–7.
87. Kuo YX, Luo TH, Wu HM. Efficacy of carbon dioxide laser and caustic agent cauterisation for the focal granular myringitis: a randomised trial. Clin Otolaryngol. 2023;48(3):451–6.
88. Griffin WL. A retrospective study of traumatic tympanic membrane perforations in a clinical practice. Laryngoscope. 1979;89:261–82.
89. Tachibana T, Kariya S, Orita Y, et al. Spontaneous closure of traumatic tympanic membrane perforation following long-term observation. Acta Otolaryngol. 2019;139(6):487–91.
90. Lou ZC. Spontaneous healing of traumatic eardrum perforation: outward epithelial cell migration and clinical outcome. Otolaryngol Head Neck Surg. 2012;147(6):1114–9.
91. Litton WB. Epithelial migration over the tympanic membrane and external auditory canal. Arch Otolaryngol Head Neck Surg. 1963;77:254.
92. Alberti PWRM. Epithelial migration on the tympanic membrane. J Laryngol Otol. 1964;78:808–30.
93. Mehta RP, Rosowski JJ, Voss SE, et al. Determinants of hearing loss in perforations of the tympanic membrane. Otol Neurotol. 2006;27(2):136–43.
94. Sheehy JL, House WF. Tympanosclerosis. Arch Otolaryngol. 1962;76:151–7.
95. Bhaya MH, Paparella MM, Morizono T, et al. Pathogenesis of tympanosclerosis. Otolaryngol Head Neck Surg. 1993;109:413–9.
96. Tos M, Stangerup SE. Hearing loss in tympanosclerosis caused by grommets. Arch Otolaryngol Head Neck Surg. 1989;115:931–5.
97. Kay DJ, Nelson M, Rosenfeld RM. Meta-analysis of tympanostomy tube sequelae. Otolaryngol Head Neck Surg. 2001;124:374–80.
98. Sade J, Berco E. Atelectasis and secretory otitis media. Ann Otol Rhinol Laryngol. 1976;85(suppl 25):66–72.
99. Danner CJ. Middle ear atelectasis: what causes it and how is it corrected? Otolaryngol Clin N Am. 2006:1211–9.
100. Ramakrishnan Y, Kotecha A, Bowdler DA. A review of retraction pockets: past, present and future management. J Laryngol Otol. 2007;121:521–5.
101. Sade J. Atelectatic tympanic membrane: histologic study. Ann Otol Rhinol Laryngol. 1993;102:712–6.
102. Ostrowski VB, Bojrab DI. Minimally invasive laser contraction myringoplasty for tympanic membrane atelectasis. Otolaryngol Head Neck Surg. 2003;128:711–8.

Malignant Otitis Externa and Osteomyelitis of the Temporal Bone

32

Kyle Allen and Alexander Malone

Introduction

Malignant otitis externa (MOE) is a severe, progressive infectious process of the external auditory canal with osteomyelitis of the temporal bone. MOE is not a neoplastic process, and the use of the word "malignant" refers, rather, to the significant morbidity and potential mortality associated with the condition. Meltzer [1] had originally reported on temporal bone osteomyelitis in 1959, but it was Chandler who coined the term "malignant otitis externa" to describe its aggressive clinical course [2]. In his original paper, he described 13 cases in which *Pseudomonas aeruginosa* was the offending organism. The mainstay of his treatment was surgical, and the mortality rate was high, with 6 of the 13 patients presented succumbing to the disease.

Due to the absence of neoplasia, some have advocated for the use of the term "necrotizing otitis externa" to avoid confusion regarding neoplastic malignancy. Other authors have preferred the terminology of skull base osteomyelitis or temporal bone osteomyelitis to describe the characteristic involvement of the temporal bone. However, MOE remains the prevalent terminology and will be used in the chapter. MOE is classically observed in elderly, diabetic patients, but also arises in patients who are immunocompromised for other reasons. Rarely, this condition can occur in patients for whom there is not a clear, underlying predisposition.

Predisposing Factors

The majority of patients with MOE have diabetes mellitus (DM). Case series have demonstrated 65–93% of patients with MOE are diabetics [2–7]. That being said, other conditions that lead to immunocompromise are also associated with MOE. These have included leukemia, lymphoma, human immunodeficiency virus (HIV) infection, post-transplant-related immunosuppression, chemotherapy-related aplasia, splenectomy, and neoplasia [4, 8]. The presentation in an otherwise healthy individual should trigger an evaluation for diabetes or immunodeficiency. Also, when cultures identify a fungal etiology, a workup for immunodeficiency should be considered because fungal MOE is seen more frequently in this cohort [9].

While MOE is most common in older adults, with an average age of onset in the eighth decade of life, the condition occurs in patients of all ages. Children with MOE are more likely to be immunocompromised due to malignancy or as a complication of chemotherapy. They also tend to have a more favorable prognosis than adults in terms of mortality [10, 11]. This finding may be due to a higher likelihood that their immunodeficiency is correctable, and it may be due to a relative lack of microangiopathy seen in DM and chronic vascular disease, in general.

MOE is generally identified in the external auditory canal with clinical features similar to acute or chronic otitis externa: inflammation, pain, purulence, and/or granulation tissue. Irrigation of the external auditory canal for removal of cerumen has been hypothesized to be a causative event, and in one series, 62% of cases were preceded by tap water irrigation of the ear [12]. A moist environment develops as a result of the inflammatory process, leading to skin maceration and a reduction of the skin's natural protective function [13]. While healthy individuals can mount an appropriate response to this injury, those in an immunocompromised state (such as the microangiopathy of diabetes) are unable to mount an appropriate and satisfactory response. With time, progression of the infection occurs beyond the skin of the ear canal into the temporal bone itself.

K. Allen (✉)
Tampa Bay Hearing and Balance Center, Tampa, FL, USA
e-mail: kallen@tampabayhearing.com

A. Malone
Florida ENT and Allergy, Tampa, FL, USA

A. D. Sweeney et al. (eds.), *Haynes-Glasscock-Shambaugh Surgery of the Ear*, https://doi.org/10.1007/978-3-032-18264-7_32

Pathways of Spread

Once established within the external auditory canal, the infection can then spread to surrounding tissues through multiple pathways (Fig. 32.1). Anteriorly and inferiorly, infection can spread through the fissures of Santorini toward the parotid gland and temporomandibular joint (TMJ). This pathway provides minimal resistance to spread, which is why infiltration of the retrocondylar fat of the TMJ is one of the most common sites of invasion demonstrated on magnetic resonance imaging (MRI) [14]. Spread inferiorly at the osseocartilaginous junction can allow for extension to the stylomastoid foramen, which can cause facial nerve injury. Spread through the tympanomastoid suture toward the jugular foramen is possible and can lead to involvement of the lower cranial nerves. Posterior spread leads to involvement of the mastoid process, which can eventually lead to injury of the vertical segment of the facial nerve, the sigmoid sinus, and the posterior fossa.

Unlike acute mastoiditis, rapid spread of infection through pneumatized spaces of the temporal bone is less common than insidious spread through venous channels and fascial planes. The compact bone along the middle and posterior fossa can be frequently affected, while the otic capsule and middle ear are rarely involved by initial, direct extension [15]. Reactive changes in chronic, progressive MOE, however, provoke middle ear mucosal disease, and otologists must be discerning to recognize the contrasts between patients with a middle ear effusion from acute dysventilation versus those with MOE. Advancement of infection within the skull base leads to the formation of granulation tissue and osseous destruction. With medial spread, the petrous apex may become involved. If Dorello's canal becomes involved, an abducens nerve palsy can result. Anterior and medial spread can lead to involvement of the sphenoid sinus, clivus, and nasopharynx. In some cases, the orbital apex and even the optic nerve may be affected, as well as the contralateral temporal bone [16].

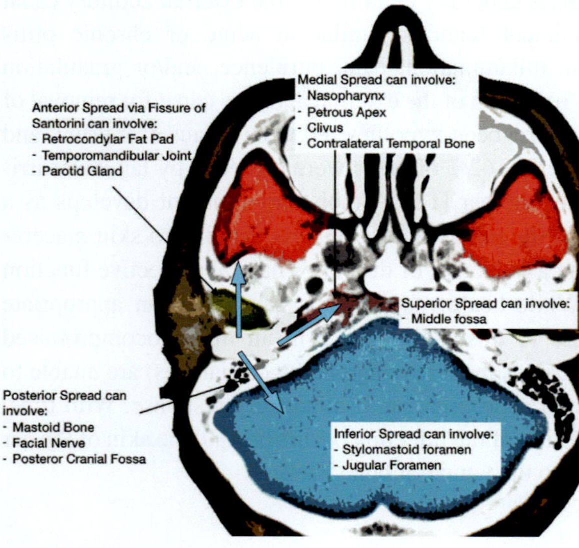

Fig. 32.1 The various routes of spread of infection from malignant otitis externa

Pathogens

Pseudomonas aeruginosa (*P. aeruginosa*) is the most common organism resulting in MOE. A 1988 review showed *Pseudomonas* to be responsible for 99% of 260 cases of MOE [17]. This gram-negative, mobile bacillus is ubiquitous in soil and water, but it is not part of the normal flora of the external auditory canal. *Pseudomonas* is frequently associated with opportunistic infections, implicated in 10% of hospital-acquired infections [18]. It may be introduced to the ear canal by water exposure or after trauma. *Pseudomonas* is also a common cause of acute otitis externa. A reduced host response allows the bacteria to develop into a more severe infection.

There are multiple features of *P. aeruginosa* infections that explain its relevance to MOE. Secreted factors include proteases, elastase, and exotoxins which can lead to tissue destruction, allow invasion, and prevent a host phagocytic response [19]. This species of bacteria also has a large genome that encodes many proteins that contribute to regulation, transport, and virulence functions. There is also an intrinsic ability to acquire mobile genetic elements that encode genes for antibiotic resistance [20]. The incidence of multidrug resistant *Pseudomonas* is on the rise, and there is concern that this may lead to difficulty treating *Pseudomonas* infection in the future [21].

When the term MOE was first coined, *Pseudomonas* was ubiquitous in affected patients [2]. It was also part of the original "Cohen Criteria" (Table 32.1), but a number of reports since then have demonstrated the role of other pathogens may also lead to MOE [22]. One series noted that *Staphylococcus aureus* (*S. aureus*) was found to be responsible for 15% of cases of MOE [23]. *S. aureus* was found to be associated with a lower rate of diabetes mellitus and immunocompromise when compared to patients in which *P. aeruginosa* was the causative pathogen. Other pathogens have included *Enterobacteriaceae, S. epidermidis, Proteus mirabilis, Klebsiella oxytoca, and P. cepacia*, among others [3, 8]. While it is possible that some of these cultures may have been the result of colonization or a polymicrobial infection, it is clear that not all MOE is caused by *Pseudomonas*.

An increasing rate of fungal lateral skull base infections has also been observed. The first case of fungal MOE was reported in 1985 and was the result of an *Aspergillus fumigatus* infection in a patient with acute myelogenous leukemia [24]. The most commonly reported fungal organ-

Table 32.1 The major and minor signs of MOE as defined by and adapted from Cohen et al. [22]

Cohen criteria
Major signs
Otalgia
Exudate
Edema
Granulation tissue
Microabscess
Positive scintigraphy *or* failure of local treatment
Minor
Pseudomonas on culture
Positive CT
Diabetes mellitus
Cranial nerve involvement
Debilitating condition
Old age

ism is *Aspergillus fumigatus,* but other species are noted such as *A. niger*, *A. flavus*, and *Scedosporium apiospermum* [8, 9]. Mucor is not reported as a common pathogen, distinct from what is seen in invasive fungal disease of the anterior skull base. The treatment of choice for invasive *Aspergillus* infections was initially intravenous amphotericin, but this medication has been largely replaced by voriconazole due to a more favorable side effect profile [25]. Though also reported in diabetics, fungal MOE is most frequently observed in patients with acquired immunodeficiency syndrome [9]. As noted above, an immune workup should be considered in patients primarily affected by fungal pathogens.

Clinical Presentation

MOE may have an insidious onset, which can lead to a delay in diagnosis. As noted above, the most common presenting symptoms are otalgia and otorrhea, which is not distinct from common acute otitis externa [4, 26]. Severe pain out of proportion to exam findings is frequently noted in MOE, however, and may last for months. Patients have often failed outpatient treatment of topical and/or systemic antibiotics prior to a MOE diagnosis. A delay in diagnosis has been reported from 2–21 months in patients referred for specialty care from otolaryngologists [26]. A high index of suspicion in diabetics and other immunocompromised patients presenting with signs of more benign disease is necessary, and close follow-up in these individuals warranted.

Other symptoms of MOE may include headache, temporomandibular joint pain, and trismus [8]. Fever is not commonly observed [27]. Hearing loss may also be present, and it is generally conductive in nature at the onset of disease, resulting from obstruction of the external auditory canal. As noted above, the middle ear space is typically spared early in the disease process. Sensorineural loss due to involvement of the otic capsule is rare initially, but it will be seen with progressive disease.

On physical examination, purulence, edema, tenderness, and granulation tissue can be seen within the external auditory canal. Edema may extend into the periauricular soft tissues and face. Granulation tissue is classically described as being located in the inferior canal at the osseocartilaginous junction. Granulation tissue or ear canal polyps have been reported in 53–96% of patients at presentation [5, 26]. A defect of the external auditory canal, if present, can be palpated with a right angle hook [28].

Cranial nerve involvement is often seen as the disease process progresses. The facial nerve is the most common nerve affected, and some degree of facial nerve involvement can be seen in 20–56% of cases [4, 29, 30]. Facial nerve involvement in MOE is largely thought to be extratemporal in nature, but there is an increased rate of mastoid involvement on computed tomography (CT), which indicates a potential vertical segment injury [2, 31]. Less frequently, the lower cranial nerves can also be affected at the jugular foramen [32]. Involvement of the trigeminal, abducens, and optic nerve is also possible with medial extension of the disease [16, 26].

Diagnosis

Differential Diagnosis

A high index of suspicion for MOE should be initially inspired by history and physical examination. The differential diagnosis includes nasopharyngeal malignancy, external auditory canal malignancy, Paget's disease, granulomatous disorders, clival lesions, and fibrous dysplasia [28]. Chandler's original report of 13 patients included a patient he later determined to have a squamous cell carcinoma [29].

Patients with MOE typically do not have leukocytosis or fever [8]. The erythrocyte sedimentation rate (ESR) is nearly universally elevated, and some use it as a marker for successful treatment of the disease [33]. C-reactive protein (CRP) levels can also be useful both for MOE diagnosis and to track treatment response.

Multiple diagnostic strategies have been developed to aid in identifying MOE. Cohen's Criteria (Table 32.1) has classically been described and is commonly used in publications [22, 34]. We performed a literature review of articles published within the past 5 years and the criteria used to define MOE (Table 32.2). Cohen's criteria were the main method of diagnosis in a third of these studies, a testament to the staying power of these criteria, though MRI findings are becoming increasingly reported, which has increased the clinical utility of MRI in these patients.

Table 32.2 Diagnostic criteria used in studies published within the last 5 years[a]

Study	Otalgia	Edema	Otorrhea	Granulation tissue	Immunosuppressed	Failure of local treatment	Culture	Microabscess	Scintigraphy	CT	MRI
Guevara et al. (2013) [59][b]									X	X	X
Lambor et al. (2013) [60]	X	X	X	X	X	X	X			X	
Le Clerc et al. (2014) [61]	X	X		X	X	X				X	X
S. Shavit et al. (2016) [3]	X	X	X	X		X		X	X	X	
Hasibi et al. (2017) [62]	X	X	X	X	X				X	X	
Glikson et al. (2017) [5]	X	X	X			X				X	

[a]Hobson [23], Lee [63], and Stevens [7] all used the Cohen criteria
[b]Guevara used clinical signs of inflammation on physical exam

On workup, culture of purulent drainage and of biopsied tissue is indicated to determine the pathogen involved. Cultures should include aerobic, anaerobic, mycobacterial, and fungal evaluations. Cultures that utilize next-generation sequencing and polymerase chain reaction (PCR) are also emerging tools. Pathologic evaluation of abnormal tissue is also important given that cancers of the ear canal and temporal bone can present similarly to MOE. Tissue sampling should include a biopsy of granulation tissue within the ear canal, abnormal nasopharyngeal tissue, and any other lesions concerning for a possible tumor. If a patient does not respond to typical antibiotic treatments, consideration should be given to repeating biopsies and cultures.

Imaging

High-resolution temporal bone CT is widely available and can usually be performed early in the evaluation of a patient with findings concerning for MOE. This modality can provide information regarding the extent of disease. CT findings in MOE typically include soft tissue inflammation and osseous erosion (Fig. 32.2). CT can have a low sensitivity for MOE, however, as early infection may not demonstrate significant osseous changes. It has been reported that more than 30% of the bone must be demineralized prior to a change becoming visible on CT [35]. Also, as noted above regarding spread through vascular and fascial channels and planes, even patients with advanced MOE and cranial neuropathies may not demonstrate any blatant osseous abnormalities. After successful treatment, the demineralized bone will slowly ossify, but the CT will remain abnormal long after the infection has resolved [36]. CT can be useful to demonstrate abscess formation and does provide useful anatomic information regarding the osseous anatomy of the temporal bone, which is poorly demonstrated on other studies.

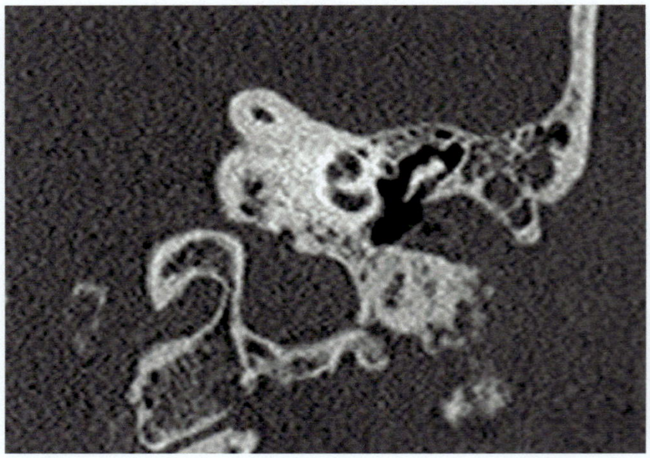

Fig. 32.2 Coronal high-resolution CT in a patient with MOE. Bone erosion is not always detected on CT until significant disease progression has occurred

MRI provides more detail as to the extent of soft tissue involvement within the skull base and also intracranially. Bone marrow can also be evaluated, and enhancement varies with the progression or regression of infection [37]. Soft tissue changes and contrast enhancement may remain abnormal following resolution of the infection. Consequently, MRI has not been thought to be an effective way to monitor for disease resolution [38]. However, a recent series noted that diffusion-weighted (DW) MRI can be useful for following infection without the use of gadolinium contrast (Fig. 32.3) [39]. In this study, it was demonstrated that the apparent diffusion coefficient (ADC) map demonstrates a high signal in the setting of active infection, and this signal reduces with the resolution of infection. Whether this option will ultimately become a standard means of monitoring treatment efficacy remains unclear, but this initial finding is promising.

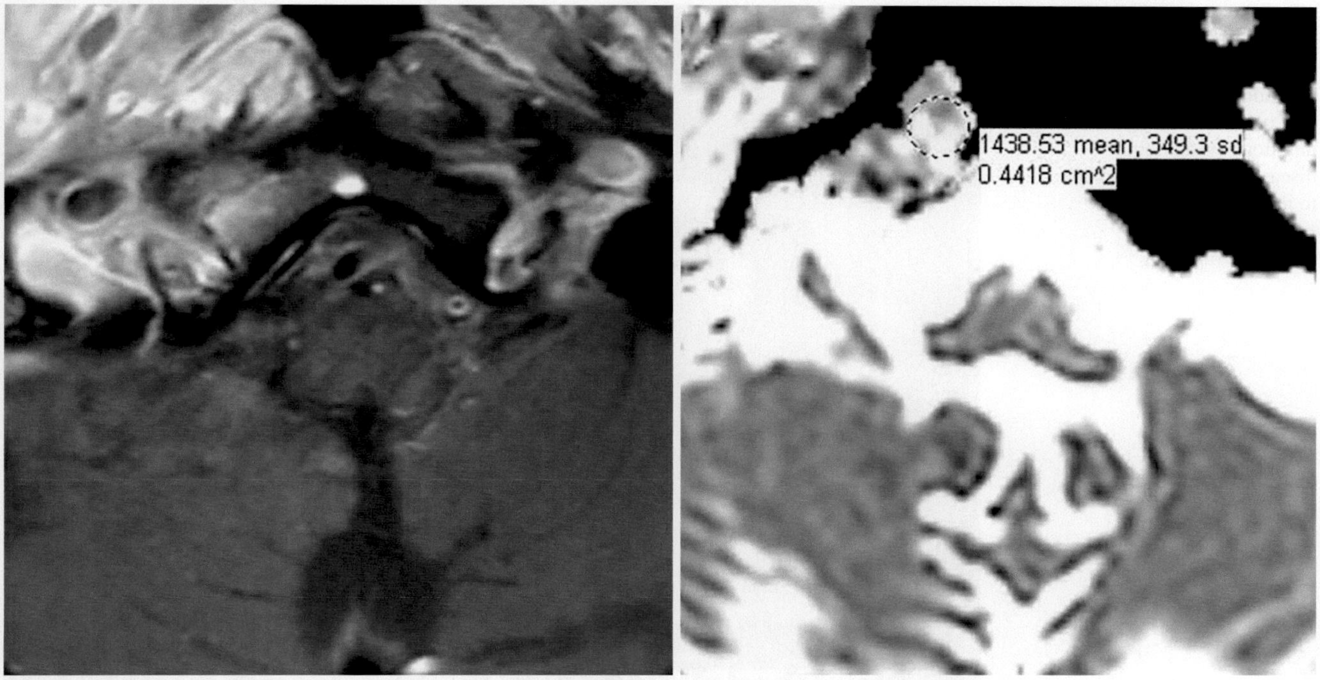

Fig. 32.3 Diffusion-weighted MRI can allow for monitoring of disease progression and resolution while avoiding the use of contrast. The T1 post-contrast MRI on the left demonstrates enhancement along the petrous apex in a patient with MOE. The diffusion-weighted MRI on the right demonstrates an elevated apparent diffusion coefficient in the same region

Nuclear medicine bone scans are a historical standard in the diagnosis of MOE. While these scans do not provide high-resolution anatomic detail, they are very useful in demonstrating osteomyelitis. Technetium-99m methylene diphosphonate (Tc-99m-MDP) scintigraphy demonstrates osteoblastic activity that occurs in the setting of osteomyelitis (Fig. 32.4). Tc-99m-MDP scintigraphy does not require demineralization of bone to demonstrate activity, so the test is positive earlier in the disease process than CT [40]. However, in terms of specificity, it has been demonstrated that technetium scintigraphy can also be positive in the setting of a severe acute otitis externa that is not MOE [41]. Therefore, differentiation between a severe acute otitis externa and MOE can be best determined by performing scintigraphy 4 and 24 h after technetium injection [42]. Osteoblasts remain active for a long duration (months to years) after infection resolution, so the Tc-99m-MDP scintigraphy is not a valid way to evaluate for treatment resolution [40, 43].

Gallium-67 binds to leukocytes and tends to accumulate in regions of active inflammation in the bone and soft tissue. This test tends to normalize more rapidly after the infection resolves and can be useful to detect resolution of MOE [40]. As Gallium-67 accumulates in sites of active infection, a positive scan in the presence of a negative Tc-99m-MDP scintigraphy would indicate acute otitis externa in the absence of osteomyelitis [44].

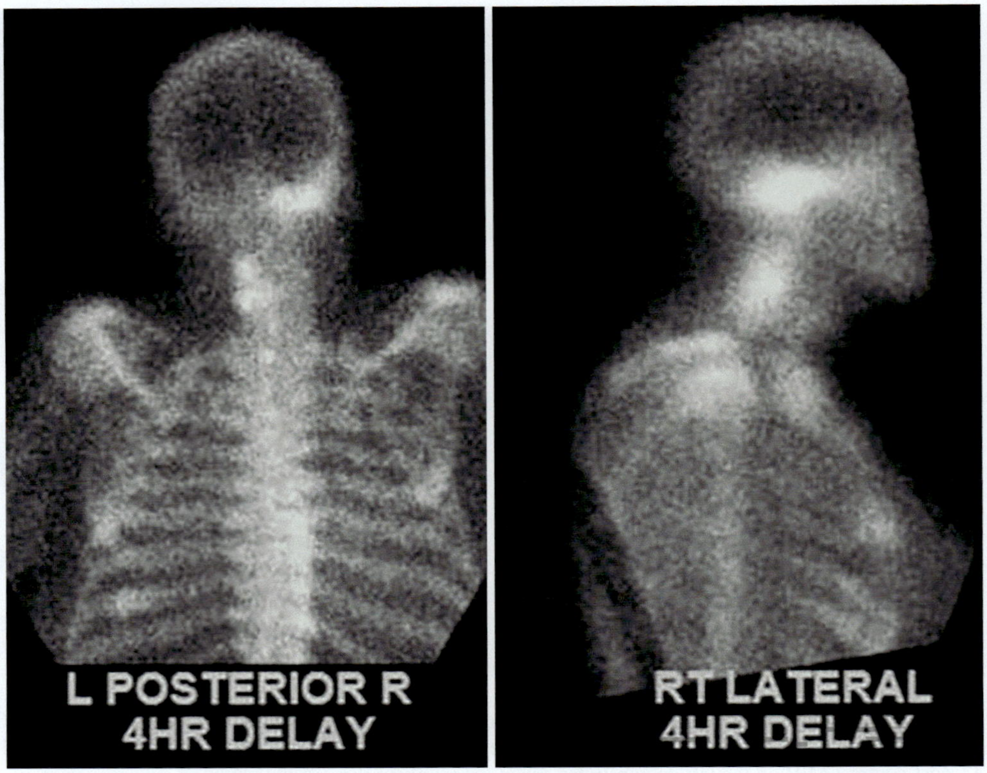

Fig. 32.4 Technetium-99m methylene diphosphonate scintigraphy of a patient with left-sided MOE. These scans stay positive for long durations even after the disease has been treated due to increased osteoblastic activity

Treatment

The treatment of MOE is largely medical. Initial reports, such as Chandler's original series, advocated for aggressive surgical intervention to remove all infected tissues [2]. Modern treatments, including improved anti-pseudomonal antibiotics, have largely pushed contemporary management away from surgical intervention. Biopsy and culture remain important, but these tasks can often be performed as an office procedure or under local anesthesia [5]. If inadequate tissue or culture material can be obtained, a procedure in the operating room under general anesthesia may be indicated. Early debridement of obstructing granulation tissue and infected cartilage may reduce the duration of antibiotic treatment [45]. Surgical intervention is indicated in the setting of abscess formation and for the removal of bony sequestra [15]. Because the facial nerve is most often involved in the extratemporal soft tissues, facial nerve decompression has not been typically recommended in the setting of MOE and facial paralysis [2]. However, a recent series suggested that a benefit in facial nerve recovery may be seen in patients undergoing operative intervention that includes facial nerve decompression, though statistical significance was not found in this study [46]. In patients undergoing facial nerve decompression, 50% have no improvement in function, and 22.9% were demonstrated to have a full recovery [47].

It is also critical that medical treatment targets the underlying predisposing condition. For diabetics, blood glucose normalization is necessary in order to maximize immune function. If a patient has a reversible immunodeficiency, improvement of immune function is vital. Renal failure should also be evaluated and managed. In many cases, it must be said that the effects of antimicrobial therapy and surgical intervention will be marginalized if the underlying, causative etiology is poorly controlled.

Culture-directed antibiotic therapy is the foundational element of MOE treatment. Antibiotics are typically planned for at least 4–8 weeks, but consideration should be given to continuing them until clinical indicators demonstrate resolution of the infection [13]. Consultation with an infectious disease specialist is advised. Aminoglycosides and anti-pseudomonal penicillins significantly helped to reduce the mortality that had been previously associated with MOE in the past [6]. As aminoglycosides require parenteral delivery and are associated with significant nephrotoxicity and ototoxicity, anti-pseudomonal cephalosporins, such as ceftazidime, are commonly employed.

Ciprofloxacin, a quinolone antibiotic, has been described as the initial drug of choice with monotherapy [6]. Ciprofloxacin has a high bioavailability when taken orally, penetrates the bone well, and does not require long-term intravenous access. Concomitant administration of magnesium significantly reduces the absorption of this drug. Ciprofloxacin and other quinolones are associated with an increased risk of tendon rupture and the development of a peripheral neuropathy, for which the FDA has issued black box warnings [48, 49]. This should be discussed with patients prior to prescribing the medication. In the setting of immunocompromise due to chronic steroid use, it should be noted that the risk of tendon rupture is higher when a quinolone is administered concomitantly with corticosteroids.

Antibiotic resistance is certainly an important consideration in the treatment of MOE. In 2002, Berenholz reported one-third of cases of MOE due to *Pseudomonas* were resistant to ciprofloxacin [50]. These findings reinforce the importance of culture-driven treatment.

Culture-negative MOE is typically presumed to be caused by *Pseudomonas*, and anti-pseudomonal antibiotics are frequently initiated. A series of eight culture-negative MOE patients were treated with a regimen of oral ciprofloxacin, intravenous ceftazidime, and topical polymyxin/neomycin/hydrocortisone drops. All patients demonstrated resolution of infection by gallium scan after 6 weeks of therapy [51]. If a patient does not have a response to therapy with such a regimen, one should suspect another pathogen, possibly fungus. Tissue biopsy with culture is important in this setting to obtain an appropriate sample for diagnosis and to determine the appropriate therapy.

Fungal MOE is most commonly related to *Aspergillus* species. As discussed earlier, voriconazole can be administered orally with a much lower side effect profile than amphotericin B. Oral itraconazole has also been successful for a *Scedosporium apiospermum* infection [52].

Hyperbaric oxygen (HBO) has been utilized in the treatment of MOE. Benefits are thought to be related to an increased partial pressure of oxygen, thereby improving leukocyte function [53]. However, there continues to be little evidence of the efficacy of this treatment in MOE. A Cochrane review found no randomized trials and could not demonstrate any evidence to support the use of HBO in MOE [54]. There are reports of successful treatment in patients with disease recalcitrant to antibiotics [55]. A systematic review of HBO use in MOE determined unproven efficacy due to a lack of strong scientific evidence but highlighted good results with few reported adverse events [56]. As the mortality rate of MOE has declined significantly with the advent of newer and better anti-pseudomonal antibiotics, HBO is not routinely offered.

Prognosis

In early reports, prior to contemporary anti-pseudomonal antibiotics, mortality rates were high. Chandler's initial report had a mortality rate of 46% [2]. Patients with cranial neuropathies were also reported to have a significantly higher mortality rate [29]. However, with improved antibiotic therapy, including anti-pseudomonal penicillins, cephalosporins, and fluoroquinolones, the mortality rate has dropped considerably. Recent reports of 46 and 25 patients have described a disease-related mortality rate of 4.4% and 8%, respectively [4, 5]. A systematic review of MOE has shown a cure rate of 87–100% in series since the 1980s [34]. Facial nerve involvement is now less predictive of mortality, and some reports show no detrimental effect on survival when these are present [32]. However, disease-specific outcomes are generally worse when cranial neuropathies exist, and lower cranial nerve involvement, in particular, does continue to portend worse outcomes, likely due to the more extensive temporal bone involvement required to jeopardize these nerves [7, 57].

Assessment for Treatment Resolution

The optimal duration of antibiotic therapy for osteomyelitis of the skull base—and even peripheral bones—has not been determined [58]. Classically, the technetium scan is used to diagnose MOE, and the resolution of the infection is determined by normalization of the gallium scan. Gallium scans are recommended to be repeated every 4 or 6 weeks [28, 51]. Until the gallium scan normalizes, antibiotics should be continued. At many institutions, a gallium scan is difficult to obtain. In these cases, clinical examination and laboratory findings may be trended to help determine when to discontinue antibiotics.

ESR is typically elevated in MOE, and reduction in this value is typically associated with a favorable response to treatment [33]. Though some report on elevated ESR and its reduction with therapeutic treatment, this is rarely the only measure utilized to terminate therapy.

MRI has been reported to be a useful tool to determine resolution of infection. Ismail reported a case in which MRI was used as the only imaging modality and presented MRI as an option to monitor treatment. However, the authors in this case do not state if clinical decision-making was based solely on the MRI. In addition, the MRI did not fully normalize, although the patient had an excellent clinical response without recurrence after antibiotic cessation [37]. Cherko reported resolution of an intense ADC map signal on DW-MRI, which was associated with resolution of infection [39]. In seven patients, the decision to stop antibiotics due to infection resolution also correlated with the resolution of the high signal on the ADC map. This technique may help MRI, which is more broadly available than nuclear medicine scans, to help determine treatment end dates.

Conclusion

In a diabetic or immunocompromised patient with severe, prolonged ear pain and otorrhea, MOE should be considered in the differential diagnosis. Confirmation of diagnosis is traditionally based on nuclear medicine studies, including technetium and gallium scintigraphy, but has increasingly been described with a combination of MRI and CT findings. Culture-directed antibiotics are the treatment of choice, and surgery is generally limited to the debridement of necrotic tissue and provision of diagnostic information. The most common pathogen in MOE is *Pseudomonas*, although fungal infections are showing increasing prevalence, especially in frankly immunosuppressed populations. Progressive cranial neuropathies and even death are the natural history of MOE, but the mortality rate has declined significantly over the past 50 years. A minimum of 6 weeks of antibiotics is recommended, and though the best practice for determining treatment efficacy is unclear, gallium scans have historically been used, when accessible.

References

1. Meltzer PE, Kelemen G. Pyocyaneus osteomyelitis of the temporal bone, mandible, and zygoma. Laryngoscope. 1959;69:1300–16.
2. Chandler JR. Malignant external otitis. Laryngoscope. 1968;78(8):1257–94. https://doi.org/10.1288/00005537-196808000-00002.
3. Stern Shavit S, Soudry E, Hamzany Y, Nageris B. Malignant external otitis: factors predicting patient outcomes. Am J Otolaryngol. 2016;37(5):425–30. https://doi.org/10.1016/j.amjoto.2016.04.005.
4. Franco-Vidal V, Blanchet H, Bebear C, Dutronc H, Darrouzet V. Necrotizing external otitis: a report of 46 cases. Otol Neurotol. 2007;28(6):771–3. https://doi.org/10.1097/MAO.0b013e31805153bd.
5. Glikson E, Sagiv D, Wolf M, Shapira Y. Necrotizing otitis externa: diagnosis, treatment, and outcome in a case series. Diagn Microbiol Infect Dis. 2017;87(1):74–8. https://doi.org/10.1016/j.diagmicrobio.2016.10.017.
6. Levenson MJ, Parisier SC, Dolitsky J, Bindra G. Ciprofloxacin: drug of choice in the treatment of malignant external otitis (MEO). Laryngoscope. 1991;101(8):821–4. https://doi.org/10.1288/00005537-199108000-00004.
7. Stevens SM, Lambert PR, Baker AB, Meyer TA. Malignant otitis externa: a novel stratification protocol for predicting treatment outcomes. Otol Neurotol. 2015;36(9):1492–8. https://doi.org/10.1097/mao.0000000000000839.
8. Carfrae MJ, Kesser BW. Malignant otitis externa. Otolaryngol Clin N Am. 2008;41(3):537–49, viii-ix. https://doi.org/10.1016/j.otc.2008.01.004.
9. Stodulski D, Kowalska B, Stankiewicz C. Otogenic skull base osteomyelitis caused by invasive fungal infection. Case report and literature review. Eur Arch Otorhinolaryngol. 2006;263(12):1070–6. https://doi.org/10.1007/s00405-006-0118-7.
10. Sobie S, Brodsky L, Stanievich JF. Necrotizing external otitis in children: report of two cases and review of the literature. Laryngoscope. 1987;97(5):598–601.
11. Rubin J, Yu VL, Stool SE. Malignant external otitis in children. J Pediatr. 1988;113(6):965–70.
12. Rubin J, Yu VL, Kamerer DB, Wagener M. Aural irrigation with water: a potential pathogenic mechanism for inducing malignant external otitis? Ann Otol Rhinol Laryngol. 1990;99(2 Pt 1):117–9.
13. Kraus DH, Rehm SJ, Kinney SE. The evolving treatment of necrotizing external otitis. Laryngoscope. 1988;98(9):934–9. https://doi.org/10.1288/00005537-198809000-00006.
14. Kwon BJ, Han MH, Oh SH, Song JJ, Chang KH. MRI findings and spreading patterns of necrotizing external otitis: is a poor outcome predictable? Clin Radiol. 2006;61(6):495–504. https://doi.org/10.1016/j.crad.2006.01.010.
15. Sreepada GS, Kwartler JA. Skull base osteomyelitis secondary to malignant otitis externa. Curr Opin Otolaryngol Head Neck Surg. 2003;11(5):316–23.
16. Holder CD, Gurucharri M, Bartels LJ, Colman MF. Malignant external otitis with optic neuritis. Laryngoscope. 1986;96(9 Pt 1):1021–3.
17. Rubin J, Yu VL. Malignant external otitis: insights into pathogenesis, clinical manifestations, diagnosis, and therapy. Am J Med. 1988;85(3):391–8.
18. Morales E, Cots F, Sala M, et al. Hospital costs of nosocomial multidrug resistant Pseudomonas aeruginosa acquisition. BMC Health Serv Res. 2012;12:122. https://doi.org/10.1186/1472-6963-12-122.
19. Balasubramanian D, Schneper L, Kumari H, Mathee K. A dynamic and intricate regulatory network determines Pseudomonas aeruginosa virulence. Nucleic Acids Res. 2013;41(1):1–20. https://doi.org/10.1093/nar/gks1039.
20. Mesaros N, Nordmann P, Plésiat P, et al. Pseudomonas aeruginosa: resistance and therapeutic options at the turn of the new millennium. Clin Microbiol Infect. 2007;13(6):560–78. https://doi.org/10.1111/j.1469-0691.2007.01681.x.
21. Sydnor ER, Perl TM. Hospital epidemiology and infection control in acute-care settings. Clin Microbiol Rev. 2011;24(1):141–73. https://doi.org/10.1128/CMR.00027-10.
22. Cohen D, Friedman P. The diagnostic criteria of malignant external otitis. J Laryngol Otol. 1987;101(3):216–21.
23. Hobson CE, Moy JD, Byers KE, Raz Y, Hirsch BE, McCall AA. Malignant otitis externa: evolving pathogens and implications for diagnosis and treatment. Otolaryngol Head Neck Surg. 2014;151(1):112–6. https://doi.org/10.1177/0194599814528301.
24. Petrak R, Portage J, Levin S. Invasive external otitis caused by Aspergillus fumigatus in an immunocompromised patient—correspondence. J Infect Dis. 1985;151(1):196.
25. Tarazi AE, Al-Tawfiq JA, Abdi RF. Fungal malignant otitis externa: pitfalls, diagnosis, and treatment. Otol Neurotol. 2012;33(5):769–73. https://doi.org/10.1097/MAO.0b013e3182565b46.
26. Jacobsen LM, Antonelli PJ. Errors in the diagnosis and management of necrotizing otitis externa. Otolaryngol Head Neck Surg. 2010;143(4):506–9. https://doi.org/10.1016/j.otohns.2010.06.924.
27. Amorosa L, Modugno GC, Pirodda A. Malignant external otitis: review and personal experience. Acta Otolaryngol Suppl. 1996;521:3–16.
28. Slattery WH, Brackmann DE. Skull base osteomyelitis. Malignant external otitis. Otolaryngol Clin N Am. 1996;29(5):795–806.
29. Chandler JR. Pathogenesis and treatment of facial paralysis due to malignant external otitis. Ann Otol Rhinol Laryngol. 1972;81(5):648–58. https://doi.org/10.1177/000348947208100505.
30. Corey JP, Levandowski RA, Panwalker AP. Prognostic implications of therapy for necrotizing external otitis. Am J Otol. 1985;6(4):353–8.
31. Soudry E, Joshua BZ, Sulkes J, Nageris BI. Characteristics and prognosis of malignant external otitis with facial paralysis. Arch Otolaryngol Head Neck Surg. 2007;133(10):1002–4. https://doi.org/10.1001/archotol.133.10.1002.
32. Mani N, Sudhoff H, Rajagopal S, Moffat D, Axon PR. Cranial nerve involvement in malignant external otitis: implications for clinical outcome. Laryngoscope. 2007;117(5):907–10. https://doi.org/10.1097/MLG.0b013e318039b30f.
33. Rubin J, Stoehr G, Yu VL, Muder RR, Matador A, Kamerer DB. Efficacy of oral ciprofloxacin plus rifampin for treatment of malignant external otitis. Arch Otolaryngol Head Neck Surg. 1989;115(9):1063–9.

34. Mahdyoun P, Pulcini C, Gahide I, et al. Necrotizing otitis externa: a systematic review. Otol Neurotol. 2013;34(4):620–9. https://doi.org/10.1097/MAO.0b013e3182804aee.
35. Stokkel MP, Boot CN, van Eck-Smit BL. SPECT gallium scintigraphy in malignant external otitis: initial staging and follow-up. Case reports. Laryngoscope. 1996;106(3 Pt 1):338–40.
36. Mendelson DS, Som PM, Mendelson MH, Parisier SC. Malignant external otitis: the role of computed tomography and radionuclides in evaluation. Radiology. 1983;149(3):745–9. https://doi.org/10.1148/radiology.149.3.6580674.
37. Ismail H, Hellier WP, Batty V. Use of magnetic resonance imaging as the primary imaging modality in the diagnosis and follow-up of malignant external otitis. J Laryngol Otol. 2004;118(7):576–9. https://doi.org/10.1258/0022215041615100.
38. Grandis JR, Curtin HD, Yu VL. Necrotizing (malignant) external otitis: prospective comparison of CT and MR imaging in diagnosis and follow-up. Radiology. 1995;196(2):499–504. https://doi.org/10.1148/radiology.196.2.7617867.
39. Cherko M, Nash R, Singh A, Lingam RK. Diffusion-weighted magnetic resonance imaging as a novel imaging modality in assessing treatment response in necrotizing otitis externa. Otol Neurotol. 2016;37(6):704–7. https://doi.org/10.1097/MAO.0000000000001022.
40. Strashun AM, Nejatheim M, Goldsmith SJ. Malignant external otitis: early scintigraphic detection. Radiology. 1984;150(2):541–5. https://doi.org/10.1148/radiology.150.2.6228955.
41. Levin WJ, Shary JH, Nichols LT, Lucente FE. Bone scanning in severe external otitis. Laryngoscope. 1986;96(11):1193–5.
42. Hardoff R, Gips S, Uri N, Front A, Tamir A. Semiquantitative skull planar and SPECT bone scintigraphy in diabetic patients: differentiation of necrotizing (malignant) external otitis from severe external otitis. J Nucl Med. 1994;35(3):411–5.
43. Parisier SC, Lucente FE, Som PM, Hirschman SZ, Arnold LM, Roffman JD. Nuclear scanning in necrotizing progressive "malignant" external otitis. Laryngoscope. 1982;92(9 Pt 1):1016–9.
44. Okpala NC, Siraj QH, Nilssen E, Pringle M. Radiological and radionuclide investigation of malignant otitis externa. J Laryngol Otol. 2005;119(1):71–5. https://doi.org/10.1258/0022215053222978.
45. Pedersen HB, Rosborg J. Necrotizing external otitis: aminoglycoside and beta-lactam antibiotic treatment combined with surgical treatment. Clin Otolaryngol Allied Sci. 1997;22(3):271–4.
46. Freeman MH, Perkins EL, Tawfik KO, et al. Facial paralysis in skull base osteomyelitis—comparison of surgical and nonsurgical management. Laryngoscope. 2023;133(1):179–83. https://doi.org/10.1002/lary.30161.
47. Marszał J, Wierzbicka M, Bartochowska A. Is facial nerve decompression justified in malignant external otitis? Literature review and own experience. J Int Adv Otol. 2023;19(3):191–8. https://doi.org/10.5152/iao.2023.22892.
48. Arabyat RM, Raisch DW, McKoy JM, Bennett CL. Fluoroquinolone-associated tendon-rupture: a summary of reports in the Food and Drug Administration's adverse event reporting system. Expert Opin Drug Saf. 2015;14(11):1653–60. https://doi.org/10.1517/14740338.2015.1085968.
49. Ciprofloxacin Hydrochloride. Food and Drug Administration. https://www.accessdata.fda.gov/drugsatfda_docs/label/2016/019537s086lbl.pdf. Accessed 6/2026.
50. Berenholz L, Katzenell U, Harell M. Evolving resistant pseudomonas to ciprofloxacin in malignant otitis externa. Laryngoscope. 2002;112(9):1619–22. https://doi.org/10.1097/00005537-200209000-00017.
51. Djalilian HR, Shamloo B, Thakkar KH, Najme-Rahim M. Treatment of culture-negative skull base osteomyelitis. Otol Neurotol. 2006;27(2):250–5. https://doi.org/10.1097/01.mao.0000181185.26410.80.
52. Yao M, Messner AH. Fungal malignant otitis externa due to Scedosporium apiospermum. Ann Otol Rhinol Laryngol. 2001;110(4):377–80. https://doi.org/10.1177/000348940111000415.
53. Saxby A, Barakate M, Kertesz T, James J, Bennett M. Malignant otitis externa: experience with hyperbaric oxygen therapy. Diving Hyperb Med. 2010;40(4):195–200.
54. Phillips JS, Jones SE. Hyperbaric oxygen as an adjuvant treatment for malignant otitis externa. Cochrane Database Syst Rev. 2013;2013(5):CD004617. https://doi.org/10.1002/14651858.CD004617.pub3.
55. Davis JC, Gates GA, Lerner C, Davis MG, Mader JT, Dinesman A. Adjuvant hyperbaric oxygen in malignant external otitis. Arch Otolaryngol Head Neck Surg. 1992;118(1):89–93.
56. Byun YJ, Patel J, Nguyen SA, Lambert PR. Hyperbaric oxygen therapy in malignant otitis externa: a systematic review of the literature. World J Otorhinolaryngol Head Neck Surg. 2021;7(4):296–302. https://doi.org/10.1016/j.wjorl.2020.04.002.
57. Hatch JL, Bauschard MJ, Nguyen SA, Lambert PR, Meyer TA, McRackan TR. Malignant otitis externa outcomes: a study of the university health system consortium database. Ann Otol Rhinol Laryngol. 2018;127(8):514–20. https://doi.org/10.1177/0003489418778056.
58. Courson AM, Vikram HR, Barrs DM. What are the criteria for terminating treatment for necrotizing (malignant) otitis externa? Laryngoscope. 2014;124(2):361–2. https://doi.org/10.1002/lary.24093.
59. Guevara N, Mahdyoun P, Pulcini C, Raffaelli C, Gahide I, Castillo L. Initial management of necrotizing external otitis: errors to avoid. Eur Ann Otorhinolaryngol Head Neck Dis. 2013;130(3):115–21. https://doi.org/10.1016/j.anorl.2012.04.011.
60. Lambor DV, Das CP, Goel HC, Tiwari M, Lambor SD, Fegade MV. Necrotising otitis externa: clinical profile and management protocol. J Laryngol Otol. 2013;127(11):1071–7. https://doi.org/10.1017/S0022215113002259.
61. Le Clerc N, Verillaud B, Duet M, Guichard JP, Herman P, Kania R. Skull base osteomyelitis: incidence of resistance, morbidity, and treatment strategy. Laryngoscope. 2014;124(9):2013–6. https://doi.org/10.1002/lary.24726.
62. Hasibi M, Ashtiani MK, Motassadi Zarandi M, et al. A treatment protocol for management of bacterial and fungal malignant external otitis: a large cohort in Tehran, Iran. Ann Otol Rhinol Laryngol. 2017;126(7):561–7. https://doi.org/10.1177/0003489417710473.
63. Lee SK, Lee SA, Seon SW, et al. Analysis of prognostic factors in malignant external otitis. Clin Exp Otorhinolaryngol. 2017;10(3):228–35. https://doi.org/10.21053/ceo.2016.00612.

33 Surgery for Congenital Aural Atresia and Stenosis

Zachary G. Schwam, Maura K. Cosetti, and Bradley W. Kesser

Introduction

Congenital aural atresia is an uncommon problem, affecting one in every 10,000–20,000 live births. It is more often unilateral, has a higher prevalence in males, and the severity of associated middle ear pathology tends to correlate with the degree of auricular deformity [1–4]. It is associated with a recognizable syndrome (most commonly Treacher Collins, Goldenhar, and hemifacial microsomia) in about 10% of patients. In about 5% of non-syndromic patients, the birth defect is inherited. As a first branchial arch anomaly, the malleus and incus are typically malformed and fused, while the stapes and inner ear are frequently preserved due to their different embryologic origins [1, 5]. During the second month of gestation, epithelium from the first branchial pouch migrates medially and is subsequently canalized in the 6th–7th months to form the external auditory canal. In congenital aural atresia there is no external auditory canal, and the distance between the temporomandibular joint (TMJ) and mastoid tip is narrowed significantly. The course of the facial nerve tends to be more anterior and lateral. In congenital aural stenosis, an ear canal is present but is diminutive and can be associated with hearing loss and cholesteatoma formation [6].

Maura K. Cosetti and Bradley W. Kesser are the senior co-authors.

Z. G. Schwam · M. K. Cosetti
Department of Otolaryngology—Head and Neck Surgery, Icahn School of Medicine at Mount Sinai, New York, NY, USA

B. W. Kesser (✉)
Department of Otolaryngology—Head and Neck Surgery, University of Virginia School of Medicine, Charlottesville, VA, USA
e-mail: Bwk2n@uvahealth.org

A. D. Sweeney et al. (eds.), *Haynes-Glasscock-Shambaugh Surgery of the Ear*, https://doi.org/10.1007/978-3-032-18264-7_33

Congenital Ear Canal Stenosis

Though the majority of this chapter focuses on congenital aural atresia (CAA), congenital aural canal stenosis (CAS) deserves special mention. Four types of ear canal stenosis were originally described by Schuknecht [7]. As discussed in greater detail below, the first two types, "A" and "B," corresponded to incomplete stenosis rather than complete canal atresia. "A" involved stenosis of the canal with relatively normal middle ear structures, while "B" involved more severe stenosis in which middle ear abnormalities were more common.

In both types of CAS described by Schuknecht, hearing loss and debris collection are relevant and distinct concerns. Debris collection, specifically, can lead to canal cholesteatoma formation, which can progress significantly before it is detected. It has been suggested that 20% of ears with CAS will develop cholesteatoma, and Cole and Jahrsdoerfer indicated that 50% of canals with a diameter less than 2 mm will develop cholesteatoma by age 20 [8, 9]. In general, high-resolution computed tomography (CT) of the temporal bone is recommended at 4–5 years of age to evaluate for cholesteatoma, if not clinically indicated by infectious symptoms and findings (otorrhea, pain, swelling, facial weakness, vertigo) before that time. Over time, surveillance scanning and close clinical evaluation are recommended into adulthood for CAS. When surgical repair of CAS is pursued, there are technical similarities between canalplasty in CAA and CAS cases, and the former is discussed in detail below. However, CAS surgery is intrinsically distinct from CAA due to the presence of residual ear canal skin, which may be sufficient to afford canalplasty without a skin graft.

History of Congenital Aural Atresia

The remainder of this chapter will focus on CAA. While atresia of the external auditory canal (EAC) had been identified in prehistoric skulls, [10] reports of surgical repair of atresia do not surface until the late 1940s and 1950s [11–17]. Nager advocated for tailoring the surgical technique to the severity of the atresia [18, 19]. For minor malformations (Group I; normal or stenotic canal with hypoplastic tympanic cleft and some malformation of the middle-ear structures), Nager described an endaural approach to widen the stenotic ear canal and address any middle ear abnormalities. For Group II malformations (fistulous tract or complete atresia of the canal with a bony atretic plate and some degree of malformation of the middle-ear structures), Nager recommended opening the mastoid antrum, aditus, and attic to expose the lateral ossicular mass, freeing the ossicular chain, and using a split-thickness skin graft to the mucoperiosteal membrane on the undersurface of the bony atretic plate. For more severe malformations (Group III; complete ear canal atresia with nonpneumatized mastoid and middle ear), he advised against surgery, or possibly a fenestration of the lateral semicircular canal [19].

Schuknecht [20] also divided congenital aural atresia (CAA) patients into three groups based on severity and reviewed three methods for surgical reconstruction: (1) fenestration of the lateral semicircular canal [12–14], (2) canalplasty [15, 16], and (3) type III tympanoplasty [11, 17]. In all of these cases, the mastoid cavity is opened to access the ossicles and middle-ear space, leaving the patient at risk for postoperative drainage and other problems associated with an open cavity.

Schuknecht later refined his classification of aural atresia and described four types: Type A was described as meatal atresia with stenosis of the fibrocartilaginous portion of the ear canal; these patients require meatoplasty or risk developing canal cholesteatoma. Type B was described as partial atresia with a stenotic ear canal (a rudimentary tympanic membrane can often be seen) and some degree of malformation of the middle ear structures; these patients require widening the canal and middle ear work, such as freeing the ossicular chain. Type C atresia was described as complete absence of the EAC with middle ear malformation; these patients require surgical creation of an ear canal and eardrum, with liberation or reconstruction of the ossicular chain. Type D atresia was described as complete absence of the EAC with poor pneumatization of the mastoid and middle ear; these patients are not candidates for canal surgery [7].

Jahrsdoerfer first described the anterior approach—avoiding opening the mastoid air cells—in 1978 [21]. This approach, the standard in modern atresia surgery, keeps the drilling anterior and superior by following the tegmen and the temporomandibular joint (TMJ) through the nonpneumatized bone of the atretic plate directly into the epitympanum and middle-ear space. The atretic bone is carefully picked away, the ossicles are freed, and temporalis fascia is used as an onlay graft with preservation of the native, now mobile, ossicular chain. Placement of a split-thickness skin graft and meatoplasty completes the procedure. With a few minor modifications, this technique is used today and continues to deliver significantly improved hearing results with fewer complications and without a mastoid cavity.

Not all patients with CAA are candidates for surgery. The introduction of high-resolution computed tomography (HRCT) of the temporal bone has allowed the otologist to better assess surgical candidacy by evaluating the aeration of the mastoid and middle ear, position of the tegmen, morphology of the ossicles, and course of the facial nerve with a high degree of accuracy. This technological development has singularly contributed to better patient selection for surgery, to more predictable surgical outcomes, and to a broadened scope of atresia surgery that includes patients with unilateral CAA [22–25].

Bellucci separated major middle-ear malformations from minor malformations, defining minor malformations as those with a normal ear canal and tympanic membrane [25]. Minor malformations include congenital stapes fixation, congenital absence of the long process of the incus, malleus bar, congenital absence of the oval window, and single stapes crus. Major malformations, discussed in this chapter, refer to aural atresia—absence of an ear canal and tympanic membrane with some degree of underdevelopment ("atresia") of the middle-ear cleft and its structures.

Surgical correction of congenital atresia is a formidable operation and demands rigorous preoperative assessment and intraoperative decision-making. The risk of facial nerve injury and sensorineural hearing loss is higher in the hands of the inexperienced surgeon. Even in the hands of the experienced otologist, stable long-term closure of the air–bone gap without canal stenosis can be difficult to achieve. However, successful surgery that achieves normal hearing with a clean, dry, well-epithelialized ear canal can be very gratifying for both the patient and otologist.

Surgery for Unilateral Versus Bilateral Atresia

For the families of children with aural atresia, education and counseling are the foundation upon which treatment decision-making is built. Patient age at the time of initial counseling is particularly important. Because aural atresia is generally less visible than the often concomitant microtia, it is common for families to focus primarily on the cosmetic treatment of the auricle. Education about the differences, timing, and implications of auricular reconstruction and atresiaplasty is often necessary. Delineation of management goals and early involvement of a plastic surgeon with experience and reliable results in auricular reconstruction are vital steps in this process. Patient discussions should broach the subjects of hearing outcomes, the use of bone conduction implants, the ultimate cosmesis of the reconstructed ear, the need for long-term follow-up related to ear cleaning and cholesteatoma surveillance, and the number of surgeries that may be needed to achieve realistic goals. Patient and family "buy-in" are critical to ensuring good follow-up and building trust.

For the otologist, a cornerstone of atresia counseling is the discussion around hearing loss and its relationship to speech development, academic performance, and quality of life. Children with aural atresia, particularly bilateral, are at high risk of speech delay and lower scholastic success [26]. Regardless of whether families choose to proceed with atresiaplasty, the importance of amplification should be emphasized at every age and stage. Hearing technology is constantly evolving, and there are myriad amplification options that are influenced by audiologic needs, patient anatomy, and family preferences.

Older literature reiterates the theme that only patients with bilateral CAA should be offered surgery [20]. The reasoning behind this philosophy was that surgery would probably not produce serviceable hearing, and the risks of facial nerve injury and sensorineural hearing loss would outweigh any potential benefit. Moreover, postoperative meatal stenosis and the failure to maintain long-term hearing were cited as arguments against operating on patients with unilateral atresia. If unilateral patients were to be operated on, it was argued, they should be operated on only when the child had reached adolescence or young adulthood and could share in the decision.

Times have changed. With refinements in preoperative imaging and surgical technique, patients with unilateral atresia may successfully undergo surgery under strict criteria. Generally, patient selection involves sorting out the high-risk (poor result) patients in whom the preoperative HRCT evaluation would indicate a low likelihood of success (defined as a postoperative speech reception threshold greater than 30 dB HL). This threshold is attainable in 75–80% of patients carefully selected for surgery.

Historically, criteria for surgical intervention (canalplasty) have been more lenient in patients with bilateral atresia in an attempt to render one ear with serviceable hearing; surgeons would operate on more marginal bilateral atresia patients. Yet, with the widespread availability, ease of surgical placement, and reliability of the osseointegrated bone conducting hearing devices, the criteria for surgery in patients with bilateral CAA should not differ from those with unilateral CAA. As in the past, poor anatomy (e.g., patients in whom there is no mastoid or middle-ear aeration, or patients in whom the course of the facial nerve places it at great risk, or patients in whom the tegmen hangs too far inferiorly, Fig. 33.1) should be avoided.

A grading system, a 10-point scale in which individual anatomic structures are given points, was developed in an effort to select those individuals who have the best chance of successful atresia surgery [22]. The system is based on a preoperative HRCT scan of the temporal bones. In addition, the appearance of the external ear prior to microtia surgery is factored in, as auricular and middle ear development are often closely correlated [4].

In our experience, to be a potential candidate, certain other criteria must be met. First, there must be audiometric evidence of normal cochlear function (normal bone conduction thresholds). Second, there must be imaging evidence of normal inner ear architecture. Since the inner ear develops embryologically from a completely separate anlage at a completely separate time from the middle and outer ear (branchial apparatus), cochlear function is typically normal in these patients. A contraindication of surgery would be a nonaerated middle ear and mastoid or a low-hanging tegmen (Fig. 33.1). If the middle ear is not aerated, we do not recommend surgery. Lack of aeration may be temporary, such as middle-ear fluid, or it may be permanent, as may be seen when the middle ear is filled with primitive mesenchymal tissue of a fibrous gelatinous nature. This tissue is found in patients with absent or poor Eustachian tube function, in whom air has never reached the middle ear or mastoid. Repeat CT scanning (generally in 1 or 2 years) may help sort out temporary fluid versus more permanent primitive mesenchymal tissue; if this soft-tissue density persists for 2 years or more, surgery is not generally recommended. Otitis media with effusion will generally clear within 1 year, revealing a well-ventilated middle ear and mastoid on subsequent HRCT scan.

We still employ the Jahrsdoerfer grading scale (Table 33.1) to assess candidacy for surgery. The stapes is assigned two points as this is the most important ossicle on which the success of the operation hinges. In approximately 4% of patients, the stapes will be fixed, and there is no way to diagnose this finding preoperatively. A fixed stapes requires that the operation be aborted or staged. If aborted, the ear is simply closed without placing the fascia or skin grafts. If staged, the first stage includes the usual atresia repair with canalplasty, tympanoplasty, split-thickness skin grafting, and meatoplasty; the second stage requires that the stapes be mobilized or a stapedectomy/stapedotomy be performed with ossicular chain reconstruction. The decision is generally made intraoperatively in consultation with the family by telephone. Anecdotally, most families in our experience have chosen to abort the operation rather than risk postoperative problems such as meatal/canal stenosis or a draining ear.

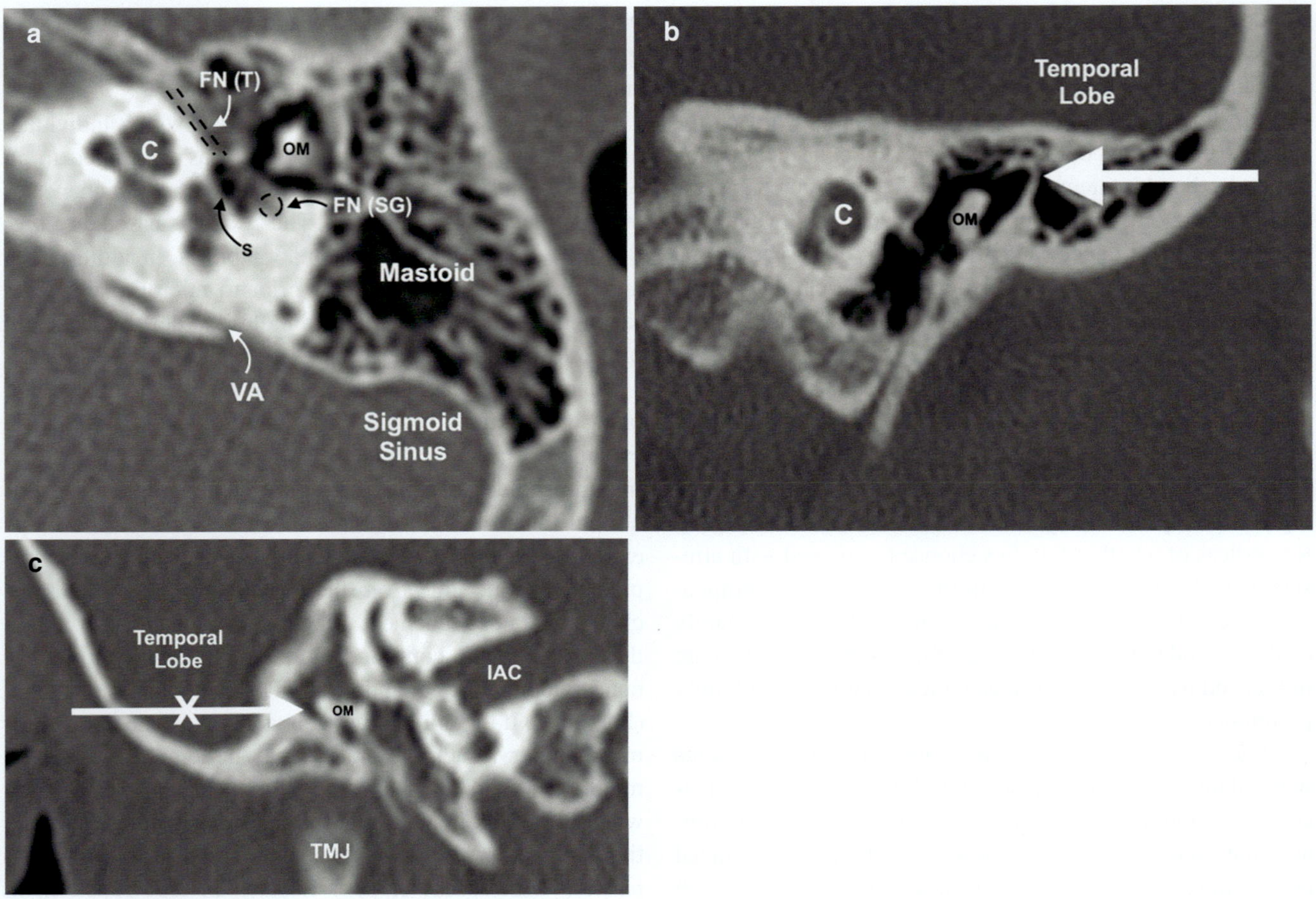

Fig. 33.1 (**a**) Axial computed tomography (CT) image of a patient with left aural atresia and favorable anatomy. The facial nerve is in a favorable location, and the mastoid and middle ear are well aerated. The ossicular mass is in continuity with the stapes. (**b**) Coronal CT of a patient with left aural atresia showing a favorable location of the tegmen in relation to the ossicular mass. The white arrow indicates the drilling corridor, which brings the surgeon into the epitympanum. (**c**) Coronal CT of a patient with right aural atresia shows a very low tegmen that completely obstructs the surgeon's path to the ossicular mass as denoted by the arrow with X through it. The middle ear space is small, constricted, and opacified. This patient is not a surgical candidate for atresiaplasty. Abbreviations: C cochlea, IAC internal auditory canal, OM ossicular mass, TMJ temporomandibular joint, FN(T) facial nerve (tympanic segment), FN(SG) facial nerve (second genu), S stapes, VA vestibular aqueduct

Table 33.1 Grading system of candidacy for surgery of congenital aural atresia from Jahrsdoerfer et al. [22]

Parameter	Points
Stapes present	2
Oval window open	1
Middle ear space	1
Facial nerve	1
Malleus/incus complex	1
Mastoid pneumatized	1
Incus-stapes connection	1
Round window	1
Appearance external ear	1
Total available points	10

Most of our patients who are candidates for surgery will be graded 7 to 8 out of 10. These scores generally translate to a reasonable chance of achieving normal or near-normal hearing (speech reception threshold ≤30 dB HL) through surgery [27]. Specifically, in their initial validation study, the creators of the grading system reported outcomes including a speech reception threshold (SRT) of <30 dB in 89.2% of those scoring ≥8/10, 72.4% for a score of 7/10, 41.1% for a score of 6/10, and 0% for a score of 5/10. It has since been suggested that patients with high scores and favorable locations of the facial nerve and temporal lobe should be considered surgical candidates. Those with scores of 6/10 have been considered to be marginal candidates, and those scoring ≤5/10 have not been considered as candidates [22].

Other Options for Atresia

As suggested above, it is important for the otologist and family to acknowledge that other options for hearing rehabilitation are available. For bilateral atresia patients, a long-term bone-conducting hearing device (such as the BAHA Softband®, Cochlear Corp., Englewood, CO) may be used, and most patients with this device develop excellent speech [28]. In general, consideration should be given to placement of a nonsurgical bone conduction hearing device such as the softband Baha®, SoundArc™ (both made by Cochlear Corp., Englewood, CO), or ADHEAR (MED-EL, Innsbruck, Austria), even within 3–6 months of life, [1] while the child awaits atresiaplasty or definitive placement of an osseointegrated bone conduction hearing device (OIBCD). An OIBCD is an excellent means of rehabilitating hearing in patients who are not candidates for atresia surgery or patients in whom atresia surgery has not significantly improved air conduction thresholds [29–33]. Both percutaneous ((BAHA System®, Cochlear Corp).; Ponto System®, Oticon Corp., Somerset, NJ) and transcutaneous (MED-EL Bonebridge®, Cochlear Osia®, and Oticon Sentio® devices exist. The newest generation of transcutaneous bone conduction devices is fully implanted under the skin but also has a significantly larger footprint than percutaneous abutments. Also, while these devices offer the benefit of hearing rehabilitation without a percutaneous abutment, they are generally MRI conditional. As it relates to the latter, care should be taken to understand the future need for MRI in a recipient due to the magnetic artifact that compromises visualization of the ipsilateral head. Regardless of patient age, the surgeon must be assured that there is sufficient bone stock for placement of an implantable device and that the device will not interfere with auricular reconstruction [34].

Deciding between atresiaplasty and bone conduction implant placement can be a complicated endeavor. On one hand, the bone conduction device intrinsically requires the use of an outwardly visible component, which could be stigmatizing, while atresiaplasty carries the possibility of hearing without amplification. For patients who have undergone atresia surgery but did not gain enough hearing to support language development or success in school, a conventional hearing aid utilizing the newly epithelialized canal may be sufficient. That being said, some evidence suggests that the audiologic outcomes after placement of a bone conduction hearing device are superior to atresiaplasty. In a meta-analysis by Nadaraja et al. examining 107 studies, postoperative SRT, PTA, and ABG were all significantly better for bone conduction devices [35]. When investigating individual devices, similarly good results were demonstrated [36, 37]. Additionally, a single-stage bone conduction device was significantly cheaper than uncomplicated atresiaplasty, not taking into account the likely need for hearing aid, complications, or missed work/school [35, 38]. However, as discussed further below, bone conduction devices may not improve sound localization, whereas atresiaplasty has been shown to improve this measure predominantly with ipsilesional stimuli [39]. As noted above, counseling should include all viable options so that patients and families can make an informed decision.

Options for Repair of Microtia

While patients with Grade I microtia (Fig. 33.2) do not require extensive reconstructive surgery, most patients with Grade III microtia and their families do elect to undergo reconstructive surgery. Fewer families choose to undergo reconstruction for Grade II microtia.

Repair of Grade II microtia (Fig. 33.3) depends on the development of the auricle, the experience, judgment, and technical expertise of the reconstructive surgeon, and, of course, the desires and expectations of the patient and their family. In some patients with Grade II microtia, the auricular cartilage is not salvageable, and the reconstructive surgeon must "start from scratch" and harvest autologous rib carti-

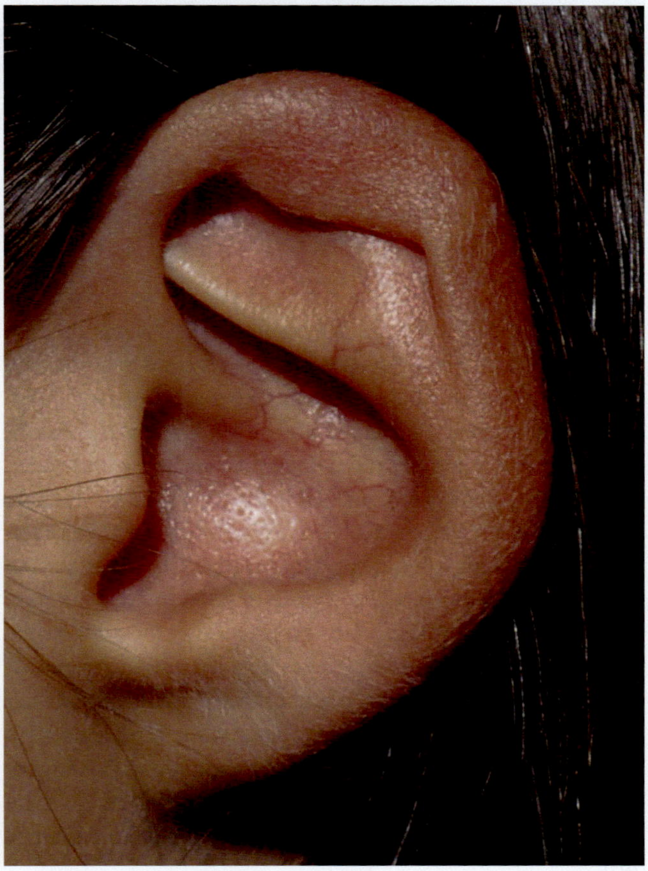

Fig. 33.2 Grade I microtia (left). The appearance of the ear is fairly well-formed but smaller. (Courtesy of Burt Brent, MD)

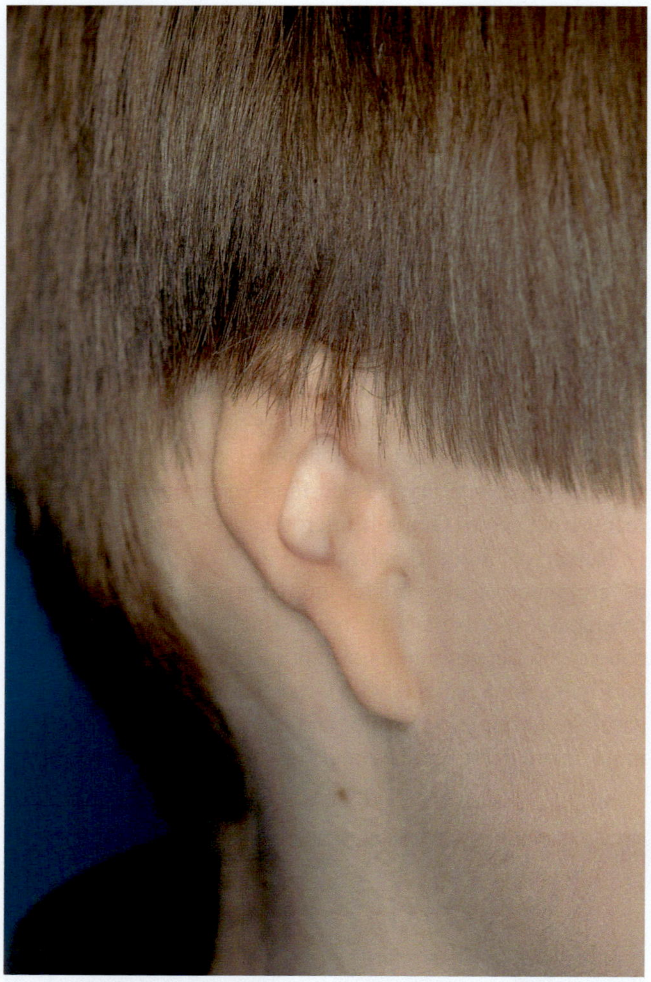

Fig. 33.3 Grade II microtia (right). The external ear remnant is about one-half of normal size and has some form. Some of the cartilaginous detail is missing. (Courtesy of Stephen S. Park, MD)

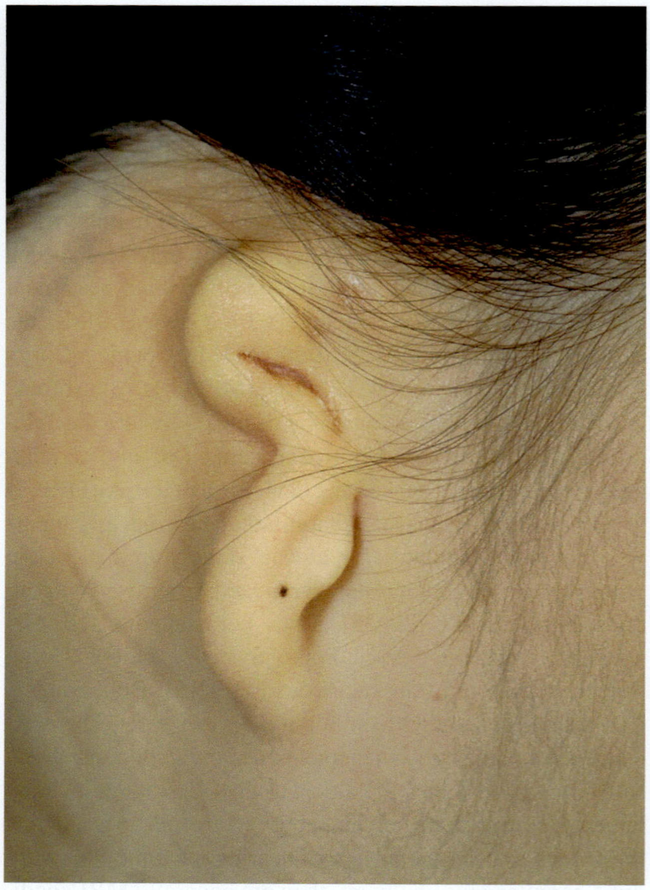

Fig. 33.4 Grade III microtia (right). Note the poorly formed ear remnant on the lateral face. Cartilage may or may not be present. (Courtesy of Stephen S. Park, MD)

lage (see below) or build a porous polyethylene implant (e.g., Medpor®, Stryker Corp., Kalamazoo, MI) to replace the cartilage remnant. It is the experience, skill, and judgment of the reconstructive surgeon as to whether the postoperative ear will be improved compared to the unoperated ear.

Options for repair of Grade III microtia (Fig. 33.4) include an auricular prosthesis that can be affixed with medical-grade tape or adhesive glue or with surgically placed titanium osseointegrated posts [32], a porous polyethylene implant (Medpor®), and autologous rib cartilage. Prostheses have the advantage of minimal morbidity with very lifelike cosmesis. Prosthetic ears have been a popular, if not preferred, method in failed surgical autogenous reconstructions, patients with severe soft-tissue/skeletal hypoplasia, patients with a low or unfavorable hairline, or patients with a total or subtotal auricular defect secondary to either trauma or malignancy [40].

Medpor® has gained considerable popularity for Grade III microtia repair over the last several years. In the hands of the experienced reconstructive surgeon, this method of microtia repair also achieves excellent cosmetic results [41, 42], and some groups advocate for early atresiaplasty with subsequent Medpor® reconstruction to facilitate critical language development [43, 44]. The procedure involves creating a template with the Medpor® implant to match the contralateral ear. A subcutaneous pocket is created at the appropriate position inferiorly for the implant. A large temporoparietal fascia (TPF) flap is elevated and delivered down over the implant. Suction is used to hold the flap to the implant. Skin grafts are used to cover the superior and posterior aspects of the implant. In the hands of the experienced surgeon, the Medpor® microtia repair affords excellent projection and definition of the auricle. Complications include fracture of the framework, framework exposure, loss of the TPF flap, and injury to the frontal branch of the facial nerve.

Microtia repair using autologous rib cartilage is a challenging series of operations that few have mastered. The first stage involves harvesting autologous rib (usually the costal cartilage of the seventh and eighth ribs, with a margin of the sixth rib cartilage) and sculpting the cartilage into the auricular framework [45, 46]. The sculpted cartilage is placed in a subcutaneous pocket at the correct location and correct orientation on the lateral skull. Small suction drains are necessary to ensure that the thin subcutaneous skin sticks down to the cartilage. Lobule transposition follows approximately 3 months later, where the soft tissue auricular remnant is translocated to the lobule position. The framework is next elevated off the lateral skull, and a relatively thick split-thickness or full-thickness skin graft is placed to create the postauricular sulcus in the third stage. Atresia repair can follow the third or fourth (and occasionally the second) stages. The tragus is created in the fourth stage.

A distinct advantage of rib graft microtia repair is that the cartilage is autologous tissue, and there is no concern for rejection. The cartilage and subcutaneous tissue also gain a robust blood supply, so there is little concern for exposure, infection, or extrusion for the atresia surgeon. In fact, the atresia surgeon must carve and remove a portion of the cartilage to ensure a wide meatus. The rib graft microtia repair has been criticized for lack of framework definition and poor projection, but in the hands of the experienced microtia surgeon, these risks are low [45–48].

Who Should Operate First?

Close communication between the reconstructive surgeon and otologist is critical to optimize the results of both surgeries [49]. Most patients with Grade I microtia do not require reconstructive surgery because this ear can rarely be improved cosmetically. As such, atresia surgery may proceed without any reconstructive work on the auricle (see Fig. 33.2).

A well-developed Grade II microtia may also not need auricular work, and atresia surgery can proceed first (see Fig. 33.3). A more poorly developed Grade II microtia is a judgment call by the reconstructive surgeon, who must decide if their skills may improve the appearance of the external ear. If auricular reconstruction is recommended, the same rules for Grade III microtia (see below) apply.

For patients with Grade III microtia, in which the external ear remnant is little more than a nub of skin or a small piece of cartilage, the reconstructive surgeon using autologous rib graft must go first (see Fig. 33.4). It is imperative that the reconstructive surgeon have a virgin field in which to place the sculpted rib cartilage; it is far easier for the reconstructive surgeon to build an ear in the absence of scar tissue and a compromised vascular bed than it is to build an ear around a hole in the side of the head. The otologic surgeon, however, drills the bony canal in the same location for every patient (see below); the reconstructed auricle may be safely moved and positioned to align with the bony canal. In fact, in approximately 50% of patients, the reconstructed auricle must be moved (usually in a posterosuperior direction) so that the meatus in the reconstructed auricle aligns with the newly created bony canal.

Atresia surgery following microtia repair with the Medpor® implant can result in exposure of the implant, infection, and even extrusion. The polyethylene implant does not acquire its own vascular supply and, therefore, if exposed during atresia surgery, will not heal or re-epithelialize. Atresia repair must be undertaken before Medpor® microtia repair. This sequence avoids the risk of exposure/extrusion of the polyethylene implant and allows the Medpor® surgeon to reconstruct the new auricle around the newly created bony canal. At the time of atresia surgery, the ear canal skin graft is simply sutured to the patient's native skin where the bony canal exits. Short-term results in patients undergoing atresia surgery *prior* to Medpor® microtia repair show comparable results to patients undergoing atresia surgery *after* rib graft microtia repair [43]. Despite this short-term success, there is concern regarding the fate of the implant if the patient undergoing Medpor® microtia repair following atresia repair needs a revision atresia operation (as many as 25–30% of atresia surgery patients will need revision surgery) [50].

Timing of Microtia and Atresia Repair

For the child with bilateral atresia, it is imperative that the hearing be tested and followed using bone conduction auditory brainstem response (ABR) testing to ensure normal cochlear function. As noted above, it is also critical that a bone-conducting hearing device be placed as soon as possible after birth so that the child will develop receptive and expressive language skills. For the child with unilateral CAA, while normal hearing in one ear is sufficient for the development of normal speech and language skills, it is becoming increasingly clear that children with unilateral hearing loss do have more subtle difficulties [51, 52]. A bone conducting hearing device for these patients can also be trialed after ensuring normal cochlear function in the atretic ear. Hearing should be followed for these children at regular intervals, usually twice/year for the first 2–3 years, then annually if the hearing remains stable.

External ear reconstruction is usually delayed until the child is about 6–7 years of age, with atresia repair following the series of operations required for rib graft microtia repair. This delay allows for growth of the rib cage, enabling sufficient costal cartilage to be harvested for sculpting the auricle. A child who is large for their age may be operated on earlier. For the child with Grade I or II microtia that does not require reconstructive external ear surgery, atresia surgery can be performed at the age of 5 if the child is cooperative. Waiting until the child is 6 or 7 allows the child to achieve a level of maturity and cooperation absolutely critical for the postoperative dressing changes, packing removal, and ear canal cleaning to ensure a good result. A potentially poor result can be salvaged postoperatively in the office but requires the cooperation of the patient.

While reconstructive surgeons using the Medpor® implant have implanted children as young as 3, we do not advocate atresia repair at that age because the child is simply too young to cooperate with the necessary postoperative packing removal and ear canal debridement. In addition, the authors feel that younger children may have a higher prevalence of Eustachian tube dysfunction or otitis media with effusion, which would jeopardize an otherwise technically successful operation. Finally, younger children may also have a higher rate of meatal or canal stenosis necessitating revision surgery. The younger child certainly is not bothered psychologically by the ear deformity and is not yet in school, where other children could tease them.

In cases of aural atresia with confirmed or suspected cholesteatoma, as in Fig. 33.5, surgical treatment of the cholesteatoma takes precedence regardless of the status of the auricle. Cholesteatoma may be present in 6.3–48% of patients with aural atresia, and any infectious symptoms or otalgia in such a patient warrants CT scan regardless of age [1, 6, 8, 53]. If the CT is suspicious for cholesteatoma, MRI with diffusion weighted imaging should be considered to confirm the need for operative intervention. Postoperative cholesteatoma formation should also be a consideration, oftentimes as a complication occurring years after the atresia and/or microtia repair.

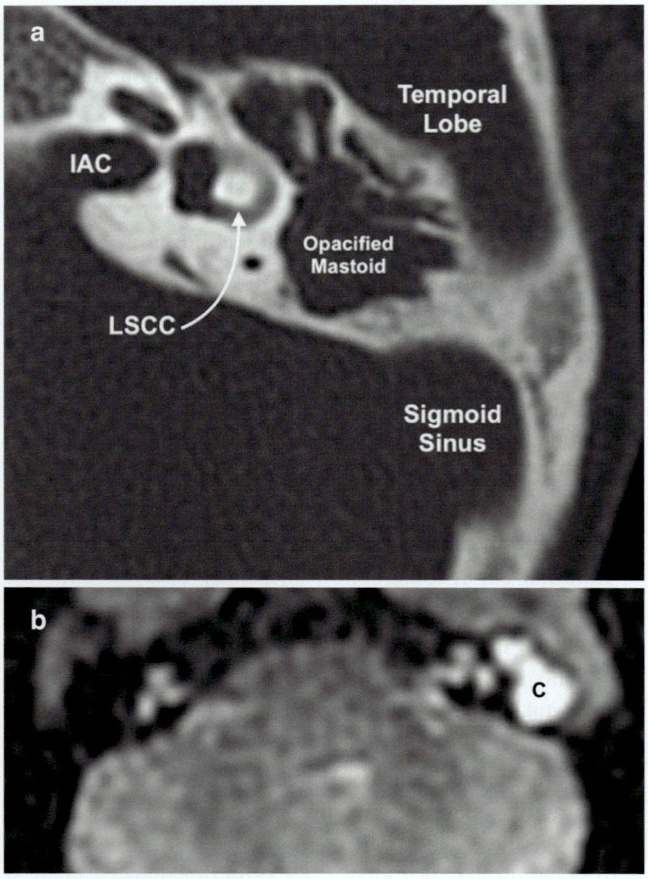

Fig. 33.5 This is a patient with left aural atresia and extensive cholesteatoma. (**a**) The middle ear and mastoid are opacified on CT scan, and this corresponds to a large area of restricted diffusion on non-echo planar diffusion weighted imaging (**b**). Abbreviations: C cholesteatoma, IAC internal auditory canal, LSCC lateral semicircular canal

Surgical Technique

Patient Preparation

The patient is placed in the supine position with the operated ear turned away. The arm on the ipsilateral side of the operated ear (split-thickness skin graft donor arm) is tucked loosely so that, in the middle of the case, the arm can be removed from under the drapes and placed on an arm board for skin grafting. No blood pressure cuff is placed on the donor arm. A half-inch swath of hair is shaved around the ear. One percent lidocaine with 1:40,000 epinephrine is injected in the postauricular area. The ear is prepped and draped in standard fashion.

Although the surgery takes 3–5 hours, urethral catheterization is not always employed, and the anesthesiologist adjusts fluid volume accordingly. A short-acting paralytic may be used for the induction of anesthesia and intubation, but no paralytic may be administered during the operation as facial nerve monitoring is mandatory for all atresia operations. The anesthesiologist is requested not to use nitrous oxide as this gas diffuses into the middle ear and can cause increased positive pressure, ballooning the fascia graft away from the ossicles.

Some surgeons find intraoperative navigation to be a useful adjunct in planning the location of the new external auditory canal and for confirming the location of the ossicular mass without surface landmarks, but this step is not necessary for surgical success [54, 55].

Incision and Drilling

A postauricular incision is made and carried down to the temporalis fascia. A quarter-sized piece of fascia is harvested, scraped, and placed on the back table to dehydrate. Mastoid periosteal incisions are made along the linea temporalis and perpendicular anteriorly, along the glenoid fossa, down toward the mastoid tip. This anterior mastoid incision allows a cuff of periosteum to remain at the glenoid fossa to which a tragal skin flap will be sutured at the end of the case to create the anterior canal wall. The mastoid periosteum is elevated and retracted posteriorly; the auricle is retracted anteriorly.

If the atresia surgery precedes the microtia repair, the incision is made just posterior to the auricular remnant and down to the mastoid tip. The meatus can be incorporated into

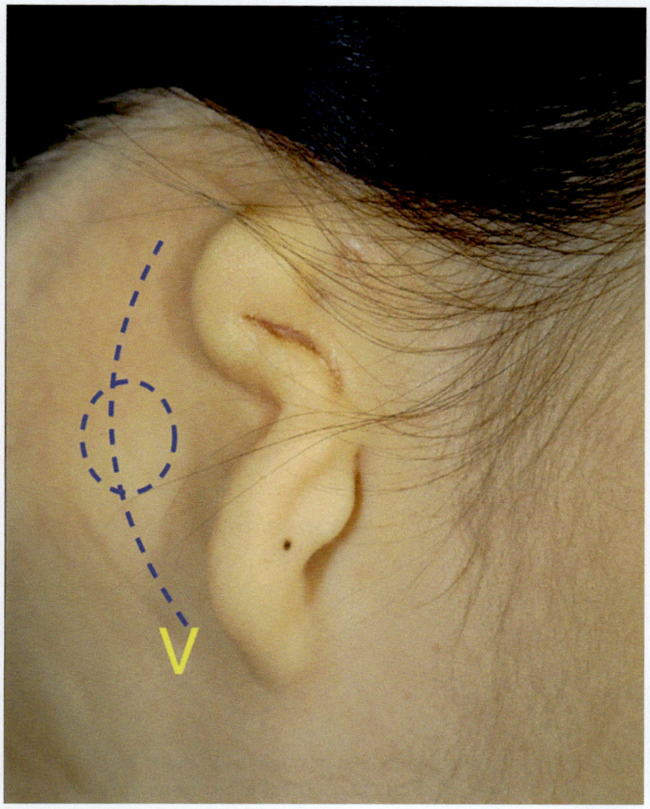

Fig. 33.6 Preoperative canalplasty picture of right Grade III microtia repair prior to Medpor® microtia reconstruction. Incision is marked out (blue dashed line) with the mastoid tip (yellow "V") and the future site of the canal (blue dashed circle) designated

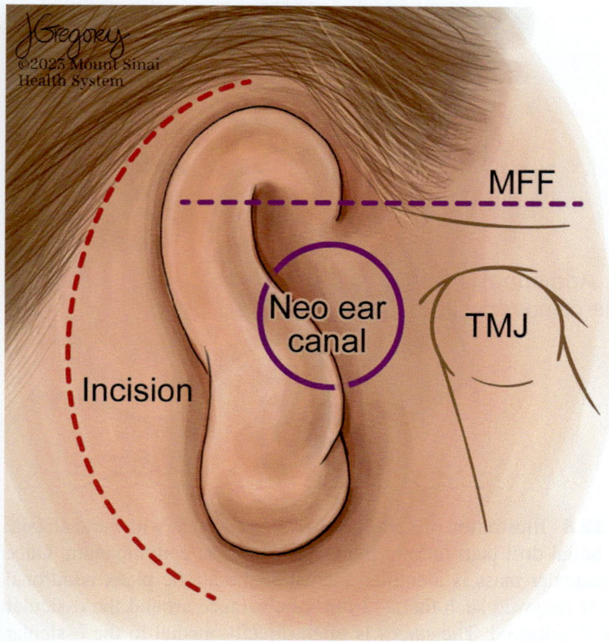

Fig. 33.7 This illustration demonstrates an anticipated incision for a patient with right atresia/microtia. In this case, the meatoplasty is conceptually planned in association with the auricular remnant, as distinct from the different technique that is shown in Fig. 33.6. The neocanal will be drilled using the middle fossa floor (tegmen) and temporomandibular joint as boundaries. Abbreviations: MFF middle fossa floor, TMJ temporomandibular joint. (Printed with permission from ©Mount Sinai Health System)

the postauricular incision at the end of the operation (Fig. 33.6). An alternative option is to plan the meatoplasty in a distinct location from the incision (Fig. 33.7). Elevation of the mastoid periosteum proceeds farther anteriorly to identify the glenoid fossa. It is critical to identify the fossa because it is an important landmark for drilling. Occasionally, there will be a dimple on the surface of the mastoid cortex to identify the site of drilling; it is important to carry the periosteal elevation anterior to this dimple to identify positively the glenoid fossa. The cribriform area is often present as a reliable surface landmark.

Using the mastoid tip, temporal line, and glenoid fossa as surface landmarks, drilling begins with a 5 mm cutting burr with continuous suction irrigation, with care taken to stay anterior and superior. The tegmen is identified superiorly and followed medially. This anterosuperior approach should hug the tegmen superiorly and the glenoid fossa anteriorly. Care is taken to avoid the mastoid antrum and to open as few mastoid air cells as possible to prevent a large cavity and the risk of postoperative infection or mucosalization of the skin graft (Fig. 33.8). As the drilling proceeds medially, dense, nonpneumatized atretic bone is encountered. This bone is carefully drilled away with progressively smaller diamond burrs, starting with a 3 mm burr. As the dissection stays superior, the goal is to enter the middle-ear cleft in the epitympanum, superior to the ossicles. This approach also avoids an aberrant facial nerve, which is common in these cases (Fig. 33.9).

At a depth of about 1.5 cm, the air space of the epitympanic middle ear is encountered, and the fused malleus–incus complex can be identified just inferiorly. The first landmark the surgeon encounters is usually the body of the incus; this can be confirmed by gentle palpation to assess mobility. The ossicular chain is typically fixed to the atretic plate medially and inferiorly at the level of the malleus neck (Fig. 33.10). With a bit more bone removal, the fused head of the malleus and body of incus are identified (Fig. 33.11).

Drilling continues on the atretic plate—with 3- and 2-mm diamond drill burrs with slow rotation—until the bone reaches eggshell thickness. The atretic bone overlying the middle ear and ossicles is carefully picked away with a Rosen needle or small dental excavator. Sharp dissection is often needed to lyse the periosteal attachments of the malleus to the underside of the atretic plate. There may also be a band of soft tissue, mostly periosteum, that courses through a bony defect in the wall separating the atretic plate from the TMJ; this band may be confused with the facial nerve. The facial nerve is most likely encountered while drilling posteriorly and inferiorly. In approximately 25% of patients, the facial nerve has a short vertical segment (sometimes nonex-

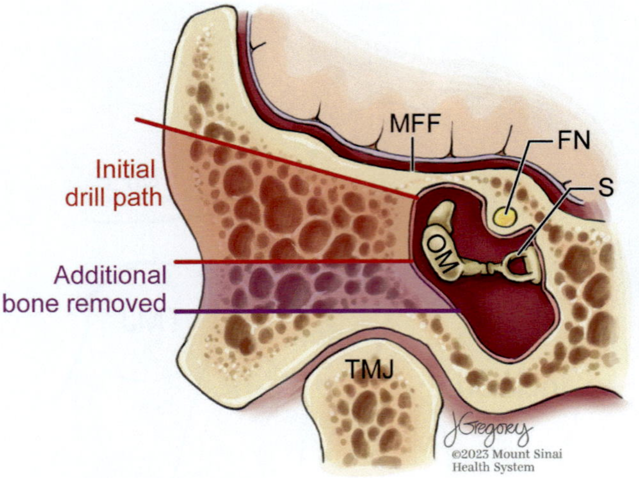

Fig. 33.8 Illustration of a coronal view of a right ear with aural atresia. The initial drill path follows the tegmen into the epitympanum. Once the ossicular mass is identified medial to the atretic plate, additional bone is removed such that 1–2 mm of clearance around the ossicular mass is achieved. The stapes is often directly medial to the ossicular mass as shown. (This image was drawn by Jill Gregory and was adapted from Kesser BW and Goddard JC, ed. by DE Brackmann, C Shelton, MA Arriaga, R Gurgel, (Elsevier, Amsterdam, Netherlands, 2022), p. 43–61. Abbreviations: FN facial nerve, MFF middle fossa floor, OM ossicular mass, S stapes, TMJ temporomandibular joint. Printed with permission from ©Mount Sinai Health System)

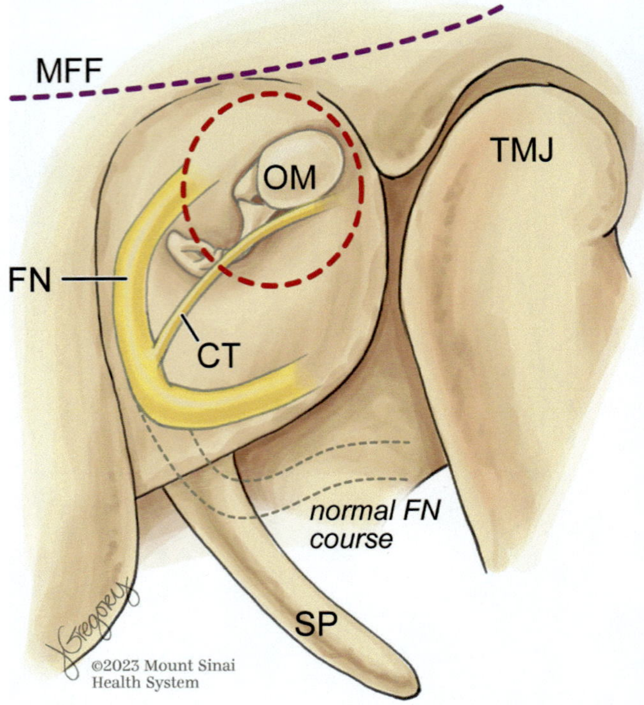

Fig. 33.9 Typical anatomic relationships in an atretic ear. The facial nerve may be quite close to the neocanal in its posteroinferior aspect and takes a much more acute, anterior turn than in patients with normal temporal bones. (This image was drawn by Jill Gregory and was adapted from Kesser BW and Goddard JC, ed. by DE Brackmann, C Shelton, MA Arriaga, R Gurgel, (Elsevier, Amsterdam, Netherlands, 2022), p. 43–61. Abbreviations: CT chorda tympani, GG geniculate ganglion, FN facial nerve, OM ossicular mass, MFF middle fossa floor, MP mastoid process, SP styloid process, TMJ temporomandibular joint. Printed with permission from ©Mount Sinai Health System)

istent). Instead, the nerve makes a sharp curve anteriorly at the second genu (Fig. 33.8). The facial nerve is most vulnerable to injury in this location [56]. Thin blood vessels coursing over the surface of the nerve seen through the thinned bone are a good clue to the location of the nerve. As mentioned, facial nerve monitoring is a necessity.

Once the atretic plate is removed, the ossicles are carefully assessed. Bone is removed 360° around the ossicular chain to maximize mobility. The incus and malleus are almost always fused, although there may be some early demarcation of an incudomalleal joint. The manubrium of the malleus is often absent (Fig. 33.11), and the neck of the malleus is usually in firm bony union with the undersurface of the atretic plate. Care must be exercised in removing the overlying fragments of bone so as not to sublux the ossicles or impart vibratory trauma to the inner ear. Bone around the fossa incudis is kept intact, and the anterior soft-tissue attachments between the malleus and anterior mesotympanic bone are also maintained to lend support to the ossicular chain. The last ligamentous attachments of the malleus to the atretic bone are incised with a #59 beaver blade or lysed with the laser.

The shape and direction of the long arm of the incus are highly variable. What is important is that the incus attaches to a stapes. The stapes superstructure may also be anomalous. In more extreme malformations, the superstructure may be monopedal with no connection to the incus. The mobility of the footplate must be determined. Congenital

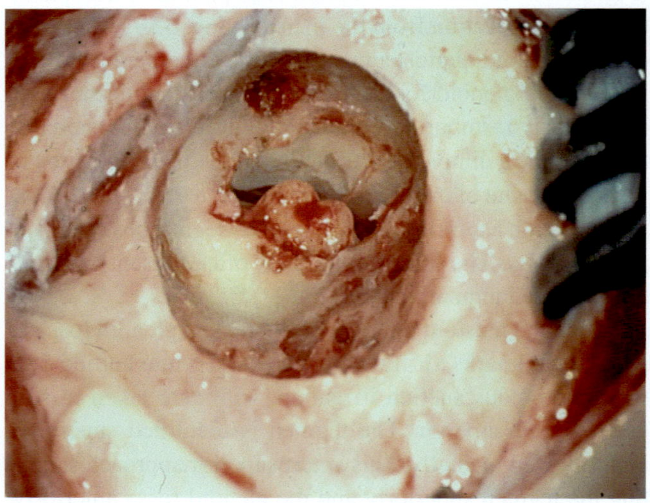

Fig. 33.10 "Buttock sign"—fused head of the malleus and body of incus as the atretic bone is removed and the epitympanum is opened (left ear)

fixation of the stapes is found in 4% of patients. It is most common in CAA to find a reasonably well-formed stapes

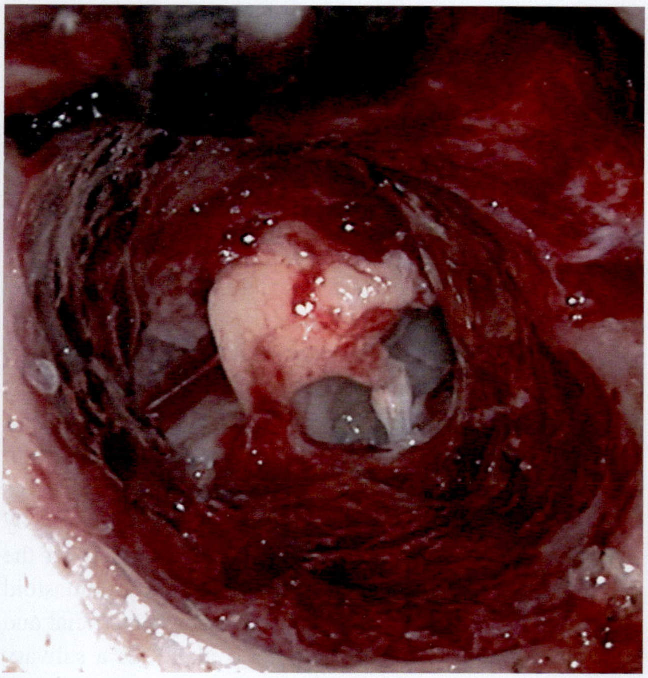

Fig. 33.11 Appearance of a typical ossicular chain after removal of all atretic bone. Note the absent malleus handle and fused malleus–incus complex (right ear). The stapes bone and the facial nerve can also be seen medial to the ossicular mass

with a mobile footplate. The oval window, in concert with the stapes footplate, may be smaller than normal, but this does not adversely affect either the reconstruction or the postoperative hearing result.

In the patient with incudostapedial joint discontinuity, the lateral ossicular mass is removed, and the ossicular chain is reconstructed with a notched partial ossicular replacement prosthesis (PORP). We have found this reconstruction to deliver superior hearing results compared to any other configuration [57].

Fascia Grafting

Prior to placing the fascia graft, the anesthesiologist is instructed to lower the expired oxygen to less than 25%. The room air fraction of inspired oxygen (21% FIO_2) is best. Lowering the expired oxygen (by lowering the inspired oxygen) reduces air diffusion into the middle ear and ballooning of the graft.

Bone must be drilled peripherally, away from the ossicular chain, to create as much room as possible for the fascia graft. In addition, the malleus-incus complex should be centered with regard to the canal and new tympanic membrane. The fascia is trimmed to size (about 1.5 cm in diameter) and placed in an overlay fashion directly onto the ossicular mass. The fascia graft should contact as much of the surface area of the malleus-incus complex as possible—the fascia graft is tucked around the ossicular chain to prevent lateralization.

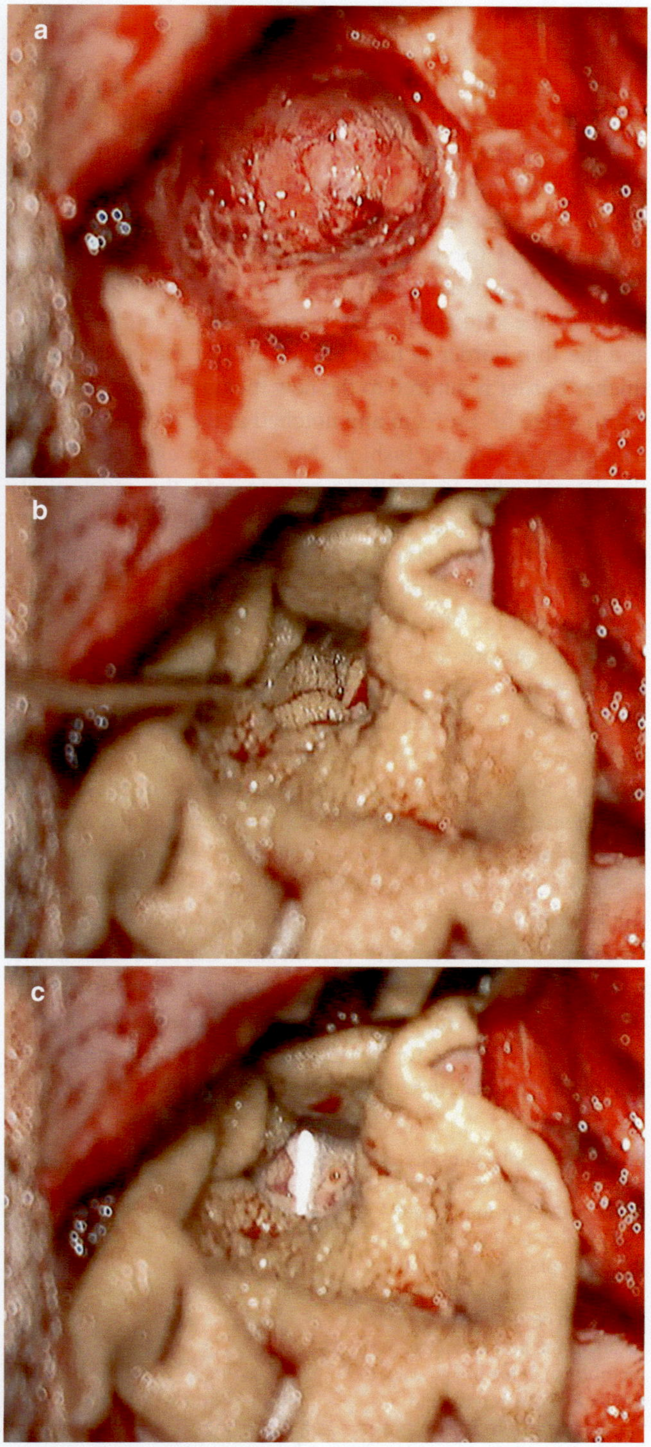

Fig. 33.12 (**a**) Thin temporalis fascia placed in an overlay fashion with approximately 1–2 mm of fascia draped up onto the canal wall. (**b**) Placement of a skin graft into the ear canal. (**c**) Placement of a Silastic® graft against the squamous epithelium that will make up the tympanic membrane

The edges of the fascia are reflected up onto the canal wall 1–2 mm in all directions (Fig. 33.12). The new eardrum will be about 1–1.5 times the diameter of a normal tympanic membrane. If large air cells have been opened, pieces of temporalis muscle are used to plug the air cells.

Skin Grafting

A split-thickness skin graft using the 2-inch dermatome blade and measuring between 0.006 and 0.015 inches is harvested from the medial aspect of the ipsilateral upper arm, contralateral upper arm, or ipsilateral thigh. A thicker graft may lead to the skin graft curling and difficult placement. Too thin, and the graft does not withstand environmental pressures (e.g., water) and can slough.

When the skin graft is harvested, the edges are freshened, and the thin border is used at the level of the eardrum; the thicker border is sutured to the new meatus. The skin graft is cut to a size of 4 × 5 cm and notched at the medial edge in a triangular or circular fashion. Notches can also be made in the lateral edge to facilitate sewing into the meatoplasty (Fig. 33.13). The graft is carefully placed down into the canal, and the notched edges are aligned over the temporalis fascia so that the entire fascia graft is covered by squamous epithelium (Fig. 33.14). The vertical slit faces anteriorly; this placement ensures that free edges will not grow into the mastoid air cells.

The key to a successful hearing result is a thin tympanic membrane and skin graft. Silastic® of 0.04 inch thickness is cut into a circular disk and placed over the new tympanic membrane to hold the notched skin edges in place and prevent blunting. The Silastic® disk also gives the surgeon something to pack against and helps prevent displacement of the skin graft.

Four to five Merocel® (Medtronic Corp., Jacksonville, FL) wicks are trimmed to 3/4 length and placed down into the ear canal onto the Silastic® disk (Fig. 33.15). The medial ear canal is packed to the level of the bony opening. The wicks are hydrated with an ototopical antibiotic solution (ofloxacin). The lateral skin graft is then folded over the hydrated wicks as the wicks hold the medial skin graft against the bony canal from which it will take its blood supply.

Meatoplasty

A hastily performed meatoplasty can ruin an otherwise flawless operation by facilitating meatal stenosis. Even a carefully constructed meatus can stenose, but if crafted with care, the risk is lower. The first priority is to ensure that the meatus and auricle align with the bony canal. The bony canal cannot move; the auricle needs repositioning to align the meatus to the bony canal in about half of patients, usually in a posterosuperior orientation. The ear can be elevated superiorly by sharply releasing the skin and subcutaneous tissue over the parotid fascia anteriorly and over the sternocleidomastoid muscle inferiorly. Care must be taken to stay superficial and not enter the substance of the parotid gland, as a salivary fistula can be created [58]. The auricle can be moved posteriorly by excising a strip of skin from the postauricular incision and suturing the auricle to the new postauricular skin edge.

One surgical technique involves making a conchal skin flap based anteriorly at the tragus. This flap is created by making a U-shaped incision in the skin of the reconstructed auricle's conchal bowl. The incision starts at the superior aspect of the tragus, extends into the skin of the concha posteriorly and curves around to the inferior aspect of the tragus. The skin is sharply elevated off the underlying cartilage and is hinged anteriorly at the tragus. The conchal skin flap is thinned and reflected anteriorly, and the underlying cartilage

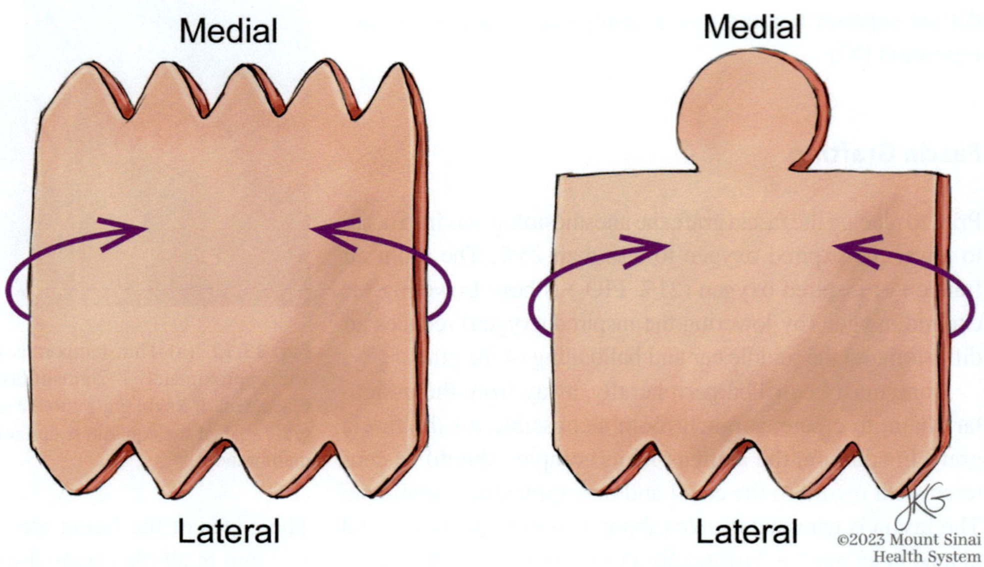

Fig. 33.13 Split-thickness skin graft with medial and lateral tabs. The four lateral tabs can be sewn into skin of the meatoplasty, and medially, triangular tabs or a circular notch can be used to cover the fascia of the new tympanic membrane. (This image was drawn by Jill Gregory and was adapted from Kesser BW and Goddard JC, ed. by DE Brackmann, C Shelton, MA Arriaga, R Gurgel, (Elsevier, Amsterdam, Netherlands, 2022), p. 43–61. Printed with permission from ©Mount Sinai Health System)

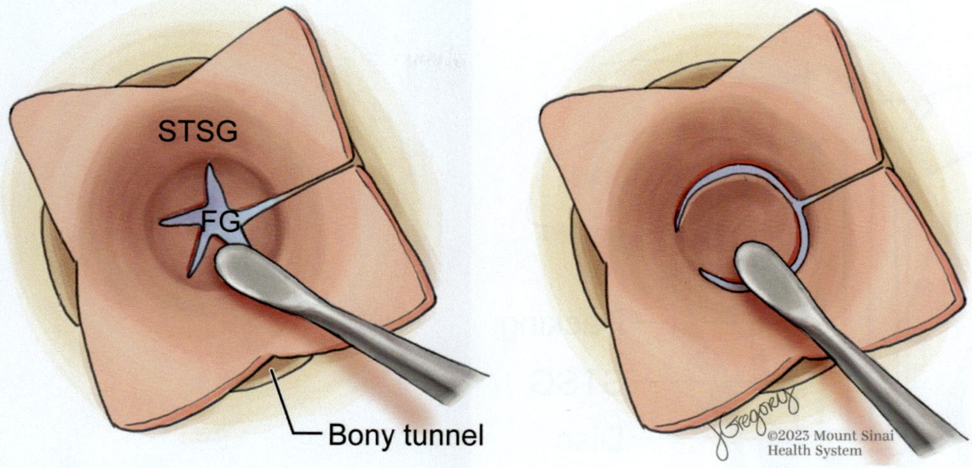

Fig. 33.14 The split-thickness skin graft is applied such that there is significant overlap with the fascia graft. The skin graft is unfurled using a duckbill elevator. The four triangular tabs will be sewn into the skin of the meatoplasty. (This image was drawn by Jill Gregory and was adapted from Kesser BW and Goddard JC, ed. by DE Brackmann, C Shelton, MA Arriaga, R Gurgel, (Elsevier, Amsterdam, Netherlands, 2022), p. 43–61. Abbreviations: FG fascia graft, STSG split-thickness skin graft. Printed with permission from ©Mount Sinai Health System)

and soft tissue are cored out with a #11 blade. The skin flap is then brought through the new meatus medially and down to the cuff of TMJ periosteum that was created at the beginning of the operation with the mastoid periosteal incisions. The conchal skin flap is sutured to this cuff of tissue with 2–3 buried 4-0 undyed Vicryl sutures to create the lateral anterior canal wall. The postauricular incision is tacked down with interrupted 3-0 undyed Vicryl sutures, and the skin graft is delivered through the meatus and sutured to the patient's native skin at the edge of the conchal bowl superiorly, posteriorly, and inferiorly (the conchal skin flap is the anterior lateral canal wall) with interrupted 5-0 fast-absorbing gut sutures. The lateral canal is packed with full-length Merocel® wicks hydrated with ofloxacin solution. After closure of the postauricular incision, a mastoid dressing is applied.

In patients having CAA repair prior to Medpor® microtia repair, the lateral skin graft is delivered through the meatus and sutured to the native skin in the postauricular area. The postauricular incision is closed around the newly created meatus (Fig. 33.16). Occasionally, anterior skin and/or cartilage is removed to ensure the meatus aligns with the bony canal. The lateral canal is packed with full ¾ length Merocel® wicks hydrated with ofloxacin solution.

Another surgical technique involves marking an "X" over the location of the neocanal, making an X-shaped incision such that there are 4 triangular flaps, and then removing the subcutaneous tissue under each individual triangular flap. The Palva flap is then horizontally split in the middle so that the periosteum is out of the way of the neocanal. The pressed fascia is then brought onto the field and placed on top of the ossicular mass; there should be a few millimeters of overlap with the bone of the neocanal. The triangular skin flaps are then sutured down to the periosteum underneath. The skin graft is brought in through the postauricular incision, ensuring complete coverage of the neocanal and with significant overlap of the fascia graft as in Fig. 33.8. A thin Silastic® disc is placed over the fascia graft to hold it in place, and the lateral triangular tabs of the skin graft are sewn into the triangular slots of the meatoplasty. Any excess skin from the graft is trimmed so there is no redundancy. In this way, the interdigitating of the meatoplasty skin and the skin graft minimizes the risk of circumferential scar formation and possible stenosis. The neocanal is then tightly packed with strips of Merocel® to stent it open (Fig. 33.15). The periosteal flaps are then sutured back down to re-suspend the ear and the postauricular incision is closed. A mastoid dressing is placed.

Postoperative Care

The patient can be discharged or admitted overnight, depending on the surgeon's preference and patient's age. Patients are given oral antibiotics (cephalexin) and pain medicine on the first postoperative day after the mastoid and skin graft dressings are removed. Antibiotic ointment is placed over the postauricular incision, and an antibiotic-soaked cotton ball is changed at the meatus daily. The patient is seen in the office 1–2 weeks after surgery, and any sutures and packing (including the Silastic® disk) are removed. A corticosteroid-antibiotic eardrop preparation is then used twice daily for 1 week with strict dry ear precautions. The canal is left open to the air. The skin graft donor site is covered with Tegaderm™ (3M, Saint Paul, Minnesota) or petroleum gauze dressing and allowed to fall off independently.

A second postoperative visit is made 1 month later, and the canal is debrided of desquamated epithelium sloughed

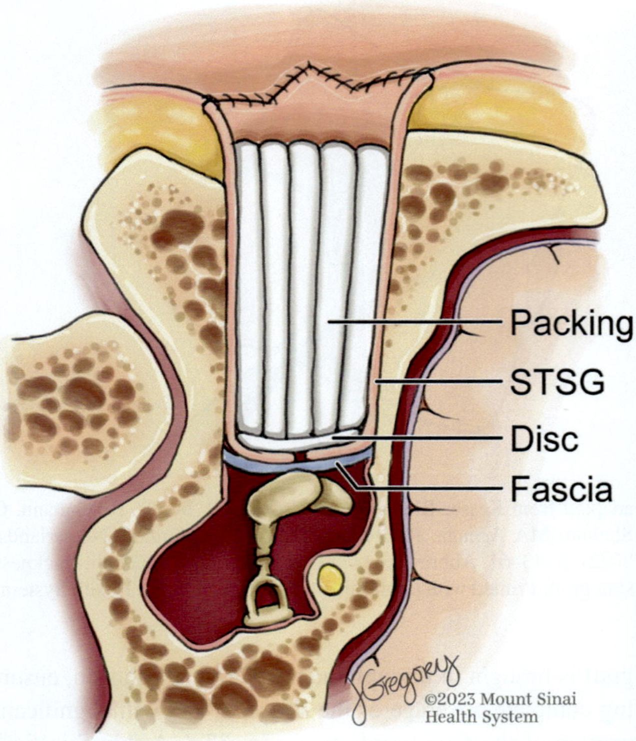

Fig. 33.15 Once the fascia and skin graft are placed, a Silastic® disc is placed on top for stabilization. Multiple Merocel® wicks are used as packing. The skin graft is sewn into the meatoplasty skin as shown. (This image was drawn by Jill Gregory and was adapted from Kesser BW and Goddard JC, ed. by DE Brackmann, C Shelton, MA Arriaga, R Gurgel, (Elsevier, Amsterdam, Netherlands, 2022), p. 43–61. Abbreviations: OM ossicular mass, STSG split-thickness skin graft. Printed with permission from ©Mount Sinai Health System)

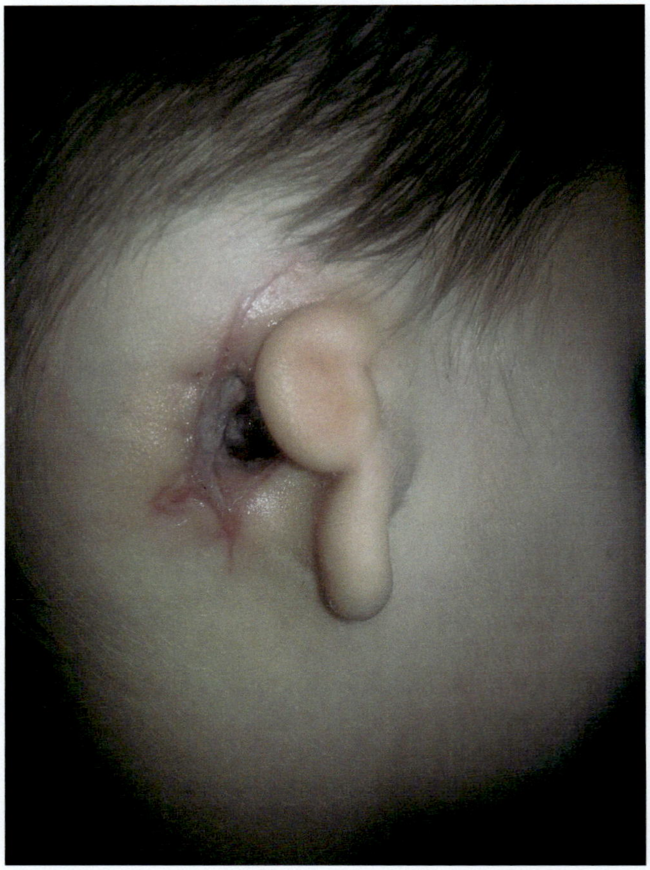

Fig. 33.16 Postoperative ear canal sits behind the auricular remnant

from the skin graft. Beneath the epithelial crust, the skin graft should be dry and healthy. The first postoperative audiogram is obtained at this visit.

It is important that the patient be followed every 6–12 months indefinitely for debridement of the desquamated epithelial crust. Although the skin graft is healthy, it is not self-cleaning. Failure to have the ear cleaned routinely may result in decreased hearing and chronic infection. There are no restrictions after the 1-month visit—patients may swim, but alcohol eardrops after swimming and once a week are advised.

Complications

Complications of atresia surgery can be minimized with proper selection of patients and with careful attention to surgical detail. Most common complications include meatal or canal stenosis in 15–20%, usually requiring revision surgery, and chronic drainage/infection in 10%, usually due to sloughing of the skin graft with "mucosalization" of the canal—requiring revision with a new skin graft or possible temporizing measures such as Gentian violet if the area is small. In Oliver and colleagues' series of 107 revision cases, 19% were for refractory otorrhea/infection, and with >3 months follow-up, 75% had achieved a dry ear canal [59]. Cholesteatoma formation, although rare, should also be considered in chronic draining ears following atresiaplasty, and this complication can occur years after the primary surgery. Thorough, careful, in-office debridement in these reconstructed ears annually is necessary to avoid keratin build-up and skin graft sloughing.

Less commonly, sensorineural hearing loss (5%) is most likely related to the high energy of the drill on the ossicular chain conducted to the cochlea; facial nerve injury has been reported to occur in 0.1% [56]. Regarding the latter, Li's meta-analysis quotes an average of 0.5% with a range of 0.0–5.0%, [60] while some of the larger series quote <1.5% [50, 56, 61]. The keys to avoiding facial nerve injury are close study of the preoperative CT scan, appropriate patient selection, and careful surgical technique. As noted above, facial nerve monitoring should be employed. As discussed below, 15–20% of patients will also lose the initial gains in hearing, due to either lateralization of the tympanic membrane or refixation of the ossicular chain. We counsel patients that approximately 15–20% will require a revision procedure at some point in the future, usually due to stenosis of the canal, loss of early hearing gains, or sloughing of the skin graft with chronic drainage [59].

Results

The two most important factors in achieving consistently good hearing outcomes in atresia surgery are careful preoperative selection of patients and meticulous surgical technique at each step of the operation. As discussed above, surgery is not recommended for patients with Jahrsdoerfer scores of 5 or below. The most important anatomic feature for successful surgery is middle-ear aeration [27, 62]; without an aerated middle-ear space, the patient is not considered a candidate for surgery.

In terms of hearing outcomes, better preoperative hearing predicts better postoperative hearing in patients undergoing canalplasty. In Nicholas and colleagues' analysis of 133 atretic ears, they found normal postoperative hearing in 66% of cases with a preoperative SRT$\leq$50 dB and only in 40% of those with preoperative SRT >60 dB [63]. One criticism of the atresia surgery case series has been the lack of long-term follow-up. Lambert examined the stability of hearing results after atresia surgery and found that almost two-thirds of patients maintained an SRT $\leq$30 dB HL for the longer follow-up (>1 year; mean, 2.8 years); about one-third required a revision procedure [50]. Similarly, De la Cruz reported a long-term ($\geq$6 months) air–bone gap (ABG) of 30 dB or less in 51% of primary cases and 39% of revisions [64]. Imbery et al. reported a decline in PTA of 8.2 dB over a mean of 4 years, and only 64% with stable hearing compared to the immediate postoperative audiogram at last follow-up. While just over 20% had a 10–20 dB decline in air conduction PTA, 15% had a decline of $\geq$20 dB [65]. Digoy and Cueva also reported on the stability of hearing in their series of atresia patients, as hearing did not change between short and long term (>1 year): 50% of patients achieved an SRT of 30 dB HL or better [66]. These authors reported no difference in hearing outcomes between patients undergoing ossiculoplasty reconstruction (53%) versus those undergoing intact native chain reconstruction [66]. Conversely, Dobratz et al. did show a significant advantage to maintaining the patient's native ossicular chain when possible [57]. Ossicular refixation is not an uncommon problem and can occur when there is insufficient bony clearance around the ossicular chain, possibly due to the close proximity of the facial nerve, forcing the surgeon to compromise on the degree of bony clearance. Low tegmen or bony exostoses/refixation can form during puberty [1]. De la Cruz reported a refixation rate of 11.5% in primary cases and 6.9% in revisions [64]. Teufert and colleagues reported improvement in refixation rates from 25% to 3.8% after changing their technique to include a laser, using a thinner skin graft, Silastic® sheeting, and Merocel® wicks [67]. Lateralization of the fascia graft may occur in 5.8–20.0% in various reports [60, 61, 68]. Having good overlap of the fascia with the bony canal, an adequately sized Silastic® disc, and tight packing can help avoid this outcome.

Revision surgery may not hold up as well long-term, as Chang et al. reported disappointing long-term hearing outcomes for patients undergoing revision atresia surgery [69]. Specifically, only 26% of cases with a poor initial result were found to benefit from revision surgery. Conversely, Oliver reported very good results for those patients undergoing revision CAA surgery for loss of early hearing gains [59]. Of Oliver's 107 revisions, 58% were for neocanal stenosis, 19% were for otorrhea/infection, and 20% were for conductive hearing loss. The majority of patients with stenosis and drainage were fixed after a single revision, and SRT had improved significantly over the preoperative value.

Surgeons 10–15 years ago counseled patients and families against repair of unilateral atresia, given the mediocre hearing gains and risk of major complications. Since the introduction of HRCT scanning with improved preoperative evaluation, the repair of unilateral atresia has become more widely accepted. Clearly, there is a learning curve for this challenging operation, and one report suggests a minimum of 32 ears to achieve proficiency in achieving good short-term hearing results, and 48 ears for good long-term hearing outcomes [70]. The anterior surgical approach as first proposed by Jahrsdoerfer has withstood the test of time and scrutiny [21]. Candidacy selection and meticulous technique are critical, as the widespread availability, ease, and reliability of osseointegrated bone conducting hearing systems can outperform atresia surgery hearing results [35, 71]. These studies, however, do not account for gains in sound localization, summation, and hearing in noise that have been demonstrated in patients undergoing surgical repair of unilateral CAA [5, 39, 72].

As the seemingly subtle deficits of unilateral hearing loss in children are further elucidated, rehabilitation of children with unilateral atresia will be more accepted and more often recommended.

Summary

While technically challenging, surgery to construct an ear canal and restore the natural sound-conducting mechanism of the middle and outer ear in patients with congenital aural atresia can be successful with careful attention to the preoperative selection of patients as candidates for the operation and with meticulous surgical technique at each step of the operation. Restoration of normal hearing in these patients is one of the most rewarding operations in our specialty.

References

1. Kesser, BW, Goddard, JC. Congenital Malformation of the External Auditory Canal and Middle Ear. In Otologic Surgery. Eds. Brackmann DE, Shelton C, Arriaga MA, Gurgel R. 4th ed. Elsevier.
2. Grundfast KM, Camilon F. External auditory canal stenosis and partial atresia without associated anomalies. Ann Otol Rhinol Laryngol. 1986;95(5 Pt 1):505–9.
3. Harada O, Ishii H. The condition of the auditory ossicles in microtia: findings in 57 middle ear operations. Plast Reconstr Surg. 1972;50(1):48–53.
4. Kountakis SE, Helidonis E, Jahrsdoerfer RA. Microtia grade as an indicator of middle ear development in aural atresia. Arch Otolaryngol Head Neck Surg. 1995;121(8):885–6.
5. Bellucci RJ. The problem of congenital auricular malformation, I: construction of the external auditory canal. Trans Am Acad Ophthalmol Otolaryngol. 1960;64:840–52.
6. Casazza GC, Jonas RH, Kesser BW. Congenital aural stenosis with cholesteatoma. Otol Neurotol. 2022;43(3):320–7.
7. Schuknecht HF. Congenital aural atresia. Laryngoscope. 1989;99(9):908–17.
8. Casale G, Nicholas BD, Kesser BW. Acquired ear canal cholesteatoma in congenital aural atresia/stenosis. Otol Neurotol. 2014;35(8):1474–9.
9. Cole RR, Jahrsdoerfer RA. The risk of cholesteatoma in congenital aural stenosis. Laryngoscope. 1990;100(6):576–8.
10. Hrdlicka A. Seven prehistoric American skulls with complete absence of external auditory meatus. Am J Phys Anthropol. 1933;17:355.
11. Pattee GL. An operation to improve hearing in cases of congenital atresia of the external auditory meatus. Arch Otolaryngol (1925). 1947;45(5):568–80.
12. Ombredanne M. [New proves of superiority of fenestration in surgery of aplasias of the ear]. Ann Otolaryngol. 1952;69(8–9):494–501.
13. Ombredanne M. [33 Operations for aplasia of the ear with atresia of the auditory canal: technic, operative establishments and results]. Acta Otolaryngol. 1952;41(1–2):69–109.
14. Woodman DG. Congenital atresia of the auditory canal; two stage operation with fenestration. AMA Arch Otolaryngol. 1952;55(2):172–81.
15. House HP. Management of congenital ear canal atresia. Laryngoscope. 1953;63(10):916–46.
16. Shambaugh GE Jr. Developmental anomalies of the sound conducting apparatus and their surgical correction. Trans Am Otol Soc. 1952;40:217–31.
17. Ruedi L. The surgical treatment of the atresia auris congenita; a clinical and histological report. Laryngoscope. 1954;64(8):666–84.
18. Nager GT. Aural atresia: anatomy and surgery. Postgrad Med. 1961;29:529–41.
19. Nager GT. Congenital aural atresia: anatomy and surgical management. Birth Defects Orig Artic Ser. 1971;07(4):33–51.
20. Schuknecht HF. Reconstructive procedures for congenital aural atresia. Arch Otolaryngol. 1975;101(3):170–2.
21. Jahrsdoerfer RA. Congenital atresia of the ear. Laryngoscope. 1978;88(9 Pt 3 Suppl 13):1–48.
22. Jahrsdoerfer RA, et al. Grading system for the selection of patients with congenital aural atresia. Am J Otol. 1992;13(1):6–12.
23. Trigg DJ, Applebaum EL. Indications for the surgical repair of unilateral aural atresia in children. Am J Otol. 1998;19(5):679–84; discussion 684–6.
24. De la Cruz A, Kesser B. Management of the unilateral atretic ear. In: Pensak M, editor. Controversies in otolaryngology-head and neck surgery. New York: Thieme Medical; 1999. p. 381–5.
25. Bellucci RJ. Congenital aural malformations: diagnosis and treatment. Otolaryngol Clin N Am. 1981;14(1):95–124.
26. Kesser BW, Krook K, Gray LC. Impact of unilateral conductive hearing loss due to aural atresia on academic performance in children. Laryngoscope. 2013;123(9):2270–5.
27. Shonka DC Jr, Livingston WJ 3rd, Kesser BW. The Jahrsdoerfer grading scale in surgery to repair congenital aural atresia. Arch Otolaryngol Head Neck Surg. 2008;134(8):873–7.
28. Hol MK, et al. The BAHA Softband. A new treatment for young children with bilateral congenital aural atresia. Int J Pediatr Otorhinolaryngol. 2005;69(7):973–80.
29. van der Pouw KT, Snik AF, Cremers CW. Audiometric results of bilateral bone-anchored hearing aid application in patients with bilateral congenital aural atresia. Laryngoscope. 1998;108(4 Pt 1):548–53.
30. Klaiber S, Weerda H. [BAHA (bone-anchored hearing aid) in bilateral external ear dysplasia and congenital ear atresia]. HNO. 2002;50(10):949–59.
31. Priwin C, et al. BAHA in children and adolescents with unilateral or bilateral conductive hearing loss: a study of outcome. Int J Pediatr Otorhinolaryngol. 2007;71(1):135–45.
32. Wazen JJ, et al. Auricular rehabilitation with bone-anchored titanium implants. Laryngoscope. 1999;109(4):523–7.
33. De la Cruz A, Linthicum FH Jr, Luxford WM. Congenital atresia of the external auditory canal. Laryngoscope. 1985;95(4):421–7.
34. Ukatu CC, Desai NK, Todd NW Jr. Site for bone-anchored hearing system for children younger than 5 years. Otolaryngol Head Neck Surg. 2015;152(2):348–52.
35. Nadaraja GS, et al. Hearing outcomes of atresia surgery versus osseointegrated bone conduction device in patients with congenital aural atresia: a systematic review. Otol Neurotol. 2013;34(8):1394–9.
36. Zernotti ME, et al. Audiological outcomes in patients with congenital aural atresia implanted with transcutaneous active bone conduction hearing implant. Int J Pediatr Otorhinolaryngol. 2019;119:54–8.
37. Bravo-Torres S, Der-Mussa C, Fuentes-Lopez E. Active transcutaneous bone conduction implant: audiological results in paediatric patients with bilateral microtia associated with external auditory canal atresia. Int J Audiol. 2018;57(1):53–60.
38. Evans AK, Kazahaya K. Canal atresia: "surgery or implantable hearing devices? The expert's question is revisited". Int J Pediatr Otorhinolaryngol. 2007;71(3):367–74.
39. Moon IJ, et al. Sound localization performance improves after canaloplasty in unilateral congenital aural atresia patients. Otol Neurotol. 2014;35(4):639–44.
40. Thorne CH, et al. Auricular reconstruction: indications for autogenous and prosthetic techniques. Plast Reconstr Surg. 2001;107(5):1241–52.
41. Reinisch JF, Lewin S. Ear reconstruction using a porous polyethylene framework and temporoparietal fascia flap. Facial Plast Surg. 2009;25(3):181–9.
42. Romo T 3rd, Presti PM, Yalamanchili HR. Medpor alternative for microtia repair. Facial Plast Surg Clin North Am. 2006;14(2):129–36. vi.
43. Roberson JB Jr, et al. Atresia repair before microtia reconstruction: comparison of early with standard surgical timing. Otol Neurotol. 2009;30(6):771–6.
44. Sharma A, Dorman MF, Spahr AJ. A sensitive period for the development of the central auditory system in children with cochlear implants: implications for age of implantation. Ear Hear. 2002;23(6):532–9.
45. Brent B. Microtia repair with rib cartilage grafts: a review of personal experience with 1000 cases. Clin Plast Surg. 2002;29(2):257–71. vii.
46. Brent B. Technical advances in ear reconstruction with autogenous rib cartilage grafts: personal experience with 1200 cases. Plast Reconstr Surg. 1999;104(2):319–34; discussion 335–8.

47. Kawanabe Y, Nagata S. A new method of costal cartilage harvest for total auricular reconstruction: part I. Avoidance and prevention of intraoperative and postoperative complications and problems. Plast Reconstr Surg. 2006;117(6):2011–8.
48. Kawanabe Y, Nagata S. A new method of costal cartilage harvest for total auricular reconstruction: part II. Evaluation and analysis of the regenerated costal cartilage. Plast Reconstr Surg. 2007;119(1):308–15.
49. Jahrsdoerfer RA, Kesser BW. Issues on aural atresia for the facial plastic surgeon. Facial Plast Surg. 1995;11(4):274–7.
50. Lambert PR. Congenital aural atresia: stability of surgical results. Laryngoscope. 1998;108(12):1801–5.
51. Kiese-Himmel C, Kruse E. [Unilateral hearing loss in childhood. An empirical analysis comparing bilateral hearing loss]. Laryngorhinootologie. 2001;80(1):18–22.
52. Wilmington D, Gray L, Jahrsdoerfer R. Binaural processing after corrected congenital unilateral conductive hearing loss. Hear Res. 1994;74(1–2):99–114.
53. Ruhl DS, Kesser BW. Atresiaplasty in congenital aural atresia: what the facial plastic surgeon needs to know. Facial Plast Surg Clin North Am. 2018;26(1):87–96.
54. Wong K, et al. Is there a role for intraoperative navigation during cochlear implantation in patients with aural atresia? Otol Neurotol. 2021;42(9):e1250–5.
55. Fan CJ, et al. Intraoperative navigation during atresiaplasty for congenital aural atresia. Int J Pediatr Otorhinolaryngol. 2021;146:110756.
56. Jahrsdoerfer RA, Lambert PR. Facial nerve injury in congenital aural atresia surgery. Am J Otol. 1998;19(3):283–7.
57. Dobratz EJ, et al. To POP or not: ossiculoplasty in congenital aural atresia surgery. Laryngoscope. 2008;118(8):1452–7.
58. Miller RS, et al. Diagnosis and management of salivary fistula after surgery for congenital aural atresia. Otol Neurotol. 2006;27(2):189–92.
59. Oliver ER, et al. Revision aural atresia surgery: indications and outcomes. Otol Neurotol. 2011;32(2):252–8.
60. Li CL, et al. A meta-analysis of the long-term hearing outcomes and complications associated with atresiaplasty. Int J Pediatr Otorhinolaryngol. 2015;79(6):793–7.
61. Moss WJ, Lin HW, Cueva RA. Surgical and audiometric outcomes for repair of congenital aural atresia and hypoplasia. JAMA Otolaryngol Head Neck Surg. 2016;142(1):52–7.
62. Oliver ER, et al. Middle ear dimensions in congenital aural atresia and hearing outcomes after atresiaplasty. Otol Neurotol. 2010;31(6):946–53.
63. Nicholas BD, et al. Does preoperative hearing predict postoperative hearing in patients undergoing primary aural atresia repair? Otol Neurotol. 2012;33(6):1002–6.
64. De la Cruz A, Teufert KB. Congenital aural atresia surgery: long-term results. Otolaryngol Head Neck Surg. 2003;129(1):121–7.
65. Imbery TE, et al. Long-term audiometric outcomes after atresiaplasty for congenital aural atresia. Otol Neurotol. 2020;41(3):371–8.
66. Digoy GP, Cueva RA. Congenital aural atresia: review of short- and long-term surgical results. Otol Neurotol. 2007;28(1):54–60.
67. Teufert KB, De la Cruz A. Advances in congenital aural atresia surgery: effects on outcome. Otolaryngol Head Neck Surg. 2004;131(3):263–70.
68. Edfeldt L, Strömbäck K. Surgical treatment of congenital aural atresia - is it still justified? Acta Otolaryngol. 2015;135(3):226–32.
69. Chang SO, Choi BY, Hur DG. Analysis of the long-term hearing results after the surgical repair of aural atresia. Laryngoscope. 2006;116(10):1835–41.
70. Patel N, Shelton C. The surgical learning curve in aural atresia surgery. Laryngoscope. 2007;117(1):67–73.
71. Yellon RF. Atresiaplasty versus BAHA for congenital aural atresia. Laryngoscope. 2011;121(1):2–3.
72. Gray L, Kesser B, Cole E. Understanding speech in noise after correction of congenital unilateral aural atresia: effects of age in the emergence of binaural squelch but not in use of head-shadow. Int J Pediatr Otorhinolaryngol. 2009;73(9):1281–7.

Part VI

Mastoid and Middle Ear Diseases

34 Eustachian Tube Dysfunction and Surgery

C. Eduardo Corrales and Dennis S. Poe

History

The Eustachian tube was first mentioned indirectly by Alcmaeon of Sparta in 400 B.C. when he proposed that goats may breathe through their ears [1], but Bartolomeus Eustachius is credited with its discovery in 1562 when he published a detailed description of its anatomy and physiologic function [2]. Valsalva later described the Eustachian tube as having cartilaginous and osseous parts and was the first to recognize the importance of the tensor veli palatini muscle in opening the Eustachian tube [3]. He also described the Valsalva maneuver, which remains clinically relevant to this day. Toynbee furthered our understanding of the Eustachian tube through extensive investigations of the peritubal muscles [4], and Politzer made important contributions in connecting the role of the Eustachian tube in middle ear pathology [5].

Anatomy

The Eustachian tube in the normal adult measures approximately 31–38 mm in length [6]. It contains a physiological functional valve that is closed in the passive resting position and is dilated open by active muscular exertion. Since the direction of mucociliary clearance within the Eustachian tube flows from the ear to the nasopharyngeal orifice, this chapter will describe the anatomy with "proximal" referring to the middle ear end and "distal" referring to the nasopharyngeal orifice. When viewing a cross-section of the tubal lumen, there are superior and inferior halves and anterolateral and posteromedial halves.

The proximal one-third is, in effect, a bony, funnel-shaped extension of the middle ear (protympanum) which becomes narrowest at the bony-cartilaginous isthmus, the smallest aperture in the entire tube. The bony portion is lined with a thin layer of cuboidal respiratory epithelium [7] and is a fixed conduit that is normally patent [8].

The distal 2/3 of the Eustachian tube is called the cartilaginous or pharyngeal portion and is composed of a cartilaginous skeleton to which is attached a complex arrangement of peritubal muscles capable of a wide range of dynamic movements. The lumen is lined by respiratory epithelium that is taller, more columnar, and more ciliated inferiorly than the cuboidal epithelium in the superior one-half. A submucosal layer of lymphatics and fat (Ostmann's fat pad) adds to the lining's thickness within the tubal lumen. The cartilaginous portion is normally closed in the resting state due to apposition of the mucosal walls. The closure occurs over a variable length (10–20 mm segment) that begins a few millimeters distal to the isthmus, where the cartilaginous skeleton becomes flexible. This portion that intermittently dilates to an open position is termed the "valve." The valve appears in the nasopharyngeal orifice as a convex bulge into the lumen of the Eustachian tube and consists of the mucosa, the submucosa, Ostmann's fat pad and the relaxed bulk of the tensor veli palatini muscle.

There are four peritubular muscles: the levator veli palatini (LVP), the salpingopharyngeus, the tensor tympani, and the tensor veli palatini (TVP). The TVP is thought to be the principal dilator of the tubal lumen [9].

The LVP is a round-bellied muscle that looks like a sling running from the base of the temporal bone at the bony Eustachian tube and passing under a groove in the inferior aspect of the medial cartilaginous lamina and membranous floor of the Eustachian tube to insert into the palatal muscu-

C. E. Corrales
Otology, Neurotology and Skull Base Surgery, Harvard Medical School, Division of Otolaryngology, Brigham and Women's Hospital, Boston, MA, USA
e-mail: ccorrales@bwh.harvard.edu

D. S. Poe (✉)
Department of Otolaryngology—Head and Neck Surgery, Boston Children's Hospital, Harvard Medical School, Boston, MA, USA
e-mail: dennis.poe@childrens.harvard.edu

A. D. Sweeney et al. (eds.), *Haynes-Glasscock-Shambaugh Surgery of the Ear*, https://doi.org/10.1007/978-3-032-18264-7_34

lature. Contraction of the LVP raises the soft palate and medially rotates the medial cartilaginous lamina.

The TVP is a flat, fan-shaped muscle with broad origins from the basisphenoid and includes dilator tubae muscle fibers originating from the membranous anterolateral wall of the Eustachian tube. It courses longitudinally along the length of the cartilaginous ET and tapers to run under the hamulus of the palatal bone and then inserts into the soft palate. The relaxed bulk of the TVP contributes to the anterolateral wall bulge into the lumen of the Eustachian tube and aids in closure of the lumen. Contraction of the TVP tenses the anterolateral membranous wall to dilate the tubal valve into the open position.

Physiology of Tubal Dilation

Intermittent brief tubal dilation is probably the principal mechanism for equilibration of middle ear pressure with the ambient atmosphere [10]. Involuntary dilation of the Eustachian tube occurs throughout the day, usually through a swallow or yawn, but it does not accompany every swallow or yawn. Barometric and chemical receptors within the middle ear are thought to provide autonomic nervous system feedback to influence the frequency of involuntary tubal opening [11, 12]. Tubal dilation occurs in normal subjects approximately 1.4 times per minute, with the duration of opening averaging 0.4 seconds [10].

Muscular contractions initiate rotational movements of the cartilaginous framework and create tension with effacement and lateral rounding of the anterolateral wall to produce active dilation of the lumen and transient opening. In other words, the convex bulge of the anterolateral wall becomes flattened or even concave to allow for dilation to an open position.

Middle ear and mastoid gas exchange is an ongoing process that continually generates a net absorption of gases, resulting in an increasingly negative pressure between tubal dilations. In a demonstration of middle ear gas exchange in humans, Pau et al. studied subjects with tympanometry while they avoided swallowing or yawning for up to 2 hours. Within 1 hour, middle ear pressures were approximately − 100 dPa and by 2 hours, − 170 dPa [13]. Failure to dilate for an extended period of time can lead to pathologically severe negative pressure and consequences of tympanic membrane retraction, atelectasis, and otitis media with effusion (OME).

Surfactants are produced within the tubal mucosa and probably aid in reducing the surface tension of the lumen and reducing the work required to dilate the tube [14]. Fluid and secretions in the middle ear are cleared by a combination of muscular pumping action associated with the tubal closing process [10] and by mucociliary activity [15]. Reflux of nasopharyngeal secretions into the middle ear is limited or prevented by the closed position of the resting pharyngeal Eustachian tube and by the trapped volume of gas in the middle ear and mastoid bone, which creates a "gas cushion." Reflux of the sounds of breathing and vocalization is also blocked by the closed resting position of the pharyngeal Eustachian tube [15].

Functions of the Eustachian Tube

In the most basic form, the Eustachian tube has three main functions [9]:

1. Ventilation function (also called pressure regulation function): It is likely the main function of the ET. Ventilation and pressure equalization lead to optimal vibration of the tympanic membrane and ossicular chain.
2. Clearance of secretions from the middle ear: The mucociliary clearance of the Eustachian tube is essential for the prevention of middle ear effusion and otitis media.
3. Middle ear protection from nasopharyngeal material and bodily sounds: The normal resting *closed* position of the Eustachian tube prevents reflux of nasopharyngeal secretions and transmission of sound into the middle ear (autophony).

Definition of Eustachian Tube Dysfunction

The fundamental concept of the Eustachian tube acting as an organ, rather than simply a tube connecting the middle ear to the nose, is critical in understanding its function and dysfunction. A definition of obstructive Eustachian tube dysfunction was published in the Clinical Consensus Statement: Balloon Dilation of the Eustachian Tube from the American Academy of Otolaryngology-Head and Neck Surgery. It stated that, "Obstructive Eustachian tube dysfunction (OETD) is a physiological disorder of the Eustachian tube (ET) that results in the inability to appropriately equalize pressure between the middle ear and the environment." [16] In an earlier international consensus statement, there was agreement to define overall Eustachian tube dysfunction as a failure of the Eustachian tube to perform its unique functions listed above and it distinguished between obstructive and patulous dysfunction [17]. Both consensus statements agreed that chronic dysfunction was defined as three or more months of persistent symptoms or signs. The concept of Eustachian tube dysfunction as a spectrum of disease that ranged between the extremes of obstructive and patulous dysfunction was introduced [17]. Patients with obstructive dysfunction may progress to normal or even patulous with time. On the mildest end of the obstructive dysfunction spectrum, patients may only have symptoms when challenged with rapid changes in ambient pressure, such as with flights or diving and this has been termed "barochallenged." [17]

The tendency to progress from obstructive to patulous dysfunction has been observed, particularly in patients with chronic allergic rhinitis [18]. Patches of atrophic mucosa or remodeled tissue showing loss of goblet cells and squamous metaplasia occur within the nose and sinuses in chronic allergic rhinitis [19–21]. It is suspected that such patches may occur within the lumen of the Eustachian tube in long-term disease, leading to failure of competence of the functional valve that results in reflux of air and sound into the middle ear through the open lumen [18]. When patients have exacerbations of chronic allergic rhinitis, they may develop obstructive dysfunction, but when their disease becomes quiescent, they could experience patulous dysfunction. Therefore, patients can alternate between obstructive and patulous on this spectrum.

In clinical practice, obstructive Eustachian tube dysfunction is commonly taken to imply an inadequate ability to open the tubal valve. When the valve fails to function properly, numerous consequences may occur within the middle ear, including otitis media with effusion and tympanic membrane retraction [9]. Obstructive Eustachian tube dysfunction with associated otitis media with effusion and/or tympanic membrane retraction has been well studied in the pediatric population [22, 23], but newer studies demonstrate an adult outpatient visit burden that extends beyond childhood [24]. In fact, obstructive Eustachian tube dysfunction with associated otitis media with effusion and/or tympanic membrane retraction is responsible for more than two million visits per year in adults over 20 years of age and more than 2.6 million visits among those less than 20 years of age [24]. The prevalence of obstructive Eustachian tube dysfunction has been estimated as 4.6% of the adult population in the United States [25].

On the other end of the spectrum of disease, patulous Eustachian tube dysfunction is due to failure of the functional valve to close, with the consequence of an abnormally open Eustachian tube. Patulous Eustachian tube dysfunction is far more common than previously believed, with estimates of approximately 7% of the normal population having some symptoms [26]. In a survey of subjects with normal ears, 2/130 (1.5%) reported habitual sniffing, a more prominent symptom and a hallmark of patulous ET [27]. Patulous ET results in internal noises being transmitted to the ear, causing autophony to breathing and voice, as well as a sense of fullness and pressure in the ear. In our recent cohort of 190 patients with patulous Eustachian tube dysfunction, 93% experienced voice autophony, 92% had breath autophony, and 57% had aural fullness [18]. In 52% of patients, the patulous state was bilateral. Classically attributed to severe and rapid weight loss, a patulous Eustachian tube is now recognized to be multifactorial in nature and newer possible risk factors include allergic disease and stress/anxiety [18].

Luminal Endoscopy and Video Endoscopy of the Eustachian Tube

Endoscopy of the human Eustachian tube has substantially increased our understanding of the functional processes in normal and pathological tubes. Initial work done by the insertion of microfiber-optic instruments into the tubal lumen yielded only limited information since the bony isthmus is only about 1.0–1.5 mm in horizontal diameter and 2–3 mm in vertical diameter [28]. In order to pass through the narrow isthmus, endoscope diameters must be restricted to 1 mm or less, which compromises image resolution, limiting it to gross structures within the middle ear such as ossicles, but fine details of movements have not been appreciated to date. This issue has limited clinical applications of trans-Eustachian endoscopy [29]. Another technical challenge is that direct contact of the endoscope lens with secretions and mucosal folds obscures inspection within the lumen such that most reports have only been able to describe gross observations such as the presence of lesions or degree of patency. Despite these limitations, there has been a lack of pathology identified within the bony Eustachian tube, even with active middle ear effusions. The evidence suggests that the principal location of pathology that causes Eustachian tube dysfunction, both obstructive and patulous, is within the cartilaginous portion [30–32].

Larger diameter (3–4 mm) fiber-optic nasopharyngoscopes or angled (30° or 45°) rigid Hopkins rod endoscopes have been used for more detailed studies of the tubal lumen. The endoscope should be carefully positioned in the nasopharyngeal orifice with the view directed superiorly approximately 45° and laterally approximately 45° to provide an optimal view into the length of the lumen. This view allows for observation of most of the pharyngeal portion of the tube as it rotates into the dilated position during the opening sequence. Careful observation of tubal dynamics has become possible with high-resolution optics. Avoidance of direct contact with the mucosa prevents interference with the dilating mechanism and limits problems with fogging of the lens. Video recordings can be made and replayed in slow motion if desired for meticulous analysis of the dilation process and study of normal physiology and pathophysiology [33, 34].

Eustachian tube endoscopy generally yields views well into the valve area during the time of maximal active dilation. The opening process can be seen endoscopically as the tube progressively dilates from the nasopharyngeal orifice up toward the isthmus, generally moving the lumen into full view of the endoscope.

Technique of Eustachian Tube Video Endoscopy

Patients are examined in the sitting position in an office setting. Topical spray anesthetic and decongestant, lidocaine (4%) topical mixed with equal parts of phenylephrine HCl 0.5% solution, is applied to both nasal cavities while the patient sniffs. Endoscopes are introduced into the nasal cavity and advanced up to the nasopharyngeal orifice of the Eustachian tube, just posterior to the inferior turbinate and identified by the anterior pillar, the lumen and the torus tubarius (Fig. 34.1). Caution must be exerted, especially in severe disease, as it is easy to pass by the torus and examine the fossa of Rosenmüller, believing it to be the Eustachian tube orifice.

The authors most commonly perform the initial endoscopic exam with a 3.7 mm diameter steerable flexible fiber-optic nasopharyngoscope EMF-P3 (Olympus, Tokyo, Japan). Careful inspection of the nasal cavity, nasopharynx, hypopharynx, and larynx is done to look for mucosal inflammation or lesions. Attention is particularly paid to evidence of nasal mucosal or turbinate disease, allergic disease, chronic rhinosinusitis, adenoid or tubal tonsil tissue hypertrophy (especially impinging on the torus tubarius) and signs of laryngo pharyngeal reflux (LPR). If the adenoid is enlarged, its proximity and degree of contact with the torus tubarius are noted. Lastly, the Eustachian tube is closely examined. The optimal fiber-optic view is most commonly obtained by introducing the endoscope along the floor of either nasal cavity and rotating it 90° to allow it to flex and steer horizontally. This permits the endoscope to be angled to view laterally deep into the lumen, allowing for evaluation of the valve dilation and closure as well as with an angled rigid endoscope. The endoscope can be passed posterior to the vomer to examine the contralateral Eustachian tube. The lumen is usually successfully viewed with a fiber-optic scope from either the contralateral or ipsilateral nasal cavity.

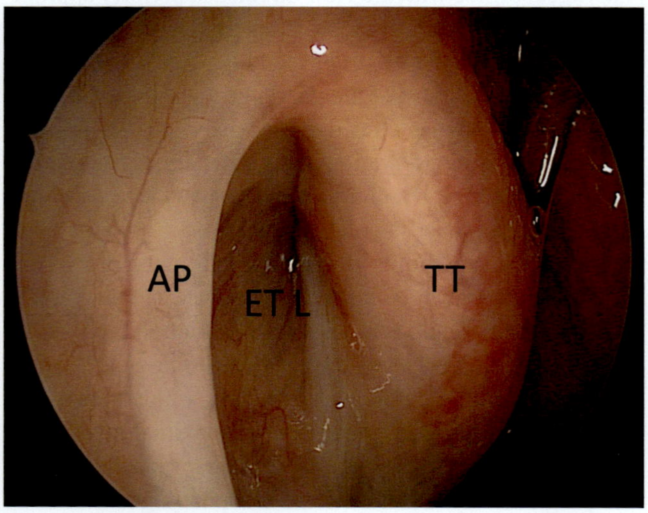

Fig. 34.1 Endoscopic view of the right Eustachian tube. AP anterior pillar, TT Torus tubarius, ET L Eustachian tube lumen. (Used with permission from Dennis Poe, MD, who retains copyright of this figure)

For a higher resolution examination, such as for video recording in normal speed or slow-motion, rigid endoscopes are preferred, generally using a 3-mm diameter, 30° or preferably 45° view angle, Hopkins rod rigid endoscope (Karl Storz, Culver City, CA). The rod endoscopes have high-resolution images but the fiber-optic endoscopes are easier to pass and can be steered deeper into the Eustachian tube lumen if desired. Distal chip-tip endoscopes provide a compromise of flexible endoscope delivery with a digital camera and resolution approximating that of a rigid endoscope, but the software technology has not yet become available to rotate the camera image 90° to correct for the rotation of the endoscope for horizontal flexion.

When using the angled rigid endoscope, it is introduced with the view angle looking directly laterally and passed along the nasal floor, following the inferior turbinate. After passing the posterior aspect of the inferior turbinate, the next landmark encountered is the anterior pillar of the Eustachian tube's nasopharyngeal orifice. Progressing posteriorly and medially, the orifice is seen next, followed by the torus tubarius. Once at the orifice, the endoscope is rotated slightly to look superiorly into the longitudinal axis of the tubal lumen. The flexible or rigid endoscope is coupled to a digital camera and images are viewed on a video monitor. Video recordings are made with a digital recording and processing module.

The patient is initially asked to vocalize "Ka" "Ka" "Ka" repeatedly to view the isolated action of the LVP. The "Ka's" stimulate palatal elevation and medial rotation of the torus tubarius and posteromedial wall of the Eustachian tube. Swallows are done to induce normal physiological tubal dilations, and forced yawns or vocalizing "Ah" are performed to cause maximal sustained dilation. The Eustachian tube is not expected to open with every swallow and yawn, and patients are coached to feel the muscular contractions in the back of their throats to generate some dilatory efforts. The procedure is repeated for the contralateral Eustachian tube orifice.

If video recording is desired, it can be reviewed and analyzed in normal time, slow motion, and even stepping through single frames that are captured at a rate of nearly 30 frames per second.

Endoscopy of the Normal Eustachian Tube

Endoscopic evaluation of the function of the Eustachian tube valve requires a dynamic exam in order to assess the degree of pathology present and also how that pathology may compromise the dilation of the anterolateral and posteromedial walls of the valve (obstructive dysfunction) or prevent its closure (patulous dysfunction). The normal dilation process was initially studied endoscopically in 30 normal subjects [33]. Normal dilation and opening were observed to have two principal consistent sequential phases during a normal swallow:

1. The soft palate was elevated by the action of the LVP muscle, medially rotating the torus tubarius and posteromedial wall. The lateral pharyngeal wall also medialized, causing transient constriction of the nasopharyngeal orifice despite the medial rotation of the posterior cushion and posteromedial wall. One hypothesis for this contrary movement could be to provide momentary protection of the Eustachian tube against reflux at the initiation of swallow.
2. The palate remained elevated, and the posteromedial wall remained medially rotated as the lateral pharyngeal wall displaced laterally to begin the dilation of the nasopharyngeal orifice.
3. The TVP began to contract, causing dilation of the lumen to propagate from the nasopharynx proximally toward the bony isthmus. The dilation occurred by displacement of the anterolateral tubal wall laterally. The LVP continued to maintain the rotation of the torus tubarius, suggesting that it may act as a scaffold to optimize the dilatory effort to the TVP, which is oriented in a relatively inefficient position in humans [35].
4. Tubal opening occurred as the functional valve of the cartilaginous tube dilated into a roughly oval aperture. The convex bulge seen in the resting anterolateral valve wall became visibly flattened or concave to produce the final opening.

Closure of the tube began with closure of the valve area and propagated distally toward the nasopharyngeal orifice. This proximal-to-distal closure has been hypothesized to have a pumping action that may protect against reflux [7]. Relaxation of the posteromedial wall, lateral pharyngeal wall, and palate occurred in variable order or even simultaneously.

The thin mucosa and subcutaneous tissues of the normal Eustachian tubes permitted viewing of the muscular contractions of the LVP and TVP. Even the ripples of distinct individual fiber contractions were often appreciated.

Alper et al. [36] performed an elegant study with healthy subjects in which electromyographic recordings were taken by hook wire electrodes placed into the LVP and TVP muscles. Sonotubometry, a technique of placing a sound emitter into the nasal cavity and recording the increase in sound amplitude by a microphone in the ear canal, was used to determine when the Eustachian tube was fully dilated to open position. The data generated during swallows showed that initiation of LVP contraction occurred first, followed by TVP contraction, followed by dilation to open. The study helps to validate that these actions can be adequately studied with ordinary endoscopic techniques.

Endoscopy of the Dysfunctional Eustachian Tube

As discussed above, in clinical practice, obstructive Eustachian tube dysfunction is commonly taken to imply an inadequate ability to open the tubal valve, causing secondary ear pathology. It may result from anatomical obstruction or physiologic failure due to: (1) hereditary factors as seen in strong family histories of ear disease, (2) mucosal inflammation with functional obstruction or failure of dilation, (3) muscular problems causing dynamic obstructive dysfunction and lastly (4) true anatomical obstruction due to neoplasms, scar or other mass lesions, the least common cause. The etiologies of tubal dilatory failure can be separated into obstructive and dynamic dysfunctions. Most obstructive problems are not true anatomical blockage; rather, they are due to functional failures to dilate the tube sufficiently or often enough to adequately aerate the middle ear.

There is increasing evidence that Eustachian tube dysfunction results from pathology within the cartilaginous portion. Slow-motion video analysis was done on 58 ears (of 40 adult patients) with pathology suggestive of tubal dysfunction [34]. All subjects had significant pathology and compromise of tubal dilation within the cartilaginous portion compared to 4/30 (13%) of normal subjects who had only mild inflammatory changes. The pathological findings are summarized in Table 34.1. All 58 tubes had significantly compromised dilation, which was judged to be: moderate opening ability—26 (45%); minimal opening—21 (36%); no opening—11 (19%).

It was noted in that study that the severity of disease in the Eustachian tube did not correlate with the severity of middle ear disease. One hypothesis is that chronic obstructive Eustachian tube dysfunction will result in retraction of the tympanic membrane due to negative middle ear pressure. If the tympanic membrane comes into contact with the mucosa of the middle ear, especially the incus or under the scutum, an inflammatory reaction can be initiated with upregulation of inflammatory mediators that cause fibroblast activity with

Table 34.1 Pathological findings in the 58 clinically dysfunctional Eustachian tubes

Mucosal edema	48 (83%)
Reduced lateral wall motion	43 (74%)
Obstructive mucosal disease	15 (26%)

Adapted from *Glasscock and Shambaugh's Surgery of the Ear*. 6th Ed. Eds Gulya, Minor, Poe. PMPH. 2010 adhesions, osteoclastic activity, epithelial proliferation and spreading, all of which may cause a biological process that causes progression of a retraction into a pocket and ultimately into cholesteatoma [37, 38]. More importantly, this biological process may continue to progress, independent of whether or not the Eustachian tube remains dysfunctional. The components of the cartilaginous Eustachian tube can be classified as the cartilaginous skeleton, tubal muscles, Ostmann's fat pad, submucosa and epithelium of the lumen, and defects were observed in each of the different components. Edema of the mucosa and submucosa was most often responsible for decreased luminal diameter and decreased ability to dilate the tube. Actual muscular dysfunction (dynamic dysfunction) as the primary problem was seen in 8%. Examples of hypofunction, hyperfunction, or lack of coordination of either the TVP, LVP, or both muscles were seen. Most commonly, reduced TVP muscle action with decreased excursion of the anterolateral wall was observed. It was unclear if the reduced motion was on the basis of chronic tension or muscular weakness. Theoretically, hypercontraction of either muscle could result in a bulky mass effect that could block the lumen.

Mucosal inflammation of the Eustachian tube lumen and associated structures is commonly seen during video endoscopy. A validated grading scale for Eustachian tube mucosal inflammation coupled with functional impairment of the valve has been developed [39]. This scale is based on the assessment of mucosal inflammation within the nasopharyngeal inlet and Eustachian tube function:

- Grade 1: Normal mucosa and normal dilation.
- Grade 2:Mildly inflamed mucosa, no apparent compromise of dilation. (Mucosa may appear slightly edematous or inflammation may be limited to a small area such as the floor. Vessels are still well seen.)
- Grade 3: Moderately inflamed mucosa, some compromise of dilation. (Mucosa appears edematous or erythematous. There may be significant cobblestoning representing lymphoid hyperplasia. Vessels are no longer sharply seen. A rounded opening of the valve does not occur.)
- Grade 4: Severely inflamed mucosa, unable to dilate open.

The scale can be used as a tool for clinicians in their assessment of mucosal inflammation for comparing future exams during clinical visits.

The most commonly encountered causes of obstructive Eustachian tube dysfunction include inflammatory disease with allergies (environmental and seasonal), adenoid hypertrophy (adenitis), reflux disease and chronic rhinosinusitis are high on the differential diagnosis. Notably, though rare, adults presenting with unilateral otitis media with effusion need to be evaluated for nasopharyngeal neoplasms with nasal endoscopy and possibly imaging for submucosal lesions easily missed on endoscopy. More commonly, adenoid hypertrophy with associated hypertrophy of the torus tubarius (posterior cushion) will cause obstructive Eustachian tube dysfunction in both children and adults. These findings are readily seen on video endoscopy during dynamic examination of the Eustachian tube [33, 34, 39–41]. During a normal swallow, the torus tubarius has a medial rotation action that is impaired in patients with adenoidal hypertrophy impinging on the torus tubarius. As the lateral adenoidal hypertrophy impinges on the torus tubarius from a posterior to an anterior vector, this causes an effective anterior displacement of the torus tubarius (the opposite effect) and effectively obstructs the Eustachian tube lumen. This is termed "anterior thrusting" of the torus tubarius and it is a common cause of obstructive Eustachian tube dysfunction, especially in children. More importantly, it should be recognized during dynamic endoscopic examination of the Eustachian tube (Fig. 34.2). On occasion, intraluminal polyps can be seen in the Eustachian tube that can cause Eustachian tube dysfunction and are easily missed if not directly visualizing the lumen (Fig. 34.3). On the other spectrum of disease, dynamic examination of the Eustachian tube can reveal a widely open tube with a longitudinal concave defect (normally convex) through the length of the valve, most frequently seen in the anterolateral wall, representing a patulous Eustachian tube (Fig. 34.4). This defect usually represents loss of tissue volume from a deficient lateral cartilaginous lamina, Ostmann's fat pad, TVP muscle bulk, submucosa or mucosa.

Risk factors for developing patulous Eustachian tube include associated comorbidities such as environmental allergy (50%), weight loss (35%), laryngopharyngeal reflux (33%) and stress and anxiety (31%) [18]. A recent study using 3-Tesla MRI demonstrated a smaller size of connective tissue surrounding the ET in patients with a patulous Eustachian tube, including the reduction of Ostmann's fat pad [42]. Paradoxically, patients with chronic sinonasal allergic disease can have both inflammation of the Eustachian tube and associated structures while at the same time have intraluminal mucosal atrophy. This combination of mucosal atrophy with surrounding inflammation needs particular attention during dynamic examination. Clinicians should be cognizant that patients with a history of chronic allergic disease with associated obstructive Eustachian tube dysfunction can convert to a patulous state secondary to mucosal atrophy or have alternating states between patulous and dysfunction.

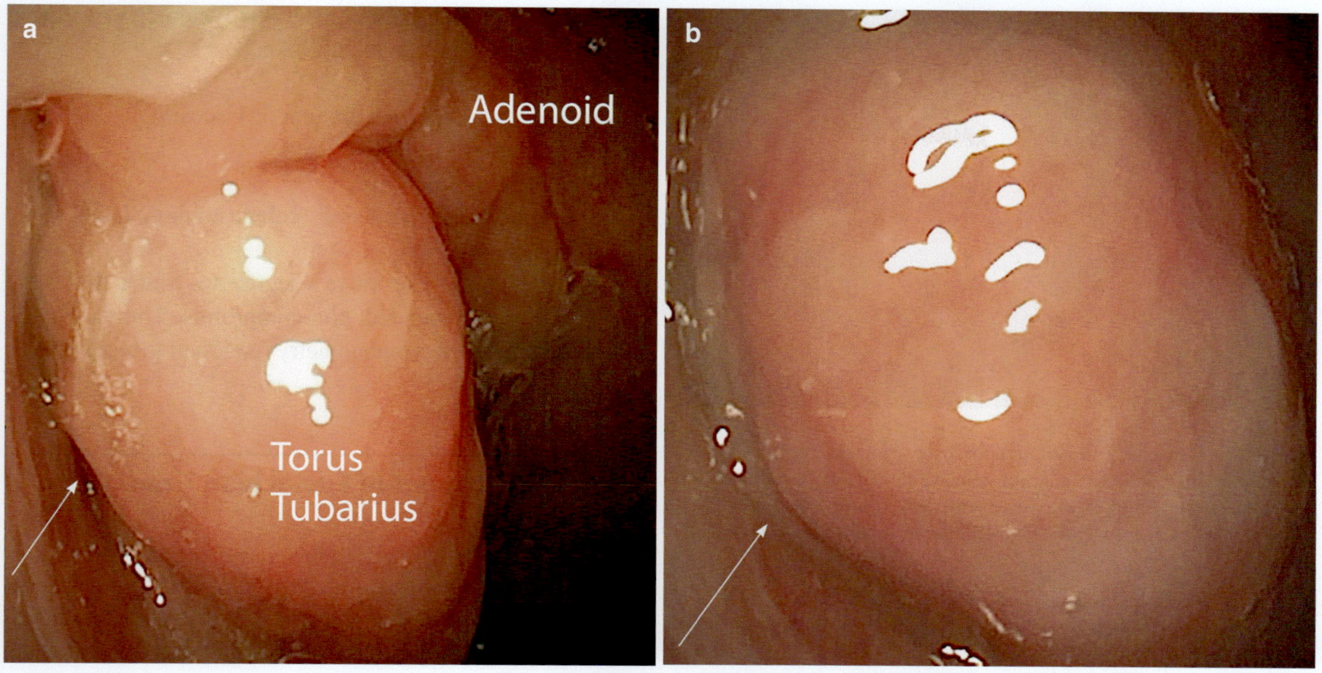

Fig. 34.2 Transnasal, 2.7 mm transnasal chip-tip flexible endoscopic view of adenoid hypertrophy with associated anterior thrusting. (**a**) Residual adenoid postadenoidectomy with hypertrophy impinging on the right Eustachian tube. White arrow indicates tubal lumen. (**b**) During swallowing, anterior thrusting of torus tubarius effectively obstructing the Eustachian tube (white arrow indicates occluded lumen during swallow). (Used with permission from Dennis Poe, MD, who retains copyright of this figure)

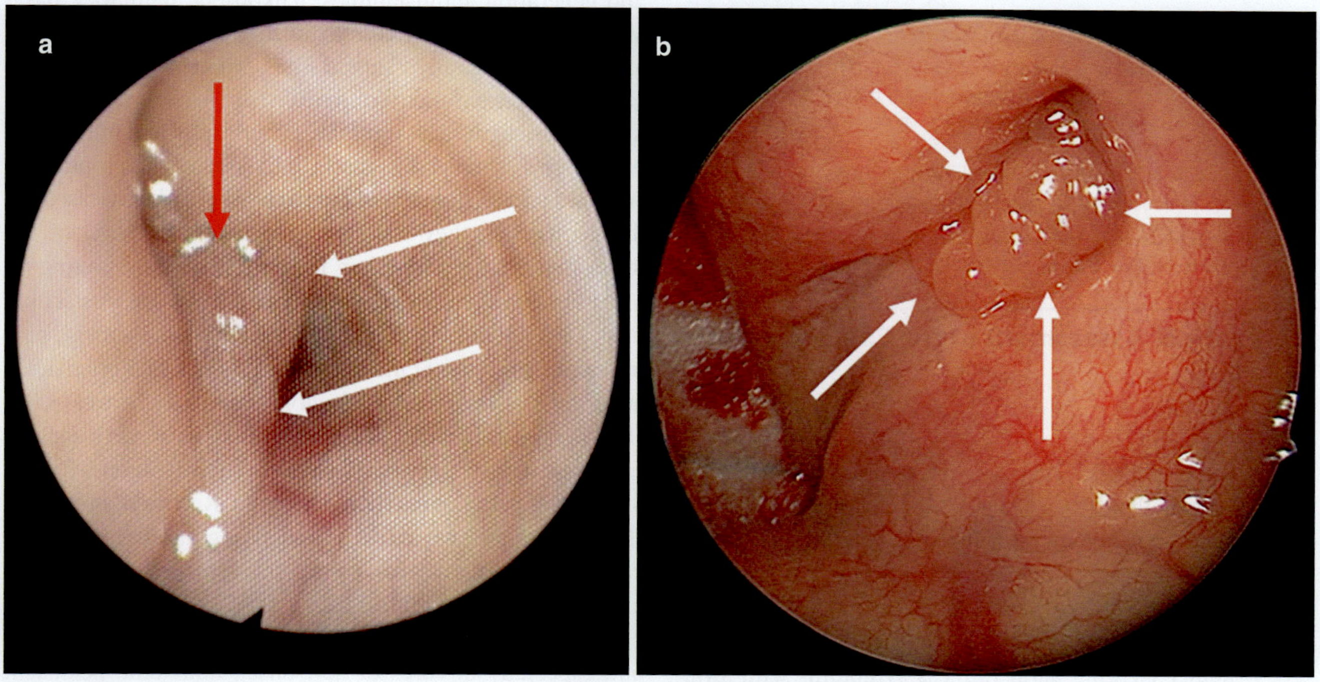

Fig. 34.3 Transnasal, 4 mm, 30 degree Hopkins rod endoscopic image of polyps (white arrows) within left Eustachian tube lumen effectively obstructing the valve

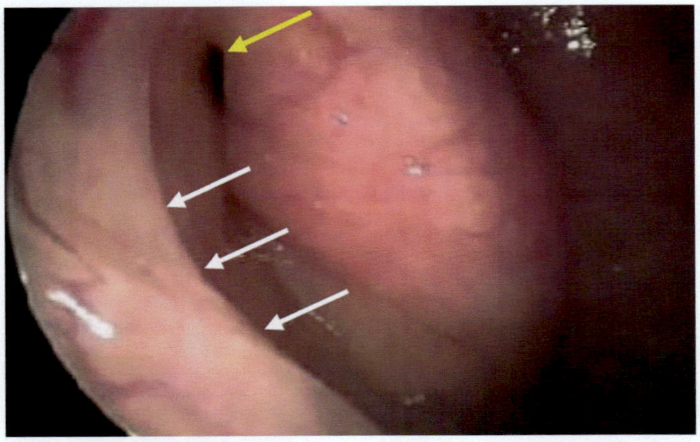

Fig. 34.4 Transnasal flexible endoscopic view of right patulous Eustachian tube. Note the anterior concave defect (white arrows) and the persistent opening of the valve superiorly (yellow arrow). (Used with permission from Dennis Poe, MD, who retains copyright of this figure)

Table 34.2 Differential diagnosis for co-morbidities associated with chronic Eustachian tube dysfunction

Allergic disease
Hypertrophied adenoid contacting torus tubarius
Tubal tonsil adenoid-like tissue compromising dilation
Chronic rhinosinusitis
Laryngopharyngeal reflux (LPR)
Tubal dynamic dysfunction
Pneumonia or chronic pulmonary disease
Primary mucosal disease Immune-deficient/suppressed Samter's (Aspirin sensitivity, Asthma, Nasal polyps) triad Granulomatosis with polyangiitis (GPA) or other granulomatous disease Other middle ear or nasopharyngeal inflammation
Anatomical obstruction with neoplasm or other lesion

Adapted from *Glasscock and Shambaugh's Surgery of the Ear*. 6th Ed. Eds Gulya, Minor, Poe. PMPH. 2010

Summary of Assessment of the Eustachian Tube [16]

1. History
   (a) Aural fullness may occur or be exacerbated by barochallenge
   (b) Hearing loss may be associated with the occurrence of fullness
   (c) May have had otitis media
   (d) Unable to perform a Valsalva maneuver or have difficulty clearing aural fullness symptoms with swallows or yawns
   (e) Autophony of voice or breath raises the possibility of a patulous Eustachian tube
2. Physical
   (a) Otoscopy for evidence of retraction, effusion
   (b) Otoscopy may include insufflation to assess for negative pressure
3. Endoscopy of the Eustachian tube (dynamic exam during swallows, yawns, vocalizing "Ah.")
   (a) MEELO assessment
   (b) Mucus—abnormal amount or viscosity
   (c) Edema
   (d) Erythema
   (e) Lymphoid hyperplasia (cobblestoning, tubal tonsil hypertrophy)
   (f) Opening of the valve (degree to which the valve opens to a rounded, non-compromised lumen)
4. Audiometry and tympanometry (conductive hearing loss, type B or C)

Medical Treatment of Eustachian Tube Dysfunction

Tubal dysfunction is predominantly due to mucosal inflammatory disease, similar to chronic sinusitis or adenoid and tubal tonsil hypertrophy, and can be managed in most cases with medical treatment. Identification of the underlying etiology is critical for success. Symptoms and signs of allergic disease should be thoroughly investigated, including testing and dietary elimination trials as indicated. Environmental measures to minimize exposure to offending allergens, oral 2nd generation antihistamines, leukotriene inhibitors, nasal antihistamines or mast cell stabilizers, nasal steroid sprays, and immunotherapy should be pursued as required. Evaluation for nasal or turbinate disease such as chronic rhinosinusitis, significant turbinate hypertrophy and other nasal pathologies should be made and treated appropriately. Adenoid and tubal tonsil hypertrophy should be assessed for the degree that they interfere with medial rotation of the torus tubarius and whether they may be contributing to inflammation that extends into the lumen of the Eustachian tube. LPR should be treated with dietary management, proton pump inhibitors if indicated, and H_2 blockers or antacids at bedtime as indicated. Refractory cases may be treated by sleeping on an inclined bed, and ultimately, surgery such as fundoplication if necessary. Careful consideration of other underlying pathologies should be done. Recurrent infections should raise the suspicion for underlying nasal or sinus disease, immunosuppression or immunodeficiency, or primary mucosal disorders (Table 34.2).

Anatomical obstruction due to neoplasm should be ruled out, especially in cases of new-onset, unilateral, persistent effusion in an adult. Contrast-enhanced imaging studies are often necessary to recognize nasopharyngeal carcinoma, submucosal lymphoma and other malignancies [43, 44].

Chronic fullness in the ear associated with a normal appearing tympanic membrane, absence of any retraction or effusion, and a normal tympanogram should not be interpreted as obstructive Eustachian tube dysfunction, especially if myringotomy fails to relieve the symptoms. Instead, a search for other causes of fullness, blockage, or otalgia is indicated. Among the differential diagnoses are obstructive Eustachian tube dysfunction, patulous Eustachian tube [18], Menière's disease [45], superior semicircular canal dehiscence [46, 47], temporomandibular disorders (including both temporomandibular joint disease and temporomandibular disorder) [48], conductive hearing loss, and migraine [49] (Fig. 34.5).

Chronic obstructive Eustachian tube dysfunction will cause negative pressure in the middle ear or effusion that should be recognizable on otologic examination and tympanometry (type C or B). An otoscopic examination might reveal a retracted or atelectatic tympanic membrane. An endoscopic examination will reveal evidence of an obstructive problem with mucosal swelling or inflammation, or a dynamic disorder with failure of muscular dilation [33]. If the symptoms of ear blockage only occur with barochallenges, the ear may appear normal or nearly so. However, the consistent pattern of ear fullness or other related complaints limited to rapid changes in ambient pressure, such as with air travel, mountain driving or diving, is important to establish the diagnosis [16]. The lumen of the Eustachian tube will usually show inflammatory disease, but to a limited degree. Most commonly, there will be a hypertrophied or pale edematous band of redundant mucosa seen running longitudinally along the floor of the lumen or along the cartilaginous wall that we term mucosal band. A minimal band in these locations can commonly be seen in normal Eustachian tubes, but when edematous and bulging prominently, it is suspected that this band may compromise the opening of the valve when barochallenged. It is known that divers with normal Eustachian tube function can experience increasing difficulty with clearing their ears over successive dives on the same day, presumably because of edema or swelling for other reasons within the mucosa and/or submucosa from the pressure challenges.

Patulous Eustachian Tube

The clinical diagnosis of a patulous Eustachian tube is made on the basis of the clinical history and pertinent features on physical examination. The diagnosis is certain when medial and lateral excursions of the TM with nasal breathing are observed; however, this is only observed in 82% of patients with a patulous Eustachian tube [18]. Otoscopy should be done with an otoscope or microscope, with the patient seated. The supine position will cause venous congestion within the Eustachian tube and often relieves symptoms temporarily. If the patient does not have autophony at the time of the examination, it may be induced by physical activity. Excursions of the tympanic membrane can be enhanced by closure of the contralateral nostril during ipsilateral nasal breathing. This is the most common means for confirming the diagnosis of a patulous Eustachian tube. However, tympanometry on the reflex decay mode can provide a more sensitive means to detect tympanic membrane impedance synchronous with ipsilateral breathing. Interestingly, many patients with patulous Eustachian tubes resort to frequent sniffing to try to control their symptoms as this maneuver creates negative pressure within the lumen that can pull the mucosal walls of the valve into a closed position, temporarily resolving their symptoms. Clinicians have referred to this common practice as "habitual sniffing," but it is not truly habitual as it is being done in response to autophony symptoms. Sniffing can generate excessive negative pressure that may cause significant tympanic membrane retraction, middle ear effusion, fixed retraction pockets and ultimately even cholesteatoma [50]. Clinicians should be aware that this does not represent a diagnosis of obstructive Eustachian tube dysfunction, but rather, of patulous Eustachian tube. Patulous Eustachian tube is likely underdiagnosed due to this scenario of negative pressure, with sequelae being interpreted as obstructive ETD. When a patient has evidence of negative pressure in the middle ear (e.g., non-adherent retraction or tympanometry measurement) and is observed to be frequently sniffing, a maneuver that would be expected to exacerbate the negative pressure, this "inappropriate sniffing" is highly suspicious of a patulous Eustachian tube.

Otic Capsule Dehiscence Syndrome

Minor's syndrome, also called otic capsule dehiscence syndrome [51], is most commonly due to superior semicircular canal dehiscence (SSCD) and should also be considered in the differential diagnosis of aural fullness and autophony [52]. Minor's syndrome can present with surprisingly similar symptoms as patulous Eustachian tube dysfunction, particularly with a sense of a blocked ear and autophony of the voice, but the autophony of breathing sounds is much more pronounced with a patulous Eustachian tube [53]. Differential diagnosis is made more challenging because Minor's syndrome may also present without vestibular symptoms and without conductive hearing loss [54]. The diagnosis is confirmed by demonstration of a bony dehiscence with high-resolution temporal bone scan (best recognized in the reconstructed Poschel and Stenvers planes), decreased thresholds on cervical vestibular evoked myogenic potential testing (cVEMP) or higher-than-normal amplitudes with ocular oVEMP. The recording of otoacoustic emission or stapedial reflexes in the presence of a conductive hearing

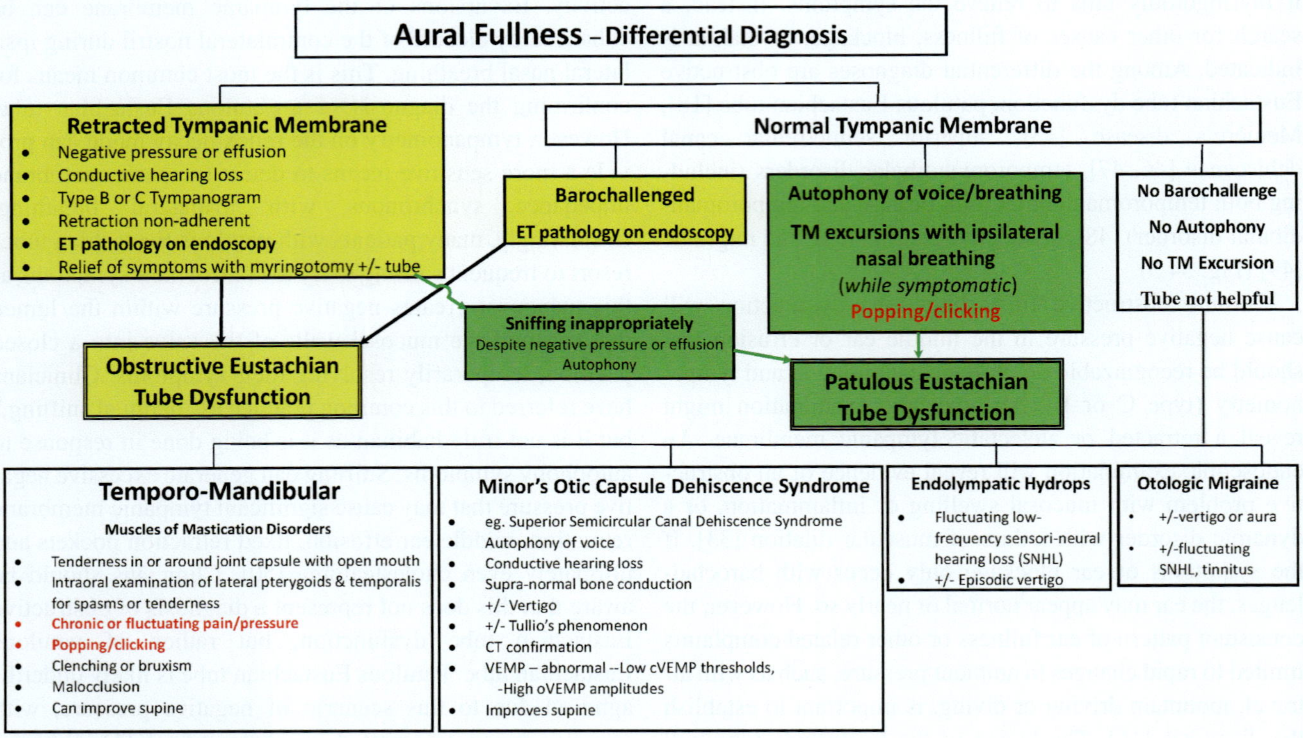

Fig. 34.5 Differential diagnosis for aural fullness. (Used with permission from Dennis Poe, MD, who retains copyright of this figure)

loss can also lead to an inner rather than middle ear source of an air-bone gap on audiometry.

Temporomandibular Disorders

Patients with aural fullness complaints but normal otoscopic exams should also be asked about and evaluated for temporomandibular disorders (TMD), including the temporomandibular joint (TMJ) and disorders involving the muscles of mastication. These disorders can cause symptoms that are erroneously attributed to obstructive Eustachian tube dysfunction. The joint capsule is examined with the patient's mouth open as wide as is comfortable, and the space between the condyle and the glenoid fossa is palpated deeply, looking for unusual tenderness, subluxation or crepitus. The patient then moves their open mandible to the right and left sides to allow for repeating the palpation for areas of tenderness, especially superiorly and posteriorly to the condyle. Deep gentle palpation is made in the temporalis and masseter muscles surrounding the TMJ, examining for spasms (palpated as a firm muscle cord), tension, hypertrophy or tenderness. Bimanual intraoral and extraoral examination is done to inspect for the same findings. The examiner's index finger is passed posteriorly into the oral cavity to locate the anterior edge of the mandibular ramus. Palpating bimanually, lateral to the ramus, the masseter muscle is thoroughly examined. Of particular importance is palpation along the origin of the muscle along the inferior border of the zygomatic arch and the normally slightly firm anterior edge of the muscle. The finger is then directed medial to the ramus and superiorly into the pterygoid space to access the insertions of the temporalis and lateral pterygoid muscle onto the coronoid process of the mandible. Some portions of the medial pterygoid may also be accessible with this palpation. If a patient does not endorse ear pain during the office visit, it is possible that no findings will be made, so the patient is coached in how to do a self-exam in the event of future episodes.

Surgical Management of Obstructive Eustachian Tube Dysfunction

Medical management is offered when a suspected underlying etiology is revealed during the work-up, but generic medical management in the absence of relevant co-morbidities has not been shown to be beneficial [16, 55]. When obstructive ETD persists chronically and if appropriate, adequate medical management has failed to resolve the dysfunction, surgical intervention may be indicated.

Tympanostomy tubes remain the principal procedure used for management of obstructive dysfunction. A myringotomy or tube is expected to relieve the symptoms as long as there is a patent opening in the tympanic membrane. However, should the symptoms and signs return after closure of the perforation, the patient may be offered a repeat procedure or an alternative. The alternative procedures may also be indicated without prior myringotomy, and with or without a tube in place [16], but failure of a tube to resolve chronic obstructive dysfunction is the most common indication for alternative procedures in our practice.

Obstructive ETD is usually due to inflammatory disease within the lumen of the cartilaginous Eustachian tube, and it is commonly associated with inflammation in other parts of the nasal cavity, sinuses, adenoid or tubal tonsil tissue on the torus tubarius of the Eustachian tubes. Nasal, turbinate, sinus surgery, adenoidectomy (including the lateral portion against or near the torus tubarius) may be indicated, depending on the pathology.

Lateral Adenoidectomy

Functional obstruction due to hypertrophic adenoid or tubal tonsil (adenoid-like tissue on the torus tubarius) that interferes with tubal dilation can be excised using monopolar suction cautery. The most common indication for this procedure is the observation of adenoid or tubal tonsil tissue preventing adequate opening of the valve of the Eustachian tube during swallows or yawns. In the more severe cases, swallowing produces compression of the torus tubarius between the adenoid and the lateral pharyngeal wall that forces the torus anteriorly to temporarily obstruct the tubal orifice at the time when the valve should be opening. Termed “anterior thrusting of the torus tubarius,” this functional obstruction is a very common cause of obstructive ETD and should be addressed in addition to considerations to treat the lumen and valve of the cartilaginous Eustachian tube. There may also be a benefit to reducing the burden of inflammation in the tissues adjacent to the Eustachian tube, even if it does not appear to be directly impairing the opening of the valve. Excision of the lateral portion of the adenoid can be accomplished with careful technique, avoiding entry into the Fossa of Rosenmüller as the internal carotid artery lies at the apex of the Fossa. Excision can be done with precision by viewing with an angled endoscope through the nasal cavity and passing the suction cautery through the mouth. The tubal tonsil (adenoid-like) tissue on the medial half of the torus tubarius may be trimmed down gently with the cautery set to low wattage. Cautery should be limited to only the medial ½ of the torus tubarius to avoid potential scarring within the lumen.

Balloon Dilation of the Cartilaginous Segment of the Eustachian Tube

Balloon dilation of the cartilaginous segment of the Eustachian tube through a transnasal endoscopic approach has gained popularity among other surgical techniques, such as laser or microdebrider, for the treatment of chronic obstructive Eustachian tube dysfunction. Kivekäs and colleagues conducted a histopathology study on the effect of balloon dilation on the mucosa of the cartilaginous Eustachian tube in patients with bilateral Eustachian tube dysfunction [56]. Biopsies taken before and directly after balloon dilation showed excoriation of the inflamed epithelium that left the basal layer intact and a “crushing” effect on the submucosal inflammatory infiltrate with flattening of lymphoid follicles. In the same study, biopsies taken at 5–12 weeks postoperatively in a subset of cases showed replacement of the crushed lymphocytic infiltrate and follicles by thin healthy fibrosis, absence of follicles and restoration of normal ciliated pseudo-columnar epithelium. Thus, balloon dilation demonstrated histological changes similar to those observed with adenoidectomy, removing possibly irreversibly inflamed epithelium and submucosa, and reducing inflammation, which may account for the reports of durable long-term results [57]. The concept of balloon dilation may be thought of as analogous to adenoidectomy in that it involves the removal of inflamed mucosa, submucosa and adenoid-like tissue from within the lumen of the Eustachian tube. As obstructive ETD often occurs in association with other diseases within the nasal cavity, sinuses, nasopharynx and adenoid, adjunctive procedures to address those issues may be indicated. When inflammation seen within the lumen of the Eustachian tube appears to be contributing to chronic obstructive ETD, balloon dilation of the Eustachian tube (BDET) may be indicated.

BDET or transnasal endoscopic balloon dilation of the cartilaginous portion has become an important approach for surgical therapy of obstructive Eustachian tube dysfunction as there is substantial accumulating evidence for efficacy, safety and durability of the procedure [57–68]. Systematic reviews and meta-analyses of studies have consistently shown improvements in multiple different assessments of Eustachian tube function after balloon dilation including: otoscopic findings (e.g., improvement in retraction of the tympanic membrane), ability to perform a Valsalva maneuver, improvement in tympanogram, reduction of mucosal inflammation within the lumen of the Eustachian tube, improvement of the validated Eustachian Tube Dysfunction Questionnaire (ETDQ-7) or other symptom scores, and tubomanometry measurements. Reported success rates ranged from 50% to 97% for the various outcomes [61–65, 68]. Significant reductions in Eustachian tube opening pressures have been demonstrated [69]. All of the studies with a mean follow-up of two or more years have shown the durability of the results [57, 65, 66, 70].

Two randomized, controlled, multicentered clinical trials have been done comparing BDET with medical management in adults. Both found statistically significant improvement in tympanograms and ETDQ-7 scores when comparing BDET with ongoing topical nasal steroid medical vs the same medical management alone at six-week follow-up [71, 72]. The first of these two FDA-mandated trials required subjects to have chronic type B or C tympanograms when entering the trial, having failed prior medical management. They were randomized to the treatment or control group and both were maintained on nasal steroids for 6 weeks. At 6 weeks a normal tympanogram (type A) was observed in 51.8% (72/139) of balloon dilation subjects vs 13.9% (10/72) of controls undergoing medical management alone [71]. Normalization of scores on ETDQ-7 was similar, with 56.2% (77/137) in the balloon dilation group vs 8.5% (6/71) in the control group. Subjects from the control group in both studies were allowed to cross over after 6 weeks, and the durability of the results in the original treatment groups was followed for 12 months in the first study [73] or beyond (mean 29 months) in the second study [70], showing durability of the results.

Another randomized-controlled trial was conducted on patients with chronic otitis media with effusion and compared the efficacy of BDET alone vs BDET with paracentesis vs paracentesis alone, with 30 subjects in each group. At one-month follow-up, endoscopic otoscopy results were better in the BDET plus paracentesis than in the BDET alone, but tympanogram results were similar. At 6 months, conversion of type B tympanograms to C or A was significantly improved in BDET alone (86.7%) and BDET plus tympanocentesis (93.3%) compared to tympanocentesis alone, which showed no significant conversion (13.4%). The authors concluded that BDET plus paracentesis may shorten the recovery period for middle ear effusion and BDET with or without paracentesis was superior to paracentesis alone in six-month results [74].

Transtympanic approaches to introduce the balloon into the cartilaginous Eustachian tube have recently been described [75–77]; however, these are not widely performed and more importantly there are no commercially available devices designed specifically for the transtympanic approach.

Balloon dilation of the bony Eustachian tube is contraindicated as the cartilaginous Eustachian tube is the most common location of inflammatory pathology [30, 78] and dilation of the bony portion carries significant risk of injury to the internal carotid artery [58].

Indications for BDET are provided in Table 34.3.

Table 34.3 Indications for balloon dilation of the cartilaginous Eustachian tube

Chronic (≥3 months) obstructive Eustachian tube dysfunction as evidenced by at least one of the following:
Barochallenge (difficulty equilibrating pressure in ears with large ambient changes)
Hearing loss or aural fullness that is relieved by auto-insufflation (after ruling out flaccid tympanic membrane or laxity in the ossicular chain as the cause of symptoms)
History of negative pressure in the middle ear or middle ear effusion
Additionally, it is generally recommended that all of the following be met:
If a potentially causal co-morbidity is present (e.g., allergic rhinitis, rhinosinusitis, and laryngopharyngeal reflux), failure to respond to appropriate medical management (e.g., 4-week trial of nasal steroid spray for allergic rhinitis, 4-week trial of antacid or proton-pump inhibitor for reflux).
Nasal endoscopy (dynamic exam, including swallows and yawns) has been performed. Findings may include pathological changes within the lumen of the Eustachian tube, but in the absence of findings, history and physical remain consistent with obstruction within the cartilaginous Eustachian tube.
If a tympanostomy tube was previously placed, it improved symptoms while patent. However, a trial of tubes is not a requirement.

Stepwise Description of Balloon Dilation of the Eustachian Tube (BDET)

The procedure is performed under local or general anesthesia and after having decongested both nasal cavities with topical oxymetazoline (Fig. 34.6). In-office anesthesia requires proper patient selection and pre-procedure medication. Dean and Pynnonen [79] published a protocol for topical anesthesia following initial placement of topical intranasal oxymetazoline. Five drops of compounded 7% tetracaine/7% lidocaine solution are placed onto the tympanic membrane in the event that some backpressure is generated during insertion of the balloon, which has been shown to be a source of discomfort [80]. Two cottonoids are then placed onto the nasal floors bilaterally and left for about 10 minutes. Approximately 0.5 ml of compounded 7% tetracaine/7% lidocaine cream is then placed into the orifice of the Eustachian tube(s), and the tetracaine-soaked cottonoids along the nasal floor are replaced and left for another 10–15 minutes. Under general anesthesia, topical oxymetazoline is placed intranasally.

Once adequately anesthetized, the nasal cavity, nasopharynx and Eustachian tubes are examined with a 0°, 4 mm diameter Hopkins rod endoscope (Karl Storz, El Segundo, CA, USA). The authors use the Acclarent balloon device (Acclarent corp., Irvine, CA, USA). The balloon is inserted into the 55° angled guide catheter, allowing the blue bulb tip to just protrude from the tip of the guide catheter. The guide and balloon are gently introduced through the nasal cavity under direct endoscopic guidance, making sure to avoid any mucosal injury that would cause bleeding and impair the view as the blood tends to drain over the Eustachian tube orifice. A 30 or 45° view with an angled endoscope is preferred in order to directly see the anterolateral wall, which leads to the lumen.

If the anatomy is favorable, the guide catheter and endoscope can be passed via the same nasal passage, or if the

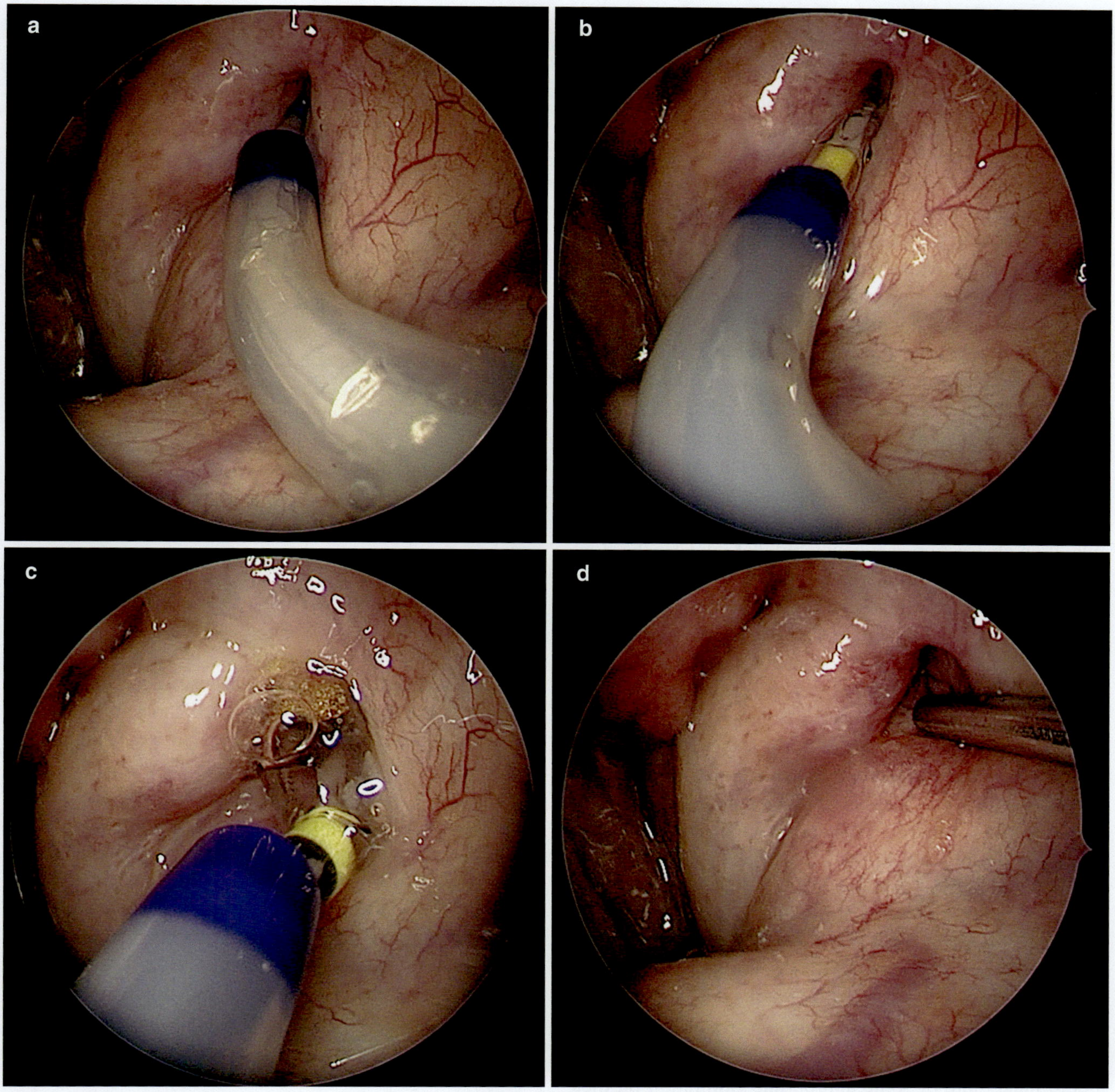

Fig. 34.6 Transnasal intraoperative endoscopic views showing balloon dilation of the left Eustachian tube using a 30° Hopkins rod. (**a**) The guide catheter is gently advanced past the inferior turbinate making sure to avoid any bleeding and inserted into the Eustachian tube. (**b**) The balloon is deployed and advanced through the catheter guide until resistance is met, and the yellow mark is at the entrance of the lumen. (**c**) The balloon is inflated under direct visualization to 12 atmospheres for up to 2 minutes. (**d**) The balloon is deflated and reinserted into the guide catheter. Inspection of the lumen is performed to evaluate for any mucosal lacerations or tears. (Used with permission from Dennis Poe, MD, who retains copyright of this figure)

nasal cavity is limited, a 45° endoscope passed through the contralateral nasal passage will usually view the lumen adequately from across the vomer. When both instruments are inserted through the same nasal cavity, the guide catheter containing the balloon is kept against the floor of the cavity and the endoscope is maintained in close contact with the guide, directly along its superior surface. The endoscope should be kept in longitudinal contact with the guide catheter, avoiding opening up an angle between the two devices as this results in uncontrolled displacement of the tips of the guide/balloon catheter and endoscope ("sword-fighting").

Upon reaching the orifice of the Eustachian tube, the guide catheter can remain on the floor of the nasal cavity, merely rotating the tip of the guide catheter to point into the lumen of the Eustachian tube. The balloon catheter is then advanced into the lumen, guiding the tip slowly and smoothly along the anterolateral wall to avoid a false passage. The lumen begins from the orifice just inside the anterior pillar and follows the anterolateral wall, passing initially in a medial direction before curving laterally toward the temporal bone. Inserting the balloon along the postero-medial wall (along the luminal side of the torus tubarius) directs the balloon catheter into the membranous anterolateral wall, missing the curvature of the lumen and risking laceration or penetration with false passage. The membranous wall is very thin and surgeons do not notice tactile feedback when a false passage has occurred. Following the anterolateral wall under direct view with an angled endoscope and with slow, smooth, non-forceful insertion will avoid the false passage issue.

At the point that the catheter reaches the laterally directed curvature of the lumen, it will pass out of sight, but the cartilaginous skeleton becomes increasingly circumferential, helping to guide the balloon superiorly up toward the isthmus. If an obstruction is encountered that impedes the slow, careful insertion, it may represent the tip catching on a mucosal fold. The balloon can be partially withdrawn and reinserted at a slightly altered angle, which will usually allow for passage. The balloon catheter should never be forcefully inserted or false passage can easily occur. Eventually, the tip of the balloon catheter will contact the isthmus, adding some resistance to the insertion. To confirm that the resistance corresponds to the isthmus and not a premature mucosal fold, there is a yellow mark on the catheter 31 mm from the tip of the Acclarent system. As the average length of an adult cartilaginous Eustachian tube is approximately 25 mm [15], the yellow mark will usually rest about 5 mm outside of the lumen of the Eustachian tube, situated approximately at the level of the anterior pillar. The yellow mark should never be allowed to pass into the lumen of the Eustachian tube in a normal sized adult as the balloon may pass into the bony portion, placing the internal carotid artery at risk. For balloon catheters that lack such a mark, surgeons should make note of some appropriate calibration on their device in order to avoid entry into the bony portion of the Eustachian tube [16]. Once in position, the balloon is inflated with saline to between 10 and 12 atmospheres for a duration typically of 2 minutes, but a shorter duration is done for lesser inflammatory disease to avoid creating a patulous Eustachian tube. For example, barochallenged Eustachian tube dysfunction may have limited pathology and 60 or 90 seconds of inflation time may be sufficient. As the balloon inflates, its tendency is to extrude from the Eustachian tube lumen. This can be prevented by bracing the guide catheter against the floor of the nasal cavity and maintaining alignment between the guide and balloon catheters. The pressure is slowly increased to 2 atm and is then stopped to check that the guide is on the floor and that the alignment is correct. Pressure is then increased to 12 atm, no faster than one atm increase in pressure per second. Excessively rapid inflation can induce profound bradycardia and, in awake patients, may cause pain. Once inflated, the balloon may protrude approximately $\frac{1}{4}$ to $\frac{1}{3}$ of its length out of the lumen. This is normal and expected. If it extrudes excessively, it can be withdrawn and a repeat dilation performed. After the allotted time, the balloon is then deflated, withdrawn into the guide catheter to prevent further excoriation of the mucosa, and the balloon and guide catheters are gently removed together. The lumen is inspected for mucosal injuries. If indicated, the procedure is repeated on the contralateral side.

Concurrent myringotomy with paracentesis, insertion of a tympanostomy tube or adenoidectomy/lateral adenoidectomy, can be performed if indicated. Generally, if there is a complete middle ear effusion, we tend to do a paracentesis or insertion of a submillimeter-sized tube.

Postoperative Instructions

Patients are instructed postoperatively to avoid nose-blowing for 1 week to avoid passing air into an unsuspected mucosal tear or false passage. There are no other restrictions in activities or precautions necessary, and antibiotics are not required, unless such measures are indicated due to adjunctive procedures. Nasal humidity (saline nasal products) can be suggested as desired.

After 1 week, patients are asked to perform a modified Valsalva maneuver several times daily (up to once hourly while awake) during the first month or until the Eustachian tube is felt to be passing air ("ear popping") spontaneously with swallows or yawns. All patients are taught the modified Valsalva maneuver (nose and mouth closed, gentle nose blow to elevate intranasal pressure and simultaneous swallow). Generally, a candidate for BDET is unable to perform this maneuver preoperatively, but should be able to do it postoperatively. The maneuver should become easier to perform as reactive swelling from the procedure subsides during the first 4–6 weeks [82]. Early aeration through the Eustachian tube may be beneficial in avoiding the accumulation of negative pressure within the middle ear that could make it increasingly difficult to open the lumen [57].

It is very important for patients with associated co-morbidities to maintain good medical control of their conditions in order to enjoy long-term success. BDET can reduce the inflammatory burden [56], but it will not protect against co-morbidities such as allergic rhinitis or laryngopharyngeal reflux from inciting inflammation again over time. Similar to adenoidectomy, the procedure gives patients a fresh start, but regrowth of disease is possible if underlying medical conditions are not controlled.

Complications and Pitfalls

1. Intraoperative bleeding—This is usually due to mucosal lacerations or false passage. If it does not stop spontaneously, control can be gained with topical oxymetazoline-soaked pledgets.
2. False passage—Inspection of the lumen is done after the dilation to make sure that a false passage has not occurred. In the event that false passage is recognized after inflation of the balloon has occurred, presumably within the false passage, repeat dilation can be done, being careful to ensure that the balloon is properly inserted into the lumen of the Eustachian tube. Passage of a catheter deep into a false passage brings the tip into increasingly close proximity to the extracranial internal carotid artery.
3. Subcutaneous emphysema and pneumomediastinum—This is a rare complication that may occur if a patient performs a nose blow or Valsalva maneuver within the first few days after BDET and is likely due to air passing into a mucosal laceration or false passage. Cases reported to date have been resolved without any necessity for treatment. Avoidance of nose blowing or Valsalva maneuver during the first week postoperatively is recommended for all patients [71, 83, 84].
4. Patulous Eustachian tube—Autophony of voice and breathing sounds has occurred in the early days postoperatively in some patients, and it is generally mild, intermittent, and self-limited, resolving within days or weeks. Patients aged 20 years and under seem to be more prone to patulous symptoms and our practice now limits the duration of inflation to no more than 90 seconds in that group. In the one-year follow-up study from the first randomized controlled trial, 2 of 143 subjects (1.4%) who had BDET developed mild autophony symptoms, one of which had resolved by the end of the study [73]. Patulous Eustachian tube can occur if BDET is performed on a patient with symptoms of aural fullness, but no evidence of obstructive ETD, signifying that another differential diagnosis is probable. Careful assessment of the history and a complete assessment for evidence of obstructive ETD is important to establish an accurate diagnosis [16]. If a patient has ever experienced autophony symptoms, which is especially common in chronic allergic rhinitis, there is an increased risk of postoperative patulous Eustachian tube. If BDET remains indicated in such a patient, a reduced balloon inflation time may be considered. It is better to undertreat and risk the need for repeat balloon dilation in the future than to cause a patulous Eustachian tube, which can be very bothersome to the patient and may not be easy to treat should it persist.
5. Synechia—There have been no reports of significant synechia or increased obstruction of the Eustachian tube after BDET. Careful attention to passing the balloon along the anterolateral wall with a slow, gentle insertion should avoid this issue.
6. Injury to the internal carotid artery—There have been no reports of such injuries. Avoidance of entry of the balloon catheter into the bony Eustachian tube should be preventive. There is an FDA recommendation for obtaining a preoperative computed tomography (CT) scan to look for possible dehiscence of the internal carotid artery into the lumen of the bony portion of the Eustachian tube. However, with careful technique to gently insert the balloon, stopping when contact is made with the isthmus and monitoring of an appropriate distance mark on the catheter, ensuring that it does not pass into the lumen of the bony Eustachian tube, the procedure can be safely performed. Surgeons may weigh the risks, benefits and potential for other diagnostic information when deciding when a CT may be appropriate for their particular patient.

Balloon Dilation of the Eustachian Tube in Pediatric Patients

There have been some retrospective series of children undergoing balloon dilation of the Eustachian tube [85–87]. A recent study compared a retrospective case series of children with two or more prior tympanostomy tubes and adenoidectomy who underwent BDET, along with placement of a submillimeter tube, in comparison to a matched-controlled group who had an additional tube placed. The treatment group showed a significant reduction in recurrence of middle ear effusion and subsequent tympanostomy tube placement [88]. The etiology of Eustachian tube dysfunction in children includes swelling of the mucosa or bulky tubal tonsil tissue around the nasopharyngeal orifice and lumen of the Eustachian tube, presence of bulky adenoid tissue in contact with the torus tubarius, and unfavorable anatomy characteristic in pediatric patients. Additionally, reflux of nasopharyngeal material and pathogens is a possible mechanism for obstructive dysfunction in younger children, raising the question as to whether dilation could exacerbate that process, which may be a cause of recurrent acute otitis media. Tympanostomy tubes remain the gold standard treatment for otitis media with effusion in children. However, early results with dilation in the pediatric population are encouraging and safety has been consistent. Additional research is needed to establish the efficacy and indications of balloon dilation in children with obstructive Eustachian tube dysfunction.

Obstructive Eustachian Tube Dysfunction Due to Pathology Within the Bony Portion

One study has estimated that 10% of cases of obstructive ETD may involve pathology within the bony portion of the Eustachian tube [57]. Soft tissue lesions within the bony portion may be suspected in cases of refractory otitis media with effusion that repeatedly recurs promptly after extrusion of a tympanostomy tube. It may be recognized on a CT scan while the middle ear is aerated with a tympanostomy tube in place. An optimal treatment for such soft tissue strictures or obstructions has not yet been developed. If accessible from the middle ear, removal may be possible using conventional microsurgical techniques. If a CT shows no evidence of dehiscence of the internal carotid artery, passing of a guidewire through a stricture has been done in an off-label use of sinus guidewires and it has been shown to benefit some of these patients. However, these patients tend not to enjoy as high a likelihood of success [57, 89]. Any dehiscence of the internal carotid artery is an absolute contraindication for this procedure, and preoperative CT is necessary to make this assessment.

Treatment of the Patulous Eustachian Tube

The main treatment objective for a patulous Eustachian tube is to reduce the abnormally wide diameter of the Eustachian tube lumen to reestablish a more competent functional valve. Conservative measures to treat a patulous Eustachian tube are first attempted before invasive procedures; thus, a stepwise approach is warranted. In fact, many patients will only require counseling and reassurance once they are informed that, despite the disturbing nature of the symptoms in some patients, the disorder causes no physiological injury. The specific trigger causing a patulous Eustachian tube should be determined, if possible, and treated accordingly. Initial treatment starts with the avoidance of triggers and behaviors that worsen symptoms. Conservative measures include discontinuing decongestants and limiting topical nasal steroids, caffeinated drinks and diuretics [53, 90]. Patients are advised to observe good hydration and to use nasal saline drops instead of sprays as they are more effective. Medications used to thicken the nasal mucosa may be effective, and these include topical estrogen drops (off-label use) and topical irritants [91, 92]. These medications must be applied properly, however, and are best administered by asking the patient to lie supine with their head hanging 15° and rotated toward the side being treated. The drops are applied in the ipsilateral nostril. In this position, gravity directs the drops to the orifice of the Eustachian tube. When the drops contact the Eustachian tube mucosa, patients should report a tickle or twinge sensation radiating to their ear. However, patients are counseled that, even though they feel the sensation in their ear, the solution is not actually entering the middle ear. A burning sensation is very common and mostly tolerated by the patients. Hypertonic saline or preparations of ascorbic acid may also be effective in alleviating the patulous symptoms. The relief may be temporary and of variable duration [93]. Consistent use of drops (3–4 drops, 2–3 times daily) for a two-month period may induce a lasting benefit in many patients. Surgery may be indicated in the event of failure of such a trial.

When patients do not improve with conservative measures, treatment is directed toward augmenting the periluminal tissue or targeting the tympanic membrane. Myringotomy with the placement of tympanostomy tubes is perhaps the most common surgical intervention, and it has been reported to aid some 50% of patients [94]. However, many patients complain of unpleasant auditory symptoms with a tube in place and may request removal of the tube if it has not helped relieve their autophony. Tympanostomy tubes may be more likely to alleviate symptoms related to middle ear pressure changes and tympanic membrane excursions, but less so for the reflux of sound [95]. Mass-loading of the tympanic membrane by placing paper patches [96], some topical ointment or Blu-Tack [97] on the posterior tympanic membrane changes its resonance qualities and has been found to provide various degrees of relief of patulous Eustachian tube symptoms. If a substantial degree of relief is attained with these transient measures, it may be prognostic that mass loading with a tympanostomy tube or cartilage graft tympanoplasty may be beneficial. In patients with floppy tympanic membrane, cartilage reinforcement of the flaccid segment significantly reduced symptoms of patulous Eustachian tube (autophony, breath sounds, and aural fullness) [98].

Another option involves insertion of an intravenous catheter into the full length of the Eustachian tube (cartilaginous and bony portions), in an off-label use (not-FDA-approved), as a shim into the tubal lumen to fill the concave defect. The use of a catheter, filled with bone wax, to block the Eustachian tube was originally described by Bluestone and others [90, 99, 100], who engaged it from the middle ear orifice and sealed the Eustachian tube around the catheter with bone wax. In a distinction of the Bluestone technique, a catheter is trimmed to the approximate length of the entire Eustachian tube and inserted transnasally so that it will become wedged into the isthmus, the narrowest segment of the Eustachian tube, to secure it in place. The flexible catheter will tend to rest within the concave defect and restore the ability of the valve to fully close. Ideally, the catheter will not entirely occlude the lumen of the Eustachian tube.

The catheter is inserted in a similar fashion to the balloon dilation described above. The nasal cavity is decongested and a Boyle-Davis gag is gently positioned. A soft red catheter is passed through the contralateral nasal passage to retract the soft palate. The nasopharynx is viewed with a

45-degree rigid telescope, introduced through the ipsilateral naris. A radio-opaque intravenous catheter, most commonly 14- or sometimes 16-gauge (2.1 or 1.7 mm diameter), is arranged. Melted bone wax (melting point is 60 °C) is drawn up into the catheter and allowed to cool. The tip is preserved and it is cut to lengths of 38–40 mm in females, 40–42 mm in males, estimated by the size of the patient's head and by the CT scan. A preoperative CT is necessary to rule out dehiscence of the internal carotid artery (ICA) into the bony Eustachian tube, which is an absolute contraindication for the procedure. The catheter is loaded into a piston-like Eustachian tube introducer (Karl Storz, El Segundo, CA, USA) so that the tip will enter the Eustachian tube orifice first. When needed, it can be maintained in place in the introducer by a small piece of bone wax protruding from the catheter that can adhere to the piston. The introducer with the catheter is passed through the oral cavity and is brought into proximity to the nasopharyngeal orifice of the Eustachian tube, under direct visualization. The Eustachian tube lumen is significantly curved, initially taking a medial course before turning laterally toward the bony Eustachian tube and the temporal bone. Accordingly, the introducer is aligned tangentially with the anterolateral wall which reliably follows the curvature of the lumen, similar to the manner of inserting a balloon catheter. Occasionally, it is necessary to medially rotate the torus tubarius to facilitate a gentle insertion. There is a natural propensity for surgeons to want to align the introducer with the torus tubarius due to its recognizable landmark, but this action steers the catheter straight into the anterolateral wall, risking mucosal laceration, which can cause a false passage. Under direct endoscopic view into the longitudinal axis of the lumen, the catheter is gently inserted slowly and smoothly through the lumen of the Eustachian tube until the engagement of the catheter into the isthmus is felt as some increased resistance. This is different from the balloon dilation, where the tip of the balloon should not enter the bony segment of the Eustachian tube. The catheter should be approximately two-thirds inserted by the time it engages the isthmus. If resistance is met earlier, the catheter may be caught in the anterolateral mucosa, in which case, it should be withdrawn and reinserted at a different angle. If it appears to be in a good position and the insertion has been smooth, the catheter is then wedged through the isthmus until the cut, proximal end of the catheter lies just within the fold of the anterior pillar, which lies at the orifice of the anterolateral wall (Fig. 34.7).

Otoscopy is performed at the end of the procedure, with a microscope or a 0-degree endoscope, to ascertain that the catheter is not at all visible within the middle ear. If it is seen within the middle ear, the catheter is withdrawn further into the nasopharynx, but making sure it is still wedged into the bony segment of the Eustachian tube. The catheter should protrude slightly from the nasopharyngeal orifice, but should not impinge into the palate, which elevates during speaking and swallowing. Ideally, the catheter will lie just inside the anterior pillar. Postoperative instructions include avoidance of nose blowing for 1 week as subcutaneous emphysema could result if an unsuspected mucosal laceration were to be present. If needed, they may irrigate the nose with saline. There are no restrictions on activities.

Otitis media with effusion (OME) occurred in 52% of our patients and tympanostomy tube may be offered concurrently with the shim procedure [93]. Rotenberg and Davidson have reported using a similar technique [101]. Rather than using an IV catheter, their shim was composed of a 19-gauge semirigid rubberized irrigation catheter, trimmed to 35 mm in length. The lumen of the catheter was similarly filled with melted bone wax. The catheter was anchored to the anterior cushion of the ET with a suture. Seven patients were operated on, and none had middle ear effusion or spontaneous

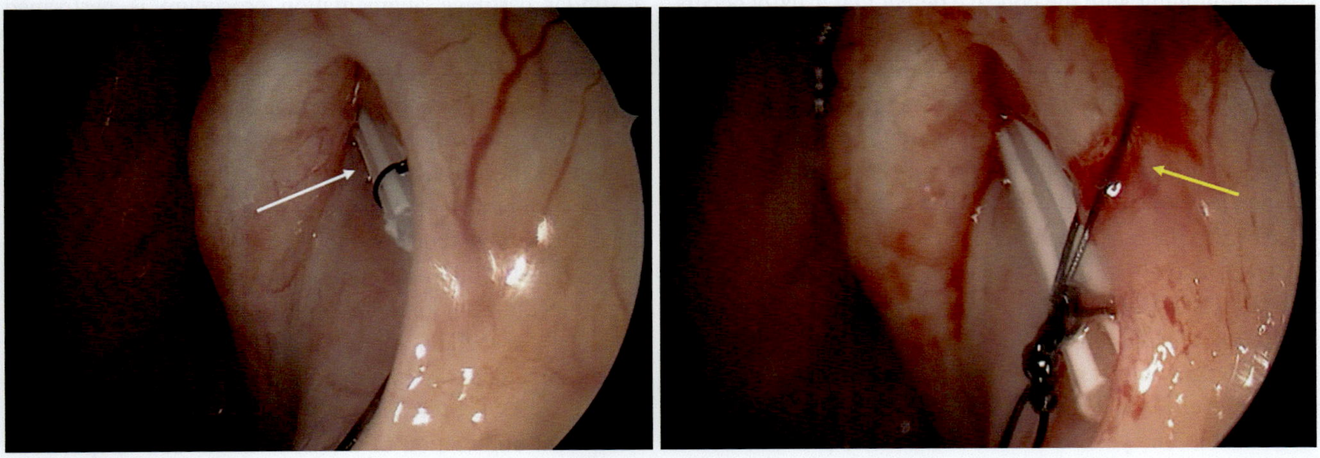

Fig. 34.7 Defect repair in the Eustachian tube. The left image shows an angio-catheter inserted into the left Eustachian tube. The catheter is filled with bone wax and rests at the anterior pillar (arrow). Right image: The catheter has been sutured to the anterior pillar (arrow). (Used with permission from Dennis Poe, MD, who retains copyright of this figure)

excursions. All patients reported complete resolution of their autophony. One patient required trimming of the catheter. No surgical complications occurred. Ward et al. recently published 12-month outcomes of Eustachian tube procedures for patients with patulous Eustachian tube, and reported that three-quarters of patients undergoing a shim placement as their first procedure on the Eustachian tube experienced resolution of symptoms 12 months later [93]. However, they also reported a 12% dislodgement rate, with extrusion of the catheter being noticed after coughing or sneezing in some cases. Due to the high rate of shim dislodgement, we have recently opted to suture the shim in place in more patients. This is especially important should the shim feel loose at the isthmus (Fig. 34.7). There is long-term experience with a comparable approach in Japan using the silicone Kobayashi Plug of 23 mm length inserted through the tympanic membrane. In a prospective multicenter study of 28 patients, patulous handicap indices were statistically significantly reduced in 27/28 patients at 6-month follow-up [102]. In an earlier retrospective series of 137 patients, long-term success was 85%. In both series, tympanic membrane perforation was reported at 17% [103].

Another means for augmenting the Eustachian tube soft tissue lumen is with calcium hydroxyapatite cement, which is used off-label [104, 105]. The Eustachian tube injection is performed as an outpatient procedure under general anesthesia using a combined endoscopic transnasal-transoral approach. The lumen of the Eustachian tube is viewed with a 45-degree endoscope through the ipsilateral nasal cavity. The authors use Prolaryn Plus® (Merz Neurosciences), an injectable calcium hydroxyapatite preloaded into a 1-mL syringe that is attached to a 20-gauge custom-made, reinforced sinus needle, bent 45° at the midpoint. It is important to introduce the needle at a very shallow angle just through the mucosa and pass it along a long superficial track (to prevent extrusion of the material from back pressure) into the submucosal space, beginning with the concave defect that usually occurs in the anterolateral wall. The injection is performed slowly, directly observing the filling of the defect. Additional injections may be performed in the opposing posteromedial wall and the floor if necessary. 1.0 ml is initially injected into the anterolateral wall and additional injections are done if deemed necessary. Most commonly a second injection more inferiorly in the cross-sectional area of the lumen and also in the anterolateral wall will be made. The usual total of the injections is 2.0 mL. Ward et al. recently published 12-month outcomes of ET procedures for patients with pET and reported that injection with hydroxyapatite had a mean symptom relief period of 7.7 months with symptom recurrence within one year of 68.4%. It tended to perform worse than shim placement or total obliteration. In fact, injecting a larger volume of filler tended to be associated with a lower likelihood of enduring symptom relief [93]. OME occurred in 11% of our patients and was usually self-limited, so tympanostomy tubes are not routinely offered unless immediate air travel is planned. Approximately 40% of the volume of the injected material is water and will absorb within 3 weeks. Patients are advised that should patulous symptoms occur within the first 3 weeks, it may be temporary as scar ingrowth is known to occur as the hydroxyapatite microspheres are absorbed over the successive 8 months, and the volume of scar may relieve the symptoms. This procedure should be reserved for small defects located favorably in the mid-portion of the membranous anterolateral wall. Defects at the 12:00 position where the mucosa is thin and tightly bound to the cartilaginous roof of the Eustachian tube will not hold a sufficient amount of material to be successful.

For failures of the above procedures or in the case of dehiscence of the internal carotid artery preventing the use of a shim, the Eustachian tube lumen may be reconstructed with cartilage implants. Multiple materials have been used, including adipose/fat graft, fascia, silicone, cadaveric acellular dermis such as AlloDerm® (Lifecell), and auto- and allograft cartilage implants to augment the defect [53]. Cartilage grafts have been shown to conserve volume better than most other graft materials. Autologous conchal cartilage or irradiated allograft rib cartilage is cut into small wedges and placed into a sub-mucoperichondrial pocket made in the posteromedial wall. An incision is made in the torus tubarius using endoscopic techniques, and sharp and blunt dissection is done to create the pocket, being careful to avoid entry into the lumen of the Eustachian tube. Tunneling is done into the valve area to a depth of 20 mm. Wedges of cartilage are packed into the pocket to create as large a bulge into the lumen of the Eustachian tube while still being able to close the defect with 4-0 Vicryl® sutures, using endoscopic suturing instruments (Karl Storz, El Segundo, CA, USA) and techniques. Patients are advised of the possibility of failure and a second-stage procedure is often necessary. In that case, a similar cartilage augmentation procedure is performed within the anterolateral wall. A tympanostomy tube is inserted in all of these patients as obstruction of the Eustachian tube is expected for at least several weeks.

Lastly, a minority of patients will require complete obliteration of the Eustachian tube lumen to control their disabling symptoms. Performing total obliteration of the Eustachian tube requires long-term tympanostomy tubes, with the possibility of complications related to the tubes or thick mucoid effusions that tend to occur in a completely occluded Eustachian tube. Thick effusions may become troublesome due to frequent plugging of the tympanostomy tubes [93, 106]. In a study by Ward et al., all patients that underwent obliteration of the Eustachian tube for patulous Eustachian tube had resolution of patulous Eustachian tube symptoms at 12 months. However, they were also likely to require subsequent tympanostomy tube or to develop otitis media with effusion, which consequently produced aural fullness and autophony of voice, but to a lesser degree than the symptoms due to patulous Eustachian tube. Autophony due to middle ear effusion can be differentiated readily by the accompanying conductive hearing loss. Thus, total Eustachian tube obliteration should be prudently contemplated only as a last alternative.

Conclusions

The Eustachian tube has defined functions that include ventilation, mucociliary clearance, and middle ear protection of nasopharyngeal secretions and sound. Eustachian tube dysfunction is a spectrum of diseases that consist of obstructive Eustachian tube dysfunction on one end and patulous Eustachian tube on the other. Obstructive dysfunction is associated with negative middle ear pressure or, at a minimum, difficulty with barochallenges. Defects in the valve causing loss of competence in the resting position are the cause of patulous dysfunction. Mucosal edema may be caused by inflammatory disease, infection, allergy, or reflux from the nasopharynx (including LPR). Particularly with chronic allergic rhinitis, patients may fluctuate from obstructive dysfunction when they are exposed to environmental challenges or patulous when their allergies are quiescent and they have residual atrophy of the mucosa and submucosa in the valve. Frequent or inappropriate sniffing to relieve autophony may result in negative pressure within the middle ear, leading to complications of retraction of the tympanic membrane, middle ear effusion or even cholesteatoma. Patulous Eustachian tube is far more common than previously believed, as it may present in this fashion with what appears at first to be an obstructive problem.

Medical treatment should be directed toward any suspected underlying etiology of inflammation whenever possible and middle ear ventilation with tympanostomy tubes is generally recommended as an initial measure when medical treatment is inadequate. However, balloon dilation of the cartilaginous Eustachian tube may be indicated even without prior tympanostomy tube placement.

Balloon dilation of the Eustachian tube (BDET) has been established as a safe and effective method for treating obstructive Eustachian tube dysfunction and has clear indications.

Similarly, treatment of a patulous Eustachian tube warrants counseling, reassurance and initial conservative measures before proceeding with surgical interventions. Interventions to manage patulous Eustachian tube include procedures that target the tympanic membrane, intraluminal shim insertion, surgical augmentation of the Eustachian tube walls with calcium hydroxyapatite or cartilage, and, as a last resort, complete obliteration of the Eustachian tube lumen.

References

1. Kühn KG. Opuscula academica medica et philologica collecta, aucta et emendata: sumtibus Leopoldi Vossii; 1828.
2. Eustachi B. Opuscula anatomica.-Venetiis, Vincentius Luchinus: De auditus organis. 1564.
3. Valsalva AM. De aure humana tractatus... Interposita est musculorum uvulae atque pharyngis nova descriptio: Pisarius, 1704.
4. Toynbee J. On the muscles which open the eustachian tube. Abstr Pap Commun R Soc Lond. 1854;6:286–7.
5. Mudry A. [Adam Politzer (1835-1920) and the Eustachian tube]. Ann Otolaryngol Chir Cervicofac. 2004;121:75–82.
6. Proctor B. Embryology and anatomy of the eustachian tube. Arch Otolaryngol. 1967;86:503–14.
7. Honjo I, Hayashi M, Ito S, Takahashi H. Pumping and clearance function of the eustachian tube. Am J Otolaryngol. 1985;6:241–4.
8. Hopf J, Linnarz M, Gundlach P, et al. [Microendoscopy of the Eustachian tube and the middle ear. Indications and clinical application]. Laryngorhinootologie. 1991;70:391–94.
9. Bluestone CD, Bluestone MB. Eustachian tube : structure, function, role in otitis media. Hamilton; Lewiston: BC Decker; 2005.
10. Honjō I. Eustachian tube and middle ear diseases. Tokyo; New York: Springer-Verlag; 1988.
11. Eden AR, Gannon PJ. Neural control of middle ear aeration. Arch Otolaryngol Head Neck Surg. 1987;113:133–7.
12. Rockley TJ, Hawke WM. The middle ear as a baroreceptor. Acta Otolaryngol. 1992;112:816–23.
13. Pau HW, Sievert U, Just T, Sade J. Pressure changes in the human middle ear without opening the eustachian tube. Acta Otolaryngol. 2009;129:1182–6.
14. Chandrasekhar SS, Mautone AJ. Otitis media: treatment with intranasal aerosolized surfactant. Laryngoscope. 2004;114:472–85.
15. Bluestone CD, Klein JO. Otitis media, atelectasis, and Eustachian tube dysfunction. In: Bluestone CD, Stool SE, Kenna MA, editors. Pediatric otolaryngology. 3rd ed. Philadelphia: WB Saunders; 1996.
16. Tucci DL, McCoul ED, Rosenfeld RM, et al. Clinical consensus statement: balloon dilation of the eustachian tube. Otolaryngol Head Neck Surg. 2019;161:6–17.
17. Schilder AG, Bhutta MF, Butler CC, et al. Eustachian tube dysfunction: consensus statement on definition, types, clinical presentation and diagnosis. Clin Otolaryngol. 2015;40:407–11.
18. Ward BK, Ashry Y, Poe DS. Patulous eustachian tube dysfunction: patient demographics and comorbidities. Otol Neurotol. 2017;38:1362–9.
19. Mygind N, Thomsen J, Jorgensen MB. Ultrastructure of the epithelium in atrophic rhinitis. Scanning electron microscopic studies. Acta Otolaryngol. 1974;77:439–46.
20. Naito K, Takeda N, Yokoyama N, et al. The distribution of eosinophil cationic protein positive eosinophils in the nasal mucosa of the nasal allergy patients. Auris Nasus Larynx. 1993;20:197–204.
21. Lim MC, Taylor RM, Naclerio RM. The histology of allergic rhinitis and its comparison to cellular changes in nasal lavage. Am J Respir Crit Care Med. 1995;151:136–44.
22. Rovers MM, Schilder AG, Zielhuis GA, Rosenfeld RM. Otitis media. Lancet. 2004;363:465–73.
23. Seibert JW, Danner CJ. Eustachian tube function and the middle ear. Otolaryngol Clin N Am. 2006;39:1221–35.
24. Vila PM, Thomas T, Liu C, Poe D, Shin JJ. The burden and epidemiology of eustachian tube dysfunction in adults. Otolaryngol Head Neck Surg. 2017;156:278–84.
25. Shan A, Ward BK, Goman AM, et al. Prevalence of eustachian tube dysfunction in adults in the United States. JAMA Otolaryngol Head Neck Surg. 2019;145(10):974–5.

26. Flisberg K, Ingelstedt S. Middle-ear mechanics in patulous tube cases. Acta Otolaryngol Suppl. 1969;263:18–22.
27. Ohta S, Sakagami M, Suzuki M, Mishiro Y. Eustachian tube function and habitual sniffing in middle ear cholesteatoma. Otol Neurotol. 2009;30:48–53.
28. Gulya AJ, Schuknecht HF. Anatomy of the temporal bone with surgical implications. 2nd ed. New York: Parthenon Pub. Group; 1995.
29. Freeman MH, Gafford JB, Fichera L, Noble J, Webster RJ 3rd, Labadie RF. Transeustachian middle ear endoscopy using a steerable distal-camera tipped endoscope. Otol Neurotol. 2022;43:206–11.
30. Chays A, Cohen JM, Magnan J. [Microfibroendoscopy of the eustachian tube]. Presse Med. 1995;24:773–4.
31. Kimura H, Yamaguchi H, Cheng SS, et al. [Direct observation of the tympanic cavity by the superfine fiberscope]. Nihon Jibiinkoka Gakkai Kaiho. 1989;92:233–8.
32. Takahashi H, Honjo I, Fujita A. Endoscopic findings at the pharyngeal orifice of the eustachian tube in otitis media with effusion. Eur Arch Otorhinolaryngol. 1996;253:42–4.
33. Poe DS, Pyykko I, Valtonen H, Silvola J. Analysis of eustachian tube function by video endoscopy. Am J Otol. 2000;21:602–7.
34. Poe DS, Abou-Halawa A, Abdel-Razek O. Analysis of the dysfunctional eustachian tube by video endoscopy. Otol Neurotol. 2001;22:590–5.
35. Bluestone CD. Impact of evolution on the eustachian tube. Laryngoscope. 2008;118:522–7.
36. Alper CM, Swarts JD, Singla A, Banks J, Doyle WJ. Relationship between the electromyographic activity of the paratubal muscles and eustachian tube opening assessed by sonotubometry and videoendoscopy. Arch Otolaryngol Head Neck Surg. 2012;138:741–6.
37. Nell MJ, Grote JJ. Structural changes in the rat middle ear mucosa due to endotoxin and eustachian tube obstruction. Eur Arch Otorhinolaryngol. 1999;256:167–72.
38. Jung JY, Pashia ME, Nishimoto SY, Faddis BT, Chole RA. A possible role for nitric oxide in osteoclastogenesis associated with cholesteatoma. Otol Neurotol. 2004;25:661–8.
39. Kivekas I, Poyhonen L, Aarnisalo A, Rautiainen M, Poe D. Eustachian tube mucosal inflammation scale validation based on digital video images. Otol Neurotol. 2015;36:1748–52.
40. Paradise JL, Bluestone CD, Rogers KD, et al. Efficacy of adenoidectomy for recurrent otitis media in children previously treated with tympanostomy-tube placement. Results of parallel randomized and nonrandomized trials. JAMA. 1990;263:2066–73.
41. Nistico L, Kreft R, Gieseke A, et al. Adenoid reservoir for pathogenic biofilm bacteria. J Clin Microbiol. 2011;49:1411–20.
42. Yoshida H, Takahashi H, Morikawa M. Anatomy of the surrounding tissue of the eustachian tube in patulous eustachian tube: 3 tesla magnetic resonance imaging approach. Otol Neurotol. 2019;40:e107–14.
43. Carlstrom LP, Van Abel KM, Carlson ML, Moore EJ, Stokken JK. Occult infratemporal fossa neurofibroma presenting with persistent unilateral tinnitus and middle ear effusion: more than meets the eye. Am J Otolaryngol. 2017;38:251–3.
44. Leonetti JP. A study of persistent unilateral middle ear effusion caused by occult skull base lesions. Ear Nose Throat J. 2013;92:195–200.
45. Lopez-Escamez JA, Carey J, Chung WH, et al. Diagnostic criteria for Meniere's disease. J Vestib Res. 2015;25:1–7.
46. Minor LB. Clinical manifestations of superior semicircular canal dehiscence. Laryngoscope. 2005;115:1717–27.
47. Minor LB, Solomon D, Zinreich JS, Zee DS. Sound- and/or pressure-induced vertigo due to bone dehiscence of the superior semicircular canal. Arch Otolaryngol Head Neck Surg. 1998;124:249–58.
48. Riga M, Xenellis J, Peraki E, Ferekidou E, Korres S. Aural symptoms in patients with temporomandibular joint disorders: multiple frequency tympanometry provides objective evidence of changes in middle ear impedance. Otol Neurotol. 2010;31:1359–64.
49. Moshtaghi O, Ghavami Y, Mahboubi H, et al. Migraine-related aural fullness: a potential clinical entity. Otolaryngol Head Neck Surg. 2018;158:100–2.
50. Takizawa Y, Mizuta K, Hamada N, et al. Relationship between tympanic membrane retraction and habitual sniffing in patients with cholesteatoma. Acta Otolaryngol. 2013;133:1030–4.
51. Wackym PA, Wood SJ, Siker DA, Carter DM. Otic capsule dehiscence syndrome: superior semicircular canal dehiscence syndrome with no radiographically visible dehiscence. Ear Nose Throat J. 2015;94:E8–E24.
52. Zhou G, Gopen Q, Poe DS. Clinical and diagnostic characterization of canal dehiscence syndrome: a great otologic mimicker. Otol Neurotol. 2007;28:920–6.
53. Poe DS. Diagnosis and management of the patulous eustachian tube. Otol Neurotol. 2007;28:668–77.
54. Mikulec AA, McKenna MJ, Ramsey MJ, et al. Superior semicircular canal dehiscence presenting as conductive hearing loss without vertigo. Otol Neurotol. 2004;25:121–9.
55. Gluth MB, McDonald DR, Weaver AL, Bauch CD, Beatty CW, Orvidas LJ. Management of eustachian tube dysfunction with nasal steroid spray: a prospective, randomized, placebo-controlled trial. Arch Otolaryngol Head Neck Surg. 2011;137:449–55.
56. Kivekas I, Chao WC, Faquin W, et al. Histopathology of balloon-dilation Eustachian tuboplasty. Laryngoscope. 2015;125:436–41.
57. Silvola J, Kivekas I, Poe DS. Balloon dilation of the cartilaginous portion of the eustachian tube. Otolaryngol Head Neck Surg. 2014;151:125–30.
58. Poe DS, Silvola J, Pyykko I. Balloon dilation of the cartilaginous eustachian tube. Otolaryngol Head Neck Surg. 2011;144:563–9.
59. Tisch M, Maier S, Maier H. [Eustachian tube dilation using the Bielefeld balloon catheter: clinical experience with 320 interventions]. HNO. 2013;61:483–7.
60. McCoul ED, Anand VK. Eustachian tube balloon dilation surgery. Int Forum Allergy Rhinol. 2012;2:191–8.
61. Randrup TS, Ovesen T. Balloon eustachian tuboplasty: a systematic review. Otolaryngol Head Neck Surg. 2015;152:383–92.
62. Huisman JML, Verdam FJ, Stegeman I, de Ru JA. Treatment of Eustachian tube dysfunction with balloon dilation: a systematic review. Laryngoscope. 2018;128:237–47.
63. Hwang SY, Kok S, Walton J. Balloon dilation for eustachian tube dysfunction: systematic review. J Laryngol Otol. 2016;130 Suppl 4:S2–6.
64. Ramakrishnan N, D'Souza R, Kadambi P. A systematic literature review of the safety and efficacy of eustachian balloon tuboplasty in patients with chronic eustachian tube dysfunction. Indian J Otolaryngol Head Neck Surg. 2019;71:406–12.
65. Luukkainen V, Kivekas I, Silvola J, Jero J, Sinkkonen ST. Balloon eustachian tuboplasty: systematic review of long-term outcomes and proposed indications. J Int Adv Otol. 2018;14:112–26.
66. Luukkainen V, Vnencak M, Aarnisalo AA, Jero J, Sinkkonen ST. Patient satisfaction in the long-term effects of Eustachian tube balloon dilation is encouraging. Acta Otolaryngol. 2018;138:122–7.
67. McMurran AEL, Hogg GE, Gordon S, Spielmann PM, Jones SE. Balloon Eustachian tuboplasty for Eustachian tube dysfunction: report of long-term outcomes in a UK population. J Laryngol Otol. 2020;134:34–40.
68. Froehlich MH, Le PT, Nguyen SA, McRackan TR, Rizk HG, Meyer TA. Eustachian tube balloon dilation: a systematic review

and meta-analysis of treatment outcomes. Otolaryngol Head Neck Surg. 2020;163(5):870–82.

69. Jansen S, Peters N, Hinkelbein J, Klussmann JP, Beutner D, Meyer MF. Subjective and objective effectiveness of eustachian tube balloon dilatation for patients with eustachian tube dysfunction-evaluation in a pressure chamber. Otol Neurotol. 2020;41:795–801.
70. Cutler JL, Meyer TA, Nguyen SA, O'Malley EM, Thackeray L, Slater PW. Long-term outcomes of balloon dilation for persistent eustachian tube dysfunction. Otol Neurotol. 2019;40(10):1322–5.
71. Poe D, Anand V, Dean M, et al. Balloon dilation of the eustachian tube for dilatory dysfunction: a randomized controlled trial. Laryngoscope. 2018;128:1200–6.
72. Meyer TA, O'Malley EM, Schlosser RJ, et al. A randomized controlled trial of balloon dilation as a treatment for persistent eustachian tube dysfunction with 1-year follow-up. Otol Neurotol. 2018;39:894–902.
73. Anand V, Poe D, Dean M, et al. Balloon dilation of the eustachian tube: 12-month follow-up of the randomized controlled trial treatment group. Otolaryngol Head Neck Surg. 2019;160:687–94.
74. Liang M, Xiong H, Cai Y, et al. Effect of the combination of balloon Eustachian tuboplasty and tympanic paracentesis on intractable chronic otitis media with effusion. Am J Otolaryngol. 2016;37:442–6.
75. Kepchar J, Acevedo J, Schroeder J, Littlefield P. Transtympanic balloon dilatation of eustachian tube: a human cadaver pilot study. J Laryngol Otol. 2012;126:1102–7.
76. Tarabichi M, Najmi M. Transtympanic dilatation of the eustachian tube during chronic ear surgery. Acta Otolaryngol. 2015;135:640–4.
77. Dean M, Chao WC, Poe D. Eustachian tube dilation via a transtympanic approach in 6 cadaver heads: a feasibility study. Otolaryngol Head Neck Surg. 2016;155:654–6.
78. Falkenberg-Jensen B, Hopp E, Jablonski GE, Pripp AH, Silvola JT. The cartilaginous Eustachian tube: reliable CT measurement and impact of the length. Am J Otolaryngol. 2018;39:436–40.
79. Dean M, Pynnonen MA. In-office balloon dilation of the eustachian tube under local anesthesia. Otolaryngol Clin N Am. 2019;52:509–20.
80. Luukkainen V, Kivekas I, Hammaren-Malmi S, et al. Balloon Eustachian tuboplasty under local anesthesia: is it feasible? Laryngoscope. 2017;127:1021–5.
81. Bluestone CDKJ. Otitis media, atelectasis, and Eustachian tube dysfunction. In: Bluestone CDSS, Kenna MA, editors. Pediatric otolaryngology. 3rd ed. Philadelphia: WB Saunders; 1996.
82. Schroder S, Lehmann M, Ebmeyer J, Upile T, Sudhoff H. Balloon Eustachian Tuboplasty (BET): our experience of 622 cases. Clin Otolaryngol. 2015;40:629–38.
83. Skevas T, Dalchow CV, Euteneuer S, Sudhoff H, Lehnerdt G. Cervicofacial and mediastinal emphysema after balloon eustachian tuboplasty (BET): a retrospective multicenter analysis. Eur Arch Otorhinolaryngol. 2018;275:81–7.
84. Shah RR, Thomas WW, Naples JG, Ruckenstein MJ. Subcutaneous emphysema and pneumomediastinum after eustachian tube balloon dilation. Otolaryngol Head Neck Surg. 2018;159:203–5.
85. Maier S, Tisch M, Maier H. [Balloon dilation of the Eustachian tube in pediatric chronic obstructive Eustachian tube dysfunction patients]. HNO. 2015;63:686–8, 690–684, 696–687.
86. Tisch M, Maier H, Sudhoff H. Balloon dilation of the eustachian tube: clinical experience in the management of 126 children. Acta Otorhinolaryngol Ital. 2017;37:509–12.
87. Leichtle A, Hollfelder D, Wollenberg B, Bruchhage KL. Balloon eustachian tuboplasty in children. Eur Arch Otorhinolaryngol. 2017;274:2411–9.
88. Toivonen J, Kawai K, Gurberg J, Poe D. Balloon dilation for obstructive eustachian tube dysfunction in children. Otol Neurotol. 2021;42:566–72.
89. Ashry Y, Kawai K, Poe D. Utility of adjunctive procedures with balloon dilation of the eustachian tube. Laryngoscope Investig Otolaryngol. 2017;2:337–43.
90. Adil E, Poe D. What is the full range of medical and surgical treatments available for patients with Eustachian tube dysfunction? Curr Opin Otolaryngol Head Neck Surg. 2014;22:8–15.
91. Oshima T, Kikuchi T, Kawase T, Kobayashi T. Nasal instillation of physiological saline for patulous eustachian tube. Acta Otolaryngol. 2010;130:550–3.
92. DiBartolomeo JR, Henry DF. A new medication to control patulous eustachian tube disorders. Am J Otol. 1992;13:323–7.
93. Ward BK, Chao WC, Abiola G, et al. Twelve-month outcomes of Eustachian tube procedures for management of patulous Eustachian tube dysfunction. Laryngoscope. 2019;129:222–8.
94. Luxford WM, Sheehy JL. Myringotomy and ventilation tubes: a report of 1,568 ears. Laryngoscope. 1982;92:1293–7.
95. Simonton KM. Abnormal patency of the Eustachian tube: surgical treatment. Laryngoscope. 1957;67:342–59.
96. Boedts M. Paper patching of the tympanic membrane as a symptomatic treatment for patulous eustachian tube syndrome. J Laryngol Otol. 2014;128:228–35.
97. Bartlett C, Pennings R, Ho A, Kirkpatrick D, van Wijhe R, Bance M. Simple mass loading of the tympanic membrane to alleviate symptoms of patulous eustachian tube. J Otolaryngol Head Neck Surg. 2010;39:259–68.
98. Brace MD, Horwich P, Kirkpatrick D, Bance M. Tympanic membrane manipulation to treat symptoms of patulous eustachian tube. Otol Neurotol. 2014;35:1201–6.
99. Bluestone CD, Cantekin EI. "How I do it"--otology and neurotology. A specific issue and its solution. Management of the patulous Eustachian tube. Laryngoscope. 1981;91:149–52.
100. Bluestone CD, Miller AE. The abnormally patulous Eustachian tube. In: Brackmann DE, Shelton C, Arriaga MA, editors. Otologic surgery. 2nd ed. Philadelphia: W.B. Saunders; 2001. p. 82–7.
101. Rotenberg BW, Busato GM, Agrawal SK. Endoscopic ligation of the patulous eustachian tube as treatment for autophony. Laryngoscope. 2013;123:239–43.
102. Ikeda R, Oshima T, Mizuta K, et al. Efficacy of a silicone plug for patulous eustachian tube: a prospective, multicenter case series. Laryngoscope. 2019;130(5):1304–9.
103. Kikuchi T, Ikeda R, Oshima H, et al. Effectiveness of Kobayashi plug for 252 ears with chronic patulous Eustachian tube. Acta Otolaryngol. 2017;137:253–8.
104. Oh SJ, Kang DW, Goh EK, Kong SK. Calcium hydroxylapatite injection for the patulous Eustachian tube. Am J Otolaryngol. 2014;35:443–4.
105. Vaezeafshar R, Turner JH, Li G, Hwang PH. Endoscopic hydroxyapatite augmentation for patulous Eustachian tube. Laryngoscope. 2014;124:62–6.
106. Doherty JK, Slattery WH 3rd. Autologous fat grafting for the refractory patulous eustachian tube. Otolaryngol Head Neck Surg. 2003;128:88–91.

Aural and Extratemporal Complications of Otitis Media

35

R. Mark Wiet, Danny Jandali, Arvind Kumar, and Richard Wiet

Introduction

As Shambaugh wrote in his preface to *Surgery of the Ear*, "no branch of medical science has been altered more profoundly, advanced more rapidly, and benefited so greatly by sulfonamide and antibiotic therapy than surgery of the ear." The senior author of this chapter recalls stories of the amazing transition Chicago witnessed as whole hospitals devoted to infectious disease began to close after the introduction of antibiotic therapy. This favorable change echoed throughout the world of otology with the development of penicillin and sulfonamide drugs.

Today, however, a much more insidious problem exists. Younger otologists are often surprised by the consequences of infection by virulent organisms. For example, a child with a ravaging otitis media can become comatose and near death within 12–24 hrs. On the other hand, complications from otitis media may present in a more occult fashion that eludes initial detection. This problem has now even led to litigation against physicians, with the accusation of "delay in diagnosis." [1].

In this chapter, the authors aim to catalog and organize current thinking on the management of the intratemporal, extradural complications of otitis media with the hope that catastrophic complications can be avoided by prompt and appropriate intervention. Intracranial complications of otitis media are covered in a subsequent chapter of this book.

Otitis media is an inflammation of part or all of the mucoperiosteal lining of the tympanomastoid compartment comprising the Eustachian tube, the tympanic cavity, the mastoid antrum, and all of the pneumatized spaces of the temporal bone. Complications of otitis media have been defined as spread of infection beyond the confines of the lining mucosa of the middle-ear cleft [2]. Both acute and chronic otitis media (COM) can cause complications (Table 35.1). In the preantibiotic era, 52% of complications were associated with virulent acute otitis media. Today, the majority of complications result from COM. Morbidity and mortality from complications can be minimized if there is a keen familiarity with the specific type of draining ear, the underlying pathology, and the early signs and symptoms of complications. These considerations are particularly significant now because the

Table 35.1 Complications of suppurative ear disease

Intratemporal extradural	Intracranial intradural
Leptomeningitis	Leptomeningitis
Acute mastoiditis	Pachymeningitis Subdural abscess
Pachymeningitis Epidural abscess Peri-sinus abscess and sigmoid sinus thrombosis	Brain abscess
Petrositis	Otitic hydrocephalus
Facial paralysis	
Labyrinthitis	

Adapted from *Glasscock and Shambaugh's Surgery of the Ear*. 6th Ed. Eds. Gulya, Minor, Poe. PMPH. 2010

R. Mark Wiet (✉)
Otology, Neurotology, and Lateral Skull Base Surgery, Neurotology and Skull Base Surgery, Northwestern Medicine Regional Medical Group, Central Dupage Hospital, Winfield, IL, USA
e-mail: Richard.wiet1@nm.org

D. Jandali
Department of Otolaryngology—Head and Neck Surgery, Duly Health and Care, Glen Ellyn, IL, USA
e-mail: Danny.jandali@duly.com

A. Kumar
Department of Otolaryngology—Head and Neck Surgery, University of Illinois – Chicago, Chicago, IL, USA

Department of Otolaryngology—Head and Neck Surgery, Northwestern University, Chicago, IL, USA

R. Wiet
Department of Otolaryngology—Head and Neck Surgery, Rush University Medical Center, Chicago, IL, USA

Clinical Otolaryngology and Neurosurgery, Feinberg School of Medicine, Northwestern University, Chicago, IL, USA

A. D. Sweeney et al. (eds.), *Haynes-Glasscock-Shambaugh Surgery of the Ear*, https://doi.org/10.1007/978-3-032-18264-7_35

rarity of complications limits the individual experience of most otologists.

Complications of Acute Otitis Media

Perforation of the Pars Tensa

Acute otitis media (AOM) of bacterial origin typically affects preschool children, and the nasopharynx is usually the source of the infection. An initial inflammation of the middle-ear cleft is followed by suppuration, and then, hopefully, treatment and resolution. However, complications of AOM usually arise as a consequence of suppuration propagation. In the inflammatory stage, hyperemia and edema of the mucoperiosteum are followed by exudation of serofibrinous fluid into the middle ear. As the fluid volume increases, pressure is exerted against the tympanic membrane (TM), and if myringotomy is not performed, the bulging TM ruptures, usually in the anterior–inferior quadrant. Pain subsides, and toxicity and fever begin to abate. In most instances, subsequent to the resolution of the inflammation, the perforation heals spontaneously. Perforation can persist in about 2% of patients. The hearing loss associated with such perforation is usually mild. The Weber generally lateralizes to the affected ear, and the Rinne may not appreciate the mild nature of the conductive hearing loss. An audiometric evaluation is generally indicated.

If the TM perforation persists, it can be surgically repaired. Eustachian tube dysfunction diminishes the chances for a successful myringoplasty. Unfortunately, an accurate preoperative evaluation of Eustachian tube dysfunction is not possible. The status of the opposite ear is not believed to be a sufficient predictor of Eustachian tube function on the ipsilateral side. The best correlate of Eustachian tube dysfunction may be mastoid pneumatization as seen on radiographic evaluation. The results of myringoplasty in an otherwise healthy ear with a well-pneumatized mastoid are generally good. Surgical techniques around this type of procedure are discussed in another chapter.

Acute Mastoiditis/Subperiosteal Abscess

In the context of AOM, acute mastoiditis is the extension of middle-ear inflammation into the antrum and mastoid air cells. Such spread occurs because the mastoid antrum and the epitympanum communicate freely with each other through the *aditus ad antrum.* According to Nager [3] "a mild form of mastoiditis regularly accompanies an AOM in which the inflammatory process is limited to the mucoperiosteum." Therefore, this early stage of inflammation of the whole middle-ear cleft is better termed as *tympanomastoiditis.* Routine computed tomography (CT) and magnetic resonance imaging (MRI) scans of the temporal bone are often reported to show "mastoiditis," even though there is no clinical evidence of pain or tenderness over the mastoid or any radiologic evidence of bone destruction. To clarify the clinical significance of such apparent inconsistencies, it is worthwhile to trace the progression of tympanomastoiditis to a subperiosteal abscess: if, during the course of tympanomastoiditis, the aditus is blocked by inflammatory tissue, mucopurulent material may become loculated within the antrum and the contiguous air cells of the temporal bone. If the infection is severe and the blockage of the aditus persists despite antibiotic therapy, retrograde thrombophlebitis may lead to edema and cellulitis of the soft tissues overlying the mastoid, causing the ipsilateral retroauricular pain, swelling, and induration of acute mastoiditis. If the pus is not drained, either spontaneously or by surgical intervention, necrosis and demineralization of the bony trabeculae occur, resulting in "coalescent mastoiditis" (Fig. 35.1). From this stage on, disease progression follows a continuum depending on the direction in which the erosive process goes:

- Most commonly, the mastoid cortex is eroded and a subperiosteal abscess develops.
- With medial progression, the abscess involves the petrous pyramid; if the apex is involved, the classic symptoms and signs of Gradenigo syndrome may develop.
- With anterior progression, the fallopian canal or the labyrinth can be compromised, resulting in facial paralysis and/or vertigo with or without sensorineural hearing loss.

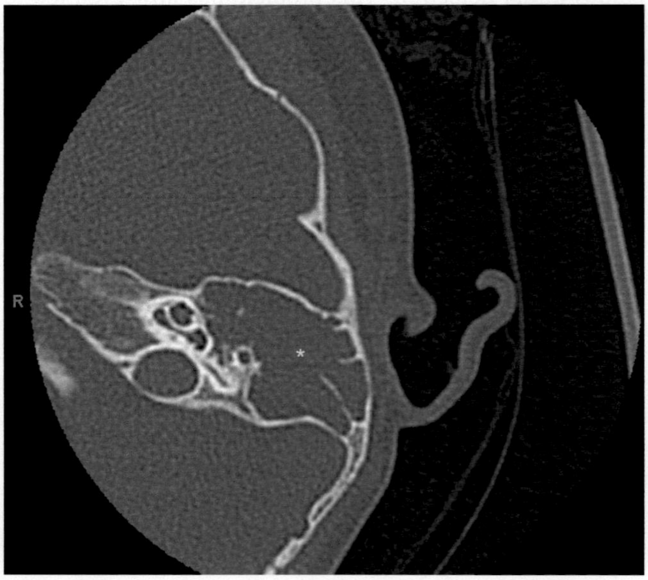

Fig. 35.1 Acute coalescent mastoiditis in the left mastoid (asterisk) shown on an axial view of a non-contrast CT scan. (Courtesy of Alex Sweeney, MD)

- If the mastoid tip is eroded, a Bezold abscess may develop.
- Progression toward the tegmen or Trautmann's triangle may result in an epidural abscess.
- Invasion of the perilymph or cerebrospinal fluid space can evolve into meningitis.

In a multicenter study of 223 consecutive cases of mastoiditis/AOM, Luntz et al. [4] found that 88% occurred in children under the age of 8 years. Upon admission to the hospital, 22% presented with one or more intratemporal or intracranial complications. The most commonly isolated organisms were *Streptococcus pneumoniae, Streptococcus pyogenes, Staphylococcus aureus, Staphylococcus* (coagulase negative), *Haemophilus influenzae,* and *Pseudomonas aeruginosa.* Cultures were positive for *Pseudomonas* spp. in 18 patients (8%), although it is important to note that, in 50% of these cases, the specimen was taken from the external auditory canal. In nearly all of these patients, recovery was uncomplicated, even though no antipseudomonal antibiotics were used in 12 of the 18 patients. These authors also found that antibiotic treatment of AOM is not a safeguard against acute mastoiditis. Early myringotomy was found to be associated with a less complicated course of mastoiditis.

Noncoalescent mastoiditis can be treated effectively using culture-specific intravenous antibiotics with myringotomy and placement of a tympanostomy tube. About 20% of patients so treated may, nonetheless, experience disease progression and ultimately need a cortical mastoidectomy. Close observation of such children is very important to anticipate and prevent serious complications of disease progression.

Coalescent mastoiditis and subperiosteal mastoid abscess formation require careful evaluation and appropriate imaging studies. This situation occurs with the breakdown of the bony septa within the mastoid and the bony destruction of the cortex. Up to 25% of patients who present with coalescent mastoiditis will have a concomitant intracranial complication [5]. *S. pneumonia* is the most common organism cultured [6]. Management includes intravenous (IV) antibiotics, myringotomy, and cortical mastoidectomy. It is important to realize that, in infants and young children, the stylomastoid foramen is located on the lateral surface of the mastoid. The postauricular incision, thus, should be modified by not extending it inferiorly below the level of the floor of the external auditory canal, and facial nerve monitoring should be used intraoperatively. Immunocompromised patients are particularly susceptible to coalescent mastoiditis [7].

Incompletely treated AOM can also lead to complications. Subacute otitis media involves the resolution of the initial symptoms of AOM, though the disease can progress to the formation of an acute mastoid abscess initially without the usual accompanying toxicity. Holt and Gates [8] reported their experience with nine patients with so-called "masked mastoiditis," in which the patient presents with an intratemporal and/or intracranial complication. The history in such cases is one of persistent, mild irritability, diarrhea, and tugging at the ear after apparent resolution of an episode of AOM following antibiotic therapy. Dormant disease has been reported by Meyerhoff et al. [9] in temporal bones with otitis media. Based on clinical studies, it is postulated that anaerobic organisms such as *Peptococcus* spp. and *Bacteroides* spp. thrive in the anaerobic environment of the mastoid in which the aditus is blocked by granulation tissue. These anaerobic organisms are of low virulence, and an indolent osteitis results, which causes little or no pain. In their series of nine cases of masked mastoiditis, Holt and Gates [8] found several associated complications, including epidural abscess (2), facial paralysis (1), meningitis and epidural abscess (1), meningitis (2), brain abscess (2), and cerebritis (1). It is important to maintain a high index of suspicion for this insidious disease and to have a low threshold for obtaining a CT scan of the temporal bones to rule out complications. When acute complications of otitis media are suspected, it is prudent to perform the CT scan with IV contrast to look for thrombophlebitis or intracranial involvement (Figs. 35.2 and 35.3). An MRI with contrast can also be useful in this situation, as can venogram if venous thrombosis is

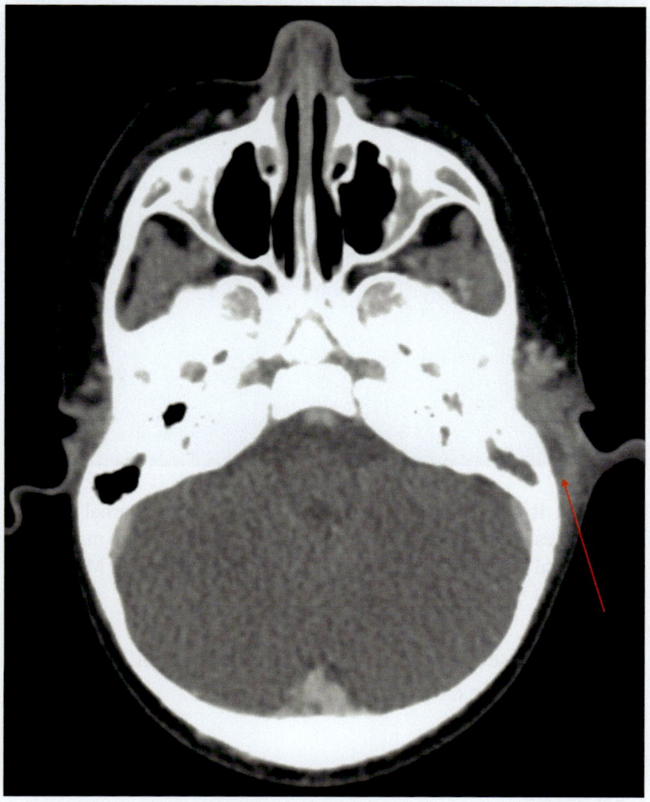

Fig. 35.2 Subperiosteal abscess (red arrow) in the setting of left acute mastoiditis on an axial view of a contrasted CT scan. (Courtesy of Alex Sweeney, MD)

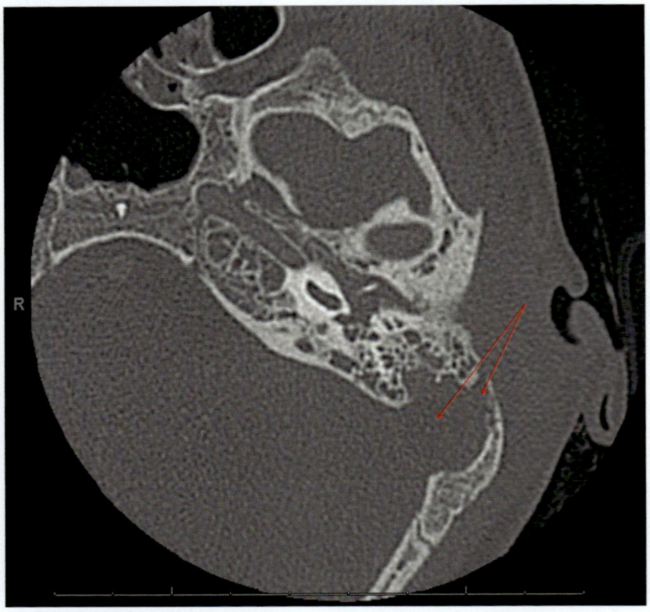

Fig. 35.3 Bony erosion of the mastoid cortex and sigmoid bone plate (red arrows) in the setting of left-sided acute mastoiditis as shown on an axial view of a non-contrast CT scan. (Courtesy of Alex Sweeney, MD)

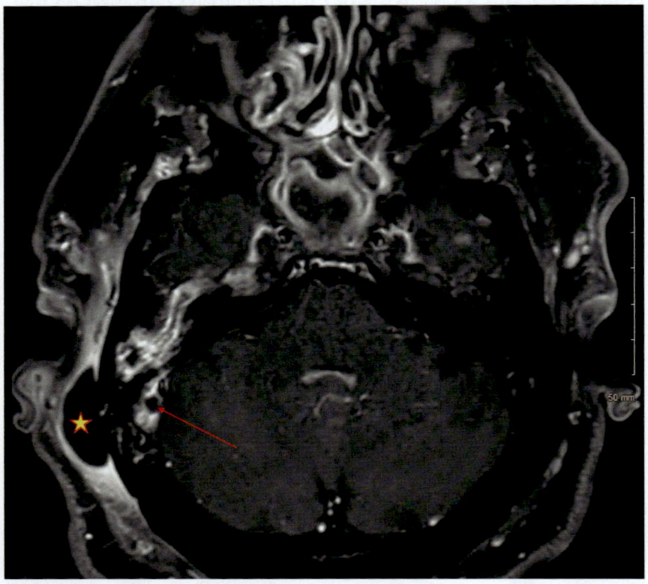

Fig. 35.4 Right subperiosteal abscess (star) and intraluminal sigmoid sinus abscess (red arrow) in the setting of right-sided acute mastoiditis on an axial view of a T1-weighted, contrast-enhanced MRI scan. (Courtesy of Alex Sweeney, MD)

suspected based on the patient's clinical presentation or the CT findings (Figs. 35.4).

Petrositis

Petrositis (also known as petrous apicitis) is an inflammation of the pneumatized spaces of the petrous portion of the temporal bone and is a rare complication of AOM. In most individuals, the petrous apex is poorly pneumatized, but when pneumatization does occur, air cells extend into the petrous pyramid in two main groups:

1. A posterior group of cells that are in continuity with the mastoid antrum and epitympanum, that cluster around the semicircular canals at the base of the pyramid, and that extend medially to the petrous apex
2. An anterior group of cells that extends from the mesotympanum, hypotympanum, and protympanum and passes around the cochlea to the petrous apex

Schuknecht [10] classified petrositis as *acute* and *chronic*.

Acute Petrositis The pathology of acute petrositis is the same as that of acute tympanomastoiditis described above. In the majority of instances, the inflammation resolves without producing any symptoms. If the products of inflammation are retained, the involved ear drains and osteitis may develop at the apex of the petrous pyramid, leading to diplopia and retro-orbital pain. The abducens nerve is compressed as it traverses Dorello's canal under Gruber's (the petroclinoid) ligament, causing paralysis of the ipsilateral lateral rectus muscle. The ipsilateral trigeminal nerve, located at the petrous apex, is also inflamed, leading to retro-orbital pain. The triad of a draining ear with ipsilateral retro-orbital pain and abducens nerve palsy is known as Gradenigo syndrome. The diagnosis is confirmed by a high-resolution temporal bone CT scan, and MRI can also be helpful to further evaluate the extent of disease (Fig. 35.5).

Chronic Petrositis In addition to inflammatory changes, there is new bone formation and resorption. Osteitis adjacent to the otic capsule, dura, or veins may cause labyrinthitis, meningitis, epidural abscess, and brain abscess.

Management of petrous apicitis primarily consists of myringotomy if the middle ear is also involved with the infection and administration of systemic antibiotics. Given the complex anatomy of the petrous apex, the risk to hearing and facial function with transtemporal approaches, and the risk to the brain with a middle fossa approach in the context of an acute infection, systemic antibiotic therapy is a mainstay of petrous apicitis treatment. However, surgical drainage can be pursued in the setting of failed medical management, and it is generally facilitated by the existence of an anatomic corridor to the petrous apex. In other words, the petrous apex can be approached by several routes, depending on the location of the infection, the pneumatization of the temporal bone, and the status of the hearing. In a non-hearing ear, the translabyrinthine and transotic approaches are the easiest and offer excellent exposure of the petrous apex. Sacrifice of hearing may be justified if the clinical con-

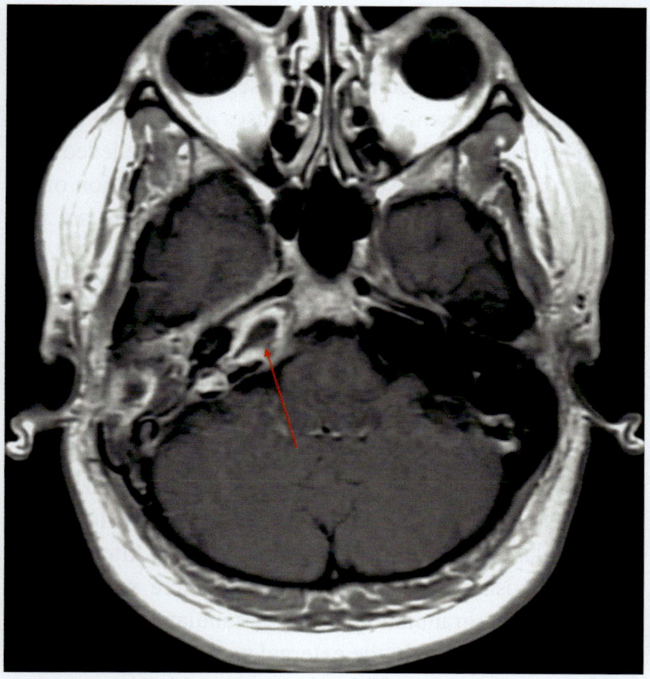

Fig. 35.5 Right-sided acute petrous apicitis (red arrow) in the setting of acute mastoiditis as shown on an axial view of a T1-weighted, contrast-enhanced MRI scan. (Courtesy of Alex Sweeney, MD)

dition endangers the patient's life, and this approach is deemed to offer the best and safest means for management. If more anterior exposure is required, the transcochlear approach is the best option. In a hearing ear, a subtemporal or an infracochlear approach affords access to anteriorly located disease. The retrolabyrinthine or subarcuate routes allow drainage of posterior apicitis with preservation of hearing. CT scans can help determine the optimal access corridor in this setting.

Facial Paralysis

Children are most susceptible to facial paralysis secondary to AOM. In this setting, paralysis of the face is rarely the initial symptom. Most commonly, the first symptoms are those of AOM, and facial paralysis follows several days later. As with other complications mentioned in this chapter, antibiotics have reduced the incidence of facial paralysis associated with an ear infection.

Pathophysiology The routes of spread of infection to the facial nerve are

1. Via natural dehiscences in the fallopian canal, most often in its tympanic segment
2. Via natural pathways that connect the middle ear and the lumen of the fallopian canal, such as the canal for the stapedius muscle, neurovascular connections, and mastoid air cells in close contact with the fallopian canal
3. Via direct infection of the bone around the fallopian canal (localized osteitis)

The organisms that cause facial paralysis are the same that cause AOM. Pus or osteitis around the dehiscent facial nerve most likely leads to inflammation and swelling of the nerve. Toxins and ischemia probably have an ancillary role.

Management

1. The management aims to treat the underlying AOM with appropriate antibiotics for at least 10 days. At the same time, myringotomy, and if appropriate, insertion of a tympanostomy tube is helpful.
2. An intact canal wall mastoidectomy is indicated if coalescent mastoiditis develops or the response to conservative treatment (step 1 above) is not satisfactory. Facial nerve decompression is not necessary in the vast majority of cases, particularly as complete facial recovery occurs in >95% of cases of paralysis secondary to AOM. However, the clinical exam, history and radiologic exam should be carefully analyzed for the possibility of underlying cholesteatoma or neoplasm in these cases.

Labyrinthitis

Schuknecht [11] described three types of labyrinthitis:

1. Serous labyrinthitis
2. Otogenic suppurative labyrinthitis
3. Meningitic suppurative labyrinthitis

Serous labyrinthitis occurs during the course of acute or chronic otitis media. It is presumed that bacterial exotoxins enter the inner ear via the oval or round window or a labyrinthine fistula. As a complication of AOM, the first two routes are more likely. According to Schuknecht [11], in the acute phase, there is no clinical method for differentiating serous from suppurative labyrinthitis. The diagnosis is retrospective. If vestibular and auditory functions are partially or completely retained, it can be assumed that the infection was serous.

Otogenic suppurative labyrinthitis is due to bacterial invasion of the inner ear from a suppurative process within the middle ear. This diagnosis generally leads to vertigo and sensorineural hearing loss. Margolis et al. [12] tested high-frequency hearing in children with a history of AOM and in a matched control group. They found a higher incidence of high-frequency hearing loss in the AOM group.

Suppurative labyrinthitis can further be complicated by meningitis. Bacterial infection within the labyrinth can gain

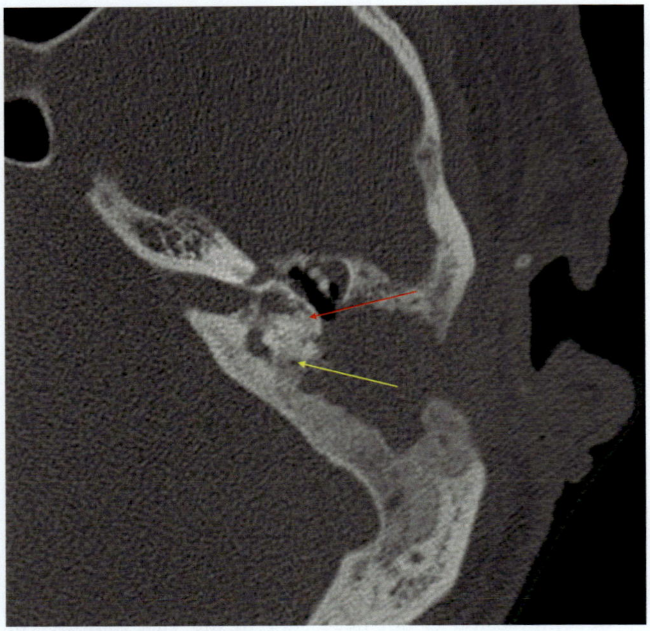

Fig. 35.6 Right-sided labyrinthitis ossificans evident on an axial view of a non-contrast CT scan years after an episode of acute mastoiditis that caused bacterial labyrinthitis. The red arrow points towards the expected location of the anterior limb of the lateral semicircular canal, and the yellow arrow points towards the expected location of the posterior limb. (Courtesy of Alex Sweeney, MD)

access to the subarachnoid space via the fundus of the cochlea or the cochlear aqueduct [5]. Labyrinthitis ossificans, or ossification of the labyrinth as the name implies, is frequently seen following suppurative labyrinthitis. It is generally due to S. pneumoniae and can complicate cochlear implantation [13] (Fig. 35.6).

In addition to antibiotic treatment of AOM, adjuvant corticosteroid therapy should be considered when labyrinthitis is suspected or diagnosed.

Complications of Chronic Otitis Media

In the antibiotic era, complications of otitis media are more commonly seen in the setting of chronic otitis media. Orji et al. [14] compared complications of chronic suppurative otitis media (CSOM) between two eras. They compared patients from the early 1990s and 2009–10. They did not show a significant change in the rates of complications but did show a shift toward predominantly extracranial complications. They explained this shift due to the improvement in antibiotic therapy targeting the usual gram-negative bacteria implicated in CSOM. A good understanding of the pathophysiology of COM enables an appreciation of which forms of COM lead to complications. Smyth [15] proposed that "middle-ear effusion (MEE) is the underlying cause of virtually all forms of chronic suppurative otitis media, ranging from benign uncomplicated perforations of the tympanic membrane, through atelectasis of the middle ear, to life-threatening cholesteatomatous disease of the petrous bone." The long-term presence of MEE causes a portion of the TM to lose its fibrous and elastic layers; this loss is believed to be caused by enzymes present in the MEE. This portion of the TM appears thin and atrophic. Subsequently there are four possible outcomes:

1. The condition of the TM remains stable for many years, and on examination, a "healed scar" is seen.
2. The weak area breaks down during a subsequent episode of AOM, leading to a permanent perforation of the pars tensa of the TM. The status of the middle ear can often be assessed by viewing it through the perforation. When there is no mucosal disease, discharge, or evidence of ossicular erosion, the ear can remain stable. Alternatively, the mucosa may appear boggy and there may be discharge and granulation tissue. Granulation tissue may present as a polyp in the external auditory canal (EAC).
3. If a large area of the TM becomes atrophic, the persistent negative middle-ear pressure can cause the atrophic TM to drape over the medial wall of the middle ear, the incus, and the stapes. The appearance of such an atelectatic TM is much like that of the thin plastic wrap used to protect food.
4. With atrophy of the posterior–superior quadrant of the TM, a retraction pocket develops. Enlargement of the pocket can result in erosion of the long process of the incus. With the development of adhesions that anchor the pocket to the middle-ear mucosa, the retraction pocket is no longer reversible. With loss of self-cleansing ability, the pocket accumulates squamous debris and becomes a cholesteatoma, which, with further enlargement, can extend medial to the body of the incus and the head of the malleus.

Therefore, there are differences among draining ears, and successful management requires an understanding of the underlying pathology and its clinical presentation. Two main types of chronic suppuration, based on the embryology of the middle-ear cleft, have been described in the British literature:

1. Tubotympanic disease (safe or benign type)
2. Atticoantral disease (unsafe or malignant type)

Tubotympanic Disease

The tubotympanic recess is derived from the first branchial pouch, which is lined by respiratory epithelium. This form of disease is characterized by a perforation of the pars tensa in which the margins of the perforation are surrounded by a rim of the pars tensa or the annulus. Disease in the middle-ear cleft is confined to the mucosa, and it is *rarely* the seat of complications. In our experience we have noted three types of tubotympanic disease:

1. A TM perforation is noted on a routine physical examination, and the patient is completely asymptomatic. Mawson and Ludman [16] have termed such a perforation as "inactive."
2. There is a TM perforation with intermittent otorrhea that readily responds to conservative treatment with aural toilet and antibiotic drops.
3. There is intractable drainage through a perforation that resists all conservative management. It is in such cases that florid granulation tissue occupies the entire middle-ear cleft, and if not treated surgically, a polyp may protrude into the EAC or other complications may develop.

Can otogenic complications, such as brain abscess, occur in "safe" and noncholesteatomatous ears? Samuel et al. [17], Rupa and Raman [18], and Browning [19] reported a series of cases in which complications occurred even though there was no cholesteatoma noted at surgery. A review of these articles shows that complications occurred in neglected cases of COM in which the underlying pathology seen at the time of surgery was florid granulation tissue in the middle-ear cleft [19]. Thus, it can be concluded that complications can occur in neglected cases of tubotympanic disease and that cholesteatoma is not typically associated with pars tensa perforations, even when complications occur.

Atticoantral Disease

The further embryologic development of the middle-ear cleft superior to the chorda tympani nerve occurs by penetration of the primordial mesoderm of the epitympanum and antrum by pavement epithelium. Chronic infection in this region is designated as atticoantral disease, is associated with cholesteatoma, and often leads to complications. In atticoantral disease, there are two types of presentation with their associated surgical implications:

1. A "perforation" in the pars flaccida
2. A "perforation" of the posterior–superior quadrant of the pars tensa

The "perforation" is, in reality, a retraction pocket and can be likened to the cut finger of a surgical glove. Its blind distal end lies deep in the middle-ear space, hidden from view by overlying bone. The erosive potential of cholesteatoma and its close proximity to important structures underlie the designation of "unsafe" to this disease.

Pars flaccida cholesteatomas enlarge laterally to the head of the malleus and the body of the incus and cause erosion of the scutum and medialization of the malleus and incus. Pars tensa cholesteatomas erode the long process of the incus or stapes early and then enlarge medial to the annulus, the body of the incus and the head of the malleus, sometimes causing lateralization of the malleus and incus. There is no erosion of the scutum as seen with pars flaccida cholesteatomas [20]. Our current understanding of the initial cause of these retraction pockets is negative pressure in the middle ear. It is for this reason that a shallow retraction pocket can be reversed with the placement of a tympanostomy tube. On the other hand, deep retraction pockets do not respond to tympanostomy tube placement and may continue to deepen, despite normal middle-ear pressure. For this reason, it is suspected that an ongoing inflammatory process may play a role in the progression of retraction pockets. Deeper pockets tend to collect keratin. When infected, these cysts drain and granulation tissue develops around the sac. The stage is now set for bone erosion and possible complications. The predominant bacterial organisms associated with atticoantral COM are *Staphylococcus aureus,* gram-negative bacilli such as *Proteus* spp. and *P. aeruginosa, Klebsiella* spp. and *E. coli. Bacteroides fragilis* is cultured when the discharge is fetid. These two forms of COM have distinctive histopathological findings, as detailed by Nager [3].

Subperiosteal Abscess

Similar to AOM, with bony erosion, the mastoid cortex can be breached, most commonly at Macewen's triangle. Pus then accumulates under the periosteum, resulting in pain, postauricular swelling and tenderness. Blunting of the postauricular crease and anterior–inferior displacement of the pinna are early signs of this complication. The postauricular area is tender and swollen, and the patient may have a fever. When the tip of the mastoid is eroded, swelling and tenderness occur in the upper neck. A Bezold abscess develops when the abscess forms deep to the sternocleidomastoid muscle. These complications occur through direct extension by bone erosion, by venous propagation, or by both [5]. In such cases, the patient complains of stiffness and tenderness of the neck. In some cases, the abscess bursts through the periosteum and skin, manifesting in a draining, postauricular fistula.

Diagnosis Diagnosis is easily confirmed with a non-contrast-enhanced temporal bone CT scan using bone windows. Simultaneously, a contrast-enhanced CT scan of the brain or MRI with contrast should be obtained to rule out concurrent intracranial complications. More than one complication has been reported in as many as 44% of cases.

Management Once the diagnosis is confirmed, IV antibiotic treatment directed against gram-negative and anaerobic bacilli is initiated. A mastoidectomy can provide treatment for the acute phase of the disease, though the definitive treatment may ultimately involve engagement of the middle ear through tympanomastoidectomy, which can be either a canal wall down procedure (CWD) or a canal wall up (CWU) procedure. Staging these procedures is not unreasonable, nor is definitive surgery in the acute setting, depending on the circumstances.

Labyrinthine Fistula

Erosion of the labyrinth occurs in 7% of cases of COM [21] and is considered the most common intratemporal complication of this disease. Cholesteatoma, particularly of the posterior–superior pars tensa variety, is the most frequent cause of lateral canal fistulae. The lateral semicircular canal is particularly susceptible to erosion because of its prominence in the *aditus* and because it frequently lies in the path of an enlarging cholesteatoma. Furthermore, one should distinguish between a bony erosion and a true fistula. Erosion occurs when the endosteal layer of bone remains intact overlying the semicircular canal, while a true fistula occurs when the endosteal layer of bone is eroded, leaving only an endosteal membrane separating the cholesteatoma from the perilymphatic space [22]. The most frequent symptom of a labyrinthine fistula is vertigo, often induced by straining against a closed glottis. Sheehy and Brackmann [23] reported on 97 cases of labyrinthine fistula and noted that almost two-thirds of the patients experienced some form of dizziness. Sensorineural hearing loss is another common associated symptom. Sheehy and Brackmann [23] found that half of the patients with a fistula had sensorineural hearing loss. Ipsilateral facial paresis/paralysis and otalgia are frequently associated symptoms.

Diagnosis The characteristic symptoms and the presence of spontaneous nystagmus should alert the surgeon to the presence of a fistula. The spontaneous nystagmus usually beats towards the nondiseased, contralateral ear. A fistula test should be performed while observing the eyes for nystagmus. If the fistula is located on the nonampullated arc of the horizontal canal, positive pressure will cause cupular deviation toward the utricular sac; e.g., with a fistula in the right ear, the nystagmus will beat toward the right. Tulio phenomenon can also be seen, which is vertigo secondary to auditory stimuli. The definitive diagnosis of a fistula is made by a thin-section bone window CT scan of the temporal bone in both the axial and coronal planes (Fig. 35.7). MRI can also be useful in these cases to assess the fluid signal in the labyrinth. Specifically, a poor prognosis is probable when there is enhancement or a loss of T2-weighted signal in the portion of the labyrinth that corresponds with the point of erosion seen on CT.

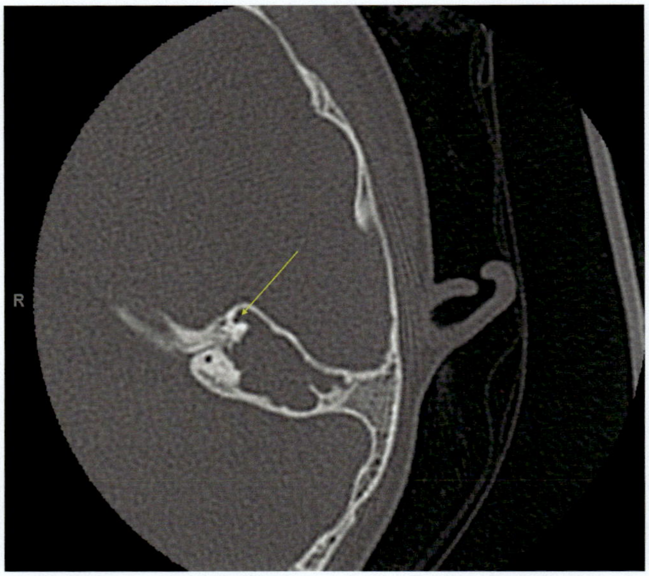

Fig. 35.7 A fistula into the anterior limb of the left superior semicircular canal is demonstrated on an axial view of a non-contrast CT. In this case, the fistula occurred in association with cholesteatoma and acute mastoiditis. (Courtesy of Alex Sweeney, MD)

Management With concurrent antibiotic therapy as described above, a tympanomastoidectomy, either CWD or CWU, comprises definitive treatment. The decision to perform CWD versus CWU mastoidectomy, and whether to remove the entire cholesteatoma matrix versus leaving some intact, remains controversial. Walsh and Baron first commented on this controversy in 1953. Walsh recommended removing the cholesteatoma matrix in its entirety as he believed it had an osteolytic effect on the underlying bone [22]. Several general principles are advocated by most authors. First, if a cholesteatoma is found within the mastoid, it should be opened and thoroughly cleaned. Second, once a labyrinthine fistula is identified, a small amount of matrix can be left over the fistula site to protect it. Third, if the matrix is planned to be removed in its entirety during the initial procedure, then any portion over a possible fistula should be the last step of the procedure. Finally, when the fistula is exposed, it should be covered with a sealant, such as fascia, perichondrium or bone dust. In terms of the nuances of the procedure, different authors recommend different approaches. Ritter recommends performing a CWD mastoidectomy and leaving the matrix intact, as this reduces the risk of damage to the inner ear [24]. On the other hand, Farrior prefers a CWD mastoidectomy and removal of the matrix at the initial operation [25]. The rationale behind this is that they noted persistent vertigo and otorrhea after manipulation of the fistula postoperatively in cases in which matrix was left behind. Manolidis et al. [21] and Sanna et al. [26] *advocate* CWU mastoidectomy and no manipulation of the cholesteatoma matrix. In a second-stage procedure, the matrix, which turns into a small cyst, may be more easily removed. In more than 96% of their patients a sensorineural hearing loss was thus avoided. Surgeons who advocate removal of cholesteatoma matrix at the initial surgery report on average sensorineural hearing loss in 10% of cases [21]. Several investigators have based the decision regarding whether or not to remove the cholesteatoma matrix on the intraoperative determination of the size or depth of the fistula. Gacek described several factors in determining whether or not to remove the entirety of the matrix [27]. First, the ability of the surgeon should be taken into account. If the surgeon is inexperienced or uncomfortable in removing the matrix, then it should be left alone. Second, the location and size of the fistula should be taken into account. Lateral canal fistulas less than 2 mm are safe to remove the matrix, as there is minimal risk of damage to the inner ear. Third, the hearing status/function of the pathologic ear should be taken into account. When there is profound hearing loss in the fistulous ear, there is no further risk to the hearing function and thus the matrix can be completely removed. In a significantly better hearing or only hearing ear, one should leave the matrix intact, especially if the fistula is greater than 2 mm. Even if the matrix is removed, a surgeon should be careful when using irrigation and suction in the area of the fistula. Farrior believes that using suction and irrigation in the area of the fistula leads to further damage to the labyrinth [25].

Overall, though there is controversy on the issue of matrix removal from a fistula in the labyrinth, it is important to remember that, regardless of the technique used, the ultimate goal is to create a safe ear. In this context, hearing should be preserved as best as possible. Surgeons should use meticulous surgical techniques, such as those listed above, and should ask for assistance when inexperienced with labyrinthine fistulae.

Labyrinthitis

The spread of infection into the labyrinth is most often associated with the bone-eroding, atticoantral type of COM. The inflammatory process reaches the vestibule or cochlea via a fistula. The presenting symptoms are vertigo, pain, hearing loss, nausea, and vomiting. Third-degree nystagmus is initially present. The initial treatment of suppurative labyrinthitis is prompt initiation of antibiotic therapy to avoid progression to meningitis. Once antibiotic treatment has been initiated, surgical management is considered. The prognosis for recovery of either vestibular or auditory function is generally poor in these cases. The management of unilateral loss of vestibular function is achieved with physical therapy, and unilateral deafness can be managed with a Contralateral Routing of Signal (CROS) hearing system, an osseointegrated implant, or a cochlear implant. The use of the latter can only occur once the infection has been resolved and the risk of future infection mitigated where possible.

Of note, a noteworthy organism that can cause labyrinthitis in the setting of COM and would potentially evade detection with routine culture is *Mycobacterium tuberculosis*. Robertson and Kumar [28] reported such an infection in a series of cases, and mycobacterial cultures should be considered during the surgical management of a chronic draining ear with labyrinthitis.

Facial Paralysis

When an infranuclear facial paralysis occurs with COM, in most cases, the underlying problem is atticoantral disease. In such cases, the exact cause or mechanism of the paralysis is unknown, largely because we have no histopathological data regarding the nerve. In the majority of cases, the paralysis is associated with cholesteatoma, but as mentioned above, tubercular otitis media should also be kept in mind [28]. It is an uncommon complication with an incidence reported between 1% and 3% in the literature [29]. In nontubercular ears, the infectious process is believed to cause bony erosion of the fallopian canal, adjacent osteitis, direct infection of the nerve, and edema. The role of pressure by the cholesteatoma is less certain.

Diagnosis Facial nerve paralysis can either present abruptly or evolve over time. When present, the otologic surgeon should have a high index of suspicion for a labyrinthine fistula since the two structures are adjacent to each other. To assess the site and extent of involvement of the facial nerve and to identify other associated complications, both a temporal bone CT scan and contrast-enhanced MRI of the brain and temporal bones should be obtained. The MRI scan delineates the extent of involvement of the nerve and provides guidance for surgical decompression, if indicated. The need for electrodiagnostic tests is guided by the mode of onset of the paralysis and its duration.

Management Prompt intervention is usually indicated when an individual with COM presents with facial nerve dysfunction. In many cases, antibiotics and corticosteroids can be started to control the inflammatory process and to reduce facial nerve edema. That being said, the use of corticosteroids can be controversial and should be carefully considered in some settings, such as the presence of poorly controlled diabetes. In contrast to the nonsurgical management of facial paralysis due to AOM, the definitive treatment for paralysis due to COM focuses on the eradication of the cholesteatoma and facial nerve decompression or repair. Four different types of damage to the facial nerve can be identified: (1) A compressed but normal segment;

(2) A reddish edematous segment; (3) A fibrosed segment; (4) An interrupted segment [30]. There is controversy regarding surgical decompression of the facial nerve, epineural incision, and maintenance of the canal wall. Most recent studies suggest that a CWD mastoidectomy is preferred by most otologists [29]. The nuances of the procedure, however, differ. Some prefer decompressing the nerve only along the injured portion, which may be only millimeters. In addition, some prefer leaving the epineurium intact, as they believe it prevents the spread of the infection. Other otologists prefer to decompress the entire length of the facial nerve from the geniculate ganglion to the stylomastoid foramen as well as incising the epineurium [30]. Complete nerve destruction or interruption is rarely encountered. If a segment is truly missing from the nerve, it is best to perform a CWD mastoidectomy with end-to-end anastomosis using a nerve graft versus redirecting the facial nerve, depending on the length of the damaged nerve. Recovery of facial nerve function is not as likely as it is in a paralysis secondary to AOM. The grade of recovery will depend on the mode of onset of paralysis, the duration of paralysis, and the extent of disease.

It is important to note that, while only 1–3% of patients with COM and cholesteatoma present with a facial nerve paralysis, a much higher percentage will have a fallopian canal dehiscence, putting the nerve at risk during a mastoidectomy for eradication of the cholesteatoma. The percentage of dehiscence varies between 19% and 33% [29]. Thus, one can infer that while the fallopian canal is at risk for erosion, the facial nerve is somewhat resistant to damage.

Meningoencephaloceles

Meningoencephaloceles (ME) are a herniation of dura mater (meningocele) and/or brain tissue (encephalocele) into the mastoid or middle ear. ME can be associated with chronic otitis media and/or cholesteatoma, leading to tegmen erosion or iatrogenic tegmen defect from mastoid surgery to eradicate the cholesteatoma. While ME are uncommon in the setting of COM, the importance of early diagnosis cannot be understated. The complications of ME can be devastating and include meningitis, intracranial abscesses, hemorrhage, venous infarction, and seizures [31].

A bony defect is required to allow for dura or brain tissue to herniate into the temporal bone; however, the dura mater overlying the middle cranial fossa can support the intracranial contents over a large defect in most patients [31] Interestingly, several anatomic studies have shown that 20–33% of adult temporal bones have one or more defects in the tegmen, but the incidence of encephaloceles is significantly lower than this [32].

Diagnosis Meningoencephaloceles often present nonspecifically. A common presenting symptom is CSF otorrhea. CSF leakage is thought to be related to the presence of aberrant arachnoid granulations found on the dural surface of the temporal bone [33]. High intracranial pressure can cause progressive enlargement with time, leading to the herniation of brain tissue. Beta-2 transferrin testing can be helpful, though it can be difficult to obtain an adequate amount for testing. Physical exam findings of a pulsatile mass or middle ear effusion are nonspecific. Audiometry typically reveals a conductive hearing loss. Patients with pseudotumor cerebri, or elevated intracranial pressure, are at increased risk. Encephaloceles due to cholesteatoma are thought to arise from local bone resorption associated with direct pressure ischemia or due to enzymatic degradation [31].

Imaging is critical to diagnosis because the initial presentation for this type of patient can be non-specific. Tegmen defects can be appropriately identified on CT imaging, and thus, a high-resolution CT temporal bone should be the initial imaging modality of choice. CT, however, cannot delineate brain tissue from cholesteatoma or granulation tissue. Hence, MRI provides additional utility for diagnosis and surgical planning. Herniation of brain tissue with interruption of the dural line, known as the teardrop sign, can often be seen on MRI. Additionally, the use of non-echo-planar diffusion-weighted imaging can be helpful to distinguish between cholesteatoma and the brain. In cases that involve the combination of a brain hernia and cholesteatoma, counseling should reinforce the potential need for multiple surgeries and multiple surgical approaches.

Management Several surgical approaches have been described for repair of tegmen defects and cholesteatoma. Regardless of the technique, the goals of repair are the same, including management of the herniated brain, restoration of dural integrity, and eradication of the mastoid infection and cholesteatoma [31]. The three approaches include a transmastoid approach from below, a middle fossa approach from above, and a combined approach. In cases involving a large meningoencephalocele, dural violation and cholesteatoma, disease resection can also be performed in conjunction with a subtotal petrousectomy and ear canal closure. In the latter situation, the resulting conductive hearing loss can be rehabilitated with bone conduction aid, though percutaneous or nonsurgical aids are favored, when audiologically appropriate, given the need for surveillance imaging and the concern for MRI artifact when an MRI conditional implanted magnet is present. Focusing on smaller (<1 cm) defects, a transmastoid approach is generally favored. Many options are used for dural closure; Jeevan et al. [31] preferred using temporalis fascia. However, fascia alone may not be sufficient to hold the intracranial contents and can lead to recurrence. The addition of a rigid (bone) or semi-rigid (tragal cartilage) material is important to prevent recurrence of the meningoencephalocele [34]. Synthetic material used as bony grafts to repair the bony defect is not routinely used due to the high incidence of extrusion, recurrence and infection [31]. Hydroxyapatite cement has been reported for successful repair of the bony defect, but again, as this material is synthetic, it should not be used in the presence of infection [35]. The core principle is that a layered closure of the defect gives the strength needed to support the intracranial contents.

Conclusions

As compared to versions of this chapter that accompanied earlier editions of this book, the work of contemporary otologists is facilitated by a far more advanced diagnostic and therapeutic armamentarium. However, the lessons of the past cannot be forgotten; rather, we must build on them and expect that, in the years to come, more advanced systems will replace those of the present. Hopefully, with better diagnostic tools and greater accumulated experience managing complications, outcomes can continue to improve for patients with significant complications of otitis media.

References

1. Matthew R, Asimacopoulos E, Valentine P. Toward safer practice in otology: a report on 15 years of negligence claims. Laryngoscope. 2011;121(10):2214–9.
2. Neely JG. Facial nerve & intracranial complications in otitis media. In: Jackler R, Brackmann BE, editors. Neurotology. 2nd ed. Philadelphia: Mosby; 2005. p. 912–25.
3. Nager GT. Pathology of the ear and temporal bone. Baltimore: Williams & Wilkins; 1993. p. 220–97.
4. Luntz M, Brodsky A, Nusem S, et al. Acute mastoiditis—the antibiotic era: a multicenter study. Int J Pediatr Otorhinolaryngol. 2001;57:1–9.
5. Arts HA, Adams ME. Intratemporal and intracranial complications of otitis media. In: Johnson JT, Rosen CA, editors. Bailey's head and neck surgery—otolaryngology, vol. 2. 5th ed. Philadelphia: Lippincott Williams & Wilkins; 2014. p. 2399–407.
6. Zevallos JP, Vrabec JT, Williamson RA, et al. Advanced pediatric mastoiditis with and without intracranial complications. Laryngoscope. 2009;119(8):1610–5.
7. Soucek S, Michaels L. The ear in acquired immunodeficiency syndrome: II. Clinical and audiological investigation. Am J Otol. 1996;17:35–9.
8. Holt GR, Gates GA. Masked mastoiditis. Laryngoscope. 1983;93(8):1034–7.
9. Meyerhoff WL, Kim CS, Papparella MM. Pathology of chronic otitis media. Ann Otol Rhinol Laryngol. 1998;87:749–60.
10. Schuknecht HF. Infections. In: Pathology of the ear. Philadelphia: Lea & Febiger; 1993. p. 218–20.
11. Schuknecht HF. Infections. In: Pathology of the ear. Philadelphia: Lea & Febiger; 1993. p. 211–6.
12. Margolis RH, Saly GL, Hunter L, Lisa L. High frequency hearing loss and wideband middle ear impedance in children with otitis media histories. Ear Hear. 2000;21(3):206–11.
13. Durisin M. Cochlear osteoneogenesis after meningitis in cochlear implant patients: a retrospective analysis. Otol Neurotol. 2010;31(7):1072–8.
14. Orgi FT, Ukaegbe O, Alex-Okoro J, et al. The changing epidemiological and complications profile of chronic suppurative otitis media in a developing country after two decades. Eur Arch Otorrinolaringol. 2016;273:2461–6.
15. Smyth GDL. Etiology of chronic suppurative otitis media. In: Smyth GDL, editor. Chronic ear disease. New York: Churchill Livingstone; 1980. p. 1–20.
16. Mawson S, Ludman H. Otitis media. In: Diseases of the ear: a textbook of otology. 4th ed. London: Arnold; 1979. p. 301–65.
17. Samuel J, Fernandes CM, Steinberg JL. Intracranial otogenic complications: a persisting problem. Laryngoscope. 1986;96(3):272–8.
18. Rupa V, Raman R. Chronic suppurative otitis media: complicated versus uncomplicated disease. Acta Otolaryngol. 1991;111(3):530–5.
19. Browning GG. The unsafeness of "safe" ears. J Laryngol Otol. 1984;98(1):23–6.
20. Valvassori GE. Imaging of the temporal bone. In: Mafee MF, Valvassori GE, Becker M, editors. Imaging of the head and neck. 2nd ed. New York; Stuttgart, Germany: Thieme; 2005. p. 74–89.
21. Manolides S. Complications associated with labyrinthine fistula in surgery of chronic otitis media. Otolaryngol Head Neck Surg. 2000;123:733–7.
22. Wiet RJ, Harvey SA, Bauer GP. Management of complications of chronic otitis media. In: Brackmann DE, Shelton C, Arriaga MA, editors. Otologic surgery. Philadelphia: W.B. Saunders; 1994. p. 257–76.
23. Sheehy JL, Brackmann DE. Cholesteatoma surgery: management of the labyrinthine fistula—a report of 97 cases. Laryngoscope. 1979;89:78–87.
24. Ritter FN. Chronic suppurative otitis media and the pathologic labyrinthine fistula. Laryngoscope. 1970;80:1025–35.
25. Farrior JB. Surgery for cholesteatoma. In: Wiet RJ, Causse JB, editors. Complications in otolaryngology—head and neck surgery, vol. 1. Philadelphia: BC Decker; 1986. p. 228–47.
26. Sanna M, Zini C, Gamoletti R, et al. Closed versus open technique in the management of labyrinthine fistulae. Am J Otol. 1988;9(6):470–5.
27. Gacek RR. The surgical management of labyrinthine fistulae in chronic otitis media with cholesteatoma. Ann Otol Rhinol Laryngol. 1974;83(10):3–19.
28. Robertson K, Kumar A. Atypical presentations of aural tuberculosis. Am J Otolaryngol. 1995;16:294–302.
29. Prassad SC, Shin SH, Russo A, et al. Current trends in the management of the complications of chronic otitis media with cholesteatoma. Curr Opin Otolaryngol Head Neck Surg. 2013;21(5):446–54.
30. Kim J, Jung GH, Park SY, Lee WS. Facial nerve paralysis due to chronic otitis media: prognosis in restoration of facial function after surgical intervention. Yonsei Med J. 2012;53:642–8.
31. Jeevan DS, Ormond DR, Kim AH, et al. Cerebrospinal fluid leaks and encephaloceles of temporal bone origin: nuances to diagnosis and management. World Neurosurg. 2015;83(4):560–6.
32. Kapur TR, Bangash W. Temporal and petromastoid defects in the temporal bone. J Laryngol Otol. 1986;100:1129–32.
33. Gulya AJ, Schuknecht HF. Anatomy of the temporal bone with surgical implications. New York: Parthenon Publishing Group; 1995.
34. Semaan MT, Gilpin DA, Hsu DP, et al. Transmastoid extradural-intracranial approach for repair of transtemporal meningoencephalocele: a review of 31 consecutive cases. Laryngoscope. 2011;121(8):1765–72.
35. Nahas Z, Tatlipinar A, Limb CJ, Francis HW. Spontaneous meningoencephalocele of the temporal bone: clinical spectrum and presentation. Arch Otolaryngol Head Neck Surg. 2008;134:509–18.

Intracranial Complications of Otitis Media

36

Samuel C. Levine, Meredith E. Adams, and Elizabeth A. Kelly

Introduction

Intracranial complications of acute and chronic otitis media include meningitis, epidural, subdural and intraparenchymal abscesses, lateral sinus thrombosis, and otitic hydrocephalus. These complications are associated with significant morbidity and mortality if there are delays in appropriate diagnosis and management. The incidence, presentation, and management of these complications have evolved over time with the introduction of new antibiotics, vaccinations, and surgical approaches. Herein is a presentation of this historical perspective as well as factors that influence the development of intracranial complications, followed by detailed presentations of the pathophysiology, diagnosis, and management of each one.

Historical Perspective

Hippocrates noted in 460 BC that "acute pain in the ear with continued high fever is to be dreaded for the patient may become delirious and die" [1]. In the preantibiotic era, the Roman physician Celsus (25 AD) and the Arabian physician Avicenna (980–1037 AD) recognized that complications from otitis media occurred abundantly and were accompanied by a high morbidity. Morgagni (1682–1771 AD) noted that the ear infection presented initially and the brain abscess was secondary [2].

Brain abscess was the first complication of otitis media to be recognized and the first one successfully treated by an operation by Morand in 1768 [3]. In 1856, Lebert accurately described the pathology of brain abscess, confirming that it follows an otologic infection [4]. Almost 30 years later, MacEwen reported a successful series of operative brain abscesses [5]. In 1908, Körner reported another series of operations for brain abscesses with a 50% recovery rate [6].

Surgical intervention for brain abscess had reached its peak of otologic interest in the 1920s [7]. The management of this relatively common complication of otitis media remained chiefly in the hands of the otologic surgeon until sulfonamides began to be used for acute otitis media (AOM) in 1935 and penicillin was introduced in 1942. Thereafter, the incidence of brain abscess, which may already have begun to decline, decreased abruptly. The relative success of surgery for brain abscess remained in sharp contrast for many years to the almost invariably fatal outcome of purulent meningitis, the most dreaded complication of otitis media and the most frequent cause of death. Treatment for generalized otitic meningitis was rarely successful; therefore, the efforts of the otologic surgeon were directed toward prevention. Whenever possible, bone-invading types of AOM and chronic otitis media (COM) were operated on before a complication had occurred. Careful clinical observation of patients with middle ear infections would frequently permit the detection of the earliest stages of meningeal involvement. With prompt and thorough surgical drainage of the suppurative focus in the temporal bone, considerable success was achieved in arresting the meningeal invasion, in many cases while it was still localized, preventing the development of otherwise fatal generalized meningitis [8]. Despite these advances, meningitis remained the most frequent cause of death in otitis media, and otitis media was by far the most frequent cause of meningitis from pathogens other than *Neisseria meningitidis*.

S. C. Levine
Department of Otolaryngology—Head and Neck Surgery, University of Minnesota, Minneapolis, MN, USA
e-mail: levin001@umn.edu

M. E. Adams
Department of Otolaryngology—Head and Neck Surgery, University of Michigan, Ann Arbor, MI, USA
e-mail: meadams@umich.edu

E. A. Kelly (✉)
Department of Otolaryngology, Boys Town National Research Hospital, Omaha, NE, USA
e-mail: elizabeth.kelly@boystown.org

A. D. Sweeney et al. (eds.), *Haynes-Glasscock-Shambaugh Surgery of the Ear*, https://doi.org/10.1007/978-3-032-18264-7_36

Infective thrombosis of the lateral sinus, the last of the three major intracranial complications of otitis media, was first described in 1826. Thirty years later, Lebert accurately described the pathology of otitic sinus thrombosis [9]. In 1880, Zaufal proposed an operation for this complication and first attempted it in 1884; however, it still ended in patient mortality [10].

The surgical treatment of sinus thrombosis was further established by the publications of Lane in 1889 and Ballance in 1890 [11, 12]. However, a controversy over whether, as part of the surgical management, to ligate the jugular vein in all cases, in some cases, or in no case continued for many years, only to be resolved by the introduction of effective antibacterial and anticoagulant medication in favor of nonligation for most cases.

The two complications of otitis media caused by expansion within the temporal bone that often lead to a fatal intracranial extension, namely, purulent labyrinthitis and petrositis, were the last serious complications to be defined and effectively treated. A technique for draining the infected labyrinth was first described in 1895 by Jansen [13]. In 1904, Gradenigo described the syndrome of continuing aural discharge, severe fifth cranial nerve pain, and sixth nerve paralysis caused by infection of pneumatic cells in the petrous portion of the temporal bone with adjacent meningitis [14]. Kopetsky and Almour in 1930 and Eagleton in 1931 described the first systematic attempts to drain an abscess of the petrous apex [15, 16]. Other methods for reaching this relatively inaccessible area were soon described. For a few years, the literature contained numerous reports of successful operations for petrositis, many of them in patients with early meningitis. Just at the time that this frequent cause of otitic meningitis began to yield to surgical therapy, it virtually disappeared from the scene of otologic experience as a result of effective antibacterial medication for AOM.

The frequency of otitis complications changed dramatically with the introduction of effective antibiotics. In the 5-year period immediately preceding the introduction of these agents, from 1928 to 1933, approximately 1 in every 40 deaths in a large general hospital was caused by an intracranial complication of otitis media, with meningitis as the most common cause, sinus thrombosis second, and then brain abscess [17]. In a subsequent 5-year period (from 1949–1954), only 1 in every 400 deaths was the result of otologic disease—an amazing ten-fold reduction in less than 20 years. The introduction of pneumococcal conjugate vaccines has also resulted in a decline of pneumococcal meningitis [18]. Recently a new pneumococcal conjugate vaccine (PCV 20) was released with coverage of more serotypes; however, the impact of this vaccine on invasive pneumococcal infections has not yet been determined.

Of the three major intracranial complications of otitis media, the reduction in mortality has been greatest for thrombophlebitis of the lateral sinus, which has nearly disappeared as a cause of death [17]. This fact is easily understood because infection of the vasculature was the usual mechanism of death from sinus thrombosis, a site where antibiotics are most effective. The incidence of brain abscess was also greatly reduced by antibiotics. Purulent meningitis, though reduced, persists today as by far the most frequent intracranial complication of otitis media. However, it has changed from a nearly 100% fatal disease to one in which recovery can be expected in the majority of instances if diagnosed early and treated adequately.

Primary care clinicians often rely on medications to manage ear disease. Intracranial complications are now observed in patients who received antibiotics considered adequate for typical AOM prior to presentation, and thus, the use of antibiotics does not completely safeguard against the development of complications [19]. Multiple series report intracranial complications occurring in patients already on oral antibiotics combined with a high proportion of negative cultures at the time of surgical intervention (33–51%). Incompletely treated OM, or selection for resistant bacteria, likely delays the time course of disease and alters symptom presentations [20]. The neurosurgeon may be the first to be called in consultation for intracranial complications. Most otologists work in combination as a team with a neurosurgeon as treatment involves both specialties.

Although the incidence of otitis media complications has declined, and a whole new range of antibiotics has been introduced, complications have not been eradicated completely. One or more prior courses of antibiotic therapy may obscure early identification and timely intervention for complications. One cannot reliably distinguish patients with and without intracranial complications based solely on clinical presentation, including specific presenting symptoms, signs, or laboratory indices. Diagnostic imaging remains essential for patients presenting with acute mastoiditis [19, 21]. The clinician should maintain a high index of suspicion in all patients with COM with accompanying symptoms of pain, including headache and otalgia, fever, neck stiffness (nuchal rigidity), and mental status changes; such symptoms are unusual from uncomplicated COM and, given the morbidity of delayed intervention, should prompt imaging evaluation with high resolution computed tomography (CT) and magnetic resonance imaging (MRI) [22]. Awareness of the significance of the symptoms and signs results in earlier diagnosis, prompt treatment, and further reduction in mortality.

We are entering a period in otology characterized by a higher threshold for aggressive surgical intervention for complications of OM, with some physicians advocating purely medical approaches for primary management. While radical mastoidectomy used to be considered the most appropriate operation for OM complications in prior years, it is apparent that many complications can be managed well with canal wall up or modified radical operations, even in the setting of COM [23]. Even so, while using best judgment, the surgeon should work to avoid surgical under-treatment. Surgical care of OM complications can require visualization (through thin bone) or exposure of the sigmoid sinus and/or dura of the middle and posterior cranial fossae. In cases where these measures are necessary, failure to perform them can result in under-treatment of intracranial complications.

Factors That Influence the Development of Complications

Intracranial complications occur as a result of many factors, often acting simultaneously, causing the infection to spread from the ear and into the intracranial cavity. The tendency of middle ear infection to spread beyond the confines of the middle ear and its adjacent spaces is influenced by the virulence of the infecting organism and its sensitivity to antibiotics, host resistance, the adequacy of antibiotic therapy, the anatomic pathways and barriers to spread, and the drainage of the pneumatic spaces, both natural and surgical. In general, intracranial complications occur when OM is either uncontrolled or inadequately treated. While acute otitis media is most common in pediatric patients, there is a greater rate of complications in adult patients [24].

The microbiology of middle ear infections remains relatively constant over time. *Streptococcus pneumoniae*, *Haemophilus influenzae*, and *Moraxella catarrhalis* cause most acute infections [25, 26]. The introduction of *H. influenzae* and *S. pneumoniae* vaccines has decreased the virulence within the bacterial species. As different antibiotics are used, the patterns of antibiotic resistance seem to change and may vary from one location to another [27]. Complications continue to occur despite the presence of vaccines [28].

The microbiology of chronic infection is different from the acute process. Organisms such as *Pseudomonas aeruginosa* are much more common [29]. The treatment of a *Pseudomonas* infection requires a higher dosage of less routinely used antibiotics. The benign type of chronic otorrhea with mucoid discharge coming from a central perforation does not, by itself, invade bone and cause complications. There is, however, nothing to prevent a virulent organism from entering such an ear and causing an acute exacerbation and a complication by the same mechanism as in any case of AOM. Unfortunately, the new organism is likely to display some greater resistance to antibiotics since the patient is likely to have received treatment for the otorrhea.

Immunocompromised individuals are at risk of developing not only otitis media but also complications of otitis media. The organisms causing the infection are more likely to be atypical pathogens. Individuals may be taking immunosuppressive medications, rendering them immunocompromised and susceptible to infection, or have other infectious, congenital, or acquired immunodeficiencies.

Intracranial extension of AOM occurs somewhat more often from poorly pneumatized than well-pneumatized temporal bones and even ears with a history of previous attacks of otitis media. The likelihood of a complication arising from chronic middle ear infections depends on the pathologic lesion causing the chronic otorrhea. The middle ear cleft has bony barriers that prevent the middle ear infection from extending intracranially. However, these barriers may be eroded by antecedent infections, granulation tissue, or cholesteatoma, thus allowing infection to spread into the cranial cavity from the middle ear. Trauma with fracture can create passages that allow infections to bypass these natural defenses.

The natural drainage of the mastoid cavity (approximately 5 cc in volume) is into a relatively smaller space, the middle ear cavity (capacity approximately 0.9 cc), which then drains through the Eustachian tube. Drainage may be inadequate, allowing infected secretions to accumulate and then erode through the middle ear cleft to extend intracranially [30].

Pathway of Spread in the Production of a Complication

Uncontrolled or poorly controlled infection in the middle ear cleft may enter the intracranial cavity through any of three routes.

Bone Erosion

Extension by bone erosion is the most frequent manner of spread, leading to a complication in cases of AOM in well-pneumatized temporal bones. This route is nearly always the manner of spread in cases of chronic suppurative otitis media. In AOM, bone erosion is the result of coalescent mastoiditis. In COM, the bone erosion is usually caused by a cholesteatoma; less often, it is caused by chronic osteomyelitis.

The bone-eroding process first exposes the soft tissue of a neighboring structure. Protective granulations form on the structure as a last line of defense. Then, after a period of time that varies with the virulence of the organism, the pus under pressure finally penetrates the wall of protective granulations by pressure necrosis. Bone erosion as the pathway of spread may be recognized by the following characteristics:

- The complication occurs several weeks or more after the onset of AOM or in chronic otitis of long duration.
- A prodromal period of partial or intermittent involvement of the structure frequently precedes the diffuse involvement. Thus, a milder, intermittent facial weakness may

precede complete facial paralysis; recurrent mild vertigo may precede diffuse purulent labyrinthitis, and localized meningitis (meningismus) may precede diffuse purulent meningitis.
- At operation, a dehiscence of the bone barrier is found between the suppurative focus and the neighboring structure. A layer of granulation tissue covers the exposed soft tissue of the neighboring structure.
- The treatment of a complication by bone erosion is directed toward the complication and always includes surgical removal of the suppurative, bone-eroding focus in the temporal bone. If such removal is neglected, the complication is likely to recur or respond poorly to treatment.

Direct Extension Along Preformed Pathways

Extension by preformed pathways may occur in either acute exacerbations of COM or AOM. The preformed pathway may be a normal anatomic opening in the bony wall, such as the oval or round window, internal auditory canal, cochlear aqueduct, or endolymphatic duct and sac. The pathway may be a developmental dehiscence, such as a patent suture or a dehiscent floor of the hypotympanum over the jugular bulb. The preformed pathway may be the result of a skull fracture or previous surgery. A perilymph fistula, either congenital or acquired, can also serve as a pathway. Occasionally, previous otitis media with coalescent mastoiditis heals but leaves a scar tissue tract to a neighboring structure. This tract acts as a preformed pathway for infections. Extension via a preformed pathway is not always easily diagnosed preoperatively. The diagnosis is suggested by the following characteristics:

- There is a history of skull fracture, operation on the temporal bone, previously healed otitis media, or repeated attacks of meningitis.
- The complication occurs early in the acute infection, thus resembling extension by thrombophlebitis.
- At operation, a dehiscence of the bone barrier not caused by bone erosion is found.
- The patient has an intracranial complication following suppurative labyrinthitis.

The treatment of a complication by a preformed pathway is directed toward the complication itself, closure of the pathway and surgical evacuation of any collection of pus within the temporal bone. An example is in treating meningitis acquired via the internal auditory canal from suppurative labyrinthitis, in which case the labyrinth should be drained at the same time that the meningitis is treated by antimicrobial medication.

Thrombophlebitis

In 1902, Körner demonstrated by histopathologic studies that it is possible for infection to pass from the lining mucosa of the middle ear and mastoid through intact bone by means of a progressive thrombophlebitis of small venules [6]. This manner of spread may occur in acute middle ear infections or acute exacerbations of a chronic infection, and in either case, it spreads through veins contiguous with either the infected pneumatized spaces of the temporal bone or the previously thrombosed dural venous sinus. There is a rich network of veins that directly communicate within the temporal bone, and in turn, directly communicate with the extracranial, intracranial, and cranial diploic veins. The extracranial veins are closely associated with the arterial supply of the temporal bone. The extracranial and intracranial venous systems anastomose through the mastoid emissary veins that enter the sigmoid sinus, which drain the superior and inferior petrosal sinuses. All of the dural venous sinuses are interconnected. Thus, sigmoid sinus thrombosis can lead to thrombophlebitis of other sinuses as well.

A complication caused by thrombophlebitis may be recognized by the following characteristics:

- The complication occurs early in the acute infection, sometimes within a day or two of the onset, usually within the first 10 days.
- In certain complications, such as purulent meningitis, the prodromal period of beginning invasion with localized meningitis, commonly called meningismus, such as is usually seen in extension by bone erosion, is absent.
- At operation, the bony walls of the middle ear and mastoid cells are intact. The bone and mucoperiosteum lining of the mastoid cells may be inflamed and bleed easily, but there is no coalescent abscess, and the bone is not dehiscent.
- Hematogenous spread of infection usually results in meningitis. Whereas venous thrombophlebitis usually leads to cerebellar abscesses, arterial spread leads to temporal lobe abscesses and diffuse septicemia.

Specific Complications

It is uncommon for an intracranial complication to occur without a temporal bone complication occurring first. Common symptoms of an impending intracranial complication are as follows:

- Persistence of otorrhea. The otorrhea is particularly foul-smelling, and the pus becomes more viscous. The pus is thicker and creamier and may be blood-stained. When intracranial complication is imminent, the discharge becomes scanty, indicative of poor drainage.

- Pain is an ominous sign that an intracranial complication is imminent. The pain is typically of a deep, boring nature and is accompanied by a change in the quality of the pus emanating from the ear. Patients may also complain of a generalized headache that is "the worst headache" they have ever had.
- High-grade fever, altered sensorium, toxemia, photophobia, and irritability are other signs of impending intracranial complications.
- Neck stiffness and generalized malaise are signs that the organism has reached the cerebrospinal fluid (CSF) space.

The principles of ear surgery remain unchanged in these complications:

- Eradication of disease
- Establishment of adequate drainage for accumulated material

Eradication of disease requires a thorough and complete mastoidectomy. All of the diseased air cells are exenterated. Pus, wherever it is encountered, is drained. All diseased or dead tissue is removed. There are some general remarks that can be made concerning all complications of mastoid disease. Specific recommendations are made in the following sections concerning each complication. Creating adequate drainage usually requires a mastoidectomy approach, with exceptions in certain situations. In the presence of AOM that has caused meningitis, usually antibiotics and a myringotomy with tube insertion suffice to provide adequate drainage. In the presence of overwhelming disease and cholesteatoma, most reports advocate canal-wall-down techniques in order to make the ear disease-free. Equally important is creating a wide meatoplasty. A wide meatoplasty permits adequate drainage and allows easy inspection and cleansing of the mastoid cavity.

Each diagnosis of intracranial disease is defined and discussed individually. Meningitis is the most common complication in this group of diagnoses in most traditional articles. Brain abscess and lateral sinus thrombosis are the next most common. Finally, other diagnoses, including otitic hydrocephalus, and subdural and epidural processes are reviewed. Pathophysiology, including microbiology, unique symptoms, specific evaluation methods, and treatment, is outlined.

Meningitis

Generalized bacterial meningitis is defined as an inflammatory response to bacterial infection of the pia-arachnoid and the CSF of the subarachnoid space. Since the subarachnoid space is continuous around the brain, spinal cord, and optic nerves, infections of this space usually involve the entire cerebrospinal axis.

Localized meningitis may be defined as a localized inflammation of the dura and pia-arachnoid confined to the region adjacent to a suppurative focus or dural irritation, without viable organisms in the CSF.

Meningitis was the most frequent intracranial complication of otitis media in the preantibiotic era. With the introduction of antimicrobial drugs, recovery from meningitis improved from 10% to 86% whereas recovery from otogenic meningitis was 59% [31, 32]. Currently, community-acquired meningitis caused by *S. pneumoniae* has fatality rates from 8% to 37% [33–36]. Other clinicians have confirmed that meningitis continues to be the most common intracranial complication of AOM [37]. AOM is often the predominant cause of meningitis compared with COM [38].

Pathophysiology

S. pneumoniae is one of the major pathogens associated with AOM [36, 39, 40]. With increased use of antibiotics, there is a growing rate of multidrug-resistant *S. pneumoniae* strains [41, 42]. Introduction of vaccinations against certain serotypes of *S. pneumoniae* have decreased the rate of meningitis related to this organism as well as rates of *H. influenzae* type B, however there is concern for increasing disease caused by non-vaccine pneumococci or other otologic pathogens [27, 36]. Anaerobic pathogens may cause more severe infections in these patients and support the initial use of broad coverage antibiotics and obtaining cultures [42]. Recovery of anaerobic organisms from the CSF may suggest intraventricular rupture of a brain abscess. Polymicrobial infection of CSF resulting from otogenic complications is uncommon.

Meningitis may result from infection spreading from the ear via retrograde thrombophlebitis, bone erosion, and preformed pathways. An important route through which infection can gain access to the CSF is via the labyrinth through the round and oval windows. Nager and Kaplan stressed that this mode of extension is via the perineural spaces to the internal auditory canal and less frequently via the endolymphatic ducts [43, 44]. Proctor postulated that otitic meningitis occurs as a result of infection spreading via the labyrinth and petrous apex [45]. Meningitis can also occur following any middle ear and mastoid surgery. Additionally, CSF leak of the temporal bone carries a risk of developing meningitis. A CSF leak is defined as any abnormal communication between the subarachnoid space and air-filled spaces of the temporal bone [46]. There are a number of different etiologies, including complications of chronic ear disease, iatrogenic pathways, temporal bone fractures, or following irradiation of tumors involving the temporal bone. Also, a leak can begin spontaneously and without any prior ear disease, as may be the case in idiopathic intracranial hypertension (IIH), or it can occur as the result of a congenital malformation. Once detected, repair is often recommended. However, there is a paucity of data to describe the duration of exposure that may increase the risk of meningitis development [47].

There are a number of neurological sequelae associated with bacterial meningitis, including hearing loss, seizures, and cognitive impairment [48]. Of all patients surviving bacterial meningitis, 5–35% experience bilateral sensorineural hearing loss [49]. Hearing loss is often associated with pneumococcal meningitis [39, 48]. Paparella described the pathophysiology of suppurative meningogenic labyrinthitis as having three phases. The acute phase involves infiltration of leukocytes and is followed by the fibrous stage, characterized by fibrous proliferation within perilymph spaces. The ossification stage ensues, with the most significant disease in the basal turn of the cochlea near the round window. He stated that the pathologic features of meningogenic suppurative labyrinthitis are essentially the same as tympanogenic labyrinthitis [50]. In a human temporal bone study, Merchant verified the hypothesis that the cochlear modiolus and the cochlear aqueduct can serve as potential pathways for the spread of infection from the meninges to the inner ear [51].

Clinical Presentation

Otogenic meningitis often goes unrecognized. Most physicians will suspect an otologic cause in the presence of otorrhea or obvious long-standing ear disease. It is imperative to rule out otitis media in the patient who does not have these characteristics.

Symptoms tend to develop rapidly when associated with AOM [52, 53]. The earliest symptoms are headache, fever, vomiting, photophobia, irritability, and restlessness. Infants may have seizures. As the infection progresses, the headache increases, and vomiting becomes more pronounced. Neck stiffness, with resistance to flexing the neck so that the chin does not touch the chest, may start with minimal discomfort and progress. Brudzinski's sign, the inability to flex the leg without moving the opposite leg (or flexion of the neck resulting in flexion of the hip and knee), is a sign of meningitis. Kernig's sign, an inability to extend the leg when lying supine with the thigh flexed toward the abdomen, is also a sign of meningitis. While these are classic physical exam findings for meningitis, they have been shown to have variable diagnostic accuracy and should be interpreted in combination with other forms of assessment [39, 54].

Management

CT and/or MRI should be obtained when an intracranial complication of otitis media is suspected. Often high-resolution CT of the temporal bones is the first management step in evaluation for suspected meningitis. A high-resolution CT scan is very useful and is typically the imaging modality of choice. Bony details are best visualized with CT. Either CT or MRI is generally recommended to evaluate for intracranial hypertension and mass effect prior to lumbar puncture to prevent brain herniation. However, there is some debate with this recommendation, as obtaining imaging first may delay lumbar puncture and initiation of antibiotic treatment, which can subsequently result in increased mortality. Some recommend obtaining CT scan in those individuals whose presentation and history are most concerning for brain herniation, such as those who present with focal neurologic signs, new-onset seizures, severely altered mental status, and a severely immunocompromised state [39, 55]. Rapid CT scanning is now available, which reduces the time to take a high-resolution scan of the temporal bones, which is particularly important in children in whom a congenital malformation of the ear needs to be ruled out. CT scans help rule out the presence of congenital ear malformations that permit leakage of CSF through an associated inner ear fistula or other potential routes for spread of infection.

Magnetic resonance imaging (MRI) provides better resolution of the intracranial tissue and shows middle ear fluid and inflammatory changes in the brain and meninges. It is an ideal modality for the assessment of intracranial complications [56]. However, no bone detail is possible, and as such, the relationship of middle ear disease with the surrounding bone is not well visualized. Often, both MRI and CT scans are obtained for optimal management and to evaluate for coexisting complications [57]. In order to minimize contrast burden, one consideration for patients in whom an intracranial complication is suspected is to pursue both a non-contrast CT and a contrasted MRI using a high-resolution temporal bone or internal auditory canal protocol.

It is imperative to identify the causative organism and the source of infection. In meningitis, the CSF analysis and culture via lumbar puncture are often the diagnostic gold standard. It is often cloudy or yellow (xanthochromic), and an elevated white blood cell count, low glucose, and high protein are expected. The pathogen is identified by microscopic examination of Gram-stained fluid with confirmation by culture; sensitivity testing aids in the selection of a suitable antimicrobial drug. A sample should be taken from the ear as well if pus is present. Unfortunately, if antibiotics are given prior to obtaining culture, only 44% will have growth on culture. Blood cultures are often recommended prior to antibiotics, especially if a lumbar puncture is delayed. This low rate of culture growth has resulted in the development of some molecular techniques for bacterial identification. Polymerase chain reaction (PCR) has the ability to detect bacteria in the blood or CSF a few days after initiation of antibiotics with a sensitivity of 87–100% and specificity of 98–100%. Additionally, detection of 16s rRNA has also shown a high sensitivity and specificity [39].

Treatment

Antimicrobial drugs are essential in the treatment of meningitis. Empiric antibiotic therapy can consist of a third-generation cephalosporin plus vancomycin [35]. The advantages of third-generation cephalosporins are their bactericidal activity, their ability to penetrate the blood-brain barrier and enter the CSF, their expanded activity against β-lactamase-producing organisms and gram-negative organisms, and their low toxicity [58]. Vancomycin is now recommended secondary to the increase in prevalence of penicillin-resistant pneumococci [35].

In a Cochrane review, corticosteroids significantly reduced rates of hearing loss and short-term neurologic sequelae associated with acute bacterial meningitis [59]. There was a non-significant decrease in the rate of mortality, with a greater reduction in mortality in those infected by *S. pneumoniae*. In children with acute bacterial meningitis, corticosteroids reduced the rate of severe hearing loss from 11% to 7.3%. In adults with acute bacterial meningitis, corticosteroids reduced the hearing loss rate from 21.9% to 15.7%. A 4-day regimen of dexamethasone—0.6 mg/kg/day divided into four daily doses—was primarily used in these studies and recommended. Authors suggest that dexamethasone should be started before or with the first dose of antibiotics [59, 60].

Role of Surgery

In AOM with an intact tympanic membrane, surgery consists of myringotomy with evacuation of the fluid from the middle ear, which is sent for examination and culture.

For the patient with coalescent mastoiditis or with a history of ear trauma and precipitous meningitis, a complete mastoidectomy with middle ear exploration should be performed. In the latter circumstance, the surgeon should look for and repair the route of CSF leakage after resolution of infection, if persistent. CT scanning usually reveals the fracture line or area of tegmen dehiscence, allowing the surgeon to identify the site of the leak.

If cholesteatoma is present, mastoid surgery is needed with the goal of making the ear disease-free and providing adequate drainage. Intact canal-wall versus canal wall down mastoidectomy approaches are considered on a case-by-case basis. In some cases, patients are critically ill, and a surgical balance can be sought between removal of the offending bulk of disease versus complete disease eradication in the acute setting.

Brain Abscess

A brain abscess is a focal suppurative process within the brain parenchyma surrounded by a region of encephalitis [40].

Brain abscesses secondary to otitis media display a bimodal age distribution, with peaks in the pediatric age group and in the fourth decade [61–63]. In most series, the male-to-female ratio has been nearly 3:1 [63–66]. Otitis media was an important cause of brain abscess in the past but has a much less significant role in developed countries as AOM and COM have been more aggressively managed [67]. COM is much more likely to cause brain abscess than AOM, and cholesteatoma now accounts for most cases [62, 63, 68, 69]. Most authors report that otogenic brain abscesses are more likely to be located in the cerebrum (temporal lobe) than in the cerebellum; however, the majority of cerebellar abscesses are associated with middle ear infections [22, 40, 53, 70]. Several studies found that otogenic abscesses occurred more frequently in the cerebellum [65, 71–73]. Brain abscesses typically occur on the same side as the otologic disease [62]. Cerebellar abscesses have a greater likelihood of a fatal outcome [74]. The mortality associated with brain abscess of otogenic origin in the antibiotic era continues to decline [63]. Several groups have reported a number of patients with cerebral or cerebellar abscess without mortality [37, 69, 75]. Permanent neurologic sequelae, including hemiparesis, decreased cognitive function, dysmetria, and dysarthria, are more commonly associated with brain abscesses [53].

Pathophysiology

Multiple organisms are often present in brain abscesses [22, 76]. Polymicrobial cultures with a high incidence of anaerobes are reported [77]. *Streptococcus* and *Staphylococcus* are common gram-positive organisms that are isolated from brain abscesses. *Escherichia coli, Proteus*, *Klebsiella*, and *Pseudomonas* species are typical gram-negative isolates. The microbiology of a brain abscess is influenced by the immune status of the host. It is interesting to note that *H. influenzae* is rarely found in otogenic brain abscesses [66].

Brain abscess can result from any of the following processes: (1) a contiguous focus of infection, such as otitis media (Fig. 36.1); (2) hematogenous spread from a distant focus of infection, such as chronic pyogenic lung disease (3) head injury or cranial surgery; and (4) an immunocompromised state.

Otogenic brain abscesses are often the result of venous thrombophlebitis or direct dural extension through the tegmen or posterior fossa bone [22, 78]. Osteitis or granulation tissue causes retrograde thrombophlebitis of dural vessels that terminate in the white matter of the brain, producing encephalitis [79]. This localized encephalitis progresses to necrosis and liquefaction of brain tissue (focal suppuration) with surrounding edema [80]. Within approximately 2 weeks, an abscess capsule surrounded by granulation tissue forms. Brain abscess formation is a continuum from cerebritis to a well-encapsulated necrotic focus; nonetheless, many authors

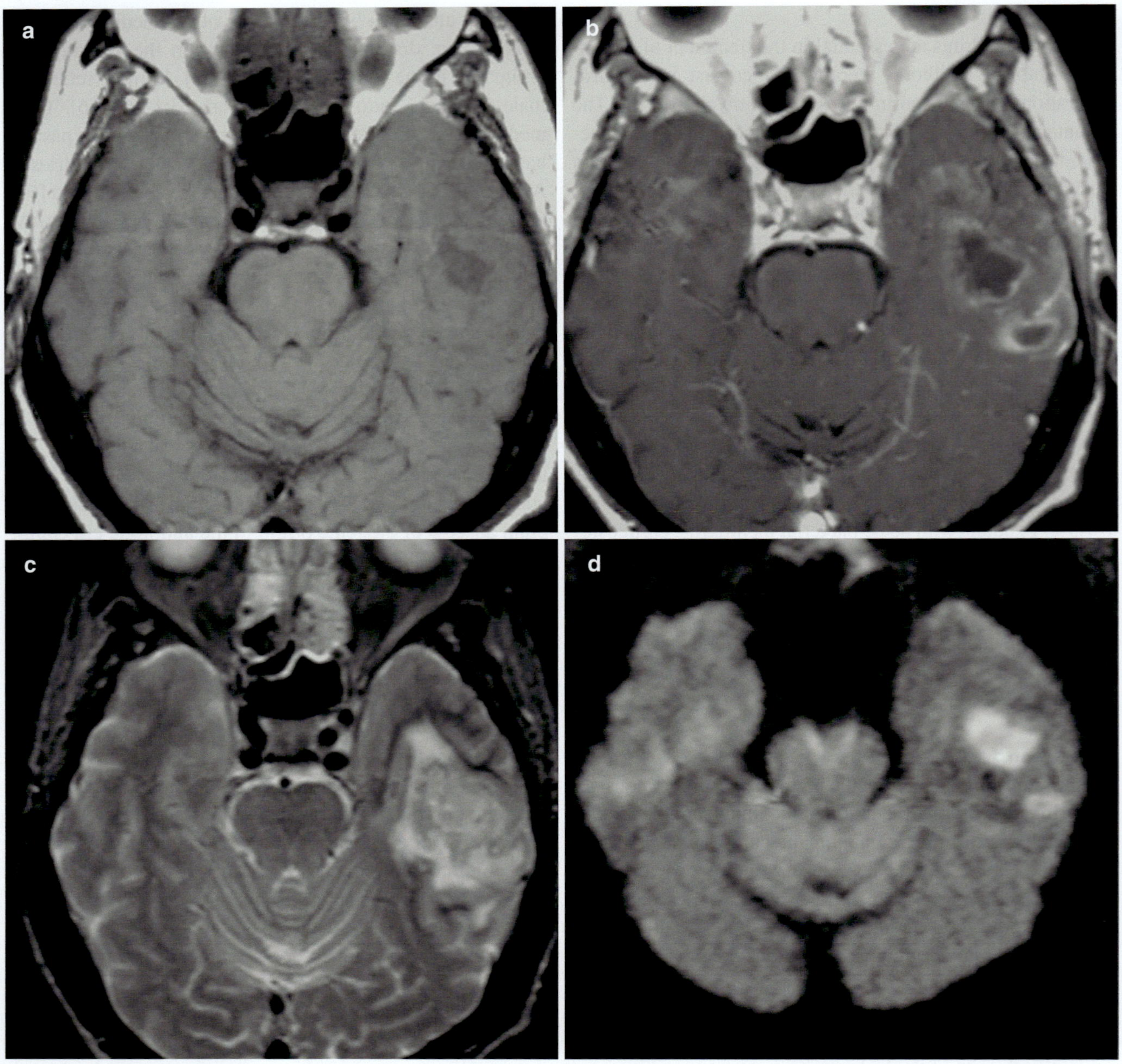

Fig. 36.1 A well-encapsulated brain abscess complicating otitis media. Magnetic resonance imaging demonstrating a peripherally enhancing and centrally nonenhancing brain abscess in the left temporal lobe. (**a**) Axial section T1 image. (**b**) Postcontrast axial section T1 image. (**c**) Axial section T2 image with surrounding edema of abscess. (**d**) Axial diffusion weighted image with central restricted diffusion due to purulent contents

have described stages of the formation of a brain abscess (Fig. 36.2) [45, 81–83]. Proinflammatory mediators are released, which may result in damage to tissue surrounding the abscess. Encapsulation is more well defined on the cortical side as compared with the ventricular side, perhaps explaining the propensity of abscesses to rupture medially into the ventricular system rather than into the subarachnoid space [82]. The maturity of the brain abscess depends on the local oxygen concentration, the offending organism, and the host's immune response.

Clinical Presentation

On presentation, patients may appear "toxic" and drowsy, complaining of deep bony otologic pain [70]. As this complication is more commonly related to chronic suppurative otitis media, patients may have a history of prolonged otorrhea

Fig. 36.2 Stages of formation of brain abscess. (Adapted from *Glasscock and Shambaugh's Surgery of the Ear*. 6th Ed. Eds. Gulya, Minor, Poe. PMPH. 2010)

Stages	Duration (days)	Disease progression
Early cerebritis (invasion)	Days 1-3 following inoculation	Perivascular inflammatory response surrounding a developing necrotic center with edema
Late cerebritis (localization)	4-10 days	Well-formed necrotic center, neovascularity in the periphery of the necrotic center
Early capsule formation	10-13 days	Well-developed layer of fibroblasts with persistent cerebritis and neovascularity
Late capsule formation	14 days	Thickening of capsule

suggesting a fulminant, destructive process [62, 63]. Brain abscess formation can be indicated by the presence of (1) headache, (2) high-grade fever, and (3) focal neurologic deficits, although this complete triad is not always present [66]. Symptoms may be present for 2 weeks before the brain abscess is fully formed [40]. Focal deficits depend on the location of the abscess. Cerebellar abscesses provoke dizziness, ataxia, nystagmus, and vomiting. Temporal lobe lesions may result in seizures. Associated signs of meningitis are usually present, including nausea/vomiting, photophobia, nuchal rigidity and hearing loss [22, 65]. Papilledema is frequently seen in stage 3 of abscess formation [84].

Imaging

Imaging is very useful in the evaluation of the patient suspected of having an otogenic brain abscess. CT scans may allow for earlier detection of abscesses and improved outcomes. The brain abscess appears as a hypodense area surrounded by an area of edema, a configuration known as the "ring" sign. In non-contrast CT, there may be areas of low attenuation with the development of a peripheral rim in later stages. In CT with contrast, uniform ring enhancement is almost always visualized [85].

MRI has also proven to be useful because it is superior to CT in detecting subtle changes in the brain parenchyma and in identifying extension into the subarachnoid space or into the ventricle [86]. On T1-weighted images, areas of central liquefaction are represented by a low signal center surrounded by a hyperintense capsule. T2-weighted images will show a high signal in any area of necrosis. Diffusion-weighted imaging (DWI) also helps to distinguish from other pathology, including necrotic tumors. Patients with brain abscesses will have a hyperintense signal on DWI with low apparent diffusion coefficient due to the viscous purulent material [66, 85, 87]. One limitation of MRI is that it cannot provide detailed information about the temporal bone; thus, a separate CT scan is required to assess the temporal bone.

Serial CT scans or MRI can be used to follow the effects of treatment, determine if the abscess is resolving, and assist in the timing of surgical intervention [22, 85, 88]. It is suggested to reimage every 2 weeks by some authors, as additional complications may arise over time, while others wait and reimage at 6 weeks and/or if symptoms worsen. Patients typically report symptom improvement weeks before the MRI appearance improves; therefore, antibiotics can be discontinued if resolution of the disease is seen on imaging [22].

Management

The patient must be hospitalized and treated with appropriate, high-dose antimicrobial medication immediately. Often empiric broad-spectrum therapy, including cefotaxime/ceftriaxone/ceftazidime, vancomycin, and metronidazole, is initiated. Metronidazole is effective against anaerobes, which are commonly found [85]. Six-week courses of antibiotics are typically recommended depending on findings with reimaging [22].

Improved imaging and more effective antibiotics have decreased the mortality rates associated with these infections [66]. The management of brain abscesses is a controversial issue. The rarity of these complications precludes the development of a standardized evidence-based management algorithm. Often patients are started on empiric antibiotic therapy and these medications are further modified to culture-directed therapy if possible [22]. However, surgical intervention recommendations often vary. There is controversy as to whether neurosurgical intervention is necessary due to newer and more effective intravenous (IV) antibiotics, which can result in the complete resolution of small brain abscesses, obviating neurosurgical intervention. Some have advocated close monitoring of the clinical and radiological response to IV antibiotics of these small abscesses. If there is no improvement or there is further expansion or mass effect from the abscess, then neurosurgical intervention is often indicated.

Additionally, as more abscess development has been associated with chronic ear disease, some have shown benefits with simply IV antibiotics and tympanomastoidectomy to address the chronic inflammation or cholesteatoma [22]. The decision to incise or aspirate a brain abscess is another controversy. Williams recommends aspiration with high doses of appropriate antibiotics because he finds that this regimen is associated with fewer permanent neurologic sequelae [89]. The advanced technology and use of image guidance have contributed to improved outcomes in these patients [66]. Others recommend total excision because they find that this leads to lower mortality and a decreased rate of recurrence. However, concern can exist surrounding a complete excision of the abscess and risk for injury to the surrounding cortical tissue [90, 91]. Neurosurgical consultation is essential in these cases.

Otogenic Suppurative Thrombophlebitis

Otogenic suppurative thrombophlebitis is defined as the simultaneous presence of venous thrombosis and suppuration in the mastoid cavity. Formation of a thrombus occurs after infection or inflammation spreads to the intima. The mural thrombus may propagate and occlude the sinus lumen as it increases in size. Embolization of septic thrombi and/or extension into adjacent sinuses and tributary vessels produces further disease.

Suppurative thrombophlebitis of the sigmoid sinus (also referred to as lateral sinus thrombophlebitis) is a potentially devastating intracranial complication of otitis media. The advent of antibiotics reduced both the frequency of this condition and the mortality rate, which declined from 100% in the pre-antibiotic era to 0–25% over the last 30 years [22, 92–95]. Suppurative thrombophlebitis of the sigmoid and adjacent venous sinuses can result from AOM or COM [96, 97].

Pathogenesis

As with other intracranial complications of OM, bacteriology has shifted over time from a predominance of *β-hemolytic streptococcus* to include *Streptococcus pneumoniae*, *Staphylococcus aureus,* including strains with methicillin resistance (MRSA), *Enterococcus*, *Pseudomonas, Klebsiella, Proteus, Bacteroides*, and other anaerobes [41, 94, 96]. Cultures commonly yield mixed flora, particularly in the setting of COM [96]. Associated drug-resistant strains are increasingly prevalent, particularly in the U.S. For example, in their review of patients with complications of AOM at a single institution, Mattos et al. observed that the frequency of culture-positive *S. pneumoniae* was similar (33%) over 2 contiguous 15 year periods, but the frequency of multidrug-resistant *S. pneumoniae* increased from 13% prior to 1998 to 55% between 1998 and 2013 [41]. The frequent use of antibiotics has also resulted in more negative intraoperative cultures. In modern series, cultures are negative in 25–80% of the reported cases [96–100].

Two pathophysiologic mechanisms for the formation of suppurative thrombophlebitis are depicted in Fig. 36.3. Overlying infection, granulation tissue, peri-sinus abscesses, or cholesteatoma incite sinus wall inflammation, either by direct extension through an eroded bony plate or via hematogenous spread from thrombophlebitic emissary veins. The sigmoid sinus is most susceptible because of its position adjacent to the mastoid air cells. The mural thrombus may progress to an occlusive thrombus and/or may propagate in a

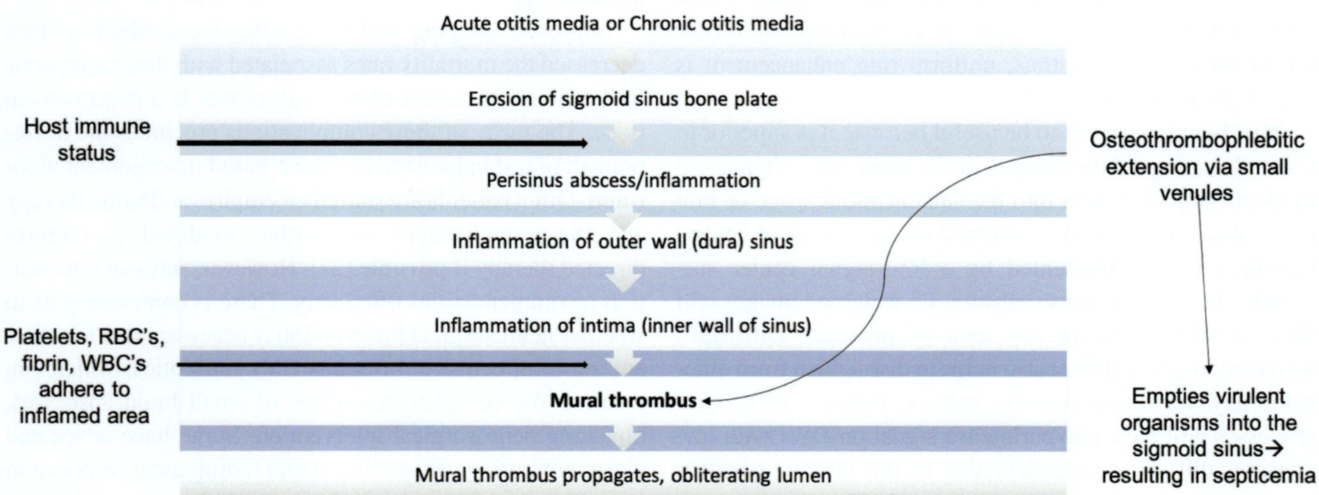

Fig. 36.3 Pathogenesis of thrombophlebitis in the sigmoid sinus. AOM acute otitis media, COM chronic otitis media, RBC red blood cell, WBC white blood cell. (Adapted from *Glasscock and Shambaugh's Surgery of the Ear*. 6th Ed. Eds. Gulya, Minor, Poe. PMPH. 2010)

retrograde fashion to adjacent intracranial sinuses (transverse, petrosal, sagittal, and cavernous) and veins (Labbé), and/or distally into the jugular vein and the right atrium of the heart. Intracranial extension may result in brain abscess, intracranial hypertension, papilledema, and infarcts with their attendant sequelae [101]. Distal spread may result in jugular foramen syndrome and lower cranial nerve deficits. Septic emboli give rise to widespread dissemination of infection and fulminant septicemia [95].

Patients who develop lateral sinus thrombosis may have an elevated prevalence of prothrombotic disorders compared to the general population. Findings among patients with lateral sinus thrombosis secondary to AOM have included elevated levels of lipoprotein apolipoprotein, factor V Leiden mutations, and antibodies against β 2-glycoprotein and cardiolipin [98, 102, 103].

Clinical Presentation

The clinical presentation of otogenic suppurative thrombophlebitis has changed markedly with widespread antibiotic availability and use. Consequently, diagnosis of this complication is often delayed and a high index of suspicion and knowledge of prior care is required to ensure proper evaluation. In resource-poor or constrained settings, patients are more likely to present as they did in the pre-antibiotic era, with a rapid onset of acute otomastoiditis accompanied by otorrhea, severe otalgia, headache, fever, and leukocytosis. Otorrhea is usually foul-smelling and blood-stained. Otalgia is described as a deep, boring pain and usually heralds worsening neurologic status. The fever curve may reveal persistent high-grade temperatures or a "picket fence" pattern, secondary to periodic release of septic emboli [95, 104].

The clinical picture of otogenic suppurative thrombophlebitis is more variable in resource-rich settings because early antibiotic therapy may mask the classic symptoms. Chronic otitis media is a more common precipitant in settings with good access to care [95]. When preceded by AOM, otologic symptoms and signs may be mild and symptom duration may be longer (more than 2 weeks, or even 2 months) prior to presentation or, in some cases, symptoms may have already resolved [97, 98]. Less than one third of affected patients present with fever and the "picket fence" pattern is rarely observed [22, 96]. White blood cell counts may be normal [97].

Instead of the classic otologic symptoms, neurologic symptoms may predominate. Headache is the most common presenting symptom reported in multiple series [97, 98, 105]. Other associated neurologic symptoms and signs include diplopia (from cranial nerve VI paresis), cranial nerve VII paresis, lethargy, and other indicators of increased intracranial pressure and dural inflammation (e.g., papilledema, nausea, vomiting, photophobia, phonophobia, nuchal rigidity, ataxia) [70, 96, 97].

Propagation of the thrombus may lead to additional localizing symptoms. Ocular proptosis, ptosis, chemosis, and ophthalmoplegia indicate that the thrombus has spread to the cavernous sinus. Tenderness, erythema and edema over the mastoid (Griesinger's sign) are pathognomonic for suppurative thrombophlebitis of the sigmoid sinus and reflect thrombosis of the mastoid emissary veins that travel to the subcutis. Propagation of the thrombus into the internal jugular vein causes it to become firm, cord-like, and very tender to palpation, and results in a stiff neck. The lymph nodes along the internal jugular vein may be enlarged and tender. Paresis of the ipsilateral lower cranial nerves (IX, X, XI) may herald occlusion of the jugular bulb. Proximal propagation can result in otitic hydrocephalus, as described elsewhere in this chapter. If *β-hemolytic streptococci* are responsible for the infection, the patient may present with anemia/low hemoglobin levels, manifesting in pallor [95].

Imaging and Other Investigations

CT scanning and MRI are the current imaging tools of choice in making the diagnosis and for following patients for evidence of thrombus progression. Before the advent of these imaging tools, cerebral angiography with observation of the venous phase was used to determine if thrombosis was present; however, cerebral angiography is no longer routinely performed because of its potential to dislodge the clot [95].

In addition to showing coalescent mastoiditis and erosion of the sigmoid sinus plate, a contrast-enhanced temporal bone CT scan may demonstrate the "delta sign"—an empty triangle at the level of the sigmoid sinus, consisting of the clot surrounded by a high-intensity rim of contrast-enhanced dura and surrounding collateral veins, in up to one third of cases [106]. However, this sign is not always detectable, and not all thrombi can be documented by CT scanning [107].

MRI is more sensitive than CT in detecting sinus thrombosis. When compared to MRI as the gold standard, CT scanning sensitivity ranges from 72% to 84% [96, 108]. On gadolinium-enhanced MRI, the thrombus appears as a soft tissue signal contrasted against a vascular and bright appearance of the dural walls [108, 109]. Early thrombus, as it is rich in deoxyhemoglobin, has an intermediate density on T1-weighted MRI images and a low intensity on T2-weighted images. As the clot matures, methemoglobin forms and the MRI appearance changes so that the clot is hyperintense on both T1- and T2-weighted images. The addition of magnetic resonance venography (MRV) permits distinction between slow venous flow and occlusive thrombus in the sigmoid and collateral venous circulation, which can be challenging to discern from traditional MRI sequences (Fig. 36.4) [98, 109]. MRI with MRV thus allows for earlier and more precise diagnosis of sinus thrombosis, delineates the patency of collateral circulation, and also offers the advantage of simultaneously identifying other intracranial complications.

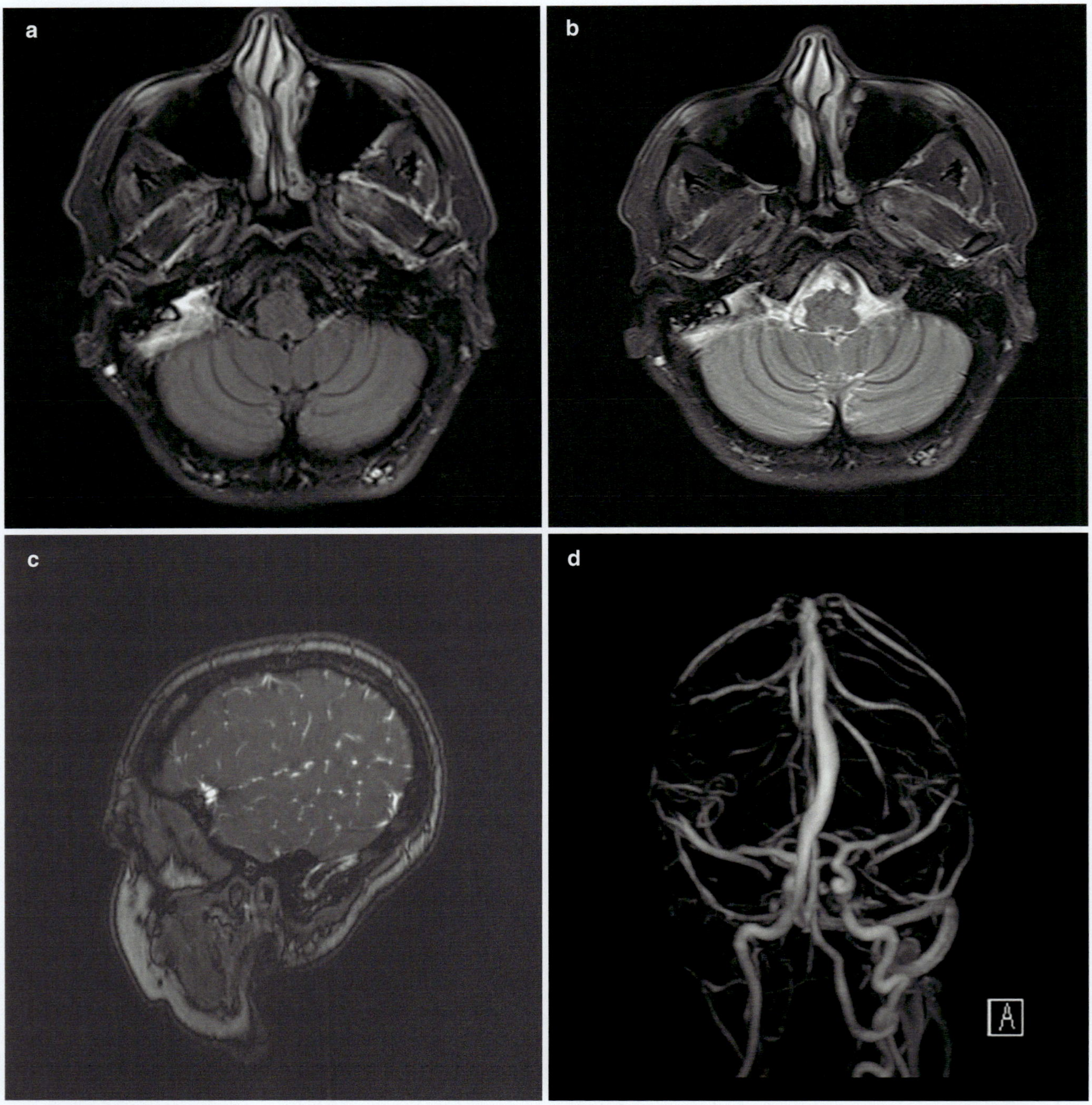

Fig. 36.4 Magnetic resonance imaging of brain demonstrating sigmoid sinus thrombosis. (**a**) Axial section on FLAIR with loss of signal void of the right sigmoid sinus. (**b**) Axial section on T2 with loss of signal void of the right sigmoid sinus. (**c**) Sagittal section of postcontrast venogram demonstrating a filling defect in the sigmoid sinus. (**d**) Maximum intensity projection demonstrating lack of signal in the right sigmoid and transverse sinuses. Enhancement of the contralateral sigmoid sinus and transverse sinus represents sinus patency on the left side

Prior to the advent of modern imaging, clinicians also used Queckenstedt's (or the Tobey-Ayer) test to detect lateral venous sinus thrombosis. It is presented here for historical interest. The test is performed as follows: a spinal needle is inserted into the subarachnoid space, a manometer is attached, and the resting CSF pressure is recorded. The change in pressure produced by digital compression of first one internal jugular vein and then the other, and then both at the same time, is noted. When the pressure fails to rise after compression of the internal jugular vein on the side of the diseased ear and fails to fall when the vein is released, with a prompt contralateral response, the test is positive. A positive Queckenstedt's test is very strong evidence in favor of occlusion of the sigmoid sinus; however, it is not infallible. A false-positive test occurs when one sigmoid sinus is smaller than the other (more commonly, the left side). A false-negative test occurs when there is unusually good collateral circulation around the obstructed sigmoid sinus via the mastoid emissary vein and the inferior petrosal sinus. Any contraindication to performing a lumbar puncture is also a contraindication to performing Queckenstedt's test.

The presence of lateral sinus thrombosis mandates (1) serial imaging to monitor for thrombus progression and (2) further investigation for additional intracranial and extracranial complications of OM [106]. The rate of coexistent intracranial complications was 80% during the pre-antibiotic era [110]. While this rate has decreased, it remains high, with modern series reporting rates of 40% or greater [96]. Common co-occurring complications are meningitis, epidural abscess, intracranial abscess, otitic hydrocephalus, and internal jugular vein thrombosis [96, 97]. It is also advisable to perform a blood culture in those suspected of having sinus thrombophlebitis, as is the case with other suspected OM complications. Evaluation for hypercoagulable states may be considered in consultation with a hematologist, given that some abnormalities are heritable and may require long-term anticoagulation [103].

Treatment

The optimal management of otogenic suppurative thrombophlebitis remains a matter of debate. In part because of the low incidence of disease, there are no evidence-based guidelines or targeted clinical consensus statements. Rather, published guidance addresses an amalgam of causes of cerebral venous thromboembolism, most of which are non otogenic and non infectious, limiting their direct applicability to this specific subgroup [107, 111]. Treatment options include antibiotic therapy, surgery, and anticoagulation. Practices vary between clinicians and by disease severity and, given the state of equipoise, shared decision making is encouraged.

It is prudent to initiate empiric parenteral antibiotic therapy upon diagnosis of otogenic sinus thrombosis [100]. As the range of potential pathogens is broad, the most commonly reported empiric regimen is ceftriaxone, vancomycin, and metronidazole, but other regimens providing broad coverage may be used [100]. Culture-directed therapy is best but often is not possible due to negative cultures. Six weeks of parenteral antibiotic therapy are usually recommended. However, some clinicians prescribe shorter courses and/or transition to oral therapy based on disease severity and the rate of clinical improvement [70, 100, 112–114].

Surgical management of lateral sinus thrombophlebitis is evolving. Ongoing areas of debate include the appropriate extent of surgery, which may range from myringotomy and mastoidectomy to thrombectomy and internal jugular vein ligation. Currently, most surgeons perform an urgent mastoidectomy with myringotomy and tube placement [100, 103]. The goals of this surgery are to remove thrombogenic perisinus inflammation, granulation tissue and abscesses and to prevent thrombus propagation and intracranial spread [22, 100]. The sigmoid sinus is decompressed (i.e., unroofed) in part or in whole, and the exposed sinus wall is inspected and palpated. A soft, pliable sinus should be left alone. If one finds that the sinus wall has already been eroded by inflammatory tissue and is, thus, open, the infected clot may be debrided [22, 106]. If rubbery clot is felt under an intact sinus wall, some surgeons carefully aspirate the sinus with a small-gauge needle and syringe. Lack of blood flow indicates that a clot is present. Venotomy may then be performed, taking care not to traumatize the medial dural wall, and the clot evacuated. While common in the pre-antibiotic era, such routine venotomy and thrombectomy are falling out of favor; they were performed in less than half of the cases reported in the last 25 years [22, 100, 103, 115], and the authors do not advocate this approach. Venotomy and thrombectomy have attendant risks, including distal propagation of thrombus, release of emboli and intracranial sinus rupture [20, 106]. Further, there is also no clear evidence that this approach improves outcomes, including rates of recanalization or symptom resolution [21, 100, 116]. Ligation of the internal jugular vein is also no longer routinely recommended but may be considered in cases with persistent sepsis and/or septic pulmonary emboli [100, 106]. Recently, cases have appeared in the literature that were successfully managed with antibiotics and myringotomy and tube placement alone [112–114, 117]. While this approach may be sufficient for select cases, mastoidectomy remains appropriate when thrombophlebitis is associated with chronic otitis media with cholesteatoma, coalescent mastoiditis, bone erosion over the sigmoid, aggressive infections, neurologic symptoms, and other intracranial complications [100, 115].

The use of anticoagulation for otogenic suppurative thrombophlebitis also varies in the literature and in practice. The goal of anticoagulation following surgical intervention is to improve clinical outcomes by expediting sinus recanalization and preventing thrombus propagation and septic embolization [118]. Common strategies include initial use of unfractionated or low molecular weight heparin (LMWH) and/or aspirin in the perioperative period and continuation of LMWH or transition to oral warfarin thereafter [22, 41, 103, 119]. Reported durations of treatment range from 3 weeks to 12 months, based on timing of clinical recovery and/or imaging evidence of recanalization [98, 100, 112, 115, 120]. There is no current evidence describing the role of direct oral anticoagulants [121].

Opponents of anticoagulation raise concerns about hemorrhagic complications [112, 122] and note that reported rates of recanalization and clinical recovery do not differ between those treated with and without anticoagulation. Completely thrombosed sinuses have been observed to recanalize without anticoagulation in as few as 6 weeks after surgical removal of perisinus inflammation and targeted antibiotic therapy [20, 120]. Further, recanalization is not essential for clinical recovery. Patients with persistent thrombus have reported complete symptom resolution, suggesting that the development of collateral venous circulation over time may be more important to recovery and survival [97, 115, 119, 122]. Advocates of anticoagulation note that the clinical risk of anticoagulation is relatively low, with bleeding complications occurring in 7% or less of treated cases, and point to its potential efficacy in preventing propagation, embolization, and reducing neurologic sequelae [97, 103, 107, 113, 123]. Thus, anticoagulation may be most appropriate for patients at higher risk of infarct or persistent septic thrombus or embolus: those with clot burdens extending beyond the sigmoid sinus (transverse, cavernous sinus, IJ), neurologic changes, known embolic events, and persistent fevers [106]. Evidence supporting anticoagulation is limited and primarily involves case series [121].

Otitic Hydrocephalus

Patients with acute or chronic otitis media may develop symptoms of increased intracranial pressure in the absence of meningitis, intracranial abscess, or other abnormalities of CSF composition. As there is no accompanying dilation of the ventricles, this condition may be best described as otitis-associated intracranial hypertension. Nevertheless, it is widely referred to as otitic hydrocephalus, a potentially confusing misnomer coined by Symonds before the advent of modern imaging [124, 125]. Otitic hydrocephalus typically arises in the setting of sigmoid sinus thrombophlebitis, but not all patients with sigmoid sinus thrombophlebitis develop otitic hydrocephalus [126].

Pathophysiology

The precise mechanism underlying the development of otitic hydrocephalus is unknown. It is commonly attributed to reduced CSF absorption in the setting of lateral sinus thrombophlebitis [127, 128]. Symonds postulated that a mural thrombus extending from the lateral sinuses into the sagittal sinus raises intracranial pressure by impeding the transfer of CSF from the subarachnoid space into the venous system through arachnoid villi (Fig. 36.5) [124, 125]. He predicted that the sagittal sinus thrombus would be only partially obstructive, as complete sagittal sinus occlusion is associated with greater neurological compromise [117]. With improvements in imaging, however, it now appears that propagation of thrombus into the sagittal sinus is not essential for the development of otitic hydrocephalus [116]. Rather, thrombosis of a lateral sinus alone may impair venous drainage enough to raise CSF pressure, particularly when the obstruction involves the dominant venous outflow tract and collateral circulation is inadequate (e.g., when cross-communication at the torcula is lacking) [117, 129]. The wide anatomical variation in cerebral venous outflow patterns (and, hence, variation in collateral tracts) may explain why not all episodes of lateral sinus thrombosis lead to otitic hydrocephalus [128].

Clinical Presentation

The onset of symptoms may be weeks after an episode of AOM or years after the onset of COM [126]. The clinical features of otitic hydrocephalus are those shared by all causes of increased intracranial pressure. Symptoms may include headache, nausea and vomiting, drowsiness, blurring of vision, and diplopia. On examination, diplopia is found to result from abducens nerve (cranial nerve VI) palsy. Intracranial pressure changes displace the brainstem, stretching one or both abducens nerves as they course between the pons and Dorello's canal [130]. Papilledema is also frequently evident and can result in optic nerve atrophy and permanent vision loss if left untreated [127]. Thus, neuroophthalmologic examination is mandatory. If lumbar puncture is considered safe after review of imaging, the opening pressure will be elevated and the cytological and biochemical composition of the CSF will be normal [128]. MRI with MRV is the imaging modality of choice as it allows for superior evaluation of the venous sinuses. In addition to complete occlusion of the lateral sinuses, diffuse brain edema without ventricular dilation is typically observed [107, 127].

Management

The goals of therapy are the eradication of ear disease and lowering of elevated intracranial pressure, both to reduce symptoms and to prevent permanent visual impairment. Multidisciplinary care is necessary, including otolaryngology, neuroophthalmology, neurosurgery and/or neurology. Management of sigmoid sinus thrombophlebitis and considerations surrounding the use of anticoagulation are discussed

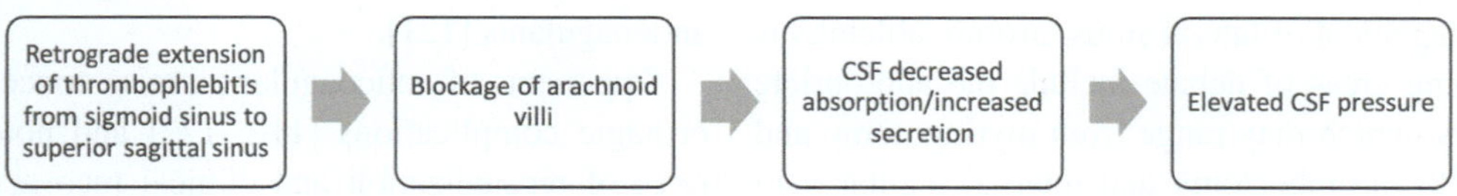

Fig. 36.5 Symonds' proposal for the pathophysiology of otitic hydrocephalus. However, sagittal sinus thrombosis is no longer considered essential for the development of otitic hydrocephalus. CSF cerebrospinal fluid. (Adapted from *Glasscock and Shambaugh's Surgery of the Ear*. 6th Ed. Eds. Gulya, Minor, Poe. PMPH. 2010)

above. In the setting of otitic hydrocephalus, surgical decompression of the diseased sinus and dura with removal of excess granulation tissue is recommended [118, 126, 131]. Notably, symptom resolution has been observed in patients who fail to recanalize the thrombosed lateral sinus, suggesting that recovery may result from the development of collateral circulation; however, this process may take months following surgical management [116, 117]. Medical therapy aimed at temporarily reducing intracranial pressure may include diuretics such as mannitol, furosemide, or acetazolamide [107]. When intracranial hypertension is persistent, serial lumbar punctures may be necessary on a short-term basis, followed by ventriculoperitoneal shunt placement for refractory cases. Close monitoring of visual fields and the severity of papilledema is essential. Optic nerve sheath fenestration may be required to halt progressive visual loss [107, 127].

Subdural Empyema

A subdural empyema is a collection of pus in the space between the dura mater and the arachnoid membrane. This condition was almost always fatal prior to the advent of antibiotic therapy. Today, subdural empyema is the rarest of the complications of otitis media [132, 133].

Pathophysiology

The subdural space, normally a potential space rather than an actual one, is divided into several large compartments by the foramen magnum, tentorium cerebelli, base of the brain, and the falx cerebri. Since these spaces are anatomically confined, a developing empyema can quickly evolve into a fatal mass lesion (Figs. 36.6 and 36.7).

Clinical Presentation

Headache of abrupt onset and unusually severe nature is typical of subdural empyema. Fever and vomiting are other symptoms that accompany this disease. The rapidity with which the patient deteriorates points to a subdural empyema.

MRI is the imaging modality of choice [134]. It has been found to be superior at detecting the presence and extensions of the infection and can also distinguish between epidural and subdural infection. Multiple, discrete, loculated subdural collections may occasionally be seen. MRI is particularly useful because of the absence of bone artifact, heightened contrast between bone, CSF, and brain parenchyma, and its multiplanar imaging capability [135]. MRI can also characterize subdural collections, allowing differentiation of sterile, bloody, and infected collections. CT is unable to perform these functions.

Treatment

Subdural empyema is a surgical emergency, and prognosis is related to the promptness of diagnosis and drainage. Lumbar puncture is contraindicated as it could precipitate herniation of the cerebellar tonsils. Emergency neurosurgical drainage alongside high-dose, intravenous antimicrobial medication is the treatment of choice. If the patient is neurologically stable, the underlying ear disease can be surgically managed [22].

Epidural (Extradural) Abscess

The epidural (extradural) space is a potential space between the dura mater and the bone delimiting the intracranial cavity. Infection here usually first manifests as granulation tissue that is in direct continuity with the suppurative process of acute or chronic otitis media, with or without cholesteatoma [70]. At surgery, granulation along the dura mater is seen more commonly than an actual abscess. OM-associated epidural granulation and abscesses most commonly occur in the posterior fossa, adjacent to or overlying the sigmoid sinus (a "perisinus abscess"), followed by the middle fossa above the

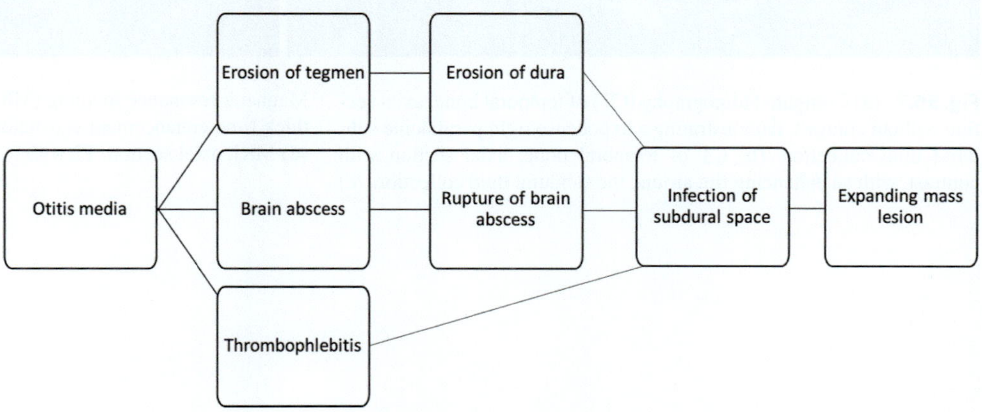

Fig. 36.6 Pathology of subdural empyema. (Adapted from *Glasscock and Shambaugh's Surgery of the Ear*. 6th Ed. Eds. Gulya, Minor, Poe. PMPH. 2010)

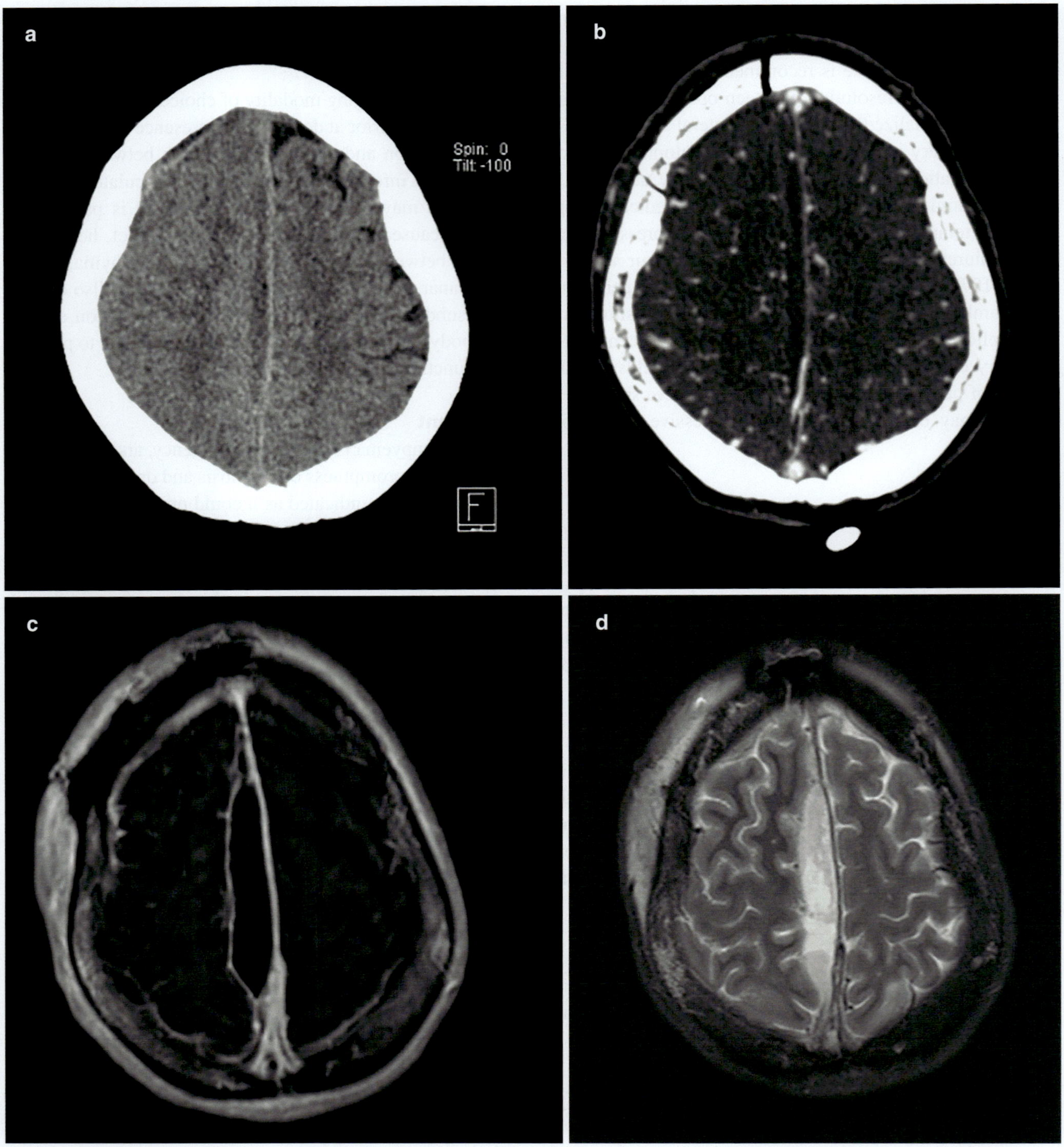

Fig. 36.7 (**a**) Computed tomography (CT) of temporal bone, axial section without contrast, demonstrating a hypodense right parafalcine subdural fluid collection. (**b**) CT of temporal bone, axial section with contrast, with an enhancing rim around the subdural fluid collection. (**c**) Magnetic resonance imaging (MRI) of the brain, postcontrast T1, with thick time enhancement surrounding a right subdural fluid collection. (**d**) MRI, axial section, T2 with hyperintense subdural fluid collection

tegmen and petrous apex [70, 136, 137]. Thus, coexistent complications should be sought if epidural granulation tissue or abscess is identified.

Pathogenesis

Acute coalescent mastoiditis may result in erosion of the bone of the sigmoid sinus plate, Trautmann's triangle, and tegmen [70, 136, 137]. As these areas of bone give way, a pocket of granulation tissue or pus can expand along the face of the sinus and posterior and middle cranial fossae. Chronic otitis media with or without cholesteatoma may be associated with granulation tissue that invades the perisinus and tegmen air cells [138]. An acute exacerbation of infection may cause silent extradural granulation tissue to progress into a more serious complication.

Clinical Presentation

Epidural granulation tissue and abscesses may present with fever, otalgia, and persistent low grade headache. However, they may be clinically silent and are rarely symptomatic unless they are large [70, 139, 140]. As such, they may be noted as incidental findings during surgery performed for another complication, but can often be visualized prior to surgery using modern imaging techniques. The common absence of localizing symptoms emphasizes the need for imaging in cases of acute mastoiditis [21].

Imaging

Erosion of the bone of the tegmen, sigmoid sinus plate, or posterior fossa is best viewed with a thin-cut temporal bone CT. The addition of contrast to CT imaging may permit visualization of dural enhancement and, if the epidural abscess is of sufficient size, a rim-enhancing lentiform collection of low-attenuation fluid. Gadolinium-enhanced MRI demonstrates dural enhancement and epidural abscesses with greater sensitivity (Fig. 36.8). An epidural abscess will appear as a circumscribed fluid collection with a signal intensity between CSF and white matter on T1-weighted sequences and similar or slightly higher intensity than CSF on T2-weighted sequences [134].

Management

The discovery of granulation tissue over the sigmoid sinus or penetrating the bone of the middle or posterior fossae should prompt further exploration during mastoidectomy. The surrounding bone should be gently removed until normal-appearing dura is encountered, and the abscess should be drained through the mastoidectomy approach. Excessive granulation tissue should be gently scraped off, working parallel to the plane of the dura, or trimmed. Care should be taken not to perforate the dura, which could result in a CSF leak and allow the infection to spread directly into the brain. Craniotomy is unnecessary for drainage of most otogenic epidural abscesses due to their location adjacent to the mastoid. All patients should receive culture-directed antibiotics. While most cases are managed surgically, as described, there are reports of successful management of small epidural abscesses with culture-directed IV antibiotics and tympanovstomy tube placement alone, and others have resolved following cortical mastoidectomy without dural manipulation or abscess drainage [21, 70].

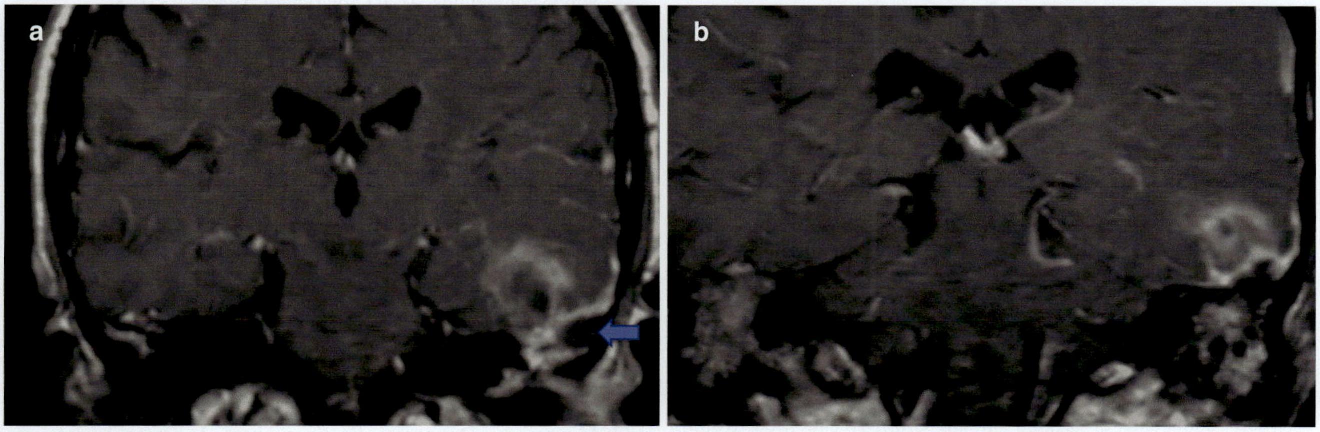

Fig. 36.8 (**a**) Magnetic resonance imaging (MRI) brain, coronal section postcontrast T1, demonstrating left temporal lobe abscess and inferior epidural abscess (arrow). (**b**) MRI brain, coronal section, postcontrast, T1 with temporal lobe abscess, epidural abscess, and mastoid opacification

Conclusions

Intracranial complications of otitis media, though increasingly rare in the present era due to the availability and efficacy of antibiotics, remain a legitimate concern for otologic surgeons. Patients are often critically ill, and significant risks for morbidity and mortality exist. A high index of suspicion for an intracranial complication should be employed for patients who have an ear infection and neurologic symptoms, symptoms that have not improved on antibiotic therapy or symptoms that have plateaued after initial improvement. Immunosuppressive conditions can also facilitate more severe infections with fewer objective signs of severity. Surgical intervention can be critical in many patients with an intracranial complication, and close follow-up is necessary to ensure complete disease resolution.

Acknowledgment A special thanks to Zuzan Cayci, MD and the neuroimaging section at the University of Minnesota for permission to use their images.

References

1. Cawthorne T. The surgery of the temporal bone. I. J Laryngol Otol. 1953;67(7):377–91.
2. Heine BBJ. Handbuch der Hals-Nassen-Ohrenheilkunde. Berlin: Springer; 1927.
3. Morand S. Opuscules de chirurgie. Paris : Chez Guillaume Desprez; 1768.
4. Lebert. Ueber Entzundung der Hirn-Sinus. Virchows Arch. 1856;9(381).
5. MacEwen W. Pyogenic infective diseases of the brain and spinal cord. Glasgow: James Maclehose; 1893.
6. Korner O. Otitischen Erkrankungen des Hirns, der Hirnhaute und der Blutleiter. Wiesbaden: Bergmann; 1908.
7. Eagleton WP. Brain abscess: its surgical pathology and operative technique. New York: Macmillan; 1922.
8. Shambaugh GJ. The surgical treatment of meningitis of otitic and nasal origin. JAMA. 1937;108(696).
9. Lebert. Ueber Gehirnabscesse. Virchows Arch. 1856;10(78).
10. Zaufal E. Operation der Sinusthrombose und Versuche mit Cocain am Gehororgane. Prag Med Wochenschr. 1884;9:474.
11. Lane W. Middle ear suppurations and their complications. BMJ. 1889;1:998.
12. Ballance C. Pyemic thrombosis of the lateral sinus. Lancet. 1890;1:1057.
13. Jansen A. Referat die Operations methoden bei den verschiedenen otitischen Gehirnkomplikationen. Verhandl Deutsch Otol Gesellsch. 1895;4:96.
14. Gradenigo G. Sulla leptomeningite circoscritta e sula paralisi dell' adducente di origine otitica. Giorn Accad Med Torino. 1904;10:59.
15. Kopetsky SJ, Almour R. Suppuration of the petrous pyramid. Ann Otol Rhinol Laryngol. 1931;39:996.
16. Eagleton WP. Unlocking the petrous pyramid for localized bulbar meningitis secondary to suppuration of the petrous apex. Arch Otolaryngol. 1931;13:386.
17. Courville CB. Intracranial complications of otitis media and mastoiditis in the antibiotic era. I. Modification of the pathology of otitic intracranial lesions by antibiotic preparations. Laryngoscope. 1955;65(2):31–46.
18. Hsu HE, Shutt KA, Moore MR, Beall BW, Bennett NM, Craig AS, et al. Effect of pneumococcal conjugate vaccine on pneumococcal meningitis. N Engl J Med. 2009;360(3):244–56.
19. Luntz M, Bartal K, Brodsky A, Shihada R. Acute mastoiditis: the role of imaging for identifying intracranial complications. Laryngoscope. 2012;122(12):2813–7.
20. Agarwal A, Lowry P, Isaacson G. Natural history of sigmoid sinus thrombosis. Ann Otol Rhinol Laryngol. 2003;112(2):191–4.
21. Mallur PS, Harirchian S, Lalwani AK. Preoperative and postoperative intracranial complications of acute mastoiditis. Ann Otol Rhinol Laryngol. 2009;118(2):118–23.
22. Wanna GB, Dharamsi LM, Moss JR, Bennett ML, Thompson RC, Haynes DS. Contemporary management of intracranial complications of otitis media. Otol Neurotol. 2010;31(1):111–7.
23. Singh B, Maharaj TJ. Radical mastoidectomy: its place in otitic intracranial complications. J Laryngol Otol. 1993;107(12):1113–8.
24. Ren Y, Sethi RKV, Stankovic KM. Acute otitis media and associated complications in United States emergency departments. Otol Neurotol. 2018;39(8):1005–11.
25. Bluestone CD, Stephenson JS, Martin LM. Ten-year review of otitis media pathogens. Pediatr Infect Dis J. 1992;11(8 Suppl):S7–11.
26. Ngo CC, Massa HM, Thornton RB, Cripps AW. Predominant bacteria detected from the middle ear fluid of children experiencing otitis media: a systematic review. PLoS One. 2016;11(3):e0150949.
27. Fortanier AC, Venekamp RP, Boonacker CW, Hak E, Schilder AG, Sanders EA, et al. Pneumococcal conjugate vaccines for preventing otitis media. Cochrane Database Syst Rev. 2014;(4):CD001480.
28. Davis S, Feikin D, Johnson HL. The effect of Haemophilus influenzae type B and pneumococcal conjugate vaccines on childhood meningitis mortality: a systematic review. BMC Public Health. 2013;13 Suppl 3:S21.
29. Feinmesser R, Wiesel YM, Argaman M, Gay I. Otitis externa - bacteriological survey. ORL J Otorhinolaryngol Relat Spec. 1982;44(3):121–5.
30. Neely G. Complications of suppurative otitis media, parts 1 and 2. Washington, DC: AAO-HNS; 1978.
31. House HP. Otitis media; a comparative study of the results obtained in therapy before and after the introduction of the sulfonamide compounds. Arch Otolaryngol. 1946;43:371–8.
32. McLay K. Otogenic meningitis. J Laryngol Otol. 1954;68(3):140–6.
33. Grindborg O, Naucler P, Sjolin J, Glimaker M. Adult bacterial meningitis-a quality registry study: earlier treatment and favourable outcome if initial management by infectious diseases physicians. Clin Microbiol Infect. 2015;21(6):560–6.
34. Thigpen MC, Whitney CG, Messonnier NE, Zell ER, Lynfield R, Hadler JL, et al. Bacterial meningitis in the United States, 1998–2007. N Engl J Med. 2011;364(21):2016–25.
35. van de Beek D, de Gans J, Tunkel AR, Wijdicks EF. Community-acquired bacterial meningitis in adults. N Engl J Med. 2006;354(1):44–53.
36. Castelblanco RL, Lee M, Hasbun R. Epidemiology of bacterial meningitis in the USA from 1997 to 2010: a population-based observational study. Lancet Infect Dis. 2014;14(9):813–9.
37. Migirov L, Duvdevani S, Kronenberg J. Otogenic intracranial complications: a review of 28 cases. Acta Otolaryngol. 2005;125(8):819–22.
38. Ibrahim SI, Cheang PP, Nunez DA. Incidence of meningitis secondary to suppurative otitis media in adults. J Laryngol Otol. 2010;124(11):1158–61.
39. McGill F, Heyderman RS, Panagiotou S, Tunkel AR, Solomon T. Acute bacterial meningitis in adults. Lancet. 2016;388(10063):3036–47.

40. Scheld W. Bacterial meningitis and brain abscess. In: Harrison's principles of internal medicine. New York: McGraw-Hill; 1994.
41. Mattos JL, Colman KL, Casselbrant ML, Chi DH. Intratemporal and intracranial complications of acute otitis media in a pediatric population. Int J Pediatr Otorhinolaryngol. 2014;78(12):2161–4.
42. Zevallos JP, Vrabec JT, Williamson RA, Giannoni C, Larrier D, Sulek M, et al. Advanced pediatric mastoiditis with and without intracranial complications. Laryngoscope. 2009;119(8):1610–5.
43. Nager GT. Mastoid and paranasal sinus infections and their relation to the central nervous system. Clin Neurosurg. 1966;14:288–313.
44. Kaplan RJ. Neurological complications of infections of head and neck. Otolaryngol Clin N Am. 1976;9(3):729–49.
45. Proctor CA. Intracranial complications of otitic origin. Laryngoscope. 1966;76(2):288–308.
46. Stenzel M, Preuss S, Orloff L, Jecker P, Mann W. Cerebrospinal fluid leaks of temporal bone origin: etiology and management. ORL J Otorhinolaryngol Relat Spec. 2005;67(1):51–5.
47. Rao N, Redleaf M. Spontaneous middle cranial fossa cerebrospinal fluid otorrhea in adults. Laryngoscope. 2016;126(2):464–8.
48. Lucas MJ, Brouwer MC, van de Beek D. Neurological sequelae of bacterial meningitis. J Infect. 2016;73(1):18–27.
49. Wellman MB, Sommer DD, McKenna J. Sensorineural hearing loss in postmeningitic children. Otol Neurotol. 2003;24(6):907–12.
50. Paparella MM, Sugiura S. The pathology of suppurative labyrinthitis. Ann Otol Rhinol Laryngol. 1967;76(3):554–86.
51. Merchant SN, Gopen Q. A human temporal bone study of acute bacterial meningogenic labyrinthitis. Am J Otol. 1996;17(3):375–85.
52. Cawthorne T. Otogenic meningitis. J Laryngol Otol. 1939;54:444–70.
53. Penido Nde O, Chandrasekhar SS, Borin A, Maranhao AS, Gurgel Testa JR. Complications of otitis media - a potentially lethal problem still present. Braz J Otorhinolaryngol. 2016;82(3):253–62.
54. Brouwer MC, Thwaites GE, Tunkel AR, van de Beek D. Dilemmas in the diagnosis of acute community-acquired bacterial meningitis. Lancet. 2012;380(9854):1684–92.
55. van de Beek D, Cabellos C, Dzupova O, Esposito S, Klein M, Kloek AT, et al. ESCMID guideline: diagnosis and treatment of acute bacterial meningitis. Clin Microbiol Infect. 2016;22 Suppl 3:S37–62.
56. Saat R, Laulajainen-Hongisto AH, Mahmood G, Lempinen LJ, Aarnisalo AA, Markkola AT, et al. MR imaging features of acute mastoiditis and their clinical relevance. AJNR Am J Neuroradiol. 2015;36(2):361–7.
57. Yorgancilar E, Yildirim M, Gun R, Bakir S, Tekin R, Gocmez C, et al. Complications of chronic suppurative otitis media: a retrospective review. Eur Arch Otorhinolaryngol. 2013;270(1):69–76.
58. Jacobs RF, Wells TG, Steele RW, Yamauchi T. A prospective randomized comparison of cefotaxime vs ampicillin and chloramphenicol for bacterial meningitis in children. J Pediatr. 1985;107(1):129–33.
59. Brouwer MC, McIntyre P, Prasad K, van de Beek D. Corticosteroids for acute bacterial meningitis. Cochrane Database Syst Rev. 2015;(9):CD004405.
60. van de Beek D, de Gans J, McIntyre P, Prasad K. Corticosteroids for acute bacterial meningitis. Cochrane Database Syst Rev. 2007;(1):CD004405.
61. de Souza CE. Complications of otitis media in children. In: Pediatric otorhinolaryngology head and neck surgery. San Diego, London: Singulair; 1999.
62. Sennaroglu L, Sozeri B. Otogenic brain abscess: review of 41 cases. Otolaryngol Head Neck Surg. 2000;123(6):751–5.
63. Menon S, Bharadwaj R, Chowdhary A, Kaundinya DV, Palande DA. Current epidemiology of intracranial abscesses: a prospective 5 year study. J Med Microbiol. 2008;57(Pt 10):1259–68.
64. Yen PT, Chan ST, Huang TS. Brain abscess: with special reference to otolaryngologic sources of infection. Otolaryngol Head Neck Surg. 1995;113(1):15–22.
65. Sengupta A, Ghosh D, Basak B, Anwar T. Clinicopathological study of otogenic brain abscess. Indian J Otolaryngol Head Neck Surg. 2009;61(4):291–6.
66. Brouwer MC, Coutinho JM, van de Beek D. Clinical characteristics and outcome of brain abscess: systematic review and meta-analysis. Neurology. 2014;82(9):806–13.
67. Carpenter J, Stapleton S, Holliman R. Retrospective analysis of 49 cases of brain abscess and review of the literature. Eur J Clin Microbiol Infect Dis. 2007;26(1):1–11.
68. Myers EN, Ballantine HT Jr. The management of otogenic brain abscess. Laryngoscope. 1965;75:273–88.
69. Szyfter W, Kruk-Zagajewska A, Borucki L, Bartochowska A. Evolution in management of otogenic brain abscess. Otol Neurotol. 2012;33(3):393–5.
70. Isaacson B, Mirabal C, Kutz JW Jr, Lee KH, Roland PS. Pediatric otogenic intracranial abscesses. Otolaryngol Head Neck Surg. 2010;142(3):434–7.
71. Murthy PS, Sukumar R, Hazarika P, Rao AD, Mukulchand, Raja A. Otogenic brain abscess in childhood. Int J Pediatr Otorhinolaryngol. 1991;22(1):9–17.
72. Dubey SP, Larawin V. Complications of chronic suppurative otitis media and their management. Laryngoscope. 2007;117(2):264–7.
73. Nathoo N, Nadvi SS, Narotam PK, van Dellen JR. Brain abscess: management and outcome analysis of a computed tomography era experience with 973 patients. World Neurosurg. 2011;75(5-6):716–26; discussion 612–7.
74. Quijano M, Schuknecht HF, Otte J. Temporal bone pathology associated with intracranial abscess. ORL J Otorhinolaryngol Relat Spec. 1988;50(1):2–31.
75. Bento R, de Brito R, Ribas GC. Surgical management of intracranial complications of otogenic infection. Ear Nose Throat J. 2006;85(1):36–9.
76. Ingham HR, Slekon JB, Roxby CM. Bacteriological study of otogenic cerebral abscesses: chemotherapeutic role of metronidazole. Br Med J. 1977;2(6093):991–3.
77. Brook I. Bacteriology of intracranial abscess in children. J Neurosurg. 1981;54(4):484–8.
78. Nissen AJ. Intracranial complications of otogenic disease. Am J Otol. 1980;2(2):164–7.
79. Maniglia AJ, VanBuren JM, Bruce WB, Bellucci RJ, Hoffman SR. Intracranial abscesses secondary to ear and paranasal sinuses infections. Otolaryngol Head Neck Surg (1979). 1980;88(6):670–80.
80. Kornblut AD. Cerebral abscess--a recurrent otologic problem. Laryngoscope. 1972;82(8):1541–56.
81. Ward PH, Setliff RC, Long W. Otogenic brain abscess. Trans Am Acad Ophthalmol Otolaryngol. 1969;73(1):107–14.
82. Erdogan E, Cansever T. Pyogenic brain abscess. Neurosurg Focus. 2008;24(6):E2.
83. Britt RH, Enzmann DR. Clinical stages of human brain abscesses on serial CT scans after contrast infusion. Computerized tomographic, neuropathological, and clinical correlations. J Neurosurg. 1983;59(6):972–89.
84. Buchheit WA, Ronis ML, Liebman E. Brain abscesses complicating head and neck infections. Trans Am Acad Ophthalmol Otolaryngol. 1970;74(3):548–54.
85. Muzumdar D, Jhawar S, Goel A. Brain abscess: an overview. Int J Surg. 2011;9(2):136–44.
86. Maniglia AJ, Goodwin WJ, Arnold JE, Ganz E. Intracranial abscesses secondary to nasal, sinus, and orbital infections in adults and children. Arch Otolaryngol Head Neck Surg. 1989;115(12):1424–9.

87. Sarrazin JL, Bonneville F, Martin-Blondel G. Brain infections. Diagn Interv Imaging. 2012;93(6):473–90.
88. Prashanth V, Pandya VK. Role of CT scan in diagnosis and management of otogenic intracranial abscess. Indian J Otolaryngol Head Neck Surg. 2011;63(3):274–8.
89. Maurice-Williams RS. Open evacuation of pus: a satisfactory surgical approach to the problem of brain abscess? J Neurol Neurosurg Psychiatry. 1983;46(8):697–703.
90. Le Beau J, Creissard P, Harispe L, Redondo A. Surgical treatment of brain abscess and subdural empyema. J Neurosurg. 1973;38(2):198–203.
91. Zhai Y, Wei X, Chen R, Guo Z, Raj Singh R, Zhang Y. Surgical outcome of encapsulated brain abscess in superficial non-eloquent area: a systematic review. Br J Neurosurg. 2016;30(1):29–34.
92. Samuel J, Fernandes CM. Lateral sinus thrombosis (a review of 45 cases). J Laryngol Otol. 1987;101(12):1227–9.
93. Singh B. The management of lateral sinus thrombosis. J Laryngol Otol. 1993;107(9):803–8.
94. Ooi EH, Hilton M, Hunter G. Management of lateral sinus thrombosis: update and literature review. J Laryngol Otol. 2003;117(12):932–9.
95. Teichgraeber JF, Per-Lee JH, Turner JS Jr. Lateral sinus thrombosis: a modern perspective. Laryngoscope. 1982;92(7 Pt 1):744–51.
96. Manolidis S, Kutz JW Jr. Diagnosis and management of lateral sinus thrombosis. Otol Neurotol. 2005;26(5):1045–51.
97. Bales CB, Sobol S, Wetmore R, Elden LM. Lateral sinus thrombosis as a complication of otitis media: 10-year experience at the children's hospital of Philadelphia. Pediatrics. 2009;123(2):709–13.
98. Ghosh PS, Ghosh D, Goldfarb J, Sabella C. Lateral sinus thrombosis associated with mastoiditis and otitis media in children: a retrospective chart review and review of the literature. J Child Neurol. 2011;26(8):1000–4.
99. Garcia RD, Baker AS, Cunningham MJ, Weber AL. Lateral sinus thrombosis associated with otitis media and mastoiditis in children. Pediatr Infect Dis J. 1995;14(7):617–23.
100. Au JK, Adam SI, Michaelides EM. Contemporary management of pediatric lateral sinus thrombosis: a twenty year review. Am J Otolaryngol. 2013;34(2):145–50.
101. Ozer E, Sivasli E, Bayazit YA, Sirikci A, Gok A, Mumbuc S, et al. Otogenic cerebral venous infarction: a rare complication of acute otitis media. Int J Pediatr Otorhinolaryngol. 2003;67(9):1019–21.
102. Oestreicher-Kedem Y, Raveh E, Kornreich L, Yaniv I, Tamary H. Prothrombotic factors in children with otitis media and sinus thrombosis. Laryngoscope. 2004;114(1):90–5.
103. Wong BY, Hickman S, Richards M, Jassar P, Wilson T. Management of paediatric otogenic cerebral venous sinus thrombosis: a systematic review. Clin Otolaryngol. 2015;40(6):704–14.
104. Wolfowitz BL. Otogenic intracranial complications. Arch Otolaryngol. 1972;96(3):220–2.
105. Kaplan DM, Kraus M, Puterman M, Niv A, Leiberman A, Fliss DM. Otogenic lateral sinus thrombosis in children. Int J Pediatr Otorhinolaryngol. 1999;49(3):177–83.
106. Bradley DT, Hashisaki GT, Mason JC. Otogenic sigmoid sinus thrombosis: what is the role of anticoagulation? Laryngoscope. 2002;112(10):1726–9.
107. Saposnik G, Barinagarrementeria F, Brown RD Jr, Bushnell CD, Cucchiara B, Cushman M, et al. Diagnosis and management of cerebral venous thrombosis: a statement for healthcare professionals from the American Heart Association/American Stroke Association. Stroke. 2011;42(4):1158–92.
108. deVeber G, Andrew M, Adams C, Bjornson B, Booth F, Buckley DJ, et al. Cerebral sinovenous thrombosis in children. N Engl J Med. 2001;345(6):417–23.
109. Davison SP, Facer GW, McGough PF, McCaffrey TV, Reder PA. Use of magnetic resonance imaging and magnetic resonance angiography in diagnosis of sigmoid sinus thrombosis. Ear Nose Throat J. 1997;76(7):436–41.
110. Syms MJ, Tsai PD, Holtel MR. Management of lateral sinus thrombosis. Laryngoscope. 1999;109(10):1616–20.
111. Chalmers E, Ganesen V, Liesner R, Maroo S, Nokes T, Saunders D, et al. Guideline on the investigation, management and prevention of venous thrombosis in children. Br J Haematol. 2011;154(2):196–207.
112. Funamura JL, Nguyen AT, Diaz RC. Otogenic lateral sinus thrombosis: case series and controversies. Int J Pediatr Otorhinolaryngol. 2014;78(5):866–70.
113. Novoa E, Podvinec M, Angst R, Gurtler N. Paediatric otogenic lateral sinus thrombosis: therapeutic management, outcome and thrombophilic evaluation. Int J Pediatr Otorhinolaryngol. 2013;77(6):996–1001.
114. Tov EE, Leiberman A, Shelef I, Kaplan DM. Conservative nonsurgical treatment of a child with otogenic lateral sinus thrombosis. Am J Otolaryngol. 2008;29(2):138–41.
115. Zanoletti E, Cazzador D, Faccioli C, Sari M, Bovo R, Martini A. Intracranial venous sinus thrombosis as a complication of otitis media in children: critical review of diagnosis and management. Int J Pediatr Otorhinolaryngol. 2015;79(12):2398–403.
116. Neilan RE, Isaacson B, Kutz JW Jr, Lee KH, Roland PS. Pediatric otogenic lateral sinus thrombosis recanalization. Int J Pediatr Otorhinolaryngol. 2011;75(6):850–3.
117. Doyle KJ, Brackmann DE, House JR 3rd. Pathogenesis of otitic hydrocephalus: clinical evidence in support of Symonds' (1937) theory. Otolaryngol Head Neck Surg. 1994;111(3 Pt 1):323–7.
118. Kuczkowski J, Dubaniewicz-Wybieralska M, Przewozny T, Narozny W, Mikaszewski B. Otitic hydrocephalus associated with lateral sinus thrombosis and acute mastoiditis in children. Int J Pediatr Otorhinolaryngol. 2006;70(10):1817–23.
119. Sitton MS, Chun R. Pediatric otogenic lateral sinus thrombosis: role of anticoagulation and surgery. Int J Pediatr Otorhinolaryngol. 2012;76(3):428–32.
120. Wong I, Kozak FK, Poskitt K, Ludemann JP, Harriman M. Pediatric lateral sinus thrombosis: retrospective case series and literature review. J Otolaryngol. 2005;34(2):79–85.
121. Mather M, Musgrave K, Dawe N. Is anticoagulation beneficial in acute mastoiditis complicated by sigmoid sinus thrombosis? Laryngoscope. 2018;128(11):2435–6.
122. Shah UK, Jubelirer TF, Fish JD, Elden LM. A caution regarding the use of low-molecular weight heparin in pediatric otogenic lateral sinus thrombosis. Int J Pediatr Otorhinolaryngol. 2007;71(2):347–51.
123. Ropposch T, Nemetz U, Braun EM, Lackner A, Walch C. Low molecular weight heparin therapy in pediatric otogenic sigmoid sinus thrombosis: a safe treatment option? Int J Pediatr Otorhinolaryngol. 2012;76(7):1023–6.
124. Symonds C. Otitic hydrocephalus. Brain. 1931;54:55–71.
125. Symonds C. Hydrocephalic and focal cerebral symptoms in relation to thrombophlebitis of the dural sinuses and cerebral veins. Brain. 1937;1937(60):531–50.
126. Sadoghi M, Dabirmoghaddam P. Otitic hydrocephalus: case report and literature review. Am J Otolaryngol. 2007;28(3):187–90.
127. Durairaj VD, Andrews B, Rao RR, Chan KH. Morbid complications of otitic hydrocephalus. Orbit. 2008;27(1):51–4.
128. Tomkinson A, Mills RG, Cantrell PJ. The pathophysiology of otitic hydrocephalus. J Laryngol Otol. 1997;111(8):757–9.
129. Koitschev A, Simon C, Lowenheim H, Kumpf M, Besch D, Ernemann U. Delayed otogenic hydrocephalus after acute otitis media in pediatric patients: the changing presentation of a serious otologic complication. Acta Otolaryngol. 2005;125(11):1230–5.
130. Azarmina M, Azarmina H. The six syndromes of the sixth cranial nerve. J Ophthalmic Vis Res. 2013;8(2):160–71.
131. O'Connor AF, Moffat DA. Otogenic intracranial hypertension. Otitic hydrocephalus. J Laryngol Otol. 1978;92(9):767–75.

132. Wu JF, Jin Z, Yang JM, Liu YH, Duan ML. Extracranial and intracranial complications of otitis media: 22-year clinical experience and analysis. Acta Otolaryngol. 2012;132(3):261–5.
133. Penido Nde O, Borin A, Iha LC, Suguri VM, Onishi E, Fukuda Y, et al. Intracranial complications of otitis media: 15 years of experience in 33 patients. Otolaryngol Head Neck Surg. 2005;132(1):37–42.
134. Weingarten K, Zimmerman RD, Becker RD, Heier LA, Haimes AB, Deck MD. Subdural and epidural empyemas: MR imaging. AJR Am J Roentgenol. 1989;152(3):615–21.
135. Baum PA, Dillon WP. Utility of magnetic resonance imaging in the detection of subdural empyema. Ann Otol Rhinol Laryngol. 1992;101(10):876–8.
136. Minks DP, Porte M, Jenkins N. Acute mastoiditis--the role of radiology. Clin Radiol. 2013;68(4):397–405.
137. Horowitz G, Fishman G, Brenner A, Abu-Ghanem S, Derowe A, Cavel O, et al. A novel radiographic sign and a new classifying system in mastoiditis-related epidural abscess. Otol Neurotol. 2015;36(8):1378–82.
138. Jang CH, Choi YH, Jeon ES, Yang HC, Cho YB. Extradural granulation complicated by chronic suppurative otitis media with cholesteatoma. In Vivo. 2014;28(4):651–5.
139. Greenberg JS, Manolidis S. High incidence of complications encountered in chronic otitis media surgery in a U.S. metropolitan public hospital. Otolaryngol Head Neck Surg. 2001;125(6):623–7.
140. Bizakis JG, Velegrakis GA, Papadakis CE, Karampekios SK, Helidonis ES. The silent epidural abscess as a complication of acute otitis media in children. Int J Pediatr Otorhinolaryngol. 1998;45(2):163–6.

Chronic Ear Disease and Cholesteatoma

37

Michael B. Gluth and Peter L. Santa Maria

Introduction

Among otologic surgeons, the colloquial term "chronic ear disease" generally refers to a long-term inflammatory state occurring within the tympanic cleft as well as the communicating pneumatized air cell system of the temporal bone. Because this is a condition wherein numerous pathophysiological mechanisms overlap to project a variable disease spectrum, it is also a condition that is challenging to define and categorize. Thus, it may be said that ear surgeons often understand what a chronic ear is better than they are able to neatly verbalize. Infectious otorrhea, tympanic membrane deficiency, conductive hearing loss, and impaired ventilation of the middle ear and mastoid are hallmarks that are evident in most chronic ears, but certainly there are instances when one or several of these elements may be absent. In addition, the unique association with cholesteatoma further complicates the scope and complexity of chronic ear disease. In the following sections, an overview is made of this peculiar entity that, not only has plagued mankind for centuries, but also comprises a major segment of modern surgical otology.

Pathologic Description and Classification of Middle Ear Disease

Otitis media is inflammation of the middle ear cavity due to any disease process, although infection is most common. The subtypes of otitis media have long been viewed as stages in a continuum of events dating back to the classic, but now controversial, *ex vacuo* theory of middle ear disease proposed by Politzer in 1867 [1], whereby Eustachian tube dysfunction leads to negative middle ear pressure, which in turn yields effusion and possibly infection. Stages of middle ear disease begin with an acute stage that can either lead to a chronic stage or resolve; furthermore, as an ear progresses through the phases of one pathologic process, it is common that it may offshoot into another associated process simultaneously (Fig. 37.1). Consequently, a great deal of overlap exists in the labeling used to describe a given chronic ear based on the status of multiple factors such as middle ear aeration, tympanic membrane integrity, infection status, and cholesteatoma presence.

The Spectrum of Otitis Media with an Intact Tympanic Membrane

The classification used to portray otitis media relates to the timing of symptoms as well as the manifestations involved. Otitis media with an intact tympanic membrane is primarily subdivided into three conditions: Eustachian tube dysfunction, otitis media with effusion, and acute otitis media (Fig. 37.2). Eustachian tube (dilatory) dysfunction refers to a disorder with negative middle ear pressure and associated symptoms such as hearing loss, ear fullness, or pressure [2]. Otitis media with effusion presents with similar symptoms as Eustachian tube dysfunction; however, a middle ear effusion is present, which is usually not culture positive for bacteria. However, systemic disease symptoms are not present in otitis media with effusion, and this terminology has replaced designations such as serous otitis media or secretory otitis media. In otitis media with effusion, mucosal edema with widening of the subepithelial space, vascular dilation, and infiltration of leukocytes is observed. However, the exact mechanism that prompts these pathologic changes, be it negative pressure or microbial colonization, is not definitively understood [3]. Eventually, proliferation of mucosal goblet cells with associated shift in mucin production, as well as reabsorption of water, will render an effusion

M. B. Gluth (✉)
Ear Sciences Centre, University of Western Australia and Ear Science Institute Australia, Perth, WA, Australia

P. L. Santa Maria
Department of Otolaryngology—Head and Neck Surgery, University of Pittsburgh, Pittsburgh, PA, USA

A. D. Sweeney et al. (eds.), *Haynes-Glasscock-Shambaugh Surgery of the Ear*, https://doi.org/10.1007/978-3-032-18264-7_37

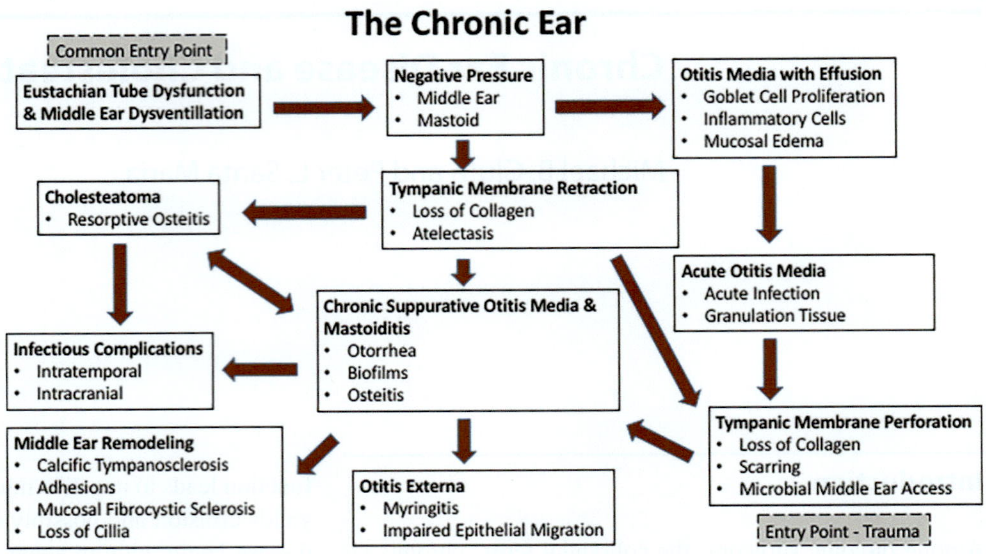

Fig. 37.1 Complexity of the chronic ear. Chronic ear disease is an overlapping spectrum of numerous related processes

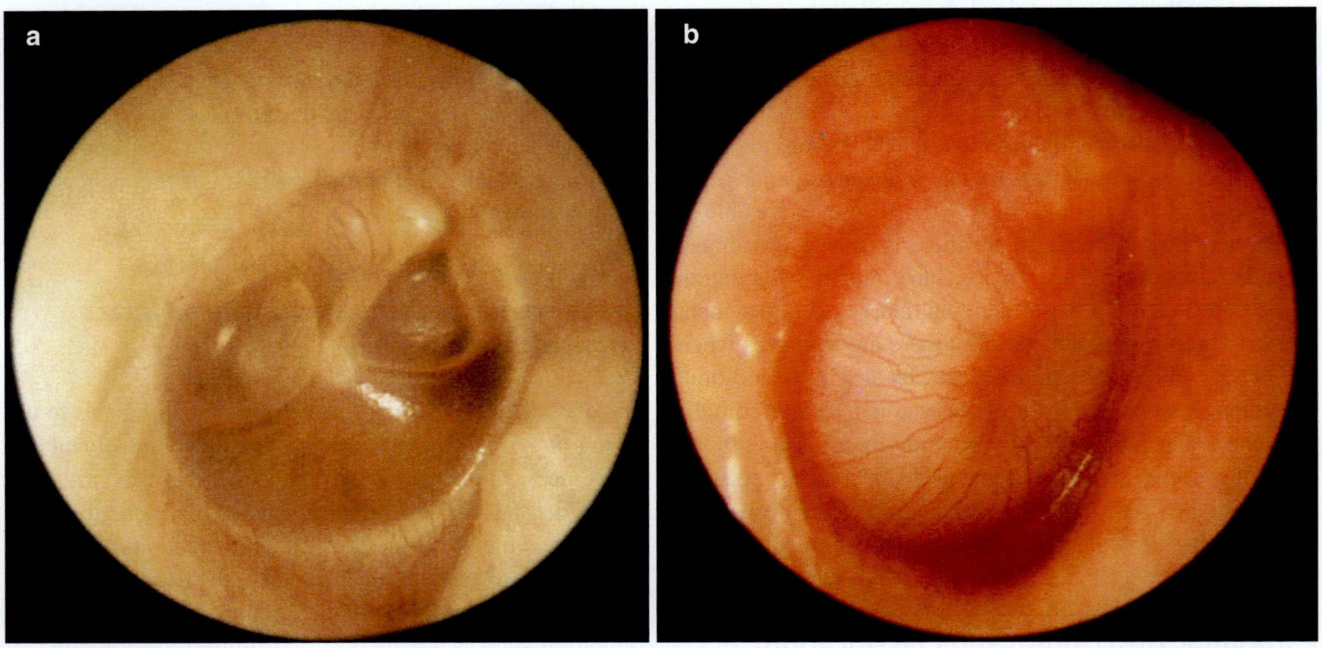

Fig. 37.2 Otitis media with an intact tympanic membrane. (**a**) Otitis media with effusion is noted with right ear serous effusion and air-fluid meniscus; however, signs of acute inflammation are not noted. (**b**) Acute otitis media presenting with right bulging inflamed tympanic membrane with prominent hyperemia, vascularity, and purulent effusion

mucoid and viscous, further impairing the middle ear clearance mechanisms [4].

Acute otitis media refers to inflammation of the middle ear that is associated with rapid onset of one or more systemic symptoms including, but not limited to, otalgia, fever, and irritability. Suppurative otorrhea can be seen in the event that tympanic membrane perforation occurs. Although most cases of acute otitis media are viral or bacterial infections, it is common for a bacterial infection to occur as a superinfection of a viral-originated process, especially if *respiratory syncytial virus* is involved [5]. The phases of otitis media have been described as *hyperemic* as the middle ear is inoculated and reacts to a pathogen, *exudative* as leukocytes release cytokines that trigger capillary leakage, *suppurative* if the infection is bacterial and the pyogenic process unfolds, and *resolution* as the inflammatory process subsides—either resulting in recovery to baseline or progression to otitis media with effusion. A temporal classification also exists for otitis media, with an acute state lasting less than three weeks, subacute from 3 weeks to 3 months, and chronic for greater than 3 months.

Chronic Suppurative Otitis Media

A severe bout of acute otitis media may result in a spontaneous tympanic membrane perforation, and the natural history of an acute perforation can follow several pathways. The perforation can heal spontaneously, the inflammation of the middle ear can resolve with the perforation failing to close and becoming a chronic dry perforation, or the perforation can be associated with ongoing middle ear infection and otorrhea. When both the perforation and infection are present for at least 3 months, an ear may be classified as having chronic suppurative otitis media (Fig. 37.3). Chronic suppurative otitis media is best thought of as a spectrum of infectious disease of bacterial persister cells that relapse between inactive and active states depending on the interactions with the immune system, antimicrobial therapies and food sources to "awaken" the bacteria [6, 7]. Common middle ear histopathologic findings associated with this condition include granulation tissue, osteitis, loss of cilia, fibrocystic sclerosis of the mucosa, and osteogenic formation of tympanosclerotic plaque. These processes can result in permanent remodeling of the middle ear cleft (Fig. 37.4). Antimicrobial and antiseptic therapies are successful at killing metabolically active bacteria, leading to periods of inactivity; however, the patient is prone to long-term relapse as the persister cells repopulate the niche [7, 8] (Fig. 37.5). Repeated antimicrobial therapy eventually leads to antimicrobial resistance and failure to convert the disease to an inactive state [9].

Chronic suppurative otitis media had been traditionally sub-typed according to several unofficial indicators, and although attempts at formal classification have been made, none have been universally adopted [10]. One distinction made depends on whether or not cholesteatoma is present. A traditional classification categorized the disease as tubotympanic, atticoantral, or mixed based on the segments of the tympanic membrane and middle ear space that are most prominently implicated. Tubotympanic chronic otitis media tends to be typified by disease of the pars tensa and mesotympanum whereas atticoantral disease primarily involves the pars flaccida and epitympanum. This categorization oversimplifies the process given that cholesteatoma can involve areas preserving the attic, may occur in the presence of Eustachian tube dysfunction and also has bacteria present [11].

Chronic ear disease has also been classified and, more importantly, graded according to disease severity. Bellucci introduced a popular grading scale based on the frequency of otorrhea and whether or not the patient had a cleft palate [12]. Austin described a classification based on the underlying ossicular status [13] that was modified by Kartush by merging it with Bellucci's classification to create the popular Middle Ear Risk Index [14] (Table 37.1). Because the results of functional reconstruction of the tympanic membrane and ossicular chain are heavily dependent on the status of the middle ear, the application of middle ear grading is an essential step in framing outcomes—without which, interpretation of hearing results cannot be meaningfully achieved [15].

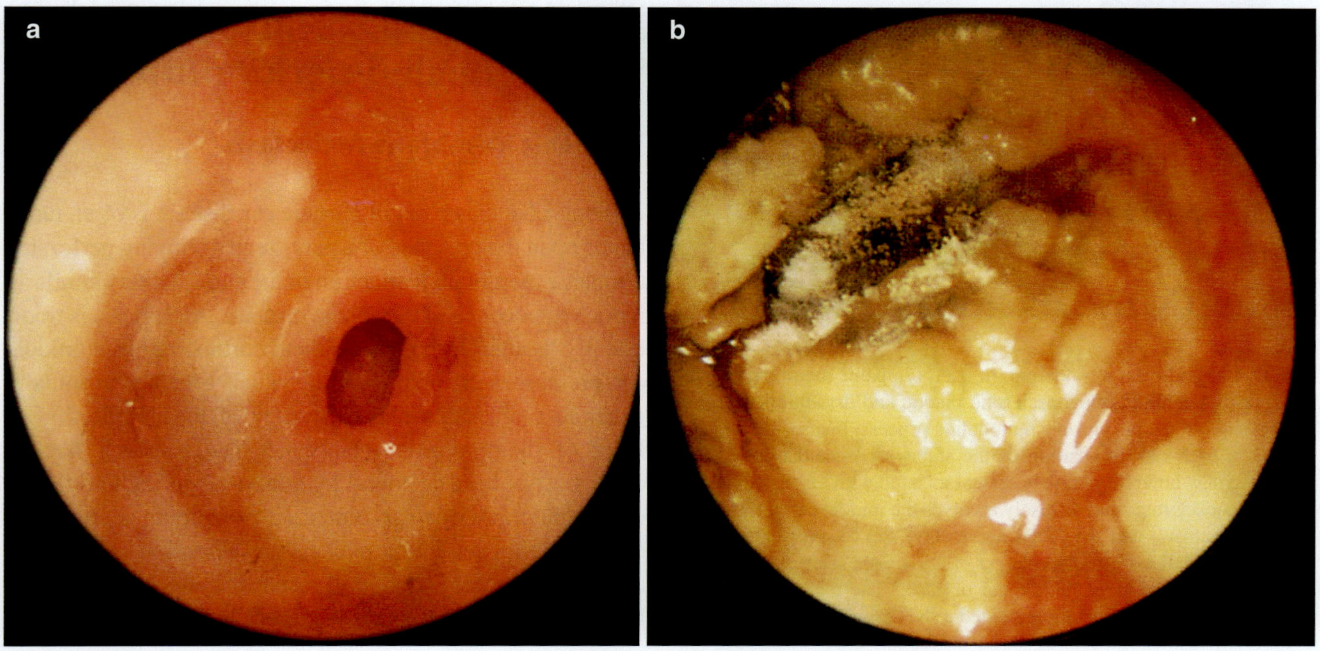

Fig. 37.3 Chronic suppurative otitis media: (**a**) Egress of pus is seen via a granulating perforation. *S. aureus* and *P. aeruginosa* are the most commonly cultured pathogens. (**b**) Polymicrobial infection with obvious fungal elements is noted, especially in ears that have been treated long-term with antibiotic and steroid-containing drops

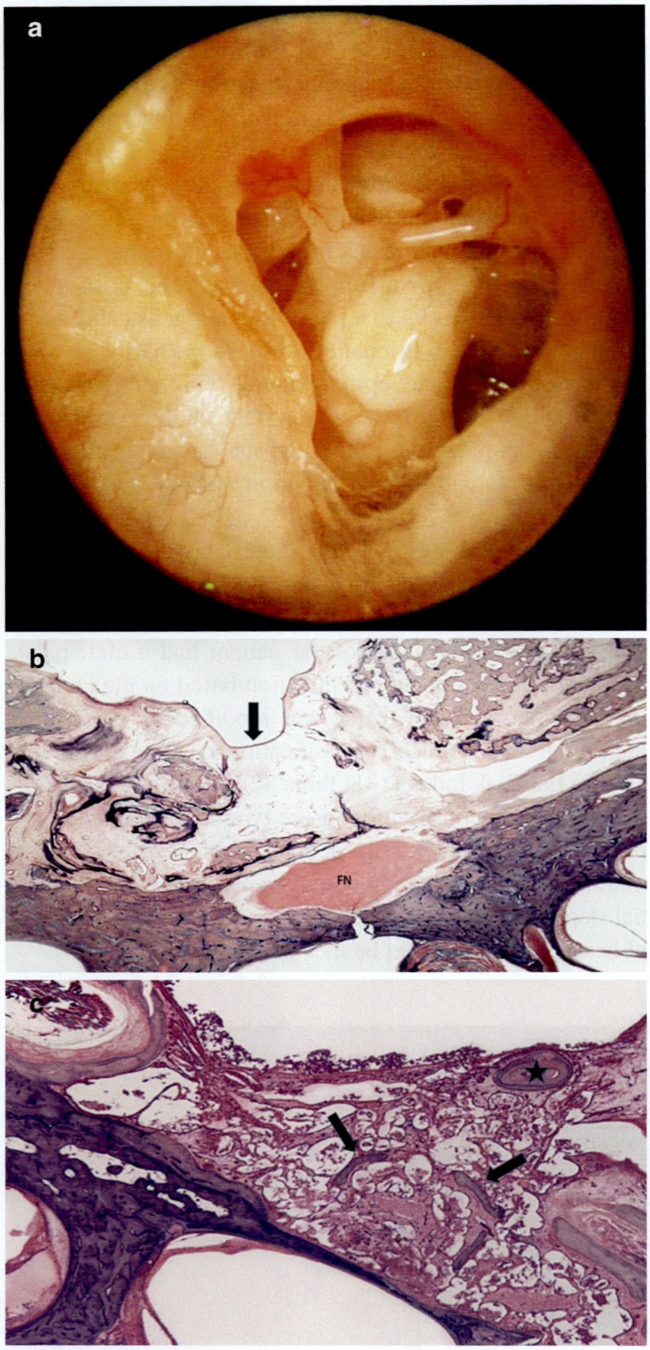

Fig. 37.4 Middle ear remodeling. (a) Left tympanic membrane perforation with calcified tympanosclerotic plaque and dry fibrotic mucosa depicts a quiescent but chronic remodeling process. Incus is eroded and there is a high risk of fixation of the stapes or ossicular heads. (b) Extensive new bone formation is seen associated with extensive middle ear tympanosclerosis that diffusely involves the middle ear between the drumhead (arrow) and the facial nerve (FN). (c) Severely remodeled middle ear cleft demonstrates changes of fibrocystic sclerosis that could be considered "end-stage middle ear disease." The malleus (star) and remnant stapes superstructure are noted to be densely embedded

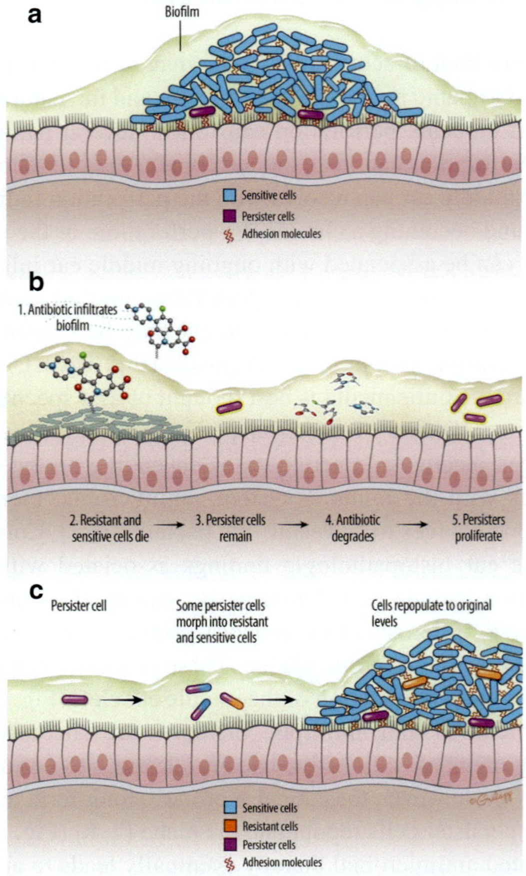

Fig. 37.5 Biofilm community in chronic suppurative otitis media: (a) Biofilm populations typically contain metabolically active and non-active or persister cells. (b) Antibiotic therapies eradicate metabolically active bacteria, leaving only persister cells. (c) Persister cells later repopulate the niche. Over time persister cells can morph into resistant cells. (© Peter Santa Maria, MD. Used with permission)

Tympanic Membrane Atelectasis

Although the diagnosis of chronic ear disease is often made based upon the presence of a persistently draining perforated tympanic membrane, retraction of the eardrum may similarly induce a sequence of chronic symptoms. Atelectasis is traditionally thought to be the result of chronic negative middle ear pressure and inflammation, which together eventually generate a retraction and deficiency of the middle fibrous layer of the tympanic membrane. The resulting flaccid, dimeric drumhead is bound by adhesions to the middle ear cleft, and this irregular tympanic membrane architecture often includes retraction pockets and retention of moisture and squamous debris that will result in focal areas of granular myringitis, impart forces that erode the ossicular chain, or

Table 37.1 Middle ear risk index

Risk factor	Status	Risk value
Otorrhea		
	Dry	0
	Occasionally wet	1
	Persistently wet	2
	Wet with cleft palate	3
Perforation		
	No	0
	Yes	1
Cholesteatoma		
	None	0
	Present	1
Ossicular status		
	All intact	0
	M+ S+	1
	M+ S-	2
	M- S+	3
	M- S-	4
	Ossicular head fixation	2
	Stapes fixation	3
Granulation or effusion		
	No	0
	Yes	2
Previous surgery		
	None	0
	Staged	1
	Revision	2
Smoker		
	No	0
	Yes	2

Adapted from reference [14]
M malleus, *S* stapes superstructure

at worst evolve into a cholesteatoma (Fig. 37.6). A theory of selective epitympanic dysventilation has been hypothesized to explain isolated retraction of the pars flaccida wherein Eustachian tube function is competent, but ventilation of the middle ear and mastoid is impaired due to blockage of the tympanic isthmus in the setting of baseline restrictions of the epitympanic diaphragm—particularly the presence of a completely closed tensor fold [16] (Fig. 37.7). Ventilation theories have been challenged recently given the presence of retraction in normally ventilated middle ears, with the explanation provided by mucosal traction between mucosal layers [17].

Several classification systems exist for tympanic membrane retraction depending on the site of tympanic membrane involvement, and those proposed by Sade [18] and Tos [19] for pars tensa and pars flaccida retractions, respectively, are noteworthy (Table 37.2). Such classifications are useful in clinical surveillance of retraction pockets over time. However, a practical classification of eardrum collapse has also been described by Black [20] to intuitively connect classification with surgical decision-making wherein:

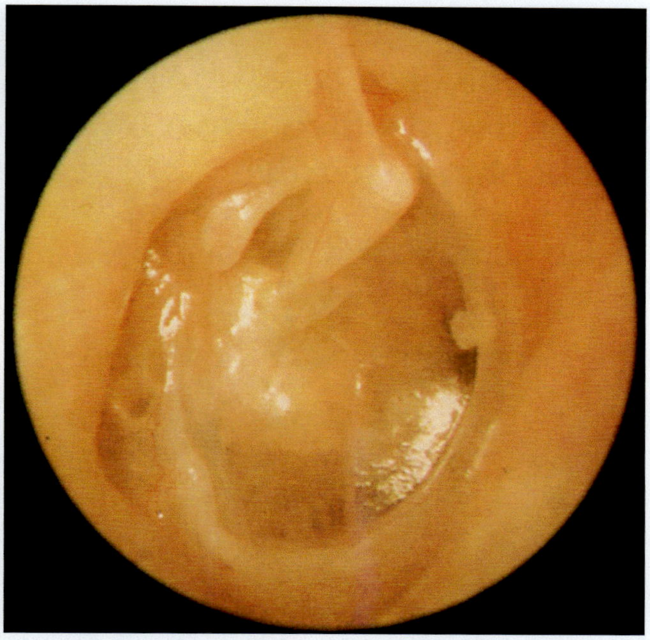

Fig. 37.6 Atelectasis with middle ear aeration: The presence of air in the protympanum of this right ear suggests recovered Eustachian tube function and a likelihood that persisting eardrum collapse is primarily due to fibrotic adhesions rather than underlying negative middle ear pressure. Although adhesive change and incudostapedial joint erosion are noted in this right ear, the lack of an effusion renders this a favorable surgical candidate for hearing restoration surgery

- Stage I is drum collapse without hearing loss, treated by observation or tympanostomy.
- Stage II is drum collapse with hearing loss but no ossicular dysfunction, treated by tympanoplasty to reinforce the drumhead.
- Stage III is drum collapse with hearing loss and ossicular dysfunction, treated by tympanoplasty with ossiculoplasty.
- Stage IV is acquired cholesteatoma, treated by definitive cholesteatoma surgery.

Risk Factors for Chronic Ear Disease

Studies linking risk factors to the incidence of chronic suppurative otitis media are lacking, and most of the data are inferred from risk factors for acute otitis media. Although chronic suppurative otitis media is much less common than acute otitis media, the latter likely predisposes an individual to the former [21]. Age is a well-recognized risk factor for acute otitis media due to the short length, small caliber, and horizontal orientation of a child's Eustachian tube. Also, children are more likely to have an immune system that has not yet been exposed to many viral and bacterial pathogens, making them more susceptible to infection [22]. A history of childhood middle ear

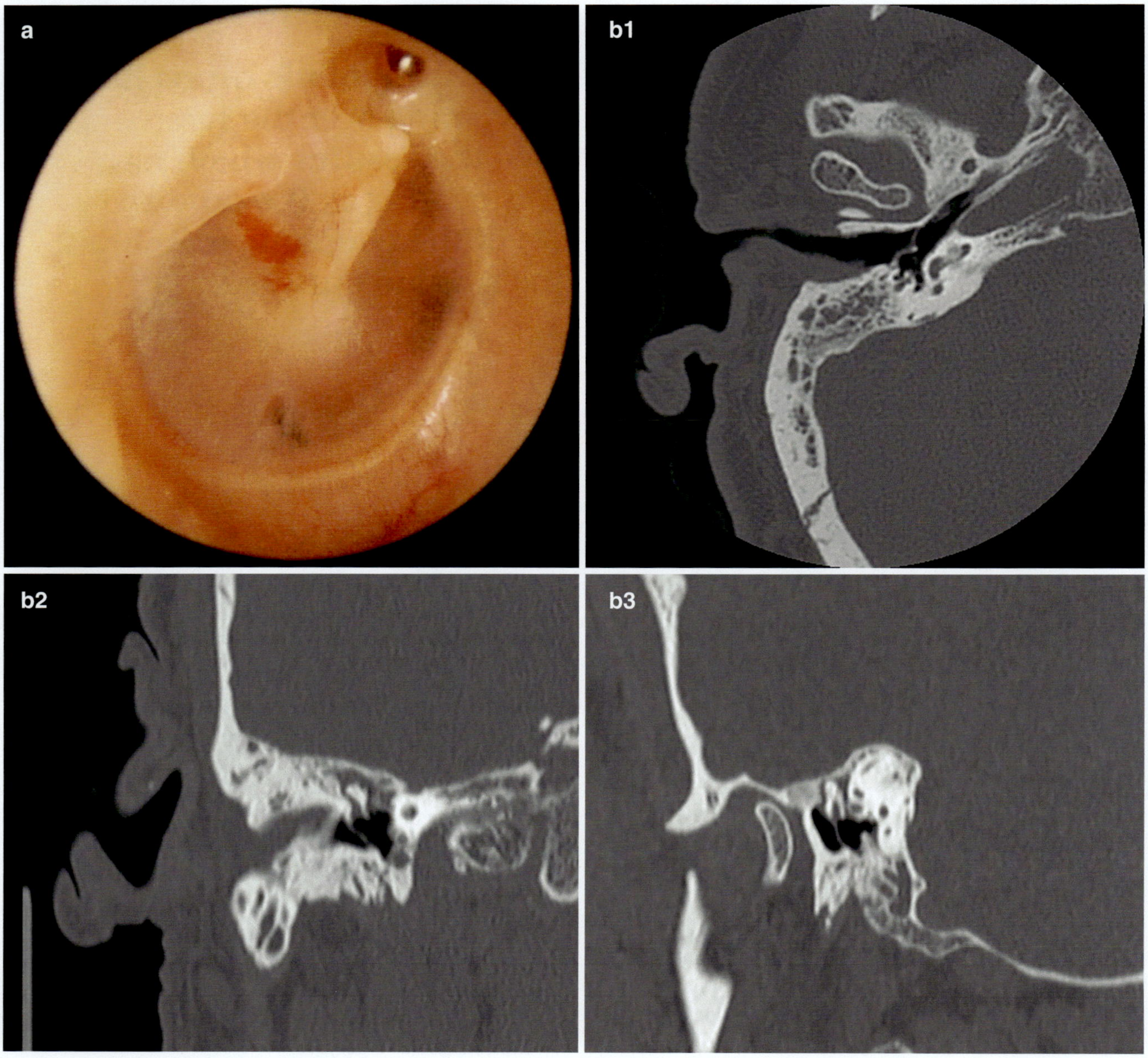

Fig. 37.7 Selective epitympanic dysventilation. (**a**) When there is an isolated retraction of the pars flaccida and postobstructive change within the mastoid, complete blockage of the epitympanic diaphragm may be the underlying cause. Here the right pars tensa is normal and the mesotympanum is ventilated. (**b**) CT scan images in the axial (1), coronal (2), and sagittal (3) planes demonstrate failed aeration and opacification of the epitympanum and mastoid with normal aeration of the mesotympanum

disease is a risk factor for having chronic otitis media as an adult. Other risk factors include craniofacial anomalies and cleft palate, frequent upper respiratory tract infections, immunodeficiency, allergic rhinitis, head and neck radiation exposure, and family history of otitis media. Social and environmental influences such as exposure to tobacco smoke, maternal breastfeeding and day care attendance are also important risk factors. The improvement of housing, hygiene, nutrition, and other social factors has been shown to result in a significant decrease in the prevalence of chronic suppurative otitis media in some societies. Several ethnic groups have been found to have a high risk of developing chronic ear disease, including indigenous peoples of Australia, Southwestern North America, Greenland and Alaska [23].

Table 37.2 Classification of tympanic membrane retractions

Grade	Description
Pars tensa retraction per Sade [18]	
1	Retracted tympanic membrane, which does not touch any middle ear structures
2	Retracted tympanic membrane touches the stapes or incus
3	Retracted tympanic membrane down to promontory
4	Retracted tympanic membrane with collected keratin
Pars Flaccida Retraction per Tos [19]	
1	Slight dimpling of the pars flaccida
2	Retraction to malleus neck; entire pocket is visible
3	Partly hidden retraction with possible erosion of the scutum
4	Deep retraction with definite scutum erosion; pocket is not entirely visualized

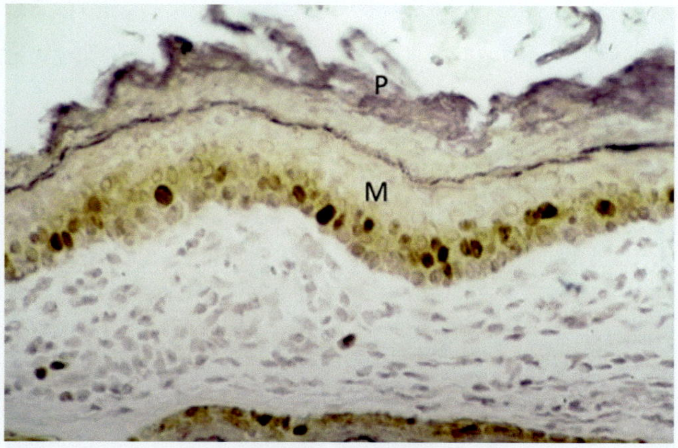

Fig. 37.8 Cholesteatoma histopathology. Note the presence of cholesteatoma matrix (M), which has the typical layers of epithelium, and also the perimatrix (P). Sloughed keratinocytes are present within the lumen of the sac

Cholesteatoma

Cholesteatoma is a "pseudo-neoplasm" comprised of keratinizing squamous epithelium that occurs in the tympanic cavity and mastoid, often in the form of an erosive cyst. Cholesteatomas have two layers, a matrix and a perimatrix (Fig. 37.8). The microanatomy of the matrix is quite similar to skin, with a stratum basale, stratum superficiale, and stratum corneum, which are oriented such that keratinized debris is sloughed into the lumen of the cholesteatoma sac. The perimatrix, located on the exterior aspect of the sac, consists of loose connective tissue, inflammatory cells, and blood vessels. The extent of the matrix and perimatrix varies tremendously from one part of a given cholesteatoma to another and in tissues affected by cholesteatoma, papillary infiltration of the matrix can be observed. The keratin of cholesteatoma is highly immunogenic in the middle ear and mastoid, prompting a foreign body-like reaction and influx of Langerhans cells as well as generation of aural inflammatory polyp, the observation of which should raise the index of clinical suspicion for cholesteatoma (Fig. 37.9). One feature of cholesteatoma that is responsible for many of its complications is the tendency to destroy bone via a process of absorptive osteitis. This is an inflammatory-mediated process that is triggered by pro-osteoclastic cytokines, ultimately leading to osteoclastic degradation of adjacent bone [24]. Active bacterial superinfection can drive cholesteatomas to behave more aggressively. This observation is supported by data from experimental animals, in which induced cholesteatomas that were inoculated with *Pseudomonas aeruginosa* were larger and demonstrated more bone resorption than uninfected cholesteatomas [25].

In 2017, the European Academy of Otology and Neurotology and the Japanese Otological Society published a joint consensus on the definition, classification, and staging of cholesteatoma [26], around which the following descriptions are framed (Table 37.3).

Congenital Cholesteatoma

Congenital cholesteatoma accounts for up to 5% of all cholesteatomas. These lesions are assumed to be present at birth and classically these are encountered in children in the anterior mesotympanum behind an intact tympanic membrane, but, in reality, numerous other locations are possible. Diagnosis requires having a normal tympanic membrane and no past history of tympanic membrane perforation, otorrhea, or otologic surgery. Past acute otitis media or middle ear effusion does not preclude the diagnosis. Congenital cholesteatoma is generally accepted to develop out of embryonic cell nests that fail to involute; however, an alternate theory implicates reflux of amniotic cells into the middle ear space [27]. An undiagnosed congenital cholesteatoma can eventually generate a perforation of the eardrum if allowed to grow into a far-advanced stage, which may then be difficult to differentiate from acquired disease. From a histologic perspective, the congenital cholesteatoma matrix cannot be distinguished from acquired cholesteatoma.

Acquired Cholesteatoma

Many theories exist to account for the development of an acquired cholesteatoma. The *retraction pocket theory* implicates progression from a retracted segment of the tympanic membrane secondary to poor middle ear ventilation, which eventually evolves into a trapped debris-filled compartment that is unable to maintain a self-cleansing mechanism. The *proliferation theory* proposes that chronic tympanic inflammation stimulates the basal keratinocytes to penetrate small breaks in the basement membrane, resulting in papillary ingrowth and formation of a viable colony of trapped epithelium. The *immigration theory* proposes that squamous epi-

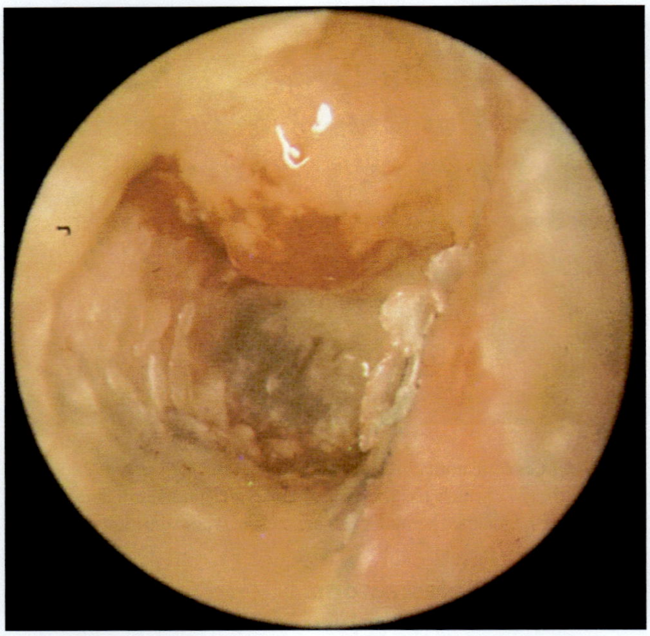

Fig. 37.9 Aural polyp due to cholesteatoma: Aural polyp is generated by chronic middle ear mucosal irritation, especially a foreign body reaction to retained keratin; thus, the presence of polyp such as this in the superior quadrant should heighten clinical suspicion for underlying cholesteatoma

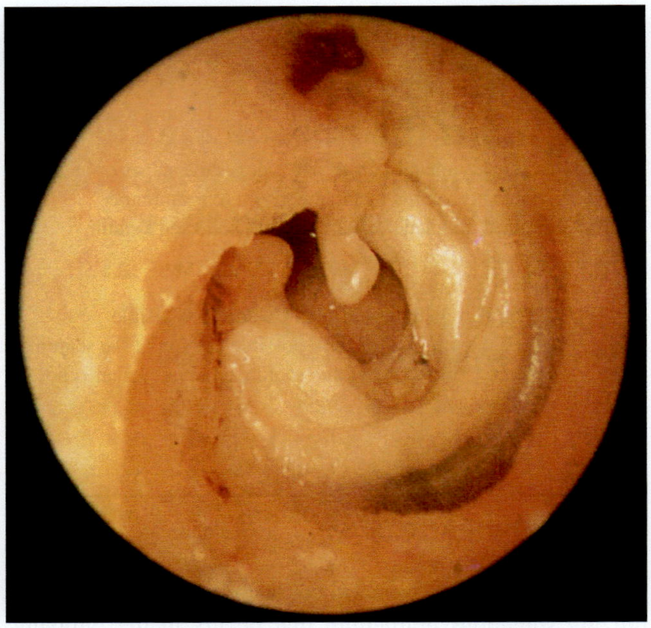

Fig. 37.10 Non-retraction pocket cholesteatoma: The pars tensa is retracted and perforated. Note the growth of skin around the margins of the perforation, which can be most easily appreciated in this case at the inferior aspect of the tympanic membrane

Table 37.3 EAONO/JOS 2017 classification and staging of cholesteatoma

Classification:	
Congenital	
Acquired	
Retraction pocket	
Pars flaccida	
Pars tensa	
Combination	
Non-retraction pocket	
Due to perforation	
Iatrogenic	
Unclassifiable	
Staging	
Stage	Description
1	Cholesteatoma localized at the site of origin (mesotympanum or epitympanum)
2	Cholesteatoma at more than one STAM subsite
3	Cholesteatoma with extracranial complication OR complete eardrum atelectasis OR erosion of more than half of the bony canal wall OR large tegmen defect requiring surgical repair
4	Cholesteatoma with intracranial complication

Adapted from reference [26]

thelium grows into the middle ear space around the margins of a perforation, and this is the basis for non-retraction pocket cholesteatoma. It does not explain cholesteatomas that develop with an intact tympanic membrane. When a cholesteatoma occurs in the presence of a tympanic perforation, it usually consists of a sheet of epithelium on the undersurface of the drumhead, the promontory of the cochlea, or the ossicular chain, as opposed to a cholesteatoma sac (Fig. 37.10). The *metaplasia theory* proposes that otitis media stimulates the middle ear mucosa into hyperplastic transformation and dedifferentiation that generates squamous epithelium, which in turn will epidermalize. Evidence is lacking for the *metaplasia theory* and current evidence points to cholesteatoma being of ectodermal origin. Recently, a *mucosal traction theory* has been proposed to address the shortcomings of traditional theories [17]. It proposes that mucosal coupling occurs between migrating opposing surfaces of mucosa, generating traction inwards. Finally, an alternate form of cholesteatoma is the implantation cholesteatoma, which develops secondary to the displacement of unwanted epithelial tissue into the middle ear space during surgery or trauma.

Spread of Retraction Pocket Cholesteatoma in the Temporal Bone

The most widely accepted sites of origin for retraction pocket cholesteatoma are, in order of descending frequency, posterior pars flaccida, posterior pars tensa, and anterior pars flaccida [28] (Fig. 37.11). However, a single cholesteatoma may have elements of several of these subtypes simultaneously. Retraction pocket cholesteatoma has a tendency to spread according to planes of embryologic origin that are defined by the ligaments and mucosal folds of the middle ear [29]. Also,

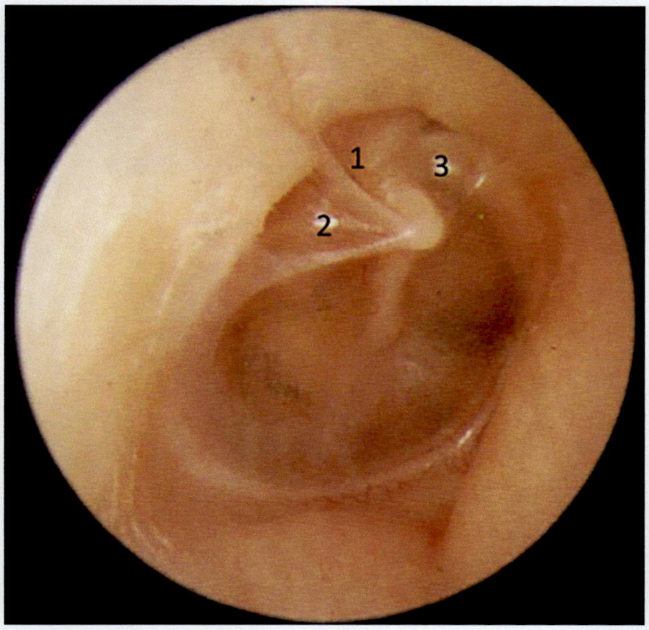

Fig. 37.11 Cholesteatoma sites of origin. The most common sites of cholesteatoma origin are (1) posterior pars flaccida, (2) posterior pars tensa, and (3) anterior pars flaccida

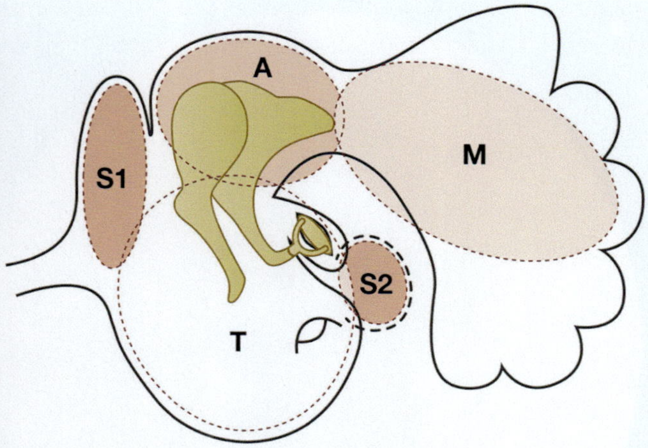

Fig. 37.12 STAM system of sites of tympanomastoid cholesteatoma involvement [26]: S1 (supratubal recess tympani) and S2 (sinus tympani) are designated difficult. *S*ites *T*ympanic cavity, *A*ttic, and *M*astoid (includes antrum) are the other subsites

connective and granulation tissue present during otitis media with effusion may act as scaffolding for the ingrowth of cholesteatoma [30]. The referenced 2017 consensus staging system [26] divides the tympanomastoid space into subsites according to the STAM system (Fig. 37.12). This system assigns the sinus tympani (S1) and the supratubal recess (S2) as two distinctly difficult cholesteatoma access *sites*. The remaining subsites are the *T*ympanic cavity, the *A*ttic, and the *M*astoid, which also includes the antrum. Stage I cholesteatoma is confined to the primary site of origin and Stage II involves multiple sites. Stage III refers to disease with extracranial complications, complete tympanic membrane atelectasis, destruction of more than half of the bony canal wall, or major tegmen destruction requiring repair. Stage IV is reserved for cases with intracranial complications.

Pars Flaccida Cholesteatoma

Pars flaccida cholesteatoma usually originates from the posterior pars flaccida into the lateral epitympanic (Prussak's) space (Fig. 37.13). These often spread posteriorly with penetration into the superior incudal space and then into the mastoid antrum by a route that extends lateral to the body of the incus. There is also the possibility of extension inferiorly into the mesotympanum and, in turn, the sinus tympani by expansion through the posterior pouch of Von Troeltsch. Passage through this pathway generally involves erosion of the long process of the incus. As the epitympanum is filled, anterior extension to the supratubal recess is commonly seen.

A less common form of pars flaccida cholesteatoma originates from the anterior pars flaccida. These may erode the head of the malleus and extend through the anterior epitympanic wall into the supratubal recess at an early stage. Inferior extension into the mesotympanum may occur by expansion in the anterior pouch of Von Troeltsch, with subsequent passage anterior to the tensor tympani tendon into the protympa-

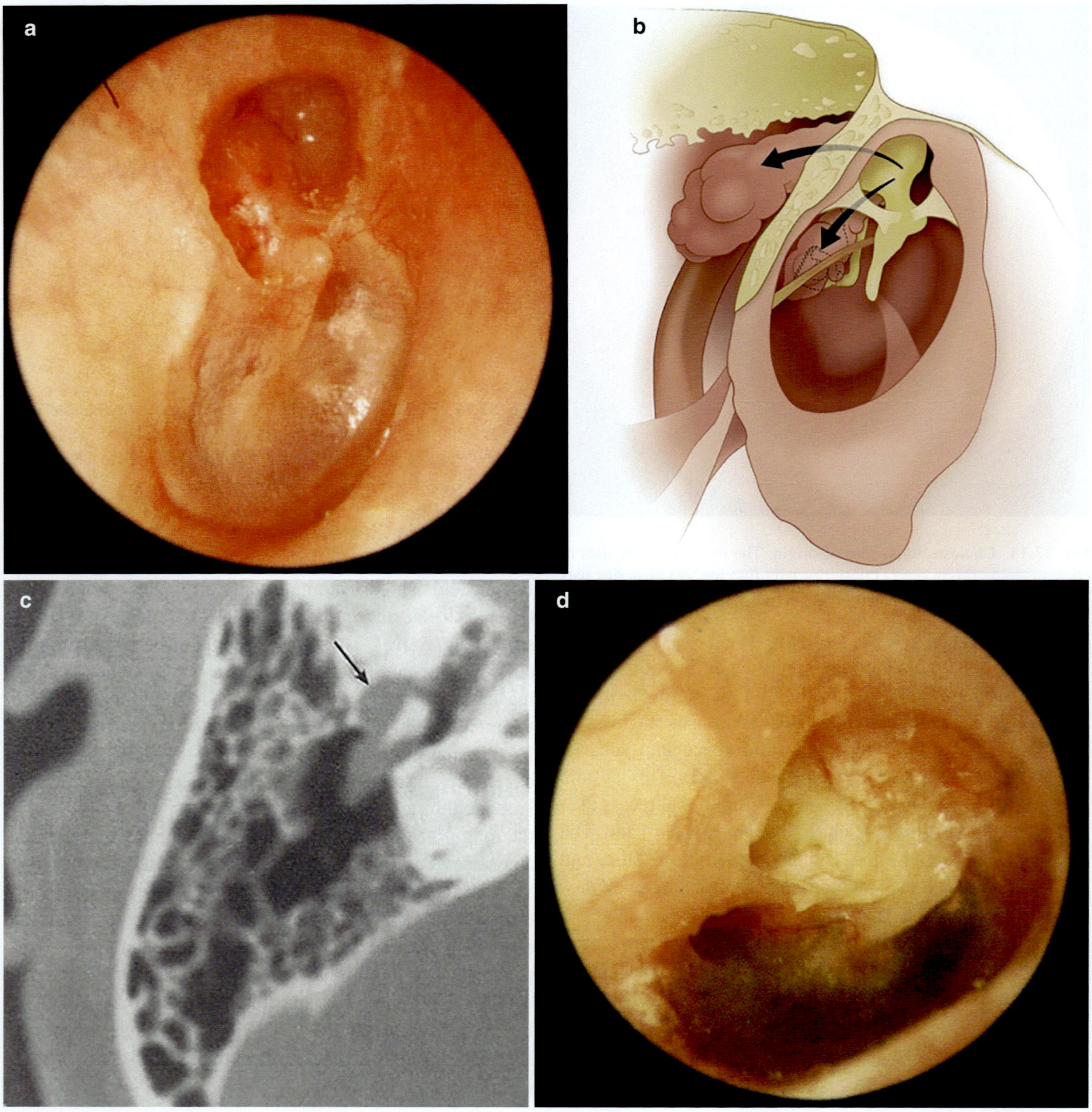

Fig. 37.13 Pattern of spread of pars flaccida cholesteatoma: (**a**) Pars flaccida cholesteatoma usually originates from a deep retraction into the lateral epitympanic (Prussak's) space. (**b**) These typically spread into the mastoid antrum by expanding into the superior incudal space and into the middle ear lateral to the incus. (**c**) Here cholesteatoma is noted lateral to the incus body as shown on the right ear axial cut CT (arrow) with extension just into the mastoid and rounded expansion of the lateral epitympanic wall. (**d**) As these expand, the canal wall bone of the scutum here in the right ear becomes eroded. (**e**) Pars flaccida cholesteatoma will secondarily extend into the mesotympanum through the posterior pouch of Von Troeltsch and can be seen here as a white mass behind a left intact pars tensa and aerated middle ear, and the hearing reconstruction prognosis in such cases is excellent

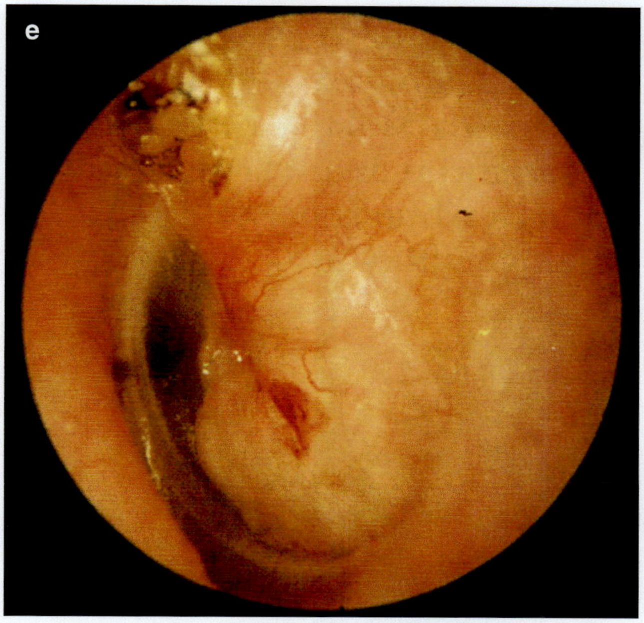

Fig. 37.13 (continued)

num. Anterior pars flaccida cholesteatoma is also known to potentially extend into the medial epitympanic wall through the anterior supralabyrinthine air cells, with involvement of the perigeniculate aspect of the facial nerve [31].

Pars Tensa Cholesteatoma

Pars tensa cholesteatoma is usually derived from the posterior aspect of the pars tensa into the mesotympanum (Fig. 37.14). These cholesteatomas may be associated with early erosion of the long process of the incus and also the stapes superstructure, with frequent deep penetration into the retrotympanum to involve the sinus tympani at an early stage. If large, these cholesteatomas often involve the round window niche and hypotympanic air cells. Superior extension of pars tensa cholesteatoma into the epitympanum usually through the posterior tympanic isthmus, with subsequent passage into the mastoid antrum medial to the body of the incus and growth over the tympanic segment of the facial nerve. A general rule of thumb is that pars tensa cholesteatoma leads to higher rates of recidivism and is associated with a worse hearing reconstruction prognosis than pars flaccida cholesteatoma.

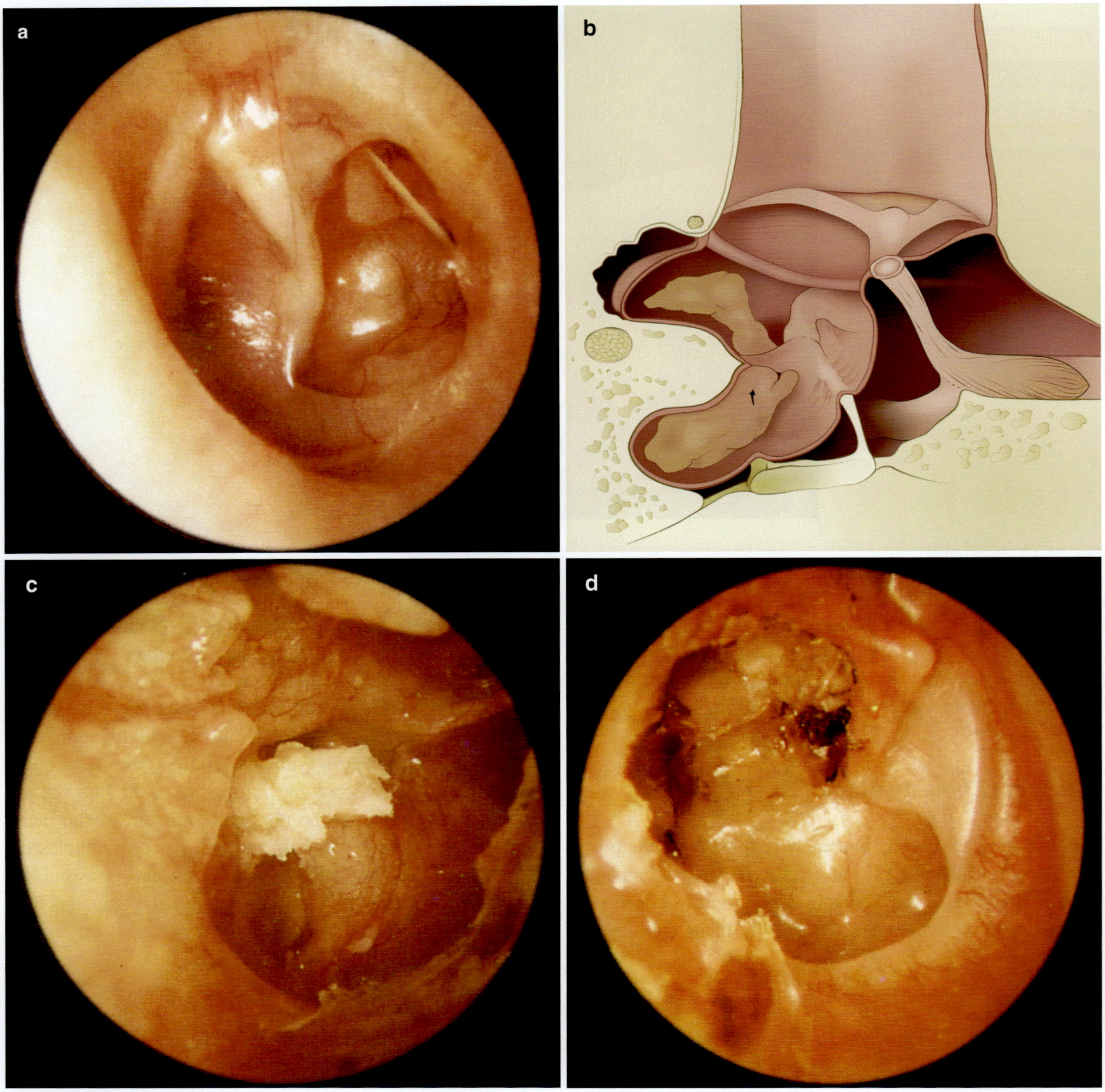

Fig. 37.14 Pattern of spread of pars tensa cholesteatoma: (**a**) Pars tensa cholesteatoma usually develops from a deep posterior retraction pocket, shown here in the left ear. (**b**) These will drape over the incudostapedial joint and stapedius tendon and they are known for early and deep penetration into the sinus tympani. (**c**) On exam, a collection of squamous debris can be seen accumulating in the posterior mesotympanum of the right ear. (**d**) Pars tensa cholesteatoma will secondarily spread to the epitympanum via a route that extends immediately over the oval window niche and fallopian canal and medial to the incus body. Here, diffuse retraction is present in the right ear and cholesteatoma is noted medial to the remnant of the malleus, while extending into the epitympanum. The hearing reconstruction prognosis for these cases is generally less favorable than that of pars flaccida cholesteatoma

Microbiology

It must be emphasized that microbial cultures do not detect the presence of an infection, only the presence of a certain threshold of metabolically active planktonic bacteria able to grow within the conditions of a clinical laboratory. Polymerase chain reaction detects bacterial DNA but cannot determine whether the bacteria are living and relevant. Acknowledging these limitations, it is noteworthy that cultures from chronic middle ear specimens typically demonstrate *P. aeruginosa, Staphylococcus aureus* and coagulase-negative *Staphylococci* [32–35]. Other bacteria occasionally cultured include *Enterobacter, Proteus, Escherichia coli, Acinetobacter, Klebsiella, Alcaligenes, Serratia, Streptococcus, Corynebacterium Peptostreptococcus* spp., *Bacteroides fragilis, Fusobacterium* spp., *Prevotella* spp., and *Porphyromonas* spp. The bacterial profile of infected cholesteatoma is similar to chronic suppurative otitis media. When an infected canal wall-down mastoidectomy cavity is present, *S. aureus* is the most common pathogen cultured, more than twice as common as *P. aeruginosa* [36]. The nasopharynx has been proposed as a reservoir of pathogenic bacteria for ear disease; however, one study comparing cultures from the middle ear and nasopharynx only found that cultured bacteria were the same 26% of the time [37].

Atypical pathogens in chronic ear disease include fungi and mycobacteria, with fungi implicated as the sole cultured pathogen in approximately 5% of cases [38]. *Aspergillus* species, including *niger* and *fumigatus*, and *Candida* species, including *albicans* and *parapsilosis*, are the most commonly cultured isolates [39]. Secondary fungal growth is common in ears that have been treated long-term with combination antibiotic and steroid ototopical medications. Tuberculous otitis accounts for less than 1% of chronic ear infections and it may be challenging to diagnose because clinical signs and symptoms are variable, there is not always an association with pulmonary or systemic tuberculosis, and mycobacteria are difficult to culture [40]. Symptoms of tuberculous otitis include otorrhea, hearing loss, otalgia, tinnitus, dizziness, and facial palsy. Large tympanic membrane perforations are typical, which may be uniquely multiple and marginal, as is erosion of the ossicular chain, most commonly the long process of the incus. Correctly diagnosing tuberculous otitis is important because multidrug regimens of anti-tuberculous medication alone without surgery are usually successful in treating uncomplicated cases [41].

Biofilms in Chronic Ear Disease

Chronic, refractory middle ear infections, cholesteatoma, otitis media with effusion, and Eustachian tube dysfunction have all been associated with bacterial biofilms, and the most common chronic ear pathogenic bacteria have been identified as being able to form them [42]. Biofilm refers to a colony of bacteria growing within an extracellular matrix structure that has enhanced abilities to resist antibiotics and to adhere to surfaces [43]. Bacteria in biofilms are able to resist antibiotics by several strategies, including an extracellular matrix that impedes most antibiotic diffusion, metabolically inactive bacterial cells, persister cells, that are tolerant to traditional antimicrobial strategies that can repopulate if antibiotics kill the active cells (Fig. 37.5) [7, 44]. Ototopicals, including antiseptics and antimicrobials, can inhibit growth but fail to eradicate biofilms in vitro [7, 45, 46]. The exception is povdone-iodine, which eliminates biofilms in vitro; however, diffusion concerns and ototoxicity potential limit its in vivo utility [8]. Treatment of biofilms ultimately requires removal and debridement, which is currently most thoroughly achieved through surgery.

Concepts of Disease Management

Management of Chronic Suppurative Otitis Media

The general scheme of treating chronic suppurative otitis media first involves applying medical management to convert active disease to inactive, therefore minimizing the purulent secretions and granulation tissue, followed by surgical correction of any residual disease sequelae such as a deficient tympanic membrane or a dysfunctional ossicular chain. Basic medical treatment typically consists of evacuation of aural secretions and debris followed by application of an ototopical medication in the form of a drop or a powder, which generally consists of some version of antimicrobial, acidifying, and/or corticosteroid component. The goal is to suppress the infection to a level of inactivity so the local immune system can rid the remaining infection or to reduce the infection to only metabolically inactive bacteria and then prevent them from "awakening" and reestablishing active disease. Fluoroquinolones are the most commonly applied ototopical antibiotics due to their favorable ototoxicity profile. Ototoxicity is a concern with several ototopicals such as those containing aminoglycosides, but when the ear is inflamed, penetration through the round window is likely reduced, leaving the individual clinician to decide if the risk-to-benefit ratio is acceptable.

Some chronic ears may respond promptly to medical therapy and easily move into a durable inactive phase, while others may follow a pattern of recurring flare-ups that require intermittent attention. Ears in either of these categories are at extremely low risk of developing a short-term complication. Surgical intervention is recommended if hearing restoration is sought or if there is intolerance to water exposure or inability to wear a hearing aid. The risk of long-term sensorineural hearing loss must not be ignored in patients with relapsing chronic ear disease [9]. Cases with persisting otorrhea that do not fully respond to medical therapy indicate a bacterial niche has transformed to include resistant bacteria and may have a higher risk of complications. However, in an immunocompetent host, the risk of a severe complication for a non-cholesteatoma chronic ear is still relatively low.

The mainstay of surgery for chronic ear disease is tympanic membrane repair, with a goal of providing barrier separation between the middle ear and the external surface open to the environment. Closure of the tympanic membrane alone is often sufficient to eliminate otorrhea and to facilitate resolution of infection. Because chronic suppurative otitis media is considered to be part of a spectrum of chronic oto-mastoiditis, mastoidectomy has also been frequently employed, and inadequate mastoidectomy has been blamed for surgical failures, with some surgeons citing particular neglected air cell tracts as significant [47]. Histopathology seems to support this concept in that diseased mucosa, osteitis, and micro-abscesses can be observed throughout the mastoid in archived temporal bone specimens. Post-obstructive phenomena, such as cholesterol granuloma and air cell effusion, are also regularly encountered during mastoid surgery. On the other hand, indicators of mastoiditis are frequently observed upon radiologic imaging of ears that have been rendered asymptomatic after tympanoplasty alone; thus, the clinical significance of these findings is questionable.

Otologic surgical tradition notwithstanding, a critical review argues against the therapeutic role of routine mastoidectomy in chronic suppurative otitis media. Albu et al. reported results of the only existing statistically powered prospective randomized trial comparing Type I tympanoplasty alone to tympanoplasty with canal wall–up mastoidectomy for ears with non-cholesteatoma chronic suppurative otitis media [48]. In this study, 282 ears that had been actively draining within 6 months of surgery were followed postoperatively for 12 months. No statistically significant benefit was detected from the addition of mastoidectomy in terms of eardrum closure or hearing. Of note, the two treatment arms were equally stratified according to the Middle Ear Risk Index, perforation size, perforation location, preoperative hearing, age, and gender. Additionally, Eliades and Limb published an exhaustive review and analysis of the existing literature pertaining to therapeutic mastoidectomy in chronic ear disease, which included 26 articles [49]. They concluded "the available literature shows no additional benefit to performing mastoidectomy with tympanoplasty for uncomplicated tympanic membrane perforations." It must be recognized that the outcomes of chronic ear disease in the literature are short-term and often focus on tympanic repair and air-bone gap closure. The current literature lacks long-term follow-up and fails to capture the potential for long-term relapse [9]. At present, it seems both reasonable and generalizable to say that surgical treatment of the mastoid should routinely be considered in decision-making for cases involving chronic otitis media, but it should not be performed simply as a matter of routine. Situations where mastoidectomy may yet impart potential benefit include refractory infection with antimicrobial-resistant pathogens, past surgical failures with radiologic evidence of extensive osteitis, or cases that involve an infectious complication, although there is yet insufficient evidence to make strong recommendations for any of these indications

In lieu of tympanoplasty and the selective application of mastoidectomy, some severely distressed ears may benefit from blind sac closure of the external auditory canal, which is often applied in combination with aggressive air cell extirpation such as subtotal petrosectomy with or without Eustachian tube plugging. This robust approach may be sensible in cases with no hearing or those with so-called "end-stage middle ear disease" that is typified by fibrocystic sclerosis and extensive calcific tympanosclerosis throughout the middle ear cleft, wherein the outlook for functional hearing reconstruction is dismal. After this procedure is undertaken and infection is definitively cleared, hearing restoration via placement of an implantable device should be safe, though in terms of the latter, consideration should be given to how an implanted magnet will affect surveillance with MRI. While MRI-conditional devices exist, the artifact created by such a device during an MRI may complicate the ability to thoroughly evaluate the ipsilateral temporal bone.

Management of Negative Middle Ear Pressure and Atelectasis

Eustachian tube dysfunction and negative middle ear pressure likely play a role in the pathophysiology of most chronic ears, at least at some point in a patient's disease history. Eustachian tube dysfunction might be due to craniofacial abnormalities, rhinologic disease, neuromuscular disease, extra-esophageal reflux, or even socioeconomic factors such as smoking. Conversely, wholly attributing chronic ear disease to Eustachian tube dysfunction alone may be an erroneous oversimplification in cases where underlying systemic disease, biofilms, and middle ear remodeling may be continuously in play, even after the Eustachian tube has attained functionality. Accordingly, the first step in managing the effects of negative middle ear pressure and resultant tympanic membrane atelectasis should start in the nose, while also considering the patient's health entirely.

Nasal steroids are the mainstay of rhinologic disease management via inflammatory cascade suppression, and this may promote optimized Eustachian tube function in patients with sinonasal disease; however, nasal steroids have less Eustachian tube utility in those without nasal inflammatory pathology [50]. Oral antihistamines and leukotriene antagonists may indirectly impart a favorable effect on tubal function in patients with established allergic rhinitis, but have little direct impact on the Eustachian tube otherwise. In the worst cases of allergic rhinitis, immunotherapy may be needed. Likewise, elimination or suppression of chronic paranasal sinus disease with appropriate dosing of systemic antibiotics or corticosteroids is desirable for similar reasons. Treatment of extra-esophageal reflux with acid suppressant medications has an uncertain indirect effect on tubal function. Topical or oral decongestant medications do not impart any measurable impact on Eustachian tube function, although they are still commonly prescribed [51, 52].

Surgery may also promote middle ear ventilation. Adenoidectomy can be supportive to improve Eustachian tube function by elimination of tubal blockage, microbial colonization, and chronic nasopharyngitis [53]. Endoscopic balloon Eustachian tuboplasty is gaining momentum as a possible method to directly address tubal insufficiency, and short-term results on properly selected patients appear promising [54]. Tympanostomy is a means of ventilating the middle ear cleft that is routine in otologic practice. However, this must be judiciously applied after weighing the risk of relapsing otorrhea in a patient with a chronic ear, especially if hearing aid use is planned or a canal wall-down cavity is present. When desired, long-term intubation can be achieved with the application of a T-style tympanostomy tube passed through a cartilage graft, which also has the advantage of concurrently providing eardrum support that otherwise can become eroded with serial intubation.

Surgical decision making for tympanic membrane atelectasis has already been alluded to in the presentation of Black's classification, whereby tympanoplasty for eardrum reinforcement and ossiculoplasty are applied incrementally to more severely affected cases to prevent disease stage progression and to restore hearing [20]. However, the decision to proceed with surgery must be counterbalanced by the risk of iatrogenic cholesteatoma in severe cases that involve deep retraction into the hypotympanum and retrotympanum, which can be technically challenging to evert. In truth, many severely atelectatic eardrums may be observed indefinitely, and it is often surprising that hearing status in advanced cases may be better than expected.

The role of mastoidectomy in managing negative middle ear pressure is controversial as the physiologic role of the mastoid air cell system in regulating middle ear gas pressure is not well understood. Contradictions exist in the literature, with some advocating a vital role of healthy intact mucosa in the mastoid antrum and epitympanum in maintaining minute-to-minute tympanic gas homeostasis in the reconstructed ear, whereas others suggest that mucosal gas absorption in these areas is partially responsible for recurrent retraction cholesteatoma [55–57]. The proposition of mastoidectomy to counteract negative middle ear pressure is based on the theory that expansion of tympanomastoid volume, according to Boyle's Law, will generate an effectual volumetric pressure buffer [58]. This concept has been particularly championed in ears having a sclerotic mastoid.

Although the creation of a volumetric pressure buffer is an intellectually satisfying concept, evidence to support therapeutic mastoidectomy for this indication is also lacking, similar to what has been outlined for therapeutic mastoidectomy to treat chronic infection. It is unclear whether this lack of evidence is due to an inherently flawed theory regarding the pressure buffer effect or inadequacy in the design and execution of clinical trials to test this hypothesis. Also, maintaining patency of surgically augmented communications between the middle ear and mastoid may be problematic due to blockage from new bone formation and mucosal webbing.

Management of Cholesteatoma

The preferred treatment modality for cholesteatoma is surgery unless the projected risk of a perioperative complication is higher than the risk of developing a cholesteatoma-related complication. The goals of cholesteatoma surgery (in descending order) are to create a safe ear that is not at risk of complications, to render the ear dry, and to facilitate hearing function. The latter of these is ideally achieved by reconstruction of the tympano-ossicular mechanism, but sometimes surgery facilitates amplification via a conventional hearing aid or implantable hearing device. It is also desirable to construct an ear that does not place undue strain on a patient's lifestyle due to the impact of caloric effect vertigo, burdensome ear care, or strict water precautions; however, this is not always possible. A final aim is also to render the ear resistant to the development of future recurrent cholesteatoma by reinforcing the drumhead or taking measures to promote middle ear ventilation.

Numerous surgical techniques have evolved to manage cholesteatoma, and the details of many of these are covered elsewhere in this textbook. Historically, these have been divided into two general categories. The first category includes procedures that preserve the intact status of the bony ear canal wall by addressing cholesteatoma via an epitympanectomy (atticotomy) approach or by a "combined approach" that merges epitympanectomy with some form of a canal wall-up mastoidectomy [59, 60]. This category is favored for preserving natural ear anatomy and for generally being associated with better hearing reconstruction results. However, intact canal-wall surgery may be very difficult to execute properly in a sclerotic temporal bone and is associated with higher residual disease rates, which in turn may result in multiple surgical procedures. The second category of operations includes the "open" procedures that involve removing the superior and posterior bony canal wall and exteriorizing all or part of the tympanomastoid space. These canal wall-down procedures are praised for the wide access they provide for dissection, and they are still considered the gold standard for cholesteatoma control with low published residual disease rates, but they also permanently alter the ear by reducing middle ear volume and by creating an open cavity that requires a lifetime of office care. A reported range of 10–50% of mastoid cavities will become infected at some point in time, and cavity instability is heavily dependent on eardrum integrity and cavity contour with respect to retention of debris [61–63]; the reality of otorrhea in some percent of open cavity cases cannot be fully avoided, even by experienced experts. Open procedures may also marginally impair the outlook for hearing reconstruction, but not overwhelmingly so if the middle ear environment is otherwise favorable. A newer third category of "hybrid" procedures has emerged that involves removal of the bony canal wall for optimized cholesteatoma dissection but then acts to restore natural anatomy by either restoring the canal wall or obliterating the mastoid and epitympanic spaces [56, 64, 65]. Published recidivism rates with most hybrid procedures are comparable to canal wall-down surgery, while hearing outcomes are generally superior. However, there is still some uncertainty about the long-term complication rates for some hybrid techniques. While these procedures seem to offer the "best of both worlds," they may be time-consuming and difficult to teach or learn.

With respect to surgical treatment of the cholesteatoma sac itself, either surgical excision or exteriorization may be used. Without question, complete removal of cholesteatoma is the best-case scenario and the goal, most often. Common sites where recurrent cholesteatoma is encountered due to incomplete removal are the sinus tympani, the oval window niche, the supratubal recess, the protympanum, and the epitympanum, whereas residual cholesteatoma within the mastoid itself is not common [60]. Improved microscopic and endoscopic visualization, skilled application of the high-speed drill, and usage of specialized instrumentation such as otologic lasers have been applied with the goal of reducing residual disease rates by facilitating complete cholesteatoma excision (Fig. 37.15). A sound approach to cholesteatoma resection generally requires sufficient access to remove the sac either as a single self-contained specimen, or in a deliberate segmented approach of delivering a series of complete specimens from given anatomic regions. Furthermore, planned surgical second-look or radiologic surveillance with diffusion-weighted MRI imaging may allow detection of residual cholesteatoma in the early postoperative period so that ultimate removal and cure may still be achieved [66]. Nevertheless, situations do still occur when the safety or feasibility of complete cholesteatoma removal is in doubt. Examples of this might be circumferential facial nerve involvement or a complex labyrinthine fistula. In such instances, disease is removed as far as is reasonable, and the affected sites are exteriorized in an open cavity so that they can be maintained by serial office debridement.

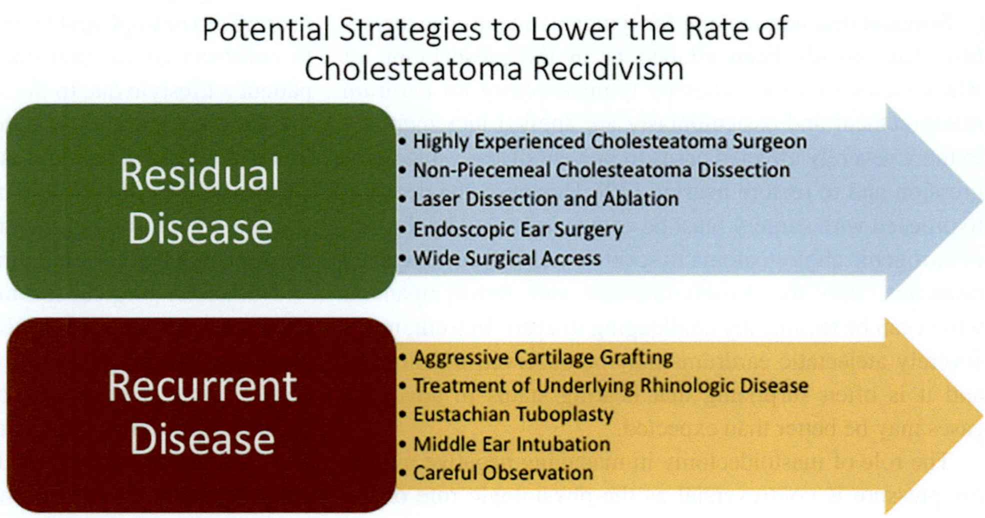

Fig. 37.15 Cholesteatoma recidivism: Recidivistic disease refers to either residual cholesteatoma that is incompletely treated during surgery or recurrent cholesteatoma that forms again *de novo* after past surgery. Potential strategies for lowering recidivism are shown

Special Situations

Systemic Disease

Occasionally, there will be clues that an underlying systemic condition is responsible for chronic ear disease; however, resistance to standard treatment usually triggers clinical suspicion. Patients with treatment-resistant disease require a comprehensive general medical workup. The differential diagnosis in these situations includes granulomatous diseases such as Sarcoidosis or one of the autoimmune vasculitides such as Churg-Strauss Syndrome, currently known as eosinophilic granulomatosis with polyangiitis (EGPA) or Granulomatosis with Polyangiitis (GPA, formerly Wegener's), which are covered elsewhere in this textbook. Laboratory workup for immunodeficiency, especially immunoglobulin subclass deficiency or HIV, is also considered. Other unusual pathologies to consider are an atypical pathogen, an underlying temporal bone neoplasm, or Langerhans Cell Histiocytosis; thus, a biopsy may be undertaken for tissue culture and histopathology.

Eosinophilic Otitis Media

Eosinophilic otitis media is characterized by chronic otitis media with effusion that is resistant to conventional treatment. It is typically bilateral and is often found in association with adult-onset bronchial asthma or nasal polyposis [67]. Clinical suspicion should be raised during myringotomy upon encountering extraordinarily viscous eosinophilic mucin that is difficult to suction. The underlying middle ear mucosa is thickened with eosinophil-rich granulation tissue. The cause of this condition is unknown; however, a significant number of these patients have patulous Eustachian tubes, driving speculation that the pathogenesis is related to aspiration of antigenic material into the middle ear, causing a localized eosinophilic inflammatory reaction. Definitive diagnosis must first rule out Churg-Strauss Syndrome and Hypereosinophilic Syndrome. This condition responds to high-dose systemic steroids, but optimal long-term management is uncertain. Tympanostomy tubes tend to be of little benefit as they promptly plug after placement. One notable characteristic of this condition is the high incidence of sensorineural hearing loss [68].

Myringitis

Sometimes the spectrum of chronic ear disease extends to the outer ear in the form of myringitis or otitis externa. Granular myringitis is a poorly understood condition wherein the epithelium of the tympanic membrane is replaced by granulation tissue and inflammatory cells, while the underlying lamina propria remains intact. This process can extend to involve the skin of the external auditory canal in a more diffuse form of canal wall epithelitis and otitis externa (Fig. 37.16). Myringitis is thought to be a common pathway of epithelial reaction to chronic irritation that is sufficient to cause a break through the epithelial basement membrane.

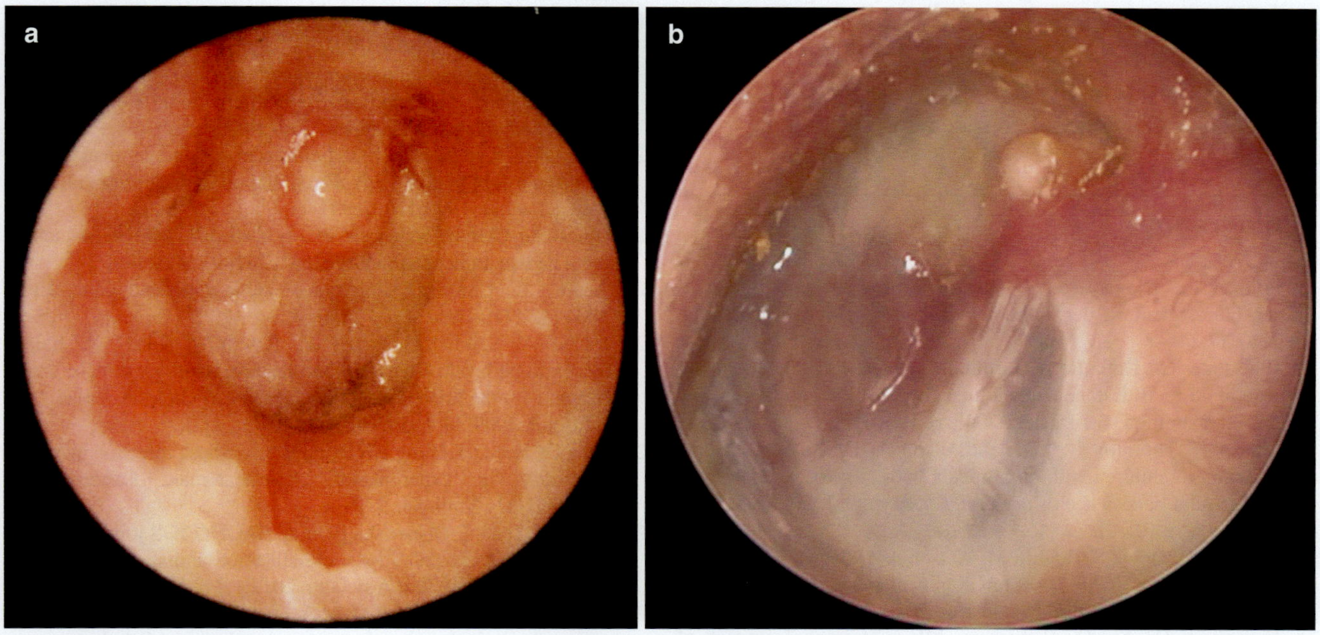

Fig. 37.16 Myringitis. (**a**) Granular myringitis and epithelitis of the right medial ear canal skin is often associated with retained debris, excessive moisture, and impaired epithelial migration. (**b**) Myringitis persisting after left lateral graft tympanoplasty may signify the need to resect or laser ablate unhealthy soft tissue including remnant eardrum and apply a small split skin graft

Common sources of irritation include long-term excessive exposure to moisture, infection, or retention of debris [69]. Normally the tympanic membrane and ear canal have a unique centrifugal epithelial migration pattern that works as a self-cleaning mechanism [70], and some cases of myringitis are hypothesized to occur as a result of this mechanism being disrupted. Ears that underwent tympanoplasty for large defects, especially when the malleus is absent, or the general condition of the remnant ear canal and eardrum skin is poor, may be at particular risk of acquiring this condition postoperatively. This is because the malleus functions as the epicenter of tympanic membrane re-epithelialization as a source of keratinocyte progenitor cells and the starting point for migration [71]; its absence in tympanoplasty is known to result in slower tympanic membrane healing and epithelialization, possible eardrum lateralization, as well as worse hearing outcomes. Treatment of myringitis is not standardized, but typically involves removing the offending source of irritation and application of medications that eliminate granulation tissue, namely corticosteroids and cauterizing agents. When medical therapy fails, surgical intervention may be required in the form of laser ablation, split skin grafting, or revision of tympanoplasty with resection of the affected segment of the eardrum.

Conclusions

Chronic ear disease is an umbrella term that encompasses a large array of pathologies that, in turn, comprise the majority of historical and contemporary otologic patient care. While debates still exist regarding the pathophysiology and management of chronic ear disease, it is important both for surgeons and patients to work, first and foremost, towards the goal of a safe ear. In this effort, both medical and surgical interventions are worthy of consideration.

Bibliography

1. Politzer A. Diagnose und Therapie der Ansammlung seröeser Flüessigkeit in der Trommelhöhle. Wien Med Wochenschr. 1867;17:244–7.
2. Bluestone C. Definitions, terminology, and classification. In: Rosenfeld R, Bluestone CD, editors. Evidence-based otitis media. 2nd ed. Hamilton: BC Decker; 2003. p. 120–35.
3. Coates H, Thornton R, Langlands J, et al. The role of chronic infection in children with otitis media with effusion: evidence for intracellular persistence of bacteria. Otolaryngol Head Neck Surg. 2008;138(6):778–81.
4. Preciado D, Goyal S, Rahimi M, Watson AM, Brown KJ, Hathout Y, Rose MC. MUC5B Is the predominant mucin glycoprotein in chronic otitis media fluid. Pediatr Res. 2010;68(3):231–6.
5. Verhoeven D, Xu Q, Pichichero ME. Differential impact of respiratory syncytial virus and parainfluenza virus on the frequency of acute otitis media is explained by lower adaptive and innate immune responses in otitis-prone children. Clin Infect Dis. 2014;59(3):376–83.
6. Khomtchouk KM, Kouhi A, Xia A, Bekale LA, Massa SM, Sweere JM, Pletzer D, Hancock RE, Bollyky PL, Santa Maria PL. A novel mouse model of chronic suppurative otitis media and its use in preclinical antibiotic evaluation. Sci Adv. 2020;6(33):eabc1828.
7. Santa Maria PL, Kaufman AC, Bacacao B, Thai A, Chen X, Xia A, Cao Z, Fouad A, Bekale LA. Topical therapy failure in chronic suppurative otitis media is due to persister cells in biofilms. Otol Neurotol. 2021;42(9):e1263–72.
8. Kaufman AC, Bacacao BS, Berkay B, Sharma D, Mishra A, O'Toole GA, Saunders JE, Xia A, Bekale LA, Santa Maria PL. Povidone-iodine fails to eradicate chronic suppurative otitis media and demonstrates ototoxic risk in mice. Otol Neurotol. 2022;43(10):e1121–8.
9. Thai A, Aaron KA, Kaufman AC, Santa Maria PL. Long-term health utilization and outcomes in chronic suppurative otitis media. Otolaryngol Head Neck Surg. 2022;167(2):341–9.
10. Nadol J. The chronic draining ear. Curr Ther Otolaryngol Head Neck Surg. 1987;18:18–22.
11. Weiss JP, Antonelli PJ, Dirain CO. Microbiome analysis of cholesteatoma by gene sequencing. Otol Neurotol. 2019;40(9):1186–93.
12. Bellucci R. Selection of cases and classification of tympanoplasty. Otolaryngol Clin N Am. 1989;22(5):911–26.
13. Austin DF. Reporting results in tympanoplasty. Am J Otol. 1985;6(1):85–8.
14. Kartush JM. Ossicular chain reconstruction. Capitulum to malleus. Otolaryngol Clin N Am. 1994;27(4):689–715.
15. Gluth MB, Moore PC, Dornhoffer JL. Method and reproducibility of a standardized ossiculoplasty technique. Otol Neurotol. 2012;33(7):1207–12.
16. Marchioni D, Alicandri-Ciufelli M, Molteni G, Artioli FL, Genovese E, Presutti L. Selective epitympanic dysventilation syndrome. Laryngoscope. 2010;120(5):1028–33.
17. Jackler RK, Santa Maria PL, Varsak YK, Nguyen A, Blevins NH. A new theory on the pathogenesis of acquired cholesteatoma: mucosal traction. Laryngoscope. 2015;125 Suppl 4:S1–S14.
18. Sade J, Berco E. Atelectasis and secretory otitis media. Ann Otol Rhinol Laryngol. 1976;85(2 Suppl 25 Pt 2):66–72.
19. Tos M, Poulsen G. Attic retractions following secretory otitis. Acta Otolaryngol. 1980;89(5–6):479–86.
20. Black B. The collapsed pars tensa: surgical classification and management. Paper presented at: Sixth International Conference on Cholesteatoma and Ear Surgery. 2001; Marseille.
21. Fliss DM, Dagan R, Houri Z, Leiberman A. Medical management of chronic suppurative otitis media without cholesteatoma in children. J Pediatr. 1990;116(6):991–6.
22. Bluestone CD. Pathogenesis of otitis media: role of eustachian tube. Pediatr Infect Dis J. 1996;15(4):281–91.
23. Acuin J. Chronic suppurative otitis media. Clin Evid. 2004;(12):710–29.
24. Juhasz A, Sziklai I, Rakosy Z, Ecsedi S, Adany R, Balazs M. Elevated level of tenascin and matrix metalloproteinase 9 correlates with the bone destruction capacity of cholesteatomas. Otol Neurotol. 2009;30(4):559–65.
25. Jung JY, Lee DH, Wang EW, et al. P. aeruginosa infection increases morbidity in experimental cholesteatomas. Laryngoscope. 2011;121(11):2449–54.
26. Yung M, Tono T, Olszewska E, et al. EAONO/JOS joint consensus statements on the definitions, classification and staging of middle ear cholesteatoma. J Int Adv Otol. 2017;13(1):1–8.
27. Persaud R, Hajioff D, Trinidade A, et al. Evidence-based review of aetiopathogenic theories of congenital and acquired cholesteatoma. J Laryngol Otol. 2007;121(11):1013–9.

28. Black B, Gutteridge I. Acquired cholesteatoma: classification and outcomes. Otol Neurotol. 2011;32(6):992–5.
29. Jackler RK. The surgical anatomy of cholesteatoma. Otolaryngol Clin N Am. 1989;22(5):883–96.
30. Goycoolea MV, Hueb MM, Muchow D, Paparella MM. The theory of the trigger, the bridge and the transmigration in the pathogenesis of acquired cholesteatoma. Acta Otolaryngol. 1999;119(2):244–8.
31. Chu FW, Jackler RK. Anterior epitympanic cholesteatoma with facial paralysis: a characteristic growth pattern. Laryngoscope. 1988;98(3):274–9.
32. Ahn JH, Kim MN, Suk YA, Moon BJ. Preoperative, intraoperative, and postoperative results of bacterial culture from patients with chronic suppurative otitis media. Otol Neurotol. 2012;33(1):54–9.
33. Yeo SG, Park DC, Hong SM, Cha CI, Kim MG. Bacteriology of chronic suppurative otitis media—a multicenter study. Acta Otolaryngol. 2007;127(10):1062–7.
34. Choi HG, Park KH, Park SN, Jun BC, Lee DH, Yeo SW. The appropriate medical management of methicillin-resistant Staphylococcus aureus in chronic suppurative otitis media. Acta Otolaryngol. 2010;130(1):42–6.
35. Shim HJ, Park CH, Kim MG, Lee SK, Yeo SG. A pre- and postoperative bacteriological study of chronic suppurative otitis media. Infection. 2010;38(6):447–52.
36. Gluth MB, Tan BY, Santa Maria PL, Atlas MD. Unique microbiology of chronically unstable canal wall down tympanomastoid cavities: considerations for surgical revision. J Laryngol Otol. 2013;127(5):458–62.
37. Chang J, Lee SH, Choi J, Im GJ, Jung HH. Nasopharynx as a microbiologic reservoir in chronic suppurative otitis media: preliminary study. Clin Exp Otorhinolaryngol. 2011;4(3):122–5.
38. Weckwerth PH, de Magalhaes Lopes CA, Duarte MA, et al. Chronic suppurative otitis media in cleft palate: microorganism etiology and susceptibilities. Cleft Palate Craniofac J. 2009;46(5):461–7.
39. Saunders JE, Raju RP, Boone JL, Hales NW, Berryhill WE. Antibiotic resistance and otomycosis in the draining ear: culture results by diagnosis. Am J Otolaryngol. 2011;32(6):470–6.
40. Vaamonde P, Castro C, Garcia-Soto N, Labella T, Lozano A. Tuberculous otitis media: a significant diagnostic challenge. Otolaryngol Head Neck Surg. 2004;130(6):759–66.
41. Cho YS, Lee HS, Kim SW, et al. Tuberculous otitis media: a clinical and radiologic analysis of 52 patients. Laryngoscope. 2006;116(6):921–7.
42. Chole RA, Faddis BT. Evidence for microbial biofilms in cholesteatomas. Arch Otolaryngol Head Neck Surg. 2002;128(10):1129–33.
43. Bjarnsholt T. The role of bacterial biofilms in chronic infections. APMIS Suppl. 2013;(136):1–51.
44. Post JC, Hiller NL, Nistico L, Stoodley P, Ehrlich GD. The role of biofilms in otolaryngologic infections: update 2007. Curr Opin Otolaryngol Head Neck Surg. 2007;15(5):347–51.
45. Wang EW, Agostini G, Olomu O, Runco D, Jung JY, Chole RA. Gentian violet and ferric ammonium citrate disrupt Pseudomonas aeruginosa biofilms. Laryngoscope. 2008;118(11):2050–6.
46. Zenga J, Gagnon PM, Vogel J, Chole RA. Biofilm formation by otopathogenic strains of Pseudomonas aeruginosa is not consistently inhibited by ethylenediaminetetraacetic acid. Otol Neurotol. 2012;33(6):1007–12.
47. Nadol JB Jr. Causes of failure of mastoidectomy for chronic otitis media. Laryngoscope. 1985;95(4):410–3.
48. Albu S, Trabalzini F, Amadori M. Usefulness of cortical mastoidectomy in myringoplasty. Otol Neurotol. 2012;33(4):604–9.
49. Eliades SJ, Limb CJ. The role of mastoidectomy in outcomes following tympanic membrane repair: a review. Laryngoscope. 2013;123(7):1787–802.
50. Gluth MB, McDonald DR, Weaver AL, Bauch CD, Beatty CW, Orvidas LJ. Management of eustachian tube dysfunction with nasal steroid spray: a prospective, randomized, placebo-controlled trial. Arch Otolaryngol Head Neck Surg. 2011;137(5):449–55.
51. Jensen JH, Leth N, Bonding P. Topical application of decongestant in dysfunction of the Eustachian tube: a randomized, double-blind, placebo-controlled trial. Clin Otolaryngol Allied Sci. 1990;15(3):197–201.
52. van Heerbeek N, Ingels KJ, Zielhuis GA. No effect of a nasal decongestant on eustachian tube function in children with ventilation tubes. Laryngoscope. 2002;112(6):1115–8.
53. Park K. Otitis media and tonsils—role of adenoidectomy in the treatment of chronic otitis media with effusion. Adv Otorhinolaryngol. 2011;72:160–3.
54. Silvola J, Kivekas I, Poe DS. Balloon dilation of the cartilaginous portion of the eustachian tube. Otolaryngol Head Neck Surg. 2014;151(1):125–30.
55. Takahashi H, Honjo I, Naito Y, et al. Gas exchange function through the mastoid mucosa in ears after surgery. Laryngoscope. 1997;107(8):1117–21.
56. Gantz BJ, Wilkinson EP, Hansen MR. Canal wall reconstruction tympanomastoidectomy with mastoid obliteration. Laryngoscope. 2005;115(10):1734–40.
57. Doyle WJ. The mastoid as a functional rate-limiter of middle ear pressure change. Int J Pediatr Otorhinolaryngol. 2007;71(3):393–402.
58. Cinamon U, Sade J. Mastoid and tympanic membrane as pressure buffers: a quantitative study in a middle ear cleft model. Otol Neurotol. 2003;24(6):839–42.
59. Dornhoffer JL, Friedman AB, Gluth MB. Management of acquired cholesteatoma in the pediatric population. Curr Opin Otolaryngol Head Neck Surg. 2013;21(5):440–5.
60. Wilson KF, London NR, Shelton C. Tympanoplasty with intact canal wall mastoidectomy for cholesteatoma: long-term hearing outcomes. Laryngoscope. 2013;123(12):3168–71.
61. Sade J, Weinberg J, Berco E, Brown M, Halevy A. The marsupialized (radical) mastoid. J Laryngol Otol. 1982;96(10):869–75.
62. Youngs R. The histopathology of mastoidectomy cavities, with particular reference to persistent disease leading to chronic otorrhoea. Clin Otolaryngol Allied Sci. 1992;17(6):505–10.
63. Gluth MB, Metrailer AM, Dornhoffer JL, Moore PC. Patterns of failure in canal wall down mastoidectomy cavity instability. Otol Neurotol. 2012;33(6):998–1001.
64. Dornhoffer JL. Retrograde mastoidectomy with canal wall reconstruction: a follow-up report. Otol Neurotol. 2004;25(5):653–60.
65. Takahashi H, Iwanaga T, Kaieda S, et al. Mastoid obliteration combined with soft-wall reconstruction of posterior ear canal. Eur Arch Otorhinolaryngol. 2007;264(8):867–71.
66. Li PM, Linos E, Gurgel RK, Fischbein NJ, Blevins NH. Evaluating the utility of non-echo-planar diffusion-weighted imaging in the preoperative evaluation of cholesteatoma: a meta-analysis. Laryngoscope. 2013;123(5):1247–50.
67. Iino Y, Tomioka-Matsutani S, Matsubara A, Nakagawa T, Nonaka M. Diagnostic criteria of eosinophilic otitis media, a newly recognized middle ear disease. Auris Nasus Larynx. 2011;38(4):456–61.
68. Iino Y, Usubuchi H, Kodama K, Takizawa K, Kanazawa T, Ohta Y. Bone conduction hearing level in patients with eosinophilic otitis media associated with bronchial asthma. Otol Neurotol. 2008;29(7):949–52.
69. Wolf M, Primov-Fever A, Barshack I, Polack-Charcon S, Kronenberg J. Granular myringitis: incidence and clinical characteristics. Otol Neurotol. 2006;27(8):1094–7.
70. Litton WB. Epithelial migration over tympanic membrane and external canal. Arch Otolaryngol. 1963;77:254–7.
71. Knutsson J, von Unge M, Rask-Andersen H. Localization of progenitor/stem cells in the human tympanic membrane. Audiol Neurootol. 2011;16(4):263–9.

Myringoplasty Techniques

38

Matthew L. Bush, Beth N. McNulty, and Kenneth C. Iverson

Introduction

Perforations of the tympanic membrane can be repaired surgically through either *myringoplasty* or *tympanoplasty*. Myringoplasty refers to the repair of a tympanic membrane perforation, which is limited to the membrane surface. This technique typically involves placing graft materials either on the outer surface of the tympanic membrane or within the perforation without elevating the annulus of the tympanic membrane. This procedure can be performed in either an operating room or an ambulatory clinic setting, depending on the technique. Conversely, tympanoplasty refers to elevation of the annulus and may involve removal of pathologic tissue from the middle ear, repair of the ossicular chain, and/or repair of a tympanic membrane perforation. Tympanoplasty will be described in separate chapters.

History of Tympanic Membrane and Middle Ear Surgery

Descriptions of methods to repair the tympanic membrane date back to the sixteenth century [1]. Banzer described the first myringoplasty using a ring-shaped piece of elkhorn covered in pig's bladder in 1640 [2]. Berthold introduced the term myringoplasty in his repair of a tympanic membrane with a full-thickness skin graft in 1878 [3]. The term tympanoplasty was coined in 1953 by Wullstein to describe surgical techniques for reconstruction of the middle-ear hearing mechanism that had been impaired or destroyed by chronic ear disease [4]. The same year Zöllner reported on surgical techniques for improving the sound conduction mechanism of the middle ear following surgery for chronic ear disease [5]. One year earlier Wullstein had described an operation for repairing tympanic membrane perforations with split-thickness skin grafts [6]. Another major contribution of these two otologists was the introduction of the operating microscope in performing otologic surgery, which improved their results significantly.

Repair of the tympanic membrane can be considered the final step in the surgical conquest of conductive hearing loss and represents the culmination of over 100 years of evolution of surgical procedures on the middle ear to improve hearing. The first of these procedures was the stapes mobilization of Kessel in 1878, soon followed by Berthold's plastic repair of a perforated tympanic membrane in the same year and Kiesselbach's attempt in 1883 to correct a congenital meatal atresia. These very eventful years might well have been the beginning of a fruitful development of operations for conductive hearing loss, for the mechanics of the middle ear had been defined clearly by Helmholtz shortly before, in 1868. However, despite the early successes with stapes mobilization reported by Boucheron in 1888 and Miot in 1890, the new surgery for deafness declined and by the end of the nineteenth century died out, as determined opposition by the leaders in otology had arisen against all attempts to improve hearing by operations on the middle ear.

The strong opposition to surgery for deafness was reflected in the standard texts of otology and otologic surgery, which scarcely mentioned, or mentioned only to condemn, such operations. For example, Kerrison's 627-page *Diseases of the Ear*, published in 1930, devoted less than a single page to "Surgical Measures for Relief of Deafness,"

M. L. Bush (✉)
Department of Otolaryngology—Head and Neck Surgery, University of Kentucky Medical Center, Lexington, KY, USA
e-mail: matthew.bush@uky.edu

B. N. McNulty
Division of Otology, Neurotology, and Cranial Base Surgery, Department of Otolaryngology—Head and Neck Surgery, University of Kentucky Medical Center, Lexington, KY, USA
e-mail: beth.mcnulty@uky.edu

K. C. Iverson
Division of Pediatric Otolaryngology, Department of Otolaryngology—Head and Neck Surgery, University of Kentucky Medical Center, Lexington, KY, USA
e-mail: Kenneth.iverson@uky.edu

A. D. Sweeney et al. (eds.), *Haynes-Glasscock-Shambaugh Surgery of the Ear*, https://doi.org/10.1007/978-3-032-18264-7_38

concluding that: "These operations, mentioned for their place in otological history, are quite obsolete today." It is even more surprising that Sir Charles Ballance, in his two-volume text, fails to mention any sort of operation to improve hearing.

Reasons for the opposition to reconstructive surgery of the middle ear were no doubt the lack of surgical microscopes, imperfect sterilization techniques, and the absence of protective antibiotics, possibly resulting in infections and other iatrogenic injuries. There were few reports of serious infections following the early operations, but one can surmise that some very unfortunate unreported results contributed to the opposition. An additional reason for the skepticism about operations to improve hearing may have been the lack of audiometers for quantitative measurements of hearing before and after surgery.

Probably the greatest reason for the lack of interest in reconstructive operations on the ear was the intense preoccupation of the otologists of those days with infections of the ear and their complications. It is interesting that Schwartze [7] described the simple mastoid operation just 3 years before Kessel mobilized the stapes, and Kuster [8], Zaufal [9], and Stacke [10] described the radical mastoidectomy at exactly the time that Boucheron and Miot were reporting successes with stapes mobilization. It is evident that the climate of otologic thought was favorable toward procedures to control infection and quite unfavorable toward operations on the ear to improve hearing.

The revival of interest in the surgery of hearing loss began when Holmgren [11], with considerable courage in the face of the concerted opposition, began his long series of operations on the labyrinth for otosclerosis, demonstrating that, with modern methods of aseptic technique, the non-infected mastoid process and labyrinth could, after all, be opened safely. The surgical application of the operating microscope, first by Nylen [12] in 1921 as a monocular instrument, and then by Holmgren, who introduced the binocular operating microscope in 1922, was an important advance destined to play an increasing role in the perfection of fenestration, stapes operations, and tympanoplasty. Sourdille's [13] ingenious and successful tympanolabyrinthopexy for otosclerosis added to the reviving interest in surgery for deafness.

The real turning point in the reorientation of otologic surgery away from operations for infection toward reconstruction of the hearing mechanism occurred when Lempert [14] combined Sourdille's several-stage operation into a more practical one-stage fenestration operation. At this time, sulfonamide therapy of acute otitis media and otitic complications had begun to lessen the urgency and frequency of operations for acute mastoiditis. Lempert emphasized careful aseptic technique in the intra- and postoperative periods. This shift, along with the later addition to sulfonamides of prophylactic penicillin, rendered postoperative infections rare. Lempert taught his operation to otologists from all parts of the world, and the number of patients successfully treated by Lempert and his pupils increased to hundreds and then thousands. Thanks to Lempert, the climate of otologic thought finally became favorable toward surgery for hearing loss. This evolution led, first, to the successful operations for congenital meatal atresia in 1947 by Patte [15] and Ombredanne [16], and finally, to the revival of stapes mobilization by Rosen in 1953 [17].

It is a remarkable fact that, during all these years, clinicians and surgeons failed to clearly see the applications of new surgical techniques to the principles of the middle-ear sound-pressure transformer, as described by Helmholtz. Holmgren, Sourdille, and Lempert had no clear idea of how the fenestrated ear functioned and why the fenestration operation could not restore hearing to normal. Likewise, Pattee and Ombredanne failed to appreciate the need to restore sound-pressure transformation by placing the substitute tympanic membrane in contact with the mobile stapes.

The mechanics of the fenestrated ear remained obscure until Bekesy and Juers began to study the problem. Juers [18] in 1948 noted that the tympanic membrane of the fenestrated ear must be intact "to protect the round window somewhat from sound pressure." Two years later, Davis and Walsh [19] defined the residual conductive hearing loss after successful fenestration as being "due to loss of the impedance-matching mechanism of the tympanic membrane, ossicular chain and oval window." The two basic principles of tympanoplasty had now been defined; namely, sound protection for the round window and sound-pressure transformation for the oval window.

It is interesting and surprising that tympanoplasty techniques for chronic otitis media began in Germany rather than in the United States, where fenestration surgery had reached a high degree of maturity and perfection. In 1950, Moritz first described the use of pedicled flaps to construct a closed middle-ear cavity in cases of chronic suppuration, to provide sound shielding or protection for the round window in preparation for a later fenestration of the horizontal semicircular canal [20]. The principles of Moritz's procedure were immediately apparent. Zöllner in 1951, and Wullstein in 1952, began to report on similar operations to provide sound protection for the round window and to reconstruct sound-pressure transformation for the oval window. Early on, Wullstein advocated free skin transplants rather than the pedicled grafts used by Moritz, and Zöllner soon after changed from pedicled to free grafts as well [6, 21].

The subsequent development of tympanoplasty techniques has continued to evolve. Soon after the introduction of split-thickness grafts, it was realized that the accumulation of keratin debris and associated infections resulting in failures made their use impractical. Zöllner replaced free distant skin grafts with meatal skin, removed as free full-thickness grafts. Vein as grafting material was reported independently by Shea and Tabb in 1960 [22, 23]. Temporalis fascia was described by Heermann in 1961 and was introduced in the United States by Storrs in 1963 [24, 25]. Plastic prostheses for reconstruction of the ossicular chain were tried early on and abandoned by Zöllner and Wullstein; however, they continued to be used in the United States both for tympanoplasty and stapedectomy. Soon after, the tendency toward rejection and extrusion of the plastic prostheses used in tympanoplasties and stapedectomies became evident. Following these initial failures, it was soon realized that wire prostheses made of stainless steel, platinum, or tantalum were better tolerated in the middle ear. Ossicular repositioning was described by Hall and Rytzner in 1957 [26]. Homograft ossicles for reconstructing the ossicular chain in tympanoplasty became popular in the early 1960s [27]. Glasscock and House reported the first large series of homograft tympanic membrane procedures in 1968 [28]. Biocompatible ossicular prostheses such as total ossicular replacement prostheses (TORPs), acting as a columella from the tympanic membrane to the oval window, and partial ossicular replacement prostheses (PORPs), connecting the stapes head to the tympanic membrane, have been in everyday use during the past 25 years [29]. During the past 25 years, otologists have used numerous types of ossicular prostheses made of various alloplastic materials such as Plastipore®, Proplast®, polyethylenes, polytetrafluoroethylene, ceramics, Teflon®, titanium and hydroxylapatite. Ossicular chain reconstruction is discussed further in a different chapter.

Goals of Myringoplasty

The primary goal of myringoplasty is to achieve complete closure of a tympanic membrane perforation, which may lead to eradication and/or prevention of aural drainage along with improvement of conductive hearing loss related to the perforation. Additionally, the closure of a perforation may prevent the development of a secondary acquired cholesteatoma. This procedure may be performed in the setting of an acute or chronic perforation or may be performed concurrently with retained ventilation tube removal. Although up to 90% of acute tympanic membrane perforations heal spontaneously [30–32], there is evidence suggesting that myringoplasty may increase successful closure in acute perforations [33]. Myringoplasty following ventilation tube removal is also effective at improving the rate of closure [34, 35]. Although less effective than the gold standard of tympanoplasty, myringoplasty can successfully close chronic tympanic membrane perforations [33].

Preoperative Evaluation

Tympanic membrane perforation can result from a variety of different pathological conditions. Myringotomy with ventilation tube placement is one of the most common causes of a persistent perforation of the tympanic membrane [36]. Perforations may also occur as a complication of an acute otitis media. In this scenario, patients often describe intense otalgia followed by a relief of pressure and otorrhea, which correspond with the rupture of the tympanic membrane and the passage of middle ear contents through the perforation. Perforations may also occur after blunt trauma to the ear, such as what may occur directly from cotton-tipped applicator use in the ear canal or indirectly through pressure created by a slap to the external ear. Forceful water compression can cause a similar injury, which may occur when diving or waterskiing. Iatrogenic tympanic membrane perforations may occur during cerumen impaction removal via irrigation or instrumentation.

Elements of the history and physical exam have significant implications on the selected technique and potential outcome of repair of the tympanic membrane. While obtaining the history of patients with tympanic membrane perforation, attention should be directed toward the etiology and the duration of the perforation. Additionally, the presence of otorrhea [37, 38] and subjective hearing loss are also important elements in the history. Prior surgical history, including myringotomy and ventilation tube placement and any prior attempt to repair the perforation should be noted [39]. Other important medical and social history elements include a history of craniofacial abnormalities and/or a history of smoking [40]. During the physical exam of the patient, otomicroscopy should be utilized to inspect the tympanic membrane and assess the size and location of the perforation, along with the relationship of the perforation to the annulus (i.e., central versus marginal) [38]. Care should be taken to assess for squamous epithelial growth through the perforation and signs of cholesteatoma. The status of the middle ear mucosa [41] and the presence of drainage through the perforation should be assessed. Evaluation of the contralateral ear in regard to perforation, retraction or effusion is also important as these factors can influence the outcomes of tympanic membrane repair [42–45]. Tuning fork and comprehensive audiometry are also critical in pre-operative assessment of these patients. Patients with chronic otorrhea may benefit from medical management with antibiotic- and steroid-containing topical drops to decrease inflammation and infection and maximize the potential for successful closure.

Indications for Myringoplasty

Two primary clinical scenarios may direct a clinician toward myringoplasty. Patients who have chronically retained tympanostomy ventilation tubes present for 2 or more years and who have had no episodes of otitis media during the preceding 12 months are eligible for concurrent myringoplasty at the time of ear tube removal [33]. Patients with chronic tympanic membrane perforations (>8 weeks in duration) that are less than 25% of the tympanic membrane perforation and central in location are also candidates for myringoplasty [33]. It may also be performed for patients with residual perforations following tympanoplasty [46].

Contraindications for Myringoplasty

Advances in surgical technique and grafting materials are expanding the role of myringoplasty, which will be further discussed in this chapter. The classic contraindications for myringoplasty include the presence of middle ear cholesteatoma, pathological conditions extending into the mastoid, marginal perforations involving the annulus, severe to profound sensorineural hearing loss in the contralateral ear, poor Eustachian tube function with middle ear atelectasis in the contralateral ear, and chronic otorrhea. The presence of significant soft tissue or bony stenosis of the external auditory canal is a relative contraindication for myringoplasty since the surgical approach is typically transcanal.

Principles Guiding Myringoplasty Technique

Kartush describes three guiding principles for office repair of perforations [47]. First, the edges of the perforation must be everted and deepithelialized. Second, chemical and mechanical irritants create an inflammatory response, which promotes epithelial proliferation. Third, material laid over or within the perforation will act as a scaffold to support epithelial migration. Myringoplasty may be performed in the outpatient clinic setting in an agreeable patient who meets the appropriate criteria. Santa Maria and Oghalai present a clinical algorithm for considering office-based myringoplasty [48]. After informed consent is obtained, the patient is placed in the supine position and the operating microscope is used to inspect the external auditory canal. Cerumen is debrided as necessary. A four-quadrant canal injection with topical anesthesia is next performed. The edges of the perforation are inspected, and a rim of tissue is removed to freshen the edges. Performing a series of small puncture holes with a Rosen needle or a sharp straight pick circumferentially around the perforation may facilitate this. This rim of tissue is gently separated from the remainder of the tympanic membrane using caution to avoid significantly enlarging the perforation. A cup forceps can then be used to remove this rim of tissue. There are various methods for inducing an inflammatory/epithelial growth response within the perforation, along with the use of multiple types of graft materials that will be discussed.

Surgical Technique

Cauterization

Chemical cauterization of the tissue within the lumen of the perforation may stimulate epithelial growth. Trichloroacetic (TCA) acid cauterization has been used for many decades, but more recently, this cautery technique was combined with a cotton pledget soaked in Euthymol otic (described as a mix of eucalyptol, methylsalicylate, menthol, thymol, oil of orange, sodium borate, boric acid, Ethyl alcohol 95% and sterile water) placed over the perforation with a reported perforation closure rate of 84% [49]. Multiple cauterizations may be required with this technique. Similarly, silver nitrate cauterization may be applied to the margins of a perforation to promote healing [50]. This acts to de-epithelialize the edges of the perforation and stimulate an inflammatory cascade. This generally requires reapplication of cautery with debridement every 2 weeks and may take up to a year for successful closure [50]. Both of these cautery methods may utilize a synthetic patch to cover the perforation.

Paper Patch and Synthetic Material Myringoplasty

Foreign materials have been used to cover perforations since the nineteenth century, starting with Toynbee's use of a rubber disk in 1857. This technique has a closure rate of about 43–67% [51–54]. In a cohort of 43 subjects with chronic perforations Park et al. found that the only predictor of treatment outcome was perforation size and suggested that a paper patch be first line for perforations smaller than 5% of the total surface area of the tympanic membrane [55]. This technique involves debriding the perforation edges as described above with or without cauterization of the tissue rimming the perforation. A small paper patch that is slightly larger than the perforation and overlaps the perforation is then applied to the lateral surface of the tympanic membrane to act as a scaffold for the regenerating epithelium. The material used is often either cigarette or filter paper. A commercially available paper hole punch may be used for sizing the patch. One may consider applying Mastisol® (Eloquest Healthcare) or iodine solution to the patch to secure its location [52]. Synthetic materials, such as a silicone patch, may also be used. This patch is made of very soft silicone in the shape of a sealed tympanostomy tube and is available in 3, 5, and 7 mm sizes, which may be trimmed [47]. In general, cauterization and patching techniques are not likely to be successful in perforations larger than 25% of the total surface area of the tympanic membrane. The patient is typically seen at weekly intervals for recauterization and patch refreshing until the perforation is closed.

Fat Graft Myringoplasty

Ringenberg was the first to use autologous fat as a plug placed within a tympanic membrane perforation in 1962 [56]. The fat plug technique is accepted as a good alternative for smaller perforations, with a closure rate of 80–90% [56–58]. Fat may be harvested at the posterior lobule or a few millimeters posterior to the postauricular crease. The incision needs to be only a few millimeters in length. If the posterior lobule is used as the harvest site, close attention must be paid not to interfere with a piercing site if present. An obvious advantage of the lobule or postauricular crease is the proximity to the surgical field [56]. The amount of adipose tissue necessary will depend on the size of the perforation, but generally a small piece is all that is necessary. It is important to be sure that no epidermis is included in the harvested tissue. Once harvested, the fat graft is kept in saline until the surgeon is prepared to place the graft. It may be sized slightly larger than the perforation and be loaded onto a Rosen needle or alligator forceps. It is then placed to span the perforation in a dumbbell conformation. A small patch is often placed over the fat, which may be a piece of Gelfilm® (Pfizer), small pieces of antibiotic-soaked Gelfoam® (Pfizer), or a synthetic patch. The reported rate of successful tympanic membrane closure with this technique has been reported as high as 87% in small perforations (3 mm or less) [52]. Recently, a combination of a fat graft with hyaluronic acid has been described to treat small to subtotal perforations with a closure rate of 81% [59]. The addition of hyaluronic acid to the fat graft is hypothesized to promote an environment within the perforation that would facilitate epithelialization.

Gelfoam Myringoplasty

While first reported in 1995, Gelfoam® plugging after tympanostomy tube extrusion has become a popular method of myringoplasty since no incisions are necessary [35, 60]. Although the use of Gelfoam® in the middle ear has been reported to be associated with increased fibrosis in rats and dogs [61, 62], it is has been used as the standard stabilizing grafting material in middle ear surgical procedures in most institutions. In 2011, Niklasson and Tano reported a closure rate of 83% in 17 patients with chronic perforations (greater than 1 year) that were less than 4 mm in size [63]. Hekkenberg reported a perforation closure rate of 95.5% with the use of a Gelfoam® graft at the time of tympanostomy tube removal compared to a closure rate of 89.7% in tube removal procedures with no Gelfoam [35]. This technique is demonstrated during a tympanostomy tube removal in Figs. 38.1, 38.2, and 38.3.

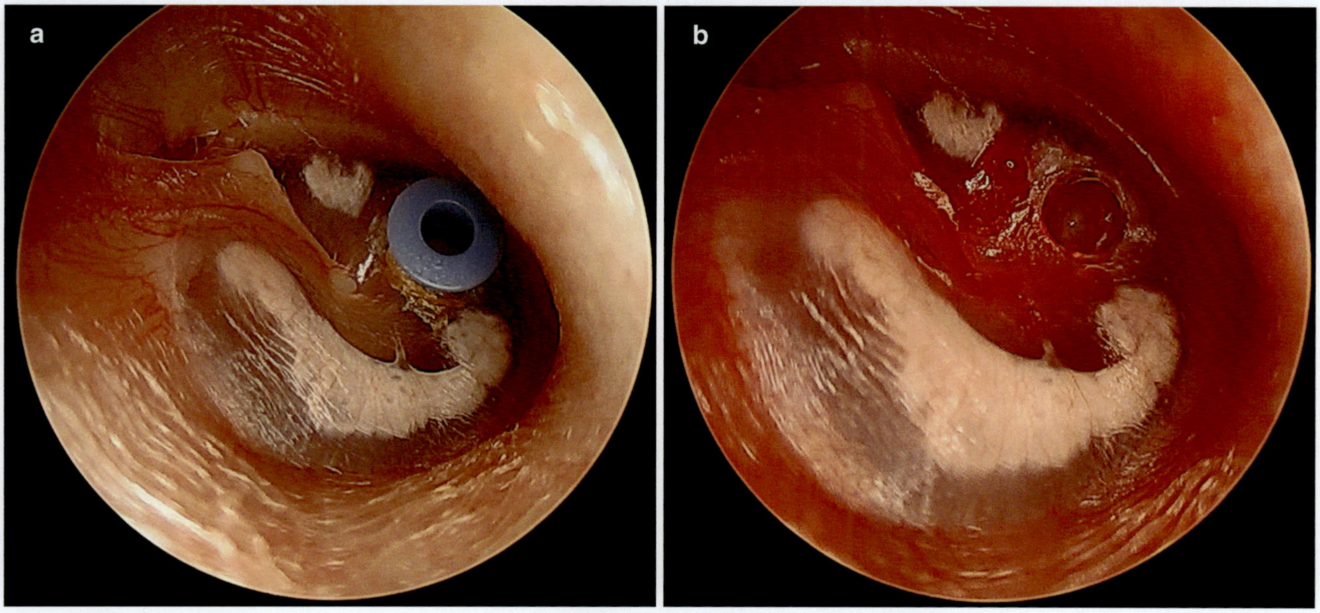

Fig. 38.1 Initially, the tympanostomy tube is visualized (**a**) and carefully removed with alligator forceps (**b**)

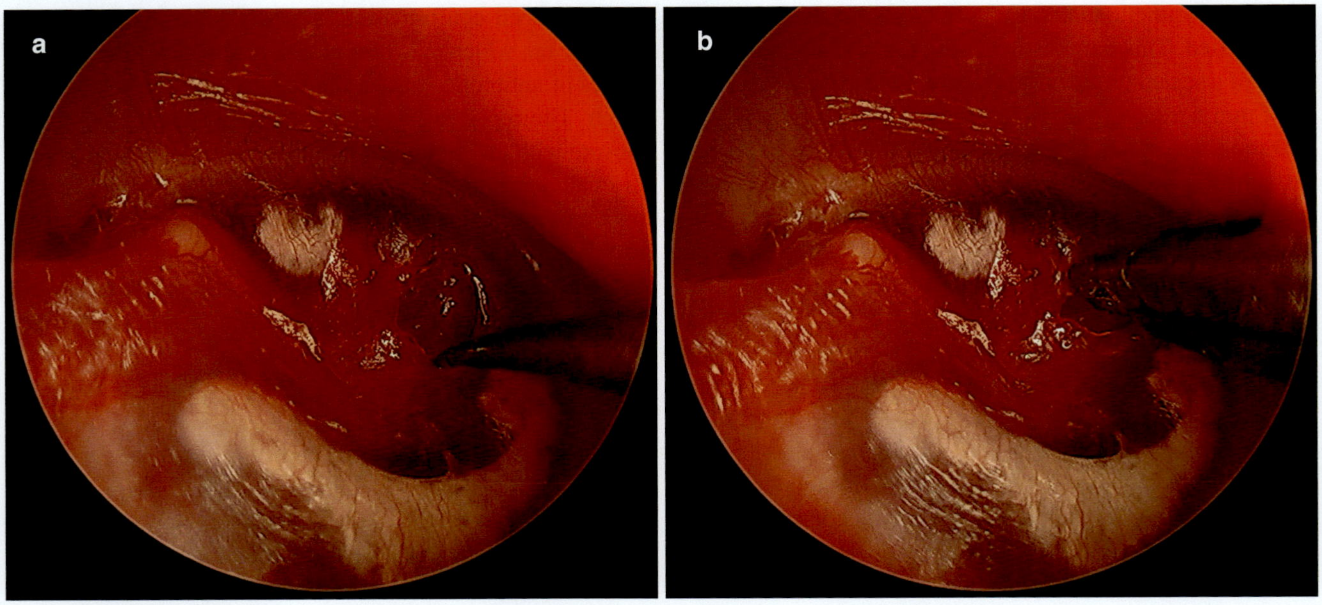

Fig. 38.2 The rim of the perforation is separated with a Rosen needle (**a**) and a cup forceps is used to remove the tissue (**b**)

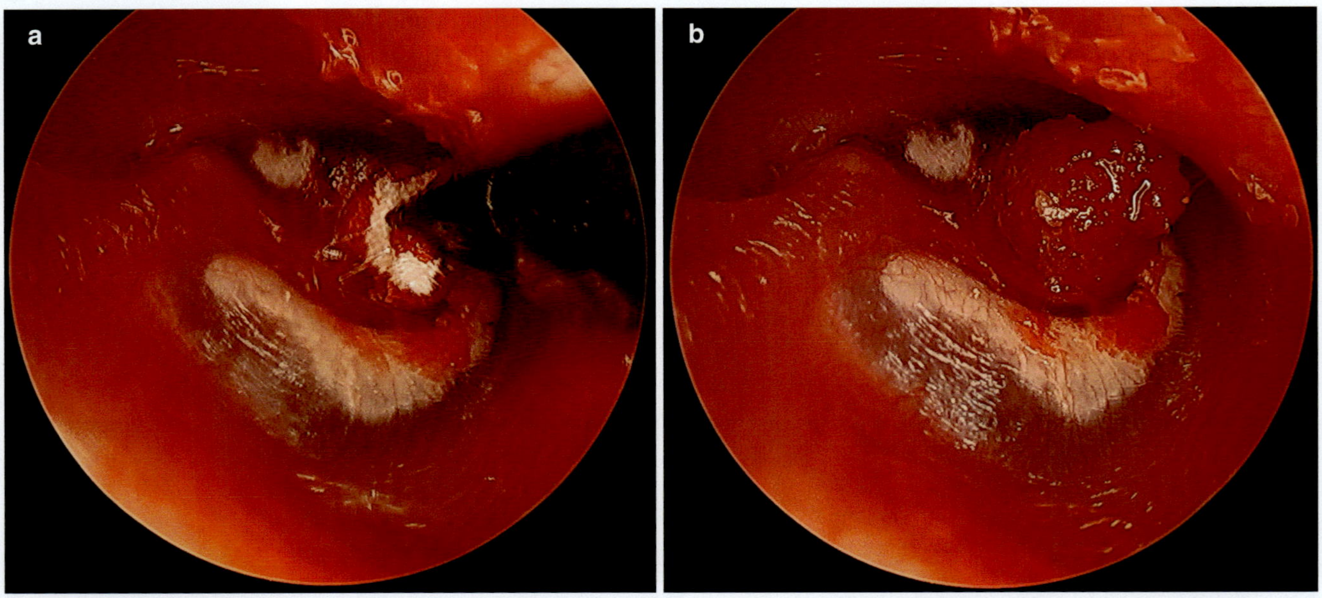

Fig. 38.3 Gelfoam® (either dry or moistened with saline or antibiotic solution) is gently packed into the perforation (**a**), resulting in a dumbbell configuration with excess extending laterally to the perforation (**b**)

Cartilage Myringoplasty

The use of cartilage for transcanal myringoplasty was initially described by Eavey in 1998 for small perforations with a 100% closure rate in 11 patients [64]. Since then, this technique has been widely used in perforations of all sizes [65, 66]. This technique involves harvesting a tragal cartilage graft and fashioning it into a "butterfly" shaped interlay graft that is 2 mm larger than the perforation. The graft is placed within the perforation so that the edge of the tympanic membrane perforation is within a groove between the two wings of the graft. This method has a reported perforation closure rate of greater than 90% with a significant improvement in hearing [64–66].

Endoscopic Myringoplasty

Once experimental, endoscopic tympanoplasty has become an accepted alternative in the management of tympanic membrane perforations [67]. While the success rate for microscopic myringoplasty is high, similar success rates of 80–100% are now reported for endoscopic myringoplasty [67–69]. An advantage of the endoscope is the wide field of view. A 4-mm angled endoscope allows the surgeon to see around anatomical obstructions, thus limiting the necessary surgical exposure. This may provide an advantage over the microscope in far anterior perforations or cases in which there is a prominent anterior bony overhang, allowing for a transcanal repair and thus avoiding a postauricular incision [70]. The gained visualization may also allow for a true myringoplasty, alleviating the need for raising a tympanomeatal flap or performing a canalplasty.

The Use of Growth Factors in Myringoplasty

In spite of the high rate of spontaneous closure of acute tympanic membrane perforations and successful closure rates from myringoplasty and/or tympanoplasty, there is a subset of patients that have treatment refractory tympanic membrane perforations. Additionally, there is a need to develop low-cost, nonsurgical, or at least minimally invasive options for tympanic membrane perforations [71]. Research within the field of tissue engineering proposes that healing of chronic wounds requires cells, scaffolds, and regulatory factors [72]. There is evidence that the use of growth factors may promote epithelialization and healing of tympanic membrane perforations. Kanemaru reported 96% successful closure of small and large chronic tympanic membrane perforations with the application of gelatin sponge infused with basic fibroblast growth factor [73]. Other researchers have investigated the role of epidermal growth factor to treat perforations in an animal model with promising results [74, 75]. Further work in a mouse model using heparin-binding epidermal growth factor demonstrates not only regeneration of the tympanic membrane but also the return of membrane vibratory properties similar to those of unperforated tympanic membranes [76].

Postoperative Management

Standard postoperative otology instructions are used, including the avoidance of nose blowing and sneezing and dry ear precautions. Patients undergoing myringoplasty do not typically require oral antibiotics or narcotic pain medications. Antibiotic otologic drops may be prescribed for 1 week postoperatively. The patient is evaluated 7–10 days after the surgery to assess graft integrity. A postoperative audiogram is obtained 8–12 weeks after surgery.

Complications

There is a low rate of complications with myringoplasty. The greatest risk is graft failure with persistent perforation. Infection after myringoplasty has been reported as high as 4.3% [46]. The risk of infection can be minimized with the use of sterile operative technique, postoperative antibiotic otologic drops, and the use of antibiotic ointment applied to the harvest site at the time of surgery. Infection may occur in the form of otitis media, otitis externa or a postoperative graft harvest site wound infection. In the case of otitis media, this may lead to graft failure. The chorda tympani nerve could be injured as it traverses the middle ear, resulting in taste disturbance, although this risk is low with a reported rate of 0.5%. Facial Nerve injury is very unlikely since there is no flap elevation or middle ear dissection. If lidocaine is used as the local anesthetic and it is allowed to enter the middle ear space, there is a risk for a temporary paralysis of a dehiscent facial nerve at the tympanic segment [46]. Vestibular symptoms can also be seen in these cases, which are generally self-limited. Tinnitus (1.2%) has also been described [46]. Hearing may be decreased during the initial postoperative period secondary to middle ear packing, hemotympanum, or effusion. This decrease generally improves over the course of 6–8 weeks. More severe forms of hearing loss could occur if the ossicular chain is traumatized.

Outcomes

Multiple factors may affect myringoplasty outcomes. A recent large study from Sweden examined a national health registry and reported the results on 3775 procedures described as underlay tympanoplasty and fat-graft myringoplasty [46]. When comparing techniques for closure of tympanic membrane perforations, underlay tympanoplasty had a higher closure rate (89%) compared with fat-graft myringoplasty (82%). Patients undergoing a reoperation or experiencing a postoperative infection had significantly lower odds of successful closure. In a study by Sckolnick et al., factors affecting myringoplasty outcomes were assessed [33]. This study found that patients undergoing myringoplasty for traumatic perforations or following myringotomy or myringotomy with tube placement had a greater than 90% closure rate compared with myringoplasty for chronic perforation, which had a 60% closure rate. There was also evidence suggesting that perforation closure was lower in patients with Down syndrome. The duration of time the retained tube was present also had a significant effect on the outcomes, with the odds of perforation closure decreasing by 15% for each year the tube is present. Regarding tympanostomy tube factors, those with multiple tubes placed had poorer outcomes than those with a single set of tubes and patients with t-tubes had poorer outcomes than those with grommet tubes. Age also affected outcomes in this study, with a decrease in successful closure by 9% with each year of age. Gelfoam myringoplasty was the most successful graft material (90.8%) compared with paper (82.6%) and fat (77.4%). Perforation location, history of otorrhea, season of repair, and graft position (plug versus lateral) were found to be non-significant factors in the outcome of myringoplasty in this study.

Conclusions

Myringoplasty is an important technique for the otologic surgeon. Though presently limited by the extent of tympanic disease, its value is sustained by cases of symptomatic, small perforations that can potentially be spared a larger surgery. Furthermore, improvements in tissue and growth factor engineering as well as applications of the endoscope to otologic surgery are promising developments that may eventually inspire a broadening of the indications for myringoplasty.

References

1. Srinivasan V, Toynton SC, Mangat KS. Transtympanic myringoplasty in children. Int J Pediatr Otorhinolaryngol. 1997;39:199–204.
2. Banzer M. Disputatio de Auditione laesa, Wittebergae, 1640, as cited by House. Trans Am Acad Ophthalmol Otolaryngol. 1963;67:233–59.
3. Berthold E. Uber myringoplastik. Medicinisch-Chirurgisches Centralblatt. 1879;14:195–207.
4. Wullstein H. [Technic and early results of tympanoplasty.]. Monatsschr Ohrenheilkd Laryngorhinol. 1953;87(4):308–11.
5. Zollner F. [Surgical techniques for the improvement of sound conduction after radical operation.] Arch Ital Otol Rinol Laringol. 1953;64(4):455–68.
6. Wullstein H. Funktionelle operationen im mittelohr mit hilfe des freien spaltlappen-transplantates. Arch Ohren-Nasen- u Kehlkopfh. 1952;161:422.
7. Schwartze HH, Eysell CG. ueber die kunstliche eroffnung des warsenfortsatzes. Arch Ohrenh. 1873;7:157.
8. Kuster E. Ueber die grundsatze der behandlung von eiterungen in starrwandigen hohlen, mit besonderer berucksichtigung des empyems der pleura. Deutsche med Wchnschr. 1889;15:254.
9. Zaufal E. des trepanation des proc. mastoid nach kusterschen grundsatzen. Arch Ohrenh. 1890;30:291.
10. Stacke L. Stacke's operations methode. Arch Ohrenh. 1893;35:145.
11. Holmgren G. Some experiences in surgery for otosclerosis. Acta Otolaryngol. 1923;5:460.
12. Nylen CO. The microscope in aural surgery, its first use and later development. Acta Otolaryngol, Suppl. 1954;116:226–40.
13. Sourdille M. New technique in the surgical treatment of severe and progressive deafness from otosclerosis. Bull N Y Acad Med. 1937;13:673.
14. Lempert J. Improvement of hearing in cases of otosclerosis: new one-stage surgical technique. Arch Otolaryngol. 1938;28:42.
15. Pattee GL. An operation to improve hearing in cases of congenital atresia of the external auditory meatus. Arch Otolaryngol (1925). 1947;45:568.
16. Ombredanne M. Surgery of deafness: fenestration in cases of congenital atresia of the external auditory canal. Oto-rhino Laryng Int. 1947;13:229.
17. Rosen S. Mobilization of the stapes to restore hearing in otosclerosis. N Y State J Med. 1953;53(22):2650–3.
18. Juers AL. Observations on bone conduction in fenestrated cases. Ann Otol Rhinol Laryngol. 1948;57:28.
19. Davis H, Walsh TE. The limits of improvement of hearing following the fenestration operation. Laryngoscope. 1950;60:273.
20. Moritz W. Horverbessernde operationen bei chronisch-entzundlichen prozessen beider mittelohren. Ztschr Laryng Rhin Otol. 1950;29:578.
21. Zollner F. Radical operation with special reference to auditory function. Z Laryngol Rhinol Otol. 1951;30(3):104–11.
22. Shea JJ Jr. Vein graft closure of eardrum perforations. J Laryngol Otol. 1960;74:358–62.
23. Tabb HG. Closure of perforations of the tympanic membrane by vein grafts. A preliminary report of twenty cases. Laryngoscope. 1960;70:271–86.
24. Storrs LA. Temporalis muscle fascia and denatured fat grafts in middle-ear surgery. Laryngoscope. 1963;73:699–701.
25. Heermann H. Tympanoplasty with fascial tissue taken from the temporal muscle after straightening the anterior wall of the auditory meatus. HNO. 1961;9:136–7.
26. Hall A, Rytzner C. Stapedectomy and autotransplantation of ossicles. Acta Otolaryngol. 1957;47(4):318–24.
27. House WJ, Patterson ME, Linthicum FH Jr. Incus homografts in chronic ear surgery. Arch Otolaryngol. 1966;84(2):148–53.
28. Glasscock ME III, House WF. Homograft reconstruction of the middle ear. A preliminary report. Laryngoscope. 1968;78(7):1219–25.
29. Shea JJ, Homsy CA. The use of proplast TM in otologic surgery. Laryngoscope. 1974;84(10):1835–45.
30. Farrior JB. Incisions in tympanoplasty: anatomic considerations and indications. Laryngoscope. 1983;93:75–86.
31. Berger G. Nature of spontaneous tympanic membrane perforation in acute otitis media in children. J Laryngol Otol. 1989;103:1150–3.
32. Lindeman P, Edstrom S, Granstrom G, et al. Acute traumatic tympanic membrane perforations. Arch Otolaryngol. 1987;113:1285–7.
33. Sckolnick JS, Mantle B, Chi DH. Pediatric myringoplasty: factors that affect success—a retrospective study. Laryngoscope. 2008;118:723–9.
34. Saito T, Iwaki E, Kohno Y, et al. Prevention of persistent ear drum perforation after long-term ventilation tube treatment for otitis media with effusion in children. Int J Pediatr Otorhinolaryngol. 1996;38:31–9.
35. Hekkenberg RJ, Smitheringale AJ. Gelfoam/Gelfilm patching following the removal of ventilation tubes. J Otolaryngol. 1995;24:362–3.
36. Lentsch EJ, Goudy S, Ganzel TM, Goldman JL, Nissen AJ. Rate of persistent perforation after elective tympanoplasty tube removal in pediatric patients. Int J Pediatr Otorhinolaryngol. 2000;54:143–8.
37. Pignataro L, Grillo Della Berta L, Capaccio P, Zaghis A. Myringoplasty in children: anatomical and functional results. J Laryngol Otol. 2001;115:369–73.
38. Onal K, Uguz MZ, Kazikdas KC, Gursoy ST, Gokce H. A multivariate analysis of otological, surgical and patient-related factors in determining success in myringoplasty. Clin Otolaryngol. 2005;30:115–20.
39. Knapik M, Saliba I. Pediatric myringoplasty: a study of factors affecting outcome. Int J Pediatr Otorhinolaryngol. 2011;75(6):818–23.
40. Becvarovski Z, Kartush JM. Smoking and tympanoplasty: implications for prognosis and the Middle Ear Risk Index (MERI). Laryngoscope. 2001;111:1806–11.

41. Denoyelle F, Roger G, Chauvin P, Garabedian EN. Myringoplasty in children: predictive factors of outcome. Laryngoscope. 1999;109:47–51.
42. Collins WO, Telischi FF, Balkany TJ, Buchman CA. Pediatric tympanoplasty: effect of contralateral ear status on outcomes. Arch Otolaryngol Head Neck Surg. 2003;129:646–51.
43. Aviles Jurado FJ, Meran Gil JL, Tobed Secall M, et al. Myringoplasty: auditory follow-up and study of prognostic factors. Acta Otorrinolaringol Esp. 2009;60:169–75.
44. Skotnicka B, Hassmann-Poznanska E. Myringoplasty in children—success factors. Otolaryngol Pol. 2008;62:65–70.
45. Santa Maria PL, Atlas MD, Ghassemifar R. Chronic tympanic membrane perforation: a better animal model is needed. Wound Repair Regen. 2007;15:450–8.
46. Berglund M, Florentzson R, Fransson M, Hultcrantz M, et al. Myringoplasty outcomes from the Swedish National Quality Registry. Laryngoscope. 2017;127(10):2389–95.
47. Kartush JM. Tympanic membrane patcher: a new device to close tympanic membrane perforations in an office setting. Am J Otol. 2000;21:615–20.
48. Santa Maria PL, Oghalai J. Is office-based myringoplasty a suitable alternative to surgical tympanoplasty? Laryngoscope. 2014;124:1053–4.
49. Scaramella LF, Farrell BP, Kooiker PD, Marra S. Effectiveness of nonsurgical office closure of tympanic membrane pars tensa perforations. Ear Nose Throat J. 2002;81:556–8, 560.
50. Stenfors LE, Carlsöö B, Salen B, et al. Repair of experimental tympanic membrane perforations. Acta Otolaryngol. 1980;90(5–6):332–41.
51. Juers AL. Office closure of tympanic perforation: a new approach. Laryngoscope. 1958;68:120–1.
52. Dursun E, Dogru S, Gungor A, Cincik H, Poyrazoglu E, Ozdemir T. Comparison of paper-patch, fat, and perichondrium myringoplasty in repair of small tympanic membrane perforations. Otolaryngol Head Neck Surg. 2008;138:353–6.
53. Golz A, Goldenberg D, Netzer A, et al. Paper patching for chronic tympanic membrane perforations. Otolaryngol Head Neck Surg. 2003;128:565–70.
54. Laurent C, Söderberg O, Annika M, Hartwig S. Repair of chronic tympanic membrane perforations using applications of hyaloronan or rice paper prostheses. ORL J Otorhinolaryngol Relat Spec. 1991;53:37–40.
55. Park SN, Kim HM, Jin KS, Maeng JH, Yeo SW, Park SY. Predictors for outcome of paper patch myringoplasty in patients with chronic tympanic membrane perforations. Eur Arch Otorhinolaryngol. 2015;272(2):297–301.
56. Ringenberg JC. Fat graft tympanoplasty. Laryngoscope. 1962;72:188–92.
57. Michell RB, Pereira KD, Lazar RH. Fat graft myringoplasty in children—a safe and successful day-stay procedure. J Laryngol Otol. 1997;111:106–8.
58. Landsberg R, Fishman G, DeRowe A, Berco E, Berger G. Fat graft myringoplasty: results of a long-term follow-up. J Otolaryngol. 2006;35:44–7.
59. Saliba I, Knapik M, Froehlich P, Abela A. Advantages of hyaluronic acid fat graft myringoplasty over fat graft myringoplasty. Arch Otolaryngol Head Neck Surg. 2012;138:950–5.
60. Puterman M, Leiberman A. Gelfoam plug tympanostomy concomitant with removal of retained ventilation tubes. Int J Pediatr Otorhinolaryngol. 2005;69:57–60.
61. Hellstrom S, Salen B, Stenfors LE. Absorbable sponge (gelfoam) in otosurgery: one cause of undesirable postoperative results? An experimental study. Acta Otolaryngol. 1983;96:269–75.
62. Joseph RB. The effect of absorbable gelatine sponge preparations and other agents on scar formation in the dog's middle ear. An experimental histopathologic study. Laryngoscope. 1962;72:1528–48.
63. Niklasson A, Tano K. The Gelfoam® plug: an alternative treatment for small eardrum perforations. Laryngoscope. 2011;121(4):782–4.
64. Eavey RD. Inlay tympanoplasty: cartilage butterfly technique. Laryngoscope. 1998;108:657–61.
65. Ghanem MA, Monroy A, Alizade FS, et al. Butterfly cartilage graft inlay tympanoplasty for large perforations. Laryngoscope. 2006;116:1813–6.
66. Alain H, Esmat NH, Ohad H, Yona V, et al. Butterfly myringoplasty for total, subtotal, and annular perforations. Laryngoscope. 2016;126:2565–8.
67. El-Guindy A. Endoscopic transcanal myringoplasty. J Laryngol Otol. 1992;106(6):493–5.
68. Karhuketo TS, Ilomäki JH, Puhakka HJ. Tympanoscope-assisted myringoplasty. ORL J Otorhinolaryngol Relat Spec. 2001;63(6):353–7.
69. Yadav SP, Aggarwal N, Julaha M, Goel A. Endoscope-assisted myringoplasty. Singapore Med J. 2009;50(5):510–2.
70. Tseng CC, Lai MT, Wu CC, Yuan SP, Ding YF. Endoscopic transcanal myringoplasty for anterior perforations of the tympanic membrane. JAMA Otolaryngol Head Neck Surg. 2016;142(11):1088–93.
71. Jackler RK. A regenerative method of tympanic membrane repair could be the greatest advance in otology since the cochlear implant. Otol Neurotol. 2012;33:289.
72. Lokmic Z, Mitchell GM. Engineering the microcirculation. Tissue Eng Part B Rev. 2008;14:87–103.
73. Kanemaru S, Umeda H, Kitani Y, Nakamura T, Hirano S, Ito J. Regenerative treatment for tympanic membrane perforation. Otol Neurotol. 2011;32:1218.
74. Chauvin K, Bratton C, Parkins C. Healing large tympanic membrane perforations using hyaluronic acid, basic fibroblast growth factor, and epidermal growth factor. Otolaryngol Head Neck Surg. 1999;121:43–7.
75. Seonwoo H, Kim SW, Kim J, Chunjie T, et al. Regeneration of chronic tympanic membrane perforation using an EGF-releasing chitosan patch. Tissue Eng Part A. 2013;19(17–18):2097–107.
76. Santa Maria PL, Gottlieb P, Santa Maria C, Kim S, et al. Functional outcomes of heparin-binding epidermal growth factor-like growth factor for regeneration of chronic tympanic membrane perforations in mice. Tissue Eng Part A. 2017;23(9–10):436–44.

Tympanoplasty: Underlay Technique

39

Nicholas L. Deep and Sean O. McMenomey

Introduction

The term tympanoplasty was introduced in 1953 by Wullstein to describe surgical techniques for reconstruction of the middle-ear hearing mechanism that had been impaired or destroyed by chronic disease [1]. That same year Zöllner reported on surgical techniques for improving the sound conduction mechanism of the middle ear following surgery for chronic ear disease [2]. In 1965 the American Academy of Ophthalmology and Otolaryngology Subcommittee on Conservation of Hearing defined tympanoplasty as "a procedure to eradicate disease in the middle ear and to reconstruct the hearing mechanism, with or without tympanic membrane grafting" [3]. This is in contrast to "myringoplasty" which implies surgery confined to the drum head itself, without the elevation of the eardrum or manipulation of the ossicles.

A tympanoplasty, therefore, includes all procedures when the drum is lifted from its position in the ear canal. It may be combined with a mastoidectomy to eradicate disease from the mastoid and/or with an ossiculoplasty to restore ossicular chain continuity. Several tympanoplasty techniques have been described. Broadly, these are categorized into underlay or overlay tympanoplasty, depending on if the graft is placed under or over the remnant tympanic membrane, respectively [4]. This chapter will detail the underlay tympanoplasty technique.

N. L. Deep
Department of Otolaryngology—Head and Neck Surgery, Division of Otology and Neurotology, Mayo Clinic, Phoenix, AZ, USA

S. O. McMenomey (✉)
Department of Otolaryngology—Head and Neck Surgery, New York University School of Medicine, NYU Langone Health, New York, NY, USA
e-mail: Sean.McMenomey@nyulangone.org

General Principles

Conceptually, the purpose of tympanoplasty is to bridge a tympanic membrane perforation with a scaffold on top of which the epithelium from the edges of the remnant drumhead or external canal wall can laterally migrate. Various graft materials have been used as scaffolds for tympanoplasty, all with the aim of reconstructing the deficient middle fibrous layer of the tympanic membrane.

The primary goal of tympanoplasty is to create a safe, dry ear by reconstructing the tympanic membrane and eradicating any middle-ear disease, most commonly of which is a retraction pocket cholesteatoma. Reconstructing the tympanic membrane provides a barrier between the dry lateral epithelialized compartment of the external auditory canal and the moist medial mucosalized compartment of the middle ear. This prevents recurrent otorrhea or secondary cholesteatoma, which may occur from the two compartments interacting. It also permits patients to safely resume water activity without restriction and improves the quality of life.

A secondary goal is to improve hearing through tympanic membrane grafting and, if needed, ossicular chain reconstruction. An intact tympanic membrane in continuity with the stapes footplate restores the most significant mechanism by which the middle ear transformer increases sound pressure delivered to the inner ear: the hydraulic lever. The hydraulic lever describes how pressure gathered over the large tympanic membrane is transmitted to the small stapes footplate through ossicular coupling. It is responsible for an approximate 17-fold increase in total pressure at the oval window. An intact tympanic membrane also "protects" the round window from competitive sounds—which act through acoustic coupling—partly by damping and partly by phase difference.

Lastly, in some cases the underlying pathology—such as Eustachian tube dysfunction—is an ongoing threat even after repair. Therefore, an additional goal of tympanoplasty is to reinforce the tympanic membrane's structural integrity. This

A. D. Sweeney et al. (eds.), *Haynes-Glasscock-Shambaugh Surgery of the Ear*, https://doi.org/10.1007/978-3-032-18264-7_39

is often achieved using cartilage to augment and strengthen the drumhead to resist future recurrent retraction pockets, atelectasis, or perforation.

Indications and Contraindications

Tympanoplasty is indicated in the setting of a tympanic membrane perforation or other middle ear pathology that results in hearing loss and/or chronic otorrhea. Such pathology includes a cholesteatoma, retraction pocket, atelectasis, tympanosclerosis, or ossicular discontinuity. The benefits of surgery should be weighed against the complications that might arise. Realistic goals should be discussed with the patient. In certain patients, a tympanoplasty may be destined to fail or the ear may be safer if left open. Ultimately, exercising restraint and realizing when not to do a given procedure comes with experience and constitutes good clinical judgment.

Absolute contraindications include poor general health, which prohibits anesthesia, malignant tumors of the external/middle ear, or complications of chronic ear disease such as meningitis, brain abscess, or lateral sinus thrombosis [5].

Several relative contraindications deserve mention along with their exceptions. Operating on a significantly better hearing ear or only-hearing ear is discouraged in order to avoid the risk of irreversible sensorineural hearing loss. Occasionally, however, the benefits of surgery outweigh the risks, as in the case of a large, destructive cholesteatoma in an only-hearing ear. The status of the contralateral ear and whether it may benefit from a hearing aid is helpful in weighing the relative risks.

Actively draining ears in the setting of an acute exacerbation of chronic otitis media, allergic rhinosinusitis, or chronic otitis externa should be managed with appropriate treatment prior to tympanoplasty. However, while most surgeons prefer to operate on a "dry" ear, there is no contraindication to performing a tympanoplasty in the face of an active infection. In fact, cholesteatomas must be treated surgically in order to attain a dry ear.

A chronic perforation without cholesteatoma in an ear with profound sensorineural hearing loss may be safely observed. However, tympanoplasty may be done to create a safe ear for water activity and to obviate routine water precautions.

A nonfunctioning Eustachian tube is considered a relative contraindication to tympanoplasty, though this is not always easily determined preoperatively. Oftentimes, poor Eustachian tube function improves following tympanoplasty by removing middle-ear disease processes such as polyps, granulation tissue, and infection. Patients with craniofacial anomalies such as cleft palate have known Eustachian tube dysfunction, and in these patients a small dry perforation may be safely followed. However, tympanoplasty should be offered in the setting of larger perforations with associated otorrhea or cholesteatoma. A ventilation tube may provide a controlled method of establishing pressure equalization [6]. Patients with nonfunctioning Eustachian tubes, repeated surgical failures, and prosthesis extrusions should be counseled on alternative options for hearing restoration, such as a hearing aid or bone conduction device.

Indications for tympanoplasty in the elderly should be individualized. Elderly patients who are infirm may be better treated conservatively. However, with modern anesthetic techniques, elderly patients in relatively good health may safely undergo surgery without significant morbidity [7].

Tympanoplasty in children is often delayed until 8–10 years of age when the Eustachian tube has reached anatomic and physiologic maturity and the incidence of otitis media has lessened. A meta-analysis found that age was a significant factor influencing the success in pediatric tympanoplasty, with outcomes improving every year up to 13 years old [8]. The status of the contralateral ear (e.g., presence of otitis media with effusion or negative middle ear pressure) may be a useful indicator to assess Eustachian tube maturity when deciding when it is safe to operate [9, 10]. Exceptions to waiting include if the child has evidence of cholesteatoma or bilateral tympanic membrane perforations with large conductive hearing losses.

Preoperative Evaluation

History

A complete neurotologic history is obtained, including the etiology of the perforation, frequency and characteristics of drainage, and any associated symptoms such as hearing loss, vertigo, tinnitus otalgia, or facial weakness. Careful review of any past otologic procedures, including ventilation tubes or prior attempts at repair, is important to elicit.

Otologic Exam

A complete head and neck examination is performed. A recent audiogram within 3 months of surgery is recommended and should include pure-tone air- and bone-conduction thresholds and speech discrimination scores. The audiogram should be verified with tuning fork testing (Weber and Rinne).

An otologic microscope is preferred when examining the ear. The size and location of a tympanic membrane perforation or retraction pocket and evidence of cholesteatoma or suspected cholesteatoma (e.g., inflammatory polyp or crusting on the tympanic membrane) are documented. The edges of the perforation should be inspected. Sharp, crisp, dry perforation margins are less worrisome compared to thickened, irregular, moist margins with heaped-up keratin debris that appears to roll over the border onto the medial surface of the tympanic membrane. Small, dry perforations may be amenable to office-based myringoplasty.

A draining ear should be optimized as best as possible prior to surgery. While in the office, any active drainage should be cleaned under the microscope. Mucoid otorrhea is less worrisome and may originate from the Eustachian tube or exposed middle ear mucosa. Purulent otorrhea may signify the need for a mastoidectomy. The patient should be instructed to take water precautions. A 1.5% acetic acid solution at body temperature may be applied using a bulb syringe twice a day prior to surgery. Afterward, topical antibiotic drops covering *Pseudomonas aeruginosa* should be instilled and tragal pressure should be applied several times to force the antibiotic solution deeper into the ear canal and middle ear. Oral antibiotics may also be considered for patients not responding to local treatment. Obtaining a dry ear is not always possible prior to surgery, especially in cases of cholesteatoma, but decreasing inflammation to the extent possible may optimize the odds of success.

Imaging Studies

Preoperative imaging is controversial and should be determined on an individualized basis. In general, dry, chronic perforations do not require preoperative imaging. A high-resolution temporal bone computed tomography (CT) of the temporal bone is indicated in cases of chronic drainage that has not responded to medical treatment or in cases of known cholesteatoma for surgical planning. Unusual symptoms such as otalgia, vertigo, sensorineural hearing loss, tinnitus, and facial nerve symptoms (weakness, twitching, or spasm) warrant imaging. This will help rule out complications of cholesteatoma such as a labyrinthine fistula or other etiologies (e.g., congenital malformation, intracranial disease, middle ear tumors). A CT may also be obtained in patients with prior surgery and in those with a craniofacial syndrome in whom there may be an aberrant facial nerve. Specific review of the extent of disease, degree of mastoid pneumatization, and involvement of critical structures (fallopian canal, lateral semicircular canal, tegmen) provides information on surgical approach and planning. A magnetic resonance imaging (MRI) study of the temporal bone with T2-weighted coronal imaging is obtained if there is a tegmen defect with concern of brain herniation.

Informed Consent

Prior to surgery, patients should be informed regarding the nature of their disease process, treatment options, proposed surgical procedures, expected outcomes, the risks and complications. Patients should be alerted to the potential need for a mastoidectomy based on intraoperative findings (including canal wall down mastoidectomy in cases of severe disease). Additionally, the possibility of a second-stage procedure should be discussed.

Graft Materials

Various grafts have been used for tympanoplasty. In the 1950s, full- and split-thickness skin grafts were used, followed by the use of canal skin or vein [11, 12]. Later temporalis fascia and tragal perichondrium were popularized and have remained the mainstay of tympanoplasty ever since [13, 14].

In 1970, Moon introduced the use of the loose areolar tissue ("fool's fascia"), which overlies the true temporalis fascia [15]. This grafting material was used extensively by Michael Glasscock, who cited several of its benefits. First, it is thin and easily manipulated when rehydrated. Second, the temporalis muscle is not violated and therefore, there is virtually no bleeding from the graft site, and extra time is not required to remove remnants of muscle or adipose tissue. Third, there is less pain with chewing since the temporalis muscle is not exposed. Finally, and perhaps most importantly, the true temporalis fascia is still available should the initial graft fail. Retrospective series have demonstrated comparable graft-take between the true temporalis fascia and fool's fascia [16].

Cartilage was introduced in the 1980s initially as a way of augmenting the structural integrity of the tympanic membrane in the setting of atelectasis and ongoing Eustachian tube dysfunction [17]. Today, many surgeons incorporate cartilage routinely in their repair owing to higher closure rates than with fascia alone. In transcanal tympanoplasty, a tragal cartilage-perichondrium composite graft is frequently used since it can provide sufficient material to repair perforations of all sizes and obviates the need to make a postauricular incision to harvest fascia.

In revision cases where fascia and perichondrium are not available, AlloDerm® (an acellular dermal homograft by LifeCell Corporation, Branchburg, NJ) or Biodesign® (a porcine intestinal submucosa by Cook Medical, Bloomington, Indiana) has shown efficacy in tympanoplasty and may be used [18, 19].

Tympanoplasty Approaches

Tympanoplasty surgery is primarily performed through a transcanal or postauricular approach. The endaural approach is less commonly used but may be the preferred approach for some surgeons. The choice of approach depends on the size and location of the perforation, the size of the ear canal (including degree of obstruction by the anterior bony canal wall), the need for performing a mastoidectomy, and the surgeon's preference, among other factors (Table 39.1). Remaining flexible is necessary as intraoperative factors often determine which approach is optimal. The postauricular approach is technically easier and provides wide exposure. However, the transcanal approach is quicker, more direct and may lead to less postoperative discomfort. Experienced otologic surgeons who are adept at manipulating the speculum and working with both hands are able to repair virtually any size perforation through the transcanal approach, so long as the bony ear canal is not overly narrow.

Over the last decade, the use of an endoscope in otologic surgery has become popular. Wide visualization through the transcanal corridor obviates the need to make a postauricular incision for exposure. Endoscopic ear surgery, however, requires one-handed dissection and denies the surgeon binocular vision. This learning curve may be overcome with practice, and proponents of the technique believe the benefits of enhanced visualization overshadow its drawbacks. Future innovations in endoscopic ear surgery may drive greater adoption.

Table 39.1 Comparison of transcanal and postauricular surgical approaches for tympanoplasty

	Indications	Advantages	Disadvantages
Transcanal approach	Small, posterior perforation[a] Large ear canals Endoscopic cases	Faster Less postoperative discomfort	Technically more demanding (requires using both hands while manipulating and stabilizing the otologic speculum or using a speculum holder)
Postauricular approach	Anterior perforations (especially large and/or marginal) Large anterior canal wall bulge obstructing the view of the anterior sulcus Narrow ear canal precluding good exposure via transcanal approach. Mastoidectomy is necessary	Technically easier Greater exposure Access to temporalis fascia or conchal cartilage without an additional incision Easily perform canalplasty for greater exposure	Slightly greater postoperative pain and swelling Risk of wound infection (<1%)

[a]Note: Experienced otologic surgeons adept with working through speculum (or endoscope) can repair large perforations (even near-total perforations) via the transcanal approach. A limited canalplasty may be done with a drill through the speculum to improve visualization

Surgical Technique

Anesthesia

Tympanoplasty is typically performed on an outpatient basis under general anesthesia. When possible, laryngeal mask anesthesia (LMA) is preferred as it avoids tracheal irritation, allows the patient to breathe spontaneously, and facilitates a smoother and quicker extubation without severe coughing or retching. The blood pressure cuff should be placed on the arm opposite the ear undergoing surgery so that it does not interfere with the surgeon. A single dose of perioperative antibiotics is given for patients with cholesteatoma or chronic drainage but is not necessary in clean, dry perforations [20]. Facial nerve monitoring is typically performed, and therefore, communication with the anesthesiologist to withhold any long-acting muscle paralytic is essential.

Patient Positioning

The patient is placed close to the edge of the table in order to prevent the surgeon from hyperextending their arms. In adults, the head is placed in a donut and rotated away from the surgeon. Slight flexion of the head, such that the chin is tucked and pointing to the contralateral shoulder, is helpful. The postauricular skin is degreased with an alcohol wipe. Long hair may be pulled back with adhesive tape and rarely is shaving required. The patient is secured with at least two straps. A time-out is performed and the ear to be operated on is confirmed.

Hemostasis and Prepping of the Surgical Area

Complete hemostasis is imperative in otologic surgery as it facilitates an unobstructed view and allows for efficiency of movement. Aspirin or other anticoagulation medications are discontinued prior to surgery and should be cleared by the patient's primary care physician. 1% lidocaine with 1:100,000 epinephrine is injected into the postauricular incision and in four quadrants at the external meatus, using a total of approximately 6 mL. The tragal skin is also routinely injected, should tragal cartilage or perichondrium be desired. Additional injection is available on the sterile field for the vascular strip. Gelfoam® soaked in undiluted (1:1000) epinephrine is also available for hemostasis as needed during the case.

The surgical area is prepped with an iodine-based antiseptic solution (Betadine) and blotted dry with a sterile towel. It is not permitted to use chlorhexidine or alcohol due to potential ototoxicity [21]. The patient is draped in standard fashion for otologic surgery.

Under the microscope, a vascular strip injection of 1% lidocaine with 1:100,000 epinephrine is performed with a 27-gauge needle. The needle is inserted into the posterosuperior lateral third of the external ear canal, at approximately the junction of the hair-bearing and non-hair-bearing skin. Once the bony ear canal is palpated, a slow injection is performed to avoid blebs. Blanching of the vascular strip and blood vessels along the tympanic membrane will be seen. Additional canal injections are performed inferiorly and anteriorly.

Preparing the Drumhead

While the injection is taking effect, the rim of the perforation is freshened by conservatively denuding the squamous epithelium. A Rosen needle is used to incise circumferentially around the margin of the perforation, followed by removing the rim with cup forceps (Fig. 39.1). Alternatively, a laser may be used. Care is taken not to over-freshen the margin as this leads to a larger perforation and a more difficult repair, which is particularly true when perforations approach the anterior margin of the tympanic membrane. The medial surface of the drum is roughened with a right-angle pick placed through the perforation. Scarifying the mucosa is thought to encourage vascularization of the graft. Large areas of tympanosclerotic (calcified) plaques may also be removed from the remnant tympanic membrane at this time. These areas have poor blood supply and therefore risk graft failure.

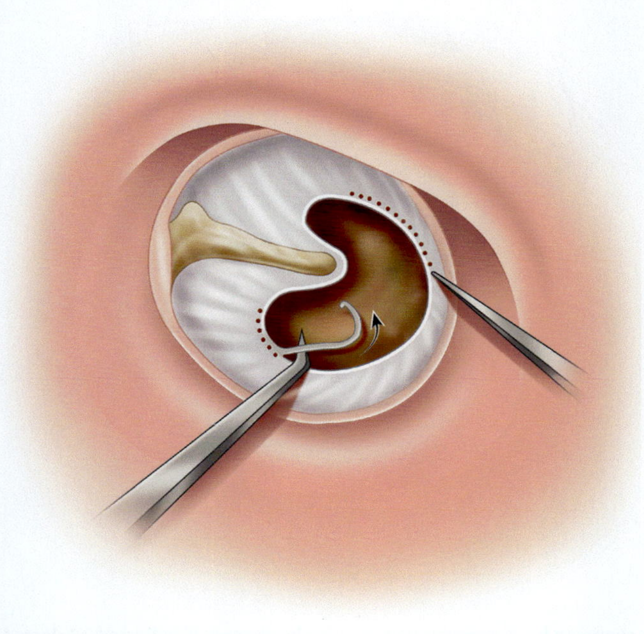

Fig. 39.1 Freshening the edges of the perforation. (Adapted from Jackler RK. *Ear Surgery Illustrated: A Comprehensive Atlas of Otologic Microsurgical Techniques*. Illustrated by Gralapp C. Thieme. 2019)

Canal Incisions

A variety of tympanomeatal flaps may be designed based on different canal incisions. Broadly, canal incisions differ depending on if a transcanal or postauricular-transcanal approach is taken.

Transcanal approach In the transcanal approach, it is imperative to use the largest speculum that may be atraumatically inserted. A tympanomeatal flap similar to one used in a stapedectomy is created (Fig. 39.2a). Two longitudinal incisions are made using a disposable sickle knife (7300 Beaver®). The first begins adjacent to the short process of the malleus (12 o'clock) and follows the tympanosquamous suture line laterally. The second incision is adjacent to the tympanic annulus starting around 7 o'clock (in the right ear) and extending laterally. Next, a disposable round knife (7200 Beaver®) is used to connect these incisions at their lateral extent with a transverse incision made approximately 6 mm from the annulus. This can be approximated by measuring two diameters of a standard 3 mm round knife. It is important that the flap have sufficient length in case the scutum requires curettage for exposure. Subsequently, the tympanomeatal flap is elevated to expose the middle ear (described below) (Fig. 39.2b).

Postauricular approach If a postauricular approach is planned, a vascular strip incision is made. Working transcanally through a speculum, the vascular strip is outlined by making longitudinal incisions along the tympanosquamous and tympanomastoid suture lines using a disposable miniblade (6700 Beaver®). These incisions should extend laterally into the cartilaginous ear canal to facilitate easy identification during the postauricular exposure. The longitudinal incisions are connected with a transverse incision a few millimeters lateral to the tympanic annulus using a disposable round knife (7200 Beaver®). In the original description of the technique by Glasscock in 1973, this transverse incision is made very close to the annulus (Fig. 39.3a) and an additional incision is made at the lateral extent of the inferior (tympanomastoid) incision at a right angle along the floor of the ear canal for 4–6 mm. This facilitates elevation of an inferior flap (Fig. 39.3b) [22]. A superior flap can also be elevated with an additional incision if required. In a modification of this technique, the transverse incision can be made

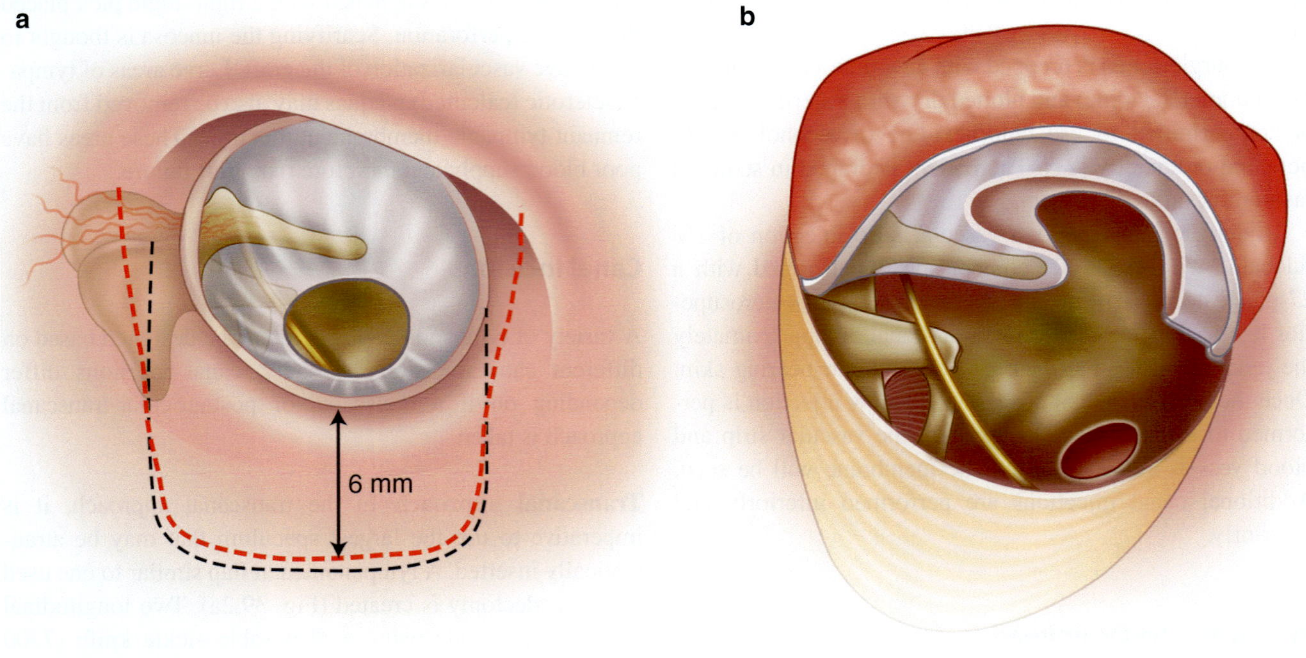

Fig. 39.2 (**a**) Tympanomeatal flap design for a transcanal approach. Traditionally, the medial end of these cuts is made tangential to the annulus (seen in black). If a larger flap is desired (e.g., 270°), then the medial ends of the incisions remain lateral and parallel to the annulus (shown in red), which facilitates extending the incisions and raising a more circumferential flap. (**b**) View of the middle ear after the tympanomeatal flap has been elevated as a single unit. (Adapted from Jackler RK. *Ear Surgery Illustrated: A Comprehensive Atlas of Otologic Microsurgical Techniques*. Illustrated by Gralapp C. Thieme. 2019)

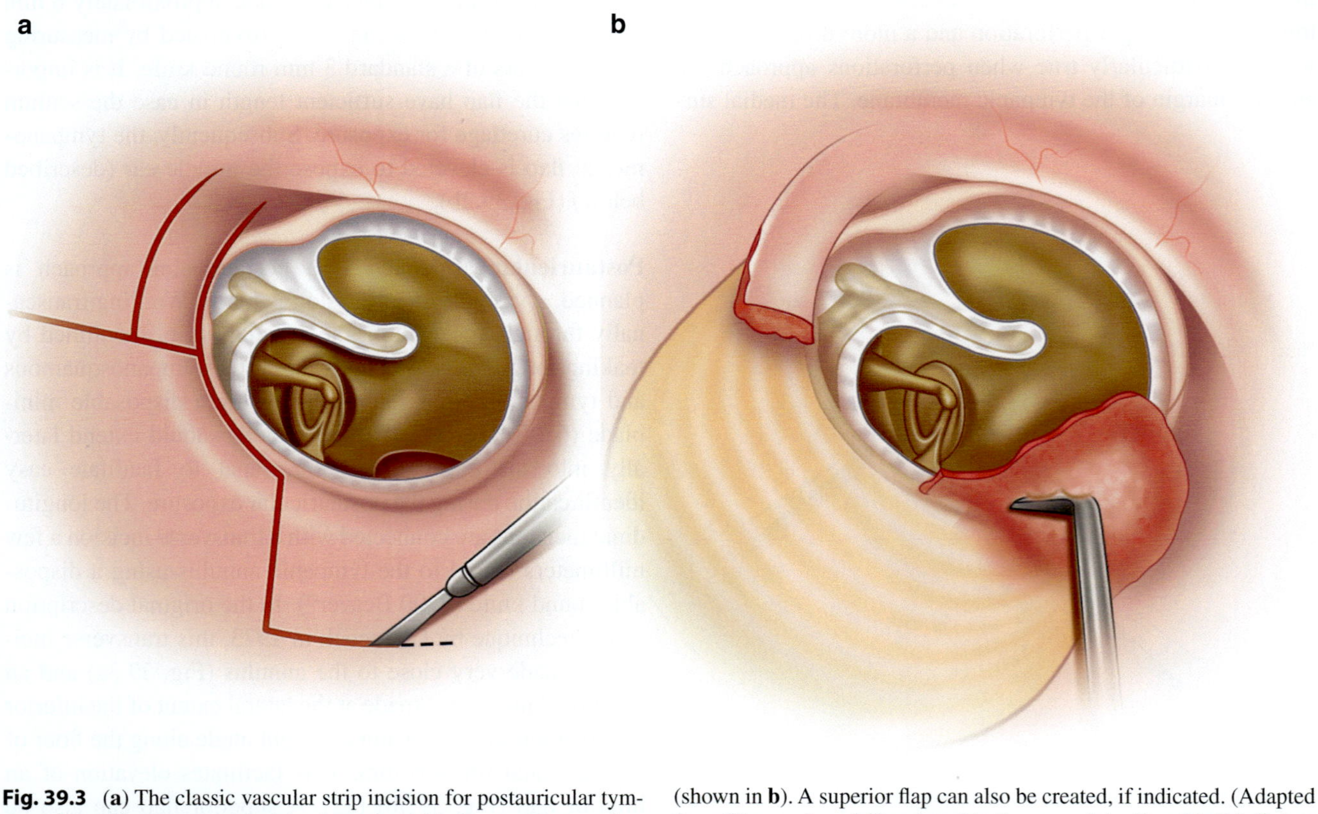

Fig. 39.3 (**a**) The classic vascular strip incision for postauricular tympanoplasty. The transverse incision is made within 2 mm of the annulus. There is an additional limb extending off the inferior longitudinal incision that serves to facilitate raising an inferior canal wall skin flap (shown in **b**). A superior flap can also be created, if indicated. (Adapted from Glasscock and Shambaugh's *Surgery of the Ear*. 6th Ed. Gulya, Minor. Poe. PMPH. 2010)

slightly more lateral (3–6 mm) to the annulus. This provides a more vascular tympanomeatal skin flap, which may be elevated as a single unit or may be split to create "swinging door" flaps (Fig. 39.4) [23].

Postauricular Incision

The postauricular incision is then made using a No. 15 blade approximately 1 cm away from the postauricular sulcus (Fig. 39.5a). The auricle is firmly grasped and forcibly pulled forward and outward as the incision is made in one sweep of the knife. Keeping tension on the auricle stretches the loose areolar tissue over the temporalis fascia and allows the surgeon to free up the area with little blood loss. Bleeding points are controlled with electrocautery. A Weitlaner retractor is placed to hold the ear forward.

Temporalis Fascia Harvest

The retractor is used to expose the loose areolar tissue overlying the temporalis fascia. Separation of the loose areolar tissue ("fool's fascia") from the true temporalis fascia is facilitated by injecting local anesthetic solution to hydrodissect the plane between the two layers. An incision is made at the level of the linea temporalis and carried down to the level of the temporalis fascia (if fool's fascia is desired) or down to the level of the temporalis muscle (if true temporalis fascia is desired). A Freer is used to gently sweep and develop the plane on either side of the fascia to be removed. The graft is dissected free with Metzenbaum scissors (Fig. 39.5b). Approximately 3 × 2 cm graft is harvested for large perforations. The fascia is cleaned of adipose or muscle tissue, then pressed onto a polytef (Teflon) block, and placed on the back table under a lamp to dehydrate.

Exposing the Ear Canal

A T-shaped incision is made in the musculoperiosteal tissue overlying the mastoid cortex with the horizontal component in the avascular plane of the linea temporalis and the vertical component between the mastoid tip and the midportion of the horizontal incision (Fig. 39.5b). The musculoperiosteal (Palva) flap is mobilized to the level of the ear canal with a Lempert periosteal elevator. Returning under the operating microscope, the posterior canal skin is elevated. The vascular strip flap (also referred to as Körner's flap) is identified and grasped with Adson forceps and rotated out of the ear canal and held forward in the blade of a Weitlaner retractor along with Palva flap. A second self-retaining retractor may be placed vertically between the temporalis muscle and mastoid tip to enhance exposure.

Occasionally, a prominent tympanosquamous suture line makes it difficult to elevate the vascular strip out of the ear canal. In such instances, sharp dissection with a 6700 Beaver® blade will release the attachments of the vascular strip from the suture line. Failure to recognize this situation may result in disruption of the vascular strip during elevation. Next, the external auditory canal is freely irrigated with physiologic solution to remove any clots. The table is tilted away from the surgeon in order to visualize the anterior drum remnant and annulus.

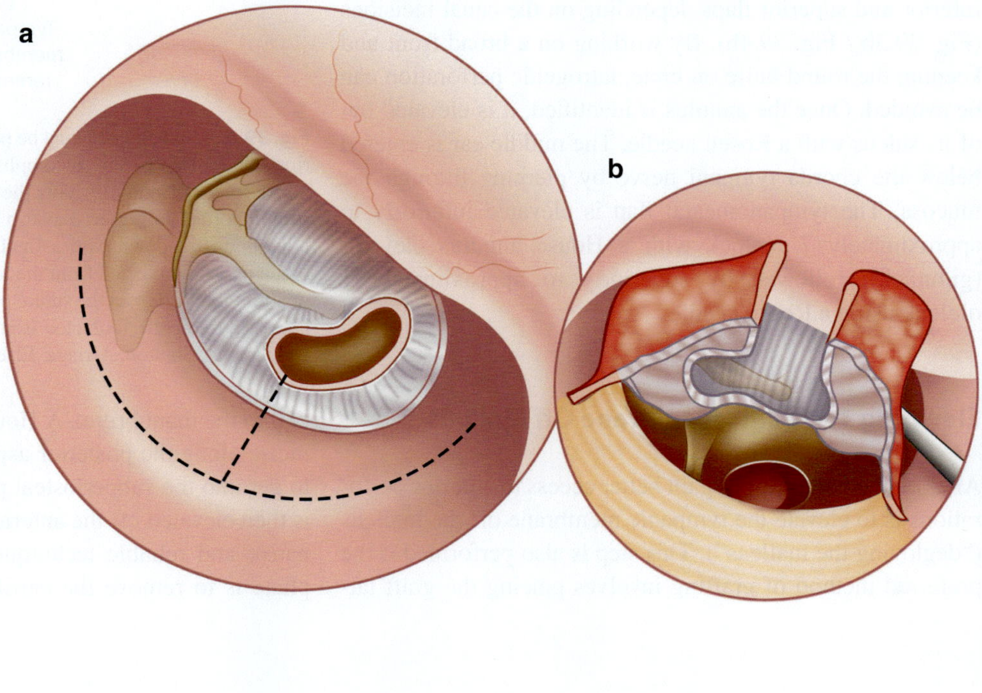

Fig. 39.4 The "swinging-door" tympanomeatal flap. This modification may be used in transcanal or postauricular approaches. A transverse incision is made more lateral (3–6 mm) to the annulus and the development of superior and inferior flaps is created with an incision around 9 o'clock through the canal skin, annulus, and tympanic membrane into the perforation. This provides wide access and ease of grafting, especially for anterior perforations. (Adapted from *Bailey's Head & Neck Surgery Otolaryngology*. 5th Ed. Eds. Johnson JT, Rosen CA. LWW. 2013)

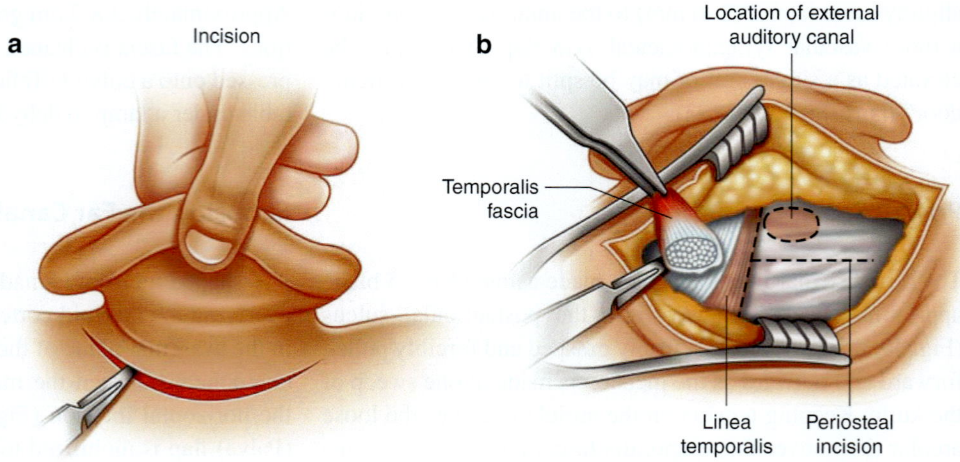

Fig. 39.5 (**a**) The postauricular incision is made approximately 1 cm from the sulcus to aid with closure. (**b**) Fascia is harvested early in the case to provide time for it to dry. The periosteal "T" incision is made with a monopolar cautery and exposes the ear canal just past its superior extent (i.e., 12 o'clock). (Adapted from *Otologic Surgery*. 4th Edition. Eds. Brackmann, Shelton, Arriaga. Elsevier. 2015)

Canalplasty

A canalplasty may be performed at this time if visualization of the anterior sulcus is limited by a prominent anterior wall (Fig. 39.6). A small square of anterior canal skin can be removed, starting about 4 mm lateral to the annulus. It is kept moist with physiologic saline solution on the back table for later replacement as a free skin graft near the end of the case. The anterior bony bulge is removed with a small diamond bur, which maximizes visualization for middle ear dissection, grafting, and postoperative monitoring.

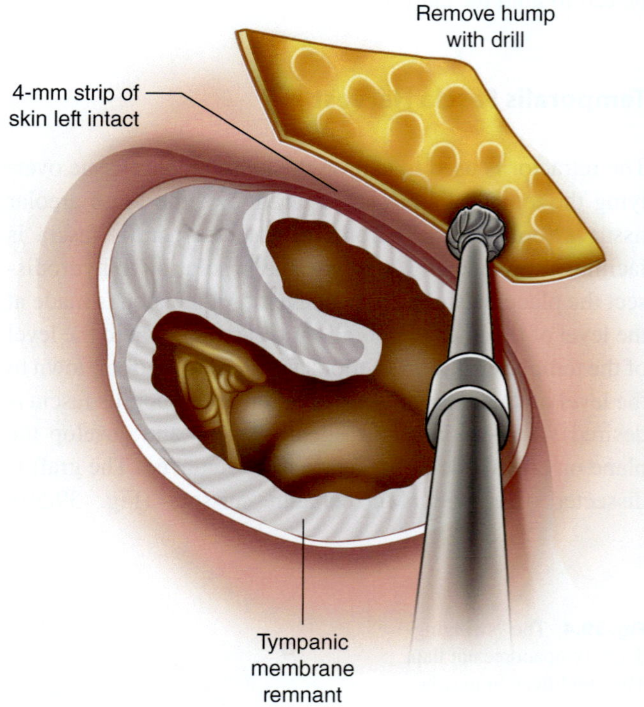

Fig. 39.6 A canalplasty may be performed to better visualize the anterior sulcus. This can be accomplished by removing a square or "doghouse" piece of skin overlying the prominent anterior canal wall hump. It is important to preserve a strip of skin attached to the annulus. The bone is drilled down with a small diamond bur. The tympanic membrane may be protected from the rotating bur with a thin disc of silastic or aluminum foil from the suture package material. The skin is replaced later as a free graft. (Adapted from *Otologic Surgery*. 4th Edition. Eds. Brackmann, Shelton, Arriaga. Elsevier. 2015)

Tympanomeatal Flap Elevation

The tympanomeatal flap is elevated toward the tympanic annulus using a regular round knife and 20-gauge suction. This is elevated as a single flap (Fig. 39.2b) or as separate inferior and superior flaps depending on the canal incisions (Fig. 39.3b / Fig. 39.4b). By working on a broad front and keeping the round knife on bone, iatrogenic perforation can be avoided. Once the annulus is identified, it is elevated out of its sulcus with a Rosen needle. The middle ear is entered below the chorda tympani nerve by piercing through the mucosa. The tympanomeatal flap is elevated inferiorly to approximately 7 o'clock with a House annulus elevator (gimmick), followed by superiorly to approximately 1 o'clock using a Rosen needle.

Elevating Tympanic Membrane Off Malleus

An optional maneuver to gain better access to anterior perforations is to elevate the tympanic membrane off the malleus ("degloving the malleus"). This step is also performed if the preferred method of grafting involves placing the graft lateral to the manubrium. A House No. 1 sickle knife is used to incise along the posterior aspect of the manubrium in order to get into the subperiosteal plane. The tympanic membrane is then elevated off the anterior face of the malleus. An alternative and reliable technique to get into the subperiosteal plane is to remove the cartilage cap of the lateral process

[24]. The remnant drumhead is elevated off the manubrium down to the umbo by working from superior to inferior. By staying within the subperiosteal plane, iatrogenic perforation is avoided, as is the risk of leaving behind remnant epithelium, which may form an epithelial pearl postoperatively. The fibrous adhesions at the umbo are cut sharply with microscissors, which then allows the drum remnant to be completely freed of the malleus.

Removal of Middle Ear Disease

The middle ear is entered, the status of the ossicular chain is determined, and any middle ear pathology is removed. A mastoidectomy is performed if necessary. Prior to grafting, the middle ear is copiously irrigated with an antibiotic solution. If diseased mucosa has been removed from the middle ear and there is significant bone exposure, Gelfilm® is placed over the medial wall of the middle ear to prevent adhesion formation. Epinephrine-soaked Gelfoam® is temporarily placed to maintain hemostasis while the surgeon prepares the graft. Harvesting of a cartilage graft is also performed at this time, if part of the surgical plan. The surgical technique of cartilage harvest and grafting is discussed in the next section.

Grafting

A large piece of Gelfoam®, which has been soaked in antibiotic solution (Ofloxacin) and pressed dry, is placed anteriorly in the Eustachian tube orifice. Smaller pieces of Gelfoam® are placed in the middle ear and circumferentially around the annulus. Overpacking is avoided as it makes it difficult to place the graft. If necessary, after grafting, additional packing may be placed medial to the graft.

For repairing large, near-total perforations, the dried fascia is shaped to approximately 2.5 × 1.5 cm and a slit is made in the fascia to accommodate the malleus. The graft is held with cup forceps and rehydrated in saline solution and then placed into the middle ear medial to the manubrium of the malleus. With a 24-gauge suction and a House annulus elevator (gimmick), the graft is advanced anteriorly into the protympanum and hypotympanum for several millimeters (Fig. 39.7a). This overlap is imperative because fascia may contract, leaving a persistent perforation anteriorly. Posteriorly, the graft is draped onto the posterior canal wall. A right-angle pick is used to manipulate the graft into position around the malleus and anchor it to the lateral epitympanic bone, which is later covered by the superior canal skin flap. Later, the vascular strip and tympanomeatal flaps are lowered, which stabilize the graft posteriorly (Fig. 39.7b).

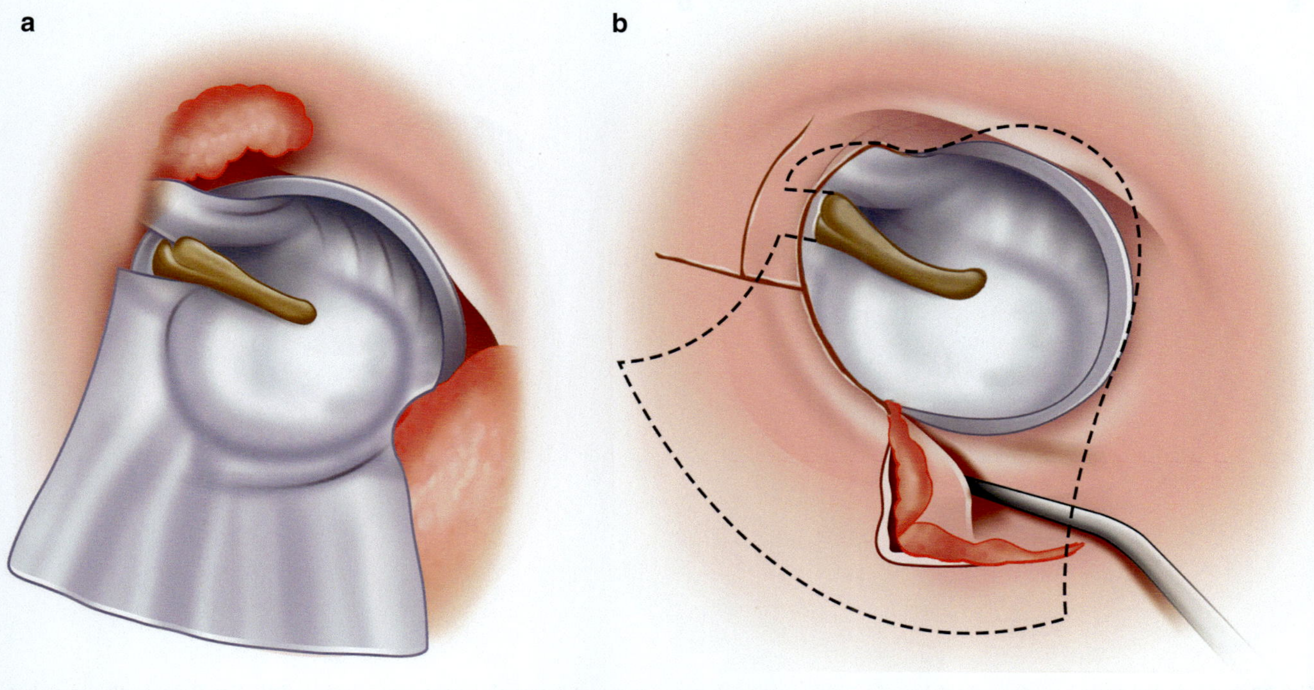

Fig. 39.7 Underlay grafting for near-total tympanic membrane perforations involves (**a**) placing the graft medial to the manubrium and advancing it anteriorly into the protympanum. In some cases, the graft can also be placed lateral to the malleus. (**b**) The ear canal skin is then replaced over the graft. The position of the graft is emphasized with a dashed line in this illustration. (Adapted from Glasscock and Shambaugh's *Surgery of the Ear*. 6th Ed. Gulya, Minor. Poe. PMPH. 2010)

For subtotal perforations not involving the manubrium, a smaller graft may be fashioned. It is placed in a similar fashion, medial to the malleus and advanced past the anterior edge of the perforation (Fig. 39.8). Various technical maneuvers may be employed to ensure the graft advances anteriorly. A piece of cartilage or Gelfilm® may be placed on top of the middle ear Gelfoam®, which serves as a platform to drag the graft across. Alternatively, the fascia graft may be placed prior to middle ear Gelfoam®, followed by placing a medium-to-large dry pressed Gelfoam® medial to it and advancing it anteriorly with a gimmick. This has the effect of dragging the graft anteriorly. Further packing of Gelfoam® medial to the graft will elevate the graft and bring it into contact with the remnant tympanic membrane. Lastly, a "swinging-door flap" may be performed to provide wide access and direct placement of the graft onto the Gelfoam® in its final position.

Lowering the Canal Wall Skin Flaps and Closing

The tympanomeatal flap (or separate inferior and superior flaps) is lowered, checking to ensure the graft is covering the perforation (Fig. 39.7b). The gimmick is used to even all edges of the flap and smooth out the graft. By ensuring a smooth transition between the graft, skin flaps and canal wall, there is less risk of iatrogenic epithelial pearl formation as the contour is favorable for outward keratin debris migration. Small pieces of Gelfoam® are placed over the graft for stabilization.

For cases done completely transcanal, the remainder of the external ear canal is packed with antibiotic-soaked Gelfoam® pressed dry, followed by antibiotic ointment (such as polymyxin B and bacitracin [Polysporin]) in the lateral third of the ear canal. A cotton ball is placed in the ear and may be removed the following day.

For cases done through the postauricular approach, the Körner's flap is rotated back into the ear canal and overlies the graft on the posterior canal wall. If a mastoidectomy was performed, it is important that the Körner's flap does not get pulled back into the mastoid cavity while the Palva flap is being closed. This can result in a fistula with the mastoid with subsequent cholesteatoma formation. Avoiding this complication is best done by ensuring a sufficiently long vascular strip and maintaining the height of the posterior canal wall when drilling the mastoidectomy. The postauricular incision is closed with 4–0 Vicryl in the deep dermal layer. Returning transcanal, a speculum is used to inspect the ear canal and ensure proper positioning of the canal skin flaps. The remainder of the external ear is packed with Gelfoam® as previously described. A mastoid dressing is applied at the end of the procedure and may be removed the following day.

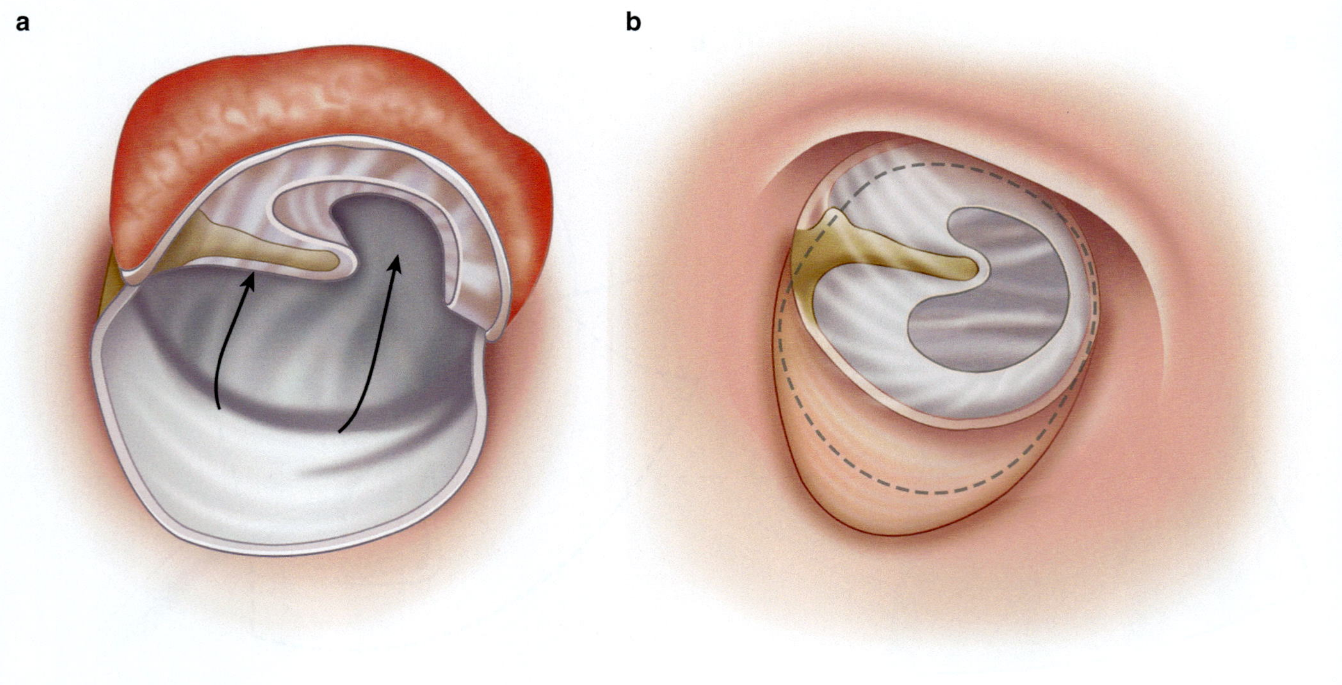

Fig. 39.8 Underlay technique for subtotal perforations not involving the manubrium. The graft is placed medial to the malleus in this example and advanced sufficiently anteriorly to provide overlap with the remnant tympanic membrane. (Jackler RK. *Ear Surgery Illustrated: A Comprehensive Atlas of Otologic Microsurgical Techniques*. Illustrated by Gralapp C. Thieme. 2019)

Cartilage Tympanoplasty

The use of cartilage in tympanic membrane reconstruction was first described by Glasscock and associates in 1982, when they used a cartilage-perichondrial composite graft for repairing retraction pockets and atelectatic tympanic membranes [17]. The rigidity of cartilage augments the overall repair of the eardrum and helps prevent future retraction or reperforation in the setting of chronic Eustachian tube dysfunction. It is also used to reconstruct the attic after it has been eroded by cholesteatoma. Over time, other authors have reported success with this technique and the rate of reperforation was lower when cartilage was used [23, 25, 26].

Cartilage Harvest

When harvesting tragal cartilage, a cut is made using a 15-blade on the medial side of the tragus to conceal the incision (Fig. 39.9a). A 2 mm strip of cartilage in the dome of the tragus may be preserved for cosmesis. Alternatively, the tip may also be removed in order to maintain the continuity of the perichondrium between the two sides. In this latter technique, after trimming the cartilage, the extra pieces are reinserted into the tragal pouch on a bed of Gelfoam® to restore the cosmesis and functional rigidity of the tragus.

The cartilage and attached perichondrium are freed from the overlying soft tissue using Metzenbaum scissors to spread. The inferior incision is made first with a cut as low as possible to maximize the size of the graft. The graft is gently held with Brown-Adson forceps and rotated outward and superiorly. A medial cut is made, and finally, the cartilage is freed superiorly from the incisura. Typically, 1.5 × 1.0 cm graft or larger is obtainable, which is large enough to reconstruct the entire tympanic membrane if needed.

Conchal cartilage may also be harvested, particularly if used as mosaic pieces during reconstruction. During a postauricular approach, the conchal cartilage is exposed by elevating the subcutaneous tissue and muscle off the conchal perichondrium using a 15-blade. The cymba cartilage, seen as a prominent bulge at the superior aspect of the concha, is often harvested. An incision is then made through the cartilage but avoiding transecting the anterior skin. With a combination of blunt dissection using a duckbill and sharp dissection using a 15-blade, the cartilage is removed from the postauricular side.

The cartilage is then fashioned on the cutting block in various ways, depending on the surgical plan. Broadly, the two cartilage grafting techniques commonly employed are: (1) the perichondrium-cartilage island flap, which uses tragal cartilage, and (2) the mosaic or palisading technique, which uses cartilage from the tragus or concha cymba.

Perichondrium and Cartilage Island Flap Technique

In the perichondrium-cartilage island flap technique, perichondrium is reflected off one side of the cartilage but left attached like a tail (Fig. 39.9b, c). It is easier to elevate the perichondrium on the side farthest from the ear canal. This creates a cartilage graft that is eccentrically positioned on the underlying perichondrium. The round knife is used to trim and shape the cartilage to the appropriate size, taking care to keep the underlying perichondrium intact. The graft is placed into the middle ear with the perichondrium facing laterally, and the cartilage is centered in the defect (Fig. 39.10). The perichondrium is checked to ensure full coverage of the defect, and the tail of the perichondrium comes onto the posterior canal wall for stability. If the

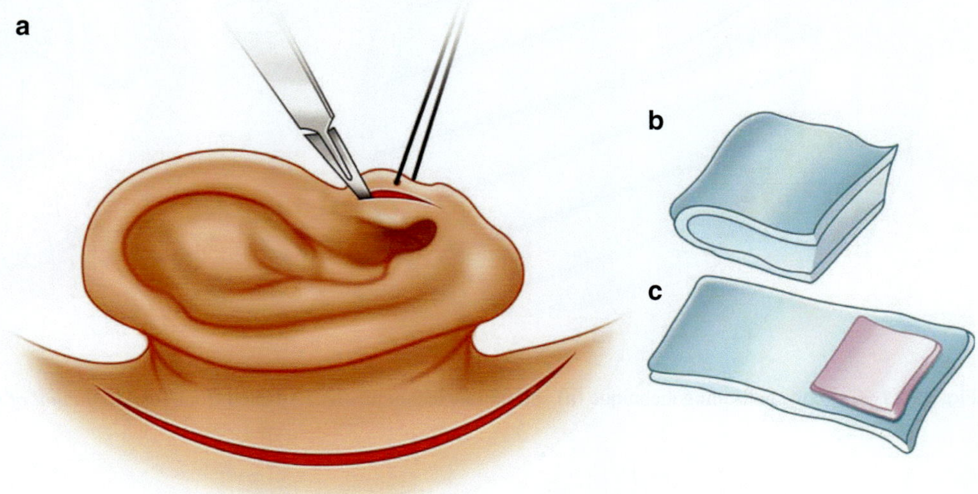

Fig. 39.9 Tragal cartilage-perichondrial graft. (**a**) The graft is harvested by making an incision along the posteromedial aspect of the tragus. (**b**) The cartilage with perichondrium on either side is harvested. (**c**) The perichondrium is elevated off the cartilage but left attached as a tail. The cartilage is eccentrically positioned on the bed of perichondrium. The cartilage is trimmed to the desired size. (Adapted from *Otologic Surgery*. 4th Edition. Eds. Brackmann, Shelton, Arriaga. Elsevier. 2015)

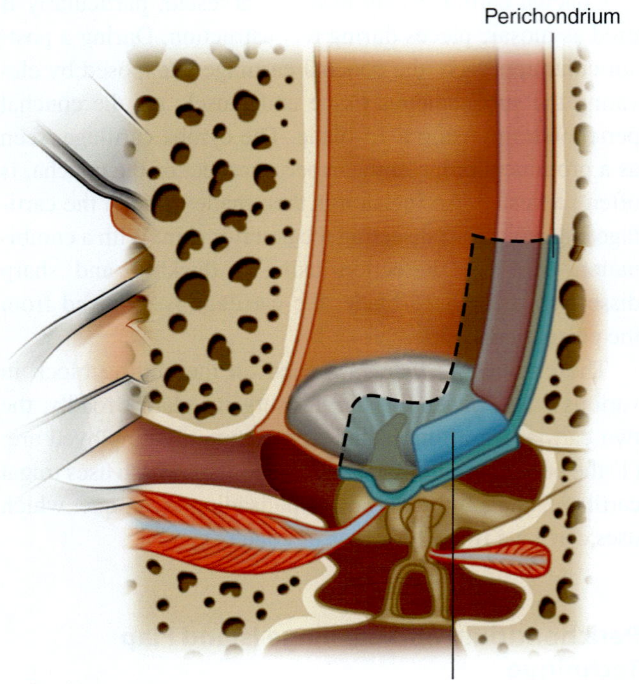

Fig. 39.10 Cartilage tympanoplasty using the perichondrial-cartilage island flap technique. A lateral view demonstrates the graft medial to the remnant drum. The perichondrial tail comes onto the posterior canal wall. This graft may be placed such that the perichondrium sits medial or lateral to the malleus, based on the surgeon's preference. (Adapted from *Otologic Surgery*. 4th Edition. Eds. Brackmann, Shelton, Arriaga. Elsevier. 2015)

malleus is involved, a wedge is cut out to accommodate it. Alternatively, for total tympanic membrane reconstruction, two cartilage islands may be fashioned by taking a central strip of cartilage out, which accommodates the malleus handle, as described by Dornhoffer [27]. The perichondrium-cartilage island flap technique is particularly useful during transcanal tympanoplasty as it avoids the need to make an additional incision to harvest fascia. The tragal cartilage with overlying perichondrium is sufficient to permit reconstruction of the entire tympanic membrane if needed.

Palisading or Mosaic Technique

The palisade technique involves removing perichondrium from both sides of the cartilage, followed by cutting the cartilage into multiple strips and laying them down onto a bed of Gelfoam® (Fig. 39.11a) [27, 28]. The theory is that strips are able to conform better to the individual anatomy and are easier to place. A similar technique is to use mosaic pieces of cartilage, which are assembled like a jigsaw puzzle to reconstruct the tympanic membrane [27]. Typically, there is one large "keystone" piece of cartilage followed by smaller pieces of cartilage to fill in the gaps (Fig. 39.11b). Lateral to the cartilage, perichondrium or fascia is placed. During the healing process, the cartilage becomes incorporated into the substance of the neo-tympanic membrane. This technique is particularly useful when ossiculoplasty is

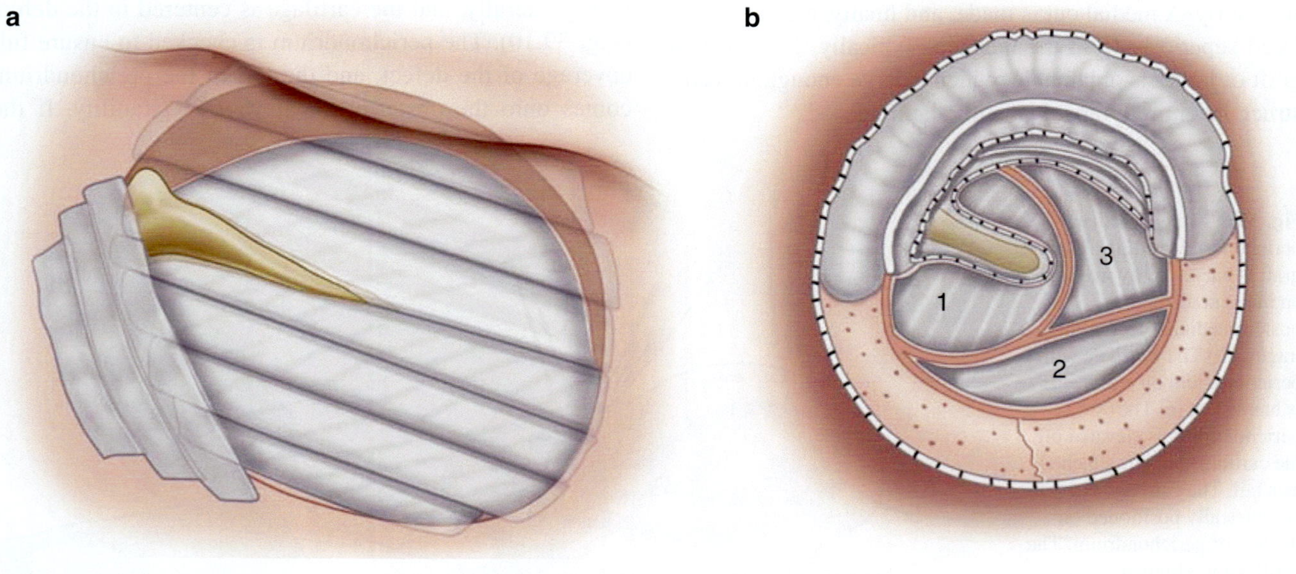

Fig. 39.11 Cartilage palisading technique (**a**) and mosaic technique (**b**). (Adapted from Tos M. *Manual of Middle Ear Surgery*. Thieme. 1993)

being performed because, in addition to reinforcing the tympanic membrane, the cartilage graft acts to prevent prosthesis extrusion.

Some surgeons prefer to thin the cartilage, which makes it more pliable and easier to manipulate. Thinning the cartilage to 0.5 mm (normally it is slightly less than 1 mm thick) may provide acoustic benefits according to some studies, though other middle ear mechanics models have refuted this theory [29, 30].

Additional Grafting Techniques

Lateral-to-Malleus (Over-Under) Tympanoplasty

An alternative grafting technique is to place the graft lateral to the malleus. This is also referred to as the "over-under technique" because the graft goes over the manubrium but under the remnant tympanic membrane and annulus [31]. The technique requires completely elevating the remnant tympanic membrane off the manubrium and umbo (as described above). Leaving behind epithelial debris risks iatrogenic pearl formation since this will be covered by the graft. The technique makes grafting technically easier in chronic perforations, whereby the malleus is often medialized. Greater graft stabilization is achieved because it is compressed between the remnant drumhead and the manubrium, providing an additional point of fixation [31, 32]. Ossiculoplasty (including an incus interposition), which incorporates the malleus, is simpler since the medial side of the malleus is free. Though there is a theoretical risk of graft lateralization, this is not typically observed in practice [32]. The technique works well with the composite perichondrial-cartilage graft by centering the cartilage in the perforation and draping the perichondrial tail lateral to the manubrium and onto the posterior canal wall.

Anterior Graft Stabilization

Anterior marginal perforations present the greatest reconstructive challenge. Reasons for this include reduced vascular supply, poor visualization, insufficient packing and inadequate graft stabilization. Failure to pack Gelfoam® sufficiently anteriorly will result in graft failure as the graft may fall away from the annulus during the postoperative period. Fascia has a tendency to retract during healing, so it is imperative that there is sufficient overlap between the graft and remnant drum. Scoring the mucosa of the protympanum aids with graft healing by promoting vascular ingrowth.

One technique employed for anterior marginal perforations is to combine the swinging-door canal wall flaps with anterior advancement of the canal flaps. The swinging-door flaps (as described previously, Fig. 39.7) can be reflected such that the surgeon has wide access and good visualization. This makes it technically easier to place the graft with precision and to ensure appropriate overlap. Once the graft is in position, the flaps are lowered and advanced inward. This effectively covers any area of deficiency from the graft, stabilizes the graft, and provides increased vascularity to the graft. It also makes the size of the perforation smaller, which aids with faster healing since it is borrowing the canal wall skin for epithelializing the tympanic membrane.

Another technique for anterior graft stabilization is to anchor the graft under the anterior canal wall skin (termed the "anterior-hitch" or "hammock technique") [33, 34]. This is accomplished by "reverse elevating" the anterior annulus such that 1–2 mm of anterior canal wall bone is exposed (Fig. 39.12a) or by designing a large 270° superiorly-based tympanomeatal flap which exposes the anterior canal wall bone (Fig. 39.12b). The graft may then be placed onto the anterior canal wall directly and is locked into place once the anterior canal skin and annulus are lowered back into place. Combining this technique with the lateral-to-malleus placement of the graft effectively provides three points of graft fixation: posteriorly under the vascular strip, centrally

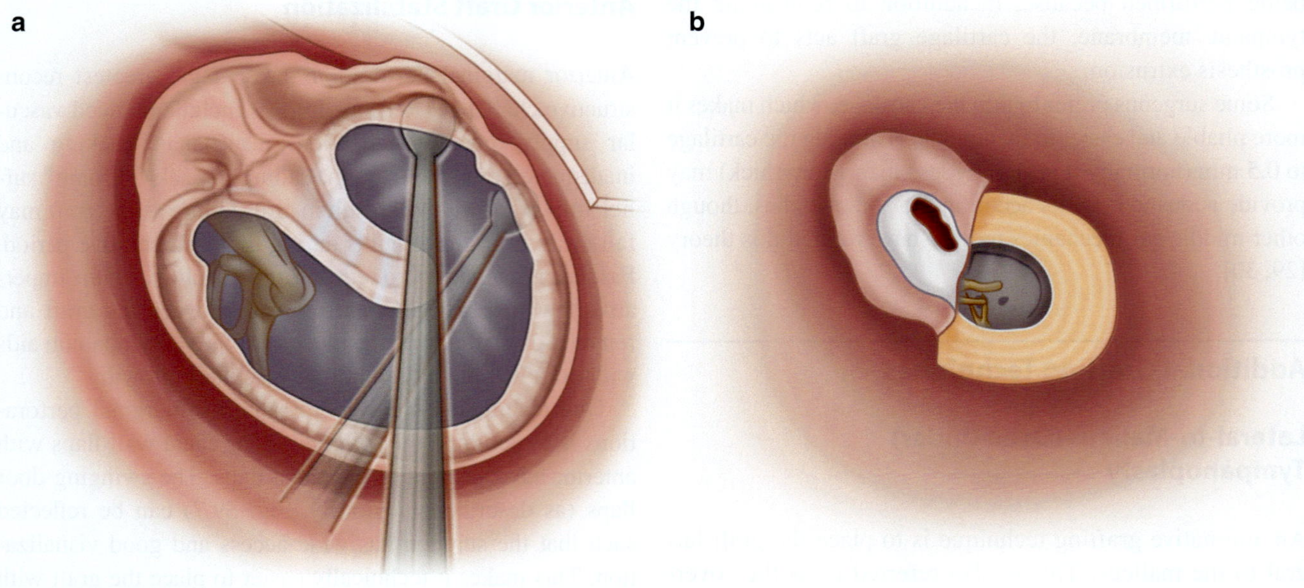

Fig. 39.12 Stabilizing the anterior graft may be achieved by (**a**) reverse elevating the anterior annulus to expose a bony ledge to anchor the graft or by (**b**) elevating a large 270° superiorly based tympanomeatal flap, which exposes the anterior bony ledge ("hammock technique"). ((**a**) Adapted from *Otologic Surgery*. 4th Edition. Eds. Brackmann, Shelton, Arriaga. Elsevier. 2015. (**b**) Adapted from Lalwani AK, Peng R. Efficacy of "hammock" tympanoplasty in the treatment of anterior perforations. *Laryngoscope*. 2013. 123(5);1236–40)

between the manubrium and remnant drumhead, and anteriorly under the canal wall skin.

Postoperative Care

Patients undergoing tympanoplasty with or without mastoidectomy are typically discharged home the day of surgery. Written and verbal discharge instructions are given. The mastoid dressing may be removed the day after surgery. Showering is permitted provided that the patient places a cotton ball impregnated with petroleum ointment in the outer-ear canal. However, the postauricular incision should be kept away from water for 2 days. Nose blowing is avoided. Oral antibiotics are given only to ears with purulent otorrhea at the time of surgery. Pain control is achieved by alternating acetaminophen and a non-steroidal anti-inflammatory. Rarely are narcotic medications required. In patients at risk for nausea and vomiting, promethazine (Phenergan®) is prescribed to be used as needed. Ear drops such as Ciprodex® are prescribed, and the patient is instructed to start these 2 weeks after surgery, using four drops twice a day.

The first postoperative visit is in 3 weeks. The remaining Gelfoam®, if any, over the graft is gently suctioned away. The second postoperative visit is approximately 3 weeks later. Persisting granulations of the ear canal are cauterized with a 25% solution of silver nitrate to promote healing. Hearing improvements may be noticed within 6–12 weeks following surgery. An audiogram is obtained 3–6 months after surgery. If cartilage was used in the reconstruction, it is normal to have a type B tympanogram due to the noncompliant nature of the graft.

Outcomes

Graft-Take Rate

Success rates with tympanoplasty depend on several factors. A favorable outcome is more likely in cases involving a benign central perforation compared to perforations associated with cholesteatoma, poor Eustachian tube function, severe mucosal disease, total loss of the ossicular chain, or those that have failed prior tympanoplasty. Certain patient factors may negatively influence tympanoplasty outcomes, including prior radiation to the temporal bone, immunodeficiencies, and craniofacial anomalies such as cleft palate [6, 26, 35]. Smoking has also been reported to be a negative prognostic factor with a threefold increase in long-term graft failure [36, 37]. These multiple factors make it difficult to compare tympanoplasty results reported in the literature.

In 1982, Glasscock and associates reported a 93% overall graft success rate in their series in 1556 cases of tympanic membrane perforation repair using the postauricular underlay grafting technique [17]. Of the 110 failures, 19 occurred within 3 weeks of surgery, 31 occurred by 3 months, 19 occurred by 6 months, and 41 occurred after 1 year. The use of cartilage grafts has been associated with even higher rates of closure [38]. Dornhoffer reported a 97.6% success rate on 533 cartilage tympanoplasties [27]. Glasscock reported a 96% success rate with cartilage tympanoplasty done for atelectasis [39].

Complications

The most common complication of tympanoplasty is reperforation, which occurs in 5–10% of cases. For these patients, revision tympanoplasty may be offered, and the results are satisfactory. Gustatory changes may occur due to manipulation of the chorda tympani nerve. Stretching of the nerve typically results in more symptoms than transection. Complete recovery has been reported in 76% of cases [40]. Conductive hearing loss may occur and is at greater risk in patients who have small conductive hearing losses preoperatively, especially in the setting of cholesteatoma, whereby the mass itself is the conduit for sound conduction. Otorrhea may occur in 6% of cases and varies from a mild otitis externa to a middle ear infection that results in loss of the graft [17]. Serous otitis media may occur in 2–6% of cases, which may benefit from a ventilation tube if it does not resolve spontaneously [17, 39]. Sensorineural hearing loss and vertigo are risks, occurring in less than 1% and associated with cases involving cholesteatoma, particularly around the stapes [17]. Should the stapes be partially avulsed, it should be repositioned in its original position and stabilized with a tissue graft. Other uncommon complications (all <1%) include delayed (temporary) facial weakness, perichondritis, canal stenosis, mucosalization of the tympanic membrane, and postauricular wound infection [17].

Conclusions

Tympanoplasty is a foundational procedure in otologic surgery. There are many techniques that can be used, and the underlay technique permits good outcomes while minimizing disruption of the native ear canal and tympanic membrane skin relative to lateral graft techniques. Technical nuances are noteworthy in this procedure, as are management nuances in the pre- and postoperative periods.

References

1. Wullstein H. [Technic and early results of tympanoplasty]. Monatsschr Ohrenheilkd Laryngorhinol. 1953;87:308–11.
2. Zöllner F. [Surgical technics for the improvement of sound conduction after radical operation]. Arch Ital Otol Rinol Laringol. 1953;64:455–68.
3. Lierle DM. Standard classification for surgery of chronic ear infection: I. Of the technical procedures in surgery for chronic ear infection * II. Of the gross pathology found at such operations * III. For the reporting of postoperative results of the surgical procedures mentioned. Arch Otolaryngol Head Neck Surg. 1965;81:204–5.
4. Rizer FM. Overlay versus underlay tympanoplasty. Part I: historical review of the literature. Laryngoscope. 1997;107:1–25.
5. Glasscock ME. Symposium: contraindications to tympanoplasty: II. An exercise in clinical judgment. Laryngoscope. 1976;86:70–6.
6. Russell JS, Cox MD, Anderson SR, Dornhoffer JL. Pediatric cartilage tympanoplasty with primary intubation. Otol Neurotol. 2015;36:453–6.
7. Saito T, et al. Recent outcome of tympanoplasty in the elderly. Otol Neurotol. 2001;22:153–7.
8. Vrabec JT, Deskin RW, Grady JJ. Meta-analysis of pediatric tympanoplasty. Arch Otolaryngol Head Neck Surg. 1999;125:530.
9. Collins WO, Telischi FF, Balkany TJ, Buchman CA. Pediatric tympanoplasty: effect of contralateral ear status on outcomes. Arch Otolaryngol Head Neck Surg. 2003;129:646.
10. Hartzell LD, Dornhoffer JL. Timing of tympanoplasty in children with chronic otitis media with effusion. Curr Opin Otolaryngol Head Neck Surg. 2010;18:550–3.
11. House WF, Sheehy JL. Myringoplasty: use of ear canal skin compared with other techniques. Arch Otolaryngol. 1961;73:407–15.
12. Shea JJ. Vein graft closure of eardrum perforations. Arch Otolaryngol. 1960;72:445–7.
13. Sheehy JL, Glasscock ME. Tympanic membrane grafting with temporalis fascia. Arch Otolaryngol. 1967;86:391–402.
14. Storrs LA. Myringoplasty with the use of fascia grafts. Arch Otolaryngol. 1961;74:45–9.
15. Moon CN. Loose areolar connective tissue: a graft for otologic surgery. Laryngoscope. 1973;83:771–7.
16. Cueva RA. Areolar temporalis fascia: a reliable graft for tympanoplasty. Am J Otol. 1999;20:709–11.
17. Glasscock ME, Jackson CG, Nissen AJ, Schwaber MK. Postauricular undersurface tympanic membrane grafting: a follow-up report. Laryngoscope. 1982;92:718–27.
18. D'Eredità R. Porcine small intestinal submucosa (SIS) myringoplasty in children: a randomized controlled study. Int J Pediatr Otorhinolaryngol. 2015;79:1085–9.
19. Downey TJ, Champeaux AL, Silva AB. AlloDerm tympanoplasty of tympanic membrane perforations. Am J Otolaryngol. 2003;24:6–13.
20. Patel PN, Jayawardena ADL, Walden RL, Penn EB, Francis DO. Evidence-based use of perioperative antibiotics in otolaryngology. Otolaryngol Head Neck Surg. 2018;158:783–800.
21. Singh S, Blakley B. Systematic review of ototoxic pre-surgical antiseptic preparations - what is the evidence? J Otolaryngol Head Neck Surg. 2018;47:18.
22. Glasscock ME. Tympanic membrane grafting with fascia: overlay: vs. undersurface technique. Laryngoscope. 1973;83:754–70.
23. Schwaber MK. Postauricular undersurface tympanic membrane grafting: some modifications of the "swinging door" technique. Otolaryngol Head Neck Surg. 1986;95:182–7.
24. Michaelides E, Kansal A, Rutter S, Schutt CA. The malleus cap: anatomic description of cartilage of the lateral process of the malleus. Am J Otolaryngol. 2017;39:208–11.
25. Levinson RM. Cartilage-perichondrial composite graft tympanoplasty in the treatment of posterior marginal and attic retraction pockets. Laryngoscope. 1987;97:1069–74.
26. Tan HE, Maria PLS, Eikelboom RH, Anandacoomaraswamy KS, Atlas MD. Type I tympanoplasty meta-analysis. Otol Neurotol. 2016;37:838–46.
27. Dornhoffer J. Cartilage tympanoplasty: indications, techniques, and outcomes in a 1,000-patient series. Laryngoscope. 2003;113(11):1844–56.

28. Jeffery CC, Shillington C, Andrews C, Ho A. The palisade cartilage tympanoplasty technique: a systematic review and meta-analysis. J Otolaryngol Head Neck Surg. 2017;46:48.
29. Zahnert T, Huttenbrink K, Murbe D, Bornitz M. Experimental investigations of the use of cartilage in tympanic membrane reconstruction. Am J Otol. 2000;21:322–8.
30. Aarnisalo AA, et al. Middle ear mechanics of cartilage tympanoplasty evaluated by laser holography and vibrometry. Otol Neurotol. 2009;30:1209–14.
31. Kartush JM, Michaelides EM, Becvarovski Z, LaRouere MJ. Over-under tympanoplasty. Laryngoscope. 2002;112:802–7.
32. Yawn RJ, Carlson ML, Haynes DS, Rivas A. Lateral-to-malleus underlay tympanoplasty: surgical technique and outcomes. Otol Neurotol. 2014;35:1809–12.
33. Peng R, Lalwani AK. Efficacy of 'hammock' tympanoplasty in the treatment of anterior perforations. Laryngoscope. 2013;123:1236–40.
34. Jung TTK, Park SK. Mediolateral graft tympanoplasty for anterior or subtotal tympanic membrane perforation. Otolaryngol Head Neck Surg. 2005;132:532–6.
35. Boronat-Echeverría NE, Reyes-García E, Sevilla-Delgado Y, Aguirre-Mariscal H, Mejía-Aranguré JM. Prognostic factors of successful tympanoplasty in pediatric patients: a cohort study. BMC Pediatr. 2012;12:67.
36. Becvarovski Z, Kartush JM. Smoking and tympanoplasty: implications for prognosis and the middle ear risk index (MERI). Laryngoscope. 2001;111:1806–11.
37. Uguz MZ, Onal K, Kazikdas KC, Onal A. The influence of smoking on success of tympanoplasty measured by serum cotinine analysis. Eur Arch Otorhinolaryngol. 2007;265:513–6.
38. Mohamad SH, Khan I, Hussain SSM. Is cartilage tympanoplasty more effective than fascia tympanoplasty? A systematic review. Otol Neurotol. 2012;33:699–705.
39. Glasscock ME, Hart MJ. Surgical treatment of the atelectatic ear. Oper Tech Otolaryngol Head Neck Surg. 1992;3:15–20.
40. Michael P, Raut V. Chorda tympani injury: operative findings and postoperative symptoms. Otolaryngol Head Neck Surg. 2007;136:978–81.

Tympanoplasty: Overlay Technique

40

Nicholas L. Deep and Peter A. Weisskopf

Introduction

Overlay tympanoplasty (also known as lateral graft tympanoplasty) is one of the two major tympanoplasty techniques. It involves placement of the graft lateral to the fibrous annulus but medial to the manubrium of the malleus to prevent lateralization. The remnant tympanic membrane is completely deepithelialized in order to avoid iatrogenic cholesteatoma formation. Superior visualization is achieved by drilling of the bony anterior canal wall, which is necessary for proper placement and healing of the graft. Executing the technique successfully requires meticulous attention to detail, but a high success rate with graft take and restoration of function can be achieved, even in the chronically draining ear. Indications for overlay tympanoplasty, details of the surgical steps and technical nuances, and postoperative complications are discussed.

History

Initial experiences with overlay tympanoplasty were reported by Wullstein and Zollner, who placed split- or full-thickness skin grafts on the denuded tympanic membrane remnant [1, 2]. Unfortunately, postoperative complications were commonly encountered, including a poor graft-take rate (71%), excessive desquamation, inflammation, graft eczema, and secondary perforation [3]. In 1956, Sooy described using a pedicle graft of canal skin to close marginal perforations [4]. In 1961, House described using a free graft using canal skin with the underlying periosteum intact, which was placed over the deepithelialized remnant drum [3]. Initial results with this technique were promising; however, actively draining ears still demonstrated poor graft take and total perforations could not be repaired. In 1964 an article by James Sheehy at the Otologic Medical Group (to become the House Ear Clinic) described the early results using fascia and what he described as the "outer surface technique." The early results demonstrated a 96% graft take rate, and they began using fascia in the majority of their cases [5]. By the mid-1960s, skin grafts were abandoned as the use of temporalis fascia, described by Storrs, resulted in dramatic improvement in healing rates of overlay grafts, which exceeded 90% [5–7]. Today, overlay tympanoplasty remains the preferred technique of the surgeons at the House Clinic.

Indications

The goal of tympanoplasty is to achieve a safe, dry ear by eradicating middle-ear disease and to improve hearing by closing the tympanic membrane perforation and/or reconstructing the ossicular chain. The general indications, contraindications and preoperative considerations for tympanoplasty have been previously discussed 38.

The overlay technique is primarily indicated in cases of total or near-total tympanic membrane perforations, large anterior perforations or those with obstructed visualization due to a prominent anterior canal wall bulge, extensive middle ear mucosal disease, previous tympanoplasty failure, or chronic otitis with an actively draining ear despite medical treatment. The lateral graft is particularly useful in retracted "floppy" tympanic membranes and will often restore middle ear aeration in ears that have been chronic problems for many years.

N. L. Deep
Department of Otolaryngology—Head and Neck Surgery, Division of Otology and Neurotology, Mayo Clinic, Phoenix, AZ, USA
e-mail: deep.nicholas@mayo.edu

P. A. Weisskopf (✉)
Division of Otology and Neurotology, Departments of Otolaryngology and Neurosurgery, Mayo Clinic, Phoenix, AZ, USA
e-mail: weisskopf.peter@mayo.edu

A. D. Sweeney et al. (eds.), *Haynes-Glasscock-Shambaugh Surgery of the Ear*, https://doi.org/10.1007/978-3-032-18264-7_40

Advantages and Disadvantages

There are several advantages of the overlay technique compared to the underlay technique. First, the anterior bulge of the external canal is removed as a normal part of the procedure, which provides excellent exposure of the entire tympanic membrane both intraoperatively and postoperatively. Second, the middle ear space is preserved because the graft is placed lateral to the tympanic annulus. This improves aeration and reduces the risk of postoperative adhesions from forming between the promontory and drum, particularly in cases of extensive middle ear mucosal disease with a retracted malleus. Third, the overlay technique does not depend on the amount or viability of the remnant tympanic membrane. As little or as much of the remnant drum may be removed as necessary to eliminate disease, without affecting the ability of the graft to heal. In experienced hands, this leads to a high graft-take rate, which, by some reports, is higher than what is seen with an underlay technique, which has a more limited graft bed and is more dependent on vascularity from the remnant drum [8]. Lastly, since this technique replaces the entire drum, it may be used in essentially all cases, irrespective of preoperative condition of the drum. Additionally, the new tympanic membrane has a new and robust blood supply, which may help decrease future perforation due to a previously diseased drum that has simply been "patched" with an underlay graft.

The primary disadvantages include difficulty with learning the technique and the precision in execution required for proper healing. In addition, epithelial cysts or iatrogenic cholesteatoma may form as a result of incomplete removal of squamous epithelium. Anterior sulcus blunting or graft lateralization may result in worse hearing. In addition, the overlay graft generally takes longer to heal (upwards of 6–8 weeks) compared to the underlay technique.

Surgical Technique

General Considerations

The overlay tympanoplasty is typically performed on an outpatient basis under general anesthesia. Local anesthesia may also be considered in adult patients who are cooperative and in cases not requiring a mastoidectomy. When possible, laryngeal mask anesthesia (LMA) is preferred as it avoids tracheal irritation, allows the patient to breathe spontaneously, and allows for a smoother and quicker extubation without severe coughing or retching. If facial nerve monitoring is being performed, communication with the anesthesiologist to withhold any long-lasting muscle paralytic is essential.

Patient Prep and Positioning

Lidocaine with 1:100,000 epinephrine is injected into the postauricular incision and into four quadrants at the external meatus. The remainder of the local anesthetic is dispensed onto the sterile field for injection of the vascular strip under the microscope. The hair is shaved approximately 3 cm behind the ear. The patient's head should be in a neutral position with the body, which may necessitate placement of a towel or donut. The head should then be rotated away from the surgeon and slightly flexed such that the chin is tucked and pointing to the contralateral shoulder. The patient should be strapped to the operating table to ensure stability. A slight Trendelenburg position (head down) is helpful. The patient is then prepped in standard fashion for otologic surgery.

Injection Under the Microscope

The vascular strip is identified between the tympanomastoid and tympanosquamous suture lines. In a slow, controlled fashion, the vascular strip is infiltrated with lidocaine with 1:100,000 epinephrine. Injection of the anterior canal skin is also performed to avoid troublesome bleeding, which may occur when this area is incised early in the procedure. Unlike a transcanal procedure, swelling or blebbing of the canal skin is of no consequence as the retroauricular approach allows excellent visualization.

Transmeatal Canal Incisions

Using a Beaver blade (6900) or a No.1 (sickle) knife, vascular strip incisions are made starting superiorly approximately 2–3 mm lateral to the bony annulus along the tympanosquamous suture line, which is roughly in line with the short process of the malleus. The second (inferior) canal incision is made along the tympanomastoid suture line (Fig. 40.1). These incisions should extend laterally into the cartilaginous ear canal to facilitate easy identification during the postauricular exposure. Undercutting the skin incision laterally will facilitate finding the flap without extending the incision into the conchal bowl. Using a large round knife and 5 Fr suction, these incisions are connected at their medial end (approximately 2 mm lateral to the annulus) and the vascular strip is back-elevated off the bone in a medial to lateral direction (Fig. 40.2).

Postauricular Exposure

The postauricular incision is then made using a No. 15 blade approximately 1 cm away from the postauricular sulcus (Fig. 40.3). The superior aspect of the skin incision should

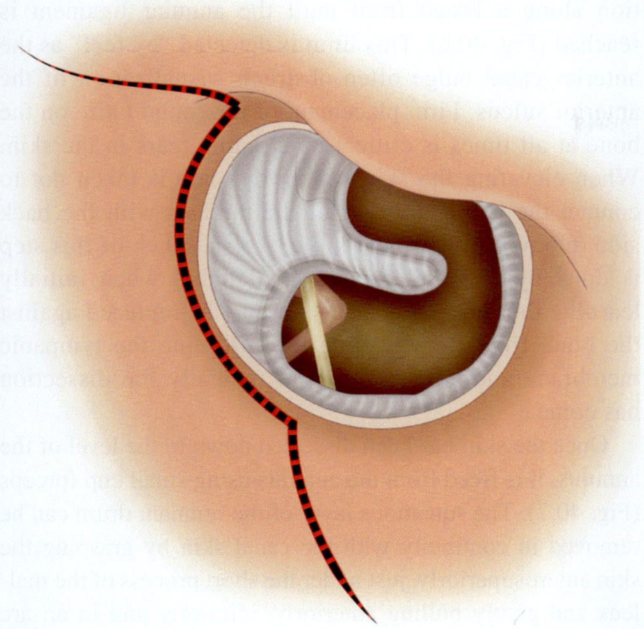

Fig. 40.1 Vascular strip incisions. (Adapted from *Otologic Surgery*. 4th Ed. Eds. Brackmann D, Shelton C, Arriaga MA. Elsevier. 2015)

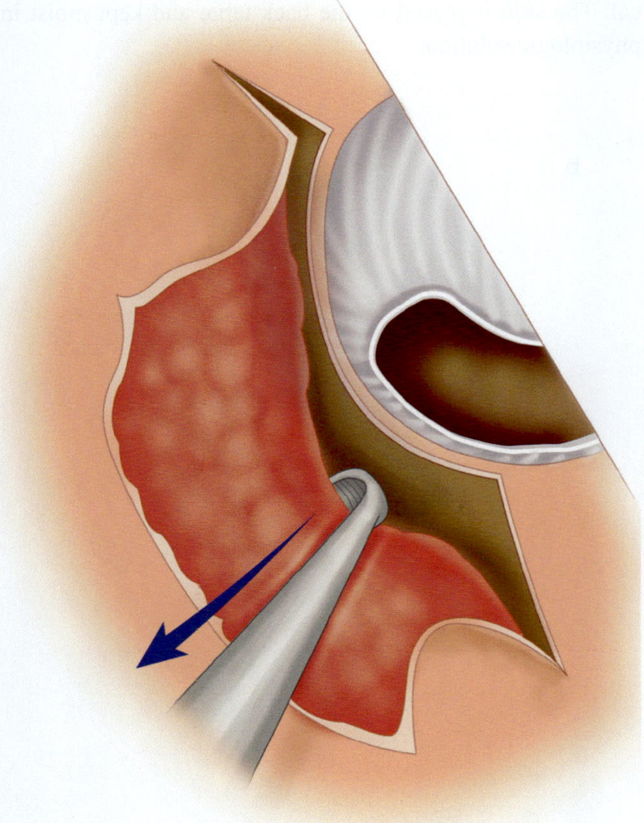

Fig. 40.2 Back-elevation of vascular strip. (Adapted from *Otologic Surgery*. 4th Ed. Eds. Brackmann D, Shelton C, Arriaga MA. Elsevier. 2015)

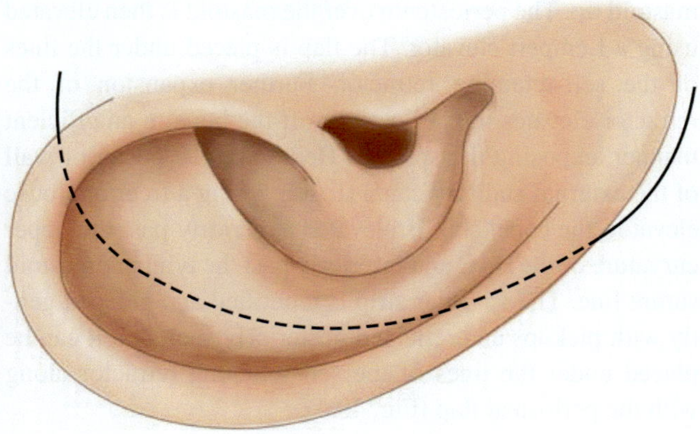

Fig. 40.3 Postauricular incision. The dotted line indicates where the incision would be cosmetically hidden by the auricle. (Adapted from Riser FM. Overlay versus underlay tympanoplasty. Part 1: Historical Review of the Literature. *Laryngoscope*. 1997. 107(12 Pt 2): 1–25)

extend sufficiently anteriorly and approximately in line with the anterior edge of the ear canal in order to facilitate good visualization once the ear is turned forward. The inferior aspect of the incision should extend at least to the floor of the external auditory canal. Dissection should come down onto the temporalis fascia superiorly. A self-retaining retractor is then placed.

Harvest of Fascia

An assistant places a Senn Rake to retract the superior skin margin, exposing the temporalis fascia. Finger dissection can quickly and efficiently clear the loose areolar connective tissue from the temporalis fascia. An incision is made with a No. 15 blade through the fascia only, approximately 1 cm above the inferior border of the muscle. Preserving a cuff of muscle with overlying fascia will facilitate closure at the end of the case. Next, using Adson-Brown forceps and baby Metzenbaum scissors, a 2 × 2 cm piece of temporalis fascia is retrieved. This is placed on a cutting block and the edges are unfurled. Any adherent muscle or fat is gently removed and subsequently placed under a heat lamp to be dehydrated.

Retracting the Vascular Strip

The zygomatic ridge is then palpated. Using monopolar cautery, a horizontal incision through the periosteum is made starting from the root of the zygoma along the linea temporalis posteriorly to the level of the skin incision. The incision is then continued in an anterior-inferior direction towards the mastoid tip. The periosteum over the mastoid is then elevated using a Lempert elevator. The flap is placed under the tines of the self-retaining retractor. Further expansion of the retractor elevates the periosteum off the bone in an efficient manner, exposing the spine of Henle and the posterior wall of the external auditory canal (EAC). Using a freer or House elevator, the canal skin is elevated superiorly past the upper curvature of the EAC and inferiorly past the tympanomastoid suture line. The vascular strip is identified and grasped gently with pickups and reflected posteriorly such that it can be placed under the tines of the self-retaining retractor along with the periosteal flap (Fig. 40.4).

Removing the Canal Skin

Using a Beaver blade, a semilunar incision is made at the anterior canal skin just medial to the bony-cartilaginous junction. The incision extends to connect the lateral ends of the two vascular strip incisions (Fig. 40.5). When making this cut, it is helpful to bevel the edge toward the bony canal, such that a sliver of cartilage remains attached to the skin, thereby enlarging the cartilaginous canal slightly as well.

Using a round knife and a 3 Fr suction, the canal skin and periosteum is elevated from a lateral to medial direction along a broad front until the annular ligament is reached (Fig. 40.6). This limit is detected "by feel" as the anterior canal bulge often obstructs visualization of the anterior sulcus. Firm placement of the round knife on the bone at all times is critical to avoiding tears in the skin. When elevating the skin superiorly, care is taken not to contact the lateral process of the malleus with the back side (elbow) of the round knife. Again, much of this step is done by feel and can be challenging when initially learning the procedure. The skin may be replaced against the bone from time to time to reexamine the tympanic membrane and confirm how far medially the dissection has come.

Once the skin has been dissected down to the level of the annulus, it is freed from the annulus using small cup forceps (Fig. 40.7). The squamous layer of the remnant drum can be removed in continuity with the canal skin by grasping the skin anterosuperiorly, just under the short process of the malleus and gently pulling anteriorly, inferiorly and in an arc motion paralleling the annulus. A round knife is used to scrape the annulus to ensure the removal of all epithelium. If possible, the annulus is preserved within its sulcus, which serves as support for the new graft; however, this is not critical. The skin is placed on the back table and kept moist in physiologic solution.

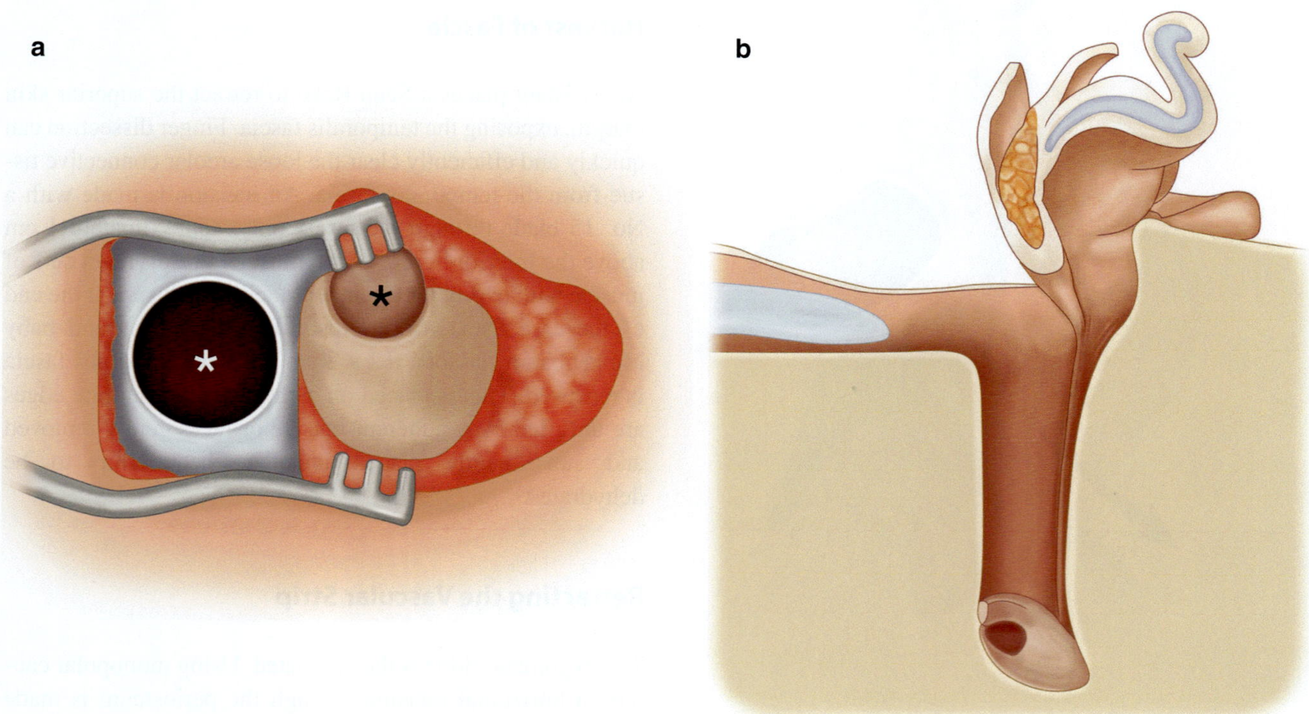

Fig. 40.4 (**a**) Surgeon's view and (**b**) side view after a postauricular approach with anterior reflection of vascular strip. In (**a**), a black asterisk identifies the ear canal, and a white asterisk identifies the temporalis muscle through a defect in the temporalis fascia, from which a graft has been harvested. (Adapted from Sheehy JL, Glasscock 3rd ME. Tympanic membrane grafting with temporalis fascia. *Arch Otolaryngol*. 1967. 86(4): 391–402)

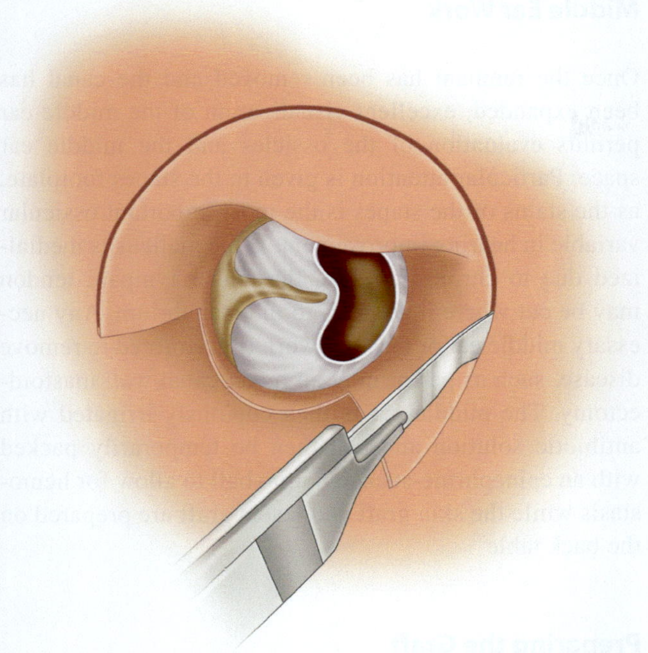

Fig. 40.5 Semilunar incision to connect the lateral ends of the vascular strip incisions. (Adapted from Riser FM. Overlay versus underlay tympanoplasty. Part 1: Historical Review of the Literature. *Laryngoscope*. 1997. 107(12 Pt 2): 1–25)

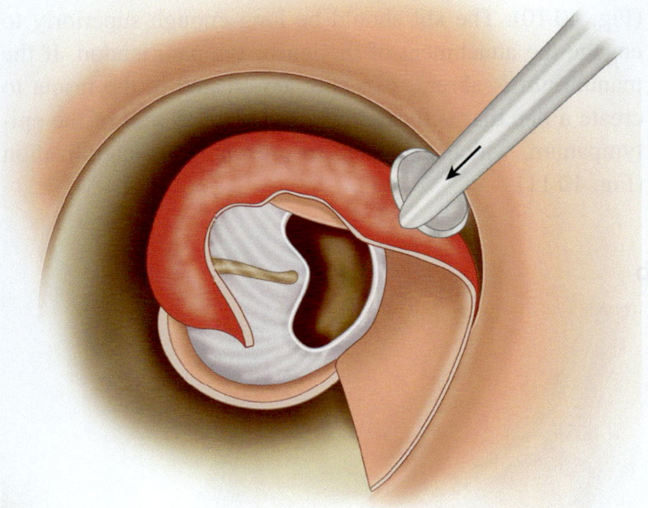

Fig. 40.6 Elevating ear canal skin. (Adapted from Riser FM. Overlay versus underlay tympanoplasty. Part 1: Historical Review of the Literature. *Laryngoscope*. 1997. 107(12 Pt 2): 1–25)

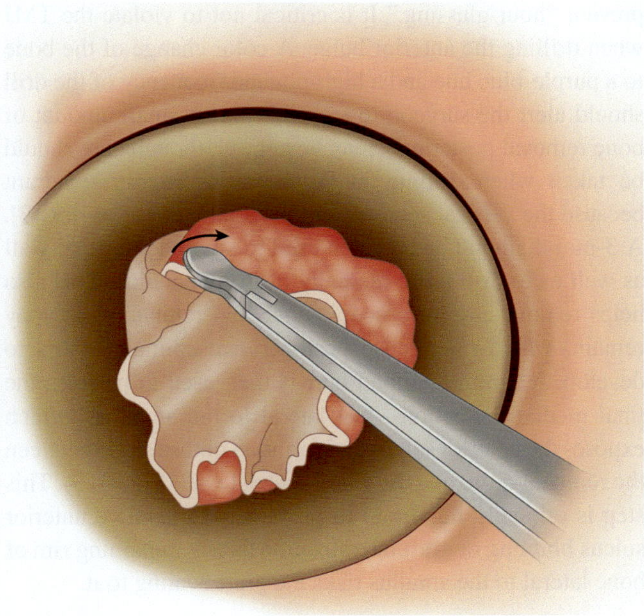

Fig. 40.7 De-epithelializing the remnant tympanic membrane and removing ear canal skin. (Adapted from *Otologic Surgery*. 4th Ed. Eds. Brackmann D, Shelton C, Arriaga MA. Elsevier. 2015)

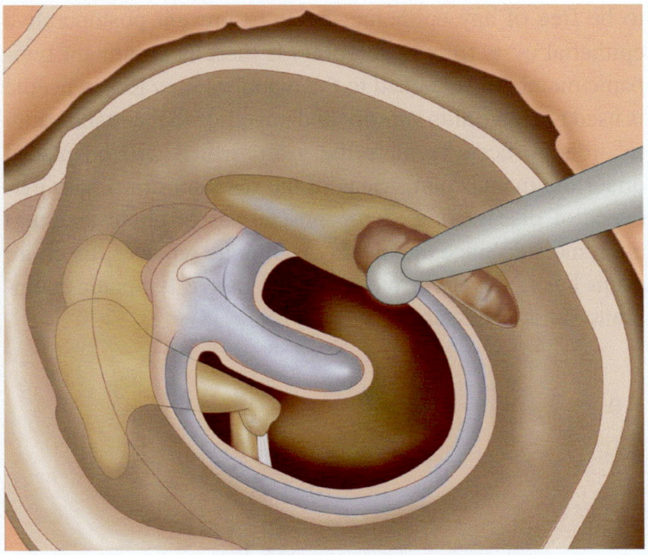

Fig. 40.8 Canaloplasty in which the anterior hump of the canal is being removed. (Adapted from *Otologic Surgery*. 4th Ed. Eds. Brackmann D, Shelton C, Arriaga MA. Elsevier. 2015)

Canaloplasty

The canal is enlarged in order to maximize visualization for middle ear dissection as well as to improve postoperative monitoring of the ear, particularly at the anterior sulcus (Fig. 40.8). The goal of the canaloplasty is to see the entire annulus and to create a funnel-shaped EAC, with its narrowest point at the annulus, and gradually widening laterally. Using a 4-mm cutting burr and continuous irrigation, the spine of Henle is smoothed down if necessary, followed by gradual enlargement of the canal starting at the bony-cartilaginous junction and progressing medially. Superior and inferior troughs are drilled first, followed by skeletonizing the mid-portion of the canal wall over the temporomandibular joint (TMJ) in order to maximize the diameter of the canal and to prevent "hour-glassing." It is critical not to violate the TMJ when drilling the anterior bulge. A color change of the bone to a purple-blue hue and a high-pitched frequency of the drill should alert the surgeon to stop drilling. A small amount of bone removal posteriorly may be helpful, though care should be taken when drilling in the posterior-inferior quadrant because the vertical segment of the facial nerve is at risk [9]. A 3-mm diamond burr is then used to smooth the canal wall as well as to drill more medially near the annulus. This also helps remove any microscopic epithelial remnants that may remain, which may cause postoperative epithelial cysts to develop. A 2-mm diamond burr is then used to perform the final medial dissection—just lateral to the annulus—which exposes the anterior sulcus and forms an obtuse angle between the remnant drum and the anterior canal wall (Fig. 40.9). This step is critically important to prevent postoperative anterior sulcus blunting or graft lateralization as any remaining rim of bone lateral to the annulus risks the graft healing to it.

Inspecting the Tympanic Membrane Remnant

The remnant tympanic membrane is evaluated and ensured to be free of any epithelial debris to prevent postoperative epithelial cysts from developing. If there is a remnant tympanic membrane attached to the manubrium, a Rosen needle is used to create slits anterior and posterior to the manubrium in order to accommodate the graft, which will be placed under the manubrium. Areas of the remnant drum with evidence of disease (e.g., tympanosclerosis or cholesteatoma) are removed. Since the overlay technique replaces the entire drum head, salvaging pieces of the native tympanic membrane is not necessary.

Middle Ear Work

Once the remnant has been removed and the canal has been expanded, excellent visualization of the middle ear permits evaluation of the ossicles and the middle ear space. Particular attention is given to the stapes footplate, as the status of the stapes is the most important ossicular variable in hearing improvement. If the malleus is medialized due to chronic disease, the tensor tympani tendon may be cut where it attaches to the manubrium. Any necessary middle ear or mastoid work is performed to remove disease, such as performing an intact canal wall mastoidectomy. The middle ear is then copiously irrigated with antibiotic solution and can then be temporarily packed with an epinephrine-soaked cotton ball to allow for hemostasis while the skin graft and fascia graft are prepared on the back table.

Preparing the Graft

The dried fascia graft is trimmed to an oval shape, measuring approximately 1.3 × 1.5 cm. The fingernail on the surgeon's index finger or ring finger is commonly used as a rough size guide. The anterior edge should be rounded to fit the annular sulcus. A slit is made along the superior aspect of the fascia to allow the graft to be placed under the manubrium (Fig. 40.10). The slit should be long enough superiorly to engage the attachment of the tensor tympani tendon. If the manubrium is absent, two slits are created in the fascia to create a flap that is tucked under the lateral wall of the epitympanum, which may help to prevent graft lateralization (Fig. 40.11).

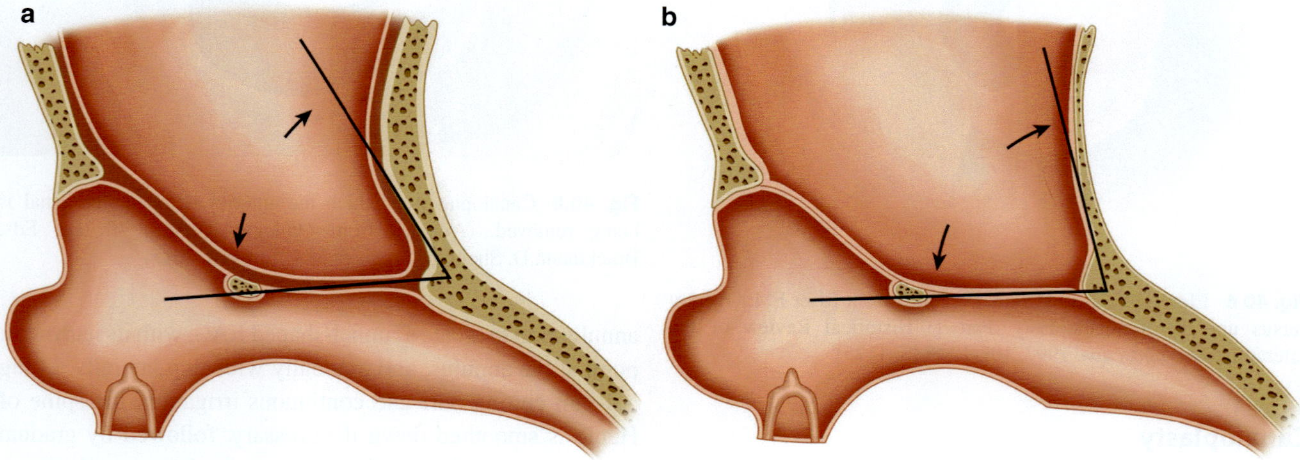

Fig. 40.9 Anterior tympanomeatal angle formed by the tympanic membrane and anterior canal wall (**a**) before and (**b**) after canaloplasty. (Adapted from Farrior JB. The anterior tympanomeatal angle in tympanoplasty: surgical techniques for the prevention of blunting. *Laryngoscope*. 1983. 93(8): 992–7)

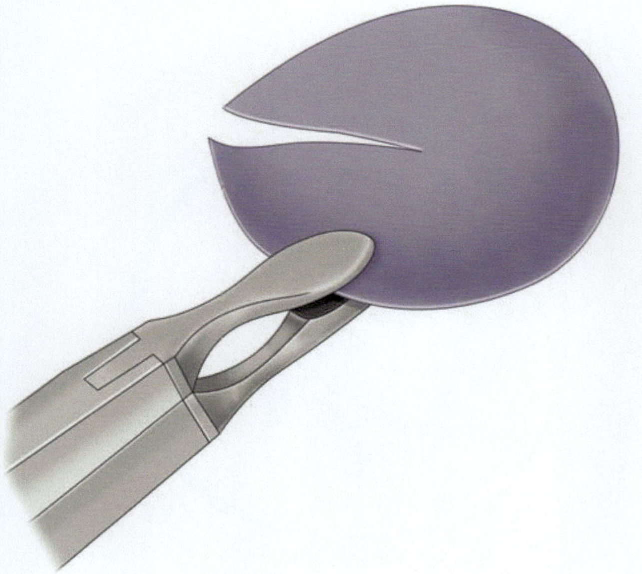

Fig. 40.10 Preparing fascia when the malleus is present. A notch has been incorporated into the fascia for the malleus. (Adapted from Sheehy JL, Glasscock 3rd ME. Tympanic membrane grafting with temporalis fascia. *Arch Otolaryngol*. 1967. 86(4): 391–402)

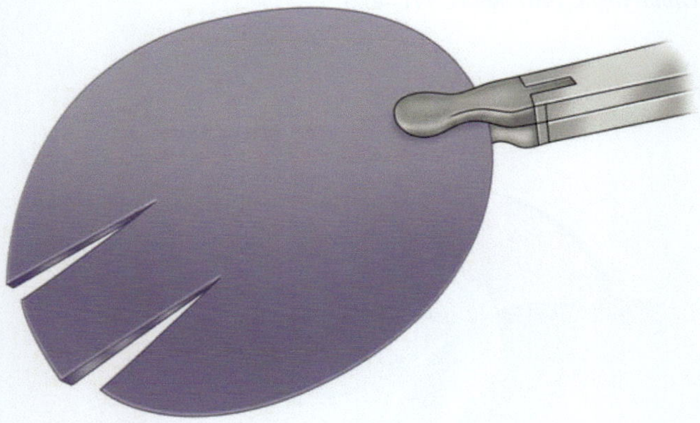

Fig. 40.11 Preparing fascia when the malleus is absent. (Adapted from *Otologic Surgery*. 4th Ed. Eds. Brackmann D, Shelton C, Arriaga MA. Elsevier. 2015)

Packing of Middle Ear

The scrub tech should have compressed pieces of Gelfoam of multiple sizes previously soaked in an antibiotic (ofloxacin) solution that are now only slightly damp. The cotton ball is removed and Gelfoam is used to pack the middle ear to support the graft. The protympanum is packed to block off the Eustachian tube and minimize postoperative pressure changes, which may disturb the graft. Care is taken not to pack medial to the umbo, as this will interfere with the placement of the fascia graft.

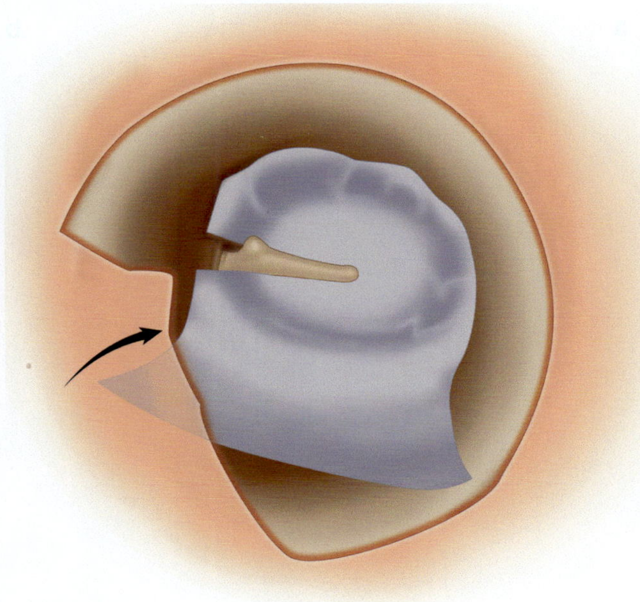

Fig. 40.12 Placing fascia graft medial to the malleus. (Adapted from *Otologic Surgery*. 4th Ed. Eds. Brackmann D, Shelton C, Arriaga MA. Elsevier. 2015)

Grafting

The fascia is grasped with alligator forceps and gently rehydrated for a couple of seconds in a physiologic solution such that it becomes less stiff. It is then placed into position, medial to the manubrium, with the slit of the graft on either side of the manubrium (Fig. 40.12). It is then pulled superiorly to tuck the apex of the slit against the tensor tympani tendon (or to the point where the tensor tendon was previously attached in cases where it is cut). The anterior edge of the graft should sit at the annular sulcus, particularly anteroinferiorly. If a remnant tympanic membrane exists anteriorly, this will support the graft and it can be placed such that the graft does not extend along the anterior canal wall, which may result in postoperative blunting. If no remnant exists, approximately 1 mm of overlap with the anterior canal wall is acceptable.

The posterior part of the graft should be long enough to be draped over the posterior canal wall, where it will be covered by the vascular strip. The graft is inspected and confirmed to be covering the perforation. Next, the two free edges of the graft are folded over the manubrium to cover it (Fig. 40.13). This helps prevent separation of the graft from the malleus handle, provides an improved appearance of the membrane postoperatively, and reinforces the pars flaccida region against developing a retraction pocket.

If an ossicular chain reconstruction is indicated, it may be performed at this time. However, the authors believe that

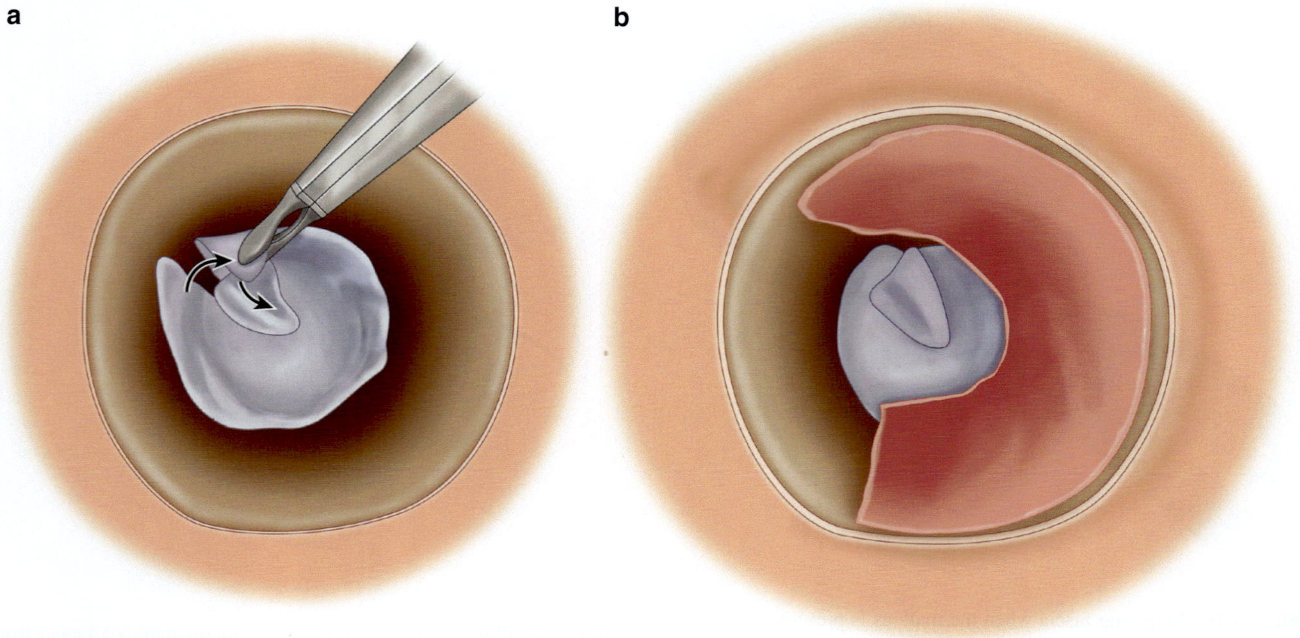

Fig. 40.13 Covering the manubrium of the malleus. (**a**) The anterior edge of the graft is folded over manubrium. (**b**) The posterior edge of the graft is folded over the superior aspect of manubrium, securing graft into place. In (**b**), previously removed ear canal skin has been replaced over the graft anteriorly. (Adapted from Sheehy JL, Glasscock 3rd ME. Tympanic membrane grafting with temporalis fascia. *Arch Otolaryngol*. 1967. 86(4): 391–402)

ossicular reconstruction is better served in a staged fashion, such as during a second-look procedure. At that time, the graft will have healed into position and a more accurate determination of the appropriate prosthesis length can be made.

Replacing Canal Skin

The external canal skin is then trimmed to square off the ragged edges and replaced to cover the exposed bone. In patients with extensive disease that involves the canal skin or a history of radiation to the area, a split-thickness skin graft may be required, which is typically taken from the lower abdomen or thigh in a cosmetically inconspicuous location. The free skin graft is placed such that it just contacts the fascia at the junction of the annulus and bony canal wall, providing a sharp angle between the two, which helps prevent anterior blunting (Fig. 40.14). A slight overlap of the free skin graft on top of the fascia graft by 1 mm is acceptable and may help promote epithelialization of the new drum head. Care should be taken to evert all skin edges to prevent postoperative epithelial cysts from developing. This may be accomplished by placing the medial aspect of the skin on the fascia graft and then dragging it laterally into position, which allows the edges to evert.

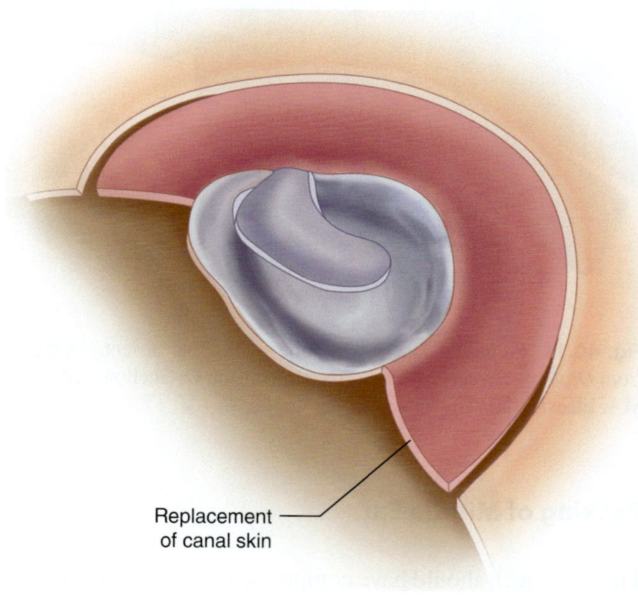

Fig. 40.14 The previously removed ear canal skin has been replaced over the anterior ear canal and graft. (Adapted from *Otologic Surgery*. 4th Ed. Eds. Brackmann D, Shelton C, Arriaga MA. Elsevier. 2015)

Packing and Closure

A tightly rolled piece of Gelfoam is placed into the anterior sulcus to preserve the obtuse angle between the new drum and the anterior canal wall. Several other pieces of moist

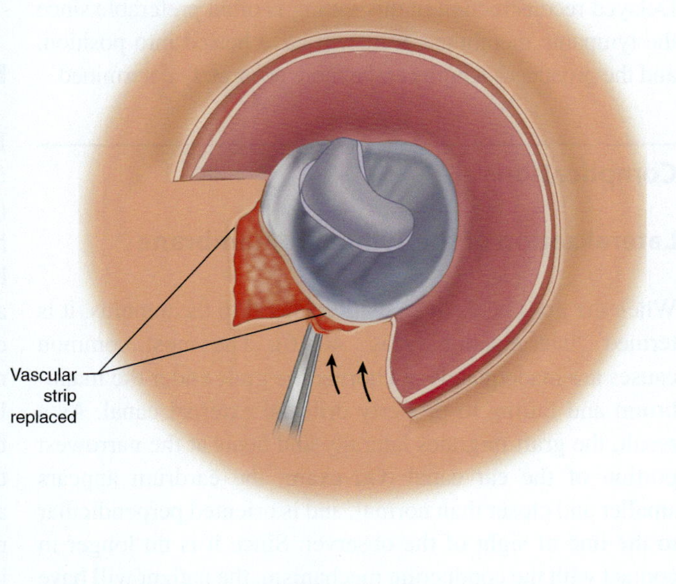

Fig. 40.15 The vascular strip is being replaced over the posterior ear canal. Medially, the vascular strip covers the graft. (Adapted from *Otologic Surgery*. 4th Ed. Eds. Brackmann D, Shelton C, Arriaga MA. Elsevier. 2015)

Gelfoam are tightly packed along the graft and medial canal, leaving room for the vascular strip to be laid down posterosuperiorly (Fig. 40.15). It should be noted that packing the canal cannot rectify the problem of lateralization that may occur if the ear canal is not properly drilled. The vascular strip is then replaced, ensuring that it is laid on top of the fascia graft posteriorly. Returning to the transmeatal view, the vascular strip is grasped with forceps and pulled medially, such that the skin edges are unfurled to avoid burying epithelium. The remainder of the external canal is packed with moist Gelfoam, followed by a cotton ball in the outer meatus. A three-layered closure of the postauricular incision (periosteal flap, subcutaneous layer, skin) is performed in customary fashion. Finally, a mastoid dressing is applied.

Postoperative Care

Routine Care Instructions

Patients are instructed to remove their mastoid dressing the day after surgery. Routine postoperative chronic ear surgery precautions are given in written form, including avoidance of nose blowing, popping ears, bending over, submerging the head under water, lifting weight greater than 10 pounds, heavy activity, and using cotton swabs to attempt to clean the ear. Patients should be instructed not to get water in the ear until cleared by their surgeon that the ear is healed. Showering is permissible 24 hours after surgery; however, the patient should place a cotton ball in the ear and cover it with Vaseline to repel the water. Mild, intermittent pain, particularly while chewing, is expected. A satisfactory postoperative pain regimen can be achieved with acetaminophen plus a nonsteroidal anti-inflammatory medication. The authors do not routinely prescribe antibiotics postoperatively, given that the disease was removed and the ear was thoroughly irrigated with an antibiotic solution during the surgery.

Postoperative Appointments

The first postoperative appointment is made 3 weeks after surgery. The goals of this appointment are to ensure the postauricular incision is healed and there are no signs of infection or complication. At this stage, the ear canal is still packed and the majority of this is left undisturbed, with the exception of any large obstructive pieces at the meatus, which would prevent eardrops from getting in. A prescription for eardrops, an antibiotic, and a steroid is given to the patient to begin using as follows: 3 drops, 3 times a day for 4 weeks. Typically, lower-potency steroid preparations are used to avoid delayed healing. Patients are instructed to continue with dry ear precautions until the next visit.

The second postoperative appointment is made 6 weeks after the first appointment (or 9 weeks after the date of surgery). At this time, the ear should be 80–90% healed. The remainder of the packing is removed from the ear canal, and the graft is inspected for integrity, graft take, position, and to assess for any complications (*discussed below*). Typically, water precautions may be stopped at this time as well.

The third visit is planned for 2–3 months later with an audiogram, which serves as a baseline after surgery. The audiogram is obtained even in patients with ossicular discontinuity awaiting reconstruction, as assessing bone conduction thresholds is beneficial prior to proceeding with the reconstruction. A second-look procedure, with or without reconstruction, is planned for no less than 6 months from the initial operation. Delayed reconstruction in this setting is often preferable since the tympanic membrane graft will have healed into position, and the prosthesis length can be more accurately determined.

Complications

Lateralization of the Tympanic Membrane

When the graft heals in a position lateral to the annulus, it is termed "lateralization" (Fig. 40.16). The most common causes are inadequately anchoring the graft under the manubrium and failing to properly drill the external canal. As a result, the graft migrates laterally and heals at the narrowest portion of the ear canal. On exam, the eardrum appears smaller and closer than normal, and is oriented perpendicular to the line of sight of the observer. Since it is no longer in contact with the conducting mechanism, the patient will have a poor hearing result. Lateralization is typically detected 6–12 months after surgery [10]. Risk factors for lateralization include the presence of a well-aerated middle ear, an unsecured graft, or a prominent anterior bulge at the TMJ. Treatment requires reoperation and replacement of a new graft under the manubrium.

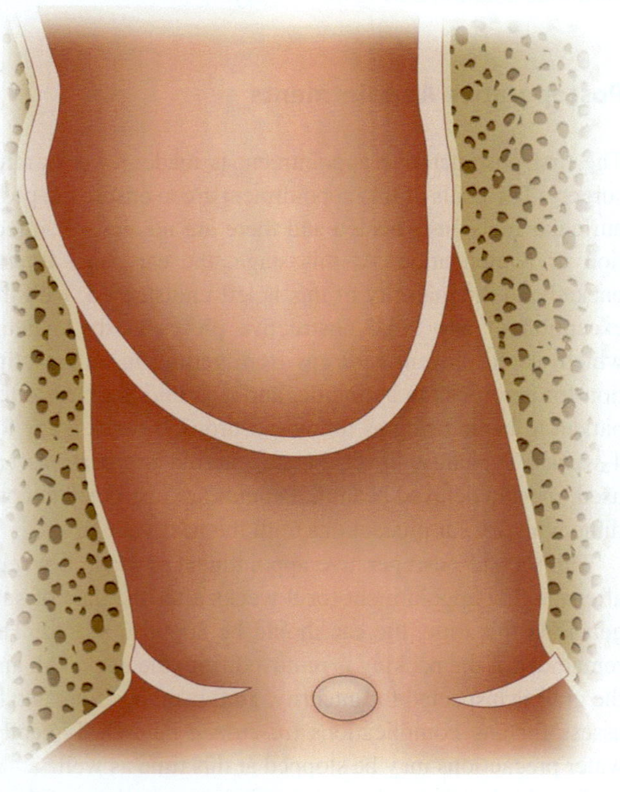

Fig. 40.16 Lateralization of tympanic membrane. The natural location of the membrane (perforated) is shown medial to the neo-tympanic membrane. (Adapted from *Otologic Surgery*. 4th Ed. Eds. Brackmann D, Shelton C, Arriaga MA. Elsevier. 2015)

Blunting in the Anterior Sulcus

Blunting at the anterior sulcus is one of the most common and frustrating complications after overlay tympanoplasty (Fig. 40.17). Minor blunting is usually of no consequence; however, severe blunting may result in a large conductive hearing loss due to the reduced vibratory portion of the drum and potential immobilization of the malleus. The anterior drum appears immobile and indistinguishable from the anterior canal wall. A slightly concave appearance is seen. Postoperative blunting can be minimized by careful surgical technique, including: (1) drilling the anterior canal bulge and the area just lateral to the annulus which converts the acute anterior tympanomeatal angle into an obtuse angle; (2) minimizing graft overlap with the anterior canal wall (as described in the "Grafting" section); (3) replacing the canal skin such that it overlaps the graft by 1 mm, particularly anterosuperiorly; and (4) tightly packing the anterior sulcus with a dried rolled-up piece of Gelfoam [11]. Reoperation is required to fix anterior blunting and may be indicated in cases with a poor hearing outcome. However, if a second-look ossicular reconstruction is planned, the problem may be mitigated by a slightly longer prosthesis.

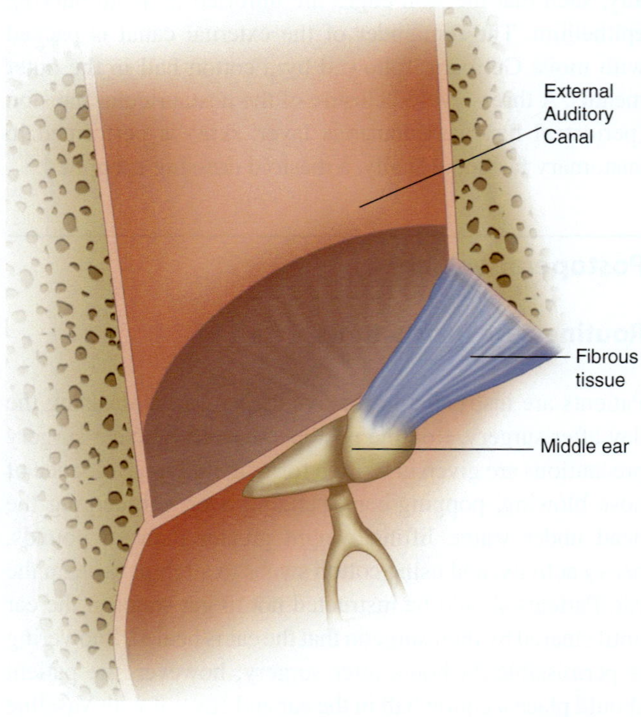

Fig. 40.17 Anterior sulcus blunting. (Adapted from *Otologic Surgery*. 4th Ed. Eds. Brackmann D, Shelton C, Arriaga MA. Elsevier. 2015)

Epithelial Cysts

Epithelial cysts may develop in the ear canal or at the margin of the eardrum where the skin graft contacts the fascia graft. This results when the skin edges are not properly everted during replacement of the canal skin. Epithelial cysts may also develop between the remnant tympanic membrane and the graft as a result of inadequate deepithelialization of the remnant drum (Fig. 40.18). These cysts most commonly occur anteroinferiorly and slowly grow over the years, ultimately resulting in a convex appearance of the anterior sulcus. Cysts may spontaneously rupture or may be marsupialized in office. Occasionally, these may become large and obstructive and require a formal surgical procedure up to and including replacing the initial graft.

Excessive Membrane Thickening

A thickened graft obscures middle ear landmarks, reduces the ability to monitor the ear, and may change the vibratory properties of the drum. This may be caused by the development of fibrous tissue between the middle fibrous layer of the remnant drum and the graft, which may be avoided by removing the majority of the remnant drum prior to grafting. Other factors that may result in a thickened graft are postoperative infection, poor Eustachian tube function, or a thick graft at the beginning. If the fascia graft is thick upon harvesting, it is essential to remove all underlying muscle attached to the graft and adequately dehydrate it with the fascia press and heat lamp to sufficiently thin the graft. Often, a thickened graft will thin over time, so watchful waiting over the course of a year may be reasonable.

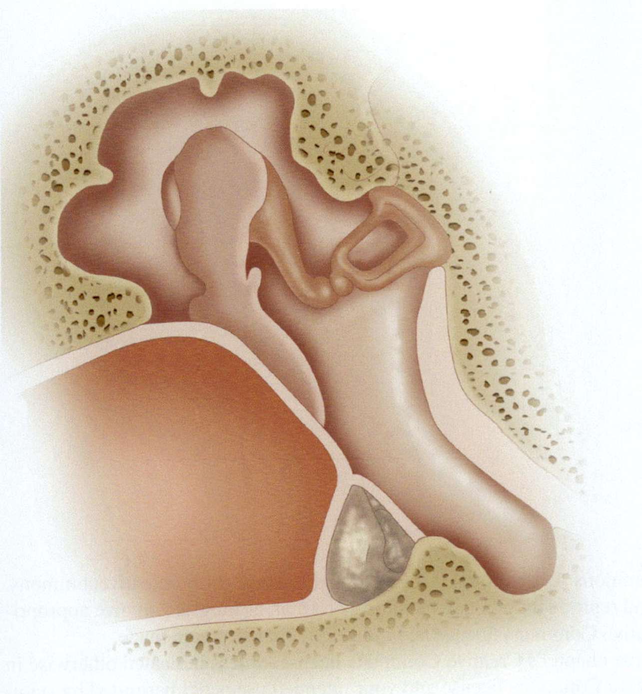

Fig. 40.18 A postoperative epithelial cyst is in the inferior ear canal (asterisk). (Adapted from *Otologic Surgery*. 4th Ed. Eds. Brackmann D, Shelton C, Arriaga MA. Elsevier. 2015)

External Canal Soft Tissue Stenosis

By the second or third postoperative visit, stenosis or webbing along the mid canal may be evident from the healing skin graft. This is managed by incising the stenosis and placing 1 or 2 ear wicks to dilate the canal. Patients tolerate this without local anesthesia since they lose sensation to the medial EAC after the overlay tympanoplasty procedure. The patient is sent home with ear drops to use twice a day to keep the ear wick fresh and dilated, and seen back in one week for reevaluation.

Outcomes

Results of tympanoplasty are measured in terms of the success or failure of graft-take and hearing improvement. These metrics depend upon multiple factors. Negative prognostic factors include Eustachian tube dysfunction, presence of cholesteatoma or atelectasis, previous tympanoplasty failure, a lateralized tympanic membrane, and smoking. As a result of these multiple patient factors and diverse clinical presentations, a direct comparison of long-term outcomes with overlay versus underlay techniques is difficult. Furthermore, the overlay technique is commonly employed in more challenging situations, such as revision tympanoplasty, extensive cholesteatoma with ossicular erosion, advanced mucosal disease, or in the setting of active chronic otitis. Therefore, it is essential to analyze outcomes from these cases separately from cases involving a small, dry central perforation, which are more likely to be treated using an underlay technique.

In experienced hands, success rates with overlay tympanoplasty are high. In a large series of 472 patients published by Sheehy, the graft-take rate was 97% and postoperative air-bone gap (ABG) was closed to <10 dB in 88% of cases [12]. Similarly, in another series of 158 patients published by Rizer, the graft-take rate was 95.6% and closure of the ABG to <10 dB in 80.4% of patients [8]. By comparison, Rizer reported the results of 554 patients undergoing the underlay technique and found a statistically significant lower graft-take rate at 88.8%. Hearing outcomes were not statistically different from the overlay technique, as closure to <10 dB ABG was achieved in 84.9% of patients [8]. These results are in contrast to Glasscock, who reported improved graft-take rate with the underlay technique (96%) compared to the overlay method (91%) [13].

Conclusions

Ultimately, high success with graft healing and acceptable hearing results can be achieved with either lateral or medial grafting tympanoplasty, and the technique employed largely depends on the skills and preferences of the surgeon. The overlay technique is a reliable method for reconstructing the tympanic membrane in essentially all cases of chronic otitis media. It provides maximal exposure of the EAC and middle ear, both during surgery and postoperatively. Potential postoperative complications may be mitigated by meticulous attention to proper surgical technique.

References

1. Wullstein H. Theory and practice of tympanoplasty. Laryngoscope. 1956;66(8):1076–93.
2. Zöllner F. The principles of plastic surgery of the sound-conducting apparatus. J Laryngol Otol. 1955;69(10):637–52.
3. House WF, Sheehy JL. Myringoplasty. Use of ear canal skin compared with other techniques. Arch Otolaryngol. 1961;73:407–15.
4. Sooy FA. A method of repairing a large marginal tympanic perforation. Ann Otol Rhinol Laryngol. 1956;65(4):911–4.
5. Sheehy JL. Tympanic membrane grafting: early and long-term results. Laryngoscope. 1964;74:985–98.
6. Storrs LA. Myringoplasty with the use of fascia grafts. Arch Otolaryngol. 1961;74(1):45–9.
7. Sheehy JL, Glasscock ME 3rd. Tympanic membrane grafting with temporalis fascia. Arch Otolaryngol. 1967;86(4):391–402.
8. Rizer FM. Overlay versus underlay tympanoplasty. Part II: the study. Laryngoscope. 1997;107(12 Pt 2):26–36.
9. Adad B, Rasgon BM, Ackerson L. Relationship of the facial nerve to the tympanic annulus: a direct anatomic examination. Laryngoscope. 1999;109(8):1189–92.
10. Sperling NM, Kay D. Diagnosis and management of the lateralized tympanic membrane. Laryngoscope. 2000;110(12):1987–93.
11. Farrior JB. The anterior tympanomeatal angle in tympanoplasty: surgical techniques for the prevention of blunting. Laryngoscope. 1983;93(8):992–7.
12. Sheehy JL, Anderson RG. Myringoplasty. A review of 472 cases. Ann Otol Rhinol Laryngol. 1980;89(4 Pt 1):331–4.
13. Glasscock ME 3rd. Tympanic membrane grafting with fascia: overlay vs. undersurface technique. Laryngoscope. 1973;83(5):754–70.

Ossicular Chain Reconstruction

41

John L. Dornhoffer and Robert Saadi

Introduction

The goal of ossicular chain reconstruction is to restore the sound-conducting connection between the inner ear and tympanic membrane. This reconstruction should have immediate stability and long-term durability. It should also comply with as many of the gain-benefit principles of ossicular acoustic mechanics as is practical. Several factors influence the results in ossiculoplasty, including the middle ear environment, the qualities of the prosthesis, and the surgical technique, all of which will be addressed in this chapter.

There is no question that the first of these factors, the middle ear environment, is the most important determinant of long-term hearing outcomes with ossicular chain reconstruction. By considering prognostic features of the middle ear environment during the preoperative assessment, patient stratification, realistic expectations, and informed consent are facilitated. The next most important factor influencing results is surgical technique. Even when operating on a diseased middle ear, the surgeon can maintain predictable and reliable outcomes by demonstrating both a fundamental understanding of middle ear mechanics, including the concept of mechanical gain, and a utilization of consistent anatomical relationships. Conversely, the variations in composition and design of the modern prosthesis prove to be least important in predicting outcomes.

Types of Ossicular Reconstruction

Tympanoplasty techniques were classically outlined by Zollner [1] and Wullstein [2] based on underlying tympanic and ossicular pathology. Subsequent modifications of the Wullstein classification have been based on the underlying properties of acoustic mechanics associated with each tympanoplasty type. Understanding this classification system is helpful, not only for purposes of grasping a global and historical view of tympanic membrane and ossicular chain reconstruction, but also for understanding basic principles of middle ear acoustic mechanics.

Type I Tympanoplasty

This procedure involves repair of the tympanic membrane in the setting of an intact native ossicular chain. At most, manipulation of the ossicular chain is limited to interventions aimed at improving mobility, such as lysis of tympanic adhesions or removal of tympanosclerotic foci.

Type II Tympanoplasty

This procedure involves repair of the tympanic membrane in combination with any type of ossiculoplasty procedure that preserves the integrity of the malleoincudal lever mechanism. The most common example of this is repair of a dysfunctional (eroded) incudostapedial articulation. Tympanoplasty with delayed staged ossiculoplasty consisting of an incus-grip stapedotomy could also be considered a subgroup within this category.

It is perhaps worth noting that these modern depictions of type II tympanoplasty differ somewhat from the classic description that was devised to deal with the uncommon scenario of isolated malleus erosion, wherein tympanic membrane grafting is applied directly upon the intact long process of the incus.

J. L. Dornhoffer (✉) · R. Saadi
Department of Otolaryngology—Head and Neck Surgery, University of Arkansas for Medical Sciences, Little Rock, AR, USA
e-mail: dornhofferjohnl@uams.edu

A. D. Sweeney et al. (eds.), *Haynes-Glasscock-Shambaugh Surgery of the Ear*, https://doi.org/10.1007/978-3-032-18264-7_41

Type III Tympanoplasty

This procedure involves repair of the tympanic membrane in combination with any type of ossiculoplasty procedure that does not preserve the integrity of the malleoincudal lever mechanism. These surgeries include removal of the incus and use of a graft or prosthesis to span the defect in the ossicular chain. Type III tympanoplasty includes the vast majority of techniques described for routine ossicular chain reconstruction. Accordingly, type III tympanoplasty classification has been further subdivided according to ossiculoplasty technique.

Stapes Columella Subtype

This type III tympanoplasty involves placement of a tympanic membrane graft directly onto the superstructure of the stapes *without* the use of a prosthesis or any other substantial interposition material.

Minor Columella Subtype

This involves the use of an interposition graft or prosthesis to establish continuity between the tympanic membrane and the superstructure of the stapes. Examples of this include the use of a synthetic partial ossicular replacement prosthesis (PORP) or sculpted ossicular (incus or malleus head) autograft. Interposition prostheses may employ a lateral contact point with the malleus manubrium or may make direct contact with the reconstructed tympanic membrane when the malleus is absent.

Major Columella Subtype

Similar to the minor columella subtype, the major columella subtype also involves interposition ossiculoplasty; however, in this procedure the stapes superstructure is absent. Thus, with a major columella subtype, the interposition graft or prosthesis is set directly upon the stapes footplate. An example is the use of a synthetic total ossicular replacement prosthesis (TORP). Tympanoplasty with delayed staged ossiculoplasty that consists of a malleus-grip stapedotomy could also be considered to fall within this subtype.

Type IV Tympanoplasty

This procedure involves repair of the tympanic membrane in such a manner that the boundary between the mucosalized middle ear space and the epithelialized lateral compartment (external auditory canal, open mastoid cavity, epitympanum) is shifted in a way that renders the stapes footplate externalized as part of the latter. As a result, the tympanic cavity is divided into a smaller-than-normal aerated space in continuity with the Eustachian tube, termed the cavum minor, in which the round window is acoustically shielded, and an external component, in which the mobile stapes footplate is covered by a thin epithelial layer and is directly exposed to incoming sound energy.

Type V Tympanoplasty

Type V tympanoplasty includes the need to address an underlying immobile stapes footplate. It is generally performed in a staged manner once active infectious disease is controlled. Historically, fenestration of the lateral semicircular canal was described as part of this procedure to counteract stapes fixation; however, total footplate removal and a soft tissue seal have generally replaced fenestration.

Preoperative Assessment

When a patient is considered for ossiculoplasty, a thorough history, examination, and audiometric evaluation should be performed on both ears. Following careful removal of cerumen and debris, otoscopy and auto-insufflation with the Valsalva maneuver under binocular microscopy provide a wealth of information. The results of the audiogram should always be correlated with the physical exam, including Weber and Rinne tuning fork tests, especially when a masking dilemma is present due to bilateral conductive hearing loss. If the audiogram and tuning fork exam do not agree, surgery should not be performed until this is reconciled.

A preoperative audiogram can be helpful in suggesting underlying pathology. Generally, a perforation will cause a conductive hearing loss between 5 and 40 dB depending on its characteristics [3]. When the tympanic membrane is intact, a conductive hearing loss greater than 35–40 dB strongly suggests the possibility of ossicular chain dysfunction. Furthermore, the pattern of hearing loss may be typical of particular scenarios; for example, fixation of the lateral ossicular chain generally causes a low-tone conductive hearing loss, with an air-bone gap (ABG) that partially closes in the middle and high frequencies. In contrast, stapes fixation tends to affect the middle and high frequencies to a relatively greater degree [4].

Although the status of the Eustachian tube will impact surgical outcomes, there is no current consensus on the optimal way to reliably assess its function. Auto-insufflation using the Valsalva or Toynbee maneuver is a helpful, albeit non-physiologic, test of tubal patency. The clinical status of the contralateral ear likewise can provide insight into tubal maturity and function in the diseased ear [5]. As part of the Eustachian tube evaluation, the nose should be examined so that allergy, adenoiditis, and rhinosinusitis can be treated in an effort to promote optimized tubal function. Furthermore, aggressive medical treatment of infection involving the ear itself should be undertaken prior to surgery, including aural toilet, and ototopical agent application.

Once patient assessment is complete, a few general rules should be applied to surgical candidacy. First, one should avoid elective surgery on an only-hearing ear as much as is reasonably possible. Second, when bilateral disease is present, surgery should be undertaken on the worse-hearing ear in the absence of any other compelling reason to do otherwise on account of underlying disease. Finally, special consideration should be given to the timing of surgery in the pediatric patient. Potential exceptions to these general rules include the following: surgery on an only-hearing ear to address progressive chronic otitis externa or cholesteatoma is not unreasonable but should be undertaken with extreme caution, and in rare cases of bilateral disease, a better-hearing ear containing more advanced and aggressive disease may need to be addressed first.

Age as a prognostic factor in tympanoplasty is controversial, with contradictory reports present in the literature [6, 7]. The authors' approach to pediatric patients is to avoid repairing the tympanic membrane during the otitis-prone years (≤3 years). If the contralateral ear is normal, routine tympanoplasty is considered at age 4 years for an ear that is dry or only occasionally drains with water contamination [8]. However, if the contralateral ear is abnormal at this time, adenoidectomy is considered and tympanoplasty is deferred until the contralateral ear reaches stable quiescence or the patient reaches age 7 years. If contralateral disease is still present at this time, a more aggressive technique, such as cartilage tympanoplasty, is performed on the worse-hearing ear. The second ear is repaired several months later, but only after the first ear is documented to have a stable satisfactory outcome and is not expected to require further surgery. Of note, other authors' perspectives on this issue are presented in the chapters on tympanoplasty and myringoplasty.

Qualities of the Prostheses

Materials

Numerous synthetic materials have been used in ossicular implants, such as porous high-density polyethylene, plastics, bioactive glass, stainless steel, gold, titanium, and hydroxylapatite. Promising short-term results continue to be published for most of these materials [9], but the long-term histological fate is uncertain in many instances. Each of the two most commonly used materials, hydroxylapatite and titanium, has advantages and disadvantages. Hydroxylapatite is produced by molding, resulting in smooth edges and grooves that have benefit when placed against the tympanic membrane and notched under the malleus, compared to the sharp stamped edges of titanium. Titanium, however, is lighter and more malleable, which makes it possible to change the angle of the prosthesis to facilitate the conical shape of the drum and to create a cradle for secure fit to the stapes. As such, the choice of prosthesis is largely dependent on the philosophy of the surgeon but can also be dictated by the operative technique used. Regardless, there seems to be no clear acoustic advantage of one prosthesis material over the other [10].

Prosthesis Design

Much has been discussed with regard to prosthesis design, including ideal weight, length, and general shape. However, most studies have been performed with laser vibrometry in non-diseased cadaver bones, and whether or not these results can be extrapolated to the diseased ear is yet to be appreciated. The ideal weight of the prosthesis has been examined by a number of investigators. Some researchers suggest that a lighter prosthesis in the range of 3–4 mg functions more effectively (Huttenbrink [11]) whereas others have suggested a weight between 10 and 35 mg to yield the best acoustic response with the vibrometer (Goode and Nishihara [12]). In the latter study, prostheses above this weight would cause low-frequency displacements to fall out of acceptable ranges, and prostheses below this weight would lead to high-frequency losses. Interestingly, the human incus normally weighs 30–40 mg. Realistically, prosthesis weight is probably not of critical importance in the diseased middle ear as long as it falls within these acceptable ranges. Cartilage is usually placed on top of the prosthesis head to prevent extrusion in most cases, and the added weight to the reconstruction appears to have no detrimental effect on the hearing result regardless of which material is used.

There are a myriad of prosthesis shapes available and an equal number of surgeons advocating one over the other. Suffice it to say that the goal of ossiculoplasty is to provide a reconstruction with immediate stability and long-term durability. It should comply with as many of the gain-benefit principles of ossicular acoustic mechanics as is practical. As such, the more stable the initial reconstruction, the higher likelihood of a good long-term outcome. Most synthetic prostheses are divided into Partial Ossicular Replacement Prostheses (PORPs), to be used with an absent incus but present stapes superstructure, and Total Ossicular Replacement Prostheses (TORPs), which are used when both the incus and stapes superstructure are absent or in poor anatomical position. The former usually consists of a head to make contact to the tympanic membrane and/or malleus and a shaft or cradle to facilitate the stapes capitulum and superstructure. These can be further subdivided into designs that are intended to directly impact the undersurface of the drumhead and those that are intended to engage the manubrium of the malleus.

Most ossicular prosthesis designs are inherently unstable in that they are top-heavy and will tend to tip unless adequately supported by the reconstruction technique. This effect can be negated somewhat with a design that is very light, such as titanium, or a head design that shifts the center of gravity over the shaft, as used in some molded hydroxylapatite designs. Short-term stability is likewise facilitated by effective two-point (preferably bony) fixation. Thus, any design that incorporates the malleus should offer improved stability in that the prosthesis may be "locked" into place between the malleus manubrium and stapes. Furthermore, recent basic science research using infrared laser vibrometry as well as retrospective clinical studies on ossiculoplasty suggest that incorporating the malleus in the reconstruction provides increased acoustic gain, discussed in further detail below [13].

Surgical Technique

Understanding the mechanisms of acoustic gain in the middle ear can be an important key for obtaining successful surgical results when performing ossicular reconstruction. Therefore, the concepts of middle ear acoustics are discussed in the following section.

Mechanisms of Gain

The modern view of middle ear acoustic science involves two basic pathways by which sound is able to stimulate the inner ear: [14, 15] ossicular coupling and acoustic coupling. The first involves transmission of sound pressure through the tympanic membrane and ossicular chain via the oval window whereas the second involves direct passage of sound pressure via the oval and round windows, with no involvement of the tympanic membrane or ossicular chain.

Ossicular Coupling

This mechanism is the primary means by which the state of impedance mismatch that exists between the air in the ear canal (low impedance) and the fluid within the cochlea (high impedance) is overcome. In such a state, sound pressure is deflected during passage through the air–fluid interface, resulting in a loss of gain in the realm of 30 dB. The coupling effect of the tympanic membrane and ossicles almost overcomes this loss.

Ossicular coupling has been attributed to the collective effect of three characteristics of the tympano-ossicular mechanism, traditionally known as the *acoustic transformer theory* [16]. The first and most significant of these characteristics is the *hydraulic lever effect* that results from the difference between the surface area of the tympanic membrane relative to that of the oval window (usually a ratio of nearly 17:1). This effect results in compression of sound energy and increase in force at the oval window, equating to a theoretical approximate increase in gain of 26 dB. The second characteristic is the *malleoincudal lever effect* that results from the difference in length between the malleus manubrium relative to that of the long process of the incus along the axis of ossicular rotation (a ratio of 1.3:1). However, theoretically, this effect only accounts for an additional 2-dB increase in gain. The final factor is the so-called *catenary lever effect*, which is generated by the elastic stretching of the tympanic membrane from the annulus to the malleus manubrium—somewhat akin to the stretched strings across a tennis racquet. The specific degree of acoustic benefit derived from the catenary effect is not well understood but probably lies within a range similar to that of the malleoincudal lever.

It is important to recognize that, in reality, ossicular coupling is a much more complex phenomenon than what is suggested by these simplified traditional models as they do not account for factors such as variation in efficiency with changes in frequency or inefficiencies in sound transmission through the tympanic membrane and ossicular chain attributed to the inherent tension or laxity of the ossicular ligaments. Thus, it is perhaps not surprising that the 25–30 dB of gain that is predicted by the acoustic transformer theory does not equate well with experimental measurements, which suggest an actual more modest increase of just over 20 dB [17–19].

Acoustic Coupling

The second pathway of sound stimulation of the inner ear involves direct passage of sound pressure via the oval and round windows [15]. Given an intact tympanic membrane and functional ossicular chain, this pathway is of only minor importance. However, in the various conditions of a diseased ear, acoustic coupling can be important. This is why, for example, a conductive hearing loss will be greater in the case of ossicular discontinuity and an intact tympanic membrane (60 dB) compared with ossicular discontinuity and an absent tympanic membrane (40–50 dB). With the former, the intact tympanic membrane restricts the acoustic coupling pathway by blocking direct access of sound pressure to the oval and round window membranes.

Phase

A final relevant consideration in middle ear acoustic mechanics is that of *phase*. A sound stimulus to the inner ear is detected as the net difference in sound pressures applied to the round and oval windows that results in movement of intracochlear fluids. If these sound pressures are simultaneously applied to the round and oval windows with equal amplitude and phase, they will counteract each other and no resultant intracochlear fluid displacement will occur. In the normal situation, this does not occur due to the unbalanced selective effect of ossicular coupling upon the oval window, the acoustic shielding effect of the tympanic membrane upon the round window, and the uneven anatomical positioning of the round window versus the oval window relative to incoming sound. However, when the tympano-ossicular mechanism is absent and acoustic coupling is primarily relied upon (as in the case of a type IV or V tympanoplasty), an unshielded round window can yield significant negative acoustic consequences due to phase cancellation [15].

Applying Mechanisms of Gain to Surgical Technique

By far the most important mechanism of acoustic gain will come from reestablishment of the hydraulic lever effect. Therefore, the primary goal of ossicular reconstruction is to maximally couple the stapes footplate to the tympanic membrane. The resulting acoustic gain is due to the difference between the surface area of the tympanic membrane relative to that of the oval window. Reestablishment of the catenary lever is also often possible by utilizing the manubrium of the malleus in the reconstruction of both the tympanic membrane and ossicular chain. Basic science research using infrared laser vibrometry as well as retrospective clinical studies on ossiculoplasty suggest that incorporating the malleus in the reconstruction provides increased acoustic gain [13]. However, since gain derived from catenary effects is several-fold less than that derived from the hydraulic lever, these theoretic benefits should be kept in proper perspective during surgical planning. Similarly, the malleoincudal lever provides such a small theoretical increase in gain (2–3 dB) that it does not constitute a compelling reason to favor a type II reconstructive mechanism over one of the type III subtypes.

Specific surgical techniques that maximize acoustic gain, and thus achieve the best outcomes for the patient, can best be illustrated by addressing situations encountered in chronic middle ear surgery. The prostheses used in the examples to follow are a combination of hydroxylapatite and titanium of the senior author's design, but the surgical technique and anatomical relationships extrapolate to many other synthetic PORPs and TORPs being used today.

Incus Erosion

Due to its location relative to the common pathways of development of cholesteatoma and tympanic membrane atelectasis, as well as its rather tenuous blood supply suspended between the stapes and malleus, erosion of the incus long process is the most common ossicular defect. Long process erosion can be encountered in roughly one-third of cases involving a chronic posterior tympanic membrane perforation due to a variety of factors, such as pressure necrosis, inflammation, and hydrolytic enzymes produced by cholesteatoma matrix.

While an eroded incus is usually obvious during middle ear exploration, in some cases palpation is required to uncover the presence of a more subtle fibrous union between the stapes and incus. The key factor in this situation is the degree of bony contact remaining. If bone of the incudostapedial joint is present to some reasonable degree, it may compel the surgeon to leave the incus untouched. However, if contact is deficient and movement with palpation is incomplete, reconstruction is recommended.

There are basically two options for reconstruction when incus erosion is present. The first involves an attempt to reconstruct the incudostapedial joint with a type II. All of the type II reconstructive techniques share many of the same theoretical advantages and disadvantages. On the positive side, they reestablish the natural malleoincudal lever with minimal disruption of the normal anatomical relationships and native ossicular connections. The primary disadvantages relate to uncertain long-term durability as little is known about the pathophysiology and natural history of incus necrosis. If erosion is related to avascular necrosis, one may speculate that the remnant of the lenticular process, if used in ossicular reconstruction, may be subject to future loss. Given the relatively small acoustic gain afforded by preservation of the malleoincudal lever, type II reconstruction of the diseased middle ear (2–3 dB) might not be worth the risk of possible revision.

The most commonly used reconstructive option for incus necrosis involves removal of the incus remnant and reconstruction between the stapes and malleus (or tympanic membrane), generally as a type III minor columella mechanism. The fundamental anatomic principles governing this reconstruction are the same regardless of the graft or prostheses used. Some key relationships include the vertical height from the stapes capitulum to the plane of the neck of the malleus (2–2.5 mm) at the attachment of the tensor tympani tendon and the horizontal or translational distance from the capitulum to this same point (3–3.5 mm). The malleus manubrium can become rotated medially as an effect of middle ear disease processes, especially along its distal aspect at the umbo. However, in the senior author's experience, the malleus neck is spared from major rotational variation due to its anchoring attachments, which allow it to be used as a consistent prosthesis target in ossicular reconstruction (Fig. 41.1). This is due to the fact that the axis of malleus medial rotation lies at the attachment of the fan-shaped anterior malleolar ligament to the anterior tympanic spine as well as to the underlying tensor tympani tendon, which anchors the malleus to the cochleariform process. In the rare instance where the neck of the malleus is pathologically displaced to an extreme degree, it may be necessary to translocate it.

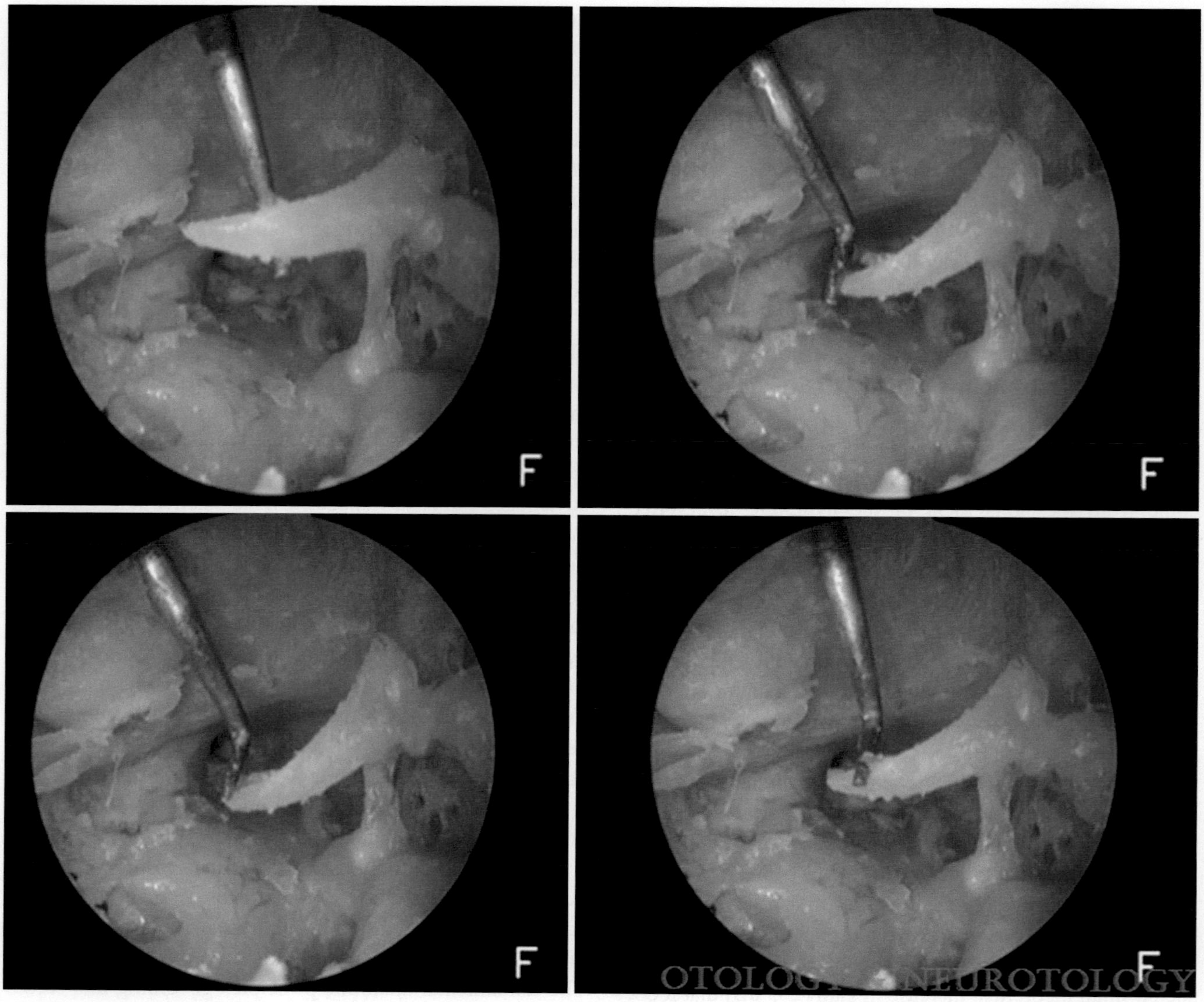

Fig. 41.1 The variable rotation of the malleus in a left ear on an axis at a point near the attachment of the anterior malleal ligament and tensor tympani tendon at the neck. Although the orientation of the distal aspect of the manubrium can vary significantly, the position of the neck is relatively constant, thereby rendering it the ideal target to engage standard length ossiculoplasty prosthesis. (Used with permission from Gluth et al. [27])

If the incus is deemed unusable or if the time and work involved with autograft preparation are not embraced, most surgeons opt for the use of a synthetic PORP. The recommended surgical technique utilizing a PORP as a minor columella is based on the principle that the vertical height to the malleus should be 2–2.5 mm and the horizontal reach should be 3–3.5 mm. While many commercially prepared prostheses are produced with a wide range of lengths or are adjustable, if reconstruction is made to the malleus neck, adjustments are not often necessary. It has been the senior author's experience that similar consistency in measurements to what is encountered in stapes surgery is seen in incus replacement if the proper site at the malleus neck is utilized and the ligamentous malleus attachments have not been severely disrupted. Although it is sensible to confirm by measuring, a prosthesis with a vertical height of 2–2.5 mm and a horizontal reach of 3 mm can be used in the vast majority of cases as long as it is designed to engage the malleus handle and there is no stapes capitulum erosion or exaggerated inferior rotation onto the promontory. It is also this author's opinion that improper prosthesis sizing and failed reconstruction are much more likely if the surgeon attempts to measure the distance from the stapes capitulum to the estimated undersurface of the posterior-superior drumhead as opposed to utilizing the relatively consistent relationship between the stapes and malleus that is outlined above.

Another important point to consider when using a PORP is that many of them have broad heads that contact the tym-

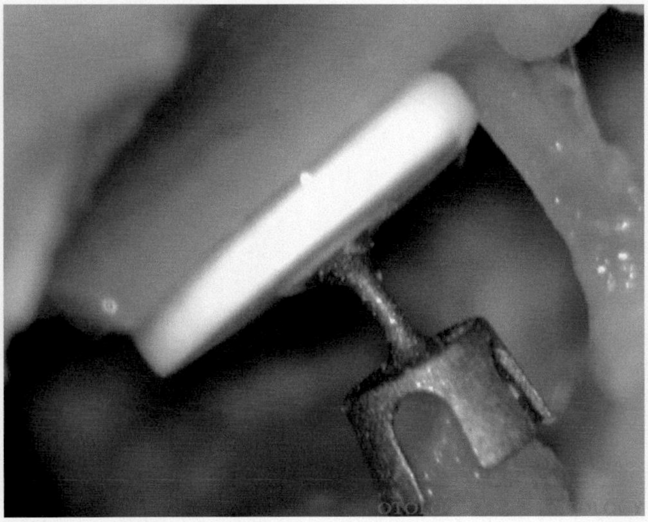

Fig. 41.2 Contour of prosthesis to malleus handle. View of a PORP from the vantage point of the facial recess in a left ear. The prosthesis is freestanding and securely stabilized by the tensor tympani tendon to the right, the medial projection of the malleus manubrium to the left, the cartilage graft cap laterally, and the stapes cradle medially. Note the bend in the prosthesis at the junction between the shaft and head to fit the contour of the malleus and tympanic membrane. (Used with permission from Gluth et al. [27])

panic membrane in addition to the malleus (in contrast to the "strut-like" structure of a sculpted incus autograft, which has no tympanic membrane contact). Since the tympanic membrane is a conical structure and not a flat disk, it is desirable to use a prosthesis that can be bent approximately 30° at the junction of the shaft and head to facilitate this shape (see Fig. 41.2). Doing so will encourage the superior edge of the prosthesis head under the malleus neck to become "locked" by the acute angle defined by the attachment of the tensor tympani tendon. In the end, the goal is to create a freestanding reconstruction that fixes to the tympanic membrane and stapes head, but not to other structures, such as the tympanic ring or cochlear promontory. A limited amount of absorbable packing can be used to achieve this end, but it should be noted that its use has been implicated with postoperative middle ear fibrosis, especially when denuded mucosa is present.

To combat synthetic prosthesis extrusion, a cartilage graft cap is recommended at the interface between the tympanic membrane and the adjacent prosthesis head. Although it has been suggested that this barrier may be optional with a prosthesis that features a hydroxylapatite head with smooth edges, cartilage is essential with sharper titanium prosthesis heads. As opposed to host incompatibility and lateral prosthesis migration beyond the tympanic membrane, the pathophysiology of prosthesis extrusion with an appropriate-length prosthesis more often seems to involve postoperative medial retraction of the tympanic membrane around the prosthesis. Cartilage can be placed in conjunction with reconstruction of the posterior half of the tympanic membrane in order to prevent retractions or cholesteatoma formation. When the cartilage graft is reconstructed exactly in piecemeal fashion, it is known as the mosaic technique. It would also appear that the size of the cartilage between the prosthesis and tympanic membrane has little effect on the hearing result. As long as the malleus is incorporated in the reconstruction, the probability of adequate coupling is maximized.

Incus and Stapes Absent

When both the incus and stapes superstructure are absent, common options for reconstruction include a type III major columella mechanism or a type IV tympanoplasty, the latter being suitable only in certain advanced cases of chronic ear disease involving a canal-wall-down mastoidectomy. A synthetic TORP is typically what is used as a major columella. The same basic principles of reconstruction and recognition of anatomical consistencies discussed with the use of a PORP apply to a TORP. To account for the absence of the stapes superstructure, an additional 2–2.5 mm is added to the vertical height recommendation. Thus, the desired TORP dimensions will be approximately 4.5 mm in height, with 3 mm of reach in order to reconstruct to the malleus neck while maintaining the shaft oriented 90° to the footplate.

One of the real challenges in this type of reconstruction relates to the lack of stability at the level of the footplate. Although the presence of the stapes superstructure offers no mechanism for acoustic gain, it does provide a convenient point for stable prosthesis fixation. The literature often shows superior hearing outcomes with a PORP versus a TORP, which is likely due to this difference in stability as opposed to acoustic advantage imparted by the presence of the superstructure. The same 30° angled interface with the neck of the malleus and tympanic membrane is utilized for lateral stability, as described earlier. However, this alone does not ensure a stable centered footplate contact point because the forces exerted by the tympanic membrane and malleus onto the TORP head encourage the shaft to displace. Several techniques have been introduced to counteract this phenomenon, including the use of footplate-stabilizing "shoes" made of titanium, hydroxylapatite, or cartilage (see Fig. 41.3). Related techniques that utilize small oval-shaped pieces of cartilage with a central hole have also been described [20].

While it is advisable to utilize the stapes superstructure when present, inferior rotation toward the promontory due to disease or previous surgery can make a minor columella reconstruction unsuitable. In such instances, a PORP or incus interposition may produce rocking of the stapes toward the promontory instead of the desired piston motion. A TORP placed on the footplate superior to the rotated superstructure is a more suitable alternative that tends to rotate the stapes superiorly into a more favorable position [21]. In other rare cases the superstructure may be deemed at risk of partial

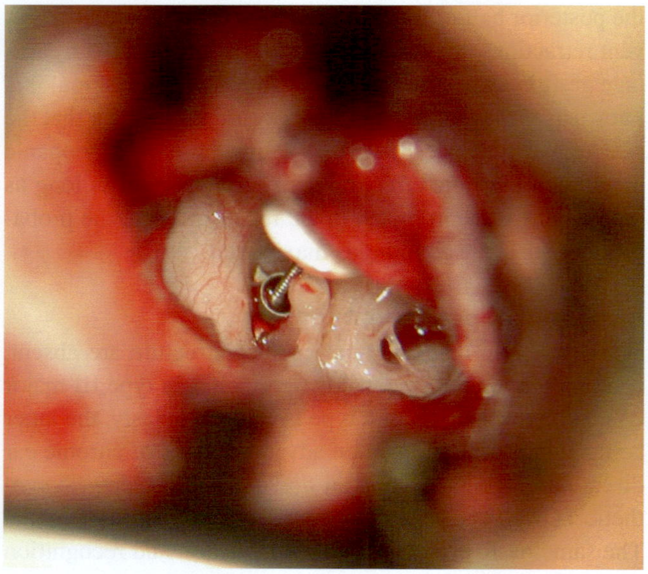

Fig. 41.3 TORP with footplate shoe for rotated stapes. When unfavorable inferior rotation of the stapes superstructure is present, a TORP is often preferable to maintain an approximate perpendicular orientation between the tympanic membrane and prosthesis shaft. In this case, the TORP is stabilized at the level of the footplate by a titanium shoe. (Used with permission from Cox et al. [30])

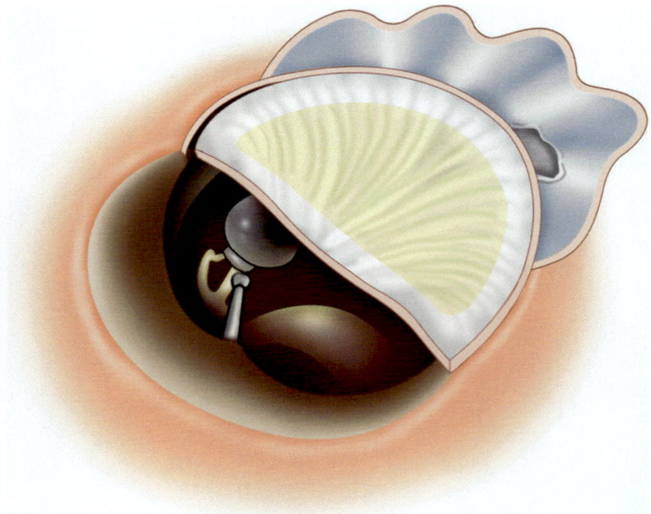

Fig. 41.4 Tympano-ossicular reconstruction without malleus. When the malleus handle is absent, the folded ridge generated by opposing edges of a composite perichondrium–cartilage island graft (indicated by yellow shading in this illustration) can be used as a pseudo-malleus to support a prosthesis that has a notch intended for the malleus handle. (Adapted from Gluth et al. [27])

fixation if the adjacent middle ear structures are fibrotic or involved with tympanosclerosis, in which case careful removal of the superstructure and placement of a TORP may be desirable [21].

Malleus Absent

The techniques previously described emphasize the use of the malleus for prosthesis stability and as an anatomical landmark for consistent length measurements; however, the malleus manubrium is not always present. Some otologists believe that the malleus is such a tremendous benefit in ossiculoplasty that techniques have been developed to create a "neo-malleus" from a piece of bone or a synthetic implant that is grafted into the tympanic membrane to be used later in staged ossicular reconstruction [22]. Nonetheless, several options do exist for single-stage ossicular reconstruction in the absence of a malleus manubrium [21].

The simplest of these single-stage techniques is reconstruction directly between the drumhead and stapes superstructure with a type III stapes columella mechanism (especially in a canal-wall-down procedure). When a wider gap between the stapes and drumhead is present or when the superstructure is absent, the use of a PORP or TORP that directly contacts the drumhead (with or without the cartilage cap, depending on the prosthesis material used) is generally required. These techniques can be effective, but great care should be exercised in measuring the correct prosthesis length. It is recommended that the reconstructed drumhead be slightly tented by the prosthesis; however, a major reason for prosthesis extrusion, regardless of material, is excessive length. Because these cases involving an absent malleus harbor the potential for graft/prosthesis adherence to the undersurface of the reconstructed tympanic membrane and ossiculoplasty failure due to delayed lateralization of the capitulum or footplate as the reconstructed tympanic membrane heals and matures, many surgeons favor staged ossiculoplasty. One innovative way to accomplish this during the second stage is to perform an ossiculoplasty via the facial recess so that elevation of a tympanomeatal flap is avoided and a stable tympanic membrane measurement is afforded [23].

Finally, an alternative single-stage technique favored by the authors involves creation of a "pseudo-malleus" by reconstructing the tympanic membrane with a composite perichondrium–cartilage island graft that forms a creased midline ridge to act in place of the manubrium (Fig. 41.4). This is achieved by creating a circular cartilage island graft measuring 8–9 mm in diameter, with a 1-mm midline strip of cartilage removed from the perichondrium, bisecting the island into two half-circles. The anterior half-circle is inserted as an underlay below the tympanic ring inferiorly and anterior tympanic spine superiorly while supported medially with absorbable packing in the anterior mesotympanum. The posterior half-circle is then lifted to expose the posterior edge of the anterior island, which is placed near the position of the absent malleus handle. This pseudo-malleus ridge can then be used for ossicular reconstruction using the same length of prostheses described earlier.

Fixed Ossicular Chain

Tympanosclerosis involving the tympanic membrane and middle ear is common when significant otitis media has been present. When these chalky white plaques involve the tympanic membrane, little or no conductive loss is expected unless the ossicular chain is also affected. Hearing loss due to tympanosclerotic fixation can occur secondary to involvement with any component of the ossicular chain.

An isolated malleus head or incus fixation with a mobile stapes can be dealt with in two ways [4]. The most common technique involves disarticulation of the incudostapedial joint followed by removal of the incus and amputation of the malleus head just above the insertion of the tensor tympani. Rarely, the malleus head is so fixed that it must be left in place; thus, a 1-mm gap is drilled between the fixed head and the mobile remnant to prevent re-fixation. Reconstruction is then accomplished with a type III minor columella, as described previously.

The second technique for correcting malleus fixation involves mobilization through an atticotomy by carefully releasing the point of fixation with a diamond drill bur. While good results have been reported with this technique, great care must be taken not to contact the ossicular chain with the bur as high-frequency sensorineural hearing loss can result. Due to this and the risk of re-fixation with new bone growth, mobilization techniques are only recommended for low-complexity ossicular fixation. Stapes fixation from tympanosclerosis represents a more complicated problem that often requires a staged approach.

Revision Ossiculoplasty

It is worth considering the difficulties associated with revision ossiculoplasty as a separate entity from primary surgery. Inherent challenges include scarring of the middle ear environment often involving the prior reconstruction, medialization or lateralization of the reconstructed drum, and alteration of landmarks. In approaching revision cases, it is important to recognize common patterns of failure of previous ossiculoplasties while still maintaining adherence to principles of mechanical gain and realistic expectations.

When performing primary surgery, it is of utmost importance to treat and document each case as though a revision surgery may be needed in the future. Taking note of the middle ear environment and clearly articulating decision-making with regard to the method for reconstruction will help substantially in the event that a hearing loss occurs in the future and revision surgery is necessary. Not having this information will be an inherent challenge in performing a revision procedure, particularly if the primary surgery was performed at another facility or by another surgeon.

Careful evaluation of the preoperative hearing test can provide significant aid in identifying the likely issue with the primary reconstruction and point to the appropriate method for reconstruction. Imaging with high-resolution computed tomography (CT) is always advisable when approaching a revision as it will help to identify more obvious causes of failure, such as displacement of the prosthesis. Regardless of technique utilized previously, any surgeon will be capable of performing revision ossiculoplasty by maintaining consistent principles and techniques, as previously described, and knowing what types of failures to expect preoperatively.

When evaluating the preoperative audiogram following a primary ossiculoplasty, it is most helpful to start with evaluation of the air and bone conduction at 2 kHz. If there is closure of the ABG at this frequency, the primary reconstruction is in good continuity. This can also be helpful to determine any degree of effusion in a patient with a prior cartilage tympanoplasty as no native drum can be examined to identify an effusion in the clinic. If the ABG is present at low frequencies, such as 500 Hz, but there is closure at 2 kHz, there is likely a stiff system due to scarring from the initial procedure. Revision will be very difficult to afford a hearing benefit in this scenario as lysis of scar may still be associated with further scarring in the future. Alternatively, if there is a 15–20 dB ABG at 2 kHz, one would expect an effusion to be present and intervention should be considered. If the ABG is greater than 20 dB at 2 kHz, then the likely issue is discontinuity, including displacement of the prosthesis. As discussed with incus necrosis, if a prior type II tympanoplasty was performed and a recurrent or worsening ABG has occurred, one should have a high suspicion for further incus necrosis causing ossicular discontinuity, in which case the surgical plan should be to convert to a type III tympanoplasty with incus removal.

If incus autograft interposition was performed previously, there are generally two patterns of failure. If the patient had an initial good outcome, followed by a maximum conductive loss with opening of the ABG at 2 kHz, then the graft has likely been resorbed. This is fairly straightforward to address, as placing a synthetic prosthesis can likely be performed without significant effort to remove a remnant graft. However, if the patient has a stiff system, with opening of the ABG at 500 Hz and closure at 2 kHz, bony fixation of the graft has likely occurred. It can be challenging to remove the graft from the facial canal or off of the stapes capitulum. Although the laser may be helpful in removal of the graft, one may also consider observation in this scenario.

Following placement of a synthetic prosthesis, causes of poor outcome can include incomplete coupling to the tympanic membrane, poor length, or poor position. If the stapes capitulum is present, the PORP may have incomplete coupling to the drum by not incorporating the malleus handle. Instead, the prosthesis may only make contact to the drum by a small cartilage cap that does not couple well to the rest of the surface area of the drum. This can be corrected by using a 2-mm PORP coupled to the neck of the malleus. If the malleus is absent, a total perichondrium–cartilage island flap can reconstitute good coupling to the entire surface area of the drum if the PORP contacts both the posterior and anterior island in the original position of the neck of the malleus. If the previously placed prosthesis was too long, it will likely demonstrate posterior displacement and make contact with the scutum, causing a stiffness tilt on the preoperative audiogram. Over time the pressure exerted by an overlong prosthesis may displace the stapes superstructure inferiorly toward the promontory. A better fit can be afforded by placing a TORP rather than trying to fit a PORP between a malleus handle and an angulated stapes superstructure.

If a TORP was previously used in the primary reconstruction, the most common cause for revision will be posterior displacement of the shaft of the TORP due to pressure on the front of the prosthesis from the malleus handle anteriorly. Often this results in a stiff system with closure of the ABG at 2 kHz due to the shaft making contact with the annular ligament of the oval window. Utilization of a footplate shoe and coupling the posterior surface of the head of the TORP to a posterior mosaic cartilage graft will increase stability.

When both the malleus and incus have been removed or have eroded over time, the choice of length of the prosthesis is often more uncertain. The drum may be inclined to lateralize and pull the prosthesis laterally off the capitulum or footplate, causing a maximum conductive loss. Rather than increase the length of the prosthesis, utilizing a more stable reconstruction of the drum can recreate the standard anatomic relationships. The same applies for a too-long prosthesis causing tenting of the tympanic membrane and leading to a stiffness tilt and later extrusion with a maximum conductive loss over time. The perichondrium–cartilage island flap anchors anteriorly to the anterior malleolar spine, and the posterior apron drapes onto the posterior bony canal. A 2-mm PORP and a 4.5-mm TORP can be used reliably with this graft technique.

Postoperative Care

With either primary or revision ossiculoplasty, the packing is removed 7–10 days after the surgery and ototopical drops prescribed for 10 days. The patient is instructed to perform the Valsalva maneuver three times a day, starting 2 weeks after the surgery. The Otovent (Abigo Medical, Sweden) has been used in children who are unable to perform this maneuver. The first postoperative audiogram is obtained 6–8 weeks post-surgery. If the patient is unable to perform the Valsalva maneuver or if the postoperative period is complicated by an effusion or retraction of the reconstructed tympanic membrane, a ventilation tube is placed 3–4 months after the surgery. Primary ventilation tube insertion is generally avoided.

Outcomes

Short-Term Results

Traditionally, ossiculoplasty "success" has been roughly judged to be a pure-tone average ABG less than 30 dB for a major columella (TORP) and less than 20 dB for a minor columella (PORP) [24]. However, in the authors' opinion, these benchmarks are only indicative of what is minimally acceptable without the need for revision and do not necessarily portray excellence in ossiculoplasty. Because the qualities of the underlying middle ear environment have the greatest impact on hearing outcomes, the results of ossiculoplasty must be reported in the context of the middle ear environment in which it is performed. Outcomes for the standardized technique of ossiculoplasty described in this chapter have been extensively reported in the literature with typically excellent results [25]. Furthermore, this technique has been analyzed within the framework of middle ear risk and has been published as the Ossiculoplasty Outcome Parameter Staging (OOPS) index (Table 41.1) [26]. As depicted in Fig. 41.5, on average, an expected postoperative ABG of approximately 10 dB is expected using this technique if the middle ear environment is ideal, compared to roughly a 20-dB ABG if the middle ear is extremely hostile. Furthermore, this standardized ossiculoplasty technique has been further validated by a second surgeon in a study that confirmed the short-term reproducibility of these results. An average postoperative ABG of 15.3 dB was noted to fall within the narrow expected hearing range that had been calculated based on underlying middle ear risk [27].

Table 41.1 Ossiculoplasty Outcome Parameter Staging (OOPS) index

Risk factor		Risk value
Middle ear factors		
Drainage	None	0
	present >50% of time	1
Mucosa	Normal	0
	Fibrotic	2
Ossicles	Normal	0
	Malleus +	1
	Malleus –	2
Surgical factors		
Type of surgery	No mastoidectomy	0
	Canal-wall-up mastoidectomy	1
	Canal-wall-down mastoidectomy	2
Revision surgery	No	0
	Yes	2

Adapted from Dornhoffer and Gardner [26]

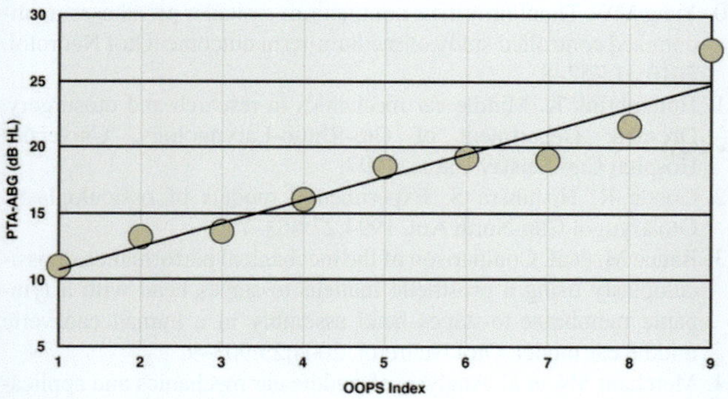

Fig. 41.5 Short-term hearing results stratified by OOPS score. (Used with permission from Cox et al. [28])

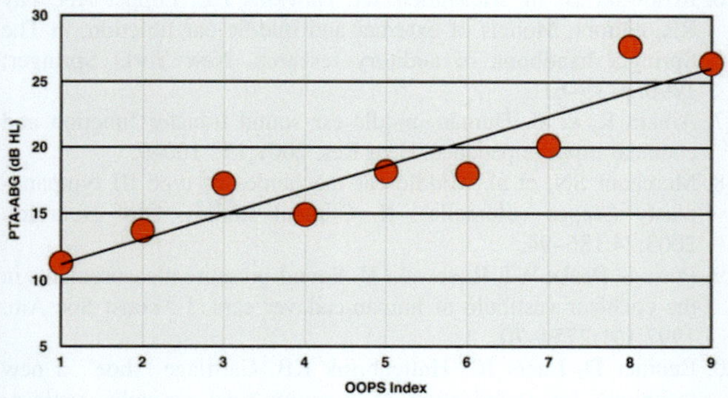

Fig. 41.6 Long-term hearing results stratified by OOPS score. (Used with permission from Cox et al. [28])

Long-Term Results

Although the OOPS index was created as a tool for predicting ossiculoplasty hearing results in the short term, it has also been shown to be predictive of long-term results (measured 5 or more years after surgery; Fig. 41.6) [28]. In patients stratified as low-risk (OOPS score ≤3) or intermediate-risk (OOPS score = 4–6), hearing results remain stable in the long term following ossiculoplasty. As noted in Fig. 41.7, the tendency to observe a slowly progressive worsening of conductive hearing loss in the years after middle ear surgery with ossiculoplasty may be most common in those patients stratified as high-risk (OOPS score ≥7). Ideally, a satisfactory hearing result would be achieved and sustained indefinitely in every patient who requires ossiculoplasty. While this goal is unrealistic, identification of those patients at increased risk for suboptimal hearing results can help the surgeon establish realistic expectations preoperatively, which may improve patient satisfaction.

Probably the most significant limitation of any otologic surgery outcomes study is related to long-term follow up. Over half of the patients in many case series do not follow up over 5 years, which raises the question as to what is the reason for their loss to follow up. It has been suggested that many patients who do not follow up as recommended are happy with their outcomes and do not feel a compelling need to continue to

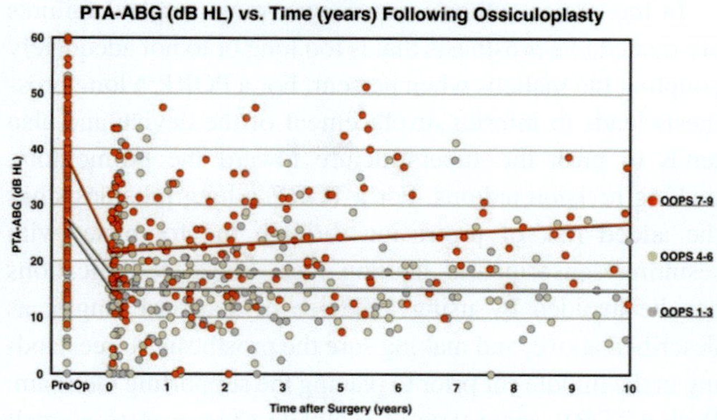

Fig. 41.7 Preoperative, postoperative, and final pure-tone average (PTA) air-bone gap (ABG) for patients based on low- (1–3), intermediate- (4–6), and high-risk (7–9) OOPS scores. (Used with permission from Cox et al. [28])

return [29]. Interestingly, upon comparison of postoperative audiometry (obtained 2–12 months after surgery) between patients who continued to follow up as recommended (for more than 5 years) and those who did not, the latter had significantly better early hearing results [28]. While this finding certainly supports the notion that many of the patients lost to follow-up are satisfied with their hearing status and thus have no desire for continued office visits, this is mere speculation.

The importance of realizing the barriers to long-term follow-up cannot be overemphasized. Failures of ossiculoplasty, including complications and recurrence of conductive hearing loss, may occur early or late and irrespective of risk stratification. In our series, half of all surgical failures occurred more than 4 years postoperatively. Additionally, we have observed patients who required a subsequent surgery more than 10 years after the first operation.

Complications

Complications or failures of ossiculoplasty are generally divided into those caused by patient factors (prosthesis extrusion) and those related to surgical technique (prosthesis displacement). In a hostile middle ear environment with continued Eustachian tube dysfunction, even a well-executed ossiculoplasty using a well-designed prosthesis is at risk of long-term failure. If the same pathologic process that made the surgery necessary in the first place is not alleviated, then the reconstructed tympanic membrane can retract around the prosthesis, leading to extrusion of the device. Methods utilized to minimize this risk would be to (1) treat the underlying Eustachian tube dysfunction/sinonasal disease prior to surgical intervention, (2) utilize the malleus when possible for bone-to-bone reconstruction, (3) use cartilage reconstruction techniques lateral to the prosthesis with good approximation to the posterior canal wall, and (4) consider long-term ventilation of the middle ear space with a tube in the postoperative period if effusion or retraction occurs.

In the senior author's experience, most surgical failures are related to a prosthesis that is too long or to not adequately coupling the malleus when present. For a PORP, a long prosthesis leads to inferior displacement of the device and also tends to push the superstructure toward the promontory, making revision tedious. For a TORP, a long prosthesis has the added risk of protrusion through the footplate, with resulting sensorineural hearing loss. These complications can be avoided by using a device of standard length, as described above, and making sure the prosthesis is freestanding in the middle ear prior to placing the supporting Gelfoam. With a TORP, some type of footplate shoe or even a small piece of fascia can be very useful, not only for prosthesis stability, but also to prevent perforation.

Conclusions

The success of ossicular reconstruction is not entirely within the surgeon's hands. Specifically, a multitude of patient factors, such as those described by the OOPS index, play an important role in the ultimate outcome of ossiculoplasty. That being said, a wealth of knowledge regarding patient selection, surgical technique, and ossicular replacement exists and should generally be employed by surgeons to optimize outcomes.

References

1. Zollner F. The principles of plastic surgery of the sound-conducting apparatus. J Laryngol Otol. 1955;69:637–52.
2. Wullstein H. The restoration of the function of the middle ear, in chronic otitis media. Ann Otol Rhinol Laryngol. 1956;65:1021–41.
3. Mehta RP, et al. Determinants of hearing loss in perforations of the tympanic membrane. Otol Neurotol. 2006;27:136–43.
4. Vincent R, Lopez A, Sperling NM. Malleus ankylosis: a clinical, audiometric, histologic, and surgical study of 123 cases. Am J Otol. 1999;20:717–25.
5. Collins WO, et al. Pediatric tympanoplasty: effect of contralateral ear status on outcomes. Arch Otolaryngol Head Neck Surg. 2003;129:646–51.
6. Dornhoffer JL. Surgical management of the atelectatic ear. Am J Otol. 2000;21:315–21.
7. Dornhoffer JL. Hearing results with cartilage tympanoplasty. Laryngoscope. 1997;107:1094–9.
8. Bellucci RJ. Dual classification of tympanoplasty. Laryngoscope. 1973;83:1754–8.
9. Coffey CS, Lee FS, Lambert PR. Titanium versus nontitanium prostheses in ossiculoplasty. Laryngoscope. 2008;118:1650–8.
10. Yung MW. Titanium versus nontitanium ossicular prostheses-a randomized controlled study of medium-term outcome. Otol Neurotol. 2010;31:752–8.
11. Huttenbrink K. Middle ear mechanics in research and otosurgery. Dresden: Department of Oto-Rhino-Laryngology, University Hospital Carl Gustav Carus; 1997.
12. Goode R, Nishihara S. Experimental models of ossiculoplasty. Otolaryngol Clin North Am. 1994;27:663–75.
13. Bance M, et al. Comparison of the mechanical performance of ossiculoplasty using a prosthetic malleus-to-stapes head with a tympanic membrane-to-stapes head assembly in a human cadaveric middle ear model. Otol Neurotol. 2004;25:903–9.
14. Merchant SN, et al. Analysis of middle ear mechanics and application to diseased and reconstructed ears. Am J Otol. 1997;18:139–54.
15. Merchant SN, et al. Toynbee Memorial Lecture 1997. Middle ear mechanics in normal, diseased and reconstructed ears. J Laryngol Otol. 1998;112:715–31.
16. Rosowski JJ. In: McMullen TA, Hawkins HL, Popper AN, Fay RR, editors. Models of external and middle ear function, in The Springer handbook of auditory research. New York: Springer; 1996. p. 15–61.
17. Aibara R, et al. Human middle-ear sound transfer function and cochlear input impedance. Hear Res. 2001;152:100–9.
18. Merchant SN, et al. Middle ear mechanics of type III tympanoplasty (stapes columella): II. Clinical studies. Otol Neurotol. 2003;24:186–94.
19. Puria S, Peake WT, Rosowski JJ. Sound-pressure measurements in the cochlear vestibule of human-cadaver ears. J Acoust Soc Am. 1997;101:2754–70.
20. Beutner D, Luers JC, Huttenbrink KB. Cartilage 'shoe': a new technique for stabilisation of titanium total ossicular replacement prosthesis at centre of stapes footplate. J Laryngol Otol. 2008;122:682–6.
21. Vincent R, et al. Ossiculoplasty with intact stapes and absent malleus: the silastic banding technique. Otol Neurotol. 2005;26:846–52.
22. Black B. Neomalleus ossiculoplasty. Otol Neurotol. 2002;23:636–42.
23. Blevins NH. Transfacial recess ossicular reconstruction: technique and early results. Otol Neurotol. 2004;25:236–41.
24. Jackson CG, et al. Ossicular chain reconstruction: the TORP and PORP in chronic ear disease. Laryngoscope. 1983;93:981–8.
25. Dornhoffer JL. Hearing results with the Dornhoffer ossicular replacement prostheses. Laryngoscope. 1998;108:531–6.
26. Dornhoffer JL, Gardner EK. Prognostic factors in ossiculoplasty: a statistical staging system. Otol Neurotol. 2001;22:299–304.
27. Gluth MB, Moore PC, Dornhoffer JL. Method and reproducibility of a standardized ossiculoplasty technique. Otol Neurotol. 2012;33:1207–12.
28. Cox MD, Trinidade A, Russell JS, Dornhoffer JL. Long-term hearing results after ossiculoplasty. Otol Neurotol. 2017;38:510–5.
29. Yung M. Long-term results of ossiculoplasty: reasons for surgical failure. Otol Neurotol. 2006;27:20–6.
30. Cox MD, et al. TORP ossiculoplasty outcomes with and without a stapes footplate prosthesis. Otolaryngol Head Neck Surg. 2015;152(3):501–5.

Canal Wall Up Mastoidectomy

42

Ashley M. Nassiri, Matthew L. Carlson, Neil S. Patel, and David S. Haynes

Introduction

Tympanomastoidectomy is a versatile procedure that allows access to the mastoid and middle ear, most commonly to address chronic otitis media with or without cholesteatoma. In adapting surgical approaches to each patient's specific disease process, mastoidectomy can be tailored to either preserve or remove the posterior portion of the external auditory canal (EAC). The former approach, referred to as canal wall up (CWU) or intact canal wall mastoidectomy, will be the focus of this chapter. The canal wall down (CWD), or open cavity, mastoidectomy will be discussed in detail elsewhere.

Almost 150 years have passed since the first cortical mastoidectomy was described by Hermann Schwartze of Halle University in Germany in 1873 [1]. During that time, opening of the mastoid was controversial, as prior attempts of mastoid "perforation" had resulted in patient mortality. Although Schwartze's first mastoidectomy was performed for acute infection, he suggested that curettage to uncover the antrum might also be useful for chronic infection. Shortly after this, William MacEwen of Scotland and William J. Mayo of Rochester, Minnesota, were among the first to use various drills to perform mastoidectomy [2]. The need for greater exposure led to the development of the radical mastoidectomy in the late nineteenth century, followed by the modified radical mastoidectomy [3, 4].

Technologic advances, including the application of the operative microscope and refined use of surgical drills, set the stage for expansion of the field [5, 6]. The advent of antibiotics in the 1930s and more widespread availability circa World War II established the feasibility of medical management of acute otologic infections, leaving surgery for persistent or advanced disease [3]. With improved outcomes supported by antibiotic treatment, the focus of surgery shifted from reducing mortality to minimizing morbidity. Jansen and Sheehy reported the first cases of the CWU mastoidectomy as part of a combined approach to the tympanomastoid cavity in the 1950s [7, 8]. Today, this safe, typically outpatient procedure is the workhorse of otologic surgery for a variety of indications and remains the primary surgical corridor to access the middle ear and mastoid process.

Pathophysiology

Acute Mastoiditis

Acute mastoiditis is defined as infection and inflammation involving the mastoid cavity, which generally develops as an extension of acute otitis media (AOM). While most cases of AOM can be treated with antibiotic therapy alone, untreated infections or those that have failed antibiotic therapy may develop into acute mastoiditis. Coalescent mastoiditis represents a more advanced disease characterized by destruction of the mastoid bony septa caused by an accumulation of purulence under pressure. In some cases, this infection leads to erosion of the cortical mastoid bone, resulting in a subperiosteal abscess. Postauricular edema, phlegmon, or subperiosteal abscess resulting from direct extension or thrombophlebitis often results in proptosis of the ear. Griesinger's sign—postauricular pain, edema, and erythema—may indicate thrombosis of the mastoid emissary

A. M. Nassiri
Department of Otolaryngology—Head and Neck Surgery, University of Colorado School of Medicine, Aurora, CO, USA

M. L. Carlson
Department of Otolaryngology—Head and Neck Surgery, Mayo Clinic, Rochester, MN, USA

N. S. Patel
Department of Otolaryngology—Head and Neck Surgery, University of Utah, Salt Lake City, UT, USA

D. S. Haynes (✉)
Department of Otolaryngology—Head and Neck Surgery, Vanderbilt University Medical Center, Nashville, TN, USA
e-mail: david.haynes@vumc.org

A. D. Sweeney et al. (eds.), *Haynes-Glasscock-Shambaugh Surgery of the Ear*, https://doi.org/10.1007/978-3-032-18264-7_42

vein or associated lateral dural venous sinuses. While difficult to conceive of today, complications from AOM were a major source of morbidity and mortality prior to the widespread availability of antibiotics, and, as a result, radical mastoidectomy was among the most common procedures performed by otolaryngologists prior to the 1950s [3].

Because AOM is the antecedent disease process, the microbial pathogens responsible for acute mastoiditis mirror those of AOM. *Streptococcus pneumoniae* is most common, followed by *Pseudomonas aeruginosa* and non-typeable *Haemophilus influenzae* [9, 10]. *Staphylococcus aureus*, *Streptococcus pyogenes*, and *Moraxella catarrhalis* are less commonly responsible for acute mastoiditis. Interestingly, recent trends have suggested an uptick in *Fusobacterium*-related acute mastoiditis (the bacterial genus associated with Lemierre's syndrome, acute thrombophlebitis of the internal jugular vein), which has been associated with increased rates of complications requiring surgical intervention [11, 12].

Chronic Suppurative Otitis Media

Chronic otitis media (COM) encompasses a wide spectrum of disease that may present with or without tympanic membrane perforation or retraction, otorrhea, cholesteatoma, effusion, and dysventilation. While there is no succinct, all-encompassing definition for this group of diseases, chronic inflammation drives most of the presenting signs and symptoms. For the purposes of this chapter, we will focus on chronic suppurative otitis media (CSOM) as a representative of this group in discussing the role of CWU tympanomastoidectomy in chronic ear disease management. CSOM is defined as purulent middle ear drainage through a perforated tympanic membrane (or tympanostomy tube) that persists beyond 2–6 weeks [13, 14]. This is distinctly different from a chronic otitis media with effusion (COME), in which there is an intact tympanic membrane with non-purulent fluid in the middle ear space. CSOM can occur with or without cholesteatoma.

Chronic infection and inflammation precipitate the majority of pathologic findings in CSOM including the development of granulation tissue, inflammatory polyps, osteitis, tympanosclerosis, and cholesterol granulomas [15, 16]. In persistent disease, the maturation of granulation tissue leads to fibrosis and adhesions, which compromise middle ear function [17]. Importantly, granulation tissue can also obstruct the antrum and ventilation pathways of the middle ear, precluding normal aeration of the tympanic cavity and mastoid. Over time, inflammatory osteitis can lead to ossicular chain erosion or fixation and exposure of the middle or posterior fossa dura. In a cadaveric study, Meyerhoff et al. identified tympanosclerosis in chronic otitis media predominantly involving the tympanic membrane followed by the tympanic cavity and ossicular chain [17].

Etiology of Chronic Suppurative Otitis Media

There exists no definitive consensus on the etiology of CSOM. One theory suggests that CSOM without cholesteatoma is initiated by an episode of acute infection with tympanic membrane perforation that leads to chronic inflammation of the middle ear mucosa [13]. Alternatively, it has been proposed that Eustachian tube dysfunction leading to middle ear effusion can undergo bacterial seeding from a tympanic membrane perforation, tympanostomy tube placement, or Eustachian tube reflux. Although the data supporting both routes of inoculation are inconclusive, it should be noted that the most common pathogenic bacteria in CSOM are those commonly found within the EAC [18].

The acute infection results in an ongoing inflammatory response that leads to mucosal edema and destruction of the epithelial lining. Over time, the persistent inflammatory response leads to long-term fibrosis, adhesions, and bony destruction [17]. Although CSOM is more prevalent in lower socioeconomic areas, specific ethnic groups, and those prone to recurrent upper respiratory tract infections, consistent risk factors that explain the development of a chronic process in certain people have not been identified [13, 19, 20].

Diagnosis and Treatment

Acute Mastoiditis

A thorough clinical history of the patient's symptoms can be very informative in diagnosing acute mastoiditis. Patients will generally describe AOM as the inciting event, with worsening otalgia over time. In some cases, patients will describe a brief period of improvement, with a relapse of symptoms, indicating an unresolved infection. Otologic examination most commonly reveals an erythematous, bulging tympanic membrane with middle ear purulence or otorrhea in the case of perforation. Patients may also have edema along the posterior aspect of the EAC along the vascular strip. Patients with acute mastoiditis usually exhibit postauricular tenderness to palpation, while those with coalescent mastoiditis with subperiosteal abscess generally present with fluctuance over the mastoid prominence associated with erythema and edema of the overlying skin. Fevers and leukocytosis are common. While clinical history and examination are generally adequate for diagnosis, computed tomography (CT) is useful in more advanced cases to evaluate for bony erosion, presence of coalescent mastoiditis, subperiosteal abscess, or other advanced temporal or intracranial complications. Early diagnosis and treatment of coalescent mastoiditis is important, as up to 16% of these patients have concomitant intracranial complication at presentation [21]. Importantly, as a clinician who may be consulted to address incidental mastoid opacification on MRI (magnetic resonance imaging) or CT, one must remember that the diagnosis of acute mastoiditis is chiefly based upon clinical findings, whereas imaging is mainly used to understand the extent of infection and to identify any concomitant complications.

The diagnosis of acute mastoiditis alone does not necessarily warrant surgical intervention; however, specific signs and symptoms may preclude more conservative measures. In the case of acute mastoiditis without abscess or intracranial complication, a trial of medical treatment is reasonable. Recent studies have shown increased rates of multidrug-resistant pathogens, which underscores the importance of using broad-spectrum antibiotics and culture data when available [22]. In mild or early cases, treatment with oral antibiotics may be sufficient. Ototopical antibiotics are added in cases with tympanic membrane perforation. Patients who have failed a trial of oral antibiotics, have evidence of sepsis, or uncontrolled pain warrant an admission to the hospital for intravenous broad-spectrum antibiotics and placement of a tympanostomy tube if no perforation is present. In patients with coalescent mastoiditis or subperiosteal abscess, surgical intervention plays an important role.

Chronic Suppurative Otitis Media

Most patients with CSOM present with intermittent or persistent otorrhea and hearing loss. CSOM is generally insidious in onset; however, patients may experience superimposed AOM, which may be associated with episodic pain and worsening drainage. Otherwise, otalgia, fevers, and headache are uncommon in CSOM, and should prompt a work-up for intracranial involvement or alternative diagnoses. While vertigo is rare, it raises suspicion of labyrinthine fistula when present.

Otologic examination reveals otorrhea, inflammation of the tympanic membrane and middle ear mucosa, and commonly a central tympanic membrane perforation. Frequently, there will be surrounding mucosalization of the remnant tympanic membrane and medial EAC. Examination of the tympanic membrane or the middle ear may be obstructed by granulation tissue or large inflammatory polyps. In cases with cholesteatoma, there may be evidence of a retraction pocket or skin debris. Although facial nerve weakness in CSOM is rare, it may be indicative of more advanced disease or alternative diagnosis such as malignancy.

Work-up in CSOM should include complete audiometric evaluation, including pure tone thresholds, tympanometry, and speech discrimination testing. Conductive hearing loss is commonly due to a combination of tympanic membrane perforation, effusion, mucosal edema, middle ear adhesions, and ossicular chain erosion or fixation. A conductive hearing loss greater than 30 dB can be suggestive of ossicular chain discontinuity. Sensorineural hearing loss may also occur less commonly, although causality has not been definitively elucidated [23–25]. Thin-cut CT of the temporal bone is useful in determining the extent of involvement and evaluating bony erosion in cases of cholesteatoma. Magnetic resonance imaging (MRI) of the temporal bone and internal auditory canal may be considered if intracranial extension of cholesteatoma or encephalocele is suspected.

CSOM without cholesteatoma can respond to medical treatment aimed to dry the ear and limit inflammation with aural toilet, dry ear precautions, and ototopical with or without systemic antibiotics. While untreated CSOM usually continues to produce otorrhea, a small portion of CSOM without cholesteatoma spontaneously resolves [26]. In some cases, microbial data may be useful in guiding antibiotic selection. Surgical management, generally tympanomastoidectomy, is indicated in patients whose symptoms persist through medical management, those with more concerning symptoms such as vertigo or severe pain, or those with CSOM with cholesteatoma. When possible, eradication of any superimposed acute infection with ototopical treatments should be attempted prior to surgical intervention.

Surgical Theory and Practice

The decision to perform a CWU mastoidectomy considers several factors including extent and location of disease, prior surgical history, hearing status in both ears, patient goals and comorbidities, and surgeon experience and preferences. A CWU tympanomastoidectomy can be used to eradicate disease, provide surgical access to the middle ear, and re-establish mastoid aeration. While the latter factor was more heavily weighted previously, recent studies suggest that maintenance of mastoid aeration postoperatively does not always correlate with clinical outcomes [27, 28]. The decision to include mastoidectomy when performing tympanoplasty in the management of CSOM varies by surgeon and heavily relies on surgeon experience and preference. Prior tympanoplasty failures, persistent tympanic membrane perforation, refractory otorrhea, and cholesteatomas limited to the middle ear space are not absolute indications for mastoidectomy, and they may be treated effectively with a tympanoplasty alone in some cases.

Once it is determined that tympanomastoidectomy will be beneficial in treating the patient, the next consideration is whether to perform a CWU or CWD mastoidectomy. CWD mastoidectomy has several advantages including improved access and visualization of the epitympanum and middle ear, which are thought to be associated with decreased recidivism in cholesteatoma surgery (Table 42.1, Fig. 42.1) [29, 30]. This discrepancy, however, can be mitigated with a planned second surgery, referred to as a "second-look" procedure, in CWU cases

Table 42.1 Pros and Cons of CWU mastoidectomy compared to CWD mastoidectomy

CWU mastoidectomy	
Pros	Cons
Rapid recovery	May require second-look procedure
Preservation of normal auricular anatomy	Limited visualization of ME (epitympanum)
Preservation of normal aural toilet	Limited postoperative exam of mastoid and ME
	Requires consistent postoperative follow-up
CWD mastoidectomy	
Pros	*Cons*
Single-stage surgery	Enlarged conchal bowl
Complete visualization of epitympanum and ME	Long-term in-office debridements
Postoperative exam of mastoid and ME in clinic	Difficulty with hearing aid fitting
Creates a "safe ear" in situations with poor follow-up	Restriction of water exposure
	At risk for caloric-induced vertigo

ME middle ear

[31]. A two-staged approach is obviated after CWD mastoidectomy, since the middle ear and mastoid cavities can be examined in clinic. While CWD mastoidectomy has some advantages, some associated disadvantages include long-term in-office debridements, difficulty with hearing aid fitting, caloric-induced vertigo, and water exposure restrictions [32]. CWD also adds complexity to future placement of a cochlear implant if needed. Despite this, several studies have demonstrated equivalent disease-specific quality of life outcomes in patients who have undergone CWU and CWD mastoidectomies [33, 34].

Conversely, a CWU mastoidectomy preserves normal auricular anatomy and is associated with a shorter recovery period. While hearing outcomes were previously reported to be improved in CWU surgery, more recent data suggest that the extent of disease, volume of the reconstructed middle ear space, and ossicular chain involvement, rather than approach, are the main factors impacting hearing outcomes [35–37]. Importantly, retrospective studies comparing clinical outcomes in CWU and CWD approaches will have some level of selection bias, as CWD mastoidectomy is generally reserved for more extensive disease. In cases with more extensive cholesteatoma, a second-look procedure 6–12 months postoperatively may be beneficial to evaluate for disease recurrence and reconstruct the ossicles. A transcanal endoscopic approach provides a minimally invasive alternative for second-look procedures and ossicular chain reconstruction [38].

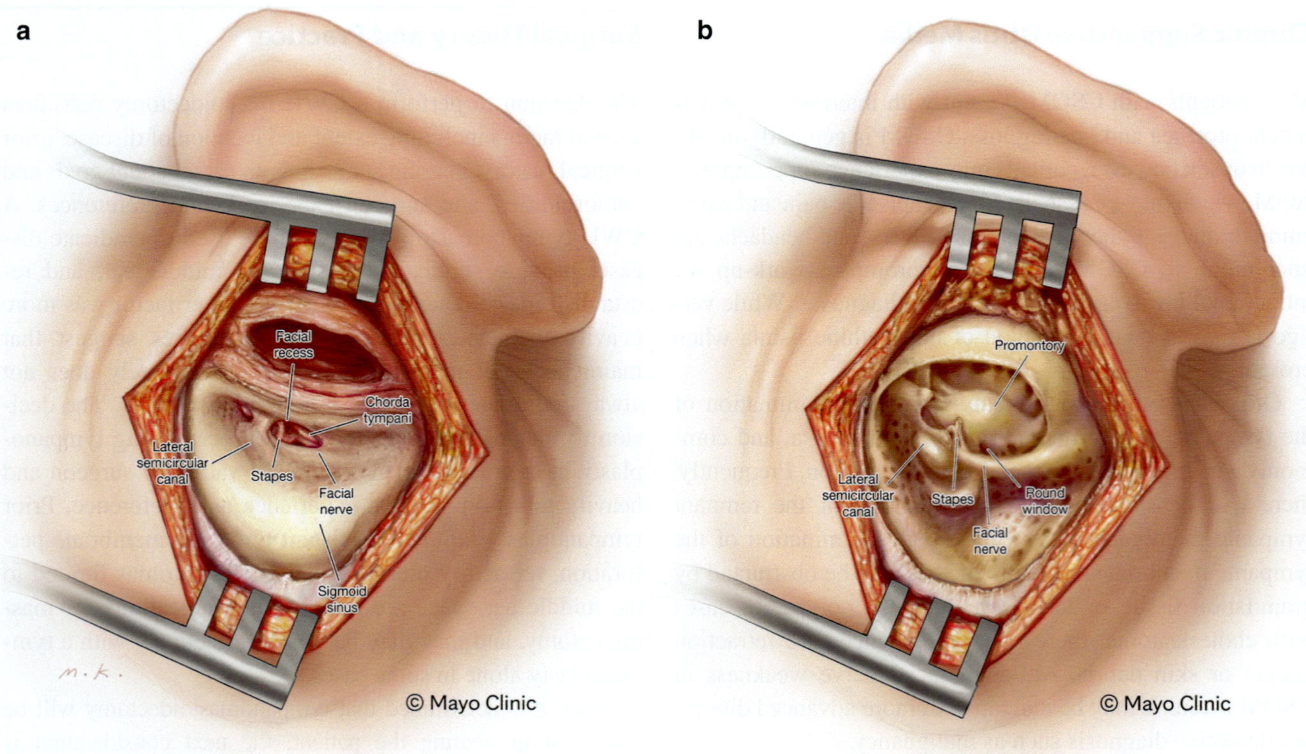

Fig. 42.1 Examples of access and visualization with a canal wall up mastoidectomy with facial recess (**a**) and canal wall down with removal of the lateral ossicular chain (**b**). (Used with permission from Mayo Foundation for Medical Education and research; all rights reserved)

Whether to perform primary CWD versus CWU mastoidectomy in COM with more extensive cholesteatoma is disputed. Preservation of the canal wall is preferred in our practice, and we approach most cases with the intention of doing a CWU mastoidectomy. The decision to perform a CWD mastoidectomy is generally made intraoperatively when the extent of disease is fully appreciated. Intraoperative findings that may be indications for CWD mastoidectomy include large or complex labyrinthine fistulae, unresectable disease on the facial nerve or stapes footplate, a low-lying tegmen that limits access to the attic, or a large posterior canal wall defect that cannot be reconstructed. For smaller labyrinthine fistulas, removal of the cholesteatoma matrix overlying the defect with autologous graft repair can be performed as part of a primary or staged CWU mastoidectomy. Although rare, the decision to proceed with CWD mastoidectomy is made preoperatively if a large labyrinthine fistula or large posterior wall erosion is identified on preoperative imaging, or if a patient's comorbidities preclude a second procedure. Many patients who have undergone one or more CWU procedures may be inclined to pursue a more "definitive" operation such as CWD mastoidectomy. Importantly, these factors are all discussed with the patient preoperatively, so the patient's preferences can guide the surgeon in intraoperative decision-making.

Finally, it is worth noting that the options for accessing the tympanomastoid cavity for chronic ear disease should not be viewed as a strict dichotomy between CWU and CWD tympanomastoidectomy. Practically speaking, transcanal surgery with atticotomy, reversible canal wall down tympanomastoidectomy (e.g., bone pâté obliteration or replacement of bony EAC), and also subtotal petrosectomy with EAC closure are options that may be employed depending upon the clinical circumstance.

Contraindications

Unresectable cholesteatoma involving the labyrinth, stapes footplate, facial nerve, carotid, dura, or sinus tympani is a contraindication to CWU tympanomastoidectomy (Table 42.2). Similarly, a large posterior canal wall defect that cannot be repaired intraoperatively is also a contraindication. A CWD mastoidectomy may be a safer option in patients who are unlikely to follow-up postoperatively, as a CWU mastoidectomy requires postoperative monitoring. While active infection is not a contraindication to this procedure, the surgeon should attempt to treat infection and dry the ear prior to surgery. Notably, conventional teaching suggested that extensive cholesteatoma in an only-hearing ear was a contraindication to CWU mastoidectomy (that is, the surgeon should perform a CWD mastoidectomy); however, most have abandoned this approach due to favorable hearing outcomes with CWU mastoidectomy, ability to surveil the ear with second-look procedures or MRI, and the increased use of cochlear implantation as a salvage option.

Table 42.2 Relative indications and contraindications of performing CWU and CWD mastoidectomy

CWU mastoidectomy	
Indications	Contraindications
Resectable cholesteatoma	Low-lying tegmen limiting access to attic
Small, resectable labyrinthine fistula	Irreparable posterior EAC wall defect
Patient likely to comply with postoperative follow-up	Comorbidities/preferences precluding second surgery
	Unresectable cholesteatoma
CWD mastoidectomy	
Indications	*Contraindications*
Low-lying tegmen limiting access to attic	Patient preference
Irreparable posterior EAC wall defect	
Comorbidities/preferences precluding second surgery	
Unresectable cholesteatoma of the stapes footplate, labyrinth, and facial nerve	

Note: These are *relative* indications and contraindications, as patient preference, situational factors, and surgeon skill and preferences play a large role in decision-making on a case-by-case basis. *EAC* external auditory canal

Preoperative Management and Surgical Planning

As discussed in prior sections, a thorough history and otologic examination with binocular otomicroscopy are critical in initial patient evaluation. Although CT scans are not obtained in every patient, they may be especially helpful in patients with advanced disease or signs and symptoms including vertigo, significant pain, facial paresis, or evidence of EAC erosion. Knowledge of erosion of the facial nerve canal, labyrinthine fistula, and tegmen and sigmoid dehiscences are particularly useful for preoperative planning. For revision surgeries, which can encompass a significant portion of an otologist's practice, imaging is helpful when the initial procedure was performed by a different surgeon.

Operative Techniques

Preparation

In developed countries, mastoidectomy surgeries are usually performed under general anesthesia without the use of long-acting paralytics to allow for continuous intraoperative facial nerve monitoring via electromyography. Preoperative antibiotics that cover skin flora are typically administered prior to incision. Depending upon the preference of the surgeon, saline irrigation used in the case may be mixed with ciprofloxacin or bacitracin. Facial nerve monitoring electrodes are placed, and, if necessary, a small amount of postauricular hair is trimmed. The ear and surrounding skin are "prescrubbed" with a betadine scrub, ensuring that the hair is cleaned. Next, the postauricular incision site, ear canal, and the tragal skin are injected with 1% lidocaine with 1:100,000 epinephrine. Care is taken to not over-inject the tragal site to avoid temporary facial nerve block. The surgical field is then prepped and draped in sterile fashion.

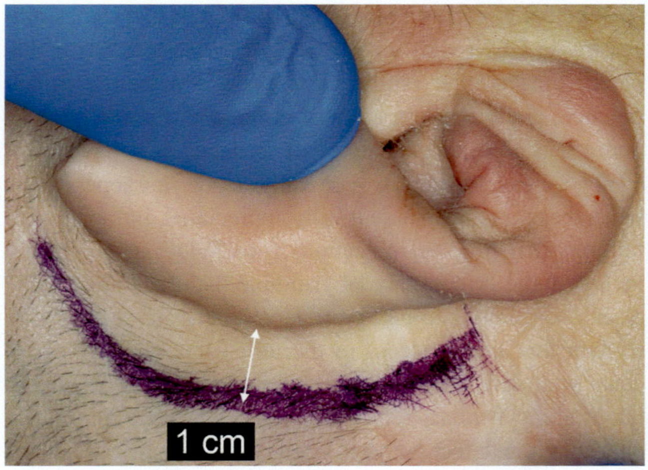

Fig. 42.2 Postauricular incision used for tympanomastoidectomy extending from the helical root to the mastoid tip

Incisions

Since a CWU mastoidectomy is frequently performed in conjunction with a tympanoplasty, we will briefly discuss the general order of steps and incisions for a tympanomastoidectomy. Further details about tympanoplasty technique have been discussed in a previous chapter.

First, the EAC and tympanic membrane are irrigated, cleaned, and examined. If the patient is additionally undergoing tympanoplasty, canal injections with 1% lidocaine with 1:50,000 or 1:100,000 epinephrine are carefully infiltrated into the posterior, inferior, and superior quadrants of the ear canal. Next, vascular strip incisions are made to create a vascular strip and tympanomeatal flap, and a large absorbable gelatin sponge (Gelfoam, Pfizer) is placed into the EAC while the mastoidectomy is performed. While this chapter will focus on a postauricular approach for mastoidectomy, the endaural approach can be utilized for transmastoid procedures.

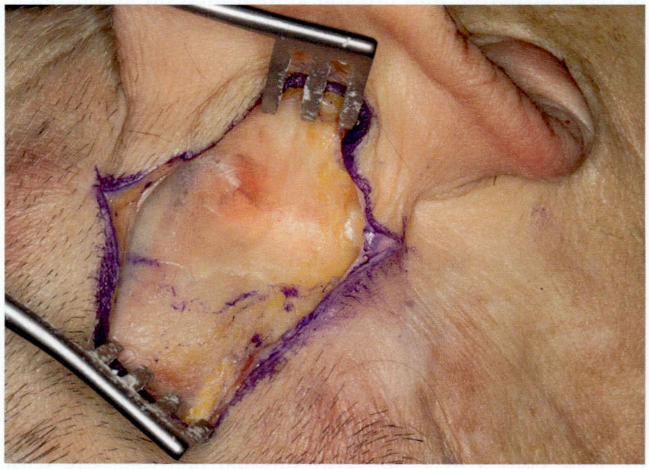

Fig. 42.3 Elevation of pinna in loose areolar plane

Next, attention is turned to the postauricular incision (Fig. 42.2). A curvilinear incision, 0.5–1 cm posterior to the postauricular sulcus, is carried from the helical root inferiorly to the mastoid tip. The incision is not made directly in the sulcus as this complicates closure and encourages scar depression. In children, the facial nerve is more lateral distally; consequently, the inferior end of the incision is directed more posteriorly to avoid facial nerve injury. The skin incision is deepened through the dermis and subcutaneous fat to the layer of loose areolar tissue (otherwise known as "fool's fascia") overlying the true temporalis fascia (Fig. 42.3). This plane is notably avascular, and, in primary cases, provides a natural plane for dissection. It is easiest to find this plane superiorly, as it sits over the temporalis muscle; once identified, the depth can be carried inferiorly and anteriorly, and the auricle can be reflected forward. The meatal cartilage is the limit of anterior dissection in this plane. In tympanomastoidectomy, the loose areolar tissue is harvested as a fascia graft (Fig. 42.4); in our practice, true temporalis fascia is

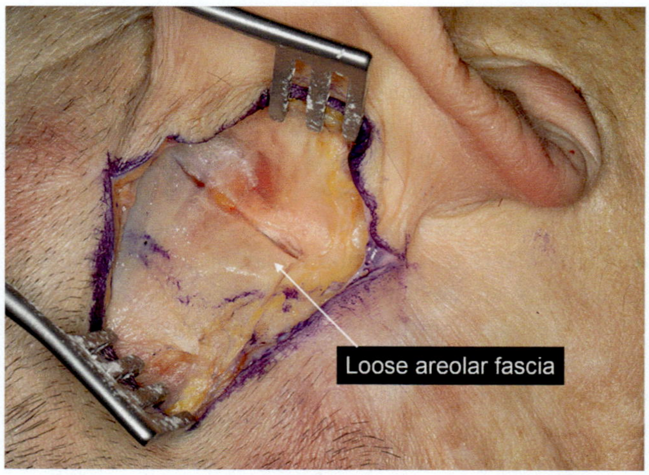

Fig. 42.4 Harvest of loose areolar fascia graft. Temporalis fascia or periosteum can be harvested through this approach by retracting the skin edge at the superior end of the incision

rarely used for tympanic membrane reconstruction, except in revision cases where the loose areolar tissue or scar is inadequate.

Once the fascia graft has been harvested, the periosteal incisions are made. In a primary case, a T-shaped incision is made through the mastoid periosteum and temporalis muscle using monopolar electrocautery. The horizontal portion of the T-shaped incision follows the linea temporalis, and the vertical limb is carried inferiorly to the mastoid tip. Small branches of the superficial temporal artery are frequently encountered superficial to the zygomatic root and require control with electrocautery. In revision mastoidectomy, a C-shaped periosteal incision placed just posterior to the posterior edge of the mastoid bowl allows for careful elevation of the periosteum off exposed structures such as the sigmoid sinus and middle fossa dura.

A Lempert elevator is used to elevate the periosteal flap anteriorly, being careful not to violate the EAC skin. The superior and posterior periosteum is also elevated to avoid tension during closure. Once the subperiosteal plane has been developed, the surgeon may elect to use a sponge over their thumb to elevate the flap anteriorly; this maneuver gently releases the periosteum approaching the EAC and avoids damage to the vascular strip. At this point, the entire mastoid cortex should be exposed, including the zygomatic root superior to the EAC (Fig. 42.5). If needed, adjustments or additional elevation should be undertaken at this point to achieve adequate exposure, as this is critical for visualization during drilling. A Weitlaner retractor is positioned to reflect the periosteum anteriorly and to visualize the mastoid and posterior external auditory meatus.

In a tympanomastoidectomy, we prefer to assess the middle ear disease and status of the ossicular chain prior to performing a mastoidectomy. Under the microscope, the vascular strip is elevated, and nested Perkins and Weitlaner retractors are used to reflect the vascular strip anteriorly in the EAC (Fig. 42.6). At this time, the tympanomeatal flap is elevated and reflected anteriorly, exposing the middle ear. The middle ear is inspected for the extent of disease, cholesteatoma, and ossicular chain erosion or fixation. We favor canalplasty to facilitate both middle ear dissection and postoperative clinical examinations in the office. If a canalplasty is performed, it is generally performed just after the elevation of the tympanomeatal flap. Importantly, if a mastoidectomy is performed prior to canalplasty, the posterior canal wall is not thinned significantly to avoid a through-and-through defect of the canal wall during canalplasty later in the case. Although an in-depth discussion of middle ear dissection and canalplasty is not within the scope of this chapter, these topics are reviewed in detail in previous chapters.

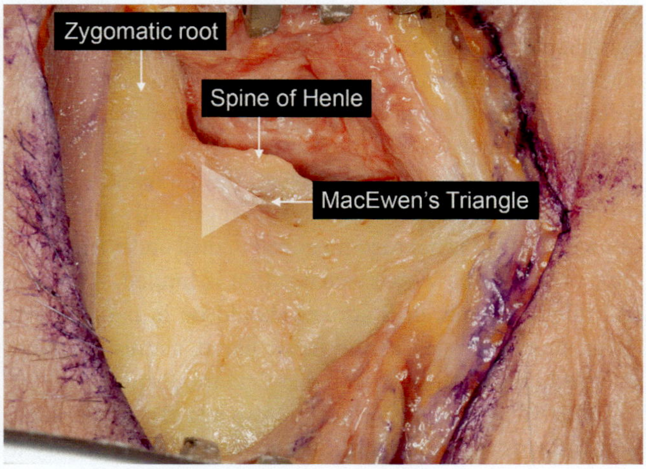

Fig. 42.5 Exposure of mastoid cortex for tympanomastoidectomy, including spine of Henle and root of zygoma. MacEwen's triangle estimates the location of the mastoid antrum medially

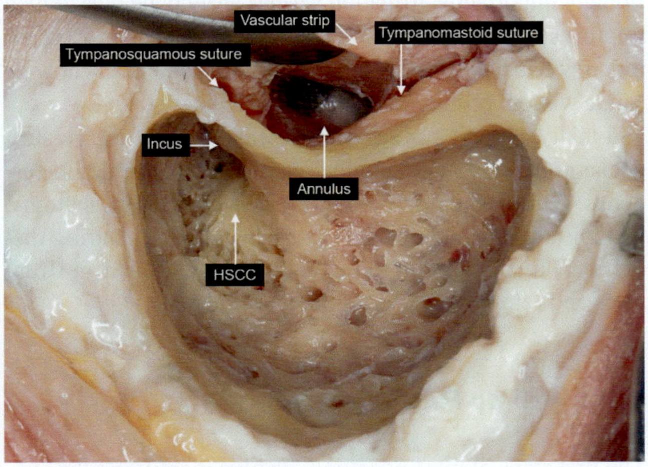

Fig. 42.6 Location of canal incision, demonstrating view of tympanic membrane. HSCC horizontal semicircular canal

Mastoidectomy Basics

Safe dissection in CWU mastoidectomy requires thorough anatomical knowledge and adequate visualization. The mastoidectomy approach utilizes a cone-shaped corridor to allow for adequate lighting of deeper structures. Bony removal to reveal desired structures is completed under binocular otomicroscopy using a high-speed otologic drill (typically 70,000–75,000 revolutions per minute) and saline irrigation. In our practice, we use both cutting burrs, which quickly remove bony portion, and coarse diamond burrs, which are reserved for more delicate dissection around critical structures such as the facial nerve. For efficiency, larger cutting burrs are used initially to remove cortical bone, with a sequential decrease in the size of burrs as the dissection progresses to narrower areas. Importantly, the largest possible burr should be used for each task for two reasons: (1) larger burrs remove bone more quickly, and (2) larger burrs remove a flatter surface area, making inadvertent penetration of underlying structures less likely. Since otologic burrs cut circumferentially, the surgeon must pay attention to all structures in contact with the burr in all directions. Consequently, it is not recommended to drill under a ledge of bone or in an area where visualization is limited. As a general rule of thumb, drill strokes should be in parallel with linear structures such as the facial nerve, as this promotes safe structural identification rather than transection.

Effective irrigation is critical to safe and efficient drilling. Constant irrigation during drilling prevents thermal injury to both bone and nerves, and it is recommended that irrigation be present in all areas actively being drilled. There is one exception to this rule; irrigation is not required when a diamond burr is being used to control small vessel bleeding within bone. Equally importantly, irrigation washes away bone dust, which improves visualization. Efficient use of a suction-irrigator requires hand positioning that allows for a constant flow of saline without obstructing the surgeon's view.

Finally, chronic ear surgery presents some of the greatest decision-making and technical challenges for otologic surgeons. At times, chronic inflammation can distort anatomy, making identification of structures challenging. During dissections, it is important to be on high alert for critical structures and return to known anatomy frequently.

Canal Wall Up Mastoidectomy

The first steps of mastoidectomy involve identifying the anatomical landmarks that define the anterior, superior, and posterior borders of the dissection: the EAC, middle fossa tegmen, and sigmoid sinus, respectively. The extent of dissection during mastoidectomy can be tailored to the needs of the patient; namely, a CWU mastoidectomy completed for cochlear implantation may not require identification of the sigmoid sinus. For the purposes of this chapter, we will describe a complete mastoidectomy employed for chronic ear disease, which opens the mastoid, tegmental, and sinodural air cells (Fig. 42.7a). Initially, the surgeon uses a 5-mm cutting burr to outline the estimated borders of the dissection along the linea temporalis and posterior wall of the EAC. Next, the tegmen is identified with long, broad strokes in parallel with the dura. Upon reaching the middle fossa tegmen, the pink dura with overlying vessels is visualized through the bone, and the sound quality of the drill becomes more high-pitched. The tegmen may be obscured by overlying bone marrow, which is especially common in children. Early identification of the middle fossa tegmen is critical in avoiding facial nerve injury and directing the remainder of the dissection. Unless involved with disease, the tegmen is left intact. Please see below for considerations in the setting of tegmen injury.

Once the tegmen is identified, the cortical bone posterior to the EAC is removed, taking care to identify the sigmoid sinus and mastoid tip. Again, identification of the sigmoid sinus requires long, broad strokes in parallel with the structure; a bluish hue is visualized through the bone overlying the sinus. Next, the sinodural angle is developed, and the remainder of the cortex is removed down to the mastoid tip. To identify the antrum, the tegmen is followed anteriorly to the superior EAC. Medial dissection through Körner's septum, the embryologic remnant of the fusion plane between the petrous and squamosal portions of the temporal bone, opens up the antrum (Fig. 42.7b). Within the antrum, the

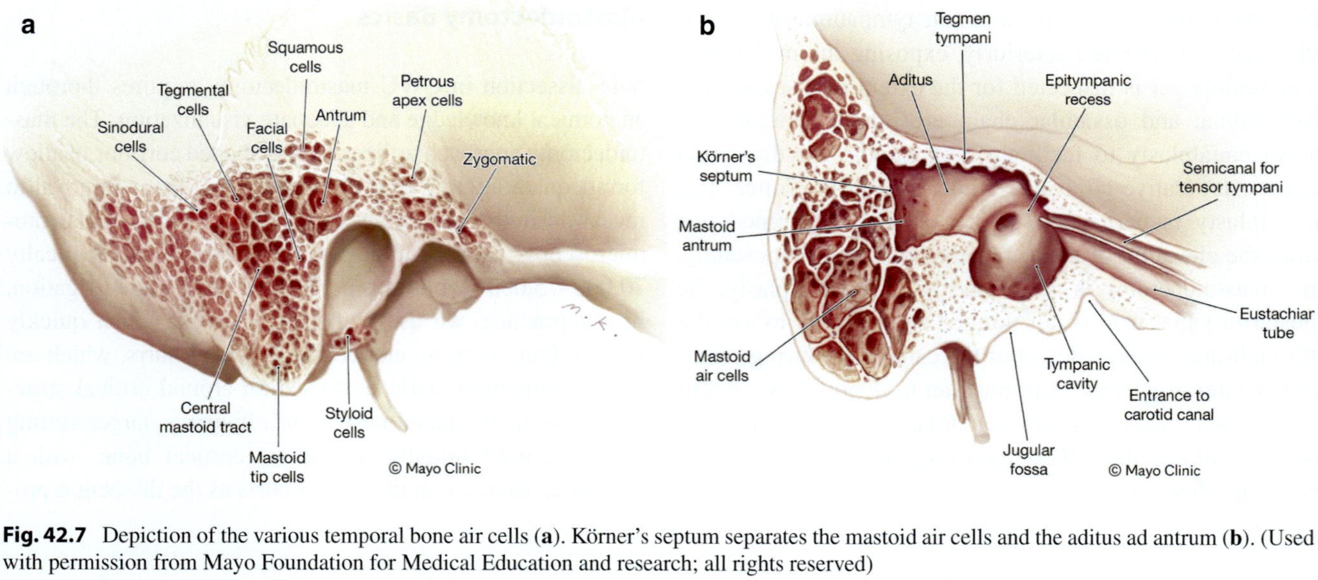

Fig. 42.7 Depiction of the various temporal bone air cells (**a**). Körner's septum separates the mastoid air cells and the aditus ad antrum (**b**). (Used with permission from Mayo Foundation for Medical Education and research; all rights reserved)

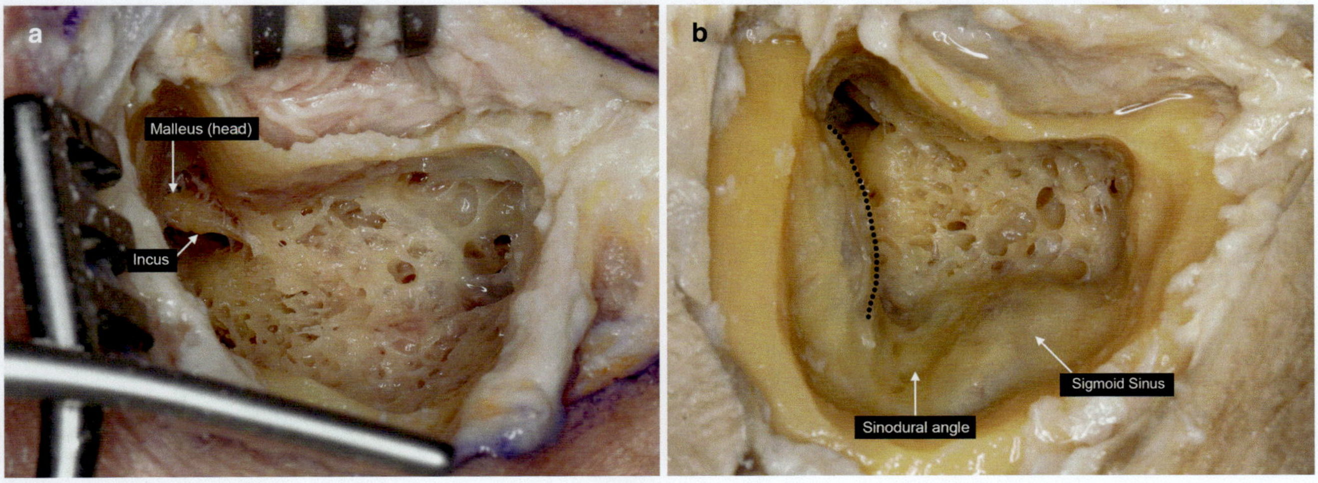

Fig. 42.8 Mastoidectomy with antrotomy demonstrating edge of Körner's septum, incus, and horizontal semicircular canal (panel **a**) and complete mastoidectomy with skeletonization of tegmen and sigmoid sinus and exenteration of air cells (panel **b**). Note the relatively low (or inferior) tegmen mastoideum (dotted line)

horizontal semicircular canal can be identified with its characteristic smooth and compact otic capsule bone. In patients with CSOM, granulation tissue, cholesteatoma, or inflamed mucosa may obstruct the antrum. The remainder of Körner's septum is removed posteriorly to fully expose the antrum (Fig. 42.8).

Next, attic dissection and exposure of the short process of the incus is achieved by following the tegmen anteriorly and thinning the bone of the superior EAC. The angle between the tegmen and EAC is developed from lateral to medial, and in most cases requires a 3-mm burr. It may be difficult to visualize this area well if the periosteum was not adequately elevated anteriorly. The short process of the incus is found at the depth of the horizontal semicircular canal. In cases with epitympanic disease, a posterior atticotomy improves access for disease removal. Access to the anterior epitympanum requires additional anteromedial dissection, and removal of the cog—a flat, bony projection from the tegmen that separates the anterior and posterior epitympanum.

Although the facial nerve is not yet encountered at this point of the procedure, the surgeon must be knowledgeable of its location within the surgical field at all times. Distal to the geniculate ganglion, the tympanic segment of the facial nerve passes superiorly to the oval window, reaching the second genu, where it turns inferiorly through the mastoid. The short process of the incus points to the second genu of the facial nerve, which is just inferior to the horizontal semicircular canal. While the proximal portion of the mastoid segment is generally medial to the horizontal semicircular canal, the distal portion becomes more lateral as it travels inferiorly toward the stylomastoid foramen; the relationship between the facial nerve and the horizontal semicircular canal can be examined on preoperative imaging when available. In our practice, the mastoid segment of the facial nerve is not routinely localized during chronic ear surgery. Rather, the mastoid segment is identified when involved with disease or if a facial recess approach is required. In most cases, however, this is not necessary, and the risk of damage to the nerve from drilling outweighs the benefit of isolating the nerve.

The extent of mastoid dissection is dependent upon the extent of disease and the goals of the procedure. In CSOM with cholesteatoma, it is important to provide access for disease removal and to restore ventilation pathways of the middle ear. In our practice, the mastoid tip is generally left intact unless involved by cholesteatoma. In thinking ahead, should the patient require a CWD mastoidectomy in the future, a smaller mastoid cavity results in a smaller, more functional, and cosmetically appealing mastoid bowl.

Soft Tissue Dissection

Middle ear disease extends into the mastoid antrum frequently, and concurrent soft tissue and bony dissection may be necessary. In cases with an epitympanic cholesteatoma that extends into the mastoid antrum, dissection of the cholesteatoma may be necessary to adequately visualize the horizontal semicircular canal and ossicles. If the cholesteatoma is contained within a squamous epithelial sac, keeping the sac intact during dissection ensures complete removal of the disease. This can be done by pulling the sac away from the abutting bone and carefully removing that bone until the mastoidectomy is complete. In large cholesteatoma, internal decompression provides the surgeon with additional working space and visualization. Depending on the size of the cholesteatoma and status of the middle ear and ossicles, the cholesteatoma can be removed *en bloc* through the middle ear or through the mastoid.

While granulation tissue in the mastoid should also be removed, normal mucosa is left intact to promote postoperative healing. Granulation tissue, however, can be adherent to delicate structures such as the facial nerve, ossicles, or dura. Granulation tissue should be bluntly dissected in parallel with the nerve to avoid avulsion injury; facial nerve monitoring can be helpful in identifying traction on the nerve; however, injury can occur without indication from the monitor. When granulation tissue is too adherent, and removal will cause damage to underlying structures, sharp dissection or trimming is recommended.

Facial Recess

Although infrequently required in chronic ear disease, the facial recess approach (posterior tympanotomy) with CWU mastoidectomy is used when additional access to the mesotympanum or hypotympanum is required. The facial recess is a triangular area defined by the incus buttress superiorly, the mastoid segment of the facial nerve posteriorly and medially, and the chorda tympani nerve anteriorly and laterally. For greater access to the hypotympanum, the chorda tympani can be divided to perform an extended facial recess.

To start, the EAC is thinned to allow access anteriorly. Next, the air cells lateral to the facial recess are removed to the level of the horizontal semicircular canal using a 3-mm cutting or coarse diamond burr. As the surgeon approaches the facial nerve, a 3-mm coarse diamond burr is used to remove the air cells overlying the nerve with long strokes in parallel with the course of the nerve. Constant and copious irrigation over the nerve helps prevent thermal injury from the drill. The surgeon may encounter small vessels overlying the nerve that can bleed during dissection; these are easily controlled with topical epinephrine on Gelfoam. These vessels serve as a useful clue to the proximity of the facial nerve, which appears as a dense, white band within the bone. The chorda tympani nerve is identified anterior and lateral to the facial nerve, using the same technique. In some cases, it is helpful to find its branching point from the facial nerve inferiorly and trace it superiorly (Figs. 42.1a and 42.9).

Once the borders of the recess have been identified, the recess is opened using a 2-mm coarse diamond burr. In a well-aerated mastoid, there is frequently an air cell tract through the facial recess. When preserving the ossicles, it is important to keep a small rim of the incus buttress intact to prevent drilling on the incus. Keeping in mind that the superior-most portion of the recess is the widest, the recess is opened superiorly to inferiorly. In narrow facial recesses, it may be helpful to briefly switch to a 1-mm diamond burr to open into the middle ear before expanding the opening with a 2-mm burr; this technique, however, is presented with caution, as a 1-mm burr can carry a higher risk of injury if it comes into contact with the nerve. In an extended facial recess approach, the chorda tympani is sharply transected at its branching point, and the tympanic membrane annulus becomes the anterior border of the recess (Fig. 42.10).

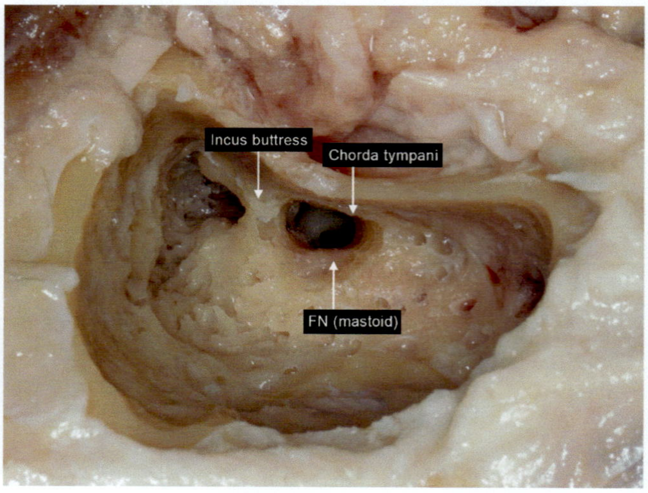

Fig. 42.9 View of middle ear through facial recess

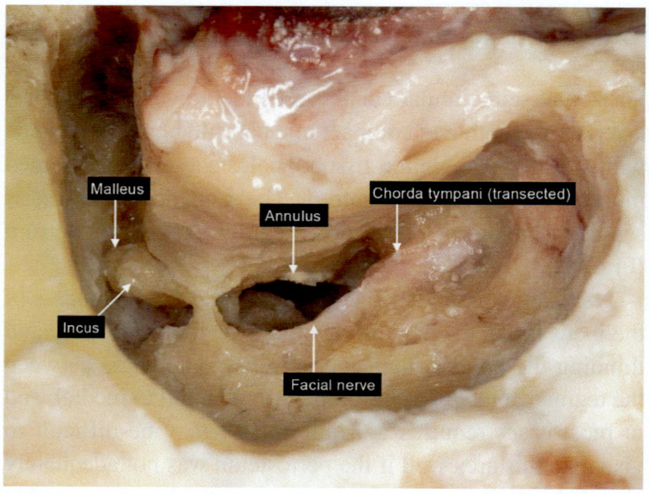

Fig. 42.10 Extended facial recess approach. Note tympanic membrane annulus as anterior limit of dissection

Acute Mastoiditis

The goals of mastoidectomy in acute mastoiditis with abscess differ significantly when compared to mastoidectomy in CSOM. In acute mastoiditis, surgical intervention aims to evacuate pus from the mastoid and any associated abscesses. Preoperative imaging should specifically be evaluated for tegmen or sigmoid sinus dehiscence and the relative location of the coalescent cavity. In general, an incision and drainage with cortical mastoidectomy is performed in conjunction with tympanostomy tube placement. In most cases, a cortical mastoidectomy is sufficient to allow for egress of infectious drainage, while avoiding the risks of complete mastoidectomy in the setting of active mastoiditis. The cortical mastoidectomy is performed with a 5-mm cutting burr as above, until pus is encountered, and the coalescent cavity is widely opened. The sigmoid sinus is frequently dehiscent, and therefore drilling posteriorly is done cautiously only when necessary. Once the cavity is opened, it is copiously irrigated with antibiotic-containing saline, and a passive drain may be placed at the discretion of the surgeon.

Closure

Once the middle ear and mastoid have been cleared of disease, both cavities are copiously irrigated with saline. In a tympanomastoidectomy, a large epinephrine-soaked Gelfoam is temporarily placed in the mastoid for hemostasis while the tympanic membrane is reconstructed, and the vascular strip is reflected back onto the posterior EAC. The postauricular incisions are closed after the EAC is packed. The periosteal layer is reapproximated using interrupted 3-0 Vicryl sutures (Ethicon), being careful to limit excess posterior pulling that may displace a shorter vascular strip into the mastoid cavity. The dermis is also closed with interrupted Vicryl sutures. The incision is covered with antibiotic ointment, and a Glasscock ear dressing (Otomed) is applied.

Postoperative Care

After surgery, patients are discharged home with 1 week of antibiotics and pain medication. If a tympanomastoidectomy was performed, and there was evidence of frank purulence during the case, 1 week of ototopical antibiotics are prescribed as well. A normal follow-up schedule involves a clinic examination 3 weeks after surgery, and a second examination and audiogram 12 weeks after surgery. Of course, if there is evidence of postoperative infection or complication, patients are followed more closely.

Complications

Most intraoperative complications result from unrecognized anatomical variations or poor visualization due to inadequate surgical exposure, bleeding, or granulation tissue. A strong grasp of both normal anatomy and potential variations is key to avoiding pitfalls in chronic ear disease. In cases of poor visualization, expanding surgical exposure remains one of the most useful tactics in a surgeon's armamentarium. Identification of landmarks such as the tegmen, horizontal semicircular canal, facial nerve, and ossicles and frequent reassessment of orientation within the surgical field can prevent injury to critical structures. Postoperative complications can generally be managed in a clinic setting with close follow-up.

Bleeding

Chronic inflammation, granulation tissue, and injury to vessels can present with significant bleeding that obscures visualization. In order to avoid injury to underlying structures, bleeding should be controlled as best possible. In cases of diffuse bleeding from granulation tissue, copious irrigation during drilling or temporary placement of a large epinephrine-soaked Gelfoam can improve visualization. Small blood vessels within the mastoid bone can be controlled with a diamond burr, while larger vessels may require bipolar electrocautery or bone wax. Electrocautery is not recommended for vessels directly overlying the facial nerve.

Injury to the sigmoid sinus can result in significant bleeding. In small defects, the first step is to gently place a postage stamp sized Gelfoam over the defect without compressing the sinus. This effectively stops the bleeding in most cases and avoids thrombus formation. Bipolar electrocautery can also be used. For larger defects, a finger is gently placed over the tear to stop bleeding and avoid the rare but dreaded complication of air embolus. It is good practice to inform the anesthesia team of the injury, so that they may monitor for hemodynamic signs of an air embolus and place the patient in Trendelenburg position. Depending on the size of the defect, various methods of repair can be used including holding pressure with a large Gelfoam and small cotton pledget (cotton must be removed prior to closure) or primary closure. As a last resort, the sigmoid sinus can be tied off with suture ligation, which requires exposure of both the pre- and post-sigmoid dura.

Facial Nerve Injury

Facial nerve injury is one of the most devastating complications of otologic surgery. While facial nerve monitoring is helpful, it is not a replacement for sound knowledge of facial nerve anatomy. The facial nerve exam should be documented preoperatively in the initial history and physical, and an exam should be completed postoperatively after extubation in the operating room.

Whether or not the facial nerve remains in continuity after an injury determines management options. In cases of complete transection of the nerve, immediate reconstruction with anastomosis of free nerve ends or an interposition cable nerve graft should be performed. The free nerve ends require freshening, decompression, and release from the surrounding bone to allow for neurorrhaphy using 9-0 nylon sutures or fibrin glue. A cable nerve graft used for a tension-free anastomosis can be obtained from the great auricular or sural nerve. Studies have shown that at best, a neurorrhaphy results in a score of III or IV on the House-Brackmann scale in the long term [39].

In partial transection, with some nerve fibers still intact, the facial nerve has the potential for reasonable recovery. Consequently, these nerves are not intentionally divided and reanastomosed, in hopes that functional recovery will surpass a score of III or IV on the House-Brackmann scale. Intraoperative facial nerve responses may be tested with direct stimulation, although even patients without responses can have functional recovery. Nerve decompression is performed in patients without responses to direct stimulation, while all patients receive postoperative oral steroids to discourage nerve edema. Close follow-up for facial nerve function is necessary for these patients, as those with persistent paralysis may require additional procedures.

Rarely, patients with no intraoperative concern for facial nerve injury present with postoperative facial paralysis. In cases of immediate postoperative paralysis, it is important to monitor the patient for at least 4 hours postoperatively, to rule out local anesthesia as a cause of paralysis. If a patient has a persistent paralysis after 4–6 hours, urgent surgical exploration is warranted. Intraoperatively, the length of the facial nerve from the geniculate ganglion to the stylomastoid foramen is examined, and suspected areas of injury are decompressed. In cases of delayed postoperative paralysis that may manifest a week or more after surgery, patients should be managed for a presumed latent herpes zoster virus activation [40, 41]. Treatment of delayed facial paralysis is nonsurgical, and includes high-dose oral steroids, with the addition of antivirals if a viral etiology is suspected.

Sensorineural Hearing Loss and Vertigo

While severe sensorineural hearing loss is rare after mastoidectomy, it can occur as a complication of opening the labyrinth or acoustic trauma from manipulation or drilling of the ossicles [42, 43]. Postoperative vertigo can be immediate or delayed and can be attributed to ossicular chain manipulation, labyrinthitis, benign paroxysmal positional vertigo (BPPV), or perilymphatic fistula. Serous labyrinthitis leads to both sensorineural hearing loss and vertigo and is associated with intralabyrinthine inflammation caused by bacterial exotoxins. Serous labyrinthitis is managed with early steroid treatment. In untreated or severe cases, bacterial (or suppurative) labyrinthitis can develop and may result in sudden hearing loss and vertigo without significant functional recovery [44]. Patients with CSOM or acute mastoiditis are at higher risk for these complications, as bacteria can be seeded if the inner ear is opened intraoperatively. Treatment involves antibiotics, steroids, and supportive measures.

Infection

Early postoperative infection impedes proper healing of incisions and can cause prolonged surgical recovery. If a patient experiences postoperative infection despite the use of topical antibiotic treatment to the postauricular incision, oral antibiotics are recommended. Close follow-up is required to monitor for incisional dehiscence.

Intracranial Injury

Intraoperative dural exposure is relatively common in mastoidectomy and generally does not lead to postoperative complications. As a preventative measure, tegmen defects can be reconstructed with autologous bone pâté to promote bony regrowth. Dura can be damaged by drilling with a cutting burr, monopolar electrocautery, or extension of cholesteatoma. Reconstruction is required in cases of dural defect with cerebrospinal fluid leak or exposed brain parenchyma. A multilayered reconstructive technique utilizes fascia, cartilage, bone pâté, and sometimes fibrin glue. Importantly, if the defect contains cholesteatoma, it is imperative to remove all skin debris before repair to avoid cholesteatoma cranialization. If an encephalocele is present, gentle bipolar cautery of the tissue will help with retraction intracranially so the repair can be completed. If the defect is large (>5 mm), it may not be possible to repair from a mastoidectomy approach alone and might require a separate middle fossa craniotomy for repair.

Conclusion

Acute and chronic otologic infections may both require CWU mastoidectomy prior to resolution. In both cases, inflammation and bleeding can make visualization difficult. Consistent use of anatomical landmarks and surgical principles to improve visualization will promote a safe surgical approach. A CWU mastoidectomy is a highly versatile workhorse of otologic surgery, and mastery of this approach is critical to treating acute and chronic ear disease.

References

1. Mawson SR. Surgery of the mastoid: the first centenary. Proc R Soc Med. 1975;68(6):391–5.
2. Mayo W. Mastoid abscess: opening of mastoid cells. Northwest Lancet. 1886;
3. Carlson ML. The history of otologic surgery at Mayo Clinic, 1883 to present. Mayo Clin Proc. 2019;94(2):e19–33.
4. Sunder S, Jackler RK, Blevins NH. Virtuosity with the Mallet and Gouge: the brilliant triumph of the "modern" mastoid operation. Otolaryngol Clin N Am. 2006;39(6):1191–210.
5. Mudry A. The history of the microscope for use in ear surgery. Am J Otol. 2000;21(6):877–86.
6. Mudry A. History of instruments used for mastoidectomy. J Laryngol Otol. 2009;123(6):583–9.
7. Sheehy JL, Patterson ME. Intact canal wall tympanoplasty with mastoidectomy. A review of eight years' experience. Laryngoscope. 1967;77(8):1502–42.
8. Jansen C. The combined approach for tympanoplasty (report on 10 years' experience). J Laryngol Otol. 1968;82(9):779–93.
9. Butbul-Aviel Y, Miron D, Halevy R, Koren A, Sakran W. Acute mastoiditis in children: pseudomonas aeruginosa as a leading pathogen. Int J Pediatr Otorhinolaryngol. 2003;67(3):277–81.
10. Laursen BB, Danstrup CS, Hoffmann S, Norskov-Lauritsen N, Christensen ALB, Ovesen T. The effect of pneumococcal conjugate vaccines on incidence and microbiology associated with complicated acute otitis media. Int J Pediatr Otorhinolaryngol. 2017;101:249–53.
11. Stern Shavit S, Raveh E, Levi L, Sokolov M, Ulanovski D. Surgical intervention for acute mastoiditis: 10 years experience in a tertiary children's hospital. Eur Arch Oto-rhino-laryng. 2019;276(11):3051–6.
12. Coudert A, Fanchette J, Regnier G, et al. Fusobacterium necrophorum, a major provider of sinus thrombosis in acute mastoiditis: a retrospective multicentre paediatric study. Clin Otolaryngol. 2020;45(2):182–9.
13. Acuin J. Chronic suppurative otitis media. BMJ Clin Evid. 2007;2007:0507.
14. Senturia B, Bluestone C, Lim D, Klein J, Paradise J. Report of the ad hoc committee on definition and classification of otitis media and otitis media with effusion. Ann Otol Rhinol Laryngol. 1980;89(3):2.
15. Wright CG, Meyerhoff WL. Pathology of otitis media. Ann Otol Rhinol Laryngol Suppl. 1994;163:24–6.
16. Wang B, Cheng Y, Xu M. Characterization of the T-cell subpopulations in the granulation tissues of chronic suppurative otitis media. Biomed Rep. 2016;4(6):694–8.
17. Meyerhoff WL, Kim CS, Paparella MM. Pathology of chronic otitis media. Ann Otol Rhinol Laryngol. 1978;87(6 Pt 1):749–60.
18. Mittal R, Lisi CV, Gerring R, et al. Current concepts in the pathogenesis and treatment of chronic suppurative otitis media. J Med Microbiol. 2015;64(10):1103–16.
19. van der Veen EL, Schilder AG, van Heerbeek N, Verhoeff M, Zielhuis GA, Rovers MM. Predictors of chronic suppurative otitis media in children. Arch Otolaryngol--Head Neck Surg. 2006;132(10):1115–8.
20. Vikram BK, Khaja N, Udayashankar SG, Venkatesha BK, Manjunath D. Clinico-epidemiological study of complicated and uncomplicated chronic suppurative otitis media. J Laryngol Otol. 2008;122(5):442–6.
21. Zevallos JP, Vrabec JT, Williamson RA, et al. Advanced pediatric mastoiditis with and without intracranial complications. Laryngoscope. 2009;119(8):1610–5.
22. Ongkasuwan J, Valdez TA, Hulten KG, Mason EO Jr, Kaplan SL. Pneumococcal mastoiditis in children and the emergence of multidrug-resistant serotype 19A isolates. Pediatrics. 2008;122(1):34–9.
23. Redaelli de Zinis LO, Campovecchi C, Parrinello G, Antonelli AR. Predisposing factors for inner ear hearing loss association with chronic otitis media. Int J Audiol. 2005;44(10):593–8.
24. Kaplan DM, Fliss DM, Kraus M, Dagan R, Leiberman A. Audiometric findings in children with chronic suppurative otitis media without cholesteatoma. Int J Pediatr Otorhinolaryngol. 1996;35(2):89–96.
25. Dumich PS, Harner SG. Cochlear function in chronic otitis media. Laryngoscope. 1983;93(5):583–6.
26. Jensen RG, Koch A, Homoe P. Long-term tympanic membrane pathology dynamics and spontaneous healing in chronic suppurative otitis media. Pediatr Infect Dis J. 2012;31(2):139–44.
27. Toros SZ, Habesoglu TE, Habesoglu M, et al. Do patients with sclerotic mastoids require aeration to improve success of tympanoplasty? Acta Otolaryngol. 2010;130(8):909–12.
28. Kwon OJ, Sung JM, Jung HK, Kim CW. Postoperative mastoid aeration following canal wall up mastoidectomy according to preoperative middle ear disease: analysis of temporal bone computed tomography scans. J Audiol Otol. 2017;21(3):140–5.
29. Hulka GF, McElveen JT Jr. A randomized, blinded study of canal wall up versus canal wall down mastoidectomy determining the differences in viewing middle ear anatomy and pathology. Am J Otol. 1998;19(5):574–8.
30. Kerckhoffs KG, Kommer MB, van Strien TH, et al. The disease recurrence rate after the canal wall up or canal wall down technique in adults. Laryngoscope. 2016;126(4):980–7.
31. Ho SY, Kveton JF. Efficacy of the 2-staged procedure in the management of cholesteatoma. Arch Otolaryngol Head Neck Surg. 2003;129(5):541–5.
32. Khalil HS, Windle-Taylor PC. Canal wall down mastoidectomy: a long term commitment to the outpatients? BMC Ear Nose Throat Disord. 2003;3(1):1.
33. Quaranta N, Iannuzzi L, Petrone P, D'Elia A, Quaranta A. Quality of life after cholesteatoma surgery: intact-canal wall tympanoplasty versus canal wall-down tympanoplasty with mastoid obliteration. Ann Otol Rhinol Laryngol. 2014;123(2):89–93.
34. Lailach S, Kemper M, Lasurashvili N, Beleites T, Zahnert T, Neudert M. Health-related quality of life measurement after cholesteatoma surgery: comparison of three different surgical techniques. Eur Arch Oto-rhino-laryngol. 2015;272(11):3177–85.
35. Kim MB, Choi J, Lee JK, et al. Hearing outcomes according to the types of mastoidectomy: a comparison between canal wall up and canal wall down mastoidectomy. Clin Exp Otorhinolaryngol. 2010;3(4):203–6.
36. Brown JS. A ten year statistical follow-up of 1142 consecutive cases of cholesteatoma: the closed vs. the open technique. Laryngoscope. 1982;92(4):390–6.
37. Chadha NK, Jardine A, Owens D, Gillett S, Robinson PJ, Maw AR. A multivariate analysis of the factors predicting hearing outcome after surgery for cholesteatoma in children. J Laryngol Otol. 2006;120(11):908–13.
38. Manzoor NF, Nassiri AM, Rivas A. Endoscopic ossiculoplasty. Curr Otorhinolaryngol Rep. 2019;7(4):244–7.
39. Arriaga MA, Brackmann DE. Facial nerve repair techniques in cerebellopontine angle tumor surgery. Am J Otol. 1992;13(4):356–9.
40. De Stefano A, Neri G, Kulamarva G. Delayed facial nerve paralysis post middle ear surgery: herpes simplex virus activation. B-ENT. 2009;5(1):47–50.

41. Gianoli GJ. Viral titers and delayed facial palsy after acoustic neuroma surgery. Otolaryngol--Head Neck Surg. 2002;127(5):427–31.
42. Kazikdas KC, Onal K, Yildirim N. Sensorineural hearing loss after ossicular manipulation and drill-generated acoustic trauma in type I tympanoplasty with and without mastoidectomy: a series of 51 cases. Ear Nose Throat J. 2015;94(9):378–98.
43. Tos M, Lau T, Plate S. Sensorineural hearing loss following chronic ear surgery. Ann Otol Rhinol Laryngol. 1984;93(4 Pt 1):403–9.
44. Jang CH, Park SY, Wang PC. A case of tympanogenic labyrinthitis complicated by acute otitis media. Yonsei Med J. 2005;46(1):161–5.

Canal Wall Down Mastoidectomy

43

Michael H. Freeman, Eric N. Appelbaum, and Marc L. Bennett

Introduction

Open cavity mastoid operations, also known as canal wall down (CWD) mastoidectomies, can be categorized as procedures where the goal of the operation is to exteriorize the contents of the epitympanic and mastoid air cells by removing some portion of the external auditory canal (EAC) wall. Most often, this is utilized in the setting of cholesteatoma. CWD mastoidectomy operations provide the benefit of wide exposure to nearly the entire tympanomastoid space, facilitating removal of cholesteatoma and permitting access for debridement in the clinic setting.

History and General Approaches

Historically, mastoidectomy has been one of the most important methods for control of otologic infection. In the pre-antibiotic era, it represented the only method for control of complicated otitis media. The first mastoidectomy was described in 1873 by Schwartze and Eysell for control of acute mastoiditis [1]. That same year, von Tröltsch suggested that persistent otorrhea caused by cholesteatoma may require more extensive surgical management as persistent disease would result in chronic otorrhea and infection [2]. In 1890, Zaufel published the first description of a CWD mastoidectomy in which he detailed the removal of the external auditory canal wall and middle ear contents to convert the tympanomastoid space into an open, common cavity [3].

Radical Mastoidectomy

These early approaches removed the posterior ear canal as well as the tympanic membrane, ossicles, and chorda tympani, without any reconstruction of the middle ear space. This approach is termed a radical mastoidectomy. After denuding its mucosal lining, the Eustachian tube isthmus is sealed with a free tissue graft (fat, muscle, bone pâté, or fascia) to allow for formation of a dry cavity. This approach has largely fallen out of favor due to the absence of any hearing reconstruction inherent to this technique. It still has a role for some unresectable cholesteatomas or aggressive malignancies.

Bondy-Modified Radical Mastoidectomy

In 1910, Bondy offered an alternative for patients suffering from pars flaccida cholesteatoma with antral extension but an intact pars tensa and serviceable hearing [4]. In what came to be known as the Bondy-modified radical mastoidectomy, the superior medial portion of the osseous EAC was removed to expose cholesteatoma within the epitympanum. This bone removal provides access to the epitympanic space. Importantly, the middle ear and pars tensa of the tympanic membrane are left unperturbed. Typically, the medial growth of the cholesteatoma matrix is left atop the ossicles in the epitympanum to avoid need for reconstruction. This allows for maintenance of largely normal middle ear function necessary for hearing preservation while allowing access to the cholesteatoma for future debridements [5].

Tympanoplasty with CWD Mastoidectomy

Cases of CWD surgery requiring removal of disease from the middle ear may require a tympanoplasty with CWD mastoidectomy. This can occur with or without ossicular chain

M. H. Freeman · M. L. Bennett (✉)
Department of Otolaryngology—Head and Neck Surgery, Vanderbilt University Medical Center, Nashville, TN, USA
e-mail: marc.bennett@vumc.org

E. N. Appelbaum
Wellstar Medical Group, Marietta, GA, USA

A. D. Sweeney et al. (eds.), *Haynes-Glasscock-Shambaugh Surgery of the Ear*, https://doi.org/10.1007/978-3-032-18264-7_43

reconstruction. Some surgeons refer to this as a tympanoplasty with modified radical mastoidectomy. This approach allows for fairly straightforward, concurrent ossicular chain reconstruction. A variety of autologous materials can be used including cartilage, fascia, or skin grafts. An anterior tympanic membrane remnant is typically preserved at a minimum to prevent lateralization of the tympanic reconstruction.

Patient Selection

Indications

Traditionally, CWD tympanomastoidectomy has been employed in the treatment of cholesteatoma, but it may be required in a number of other situations where the posterior or superior EAC wall has eroded and cannot be easily reconstructed. While this is most commonly due to attic cholesteatoma, canal cholesteatoma, prior infection, and iatrogenic injury from prior procedures also occur and can result in a defect that is not amenable to reconstruction (Fig. 43.1). Some patients may not medically tolerate second- and third-look procedures. These patients are excellent candidates for CWD surgery due to the low risk of operative disease recurrence and fairly straightforward process of in-clinic debridement. Some surgeons also advocate for CWD procedures in the setting of aggressive otitis media and mastoiditis or cholesteatoma if routine follow up is not likely.

Some patients have cholesteatoma that cannot be safely removed in its entirety, and in these cases exteriorization of disease through a CWD approach is favored. The classic example of this idea is a cholesteatoma with labyrinthine fistula without significant sensorineural hearing loss—in these cases, a layer of cholesteatoma matrix may be left to cover the dehiscent lateral semicircular canal, and the absence of a posterior–superior ear canal can facilitate debridement of residual and recurrent disease in the clinic. Furthermore, CWD can be indicated in cases of an only-hearing ear with severe cholesteatoma, as the presence of recidivistic cholesteatoma can increase risk of bone erosion and eventual profound sensorineural hearing loss. Lastly, in a patient with an extremely anterior sigmoid sinus or low-lying middle fossa dura, a traditional intact canal wall mastoidectomy may not safely permit thorough disease removal. In such cases, a CWD may be the safest avenue to remove cholesteatoma.

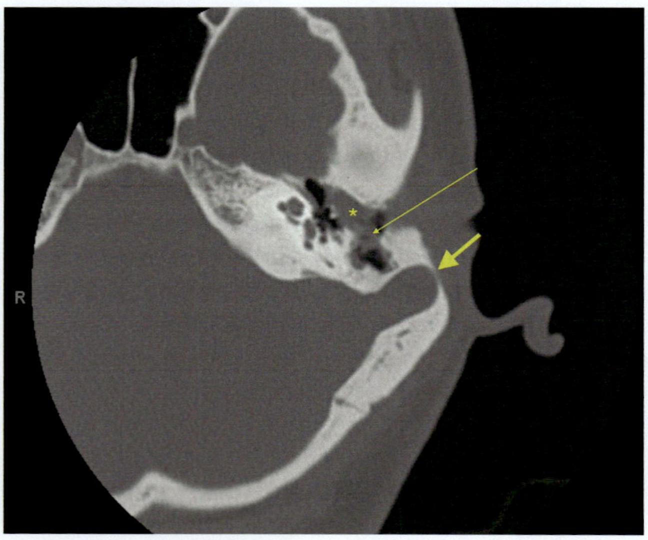

Fig. 43.1 Axial computed tomography image of a left ear with a large ear canal defect (thin arrow) and extensive, infected cholesteatoma (*) in the setting of a low tegmen and anterior-lateral sigmoid sinus (thick arrow). (Courtesy of Alex D. Sweeney, MD)

Contraindications

The presence of an otogenic cerebrospinal fluid (CSF) leak at the time of surgery is an absolute contraindication to CWD surgery for some surgeons. In essence, concerns exist in such a case that intracranial contents can be "exteriorized," thus facilitating the development of an intracranial infection. Though CWD surgery can be performed in the setting of a canal wall defect, a relative contraindication to CWD surgery exists when the defect is relatively reparable. One common example of this is a pars flaccida cholesteatoma that is treatable with an atticotomy—in these cases, the defect in the medial ear canal can often be reconstructed successfully while avoiding the morbidity of an open mastoid cavity.

Anatomy around the ear canal is also relevant to the subject of when a CWD should be avoided. Surgeons must be conscious of broad exposure of the sigmoid, dura, and labyrinth when deciding to proceed with CWD surgery, as these areas can be pitfalls when debriding the mastoid bowl in the clinic setting. Another important consideration prior to performing a CWD surgery is a patient's ability to regularly follow-up, as noted above. Decision-making in surgery is made challenging when reconciling objective findings and surgeon experience with patient preferences and social determinants of health. The concept of CWD cavity maintenance is an important factor to discuss with patients and family prior to performance of this procedure, if possible. The frequency of CWD maintenance visits needed to maintain a healthy cavity can ultimately depend on how the cavity heals, but, in general, these visits need to occur regularly for the rest of the patient's life to prevent an accumulation of debris that can foster infection and drainage. In some cases, patients are unable to tolerate such debridement, which is not uncommonly the case in the pediatric population. Though performance of a CWD procedure may ultimately be the most medically appropriate option in such a patient, a point of good counseling may involve the consideration of a CWD procedure as relatively contraindicated until the patient and family have a clear understanding of the need for regularly cleaning, and, potentially, the occasional use of anesthesia to facilitate these efforts if a patient cannot tolerate them. An alternate to a traditional CWD procedure and meatoplasty in these cases can be an otic capsule sparing subtotal petrosectomy with ear canal closure, which can obviate the need for routine, in-clinic debridement in favor of the potential for subsequent surgery if residual skin is trapped beneath the closure. While factors such as tobacco use, diabetes mellitus, prior external beam radiation therapy, and malnutrition may all complicate healing following CWD surgery, they are not technically contraindications. Patients in professions requiring frequent water exposure can also be poor candidates for CWD surgery, as water exposure is likely to lead to issues with infection due to moisture trapping or vertigo due to caloric responses of the lateral semicircular canal. If these relative contraindications are significant considerations for a patient, EAC overclosure with or without CWD may be favorable over a traditional CWD approach.

Preoperative Evaluation

Detailed microscopic evaluation of the ear should be performed, taking care to remove purulence and debris that can cloud evaluation of the EAC wall defect. A preoperative audiogram is important for establishing the baseline hearing function of the ear. This measure can help outline the role of ossicular reconstruction and can help guide patients regarding the downstream possibility of implantable bone conducting hearing devices or cochlear implantation. Computed tomography (CT) imaging is also important to help surgeons better understand the natural history of the disease that led to surgical consultation, any potential ear canal defect, and the position of the facial nerve, and can highlight potential areas of procedural complexity, such as dehiscence in the semicircular canals, sigmoid sinus, or posterior fossa bone plate or tegmen. The audiogram combined with high-resolution temporal bone CT imaging can also help surgeons determine the optimal type of CWD surgery to perform as well as the role for ossicular reconstruction or bone conducting devices. Magnetic resonance imaging (MRI) is generally not necessary prior to pursuing more routine tympanomastoidectomy surgery, but it can be useful to evaluate the presence of fluid or inflammation in the inner ear when an otic capsule dehiscence is noted, to evaluate concerns for concomitant meningoencephalocele, and to evaluate soft tissue densities seen on CT that need further characterization.

Procedure Goals

The goals of CWD tympanomastoidectomy are:

1. *Elimination of cholesteatoma (if present)*: Removal of the posterior EAC wall provides access to dissection within the anterior epitympanum, the protympanum, and the supratubal and supralabyrinthine air cells. Some areas of the posterior epitympanum and mesotympanum, especially the sinus tympani, are difficult to directly visualize with a microscope during intact canal wall surgery, even if the facial recess is opened. Dissection of cholesteatoma is particularly difficult in the latter location, and it is a frequent site of disease recurrence [6–8]. Instrument access is improved after removal of the canal wall, as well, allowing for easier dissection of cholesteatoma. For many surgeons, the use of angled endoscopes has reduced the rate of CWD approaches [9]. That said, in the long term, the ability to debride small, residual, or recurrent cholesteatoma in the clinic setting provided by a CWD cavity can be quite helpful for refractory cases involving difficult-to-access disease.
2. *Creation of a stable mastoid cavity*: The second goal of CWD tympanomastoidectomy is the creation of a stable mastoidectomy cavity. The design of the mastoid cavity and anticipation of how it will heal are vitally important to prevention of recurrent infection and drainage. The most important consideration in mastoid cavity design is the size of the mastoid cavity relative to the opening at the newly created meatus. Those cavities that are relatively large with a comparatively small meatus will retain heat and moisture alongside poorer auto-elimination of squamous debris—increasing risk of bacterial and fungal growth. The tradeoffs in this instance are a cosmetic outcome that is closer in appearance to the native meatus and a relatively smaller amount of temperature change and moisture that can pass into the cavity. Conversely, a small cavity with a relatively larger meatus will have less debris accumulation, more debris clearance ability, and decreased potential for bacterial and fungal growth. The tradeoffs in this instance are a cosmetic outcome that is more distinct from the native appearance of the meatus and a relatively higher probability that external entities (i.e., water, foreign objects, wind) can penetrate the cavity and lead to infection, injury, and/or caloric activation of the labyrinth.
3. *Maximize hearing outcomes*: Another goal of CWD tympanomastoidectomy is maximization of hearing. Good

hearing outcomes are difficult to achieve in CWD surgery due to the intrinsic severity and destructive action of the disease that leads to consideration of this procedure, and also because of the destructive nature of the surgery itself. In cholesteatoma and chronic otomastoiditis, erosion of the ossicles and impedance of tympanic membrane vibration produce a conductive hearing loss. Cases of chronic ear disease also frequently involve associated tympanosclerosis, which can contribute to conductive hearing loss. Paradoxically, conductive hearing loss may worsen after cholesteatoma removal if the cholesteatoma was, itself, conducting sound to the cochlea. Sensorineural hearing loss may occur through repeated infections or violation of the otic capsule, though hearing losses in these circumstances are typically mixed.

Restoration of an air-conducted hearing pathway with ossicular reconstruction is often difficult in these scenarios. CWD approaches generally necessitate removal of the incus and malleus. Having an intact stapes superstructure allows for placement of a very short partial ossicular replacement prosthesis (PORP) versus a cartilage cap directly atop the stapes. If the stapes is absent, a total ossicular replacement prosthesis (TORP) may be sized and placed. In general, CWD approaches have worse hearing outcomes than intact canal approaches [10]. In patients with poor hearing after reconstruction, options range from conventional hearing aids to bone conducting hearing devices or cochlear implantation when sensorineural loss is pronounced. The technical considerations for these rehabilitation options are beyond the scope of this chapter and are discussed elsewhere in this book.

Operating Room Setup

Prior to the induction of anesthesia, the operative plan, correct surgical site, patient positioning, and special surgical needs should be reviewed with the Anesthesia team. At our institution, we turn the patient's head 180° away from the Anesthesia team for the procedure, and the surgical scrub team and instrument tables are positioned on the opposite side of the patient from the surgeon. The patient is positioned supine on the bed with the head turned away from the operative side in order to fully expose the ear. Any hair close to the planned postauricular incision site may be trimmed. The authors prefer a curvilinear, "C"-shaped incision 2–3 mm posterior to the postauricular crease. This planned incision may be injected with local anesthetic to reduce bleeding when opening.

Due to the extensive amount of dissection and drilling that may take place around the facial nerve, we use a facial nerve monitor for these cases with electrodes placed in the ipsilateral orbicularis oculi and oris. The ground electrode is placed in the contralateral deltoid, and the system is set to 100 μV threshold limits. Anesthesia should be asked to avoid long-acting paralytics to ensure that facial monitoring is reliable. The operative field should be sterilized according to institutional guidelines and draped to expose the postauricular skin and auricle.

Operative Technique

The procedure should begin with thorough examination of the EAC and middle ear space with use of the operative microscope. In situations where the necessity of a CWD surgery is uncertain, this initial examination may facilitate early decision-making. During this initial transcanal examination, debridement of cholesteatoma should be performed with caution. This is especially relevant if the location of the stapes or facial nerve is unclear, if preoperative imaging has shown the cholesteatoma to involve the stapes footplate, or if there is concern for a labyrinthine fistula.

Surgery proceeds with ear canal incisions to outline the vascular strip and tympanomeatal flap. This step allows for preservation of as much healthy canal skin as possible, which can be important later when reconstructing the mastoid cavity. The canal skin is infiltrated with local anesthetic and vasoconstrictant (2% lidocaine with 1:50,000 epinephrine solution is used at the senior author's center) at the 12 o'clock and 6 o'clock positions to mitigate bleeding from the tympanic suture vasculature and to provide additional anesthesia to a sensitive portion of the surgical field. The medial soft tissue cut is then defined along the posterior EAC wall just lateral to the annulus. If cholesteatoma is present, the skin between this cut and the cholesteatoma can be assumed to be unsalvageable and will eventually be replaced by a soft tissue graft. The vascular strip incisions should be designed in such a way that the flap is trapezoidal to maximize blood supply.

The postauricular incision is then performed to obtain soft tissue for grafting and to expose the mastoid bone. The incision may be similar to the standard "C"-shaped incision of otologic surgery with few modifications. The superior limb of the incision may require anterior extension to fully access the anterior epitympanum and anterior portions of the tegmen tympani and mastoideum. The inferior extent of the incision should be dictated by the size and shape of the patient's mastoid bone and auricle. It is uncommon for cholesteatoma to extend to the mastoid tip, and eviscerating it should be avoided in the design and creation of the mastoid cavity to prevent formation of a dependent, debris-accumulating site.

Following incision of the dermis and subcutaneous tissue, the surgeon should obtain a serviceable fascia tissue graft.

Due to their thin, pliable nature, fascia grafts are an excellent reconstructive medium for the neotympanum and lining for the remainder of the middle ear and mastoid cavities. Fascia may also be used for reconstruction of tegmen and dural defects, or to cover a labyrinthine fistula. The loose areolar tissue covering the temporalis fascia and mastoid periosteum is an excellent graft donor site but may be absent due to prior surgeries. In such cases where a loose areolar tissue or temporalis fascia graft is not available, the existing incision may be extended to reveal available fascia or a secondary donor site may be utilized. True temporalis fascia, perichondrium, and periosteum medial to the temporalis are usually accessible in a standard surgical field.

Creation of the periosteal flaps in CWD tympanomastoidectomy carries extra importance. In standard mastoidectomy approaches, the Palva flap is often kept long to facilitate reapproximation of this layer during closing. This avoids creation of a visible postauricular depression as well as formation of a mastoid-cutaneous fistula. In CWD surgery, however, a short, anteriorly based Palva flap helps to not only limit the size of the mastoid cavity, but also to maintain healthy blood supply to the remaining cortex. Alternatively, a long posteriorly based periosteal flap or a temporalis muscle flap may be utilized to fill the cavity at the sinodural angle. Restricting the mastoid cavity to only the size required for cholesteatoma removal increases the ratio of meatoplasty opening width to cavity volume—increasing ventilation and limiting bacterial growth and risk of chronic otorrhea.

The posterior EAC skin is gently elevated forward from its attachments at the spine of Henle, which may be done with a blunt instrument such as a Freer elevator. The posterior EAC skin is then elevated anteriorly with care not to damage the anterior canal skin. If the vascular strip incisions were previously made, they may be identified at this point and opened completely.

Mastoidectomy

Once the mastoid cortex and posterior EAC wall have been exposed, the surgery may proceed with removal of bone to expose the cholesteatoma. As this process is ongoing, consideration should be given toward the ultimate conformation of the mastoid cavity. In some cases, the decision to create a CWD cavity is known preoperatively, and the surgeon can remove the ear canal early in the procedure to facilitate efficient and safe dissection. In other cases, the decision to perform a CWD procedure is made intraoperatively, and the standard techniques for intact canal wall mastoidectomy can be followed until the decision is made to convert. In either case, there are a handful of special considerations for CWD tympanomastoidectomy.

The operating surgeon should be aware of any potential areas of tegmen thinning, complete dehiscence, or meningoencephalocele existence during mastoidectomy. Iatrogenic exposure of dura and/or creation of a CSF leak, or the existence of the aforementioned issues due to previous surgery, idiopathic intracranial hypertension, or bony erosion, is particularly problematic in CWD mastoidectomy surgery due to the associated predisposition to intracranial infection. Definitive tegmen identification is essential for safe entry into the aditus ad antrum, especially in the setting of a contracted or sclerotic mastoid, often seen in patients with chronic ear disease. Avoidance of routine skeletonization of the sigmoid sinus, posterior fossa dura, and digastric ridge aids in preventing an oversized mastoid cavity.

Cholesteatoma Dissection

Once the posterior and lateral extent of the cholesteatoma is identified, attention should be turned to the anteromedial extent toward the tympanic space. The remaining cholesteatoma matrix and debris should be identified and carefully elevated from the surrounding bone. Identification of areas of concern on pre-procedural imaging, such as a labyrinthine fistula or tegmen dehiscence, should guide the operative surgeon in the order of dissection. If erosion is anticipated or suspected, the matrix may be left intact over the area of concern initially to prevent accidental exposure of the fistula "early" in the procedure. In general, if these areas will be engaged in an attempt to completely remove the matrix, this step should be the final step in the operation prior to reconstruction, and it is recommended that reconstructive substrate be available to address any outcome in this type of effort. Even if preoperative imaging shows no sign of potential cranial or labyrinthine extension, care should be taken when dissecting matrix in areas particularly prone to erosion: the tegmen tympani, the lateral semicircular canal, the facial nerve, and the oval window footplate.

Dissection of the middle ear space should be approached in a systematic and stepwise fashion, which, initially, should follow the same principles of dissection employed in canal wall up (CWU) tympanomastoidectomy. The first part of dissection identifies healthy tissue and separates it from disease. In doing so, the tympanic membrane is elevated from the tympanic ring, initially posteriorly but proceeding inferiorly, superiorly, and anteriorly, as needed, to get a full assessment of the middle ear. Regarding the malleus, the tympanic membrane is generally separated to isolate the ossicular chain. Regarding the tympanic membrane, healthy portions uninvolved with cholesteatoma can be preserved. Regarding the ossicular chain, the incus and malleus often require removal for dissection of the anterior epitympanum and supratubal recess, frequent sites of residual cholesteatoma when performing revision surgery, and also for complete separation of the tympanic space and the mastoid cavity. The resulting visualization and access represent a distinct advantage provided by the CWD procedure versus an intact canal wall approach. That being said, the manubrium, along with the tensor tendon and fibrous connection at the umbo, may be preserved depending on the cholesteatoma extent. Preservation of these structures allows for increased stability of the tympanic membrane reconstruction and may aid in ossicular reconstruction.

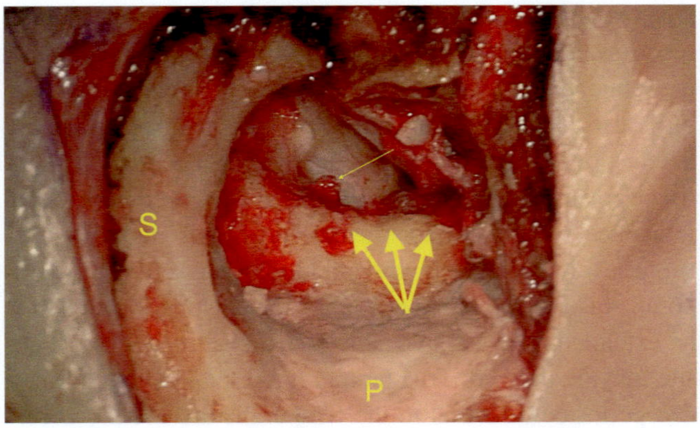

Fig. 43.2 Postauricular anatomy of an intraoperative (right ear) canal wall down cavity. The incus and malleus have been removed. The stapes is marked with a thin arrow. The facial ridge has been lowered (thick arrows). *P* posterior, *S* superior. (Courtesy of Alex D. Sweeney, MD)

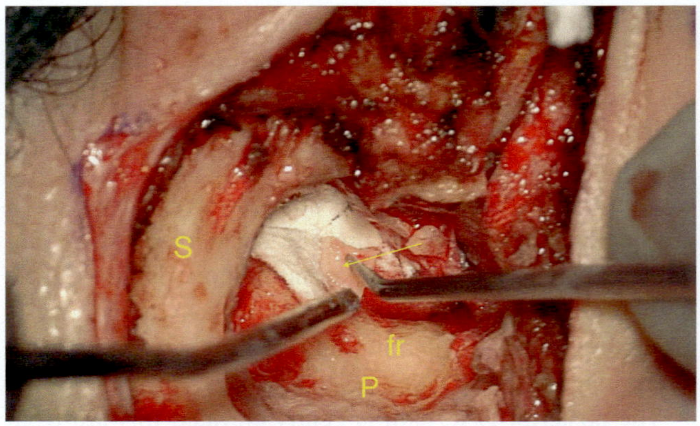

Fig. 43.3 Postauricular anatomy of an intraoperative (right ear) canal wall down cavity. The ossicular graft has been placed and is covered by cartilage (thin arrow). Gelfoam fills the middle ear cavity. *P* posterior, *S* superior, *fr* facial ridge. (Courtesy of Alex D. Sweeney, MD)

Preparation of Cavity

If the posterior EAC wall has not already been removed by this point of the procedure, this should be completed to facilitate removal of disease from the tympanic space. The lateral portion of the EAC wall may be removed with a cutting burr for ease and efficiency, but a diamond burr should be considered once the medial bony canal is reached to avoid inadvertent injury to the facial nerve, ossicular injury, or disruption of the cholesteatoma capsule. Medial dissection should proceed first into the antrum, superior to the lateral semicircular canal, to avoid injury to the facial nerve. If incus will be removed, early separation of the incudostapedial joint and removal allow for more efficient surgery while maintaining safety with respect to hearing.

The bone overlying the facial nerve in its mastoid segment, known as the facial ridge, serves as the boundary between the tympanic cavity and mastoid bowl. It is extremely important to lower the facial ridge to the level of the chorda tympani or facial nerve proper while preserving a thin layer of protective bone (Figs. 43.2 and 43.3). It is important to note that the facial nerve course typically becomes more superficial in the inferior descending segment, increasing risk of iatrogenic nerve exposure and injury. The importance of this maneuver cannot be overstated, as a high facial ridge can trap debris, make debridement challenging in the clinic, and serve as a locus for cholesteatoma regrowth beyond what is immediately apparent on exam. That said, some cases exist where the ridge is deliberately left higher than the level of the facial nerve in order to facilitate ossicular reconstruction with a prosthesis, though this maneuver should only be considered when a dependent area will not consequently form—hearing outcomes are secondary to safety, and no good hearing outcome is as durable or useful in a chronically infected cavity.

After removal of all diseased air cells, it is important to smooth the edges of the mastoidectomy bowl, a process known as saucerization. In CWD approaches, properly saucerizing the cavity allows for better view of the entirety of the cavity for cleaning while also allowing for maximal prolapse of soft tissue into the cavity, providing a route for autoobliteration of the ultimate cavity. Bone material can also be collected during the process of drilling and reutilized to shape the cavity once disease has been eradicated. Specifically, bone dust can be collected, strained, impregnated with a non-ototoxic topical antibiotic, and mixed with a small amount of fibrin sealant to form dense sheets of bone graft that are malleable enough to be shaped into the cavity, as discussed below (Fig. 43.4).

To complete a tympanoplasty with CWD mastoidectomy, ossicular reconstruction is performed or the stapes can be left in contact with a cartilage graft beneath the tympanic membrane. A fascia graft is used to reconstruct the tympanic membrane, and residual tympanic membrane is draped over the graft (Fig. 43.5). However, the meatoplasty, discussed below, is usually performed immediately before completion of this procedure.

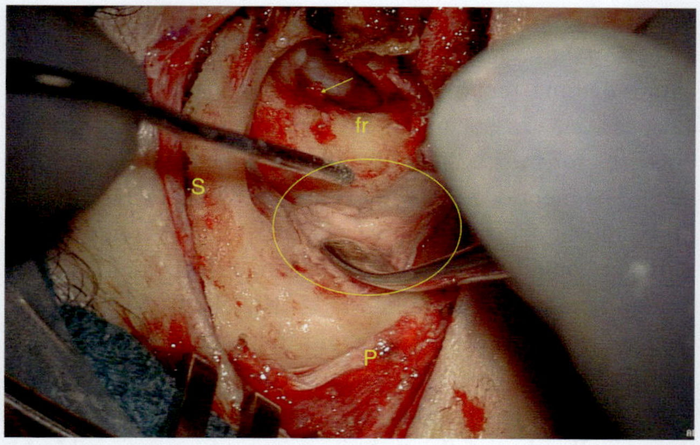

Fig. 43.4 Placement of bone graft material (pate) in the posterior aspect of the mastoid cavity (circled). The stapes is marked by a thin arrow. *P* posterior, *S* superior, *fr* facial ridge. (Courtesy of Alex D. Sweeney, MD)

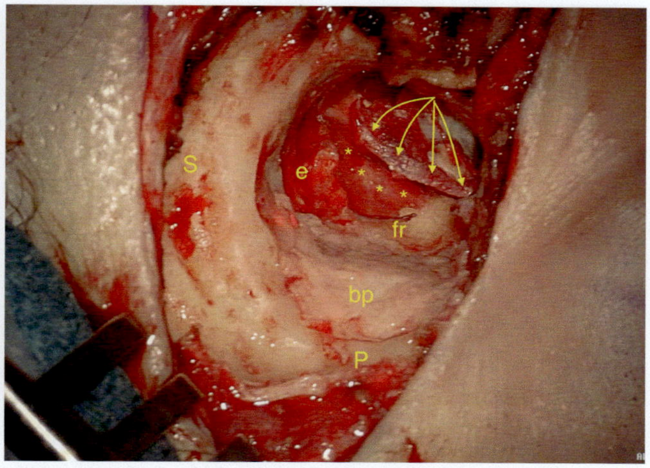

Fig. 43.5 Completion of a right tympanoplasty with CWD mastoidectomy, immediately after meatoplasty. The arrow represents replacement of the residual ear drum skin. The * marks the fascia graft used to repair the tympanic membrane. *S* superior, *P* posterior, *fr* facial ridge, *e* epitympanum, *bp* bone pate. (Courtesy of Alex D. Sweeney, MD)

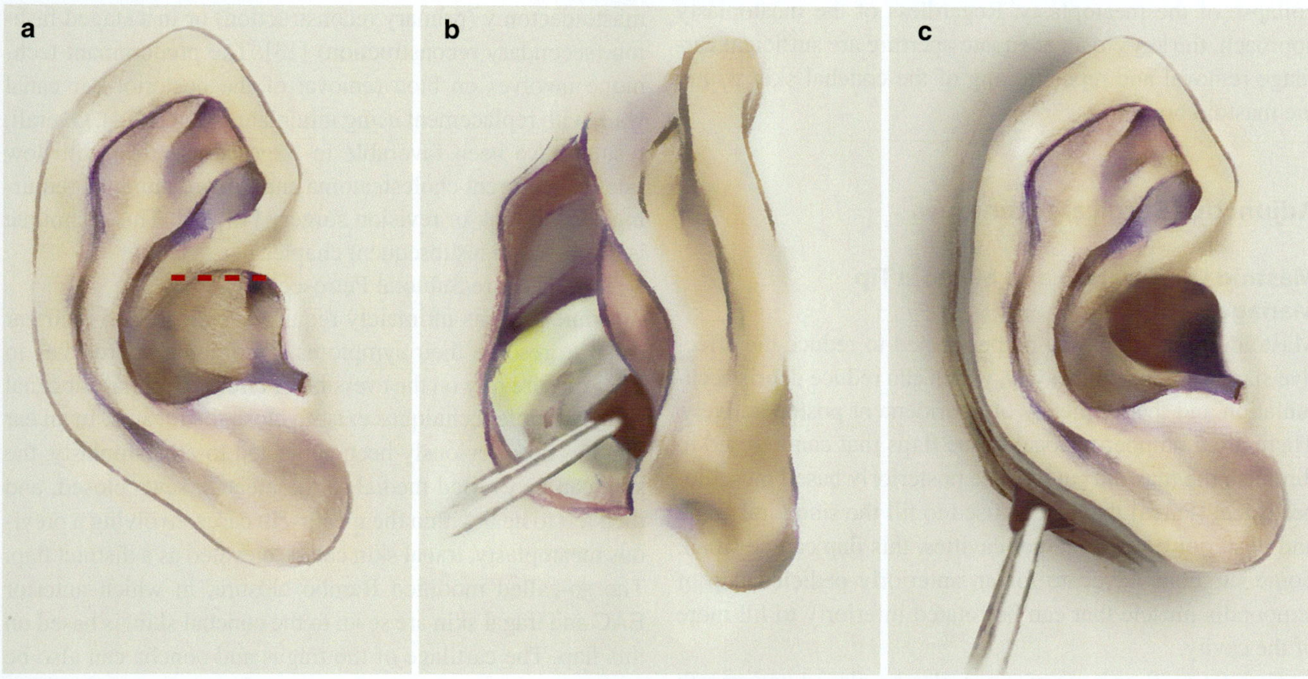

Fig. 43.6 Demonstration of the one-cut meatoplasty (**a**) incision line. The vector of tension on the meatoplasty is posterior (**b**), resulting in an open final appearance of the meatoplasty (**c**). (Used with permission from Hovis et al. [11])

Meatoplasty

Effective meatoplasty is essential to a dry and healthy mastoidectomy cavity. The goal of meatoplasty is to create a size match between the mastoid cavity and the external meatus. However, as previously mentioned, a balance should be struck between an opening that is wide enough to maximize self- and manual-cleaning, and small enough to minimize caloric activation and cosmetic dissatisfaction. Multiple techniques have been published and utilized for this process, all of which involve removal of the anteromedial portion of the conchal cartilage and creation of a series of incisions in the lateral canal and conchal skin to allow retraction into the cavity. It is important to remove sufficient conchal cartilage to allow for a tension-free opening. The "one-cut" meatoplasty technique is a safe, simple, and expedient technique that provides an improved cosmetic outcome (Figs. 43.6 and 43.7) [11]. The conchal skin flap is split with a single axial

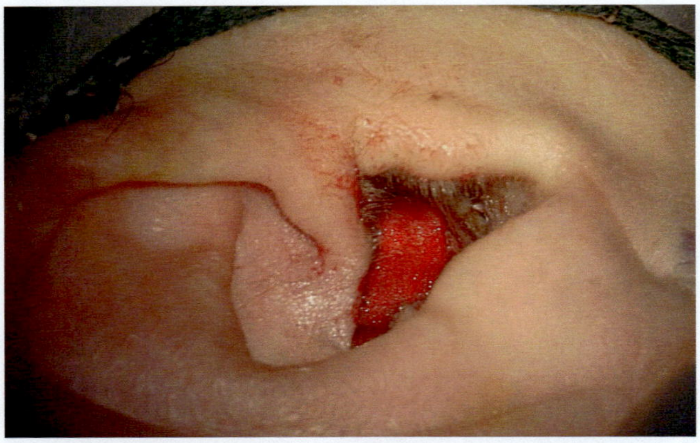

Fig. 43.7 A completed "one-cut" meatoplasty on a right ear. Gelfoam is noted within the opened meatus. (Courtesy of Alex D. Sweeney, MD)

cut through the incisura. A more traditional meatoplasty approach involves two or more endaural incisions. Vicryl™ retention sutures may be placed at the procedure end to attach the skin flaps to the mastoid periosteum and prevent collapse of the meatoplasty. Regardless of the meatoplasty approach, the keys to an adequate aperture are sufficient cartilage removal and repositioning of the conchal skin within the mastoid bowl.

Adjunctive Surgical Techniques

Mastoid Obliteration and Mastoid Tip Management

Mastoid obliteration may be performed to reduce the effective size of the mastoid cavity, which can reduce debris accumulation and the frequency of debridement postoperatively. There are a number of local tissue flaps that can be used to diminish the mastoid cavity. The posteriorly based musculoperiosteal (Palva) flap can be used to fill the sinodural angle and posterior bowl. In larger cavities, this flap can be small. Some surgeons advocate for an anteriorly pedicled flap of temporalis muscle that can be rotated inferiorly to fill more of the cavity.

Free fat graft or bone pâté can also be placed underneath these flaps to obliterate some of the dead space of the mastoid—care must be taken, however, to ensure that no residual cholesteatoma remains below this obliteration and that the bone pâté is harvested prior to encountering any cholesteatoma to avoid contamination. Also, it is important to consider that the complete survival of a non-vascularized graft, fat or bone, is not assured, and if this graft is designed as a foundational part of the cavity's structure and function, a poor long-term outcome can follow the initial appearance of success. When successful, however, obliteration can lead to a cavity that favors a native external auditory with minimal rates of cholesteatoma recurrence [12]. Use of synthetic materials such as bone cement are not favored in our experience due to concerns for infection and healthy epithelialization. Also, it should be mentioned that revision surgery is always a possibility in the setting of cholesteatoma, and techniques that will significantly complicate a revision effort, such as those that obliterate critical landmarks such as the facial nerve, the tegmen, and the otic capsule with bone or bone-substitute, should be only employed with extreme caution. Even if obliteration in these cases reduces the risk of a recurrence, the overall value of the technique is made questionable by the rarer recurrence being relatively more catastrophic.

Posterior Ear Canal Reconstruction

Posterior canal wall reconstruction has been developed as a technique to bridge between intact canal wall and CWD mastoidectomy. There are a variety of styles of this procedure used, and they can be employed at the time of initial mastoidectomy (primary reconstruction) or in a staged fashion (secondary reconstruction) [13]. The predominant technique involves en bloc removal of the posterior ear canal wall, with replacement using miniplate fixation [14]. Overall, results have been favorable in large case series, with low rates of recurrent cholesteatoma and limited numbers requiring second look or revision surgery [13, 14]. This technique is discussed in a subsequent chapter.

EAC Closure/Subtotal Petrosectomy

Some patients ultimately require overclosure of their ear canal to resolve their symptoms. Traditional approaches to EAC closure rely on the eversion of circumferential ear canal skin. Multiple techniques exist to close the meatus. In an ear that has not previously been subjected to a meatoplasty, the skin can be everted medial to the meatus, sewn closed, and then left to heal within the meatus. In cases involving a previous meatoplasty, tragal skin can be elevated as a distinct flap. The so-called modified Rambo closure, in which anterior EAC and tragal skin are sewn to the conchal skin, is based on this flap. The cartilage of the tragus and concha can also be approximated in this technique for reinforcement of the closure. In these approaches, it is extremely important to remove all keratinizing material within the mastoid cavity and tympanic space before overclosure to prevent cholesteatoma growth beneath the closure. Diffusion-weighted MRI may be used to surveil the cavity for disease recurrences when the ear canal is closed, and the use of this modality should be considered when weighing options for bone conduction hearing given that an implantable magnet will complicate efforts to visualize the cavity.

Postoperative Care

Saline-dampened Gelfoam is used to fill the mastoidectomy bowl at the conclusion of surgery. The Glasscock ear dressing and the cotton ball placed in the meatoplasty can be removed the day after surgery. Significant bloody drainage from the exposed incision lines and meatus is expected for at least 2 weeks after surgery and can be managed, as needed, with replacement of a cotton ball coated with petroleum jelly into the meatus. Fluoroquinolone ototopical drops are started the week after surgery to help break down any absorbable packing material in the meatus and to prevent bacterial colonization. Oral antibiotics are not always utilized during the early recovery period, though particularly severe or atypical infections may necessitate their use. Low-dose narcotic pain medication may be required in addition to Tylenol and anti-inflammatory medication. The first postoperative visit is generally scheduled for 2–3 weeks after surgery, at which time most of the residual packing may be removed. Intermittent drainage or blood spotting may be expected for months until the entirety of the cavity re-epithelializes. Patients are seen on a variable follow-up schedule until the cavity stabilizes, at which point they can generally be seen every 6 or 12 months depending on their rate of mastoid debris accumulation.

Long-term cavity maintenance varies, but intermittent drainage often requires treatment with a course of topical antibiotic–steroid combination drops. Some patients prone to moisture development can use a hair dryer on its lowest cool air setting to address residual water and sweat in the cavity, which can precipitate microbial growth and cavity mucosalization. Mucosa and granulation tissue formation may be treated either with topical silver nitrate or gentian violet, as well as a variety of compounded powders. Care should be taken when using these substances, however, to avoid the exposure of ototoxic substances to the middle ear.

One of the benefits of canal wall down approaches is that they generally minimize the likelihood of additional surgery. Cholesteatomas can still occur in a manner that warrants further surgery, but a significant portion of disease that would otherwise require surgery with an intact canal wall can be diagnosed and managed in office. CT is not always required for surveillance in a canal wall down cavity, though it can be useful if drainage persists.

Complications of CWD Surgery

Open mastoid cavity surgery has many of the same complications as traditional intact canal wall mastoidectomy, including facial paralysis, CSF leak, hearing loss (conductive and sensorineural), vestibular injury, bleeding, chronic otorrhea, and recurrent cholesteatoma.

Recurrent cholesteatoma requiring surgery generally occurs at a lower incidence in CWD procedures, as many recurrences that occur can be debrided in the clinic, as noted above. Rates of recurrent/residual cholesteatoma range from 0% to 13% after CWD, as compared to 17% to 61% of intact canal wall procedures [15]. While it is not uncommon to have persistent cholesteatoma after a CWD procedure, recurrent cholesteatoma developing de novo is quite rare, with one series suggesting a 1% incidence [16].

Conductive loss following the CWD approach can result from altered sound mechanics attributable to anatomical changes. Hearing loss can also be exacerbated by cholesteatoma or chronic inflammatory ear disease, which can independently impede vibration. Sensorineural hearing loss following CWD surgery is fairly rare but can be a concern in the setting of a cochlear or labyrinthine fistula.

"Mastoid cavity instability" is a term applied to a chronically draining mastoid bowl. While this situation can arise even in a perfectly constructed mastoid bowl, it is more common in cases of poor saucerization, an insufficient meatoplasty, or a high facial ridge. If not medically manageable with topical agents, revision surgery may be necessary. The high facial ridge, in particular, frequently requires revision surgery [17].

Also, as noted above, caloric activation can be problematic after CWD procedures. In CWD approaches, the lateral semicircular canal is only shielded from the outside world by a 1–2 mm layer of otic capsule bone, and in the setting of a preexisting labyrinthine fistula, even less. This relative lack of insulation can cause rotatory vertigo in response to temperature changes that can occur with wind blowing into the ear as well as cold and warm water exposure. As previously discussed, intraoperative techniques that can mitigate this risk include avoidance of an excessive meatoplasty and obliteration of the mastoid cavity. The use of earplugs or ear coverings can help to mitigate this issue postoperatively.

Excessive thinning of the middle fossa plate, especially in cases of idiopathic intracranial hypertension, can result in the formation of a meningoencephalocele within the open mastoid cavity. If a CSF leak is not present, these patients can be observed, taking care not to injure the sac during routine debridement of the mastoid bowl. Repair of a large encephalocele, especially in the setting of a CSF leak, can be challenging and sometimes requires EAC overclosure.

Revision CWD surgery can proceed similarly to primary CWD approaches, with a few notable suggestions. The periosteal incision should be made carefully to ensure that entry into the cavity is controlled. As with any revision surgery, preoperative clinical and radiographic analysis can facilitate safe dissection. Care should also be taken to minimize traction on the tegmen and facial ridge, as prior surgery could cause dehiscence and fibrosis that facilitate injury with blunt dissection.

Summary

Canal wall down surgery, when performed properly, can result in a safe, dry ear with reasonable hearing and vestibular function. Cholesteatoma recurrence rates are low with this technique as are complication rates. Obliteration of a CWD cavity can be a useful adjunct toward minimizing its volume, but these techniques should be carefully considered in terms of risks for recurrent or residual disease, foreign body inflammation or infection, and the possible need for revision surgery. Overall, CWD approaches are a mainstay of the management of chronic ear disease.

References

1. Schwartze E. Ueber die künstliche Eröffnung des Warzenfortsatzes. Archiv f Ohrenheilkunde. 1873;7(1):157–62. https://doi.org/10.1007/BF01803976.
2. von Tröltsch AF. Lehrbuch Der Ohrenheilkunde Mit Einschluss Der Anatomie Des Ohres. FCW Vogel; 1873.
3. Zaufal E. Technik der Trepanation des Processus mastoideus nach Küsterschen Grundsätzen. Arch Ohrenheilk 1890;291.
4. Bondy G. Totalufmelsselung mit Erhaltung von Trommelfell and Gehorknochelchen. Mschr Ohrenheilk. 1910;44:15–28.
5. Berrettini S, Ravecca F, de Vito A, Forli F, Valori S, Franceschini SS. Modified Bondy radical mastoidectomy: long-term personal experience. J Laryngol Otol. 2004;118(5):333–7. https://doi.org/10.1258/002221504323086499.
6. McRackan TR, Abdellatif WM, Wanna GB, et al. Evaluation of second look procedures for pediatric cholesteatomas. Otolaryngol Head Neck Surg. 2011;145(1):154–60. https://doi.org/10.1177/0194599810396624.
7. Volgger V, Lindeskog G, Krause E, et al. Identification of risk factors for residual cholesteatoma in children and adults: a retrospective study on 110 cases of revision surgery. Braz J Otorhinolaryngol. 2020;86(2):201–8. https://doi.org/10.1016/j.bjorl.2018.11.004.
8. Roger G, Denoyelle T, Chauvin P, Schlegel-Stuhl N, Garabedian EN. Predictive risk factors of residual cholesteatoma in children: a study of 256 cases. Otol Neurotol. 1997;18(5):550–8.
9. da Silva MNL, da Costa SS, Selaimen FA, et al. Residual cholesteatoma after endoscopic-assisted canal wall-up tympanomastoidectomy: a randomized controlled trial. Otol Neurotol. 2022;43(7):803–7. https://doi.org/10.1097/MAO.0000000000003575.
10. Chadha NK, Jardine A, Owens D, Gillett S, Robinson PJ, Maw AR. A multivariate analysis of the factors predicting hearing outcome after surgery for cholesteatoma in children. J Laryngol Otol. 2006;120(11):908–13. https://doi.org/10.1017/S0022215106002179.
11. Hovis KL, Carlson ML, Sweeney AD, Haynes DS. The one-cut meatoplasty: novel surgical technique and outcomes. Am J Otolaryngol. 2015;36(2):130–5. https://doi.org/10.1016/j.amjoto.2014.10.002.
12. Yamamoto Y, Takahashi K, Morita Y, Ohshima S, Takahashi S. Long-term follow-up results of canal wall down tympanoplasty with mastoid obliteration using the bone pate plate for canal wall reconstruction in cholesteatoma surgery. Otol Neurotol. 2014;35(6):961–5. https://doi.org/10.1097/MAO.0000000000000414.
13. Stevens SM, Walters ZA, Babo K, Peddireddy N, Tawfik KO, Samy RN. Canal reconstruction mastoidectomy: outcomes comparison following primary versus secondary surgery. Laryngoscope. 2019;129(11):2580–7. https://doi.org/10.1002/lary.27558.
14. Walker PC, Mowry SE, Hansen MR, Gantz BJ. Long-term results of canal wall reconstruction tympanomastoidectomy. Otol Neurotol. 2014;35(6):954–60.
15. Kerckhoffs KP, et al. The disease recurrence rate after the canal wall up or canal wall down technique in adults. Laryngoscope. 2016;126(4):942–6. https://onlinelibrary-wiley-com.proxy.library.vanderbilt.edu/doi/full/10.1002/lary.25591. Accessed 23 Apr 2023.
16. Pareschi R, Lepera D, Nucci R. Canal wall down approach for tympano-mastoid cholesteatoma: long-term results and prognostic factors. Acta Otorhinolaryngol Ital. 2019;39(2):122–9. https://doi.org/10.14639/0392-100X-2237.
17. Gluth MB, Metrailer AM, Dornhoffer JL, Moore PC. Patterns of failure in canal wall down mastoidectomy cavity instability. Otol Neurotol. 2012;33(6):998–1001. https://doi.org/10.1097/MAO.0b013e31825f2346.

Further Reading

Zöllner F. Die Radikal-Operation mit besonderem Bezug auf die Horfunktion. Z Laryngol Rhinol Otol. 1951;30(3):104–11.

Wullstein H. Funktionelle Operationen im Mittelohr mit Hilfe des freien Spaltlappen-Transplantates. Archiv f Ohren-, Nasen- u Kehlkopfheilkunde. 1952;161(2):422–35. https://doi.org/10.1007/BF02129204.

Jansen C. Ulur Radikaloperation Und Tympanoplastik. Sitz Ber Fontbild Arztekamm Ob.v. 18, 1958.

Sadé J, Ar A. Middle ear and auditory tube: middle ear clearance, gas exchange, and pressure regulation. Otolaryngol Head Neck Surg. 1997;116(4):499–524. https://doi.org/10.1016/S0194-59989770302-4.

Reversible Canal Wall Down Surgery and Mastoid Obliteration

44

Bruce J. Gantz and Daniel Q. Sun

Introduction

The primary goal in the surgical management of chronic otitis media with cholesteatoma is the creation of a dry, safe ear through the removal of disease and subsequent alteration of anatomy to prevent recurrence. This goal can be accomplished effectively with tympanomastoidectomy procedures that preserve (closed cavity, canal wall up [CWU]) or remove (open cavity, canal wall down [CWD]) the posterior ear canal wall, both described in previous chapters. In this chapter, we describe the technique of canal wall reconstruction (CWR) tympanomastoidectomy with mastoid obliteration. CWR combines elements of the canal wall up (CWU) and canal wall down (CWD) procedures to optimize surgical exposure for removal of disease and creates a blockage of the attic that minimizes the risk of recurrent retraction pockets extending beyond clinical visualization.

History

Obliteration of the mastoid and/or reconstruction of the posterior canal wall have been practiced since the 1970s, and these techniques were initially developed as a second-stage procedure to address a preexisting open mastoid cavity and its associated problems of cleaning and drainage. Palva [1] proposed the use of the soft tissue flap in 1973 and studies [2–4] on the use of other autologous materials soon followed. Biocompatible materials were also studied [5, 6] but the failure rates were high—up to 50% in some reports [5]. In 1987, Mercke [7] published the outcomes of 57 patients with middle ear cholesteatoma treated with a single-stage mastoid obliteration and posterior canal wall reconstruction procedure using autologous bone, demonstrating a success rate of 98% in achieving a dry, disease-free ear at a second-look procedure performed at a 1-year interval. Although the removal of the posterior canal wall was first performed by Wullstein [8], Mercke combined this maneuver with blocking attic and obliterating the mastoid. These techniques form the foundation on which canal wall reconstruction is based. Important modifications to the Mercke technique have been published by the senior author [9] and are described in detail below. The long-term results using the technique in 273 children and adults have also recently been published [10]. Reports of mastoid obliteration have been published, although many studies focus on the use of synthetic materials [11–15].

Pathophysiology and Indications for CWR

The pathophysiologic features of cholesteatoma and indications for its surgical management have been discussed in previous chapters. We will focus on the specific role of CWR approach in the surgical management of cholesteatoma.

Advantages and Disadvantages of CWU and CWD Techniques

CWD tympanomastoidectomy is the "gold standard" for surgical management of cholesteatoma [16, 17]. The enhanced exposure to the attic, antrum, and middle ear afforded by removal of the posterior canal wall provides for optimal visualization and removal of disease. Removal of the canal wall and lateral attic also prevents retraction pocket and recurrent cholesteatoma formation. In addition, all nitrogen-absorbing mucosa of the mastoid cavity and epitympanum is

B. J. Gantz
Department of Otolaryngology—Head and Neck Surgery,
University of Iowa Hospitals and Clinics, Iowa City, IA, USA
e-mail: bruce-gantz@uiowa.edu

D. Q. Sun (✉)
Department of Otolaryngology—Head and Neck Surgery,
University of Cincinnati, Cincinnati, OH, USA
e-mail: daniel.sun@uc.edu

A. D. Sweeney et al. (eds.), *Haynes-Glasscock-Shambaugh Surgery of the Ear*, https://doi.org/10.1007/978-3-032-18264-7_44

removed and will be ultimately replaced by stratified squamous epithelium after healing has occurred. When performed properly, the CWD procedure can result in a recidivism rate as low as 2% [16].

Disadvantages of the CWD technique include the accumulation of debris in the mastoid cavity, necessitating periodic debridement and, potentially, the need for ongoing water restrictions to help avoid infections. Furthermore, the middle ear space that results after CWD is narrower than that created by CWU surgery, which can make ossicular reconstruction more difficult. However, if the middle ear does not aerate, the hearing results are similar with CWD and CWU. The wide meatoplasty that is a critical component of the CWD technique can also present difficulties in the placement of a hearing aid and may have an unacceptable aesthetic appearance to some patients.

Preservation of the posterior canal wall in cholesteatoma surgery has a number of advantages, including the elimination of the need for periodic cleaning and water restrictions, as well as preservation of a middle ear cleft to facilitate ossicular reconstruction and hearing restoration. However, the recidivism rate has been reported to be as high as 36% in adults and 67% in children [18], higher by many reports than the incidence of recurrent disease seen with CWD procedures [17, 19]. The high rate of recidivism seen in CWU procedures can be due to a number of factors. First, exposure of the attic, antrum, and facial recess is more limited in CWU procedures when compared with CWD approaches, which may lead to difficulty in complete removal of all involved air cell tracts and increase the likelihood of leaving residual cholesteatoma at the initial procedure. Access is further obscured when a low temporal mastoideum reduces visualization of the tegmen tympani. Second, the epitympanum and mastoid cavity are ultimately relined with nitrogen-absorbing cuboidal mucosal epithelium after CWU procedures. The presence of this nitrogen-absorbing mucosa is thought to lead to negative middle ear and mastoid pressures, especially when continued inflammation with associated hypervascularity affects the mucosal layer [20]. This large surface area of nitrogen-absorbing epithelium, along with underlying Eustachian tube dysfunction, can lead to progressive retraction of the tympanic membrane postoperatively into the attic and mastoid, and, ultimately, recurrence of cholesteatoma [9]. Eustachian tube dysfunction exacerbates this scenario, especially in children.

Rationale for the CWR Approach

The CWR approach seeks to achieve the low recurrence rates of the CWD approach gained by improved operative exposure, while maintaining the benefits of an intact ear canal. The posterior canal wall is removed en bloc using a microsagittal saw and special thin blade (Medtronic, Stryker, Anspach), to provide CWD-like exposure, thereby optimizing visualization and facilitating the complete removal of cholesteatoma. The canal wall is replaced after the disease has been removed. The attic and mastoid cavity are then isolated from the middle ear using pieces of cortical bone and obliterated using bone pâté. Replacement of the posterior canal wall allows for preservation of near-normal middle ear anatomy, which can aid with ossicular reconstruction and avoid the need for routine cavity cleanings. Furthermore, physically blocking the attic and mastoid cavities decreases re-retraction of the tympanic membrane by eliminating the negative pressure associated with a nitrogen-absorbing mucosa lining the cavity and limits tympanic membrane retraction into the middle ear only, thereby still allowing the ear to be self-cleaning. Therefore, CWR is a systematic approach that can be used to provide patients of all ages with a safe, dry ear regardless of the degree of Eustachian tube dysfunction.

Patient Selection

Indications for CWR include patients of all ages with congenital or acquired cholesteatoma of the middle ear with extension to the attic, antrum, or mastoid not amenable to simple tympanoplasty or atticotomy. CWR can be performed in patients who have had prior mastoid surgery unless the posterior canal wall has been removed or destroyed, or the lateral portion of the posterior canal wall drilled away in a prior CWU procedure. The procedure is not contraindicated in patients with facial paralysis, labyrinthine fistula, or an encephalocele. CWR can be performed in patients with extensive scutum erosion or destruction of the medial aspect of the posterior canal wall from cholesteatoma or prior surgery, though there are additional reconstructive considerations in these circumstances.

Contraindication

CWR is contraindicated in patients with severe mastoid cholesteatomas that cannot be cleared from all mastoid air cell tracts, as sometimes occurs in young children. Care should be taken in the use of the CWR technique in patients with an extensive infectious component of their disease, though infection, in general, is not a contraindication to the procedure. In these cases, it is suggested that the patient be treated with salt water irrigation and antibiotic topical drops for a period of 4–6 weeks prior to the procedure if there are no contraindications to doing so, including a potential delay in care.

Operative Techniques

Patient Preparation

The patient is placed in the supine position on the operating room table with the head turned away from the side to be operated upon, and facial nerve monitoring electrodes are applied to the orbicularis oris and orbicularis oculi muscles. Hair is clipped from the postauricular area, and a C-shaped incision is marked 3–4 cm behind the pinna and within the hairline. One percent lidocaine with 1:100,000 epinephrine is injected, and then, povidone-iodine solution is applied to the area, including the external auditory canal.

Sterile towels are placed around the prepared area being careful to include the face on the involved side in the field. A large sterile adhesive drape is then applied over the field and surrounding towels followed by application of a split drape to the torso and surrounding area. A sterile irrigation/drainage bag is applied after trimming the adhesive drape around the auricle and postauricular area.

Mastoidectomy and Canal Wall Removal

A postauricular incision is made approximately 2 cm behind the hairline and carried to the level of the temporalis fascia superiorly. Dissection of the skin flap is carried anteriorly to within 2–3 mm of the external auditory canal. A wide (3–4 cm) anteriorly based musculoperiosteal (Palva) flap is then incised, elevated, and retracted anteriorly with the pinna. Bone pâté is then collected from the squamous temporal bone using a large cutting burr and suction with an attached bone pâté collector (Otomed Corporation, Lake Havasu City, AZ, or Anspach, Palm Beach Gardens, FL). Bone pâté is then collected from the cortical bone of the temporal and retrosigmoid areas. Bone pâté collection from the mastoid is avoided due to the possible presence of mucosal disease or cholesteatoma, which may increase the risk of disease re-implantation during reconstruction. After collection, the bone pâté is soaked in bacitracin solution and placed aside until the reconstruction. The mastoid tip is isolated lateral to the digastric ridge. An osteotome and mallet can then be used to remove the mastoid tip and inferior cortical bone. The mastoid tip is later used to fashion complete blocks of the attic and facial recess.

An intact canal wall mastoidectomy and posterior tympanotomy are then performed. Care is taken to maintain adequate posterior canal wall bone thickness and to avoid lowering (medializing) the lateral portion of the bony canal, both of which are important considerations in the canal wall reconstruction to come. Cholesteatoma that is encountered in the mastoid or facial recess is removed as exenteration of air cells in these areas progresses. Meticulous removal of all air cells in the sinodural angle, mastoid tip, and retrofacial areas is of the utmost importance. The facial recess is opened widely and extended inferior to the floor of the external auditory canal. The chorda tympani nerve is removed to extend the facial recess. Disarticulation and removal of the incus and head of malleus are then performed. The tensor tympani is cut. The skin of the posterior, inferior, and superior external auditory canal is elevated off of the underlying bone without any prior canal skin incisions (Fig. 44.1). In contrast to standard tympanomastoidectomy procedures, it is important in canal wall reconstruction to keep the posterior canal skin intact. The annulus is elevated, which allows the tympanic membrane and canal skin to be reflected anteriorly as an intact sleeve. The tympanic membrane remnant is separated from the cholesteatoma sac in this process.

A microsagittal saw (Anspach, Palm Beach Gardens, FL; Jed Med Bien Air, St Louis, MO; Medtronic, Minneapolis, MN; or Stryker, Kalamazoo, MI) is then used under continuous irrigation to create superior and inferior cuts in the posterior canal wall. The cuts are performed in a self-locking fashion to help prevent collapse of the canal into the mastoid after reconstruction (Fig. 44.1). Superiorly, two cuts are made. The first is parallel to the tegmen in a posterior to anterior direction, terminating at a point just superior to the 12 o'clock position of the ear canal (Fig. 44.2a). The second cut is perpendicular to the first, made from the superior external canal to meet the posterosuperior cut at a right angle (Fig. 44.2b). The inferior cut starts medially at the inferior extent of the facial recess and proceeds laterally toward the 6 o'clock position at the lateral extent of the external auditory canal (Fig. 44.2c). While proceeding from medial to lateral,

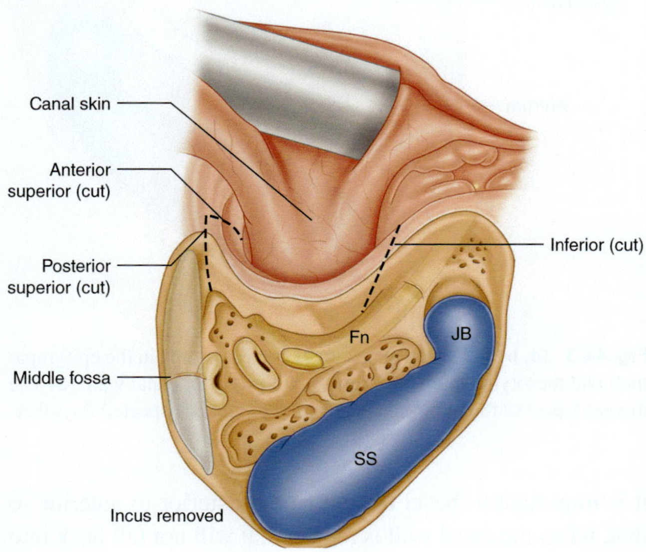

Fig. 44.1 Canal wall up mastoidectomy with facial recess with proposed external canal wall cuts. As noted, the incus has been removed. *SS* sigmoid sinus, *JB* jugular bulb, *Fn* facial nerve. (Adapted from Ref. [21])

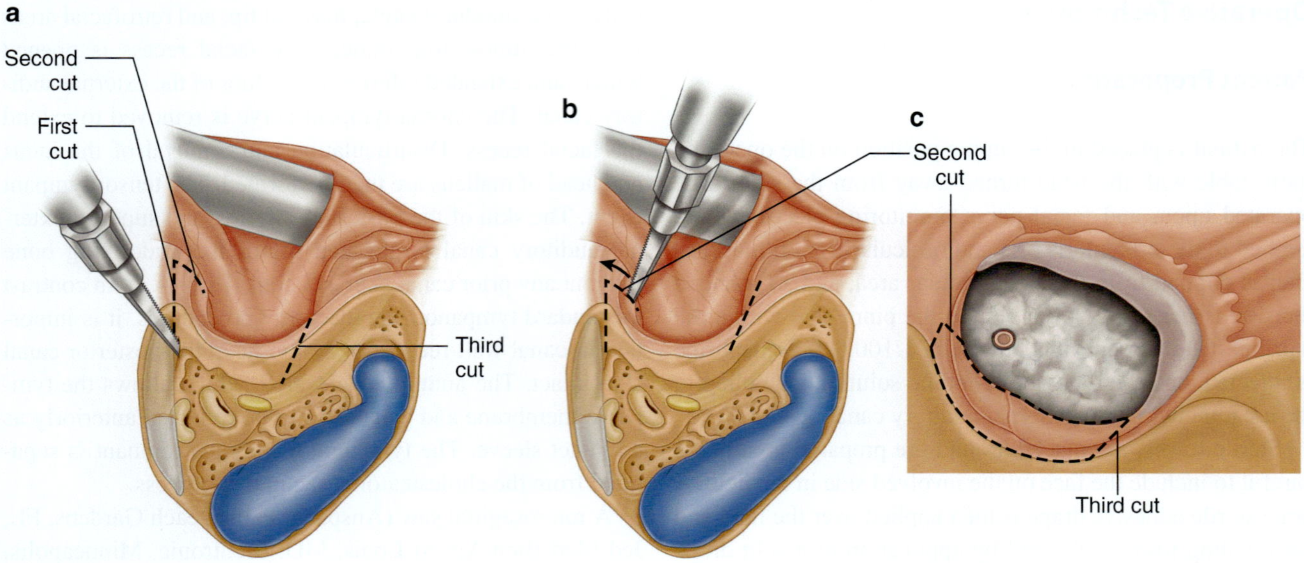

Fig. 44.2 (**a–c**) Bone cuts for ear canal removal. (**a**) The first bone cut is made with a microsagittal saw in the external canal wall. (**b**) The second bone cut is made at a right angle to the first. (**c**) The third bone cut is made from an inferior aspect of the facial recess extending laterally and beveling such that, when replaced, there is resistance to the canal wall collapsing into the mastoid cavity. (Adapted from Ref. [21])

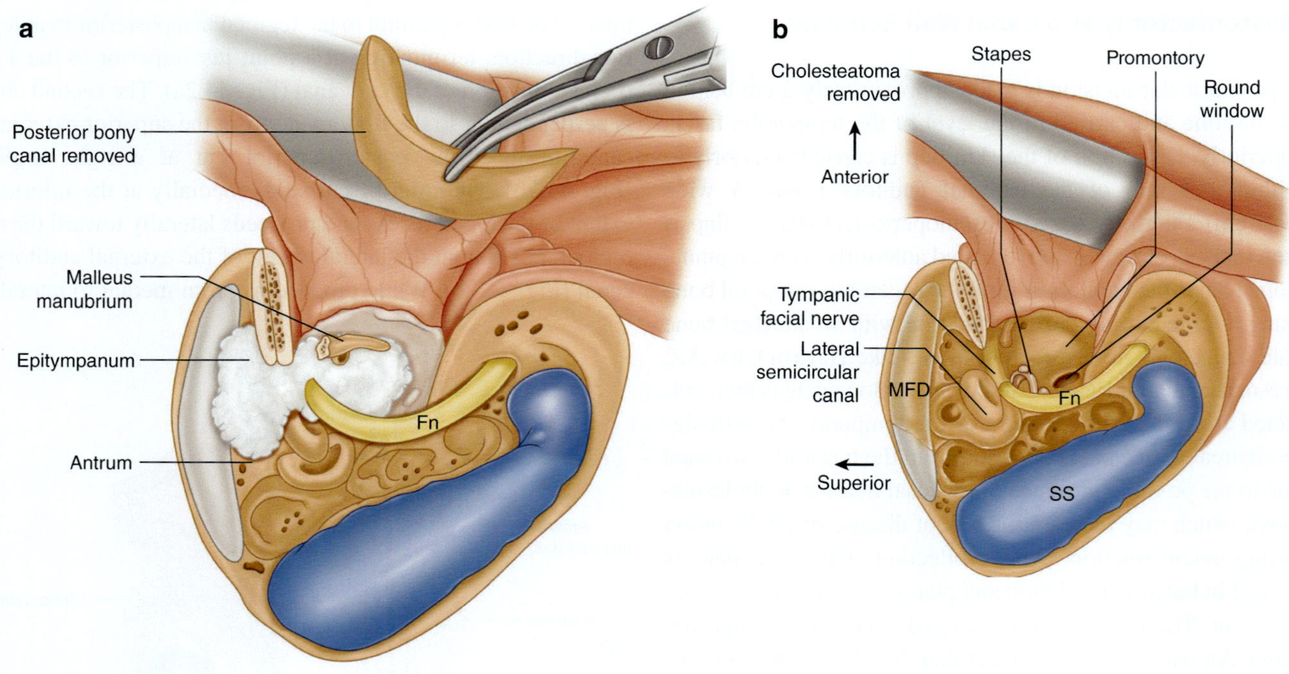

Fig. 44.3 (**a, b**) Enhanced exposure of cholesteatoma in the epitympanum and mesotympanum after removal of posterior canal wall. (**a**) The medial aspect of the removed canal wall segment is inspected for adherent squamous epithelium. Disease in the middle ear and mastoid is exposed. (**b**) Middle ear and mastoid visualization achieved with ear canal removal. (Adapted from Ref. [21])

it is important to bevel the cut from posterior to anterior so that, when the canal wall is replaced, it will not fall back into the mastoid when the canal wall skin is packed back into place. The posterior canal wall segment is then removed and the medial portion inspected (Fig. 44.3a). Any adherent squamous epithelium is removed with a diamond drill or gauze sponge. The posterior canal wall is then set aside for future reconstruction.

Using the enhanced exposure afforded by the removal of the ear canal wall, cholesteatoma is then carefully dissected from the tympanic cavity, epitympanum, antrum, and mastoid (Fig. 44.3b). The anterior attic is exposed and the anterior epitympanic space cleared of any residual disease including the cog as well as the sinus tympani. The zygomatic root air cells are drilled away similar to a CWD procedure.

Reconstruction

Reconstruction begins with the placement of a tear-drop-shaped piece of reinforced Silastic™ (0.4 mm thick) into the middle ear with the neck extending into the Eustachian tube. The Silastic™ graft rests on top of the stapes superstructure (if present) and extends into the Eustachian tube but does not extend posteriorly into the facial recess. In patients without an intact stapes superstructure, an additional wedge-shaped piece of Silastic™ is placed onto the footplate, resting underneath the larger tear-drop-shaped Silastic™ graft. This will hold a space for reconstruction during a second-look procedure. A temporalis fascia graft is then harvested. This graft must be large enough to extend beyond the margins of the posterior canal wall cuts. The temporalis fascia is placed medial to the tympanic membrane (TM) remnant, extending laterally to the bony/cartilaginous junction. Gelfoam® disks are placed between the Silastic™ graft and the underlay fascia graft to hold it in place (Fig. 44.4).

Mercke originally described blocking the attic with calvarial bone chips and bone pâté. In our experience [10], it was noted that several subjects experienced a limited attic retraction pocket that could be made self-cleaning by a secondary endaural atticotomy. Because of this finding, the attic reconstruction was altered to include a complete block of the attic with a larger piece of mastoid tip cortical bone. The bone block is fashioned with a rongeur to extend from the zygomatic root of the attic anteriorly to the posterior aspect of the lateral semicircular canal and is wide enough to span from the tympanic facial nerve in a lateral direction to beyond the scutum (Fig. 44.5). The bony posterior canal wall is then replaced, and an additional calvarial bone graft is placed in a near-coronal orientation into the facial recess (Fig. 44.6). The self-locking nature of the posterior canal wall cuts

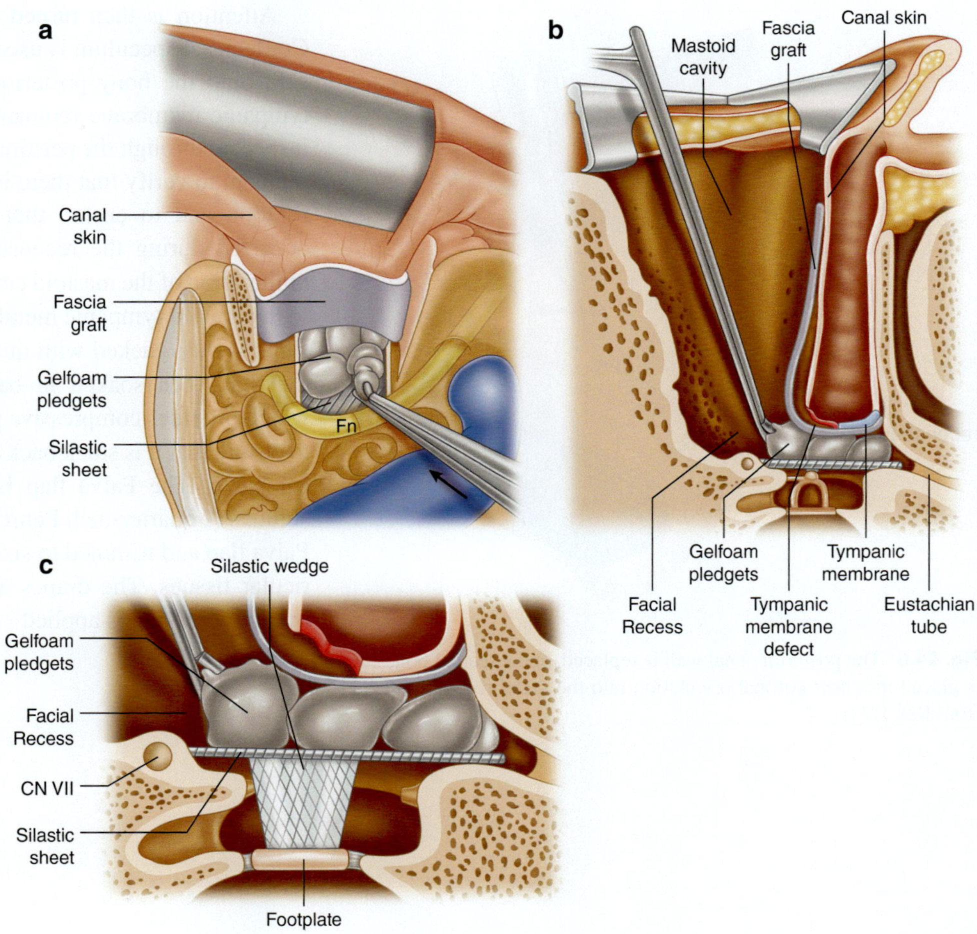

Fig. 44.4 (a–c) Reconstruction after cholesteatoma removal. (a) Surgeon's and (b) cross-sectional views of the temporal bone showing a Silastic™ sheet in the mesotympanum extending into the Eustachian tube. The fascial graft is placed medial to the tympanic membrane remnant and it extends laterally to the bony-cartilaginous junction while spanning the posterior canal wall cuts, thereby minimizing the risk of postoperative bone exposure. Gelfoam® is placed between the Silastic™ and fascial graft. (c) A Silastic™ wedge can also be placed to support the new tympanic membrane when the stapes superstructure is absent. (Adapted from Ref. [21])

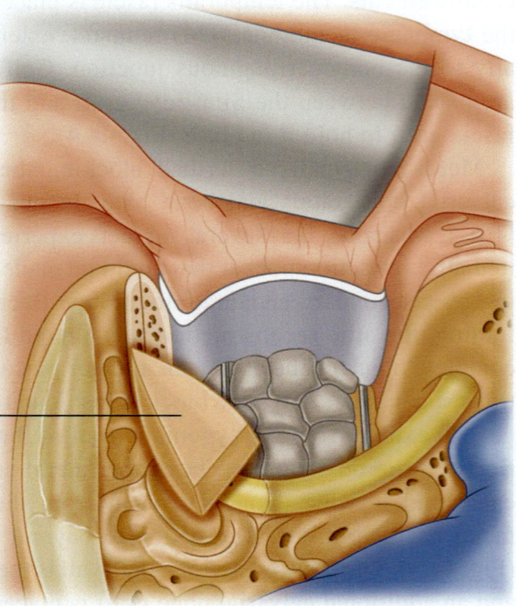

Fig. 44.5 A large bone chip is placed into the attic in the near-axial orientation, extending from the zygomatic root to the lateral semicircular canal and from the tympanic facial nerve to well beyond the scutum, to prevent postoperative tympanic membrane retraction beyond what can be seen on a standard otologic exam. (Adapted from Ref. [21]).

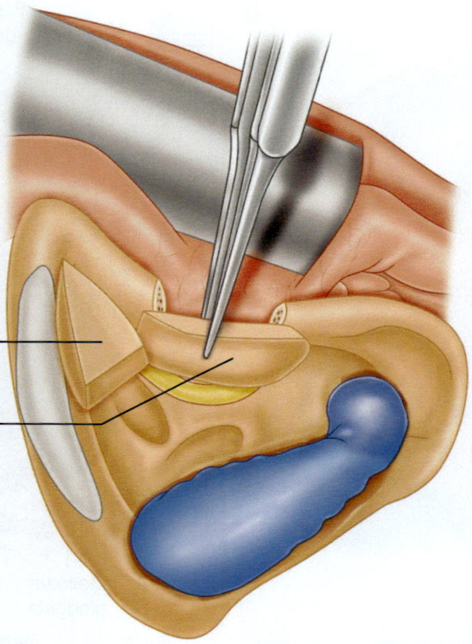

Fig. 44.6 The posterior canal wall is replaced, and a second bone chip is placed in a near-coronal orientation into the facial recess. (Adapted from Ref. [21])

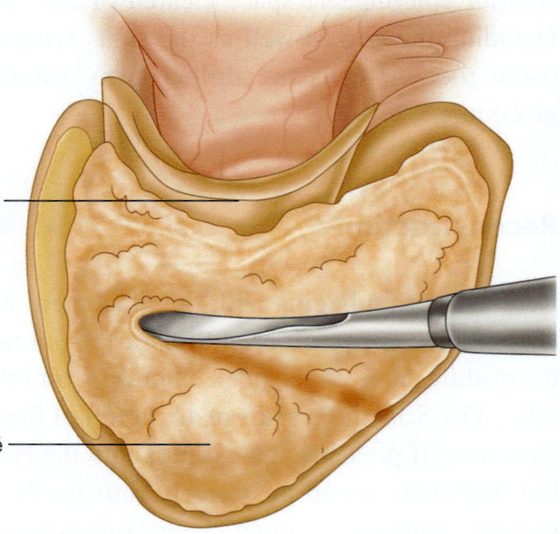

Fig. 44.7 Mastoid cavity and antrum obliterated with bone pâté. (Adapted from Ref. [21])

ensures stability of the posterior canal wall without the need of additional glue or other securing methodology. The attic, antrum, and mastoid complex are then filled with bone pâté, and dry gauze is used to compress the pâté in place and remove excess bacitracin solution from the pâté (Fig. 44.7).

Attention is then turned to the ear canal where a thin Cottle nasal speculum is used to displace the posterior canal skin onto the bony posterior canal wall and visualize the tympanic membrane remnant. The underlay fascial graft is inspected through the perforation in the tympanic membrane remnant to verify that there is complete coverage of the perforation and to ensure that no slippage of the graft had occurred during the reconstruction of the canal wall and obliteration of the mastoid cavity. Gelfoam® is placed lateral to the grafted tympanic membrane, and the external auditory canal is then packed with quarter-inch iodoform strip gauze that has been soaked in bacitracin ointment (Fig. 44.8), which provides compressive pressure on the ear canal sleeve to ensure that it is stuck back down to the reconstructed bony ear canal. The Palva flap is then closed with absorbable sutures. A quarter-inch Penrose drain is placed lateral to the Palva flap and trimmed to size prior to closure of the postauricular tissues. The drapes are then removed and a sterile mastoid dressing is applied.

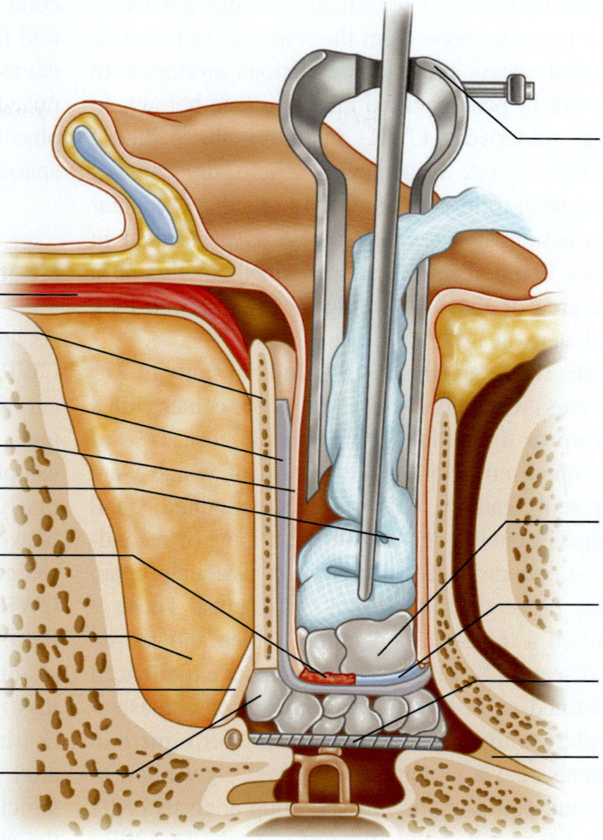

Fig. 44.8 Cross-sectional view of reconstruction in CWR, including the use of a Cottle speculum to replace the posterior canal wall skin onto the replaced bony canal wall, followed by packing with iodoform strip gauze. (Adapted from Ref. [21])

Postoperative Care

Perioperatively, patients are given antibiotics, typically piperacillin-tazobactam. Penicillin-allergic patients are typically administered clindamycin. Postoperatively, intravenous antibiotics are continued for 24 h. The Penrose drain is removed on the first postoperative day. The mastoid dressing is changed before discharge, at which time the patient is instructed to remove it in 2–3 days. Patients are discharged from the hospital with either oral levofloxacin (in adults), amoxicillin/clavulanate (in adults allergic to levofloxacin and patients under age 18), or clindamycin (in patients allergic to penicillin), to complete a 14-day course. The iodoform-bacitracin pack is removed from the external canal 1 week postoperatively and the skin sutures are removed. The patient is instructed to place ciprofloxacin drops three times a day for a month, and return for debridement of the Gelfoam and other debris.

A second-look tympanoplasty with ossiculoplasty is performed, typically 6 months after the initial tympanomastoidectomy, via a transcanal approach. Generally, there is no need to re-expose the obliterated mastoid. The status of the middle ear and tympanic membrane graft is assessed, the middle ear is examined for the presence of residual cholesteatoma following removal of Silastic™, and ossicular reconstruction is performed. Ossiculoplasty usually involves placement of a thin tragal cartilage graft over a titanium ossicular prosthesis.

CWR Outcomes

Recurrence Rate

Reports of the rate of recurrent cholesteatoma after CWU procedures vary (16–61%) [18, 22–25]; however, they are accepted as being higher than CWD procedures (2–17%) [16, 26, 27], which vary based on the age of the patient and length of follow-up. As with any mastoid obliteration procedure, complete removal of cholesteatoma and all diseased mastoid air cell tracts is of critical importance in the CWR technique. Wide saucerization, thorough removal of the retrofacial cells, and careful sharpening of the sinodural angle are critical steps in this process. Additionally, the cog is removed, providing wide exposure of the anterior epitympanum to allow for complete eradication of cholesteatoma.

In 2005, we published our initial 8-year experience with CWR [9]. Important modifications from the technique initially developed by Mercke [7] included locking canal wall cuts for stability, using bone from the mastoid tip to create antral and facial recess blocks, and various strategies to decrease the risk of postoperative infection (see below). In 130 ears that underwent CWR, including 40 pediatric patients, the success rate in achieving a safe, dry ear was 98.5%, with a mean follow-up time of 48 months. Ossicular chain reconstruction at a second stage was performed in 78.5% of cases. Ten percent of ears contained small keratin pearls in the area of the oval window at the second-look operation and were cleared.

These results were confirmed in a follow-up study of 273 patients (285 ears) who underwent CWR at our center with a mean follow-up of 4.3 years [10]. In this cohort, 14% of patients developed retraction pockets, most of which were shallow and self-cleaning; 12% of ears contained small residual disease isolated to the middle ear at time of second-look operation, which were cleared and ossicular chain reconstruction proceeded in all but 3 patients. These 3 patients required a third-look operation, which showed no evidence of disease. Overall, 8.5% of patients experienced recidivism defined as deep retraction pocket or cholesteatoma. Secondary endaural atticotomy was performed in 5.9% of patients; 2.6% of patients required conversion to CWD or subtotal petrosectomy. In subgroup analysis of 92 patients with long-term follow-up (≥5 years), 18 (20%) experienced recurrence of disease, 13 were treated with endaural atticotomy, 4 with conversion to CWD, and 1 with conversion to subtotal petrosectomy. Importantly, no patients experienced recurrent cholesteatoma in the mastoid region because of retained squamous epithelium.

Similarly low recurrence rates are also enjoyed by pediatric patients. It is often the case that children with cholesteatoma are treated with CWU procedures in the hopes of maintaining a self-cleaning ear; however, recurrent cholesteatoma is more frequent in this population and long-term recidivism rates have been as high as 46% [28]. As such, children are excellent candidates for a CWR procedure. In our cohort, 25% of whom were pediatric patients, there was an 11.6% recidivism rate in children where a secondary procedure was required, with only 2 children (2.9%) requiring conversion to CWD or subtotal petrosectomy [10].

These results, while favorable, represent a continuous evolution in technique based on our experience with CWR. For instance, originally Mercke described placing small bone chips to block the attic. The re-retraction rate improved with altering the surgical technique to include obliteration of the epitympanum with small chips of bone and a large cortical bone block from the mastoid tip (from 14% to 7.1%). It is important that a large bone chip be carefully placed in the attic to completely seal off the epitympanum from the mesotympanum (Fig. 44.6). The bone chip in the facial recess is placed in a near-coronal orientation and completely blocks this space, effectively separating the mastoid from the tympanic cavity (Fig. 44.7). These results also demonstrate that concerns regarding mastoid obliteration raised by some authors [5, 29], including altered mastoid physiology and absence of the mastoid cavity as a ventilatory space, have not been borne out in our practice.

Hearing Results

As with CWU and CWD techniques, the primary goal of the CWR tympanomastoidectomy is the creation of a dry, safe ear. Hearing reconstruction is a secondary, although important, consideration. Ongoing Eustachian tube dysfunction can predispose patients with chronic otitis media to ossiculoplasty prosthesis extrusion and secretory otitis media, both of which may contribute to conductive hearing loss. When secretory otitis media occurs in patients who have undergone CWR, the authors do not offer patients ventilation tube placement, given the high risk of chronic otorrhea that may result. Instead, the authors tolerate the conductive hearing loss that may result from secretory otitis media and prefer hearing amplification rehabilitation, if needed. In our series, after a second-look procedure with ossicular chain reconstruction, some patients had excellent gap closure, although the average air bone gap closure was small (from 28 dB to 23 dB) [10]. This variability in hearing outcome is felt to vary based on the underlying level of Eustachian tube dysfunction, with poor function leading to worse hearing outcome. More information on the influence of middle ear ventilation on hearing outcomes can be found in the chapter on ossicular chain reconstruction.

Complications

Complications of CWU procedures such as tympanic membrane perforation and extrusion of ossiculoplasty prostheses can occur with the CWR technique, but their incidence can be minimized by meticulous attention to the placement of the fascial underlay graft (Fig. 44.4) and the coverage of the titanium ossiculoplasty prosthesis with a cartilage graft. Exposed bone in the external auditory canal was observed in 17 patients (6.3%) and all but 2 were managed conservatively with topical therapy and periodic debridement. Two patients required secondary canalplasty. In contrast to CWU or CWD approaches, keeping canal skin intact without incisions and using a broad fascial underlay that covers the bony canal wall cuts help minimize this risk.

Other complications include cerebrospinal fluid (CSF) leak and facial nerve injury, which were observed in 14 (4.9%) and 4 (1.4%) of ears, respectively. CSF leak was most commonly sustained while making the superior canal cuts with the sagittal saw. All CSF leaks were recognized and repaired intraoperatively using muscle or fascial grafts. One patient experienced persistent CSF leak that was repaired secondarily via a middle fossa approach. Facial nerve paresis occurred after CWR in two cases and ossiculoplasty in another two cases. All recovered to House-Brackmann grade I or II; however, two patients required decompression of the mastoid segment.

A greater concern with the CWR procedure is the possibility of wound infection, which, theoretically, could progress to involve the mastoid bone pâté and posterior canal wall. Fortunately, careful attention to a number of details in the CWR technique can effectively reduce the incidence of infection [9]. First, perioperative antibiotics, with coverage for *Pseudomonas aeruginosa*, are an important measure in preventing wound infections. Typically, patients are given piperacillin-tazobactam intravenously prior to surgery and for 48 h postoperatively. Patients are then discharged on a 2-week course of oral levofloxacin. Pediatric patients are given piperacillin-tazobactam perioperatively and discharged on amoxicillin-clavulanate for 2 weeks. Clindamycin is used for penicillin-allergic patients. Second, bone pâté is collected from non-diseased cortical bone and is soaked in bacitracin solution prior to placement in the mastoid. Pâté collection is stopped if air cells become exposed during the drilling process. Third, placement of a Penrose drain between the postauricular skin flap and the Palva flap for 12–24 h postoperatively helps to prevent the formation of a hematoma, which may subsequently become infected. In the first 2 years of our experience with CWR, the rate of postoperative wound infection was 14% [9]. After the above protocol was instituted however, the rate of wound infection declined to 4.5% [10]. Presently, only 24 h of piperacillin-tazobactam is used with no evidence of increased infection rate. Only one patient has required conversion to a canal wall down cavity as a result of infection.

Conclusions

CWR tympanomastoidectomy combines components of CWU and CWD techniques to allow wide visualization for removal of primary and recurrent cholesteatomas with optimal preservation of near-normal external auditory canal and middle ear anatomy. Obliteration of the mastoid with blockage of the attic and facial recess in CWR tympanomastoidectomy helps to prevent recidivistic disease by removing nitrogen-absorbing mucosa and physically obstructing tympanic membrane re-retraction. Careful attention to detail in removing all mastoid and epitympanic air cells, reconstruction of the posterior canal wall and tympanic membrane, and obliteration of the mastoid and attic are of the utmost importance for success with the CWR technique.

References

1. Palva T. Operative technique in mastoid obliteration. Acta Otolaryngol. 1973;75:289–90.
2. Smith MF. Reconstruction of the open mastoidectomy ear: a six year progress report. Ann Otol Rhinol Laryngol. 1975;84:552–7.
3. Smyth GD, Dowe AC. Cartilage canalplasty. Laryngoscope. 1971;81:786–92.
4. Pappas JJ, Bailey HA Jr, McGrew RN, et al. Homograft septal cartilage for attic support in intact canal wall tympanomastoidectomy and tympanoplasty. Laryngoscope. 1981;91:1457–62.
5. Shea JJ Jr, Malenbaum BT, Moretz WH Jr. Reconstruction of the posterior canal wall with Proplast. Otolaryngol Head Neck Surg. 1984;92:329–33.
6. Reck R, Helms J. The bioactive glass ceramic Ceravital in ear surgery. Five years' experience. Am J Otol. 1985;6:280–3.
7. Mercke U. The cholesteatomatous ear one year after surgery with obliteration technique. Am J Otol. 1987;8:534–6.
8. Wullstein H. The restoration of the function of the middle ear, in chronic otitis media. Ann Otol Rhinol Laryngol. 1956;65:1021–41.
9. Gantz BJ, Wilkinson EP, Hansen MR. Canal wall reconstruction tympanomastoidectomy with mastoid obliteration. Laryngoscope. 2005;115:1734–40.
10. Walker PC, Mowry SE, Hansen MR, et al. Long-term results of canal wall reconstruction tympanomastoidectomy. Otol Neurotol. 2014;35:954–60.
11. Roberson JB Jr, Mason TP, Stidham KR. Mastoid obliteration: autogenous cranial bone pate reconstruction. Otol Neurotol. 2003;24:132–40.
12. Zini C, Quaranta N, Piazza F. Posterior canal wall reconstruction with titanium micro-mesh and bone pate. Laryngoscope. 2002;112:753–6.
13. Moffat DA, Gray RF, Irving RM. Mastoid obliteration using bone pate. Clin Otolaryngol Allied Sci. 1994;19:149–57.
14. Geyer G, Dazert S, Helms J. Performance of ionomeric cement (Ionocem) in the reconstruction of the posterior meatal wall after curative middle-ear surgery. J Laryngol Otol. 1997;111:1130–6.
15. Grote JJ, van Blitterswijk CA. Reconstruction of the posterior auditory canal wall with a hydroxyapatite prosthesis. Ann Otol Rhinol Laryngol Suppl. 1986;123:6–9.
16. Palva T. Surgical treatment of chronic middle ear disease. II. Canal wall up and canal wall down procedures. Acta Otolaryngol. 1987;104:487–94.
17. Abramson M. Open or closed tympanomastoidectomy for cholesteatoma in children. Am J Otol. 1985;6:167–9.
18. Shohet JA, de Jong AL. The management of pediatric cholesteatoma. Otolaryngol Clin N Am. 2002;35:841–51.
19. Rosenfeld RM, Moura RL, Bluestone CD. Predictors of residual-recurrent cholesteatoma in children. Arch Otolaryngol Head Neck Surg. 1992;118:384–91.
20. Ars B, Wuyts F, Van de Heyning P, et al. Histomorphometric study of the normal middle ear mucosa. Preliminary results supporting the gas-exchange function in the postero-superior part of the middle ear cleft. Acta Otolaryngol. 1997;117:704–7.
21. Brackmann D, Shelton C, Arriaga MA. Canal wall reconstruction tympanomastoidectomy. In: Otologic surgery. 4th ed. Elsevier; 2015.
22. Sheehy JL, Brackmann DE, Graham MD. Cholesteatoma surgery: residual and recurrent disease. A review of 1,024 cases. Ann Otol Rhinol Laryngol. 1977;86:451–62.
23. Syms MJ, Luxford WM. Management of cholesteatoma: status of the canal wall. Laryngoscope. 2003;113:443–8.
24. Dodson EE, Hashisaki GT, Hobgood TC, et al. Intact canal wall mastoidectomy with tympanoplasty for cholesteatoma in children. Laryngoscope. 1998;108:977–83.

25. Stangerup SE, Drozdziewicz D, Tos M. Cholesteatoma in children, predictors and calculation of recurrence rates. Int J Pediatr Otorhinolaryngol. 1999;49(Suppl 1):S69–73.
26. Cody DT, McDonald TJ. Mastoidectomy for acquired cholesteatoma: follow-up to 20 years. Laryngoscope. 1984;94:1027–30.
27. Vartiainen E. Ten-year results of canal wall down mastoidectomy for acquired cholesteatoma. Auris Nasus Larynx. 2000;27:227–9.
28. Prasad SC, La Melia C, Medina M, et al. Long-term surgical and functional outcomes of the intact canal wall technique for middle ear cholesteatoma in the paediatric population. Acta Otorhinolaryngol Ital. 2014;34:354–61.
29. Doyle WJ. The mastoid as a functional rate-limiter of middle ear pressure change. Int J Pediatr Otorhinolaryngol. 2007;71:393–402.

Endoscopic Ear Surgery

45

De'Andre A. Warren, Alexandra M. Arambula, and Alejandro Rivas

Introduction

Otologic surgery traditionally has been performed under binocular microscopy, providing the surgeon with visual depth perception critical for the fine movements required of microsurgery. However, the microscope requires a linear perspective for visualization, which is inherently limiting. In light of this issue, different surgical approaches have been developed to increase accessibility to sections of the middle ear cleft that are difficult to visualize with the microscope, most commonly the postauricular or endaural approaches. As surgical optics continued to advance, telescopes and endoscopes gained mainstream use in other surgical specialties and became part of standard practice in other areas of otolaryngologic surgery, such as endoscopic sinus surgery. Some of the earliest uses of endoscopes in otology were reported in the 1970s, describing inspection both of the tympanic membrane (TM) in the office and of the cerebellopontine angle through a translabyrinthine approach [1]. Over the last 20 years, endoscopes have been further utilized to complete not only transcanal surgical procedures, such as placement of pressure equalizing tubes, tympanoplasties and stapedectomies, but also transmastoid procedures, such as cochlear implantation, and transpromontory procedures such as vestibular schwannoma (VS) resections.

Endoscopic ear surgery (EES) has various advantages and disadvantages that should be taken into consideration for otologic surgery. Among its primary advantages, endoscopes provide a wide field of view, improving the surgeon's ability to visualize surgical anatomy that is otherwise covered by bony ledges. Consequently, endoscope use for patients with anterior perforations or unfavorable external auditory canal anatomy may provide adequate visualization without the need for a postauricular incision or significant alterations in patient or bed positioning. With the availability of 30-, 45-, and 70-degree endoscopes and angled instruments, surgeons can visualize around corners and gain access to structures of the middle ear space (i.e., the epitympanum, retrotympanum, or protympanum) via a transcanal approach that might otherwise require a postauricular incision. The surgeon may also easily adjust the display monitor to place their own cervical spine into a neutral position, improving the surgeon's ergonomics. Because of the improved visualization with ultra-high-definition technology, as well as the shared display screen, the endoscope enhances resident and medical student education regarding both anatomy and surgical technique.

While endoscopes undoubtedly offer advantages for otologic surgery, there are limitations that must be considered. First, by its very nature, EES is one-handed surgery—the surgeon must hold the endoscope in one hand and their working instrument in the other; therefore, the surgeon must switch between dissecting instruments and the suction to remove blood from the field of view. Another disadvantage of the endoscope is the loss of three-dimensional binocular vision, which may lead to loss of depth perception, though the surgeon is often able to move the endoscope in and out of the surgical field to gain a better sense of depth, similar to that of depth perception experienced during sinus surgery. Finally, while there have been limited uses of the endoscope for mastoid work, the endoscope is best suited for middle ear disease that does not extend beyond the dome of the lateral semicircular canal, as the capabilities of visualization and dissection are limited beyond this anatomic boundary. This may limit applications in certain disease processes, such as cholesteatoma that extends to the mastoid air cells, typically requiring an open transmastoid approach.

D. A. Warren · A. M. Arambula · A. Rivas (✉)
Department of Otolaryngology—Head and Neck Surgery, Case Western Reserve University/University Hospitals Cleveland Medical Center, Cleveland, OH, USA
e-mail: alejandro.rivas@uhhospitals.org

A. D. Sweeney et al. (eds.), *Haynes-Glasscock-Shambaugh Surgery of the Ear*, https://doi.org/10.1007/978-3-032-18264-7_45

Equipment and Operating Room Setup

While much of the surgical equipment and operating room (OR) setup are similar to that for microscopic ear surgery (MES), preparation for EES has some key differences. Rigid endoscopes measuring 14 cm long × 2.7–3 mm in diameter are ideal to access any middle ear cleft, allow space for the dissecting hand to introduce instruments, and minimize potential bending of the scope in curved ear canals. While most procedures can be performed only with a 0-degree scope, 30-degree or 45-degree scopes can aid in working around corners, such as the epitympanum and the sinus tympani. The 70-degree scope may be beneficial for thorough inspection of the antrum during surgery, but it is not recommended for dissection. Given the single-handed nature of EES, specialized instruments are beneficial to improve surgical efficiency while maintaining the field of view. For example, a suction elevator allows the surgeon to develop a tympanomeatal flap with one hand rather than switching between a round knife and Frazier tip suction intermittently (Fig. 45.1a). Even with the suction elevator, cotton balls or cottonoids soaked in epinephrine are helpful to assist with hemostasis (Fig. 45.1b). Finally, curved or disposable Frazier-tip suctions that can be bent are useful in suctioning out difficult-to-reach areas.

After induction of general anesthesia, the patient may be rotated 180 degrees to allow room for the equipment, display monitor, and scrub technician per the surgeon's preference. The scrub usually is seated across from the surgeon, with the display screen located at the head of the bed adjacent to the scrub (Fig. 45.2). The light source is recommended to be set to below 60% intensity to avoid thermal injuries. Ozruran et al. have shown that 50% light intensity is adequate for visualization; however, for the 4 mm-0 degree endoscope, temperatures at 100% and 50% light intensity were recorded as 48.4 and 43.2 °C, respectively. For the 2.7 mm-0 degree endoscope, temperatures recorded at 100% and 50% light intensities were 37.8 and 35.3 °C, respectively [2]. This may cause inadvertent heat injury to the structures of the middle ear such as the chorda tympani and the stapes. Given this data, the authors' preference is to maintain a light intensity less than 40%, which does not seem to have negative effects on visualization.

Prior to beginning the surgery, preparing the ear canal for visualization is paramount for EES. Canal injections with dilute epinephrine should be performed slowly, with visualization of canal wall blanching to the level of the tympanic annulus. A good canal injection will minimize bleeding during the remainder of the procedure, improving visualization and surgical efficiency. Curved iris scissors should then be used to trim canal hairs, which can otherwise smear the

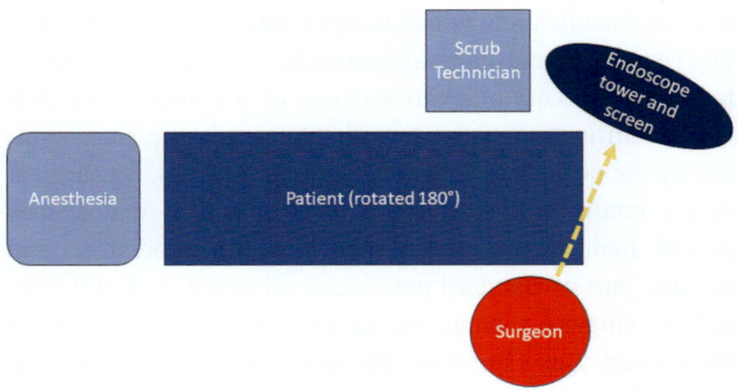

Fig. 45.2 Schematic of ideal operating room arrangement for EES

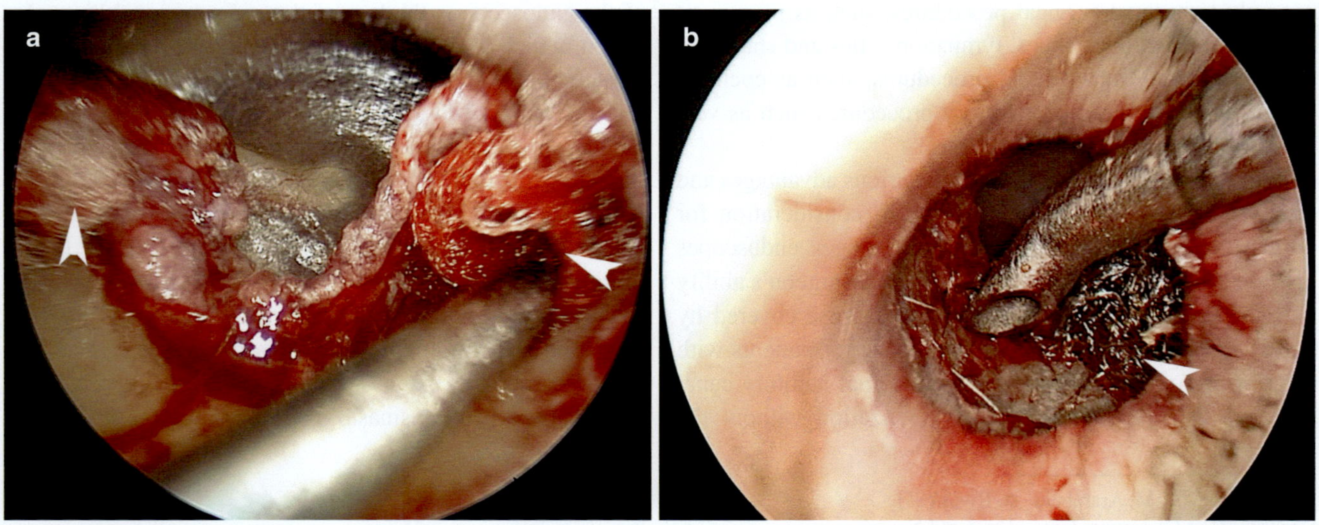

Fig. 45.1 Tympanomeatal flap elevation. (**a**) Elevation of tympanomeatal flap using cotton balls superiorly and inferiorly (arrowheads). (**b**) Elevation of tympanomeatal flap using 45 degrees suction elevator in a very narrow pediatric ear canal. Notice the cotton ball (arrowhead) keeping the flap elevated

endoscope with blood products during its movement in and out of the ear canal. Antifog solution and a wet sponge should be positioned on the drapes adjacent to the ear to allow for efficient cleaning of the endoscope throughout the procedure. The procedure can then begin, modified to specified pathologies as discussed below.

Tympanoplasty

The endoscope can be used to perform a tympanoplasty for perforations in multiple locations and clinical settings. Repairs have been described for anterior perforations as well as perforations in chronic otitis media (COM) without cholesteatoma. Here we will discuss two techniques for endoscopic tympanoplasty.

Underlay (Medial Graft)/Lateral to Malleus Underlay Technique

The first approach is the medial graft technique (underlay) (Fig. 45.3). This begins with de-epithelialization of the rim of the perforation, which can be done with a Rosen needle or a 5910 beaver blade. This creates trauma at the edges of the perforation, which in turn stimulates regrowth of the tympanic membrane (TM). Next, the tympanomeatal flap can be created. While there are many different tympanomeatal flap designs, which may be utilized for a variety of different perforations, the authors prefer a ship sail tympanomeatal flap. A vertical superior cut is made, starting anterior to the lateral process of the malleus and extending laterally and superiorly. An inferior vertical cut is usually placed at 6 o'clock, extending laterally and posteriorly. The two incisions are then connected with a horizontal incision 5 mm lateral to the annulus. The flap is then elevated using a suction elevator and cottonoids, which function as a second-hand maintaining traction and elevation of the flap (Fig. 45.3a, b). In anterior perforations, the drum should be degloved from the handle of the malleus in order to perform a lateral to malleus underlay technique (Fig. 45.3c). Placement of the tympanomeatal flap's superior, vertical incision anterior to the malleus handle aids in skeletonization of the malleus when necessary. For graft material, fascia, tragal cartilage with or without perichondrium, and artificial grafts can be utilized in a similar fashion to microsurgical techniques (Fig. 45.3d–f).

Overlay (Lateral Graft) Technique

The lateral graft technique is another method of tympanoplasty utilized most commonly for anterior perforations, large perforations, or failed prior tympanoplasties. First, a vascular strip is designed with a superior–vertical incision, inferior–vertical incision, and a horizontal incision at the level of the annulus to connect the two vertical incisions. Then, a lateral incision is made at the bony cartilaginous junction along the anterior canal wall, connecting the vertical vascular strip incisions superiorly and inferiorly. Similar to the microscopic approach, the anterior external auditory canal skin is then elevated off the bony canal to the level of the tympanic membrane, and along with the squamous layer of the tympanic membrane, it is removed and set aside for later use. The fibrous and mucosal layers of the TM are left in place. A wide canalplasty is then performed. The drill speed can be lowered to 10,000 rotations per minute as drilling progresses closer to the ossicles. The canalplasty is performed until 360 degrees of the annulus can be seen, creating an anterior shelf to minimize the risk of postoperative blunting and graft lateralization. The vascular strip must then be back elevated. Copious irrigation is important to ensure no fragments of squamous debris are left in the middle ear cleft. Temporalis fascia or tragal perichondrium can be used for reconstruction. The graft is placed medial to the malleus handle and lateral to the annulus, with a superior slit cut in the perichondrium or fascia to accommodate the neck of the malleus. Posterosuperiorly, the graft must be placed under the vascular strip. The previously removed anterior canal skin is then replaced, with a small amount of overlap of the canal skin with the graft at the anterior sulcus. The anterior sulcus needs to be packed tightly to help prevent blunting.

Endoscopic Tympanoplasty Outcomes

Studies comparing total endoscopic ear surgery (TEES) tympanoplasties to MES tympanoplasties have shown that TEES tympanoplasties have similar graft take rates and audiologic outcomes, while reducing operative time and need for a postauricular incision. *Marchioni* et al. performed a retrospective chart review of 109 patients who underwent endoscopic type 1 tympanoplasty; 86% of patients had successful graft take, 89% had improvement in their air bone gap (ABG) within 20 dB, and only 8% of patients needed revision surgery [3]. *Creighton* et al. evaluated TEES lateral graft tympanoplasties (type 1) for anterior and subtotal perforations in 20 ears and found that audiometric outcomes and graft failure rates were similar to historic data for microscopic techniques [4]. Several other studies have compared microscopic postauricular approaches to endoscopic transcanal approaches and have found similar results. However, these studies have also found that EES is associated with shorter surgical times, lesser need for a postauricular incision and canalplasty, less postoperative pain, and fewer wound healing issues [5–12]. Additionally, some studies have compared endoscopic approaches for both a lateral graft and an interlay technique, noting comparable perforation closure rates, but a slight increased incidence of iatrogenic cholesteatoma with the interlay technique [13, 14]. *Kaya* et al. examined endoscopic versus microscopic approaches for type 1 tympanoplasty in a randomized controlled trial analyzing patients who underwent an endoscopic tympanoplasty in one ear and a micro-

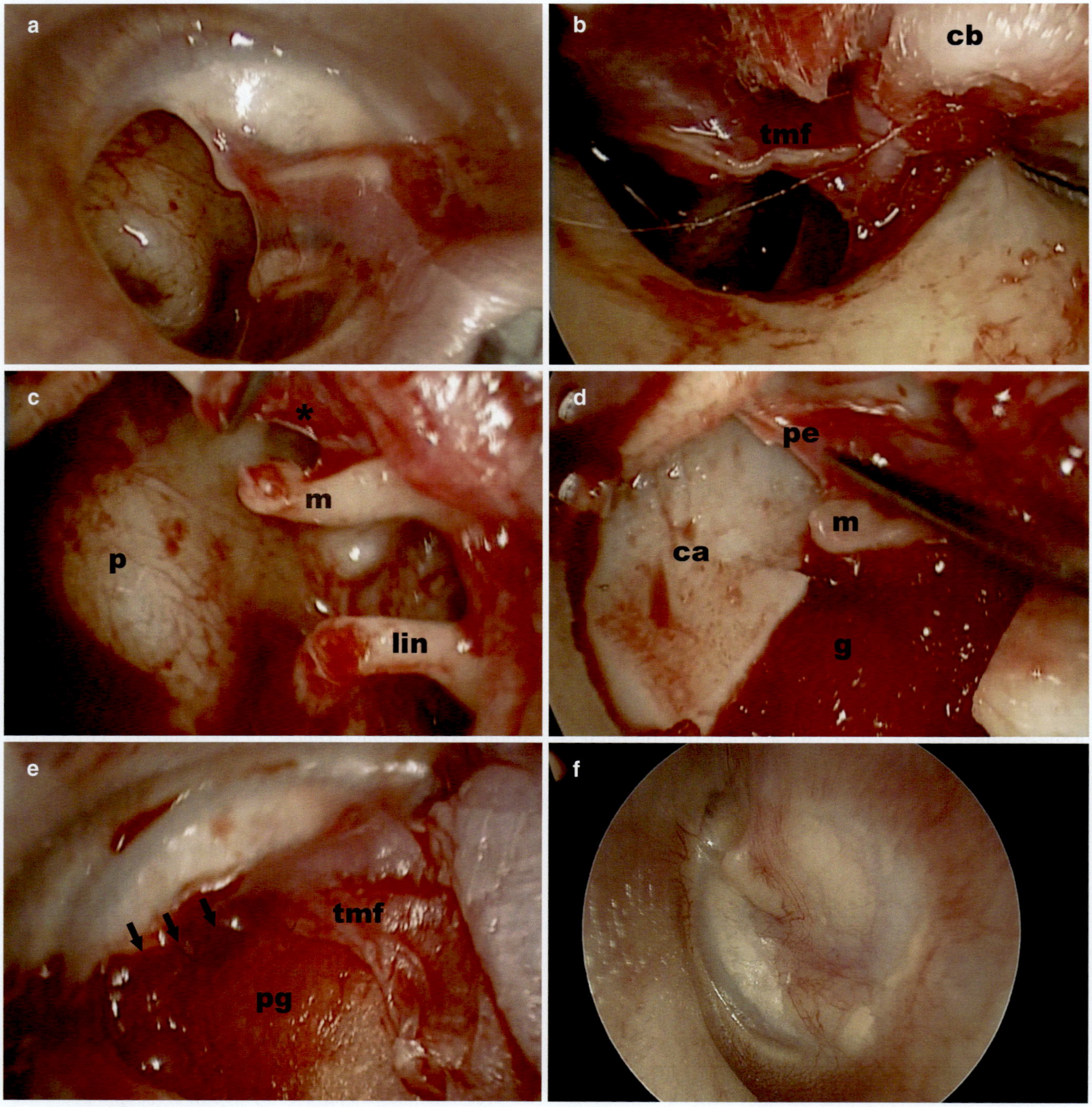

Fig. 45.3 Lateral to malleus underlay tympanoplasty (left ear), (panel **a**–**e**: surgical view, panel f: anatomic view). (**a**) Inferior, marginal tympanic membrane perforation involving the umbo. (**b**) Elevation and reflection of the tympanomeatal flap (tmf) using cotton balls (cb) with access into the middle ear cleft. (**c**) The drum is degloved from the umbo (asterisk) in order to place the graft over the manubrium (m); long process of incus (lin); promontory (p). (**d**) Placement of cartilage graft (ca) over Gelfoam® (g), around the manubrium (m) and under the perforation edges (pe). (**e**) Placement of perichondrium graft (pg) over the cartilage and manubrium, under the remaining drum and tmf repositioned. The edges of the perforation are unfurled and covered by the reconstruction (arrows). (**f**) Postoperative image of cartilage neotympanum

scopic approach in another. Their findings also supported prior findings of shorter operative time, comparable audiologic outcomes and graft take rates, and decreased pain postoperatively [15].

Perforations in chronic otitis media (COM) without cholesteatoma have perforation closure rates and audiometric outcomes comparable to those of MES [16, 17]. *Ohki* et al. published a case–control study analyzing type 1 tympanoplasty in COM without cholesteatoma, performed by either microscopic or endoscopic techniques. Their group found that in cases with increased inflammation of the middle ear space, endoscopic approaches had improved closure of the ABG compared to microsurgical technique [18]. Similar to adults, TEES tympanoplasties in the pediatric population have demonstrated no difference in perforation closure rates or closure of the ABG compared to MES, as well as shorter operative time with the TEES approach [19, 20].

Tympanoplasty can be safely performed utilizing the endoscope with multiple techniques. Overall, data on children and adults who have perforations with or without COM have demonstrated comparable surgical and audiometric outcomes when compared to MES. The main benefits of using the TEES approach include decreased operative time, decreased postoperative pain, and decreased need for a postauricular incision.

Cholesteatoma Surgery

Cholesteatomas in COM present the otologic surgeon with a unique challenge. Given the minute scale and complex anatomy of the middle ear space, cholesteatomas are able to grow into areas that are difficult to access, particularly through transcanal microscopic approaches. The sinus tympani, epitympanum, and aditus ad antrum are particularly difficult to visualize [21, 22]. Standard techniques using the microscope include canal wall up surgery with posterior atticotomy, or canal wall down tympanomastoidectomy. These approaches have additional morbidity compared to transcanal approaches, which may be as minimal as a postauricular incision or encompass more significant issues inherent to canal wall down approaches, such as need for frequent debridement, chronic otorrhea, or a significant conductive hearing loss. EES, on the other hand, provides the opportunity to remove limited cholesteatoma in a transcanal fashion, given its ability to look around corners and remove disease from difficult-to-access areas, provided the cholesteatoma does not extend into the mastoid past the dome of the lateral semicircular canal. In those cases of more extensive disease, a mastoidectomy is needed, and proceeding with a traditional microscopic tympanomastoidectomy may prove more efficient for disease management.

Technique

The initial surgical approach to cholesteatoma resection is similar to perforation repairs. A tympanomeatal flap is elevated using a suction elevator and cottonoids soaked in epinephrine. For epitympanic cholesteatomas, a wide atticotomy with either curettes or a drill can then be performed to improve visualization of the epitympanum until the posterior edge of the cholesteatoma sac is identified. The cholesteatoma must then be carefully dissected and completely removed. Lateral epitympanic cholesteatomas can be excised with complete preservation of the ossicular chain. Anterior and posterior epitympanic cholesteatomas may require removal of the incus and/or the malleus head to achieve full excision. If the cholesteatoma extends posteriorly past the dome of the lateral semicircular canal, this will likely require conversion to an open approach and a mastoidectomy in order to completely clear disease. After removal of the cholesteatoma, the 30-degree and 45-degree angled scope can be used to visualize difficult-to-see areas and confirm that there is no keratin debris remaining in the middle ear. In the event that these areas are of concern, angled instruments such as Thomassin dissectors and angled suctions can be used to remove remnant debris. During reconstruction, which is similar to a tympanoplasty as discussed above, reconstruction of the scutum is necessary and typically performed with tragal cartilage.

Cholesteatoma Resection Outcomes

Recidivism (residual or recurrent disease) is of paramount interest when assessing outcomes of cholesteatoma surgery. When comparing TEES cholesteatoma resection to MES, current literature suggests lower recidivism rates for endoscopic approaches [23–25]. Several studies have demonstrated that, when cholesteatoma surgery is started with the endoscope, there is a reduction in the need for mastoidectomies without changes in recidivism rates [26–29]. Identified predictors of residual and recurrent disease after TEES include pediatric case distribution and extension of disease to multiple middle ear compartments and the mastoid [30]. In a recent systematic review, *Nair* et al. documented recurrent disease rates of 2.5–18% compared to 5–37% in TEES versus MES, respectively, and residual disease rates of 6–33% compared to 10–40%, respectively [31]. However, the majority of published TEES studies include follow-up intervals ranging from 1 to 3 years after the initial surgery. As cholesteatomas can recur at intervals far beyond these follow-up periods, more data are needed to confirm that lower recidivism rates observed with TEES approaches are sustained over time.

Other advantages of TEES in cholesteatoma surgery, such as decreased operative time and decreased postoperative pain, were shown by *Wu* et al. in a randomized controlled trial evaluating patients with cholesteatoma limited to the epitympanum, without mastoid extension [24]. When extensive disease is encountered, conversion from endoscopic to open approaches carries a significant increase in operative time when compared to standard microscopic tympanomastoidectomy [26, 30].

Overall, cholesteatoma limited to the middle ear cleft can be addressed safely utilizing the TEES technique with improvement in short-term recidivism rates, better pain control, and avoidance of mastoidectomy. Though operative times may be shorter for TEES, if a mastoidectomy is needed due to the extent of disease, operative time significantly increases.

Ossicular Chain Reconstruction

TEES is a viable option to perform ossiculoplasty (Fig. 45.4) in indicated cases, such as cholesteatoma, erosion of the ossicular chain, traumatic disarticulation, ossicular fixation,

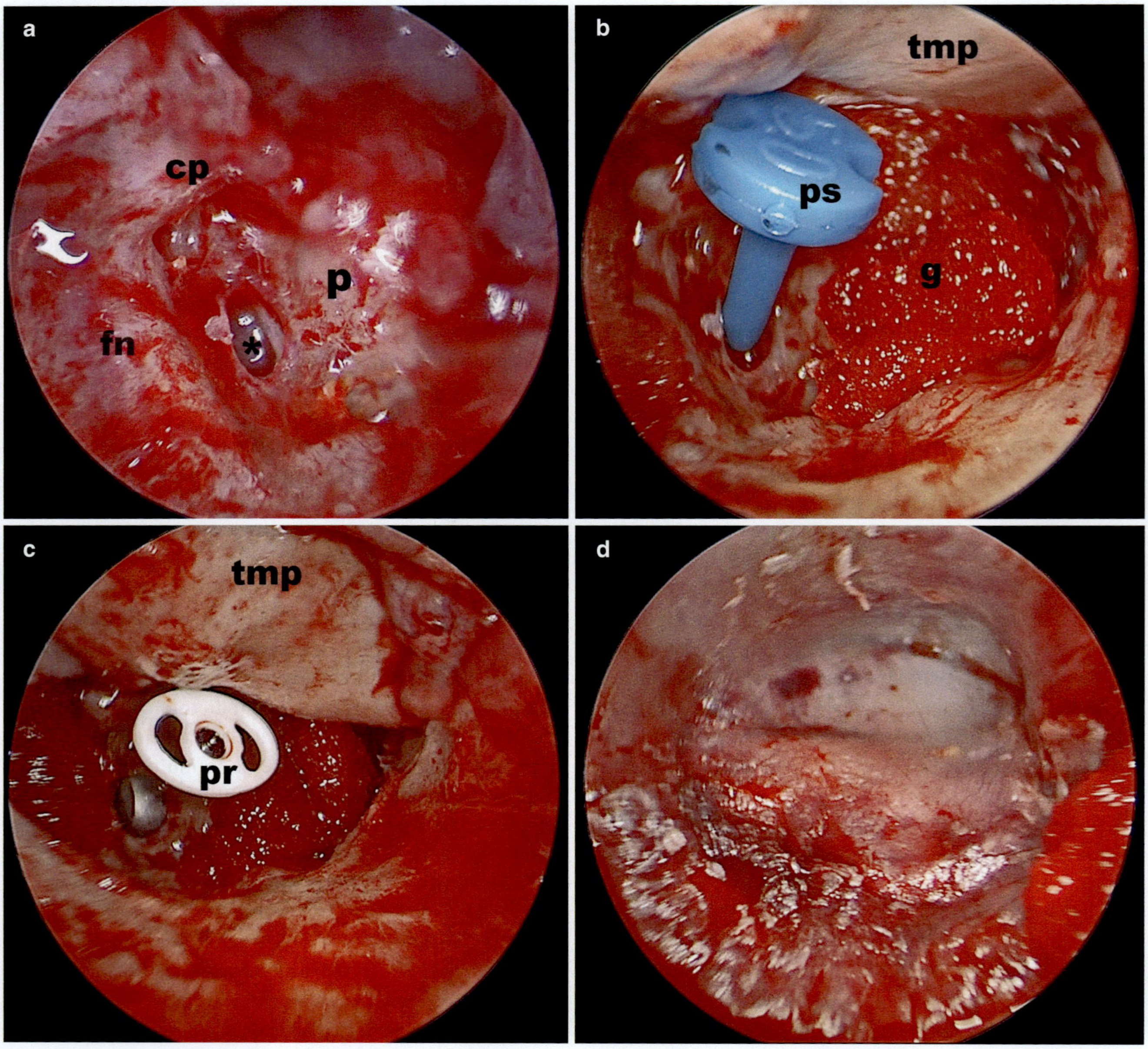

Fig. 45.4 TEES ossiculoplasty with TORP as a second look after previous cholesteatoma surgery (right ear). (**a**) The tympanic membrane (tmp) has been reflected and the middle ear is visualized with absence of the ossicular chain; footplate (asterisk), promontory (p), fn (tympanic segment of the facial nerve), cp (cochleariform process). (**b**) After the mobility of the footplate is confirmed, Gelfoam® (g) is placed over the promontory and a prosthesis sizer (ps) is used to determine the prosthesis length. (**c**) A TORP (pr) is placed standing over the footplate. (**d**) Final view after the previously reconstructed cartilage tmp (tympanic membrane) is repositioned over the prosthesis

and congenital ossicular malformations. The endoscope provides distinct advantages that include high-quality optics, wide field of view which can improve visualization of the ossicles, ability to see past the tip of the instrument, and precise prosthesis coupling.

Technique

The surgical approach is the same as in TEES tympanoplasty (Fig. 45.5). After the tympanomeatal flap is elevated, the ossicular pathology is assessed. Once the decision to proceed with ossicular chain reconstruction is confirmed (Fig. 45.5a, b), hemostasis of the middle ear space is achieved with epinephrine-soaked cottonoids. Since TEES is a one-handed technique, and there is decreased depth perception, placing a prosthesis directly over the stapes or footplate may lead to a significant amount of undesired movement of the ossicle. To prevent this from happening, a small piece of Gelfoam® is placed over the promontory and then the desired prosthesis is placed over the Gelfoam®, inferior and perpendicular to the axis of the stapes capitulum or footplate (Fig. 45.5c). When

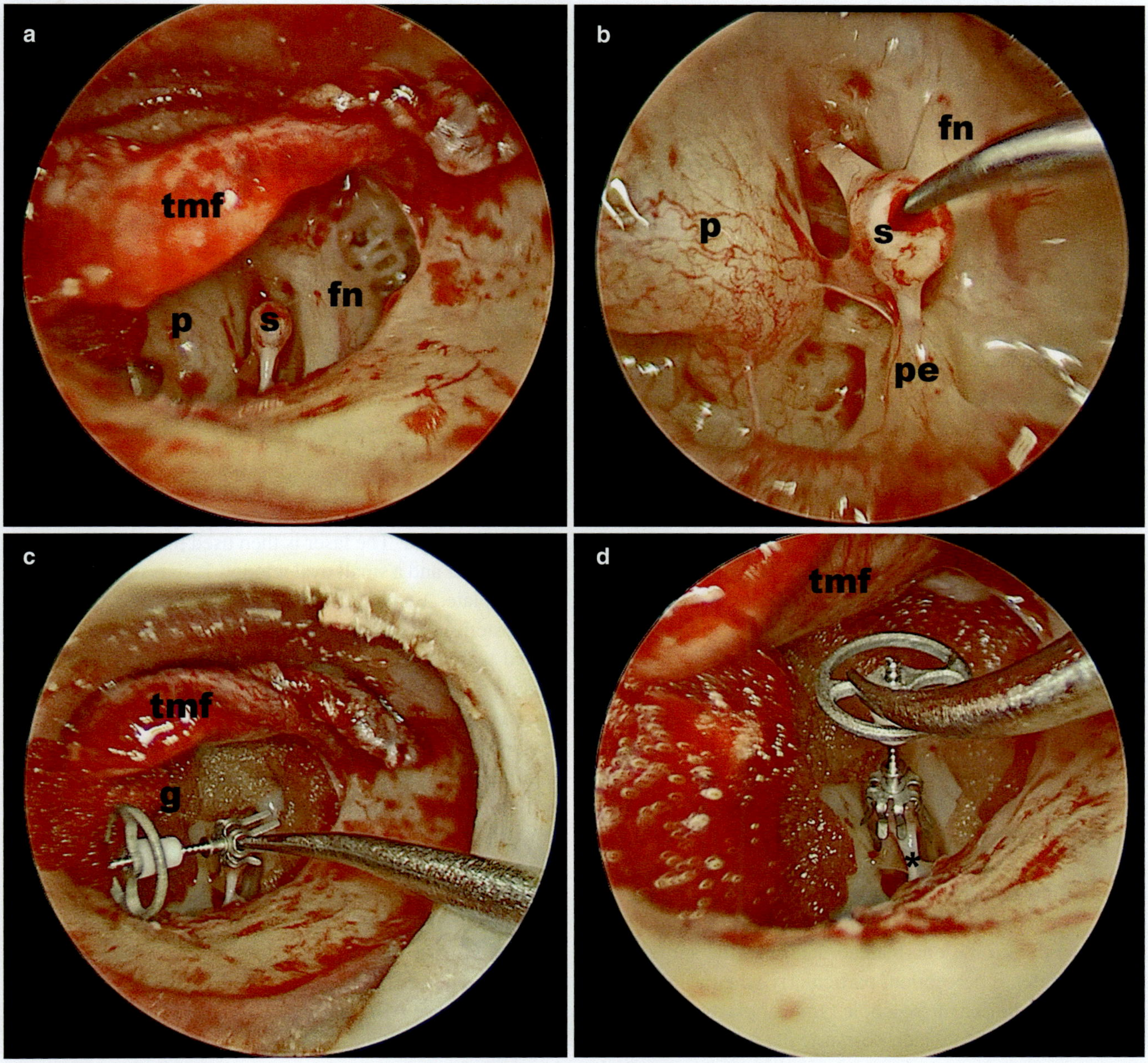

Fig. 45.5 TEES ossiculoplasty with PORP (left ear). (**a**) The tympanomeatal flap (tmf) is reflected and the middle ear has been entered, visualizing the promontory (p), stapes (s), and tympanic segment of the facial nerve (fn). (**b**) The stapes is palpated, and its mobility confirmed; pyramidal eminence (pe). (**c**) Gelfoam® (g) is placed over the promontory and the PORP is dropped inferior and perpendicular to the axis of the stapes, centering the basket of the PORP over the capitulum. (**d**) PORP is tilted over the stapes to stand and couple over the capitulum, under the tmf; stapedial tendon (asterisk)

using a partial ossicular prosthesis (PORP), the basket of the PORP is centered over the capitulum and then the prosthesis is tilted over the stapes to couple in position (Fig. 45.5d). Similarly, when using a total ossicular prosthesis (TORP), the base of the prosthesis is centered over the footplate and the head of the prosthesis is then tilted to stand over the footplate and couple in position (Fig. 45.4d). Gelfoam® is used to secure the prosthesis in place, a previously harvested tragal cartilage graft is placed over the prosthesis cap, and the tympanomeatal flap is repositioned.

Ossiculoplasty Outcomes

TEES ossiculoplasty has favorable audiometric outcomes when compared to microscopic approaches [32–34]. Comparison of audiometric outcomes between TEES and MES using PORPs and TORPs was evaluated by *Yawn* et al. The mean postoperative ABG in the TEES group was 13.8 dB compared to 16.7 dB in the MES group for PORPs. For TORPs, the postoperative ABG was 15.9 dB versus 17.2 dB in the TEES versus MES groups [35]. There was no significant difference in audiometric outcomes or complication rates, including prosthesis extrusion and postoperative tympanic membrane perforations, in either group. Studies using an autologous graft for reconstruction and those where only a pediatric population was analyzed also found similar results [36–38]. Most of these studies cite low population size as a possible explanation for lack of a statistically significant difference in audiometric outcomes between TEES and MES ossiculoplasty, particularly for PORPs. In a larger study, *Sakai* et al. looked at 198 cases where 64% required a PORP and 31.8% were reconstructed using TEES. The median ABG for TEES PORP was 12.3 dB compared with 16.3 dB for MES PORP ($p = 0.02$) [39]. This study suggests that there might be a slight audiologic benefit using TEES, likely due to better visualization of the coupling between the stapes prosthesis and the neotympanum. While the trends of TEES ossiculoplasty are overall similar to that of MES, more data is required regarding the endoscopic approach's potential for improved hearing outcomes.

Stapes Surgery

Stapedotomy or stapedectomy may be performed endoscopically, though the use of the endoscope presents a unique challenge due to the one-handed nature of the surgery and the loss of depth perception, particularly when using a drill. Additionally, unlike microscopic tympanoplasty and cholesteatoma resection, in which postauricular incisions are common, microscopic stapedotomy/stapedectomy is routinely performed transcanal; therefore, the use of the endoscope does not reduce the need for a postauricular incision. The main advantage of the endoscope with regard to stapes surgery is the excellent visualization of the oval window, which the authors have found to be beneficial, particularly in revision cases and stapes malformations.

Technique

For both stapedotomy and stapedectomy, a tympanomeatal flap is elevated utilizing techniques as described in early sections of this chapter. After entering the middle ear, fixation of the stapes is confirmed. Then, scutum removal is performed with a curette to ensure that the entire stapes is visualized and that the field is wide enough for instrument maneuvering. Scutum removal is carefully performed without injuring the chorda tympani (Fig. 45.6a). Down fracture of the stapes is then performed to expose the footplate (Fig. 45.6b). The distance from the footplate to the long process of the incus is then measured for the selection of a prosthesis.

Stapedotomy

The laser, followed by serial perforators or a 0.7 mm drill bit, is used to create a 0.7 mm fenestra (Fig. 45.6c). Although the microdrill may be more challenging to use with the endoscope because of the loss of depth perception, its use produces minimal differences in outcomes, cost, and safety when comparing TEES to MES [40]. Next, the piston prosthesis is placed in the footplate fenestra, and crimped onto the incus long process with the laser (Fig. 45.6d). A blood patch is used to seal the fenestra, followed by repositioning of the tympanomeatal flap.

Stapedectomy

Before performing a stapedectomy, a tragal perichondrium graft is harvested. The laser is then used to make a rosette in the footplate and a small oval window rasp is used to fracture the footplate. A small and large rasp are then used to remove the posterior 50–75% of the footplate. The previously harvested perichondrium graft is placed over the footplate and the prosthesis, most commonly a bucket handle prosthesis, is placed on the graft, with the handle secured on the long process of the incus. There are some disadvantages to this approach, which include creation of a larger opening into the vestibule, and associated higher risk of sensorineural hearing loss, postoperative perilymphatic fistula, and postoperative vertigo. Great care must be taken to avoid suctioning perilymph directly from the vestibule to minimize these risks.

Stapes Surgery Outcomes

Reported audiometric outcomes demonstrate that 56–91% of patients achieve ABG closure within 10 dB when undergoing a TEES approach [41–47], which is comparable to that reported for microscopic approaches [48–51]. Proposed advantages of TEES include decreased need for an endaural incision and decreased dysgeusia [48, 52, 53]. Reported rates of postoperative dysgeusia are lower in TEES versus MES at 5.9 versus 16.9%, respectively [41]. TEES revision stapes

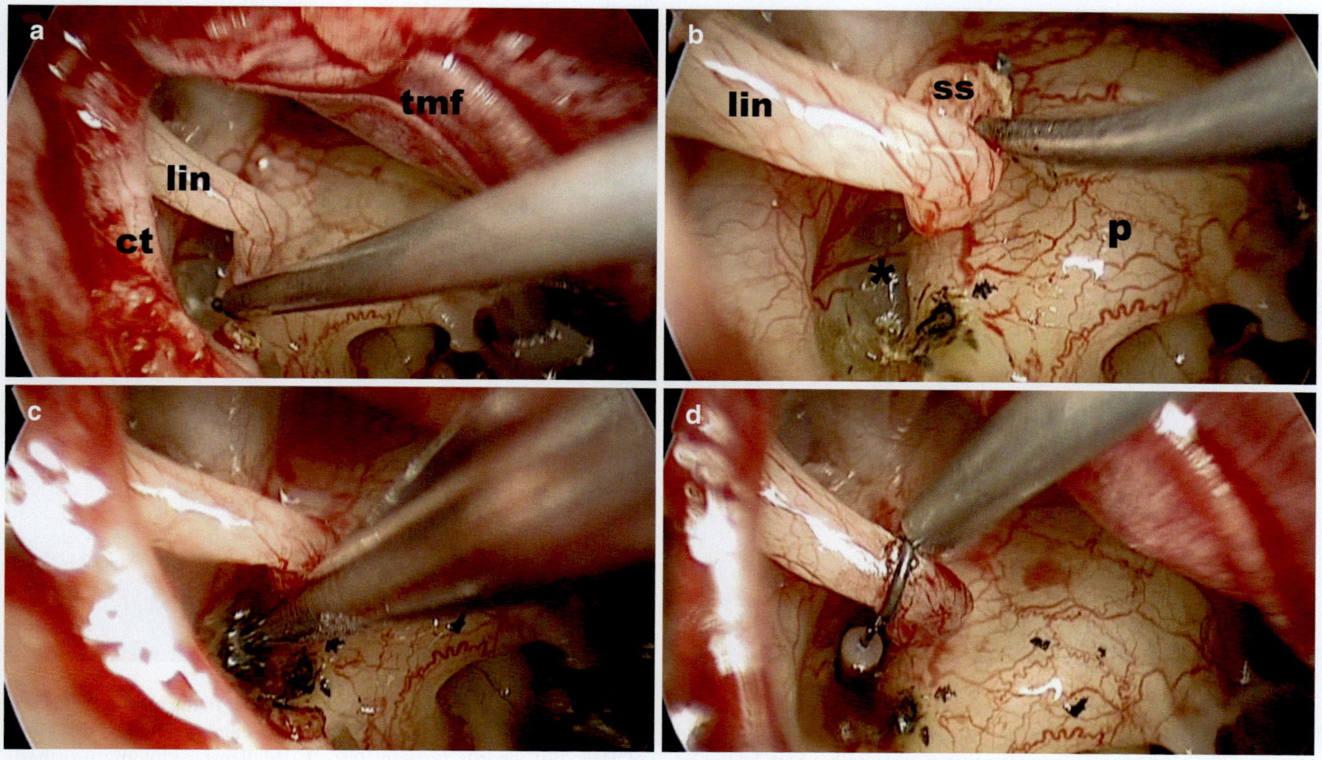

Fig. 45.6 TEES Stapedotomy (right ear). (**a**) After elevating the tympanomeatal flap (tmf), curetting the scutum, and confirming the stapes fixation, the stapedial tendon and posterior crura are divided with the CO_2 laser; chorda tympani (ct); long process of incus (lin). (**b**) After separating the incudostapedial joint, the stapes suprastructure (ss) is down fractured; promontory (p); footplate (asterisk). (**c**) The laser followed by a microdrill is used to create a 0.7 mm fenestra. (**d**) A nitinol prosthesis is placed and crimped with the CO_2 laser

surgery and pediatric stapes surgery have similar audiologic outcomes and complication rates when compared to MES [54–56], with the advantages of TEES including improved visualization of anatomic variations, malformations, and ease of identification of a displaced prosthesis (Fig. 45.7).

Lateral Skull Base Procedures and Middle Ear Tumors

As endoscopic ear surgery continues to evolve, neurotologic surgeons have expanded the use of the endoscope to address diseases of the lateral skull base. This section will provide a brief overview on the variety of procedures currently being performed utilizing endoscopes. Vestibular schwannomas (VS), historically known as acoustic neuromas, are tumors of the internal auditory canal (IAC) and cerebellopontine angle that have been traditionally managed surgically by translabyrinthine, retrosigmoid, or middle cranial fossa approaches. *Marchioni* et al. described a novel way to access the IAC to resect a VS through the ear canal, the transcanal transpromontory approach [57] (Fig. 45.8). This approach was initially described with utilization of the endoscope, which improves visualization around critical structures [58]. However, because of the need for a wide canalplasty and the advantage of tumor dissection using two hands, this initial total endoscopic approach has evolved to a combined endoscopic and microscopic approach or a solely microscopic approach [59–62]. The transcanal transpromontory approach is ideal for tumors mainly involving the IAC with minimal extension into the cerebellopontine angle. Because this approach involves drilling through the cochlea, this procedure should only be pursued in patients with non-serviceable hearing.

The procedure starts by creating a circumferential incision in the external auditory canal at the osseocartilaginous junction and removing all ear canal skin, the tympanic membrane, and the lateral ossicular chain (Fig. 45.8a, b). A wide canalplasty is then performed, with the limits of dissection being the mastoid and tympanic facial nerve (FN) segments posteriorly and superiorly, respectively, the petrous internal carotid artery anteriorly, and the jugular bulb inferiorly. The stapes is removed, and the drill is then used to connect the oval window to the round window and proceed to open the basal turn, middle turn, and apical turn of the cochlea (Fig. 45.8c). Dissection of the tensor tympani muscle is required to allow complete opening of the cochlea's apical turn. The infracochlear air cells are opened until the porus acusticus of the IAC is reached, and the IAC is skeletonized (Fig. 45.8d). Once the tumor is encountered, it is peeled away from the facial nerve and resected (Fig. 45.8e, f). The

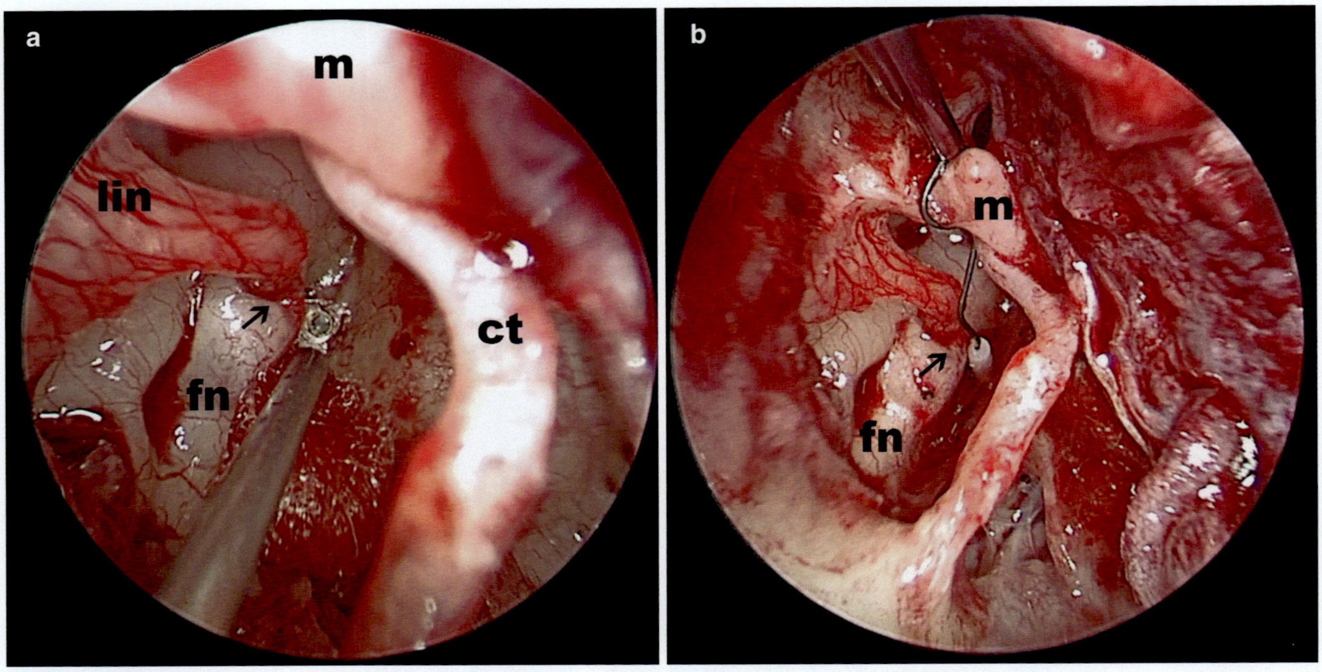

Fig. 45.7 TEES malleostapedotomy in congenital stapes malformation (right ear). (**a**) After elevating the tympanomeatal flap (tmf), and curetting the scutum, we encountered a congenitally short lenticular and long process of the incus (lin), absent stapes suprastructure, and near complete dehiscent facial nerve (fn) over the footplate (arrow). The fenestra was performed with the CO_2 laser in the most anterior portion of the footplate that could be visualized and noted to be fixed (end of laser tip); chorda tympani (ct). (**b**) Malleostapedotomy prosthesis placed from the malleus neck to the anterior footplate fenestra, adjacent to the dehiscent facial nerve (arrow)

IAC defect and middle ear space are filled with fat and the Eustachian tube packed with muscle. A Rambo overclosure of the external auditory canal is then completed. Reported outcomes with this approach have shown no postoperative cerebrospinal fluid leaks and good facial nerve (FN) outcomes [63]. In a cohort of 49 patients who underwent a transpromontory VS resection, 95.9% had FN function preserved [House-Brackmann (HB) I-II] with stable results at follow-up, and 4.1% of cases had FN function reduced, none of which were worse than a HB III [64]. The transcanal transpromontory approach is an efficient, minimally invasive option for resection of small VS without serviceable hearing. Nonetheless, with the expanded indications of cochlear implantation in single-sided deafness for patients with intact postoperative cochlear nerves, this technique might have limited application in the future given the associated requisite cochlear drilling.

Benign tumors confined to the middle ear cleft have proven to be an ideal pathology to access through TEES [65–68]. As glomus tympanicum represents the most common benign middle ear tumor, we will discuss the surgical techniques and outcomes utilized for this pathology (Fig. 45.9). Case selection is of paramount importance and can be determined based on the extent of disease. The tumor sizes that have been reported to be successfully resected via TEES have no mastoid involvement and include only tumors within the modified Fisch-Mattox classification A1, A2, and B1 [69–71]. The largest series reported 30 patients who underwent TEES glomus tympanicum resection, achieving gross total resection (GTR) in 90% of cases. When the tumor had a close relationship with the internal carotid artery, near total resection was performed. There were no reported postoperative complications and no recurrences in the GTR group [70]. Auditory outcomes have shown an improvement in the ABG that ranges from 2.84 to 5.9 dB after surgery [65, 67].

To maximize the chance for GTR, creating an appropriate tympanomeatal flap for surgical visualization is key. A superiorly based tympanomeatal flap is created with an anteroinferior and posterior vertical incision, connected inferiorly by a horizontal incision 4 mm lateral to the annulus. The tympanomeatal flap is raised to give good access to the hypotympanum. If necessary, a wide canalplasty can be performed to give further exposure of the hypotympanum. The undersurface of the TM is then separated from the tumor. When the tumor extends into the protympanum, the tympanic membrane should be degloved from the handle of the malleus to minimize the risk for intraoperative tympanic membrane perforations (Fig. 45.9a). Prior to attempting resection, the tumor can be devascularized using either bipolar cautery, a potassium titanyl phosphate (KTP) laser, or even an ultrasonic aspirator [72]. Fibrillar and thrombin-soaked Gelfoam® and cottonoids can be applied for hemostasis throughout tumor dissection, particularly to improve visualization during tumor separation from the ossicles. Although the number of cases reported in the literature is limited, the available body of evidence suggests that TEES is a viable

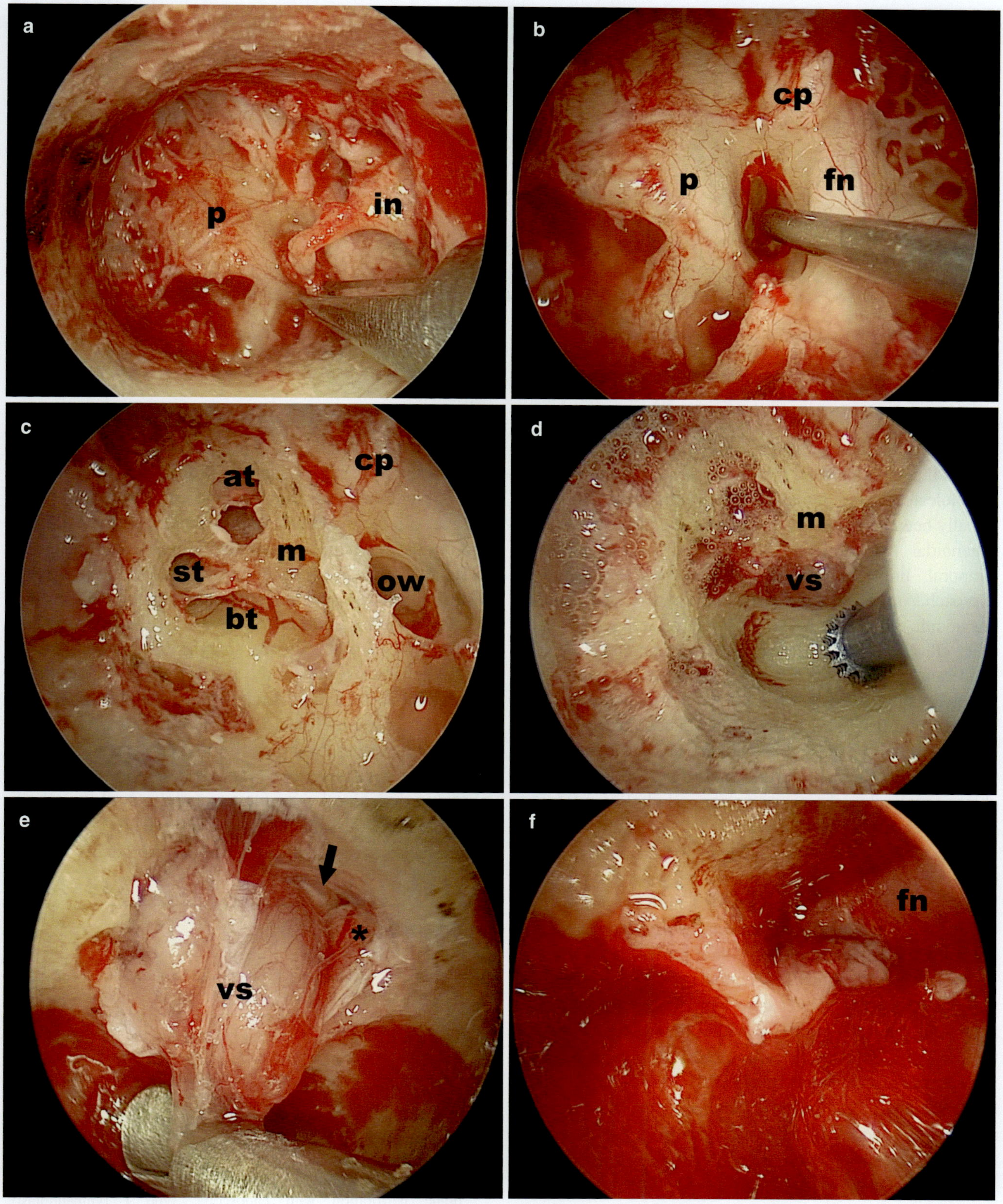

Fig. 45.8 Endoscopic transpromontorial approach for the resection of vestibular schwannoma (left ear) (**a**) Wide canalplasty performed after removal of ear canal skin, the tympanic membrane, and malleus; promontory (p); incus (in). (**b**) The incus and stapes excised; tympanic segment of the facial nerve (tfn); cochleariform process (cp). (**c**) The cochlea is drilled, and the basal turn (bt), middle turn, and apical turn (mt) are identified; modiolus (m); scala tympani (st); oval window (ow). (**d**) The infracochlear air cells are opened until the IAC is exposed starting at the fundus where the vestibular schwannoma (vs) is identified. (**e**) Tumor (vs) arising from the inferior vestibular nerve is peeled away from the facial nerve (arrow) and superior vestibular nerve (asterisk). (**f**) The tumor has been resected leaving the facial nerve (fn) intact

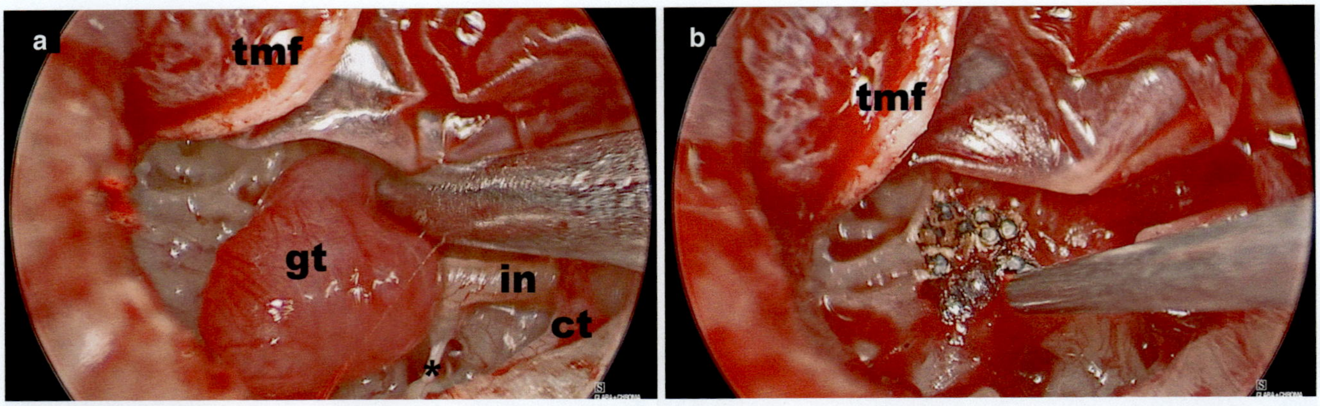

Fig. 45.9 TEES glomus tympanicum resection (left ear). (**a**) Glomus tympanicum (gt) seen emanating from the promontory, after elevating of the tympanomeatal flap (tmf), and separating the drum away from the tumor; incus (in) chorda tympani (ct); stapedial tendon (asterisk). (**b**) Control of bleeding from the tympanic plexus in the promontory with the CO_2 laser

and safe technique for the resection of glomus tympanicum tumors that do not extend into the mastoid.

Cholesterol granulomas of the petrous apex have traditionally been accessed via a middle fossa approach, a transsphenoidal approach, or in cases of well-pneumatized temporal bones, through a microscopic infracochlear approach. As this last approach is entirely performed through the middle ear, TEES is an ideal way to access this space. After elevation of a superiorly based tympanomeatal flap, a wide canalplasty is performed for adequate exposure of the hypotympanum. The cochlea and the subcochlear canaliculus are identified. The limits of the dissection include the cochlea superiorly, the jugular bulb inferiorly, and the petrous carotid artery anteriorly. By drilling and following the subcochlear canaliculus, the petrous apex and cholesterol granuloma are encountered. Once entered, the granuloma can be marsupialized and drained. The major advantage of the endoscope is its ability to visualize within the cyst, which better permits lysis of adhesions for additional cyst content eradication. In limited case reports in the literature, most patients experience resolution of their presenting symptoms, without changes in their preoperative hearing status [73, 74]. Only one reported patient case experienced recurrence of symptoms due to hemorrhage within the cyst cavity, which required revision surgery [73], similar to previous reports with the microscopic approach [75]. The TEES infracochlear approach, therefore, seems a promising avenue for minimally invasive access to the petrous apex in well-pneumatized temporal bones, with outcomes comparable to MES.

Conclusion

The increasing use of the endoscope for otologic surgery is providing a new perspective on the complex anatomy of the middle ear. Over the last 10 years, there has been an increased understanding of how the structures of the middle ear function and interact physiologically, as well as of the optimal methods for surgical intervention. Further advances in surgical optics, such as those that gave rise to endoscopic techniques, may continue to enable surgeons to remove disease in a minimally invasive fashion while restoring the natural physiologic function of the ear. Furthermore, the endoscope provides an excellent visualization tool for not only the surgeon but everyone in the OR, which can significantly aid in trainee education. To date, clinical outcome studies have demonstrated that TEES for diseases limited to the middle ear space and some skull base pathologies (limited cholesteatoma, ossiculoplasty, tympanoplasty, stapes surgery, middle ear tumors, cholesterol granulomas, and small vestibular schwannomas, among others) is an effective, safe, and comparable option to other traditional approaches.

References

1. Steiner W. Techniques of diagnostic and operative endoscopy of the head and neck. Endoscopy of ear, cerebellopontine angle, nose, paranasal sinuses, larynx, oro- and hypopharynx. Endoscopy. 1979;11(1):51–9. https://doi.org/10.1055/s-0028-1098325. PMID: 371958.
2. Ozturan O, Dogan R, Eren SB, Aksoy F. Intraoperative thermal safety of endoscopic ear surgery utilizing a holder. Am J Otolaryngol. 2018;39(5):585–91. https://doi.org/10.1016/j.amjoto.2018.07.001. Epub 2018 Jul 2. PMID: 30001978.
3. Marchioni D, Gazzini L, De Rossi S, Di Maro F, Sacchetto L, Carner M, Bianconi L. The management of tympanic membrane perforation with endoscopic type I tympanoplasty. Otol Neurotol. 2020;41(2):214–21. https://doi.org/10.1097/MAO.0000000000002465. PMID: 31663990.
4. Creighton FX Jr, Kozin E, Rong A, Cohen M, Lee D. Outcomes following transcanal endoscopic lateral graft tympanoplasty. Otol Neurotol. 2019;40(10):e989–92. https://doi.org/10.1097/MAO.0000000000002400. PMID: 31568133.

5. Crotty TJ, Cleere EF, Keogh IJ. Endoscopic versus microscopic type-1 tympanoplasty: a meta-analysis of randomized trials. Laryngoscope. 2023;133(7):1550–7. https://doi.org/10.1002/lary.30479. Epub 2022 Nov 9. PMID: 36349835.
6. Kim DJ, Lee HM, Choi SW, Oh SJ, Kong SK, Lee IW. Comparative study of endoscopic and microscopic tympanoplasty performed by a single experienced surgeon. Am J Otolaryngol. 2021;42(1):102788. https://doi.org/10.1016/j.amjoto.2020.102788. Epub 2020 Oct 23. PMID: 33171411.
7. Zhang Y, Wang W, Xu K, Hu M, Ma Y, Lin P. Comparison of clinical outcome between endoscopic and postauricular incision microscopic type-1 tympanoplasty. Acta Otolaryngol. 2021;141(1):29–33. https://doi.org/10.1080/00016489.2020.1821091. Epub 2020 Oct 6. PMID: 33019832.
8. Shakya D, Kc A, Nepal A. A comparative study of endoscopic versus microscopic cartilage type I tympanoplasty. Int Arch Otorhinolaryngol. 2020;24(1):e80–5. https://doi.org/10.1055/s--0039-1693139. Epub 2019 Nov 4. PMID: 31892962; PMCID: PMC6828568.
9. Manna S, Kaul VF, Gray ML, Wanna GB. Endoscopic versus microscopic middle ear surgery: a meta-analysis of outcomes following tympanoplasty and stapes surgery. Otol Neurotol. 2019;40(8):983–93. https://doi.org/10.1097/MAO.0000000000002353. PMID: 31348133.
10. Plodpai Y. Endoscopic vs microscopic overlay tympanoplasty for correcting large tympanic membrane perforations: a randomized clinical trial. Otolaryngol Head Neck Surg. 2018;159(5):879–86. https://doi.org/10.1177/0194599818786948. Epub 2018 Jul 10. PMID: 29986622.
11. Tseng CC, Lai MT, Wu CC, Yuan SP, Ding YF. Comparison of the efficacy of endoscopic tympanoplasty and microscopic tympanoplasty: a systematic review and meta-analysis. Laryngoscope. 2017;127(8):1890–6. https://doi.org/10.1002/lary.26379. Epub 2016 Nov 9. PMID: 27861950.
12. Kuo CH, Wu HM. Comparison of endoscopic and microscopic tympanoplasty. Eur Arch Otorhinolaryngol. 2017;274(7):2727–32. https://doi.org/10.1007/s00405-017-4570-3. Epub 2017 Apr 24. PMID: 28439691.
13. Bao JW, Zhan KY, Wick CC. Comparison of endoscopic underlay and over-under tympanoplasty techniques for type I tympanoplasty. Laryngoscope Investig Otolaryngol. 2022;7(4):1186–93. https://doi.org/10.1002/lio2.879. PMID: 36000055; PMCID: PMC9392374.
14. Ranguis SC, Leonard CG, James AL. Prospective comparison of pediatric endoscopic lateral graft and interlay tympanoplasty. Otol Neurotol. 2021;42(6):867–75. https://doi.org/10.1097/MAO.0000000000003053. PMID: 34111050.
15. Kaya I, Sezgin B, Sergin D, Ozturk A, Eraslan S, Gode S, Bilgen C, Kirazli T. Endoscopic versus microscopic type 1 tympanoplasty in the same patients: a prospective randomized controlled trial. Eur Arch Otorhinolaryngol. 2017;274(9):3343–9. https://doi.org/10.1007/s00405-017-4661-1. Epub 2017 Jul 1. PMID: 28669049.
16. Hsu YC, Kuo CL, Huang TC. A retrospective comparative study of endoscopic and microscopic Tympanoplasty. J Otolaryngol Head Neck Surg. 2018;47(1):44. https://doi.org/10.1186/s40463-018-0289-4. PMID: 29973286; PMCID: PMC6033204.
17. Yang Q, Wang B, Zhang J, Liu H, Xu M, Zhang W. Comparison of endoscopic and microscopic tympanoplasty in patients with chronic otitis media. Eur Arch Otorhinolaryngol. 2022;279(10):4801–7. https://doi.org/10.1007/s00405-022-07273-2. Epub 2022 Feb 5. PMID: 35122510; PMCID: PMC9474537.
18. Ohki M, Kikuchi S, Tanaka S. Endoscopic type 1 tympanoplasty in chronic otitis media: comparative study with a postauricular microscopic approach. Otolaryngol Head Neck Surg. 2019;161(2):315–23. https://doi.org/10.1177/0194599819838778. Epub 2019 Mar 26. PMID: 30912997.
19. Mitton TJ, Killeen DE, Momin ZK, Hunter JB, Isaacson B, Lee K, Kutz JW Jr. Endoscopic versus microscopic pediatric tympanoplasty: is there a difference between closure rates and hearing outcomes? Otol Neurotol. 2022;43(10):1205–11. https://doi.org/10.1097/MAO.0000000000003694. Epub 2022 Sep 28. PMID: 36166975.
20. Dunya G, Casazza GC, Blotter J, Park EJ, Park AH. Comparing two different techniques to repair pediatric anterior tympanic membrane perforations. Int J Pediatr Otorhinolaryngol. 2021;150:110903. https://doi.org/10.1016/j.ijporl.2021.110903. Epub 2021 Aug 30. PMID: 34479059.
21. Bennett ML, Zhang D, Labadie RF, Noble JH. Comparison of middle ear visualization with endoscopy and microscopy. Otol Neurotol. 2016;37(4):362–6. https://doi.org/10.1097/MAO.0000000000000988. PMID: 26945313.
22. Karchier EB, Niemczyk K, Orłowski A. Comparison of visualization of the middle ear by microscope and endoscopes of 30° and 45° through posterior tympanotomy. Wideochir Inne Tech Maloinwazyjne. 2014;9(2):276–81. https://doi.org/10.5114/wiitm.2014.41618. Epub 2014 May 8. PMID: 25097700; PMCID: PMC4105663.
23. Li B, Zhou L, Wang M, Wang Y, Zou J. Endoscopic versus microscopic surgery for treatment of middle ear cholesteatoma: a systematic review and meta-analysis. Am J Otolaryngol. 2021;42(2):102451. https://doi.org/10.1016/j.amjoto.2020.102451.
24. Wu L, Liu Q, Gao B, Huang S, Yang N. Comparison of endoscopic and microscopic management of attic cholesteatoma: a randomized controlled trial. Am J Otolaryngol. 2022;43(3):103378. https://doi.org/10.1016/j.amjoto.2022.103378.
25. Basonbul RA, Ronner EA, Kozin ED, Lee DJ, Cohen MS. Systematic review of endoscopic ear surgery outcomes for pediatric cholesteatoma. Otol Neurotol. 2021;42(1):108–15. https://doi.org/10.1097/MAO.0000000000002876. PMID: 33165162.
26. Hunter JB, Zuniga MG, Sweeney AD, Bertrand NM, Wanna GB, Haynes DS, Wootten CT, Rivas A. Pediatric endoscopic cholesteatoma surgery. Otolaryngol Head Neck Surg. 2016;154(6):1121–7. https://doi.org/10.1177/0194599816631941. Epub 2016 Mar 1. PMID: 26932974.
27. Cohen MS, Basonbul RA, Kozin ED, Lee DJ. Residual cholesteatoma during second-look procedures following primary pediatric endoscopic ear surgery. Otolaryngol Head Neck Surg. 2017;157(6):1034–40. https://doi.org/10.1177/0194599817729136. Epub 2017 Sep 5. PMID: 28871887.
28. Ghadersohi S, Carter JM, Hoff SR. Endoscopic transcanal approach to the middle ear for management of pediatric cholesteatoma. Laryngoscope. 2017;127(11):2653–8. https://doi.org/10.1002/lary.26654. Epub 2017 May 23. PMID: 28543174.
29. Glikson E, Yousovich R, Mansour J, Wolf M, Migirov L, Shapira Y. Transcanal endoscopic ear surgery for middle ear cholesteatoma. Otol Neurotol. 2017;38(5):e41–5. https://doi.org/10.1097/MAO.0000000000001395. PMID: 28333776.
30. Manzoor NF, Totten DJ, McLeod ME, Sherry AD, Perkins EL, Haynes DS, Rivas A. Comparative analysis of recidivism after endoscopic and microscopic-based cholesteatoma resection. Otol Neurotol. 2022;43(4):466–71. https://doi.org/10.1097/MAO.0000000000003476. PMID: 35287152.
31. Nair S, Aishwarya JG, Vasu PK, Karthikeyan A, Shalini M. Outcomes of totally endoscopic versus microscopic techniques in middle ear cholesteatoma: a systematic review and meta-analysis. Indian J Otolaryngol Head Neck Surg. 2022;74(Suppl 3):4200–11.
32. Das A, Mitra S, Ghosh D, Sengupta A. Endoscopic ossiculoplasty: is there any edge over the microscopic technique? Laryngoscope. 2020;130(3):797–802. https://doi.org/10.1002/lary.28074. Epub 2019 May 23. PMID: 32073145.

33. Tsetsos N, Vlachtsis K, Stavrakas M, Fyrmpas G. Endoscopic versus microscopic ossiculoplasty in chronic otitis media: a systematic review of the literature. Eur Arch Otorhinolaryngol. 2021;278(4):917–23. https://doi.org/10.1007/s00405-020-06182-6. Epub 2020 Jul 7. PMID: 32632614.
34. Baazil AHA, Ebbens FA, van Spronsen E, De Wolf MJF, Dikkers FG. Comparison of long-term microscopic and endoscopic audiologic results after total ossicular replacement prosthesis surgery. Otol Neurotol. 2022;43(10):1189–95. https://doi.org/10.1097/MAO.0000000000003733. PMID: 36302389; PMCID: PMC9671587.
35. Yawn RJ, Hunter JB, O'Connell BP, Wanna GB, Killeen DE, Wick CC, Isaacson B, Rivas A. Audiometric outcomes following endoscopic ossicular chain reconstruction. Otol Neurotol. 2017;38(9):1296–300. https://doi.org/10.1097/MAO.0000000000001527. PMID: 28796085.
36. Soloperto D, Laura E, Gazzini L, Cerullo R, Ferrulli G, Nocini R, Molteni G, Marchioni D. Exclusive endoscopic ossiculoplasty with autologous material: step-by-step procedure and functional results. Eur Arch Otorhinolaryngol. 2023;280(11):4869–78. https://doi.org/10.1007/s00405-023-08005-w. Epub 2023 May 9. PMID: 37160464.
37. Caloway CL, Basonbul RA, Ronner EA, Tolisano AM, Zhu AW, Suresh H, Lee DJ, Isaacson B, Cohen MS. Pediatric endoscopic ossiculoplasty following surgery for chronic ear disease. Laryngoscope. 2020;130(12):2896–9. https://doi.org/10.1002/lary.28526. Epub 2020 Feb 5. PMID: 32022283.
38. Kwinter A, Purcell PL, Leonard CG, James AL. Comparing transcanal endoscopic ear surgery to post-auricular microscope-guided surgery in pediatric ossiculoplasty: hearing outcomes and postoperative pain. Otol Neurotol. 2021;42(10):e1648–51. https://doi.org/10.1097/MAO.0000000000003235. PMID: 34172655.
39. Sakai M, Killeen DE, Ma C, Newcomer M, Hunter JB, Isaacson B, Kutz JW Jr. Audiometric outcomes comparing endoscopic versus microscopic ossiculoplasty. Otol Neurotol. 2022;43(7):820–6. https://doi.org/10.1097/MAO.0000000000003577. Epub 2022 Jul 7. PMID: 35802898.
40. Kaul VF, Chow K, Estrera SL, Schwam ZG, Wanna GB. Microdrill in endoscopic stapes surgery: is it safe? Am J Otolaryngol. 2020;41(6):102666. https://doi.org/10.1016/j.amjoto.2020.102666. Epub 2020 Aug 12. PMID: 32854042.
41. Yancey KL, Manzoor NF, Rivas A. Endoscopic stapes surgery: pearls and pitfalls. Otolaryngol Clin N Am. 2021;54(1):147–62. https://doi.org/10.1016/j.otc.2020.09.015. Epub 2020 Nov 2. PMID: 33153730.
42. Naik C, Nemade S. Endoscopic stapedotomy: our view point. Eur Arch Otorhinolaryngol. 2016;273(1):37–41. https://doi.org/10.1007/s00405-014-3468-6. Epub 2014 Dec 27. PMID: 25542249.
43. Kuo CW, Wu HM. Fully endoscopic laser stapedotomy: is it comparable with microscopic surgery? Acta Otolaryngol. 2018;138(10):871–6. https://doi.org/10.1080/00016489.2018.1490029. Epub 2018 Aug 16. PMID: 30113877.
44. Nassiri AM, Yawn RJ, Dedmon MM, Tolisano AM, Hunter JB, Isaacson B, Rivas A. Primary endoscopic stapes surgery: audiologic and surgical outcomes. Otol Neurotol. 2018;39(9):1095–101. https://doi.org/10.1097/MAO.0000000000001958. PMID: 30124621.
45. Bianconi L, Gazzini L, Laura E, De Rossi S, Conti A, Marchioni D. Endoscopic stapedotomy: safety and audiological results in 150 patients. Eur Arch Otorhinolaryngol. 2020;277(1):85–92. https://doi.org/10.1007/s00405-019-05688-y. Epub 2019 Oct 17. PMID: 31624863.
46. Hunter JB, Zuniga MG, Leite J, Killeen D, Wick C, Ramirez J, Rivas JA, Nogueira JF, Isaacson B, Rivas A. Surgical and audiologic outcomes in endoscopic stapes surgery across 4 institutions. Otolaryngol Head Neck Surg. 2016;154(6):1093–8. https://doi.org/10.1177/0194599816633654. Epub 2016 Mar 22. PMID: 27006295.
47. Bartel R, Sanz JJ, Clemente I, Simonetti G, Viscacillas G, Palomino L, Asarta I, Lao X. Endoscopic stapes surgery outcomes and complication rates: a systematic review. Eur Arch Otorhinolaryngol. 2021;278(8):2673–9. https://doi.org/10.1007/s00405-020-06388-8. Epub 2020 Oct 1. PMID: 33001293.
48. Hajiioannou J, Gkrinia E, Tzimkas-Dakis K, Palla E, Brotis A, Korais C, Saratziotis A, Lachanas V, Skoulakis C. Microscopic versus endoscopic stapes surgery: systematic review and meta-analysis. J Laryngol Otol. 2022;136(11):1014–22. https://doi.org/10.1017/S0022215121004436. Epub 2022 Jan 11. PMID: 35012693.
49. Koukkoullis A, Tóth I, Gede N, Szakács Z, Hegyi P, Varga G, Pap I, Harmat K, Németh A, Szanyi I, Lujber L, Gerlinger I, Révész P. Endoscopic versus microscopic stapes surgery outcomes: a meta-analysis and systematic review. Laryngoscope. 2020;130(8):2019–27. https://doi.org/10.1002/lary.28353. Epub 2019 Nov 12. PMID: 31714605.
50. Vaughan C, Fox R, Jufas N, Kong JHK, Patel NP, Saxby AJ. Endoscopic stapedectomy: collective experience from a large Australian center. Otol Neurotol. 2020;41(9):1198–201. https://doi.org/10.1097/MAO.0000000000002762. PMID: 32925837.
51. Nikolaos T, Aikaterini T, Dimitrios D, Sarantis B, John G, Eleana T, Konstantinos M. Does endoscopic stapedotomy increase hearing restoration rates comparing to microscopic? A systematic review and meta-analysis. Eur Arch Otorhinolaryngol. 2018;275(12):2905–13. https://doi.org/10.1007/s00405-018-5166-2. Epub 2018 Oct 16. PMID: 30327907.
52. Kojima H, Komori M, Chikazawa S, Yaguchi Y, Yamamoto K, Chujo K, Moriyama H. Comparison between endoscopic and microscopic stapes surgery. Laryngoscope. 2014;124(1):266–71. https://doi.org/10.1002/lary.24144. Epub 2013 May 13. PMID: 23670854.
53. Sproat R, Yiannakis C, Iyer A. Endoscopic stapes surgery: a comparison with microscopic surgery. Otol Neurotol. 2017;38(5):662–6. https://doi.org/10.1097/MAO.0000000000001371. PMID: 28319495.
54. Fernandez IJ, Villari D, Botti C, Presutti L. Endoscopic revision stapes surgery: surgical findings and outcomes. Eur Arch Otorhinolaryngol. 2019;276(3):703–10. https://doi.org/10.1007/s00405-019-05280-4. Epub 2019 Jan 11. PMID: 30635709.
55. Nassiri AM, Yawn RJ, Dedmon MM, Tolisano AM, Hunter JB, Isaacson B, Rivas A. Audiologic and surgical outcomes in endoscopic revision stapes surgery. Laryngoscope. 2019;129(10):2366–70. https://doi.org/10.1002/lary.27786. Epub 2019 Jan 8. PMID: 30623430.
56. Tolisano AM, Fontenot MR, Nassiri AM, Hunter JB, Kutz JW Jr, Rivas A, Isaacson B. Pediatric stapes surgery: hearing and surgical outcomes in endoscopic vs microscopic approaches. Otolaryngol Head Neck Surg. 2019;161(1):150–6. https://doi.org/10.1177/0194599819836679. Epub 2019 Mar 12. PMID: 30857467.
57. Marchioni D, Alicandri-Ciufelli M, Rubini A, Masotto B, Pavesi G, Presutti L. Exclusive endoscopic transcanal transpromontorial approach: a new perspective for internal auditory canal vestibular schwannoma treatment. J Neurosurg. 2017;126(1):98–105. https://doi.org/10.3171/2015.11.JNS15952. Epub 2016 Mar 11. PMID: 26967786.
58. Yacoub A, Wimmer W, Molinari G, Alicandri-Ciufelli M, Presutti L, Caversaccio M, Anschuetz L. Transcanal transpromontorial approach to lateral skull base: maximal area of exposure and surgical extensions. World Neurosurg. 2020;135:e181–6. https://doi.org/10.1016/j.wneu.2019.11.102. Epub 2019 Nov 26. PMID: 31778835.
59. Presutti L, Bonali M, Marchioni D, Pavesi G, Feletti A, Anschuetz L, Alicandri-Ciufelli M. Expanded transcanal transpromontorial approach to the internal auditory canal and cerebellopontine angle: a cadaveric study. Acta Otorhinolaryngol Ital. 2017;37(3):224–30. https://doi.org/10.14639/0392-100X-1258. PMID: 28516966; PMCID: PMC5463513.

60. Marchioni D, Carner M, Soloperto D, Bianconi L, Sacchetto A, Sacchetto L, Masotto B, Presutti L. Expanded transcanal transpromontorial approach: a novel surgical technique for cerebellopontine angle vestibular schwannoma removal. Otolaryngol Head Neck Surg. 2018;158(4):710–5. https://doi.org/10.1177/0194599818756592. Epub 2018 Feb 6. PMID: 29405836.
61. Marchioni D, Caiazza N, Dallari V, Sacchetto A. Expanded transcanal transpromontorial approach for vestibular schwannoma. Am J Otolaryngol. 2022;43(5):103486. https://doi.org/10.1016/j.amjoto.2022.103486. Epub 2022 May 6. PMID: 35550312.
62. Isaacson B, Tolisano AM, Patel AR, Barnett SL. Transcanal microscopic transpromontorial approach for vestibular schwannoma. J Neurol Surg B Skull Base. 2019;80(Suppl 3):S279–80. https://doi.org/10.1055/s-0039-1677843. Epub 2019 Feb 28. PMID: 31143589; PMCID: PMC6534664.
63. Wick CC, Arnaoutakis D, Barnett SL, Rivas A, Isaacson B. Endoscopic transcanal transpromontorial approach for vestibular schwannoma resection: a case series. Otol Neurotol. 2017;38(10):e490–4. https://doi.org/10.1097/MAO.0000000000001588. PMID: 29135868.
64. Marchioni D, Soloperto D, Masotto B, Fabbris C, De Rossi S, Villari D, Presutti L. Transcanal transpromontorial acoustic neuroma surgery: results and facial nerve outcomes. Otol Neurotol. 2018;39(2):242–9. https://doi.org/10.1097/MAO.0000000000001658. PMID: 29227438.
65. Quick ME, Acharya A, Friedland P, Kong JHK, Saxby AJ, Patel NP, Kadhim L. Endoscopic management of early stage middle ear paragangliomas—an Australian case series. Otol Neurotol. 2021;42(10):e1677–82. https://doi.org/10.1097/MAO.0000000000003234. PMID: 34121083.
66. Larrosa F, González-Sánchez N, Remacha J, Sandoval M, Bernal-Sprekelsen M. Nuances in transcanal endoscopic approach to benign middle ear tumours in adult patients. Acta Otorrinolaringol Esp (Engl Ed). 2022;73(5):279–85. https://doi.org/10.1016/j.otoeng.2022.08.002. Epub 2022 Aug 26. PMID: 36031112.
67. Killeen DE, Wick CC, Hunter JB, Rivas A, Wanna GB, Nogueira JF, Kutz JW Jr, Isaacson B. Endoscopic management of middle ear paragangliomas: a case series. Otol Neurotol. 2017;38(3):408–15. https://doi.org/10.1097/MAO.0000000000001320. PMID: 28192382.
68. Pollak N, Soni RS. Endoscopic excision of a tympanic paraganglioma: training the next generation of ear surgeons. World J Otorhinolaryngol Head Neck Surg. 2017;3(3):160–2. https://doi.org/10.1016/j.wjorl.2017.08.002. PMID: 29516061; PMCID: PMC5829298.
69. Marchioni D, Alicandri-Ciufelli M, Gioacchini FM, Bonali M, Presutti L. Transcanal endoscopic treatment of benign middle ear neoplasms. Eur Arch Otorhinolaryngol. 2013;270(12):2997–3004. https://doi.org/10.1007/s00405-013-2371-x. Epub 2013 Feb 3. PMID: 23377229.
70. Fermi M, Ferri G, Bayoumi Ebaied T, Alicandri-Ciufelli M, Bonali M, Badr El-Dine M, Presutti L. Transcanal endoscopic management of glomus tympanicum: multicentric case series. Otol Neurotol. 2021;42(2):312–8. https://doi.org/10.1097/MAO.0000000000002929. PMID: 33351561.
71. Fountarlis AL, Hajiioannou J, Lachanas V, Tsitiridis I, Saratziotis A, Alagianni A, Skoulakis C. Endoscopic management of glomus tympanicum tumor: report of three cases and review of the literature. J Audiol Otol. 2023;27(3):145–52. https://doi.org/10.7874/jao.2022.00276. Epub 2022 Nov 24. PMID: 36423621; PMCID: PMC10352693.
72. O'Connell BP, Hunter JB, Carlson ML, Isaacson B, Rivas A, Wanna GB. Utility of an ultrasonic aspirator in transcanal endoscopic resection of temporal bone paraganglioma. J Neurol Surg B Skull Base. 2017;78(1):96–8. https://doi.org/10.1055/s-0036-1585090. Epub 2016 Jul 26. PMID: 28180050; PMCID: PMC5289267.
73. Wick CC, Hansen AR, Kutz JW Jr, Isaacson B. Endoscopic infracochlear approach for drainage of petrous apex cholesterol granulomas: a case series. Otol Neurotol. 2017;38(6):876–81. https://doi.org/10.1097/MAO.0000000000001422. PMID: 28498267.
74. Angeletti D, Pace A, Iannella G, Rossetti V, Colizza A, Di Gioia C, Magliulo G. Tympanic cholesterol granuloma and exclusive endoscopic approach. Am J Case Rep. 2020;21:e925369. https://doi.org/10.12659/AJCR.925369. PMID: 32960877; PMCID: PMC7520131.
75. Fong BP, Brackmann DE, Telischi FF. The long-term follow-up of drainage procedures for petrous apex cholesterol granulomas. Arch Otolaryngol Head Neck Surg. 1995;121(4):426–30. https://doi.org/10.1001/archotol.1995.01890040050008. PMID: 7702817.

Primary Surgery for Otosclerosis

46

John T. McElveen Jr and J. Walter Kutz Jr

Introduction

Otosclerosis is one of the most common causes of hearing loss. It can have an autosomal dominant inheritance with an incomplete penetrance rate of 20–40% [1–3]. Originally recognized by Politzer, otosclerosis is a primary bony dysplasia affecting the endochondral otic capsule [4]. It is distinguished from the surrounding endochondral bone by its irregular woven appearance. In its active (otospongiotic) phase, it is characterized by an increased number of osteoblasts and numerous fibrovascular spaces. In its quiescent (otosclerotic) phase, the fibrovascular spaces become filled with lamellar bone. In most cases, the otosclerotic focus remains small and asymptomatic; however, in 10–12% of patients, the focus expands to encroach on the annular ligament and stapes footplate to produce a slowly progressive conductive hearing loss (stapedial otosclerosis) [5]. In some of these patients, the otosclerotic focus extends into the cochlear endosteum (cochlear otosclerosis) resulting in a concomitant sensorineural hearing loss (SNHL), which varies in severity.

The prevalence of otosclerosis varies amongst races, being more common in Caucasians, less common in Southeast Asians and Native Americans, and rare in patients of African descent. Temporal bone studies have shown that the prevalence of histologic otosclerosis is 8.3–12% in Caucasians and 1% in patients of African descent [6–8]. Although histologic otosclerosis has similar prevalence in both genders, women are 1.4–2 times more likely than men to develop clinical symptoms of the disease. In those patients clinically affected with otosclerosis, there is an 85–90% probability that the contralateral ear will eventually be involved [9].

Although multiple genetic loci associated with otosclerosis have been identified, the exact cause for the abnormal bone remodeling that produces the otosclerotic foci remains uncertain. Ultrastructural and immunohistochemical evidence of measles-like structures and antigenicity in active otosclerotic lesions published by McKenna et al. has implicated the measles virus in the formation of the otosclerotic foci [10, 11]. In addition, measles ribonucleic acid (RNA) has been demonstrated in fresh and archival footplate specimens. This hypothesis may be further strengthened by the decline in otosclerosis following the introduction of the measles vaccination [12]. In a more recent temporal bone study, the prevalence of histologic otosclerosis had decreased to 3% from 4% [13].

This chapter will explore the history of otosclerosis surgery, discuss the pathogenesis of the disease, and review the proper evaluation and management of patients suspected of having hearing loss due to otosclerosis.

History of Otosclerosis Surgery

Antonio Maria Valsalva, who was a Professor of Anatomy in Bologna, Italy is credited with first describing stapes fixation as a cause of hearing loss. Although his study of anatomy encompassed other areas of the human body, the anatomy of the ear was his favorite subject. His meticulous postmortem dissections in 1704 of an individual known to be deaf revealed fixation of the stapes as the cause of hearing loss [14].

In 1841, Toynbee's publication firmly established the link between deafness and stapes fixation [15]. In a subsequent publication, he reported stapes fixation in 39 of the 1659 temporal bones he had fastidiously dissected and concluded that "osseous ankylosis of the stapes to the fenestra ovalis was one of the common causes of deafness" [16].

J. T. McElveen Jr (✉)
Carolina Ear & Hearing Clinic, PC, Raleigh, NC, USA

Carolina Ear Research Institute, Raleigh, NC, USA

J. W. Kutz Jr
Department of Otolaryngology—Head and Neck Surgery, University of Texas Southwestern Medical Center, Dallas, TX, USA
e-mail: walter.kutz@utsouthwestern.edu

A. D. Sweeney et al. (eds.), *Haynes-Glasscock-Shambaugh Surgery of the Ear*, https://doi.org/10.1007/978-3-032-18264-7_46

It was assumed by Toynbee and others that chronic inflammatory mucosal changes in the middle ear resulted in secondary ankylosis of the stapes. However, in December 1893, Politzer described the histologic findings in 16 cases of stapes fixation. His findings indicated that the deafness, which had been attributed to "chronic interstitial middle ear catarrh" with secondary stapes fixation, was really due to a primary disorder of the labyrinthine capsule." He referred to it as "otosclerosis." His findings were initially published in Zeitschrift Für Ohrenheilkunde [4], and then translated into English and published a few months later in the Archives of Otology [17]. Despite both publications, it took almost half a century for Politzer's views to gain universal acceptance.

The evolution of the surgical treatment for otosclerosis can be divided into three distinct eras. The First Era of Stapes Surgery lasted from 1876 to 1900. This was followed by the Fenestration Era, which lasted from 1900 to 1952. The current Era of Stapes Surgery has lasted from 1952 to present.

Professor Johannes Kessel from Graz is considered by many to be the "Father of Stapes Surgery." Kessel was under the mistaken impression that the hearing loss associated with otosclerosis was caused by increased pressure in the inner ear fluids. He thought that, by removing the stapes, he could relieve that pressure. To test his hypothesis, he removed the columella (stapes equivalent) from two pigeons. Kessel reported that clear fluid drained from their ears for 8 days until a membrane formed to seal the oval window. According to Kessel, during this time, the pigeons did not experience any vertigo or hearing loss [18].

In 1878, based on these observations, he published his experience using a direct approach through the tympanic membrane to either mobilize or extract the stapes. He reported "some improvement in hearing and no serious complications" [19].

In 1890, Camille Miot of France reported on over 200 cases of stapes mobilization in which he used strict antisepsis. Fifty-nine percent of his patients experienced hearing improvement [20]. In the United States, during this same time, Blake and Jack at the Eye and Ear infirmary in Boston practiced stapes mobilization and stapes removal. They reported their results at the American Otological Society Meeting in 1892. A subsequent article by Jack would later greatly influence Dr. John Shea's technique for stapes surgery [21].

In many of these stapes mobilization and stapes removal patients, hearing improvement lasted only for a period of days to weeks, and there was always the risk of labyrinthitis with the potential for lethal intracranial complications. Consequently, stapes surgery fell into disrepute. It was vehemently criticized by the leading otologists, Politzer, Siebenmann, and Moure, who in 1899 at the sixth International Otology Congress of Otology declared that, "Stapes surgery is useless, often mutilating, and dangerous." They went on to say, "The question of surgical therapy for otosclerosis was interred with great pomp at the 1894 International Conference in Rome. There is no reason to revive it" [22, 23]. In 1900, Johannes Kessel was publicly censured for unscrupulousness. Embittered, he resigned from his position as Professor in disgrace.

Stapes surgery for otosclerosis was abruptly discontinued for over 50 years. During this time, attempts to surgically improve hearing were focused on the fenestration of the labyrinth (Fenestration Era: 1900–1960).

The concept of improving hearing by fenestrating the labyrinth once again dates to Johannes Kessel (1876) of Germany. Kessel noted a fracture through the lateral semicircular canal during a postmortem exam of a young man who had fallen off a wagon and fractured his temporal bone. Prior to dying, the man noted a marked improvement in his hearing. Kessel tried unsuccessfully to duplicate the fracture in other patients using a chisel and gouge [19].

In 1897, Passow postulated that it would be better to detour around the obstruction in the oval window rather than to mobilize or extract the stapes. He reported an operation in which he used a drill to create a fenestra in the promontory near the oval window, which he covered with mucous membrane from the middle ear resulting in a temporary improvement in hearing [24].

Floderus, in 1899, suggested an opening of the vestibular labyrinth and covering it with a skin graft [25]. George J. Jenkins had already been opening the lateral semicircular canal for the treatment of vertigo, a procedure he referred to as "fenestration." At the XVIIth International Congress of Medicine in London in 1913, he suggested doing the same for treating otosclerosis [26].

In the early 1920s, Gunnar Holmgen of Sweden made a systematic effort to fenestrate the superior or lateral semicircular canals, but he closed the fenestration to the exterior [27]. In 1924, Maurice Sourdille, of Nantes, France visited Holmgren and observed one "closed fenestration" operation and realized the shortcoming of Holmgren's technique. He returned to France and developed the three-stage exteriorized fenestra operation. In 1937, he achieved a lasting hearing improvement in 64% of 109 operated patients with his "tympano-labyrintho-pexie" [28]. In 1938, Julius Lempert, using an endaural approach, developed a single-stage fenestration procedure, which supplanted Sourdille's technique [29]. Using Lempert's single stage technique, significant and lasting hearing improvement was achieved in large series of patients.

The present era of stapes surgery began in 1952 when Rosen, unaware of the earlier work of Miot, reintroduced stapes mobilization. Dr. Rosen had made it a practice to perform exploratory tympanotomy procedures on his patients a few weeks prior to performing a fenestration operation. This was done to ensure that the patient did indeed have otosclerosis with stapes fixation. On the sixth such patient, as he was checking to make certain the stapes was fixed, he inadvertently mobilized the stapes. The patient noted a marked improvement in his hearing [30]. Thus, began the trend toward stapes mobilization. Unfortunately, many of the patients undergoing stapes mobilization eventually redeveloped stapes fixation.

In the fall of 1953, Dr. John Shea went to learn the technique of stapes mobilization from Rosen. Seeing Dr. Shea's keen interest, Rosen suggested that Dr. Shea go to Vienna to practice the mobilization technique on the abundant cadaveric material available there. During his time in Vienna, Dr. Shea reviewed the medical literature regarding stapes surgery, including an article from 1902 written by Jack of Boston. The article, "Supplementary Report on a Case of Double Stapedectomy Operated Upon 10 Years Ago" [21], made Shea realize that what was needed to make stapedectomy safe and successful was to do what had happened spontaneously in Jack's patient; seal the oval window with a tissue membrane and bridge the gap between the incus and the oval window. He returned to Memphis and initially used cortical bone to replace the stapes. The patient initially heard better, but developed a severe reaction to the cortical bone. Working with Harry Treace, a Teflon stapes prosthesis was fashioned to bridge the gap between the incus and the vein covered oval window, resulting in a hearing improvement without the formation of scar tissue.

On Thursday, May 17, 1956, with the assistance of Dr. Howard P. House, Dr. Shea presented his new stapedectomy technique before the Triological Society in Montreal, Canada. Dr. House was scheduled to moderate the panel: "Symposium-The Operation for the Mobilization of the Stapes in Otosclerotic Deafness." Just before the panel was to begin, Dr. Shea told Dr. House about his first patient who had successfully undergone a stapedectomy. Knowing that something like this would be extremely controversial, Dr. House told Dr. Shea that he would call on him as the last discussant from the audience. Dr. Shea took the opportunity to approach the podium and present his stapedectomy experience to the membership of the Triological Society. Before Dr. Shea could be unduly criticized by the audience, Dr. House explained that unfortunately the time for the symposium had expired and brought down his gavel, ending the session [31]. Within a decade, stapedectomy had become the standard operation for the treatment of otosclerosis.

Those interested in further information regarding the history of otosclerosis are encouraged to read *For the World to Hear* and *The Unreasonable Man: The Trials and Triumphs of William F. House, M.D* [32, 33]. In these two books, Dr. Howard House and Dr. William F. House, respectively, give their personal insights into the individuals and innovations associated with the development of stapes surgery.

Since Shea's revival of stapes surgery, various methods have been devised to circumvent stapes fixation. The complete removal of the footplate (once commonly practiced) is now reserved for select cases. It has been replaced by various methods to remove more limited parts of the footplate and, ultimately, precise fenestration of the fixed footplate. Since this development in the early 1960s by Shea in the United States and Marquet and Mignon in Europe, small fenestra stapedotomy is the procedure of choice for most surgery [34]. The small fenestra was originally created using a handheld or electric microdrill. However, in 1980 Perkins reported a series of 11 patients who had successfully undergone laser stapedotomy. In these patients, he used a microscope-mounted focused argon beam laser to create the fenestra. Currently, the variety of lasers continue to be used by themselves or in conjunction with a microdrill to create a fenestra in the footplate [35].

Portman and Claverie in 1957 suggested utilizing part of the superstructure of the stapes for bridging the gap from the incus to the oval window. Other variations on this theme include removal of the posterior footplate, as well as removal of the anterior fixed footplate, maintaining ossicular continuity via the posterior crus [36].

Over time, numerous types of prosthesis have been designed for stapes surgery [37]. The Schuknecht type of stapedectomy fat-wire prosthesis was developed to address both the need to seal the open vestibule and to reconstruct the ossicular chain [38]. Later, with the popularization of small fenestra surgery, additional prostheses were made available, varying mostly in the materials of construction, in the mode of attachment to the incus and in the diameter of their pistons.

Pathology

The normal otic capsule has an extremely low remodeling rate; compared to the 10% annual turnover rate of some of other bones, the rate for the normal otic capsule is no more than 2% [39]. Otosclerosis is a disease of abnormal bone remodeling occurring in the endochondral layer of the temporal bone. The normal temporal bone has embryonic cartilage rests called "globuli interossei." These rests are associated with sites of predilection in otosclerosis. The first histologic sign of otosclerosis is a change in the extracellular staining pattern that has been termed "blue mantle." This presumably unstable matrix begins to remodel giving rise to an otosclerotic focus. Immature bone is then laid and continued remodeling occurs, with prominent osteoblastic involvement ("otospongiosis"). The process is completed by maturation of the lesion into sclerotic, dense, irregularly woven and poorly vascularized bone ("otosclerosis"). The disease process is not necessarily a continuous, linear process; active areas can become inactive and reactivated later, and various stages of the disease can coexist in a single focus.

Foci of otosclerosis can occur in any portion of the otic capsule; however, there are areas of predilection. Schuknecht and Barber studied the temporal bones of patients with clinically apparent otosclerosis [40]. Stapes fixation by a focus anterior to the footplate was present in 96% of cases. Fixation is first caused by remodeling bone encroaching on the anterior footplate with subluxation of the posterior part of the footplate. As the process progresses and the lesion transgresses the stapediovestibular joint, bony fixation of the footplate occurs. The former mechanism of fixation will result in hearing loss more pronounced in low frequencies, the latter apparent in all frequencies. In 49%, there was involvement of other areas as well: the round window niche in 30%, the cochlear apex in 12%, and less frequent involvement of the walls of the internal auditory canal, around the cochlear aqueduct, semicircular canals, and the unusual disease limited to the footplate. Of special note is the involvement of the round window niche, found to be obliterated in 7% of histological specimens [40]. Obliteration of the round window niche can cause conductive loss, irrespective of the state of the stapes. Even with extensive disease, invasion of the membranous labyrinth is rare. The location and extent of the foci determine the clinical presentation: extent of the conductive loss and the presence or absence of SNHL. For a more detailed description and numerous photos of the histopathology of otosclerosis, see *Schuknecht's Pathology of the Ear* [41].

Gross appearance of otosclerotic foci is distinctly different from the normal otic capsule under the operative or examination microscope. Active, spongiotic lesions, having rich vascularization and hyperemic overlying mucosa, may be seen through the tympanic membrane as a red discoloration of the promontory. This sign is named after Hermann Schwartze. Intraoperatively, a mature focus of otosclerosis is seen as a white, well-demarcated lesion compared to the ivory color of the otic capsule.

Etiology

The exact cause for the abnormal bone remodeling seen in the otosclerotic otic capsule has yet to be determined. Research regarding the genetics of otosclerosis and potential contribution of viral infection and the immune and endocrine systems has offered new insights in the etiology of this disease [42].

Bone turnover is controlled by an intricate and complex mechanism. Cytokine factors that include osteoprotegerin (OPG), receptor activator for nuclear factor kappa B (RANK), and RANK ligand (RANK-L) play a major role in the system that directly controls bone turnover. Receptor activator for nuclear factor kappa B ligand is expressed by osteoblasts that are involved in bone turnover. Activation of its specific receptor RANK on osteoclasts promotes differentiation (in the presence of macrophage stimulating factor) [43], activation [44], and survival [45] of osteoclasts. Bone remodeling is a process of bone resorption by osteoclasts and bone deposition by osteoblasts. Osteoprotegerin is a competitive inhibitor of RANK-L. High levels of OPG inhibit bone remodeling by inhibiting the differentiation, survival, and fusion of osteoclastic precursor cells, by suppressing activation and promoting apoptosis of osteoclasts [46]. Fibroblasts of the spiral ligament are a probable source of OPG, which is found in high levels in perilymph [47]. Osteoprotegerin may be dispersed throughout the otic capsule by the perilymphatic canalicular system traversing the bone [48]. The production of OPG in the cochlea may be the reason for the extremely slow turnover of bone in the otic capsule [47, 48]. This cytokine regulatory mechanism may be influenced by genetic, endocrine, infectious, metabolic, biochemical, biomechanical, and other factors.

Otosclerosis can have an underlying genetic cause, inherited in an autosomal dominant pattern with incomplete penetration of 20–40%. Monozygotic twins have a nearly 100% concordance rate of otosclerosis [1]. However, because information does not exist on the genetic transmission of histologic otosclerosis, it is not known whether the genetic basis of inheritance is related to the formation of an otosclerotic focus within the temporal bone or the tendency for a lesion to progress once it has begun, or both. There appears to be no significant difference in the degree of clinical severity between sporadic and familial cases [2]. To date, ten loci associated with otosclerosis have been identified and are designated OTSC1-10. The tenth locus has just recently been described [49]. Association analysis has revealed a significant association between both familial and sporadic cases of clinical otosclerosis and the COL1A1 gene using multiple polymorphic markers within the COL1A1 gene [50]. A preliminary study has demonstrated that osteoporosis may be more common in patients with otosclerosis, and these two common bone diseases may share some genetic and molecular pathologic mechanisms [51]. Based on the pattern of prevalence of otosclerosis and otitis media, it has been speculated that genetic susceptibility to otosclerosis may reduce susceptibility to otitis media [52].

The evidence that has emerged thus far is suggestive of a possible persistent measles infection similar to what occurs in the central nervous system in subacute sclerosing panencephalitis [53]. Support of this hypothesis originates from ultrastructural and immunohistochemical evidence of measles-like structures and antigenicity in active otosclerotic lesions [11, 54, 55]. In addition, measles ribonucleic acid (RNA) has been found in archival and fresh footplate specimens with otosclerosis [10, 56, 57].

Elevated levels of anti-measles antibodies have also been reported in the perilymph of patients undergoing stapedectomy for otosclerosis as compared to controls [58]. Others have reported lower levels of circulating anti-measles antibodies in patients with otosclerosis as compared to healthy controls [59]. This hypothesis is further strengthened by recent evidence that the incidence of otosclerosis has declined since the introduction of measles vaccination [12].

Hormones may influence otosclerosis. Otosclerosis is more prevalent in women compared to men by a factor of 1.4–2. It has been long held that pregnancy and lactation can accelerate otosclerosis, although reliable evidence for this is lacking [60].

Diagnosis

Otosclerosis typically presents as a progressive hearing loss starting in the third or fourth decade of life. A thorough history and physical exam can generally suggest otosclerosis as the cause of hearing loss and options of treatment, including stapedotomy, can be discussed. However, it is essential that conditions that could contraindicate stapes surgery, such as semicircular canal dehiscence or Meniere's disease, are identified [61–63].

Clinical History

Patients typically describe progressive hearing loss that may be bilateral (75% of patients) and is often asymmetric. The most common age to develop hearing loss is in the third or fourth decade of life, with greater than 90% of patients presenting before the age of 50 [64]. Juvenile-onset otosclerosis is much less common and encompasses <1% of otosclerosis cases [65]. Because otosclerosis can be inherited in an autosomal dominant fashion with variable penetrance, a significant number of patients will recall having a relative with the onset of hearing loss at an early age. The diagnosis is highly suspected in patients who recall a family member undergoing surgery for otosclerosis. Rarely, otosclerosis will present with primarily progressive sensorineural hearing loss.

About 10–30% of patients with otosclerosis present with dizziness or vertigo; although severe, episodic vertigo is not characteristic of otosclerosis. Instead, patients may have unsteadiness, brief vertigo episodes, or vague dizziness. If a patient describes episodic and severe vertigo lasting greater than 20 min, a concomitant diagnosis of Meniere's disease should be considered. If Meniere's disease is a concern, a stapes operation should not be performed since the saccule may be abutting the undersurface of the footplate.

Physical Examination

Otosclerosis presents as a progressive conductive hearing loss in the setting of a normal-appearing tympanic membrane. A prior history of otologic infections or trauma would suggest other causes of conductive hearing loss such as tympanosclerosis or lateral ossicular chain problems. With active otospongiosis, a vascular blush may be seen on the cochlear promontory and is referred to as Schwartze's sign. Careful inspection of the tympanic membrane for retraction pockets, tympanosclerosis, perforations, and abnormal malleus movement is necessary to rule out other causes of conductive hearing loss. The external auditory canal should be inspected for lesions such as osteomas, exostoses, or infection that may cause problems with stapes surgery.

Verification of the audiogram with a 512 Hz tuning fork is recommended before surgery is considered. The Weber exam should lateralize to the affected ear. Many surgeons require a negative 512 Hz Rinne test (bone conduction > air conduction) before considering stapedectomy. During the Rinne exam, the tuning fork should be placed just posterior to the pinna and inferior to the temporal line to maximize bone conduction.

Audiometry

Comprehensive audiometry, including air and bone thresholds, speech discrimination, and acoustic reflexes, is essential. Although otosclerosis most often presents with conductive hearing loss, mixed hearing loss, and rarely, purely sensorineural hearing loss may be present. Low-frequency conductive hearing loss occurs early in the disease process because otosclerosis initially fixes the anterior footplate. As the disease progresses, the conductive hearing loss affects the higher frequencies. The maximum air–bone gap from stapes fixation is 55–60 dB. If the air-bone gap is greater than 60 dB, ossicular discontinuity should be considered. With otosclerosis, an increased bone-line threshold at 2000 Hz is common and is referred to as Carhart's notch. This is an artifact and may be related to the resonance frequency of the external auditory canal and middle ear in the setting of ossicular fixation [66]. The Carhart's notch often resolves after successful stapes surgery.

Superior semicircular canal dehiscence can also present with low-frequency conductive hearing loss; however, suprathreshold bone conduction (<0 dB) is often seen. In addition, acoustic reflexes are present, which is not possible in the setting of fixed ossicles such as seen in otosclerosis. Patients may often have vestibular symptoms associated with superior semicircular canal dehiscence. Thus, it is important to check suprathreshold bone conduction and acoustic reflexes in all cases of conductive hearing loss to differentiate otosclerosis, lateral ossicular chain problems, or superior semicircular canal dehiscence.

Imaging

If otosclerosis is highly suspected as the cause of conductive hearing loss in an adult, imaging is usually not necessary. That being said, a computed tomographic (CT) scan is a reasonable diagnostic tool in this setting when concerns exist that a pathology other than otosclerosis may be present, such as what is described above for superior semicircular canal dehiscence. If a CT of the temporal bone is obtained, the sensitivity for detecting an otosclerosis focus is 85–87% [67, 68]. A high-resolution CT of the temporal bone should be obtained in all children with conductive hearing loss to evaluate for middle ear and inner ear abnormalities such as X-linked gusher syndrome [69].

Surgery for Otosclerosis

Although there are multiple surgical procedures to address the conductive hearing loss associated with otosclerosis, the stapedotomy procedure is the most common. A fenestra is created in the stapes footplate, a piston prosthesis is placed though the fenestra, and the prosthesis is attached to the incus. The next most common approach would be a stapedectomy procedure where part or all of the stapes footplate is removed. A tissue graft, such as fascia, perichondrium, or vein, is placed over the vestibule. A prosthesis is then placed over the tissue graft and attaches to the incus.

Stapes surgery requires special skills and is considered advanced otologic surgery. Reliable and consistent results may take approximately 50 procedures [70, 71]. Because the number of stapes surgery procedures have declined, it may take even more time for trainees to develop proficiency [71].

Indications

Surgery for otosclerosis can be considered if the conductive component of the hearing loss is enough that the patient will notice the improvement in hearing. An air–bone gap of 25 dB or more at frequencies between 500 and 1000 Hz and a negative Rinne tuning fork exam are commonly used as guidelines to consider stapes surgery. In case of bilateral disease, the worst hearing ear should be operated on first. If the first side is successful, the second side can be operated on 6–12 months later. Concomitant sensorineural hearing loss in the ear affected by otosclerosis is not a contraindication to surgery, but patients should be counseled that hearing aids may be necessary postoperatively to correct the sensorineural component even when surgery is successful. In patients with far-advanced otosclerosis, a stapedotomy may allow the use of hearing aids and should be considered before a cochlear implant in most cases.

Contraindications

Stapes surgery is contraindicated in patients with chronic eustachian tube dysfunction, tympanic membrane perforation, or chronic otitis media [72]. Stapes surgery should be avoided in an only-hearing ear, unless a profound mixed hearing loss is present and a cochlear implant would be an option if the stapes surgery was not successful. Concomitant Meniere's disease is a contraindication to stapedectomy and should be ruled out in patients with episodic vertigo. Occupations that depend on an intact vestibular system may be a relative contraindication to stapes surgery. Age is not a contraindication; however, the likelihood of success may decrease in patients older than 70 years old [73].

Informed Consent

Since stapes surgery is elective, thorough informed consent is necessary. It is essential to discuss alternative options to stapes surgery, including conventional hearing aids and bone conducting hearing devices.

Risks of sensorineural hearing loss, including profound sensorineural hearing loss, may occur in 1% of stapes surgery. Other risks that should be discussed include tympanic membrane perforation, facial nerve paresis or paralysis, dysgeusia, tinnitus, dizziness, failure to correct conductive hearing loss, and need for further procedures. Patients with occupations that depend on chorda tympani function (e.g., chef, sommelier) should be informed of the risk of injury to the chorda tympani nerve. Pilots, scuba divers, and sky divers should be informed of the possibility of sensorineural hearing loss or vertigo due to barotrauma. House et al. concluded scuba diving was safe after stapes surgery if the patient could autoinsufflate [74].

Operative Note

The operative note should include the status of the lateral ossicular chain, presence and location of otosclerotic foci, round window patency, facial nerve location and dehiscence, and status of the chorda tympani nerve at the conclusion of the procedure. The type and size of the prosthesis are also described.

Anesthesia

Stapes surgery can be performed using local-only anesthesia, local anesthesia with sedation (monitored anesthesia care [MAC]), or general anesthesia. The selection of which type of anesthesia to utilize is surgeon, patient, and procedure dependent. Some surgeons prefer local anesthesia, with or without sedation, to assess the hearing and vestibular response intraoperatively and to avoid excessive inner ear irritation. Other surgeons, especially at teaching institutions, prefer a general anesthetic, citing patient comfort, avoidance of head movement, lack of time constraints, and resident involvement. Vital et al. in 2008 compared the incidence of a profound hearing loss between 160 operations under general anesthesia and 108 operations under local anesthesia and found a higher incidence of profound hearing loss in the general group (1.8%) compared to the local group (0%) [75]. However, in a more recent systematic review comparing local versus general anesthesia in 417 procedures, the authors concluded that there was no statistical difference in postoperative air–bone gap, worsening of SNHL, or postoperative vertigo [76].

In juvenile-onset otosclerotic patients, the surgeon is restricted to general anesthesia, whereas, in revision stapes surgery, local anesthesia is preferred, if possible, to intraoperatively monitor any vestibular symptoms during prosthesis manipulation.

Typically, in general anesthesia cases and in patients with monitored anesthesia care (MAC), the anesthesiologist is positioned at the patient's feet (Fig. 46.1). In local anesthesia cases, an ether screen is utilized to lift the drape off the patient's face and a window is cut in the drape to minimize patient claustrophobia.

Perioperative Antibiotics and Steroids

Although stapes surgery is considered “clean” otologic surgery, and the Cochrane report did not find any evidence supporting perioperative antibiotic therapy [77], most centers continue to treat their patients with prophylactic antibiotics because the risks associated with post-stapedotomy infection include deafness and labyrinthitis [78]. In addition, intraoperative and postoperative corticosteroids may be used to minimize the chance of serous labyrinthitis. However, clinical studies supporting use of perioperative corticosteroids are lacking. In one study from Germany, the use of steroids appeared to exacerbate the vestibular symptoms and had no effect on the change in bone conduction [79].

Surgical Technique

Positioning

Proper positioning of the patient is essential and allows for good visualization of the oval window niche and neighboring structures and ease of approach to the middle ear. Bringing the tympanic membrane to a near horizontal plane serves these goals. With the patient in a supine position, the patient's head is turned toward the contralateral shoulder and tilted downward 10° to 15°. This is best achieved by a surgical bed with a separate head rest. The surgeon position should be comfortable, preferably having his or her legs on the floor and back supported. The operating microscope is positioned at the head of the table.

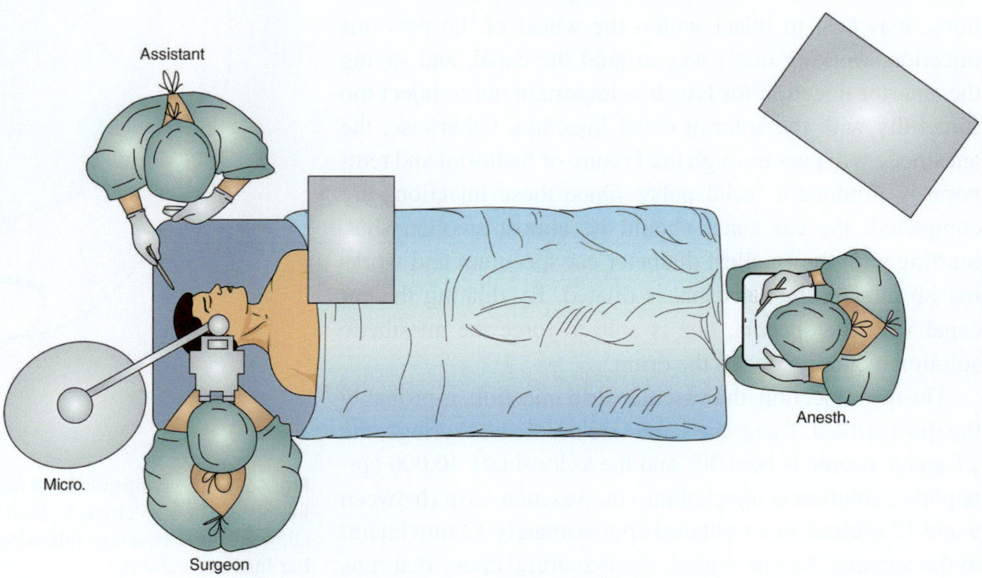

Fig. 46.1 The standard patient and personnel positioning for stapes surgery. The microscope is brought in from the head of the table, the otologic scrub technician is situated across from the surgeon, and anesthesia is located at the foot of the table. (Adapted from the House Ear Institute archives)

Exposure and Exploration

The surgical approach for stapes surgery has changed little since Shea's revival of stapes surgery in the 1950s. Typically, the tympanomeatal flap has been elevated using either a classic transcanal approach or, if more exposure is needed, an endaural approach. Traditionally, the operating microscope is used to facilitate visualization; however, more recently, endoscopes have been utilized to perform a variety of middle ear procedures, including stapedotomy.

Regardless of which approach one utilizes, it is essential that the ear be injected properly with local anesthetic including a vasoconstrictive agent to minimize bleeding and, in local anesthesia cases, avoid patient discomfort.

Prior to injecting the ear canal, the canal should be thoroughly irrigated and the microscope used to carefully inspect the tympanic membrane and remove any remaining debris or cerumen in the ear canal. The ear speculum can be stabilized by hand or with a speculum holder. Traditionally, it has been taught to perform a four-quadrant injection at the bony cartilaginous junction. However, at the bony cartilaginous junction, the skin is tightly bound to the underlying bone, making the injection more difficult to perform. By using a slightly larger ear speculum and injecting 5 mm lateral to the bony cartilaginous junction, one can easily inject the local anesthetic solution. Although xylocaine with 1:100,000 epinephrine is the stock concentration readily available and can be used for the canal injections, a solution of xylocaine with 1:40,000 epinephrine may provide better hemostasis. This can be made up intraoperatively by mixing 0.5 mL of 1:1000 epinephrine with 19.5 mL of plain xylocaine (if the patient is >65 years of age, the concentration is reduced to a 1:60,000 solution). Using a 27-gauge, 1.5-inch beveled needle and a 3 cc glass Luer lock syringe, the initial injection is placed in the posterior aspect of the canal just lateral to the bony cartilaginous junction. Instead of making four separate injections, it is best to inject within the wheal of the previous injection, working one's way around the canal, and saving the anterior injection for last. It is important not to inject too forcefully with the anterior canal injection. Otherwise, the anesthetic will pass through the Fissure of Santorini and temporarily produce a facial palsy. Once these injections are completed, the ear canal should be almost swollen shut. Starting with the smallest diameter ear speculum and working up in size, the ear canal is dilated. By dilating the ear canal with the specula, one is able to force the anesthetic solution medially toward the drum.

The next injection, the vascular strip injection, is probably the most critical. Using the same size needle and syringe, the 27-gauge needle is bent 30° and the xylocaine/1:40,000 epinephrine solution is injected into the vascular strip (between 9 and 12 o'clock in a right ear) approximately 12 mm lateral to the annulus. As one injects, the manubrial artery that runs along the handle of malleus should blanche. By injecting gently, one will avoid creating blebs in the vascular strip.

Once the ear canal has been anesthetized, a sickle knife is used to make vertical canal incisions at 6 o'clock and 12 o'clock, beginning just lateral to the annular ligament and extending 8–10 mm. The vertical incisions are connected with a horizontal incision approximately 8 mm lateral to the annulus. It is important to cut completely through the vascular strip; otherwise the persistent fibrous connections will limit flap elevation. If one is having difficulty cutting through a thick vascular strip, one can use the Rosen canal knife as an elevating instrument and gently lift the fibrous tissue off the underlying bone. Curved Bellucci scissors can then be used to complete the horizontal incision across the thick fibers, being careful to stay lateral and not compromise the posterior superior length of the tympanomeatal flap (Fig. 46.2).

Some surgeons may prefer a triangle type flap as opposed to a trapezoid one. Regardless which shape of flap one creates, it is essential that the superior portion of the flap extends far enough anteriorly and laterally to completely cover the bone defect created by curetting the posterior-superior bony canal wall. Otherwise, a gap will be present when the flap is returned to its normal anatomical position.

Once the vertical and horizontal incisions have been made, a round knife is used to elevate the flap down to the level of the annular ligament. It is important not to apply the suction directly to the flap to prevent swelling of the flap. Once the annular ligament is positively identified, a Rosen needle is used to enter the middle ear space (approximately 8

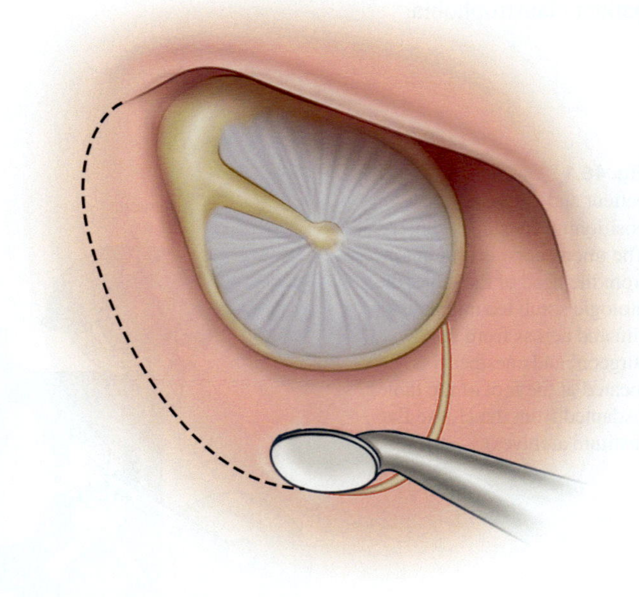

Fig. 46.2 The tympanomeatal flap (right ear) used to access the stapes footplate. The 12 o'clock, vertical incision should be anterior enough to allow adequate coverage following curetting. (Adapted from the House Ear Institute archives)

o'clock position in a right ear), just inferior to the chorda tympani nerve.

The flap is then folded anteriorly, allowing visualization of the mesotympanum. Prior to performing a stapedotomy, it is essential for the surgeon to be able to visualize the pyramidal process and the tympanic portion of the facial nerve. Bone removal from the posterior-superior bony canal wall is often necessary. The bone can be removed with a microdrill or a House curette, being careful to preserve the chorda tympani nerve and avoid downward pressure.

Next, the middle ear pathology is delineated. Patency of the round window is examined and described in the operative note. The oval window niche is surveyed for the evidence of otosclerosis. Mobility of the ossicular chain is checked. The malleus and incus are palpated and their mobility assessed. The movement of the stapes is examined by direct and gentle manipulation of the suprastructure. If the stapes is found to be fixed and the incus and malleus are mobile, the surgeon can proceed with stapedotomy.

The traditional sequence of steps for stapes surgery is as follows: A measurement is made from the long process of the incus to the footplate. The incudostapedial joint is separated with a joint knife (Fig. 46.3). The stapedial tendon is cut with scissors or with a laser as close as possible to the pyramidal eminence to minimize both visual and physical obstruction in the corridor through which the prosthesis will be introduced (Fig. 46.4). If the operating surgeon has a laser available, the posterior crus is divided as close to the footplate as possible to prevent obstruction of the view and approach to the footplate after removal of the suprastructure (Fig. 46.5). Section of the anterior crus (Fig. 46.6) is often not possible or necessary. The suprastructure is fractured downward toward the promontory and removed from the middle ear. The footplate fenestra is then created and shaped using a laser, drill and/or microdissector (Figs. 46.7 and 46.8), and the prosthesis placed onto the incus and into the fenestra. The prosthesis is then secured to the long process of the incus (Fig. 46.9).

However, as described by Fisch and subsequently others [80, 81], in many cases (where the suprastructure is angled slightly toward the promontory) the fenestra can be created prior to removing the entire suprastructure. In this technique, one can separate the incudostapedial joint, leaving the lenticular process of the incus resting on the capitulum of the stapes. The laser is then used to section the stapedius tendon and remove the posterior crus of the stapes. Using a laser or

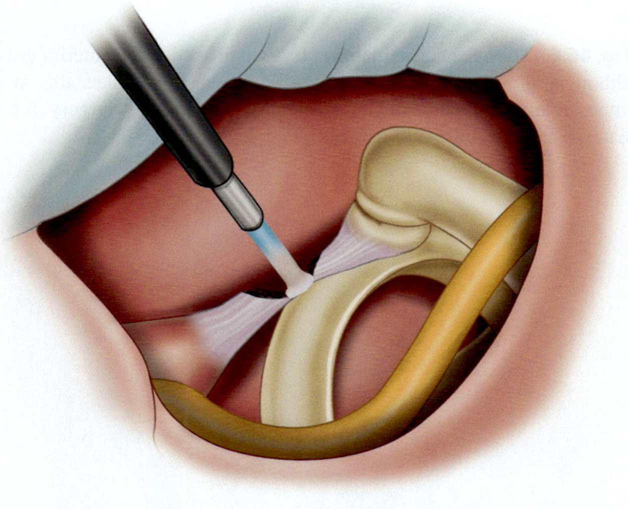

Fig. 46.4 Sectioning of the stapedial tendon with a laser or microscissors. The tendon should be sectioned as close to the pyramidal eminence as possible. (Adapted from Glasscock and Shambaugh's Surgery of the Ear, 6th Edition. Eds. Gulya, Minor, Poe. PMPH. 2010)

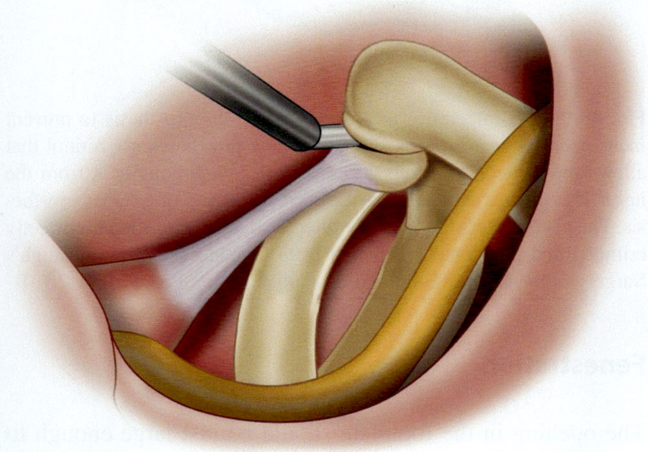

Fig. 46.3 The incudostapedial joint is sectioned with a joint knife or small right-angled pick. This step is often performed before sectioning the stapedial tendon to give more support to the stapes, and movement from a posterior to anterior direction (parallel to the tendon) optimizes stability. (Adapted from Glasscock and Shambaugh's Surgery of the Ear, 6th Edition. Eds. Gulya, Minor, Poe. PMPH. 2010)

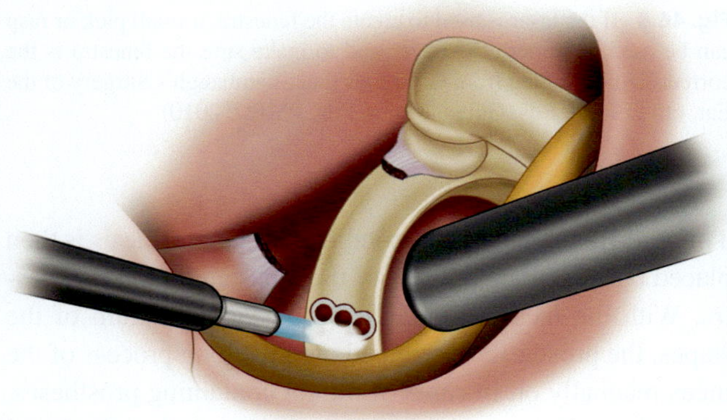

Fig. 46.5 Sectioning of the posterior crus with a laser. The posterior crus should be sectioned as close to the footplate as possible to prevent the remnant crura from obstructing the view of the footplate. Damage to the facial nerve with the laser should be avoided. (Adapted from Glasscock and Shambaugh's Surgery of the Ear, sixth Edition. Eds. Gulya, Minor, Poe. PMPH. 2010)

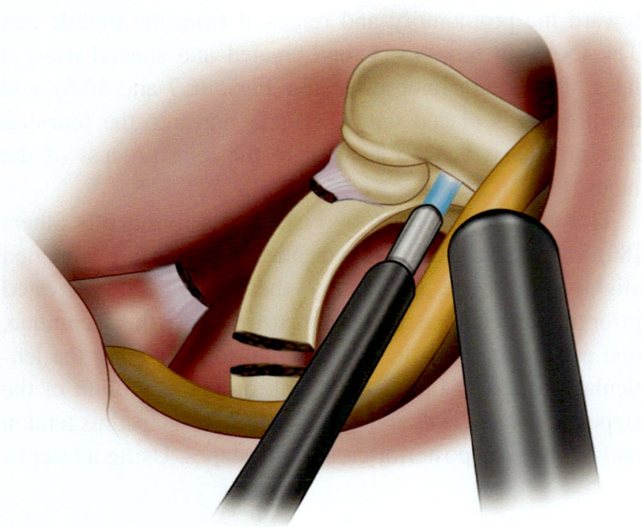

Fig. 46.6 The laser can sometimes be used to section the anterior crus; although, the position of the anterior crus usually makes this step impossible. (Adapted from Glasscock and Shambaugh's Surgery of the Ear, 6th Edition. Eds. Gulya, Minor, Poe. PMPH. 2010)

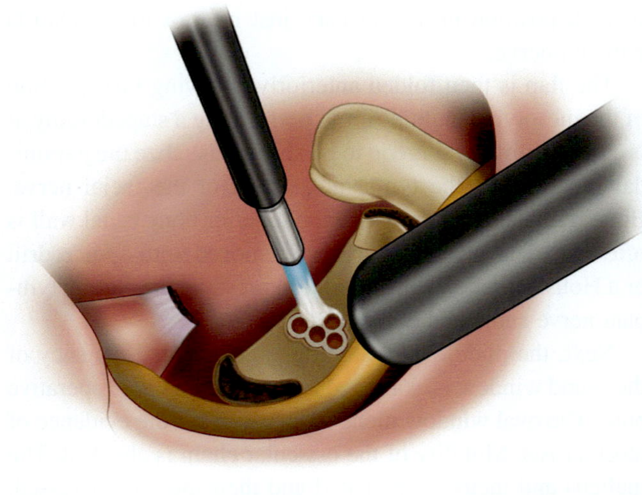

Fig. 46.7 A laser is used to obtain hemostasis of the small vessels on the footplate and to start the fenestra. A rosette is created in the location of the fenestra and consists of overlapping laser shots. A drill or perforator can be used to create the fenestra once the footplate is thinned, or the laser can be used to complete the fenestra. (Adapted from Glasscock and Shambaugh's Surgery of the Ear, 6th Edition. Eds. Gulya, Minor, Poe. PMPH. 2010)

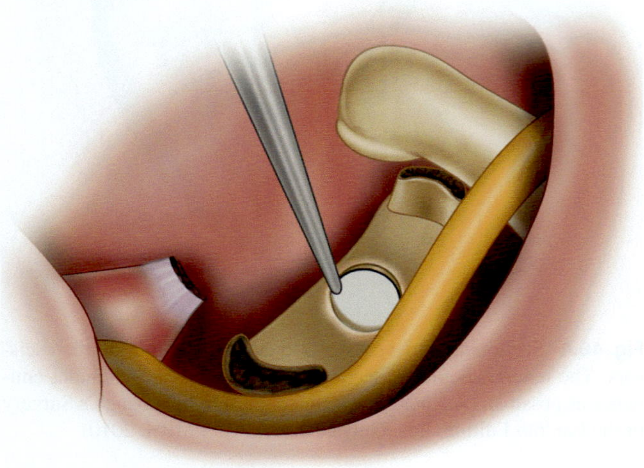

Fig. 46.8 If the laser is used to create the fenestra, a small pick or rasp can be used to smooth the edges and to make sure the fenestra is the correct size. (Adapted from Glasscock and Shambaugh's Surgery of the Ear, 6th Edition. Eds. Gulya, Minor, Poe. PMPH. 2010)

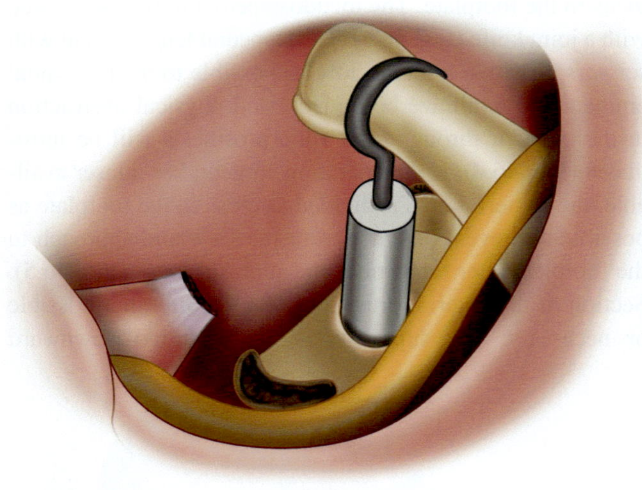

Fig. 46.9 It is imperative to properly crimp the prosthesis to prevent incus necrosis or prosthesis slippage. Many prostheses use nitinol that allows the surgeon to crimp the prosthesis by applying heat from the laser. This picture demonstrates the correct position of a stapes prosthesis. The piston enters the vestibule directly and the wire-loop is correctly crimped and positioned. (Adapted from Glasscock and Shambaugh's Surgery of the Ear, 6th Edition. Eds. Gulya, Minor, Poe. PMPH. 2010)

a microdrill, the fenestra is completed. The prosthesis is then placed onto the long process of the incus and into the fenestra. With the incus still stabilized by the capitulum of the stapes, the prosthesis is crimped onto the long process of the incus manually or, in cases of nitinol containing prostheses, with a laser. The remaining suprastructure is then fractured toward the promontory and removed from the field. The Fisch technique may be particularly useful in resident training. The resident can place and crimp the prosthesis onto a stabilized incus, minimizing the likelihood of the piston extending too deeply into the vestibule.

Fenestration

The opening in the footplate should be just large enough to accommodate the piston, so it can move freely. The fenestra can be created with an electric microdrill or a laser with similar success [82]. If one is using a microdrill, a diamond burr with a diameter slightly larger than the piston diameter should be used. The footplate can be quite thin and minimal downward pressure should be exerted when creating the fenestra.

Lasers can cut and coagulate with great precision and without generating pressure or gross movement. These qualities are desirable for stapes surgery in several applications: fenestrating a thin footplate with the reduced risk of resultant floating footplate; having the ability to fenestrate a mobile footplate; and creating a fenestra with minimal movement of the footplate or perilymph thus reducing inner ear irritation and trauma. Although there are no studies that clearly demonstrate a difference in results between the use of drill and laser, for most otologic surgeons, the laser has proven to be a most useful tool.

These advantageous qualities are shared by lasers both in the visible (argon or potassium titanyl phosphate [KTP-532]) and the invisible light range (carbon dioxide [CO_2] or erbium yttrium aluminum garnet [Er-YAG]); both types have been used with similar success and low complications rates [83].

Lasers in the visible light range are convenient in being deliverable through a flexible fiberoptic handheld piece and not requiring a separate aiming beam. Visible lasers are best absorbed by pigmented tissue and less so by clear fluids or white tissue. Because they are delivered through a fiberoptic cable, the light energy disperses rapidly after leaving the tip thus allowing for both coagulation and cutting depending upon the distance between the tip and the target. Much experience has been gained with these lasers with good results and few complications, proving that with proper use visible light lasers are efficacious and safe for creation of a small fenestra stapedotomy.

Lasers in the non-visible spectrum, such as erbium-yttrium-aluminum garnet (Er-YAG) or carbon dioxide lasers, have also been used successfully for stapedotomy [84, 85]. Carbon dioxide and Er-YAG lasers have the advantage of rapid attenuation in perilymph. In a study looking at the attenuation of seawater as a function of laser wavelength, the argon and KTP lasers traveled 229 feet before half of the energy was absorbed. Whereas the Er-YAG laser and CO_2 laser traveled 0.0007 and 0.007 mm, respectively, before half of the energy was absorbed [84]. The increased energy absorption by the perilymph results in decreased penetration of energy into the vestibule potentially reducing the risk to the structures within the vestibule.

In the past, the CO_2 laser required a microscope-attached delivery system with a direct sight line from the microscope to the footplate. Recently, handheld, flexible CO_2 delivery systems with an aiming beam have been introduced.

With both the visible and non-visible spectrum lasers, an overlapping rosette pattern is created on the footplate that will accommodate the selected piston (Fig. 46.7). The surgeon should allow 2 or 3 s to lapse between laser pulses to allow the perilymph to cool. It is better to create a slightly large fenestra than a slightly small one, as friction between the prosthesis and the bone edges of the fenestra can adversely impact the result. An oval window rasp or similar instrument can be used to ensure that the fenestra is the appropriate diameter (Fig. 46.8).

Prosthesis Choice, Placement, and Attachment

Many prosthesis designs are currently available [86]. They differ mostly in the mode of attachment to the incus, the diameter and length of the distal piston or rod, the material of construction, and weight (although the last variable has little influence on hearing results). A number of prostheses attach to the incus with a metallic loop that needs to be crimped for a stable fit around the incus; others attach without crimping. Robinson-type prostheses have a bucket that cradles the lenticular and long processes of the incus and a handle that stabilizes the prosthesis. The nitinol prosthesis makes use of the elastic memory of a nitinol metallic wire that coils around the incus in response to heating. Preliminary results reported with this prosthesis have shown equivalency in hearing results with other prostheses [87, 88]. Some surgeons have expressed concern that the nickel component of the metal may not be as biocompatible within the ear as stainless steel and platinum [87]. Self-retaining prostheses that are clipped to the incus are available as well [89]. Despite these innovations in stapes prosthesis design, platinum and titanium ribbon-type prostheses continue to be utilized. As compared to the previously used steel wire, the ribbon makes a wider and more stable contact point with the incus. Platinum and titanium are devoid of steel coiling memory and hence are easier to manually crimp. The shaft connecting the ribbon to the piston base is stiff, but malleable, and can be easily angulated after placement of the prosthesis for optimal incus to fenestra angulation.

Theoretically, larger prosthesis diameter should yield better closure of the air–bone gap, at least in low- and-middle frequencies [90, 91], although some studies have reported similar long-term results for 0.4 mm piston diameter prosthesis versus 0.6 mm [92]. Studies comparing the results with various types of commercially available prostheses are limited by confounding effects (such as the size of the fenestra and small sample size) and by ceiling effect as a reasonable air–bone gap closure is usually achieved regardless of the prosthesis size. Some surgeons prefer a 0.4-mm prosthesis to allow for the fenestration of the stapes and crimping of the prosthesis to the incus before fracture and removal of the suprastructure as with the Fisch technique [80].

As magnetic resonance imaging (MRI) scans advance to create progressively stronger magnetic fields and have wider indications for use, concern for the safety of stapes and other middle ear prostheses has grown. A magnetic field can both heat and move a ferromagnetic prosthesis. All prostheses implanted since 1989 are generally felt to be safe for MRI scanning with up to 3 T magnet strength [93, 94, 121].

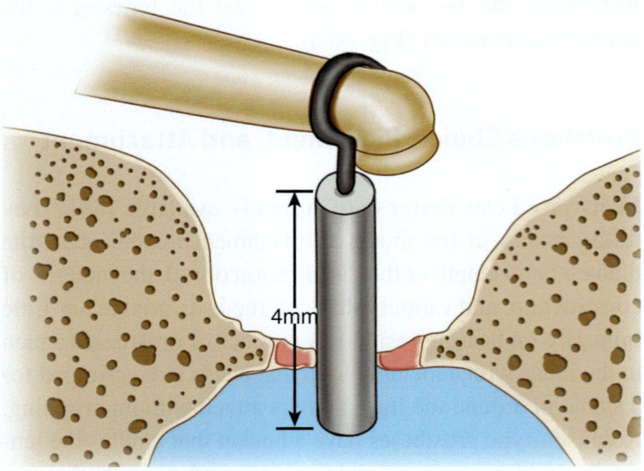

Fig. 46.10 Before creating the fenestra, the distance between the footplate and the medial aspect of the long process of the incus is measured. An additional 0.25 mm is added to the length of the prosthesis to ensure the prosthesis is in the vestibule. (Adapted from Glasscock and Shambaugh's Surgery of the Ear, 5th Edition. Eds. Glasscock, Gulya. BC Decker Inc. 2003)

Prostheses are made in various lengths to accommodate variations in anatomy and pathology. The prosthesis should protrude into the vestibule up to 0.25 mm. If measuring from the under surface of the incus to the footplate, the correct length of the prosthesis is the measured distance to the opening in the footplate plus 0.25 mm (Fig. 46.10). If one is measuring from the top of the long process to the footplate, 0.25 mm should be subtracted from the measured distance to compensate for the thickness of the long process. With either measuring technique, an additional 0.25 mm may be added if the need for bending the shaft of the prosthesis is anticipated.

A prosthesis of the appropriate length is selected based on the measurement of the fenestra diameter and the distance between the fenestra and incus. The surgeon ascertains sufficient opening of the loop of the prosthesis. The prosthesis is grasped by its loop with a smooth alligator forceps in an angle relative to the axis of the prosthesis, which allows its placement on the incus and fenestra in one movement. If the piston cannot be inserted into the fenestra in the initial effort, it is left in the oval window niche and manipulated to the fenestra in a separate maneuver. Tightening the ribbon or wire loop to the long process of the incus is done with a crimper. The crimping is done at the narrowest area of the long process, and then the prosthesis can be moved proximally along the incus to achieve a favorable angle. The crimper should be engaged with both its claws visible to the surgeon and having a deep purchase to the incus. Engagement that is too shallow or angulated backward may result in an elliptical loop around the incus that may allow differential movement of the incus against the prosthesis, which may result in a reduced hearing gain and long-term failure by erosion of the distal end of the incus. Common reasons for differential movement of the incus and the prosthesis are improper crimping or friction between the piston and the walls of the oval window niche or fenestra. The wire of the prosthesis can be manipulated with a right-angled hook to clear some obstacles and create a better and more perpendicular angle in relation to the entrance to the vestibule. Some surgeons use a vein or connective tissue graft to completely seal the fenestra prior to piston placement. Others place blood or loose connective tissue around fenestra after the prosthesis has been placed.

The tympanomeatal flap is restored to its normal anatomical position and surveyed for any perforations requiring grafting. The edges are inspected and unfurled. The flap is stabilized with a small piece of Gelfoam® and the canal filled with bacitracin ointment.

Total Stapedectomy

Although chronologically stapedotomy was introduced as an evolutionary improvement over stapedectomy, done properly both techniques can yield similar results. In certain situations, stapedotomy is not possible and stapedectomy is performed (e.g., a floating footplate, a comminuted fracture of the footplate, a footplate inadvertently removed during suprastructure dislocation through anterior crus attachment, and some revision surgeries). Stapedectomy is also a solution when the instruments required to create a small fenestra are lacking. Special care should be taken to minimize trauma to the inner ear when extracting the intact or fragmented footplate. The gap between the prosthesis and the oval window opening to the vestibule must be sealed with a tissue graft, such as fat or perichondrium. Although the hearing results for stapedectomy and stapedotomy are similar, the occurrence, duration, and severity of vestibular symptoms are greater for stapedectomy.

Alternative Therapies for Otosclerosis

Patients suffering from long-term otosclerosis may develop "far-advanced" otosclerosis with air conduction thresholds >85 dB and non-measurable bone conduction thresholds (because of the technical limitations of the audiometer). As originally advocated by House and Sheehy, the traditional recommendation for these patients who were unable to benefit from hearing aids was stapes surgery [95]. This approach is still recommended as a first line of treatment prior to cochlear implantation. The surgeon's decision to perform a stapedotomy versus going directly to cochlear implantation is made even more difficult because the patient's preoperative speech discrimination scores may be underestimated when acoustic thresholds are elevated. In Shea's far-advanced otosclerosis study [96], speech discrimination improved by 15%, and in a study by Lippy et al., speech discrimination continued to improve to reach an additional 32.7% after 2 years [97]. In light of this data, many surgeons would recommend initially attempting a stapedotomy since it may be effective and considerably less expensive than cochlear implantation. In addition, based on studies by Calmels et al. and Kabbara et al., a prior stapedotomy did not interfere with subsequent cochlear implantation outcomes [98, 99]. In Calmels' study, the four patients who underwent prior stapedotomy had postoperative speech discrimination scores ranging from 70% to 95%, with a mean of 80% [98].

Postoperative Care

Stapes surgery has changed from an inpatient procedure to an outpatient or 23-h observation procedure. Patients can often be discharged from the hospital or surgical center a few hours after surgery. To minimize postoperative symptoms of vertigo, a transdermal scopolamine patch, which is typically placed behind the contralateral ear in the preoperuptive holding area, is left in place for 3 days.

Patients are instructed to keep their ears dry, to avoid strenuous physical activities (e.g., heavy lifting, Valsalva maneuvers), to avoid nose blowing, and to sneeze with an open mouth. Air travel is permissible a couple of days after the operation.

Patients are typically seen 3 weeks postoperatively. Two nights before and the night before their postoperative visit, the patient is instructed to fill the ear canal with mineral oil and plug it with cotton before going to sleep. The cotton ball is removed the following morning. Placement of the mineral oil facilitates the removal of dried blood in the ear canal during the postoperative visit without patient discomfort.

During the 3-week postoperative visit, the ear canal and tympanic membrane are inspected and the patient's hearing tested with a 512 Hz tuning fork. If everything has healed appropriately, the patient is instructed to resume their normal activities. The patient returns 3 months postoperatively for an otologic exam and a complete audiological evaluation.

Results

Bone conduction is often improved after surgery with correction of the Carhart's notch. Hence, in evaluating the results of surgery, postoperative air–bone gap is calculated based on postoperative air and bone conduction measurements, as stipulated by the guidelines issued by committee on hearing and equilibrium of the American Academy of Otolaryngology—Head and Neck Surgery [100]. Experienced stapes surgeons can optimally achieve closure of the air–bone gap to 10 dB or less in 90% of patients with an incidence of profound SNHL of not more than 1%. In 90% of patients, closure of air–bone gap is stable for many years [101, 102].

Complications

Intraoperative Problems and Complications

Tears in the Tympanomeatal Flap

Tears in the tympanomeatal flap commonly occur when elevation is performed in a limited segment rather than in a broad plane, or when the tympanic membrane is elevated without including the annulus.

Subluxation of the Incus

Subluxation and dislocation of the incus occur most often during curettage of the bony annulus, separation of the incudostapedial joint, manipulation around the oval window, and crimping. Subluxation implies that part, but not all, of the attachments of the incus has been disrupted. In this case, chances are high for achieving a good functional result from completing the procedure with an incus attachment prosthesis, although crimping the prosthesis to a loose incus is more challenging. Some surgeons prefer to abort the procedure and attempt completion as a separate procedure after giving sufficient time for the incus to reattach to the malleus. However, if disarticulation or complete disruption of the joint occurs, as indicated by complete freedom of the incus to move in medial, lateral, anterior, and posterior directions, it is best to remove the incus and perform a malleovestibulopexy. Another option is to place a total ossicular replacement prosthesis onto a fenestra that is covered by perichondrium in a single or staged procedure, though it is worth noting that the statistical probability of success quoted above likely lowers in these cases.

Overhanging Facial Nerve

The location of the facial nerve should be visually verified as soon as the oval window area is exposed. The facial nerve can be dehiscent of its covering bone, but usually does not extend significantly out of the fallopian canal (i.e., prolapse or overhang the oval window) In a series of 1497 stapedectomy procedures, prolapse of the facial nerve was found in 40 (2.6%); in 28 (1.9%) the prolapsed nerve covered more than 50% of the oval window niche. Only four operations had to be aborted for this reason [103]. If the prolapsed nerve abuts the promontory inferior to the oval window, surgery should not be completed. In most cases, surgery can be completed by drilling a small fenestra that includes the inferior aspect of the annular ligament. It is best to drill around the midpoint of the inferior margin, where the thickness of the promontory is greatest [104]. This technique is similar to the one used for extracting a floating footplate. Generally, with an overhanging facial nerve, the prosthesis must be longer than usual to accommodate bending inferiorly to avoid the nerve and being positioned perpendicular to the fenestra.

Obliterative Otosclerosis of the Oval Window

The oval window niche can be obliterated by severe thickening of the stapedial footplate and/or the margins of the niche. In a series of 293 primary stapedectomy procedures, obliterative otosclerosis was found in 14 (4.7%) [105]. The laser is not efficient in removing such large amounts of bone. Fenestration can be achieved after first saucerizing the obliterated niche with a diamond bur. Once the oval window niche is saucerized, the remaining footplate is blue lined. However, prior to completing the fenestra with the diamond bur, the measurement for prosthesis length is repeated. This ensures that the prosthesis extends adequately into the vestibule. Measurements for prosthesis length are made just prior to fenestration. If obliterative otosclerosis is found in one ear, there is 50% chance of the same finding to be present in the other ear [105].

Otosclerosis Involving the Round Window

The round window can be partially or completely obliterated by otosclerosis. Complete obliteration is associated with significant conductive hearing loss [106]. Attempts at removing this obstruction have resulted in sensorineural hearing loss and are not recommended. During exploration of the ear, it is impossible to ascertain whether an otosclerotic obliteration is partial or complete. Even a minute opening to the round window membrane can permit a good hearing result with surgery. Hence, if the round window is thought to be obliterated, the procedure should be completed and the finding noted in the operative note. If a residual conductive loss is present following surgery, revision surgery is not recommended as the likely cause of failure is a completely obliterated round window.

Persistent Stapedial Artery

The stapedial artery develops and degenerates during the first trimester of gestation. The artery traverses the obturator foramen and after normal regression it is often seen as a small vessel running across the footplate. When the artery persists, it arises from the internal carotid artery to either replace the middle meningeal artery or to branch into three arteries accompanying the branches of the trigeminal nerve. The incidence of persistent stapedial artery recorded in surgical observations is 1 in 5000–10,000 ears (Fig. 46.11); however, based on temporal bone studies, the incidence may be higher [41]. Coagulation of a persistent stapedial artery may have consequences, and as such, routine performance of this maneuver is not recommended by the authors. That being said, this rare

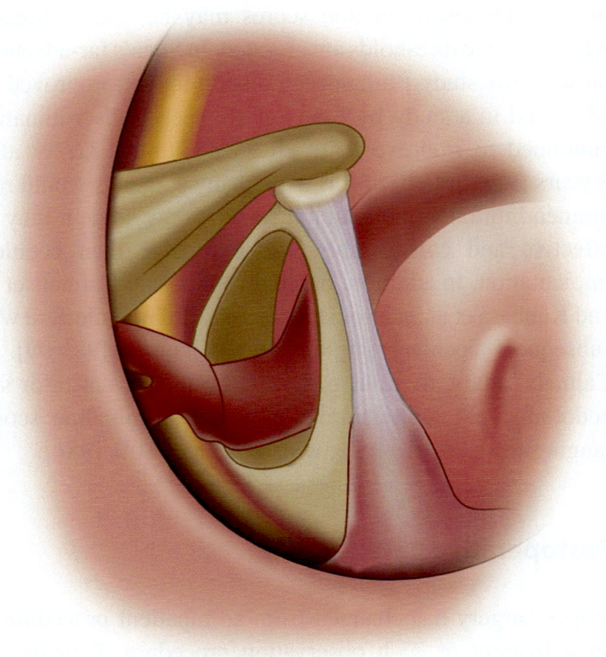

Fig. 46.11 A persistent stapedial artery. The artery should not be coagulated; however, the procedure can often be completed by creating the fenestra posterior to the artery. (Adapted from Glasscock and Shambaugh's Surgery of the Ear, 6th Edition. Eds. Gulya, Minor, Poe. PMPH. 2010)

vessel often only occupies the anterior half of the footplate, and fenestration can be completed in the posterior half. The procedure should be completed only if the space left by the artery is clearly sufficient for safe fenestration.

Malleus Ankylosis

The malleus head can be ankylosed to the wall or to the roof of the epitympanum by a spur or bar of bone. The etiology of this type of ankylosis has no association with that of otosclerosis, and may be the consequence of a developmental defect or new bone formation during inflammation of the middle ear cleft. Although malleus fixation was found in only 0.5% of the specimens at Massachusetts Eye and Ear Infirmary's temporal bone collection [107], some surgical series report a slightly higher incidence of 1–2%. Physical examination and audiometry can raise the suspicion of malleus fixation. On pneumatic otoscopy, reduced mobility of the umbo, manubrium, or lateral process of the manubrium is noticed. If suspected, the diagnosis can often be confirmed by laser Doppler vibrometry, although this technology is not routinely available.

Myringosclerosis can be associated with malleus fixation. Most cases of fixation of the malleus are unilateral in contrast to otosclerosis. During exploration of the ear, the movement of each of the ossicles should be assessed independently by gentle palpation. Fixation of the malleus can be corrected during stapes surgery by removing the incus and head of malleus and reconstruction with a malleus attachment prosthesis or by removing the area of malleus fixation after disarticulating the incudostapedial joint.

Perilymph Gushers and Oozers

Fenestration of the footplate may be followed by fluid egress from the vestibule to the middle ear. Although named perilymph gushers and oozers, this is in fact flow of cerebrospinal fluid (CSF). Schuknecht suspected that oozers were a steady trickle of fluid, associated with a persistent cochlear aqueduct, which in the great majority of humans does not allow free flow [108]. A gusher is a strong and forceful flow (Fig. 46.12) originating from a defect in the cribrose area of the fundus of the internal auditory canal. This defect is often associated with other inner ear anomalies and congenital fixation of the stapes, and although high-resolution CT may be helpful, cases of perilymph gushers may have normal appearing CT scans.

With any stapes surgery, it is prudent to inspect the round window membrane for bulging. If present, carefully inspect the footplate to ensure that it is truly fixed by otosclerosis. If not, one can abort the operative procedure.

Creating a fenestra in an ear with a defect in the cribrose area of the internal auditory canal results in the rapid release of inner ear fluids that can threaten sensorineural hearing and needs to be addressed immediately. The fenestra is packed with tissue graft or a cotton pledget. Placing a lumbar drain and lowering spinal fluid pressure can also be useful. Stapedectomy should be completed by using a perichondrium or vein tissue graft that is held in place with a stapes prosthesis. X-linked recessive stapes gusher syndrome should be suspected in male patients with childhood onset of hearing impairment [69].

Floating or Depressed Footplate

A footplate that is irretrievably depressed into the vestibule (Fig. 46.13) will almost certainly cause immediate and in some cases, long-term vertigo. Once a footplate has settled in the vestibule, there is no safe way to extract it without further jeopardizing the inner ear. If preoperative evaluation makes limited ankylosis likely, the procedure may be deferred or extreme care should be exercised while manipulating the suprastructure. Fenestration by laser reduces the chances of a footplate disarticulation as the laser exerts relatively less pressure than other methods. Another preventive measure is assessing the movement of the footplate before completing the fracturing and disengaging the suprastruc-

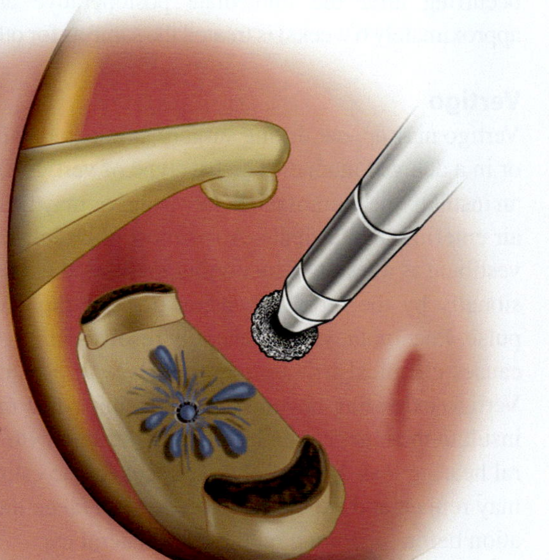

Fig. 46.12 A perilymph gusher requires prompt treatment to prevent severe to profound sensorineural hearing loss. Despite prompt treatment, profound sensorineural hearing loss often results. (Adapted from Glasscock and Shambaugh's Surgery of the Ear, 6th Edition. Eds. Gulya, Minor, Poe. PMPH. 2010)

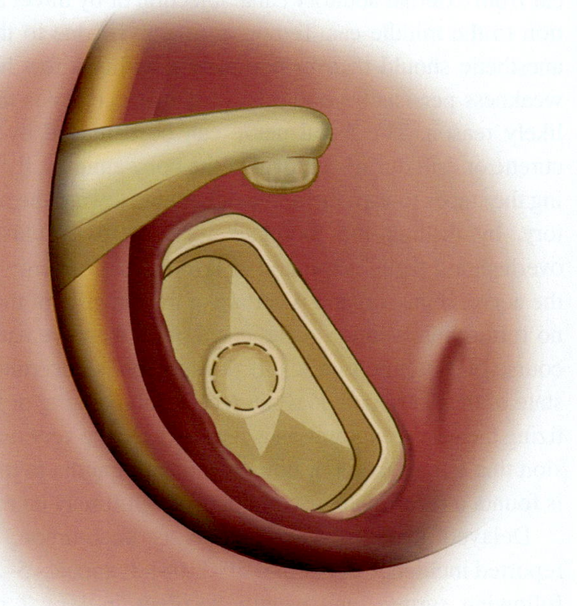

Fig. 46.13 A floating footplate in the vestibule places the membranous labyrinth at risk if an attempt is made to remove the footplate from inside the vestibule. As pictured, this footplate has been subluxed superiorly under the superior lip of the oval window. If the footplate is completely in the vestibule, it would be advisable to leave the footplate in the vestibule and complete the procedure. (Adapted from Glasscock and Shambaugh's Surgery of the Ear, 6th Edition. Eds. Gulya, Minor, Poe. PMPH. 2010)

ture. If the footplate seems to be mobilized, every effort should be made to divide the crura prior to removal.

In the case of a floating footplate, fenestration can still sometimes be made with a laser. If that instrument is unavailable or the footplate too thick for the laser to penetrate, a small burr hole can be created inferior to the annular ligament of the footplate and the footplate elevated with a small hook. The opening is then sealed with a tissue graft and an appropriately sized prosthesis is placed. If the footplate is depressed into the vestibule, it should not be extracted and the procedure is completed. However, results are highly variable. If the footplate is still attached at one end, it can sometimes be removed by a small hook engaged to a remnant of the crus on the nondepressed side. Small fragments of footplate or bone dust usually do not harm the inner ear.

Postoperative Complications

Facial Palsy

Immediate facial paralysis is most likely related to local anesthesia or intraoperative trauma to the nerve. When facial paralysis is the result of local anesthesia, it is most often related to overzealous injection in the anterior portion of the external auditory canal. Local anesthesia can also infiltrate the middle ear from external auditory canal injection or by direct application to the middle ear. Temporary paralysis due to the local anesthetic should recover completely within a few hours. If weakness persists beyond 3 h, a traumatic injury is the more likely reason. The facial nerve can be damaged by a bone curette or drill during removal of the bony annulus, by fracturing the stapes toward the nerve rather than toward the promontory, by drilling the footplate adjacent to a dehiscent or overhanging facial nerve and or through laser energy heating the nerve. If the surgeon is certain of the integrity of the nerve, no further intervention is indicated other than eye care and a course of systemic steroids. If the surgeon is uncertain of the state of the nerve and does not recall manipulating or traumatizing the nerve, exploration is required. On the very rare occasion that a transaction or other significant trauma to the nerve is found, a repair with or without cable graft may be required.

Delayed facial nerve paralysis is uncommon, with a reported incidence of about 0.5% [108]. It appears 5–20 days following surgery and usually resolves in 1 or 2 months. These patients are managed similarly to those with Bell's palsy [109, 110].

Chorda Tympani Dysfunction

The chorda tympani exits the posterior iter and typically traverses the field of stapes surgery. Injury to the nerve may result in hypogeusia and dysgeusia, with evidence of atrophy of the fungiform papillae in the denervated area. Symptoms arise more often in stapes surgery and myringoplasty compared to surgery for chronic otitis media because in the latter condition the nerve has already been damaged by the disease prior to surgery [111, 112]. It is rare that the chorda tympani nerve does not need to be manipulated to obtain proper exposure for stapes surgery, and as such, it is generally at risk. Infrequently, the nerve is situated to prohibit surgery and needs to be cut. A severed nerve will cause temporary symptoms, which improve in most patients over the course of 3–6 months. In the course of typical stapes surgery, the nerve is manipulated, stretched, or dried out. The dried nerve recuperates function quickly and completely. The stretched nerve may cause the most disturbing and potentially chronic symptoms of metallic taste, unpleasant taste, and altered taste of various foods. The stretched nerve seems to cause more disturbing symptoms compared to a severed nerve [111, 112]. Hence, if the surgeon estimates during surgery that the nerve has been significantly stretched, it may be better to sacrifice the nerve.

Otitis Media

Acute otitis media in the immediate postoperative period is worrisome as the risk of suppurative labyrinthitis and meningitis is greater. In the rare occurrence of the latter complications, the patient experiences pain and fever; management includes removal of any ear canal packing and admission to the hospital. Treatment with broad-spectrum antibiotics is initiated and adjusted according to culture if available. Steroids may be helpful to minimize inner ear damage. Acute otitis media occurring after the immediate postoperative area (lasting approximately 6 weeks) is treated the same as for other patients.

Vertigo

Vertigo may appear during surgery, immediately following it, or in a delayed manner. The first type of vertigo may indicate an insult to the membranous labyrinth, or may be the result of air entering the vestibule. Air is most often introduced to the vestibule as a result of suctioning in the oval window or occasionally by the rapid expansion of perilymph from a laser pulse. Pneumolabyrinth generally resolves in 24–48 h. Blood causes chemical irritation and resolves in a matter of days. Vertigo extending beyond that time suggests a more serious insult to the inner ear and is often associated with sensorineural hearing loss. Even if hearing recovers, a vestibular deficit may remain and should be tested for and taken into consideration before operating on the contralateral ear.

Delayed vertigo after stapes surgery is rare and can be the result of benign positional paroxysmal vertigo [113] that can be treated by physical therapy or the result of a perilymph fistula [114]. A perilymph fistula can occur in the early or late postoperative period.

Reparative Granuloma

A reparative granuloma is a mass of exuberant granulation tissue developing in reaction to surgery, a foreign body (e.g., surgical glove powder, Gelfoam® sterilized by formaldehyde, the prosthesis, fabric particles from the surgical drapes), or to perilymph [115]. It manifests in the 5th to 15th day after surgery. The associated symptoms and signs of labyrinthitis (dizziness, tinnitus, hearing loss, and nystagmus toward the nonoperated side) appear after an early period of hearing gain. Otoscopy reveals edema, thickening, and hyperemia of the skin flaps and tympanic membrane. Audiometry demonstrates a mixed hearing loss and decreased speech discrimination scores. Clinical suspicion of a reparative granuloma is an indication for immediate reexploration in an attempt to reduce the likelihood and extent of permanent inner ear dysfunction. Steroids may be useful in this setting as well. The granulation tissue and prosthesis are removed and the fenestra is sealed with a tissue graft. Early intervention may help patients recover some hearing. Vestibular symptoms usually resolve in weeks or months. Changes in surgical technique and materials may have contributed to making this complication relatively rare.

Sensorineural Hearing Loss

Slight transient depression (<5 dB) in bone conduction immediately following the procedure is a common occurrence and attributable to mild serous labyrinthitis. Permanent sensorineural hearing loss can occur immediately following surgery or appear weeks or months after. Early loss, especially at high-frequencies, is attributable to surgical trauma. Delayed sensorineural hearing loss should raise the suspicion of a perilymph fistula. A delayed fluctuating low-frequency loss may indicate post-traumatic hydrops. Up to 1% of patients undergoing stapes surgery suffer partial or even complete sensorineural hearing loss.

Conductive Hearing Loss

Conductive hearing loss after stapes surgery can appear unexpectedly immediately after the operation or more commonly delayed after initial good result. The etiology of immediate and delayed conductive loss and their respective treatment are different. Common reasons for immediate conductive loss after stapes surgery are (1) malfunctioning prosthesis (e.g., too short a prosthesis), (2) unrecognized malleus fixation, (3) unrecognized round window obliteration, (4) middle ear effusion, and (5) presence of unrecognized superior semicircular canal dehiscence (SSCD). Computed tomographic scanning can help in identifying SSCD and, at times, round window obliteration. Revision surgery may be considered after waiting for several months.

More commonly, conductive hearing loss appears at a variable time after a good initial closure or reduction of the air–bone gap. The most frequent findings for recurrent conductive hearing loss following stapes surgery are erosion or necrosis of the incus at the site of prosthesis attachment (64%), malpositioned prosthesis (41%), bony (14%) or fibrous regrowth at the oval window area, and round window obliteration (23%) [115]. Incus erosion initially manifests with a fluctuating loss intermittently improved by the Valsalva maneuver or changing head position. Eventually, complete discontinuity of the ossicular chain occurs resulting in a large air–bone gap. Incus erosion is due to resorptive osteitis from differential movement of the prosthesis and incus or foreign body reaction, as occurred with polyethylene struts. As the incus has good intraosseous blood supply, strangulation of the mucosa by crimping is not a likely cause.

Treatment of Otosclerosis with Cochlear Involvement

Sensorineural hearing loss occurs in 20–30% of patients with otosclerosis and is usually progressive. It is suspected that cochlear otosclerosis causes sensorineural hearing loss by affecting the spiral ligament [116]. A high-resolution CT may show lucency around the cochlea that is the result of demineralization of the otic capsule.

A variety of pharmaceutical agents that reduce bone resorption have been prescribed as a possible treatment for the progressive sensorineural hearing loss associated with otosclerosis. Sodium fluoride was historically used to treat cochlear otosclerosis based on studies suggesting modest reduction in the progression of sensorineural hearing loss with minimal side effects; however, its use has largely fallen out of favor due to limited and inconsistent evidence of efficacy. [117, 118]. However, currently third-generation bisphosphonates such as risedronate and zoledronate are available that demonstrate much more powerful anti-resorptive properties. In a limited retrospective pilot study of patients treated with the third-generation bisphosphonates, there was no significant progression of sensorineural hearing loss (i.e., stabilization) at an average follow-up of 13 months. Despite these encouraging results, there are greater risks associated with systemic bisphosphonates than with fluoride therapy [119, 120].

Summary

Otosclerosis is one of the more common causes of hearing loss. Multiple genetic loci associated with otosclerosis have been identified, and forms of the disease may be inherited in an autosomal dominant pattern with an incomplete penetrance rate of 20–40%. Although the precise cause for the abnormal bone remodeling that produces the otosclerotic foci remains uncertain, ultrastructural and immunohistochemical evidence of measles-like structures and antigenicity in active otosclerotic lesions has also been identified. Following the introduction of the measles vaccination, there has been a decline in the incidence of otosclerosis and improved medical treatment for otosclerosis may be available in the future.

For the time being, symptomatic otosclerotic patients can benefit from amplification in the form of hearing aids or from stapes surgery. The prostheses and techniques used in stapes surgery have continued to evolve since Shea's revival of stapes surgery in the 1950s. Currently, the most common procedure to correct stapedial fixation is small-fenestra stapedotomy with the assistance of microdrills and/or lasers.

Successful surgery reduces air–bone gaps to less than 10 dB and is achieved in 90% of patients. Noteworthy complications include sensorineural hearing loss (1%), chorda tympani nerve dysfunction, and vestibular injury. Revision surgery is technically demanding and is associated with lower success rates and slightly higher complication rates compared to primary surgery.

Patients with significant sensorineural hearing loss can still be candidates for stapes surgery even if they may require amplification after a successful operation. However, some patients with far advanced otosclerosis may require cochlear implantation.

References

1. Fowler EP. Otosclerosis in identical twins. A study of 40 pairs. Arch Otolaryngol. 1966;83(4):324–8.
2. Morrison AW. Genetic factors in otosclerosis. Ann R Coll Surg Engl. 1967;41(2):202–37.
3. Bittermann AJ, Wegner I, Noordman BJ, Vincent R, van der Heijden GJ, Grolman W. An introduction of genetics in otosclerosis: a systematic review. Otolaryngol Head Neck Surg. 2014;150(1):34–9.
4. Politzer A. Ueber primäre Erkrankung der knöchernen Labyrinthkapsel. Zeitschr Ohrenheil. 1893;25:309–27.
5. Pearson RD, Kurland LT, Cody DT. Incidence of diagnosed clinical otosclerosis. Arch Otolaryngol. 1974;99(4):288–91.
6. Weber M. Otosklerose und umbau der labyrinthkapsel. Leipzig: Poeschel und Trepte; 1935.
7. Engstrom H. Uber das vorkmmen der otosklerose nebst experimentellen studien uber chirurgische behandlung der krankheit. Acta Otolaryngol (Suppl). 1940;43:1–153.
8. Guild SR. Histologic otosclerosis. Ann Oto Rhino Laryngol. 1944;53:1045–71.
9. Nager GT. Pathology of the ear and temporal bone. 1st ed. Williams and Wilkins; 1993.
10. McKenna MJ, Kristiansen AG, Haines J. Polymerase chain reaction amplification of a measles virus sequence from human temporal bone sections with active otosclerosis. Am J Otol. 1996;17(6):827–30.
11. McKenna MJ, Mills BG. Immunohistochemical evidence of measles virus antigens in active otosclerosis. Otolaryngol Head Neck Surg. 1989;101(4):415–21.
12. Arnold W, Busch R, Arnold A, Ritscher B, Neiss A, Niedermeyer HP. The influence of measles vaccination on the incidence of otosclerosis in Germany. Eur Arch Otorhinolaryngol. 2007;264(7):741–8.
13. Declau F, van Spaendonck M, Timmermans JP, et al. Prevalence of histologic otosclerosis: an unbiased temporal bone study in Caucasians. Adv Otorhinolaryngol. 2007;65:6–16.
14. Valsalva AM. Opera, hoc est, tractatus de aure humana. Venice: Pitteri; 1735.
15. Toynbee J. Pathological and surgical observations on the diseases of the ear. Med Chir Trans. 1841;24:190.
16. Toynbee J. A descriptive catalogue of preparations illustrative of the diseases of the ear. London: Churchill; 1857.
17. Politzer A. Primary disease of the bony labyrinthine capsule. Arch Otol. 1894;23:255–70.
18. Kessel J. Über die durchschneidung des steigbügelmuskels beim menschen und über die extraction des steigbügels. respektive der Columella bie Thieren. Arch Ohrenh. 1876;11:199–217.
19. Kessel J. Über das mobilisieren des steigbügels durch ausschneiden des trommelfells, hammers und ambosses bei undurchgängigkeit der tube. Arch Ohrenh. 1978;13:69–88.
20. Miot C. De la mobilisation de l'etrier. Rev Laryngol Otol Rhinol (Bord). 1890;10:113–30.
21. Jack FL. Supplementary report on a case of double stapedectomy operated on ten years ago. Paper presented at: American Otological Society; 1902.
22. Siebenmann F. Sur le traitement chirurgical de la sclerose otique. Congr Inter Med Sec Otol. 1900;13:170.
23. Politzer A. Geschichte der otosclerose. In: Geschichte der Ohrenheilkunde, vol. 2. Stuttgart: Enke Verlag; 1913. p. 171–5.
24. Politzer A. Cited in Panse R. Discussion, Die operative Behandlung hochgradiger Schwerhörigkeit. Verh Dtsch Otol Ges. 1897;6:141–145.
25. Floderus B. Bidrag till stigbygelankylosens operative radikalbehandlung. Nord Med Ark. 1899;32:1–17.
26. Jenkins GJ. Otosclerosis: certain clinical features and experimental operative procedures. Trans XVIIth Inter Congr Med London. 1913;46:3–12.
27. Holmgren G. The surgery of otosclerosis. Ann Otol Rhinol Laryngol. 1937;46:3–12.
28. Sourdille M. New technique in the surgical treatment of severe and progressive deafness from otosclerosis. Bull N Y Acad Med. 1937;13:673.
29. Lempert J. Improvement of hearing in cases of otosclerosis: a new one stage surgical technique. Arch Otolaryngol. 1938;28:42–97.
30. Rosen S. Palpation of stapes for fixation: preliminary procedure to determine fenestration suitability in otosclerosis. AMA Arch Otolaryngol. 1952;56:610–5.
31. House HP. Symposium—the operation for the mobilization of the stapes in otosclerotic deafness. Paper presented at: The American Laryngological, Rhinological and Otological Society; Montreal, Canada; 1956.
32. Hyman S. For the world to hear: a biography of Howard P. House, M.D. Hope Publishing House; 1990.
33. Vondrak JC. The unreasonable man: the trials and triumphs of William F. House, M. D. William F. House, LLC; 2014.
34. Shea JJ Jr. A personal history of stapedectomy. Am J Otol. 1998;19(5 Suppl):S2–12.
35. Perkins RC. Laser stapedotomy for otosclerosis. Laryngoscope. 1980;90(2):228–40.
36. Silverstein H. Laser stapedotomy minus prosthesis (laser STAMP): a minimally invasive procedure. Am J Otol. 1998;19(3):277–82.
37. Gjuric M, Rukavina L. Evolution of stapedectomy prostheses over time. Adv Otorhinolaryngol. 2007;65:174–8.
38. Schuknecht HF, Mc GT, Colman BH. Stapedectomy. Ann Otol Rhinol Laryngol. 1960;69:597–609.
39. Frisch T, Sorensen MS, Overgaard S, Bretlau P. Estimation of volume referent bone turnover in the otic capsule after sequential point labeling. Ann Otol Rhinol Laryngol. 2000;109(1):33–9.
40. Schuknecht HF, Barber W. Histologic variants in otosclerosis. Laryngoscope. 1985;95(11):1307–17.
41. Schuknecht H. Pathology of the ear. Lee and Fibeger; 1993.

42. Stankovic KM, McKenna MJ. Current research in otosclerosis. Curr Opin Otolaryngol Head Neck Surg. 2006;14(5):347–51.
43. Quinn JM, Whitty GA, Byrne RJ, Gillespie MT, Hamilton JA. The generation of highly enriched osteoclast-lineage cell populations. Bone. 2002;30(1):164–70.
44. Burgess TL, Qian Y, Kaufman S, et al. The ligand for osteoprotegerin (OPGL) directly activates mature osteoclasts. J Cell Biol. 1999;145(3):527–38.
45. Lacey DL, Tan HL, Lu J, et al. Osteoprotegerin ligand modulates murine osteoclast survival in vitro and in vivo. Am J Pathol. 2000;157(2):435–48.
46. Udagawa N, Takahashi N, Yasuda H, et al. Osteoprotegerin produced by osteoblasts is an important regulator in osteoclast development and function. Endocrinology. 2000;141(9):3478–84.
47. Zehnder AF, Kristiansen AG, Adams JC, Merchant SN, McKenna MJ. Osteoprotegerin in the inner ear may inhibit bone remodeling in the otic capsule. Laryngoscope. 2005;115(1):172–7.
48. Zehnder AF, Kristiansen AG, Adams JC, Kujawa SG, Merchant SN, McKenna MJ. Osteoprotegerin knockout mice demonstrate abnormal remodeling of the otic capsule and progressive hearing loss. Laryngoscope. 2006;116(2):201–6.
49. Schrauwen I, Weegerink NJ, Fransen E, et al. A new locus for otosclerosis, OTSC10, maps to chromosome 1q41-44. Clin Genet. 2011;79(5):495–7.
50. McKenna MJ, Kristiansen AG, Bartley ML, Rogus JJ, Haines JL. Association of COL1A1 and otosclerosis: evidence for a shared genetic etiology with mild osteogenesis imperfecta. Am J Otol. 1998;19(5):604–10.
51. Clayton AE, Mikulec AA, Mikulec KH, Merchant SN, McKenna MJ. Association between osteoporosis and otosclerosis in women. J Laryngol Otol. 2004;118(8):617–21.
52. Manolidis S, Alford RL, Smith RJ, Ball C, Manolidis L. Do the genes that cause otosclerosis reduce susceptibility to otitis media? Otol Neurotol. 2003;24(6):868–71.
53. Ferlito A, Arnold W, Rinaldo A, et al. Viruses and otosclerosis: chance association or true causal link? Acta Otolaryngol. 2003;123(6):741–6.
54. McKenna MJ, Mills BG, Galey FR, Linthicum FH Jr. Filamentous structures morphologically similar to viral nucleocapsids in otosclerotic lesions in two patients. Am J Otol. 1986;7(1):25–8.
55. McKenna MJ, Mills BG. Ultrastructural and immunohistochemical evidence of measles virus in active otosclerosis. Acta Otolaryngol Suppl. 1990;470:130–9. discussion 139–140.
56. Karosi T, Konya J, Szabo LZ, Sziklai I. Measles virus prevalence in otosclerotic stapes footplate samples. Otol Neurotol. 2004;25(4):451–6.
57. Niedermeyer H, Arnold W, Neubert WJ, Hofler H. Evidence of measles virus RNA in otosclerotic tissue. ORL J Otorhinolaryngol Relat Spec. 1994;56(3):130–2.
58. Niedermeyer HP, Arnold W. Otosclerosis: a measles virus associated inflammatory disease. Acta Otolaryngol. 1995;115(2):300–3.
59. Lolov SR, Encheva VI, Kyurkchiev SD, Edrev GE, Kehayov IR. Antimeasles immunoglobulin G in sera of patients with otosclerosis is lower than that in healthy people. Otol Neurotol. 2001;22(6):766–70.
60. Lippy WH, Berenholz LP, Schuring AG, Burkey JM. Does pregnancy affect otosclerosis? Laryngoscope. 2005;115(10):1833–6.
61. Mikulec AA, McKenna MJ, Ramsey MJ, et al. Superior semicircular canal dehiscence presenting as conductive hearing loss without vertigo. Otol Neurotol. 2004;25(2):121–9.
62. Merchant SN, Rosowski JJ, McKenna MJ. Superior semicircular canal dehiscence mimicking otosclerotic hearing loss. Adv Otorhinolaryngol. 2007;65:137–45.
63. Zhou G, Gopen Q, Poe DS. Clinical and diagnostic characterization of canal dehiscence syndrome: a great otologic mimicker. Otol Neurotol. 2007;28(7):920–6.
64. Niedermeyer HP, Hausler R, Schwub D, Neuner NT, Busch R, Arnold W. Evidence of increased average age of patients with otosclerosis. Adv Otorhinolaryngol. 2007;65:17–24.
65. Vincent R, Sperling NM, Oates J, Jindal M. Surgical findings and long-term hearing results in 3,050 stapedotomies for primary otosclerosis: a prospective study with the otology-neurotology database. Otol Neurotol. 2006;27(8 Suppl 2):S25–47.
66. Katz J. Handbook on clinical audiology. 5th ed. Lippincott Williams and Wilkins; 2002.
67. Vicente Ade O, Yamashita HK, Albernaz PL, Penido Nde O. Computed tomography in the diagnosis of otosclerosis. Otolaryngol Head Neck Surg. 2006;134(4):685–92.
68. Naumann IC, Porcellini B, Fisch U. Otosclerosis: incidence of positive findings on high-resolution computed tomography and their correlation to audiological test data. Ann Otol Rhinol Laryngol. 2005;114(9):709–16.
69. Cremers CW. How to prevent a stapes gusher. Adv Otorhinolaryngol. 2007;65:278–84.
70. Hughes GB. The learning curve in stapes surgery. Laryngoscope. 1991;101(12 Pt 1):1280–4.
71. Yung MW, Oates J, Vowler SL. The learning curve in stapes surgery and its implication to training. Laryngoscope. 2006;116(1):67–71.
72. Falcone MT, Gajewski BJ, Antonelli PJ. Hearing loss with stapedotomy in otitis media. Otolaryngol Head Neck Surg. 2003;129(6):666–73.
73. Iurato S, Bux G, Mevoli S, Onori M. Stapes surgery in the elderly. Adv Otorhinolaryngol. 2007;65:231–6.
74. House JW, Toh EH, Perez A. Diving after stapedectomy: clinical experience and recommendations. Otolaryngol Head Neck Surg. 2001;125(4):356–60.
75. Vital V, Konstantinidis I, Vital I, Triaridis S. Minimizing the dead ear in otosclerosis surgery. Auris Nasus Larynx. 2008;35(4):475–9.
76. Wegner I, Bittermann AJ, Zinsmeester MM, van der Heijden GJ, Grolman W. Local versus general anesthesia in stapes surgery for otosclerosis: a systematic review of the evidence. Otolaryngol Head Neck Surg. 2013;149(3):360–5.
77. Verschuur HP, de Wever WW, van Benthem PP. Antibiotic prophylaxis in clean and clean-contaminated ear surgery. Cochrane Database Syst Rev. 2004;2004(3):CD003996.
78. Ottoline AC, Tomita S, Marques Mda P, Felix F, Ferraiolo PN, Laurindo RS. Antibiotic prophylaxis in otolaryngologic surgery. Int Arch Otorhinolaryngol. 2013;17(1):85–91.
79. Riechelmann H, Tholen M, Keck T, Rettinger G. Perioperative glucocorticoid treatment does not influence early post-laser stapedotomy hearing thresholds. Am J Otol. 2000;21(6):809–12.
80. Fisch U. Stapedotomy versus stapedectomy. Am J Otol. 1982;4(2):112–7.
81. Green JD Jr, McElveen JT Jr. Next generation shape memory prosthesis (NiTiBOND) for stapedotomy: short-term results. Laryngoscope. 2017;127(4):915–20.
82. Somers T, Vercruysse JP, Zarowski A, Verstreken M, Offeciers E. Stapedotomy with microdrill or carbon dioxide laser: influence on inner ear function. Ann Otol Rhinol Laryngol. 2006;115(12):880–5. discussion 886.
83. Buchman CA, Fucci MJ, Roberson JB Jr, De La Cruz A. Comparison of argon and CO2 laser stapedotomy in primary otosclerosis surgery. Am J Otolaryngol. 2000;21(4):227–30.
84. Lesinski SG. Revision stapedectomy. Curr Opin Otolaryngol Head Neck Surg. 2003;11(5):347–54.
85. Jovanovic S, Schonfeld U, Scherer H. CO2 laser stapedotomy with the "one-shot" technique--clinical results. Otolaryngol Head Neck Surg. 2004;131(5):750–7.
86. Fritsch MH, Naumann IC. Phylogeny of the stapes prosthesis. Otol Neurotol. 2008;29(3):407–15.
87. Harris JP, Gong S. Comparison of hearing results of nitinol SMART stapes piston prosthesis with conventional piston pros-

theses: postoperative results of nitinol stapes prosthesis. Otol Neurotol. 2007;28(5):692–5.
88. Brown KD, Gantz BJ. Hearing results after stapedotomy with a nitinol piston prosthesis. Arch Otolaryngol Head Neck Surg. 2007;133(8):758–62.
89. Wengen DF. A new self-retaining titanium clip stapes prosthesis. Adv Otorhinolaryngol. 2007;65:184–9.
90. Rosowski JJ, Merchant SN. Mechanical and acoustic analysis of middle ear reconstruction. Am J Otol. 1995;16(4):486–97.
91. Marchese MR, Cianfrone F, Passali GC, Paludetti G. Hearing results after stapedotomy: role of the prosthesis diameter. Audiol Neurootol. 2007;12(4):221–5.
92. Shabana YK, Ghonim MR, Pedersen CB. Stapedotomy: does prosthesis diameter affect outcome? Clin Otolaryngol Allied Sci. 1999;24(2):91–4.
93. Syms MJ. Safety of magnetic resonance imaging of stapes prostheses. Laryngoscope. 2005;115(3):381–90.
94. Fritsch MH. MRI scanners and the stapes prosthesis. Otol Neurotol. 2007;28(6):733–8.
95. Daher GS, Kocharyan A, Carlson ML, Dillon WP, Fischbein NJ, Jackler R, Rassner U, Gurgel RK. MRI of Stapes Prostheses: A systematic review. Otol Neurotol. 2024. 45(5): 469–474.
96. House HP, Sheehy JL. Stapes surgery: selection of the patient. Ann Otol Rhinol Laryngol. 1961;70:1062–8.
97. Shea PF, Ge X, Shea JJ Jr. Stapedectomy for far-advanced otosclerosis. Am J Otol. 1999;20(4):425–9.
98. Lippy WH, Burkey JM, Arkis PN. Word recognition score changes after stapedectomy for far advanced otosclerosis. Am J Otol. 1998;19(1):56–8.
99. Calmels MN, Viana C, Wanna G, et al. Very far-advanced otosclerosis: stapedotomy or cochlear implantation. Acta Otolaryngol. 2007;127(6):574–8.
100. Kabbara B, Gauche C, Calmels MN, et al. Decisive criteria between stapedotomy and cochlear implantation in patients with far advanced otosclerosis. Otol Neurotol. 2015;36(3):e73–8.
101. Committee on hearing and equilibrium guidelines for the evaluation of results of treatment of conductive hearing loss. American Academy of Otolaryngology-Head and Neck Surgery Foundation, Inc. Otolaryngol Head Neck Surg. 1995;113(3):186–7.
102. Aarnisalo AA, Vasama JP, Hopsu E, Ramsay H. Long-term hearing results after stapes surgery: a 20-year follow-up. Otol Neurotol. 2003;24(4):567–71.
103. Shea JJ. Stapedectomy—long-term report. Ann Otol Rhinol Laryngol. 1982;91(5 Pt 1):516–20.
104. Neff BA, Lippy WH, Schuring AG, Rizer FM. Stapedectomy in patients with a prolapsed facial nerve. Otolaryngol Head Neck Surg. 2004;130(5):597–603.
105. Saunders NC, Fagan PA. Promontory drilling in stapedectomy: an anatomical study. Otol Neurotol. 2006;27(6):776–80.
106. Ayache D, Sleiman J, Plouin-Gaudon I, Klap P, Elbaz P. Obliterative otosclerosis. J Laryngol Otol. 1999;113(6):512–4.
107. Nadol JB Jr. Histopathology of residual and recurrent conductive hearing loss after stapedectomy. Otol Neurotol. 2001;22(2):162–9.
108. Harris JP, Mehta RP, Nadol JB. Malleus fixation: clinical and histopathologic findings. Ann Otol Rhinol Laryngol. 2002;111(3 Pt 1):246–54.
109. Schuknecht HF, Reisser C. The morphologic basis for perilymphatic gushers and oozers. Adv Otorhinolaryngol. 1988;39:1–12.
110. Shea JJ Jr, Ge X. Delayed facial palsy after stapedectomy. Otol Neurotol. 2001;22(4):465–70.
111. Salvinelli F, Casale M, Vitaliana L, Greco F, Dianzani C, D'Ascanio L. Delayed peripheral facial palsy in the stapes surgery: can it be prevented? Am J Otolaryngol. 2004;25(2):105–8.
112. Clark MP, O'Malley S. Chorda tympani nerve function after middle ear surgery. Otol Neurotol. 2007;28(3):335–40.
113. Michael P, Raut V. Chorda tympani injury: operative findings and postoperative symptoms. Otolaryngol Head Neck Surg. 2007;136(6):978–81.
114. Atacan E, Sennaroglu L, Genc A, Kaya S. Benign paroxysmal positional vertigo after stapedectomy. Laryngoscope. 2001;111(7):1257–9.
115. Albera R, Canale A, Lacilla M, Cavalot AL, Ferrero V. Delayed vertigo after stapes surgery. Laryngoscope. 2004;114(5):860–2.
116. Kuhweide R, Van de Steene V, Vlaminck S, Casselman JW. Reparative granuloma related to perilymphatic fistula. Adv Otorhinolaryngol. 2007;65:296–9.
117. Doherty JK, Linthicum FH Jr. Spiral ligament and stria vascularis changes in cochlear otosclerosis: effect on hearing level. Otol Neurotol. 2004;25(4):457–64.
118. Bretlau P, Salomon G, Johnsen NJ. Otospongiosis and sodium fluoride. A clinical double-blind, placebo-controlled study on sodium fluoride treatment in otospongiosis. Am J Otol. 1989;10(1):20–2.
119. Shambaugh GE Jr, Scott A. Sodium fluoride for arrest of otosclerosis; theoretical considerations. Arch Otolaryngol. 1964;80:263–70.
120. Quesnel AM, Seton M, Merchant SN, Halpin C, McKenna MJ. Third-generation bisphosphonates for treatment of sensorineural hearing loss in otosclerosis. Otol Neurotol. 2012;33(8):1308–14.
121. McKenna M, Mansfield JC. Safety of bisphosphonates in women of child bearing age. Aliment Pharmacol Ther. 2009;29(11):1214–5. author reply 1215–1216.

Revision Surgery for Otosclerosis

47

Benjamin Lovin and Angela Peng

Introduction

Revising any type of operation typically adds an added layer of complexity compared to its primary counterpart. Revision stapes surgery may represent one of the most challenging cases in otology, considering the potential risks involved and the fact that an already difficult operation with a high learning curve is paired with higher complication rates and altered middle ear anatomy. Nevertheless, there are still objective and measurable benefits to be had with revision stapes surgery. While the absolute number of primary stapes operations is declining over time, the relative number of revision cases appears to be increasing [1–3]. As such, a complete understanding of the considerations involved in revision surgery is critical for the otologist to deliver successful outcomes.

Preoperative Workup

Indications for revision stapedectomy include unchanged or worsened hearing loss as well as vertigo [4]. The average time between primary and revision stapedectomy ranges from 7 to 11 years, [5, 6] which likely points towards the development of a new pathologic process causing the hearing loss rather than an issue with the initial technique or surgery.

History

Preoperative evaluation should start with a thorough history. Patient factors that may be associated with the need for revision surgery include younger age, smoking status, dyslipidemia, and hypertension [7].

It is important to ask the patients if they experienced any subjective hearing changes after their primary stapes surgery. If the hearing initially improved and then worsened over time, then this suggests an acquired problem with the conductive hearing mechanism, such as prosthesis displacement or incus necrosis. One should always inquire also about any history of trauma as that may cause ossicular/prosthesis discontinuity. If the patient never experienced hearing improvement following initial surgery, the clinician should consider these possibilities: initial prosthesis length was too short, there was an incomplete labyrinthine fenestration, complete round window obliteration, adhesions or fibrosis around the implant and fenestration, epitympanic fixation of the malleus or incus, or mobile third window phenomenon.

Postoperative vertigo that does not resolve should also be taken into consideration, as this may be a sign of perilymphatic fistula or sunken prosthesis. Postoperative dysgeusia is also worth discussing.

If the revision is being performed by someone who was not the primary surgeon, it is important to obtain prior operative reports, if possible, to determine the implant that was used and to see if there were potential difficulties that the previous surgeon encountered. Some findings and technical complexities noted during a primary surgery may influence decision-making around whether or not a revision procedure should be performed.

Audiogram

An audiogram helps guide the decision for revision surgery. The hearing loss may be a conductive, sensorineural hearing

B. Lovin
Department of Otolaryngology—Head and Neck Surgery, University of Virginia College of Medicine, Charlottesville, VA, USA

A. Peng (✉)
Bobby R. Alford Department of Otolaryngology—Head and Neck Surgery, Baylor College of Medicine, Houston, TX, USA
e-mail: angela.peng@bcm.edu

A. D. Sweeney et al. (eds.), *Haynes-Glasscock-Shambaugh Surgery of the Ear*, https://doi.org/10.1007/978-3-032-18264-7_47

loss, or a mixture of both. Obtaining baseline audiometry from the primary surgery is crucial for comparison. If a new audiogram shows a sensorineural component without a conductive loss, revision stapedectomy would not be beneficial for improved hearing outcomes. In this case, amplification and even possibly cochlear implantation may be warranted based on the degree of loss. Similarly, word recognition scores are also important to note, as although there are some reports of word recognition score improvements following successful stapes surgery, a cochlear implant can also be considered in cases with poor speech discrimination alongside significant mixed hearing loss. Tympanometry may also be considered, as a hypercompliant tympanic membrane may be evidence of discontinuity of the reconstruction (e.g., incus long process necrosis or slipped prosthesis), and poor tympanic membrane compliance could reflect lateral chain fixation.

Physical Examination

A physical exam will likely be unremarkable after a routine primary stapedotomy, but the clinician should always check for serous otitis media, tympanic membrane retraction, a tympanic membrane perforation, and the presence of cholesteatoma as causes for the hearing loss. In the setting of a dislodged prosthesis or collapsed tympanomeatal flap, physical exam findings can be particularly valuable (Fig. 47.1). Pneumatic otoscopy can also be performed to check the mobility of the lateral ossicular chain to ensure the absence of epitympanic fixation, as noted above.

In the rare case of a reparative granuloma captured days after primary surgery, a darkened region may be seen in the posterior mesotympanum over the prosthesis and incus [4]. Some patients, when asked to auto-insufflate or following a sneeze, may note improvement in sound distortion and speech discrimination, pointing toward loose wire syndrome [8].

Tuning fork testing should reveal persistent conductive hearing loss, which should corroborate the hearing loss seen on the postoperative audiogram. A negative Rinne test with a 512 Hz tuning fork is the most commonly used examination benchmark for determining candidacy for stapes surgery (primary or revision).

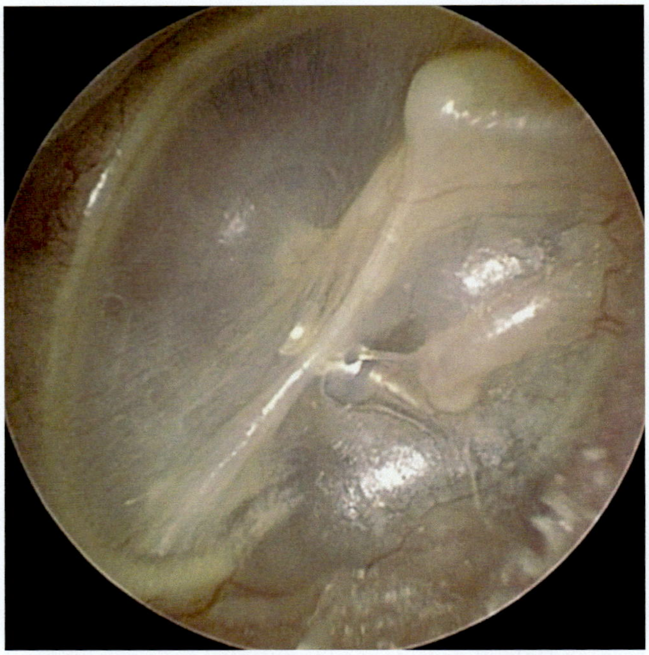

Fig. 47.1 Collapse of the tympanomeatal flap and displacement of a bucket-handle prosthesis seen on otoendoscopy of a left ear in a patient who had stapes surgery 3 decades prior. (Courtesy of Alex D. Sweeney, M.D.)

Imaging

A thin-slice temporal bone computed tomography (CT) without contrast should be obtained during the evaluation of persistent or new conductive hearing loss following stapes surgery. This modality can help evaluate the continuity of the conductive mechanism, including degradation of the ossicles, displacement of the prosthesis in relation to the incus and footplate (Fig. 47.2), re-ossification of the footplate under the prosthesis, and malleus/incus fixation.

CT imaging can also be used to measure the depth of the prosthesis within the vestibule [9]. An excessively long prosthesis will appear deeply seated, almost touching the medial wall of the vestibule. A prosthesis that is too short may appear to not completely fenestrate the footplate and may have a tip visible outside the vestibule. The clinician should confirm the patency of the round window because obliteration from the development of cochlear otosclerosis could cause a conductive loss or even mixed loss (Fig. 47.3) that

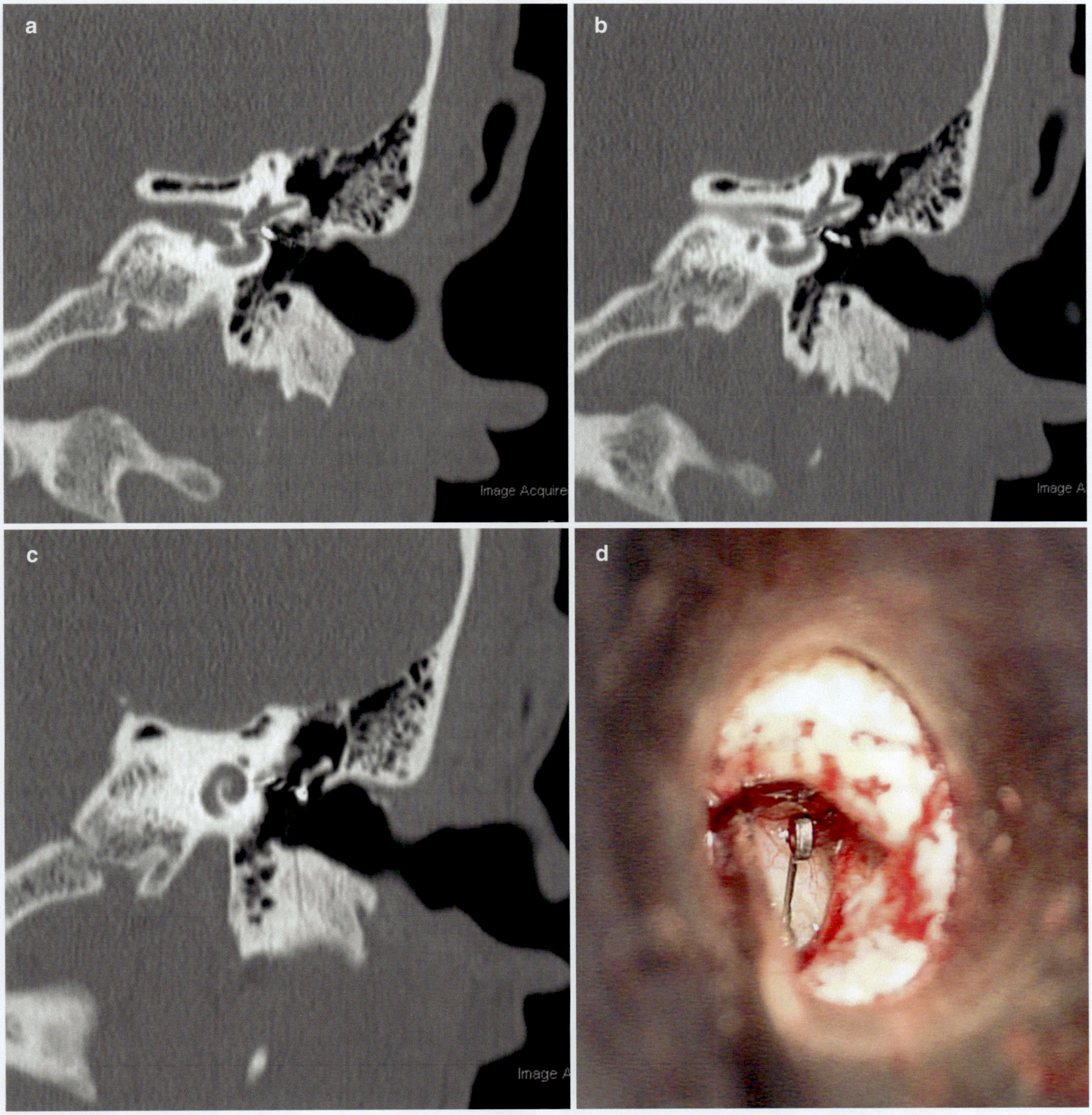

Fig. 47.2 An implant is noted appropriately on the footplate, but the long process of incus was necrosed. (**a**) Implant position at footplate. (**b**) Prosthesis extending toward incus. (**c**) Prosthesis on the incus, but there is necrosis of the long process of the incus. (**d**) Intraoperative photo confirming incus necrosis

may not improve with further surgery. In other words, patients with round window obliteration may be poor candidates for revision stapes surgery if the rest of the workup does not reveal a reparable cause of hearing loss. Thus, other aural rehabilitation options should be discussed.

Pneumolabyrinth can also be seen, which may be suggestive of a perilymphatic fistula (Fig. 47.4) [10].

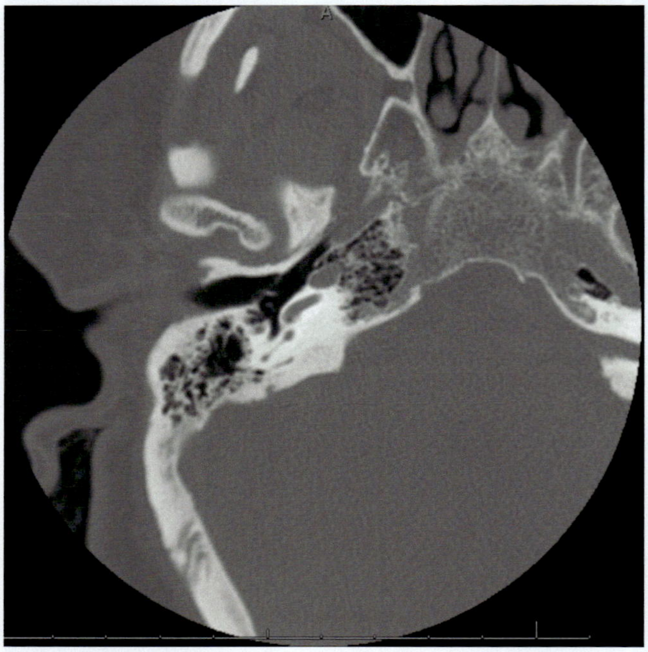

Fig. 47.3 Round window obliteration

Preparation for Surgery

Thorough patient counseling about realistic expectations and potential outcomes (discussed below) is critical. Another crucial step is ensuring that equipment is available to repair the different possibilities of what may be encountered during the surgery. The rarity of revision stapes surgery may lead to an undersupply of relevant tools or the expiration of tools previously ordered. The surgical facility should be equipped with ossicular prostheses that are standard for the surgeon, as well as those to account for incus necrosis, such as an offset prosthesis that can attach to residual incus. Another option for incus necrosis or a loose prosthesis is bone cement (hydroxyapatite cement), which may be used to better secure the prosthesis to the incus (Fig. 47.5). If utilized, the surgeon should be careful not to drip the cement around the footplate and try to bond the prosthesis to the incus by applying the cement 360° around both structures to enable better adherence. Malleovestibulopexy or total ossicular replacement prosthesis are other options in cases of far-advanced necrosis of the incus long process. In the latter, it is important to consider middle ear ventilation and any evidence of Eustachian tube dysfunction given the lack of rigid fixation on either side of the prosthesis. Overall, it is encouraged that surgeons explore their equipment options with their operating room staff and manufacturer representatives so that all bases are covered.

Due to the likelihood of adhesions, the use of laser (CO_2, KTP, argon—per surgeon preference and facility availabil-

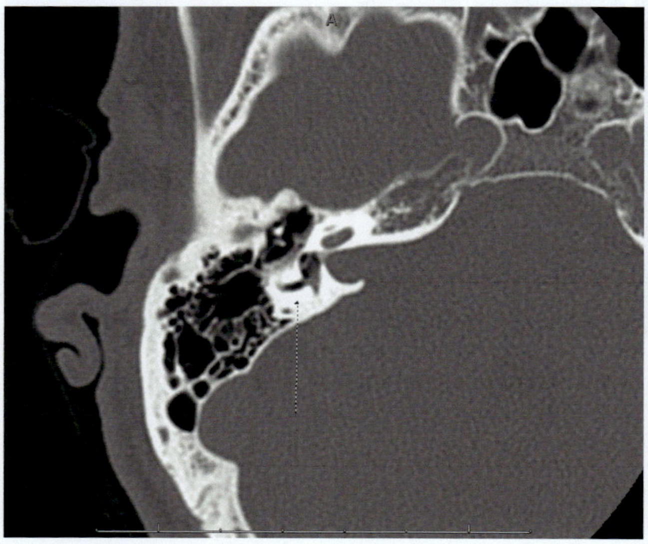

Fig. 47.4 Pneumolabyrinth demonstrated on an axial view of a CT. Air is seen in the vestibular and lateral semicircular canal (arrow). (Courtesy of Alex D. Sweeney, M.D.)

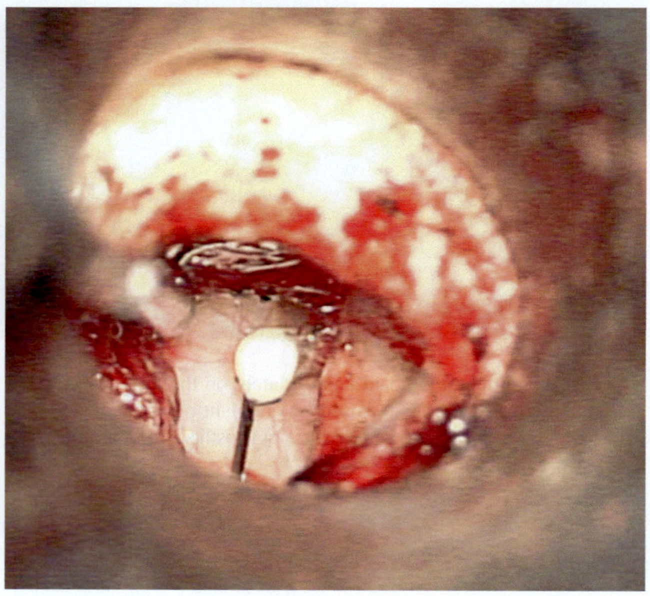

Fig. 47.5 Use of hydroxyapatite cement for incus necrosis

ity) may be helpful to minimize manipulation of the stapes footplate. In addition to lysis of the adhesions, lasers can also provide hemostasis and controlled re-fenestration of the footplate with a tightly regulated depth of heat penetrance into the perilymph. However, as with primary surgeries, if the facial nerve is dehiscent or significantly overhanging the footplate, the laser must be used carefully, or not at all, to avoid thermal injury.

Some surgeons prefer to perform revision stapedectomy under local-only anesthetic to assess for vertigo during the manipulation of the prosthesis and to verify hearing improvement intraoperatively. Other surgeons choose to utilize general anesthesia for all stapes surgeries, which can also lead to good outcomes, as discussed in the previous chapter. Ultimately, this decision comes down to surgeon preference.

Hearing Outcomes

Despite the heightened risks of revision stapes surgery, measurable audiologic benefits can still exist, thus justifying the consideration of this procedure. In a systematic review, the mean rate of air–bone gap (ABG) closure to within 10 and 20 dB was 51% and 74%, respectively [11]. Recent studies have demonstrated the mean postoperative ABG after revision cases being 7–16 dB [3, 5, 12–16]. While beneficial, it is noteworthy that these outcomes remain significantly worse than those of primary stapes surgery both in absolute and relative values [12, 15]. Furthermore, with each successive revision, the magnitude and chance of hearing improvement diminish [14, 16]. That being said, hearing improvement in revision cases does appear to be as durable over the course of the first year as compared to those after primary surgery [13].

Several patient and intraoperative factors may influence audiologic outcomes. Regarding patient selection, multiple studies have shown that those with recurrent hearing loss after initially successful primary surgery achieved better postoperative ABG than those with persistent hearing loss [3, 16, 17]. Failure to improve hearing with primary stapes surgery may denote other reasons for conductive hearing loss, such as superior canal dehiscence or round window obliteration. This patient population has independently shown worse audiologic outcomes after revision surgery [17]. Regarding intraoperative factors, there is no consistent data correlating intraoperative findings to audiologic outcomes; however, some authors have suggested that issues at the oval window (e.g., obliteration), abundant fibrous tissue, reparative granuloma, and round window obliteration present larger obstacles to hearing improvement [3, 12, 17].

Other authors have suggested that prosthesis dislocation as the primary cause for failure is associated with higher success rates [5, 18]. Schwam et al. and Lippy et al. both demonstrated an audiologic benefit of using lasers (CO_2 and Argon, respectively) in revision cases [12, 14]. Furthermore, Lippy et al. suggested the best audiologic outcomes may be achieved with the use of a Robinson prosthesis, but this has not been validated in other studies [3, 5, 12, 14]. Importantly, it does appear that audiologic outcomes are worse when the incus is not available to be utilized in reconstruction [3, 14, 18].

Regarding sensorineural hearing changes, revision cases have a higher rate of sensorineural hearing loss [3, 4, 15]. The systematic reviews by Battista et al. and Schmid et al. detail rates of sensorineural hearing loss and deafness between 0–20% and 0–14%, respectively, after revision surgery [10, 11]. Other studies have suggested that the average rates of these outcomes are 5.1% and 1.8%, respectively, which remain considerably higher than those after primary surgery [19].

Complications

Outside of audiologic outcomes as discussed above, complications after revision surgery are akin to those after primary surgery and include, but are not limited to, benign paroxysmal positional vertigo (BPPV), third window phenomena, perilymphatic fistula, dysgeusia, facial nerve paresis, endolymphatic hydrops, and reparative granuloma. Schwam et al. demonstrated a higher rate of overall otologic complications in revision cases, with the largest differences in rates of endolymphatic hydrops and reparative granuloma [12]. In contrast, other studies have reported rates of postoperative dizziness and dysgeusia similar to those after primary stapes surgery [13, 19–21].

Conclusion

Revision stapes surgery can be complex, from the review of prior medical records to the preoperative counseling and the actual technical performance of the surgery. Thus, expectations must align between the surgeon and the patient. Though outcomes in these cases can be excellent and gratifying, all cases of revision stapes surgery should involve careful patient selection, thorough counseling, and meticulous surgical technique.

References

1. Vrabec JT, Coker NJ. Stapes surgery in the United States. Otol Neurotol. 2004;25:465–9.
2. Meyer TA, Lambert PR. Primary and revision stapedectomy in elderly patients. Curr Opin Otolaryngol Head Neck Surg. 2004;12:387–92.
3. Babighian GG, Albu S. Failures in stapedotomy for otosclerosis. Otolaryngol Head Neck Surg. 2009;141(3):395–400.

4. Sakano H, Harris JP. Revision stapes surgery. Curr Otorhinolaryngol Rep. 2022;10(1):40–8.
5. Gros A, Vatovec J, Zargi M, Jenko K. Success rate in revision stapes surgery for otosclerosis. Otol Neurotol. 2005;26:1143–8.
6. Marchica C, Saliba I. The relationship between stapes prosthesis length and rate of stapedectomy success. Clin Med Insights Ear Nose Throat. 2015;24(8):23–31.
7. Normant S, Gendre A, Boucher S, Godey B, Bordure P, Michel G. Predictive factors of revision stapes surgery in otosclerosis. J Laryngol Otol. 2023;137(8):906–9.
8. McGee TM. The loose wire syndrome. Laryngoscope. 1981;91(9):1478–83.
9. Whetstone J, Nguyen A, Nguyen-Huynh A, Hamilton BE. Surgical and clinical confirmation of temporal bone CT findings in patients with otosclerosis with failed stapes surgery. AJNR Am J Neuroradiol. 2014;35(6):1195–201.
10. Battista RA, Wiet RJ, Joy J. Revision stapedectomy. Otolaryngol Clin North Am. 2006;39(4):677–97, v-vi.
11. Schmid A, Hausler R. Revision stapedectomy: an analysis of 201 operations. Otol Neurotol. 2009;30:1092–100.
12. Schwam ZG, Schettino A, Babu SC, Bojrab DI, Michaelides EM, Schutt CA. Outcomes in revision stapes surgery. Otolaryngol Head Neck Surg. 2021;165(5):705–9.
13. Andersen SA, Ohman MC, Sorensen MS. The stability of short-term hearing outcome after stapedotomy: a prospective database study. Acta Otolaryngol. 2015;135(9):871–9.
14. Lippy WH, Battista RA, Berenholz L, Schuring AG, Burkey JM. Twenty-year review of revision stapedectomy. Otol Neurotol. 2003;24:560–6.
15. Sharaf K, Grueninger I, Hilpert A, et al. Stapes and stapes revision surgery: preoperative air-bone gap is a prognostic marker. Otol Neurotol. 2021;42(7):985–93.
16. Ozuer MZ, Olgun L, Gultekin G. Revision stapes surgery. Otolaryngol Head Neck Surg. 2012;146(1):109–13.
17. Luryi AL, Schettino A, Michaelides EM, Babu S, Bojrab DI, Schutt CA. Revision stapes surgery: hearing symptoms and associations with intraoperative findings and outcomes. Otolaryngol Head Neck Surg. 2022;167(2):350–5.
18. Wegner I, Vincent R, Derks LSM, et al. An internally validated prognostic model for success in revision stapes surgery for otosclerosis. Laryngoscope. 2018;128(10):2390–6.
19. Hall AC, Mandavia R, Selvadurai D. Total endoscopic stapes surgery: systematic review and pooled analysis of audiological outcomes. Laryngoscope. 2020;130(5):1282–6.
20. Pauli N, Finizia C, Lundman L, Bjorsne A, Dahlin-Redfors Y. Are there differences in revision stapes surgery outcomes between university and county clinics? A study from the quality register for otosclerosis surgery in Sweden. Eur Arch Otorhinolaryngol. 2023;280(5):2247–55.
21. Bartel R, Sanz JJ, Clemente I, et al. Endoscopic stapes surgery outcomes and complication rates: a systematic review. Eur Arch Otorhinolaryngol. 2021;278(8):2673–9.

Part VII

Diseases of the Inner Ear and Skull Base

Pulsatile Tinnitus, Tonal Tinnitus, and Hyperacusis

48

Michael D. Seidman, Firas K. Sbeih, Syed Ahsan, and Tanya Singh

Introduction

Tinnitus is the perception of sound in the absence of an external acoustic stimulus. It is a common and potentially debilitating symptom with various etiologies. A detailed history and focused physical examination are crucial to identifying the underlying cause. There are currently no U.S. Food and Drug Administration (FDA)-approved treatments for tinnitus and it remains poorly understood. However, treatment options are available to help patients improve their quality of life and possibly mitigate the tinnitus. Tinnitus places a large economic burden on our healthcare system and is the number one cause of disability in veterans [1].

Hyperacusis may be described as a diminished tolerance to ordinary environmental sounds that leads to discomfort, distress, or disproportionate reactions [2]. Other definitions may emphasize the annoyance, phonophobia, irritability, pain, or other negative responses related to certain sounds [3]. Many patients suffer from tinnitus and hyperacusis concomitantly. Most of our understanding of hyperacusis stems from tinnitus-focused research, and therapies directed at alleviating tinnitus have shown some benefit in reducing hyperacusis.

M. D. Seidman (✉)
Otologic/Neurotologic/Skull Base Surgery, Wellness and Integrative Medicine, Advent Health, Orlando, FL, USA

Otolaryngology—Head and Neck Surgery, University of Central Florida, Orlando, FL, USA

Department of Otolaryngology—Head and Neck Surgery, University of South Florida, Tampa, FL, USA
e-mail: Michael.Seidman.MD@adventhealth.com

F. K. Sbeih · T. Singh
University of Central Florida College of Medicine, Orlando, FL, USA
e-mail: Firas_Sbeih@knights.ucf.edu; TanyaSingh@knights.ucf.edu

S. Ahsan
Otology/Neurotology, Kaiser Permanente—Southern California, Department of Otolaryngology—Head & Neck Surgery, University of California, Irvine, Irvine, CA, USA

Epidemiology of Tinnitus

Over 50 million US adults have experienced tinnitus with around one-third experiencing frequent symptoms over the past 12 months [4, 5]. The 2011–2012 results from the U.S. Centers for Disease Control National Health and Nutrition Examinations Survey estimate that 15% of US adults experienced tinnitus with 67% reporting frequent symptoms over the past year. It is more common in men and in the non-Hispanic White population, and increases with age until the seventh decade, after which the prevalence decreases with increasing age [4, 6, 7]. Tinnitus can be intermittent or continuous; the severity of which can vary across the patient population with about 2–4% reporting severe debilitating symptoms [4].

Classification of Tinnitus

There are several ways to categorize tinnitus. One method is to classify tinnitus as either subjective or objective [8]. Subjective tinnitus is much more common and represents an auditory perception only the patient hears [9]. Tonal tinnitus (non-pulsatile) is a type of subjective tinnitus in which the patient hears a well-defined sound such as ringing or hissing. Objective tinnitus is caused by somatosounds or mechanical sounds created within the body that can be detected by the subject and occasionally the examiner [10, 11].

The management of tinnitus varies depending on the type of tinnitus experienced by the patient. A thorough medical history and physical examination are required to rule out possible causes of tinnitus, as well as to guide subsequent workup. Thus, it is critical to identify the type of tinnitus the patient is experiencing. The following sections provide a detailed discussion of the different types of tinnitus and the options available for treatment.

A. D. Sweeney et al. (eds.), *Haynes-Glasscock-Shambaugh Surgery of the Ear*, https://doi.org/10.1007/978-3-032-18264-7_48

Pulsatile Tinnitus

Pulsatile tinnitus (PT) can be described as a rhythmic pulsating sound, usually synchronous with the patient's heart beat. Tinnitus that varies with movement, exertion, positional changes, or during physical examination points towards pulsatile tinnitus [12]. While pulsatile tinnitus is far less common, the associated structural pathophysiology makes it amenable to pinpointing a potential cause. The source of the tinnitus may also be audible to the examiner via a Toynbee stethoscope [13, 14]. Causes of pulsatile tinnitus are generally vascular or muscular in origin and can be classified as pulsatile, muscular, or spontaneous subtypes [15]. Pulsatile tinnitus may derive from turbulent blood flow secondary to vascular anomalies such as arteriovenous malformations (AVMs), carotid stenosis, or vascular heart disease [15]. Muscular tinnitus presents with clicking noise, and is commonly caused by palatal myoclonus, stapedius or tensor tympani muscle spasm, or a patulous Eustachian tube [16]. Another type of tinnitus, which is rare, is termed "typewriter tinnitus" and is potentially associated with vascular compression of the auditory nerve at the cerebellopontine angle (CPA)/porus acousticus by a loop of the anterior inferior cerebellar artery (AICA). These patients present with a "machine gun" or "typewriter" unilateral intermittent sounds. This is distinguished from middle ear myoclonus by abnormal finding on auditory brainstem response (ABR), lack of trigger from sound exposure, association with dizziness or facial spasm, magnetic resonance imaging (MRI) findings of vascular compression, and improvement with carbamazepine [17]. It's important to emphasize that, in some cases, the only evidence of "typewriter" tinnitus is a positive response to carbamazepine.

Table 48.1 Causes of pulsatile tinnitus

Vascular		Non-Vascular
Arterial	Venous (most common)	Glomus tumor Middle ear effusion Chronic otitis Arnold-Chiari malformation Paraganglioma Idiopathic intracranial hypertension Otosclerosis Palatal myoclonus Superior semicircular canal dehiscence Paget's disease Meningioma
Arteriosclerotic plaques (common in elderly patients) Aberrant internal carotid artery Carotid artery stenosis Carotid artery dissection Carotid artery fibromuscular dysplasia Persistent stapedial artery High cardiac output (anemia, thyrotoxicosis, or pregnancy) Carotid cavernous fistula	High-riding jugular bulb Sigmoid diverticulum Sigmoid sinus dehiscence Jugular diverticulum Large emissary vein Condylar vein abnormalities Intramastoid venous channel Transverse sinus stenosis	
Arteriovenous malformation Arteriovenous Fistula		

Mechanism

It is unclear why some patients experience pulsatile tinnitus, while others with similar underlying pathology do not. One theory is that individuals experiencing pulsatile tinnitus have alterations in the inner ear allowing them to detect normal flow sounds not audible to other people. Alternatively, the discrepancy may simply be related to the pathology of increased turbulence [18]. The exact pathophysiology is difficult to ascertain due to the various etiologies linked with pulsatile tinnitus. As noted earlier, pulsatile tinnitus can be vascular or nonvascular (Table 48.1). Vascular causes may be arterial in origin, such as carotid artery atherosclerosis, carotid artery dissection, persistent stapedial artery, or carotid artery fibromuscular dysplasia [12, 19]. Venous causes of tinnitus are congenital variants and pathologic transformations that include high jugular bulb, sigmoid sinus, and jugular vein diverticulum; sigmoid sinus dehiscence; transverse or sigmoid stenosis; and condylar vein abnormalities [12, 18, 20]. Arteriovenous anomalies such as arteriovenous malformations and dural arteriovenous fistulas (dural AVF) can also contribute [18]. Nonvascular causes of pulsatile tinnitus include neoplasms such as paragangliomas, osseous pathology such as Paget's disease, superior semicircular canal dehiscence (SSCD), and idiopathic intracranial hypertension (IIH) [19]. Unfortunately in about 30% of cases of pulsatile tinnitus, a root cause is not identified [12, 21].

Diagnosis

Patients with pulsatile tinnitus require a thorough evaluation. A sound approach to the diagnosis of tinnitus described by Ahsan et al. is to determine whether the pulsatile tinnitus is arterial, venous, or nonvascular in origin [13]. Arterial and venous tinnitus can be distinguished by compression of vasculature in the neck. Slight compression would occlude a vein and therefore decrease tinnitus of venous but not arterial origin. Dampening an arterial tinnitus, however, would require stronger compression to occlude the carotid artery (Table 48.2) [22]. Arterial causes may also manifest as a bruit that is audible on auscultation of the affected side, such as a carotid bruit. A carotid Doppler or computed tomography angiography (CTA) should be used to confirm the diagnosis [13]. If CTA is inconclusive, a four-vessel cerebral arteriography should be considered, but it may not reveal any new findings [12]. Four-vessel cerebral angiography is superior to CTA when it comes to detecting small dural arteriovenous malformations (AVMs), which supports the consideration of a four-vessel angiogram given a negative CTA when suspicion of a dural AVM is high [12,

Table 48.2 Physical exam findings which can differentiate venous from arterial pulsatile tinnitus (PT)

Physical exam maneuvers	Venous	Arterial
Ipsilateral Jugular vein compression	Reduction in tinnitus	No effect
Contralateral Jugular vein compression	Increase	No effect
Head rotation to opposite to side of PT	Increase	No effect
Head rotation towards side of PT	Decrease	No effect
Valsalva maneuver	Decrease	No effect
Firm compression of ipsilateral carotid	No affect	Decrease

23]. These imaging studies come with certain risks such as radiation exposure, contrast-induced nephropathy, and stroke. In general, the authors recommend a CTA for unilateral pulsatile tinnitus which is not audible by use of Toynbee stethoscope. The CTA can identify the more common causes of PT such as Superior Semicircular Canal (SCC) dehiscence, sigmoid sinus diverticulum/dehiscence as well as jugular bulb abnormalities. It can also be relied upon to identify a dural AVF. For bilateral pulsatile tinnitus, an MRI +/− MRA/MRV (magnetic resonance angiography/magnetic resonance venography) is recommended because one of the most common causes is benign intracranial hypertension/idiopathic intracranial hypertension (IIH). Some indirect signs of IIH are noted on MRI (T2 sequence), such as posterior globe flattening, buckling of the optic nerve, empty sella, distension of the optic nerve sheath, and transverse sinus stenosis or absence.

Nonvascular causes of pulsatile tinnitus should also be considered and could be determined through history and physical examination. Idiopathic intracranial hypertension is a common cause of pulsatile tinnitus often observed in young, overweight females [24]. These patients may also present with headaches, visual changes, neck pain, and characteristic findings of papilledema on funduscopic examination, in the latter stages. If the patient meets the Dandy criteria for IIH as demonstrated by increased intracranial pressure (ICP) without any obvious causes for the increased ICP, IIH likely explains the tinnitus [24]. More than half of the patients who suffer from IIH demonstrate symptoms of pulsatile tinnitus with the majority experiencing bilateral tinnitus [25]. IIH could be considered a venous cause of pulsatile tinnitus as it appears that the tinnitus is caused by venous stenosis, resulting in turbulent flow in the transverse venous sinus [18, 26]. Anemia and thyrotoxicosis can also lead to pulsatile tinnitus due to high cardiac output [15]. It is also important to consider the possibility of superior semicircular canal dehiscence (SSCD) as a cause of pulsatile tinnitus. SSCD was first described by Lloyd Minor, MD et al. in 1998 [27]. Patients with SSCD can experience a range of symptoms from aural fullness, dizziness often exacerbated by loud sound (Tullio sign), autophony, conductive hearing loss, and pulsatile tinnitus.

Treatment

The treatment of pulsatile tinnitus is dependent on its etiology. The infrequency of pulsatile tinnitus coupled with the lack of prospective randomized clinical trials for its treatment makes recommending treatment options more challenging. For this reason, following a thorough history and physical examination, targeted laboratory evaluation assessing for cardiovascular health via markers such as cholesterol panel and imaging is recommended to delineate the etiology and pinpoint the location of the anomaly. Pentoxifylline (trental), typically used for claudication, has the potential to improve blood flow and decrease turbulence in the inner ear. The senior author (MDS) has utilized pentoxifylline (trental®) 400 mg three times a day (t.i.d.) with up to 70% of patients noting improvement. This treatment could be offered for 3–4 months and discontinued if ineffective. More invasive approaches have also been used for the treatment of pulsatile tinnitus. In a retrospective analysis of patients who received carotid endarterectomy for severe carotid artery stenosis, 70% of patients who suffered from pulsatile tinnitus reported symptomatic improvement [28]. Stenting of the internal carotid artery in patients with pulsatile tinnitus has also been shown to be effective [29]. In patients with transverse sinus, sigmoid sinus, jugular bulb diverticula, or dural AVF as a cause of their pulsatile tinnitus, endovascular treatment with coiling has attenuated the tinnitus [18, 20, 30].

Tonal Tinnitus

Tonal tinnitus is the perception of a near-continuous sound at a well-defined frequency such as ringing, hissing, or buzzing. Tonal tinnitus is categorized as subjective tinnitus, and the patient is able to define a specific pitch to the tinnitus [31]. In certain populations such as Germany, tonal tinnitus accounts for 50% of all tinnitus cases [32].

Pathophysiology

The pathophysiology of tonal tinnitus is not clear, although several theories exist to explain the underlying mechanism. The complexity of the pathophysiology of tinnitus derives from the complexity of the auditory pathway and its robust interactions with other central systems such as the limbic system [33]. Tinnitus has been linked to a variety of etiologies such as otologic, neurologic, infectious, and drug-related causes [15]. Otologic causes include noise-induced hearing loss, presbycusis, otosclerosis, impacted cerumen, Ménière's disease (MD), as well as other causes of hearing loss [15]. Tinnitus has been linked to affective disorders such as depression and generalized anxiety disorder, and has also been associated with stress, hypertension, sleep disorders, cognitive decline, and more [34, 35].

While analyzing central and peripheral pathways to identify a cause, it is apparent that the etiology of tinnitus is multifactorial, and there are myriad factors to be considered. A comparison between those who suffer from tinnitus and those who do not may reveal more insight into the pathophysiology. Challenges with such a comparison are due to potential confounders such as age, sex, social activities, comorbid diseases, medications, stress, sleep, and various etiologies that lead to tinnitus in the first place [4].

Several studies suggest that neural hyperactivity and an imbalance between excitation and inhibition pathways may be central to many cases of tinnitus. Increased neuronal activity in the dorsal cochlear nucleus (DCN) in the absence of a physical stimulus has been demonstrated to induce phantom sound impression [36, 37]. The discordant dysfunction theory attributes DCN hyperactivity to an imbalance between damaged outer hair cells (OHCs) and better functioning inner hair cells (IHCs) [38]. Brozoski et al. have demonstrated the role of the DCN in tinnitus using animal models, but attempting ablation of the DCN in rats to extinguish tinnitus did not improve tinnitus [39]. The lack of improvement following DCN ablation may further suggest that the pathophysiology of tinnitus is not a straightforward pathway. The DCN likely plays an important role in the perception of tinnitus, but additional research is needed to delineate how the entire auditory system integrates in tinnitus patients as well as to evaluate the effects of non-auditory structures.

Other important areas in the study of tinnitus are the GABAergic input, limbic system, cochlear nerve activity, cerebellum, and comorbid etiologies. GABA deficiency has been demonstrated in the auditory cortex of tinnitus patients and could explain the presence of excessive signaling [40]. Similarly, excessive signaling was noted in the auditory midbrain of patients with decreased cochlear input when examined with functional magnetic resonance imaging (fMRI) [41]. The elevation in signaling on fMRI may instead be explained by hyperacusis. Elevation in the neural activity of the paraflocculus in the cerebellum was also linked to tinnitus [42].

The limbic system is considered to play a crucial role in tinnitus perception and assigning importance of tinnitus. The amygdala, part of the limbic system which is essential to the processing of experiences and relating emotions to various stimuli, demonstrates increased activity due to tinnitus [43]. It is not exactly clear whether the amygdala is related to the emergence of tinnitus or assigning an aversive emotion to it. The limbic system may serve a more important central role in tinnitus perception (i.e., distress) as it could be implicated in a gating mechanism that may or may not permit the tinnitus signal to be perceived [44].

Diagnostic Techniques

In 2014, The American Academy of Otolaryngology-Head and Neck Surgery (AAO-HNS) released the first evidence-based clinical guideline to help healthcare providers manage patients with tinnitus [45]. The guideline development involved extensive literature search and input from healthcare providers from various fields, such as otolaryngology, neurology, audiology, psychiatry, and radiology [45]. The guideline provides a set of key action statements on a variety of decisions typically made during the care of tinnitus patients.

History and Physical Examination

A focused history in a patient with tinnitus should include quality of the tinnitus, onset, duration, chronicity, severity, laterality, mitigating, and aggravating factors. It is also important to note the setting in which the patient experiences their symptoms and associated symptoms such as vertigo or hyperacusis.

The physician should inquire about the patient's past medical and surgical history as tinnitus could be related to medical illnesses such as hyperthyroidism or anemia [15]. Special attention should be focused on the history of hearing loss, neurological symptoms, and family history of tinnitus, vertigo, or hearing loss. All medications, supplements, and dietary habits with particular attention to salt, caffeine, sweeteners, and alcohol use need to be noted. The patient should also be asked about smoking, alcohol consumption, and recreational drug use. It is important to assess the patient's mental health and to screen for depression, anxiety, and stress.

The level of distress patients experience from tinnitus varies and may or may not affect quality of life and functionality [45]. To aid in the assessment of tinnitus, several validated questionnaires exist to help the patient scale the severity of their symptoms and the impact on quality of life. These include the Tinnitus Questionnaire (TQ), Tinnitus Handicap Inventory (THI), Tinnitus Coping Style Questionnaire, Visual Analog Scale (VAS), and the Tinnitus Functional Index (TFI) [46–49]. These questionnaires are also used in clinical trials to assess the efficacy of a treatment under investigation.

The physical examination should include a microscopic examination of the ears, pneumatic otoscopy, cranial nerve testing, and a tuning fork examination. The physician should also auscultate the heart for murmurs, the neck for bruits, and auscultate around the ears bilaterally. Compression of the neck vessels with different levels of pressure should be performed on one side at a time while asking the patient to report changes in the loudness of the tinnitus to evaluate for pulsatile tinnitus.

Audiometry

The AAO-HNS clinical guideline recommends a comprehensive audiologic evaluation for any patient with tinnitus that is unilateral, chronic (greater than 6 months), or associated with hearing impairment. Physicians may still offer a comprehensive audiologic evaluation to patients presenting with tinnitus even if they do not meet the recommendation criteria [45]. The audiologic evaluation should include pure-tone testing for both air and bone conduction to distinguish the type of hearing loss. Speech reception thresholds should also be assessed to identify the extent of the hearing deficit. Psychoacoustic measures such as tinnitus loudness, loudness match, minimal masking levels, and residual inhibition may be tested and can help in the management of patients [50]. Otoacoustic emission testing may be useful in that it provides insight into the functionality of the outer hair cells, which have been implicated in the pathophysiology of tinnitus.

Imaging

The decision to pursue diagnostic imaging depends on information gathered from the history and physical examination. Diagnostic imaging studies are not recommended in the evaluation of a tinnitus patient unless the patient's tinnitus is unilateral, pulsatile, associated with asymmetric hearing loss, or associated with focal neurologic deficits [45]. For unilateral tonal tinnitus or tonal tinnitus associated with focal neurological symptoms or signs, imaging with MRI should be recommended.

Treatment

Physician Counseling and Reassurance

Anxiety is common among patients who suffer from tinnitus. It is very important for the provider to avoid the use of negative counseling strategies that provide no hope. The physician should inform the patient that although there is currently no FDA approved treatment for tinnitus, there are interventions that could help mitigate their symptoms. The patient should be reassured that tinnitus is a symptom, not a disease and is rarely a sign of a dangerous disorder.

Patients should be advised that their tinnitus distress is likely to improve without the need for medical intervention, as evidenced by many clinical trials in which tinnitus sufferers experience significant improvements despite receiving placebo treatment. Additionally, clinical observation has noted that avoidance of salt, caffeine, alcohol, simple sugars, sweeteners, and other dietary modifications may improve a patient's tinnitus [4].

The history and physical along with the audiologic evaluation should guide the management of tinnitus. If the tinnitus seems to be related to an offending agent such as salicylates, aminoglycosides, PDE5 (phosphodiesterase-5) inhibitors or diuretics, then cessation of the offending agent is required to resolve the tinnitus [51]. Withdrawal of certain drugs such as benzodiazepines has also been implicated in tinnitus [52, 53].

The following sections will review some of the common strategies utilized in the management of tonal tinnitus. These include hearing aids, masking therapy, tinnitus retraining therapy (TRT), psychological interventions, pharmacologic, surgical, and alternative therapies. The success of these strategies varies widely, and there has not been consistent evidence to support the use of one treatment modality over another. Treatment should utilize less invasive treatment options initially followed by more invasive strategies, if initial treatment fails and the tinnitus is severe.

Hearing Aids and Masking Therapy

Hearing aids are believed to help improve tinnitus by augmenting external sounds that make the patient's tinnitus less noticeable. Hearing aids may also help offset the rewiring of neural circuits believed to take place in the auditory cortex of a patient with hearing loss; this is the basis of the neural plasticity theory of tinnitus [54].

Patients who utilized hearing aids along with counseling showed more improvement in their tinnitus handicap questionnaire results compared to patients who received counseling alone [55]. Prospective studies have also demonstrated improvements in subjective tinnitus among patients receiving hearing aids [56, 57]. The masking of tinnitus employs the concept of residual inhibition where sounds are utilized to minimize the perception of the patient's tinnitus [58].

Masking is a reasonable initial approach to help with tinnitus, and there can be some residual inhibition of the sound even after the masking sound is off [59]. It is possible to achieve residual inhibition with sounds that have a wide range of frequencies. The residual inhibition caused by masking therapy is usually transient and sometimes lasts only seconds to minutes. In addition, peripheral masking becomes less effective in chronic tinnitus cases such as those lasting longer than 4 years. In certain cases, hearing aids may exacerbate the tinnitus, especially if the hearing aids are occlusive.

Tinnitus Retraining Therapy

The neurophysiological model of tinnitus developed by Jastreboff demonstrates the complexity of the interconnections between the auditory system, limbic system, autonomic nervous system, and the auditory cortex [38]. These interconnections can explain how emotions and perceptions related to the tinnitus can exacerbate the severity of the tinnitus. Tinnitus retraining therapy (TRT), developed by Jastreboff and Jastreboff, is a therapy technique aimed at reducing the symptoms of tinnitus through habituation to the evoked responses [60]. The therapy is based on neurophysiological evidence that acoustic signals coupled with directive counseling can habituate the patient to their tinnitus, allowing for improved quality of life. This is achieved by attempting to extinguish the conditioned arc reflexes, described in the neurophysiological model, between the tinnitus perception in the auditory pathway and the emotional and physiological responses of the limbic and autonomic nervous system.

The two key components of TRT are directive counseling and sound therapy. Directive counseling is an intensive and interactive assessment of the patient's emotional and physiological responses to tinnitus. The patient is educated about the auditory pathway and how sound signals captured by the ear are translated to neuronal signals in the auditory cortex. The patient is also educated about the neurophysiology underlying tinnitus, and the potential to improve by rewiring the interconnections facilitating the negative tinnitus response. Sound therapy utilizes acoustic stimuli meant to induce reorganization of signals in the auditory pathway to eliminate or reduce the perception of tinnitus. The sound signal is set at a level that does not interfere with normal hearing, but still allows for auditory habituation. The sound signal recommended is usually broad-band and causes some masking of the tinnitus. The physician would also recommend environmental background noise exposure when the patient is not using the sound generator, and the avoidance of silence.

TRT has delivered promising results with many studies showing improvement in tinnitus results. In one study, 82% of the patients showed statistically significant improvement in their THI scores after 12 months of therapy [61]. Other studies have produced similar results [62]. In 2019, the Tinnitus Retraining Therapy Trial published their results for a randomized, placebo-controlled, multicenter study on tinnitus retraining therapy versus standard of care at several participating military hospitals [63]. The study had 151 participants with a follow-up of 18 months. The patients were divided into three groups based on TRT with conventional sound generators + counseling, placebo sound generators + counseling, or standard of care (typical information provided to patients with tinnitus at participating military medical centers based on guidelines from American Speech Language Hearing Association). The standard of care focused on the patients symptoms and aimed to reduce negative cognitive, affective, physical, and behavioral reactions to tinnitus and the patients were encouraged to use environmental sound enrichment when possible but no use of sound generators. The results of the study was that there was no difference between treatment groups with respect to tinnitus distress using TQ, TFI, THI, and Visual Analog scale (VAS). Their findings are inconsistent with those of other studies. Missed visits and smaller than planned sample size may have masked true differences between groups.

Psychological Treatment

Cognitive behavioral therapy (CBT), originally developed for the treatment of anxiety and depression, has been shown to have promising results on reducing negative perceptions related to tinnitus. CBT utilizes restructuring of negative thoughts into more helpful and positive outlooks [64]. The usual weekly therapy sessions involve interactive communication between the patient and the provider with a focus on altering the patient's negative beliefs into more optimistic views. The patient is encouraged to avoid catastrophizing and to develop alternative views that encourage improvement. Cognitive behavioral therapy has been shown to be as effective as tinnitus retraining therapy [62].

Pharmacologic Therapy

There is currently no FDA approved medical treatment for tonal tinnitus. The medications utilized in the treatment of tinnitus act to alleviate symptoms associated with tinnitus rather than affecting the tinnitus itself. For instance, antidepressants and antianxiety drugs have been used in the treatment of tinnitus to nullify the psychological aspects that exacerbate it. The lack of rigorous research combined with potential side effects precludes pharmacological therapies from being first-line options. The following sections will review some of the pharmacological treatments utilized in the management of tinnitus.

The depression and anxiety that usually accompany tinnitus have led to many investigations on the role of antidepressants and antianxiety medications in the treatment of tinnitus. In a randomized, double-blinded, placebo-controlled study, sertraline was found to be superior to placebo treatment in improving tinnitus as documented by the Tinnitus Severity Questionnaire and a visual analog scale for tinnitus loudness and annoyance [65]. However, a Cochrane review of six trials that utilized antidepressants to treat tinnitus demonstrated the need for more standardization in clinical studies. Only one study out of the six was considered to have a grade A overall quality, another one was considered grade B, and the other four were given grade C [66]. The review showed that there was not a significant benefit from the use of antidepressants in treating tinnitus, and the side-effect profile for antidepressants was not tolerable in many patients [66].

On the other hand, a randomized placebo-controlled study of alprazolam showed reduction in tinnitus and tinnitus annoyance in 76% of the patients in the treatment group compared to 5% of the patients receiving placebo [67]. Another randomized clinical trial demonstrated superiority of alprazolam over placebo in improving visual analog scale scores, but lacked statistically significant improvement in THI and tinnitus loudness scores [68]. The lack of consistency in results combined with scarcity of rigorous research makes it difficult to judge antidepressants and antianxiety medications when it comes to the treatment of tinnitus. The side-effect profile of many of these medications also makes it difficult to ensure true blinding of patients during clinical trials.

Gabapentin has been also considered as an agent to treat tinnitus. However, several randomized clinical trials have shown that gabapentin was not superior to placebo in improving tinnitus [69–71]. The physician's clinical judgement and an individualized consideration of the patient's symptoms should guide the decision of whether to utilize any of these medications.

Transtympanic therapy has also been utilized in the treatment of tinnitus. Lidocaine is one agent that could be administered transtympanically and lead to the relief of tinnitus; however, the results are usually short-lived and have significant severe vertigo side effects which are often worse for the patient than the tinnitus [72]. Gentamicin and corticosteroids can also be administered transtympanically, and both show benefits in certain patients with tinnitus. Gentamicin has been shown to reduce symptoms of tinnitus in patients suffering from Ménière's disease, but its utility in other patients is limited [73]. Corticosteroids administered transtympanically have been shown to improve hearing loss and tinnitus. The effect on tinnitus might be secondary to the improvement in hearing loss. Auris Medical is investigating two novel drugs, AM-101 for the management of tinnitus and AM-111 for sudden sensorineural hearing loss (SNHL) and tinnitus. These medications affect the caspase pathway and JNK (c-Jun N-terminal kinase) receptors with AM-101 noted to have efficacy in reducing tinnitus caused by glutamate excitatoxicity [74].

Alternative Therapies

Complementary integrative medicine has been gaining popularity lately in the treatment of many chronic conditions. Lack of rigorous research trials on the efficacy of the different alternative medicines makes it challenging to use these therapies in the treatment of tinnitus. Alternative medicines have helped a number of patients improve their tinnitus symptoms and more people are likely to benefit as we gain a better understanding of the different agents. The challenge faced by complementary-integrative medicine is the lack of interest by pharmaceutical companies to fund research into this arena as it is deemed too expensive and unlikely to be protected by a patent [75].

A double-blinded, placebo-controlled study comparing 3 mg of melatonin to placebo found that melatonin did not improve tinnitus more than placebo. However, nearly half the patients who reported sleep difficulties related to their tinnitus reported improvement after the use of melatonin compared to 20% in the placebo group [76]. Melatonin seems to help patients suffering from tinnitus with concurrent sleep difficulties.

The B-complex vitamins may also help some patients with tinnitus, but again, more research is needed to make adequate recommendations on the use of these vitamins. Patients who experienced deficiency in these vitamins were found to have tinnitus [77]. The B-complex vitamins seem to help with tinnitus by providing a stabilizing effect on the peripheral and central nervous systems [75]. Most of the evidence for the success of these vitamins is anecdotal in nature. Vitamin B12 (cobalamin) has been helpful in several patients with severe tinnitus and a significant percentage of patients (47%) complaining of tinnitus have been found to be deficient in cobalamin [78]. This information supports the assessment of vitamin B12 levels during the initial evaluation of a tinnitus patient.

Zinc has also been the subject of a lot of research in the search for a cure for tinnitus. Zinc seems to play an intimate role in auditory physiology and cochlear protection. The copper/zinc superoxide dismutase antioxidant system is considered essential for the protection of the cochlea against free radical damage [79]. Research on the efficacy of zinc in treating tinnitus has yielded mixed results. A prospective, randomized, placebo-controlled clinical trial showed that 31% of patients with tinnitus had zinc deficiency and 82% of the patients treated with zinc demonstrated a decrease in severity of their subjective tinnitus [80]. However, a Cochrane review of three trials investigating the role of zinc in the treatment of tinnitus showed that there was no evidence for the improvement in tinnitus through zinc supplementation. The trials analyzed by the review did not assess the changes in quality of life and other important psychosocial aspects after treatment with zinc [81]. Further, well-designed research is required to evaluate the true association between zinc and tinnitus.

Ginkgo biloba, used for centuries to treat a variety of medical illnesses, has demonstrated benefit in a substantial number of tinnitus patients though its use remains controversial. The active ingredient believed to have medicinal benefits in ginkgo biloba is EGb 761. In a study analyzing 19 clinical trials that used EGb 761 for tinnitus treatment, EGb 761 demonstrated appreciable improvement in tinnitus. Eight out of the 19 studies utilized a comparison drug or a placebo and those studies also showed EGb 761 to be superior to the control group [82]. Ginkgo biloba was also considered to be very tolerable with no significant difference in side effects compared to the placebo group [82]. In comparison, a double-blinded randomized prospective study, out of Birmingham University in the UK, showed that patients who received 150 mg of ginkgo biloba daily did not have better outcomes than the placebo group [83]. However, this study did not use the EGb 761 extract of ginkgo biloba and used a suboptimal dose.

Procedural Interventions

While the management of tinnitus is typically nonsurgical, advances in surgical procedures coupled with favorable results achieved through invasive approaches have led to increased adoption of procedural interventions especially in patients with severe refractory tinnitus. The following sections will discuss some of the more common procedural approaches to treating tinnitus.

The association between tinnitus and hearing loss has sparked interest in the effects of cochlear implantation for hearing rehabilitation on tinnitus. In a study assessing these effects in patients with unilateral hearing loss, all 26 patients who received the operation reported subjective improvement in their tinnitus [84]. Another study involving post-lingually profoundly deaf adults also showed significant improvement in tinnitus following implantation [85]. However, other studies have reported either worsening of tinnitus or new-onset of tinnitus following implantation [85, 86]. In addition, cochlear implantation is also not available to all patients suffering with tinnitus as they need to qualify for the procedure based on the level of hearing impairment. Shorter electrode arrays are being investigated which can reduce tinnitus and preserve existing hearing [87].

Cochlear nerve sectioning has also been considered as a treatment option for tinnitus in the past. One study of 151 patients showed that 67% of patients had complete resolution of their tinnitus, 28% had improvement, and the remainder of patients experienced no improvement after nerve sectioning [88]. However, no other studies have matched these results. A study by House and Brackmann (1981) reported the results of translabyrinthine resection of the eighth cranial nerve in 68 patients, some of whom had vestibular nerve section (VNS) and others had VNS and cochlear nerve section (CNS). Improvement was noted in 45% of patients and 55% reported no change or worsening of their tinnitus. Subsequently, in a subgroup of 17 patients with Ménière's disease (MD), 12 had preoperative tinnitus and underwent VNS and CNS. After surgery, only three patients reported improvement in their tinnitus, while three stated that their tinnitus had worsened. In their report, 32 of 39 patients who underwent middle fossa VNS (superior and inferior vestibular neurectomy) had preoperative tinnitus. About 95% of patients had resolution or improved dizziness, but the tinnitus increased significantly. They concluded that cutting the cochlear nerve has little to no effect on tinnitus in MD patients [89].

Direct electrical stimulation of the auditory cortex is an investigational surgical approach that can be utilized to alleviate tinnitus. The theory behind this procedure is that peripheral injury of the auditory pathway will lead to maladaptive changes of the auditory circuit centrally. The central auditory pathway can be directly targeted through the auditory cortex, which could affect the tonotopic organization of Heschl's gyrus [90]. Our experience with direct electrical stimulation has yielded variable results with some patients experiencing no improvement, while others experienced significant improvements [91]. More research is needed to understand why patients respond differently to direct electrical stimulation of their auditory cortex.

Another investigational surgical treatment that has been evaluated is deep brain stimulation (DBS) of auditory and nonauditory regions of the brain. Historically, DBS has been effective in many disorders including Parkinson's disease, essential tremor, chronic pain, epilepsy, and obsessive-compulsive disorder [92–94]. DBS has the potential to stimulate deep brain regions of the classical and non-classical auditory pathways. Recent human and animal studies have targeted the ventral intermediate nucleus of the thalamus (VIM) and caudate nucleus to examine the suppressive effects on tinnitus [95–97]. Preliminary findings have shown modulation of tinnitus brain activity by stimulation of non-auditory regions [96, 97].

Vagal nerve stimulation has demonstrated some success in treating patients with severe refractory tinnitus. In a case series, ten patients with severe refractory chronic tinnitus received left-sided vagal nerve stimulation while hearing tones that excluded the tinnitus matched frequency [98]. Four out of the ten patients exhibited significant clinical improvement. In a prospective randomized double-blind placebo-controlled clinical trial, vagus nerve stimulation paired with tones was compared with unpaired vagus nerve stimulation. The results of the study showed that 50% of the paired group showed improvement, while only 28% of the control group demonstrated improvement in their symptoms [99]. More research is required to understand why patients respond differently to this treatment and how to determine the ideal candidate for this procedure.

Finally, another recent treatment option involves bimodal auditory and nonauditory stimulation to modulate tinnitus-related activity along the pathway. One treatment option involves the combination of auditory and electrical stimulation utilizing the plasticity of firing patterns in the cochlear nucleus . Meanwhile the second option involves pairing auditory stimulation with vagal stimulation which is aimed at rearranging the auditory cortical maps. Both treatment modalities have shown promising results in both objective and subjective outcomes [100].

Hyperacusis

Hyperacusis is an auditory disorder that manifests as an intolerance to ordinary environmental sounds that most people deem non-threatening or non-bothersome [2]. Other definitions of hyperacusis may emphasize annoyance, fear, pain, irritability, or other responses related to the offending sound [3].

Epidemiology

Prevalence studies of hyperacusis have been limited, but it is suggested to affect millions of people. Epidemiological studies in Poland and Sweden showed a prevalence of 15.2 and 8.6%, respectively [101, 102]. Hyperacusis was also found to affect patients with a variety of medical conditions, especially tinnitus. In a survey of patients with a primary complaint of hyperacusis, 86% also complained of tinnitus [103]. Conversely, patients with tinnitus as their primary complaint demonstrated a 40% prevalence of hyperacusis [103]. This degree of association suggests that tinnitus and hyperacusis may be linked by a similar underlying mechanism. Hyperacusis is also seen in patients with Lyme disease, Williams syndrome, post-traumatic stress disorder (PTSD), depression, migraine, Bell's palsy, head injury, and perilymph fistula [104]. The association between hyperacusis and these conditions may reveal more insight the pathophysiology of hyperacusis.

Pathophysiology

Similar to tinnitus, the pathophysiology of hyperacusis is poorly understood and several theories have been proposed to explain the underlying mechanism. The strong link between tinnitus and hyperacusis has led to significant interest in identifying a common mechanism. Neural hyperactivity and an imbalance between excitation and inhibition pathways may also contribute to hyperacusis. Peripheral or central damage to the auditory system has been strongly correlated to tinnitus and hyperacusis. According to the Central Gain Model, damage to the auditory system, whether peripherally or centrally, will lead to recalibration in sensitivity to account for the decreased sensory input [105]. The neuronal recalibration can induce erroneous signaling that would be perceived as tinnitus, and/or amplification of sensory signals leading to hyperacusis. Other models explaining hyperacusis include tonotopic reorganization and limbic system interactions, both of which are also thought to contribute to tinnitus.

The high prevalence of hyperacusis in individuals with Williams syndrome poses the question of whether the underlying mechanism can be generalized to other hyperacusis patients [106]. The proposed mechanism for this association involves 5-hydroxytryptamine (5-HT) dysfunction, which plays a role in modulation of auditory gain and assigning significance to sound [107]. 5-HT dysfunction is also present in conditions such as PTSD and migraine, which are commonly associated with hyperacusis [104]. 5-HT dysfunction cannot adequately explain or account for the occurrence of hyperacusis in other individuals. Additionally, the strong association with Williams syndrome may be related to auditory gain following conductive hearing loss due to repetitive bouts of otitis media with effusion [2].

Diagnosis

The evaluation of a hyperacusis patient should start by ruling out the aforementioned diseases as a cause. The physician should perform a focused history and physical examination. The history should elicit information related to the quality of the hyperacusis and whether it is associated with other symptoms such as tinnitus or vertigo. Depending on the clinical evaluation, the physician may opt to directly treat the suspected medical illness or pursue further testing. Laboratory testing can be utilized to diagnose conditions such as Lyme disease, neurosyphilis, hyperthyroidism, and vitamin deficiencies [108]. Imaging studies may also be required depending on the differential, as hyperacusis has been linked to vascular aneurysms, vascular malformations, multiple sclerosis, and Chiari malformations along with other anatomically variable conditions [108].

The evaluation of hyperacusis may include measurement of the uncomfortable loudness levels (ULLs). ULLs are usually decreased in patients with hyperacusis, with the average being around 70 dB HL [1–3, 109]. Different studies have yielded different results on ULLs, calling into question their utility. Subjective quantification of symptoms via questionnaires and other patient-response modalities, similar to what is available for tinnitus, is another option. The Hyperacusis Questionnaire (HQ) is a two-part questionnaire that scores patients' responses. Final scores range between 0 and 42, with 28 considered the threshold for hyperacusis [110]. Other questionnaires include the Multiple Activity Scale for Hyperacusis (MASH) and the German Questionnaire on Hypersensitivity to Sound (GUF) [111, 112].

Treatment

Counseling and patient education are an important part of the management of a hyperacusis patient. Due to the diminished tolerance to sounds, some patients turn to occlusive ear devices that reduce sound entry into the ears. Paradoxically, this could worsen the hyperacusis by increasing central auditory gain due to reduced sensory input to the auditory cortex [2].

Considering the increased incidence of hyperacusis in tinnitus patients coupled with a possible common underlying mechanism, it is not surprising that many of the current hyperacusis treatment options were originally intended to treat tinnitus. For instance, tinnitus retraining therapy, discussed earlier, has also been used to treat patients with hyperacusis. In one case series, TRT was utilized to treat 45 patients that had either tinnitus or hyperacusis or both. More than 80% of the patients with hyperacusis demonstrated subjective improvement [113].

In a randomized, placebo-controlled, clinical trial, 36 patients were divided into 4 treatment groups [114]. The group that received both directive counseling and binaural sound therapy demonstrated the highest improvement from baseline pre-treatment categorical measures, while the group that received sound therapy alone had better results than the counseling-only group [114]. The combination of both treatment strategies seems to be the most efficacious approach. Other therapeutic options to consider are cognitive behavioral therapy, hearing aids, and in severe refractory cases, electrical stimulation.

Conclusion

Tinnitus and hyperacusis are common conditions that affect millions of Americans, especially veterans. The exact mechanisms underlying both conditions are still under investigation, but a few theories have been developed to try to explain the pathophysiology. There is still no cure for tinnitus or hyperacusis, but a variety of treatment options exist that can help reduce the distress caused by these symptoms. A thorough medical history and focused physical examination should guide the initial treatment. Generally, a less invasive to more invasive approach is adopted by most practitioners. Research is essential to the continued advancement of our understanding of tinnitus and hyperacusis, and is getting closer to establishing a cure.

References

1. Oleksiak M, Smith BM, St Andre JR, Caughlan CM, Steiner M. Audiological issues and hearing loss among veterans with mild traumatic brain injury. J Rehabil Res Dev. 2012;49(7):995–1004.
2. Baguley DM. Hyperacusis. J R Soc Med. 2003;96(12):582–5.
3. Tyler RS, Pienkowski M, Roncancio ER, et al. A review of hyperacusis and future directions: part I. Definitions and manifestations. Am J Audiol. 2014;23(4):402–19.
4. Shargorodsky J, Curhan GC, Farwell WR. Prevalence and characteristics of tinnitus among US adults. Am J Med. 2010;123(8):711–8.
5. Hoffman JH, Reed GW. Epidemiology of Tinnitus. In: Snow JB, editor. Tinnitus: theory and management. London: BC Decker; 2004.
6. Wiley TL, Cruickshanks KJ, Nondahl DM, Tweed TS. Self-reported hearing handicap and audiometric measures in older adults. J Am Acad Audiol. 2000;11(2):67–75.
7. Nondahl DM, Cruickshanks KJ, Wiley TL, Klein R, Klein BE, Tweed TS. Prevalence and 5-year incidence of tinnitus among older adults: the epidemiology of hearing loss study. J Am Acad Audiol. 2002;13(6):323–31.
8. Seidman MD, Standring RT, Dornhoffer JL. Tinnitus: current understanding and contemporary management. Curr Opin Otolaryngol Head Neck Surg. 2010;18(5):363–8.
9. Jastreboff PJ. Phantom auditory perception (tinnitus): mechanisms of generation and perception. Neurosci Res. 1990;8(4):221–54.
10. Herraiz C, Aparicio JM. Diagnostic clues in pulsatile tinnitus (somatosounds). Acta Otorrinolaringol Esp. 2007;58(9):426–33.
11. Chan Y. Tinnitus: etiology, classification, characteristics, and treatment. Discov Med. 2009;8(42):133–6.
12. Mattox DE, Hudgins P. Algorithm for evaluation of pulsatile tinnitus. Acta Otolaryngol. 2008;128(4):427–31.
13. Ahsan SF, Seidman M, Yaremchuk K. What is the best imaging modality in evaluating patients with unilateral pulsatile tinnitus? Laryngoscope. 2015;125(2):284–5.
14. Ahmad N, Seidman M. Tinnitus in the older adult: epidemiology, pathophysiology and treatment options. Drugs Aging. 2004;21(5):297–305.
15. Lockwood AH, Salvi RJ, Burkard RF. Tinnitus. N Engl J Med. 2002;347(12):904–10.
16. Seidman MD, Arenberg AG, Shirwany NA. Palatal myoclonus as cause of objective tinnitus: a report of six cases and a review of the literature. ENT J. 1999;78(4):292–7.
17. Sunwoo W, Jeon Y, Bae Y, et al. Typewriter tinnitus revisited: the typical symptoms and the initial response to carbamazepine are the most reliable diagnostic clues. Sci Rep. 2017;7:10615.
18. Hofmann E, Behr R, Neumann-Haefelin T, Schwager K. Pulsatile tinnitus: imaging and differential diagnosis. Dtsch Arztebl Int. 2013;110(26):451–8.
19. Pegge SA, Steens SC, Kunst HP, Meijer FJ. Pulsatile tinnitus: differential diagnosis and radiological work-up. Curr Radiol Rep. 2017;5(1):5.
20. Park Y, Kwon H. Awake embolization of sigmoid sinus diverticulum causing pulsatile tinnitus: simultaneous confirmative diagnosis and treatment. Interv Neuroradiol. 2011;17(3):376–9.

21. Sonmez G, Basekim CC, Ozturk E, Gungor A, Kizilkaya E. Imaging of pulsatile tinnitus: a review of 74 patients. Clin Imaging. 2007;31(2):102–8.
22. Sismanis A. Pulsatile tinnitus: contemporary assessment and management. Curr Opin Otolaryngol Head Neck Surg. 2011;19(5):348–57.
23. Narvid J, Do HM, Blevins NH, Fischbein NJ. CT angiography as a screening tool for dural arteriovenous fistula in patients with pulsatile tinnitus: feasibility and test characteristics. AJNR Am J Neuroradiol. 2011;32(3):446–53.
24. Markey KA, Mollan SP, Jensen RH, Sinclair AJ. Understanding idiopathic intracranial hypertension: mechanisms, management, and future directions. Lancet Neurol. 2016;15(1):78–91.
25. Wall M, Kupersmith MJ, Kieburtz KD, et al. The idiopathic intracranial hypertension treatment trial: clinical profile at baseline. JAMA Neurol. 2014;71(6):693–701.
26. Farb RI, Vanek I, Scott JN, et al. Idiopathic intracranial hypertension: the prevalence and morphology of sinovenous stenosis. Neurology. 2003;60(9):1418–24.
27. Minor LB, Solomon D, Zinreich JS, Zee DS. Sound- and/or pressure-induced vertigo due to bone dehiscence of the superior semicircular canal. Arch Otolaryngol Head Neck Surg. 1998;124(3):249–58.
28. Kirkby-Bott J, Gibbs HH. Carotid endarterectomy relieves pulsatile tinnitus associated with severe ipsilateral carotid stenosis. Eur J Vasc Endovasc Surg. 2004;27(6):651–3.
29. Ihn YK, Jung WS, Kim BS. Disappeared pulsatile tinnitus related to petrous segment stenosis of the ICA after relief of the stenosis by stenting. Interv Neuroradiol. 2013;19(1):97–101.
30. Trivelato FP, Araujo JF, Dos Santos SR, Rezende MT, Ulhoa AC, Castro GD. Endovascular treatment of pulsatile tinnitus associated with transverse sigmoid sinus aneurysms and jugular bulb anomalies. Interv Neuroradiol. 2015;21(4):548–51.
31. Turner JJ. Auditory dysfunction: tinnitus. In: Walker HK, Hall WD, Hurst JW, editors. Clinical methods: the history, physical, and laboratory examinations. Boston: Butterworth Publishers, a division of Reed Publishing; 1990.
32. Argstatter H, Krick C, Bolay HV. Music therapy in chronic tonal tinnitus. Heidelberg model of evidence-based music therapy. HNO. 2008;56(7):678–85.
33. Muhlau M, Rauschecker JP, Oestreicher E, et al. Structural brain changes in tinnitus. Cereb Cortex. 2006;16(9):1283–8.
34. Minen MT, Camprodon J, Nehme R, Chemali Z. The neuropsychiatry of tinnitus: a circuit-based approach to the causes and treatments available. J Neurol Neurosurg Psychiatry. 2014;85(10):1138–44.
35. Seidman MD, Standring RT. Noise and quality of life. Int J Environ Res Public Health. 2010;7(10):3730–8.
36. Brozoski TJ, Bauer CA, Caspary DM. Elevated fusiform cell activity in the dorsal cochlear nucleus of chinchillas with psychophysical evidence of tinnitus. J Neurosci. 2002;22(6):2383–90.
37. Levine RA. Somatic (craniocervical) tinnitus and the dorsal cochlear nucleus hypothesis. Am J Otolaryngol. 1999;20(6):351–62.
38. Jastreboff PJ. The neurophysiological model of tinnitus. In: Snow JB, editor. Tinnitus: theory and management. London: BC Decker; 2004. p. 96–106.
39. Brozoski TJ, Bauer CA. The effect of dorsal cochlear nucleus ablation on tinnitus in rats. Hear Res. 2005;206(1–2):227–36.
40. Sedley W, Parikh J, Edden RA, Tait V, Blamire A, Griffiths TD. Human auditory cortex neurochemistry reflects the presence and severity of tinnitus. J Neurosci. 2015;35(44):14822–8.
41. Melcher JR, Levine RA, Bergevin C, Norris B. The auditory midbrain of people with tinnitus: abnormal sound-evoked activity revisited. Hear Res. 2009;257(1–2):63–74.
42. Bauer CA, Kurt W, Sybert LT, Brozoski TJ. The cerebellum as a novel tinnitus generator. Hear Res. 2013;295:130–9.
43. Mirz F, Gjedde A, Sodkilde-Jrgensen H, Pedersen CB. Functional brain imaging of tinnitus-like perception induced by aversive auditory stimuli. Neuroreport. 2000;11(3):633–7.
44. Rauschecker JP, Leaver AM, Muhlau M. Tuning out the noise: limbic-auditory interactions in tinnitus. Neuron. 2010;66(6):819–26.
45. Tunkel DE, Bauer CA, Sun GH, et al. Clinical practice guideline: tinnitus. Otolaryngol Head Neck Surg. 2014;151(2 Suppl):S1–s40.
46. Newman CW, Jacobson GP, Spitzer JB. Development of the tinnitus handicap inventory. Arch Otolaryngol Head Neck Surg. 1996;122(2):143–8.
47. Kuk FK, Tyler RS, Russell D, Jordan H. The psychometric properties of a tinnitus handicap questionnaire. Ear Hear. 1990;11(6):434–45.
48. Meikle MB, Henry JA, Griest SE, et al. The tinnitus functional index: development of a new clinical measure for chronic, intrusive tinnitus. Ear Hear. 2012;33(2):153–76.
49. Budd RJ, Pugh R. Tinnitus coping style and its relationship to tinnitus severity and emotional distress. J Psychosom Res. 1996;41(4):327–35.
50. Henry JA, Meikle MB. Psychoacoustic measures of tinnitus. J Am Acad Audiol. 2000;11(3):138–55.
51. Cazals Y. Auditory sensori-neural alterations induced by salicylate. Prog Neurobiol. 2000;62(6):583–631.
52. Busto U, Fornazzari L, Naranjo CA. Protracted tinnitus after discontinuation of long-term therapeutic use of benzodiazepines. J Clin Psychopharmacol. 1988;8(5):359–62.
53. Ashton H. Benzodiazepine withdrawal: an unfinished story. Br Med J (Clin Res Ed). 1984;288(6424):1135–40.
54. Del Bo L, Ambrosetti U. Hearing aids for the treatment of tinnitus. Prog Brain Res. 2007;166:341–5.
55. Searchfield GD, Kaur M, Martin WH. Hearing aids as an adjunct to counseling: tinnitus patients who choose amplification do better than those that don't. Int J Audiol. 2010;49(8):574–9.
56. Trotter MI, Donaldson I. Hearing aids and tinnitus therapy: a 25-year experience. J Laryngol Otol. 2008;122(10):1052–6.
57. Sweetow RW, Sabes JH. Effects of acoustical stimuli delivered through hearing aids on tinnitus. J Am Acad Audiol. 2010;21(7):461–73.
58. Vernon JA, Meikle MB. Tinnitus masking: unresolved problems. Ciba Found Symp. 1981;85:239–62.
59. Feldmann H. Homolateral and contralateral masking of tinnitus by noise-bands and by pure tones. Audiology. 1971;10(3):138–44.
60. Jastreboff PJ, Jastreboff MM. Tinnitus retraining therapy (TRT) as a method for treatment of tinnitus and hyperacusis patients. J Am Acad Audiol. 2000;11(3):162–77.
61. Jastreboff PJ. Tinnitus retraining therapy. Prog Brain Res. 2007;166:415–23.
62. Grewal R, Spielmann PM, Jones SE, Hussain SS. Clinical efficacy of tinnitus retraining therapy and cognitive behavioural therapy in the treatment of subjective tinnitus: a systematic review. J Laryngol Otol. 2014;128(12):1028–33.
63. Scherer RW, Gormby C. Effect of tinnitus retraining therapy vs standard of care on tinnitus related quality of life. A randomized clinical trial. JAMA Otolaryngol Head Neck Surg. 2019;145(7):597–608.
64. Martinez Devesa P, Waddell A, Perera R, Theodoulou M. Cognitive behavioural therapy for tinnitus. Cochrane Database Syst Rev. 2007;1:Cd005233.
65. Zoger S, Svedlund J, Holgers KM. The effects of sertraline on severe tinnitus suffering--a randomized, double-blind, placebo-controlled study. J Clin Psychopharmacol. 2006;26(1):32–9.

66. Baldo P, Doree C, Molin P, McFerran D, Cecco S. Antidepressants for patients with tinnitus. Cochrane Database Syst Rev. 2012;9:Cd003853.
67. Johnson RM, Brummett R, Schleuning A. Use of alprazolam for relief of tinnitus. A double-blind study. Arch Otolaryngol Head Neck Surg. 1993;119(8):842–5.
68. Jalali MM, Kousha A, Naghavi SE, Soleimani R, Banan R. The effects of alprazolam on tinnitus: a cross-over randomized clinical trial. Med Sci Monit. 2009;15(11):Pi55–60.
69. Witsell DL, Hannley MT, Stinnet S, Tucci DL. Treatment of tinnitus with gabapentin: a pilot study. Otol Neurotol. 2007;28(1):11–5.
70. Dehkordi MA, Abolbashari S, Taheri R, Einolghozati S. Efficacy of gabapentin on subjective idiopathic tinnitus: a randomized, double-blind, placebo-controlled trial. Ear Nose Throat J. 2011;90(4):150–8.
71. Aazh H, El Refaie A, Humphriss R. Gabapentin for tinnitus: a systematic review. Am J Audiol. 2011;20(2):151–8.
72. Sakata H, Kojima Y, Koyama S, Furuya N, Sakata E. Treatment of cochlear tinnitus with transtympanic infusion of 4% lidocaine into the tympanic cavity. Int Tinnitus J. 2001;7(1):46–50.
73. Daneshi A, Jahandideh H, Pousti SB, Mohammadi S. One-shot, low-dosage intratympanic gentamicin for Ménière's disease: clinical, posturographic and vestibular test findings. Iran J Neurol. 2014;13(1):33–9.
74. Staecker H, Maxwell KS, Morris JR, van de Heyning P, Morawski K, Reintjes F, et al. Selecting appropriate dose regimens for AM-101 in the intratympanic treatment of acute inner ear tinnitus. Audiol Neurootol. 2015;20:172–82.
75. Seidman MD, Babu S. Alternative medications and other treatments for tinnitus: facts from fiction. Otolaryngol Clin N Am. 2003;36(2):359–81.
76. Newall CA, Anderson LA, Phillipson JD, editors. Herbal medicine: a guide for health-care professionals. London: Pharmaceutical Press; 1996.
77. Meyer B. Tinnitus-multicenter study: a multicentric study of the ear. Ann Otolaryngol. 1980;103:185–8.
78. Shemesh Z, Attias J, Ornan M, Shapira N, Shahar A. Vitamin B12 deficiency in patients with chronic-tinnitus and noise-induced hearing loss. Am J Otolaryngol. 1993;14(2):94–9.
79. Sha SH, Zajic G, Epstein CJ, Schacht J. Overexpression of copper/zinc-superoxide dismutase protects from kanamycin-induced hearing loss. Audiol Neurootol. 2001;6(3):117–23.
80. Arda HN, Tuncel U, Akdogan O, Ozluoglu LN. The role of zinc in the treatment of tinnitus. Otol Neurotol. 2003;24(1):86–9.
81. Person OC, Puga ME, da Silva EM, Torloni MR. Zinc supplementation for tinnitus. Cochrane Database Syst Rev. 2016;11:Cd009832.
82. Holstein N. Ginkgo special extract EGb 761 in tinnitus therapy. An overview of results of completed clinical trials. Fortschr Med Orig. 2001;118(4):157–64.
83. Drew S, Davies E. Effectiveness of Ginkgo biloba in treating tinnitus: double blind, placebo controlled trial. BMJ. 2001;322(7278):73.
84. Punte AK, Vermeire K, Hofkens A, De Bodt M, De Ridder D, Van de Heyning P. Cochlear implantation as a durable tinnitus treatment in single-sided deafness. Cochlear Implants Int. 2011;12(Suppl 1):S26–9.
85. Bovo R, Ciorba A, Martini A. Tinnitus and cochlear implants. Auris Nasus Larynx. 2011;38(1):14–20.
86. Mo B, Harris S, Lindbæk M. Cochlear implants and health status: a comparison with other hearing-impaired patients. Ann Otol Rhinol Laryngol. 2004;113(11):914–21.
87. Gantz BJ, Dunn C, Walker E, Voorst TV, Gogel S, Hansen M. Outcomes of adolescents with a short electrode cochlear implant with preserved residual hearing. Otol Neurotol. 2016;37(2):e118–25.
88. Pulec JL. Cochlear nerve section for intractable tinnitus. Ear Nose Throat J. 1995;74(7):468–470–466.
89. House J, Brackmann DE. Ciba foundation symposium 85. Yale J Biol Med. 1981;55(5-6):554–5.
90. Seidman MD, Ridder DD, Elisevich K, et al. Direct electrical stimulation of Heschl's gyrus for tinnitus treatment. Laryngoscope. 2008;118(3):491–500.
91. Swegal WC, Meklir T, Elisevich K, Bowyer SM, De Ridder D, Seidman MD. Direct electrical stimulation of the auditory cortex for tinnitus treatment. AAO-HNS and OTO EXPO; 2016.
92. Hamani C, Temel Y. Deep brain stimulation for psychiatric disease: contributions and validity of animal models. Sci Transl Med. 2012;4:142rv8.
93. McIntyre CC, Savasta M, Kerkerian-LeGoff L, Vitek J. Uncovering mechanisms of action of deep brain stimulation: activation, inhibition or both. Clin Neurophysiol. 2004;115(6):1239–48.
94. Perlmutter JS, Mink JW. Deep brain stimulation. Annu Rev Neurosci. 2006;29:229–57.
95. Shi Y, Burchiel KJ, Anderson VC, Martin WH. Deep brain stimulation effects in patients with tinnitus. Otolaryngol Head Neck Surg. 2009;141(2):285–7.
96. Cheung SW, Larson PS. Tinnitus modulation by deep brain stimulation in locus of caudate neurons (area LC). Neuroscience. 2010;169(4):1768–78.
97. Ahsan S, Luo H, Zhang J, et al. An animal model of deep brain stimulation for treating tinnitus: a proof of concept study. Laryngoscope. 2018;128(5):1213–22.
98. De Ridder D, Vanneste S, Engineer ND, Kilgard MP. Safety and efficacy of vagus nerve stimulation paired with tones for the treatment of tinnitus: a case series. Neuromodulation. 2014;17(2):170–9.
99. Tyler R, Cacace A, Stocking C, et al. Vagus Nerve Stimulation Paired with Tones for the Treatment of Tinnitus: A Prospective Randomized Double-blind Controlled Pilot Study in Humans. Sci Rep. 2017;7(1):11960.
100. Riffle T, Martel D, Jones G, Shore S. Bimodal auditory-electrical stimulation for the treatment of tinnitus: pre-clinical and clinical studies. Curr Top Behav Neurosci. 2021;51:295–323.
101. Fabijanska A, Rogowski M, Bartnik G, Skarzynski H. Epidemiology of tinnitus and hyperacusis in Poland. In: Proceedings of the Sixth International Tinnitus Seminar. London: The Tinnitus and Hyperacusis Centre; 1999. p. 569–71.
102. Andersson G, Lindvall N, Hursti T, Carlbring P. Hypersensitivity to sound (hyperacusis): a prevalence study conducted via the internet and post. Int J Audiol. 2002;41:545–54.
103. Anari M, Axelsson A, Eliasson A, Magnusson L. Hypersensitivity to sound--questionnaire data, audiometry and classification. Scand Audiol. 1999;28(4):219–30.
104. Katzenell U, Segal S. Hyperacusis: review and clinical guidelines. Otol Neurotol. 2001;22(3):321–6; discussion 326–327.
105. Auerbach BD, Rodrigues PV, Salvi RJ. Central gain control in tinnitus and hyperacusis. Front Neurol. 2014;5:206.
106. Marriage J, Barnes NM. Is central hyperacusis a symptom of 5-hydroxytryptamine (5-HT) dysfunction? J Laryngol Otol. 1995;109(10):915–21.
107. Thompson GC, Thompson AM, Garrett KM, Britton BH. Serotonin and serotonin receptors in the central auditory system. Otolaryngol Head Neck Surg. 1994;110(1):93–102.
108. Pienkowski M, Tyler RS, Roncancio ER, et al. A review of hyperacusis and future directions: part II. Measurement, mechanisms, and treatment. Am J Audiol. 2014;23(4):420–36.
109. Jastreboff PJ, Jastreboff MM. Treatments for decreased sound tolerance (Hyperacusis and Misophonia). Semin Hear. 2014;35(2):105–20.
110. Khalfa S, Dubal S, Veuillet E, Perez-Diaz F, Jouvent R, Collet L. Psychometric normalization of a hyperacusis questionnaire. ORL J Otorhinolaryngol Relat Spec. 2002;64(6):436–42.

111. Nelting M, Rienhoff NK, Hesse G, Lamparter U. The assessment of subjective distress related to hyperacusis with a self-rating questionnaire on hypersensitivity to sound. Laryngorhinootologie. 2002;81(5):327–34.
112. Dauman R, Bouscau-Faure F. Assessment and amelioration of hyperacusis in tinnitus patients. Acta Otolaryngol. 2005;125(5):503–9.
113. Madeira G, Montmirail C, Decat M, Gersdorff M. TRT: results after one year treatment. Rev Laryngol Otol Rhinol (Bord). 2007;128(3):145–8.
114. Formby C, Hawley ML, Sherlock LGP, et al. A sound therapy-based intervention to expand the auditory dynamic range for loudness among persons with sensorineural hearing losses: a randomized placebo-controlled clinical trial. Semin Hear. 2015;36(2):77–110.

Congenital Hearing Loss and Inner Ear Malformations

49

Brendan P. O'Connell, Teresa G. Vos, Jacob B. Hunter, and Kevin B. Brown

Introduction

Congenital hearing loss affects approximately 1 in 500 newborns, and 1 in 300 children by the age of 4 years [1, 2]. Congenital hearing loss can generally be grouped into genetic and non-genetic (i.e., environmental) etiologies, with the former accounting for 50–66% of reported cases [1, 3]. Genetic hearing loss is associated with specific syndromes in 30% of cases, with the remaining 70% occurring in isolation (nonsyndromic) [4]. Amplification with hearing aids is the mainstay of treatment for mild to moderately severe sensorineural hearing loss (SNHL), while cochlear implantation is the gold standard for auditory rehabilitation in children with advanced sensorineural hearing loss and poor speech perception. Given that approximately 20% of children with congenital SNHL have anatomic abnormalities of the temporal bone, understanding the implications that inner ear malformations have on cochlear implantation surgery and expected outcomes is critical [5, 6]. The objectives of this chapter are as follows: (1) review causes of genetic hearing loss with respect to both syndromic and nonsyndromic etiologies, (2) describe common cochleovestibular anomalies, and (3) review operative considerations and expected outcomes for cochlear implantation of malformed inner ears.

B. P. O'Connell (✉)
Charlotte Eye, Ear, Nose and Throat, Charlotte, NC, USA

T. G. Vos · K. B. Brown
Department of Otolaryngology—Head and Neck Surgery, University of North Carolina, Chapel Hill, NC, USA

J. B. Hunter
Department of Otolaryngology—Head and Neck Surgery, Thomas Jefferson University School of Medicine, Philadelphia, PA, USA

Genetic Causes of Hearing Loss: Nonsyndromic

Currently, over 100 gene loci have been implicated in hereditary, nonsyndromic SNHL, which can generally be classified by the mode of inheritance [3]. The majority (80%) of mutations are inherited in autosomal recessive (AR) fashion, with autosomal dominant (AD) inheritance accounting for roughly 20% of cases. A small subset of nonsyndromic hereditary hearing impairment is attributable to either X-linked or mitochondrial inheritance. A detailed list of mapped hearing loss genes can be found on the hereditary hearing loss web page (http://hereditaryhearingloss.org). The following terminology is generally used to categorize nonsyndromic SNHL genes according to inheritance pattern: DFNA for AD, DFNB for AR, and DFNX for X-linked. Below, the more common mutations and hearing loss manifestations for AR and AD patterns of inheritance are detailed.

Autosomal Recessive

Nonsyndromic AR hearing loss is usually severe and manifests early in life prior to the acquisition of language skills. Given the inheritance pattern, a family history of hearing loss is often not present. While many different mutations have been identified to cause nonsyndromic AR hearing loss, mutations in the *GJB2* (*DFNB1*) and *SLC26A4* (*DFNB4*) genes account for the majority of these cases. *GJB2* encodes connexin 26, a gap junction protein involved in potassium transport within the cochlea. Mutations in *GJB2* were initially described in the late 1990s, and have since been found to be present in approximately 50% of patients with nonsyndromic AR hearing loss [7, 8]. *SLC26A4* encodes a chloride and iodide transporter. Mutations in *SLC26A4* can also be found in association with enlarged vestibular aqueduct (EVA) and goiter; if the latter develops, Pendred syndrome is diagnosed.

A. D. Sweeney et al. (eds.), *Haynes-Glasscock-Shambaugh Surgery of the Ear*, https://doi.org/10.1007/978-3-032-18264-7_49

Autosomal Dominant

Nonsyndromic AD hearing loss is often suggested by family history. Unlike AR SNHL in which two specific gene mutations predominate, no single gene accounts for a significant proportion of AD SNHL. Hearing loss associated with AD mutations is typically progressive, variable in severity, and delayed or post-lingual.

Genetic Causes of Hearing Loss: Syndromic

As mentioned previously, approximately 20–30% of hereditary hearing loss is syndromic. In children with sensorineural hearing loss due to a congenital syndrome, the risk of cochlear and vestibular abnormalities of the temporal bone is increased [9]. Over 400 syndromes have been described in which hearing loss is a feature; the conditions that account for the majority of syndromic etiologies are detailed in Table 49.1 [3]. In general, Waardenburg, branchio-oto-renal (BOR), and CHARGE syndromes can be diagnosed with a detailed history and physical examination. In contrast, additional testing is typically needed to diagnose Usher and Pendred syndromes, which do not have the same observable characteristics that facilitate immediate diagnosis. In regard to Usher syndrome, various phenotypes (types I–III) exist that are marked by varying age of onset for SNHL/retinitis pigmentosa and the presence or absence of vestibular dysfunction [3]. The diagnosis of Usher syndrome can be made with a proven family history, development of retinitis pigmentosa, or molecular testing. As mentioned previously, Pendred syndrome is often suspected when enlarged vestibular aqueduct (EVA) is identified on imaging studies, as roughly 30% of children with EVA have mutations in *SLC26A4*.

Table 49.1 Common congenital hearing loss syndromes and associated features

Syndrome	Inheritance pattern	Hearing loss	Inner ear anomalies	Non-inner ear manifestations
Branchio-oto-renal	AD	CHL, SNHL or mixed Variable severity	Cochlear hypoplasia Large porus acousticus	EAC atresia Ossicular chain abnormalities Branchial arch defects Renal anomalies
CHARGE	AD	CHL, SNHL or mixed Variable severity	SCC aplasia Aplastic oval window Absent or deficient cochlear nerve	EAC atresia Microtia Ossicular chain abnormalities Coloboma Heart defects Choanal atresia Developmental and cognitive delay Genital hypoplasia
Waardenburg	AD	SNHL Variable severity	EVA Hypoplasia of the IAC Malformed SCCs	Pigmentary changes of the skin and eyes Dystopia canthorum
Pendred	AR	Severe SNHL	EVA and endolymphatic sac IP Enlarged vestibule	Euthyroid goiter
Usher	AR	SNHL Variable severity	EVA and endolymphatic sac IP Enlarged vestibule	Retinitis pigmentosa Vestibular abnormalities
X-linked deafness with stapes gusher	X-linked	Mixed loss progresses to profound SNHL	Lack of bone separating IAC from basal turn of cochlea Enlarged, bulbous IAC Cochlear hypoplasia	Stapes fixation

Adapted from reference [3]

AD autosomal dominant, *AR* autosomal recessive, *SNHL* sensorineural hearing loss, *CHL* conductive hearing loss, *SCC* semicircular canal, *EVA* enlarged vestibular aqueduct, *IP* incomplete partition, *IAC* internal auditory canal, *EAC* external auditory canal

Clinical Evaluation of Children with Congenital Sensorineural Hearing Loss

In light of the rapidly expanding body of literature pertaining to genetic causes of congenital hearing loss, incorporating relevant data into the clinical workup of children with hearing loss can be challenging. In addition to the routine audiometric battery of tests performed to diagnose childhood hearing loss, which are not detailed herein, history and physical examination directed at eliciting the following variables can help direct further workup: (1) evidence of an environmental cause (e.g., congenital rubella, congenital cytomegalovirus (CMV), or prematurity), (2) signs or symptoms of syndromic disease, and (3) family history of hearing loss suggestive of a genetic etiology [3].

Given the prevalence of CMV, testing for CMV in neonates that fail their newborn hearing screening is often recommended [10]. Of note, in a CMV-positive neonate with mild-to-moderate bilateral hearing loss, genetic screening may be considered due to increased risk of underlying co-morbid genetic abnormality in this population [11]. If physical examination reveals abnormalities suggestive of possible syndromic associations, then further diagnostic testing is recommended on the basis of suspected etiologies. Imaging with computed tomography (CT) and/or magnetic resonance imaging (MRI) is generally recommended to evaluate inner ear structures. Many centers are now obtaining non-contrast MRI with high-resolution T2-weighted sequences as the initial study of choice which avoids radiation exposure; if the MRI is normal, further CT imaging is obviated. If the MRI demonstrates an inner ear malformation, then CT can be obtained to better delineate the course of the facial nerve, which could become useful information if cochlear implantation becomes necessary. In cases of profound loss, or if CHARGE syndrome is suspected, MRI is always indicated to evaluate for the presence of the cochlear nerve [12, 3].

In all cases of congenital or prelingual SNHL, a thorough discussion should occur between the clinician and patient/parents such that both parties are engaged in shared decision making with respect to genetic testing. If there is no identifiable environmental cause, family history of similar hearing loss, signs of a syndrome, or imaging anomaly to explain a child's hearing loss, sequencing of *GJB2* is often advocated given the prevalence of mutations in this gene and its relatively high diagnostic yield [13]. Imaging may also inform the decision making process to perform directed genetic testing; for example, if EVA is identified, testing for *SLC26A4* mutations should be considered. If the etiology for SNHL remains unknown and mutations in *GJB2* are not present, more comprehensive genetic testing can be considered to detect mutations in all genes known to cause nonsyndromic hearing loss and all mimics [14].

Potential advantages of pursuing whole exome testing include the identification of the definitive cause for SNHL and the fact that results can assist in identifying other medical conditions associated with specific syndromes. Testing also carries potential societal benefit, in that further knowledge regarding underlying genetic defects may facilitate development and introduction of novel therapeutics. An obvious disadvantage is cost, but with the adoption of next-generation sequencing methods, a decrease in cost is anticipated in coming years. Results of genetic testing rarely change the actual management of the underlying hearing loss, but results can be helpful for projecting potential for further hearing loss. It is also helpful for providing family/patient information about risk of future progeny experiencing hearing loss. As discussed later, cochlear implantation remains the hearing rehabilitative strategy of choice for children with advanced hearing loss and poor speech recognition, regardless of etiology.

Congenital Inner Ear Anomalies

Approximately 20% of children with congenital SNHL have associated anatomic abnormalities of the temporal bone. Congenital inner ear anomalies can generally be divided into two groups: (1) those with abnormalities of both the bony and membranous labyrinth and (2) those with isolated involvement of the membranous labyrinth. The former can be detected radiographically, while anomalies isolated to the membranous labyrinth are not readily identified with temporal bone radiographs. Abnormalities of the bony labyrinth have significant implications in regard to candidacy for implantation, operative technique, and audiologic outcomes. A number of classification systems for bony labyrinthine anomalies have been described. Given the multitude of possible malformations and the lack of a universally accepted classification scheme, the nomenclature for inner ear anomalies can be confusing. The more commonly referenced classification systems will be described below.

Malformations of the Bony Labyrinth

Jackler Classification System

Before Jackler et al. published their seminal article regarding cochleovestibular anomalies in 1987, the term Mondini dysplasia had come to mean virtually any congenital malformation of the osseous labyrinth detectable on imaging [6]. As imaging techniques improved, distinct abnormalities of the inner ear were identified and the need for more detailed diagnostic criteria of cochleovestibular abnormalities became apparent. Jackler et al. proposed a classification system using images taken by polytomography, working with the premise that deformities were the result of developmental arrest that occurred at specific time points throughout the continuum of inner ear embryogenesis. Jackler et al. described the following anomalies, which are detailed in Table 49.2:

1. Complete labyrinthine aplasia (Fig. 49.1)
2. Common cavity (Fig. 49.2)
3. Cochlear aplasia (Fig. 49.3)
4. Cochlear hypoplasia (Fig. 49.4)
5. Incomplete partition (IP)

Complete labyrinthine aplasia, characterized by an absence of both the labyrinth and cochlea, is the only malformation that absolutely precludes cochlear implant (CI). It is also important to distinguish aplasia from labyrinthitis ossificans. On computed tomography (CT) imaging, bone density anterior to the internal auditory canal (IAC) in the setting

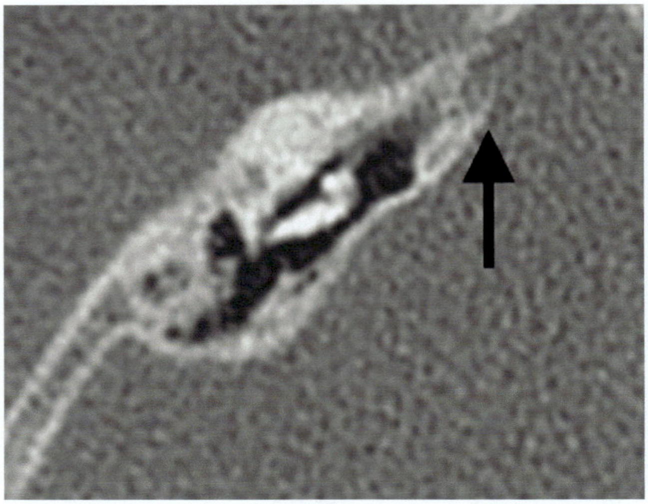

Fig. 49.1 *Complete labyrinthine aplasia*: Axial CT demonstrates absence of both the cochlea and the labyrinth (arrow)

Table 49.2 Description of cochleovestibular anomalies as classified by Jackler et al.

Cochleovestibular anomaly	Developmental arrest	Description
Complete labyrinthine aplasia (Michel deformity)	Third week	Occurs before formation of otic capsule, therefore no inner ear development Extremely rare
Common cavity	Fourth week	Cochlea and vestibule form a common cavity without internal separation Poorly differentiated membranous labyrinth
Cochlear aplasia (cochlear agenesis)	Fifth week	Absent cochlea Vestibule and semicircular canals are developed but typically malformed
Cochlear hypoplasia	Sixth week	Cochlea is present but hypoplastic (up to 1 turn) Normal or malformed vestibule and semicircular canals
Incomplete partition (classic Mondini dysplasia)	Seventh week	Cochlea has completed 1.5 turns Incomplete or absent interscalar septum between middle and apical turns Normal or malformed vestibule and semicircular canals Most common cochlear anomaly Mondini's original description also included EVA and bulbous IAC

Adapted from reference [6]
EVA enlarged vestibular aqueduct, *IAC* internal auditory canal

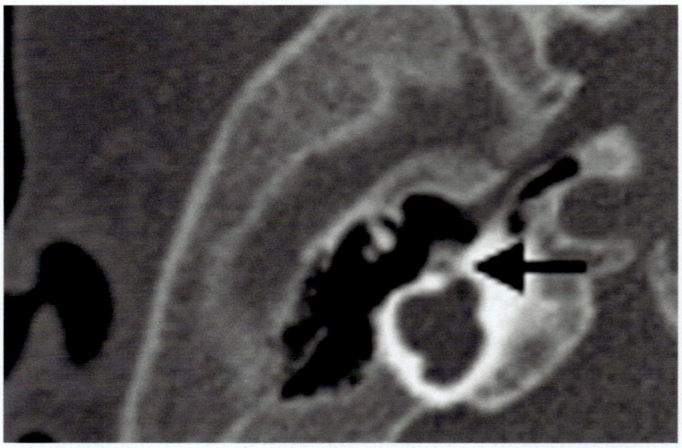

Fig. 49.2 *Common cavity*: Axial CT demonstrates a common cystic cavity with aplastic semicircular canals. A rudimentary cochlear bud is appreciated at the anterior aspect of the cavity (arrow)

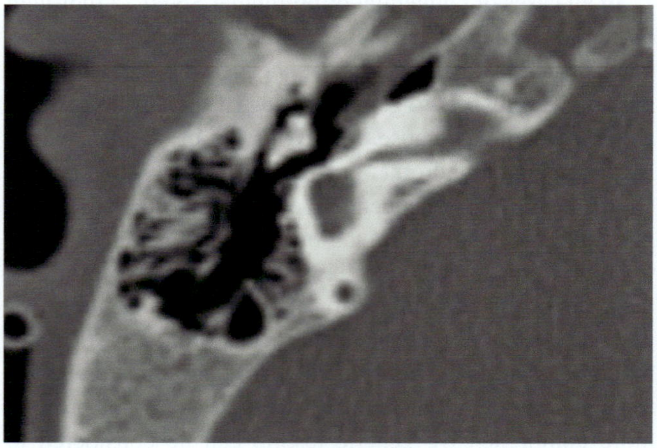

Fig. 49.3 *Cochlear aplasia*: Axial CT through the epitympanum shows a single common cystic cavity with hypoplastic semicircular canals and a narrowed internal auditory canal

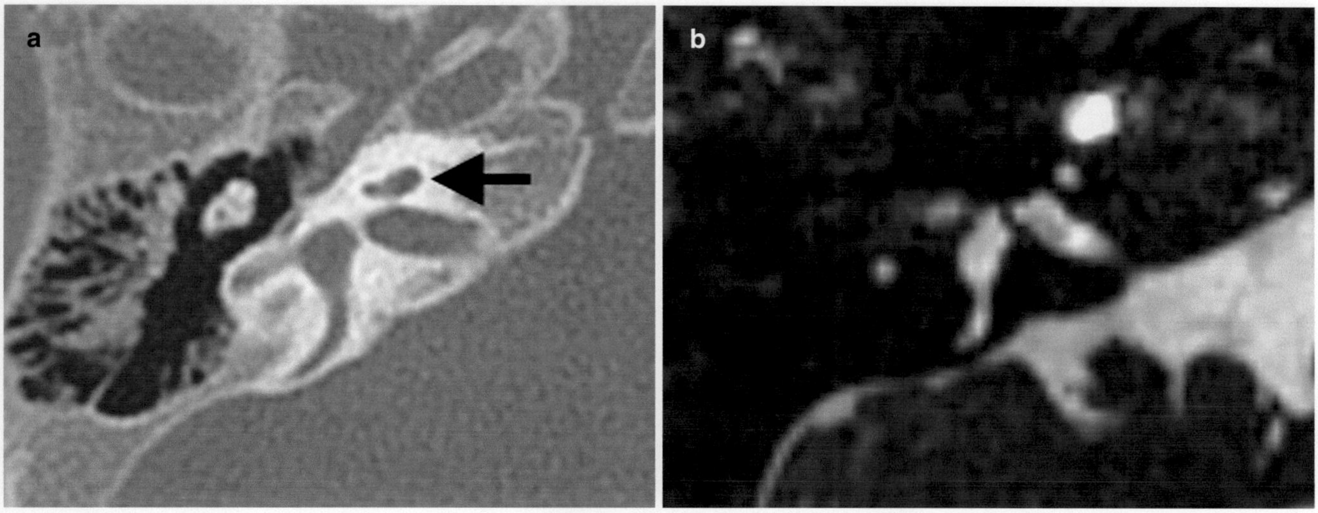

Fig. 49.4 *Cochlear hypoplasia*: (**a**) Axial CT and (**b**) axial T2-weighted MRI show an underdeveloped, bud-like cochlea (arrow). A dilated vestibule and dysmorphic lateral semicircular canal anatomy can also be appreciated

of a normal cochlear promontory indicates labyrinthitis ossificans, and not an aplastic malformation [15]. On MRI, the presence of T2-hyperintense residual perilymph also implicates labyrinthitis ossificans as the underlying pathology.

Phelps Classification System

A few years later in 1992, Phelps published a classification system based on the presence of the basal turn of the cochlea [16]. It was felt that this system would correlate better with outcomes of cochlear implantation. The following abnormalities were described:

1. Severe labyrinthine dysplasia
2. Mondini dysplasia
3. Mondini-like dysplasia
4. Incomplete partition

Severe labyrinthine dysplasia was defined as cochleae that lacked a normal basal turn. Conversely, Mondini dysplasia was used to describe cochleae in which a normal basal turn was present. The system further characterized cochlea in which the basal turn was present, but the cochlea was shortened (1.5–2 turns), as "Mondini-like" dysplasia. Lastly, their publication described a distinct type of incomplete partition (IP) occurring in patients with X-linked deafness. This deformity is characterized by a deficient lamina cribosa, which separates the lateral end of the internal auditory canal (IAC) from the basal turn of the cochlea. The Phelps schema is commonly referenced when discussing historical classification systems; however, the nomenclature is seldom used in current descriptions of inner ear malformations.

Sennaroglu Classification System

Similar to Jackler et al., Sennaroglu et al. proposed a classification scheme based on the concept of developmental arrest along a linear continuum of embryogenesis [17]. However, in contrast to Jackler et al., their group characterized cochlear aplasia as antecedent to the common cavity malformation as below.

1. Complete labyrinthine aplasia
2. Cochlear aplasia
3. Common cavity
4. Incomplete partition type I (Fig. 49.5)
5. Cochlear hypoplasia
6. Incomplete partition type II (Fig. 49.6)
7. Incomplete partition type III (Fig. 49.7)

Another notable difference when compared to the Jackler classification is the spectrum of IP abnormalities that are described. Incomplete partition type I, also referred to as cystic cochleovestibular malformation, is the most severe form of IP. In this malformation, both the cochlear and vestibular systems are enlarged with no anatomic separation between the two elements. There is also a complete absence of the modiolus and interscalar septa. Along the continuum of embryogenesis, IP type I precedes cochlear hypoplasia because separable cochlear and vestibular structures are present in the latter. IP type II is similar to the IP described by Jackler et al., in which the cochlea consists of 1.5 turns, with an incomplete separation between the middle and apical turns that results in a cystic apex. Sennaroglu et al. suggest that the term "Mondini deformity" should be reserved for

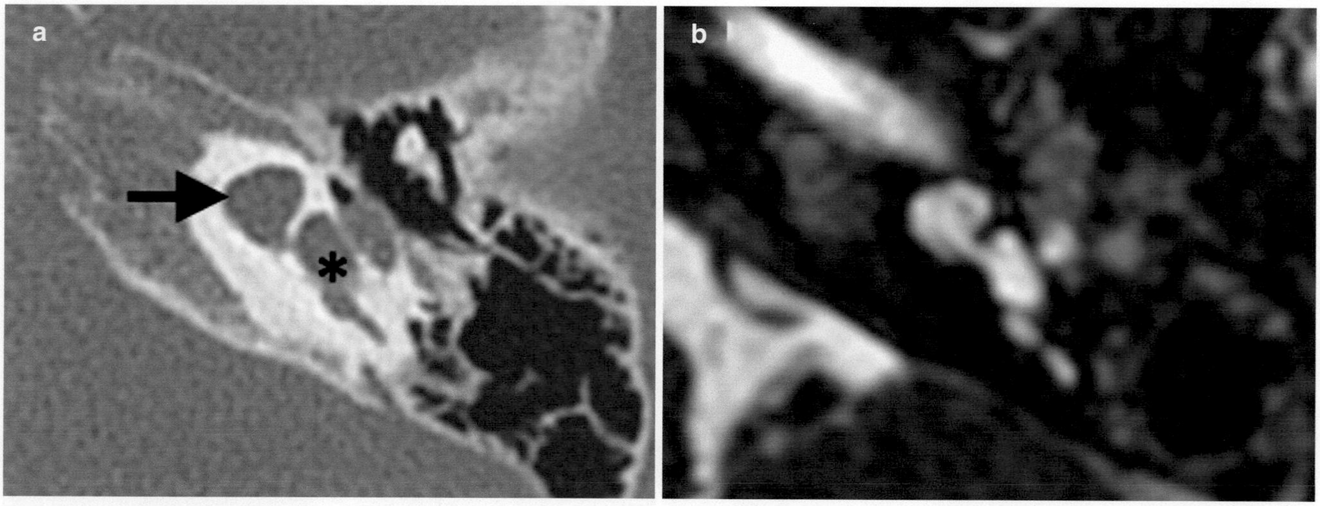

Fig. 49.5 *Incomplete partition type I*: (**a**) Axial CT and (**b**) axial T2-weighted MRI demonstrate a complete absence of the modiolus and interscalar septa in a malformed cochlea (arrow) and vestibule (asterisk) without anatomic separation between the two elements

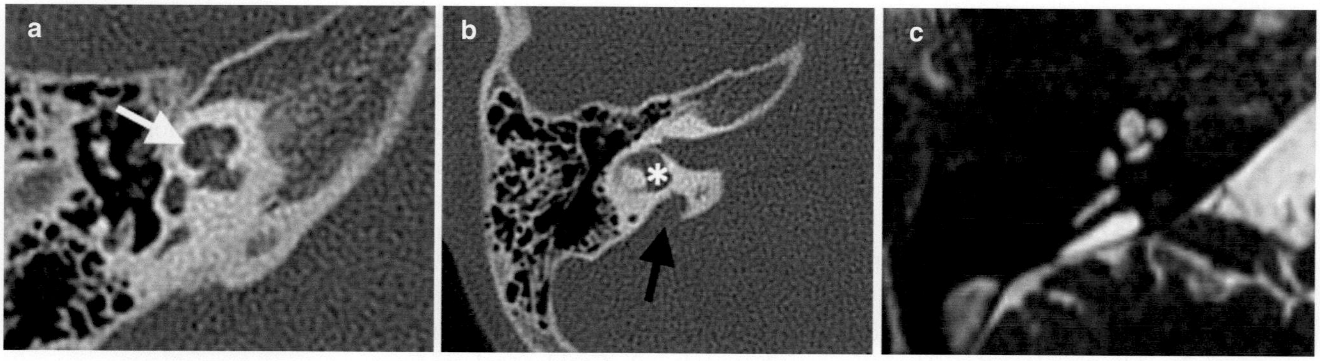

Fig. 49.6 *Incomplete partition type II*: (**a/b**) Axial CT and (**c**) axial T2-weighted MRI demonstrate an incomplete interscalar septum between the middle and apical turns of the cochlea (white arrow) in addition to a dilated vestibule (asterisk). An enlarged vestibular aqueduct can also be appreciated (black arrow)

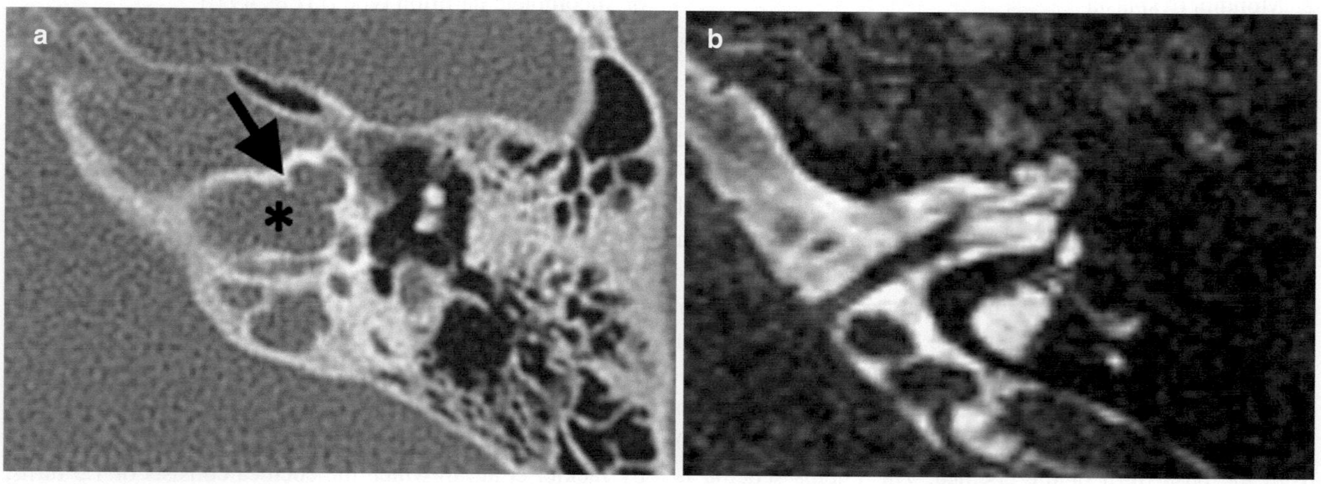

Fig. 49.7 *Incomplete partition type III*: (**a**) Axial CT and (**b**) axial T2-weighted MRI demonstrate presence of an interscalar septum (black arrow), but absence of the lamina cribrosa and modiolus (asterisk)

ears in which the triad of an IP type II, a dilated vestibule, and enlarged vestibular aqueduct are present. Lastly, IP type III is characterized by lack of the lamina cribrosa and modiolus, but presence of an interscalar septum. This malformation has considerable similarities to the X-linked IP described previously by Phelps [18].

Alternatives to Developmental Arrest Model

Despite the merits of the aforementioned classification systems, explaining all cochleovestibular malformations based on arrest of embryologic development along a linear continuum may be oversimplified. Various groups have proposed that a number of distinct anomalous paths of development do not necessarily line along a linear continuum. It is likely that other factors such as gene expression and environmental influences also impact the inner ear phenotype [19].

Malformations of the Temporal Bone Irrespective of the Bony Labyrinth

The previously described anomalies all involve the cochlea, albeit to varying degrees. It is also possible to have isolated malformations of other temporal bone structures in the setting of a normal cochlea.

Enlarged Vestibular Aqueduct

Enlarged vestibular aqueduct is the most common abnormality of the temporal bone detected on radiographic studies and can occur either as an isolated finding or in combination with other temporal bone anomalies (Fig. 49.8). In the majority of cases, EVA occurs concomitant with IP [5, 20–22]. Despite the relatively high incidence amongst patients with congenital temporal bone anomalies, criteria for diagnosis of EVA are not standardized. Some authors define EVA as the diameter of the vestibular aqueduct being larger than the diameter of the posterior semicircular canal. Others indicate that a vestibular aqueduct is enlarged if it is larger than 1.5 mm at the midpoint between the IAC and the operculum [17]. Lastly, Vijayasekaran et al. defined EVA as having a diameter $\geq$ 1.0 mm at its midpoint, or $\geq$ 2.0 mm at the operculum; this metric has since been referred to in the literature as the Cincinnati criteria [23]. As mentioned previously, MRI is often the initial diagnostic imaging study performed in order to limit radiation exposure in infants. If there are abnormalities suggesting increased likelihood of aberrant facial nerve position or findings to suggest cochlear nerve deficiency (CND), subsequent CT temporal bone should be performed. It should also be noted that in mildly dilated EVA, CT may have improved sensitivity in identifying enlargement of the aqueduct at level of the operculum [24]. According to embryologic models, EVA is the result of arrest of between weeks 5 and 8 [6]. In general, hearing is normal at birth, but progressive loss manifests in roughly 40% of patients, often leading to profound sensorineural deficits. In addition, it is generally believed that head trauma is a precipitating factor for hearing loss.

Malformations of the Membranous Labyrinth

Anomalies of the membranous labyrinth occur either concomitantly with bony malformations or in isolation (Table 49.3). Given that they cannot be detected radiographically, the incidence of such defects is not clear. It has been suggested that the development of a cerebrospinal

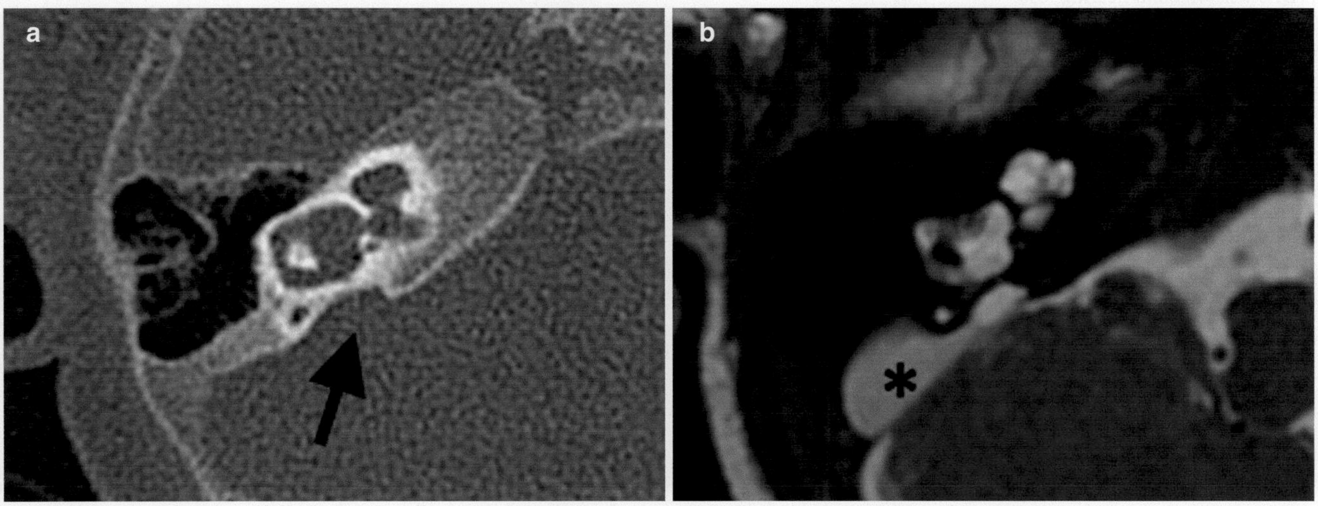

Fig. 49.8 *Enlarged vestibular aqueduct*: (**a**) Axial CT demonstrates a markedly enlarged vestibular aqueduct (black arrow), which exceeds the dimensions of the adjacent posterior semicircular canal. (**b**) Axial T2-weighted MRI demonstrates enlargement of the endolymphatic sac (asterisk) leading into the vestibular aqueduct

fluid (CSF) leak in an otherwise normal appearing ear may indicate the presence of an underlying membranous abnormality [25].

Cochlear Nerve Anomalies

Absence and hypoplasia of the cochlear nerve have been described in association with congenital SNHL. While a narrow IAC (less than 2 to 2.5 mm in diameter) on CT imaging is suggestive of cochlear nerve absence or hypoplasia, an MRI with high-resolution T2-weighted sequences in an oblique sagittal plane perpendicular to the long axis of the IAC is warranted to evaluate the contents of the IAC (Fig. 49.9). If the cochlear nerve cannot be identified, it is considered absent, while a cochlear nerve smaller in caliber than the other nerves of the IAC is considered hypoplastic; both cochlear nerve absence and hypoplasia are typically grouped together as cochlear nerve deficiency (CND) [26, 27]. In addition, other cochleovestibular anomalies are reported in up to 81% of patients with cochlear nerve deficiency, and thus studies suggest that patients with narrow IACs, common cavity malformations, and patients with CHARGE syndrome should undergo MRI evaluation to evaluate the presence of a cochlear nerve [12, 28]. MRI should also be strongly considered in all patients with congenital severe-to-profound sensorineural hearing loss or patients who demonstrate no reliable auditory thresholds with behavioral/play audiometry [29]. Historically, the absence of a cochlear nerve on MRI studies had been a contraindication to cochlear implantation. However, recent studies have suggested that the absence of a cochlear nerve does not necessarily preclude the possibility that some cochlear nerve fibers are present [30, 31]. Even if MRI suggests cochlear nerve deficiency, a full audiometric analysis should be performed to assess for the evidence of intact audition to suggest presence of a cochlear nerve [32]. Cochlear implantation in patients with cochlear nerve anomalies is indicated on the side which demonstrates better candidacy based on imaging [26]. If there is lack of benefit from a cochlear implant, it may be appropriate to proceed with auditory brainstem implantation (ABI) at centers offering approved trials as ABI is not currently approved by the U.S. Food and Drug Administration (FDA) for this indication [33]. Outcomes of implantation in the setting of cochlear nerve anomalies will be discussed later in the chapter.

Table 49.3 Membranous labyrinthine anomalies

Membranous labyrinthine anomaly	Hearing loss pattern	Description
Alexander malformation	High-frequency SNHL	Least severe membranous malformation Dysplastic basal turn Otherwise normal labyrinth
Scheibe malformation, or cochleosaccular dysplasia	Severe-to-profound SNHL	Most common membranous labyrinthine anomaly Involves cochlea and saccule Poorly developed organ of Corti and abnormal stria vascularis Associated with Usher, Jervell and Lange-Nielsen, Waardenburg, and trisomy 18 syndromes
Bing-Siebenmann	Profound SNHL	Complete membranous labyrinthine dysplasia Described as part of Usher and Jervell and Lange-Nielsen syndromes

SNHL sensorineural hearing loss

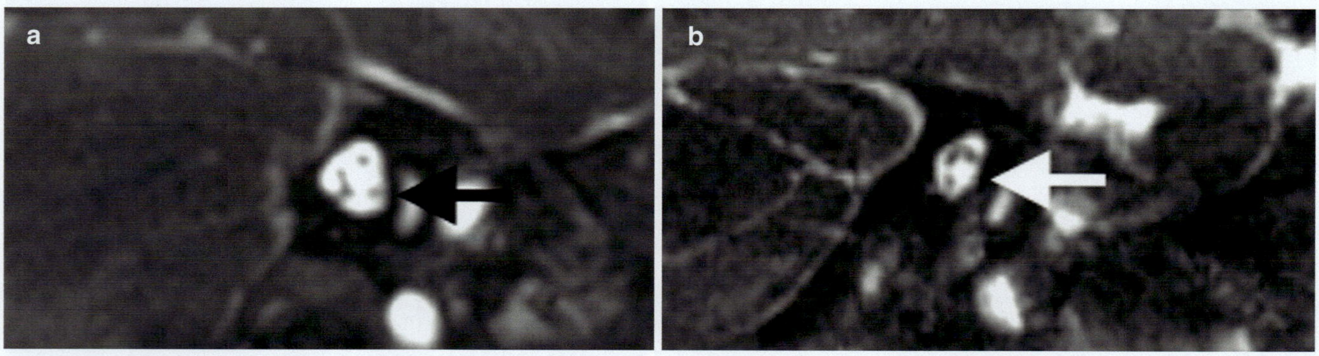

Fig. 49.9 *Cochlear nerve deficiency*: Oblique sagittal T2-weighted MRI demonstrates cross-section of the facial, superior vestibular, inferior vestibular, and cochlear nerves within the IAC. (**a**) Normal IAC: Four nerves are visible; the cochlear nerve (black arrow) is present running in the anteroinferior quadrant of the IAC. (**b**) Cochlear nerve deficiency: Only three nerves are visible; the cochlear nerve is not present in the anteroinferior quadrant of the IAC (white arrow)

Implications for Cochlear Implantation

At the beginning of the cochlear implant (CI) era, surgery was generally contraindicated in congenitally or prelingually deafened children with severely malformed inner ears. With recent advances in device technology and implantation techniques, combined with a better understanding of the benefit that these patients receive from cochlear implantation, more children with cochleovestibular anatomic malformations are now considered surgical candidates. While cochlear implantation in non-malformed ears is typically a straightforward operation, surgery in patients with temporal bone and/or cochleovestibular anomalies can be particularly challenging. Difficulties associated with cochlear implantation in malformed inner ears predominantly revolve around three issues: (1) facial nerve abnormalities requiring a modified surgical approach, (2) identifying the best location to enter the cochlea given that the round window location is not consistent, and (3) CSF leakage complicating insertion of the electrode. In addition to these primary concerns, other associated abnormalities should be considered preoperatively including the possibility of an underdeveloped mastoid or middle ear and hypoplastic or aplastic cochlear nerve [34]. Other operative variables such as the choice of electrode and role for intraoperative imaging will be reviewed.

Surgical Approach

Facial Nerve Considerations

As in all surgeries of the temporal bone, avoidance of injury to the facial nerve is of utmost importance. A recent systematic review demonstrated that 25% of patients with cochleovestibular anomalies have aberrant facial nerve anatomy noted at the time of implant surgery [5, 35]. While the authors advocate for the use of facial nerve monitoring in all patients undergoing cochlear implantation, it is imperative in patients with cochleovestibular anomalies given the high incidence of facial nerve anomalies in this patient population.

Facial nerve anomalies occur most frequently in patients with common cavities, hypoplastic cochleae, and patients with semicircular canal abnormalities in which the lateral canal does not develop normally [19, 36–38]. In fact, cochlear hypoplasia accounts for roughly 50% of all cases of anomalous facial nerve anatomy [39]. An anteromedially-displaced vertical segment of the facial nerve may preclude entry into the middle ear space through the standard transmastoid facial recess. In the tympanic segment, aberrant nerves often course inferior to the cochleariform process and across the promontory towards the round window or if the stapes is absent or malformed may course over the oval window [19, 40, 41]. It is, therefore, advocated to remove the incus and the incus buttress to visually identify the facial nerve in its horizontal tympanic segment, enabling safer tracing of nerve into bone of mastoid segment [42]. If the nerve overlies either the round window or desired cochleostomy location, a more anterior position on the promontory should be chosen to drill a cochleostomy. In patients with a hypoplastic lateral semicircular canal, the second genu of the facial nerve may also be located in an aberrant location.

Transmastoid Posterior Tympanotomy/Facial Recess Approach

The majority of patients with cochleovestibular anomalies can be successfully implanted via a facial recess approach [36]. Alternative approaches should be considered if aberrant facial nerve anatomy precludes access to the middle ear and/or cochlea, or increased exposure is needed to allow for the identification of landmarks such that an appropriately positioned cochleostomy can be made. For example, in common cavity or hypoplastic cochlea deformities, it is possible that neither the promontory nor round window can be reliably identified through the facial recess secondary to underdevelopment of cochlear structures.

Subtotal Petrosectomy with Blind Sac Closure of the External Auditory Canal Approach

Subtotal petrosectomy is a useful approach when either the facial nerve position precludes the standard facial recess approach or spinal fluid gushers do not resolve with conservative measures. One advantage of performing a subtotal petrosectomy is that it provides excellent exposure to the promontory, oval and round windows. Subtotal petrosectomy entails removal of the posterior bony ear canal wall, packing of the Eustachian tube, obliteration of the mastoid cavity, removing all squamous epithelium from the canal and tympanic membrane, and overclosing the external auditory meatus with a resultant blind sac [43–46]. Closure of the canal may risk potential development of cholesteatoma secondary to incomplete removal of squamous epithelium medial to the blind sac.

Transmastoid Retrofacial Approach

The transmastoid retrofacial approach allows access to the posterior mesotympanum and round window. If the facial nerve is displaced anteriorly and/or laterally, it may preclude safe opening of the facial recess. Removing bone medial to the nerve to access the middle ear and cochlea by a retrofacial approach provides a viable alternative to subtotal petrosectomy [47–49].

Suprameatal Approach

The suprameatal approach involves introduction of the electrode array into the middle ear by drilling the suprameatal region and exposing the antrum; a standard mastoidectomy is not necessary. A tympanomeatal flap is then elevated, the middle space is entered, and a cochleostomy with subsequent electrode insertion is performed working through the ear canal [50, 51]. Although literature pertaining to this approach specifically in patients with cochleovestibular anomalies is lacking, its utility in cases with an anteriorly displaced facial nerve and/or a small facial recess has been valuable in the senior author's experience. While most reports regarding this technique describe limited drilling in the suprameatal region, one shouldn't hesitate to perform a standard mastoidectomy for improved identification of landmarks to facilitate accessing the antrum without injury to vital anatomic structures.

Transmastoid Labyrinthotomy Approach

Lastly, the transmastoid labyrinthotomy approach, initially described by Molter et al., creates an opening into the inner ear where the lateral semicircular canal is normally located, avoiding any attempt to open the facial recess and expose the facial nerve [52]. This technique has been reported in patients with common cavities or hypoplastic cochleae [5, 53, 54]. Proponents cite the ability to avoid facial recess and promontory dissection, and implant the electrode array with maximum visualization. Furthermore, control of any potential CSF gusher is facilitated by enhanced exposure to the cochleostomy site through the mastoid, as opposed to the facial recess.

Electrode Insertion and Management of CSF Leak

Cochlear implantation and electrode insertion can be complicated by significant egress of perilymph following the cochleostomy. Given that the inner ear only contains a few microliters of perilymph, high flow fistulas encountered during CI surgery involve passage of CSF through the perilymphatic space and out via the cochleostomy. Reported rates of CSF leak in patients with cochleovestibular anomalies range between 7% and 75% [5, 19, 35, 55–57]. This wide range is likely due to varying definitions of what is considered pathologic leakage. In a recent systematic review, 32% of patients with cochleovestibular malformations had a CSF leak seen during CI surgery [39]. This study did not demonstrate a statistically significant difference in leak rates between mild/moderate and severe anomalies. Other groups, however, have suggested that CSF leak occurs most frequently in patients with common cavity malformations [19].

It is generally accepted that CSF leakage during cochlear implantation occurs due to a defect in the lamina cribosa, a small bony plate at the lateral end of the IAC, through which the cochlear nerve passes [19]. Temporal bone CT imaging is able to demonstrate the defect in the lateral IAC. However, not all patients with radiographic evidence of a defect at the level of the fundus develop CSF leakage during implant surgery [28, 36].

If a CSF leak is encountered during surgery, conservative measures, including head of bed elevation and passive suctioning of spinal fluid, are encouraged. Once the leakage slows, the electrode is inserted and muscle is used to pack the cochleostomy site around the electrode, creating a watertight seal. Small round window incisions may permit the placement of an electrode in a manner that effectively seals the opening and leak. Some authors advocate for larger than normal cochleostomies so that tighter packing can be achieved; Sennaroglu et al. reported the need for more aggressive intervention has decreased since adopting the larger cochleostomy technique [19, 36, 57]. Reinforcement with fibrin glue or gelatin packing may help slow egress of fluid [19, 35]. If significant leakage persists, consideration should be given to packing of the Eustachian tube and/or placement of a lumbar drain. As mentioned above, persistent CSF leaks can also be managed by performing subtotal petrosectomy. Lastly, Sennaroglu et al. have described using a custom electrode with a cork-type stopper at the proximal portion of the electrode; early results with this electrode seem promising, but further studies are needed to corroborate these findings [58]. For any patient with significant egress of spinal fluid during surgery, the importance of avoiding strenuous activity postoperatively should be emphasized such that the cochleostomy seal has time to heal.

Choice of Electrode Array

Choosing a suitable electrode array is critical for achieving successful outcomes and avoiding complications when implanting malformed cochleae. In general, if the cochlear interscalar septum is absent (common cavity, hypoplastic cochlea, and more severe IPs) and/or the lamina cribrosa is deficient, then pre-curved styleted electrodes should be avoided to minimize risk of insertion into the IAC. In common cavity deformities, auditory neural tissue is thought to lie peripherally along the walls of the cavity [29, 59]. For this reason, straight electrodes with fully-banded electrode contacts are more likely to reside against the lateral wall of the cavity and achieve greater contact with neural tissues. Given the smaller size of the cochlea in hypoplastic cochlear malformations, shorter electrode arrays are typically preferred. In patients with EVA or IP type II, either straight or pre-curved arrays can be used. Full insertion can usually be achieved with standard length electrodes in these patients.

IAC Insertion and Intraoperative Imaging

Although rare, there are reported cases of electrodes being inserted into the IAC [56, 60]. The risk of IAC insertion is potentially increased in patients with the following malformations: IPs type I and III/X-linked deafness, cochlear hypoplasia, and common cavity [36, 61]. Insertion into the

IAC can result in facial nerve injuries, vertigo, and suboptimal hearing outcomes [29]. Use of lateral wall electrodes can help prevent insertion into the IAC and reduce danger of repositioning if electrodes are in the IAC. Most authors suggest obtaining intraoperative imaging to confirm electrode position within the inner ear in all patients with cochleovestibular anomalies [56, 57]. There is no consensus regarding the need for, or type of imaging modality, to be obtained; plain radiographs, CT, and fluoroscopy have all been described [42, 62–64].

Audiologic Outcomes

A recent systematic review of all CI in inner ear malformations revealed that the majority of patients (80%) with cochleovestibular malformations are able to perform open-set speech perception testing [39]. This supports the notion that in general, patients with inner ear anomalies derive significant benefit from cochlear implantation [19, 21, 56, 65]. However, the development of speech perception does appear to be significantly correlated with the severity of the malformation. Specifically, patients with mild-to-moderate anomalies obtain open-set speech abilities (85%) more often than those with severe anomalies (54%) [39]. Detailed comparisons of performance between specific inner ear malformations are problematic given the lack of a standardized classification scheme and inconsistencies in reporting audiologic results [65].

In children with IP-EVA spectrum abnormalities, the prognosis for developing open-set speech perception is excellent. Studies have shown that up to 100% of children with IP-EVA achieve open-set speech understanding [5]. In fact, IP-EVA patients are expected to achieve speech perception outcomes comparable to deaf patients without cochleovestibular anomalies and the majority exclusively use oral communication [19, 66]. There is data to suggest that isolated EVA patients may expect a slight performance advantage when compared to concomitant EVA and IP; however, larger studies are needed to confirm this finding [20].

In contrast, patients with cochlear aplasia, common cavity malformations, and cochlear hypoplasia perform significantly worse than those with milder forms of cochleovestibular dysplasia [5, 19, 67]. When aggregating multiple studies, the pooled rate of development of open-set speech perception for children with hypoplastic malformations was noted to be 50% [5]. While this rate of speech perception acquisition is modest, it should be noted that even the poorest performers demonstrate gains with increased use of their implant [19].

Children with deficient cochlear nerves typically perform at a significantly lower level when compared to other cochleovestibular malformations. The prognosis for developing speech perception abilities is poor, but the majority of children with CND do acquire sound awareness after implantation [5]. Fewer patients attain closed-set perception than sound awareness, and even fewer gain open-set speech perception [68]. Although this can be considered objective benefit, patients with CND are generally considered poor candidates for cochlear implantation. If implantation is performed, the better anatomic ear should be selected. In the case of bilateral cochlear nerve deficiency or no benefit with CI, auditory brainstem implantation may be discussed as a rehabilitative option at a center offering it as part of a clinical trial. In cases of CI for CND, parents are appropriately optimistic that their child will develop spoken language. This can occur at the risk of not developing any form of communication. As such we make the rare recommendation that children undergoing CI with CND undergo rehabilitation with both visual and spoken language, such that at least one form of communication will be present for the developing child.

Conclusion

Congenital hearing loss is a common sensory impairment. With advances in molecular genetics, the potential to identify hereditary causes of pediatric hearing loss has greatly expanded. Recent data suggest that genetic hearing loss accounts for over half of all congenital or prelingual hearing loss cases. Cochlear implantation is widely accepted as a suitable intervention for children with severe to profound SNHL and most cochleovestibular malformations. Given the prevalence (20%) of cochleovestibular malformations in children with SNHL, surgeons and audiologists must be familiar with the role of cochlear implantation in these patients. While the majority of children with cochleovestibular malformations are able to obtain open-set speech perception, performance appears to correlate with severity of the underlying malformation.

References

1. Morton CC, Nance WE. Newborn hearing screening--a silent revolution. N Engl J Med. 2006;354:2151–64.
2. Alford RL, Arnos KS, Fox M, et al. American College of Medical Genetics and Genomics guideline for the clinical evaluation and etiologic diagnosis of hearing loss. Genet Med. 2014;16:347–55.
3. Carey JC, Palumbos JC. Advances in the understanding of the genetic causes of hearing loss in children inform a rational approach to evaluation. Indian J Pediatr. 2016;83:1150–6.
4. Shearer AE, Smith RJ. Genetics: advances in genetic testing for deafness. Curr Opin Pediatr. 2012;24:679–86.
5. Buchman CA, Teagle HF, Roush PA, et al. Cochlear implantation in children with labyrinthine anomalies and cochlear nerve deficiency: implications for auditory brainstem implantation. Laryngoscope. 2011;121:1979–88.

6. Jackler RK, Luxford WM, House WF. Congenital malformations of the inner ear: a classification based on embryogenesis. Laryngoscope. 1987;97:2–14.
7. Chang KW. Genetics of hearing loss--nonsyndromic. Otolaryngol Clin North Am. 2015;48:1063–72.
8. Kelsell DP, Dunlop J, Stevens HP, et al. Connexin 26 mutations in hereditary non-syndromic sensorineural deafness. Nature. 1997;387:80–3.
9. McClay JE, Tandy R, Grundfast K, et al. Major and minor temporal bone abnormalities in children with and without congenital sensorineural hearing loss. Arch Otolaryngol Head Neck Surg. 2002;128:664–71.
10. Park AH, Duval M, McVicar S, Bale JF, Hohler N, Carey JC. A diagnostic paradigm including cytomegalovirus testing for idiopathic pediatric sensorineural hearing loss. Laryngoscope. 2014;124:2624–9.
11. Peterson J, Nishimura C, Smith RJ. Genetic testing for congenital bilateral hearing loss in the context of targeted cytomegalovirus screening. Laryngoscope. 2020;130:2714.
12. Holcomb MA, Rumboldt Z, White DR. Cochlear nerve deficiency in children with CHARGE syndrome. Laryngoscope. 2013;123:793–6.
13. Preciado DA, Lawson L, Madden C, et al. Improved diagnostic effectiveness with a sequential diagnostic paradigm in idiopathic pediatric sensorineural hearing loss. Otol Neurotol. 2005;26:610–5.
14. Sloan-Heggen CM, Smith RJ. Navigating genetic diagnostics in patients with hearing loss. Curr Opin Pediatr. 2016;28(6):705.
15. Joshi VM, Navlekar SK, Kishore GR, Reddy KJ, Kumar EC. CT and MR imaging of the inner ear and brain in children with congenital sensorineural hearing loss. Radiographics. 2012;32:683–98.
16. Phelps PD. Cochlear implants for congenital deformities. J Laryngol Otol. 1992;106:967–70.
17. Sennaroglu L, Saatci I. A new classification for cochleovestibular malformations. Laryngoscope. 2002;112:2230–41.
18. Sennaroglu L, Sarac S, Ergin T. Surgical results of cochlear implantation in malformed cochlea. Otol Neurotol. 2006;27:615–23.
19. Papsin BC. Cochlear implantation in children with anomalous cochleovestibular anatomy. Laryngoscope. 2005;115:1–26.
20. Pritchett C, Zwolan T, Huq F, et al. Variations in the cochlear implant experience in children with enlarged vestibular aqueduct. Laryngoscope. 2015;125:2169–74.
21. Lee KH, Lee J, Isaacson B, Kutz JW, Roland PS. Cochlear implantation in children with enlarged vestibular aqueduct. Laryngoscope. 2010;120:1675–81.
22. Rodriguez K, Shah RK, Kenna M. Anomalies of the middle and inner ear. Otolaryngol Clin N Am. 2007;40(81–96):vi.
23. Vijayasekaran S, Halsted MJ, Boston M, et al. When is the vestibular aqueduct enlarged? A statistical analysis of the normative distribution of vestibular aqueduct size. AJNR Am J Neuroradiol. 2007;28:1133–8.
24. Connor SE, Dudau C, Pai I, Gaganasiou M. Is CT or MRI the optimal imaging investigation for the diagnosis of large vestibular aqueduct syndrome and large endolymphatic sac anomaly? Eur Arch Otorhinolaryngol. 2019;276(3):693–702.
25. Luntz M, Balkany T, Hodges AV, Telischi FF. Cochlear implants in children with congenital inner ear malformations. Arch Otolaryngol Head Neck Surg. 1997;123:974–7.
26. Kutz JW Jr, Lee KH, Isaacson B, Booth TN, Sweeney MH, Roland PS. Cochlear implantation in children with cochlear nerve absence or deficiency. Otol Neurotol. 2011;32:956–61.
27. Glastonbury CM, Davidson HC, Harnsberger HR, Butler J, Kertesz TR, Shelton C. Imaging findings of cochlear nerve deficiency. AJNR Am J Neuroradiol. 2002;23:635–43.
28. Mylanus EA, Rotteveel LJ, Leeuw RL. Congenital malformation of the inner ear and pediatric cochlear implantation. Otol Neurotol. 2004;25:308–17.
29. Coelho DH, Roland JT Jr. Implanting obstructed and malformed cochleae. Otolaryngol Clin N Am. 2012;45:91–110.
30. Thai-Van H, Fraysse B, Berry I, et al. Functional magnetic resonance imaging may avoid misdiagnosis of cochleovestibular nerve aplasia in congenital deafness. Am J Otol. 2000;21:663–70.
31. Fritzsch B, Nichols DH. DiI reveals a prenatal arrival of efferents at the differentiating otocyst of mice. Hear Res. 1993;65:51–60.
32. Freeman SR, Sennaroglu L. Management of cochlear nerve hypoplasia and aplasia. Adv Hear Rehabil. 2018;81:81–92.
33. Sennaroglu L, Bajin MD. Classification and current management of inner ear malformations. Balkan Med J. 2017;34(5):397.
34. Da Costa Monsanto R, Sennaroglu L, Uchiyama M, Sancak IG, Paparella MM, Cureoglu S. Histopathology of inner ear malformations: potential pitfalls for cochlear implantation. Otol Neurotol. 2019;40(8):e839–46.
35. Hoffman RA, Downey LL, Waltzman SB, Cohen NL. Cochlear implantation in children with cochlear malformations. Am J Otol. 1997;18:184–7.
36. Sennaroglu L. Cochlear implantation in inner ear malformations--a review article. Cochlear Implants Int. 2010;11:4–41.
37. Satar B, Mukherji SK, Telian SA. Congenital aplasia of the semicircular canals. Otol Neurotol. 2003;24:437–46.
38. Sennaroglu L, Tahir E. A novel classification: anomalous routes of the facial nerve in relation to inner ear malformations. Laryngoscope. 2020;130:E696–703.
39. Pakdaman MN, Herrmann BS, Curtin HD, Van Beek-King J, Lee DJ. Cochlear implantation in children with anomalous cochleovestibular anatomy: a systematic review. Otolaryngol Head Neck Surg. 2012;146:180–90.
40. Ito J, Sakota T, Kato H, Hazama M, Enomoto M. Surgical considerations regarding cochlear implantation in the congenitally malformed cochlea. Otolaryngol Head Neck Surg. 1999;121:495–8.
41. Zheng Y, Schachern PA, Djalilian HR, Paparella MM. Temporal bone histopathology related to cochlear implantation in congenital malformation of the bony cochlea. Otol Neurotol. 2002;23:181–6.
42. Coelho DH, Waltzman SB, Roland JT Jr. Implanting common cavity malformations using intraoperative fluoroscopy. Otol Neurotol. 2008;29:914–9.
43. Polo R, Medina MD, Aristegui M, et al. Subtotal petrosectomy for cochlear implantation: lessons learned after 110 cases. Ann Otol Rhinol Laryngol. 2015;125(6):485–94.
44. Bernardeschi D, Nguyen Y, Smail M, et al. Middle ear and mastoid obliteration for cochlear implant in adults: indications and anatomical results. Otol Neurotol. 2015;36:604–9.
45. Bendet E, Cerenko D, Linder TE, Fisch U. Cochlear implantation after subtotal petrosectomies. Eur Arch Otorhinolaryngol. 1998;255:169–74.
46. Free RH, Falcioni M, Di Trapani G, Giannuzzi AL, Russo A, Sanna M. The role of subtotal petrosectomy in cochlear implant surgery--a report of 32 cases and review on indications. Otol Neurotol. 2013;34:1033–40.
47. Rizk H, O'Connell B, Stevens S, Meyer T. Retrofacial approach to access the round window for cochlear implantation of malformed ears. Otol Neurotol. 2015;36:e79–83.
48. Liening DA, Haupert M, Kartush J. Cochlear implantation and variation of facial nerve anatomy: a case report. Ear Nose Throat J. 1994;73:667–9.
49. Huang CC, Lin CY, Wu JL. Retrofacial approach of cochlear implantation in inner ear malformation with aberrant facial nerve: a case report. Auris Nasus Larynx. 2006;33:179–82.
50. Kronenberg J, Baumgartner W, Migirov L, Dagan T, Hildesheimer M. The suprameatal approach: an alternative surgical approach to cochlear implantation. Otol Neurotol. 2004;25:41–4; discussion 44–45.
51. Postelmans JT, Tange RA, Stokroos RJ, Grolman W. The suprameatal approach: a safe alternative surgical technique for cochlear implantation. Otol Neurotol. 2010;31:196–203.

52. Molter DW, Pate BR Jr, McElveen JT Jr. Cochlear implantation in the congenitally malformed ear. Otolaryngol Head Neck Surg. 1993;108:174–7.
53. McElveen JT Jr, Carrasco VN, Miyamoto RT, Linthicum FH Jr. Cochlear implantation in common cavity malformations using a transmastoid labyrinthotomy approach. Laryngoscope. 1997;107:1032–6.
54. Zarandy MM. Transmastoid labyrinthotomy approach for cochlear implantation in a common cavity malformation: a case report. Ear Nose Throat J. 2008;87:E1–3.
55. Weber BP, Dillo W, Dietrich B, Maneke I, Bertram B, Lenarz T. Pediatric cochlear implantation in cochlear malformations. Am J Otol. 1998;19:747–53.
56. Tucci DL, Telian SA, Zimmerman-Phillips S, Zwolan TA, Kileny PR. Cochlear implantation in patients with cochlear malformations. Arch Otolaryngol Head Neck Surg. 1995;121:833–8.
57. Graham JM, Phelps PD, Michaels L. Congenital malformations of the ear and cochlear implantation in children: review and temporal bone report of common cavity. J Laryngol Otol Suppl. 2000;25:1–14.
58. Sennaroglu L, Atay G, Bajin MD. A new cochlear implant electrode with a "cork"-type stopper for inner ear malformations. Auris Nasus Larynx. 2014;41:331–6.
59. Beltrame MA, Birman CS, Cervera Escario J, et al. Common cavity and custom-made electrodes: speech perception and audiological performance of children with common cavity implanted with a custom-made MED-EL electrode. Int J Pediatr Otorhinolaryngol. 2013;77:1237–43.
60. Wootten CT, Backous DD, Haynes DS. Management of cerebrospinal fluid leakage from cochleostomy during cochlear implant surgery. Laryngoscope. 2006;116:2055–9.
61. Cosetti MK, Friedmann DR, Heman-Ackah SE, Perez R, Waltzman SB, Roland JT Jr. Surgical techniques and outcomes of cochlear implantation in patients with radiographic findings consistent with X-linked deafness. Int J Pediatr Otorhinolaryngol. 2015;79:1689–93.
62. Copeland BJ, Pillsbury HC, Buchman CA. Prospective evaluation of intraoperative cochlear implant radiographs. Otol Neurotol. 2004;25:295–7.
63. Eisenman DJ, Ashbaugh C, Zwolan TA, Arts HA, Telian SA. Implantation of the malformed cochlea. Otol Neurotol. 2001;22:834–41.
64. Fishman AJ, Roland JT Jr, Alexiades G, Mierzwinski J, Cohen NL. Fluoroscopically assisted cochlear implantation. Otol Neurotol. 2003;24:882–6.
65. Farhood Z, Nguyen SA, Miller SC, Holcomb MA, Meyer TA, Rizk AH. Cochlear implantation in inner ear malformations: systematic review of speech perception outcomes and intraoperative findings. Otolaryngol Head Neck Surg. 2017;156(5):783–93.
66. Miyamoto RT, Bichey BG, Wynne MK, Kirk KI. Cochlear implantation with large vestibular aqueduct syndrome. Laryngoscope. 2002;112:1178–82.
67. Jeong SW, Kim LS. A new classification of cochleovestibular malformations and implications for predicting speech perception ability after cochlear implantation. Audiol Neurootol. 2015;20:90–101.
68. Vesseur A, Free R, Snels C, Dekker F, Mylanus E, Verbist B, Frijns J. Hearing restoration in cochlear nerve deficiency: the choice between cochlear implant or auditory brainstem implant, a meta-analysis. Otol Neurotol. 2018;39(4):428–37.

Sudden Sensorineural Hearing Loss

50

Cameron C. Wick and Craig A. Buchman

Introduction

Approximately 14–31% of US adults (27–61 million people) suffer from hearing loss [1]. Most cases present gradually and are attributed to age-related changes (e.g., presbycusis), but a subset will suffer from a sudden loss. Sudden sensorineural hearing loss (SSNHL) is defined as a decline in hearing of at least 30 dB over three sequential frequencies that occurs within 72 hours [2]. The annual incidence of SSNHL in the United States is estimated to be 10.7 per 100,000 people, which equates to 34,000 new cases per year [3]. Other societies have reported an incidence rate ranging from 7.8 per 100,000 people in Taiwan to 160 per 100,000 people in Germany [4, 5].

Regardless of the true incidence, SSNHL imparts an economical and psychological burden through its detrimental impact on sound localization, hearing in noise, and communication abilities. This lower quality of life carries a 2.2 times higher rate of clinical depression [6]. The negative impact of SSNHL can be long-term and is particularly devastating if accompanied by persistent tinnitus or imbalance [6–8].

Etiology

Sudden sensorineural hearing loss was first reported by De Kleyn in 1944 who suggested it arose from brainstem pathology secondary to a vitamin deficiency [9]. Since then, theories about ruptured cochlear membranes, viral inflammation, and vascular insults have been popularized [10, 11]. In reality SSNHL is a heterogeneous disorder with numerous etiologies and an identifiable cause is found in only 15–29% of cases [12, 13]. The impact of finding the underlying cause can have implications on hearing prognosis, patient counseling, disease management, and prevention of systemic sequelae associated with some of the causes.

The literature describes over 100 diagnoses linked to SSNHL. In 2010, Chau et al. performed a systematic review of 23 studies with 686 SSNHL cases to summarize the most common etiologies [13]. The breakdown was 71.0% for idiopathic cases, 12.8% for infectious diseases including presumed upper respiratory illness, 4.7% for otologic diseases, 4.2% for trauma, 2.8% for vascular or hematologic problems, 2.3% for neoplastic diseases, and 2.2% for other causes. Other studies have reported an increased risk of developing SSNHL among patients with acquired cardiovascular risk factors, diabetes, migraine, systemic lupus erythematosus, psoriasis, human immunodeficiency virus, iron-deficiency anemia, obstructive sleep apnea, metabolic syndrome, osteoporosis, and chronic kidney disease [14–27]. The proposed etiologies, their relative frequencies, and the odds ratios for specific risk factors are summarized in Table 50.1.

C. C. Wick (✉)
Department of Otolaryngology—Head and Neck Surgery, University Hospitals Cleveland Medical Center, Cleveland, OH, USA
e-mail: cameron.wick@uhhospitals.org

C. A. Buchman
Department of Otolaryngology—Head and Neck Surgery, University of Utah, Salt Lake City, UT, USA

A. D. Sweeney et al. (eds.), *Haynes-Glasscock-Shambaugh Surgery of the Ear*, https://doi.org/10.1007/978-3-032-18264-7_50

Table 50.1 Sudden sensorineural hearing loss etiologies and risk factors

Etiologies	Percentage	Risk
Idiopathic	71.0	
Infectious	12.8	2.2 (1.1–4.4) [21]
Upper respiratory illness		
Meningitis		
Group A *Streptococcus*		
Epstein–Barr virus		
Mumps		
Herpes simplex virus		
Treponema pallidum		
Borrelia burgdorferi (Lyme disease)		
Human immunodeficiency virus		
Others		
Otologic	4.7	
Autoimmune inner ear disease		
Ménière's disease		
Otosclerosis		
Chronic otitis media		
Otologic surgery		
Trauma	4.2	
Traumatic brain injury		
Skull fracture		
Acoustic trauma		
Barotrauma		
Vascular	2.8	1.6 (1.3–2.1) [49]
Cardiovascular disease		1.5 (1.0–2.4) [17]
Stroke		1.0 (0.7–1.4) [17]
Diabetes		1.3 (1.1–1.6) [22]
Hypertension		1.5 (1.1–2.0) [27]
Iron deficiency anemia		
Sickle cell anemia		
Hemodialysis coagulopathy		
Neoplastic	2.3	
Vestibular schwannoma		
Meningioma		
Paraganglioma		
Endolymphatic sac tumors		
Others		
Other	2.2	1.8 (1.2–2.6) [18]
Multiple sclerosis or CNS disease		1.5 (1.2–1.9) [20]
Migraine		2.3 (1.4–3.6) [19]
Psoriasis		1.5 (1.0–2.2) [23]
Systemic lupus erythematosus		3.5 (2.0–6.4) [24]
Obstructive sleep apnea		1.8 (1.4–2.3) [25]
Metabolic syndrome		1.3 (1.1–1.6) [17]
Osteoporosis		2.2 (1.7–2.9) [17]
Smoking		
Heavy alcohol consumption		
Non-otologic surgery		

Etiology percentages as reported by Chau et al. [13]. Odds ratios and risk derived from the literature as noted

Cochlear Etiologies

Infectious

Viral infections have commonly been suggested as a mechanism for SSNHL. Nearly 25% of patients with SSNHL report a "head cold" or fever around the time of hearing loss [28]. While certain viruses like herpes simplex virus, cytomegalovirus, and rubella have well-established neurotrophic affinity in congenital sensorineural hearing loss, the pathophysiology of adult-onset, acute viral infection is less clear. Proposed mechanisms of viral insult within the cochlea and cochlear nerve include direct invasion, secondary inflammation, reactivation of latent virus in the spiral ganglion, and immune-mediated destruction [13, 29]. Viruses, including influenza A, have shown the ability to infect human Schwann cells, which could lead to demyelination and SSNHL [30]. Because sampling inner ear fluid during episodes of SSNHL is not clinically useful or indicated, the causative nature of specific viruses is largely dependent on serology studies or postmortem histology. Both methods infer a viral etiology rather than demonstrate direct causality.

Despite these limitations, serology, epidemiology, and histopathology data have identified multiple viruses potentially responsible for SSNHL [31]. The routine use of serologic testing, however, has not shown benefit and has potential to complicate the medical decision making if false-positives are present [13, 32]. Some of the data used to infer a viral etiology compared normal hearing control subjects to patients with SSNHL and found higher seroconversion rates in the SSNHL population for influenza B, enterovirus, and herpes simplex 1 virus [11, 33]. Other studies used serology to extrapolate that mumps virus and varicella-zoster virus (Ramsay Hunt Syndrome) were the offending agents [34, 35]. Even if a higher rate of viral seroconversion is present amongst SSNHL patients, the percentage of affected individuals varies across the different studies. For instance, Wilson et al. (1983) detected mumps, rubella, varicella-zoster virus, cytomegalovirus, or influenza virus seroconversion in 76 of 122 subjects (63%) [11]. On the other hand, seroconversion rates were much lower in Xenellis et al. (2007) who found 70 of 262 subjects (27%) seroconverted for Epstein–Barr virus, herpes simplex, or cytomegalovirus and Gross et al. (2007) who found only 4 of 48 subjects (8%) seroconverted for Epstein–Barr virus, enterovirus, or cytomegalovirus, respectively [36, 37]. In conclusion, there is data to support an association between viral infections and SSNHL. However, the specific type of virus often remains unknown. A thorough history and identification of associated viral symptoms may lead the clinician to a specific viral diagnosis, but otherwise routine serologic testing is not recommended.

Coronavirus disease 2019 (COVID-19) is a respiratory and vascular disease caused by the severe acute respiratory syndrome coronavirus 2 (SARS-CoV-2) virus. The virus has a known tropism for sensory neuroepithelium as demonstrated by the common symptoms of anosmia and ageusia. While audiovestibular symptoms are less frequent, the molecular mechanism for SARS-CoV-2 to infect inner ear neuroepithelium has been demonstrated and many case series exist [38]. The potential impact of the COVID-19 vaccination remains less clear. Population-based analyses from Finland and the United States failed to show an association between receiving the vaccination and an increased risk of SSNHL [39, 40]. However, a study from Israel did show a small increased risk [41]. If there is a small increased risk of SSNHL that risk must be individually weighed versus the other detriments of COVID-19, including SSNHL.

Bacterial infections, particularly meningitis, can have devastating neurologic consequences. The incidence of long-term neurologic sequelae in survivors of bacterial meningitis ranges from 10% to 30% [42]. Meningitis from *Streptococcus pneumoniae* has the highest incidence of sensorineural hearing loss [43]. A robust host immune response to the infectious organism is responsible for the acute onset of hearing loss and corresponds with improved hearing results following administration of steroids and other anti-inflammatory agents [44, 45]. When early hearing loss is present, the future progression of hearing loss is less predictable and repeated hearing tests are advised [46]. More common infections, like bacterial or viral acute otitis media and its resultant effusion, can also cause hearing loss. This loss is often conductive secondary to a middle ear effusion but sensorineural components have been reported [47].

Vascular

Vascular theories for SSNHL stem from the cochlea's blood supply off the labyrinthine artery, which is a terminal branch of the anterior inferior cerebellar artery. Occlusion of the labyrinthine artery was suggested as a SSNHL cause as early as 1949 [48]. Exactly how the labyrinthine artery becomes occluded is less clear. Theories of thrombosis, atherosclerosis, hypotension, vasospasm, and embolism have all been proposed. The impact of acquired cardiovascular risk factors and diabetes is mixed with some studies supporting a link while other studies do not [17, 49–52].

Occlusion of intracranial arteries leads to ischemic necrosis and stroke. If labyrinthine artery occlusion is the cause of SSNHL, then it might signify a predisposition for the occlusion of other intracranial arteries. This rationale has led to investigations on the relationship of strokes and SSNHL. Patients with a history of SSNHL have a 1.6 times higher risk of stroke when compared to a normal hearing cohort [53, 54]. Likewise, a nation-wide population study from Taiwan looked at 11,115 patients with a history of stroke and found a 1.7 times higher risk of SSNHL [55]. Another prospective study of 364 patients having had a posterior circulation stroke identified 8% of patients presented with sudden hearing loss as the chief complaint [56]. Other symptoms that suggest disruption of blood flow in the anterior inferior cerebellar artery include vertigo, nystagmus, facial weakness, ataxia, as well as SSNHL. Vertebral artery dissection can cause occipital headache, neck pain, vision loss, ataxia, and SSNHL. The potential for SSNHL to accompany these severe conditions highlights the importance of a detailed history and physical exam when evaluating a patient with SSNHL.

Inflammatory/Autoimmune

Sudden sensorineural hearing loss has been associated with both systemic and ear specific immune-mediated diseases. The association between autoimmunity and sensorineural hearing loss was suggested as early as 1979 [57]. In that landmark report autoimmune inner ear disease (AIED) was described as bilateral progressive, fluctuating sensorineural hearing loss. Its therapeutic response to steroids and cyclophosphamide led McCabe to assume an autoimmune etiology. Since then, the literature has been filled with case reports of SSNHL in the context of Cogan's syndrome, temporal arteritis, granulomatosis with polyangiitis (historically known as Wegener's granulomatosis), Sjogren's syndrome, relapsing polychondritis, polyarteritis nodosa, systemic sclerosis, Behçet's syndrome, systemic lupus erythematosus, and others (Fig. 50.1) [58–66]. Elevated levels of circulating immune complexes, increased expression of major histocompatibility complex (MHC) class II genes, abnormal subpopulations of T-cells, and inner ear autoantibodies have

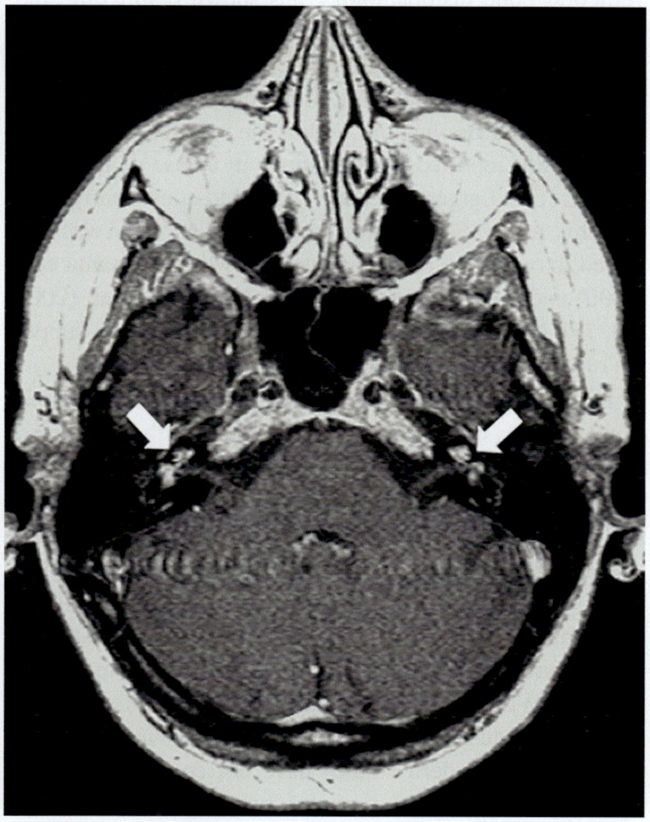

Fig. 50.1 Bilateral labyrinthitis associated with Cogan's syndrome. This T1-weighted axial magnetic resonance imaging with gadolinium contrast and without fat suppression shows bilateral enhancement within the cochlea and vestibule (arrows)

been described but the association between the pathologic immune responses and a specific inner ear structure is less well defined [67]. This link between autoimmune disease and inner ear damage continues to be a source of active investigation. Animal models have provided insight into the pathophysiology for some of the autoimmune diseases. For instance, in Cogan's syndrome the immunoglobulin G (IgG) immunoglobulins have an affinity for a supporting protein in the sensory epithelia of the inner ear Density-Enhanced Protein tyrosine phosphatase-1 (DEP-1/CD148) as well as connexin 26 that results in sensorineural hearing loss in mice [58]. Despite this insight, for most autoimmune diseases the specific target within the inner ear remains elusive. Autoimmune serology studies like antinuclear autoantibodies (ANA), rheumatoid factor, antimitochondrial autoantibodies, anti-double stranded DNA, Anti-Sjogren's Syndrome Type A (Anti-SSA; Ro), Anti-Sjogren's Syndrome Type B (Anti-SSB; La), and others yield mixed results and are not currently recommended for SSNHL. The clinician must assess for other signs of systemic autoimmunity and be aware that SSNHL may be an early manifestation of AIED or a systemic illness [68].

Histopathology

Temporal bone histopathology has shown conflicting findings regarding the previously mentioned cochlear etiologies of SSNHL, perhaps because of the varied underlying etiologies. The histologic hallmark of an inner ear vascular insult is fibrosis and ossification within the cochlea. Schuknecht et al. (1986) reported these findings in a case of idiopathic SSNHL [69]. Larger series have failed to consistently replicate this result. For instance, a vascular etiology was suggested in only 1 of 12 specimens reviewed by Vasama et al. (2000) and 1 of 17 specimens from Merchant et al. (2005) [70, 71]. Neither of these studies found evidence to support the ruptured membranes theory.

Histologic evidence for a viral etiology first stemmed from an analysis of four temporal bones with a history of upper respiratory illness preceding unilateral SSNHL. The tissues showed degeneration of the organ of Corti, loss of spiral ganglion neurons, and variable stria vascularis atrophy. There was no evidence of vascular pathology [72]. This report and follow-up studies suggested that these findings were analogous to cases afflicted with a known history of viral labyrinthitis secondary to rubella, measles, or mumps [72, 73]. While similarities may exist, the studies did not show direct causality and the relationship to viral pathology was inferred. Modern studies have not consistently found viral antigens or viral particles on electron microscopy within most SSNHL specimens [71]. Additionally, experimental models with inner ears directly inoculated with pathogenic viruses do not always show hearing loss and if they do it is often a progressive rather than sudden loss [74, 75]. Merchant et al. (2005) did replicate many of the pathologic changes initially described by Schuknecht (1962), specifically loss of hair cells and supporting cells of the organ of Corti with variable degradation of the tectorial membrane, stria vascularis, spiral limbus, and cochlear neurons [71, 72]. Merchant concluded that the SSNHL comes from activation of cellular stress pathways, including nuclear factor-κB, that causes apoptosis of the inner ear structures [71].

Retrocochlear Etiologies

Tumor

Neoplasms of the cerebellopontine angle (CPA) may cause SSNHL. Vestibular schwannomas (VS) account for 90–95% of tumors in the CPA and modern estimates show the incidence of spontaneous VS may be as high as 2 per 10,000 people (0.02%) [76]. The hearing loss associated with VS is most commonly progressive, but sudden losses with or without recovery have been described [77, 78]. SSNHL has also been described for CPA meningiomas as well as more rare pathology like metastatic disease or paraneoplastic syndromes [79–81]. The clinical importance of a neoplasm diagnosis is self-evident and therefore evaluation for retrocochlear lesions via magnetic resonance imaging (MRI) is supported by the American Academy of Otolaryngology—Head and Neck Surgery (AAO-HNS) clinical practice guideline on sudden hearing loss (Table 50.2) [32]. Workup for a retrocochlear lesion should occur even if there is recovery of hearing.

Trauma

Sudden hearing loss secondary to trauma has been well described. Creation of a perilymphatic fistula can occur from excess external or intracranial pressure. Common scenarios of external pressure include slap injuries to the ear, barotrauma from recreational diving, and blast injuries [82–85]. Other causes like whiplash and sneezing may increase intracranial pressure and result in SSNHL [86, 87]. Some inner ear pathology like enlarged vestibular aqueduct syndrome may predispose patients to sudden hearing loss, even after minor head trauma [88].

Other

Unilateral sudden hearing loss associated with Ménière's disease is accompanied by tinnitus, aural fullness, and vertigo lasting greater than 20 minutes. The hearing loss is often less severe than idiopathic SSNHL and shows a predilection for lower frequencies. The fluctuating hearing loss of Ménière's disease implies that it recovers but with repeated attacks a progressive loss may occur [89].

Ototoxicity from aminoglycoside antibiotics, platinum-based chemotherapeutics, and other medications can cause

Table 50.2 2012 AAO-HNS clinical practice guideline on sudden hearing loss

Statement number	Action statement	Recommendation strength
Diagnosis		
1	Distinguish SNHL from CHL	Strong recommendation
2	Assess for modifying factors like bilateral hearing loss, fluctuating hearing loss, or focal neurologic findings	Recommended
3	Clinicians should not order a CT head in the initial evaluation of SSNHL	Strong recommendation
4	Confirm SSNHL with audiometric evaluation; Report diagnosis as idiopathic if an underlying condition is not identified on history and physical exam	Recommended
5	Do not obtain routine laboratory tests	Strong recommendation
6	Evaluate for retrocochlear pathology using a MRI, ABR, or audiometric follow-up	Recommended
Shared decision making		
7	Educate patients on the natural history of SSNHL, benefits and risks of medical intervention, and limitations of existing data	Strong recommendation
Treatment		
8	Offer systemic steroids as initial therapy	Option
9	Offer hyperbaric oxygen therapy within 3 months of SSNHL onset	Option
10	Do not routinely prescribe antivirals, thrombolytics, vasodilators, vasoactive substances, or antioxidants	Recommended
11	Offer salvage intratympanic steroid perfusion if there is incomplete recovery after initial management	Recommended
Follow-up		
12	Obtain follow-up audiometric evaluation within 6 months of SSNHL diagnosis	Recommended
13	Counsel patients with incomplete recovery on the benefits of hearing amplification, hearing assistive technology, and other supportive measures	Strong recommendation

Table adapted from Stachler et al. [32]
AAO-HNS American Academy of Otolaryngology—Head and Neck Surgery, *CHL* conductive hearing loss, *CT* computed tomography, *MRI* magnetic resonance imaging, *SNHL* sensorineural hearing loss, *SSNHL* sudden sensorineural hearing loss

SSNHL [90]. A genetic susceptibility for aminoglycoside-induced hearing loss exists in patients that carry a mutated A1555G allele in the mitochondrial 12S ribosomal RNA [91]. Likewise, cisplatin sensitivity occurs in patients with mutated glutathione S-transferase (GST), thiopurine S-methyl transferase (TMPT), and catechol-O-methyl transferase (COMT) [90]. The genetic defects in both aminoglycoside-induced and cisplatin-induced hearing loss relate to the inner ear's ability to handle oxidative stress, although the ultimate cell death pathway differs between the offending agents.

Presentation and Evaluation

The average age of SSNHL is 50–60 years but wide variation exists. Most commonly the loss is unilateral and frequently is noticed upon awakening [92]. Common accompanying symptoms include tinnitus (80%), aural fullness (80%), and vertigo (35%) [93, 94]. Some patients may also describe a blocked sensation or periauricular numbness. The hearing loss severity and configuration vary with a roughly equal distribution between mild, moderate, and severe losses [31].

The workup for SSNHL begins with a thorough history and medical examination. Subtle associations or exam findings relevant to the previously discussed etiologies can guide the subsequent evaluation. A detailed otoscopic examination, including Weber and Rinne tuning fork tests, can distinguish between conductive and sensorineural hearing losses. Formal audiometric evaluation will confirm the type and severity of the hearing loss and should be performed in a timely manner. The neurologic examination is paramount and should include assessment of the vestibular system and cranial nerves. The low yield of laboratory tests like a complete blood count, C-reactive protein, erythrocyte sedimentation rate, and autoimmune studies had led the AAO-HNS to strongly recommend against routine blood work, unless the history or physical exam suggests a specific etiology [32]. Ruling out retrocochlear pathology is best performed with a contrasted MRI that contains thin cuts through the internal auditory canal. The yield for tumor detection in patients with SSNHL is considerably higher than it is in asymptomatic patients [95, 96]. If an MRI cannot be obtained, then an auditory brainstem response or a contrasted computed tomography of the temporal bone should be performed. Even when a tumor is not present, the MRI can find evidence of demyelinating disease, vascular pathology, inner ear inflammation, and cochlear hemorrhage [97]. The three-dimensional fluid-attenuated inversion recovery (3D-FLAIR) MRI sequence may show an abnormal inner ear in up to 27% of patients, with abnormal findings predicting worse hearing recovery (Fig. 50.2) [98].

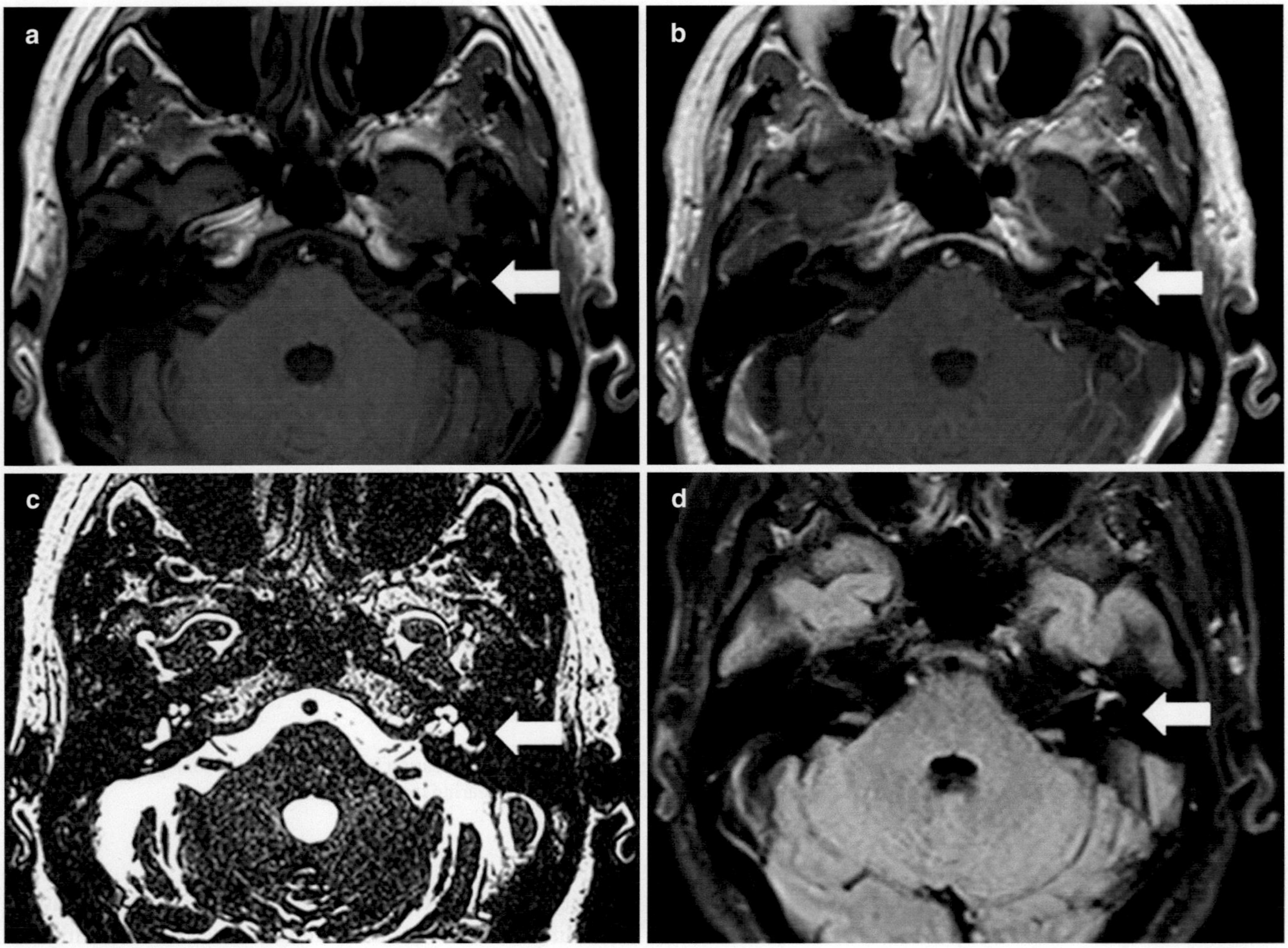

Fig. 50.2 Positive magnetic resonance imaging (MRI) findings in a case of left sudden sensorineural hearing loss and vertigo. The arrow marks the left inner ear. (**a**) T1-weighted axial MRI without contrast shows enhanced signal in the left cochlea and vestibule. (**b**) T1-weighted axial MRI with gadolinium contrast shows minor internal auditory canal enhancement and no tumor identification. (**c**) T2-heavily weighted MRI shows a patent cerebrospinal fluid (CSF) signal within the cochlea. This patency helps rule-out cochlear schwannomas and labyrinthitis ossificans. (**d**) Fluid-attenuated inversion recovery (FLAIR) sequence shows marked left inner ear enhancement consistent with inflammation or hemorrhage

Treatment

If an underlying diagnosis is found, it should guide the treatment and include referrals to appropriate specialists. Many cases will not have a known etiology and should be labeled as idiopathic SSNHL. Patients should be educated on the natural history of SSNHL, different treatment options, and limitations of the current data on this heterogeneous population.

The natural history of SSNHL was studied by Mattox et al. in 1977. They looked at 89 patients with idiopathic SSNHL that did not receive medical treatment and found that 65% spontaneously recovered to a functional hearing level [12]. The majority of patients recovered within 14 days of the hearing loss. A similar finding in 2007 from the Swedish national database reported on 90 untreated patients, of which 28% had a large (> 30 dB) spontaneous recovery and 36% had a moderate (10–30 dB) spontaneous recovery [93]. In contrast, Wilson et al. (1980) reported a recovery rate of 32% in 34 patients receiving placebo therapy [99].

A poor prognosis for hearing recovery has been identified in older patients, those with profound hearing loss, flat audiometric configurations, high-frequency loss, delayed treatment, the presence of vertigo, and cochlear enhancement on MRI [12, 98–103], The impact of diabetes and cardiovascular risk factors on recovery has shown conflicting results. A recent multivariate analysis found the absence of diabetes and hypercholesterolemia had odds ratios of 1.69 and 1.70 in favor of hearing recovery [104]. Other studies, including a review of 141 patients, have shown that recovery was independent of hypertension, diabetes, cholesterol, and smoking history [52]. In general, co-morbidities like diabetes, cardiovascular disease, and metabolic syndrome tend to predict worse hearing recovery.

Steroids

Since the 1980s corticosteroids have been the mainstay of treatment for SSNHL [99, 105]. The data to support their use is mixed and the purported mechanism of action unclear. In 2013, an updated Cochrane review found three randomized controlled trials totaling 267 patients that compared oral corticosteroid treatment versus placebo or untreated control arms [106]. Their conclusion was that the value of steroids for idiopathic SSNHL remains unclear and the results of the randomized trials were contradictory.

The three randomized trials warrant further discussion. The first study was Wilson et al. (1980). This study was a double-blinded, controlled trial with three arms: steroid treatment ($n = 33$), placebo ($n = 34$), and non-participating controls ($n = 52$). All participants received treatment within 10 days of hearing loss, but the type, duration, and dosage of the oral steroids differed between the two treatment centers. Also, details on the randomization process were lacking. The authors concluded a benefit of steroid therapy based on 61% of the treatment arm demonstrating hearing improvement, while only 32% of the placebo arm demonstrated improvement. The percentage of patients improving with steroid intervention varied widely between the two centers (73 vs. 36%). The authors further analyzed patients that fell within a "steroid effective zone" that excluded 48 patients with profound or mid-frequency hearing losses. In this analysis, only 18 patients in the treatment arm were included to produce an improvement rate of 78% compared to 56 patients in the control arm with an improvement rate of 38% [99, 106].

The next study was Cinamon et al. (2001). This prospective, double-blinded, placebo-controlled trial allocated 41 patients into four arms: steroid treatment, steroid placebo, carbogen inhalation, and inhalation placebo. The steroid was prednisone (1 mg/kg/day) for 5 days, while the carbogen inhalation contained 5% CO_2 with 95% oxygen that was inhaled for 30 minutes six times a day. All patients were treated within 9 days of hearing loss. The results showed no difference between the steroid treatment and steroid placebo arms with 80% and 81% recovery rates, respectively. The inhalation groups also showed no outcome difference [106, 107]. The authors less stringent definition of "recovery," defined as a 15 dB improvement from the initial SSNHL audiogram, may account for the higher-than-expected recovery rates.

The final randomized study was Nosrati-Zarenoe et al. (2012). This prospective, double-blinded, placebo-controlled trial had 103 patients divided between steroid treatment ($n = 51$) and steroid placebo ($n = 52$). The steroid intervention was prednisolone (60 mg/day) for 3 days followed by a 5-day taper. If hearing recovery was incomplete after 8 days, the treatment arm continued prednisolone 10 mg/day for 24 more days. All treatment started within 7 days of hearing loss. At 8-day and 30-day follow-ups, the hearing improvement for the steroid treatment were 25.5 dB and 39.0 dB compared to 26.4 dB and 35.1 dB in the placebo arm. This led the authors to conclude no difference between steroid treatment and placebo. Ten patients were excluded from the final analysis for failure to meet inclusion criteria. Another 20 patients failed to comply with the protocol leading the authors to rely on a modified intention-to-treat analysis [102, 106].

Two meta-analyses have also questioned the true benefit of steroid treatment compared to placebo, although the same heterogeneity issues limit their conclusions. One review combined data from Wilson et al. [99] and Cinamon et al. [107] to show an odds ratio favoring steroids (odds ratio [OR]: 2.47; 95% confidence interval [CI]: 0.89–6.84; $p = 0.08$). Despite the large effect size, this did not meet statistical significance leading the authors to conclude no difference between steroid treatment and placebo [108]. The next review looked at four trials using five different statistical analysis methods. Each statistical analysis favored steroid treatment but fell short of meeting statistical significance, again leading the authors to conclude no difference between steroids and placebo [109].

The potential benefit of steroids within the cochlea stems from its ability to mitigate local and systemic inflammation, inhibit pathologic host immune responses, improve fluid homeostasis, and inhibit the apoptotic cascade. The different corticosteroids have varying degrees of bioavailability and relative anti-inflammatory action (Table 50.3) [110]. Paying attention to the steroid regimen is important as it impacts how much steroid penetrates the cochlea. Validated drug delivery computer simulation models can help compare how different steroid regimens concentrate within inner ear fluid, but there remains no consensus on the optimal steroid, steroid dose, or delivery method for SSNHL [111, 112]. Drug delivery pharmacokinetics are just one key variable that influences the potential impact of steroids and the wide range of reported steroid response (35–87%) [100, 113].

Clinicians have attempted to overcome problems of steroid bioavailability by increasing the systemic dose, delivering steroids via an intratympanic route, or combining systemic and intratympanic therapies. High-dose protocols using a short pulse therapy of 300 mg oral dexamethasone (equivalent to 1875 mg prednisone) for 3 days did not show a difference in hearing recovery compared to 70 mg oral prednisone tapered over 7 days [114]. In contrast, two high-dose regimens with longer tapers (1200 mg hydrocortisone, equivalent to 300 mg prednisone, over 18 days and 600 mg hydrocortisone over 16 days) showed an impressive rate of 87% recovery [115]. Systemic steroids, and particularly the

Table 50.3 Relative actions and dosing equivalencies of corticosteroids

Corticosteroid	Anti-inflammatory activity	Mineral corticoid activity	Equivalent dose (mg)	Plasma half-life (min)
Cortisone	0.8	0.8	25	30
Hydrocortisone	1.0	1.0	20	90
Prednisone	4.0	0.8	5	60
Prednisolone	4.0	0.8	5	200
Triamcinolone	5.0	0.0	4	300
Methylprednisolone	5.0	0.0	4	180
Betamethasone	25.0	0.0	0.75	200
Dexamethasone	25–30	0.0	0.75	200

high-dose or long-term regimens, need to balance potential therapeutic benefit with adverse events. Steroid therapy is known to cause glucose intolerance, hypertension, adrenal suppression, gastrointestinal bleeding, pancreatitis, osteoporosis, cataracts, myopathy, insomnia, altered mental status, and aseptic necrosis of the femoral or humeral heads [106]. Systemic steroid use should be limited in elderly patients, diabetics, and others with medical co-morbidities. Further studies should be considered to better assess the effects of these alternative systemic steroid regimens.

The concern for steroid intolerance and the ability to deliver higher steroid concentrations via the intratympanic route led Rauch et al. (2011) to conduct a multi-institutional, prospective, randomized trial comparing oral versus intratympanic regimens. Using a non-inferiority methodology one arm (n = 121) received 60 mg prednisone for 14 days with a 5 days taper, while the other arm (n = 129) received four intratympanic doses of 40 mg methylprednisolone over 14 days. The results showed that hearing levels 2 months after treatment in the intratympanic group were not inferior to the oral therapy group. Additionally, both arms lacked serious adverse events [116]. The AAO-HNS now recommends the use of intratympanic steroids as salvage therapy or an alternative option if systemic steroids are contraindicated (Table 50.2) [32]. A literature review also supported intratympanic steroids as a salvage or alternative therapy but did not show benefit of any particular intratympanic regimen [112]. Other centers, however, have found higher concentrations (24 mg/mL dexamethasone versus 10 mg/mL dexamethasone) to deliver superior results [117]. These results also require further study to demonstrate the efficacy of one regimen over the other.

Clinicians and patients may also consider combining both systemic and intratympanic therapies to harness their complementary actions on the immune system. Use of intratympanic steroids as a salvage therapy may also miss a therapeutic window. Contradictory results again show a mixed treatment effect with some studies favoring combined therapy, while others show no additional benefit compared to systemic therapy alone [98, 118–122]. A meta-analysis analyzed 14 randomized trials to compare 756 patients with combined therapy versus 638 patients with systemic therapy alone. They found a significant benefit to combined therapy with an odds ratio of 2.50 (95% CI: 1.95–3.21; $p < 0.0001$). Using a random-effects model, this predicted a 13.0 dB pure-tone average improvement with combined therapy (CI: 9.24–16.77, $p < 0.0001$). They also report a low rate of tympanic membrane perforations following the intratympanic delivery (0.9%) [123].

For intratympanic steroids to reach their desired target within the cochlea, they must first permeate the round window. The round window is 70 μm thick in humans and composed of a tri-layered structure with inner and outer epithelial layers surrounding a middle connective tissue core [124]. Diffusion of solutes across the membrane depends on their molecular weight, concentration, liposolubility, and the electric charge within the middle ear [125]. Obstruction or obliteration of the round window niche can inhibit drug delivery to the cochlea. In a review of 202 temporal bones, 11% were found to have a fibrous plug or fat plug obstructing the niche, while another 21% had adhesions or an extraneous (false) membrane [124, 126]. This potential obstruction had led some to advocate for middle ear endoscopy and lysis of adhesions at the time of drug delivery. In review of 41 intratympanic infusions assisted by middle ear endoscopy, the round windows were partially obstructed in 17% of cases and completely obstructed in 12% of cases [127].

A second obstacle for drug delivery into the cochlea is the time needed for diffusion across the round window membrane. Dispersion of the drug in the middle ear reduces its ability to contact and therefore cross the membrane. Sealing the round window niche with a 1% sodium hyaluronate gel can help reduce drug leakage at the delivery site [128]. Novel drug delivery systems such as a dexamethasone impregnated controlled release poly(D,L-lactide-co-glycolide) (PLGA) polymer implant has potential for prolonging the drug–membrane interaction, thus increasing drug concentration within the cochlea [129]. A drug-eluting thermosensitive gels (OTO-104) showed initially promising results for dexamethasone delivery in patients with unilateral Ménière's disease, but additional testing is ongoing [130–132]. At room temperature, this solution is in a liquid state, but after intratympanic injection, it forms a viscous gel that slowly releases its drug contents. Another method of prolonging drug delivery to the round window is use of a microwick. This requires placement of a tympanostomy tube overlying the round window. A 1 mm × 9 mm microwick is then placed through the tube so that its medial end rests within the round window niche. Patients can then self-administer a steroid containing otic drops for increased drug delivery [133]. Some results of using the microwick for salvage SSNHL therapy have shown benefit compared to systemic steroids [134].

Once a drug makes it into the cochlea, it spreads through the perilymphatic space via simple diffusion [135]. The length of the human scala tympani (28.5 mm) can make drug delivery to the cochlear apex challenging. Additionally, the cochlear aqueduct's insertion at the basal turn of the cochlea may influence drug elimination from the scala tympani. This creates a substantial concentration gradient within the cochlea such that the cochlear apex may not receive much of the therapeutic drug [136–138]. An experimental drug delivery system into the cochlea apex has shown promise for reducing the basal–apical drug gradient, but its application has yet to be verified in vivo [139].

Hyperbaric Oxygen

The data in support of hyperbaric oxygen therapy (HBOT) for SSNHL is less robust than steroid therapy. Many of the studies suffer from delays in treatment and limited comparison groups. A systematic review of six randomized trials pooled data from 304 patients to show that HBOT improved hearing recovery by 25% (OR: 1.39; 95% CI: 1.05–1.84; $p = 0.02$). The authors acknowledged that the clinical significance of this recovery was unknown and did not recommend its routine use for SSNHL [140]. A Cochrane review from 2012 drew similar conclusions [141]. Isolated reports of HBOT with concurrent intratympanic steroids for salvage therapy have shown positive results but the data are limited [142]. Currently, the AAO-HNS presents HBOT as an option if started within 3 months of hearing loss onset (Table 50.2) [32].

Antivirals and Vasodilators

There is limited support for antivirals and vasodilators as adjunct therapies for SSNHL. A randomized trial of 84 patients receiving either prednisone with valacyclovir or prednisone with placebo demonstrated no additional benefit from the antiviral [143]. This study, along with three other randomized trials on antiviral therapies, was part of a systematic review that concluded there was no additional therapeutic benefit of antivirals [144]. A Cochrane review from 2012 stated that there was no evidence to support antiviral therapy with SSNHL [145]. Similarly, a systematic review and Cochrane review on vasoactive or hemodilution substances (carbogen, prostaglandin E1, naftidrofuryl, and low-molecular weight dextran) showed only weak support from poorly controlled studies for these substances [144, 146]. They both concluded their role as an adjunctive treatment for SSNHL remains unproven. Due to the poor data, the AAO-HNS strongly recommends against both antivirals and vasodilators (Table 50.2) [32].

Current Practice

When a patient presents with a chief complaint of sudden hearing loss, it is imperative to obtain an audiogram to document the degree and type of loss. At the same time, a thorough history and physical exam is performed, both focusing on factors previously discussed in this chapter. If a cause for the hearing loss can be deduced from the history and physical, then that etiology should dictate further treatment, referrals, and workup. Laboratory studies are not routinely performed unless the history suggests a particular etiology that may benefit from blood work, such as autoimmune inner ear disease. If there is no obvious diagnosis, then it is critical to assess for retrocochlear pathology. The gold standard is a gadolinium-enhanced MRI with thin slices through the internal auditory canal. If the patient is unable to obtain an MRI, then an auditory brainstem response or contrasted CT temporal bone should be obtained. If there is still no definitive diagnosis, then the patient is labeled with idiopathic SSNHL and they are counseled on the broad differential diagnosis, associated risk factors, and natural history of sudden hearing loss.

The decision to treat the patient and the treatment of choice have not been clearly defined in the literature. We believe these decisions require thorough patient education on the various treatment options and their risk–benefit profile. Additionally, the patient is counseled on the negative impact of sensorineural hearing loss. Our first-line treatment is systemic steroids prescribed as 1 mg/kg (up to 60 mg) of prednisone taken in the morning for 10 days followed by a 5-day taper. The patient is reassessed at the end of the taper. If there is no hearing improvement or only partial improvement, then a series of intratympanic dexamethasone (10 mg/mL) injections are offered as salvage therapy. Typically, two or three injections are performed spaced out 1-week apart. For the first injection, a small application of phenol or topical anesthetic is placed on the posterior tympanic membrane. The steroid solution is warmed in a 1 cc syringe with a 27-gauge needle and injected into the middle ear. Care is taken to avoid the posterior–superior quadrant where the needle could damage the incudostapedial joint. The patient is instructed to lie still without swallowing or speaking for 15 minutes. On the subsequent injections, the topical anesthetic is often not necessary.

If the patient has diabetes or a medical contraindication to systemic steroids, then intratympanic steroids are offered as first-line therapy. Increasingly patients desire maximally medical therapy and are willing to accept the risk–benefit profile of both systemic and intratympanic steroids. In these situations, or

Fig. 50.3 Management algorithm for sudden sensorineural hearing loss. MRI magnetic resonance imaging, SSNHL sudden sensorineural hearing loss

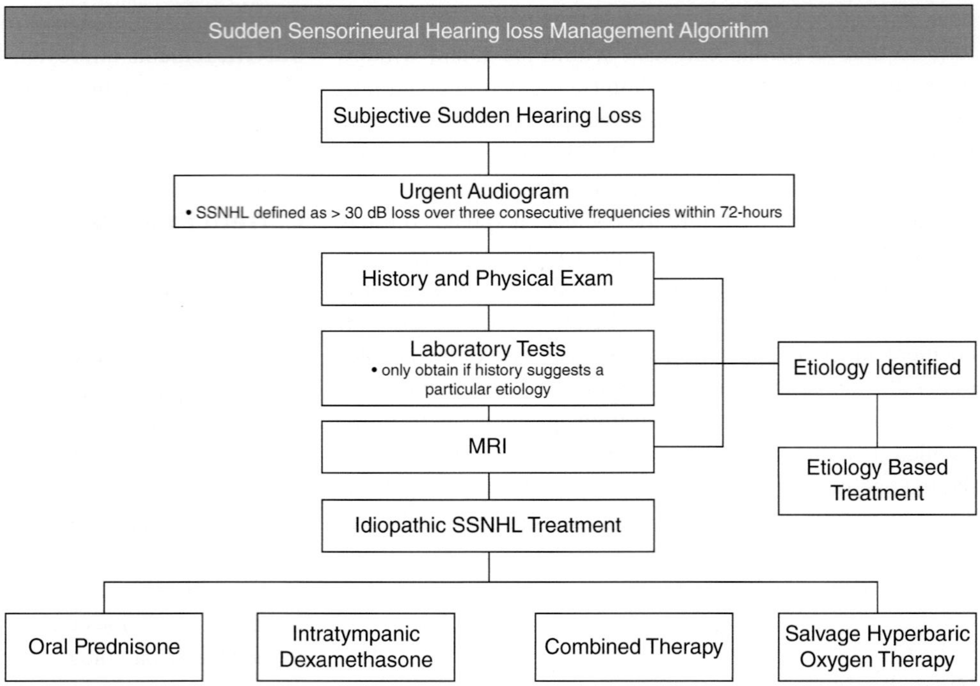

cases of a profound loss with a poor prognosis for recovery, the patient is offered combination therapy. Hyperbaric oxygen therapy is also offered as a salvage option if the previously described interventions have not worked. The variability in insurance coverage for HBOT is discussed. We do not use antivirals or anticoagulants. Our management algorithm is summarized in Fig. 50.3. Hearing should be retested 3 months later and the result is assumed to be final, but patients should be counseled on the chance for fluctuation. At this point, tinnitus management and hearing rehabilitative options are discussed in context of the patient's perceived detriment and objective testing.

References

1. Hoffman HJ, Dobie RA, Losonczy KG, Themann CL, Flamme GA. Declining prevalence of hearing loss in US adults aged 20 to 69 years. JAMA Otolaryngol Head Neck Surg. 2017;143:274–85.
2. National Institute of Health. Sudden deafness. Bethesda: National Institute of Health; 2013. NIH publication 00-4757. http://www.nidcd.nih.gov/health/sudden-deafness. Accessed 25 Mar 2017.
3. Byl FM. Seventy-six cases of presumed sudden hearing loss occurring in 1973: prognosis and incidence. Laryngoscope. 1977;87:817–25.
4. Wu CS, Lin HC, Chao PZ. Sudden sensorineural hearing loss: evidence from Taiwan. Audiol Neurotol. 2006;11:151–6.
5. Klemm E, Deutscher A, Mösges R. A present investigation of the epidemiology in idiopathic sudden sensorineural hearing loss. Laryngorhinootologie. 2009;88:524–7.
6. Tseng CC, Hu LY, Yang AC, Shen CC, Tsai SJ. Risk of depressive disorders following sudden sensorineural hearing loss: a nationwide population-based retrospective cohort study. J Affect Disord. 2016;197:94–9.
7. Harkonen K, Kivekas I, Rautiainen M, Kotti V, Vasama JP. Quality of life and hearing eight years after sudden sensorineural hearing loss. Laryngoscope. 2017;127:927–31.
8. Carlsson PI, Hall M, Lind KJ, Danermark B. Quality of life, psychosocial consequences, and audiological rehabilitation after sudden sensorineural hearing loss. Int J Audiol. 2011;50:139–44.
9. De Kleyn A. Sudden complete or partial loss of function of the octavus-system in apparently normal persons. Acta Otolaryngol. 1944;32:407–29.
10. Simmons FB. Theory of membrane breaks in sudden hearing loss. Arch Otolaryngol. 1968;88:41–8.
11. Wilson WR, Veltri RW, Laird N, et al. Viral and epidemiologic studies of idiopathic sudden hearing loss. Otolaryngol Head Neck Surg. 1983;91:653–8.
12. Mattox DE, Simmons FB. Natural history of sudden sensorineural hearing loss. Ann Otol Rhinol Laryngol. 1977;86:463–80.
13. Chau JK, Lin JR, Atashband S, Irvine RA, Westerberg BD. Systematic review of the evidence for the etiology of adult sudden sensorineural hearing loss. Laryngoscope. 2010;120:1011–21.
14. Keller JJ, Wu CS, Kang JH, Lin HC. Association of acute myocardial infarction with sudden sensorineural hearing loss: a population-based case-control study. Audiol Neurotol. 2013;18:3–8.
15. Kou CL, Shiao AS, Wang SJ, Chang WP, Lin YY. Risk of sudden sensorineural hearing loss in stroke patients: a 5-year nationwide investigation of 44,460 patients. Medicine (Baltimore). 2016;95:e4841.
16. Chang SL, Hsieh CC, Tseng KS, Weng SF, Lin YS. Hypercholesterolemia is correlated with an increased risk of idiopathic sudden sensorineural hearing loss: a historical prospective cohort study. Ear Hear. 2014;35:256–61.
17. Lin SW, Lin YS, Weng SF, Chou CW. Risk of developing sudden sensorineural hearing loss in diabetic patients: a population-based cohort study. Otol Neurotol. 2012;33:1482–8.
18. Chu CH, Liu CJ, Fuh JL, Shiao AS, Chen TJ, Wang SJ. Migraine is a risk factor for sudden sensorineural hearing loss: a nationwide population-based study. Cephalalgia. 2013;33:80–6.

19. Lin C, Lin SW, Weng SF, Lin YS. Risk of sudden sensorineural hearing loss in patients with systemic lupus erythematous: a population-based cohort study. Audiol Neurotol. 2013;18:95–100.
20. Yen YC, Lin YS, Weng SF, Lai FJ. Risk of sudden sensorineural hearing loss in patients with psoriasis: a retrospective cohort study. Am J Clin Dermatol. 2015;16:213–20.
21. Lin C, Lin SW, Weng SF, Lin YS. Increased risk of sudden sensorineural hearing loss in patients with human immunodeficiency virus aged 18 to 35 years: a population-based cohort study. JAMA Otolaryngol Head Neck Surg. 2013;139:251–5.
22. Chung SD, Chen PY, Lin HC, Hung SH. Sudden sensorineural hearing loss associated with iron-deficiency anemia: a population-based study. JAMA Otolaryngol Head Neck Surg. 2014;140:417–22.
23. Sheu JJ, Wu CS, Lin HC. Association between obstructive sleep apnea and sudden sensorineural hearing loss: a population-based case-control study. Arch Otolaryngol Head Neck Surg. 2012;138:55–9.
24. Chien CY, Tai SY, Wang LF, et al. Metabolic syndrome increases risk of sudden sensorineural hearing loss in Taiwan: a case-control study. Otolaryngol Head Neck Surg. 2015;153:105–11.
25. Yeh MC, Weng SF, Shen YC, et al. Increased risk of sudden sensorineural hearing loss in patient with osteoporosis: a population-based, propensity score-matched, longitudinal follow-up study. J Clin Endocrinol Metab. 2015;100:2413–9.
26. Lasisi OA, Salako BL, Kadiri S, et al. Sudden sensorineural hearing loss and hemodialysis. Ear Nose Throat J. 2006;85:819–21.
27. Wang IK, Wang CY, Muo CH, Yen TH, Sung FC. Risk of sudden sensorineural loss in patients with end-stage renal disease undergoing dialysis. Nephrology (Carlton). 2017;22:397–402.
28. Lindsay JR. Sudden deafness due to virus infection. Arch Otolaryngol. 1959;69:13–8.
29. Davis LE, Johnsson LG. Viral infections of the inner ear: clinical, virologic, and pathologic studies in humans and animals. Am J Otolaryngol. 1984;4:347–62.
30. Levine J, Buchman CA, Fregien N. Influenza a virus infection of human Schwann cells in vitro. Acta Otolaryngol. 2003;123:41–5.
31. Schreiber BE, Agrup C, Haskard DO, Luxon LM. Sudden sensorineural hearing loss. Lancet. 2010;375:1203–11.
32. Stachler RJ, Chandraseker SS, Archer SM, et al. Clinical practice guideline: sudden hearing loss. Otolaryngol Head Neck Surg. 2012;146(IS):S1–S35.
33. Mentel R, Kaftan H, Wegner U, Reimann A, Gurtler L. Are enterovirus infections a co-factor in sudden hearing loss? J Med Virol. 2004;72:625–9.
34. Fukuda S, Chida E, Kuroda T, Kashiwamura M, Inuyama Y. An anti-mumps IgM antibody level in the serum of idiopathic sudden sensorineural hearing loss. Auris Nasus Larynx. 2001;28:S3–5.
35. Wackym PA. Molecular temporal bone pathology: II. Ramsay Hunt syndrome (herpes zoster oticus). Laryngoscope. 1997;107:1165–75.
36. Xenellis J, Nikolopoulos TP, Stavroulaki P, et al. Simultaneous and sequential bilateral sudden sensorineural hearing loss: are they different from unilateral sudden sensorineural hearing loss? ORL. 2007;69:306–10.
37. Gross M, Wolf DG, Elidan J, Eliashar R. Enterovirus, cytomegalovirus, and Epstein-Barr virus infection screening in idiopathic sudden sensorineural hearing loss. Audiol Neurotol. 2007;12:179–82.
38. Jeong M, Ocwieja KE, Han D, et al. Direct SARS-CoV-2 infection of the human inner ear may underlie COVID-19-associated audiovestibular dysfunction. Commun Med (Lond). 2021;1(1):44.
39. Nieminen TA, Kivekäs I, Artama M, Nohynek H, Kujansivu J, Hovi P. Sudden hearing loss following vaccination against COVID-19. JAMA Otolaryngol Head Neck Surg. 2023;149(2):133–40.
40. Formeister EJ, Wu MJ, Chari DA, et al. Assessment of sudden sensorineural hearing loss after COVID-19 vaccination. JAMA Otolaryngol Head Neck Surg. 2022;148(4):307–15.
41. Yanir Y, Doweck I, Shibli R, Najjar-Debbiny R, Saliba W. Association between the BNT162b2 messenger RNA COVID-19 vaccine and the risk of sudden sensorineural hearing loss. JAMA Otolaryngol Head Neck Surg. 2022;148(4):299–306.
42. Townsend GC, Scheld WM. Adjunctive therapy for bacterial meningitis: rationale for use, current status, and prospects for the future. Clin Infect Dis. 1993;17(suppl 2):S537–49.
43. Woolley AL, Kirk KA, Neumann AM Jr, et al. Risk factors for hearing loss from meningitis in children: the children's hospital experience. Arch Otolaryngol Head Neck Surg. 1999;125:509–14.
44. Merchant SN, Gopen Q. A human temporal bone study of acute bacterial meningogenic labyrinthitis. Am J Otol. 1996;17:375–85.
45. Rappaport JM, Bhatt SM, Burkard RF, Merchant SN, Nadol JB Jr. Prevention of hearing loss in experimental pneumococcal meningitis by administration of dexamethasone and ketorolac. J Infect Dis. 1999;179:264–8.
46. Rodenburg-Vlot MB, Ruytjens L, Oostenbrink R, Goedegebure A, van der Schroeff MP. Systematic review: incidence and course of hearing loss caused by bacterial meningitis: in search of an optimal timed audiological follow-up. Otol Neurotol. 2016;37:1–8.
47. Hyden D, Akerlind B, Peebo M. Inner ear and facial nerve complications of acute otitis media with focus on bacteriology and virology. Acta Otolaryngol. 2006;126:460–6.
48. Rasmussen H. Sudden deafness. Acta Otolaryngol. 1949;37:65–70.
49. Aimoni C, Bianchini C, Borin M, et al. Diabetes, cardiovascular risk factors and idiopathic sudden sensorineural hearing loss. Audiol Neurootol. 2009;15:111–5.
50. Marucci R, Alessandrello Liotta A, Cellai AP, et al. Cardiovascular and thrombophilic risk factors for idiopathic sudden sensorineural hearing loss. J Thromb Haemost. 2005;3:929–34.
51. Rudack C, Langer C, Stoll W, Rust S, Walter M. Vascular risk factors in sudden hearing loss. Thromb Haemost. 2006;95:454–61.
52. Ciorba A, Hatzopoulos S, Bianchini C, et al. Idiopathic sudden sensorineural hearing loss: cardiovascular risk factors do not influence hearing threshold recovery. Acta Otorhinolaryngol Ital. 2015;35:103–9.
53. Lin HC, Chao PZ, Lee HC. Sudden sensorineural hearing loss increases the risk of stroke: 5-year follow-up study. Stroke. 2008;39:2744–8.
54. Lin RJ, Krall R, Westerberg BD, Chadha NK, Chau JK. Systematic review and meta-analysis of the risk factors for sudden sensorineural hearing loss in adults. Laryngoscope. 2012;122:624–35.
55. Kuo CL, Shiao AS, Wang SJ, Chang WP, Lin YY. Risk of sudden sensorineural hearing loss in stroke patients: a 5-year nationwide investigation of 44,460 patients. Medicine (Baltimore). 2016;95:e4841.
56. Lee H, Baloh RW. Sudden deafness in vertebrobasilar ischemia: clinical features, vascular topographical patterns and long-term outcome. J Neurol Sci. 2005;228:99–104.
57. McCabe BF. Autoimmune sensorineural hearing loss. Ann Otol Rhinol Laryngol. 1979;88:585–9.
58. Lunardi C, Bason C, Leandri M, et al. Autoantibodies to inner ear and endothelial antigens in Cogan's syndrome. Lancet. 2002;360:915–21.
59. Wolfovitz E, Levy Y, Brook JG. Sudden deafness in a patient with temporal arteritis. J Rhematol. 1987;14:384–5.
60. Kempf HG. Ear involvement in Wegner's granulomatosis. Clin Otolaryngol Allied Sci. 1989;14:451–6.
61. Garcia Berrocal JR, Arellano B, Vargas JA, et al. Immune-mediated inner ear disease: report of clinical cases. Acta Otorrinolaringol Esp. 1997;48:565–70.
62. Kumakiri K, Sakamoto T, Karahashi I, Mineta H, Takebayashi S. A case of relapsing polychondritis preceded by inner ear involvement. Auris Nasus Larynx. 2005;32:71–6.
63. Rowe-Jones JM, Macallan DC, Sorooshian M. Polyarteritis nodosa presenting as bilateral sudden onset cochlea-vestibular failure in a young woman. J Laryngol Otol. 1990;104:562–4.

64. Deroee AF, Huang TC, Morita N, Hojjati M. Sudden hearing loss as a presenting symptom of systemic sclerosis. Otol Neurotol. 2009;30:277–9.
65. Pollak L, Luxon LM, Haskard DO. Labyrinthine involvement in Behçet's syndrome. J Laryngol Otol. 2001;115:522–9.
66. Roverano S, Cassano G, Paira S, et al. Asymptomatic sensorineural hearing loss in patients with systemic lupus erythematosus. J Clin Rheumatol. 2006;12:217–20.
67. Yehudai D, Shoenfeld Y, Toubi E. The autoimmune characteristics of progressive or sudden sensorineural hearing loss. Autoimmunity. 2006;39:153–8.
68. Garcia Berrocal JR, Ramirez-Camacho R. Sudden sensorineural hearing loss: supporting the immunologic theory. Ann Otol Rhinol Laryngol. 2002;111:989–97.
69. Schuknecht HT, Donovan ED. The pathology of idiopathic sudden sensorineural hearing loss. Arch Otorhinolaryngol. 1986;243:1–5.
70. Vasama JP, Linthicum FH Jr. Idiopathic sudden sensorineural hearing loss: temporal bone histopathologic study. Ann Otol Rhinol Laryngol. 2000;109:527–32.
71. Merchant SN, Adams JC, Nadol JB Jr. Pathology and pathophysiology of sudden sensorineural hearing loss. Otol Neurotol. 2005;26:151–60.
72. Schuknecht HF, Benitez J, Beekhuis J, Igarashi M, Singleton G, Ruedi L. The pathology of sudden deafness. Laryngoscope. 1962;72:1142–57.
73. Schuknecht HT, Kimura RS, Naufal PM. The pathology of sudden deafness. Acta Otolaryngol. 1973;76:75–97.
74. Stokroos RJ, Albers FWJ, Schrim J. The etiology of idiopathic sudden sensorineural hearing loss: experimental herpes simplex virus infection of the inner ear. Am J Otol. 1998;19:447–52.
75. Tamura M, Ogino S, Matsunaga T, et al. Experimental labyrinthitis in Guinea pigs cause by a hantavirus. ORL J Otorhinolaryngol Relat Spec. 1991;53:1–5.
76. Lin D, Hegarty JL, Fischbein NJ, Jackler RJ. The prevalence of "incidental" acoustic neuroma. Arch Otolaryngol Head Neck Surg. 2005;131:241–4.
77. Matthies C, Samii M. Management of 1000 vestibular schwannomas (acoustic neuromas): clinical presentation. Neurosurgery. 1997;40:1–9.
78. Inoue Y, Kanzaki J, Ogawa K. Vestibular schwannoma presenting as sudden deafness. J Laryngol Otol. 2000;114:589–92.
79. Cadoni G, Ciafoni A, Agostino S, et al. Magnetic imaging findings in sudden sensorineural hearing loss. J Otolaryngol. 2006;35:310–6.
80. Uppal HS, Ayshford CA, Wilson F. Sudden onset bilateral sensorineural hearing loss: a manifestation of occult breast carcinoma. J Laryngol Otol. 2001;115:907–10.
81. Dalmau J, Porta-Etessam J. Paraneoplastic cerebral syndromes with Oto-neuro-ophthalmologic manifestations. Rev Neurol. 2000;31:1213–9.
82. Hardin MF, Barker M, Neis PR. Sensorineural hearing loss as the result of cliff jumping. J Ark Med Soc. 2003;99:327–30.
83. Whinney DJ, Parik AA, Brookes GB. Barotraumatic fracture of the stapes footplate. Am J Otol. 1996;17:697–9.
84. Rozsasi A, Sigg O, Keck T. Persistent inner ear injury after diving. Otol Neurotol. 2003;24:195–200.
85. Patterson JH, Hamernik RP. Blast overpressure induced structural and functional changes in the auditory system. Toxicology. 1997;121:29–40.
86. Segal S, Eviatar E, Berenholz L, Vaiman M, Kessler A, Shlamkovitch N. Hearing loss after direct blunt neck trauma. Otol Neurotol. 2003;24:734–7.
87. Whitehead E. Sudden sensorineural hearing loss with fracture of the stapes footplate following sneezing and parturition. Clin Otolaryngol Allied Sci. 1999;24(5):462–4.
88. Noordman BJ, van Beeck CE, Witte B, Goverts T, Hensen E, Merkus P. Prognostic factors for sudden drops in hearing level after minor head injury in patients with an enlarged vestibular aqueduct. Otol Neurotol. 2015;36:4–11.
89. Nakashima T, Pyykko I, Arroll MA, et al. Ménière's disease. Nat Rev Dis Primers. 2016;12:16028.
90. Schacht J, Talaska AE, Rybak LP. Cisplatin and aminoglycoside antibiotics: hearing loss and its prevention. Anat Rec (Hoboken). 2012;295:1837–50.
91. Casano RA, Johnson DF, Bykhovskaya Y, Torricelli F, Bigozzi M, Fischel-Ghodsian N. Inherited susceptibility to aminoglycoside ototoxicity: genetic heterogeneity and clinical implications. Am J Otolaryngol. 1999;20:151–6.
92. Oh JH, Park K, Lee SJ, Shin YR, Choung YH. Bilateral versus unilateral sudden sensorineural hearing loss. Otolaryngol Head Neck Surg. 2007;136:87–91.
93. Nosrati-Zarenoe R, Arlinger S, Hultcrantz E. Idiopathic sudden sensorineural hearing loss: results drawn from the Swedish national database. Acta Otolaryngol. 2007;127:1168–75.
94. Nakashima T, Yanagita N. Outcome of sudden deafness with and without vertigo. Laryngoscope. 1993;103:1145–9.
95. Aarnisalo AA, Suoranta H, Ylikoski J. Magnetic resonance imaging findings in the auditory pathway of patients with sudden deafness. Otol Neurotol. 2004;25:245–9.
96. Vernooij MW, Ikram MA, Tanghe HL, et al. Incidental findings on brain MRI in the general population. N Engl J Med. 2007;357:1821–8.
97. Tagaya M, Teranishi M, Naganawa S, et al. 3 Tesla magnetic resonance imaging obtained 4 hours after intravenous gadolinium injection in patients with sudden deafness. Acta Otolaryngol. 2010;130:665–9.
98. Lee JI, Yoon RG, Lee JH, et al. Prognostic value of labyrinthine 3D-FLAIR abnormalities in idiopathic sudden sensorineural hearing loss. AJNR Am J Neuroradiol. 2016;37:2317–22.
99. Wilson WR, Byl FM, Laird N. The efficacy of steroids in the treatment of idiopathic sudden sensorineural hearing loss. A double-blind clinical study. Arch Otolaryngol. 1980;106:772–6.
100. Gallo DE, Khojasteh E, Gloor M, Hegemann SCA. Effectiveness of systemic high-dose dexamethasone therapy for idiopathic sudden sensorineural hearing loss. Audiol Neurotol. 2013;18:161–70.
101. Cvorovic L, Deric D, Probst R, Hegemann S. Prognostic model for predicting hearing recovery in idiopathic sudden sensorineural hearing loss. Otol Neurotol. 2008;29:464–9.
102. Nosrati-Zarenoe R, Hultcrantz E. Corticosteroid treatment of idiopathic sudden sensorineural hearing loss: randomized triple-blind placebo-controlled trial. Otol Neurotol. 2012;33:523–31.
103. Bogaz EA, Maranhao AS, Inoue DP, Suzuki FA, Penido NO. Variables with prognostic value in the onset of idiopathic sudden sensorineural hearing loss. Braz J Otorhinolaryngol. 2015;81:520–6.
104. Lin CF, Lee KJ, Yu SS, Lin YS. Effect of comorbid diabetes and hypercholesterolemia on the prognosis of idiopathic sudden sensorineural hearing loss. Laryngoscope. 2016;126:142–9.
105. Moskowitz D, Lee KJ, Smith HW. Steroid use in idiopathic sudden sensorineural hearing loss. Laryngoscope. 1984;94:664–6.
106. Wei BP, Stathopoulos D, O'Leary S. Steroids for idiopathic sudden sensorineural hearing loss. Cochrane Database Syst Rev. 2013;7:CD003998.

107. Cinamon U, Bendet E, Kronenberg J. Steroid, carbogen or placebo for sudden hearing loss: a prospective double-blind study. Eur Arch Otorhinolaryngol. 2001;258:477–80.
108. Conlin AE, Parnes LS. Treatment of sudden sensorineural hearing loss, II: a meta-analysis. Arch Otolaryngol Head Neck Surg. 2007;133:582–6.
109. Labus J, Breil J, Stuetzer H, Michel O. Meta-analysis for the effect of medical therapy vs. placebo on recovery of idiopathic sudden sensorineural hearing loss. Laryngoscope. 2010;120:1863–71.
110. Mager DE, Lin SX, Blum RA, Lates CD, Jusko WJ. Dose equivalency evaluation of major corticosteroids: pharmacokinetics and cell trafficking and cortisol dynamics. J Clin Pharmacol. 2003;43:1216–27.
111. Liebau A, Pogorzelski O, Salt AN, Plontke SK. Hearing changes after intratympanically applied steroids for therapy of sudden hearing loss: a meta-analysis using mathematical simulations of drug delivery protocols. Otol Neurotol. 2016;38:19–30.
112. Seggas I, Koltsidopoulos P, Bibas A, Tzonou A, Sismanis A. Intratympanic steroid therapy for sudden hearing loss: a review of the literature. Otol Neurotol. 2010;32:29–35.
113. Slattery WH, Fisher LM, Iqbal Z, Liu N. Oral steroid regimens for idiopathic sensorineural hearing loss. Otolaryngol Head Neck Surg. 2005;132:5–10.
114. Westerlaken BO, de Kleine E, van der Laan B, Albers F. The treatment of idiopathic sudden sensorineural hearing loss using pulse therapy: a prospective, randomized, double-blinded clinical trial. Laryngoscope. 2007;117:684–90.
115. Aoki D, Takegoshi H, Kikuchi S. Evaluation of super-high-dose steroid therapy for sudden sensorineural hearing loss. Otolaryngol Head Neck Surg. 2006;134:783–7.
116. Rauch SD, Halpin CF, Antonelli PJ, et al. Oral vs intratympanic corticosteroid therapy for idiopathic sudden sensorineural hearing loss. JAMA. 2011;305:2071–9.
117. Alexander TH, Harris JP, Nguyen QT, Vorasubin. Dose effect of intratympanic dexamethasone for idiopathic sudden sensorineural hearing loss: 24 mg/ml is superior to 10 mg/ml. Otol Neurotol. 2015;36:1321–7.
118. Lee JB, Choi SJ. Potential benefits of combination therapy as primary treatment for sudden sensorineural hearing loss. Otolaryngol Head Neck Surg. 2016;154:328–34.
119. Arslan N, Oguz H, Demirci M, et al. Combined intratympanic and systemic use of steroids for idiopathic sudden sensorineural hearing loss. Otol Neurotol. 2011;32:393–7.
120. Jung DJ, Park JH, Jang JH, Ky L. The efficacy of combination therapy for idiopathic sudden sensorineural hearing loss. Laryngoscope. 2016;126:1871–6.
121. Ahn JH, Yoo MH, Yoon TH, et al. Can intratympanic dexamethasone added to systemic steroids improve hearing outcome in patients with hearing deafness. Laryngoscope. 2008;118:279–82.
122. Lim HJ, Kim YT, Choi SJ, et al. Efficacy of 3 different steroid treatments for sudden sensorineural hearing loss: a prospective, randomized trial. Otolaryngol Head Neck Surg. 2013;148:121–7.
123. Han X, Yin X, Du X, Sun C. Combined intratympanic and systemic use of steroids as a first-line treatment for sudden sensorineural hearing loss: a meta-analysis of randomized, controlled trials. Otol Neurotol. 2017;38:487–95.
124. Juan ID, Linthicum FJ Jr. Round window fibrous plugs. Otol Neurotol. 2010;31:1354–5.
125. Mikulec AA, Hartsock JJ, Salt AN. Permeability of the round window membrane is influenced by the composition of applied drug solutions and by common surgical procedures. Otol Neurotol. 2008;29:1020–6.
126. Goycoolea MV, Lundman L. Round window membrane: structure, function and permeability: a review. Microsc Res Tech. 1997;36:201–11.
127. Silverstein H, Rowan PT, Olds MJ, Rosenberg SI. Inner ear perfusion and the role of round window patency. Am J Otol. 1997;18:586–9.
128. Salt AN, Sirjani DB, Hartsock JJ, Gill RM, Plontke SK. Marker retention in the cochlea following injections through the round window membrane. Hear Res. 2007;232:78–86.
129. Plontke SK, Glien A, Rahne T, Mader K, Salt AN. Controlled release dexamethasone implants in the round window niche for salvage treatment of idiopathic sudden sensorineural hearing loss. Otol Neurotol. 2014;35:1168–71.
130. Salt AN, Hartsock J, Plontke S, LeBel C, Piu F. Distribution of dexamethasone and preservation of inner ear function following intratympanic delivery of a gel-based formulation. Audiol Neurotol. 2011;16:323–35.
131. Lambert PR, Nguyen S, Maxwell KS, et al. A randomized, double-blind, placebo-controlled clinical study to assess safety and clinical activity of OTO-104 given as a single intratympanic injection in patients with unilateral Ménière's disease. Otol Neurotol. 2012;33:1257–65.
132. Lambert PR, Carey J, Mikulec AA, Otonomy Ménière's Study Group. Intratympanic sustained-exposure dexamethasone thermosensitive gel for symptoms of Ménière's disease: randomized phase 2b safety and efficacy trial. Otol Neurotol. 2016;37:1669–76.
133. Silverstein H, Thompson J, Rosenberg SI, Brown N, Light J. Silverstein MicroWick. Otolaryngol Clin North Am. 2004:1019–34.
134. Zanetti D, Di Berardino F, Nassif N, Redaelli De Zinis LO. Intratympanic steroid delivery by an indwelling catheter in refractory severe sudden sensorineural hearing loss. Auris Nasus Larynx. 2018;45(2):227–33.
135. Salt AN, Plontke SK. Principles of local drug delivery to the inner ear. Audiol Neurotol. 2009;14:350–60.
136. Plontke SK, Biegner T, Kammerer B, Delabar U, Salt AN. Dexamethasone concentration gradients along scala tympani after application to the round window membrane. Otol Neurotol. 2008;29:401–6.
137. Plontke SK, Siedow N, Wegener R, Zenner HP, Salt AN. Cochlear pharmacokinetics with local inner ear drug delivery using a three-dimensional finite-element computer model. Audiol Neurotol. 2007;12:37–48.
138. Salt AN, Plontke SK. Drug diffusion to the apex of the human cochlea? A comment on "Kang WS, Nguyen K, McKenna CE, Sewell, McKenna MJ, Jung DH. Intracochlear drug delivery through the oval window in fresh cadaveric human temporal bones". Otol Neurotol. 2016;37:1462–3.
139. Lichtenhan JT, Hartsock J, Dornhoffer JR, Donovan KM, Salt AN. Drug delivery into the cochlear apex: improved control to sequentially affect finely spaced regions along the entire length of the cochlear spiral. J Neurosci Methods. 2016;273:201–9.
140. Bennett M, Kertesz T, Yeung P. Hyperbaric oxygen therapy for idiopathic sudden sensorineural hearing loss and tinnitus: a systematic review of randomized controlled trials. J Laryngol Otol. 2005;119:791–8.
141. Bennett M, Kertesz T, Perleth M, Yeung P, Lehm JP. Hyperbaric oxygen therapy for idiopathic sudden sensorineural hearing loss and tinnitus. Cochrane Database Syst Rev. 2012;10:CD004739.
142. Lam H, Muller-Kortkamp C, Warnecke A, et al. Concurrent hyperbaric oxygen therapy and intratympanic steroid application as salvage therapy after severe sudden sensorineural hearing loss. Clin Case Rep. 2016;4:287–93.

143. Tucci DL, Farmer JC Jr, Kitch RD, Witsell DL. Treatment of sudden sensorineural hearing loss with systemic steroids and valacyclovir. Otol Neurotol. 2002;23:301–8.
144. Conlin AE, Parnes LS. Treatment of sudden sensorineural hearing loss, I: a systematic review. Arch Otolaryngol Head Neck Surg. 2007;133:573–81.
145. Awad Z, Huins C, Pothier DD. Antivirals for idiopathic sudden sensorineural hearing loss. Cochrane Database Syst Rev. 2012;15:CD006987.
146. Agarwal L, Pohier DD. Vasodilators and vasoactive substances for idiopathic sudden sensorineural hearing loss and tinnitus. Cochrane Database Syst Rev. 2009;4:CD003422.

Ménière's Disease

51

Rahul Mehta and Moisés Arriaga

Ménière's Disease

Ménière's disease is an inner ear disorder manifesting as a combination of four characteristic symptoms—spontaneous episodic rotatory vertigo, fluctuating sensorineural hearing loss, tinnitus, and aural fullness. The prevalence of Ménière's disease in the United States varies from 9 per 100,000 in patients <18 years of age to 440 per 100,000 in patients ≥65 years of age [1]. In a tertiary neurotology—otology practice, Ménière's patients constitute a large proportion of patients with non-positional, spontaneous spells of episodic vertigo. Vrabec et al., in their retrospective data review done in an academic referral practice, found that in their cohort of 295 patients coded with diagnosis of Ménière's disease, 64% had definitive Ménière's disease based on the American Academy of Otolaryngology—Head and Neck Surgery (AAO-HNS) 1995 guidelines [2].

Etiology

Since its description by Prosper Meniere in 1861, this condition has been widely studied in the literature. Although we have a basic understanding of the pathophysiology behind this disease, the etiology is still a mystery. Most likely, the causation is multifactorial, and genetic predisposition, allergy, autoimmune dysfunction, and ischemia all have been proposed as potential etiologies [3]. The possible relationship of Ménière's disease with migraine-associated vertigo has also generated considerable interest [4].

Pathophysiology

The literature consistently defines the pathophysiology behind Ménière's disease as the presence of endolymphatic hydrops. This finding was originally described in temporal bones by Hallpike et al. [5]. It indicates that there is excessive fluid accumulation with an increase in pressure in the endolymphatic system of the inner ear. In cochlear hydrops, expansion of endolymphatic volume results in Reissner's membrane bulging into the scala vestibuli (Fig. 51.1).

A temporal bone study by Merchant et al. showed that temporal bones of all Ménière's patients had endolymphatic hydrops in at least one of the ears, but not all cases with hydrops in the temporal bones had Ménière's symptoms. So, they suggested that endolymphatic hydrops should be considered a histological marker for Ménière's syndrome rather than being directly responsible for its symptoms [6].

The extra endolymph accumulates because of excess production or decreased absorption. Endolymph is mainly produced in the stria vascularis with some contribution from dark vestibular cells and planum semilunatum. In the normal state, endolymph is maintained without any true "flow" as hypotheses of longitudinal, radial, and dynamic endolymph flow have not been supported in studies proffered by Salt et al. [7]. In the pathological state of excess fluid, longitudinal flow seems to contribute to endolymph metabolism, thus flowing longitudinally, slowly from duct to endolymphatic sac. Paparella suggested that obstruction in the endolymphatic sac or duct causes altered longitudinal flow and leads to backlog of endolymphatic fluid causing hydrops [8]. Gibson and Arenberg suggested that the narrowed duct gets

R. Mehta
University of Mississippi Medical Center, Jackson, MS, USA
e-mail: rmehta@umc.edu

M. Arriaga (✉)
Department of Otolaryngology—Head and Neck Surgery, Louisiana State University School of Medicine, New Orleans, LA, USA

Our Lady of the Lake Hearing and Balance Center, Baton Rouge, LA, USA
e-mail: maa@neurotologic.com

A. D. Sweeney et al. (eds.), *Haynes-Glasscock-Shambaugh Surgery of the Ear*, https://doi.org/10.1007/978-3-032-18264-7_51

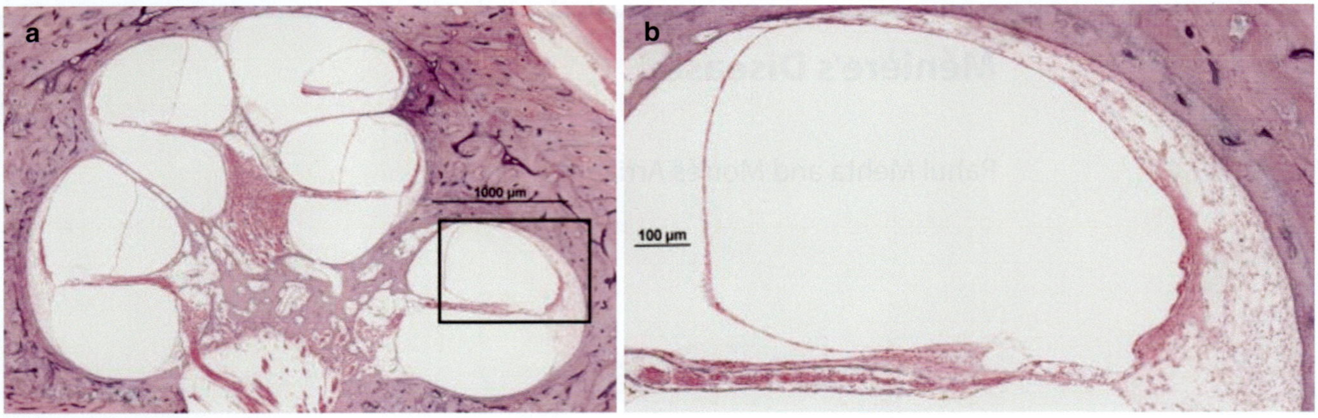

Fig. 51.1 Histopathology of Ménière's disease with excessive endolymph dilating Reissner's membrane. This is a representative temporal bone section of a patient with Ménière's disease (hematoxylin and eosin): (**a**) Mid-modiolar section (4×); squared area = basal turn of the cochlea. (**b**) Basal turn of the cochlea (20×), showing distension of the Reissner's membrane into the scala vestibuli. (Reprinted with permission from Cureoglu et al. [71])

obstructed by debris that is cleared by combination of secretion of hydrophilic protein and saccin hormone, which in turn increases endolymph production. They also proposed that, with pressure, sudden restoration of longitudinal flow initiates vertigo attacks [9]. In contrast, Schuknecht's theory proposed that ruptures in the membranous labyrinth cause leakage of potassium rich endolymph into perilymph leading to attacks of vertigo. Subsequently, healing of membranes restores normal physiology thus terminating the attack [10].

Clinical Symptoms

The characteristic presentation of Ménière's disease is recurrent episodes of spontaneous episodic rotatory vertigo with tinnitus and ipsilateral hearing loss. Patients often describe a sensation of fullness, worsening tinnitus, and decreased hearing before onset of vertigo attack. A typical attack lasts from 20 minutes to 24 hours. It can be accompanied by nausea, vomiting, or, rarely, diarrhea and sweating. Although serious vertigo usually subsides in 24 hours, light headedness or disequilibrium may persist. Patients are usually normal between the attacks, though for some patients persisting instability from a change in baseline vestibular function can be an ongoing symptom after resolution of acute attacks.

Hearing loss may fluctuate during the initial years of Ménière's disease. The loss classically starts as low-frequency sensorineural hearing loss, which improves after the attack. But eventually, hearing loss becomes permanent and flat across all frequencies. Two special manifestations of Ménière's disease are Lermoyez syndrome and Tumarkin's attacks:

- Lermoyez syndrome is a variant of Ménière's disease where hearing improves during or just after the vertigo attack.
- Tumarkin's attacks are seen with advanced Ménière's disease; patients experience sudden "drop attacks" without loss of consciousness. These are presumed to be caused by damage to otolith organs in the utricle and saccule and resulting alteration in tone in the anti-gravity musculature [11].

In a long-term (14 years) follow-up study of Ménière's patients, Green et al. found that vertiginous episodes resolved completely in 50% of patients and somewhat resolved in 28%. Hearing was absent in 48% and worse in 21%. Bilateral disease was present initially in 13% and developed subsequently in 45% patients. The data from this study signifies that, in more than three fourths of patients, vertigo can improve, and significant hearing loss is common [12]. House et al. also found bilateral disease at presentation in 11% of patients and 12% of unilateral patients becoming bilateral during follow-up. The average time interval for conversion from unilateral to bilateral disease was 7.6 years [13].

Diagnosis

For purposes of this chapter, we will consider all the diagnostic categories listed as "Ménière's disease." This distinction is important because patients may manifest stages of Ménière's disease on a clinical spectrum or as a part of a process that evolves over time. Some authors, thus, focus on distinctions between Ménière's disease and Ménière's syndrome.

The diagnosis of Ménière's disease is clinical because no single test can confirm the diagnosis. The American Academy of Otolaryngology and Head Neck Surgery published guidelines in 1972 with revisions in 1985 and 1995 for the diagnosis of Ménière's disease (Table 51.1) [14].

Recently, collaboration between the Barany Society, The Japan Society for Equilibrium Research, European Academy of Otology and Neurotology and Equilibrium Committee of AAO-HNS, and Korean Balance Society created and published a consensus document (Lopez-Escamez et al.). These were the 2015 AAO-HNS Equilibrium Committee Amendment to the 1995 AAO-HNS guidelines (Table 51.2) [15].

Differential Diagnosis

The differential diagnosis of Ménière's disease is listed in Table 51.3 [15]. Of these conditions, a detailed discussion regarding vestibular migraines and migraine associated vertigo is below.

Vestibular Migraine/Migraine-Associated Vertigo

Among the extensive list of conditions listed in the differential diagnosis of Ménière's disease, vestibular migraines deserve a specific discussion. Even though the relationship between vertigo and migraine was suspected in the 1800s, it was not until 2001 with Neuhauser's paper that the diagnostic criteria for vestibular migraine came into existence [16]. Vestibular migraine patients present with episodic vertigo lasting from seconds to days. Radtke et al., on long-term follow-up of vestibular migraine patients, found concomitant cochlear symptoms with vertigo increased from 15% initially to 49%, and 18% developed mild bilateral sensorineural hearing loss, which also involved the low-frequency range [17]. The pathophysiology behind vestibular migraine is involvement of central vestibular nuclei rather than peripheral vestibular apparatus. In a retrospective study of 147 patients, Neff et al. found one-quarter of patients had both Ménière's disease and vestibular migraine in a tertiary dizziness clinic. About 38% of their vestibular migraine patients had ear-related symptoms during vestibular episodes and headaches. Also, 49% of Ménière's patients had headaches

Table 51.1 1995 AAO-HNS guidelines for diagnosis of Ménière's disease

Certain	Definite Ménière's disease, plus histopathologic confirmation of hydrops
Definite	Two or more definitive spontaneous episodes of vertigo 20 min or longer Audiometrically documented hearing loss on at least one occasion Tinnitus or aural fullness in the treated ear Other causes excluded
Probable	One definitive episode of vertigo Audiometrically documented hearing loss on at least one occasion Tinnitus or aural fullness in the treated ear Other causes excluded
Possible	Episodic vertigo of the Ménière's disease type without documented hearing loss or sensorineural hearing loss, fluctuation or fixed, with disequilibrium but without definitive episodes Other causes excluded

Reused from reference [14] with permission

Table 51.2 Amended 2015 criteria for diagnosis of Ménière's disease

Characteristic	Definite Ménière's disease[a]	Probable Ménière's disease[a]
Number of episodes necessary for diagnosis	2 or more	2 or more
Duration of episodes	20 min–12 h	20 min–24 h
Necessary symptoms	Vertigo Audiometrically measured low-to-mid frequency sensorineural hearing loss Fluctuating aural symptoms Hearing changes Tinnitus Aural fullness	Vertigo or dizziness Fluctuating aural symptoms Hearing changes Tinnitus Aural fullness

Adapted from reference [15]

[a]Diagnosing definite or probable Ménière's disease requires that no other vestibular diagnosis better accounts for the patient's symptoms

Table 51.3 Differential diagnosis of Ménière's disease

Autosomal dominant sensorineural hearing loss type 9 (DFNA9) caused by COCH gene
Autosomal dominant sensorineural hearing loss type 6/14 Deafness Autosomal Dominant 6 (DFNA6/14) caused by WFS1 gene
Autoimmune inner ear disease
Cerebrovascular disease (stroke/ transient ischemic attack (TIA) in the vertebrobasilar system/bleeding)
Cogan's syndrome
Endolymphatic sac tumor
Meningiomas and CP angle masses
Neuroborreliosis
Otosyphilis
Susac syndrome
Third window syndromes (perilymph fistula, canal dehiscence, enlarged vestibular aqueduct)
Vestibular migraine
Vestibular paroxysmia
Vestibular Schwannoma
Vogt-Koyanagi-Harada syndrome

Reused from reference [15] with permission

with migraine features, migraine symptoms, or first-degree relatives with migraine [18]. Also, the prevalence of migraine is twice as high in MD patients than in an age and sex matched control group [19]. Hence, an overlap in symptoms in both conditions is clear. So, the biggest question at this moment is if there is an overlap in pathophysiology of both as well, or on the contrary, are these conditions different manifestations of the spectrum of the same disease. In a recent review of the relationship between vestibular migraine and Ménière's disease, Liu et al. suggested that migraines cause vestibular symptoms through effects on the inner ear from the trigeminovascular system and through central activation of vestibular centers. New theories are implicating migraine as being a common etiology between vestibular migraine and Ménière's disease. That being said, authors have also pointed out that there is not enough evidence to definitely link these two in a mechanistic way. At present, it is important to be cognizant of the blurred lines between the two disorders to assist in clinical diagnosis and treatment [4]. On a practical basis, it is important to be mindful of vestibular migraines as both a part of the differential diagnosis and as a potential contributing diagnosis in patients suspected of having Ménière's disease.

Tests

- *Audiometry*: An audiogram is the most important diagnostic study when Ménière's disease is suspected. This test confirms the presence of sensorineural hearing loss in one or both ears. Serial audiograms are advised to keep track of fluctuations in patients suspected of having Ménière's disease. Classically, low-frequency hearing loss affecting the apical turn of the cochlea is the initial expected pattern. A "peak "pattern audiogram, with low-frequency hearing loss, better hearing at 2000 Hz, and worse hearing at frequencies greater than 2000 Hz, has been described by Paparella et al. [20].
- *Vestibular testing*: While the details of vestibular testing are reviewed in another chapter, there are nuances of interpretation in Ménière's disease that influence clinical management.
  - *Caloric testing*: This test assesses the low-frequency range of horizontal vestibular ocular reflex function (i.e., lateral semicircular canal function), which in turn reflects superior vestibular nerve function. Ipsilateral vestibular hypofunction might be a significant finding on bithermal caloric testing. However, it is important to note that 50% of patients might have completely normal caloric tests even with incapacitating vertigo spells [21]. In some situations, we have found that an ear affected by Ménière's disease, but not yet permanently damaged may reveal vestibular hypersensitivity to motion, pressure (fistula testing), sound (Tullio testing), vibration, and caloric testing. Thus, the interpretation of caloric tests is performed in the context of the clinical history, audiogram, and remainder of vestibular testing.
  - *Video head impulse test (VHIT)*: VHIT is usually normal in patients with early Ménière's disease. This test assesses high-frequency function of the VOR and is unreliable in detecting canal paresis of less than 50%.
  - *Cervical vestibular evoked myogenic response* (cVEMP) It is used to assess the function of the saccule, and ocular vestibular evoked myogenic response (oVEMP) is used to assess the utricle. The cVEMP amplitude asymmetry ratio of more than 0.33 confirms an abnormal response in one ear, which can be an augmented or reduced response [22]. Augmented cVEMP can be because of saccular dilatation seen in initial stages of disease [23]. Utricular hydrops can lead to augmented oVEMP responses with an asymmetry ratio of more than 0.40.
  - *Electrocochleography (ECOG)*: The authors have found ECOG to be particularly useful in early Ménière's disease when hearing may fluctuate back to normal or the low-frequency hearing asymmetry is minimal despite suggestive clinical features of Ménière's disease. As a reflection of the relative electrical charge disparity of endolymph and perilymph, an elevated ratio of summating potential (SP) to action potential (AP) is considered to be a significant finding in favor of the diagnosis of hydrops. The exact ratio of abnormal results varies in each vestibular laboratory according to the electrode type and stimulus. Our team uses a ratio of 35% as diagnostic. Sass et al. in their study showed that sensitivity and specificity of trans-tympanic SP/AP ratio were 62 and 95%, respectively [24].
  - *Rotational chair testing (ROTO)*: In Ménière's disease, our team finds ROTO useful to identify uncompensated vestibulopathy, which is characterized by phase lag, decreased VOR (vestibular-ocular reflex) gain, and asymmetry on rotation. Vestibular hypersensitivity in the dark (VOR gain) or in the light with optokinetic stimulation (VVOR—visually enhanced vestibulo-ocular reflex) helps define a migraine or central component [25]. Findings of uncompensated vestibulopathy suggest vestibular physical therapy may be useful to the patient, and vestibular hypersensitivity findings suggest mild vestibular suppression may help instability between attacks.
- *Magnetic resonance imaging (MRI) with gadolinium*: As in any patient with asymmetric hearing loss, MRI of the internal auditory canal (IAC) and posterior fossa (with and without gadolinium) has over 99% sensitivity in

diagnosing vestibular schwannomas or other neoplasms of the auditory–vestibular nerve complex. The increasing availability of high powered 3 Tesla MRI with advanced three-dimensional (3D) protocols has generated considerable interest in direct scanning of inner ear structures with gadolinium injection (transtympanic or intravenous). Nakashima et al. described transtympanic injection of gadolinium using a 23-gauge needle followed by 3 T MRI. 3D fluid-attenuated inversion recovery (FLAIR) images in their study revealed that the gadolinium entered the perilymphatic space and delineated the perilymphatic and endolymphatic spaces of the inner ear. In patients with endolymphatic hydrops, the perilymphatic space surrounding the endolymph was small or had disappeared. Gadolinium appeared first in the scala tympani of the basal turn of the cochlea and the perilymphatic space of the vestibule. One day after the intratympanic injection of gadolinium, the gadolinium was observed in almost all parts of the perilymph. Six days after the intratympanic injection, the gadolinium had almost disappeared from the inner ear [26]. Recently Sano et al. reported that in images taken 4 h after the intravenous gadolinium injection using heavily T2 weighted 3D FLAIR technique, endolymphatic hydrops was observed in both cochlea and vestibule [27]. Although 3D inner ear imaging is not routine clinical practice yet, with ongoing technical advancement, direct imaging of the endolymphatic spaces will likely be an integral part of the investigation protocol for Ménière's disease patients in the future.

- *Computed tomography (CT)*: Temporal bone CT, especially including Poschl and Stenver views, is obtained to rule out a dehiscent superior semicircular canal if that diagnosis is being considered. A CT can also be valuable to obtain prior to any surgical intervention on the temporal bone, in general.

Treatment for Ménière's Disease

Most treatment protocols described in the literature are directed towards two goals: first, to treat acute vertigo attacks and second, to prevent recurrence. Prophylactic treatments intended to prevent recurrence are again divided into hearing/vestibular function-preserving or function-ablating treatments. Our treatment algorithm is outlined in Table 51.4 and Fig. 51.2.

Acute Vertigo

For acute episodes, we recommend benzodiazepines, especially lorazepam, which has rapid onset and is available in a sublingual form. Benzodiazepines are utilized for their gamma-aminobutyric acid (GABA) agonist properties. GABA is a central inhibitory neurotransmitter and its agonist can inhibit neural firing throughout the brain and vestibular nuclei, thus alleviating acute symptoms [28]. Mild symptoms can be treated with anti-histamines like meclizine. Vegetative symptoms are managed with anti-emetics like promethazine or even central anti-emetics like ondansetron.

Of note, vestibular suppressants provide symptomatic relief only and can be counterproductive if used for a longer term because they can delay vestibular compensation by suppressing the adaptive response.

Prevention of Recurrent Spells

Conservative Management

Lifestyle modification and diet: The importance of diet cannot be stressed enough in the management of Ménière's disease. A patient questionnaire study by Luxford et al. showed that the patients who followed diet advice more than 6 months had larger improvement in number of spells and functional rating. Due to this finding, the authors concluded that nutrition education by referral to a dietician may improve outcomes in the medical treatment of Ménière's disease [29]. A subset of patients clearly associates worsening of their symptoms after eating food with a high salt content. This association, and the eventual concept of salt manipulation causing changes in Ménière's symptoms, was first described by Furstenberg [30]. Salt restriction of less than 1.5 grams per day forms an essential component of diet and lifestyle change advice. Limiting caffeine and smoking may also be helpful adjuncts. Over time, many patients become very effective at identifying their own dietary triggers, and clinicians can adapt their initial recommendations based on clinical response.

Diuretic Therapy

For many practitioners, diuretic therapy has become a mainstay of initial Ménière's disease management. In a study of 54 patients treated with diuretics and a low salt diet for 24 months, complete or substantial vertigo control occurred in 79%, limited control in 19%, and worsening control in 2%. Hearing improved in 35%, was unchanged in 29%, was worse in 22%, and could not be classified in 14%. The authors also found a stabilization of low and mid threshold frequencies with 74 months follow-up, thus leading to a conclusion that diet and diuretic might decrease the natural progression of sensorineural hearing loss in Ménière's disease [31].

Dyazide®, which is a combination of hydrochlorothiazide and triamterene, is our preferred diuretic unless the patient is allergic to sulfa-based medication. In the latter situation, spironolactone is used. It's also important to measure

Table 51.4 Ménière's disease management algorithm and outcomes

Conservative Management			Ablative Management		
Intervention Type	Specific Intervention	Outcomes	Intervention Type	Specific Intervention	Outcomes
Medical (primary)	Diet, diuretic, vasodilator	80% vertigo improvement	Medical	Gentamicin	85% vertigo improvement 30% hearing loss progression
Medical (adjuncts)	Steroids, histamine or betahistine		Surgical	Vestibular neurectomy	95% vertigo improvement 5% hearing loss progression
Surgical	Sac decompression	65% vertigo improvement when medical treatment failed. 80% require no further intervention.	Surgical	Labyrinthectomy	99% vertigo improvement 100% hearing loss progression

serum electrolytes (especially potassium) after starting diuretics.

Betahistine or Histamine

Betahistine is a histamine analog with weak action at Histamine H1 receptors and more potent antagonist effects at Histamine H3 receptors. The mechanism of action in Ménière's disease is still not completely clear, although vascular and neurological theories have been presented by different researchers. Animal studies have confirmed increase in blood supply to vestibulocochlear apparatus, and Bertlich et al. demonstrated that the H3 receptors are a mechanism for betahistine-induced increase in cochlear blood flow [32]. In another animal study, Dziadziola et al. found increases in vestibular blood flow with betahistine administration [33]. Nonetheless, the autoregulatory characteristics of the human central nervous system (CNS) vascular system make such a mechanism controversial. Lacour et al. reported that the mechanism of action lies in the central nervous system, in particular neuronal systems / histaminergic tuberomammillary and vestibular nuclei, which are involved in recovery after vestibular loss [34]. Animal studies demonstrate that histamine analogs decrease the vestibular nuclear automatic firing rate thus supporting the central theory.

Betahistine is used frequently for many causes of dizziness worldwide, although the evidence for such use is admittedly controversial. In a multicenter double-blind randomized trial, in which 55 patients received either betahistine 48 mg/day or flunarizine 10 mg/day, betahistine was significantly superior to flunarizine for frequency and duration of vertigo attacks and the presence of vegetative symptoms [35]. Contrarily, a recent Cochrane review did not find enough evidence to conclude that betahistine is useful in Ménière's disease. Interestingly, no trial reported any serious adverse effects with betahistine [36]. In the authors' practice, betahistine or subcutaneous histamine is offered as part of the medical regimen for Ménière's disease; however, three times daily betahistine dosage leads to compliance issues, and to circumvent this issue, we prefer weekly subcutaneous Injection of histamine in a tapering schedule.

Allergy Treatment

Studies have shown that the prevalence of allergy is much higher in patients with Ménière's disease than in the general population or the population of patients visiting an otologic clinic for other symptoms. Derebery et al. showed that, out of their 734 respondents with Ménière's disease, 59.2% reported possible airborne allergy, 40.3% had or suspected food allergies, and 37% had had confirmatory skin or in vitro tests for allergy. These prevalence rates were significantly higher than those found in the control group, of which 42.7% reported having or suspecting airborne allergies and 25% had or suspected food allergies [37]. Thus, inclusion of allergy management as part of a treatment battery for Ménière's disease can be beneficial. In these patients, any allergic history, including the presence of a family history of allergy, the presence of bilateral symptoms, the presence of symptoms after exposure to a food or inhaled allergen or seasonal change, or the presence of childhood allergy could be considered as indications for allergy testing [38]. The authors refer all such patients to allergy and immunology specialists who investigate and treat the allergies with desensitization if possible.

Meniett Device

The Meniett is a device that generates a sequence of micro pressure pulses that pass via tympanostomy tube into the middle ear and against the round window. The use of this device is based on the hypothesis of decreasing endolymphatic hydrops with low pressure pulses. The device is driven by a small, handheld, computer-controlled ear piece that generates air pressure pulses within 0–20 cm of water at a frequency of 5.8–6.1 Hz for a duration of 0.6 s. The device was U.S. Food and Drug Administration (FDA) approved in

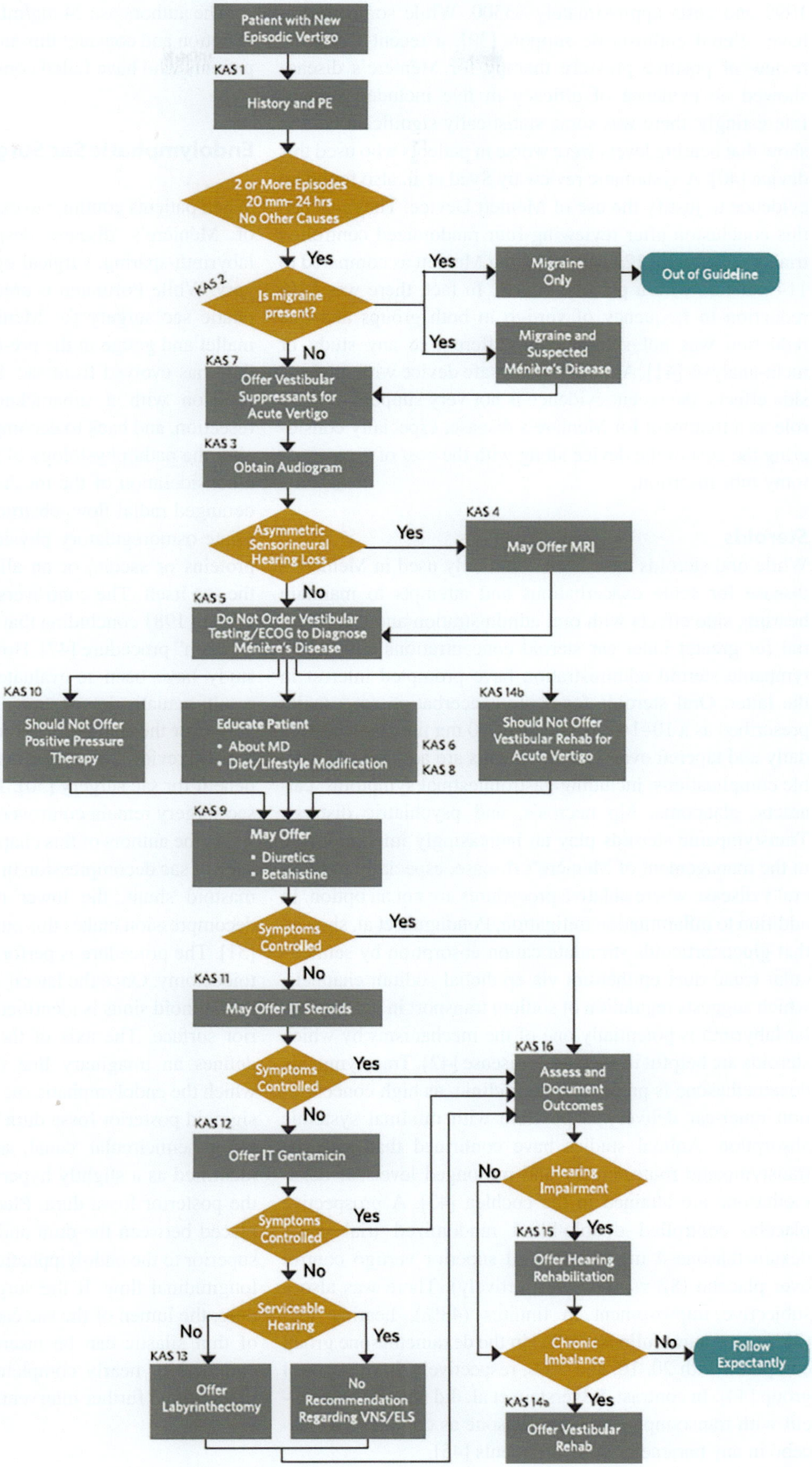

Fig. 51.2 The American Academy of Otolaryngology Head Neck Surgery Foundation revised and published Clinical Practice Guidelines for Ménière's Disease again in 2020 [70] (Reprinted with permission)

1999 and costs approximately $3500. While some studies have offered enthusiastic support [39], a recent Cochrane review of positive pressure therapy for Ménière's disease showed no evidence of efficacy in five included studies. Interestingly, there was some statistically significant data to show that hearing levels were worse in patients who used this device [40]. A systematic review by Syed et al. also found no evidence to justify the use of Meniett Device. They reached this conclusion after reviewing four randomized controlled trials (RCTs) with 123 patients using Meniett as compared to 114 patients with a placebo device. In fact, there was 61% reduction in frequency of vertigo in both groups and this reduction was not significantly different in any study or meta-analysis [41]. Although it is a safe device with minimal side effects, the recent evidence is not very supportive of its role as a treatment for Ménière's disease, especially considering the cost of the device along with the cost of tympanostomy tube insertion.

Steroids

While oral steroids have been commonly used in Ménière's disease for acute exacerbations and attempts to maintain hearing, side effects with oral administration and the potential for greater inner ear steroid concentrations with transtympanic steroid administration have prompted interest in the latter. Oral steroids for acute exacerbation are usually prescribed as a 10–14-day course of 30 mg prednisone twice daily and tapered over 3 days. Patients are advised of possible complications, including gastrointestinal symptoms, cataracts, glaucoma, hip necrosis, and psychiatric distress. Transtympanic steroids play an increasingly important role in the management of Ménière's disease, especially in bilateral v disease where ablative procedures are not an option. In addition to inflammation mitigation, Pondugula et al. showed that glucocorticoids stimulate cation absorption by semicircular canal duct epithelium via epithelial sodium channels, which suggests regulation of sodium transport in the vestibular labyrinth is potentially one of the mechanisms by which steroids are helpful in Ménière's disease [42]. Transtympanic dexamethasone is preferred in our clinic, as high concentration inner-ear delivery is possible with minimal systemic absorption. Animal studies have confirmed that with the transtympanic route, higher and prolonged levels of dexamethasone are attained in the cochlea [43]. A prospective placebo controlled double-blind randomized trial using dexamethasone 4 mg/mL showed superior vertigo control over placebo (82 vs. 57%, respectively). There was also a subjective improvement in tinnitus (48%), hearing loss (35%), and aural fullness (48%) in the dexamethasone group compared with 20, 10, and 20%, respectively, in the control group [44]. In contrast, Silverstein et al. did not find any benefit with transtympanic dexamethasone as compared to placebo in any parameter in their patients [45].

The authors use 24 mg/mL dexamethasone transtympanic injection and consider this an important option for Ménière's patients who have failed conservative management.

Endolymphatic Sac Surgery

When patients continue to experience debilitating symptoms of Ménière's disease despite medical management, a labyrinth-sparing, surgical option is endolymphatic sac surgery. While Portmann is credited with describing endolymphatic sac surgery for Ménière's disease in 1926 using a mallet and gouge in the pre-microscope era [46], the procedure has evolved from sac decompression alone to decompression with a subarachnoid or mastoid shunt, to sac resection, and back to decompression. How these procedures alter the pathophysiology of Ménière's disease goes back to a consideration of the mechanism of the disease, including deranged radial flow, obstructed longitudinal flow, inappropriate osmoregulatory physiology from secretion of glycoproteins or saccin, or an allergic/inflammatory reaction of the sac itself. The controversy was heightened by Thomsen et al. in 1981 concluding that the clinical effects were merely a "sham" procedure [47]. However, the results of the "sham" study have been re-evaluated to show that the published results actually demonstrated a significant benefit for sac surgery over the sham procedure [48] [49]. Another recent systematic review concluded that low level data does suggest a benefit for sac surgery [50]. That being said, the data around sac surgery remain controversial.

As the authors of this chapter have experienced equal efficacy of sac decompression in comparison to endolymphatic–mastoid shunt, the lower risk of hearing loss with sac decompression makes this our team's preferred sac operation [51]. The procedure is performed by first performing a mastoidectomy. Once the lateral semicircular canal is identified, the sigmoid sinus is identified and decompressed on its anterior surface. The axis of the horizontal semicircular canal defines an imaginary line (Donaldson's line), inferior to which the endolymphatic sac is situated (Fig. 51.3). The presigmoid posterior fossa dura is decompressed up to the posterior semicircular canal, and the endolymphatic sac is identified as a slightly hypervascular, whitish thickening of the posterior fossa dura. Pledgets of oxidized cellulose are placed between the dura and the petrous bone inferior and superior to the endolymphatic sac in the hopes of facilitating longitudinal flow. If the surgeon prefers a shunting procedure, the lumen of the sac can be gently opened and a piece of thin silastic can be inserted. About 67% demonstrated complete or nearly complete control of vertigo with 80% requiring no further intervention [50].

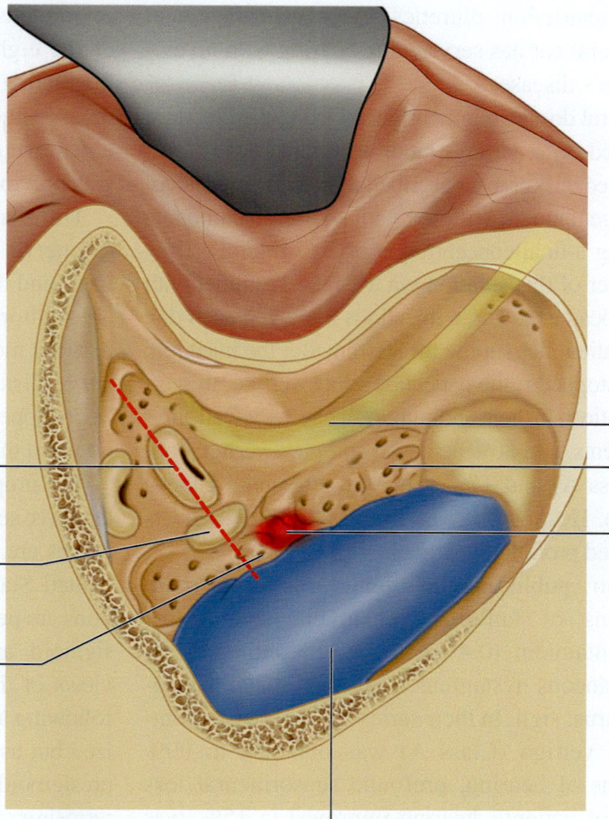

Fig. 51.3 Approach to endolymphatic sac decompression. The mastoidectomy has been completed, and the approximate location of the sac is highlighted relative to Donaldson's line. (Adapted from Otologic Surgery. 4th Ed. Eds. Brackmann D, Shelton C, Arriaga MA. Elsevier. 2015)

Ablative Therapy

Vestibular ablation for vertigo is based on the assumption that vertigo episodes occur in response to acute changes in vestibular function. As described in the general vestibular physiology chapter, an acute unilateral change in vestibular function results in acute vertigo until a combination of central vestibular suppression (cerebellar clamp) and compensatory and habituation changes facilitate accommodation. If medical and non-ablative surgical therapy, such as steroids and sac surgery, fail to stabilize vestibular function, ablating residual vestibular function is highly effective in preventing further vertigo attacks because there is no longer function which can fluctuate in the affected ear.

Vestibular ablation can be accomplished medically with transtympanic aminoglycoside (i.e., gentamicin) injection and surgically with selective vestibular nerve section or labyrinthectomy. The surgeon must carefully consider the possibility of bilateral disease, as bilateral ablation produces debilitating oscillopsia (Dandy's syndrome) [52].

Vestibular compensation and vestibular therapy: Following vestibular ablation (or any acute change in vestibular function), central compensation is necessary. A complex cascade of cerebellar suppression and release of tonic vestibular input and central adaptation to the new asymmetry is enhanced by dedicated vestibular rehabilitation maneuvers [53].

Transtympanic Gentamicin

Transtympanic gentamicin is a non-surgical option for unilateral Ménière's disease patients when conservative and non-ablative measures have failed. Gentamicin is instilled in the middle ear via transtympanic injection, through a pressure equalization (PE) tube, a T tube with a microcatheter, or a Silverstein microwick. Once injected into the middle ear, gentamicin seeps into perilymph and eventually endolymph via the round window membrane and oval window annular ligament. Aminoglycosides irreversibly enter hair cells through one-way channels, interfere with secondary cell messenger action, and even affect the integrity of the hair cell plasma membrane. Thus, the vestibulotoxic effect is achieved by damaging vestibular hair cells. Although primarily vestibulotoxic, gentamicin has cochleotoxic potential as well. Hence, the biggest drawback is its potential for sensorineural hearing loss. Some of its biggest advantages, however, are that it can be safely done in the office without general anesthesia, and it is inexpensive. It is important to understand that this option is recommended after patients have failed salt restriction, diuretics, medical management and the contralateral ear has serviceable hearing with no evidence of Ménière's disease.

There are several dosage regimens described in the literature ranging from fixed dose administration to titrated dose plans. Greenberg and Nedzelski have described a fixed dose protocol with 40 mg/mL gentamicin buffered with sodium bicarbonate to a pH 6.4 giving a final concentration of 26.7 mg/mL. They instill one milliliter of this solution via a T-tube grommet with an attached microcatheter. Three injections are given each day for 4 days. The patient lies supine for 30 min after the injection, and treatment is stopped if the patient develops vertigo, nystagmus, or deterioration in their audiogram. They reviewed their results of 30 patients, and 80% achieved complete vertigo control (Vertigo Class A) and 17% achieved substantial control (Vertigo Class B). Hearing decreased in 27% of their patients and 13% developed profound hearing loss [54].

Wu and Minor published their long-term results with weekly injections of buffered gentamicin solution of 26.7 mg/mL gentamicin (0.4 mL) injected until patients developed spontaneous nystagmus, post head shake nystagmus, or a head thrust sign. In their series of 34 patients, complete control of vertigo (Class A) was obtained in 90% patients. In terms of hearing, profound sensorineural loss occurred in 3% of patients, hearing improved in 15%, was unchanged in 68%, and was worse in 17% [55].

In a meta-analysis of intratympanic gentamicin for Ménière's disease by Cohen-Kerem et al., 15 trials with 627 patients were reviewed. None of the trials were double-blind or blinded prospectively. Complete (Class A) vertigo control was achieved in 74.7% patients and complete or substantial (Class B) control was achieved in 92.7% patients. The success rate was not affected by gentamicin treatment regimen (fixed or titration). Thus, they concluded that intratympanic gentamicin appears to be effective in the treatment of vertigo in intractable Ménière's disease [56].

Other aminoglycosides have varying degrees of vestibulotoxicity. Streptomycin was the first drug used for this purpose. Shea proposed combining it with steroids to minimize the cochleotoxic effects [57]. An application of streptomycin to vestibular ablation in this context is through intramuscular administration with a titration technique for bilateral partial vestibular ablation. Conceptually, this medication is used in an attempt to eliminate debilitating attacks but avoid the debilitating side effect of oscillopsia. It is the authors' opinion that this treatment option be considered as a last resort in a disabled patient [58].

Vestibular Nerve Section

Selective vestibular nerve section has a success rate of 95% total or substantial vertigo control in multiple retrospective series, including the authors' experience [59]. The surgical principle is that selectively sectioning the vestibular division of the eighth nerve eliminates the connection between the fluctuating peripheral vestibular end organ and the CNS; thus, in the absence of vestibular function, the ear can no longer trigger a new asymmetry in vestibular function, which was previously precipitating vertigo.

Different approaches have been proposed for sectioning the nerve based on anatomic considerations of the nerve itself and its location in the cerebellopontine angle and internal auditory canal (IAC). The vestibular portion of the eighth nerve is most distinct from the cochlear portion of the eighth nerve distally in the IAC. Histologically, even though the fibers appear to be distinct, there can be overlap of vestibular fibers in the cochlear nerve (Fig. 51.4).

In Europe, Garcia-Ibanez popularized middle fossa vestibular nerve section on the premise that the cochlear and vestibular nerves are most anatomically separate in this location. In the United States, however, most selective vestibular nerve sections are performed through the posterior fossa [60]. The retrosigmoid and retrolabyrinthine approaches provide similar views of the eighth nerve. In the retrolabyrinthine approach, following a complete mastoidectomy, the labyrinth is skeletonized but usually kept intact, and a wide decompression of the presigmoid posterior fossa dura, sigmoid sinus, and 1–2 cm of retrosigmoid dura are accomplished. The dura is incised just posterior to the posterior semicircular canal, and the superior (vestibular) division of the eighth nerve is sectioned (Fig. 51.5). In the retrosigmoid approach, the sigmoid sinus and retrosigmoid posterior fossa dura are decompressed and the dural incision is performed posterior to the sigmoid sinus. After draining cerebrospinal fluid, the eighth nerve can be identified from the root entry to the porus acousticus. Often the dissection plane between the vestibular and cochlear division is identified by a difference in color between the cochlear and vestibular divisions as well as a small vessel that often runs parallel to the plane between the two portions of the nerve.

Patients are warned of the existing risks of craniotomy including cerebellar hemorrhage, stroke, paralysis, facial paralysis, and total hearing loss. The efficacy of this approach is approximately 95% with approximately a 1% chance of serious operative side effects.

Labyrinthectomy

Complete vestibular ablation by surgical removal of the inner ear neuroepithelium in patients without serviceable hearing can be accomplished through transcanal or transmastoid labyrinthectomy.

- Transcanal labyrinthectomy: Following a tympanomeatal flap elevation, the stapes is removed, and the promontory between the round window and oval window is drilled to

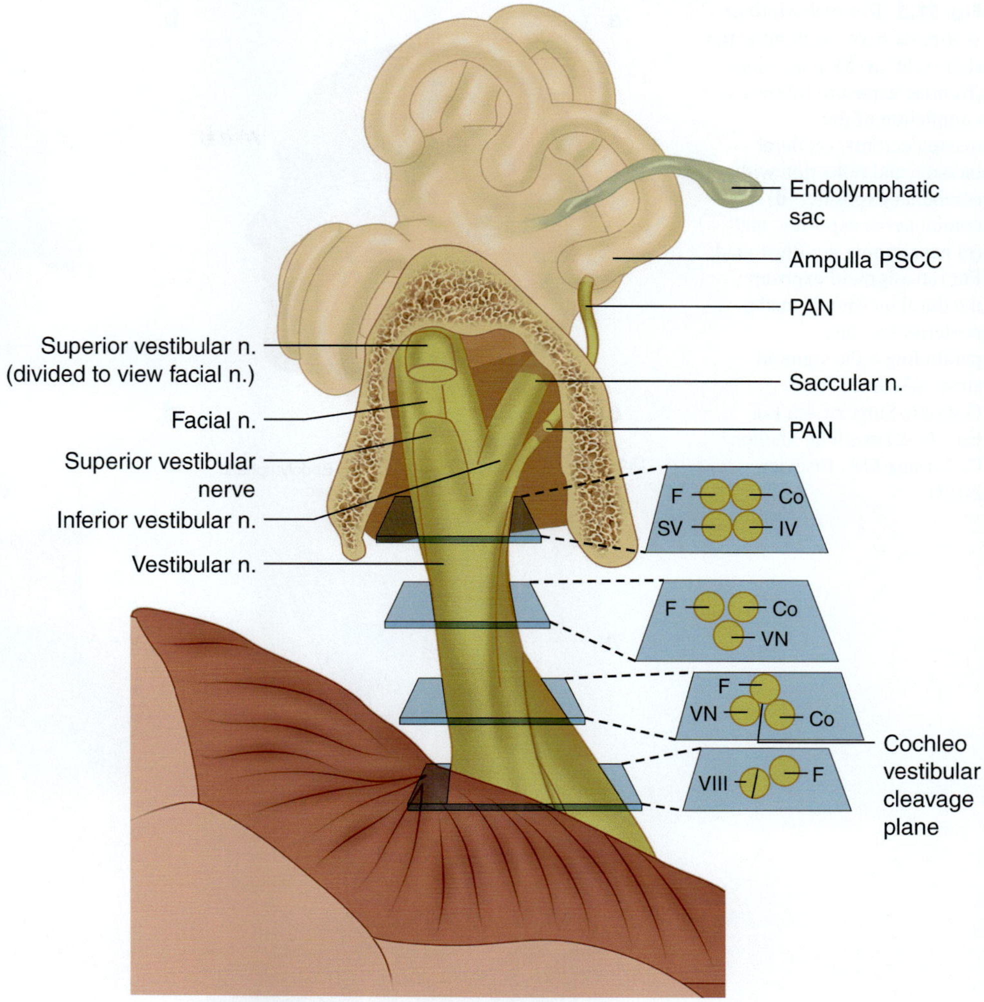

Fig. 51.4 Anatomy of the eighth cranial nerve as it rotates from root entry zone and porus acousticus to fundus of the internal auditory canal. (Adapted from Otologic Surgery. 4th Ed. Eds. Brackmann D, Shelton C, Arriaga MA. Elsevier. 2015)

create a large opening to the vestibule. The surgeon then systematically resects the five neuroepithelial structures (saccule, utricle, and three ampullae of the semicircular canals). The remaining vestibule is packed with absorbable sponge containing gentamicin. In a small percentage of patients, vertigo or persisting disequilibrium following transcanal labyrinthectomy has been blamed on traumatic vestibular neuroma, as labyrinthectomy sections vestibular input distal to Scarpa's ganglion and the selective nerve sections are usually pre-ganglionic (medial to Scarpa's ganglion which is located distally in the IAC). A translabyrinthine approach to nerve section or completion labyrinthectomy has been proposed to remedy this condition; however, the concept of symptomatic traumatic neuroma is controversial [61].

- Transmastoid labyrinthectomy: Following a complete mastoidectomy, the lateral, superior and posterior semicircular canals are drilled with care to positively identify the ampulla of each semicircular canal. The ampulla of the posterior canal is, anatomically, the most challenging because it is often medial to the vertical segment of the facial nerve. To assure safety and complete neuroepithelial removal, exposure of the vestibule after removing the lateral and superior canals allows the surgeon to drill from the vestibule toward the ampulla of the posterior canal remaining completely medial to the facial nerve. The surgeons must assure removal of the macula of the saccule and utricle also. Again, packing the vestibule with absorbable sponge soaked in gentamicin is recommended to assure chemical ablation of any residual neuro-epithelium. Transmastoid labyrinthectomy and translabyrinthine vestibular neurectomy are recognized as 99% effective at vertigo control in ipsilateral Ménière's disease, but they result in profound sensorineural hearing loss on the operative side (Figs. 51.6 and 51.7) [62].

As an otologist considers ablative therapy, they should keep in mind that, given enough time, most patients' spells spontaneously cease ("burn out"). In a classic series by Silverstein, 71% of patients who were offered but refused ablative therapy had complete control of vertigo at an average follow-up of 8.3 years. However, 93% had complete control after ablation with vestibular neurectomy [63].

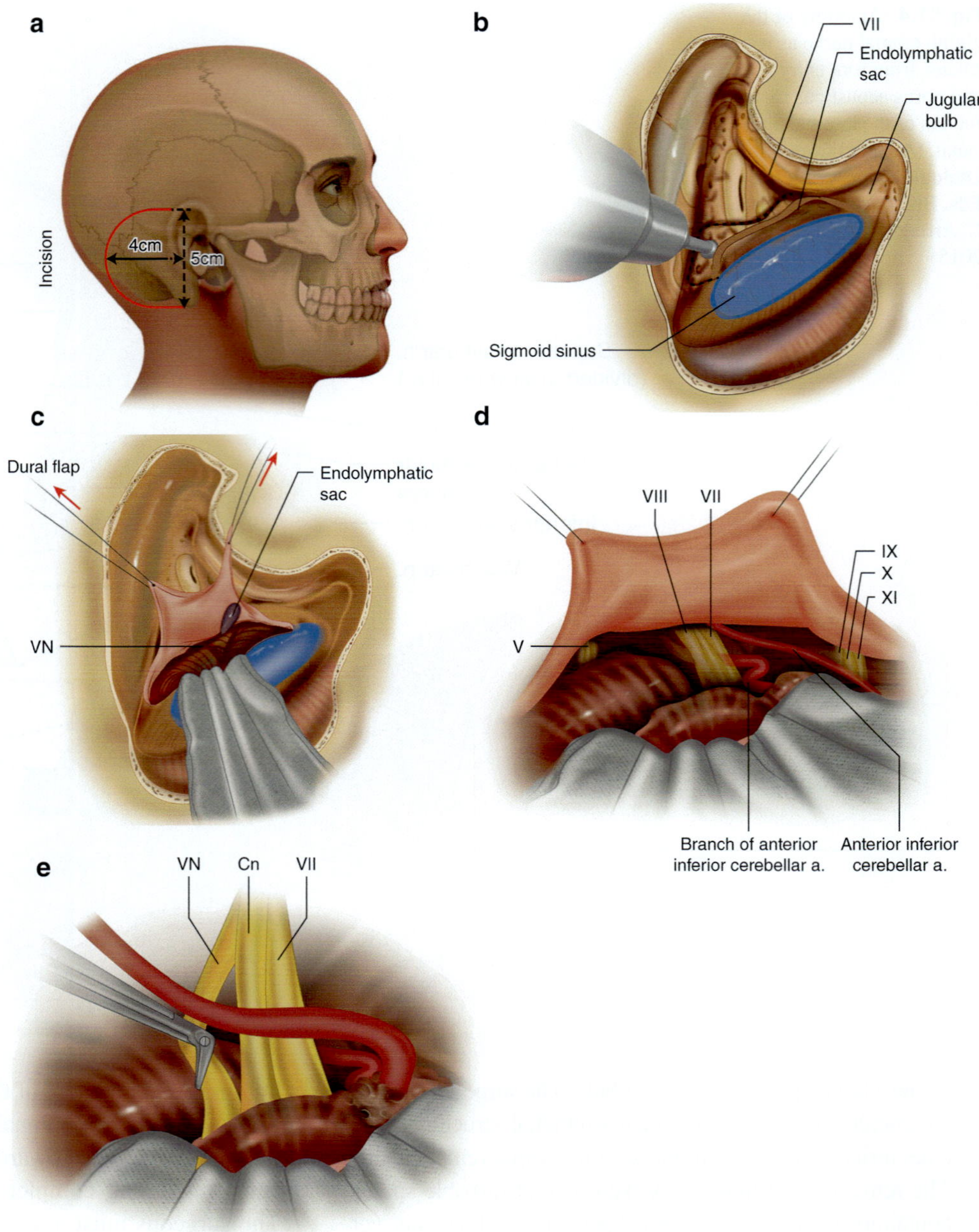

Fig. 51.5 Retrolabyrinthine vestibular nerve section on the right side. (**a**) Skin incision, (**b**) bone exposure following completion of the mastoidectomy, (**c**) dural incision and reflection with cerebellar exposure, (**d**) cranial nerve exposure, and (**e**) neurectomy are illustrated. For retrosigmoid exposure, the dural incision is made posterior to—and paralleling—the sigmoid sinus. (Adapted from Otologic Surgery. 4th Ed. Eds. Brackmann D, Shelton C, Arriaga MA. Elsevier. 2015)

Adjunctive and Experimental Considerations

Cochlear Implants

For patients with advanced bilateral disease and severe-to-profound sensorineural loss, cochlear implantation is a good option for hearing rehabilitation. A retrospective study in a tertiary academic center concluded that the patients with advanced binaural involvement may present a challenge to conventional criteria for cochlear implant candidacy because of fluctuating symptoms, but these patients in their series achieved significant benefit over baseline after implantation. They also stressed that previous vestibular surgery, including labyrinthectomy, does not contraindicate cochlear implantation [64].

Furthermore, a prospective study by Perkins et al. showed patients with unilateral Ménière's disease who underwent simultaneous labyrinthectomy and cochlear implantation experienced improvements in sound localization, speech discrimination, tinnitus severity, and quality of life with the device use [65]. Recent systematic reviews and meta-analysis support Cochlear implantation with or without labyrinthectomy as a viable option for treatment of patients with Ménière's disease. The reviews not only point towards high rates of tinnitus suppression and vertigo control but also demonstrate similar cochlear implant speech perception outcomes in patients with Ménière's disease as compared to non-Ménière's disease implant recipients [66, 67].

Vestibular Implants

Vestibular implants also deserve mention in the treatment options for Ménière's disease patients. Although still in relative infancy, these devices conceptually offer promise. There have been human trials conducted by several teams. Rubenstein et al., for example, received FDA approval to enroll 10 patients with uncontrolled Ménière's disease as part of a feasibility study. The UW (University of Washington)/Nucleus Vestibular Implant is a modified freedom cochlear implant with a receiver / stimulator attached to a trifurcating array containing three electrodes per array. The main concept involves providing patient controlled stimulus to the vestibular apparatus in the setting of a sudden loss of vestibular tonic output. This device could even be programmed to override excessive signals, assuming a situation could arise in which overstimulation could cause vertigo. Preliminary steps in surgery are similar to cochlear implant surgery. After cortical mastoidectomy, semicircular canals are blue lined and fenestrated with a dissecting pick, electrodes are inserted 2.5 mm into the perilymphatic space, and positioned adjacent to each of the 3 ampullae. Short-term results have been promising, but long-term (63 weeks after the surgery) responses diminished or were lost. Even speech discrimination dropped over time. This was contrary to the long-term results in primates. The human trial ended with four implants, but a newer implant is awaiting FDA approval [68]. Improvements include integration of a cochlear Implant with the vestibular implant, or an implant that dynamically senses head motion proposed by the Johns Hopkins group [69].

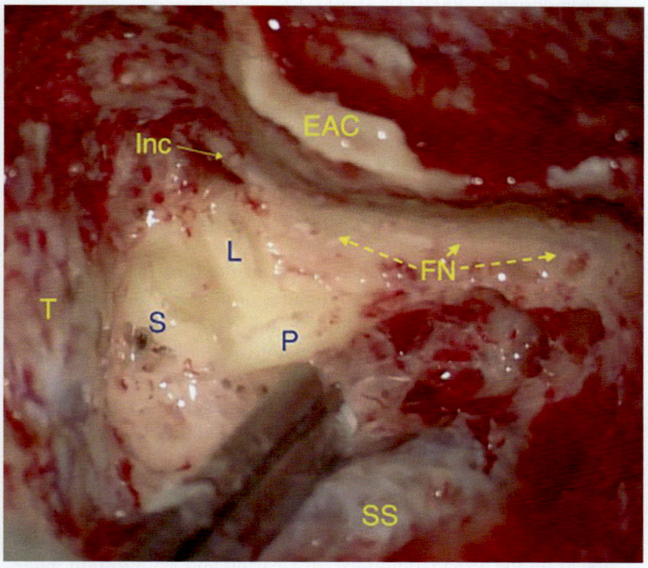

Fig. 51.6 Labyrinthectomy on a right ear. The facial nerve (FN), Tegmen (T), and sigmoid sinus (SS) have been skeletonized, and the bony ear canal (EAC) has been thinned. The incus (Inc) is exposed. The lateral (L), posterior (P), and superior (S) semicircular canals have been blue-lined. (Image courtesy of Alex D. Sweeney, MD)

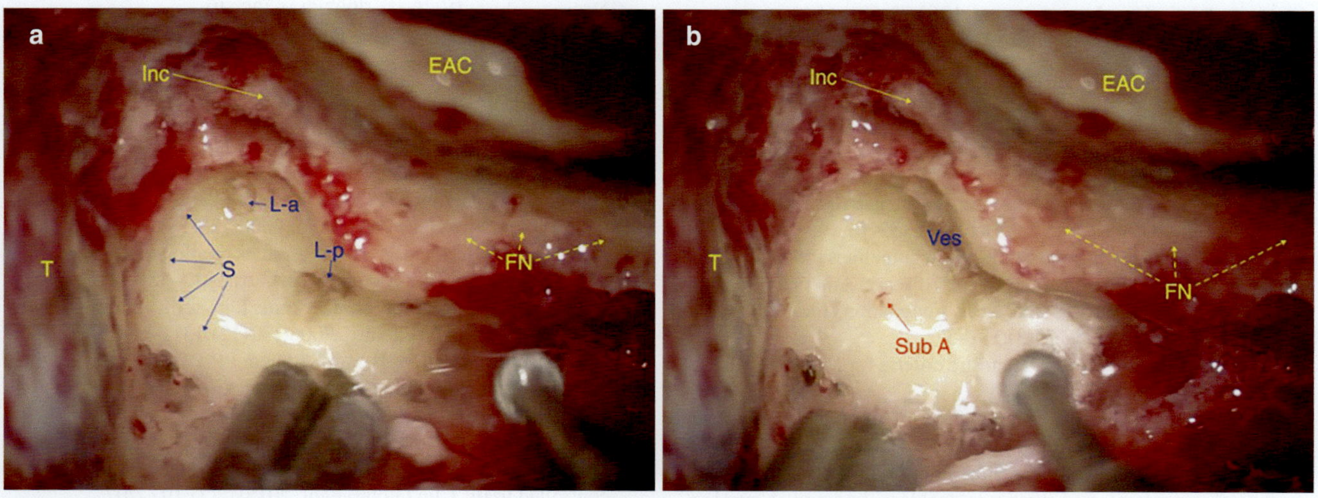

Fig. 51.7 Sequential picture of a right ear labyrinthectomy. (**a**) Opening and partial removal of all three semicircular canals with the anterior (L-a) and posterior (L-p) limbs of the lateral semicircular canal labeled. The superior canal has also been opened and is labeled (S) with arrows). (**b**) The vestibule has been exposed (Ves), as has the subarcuate artery (Sub A). FN Facial nerve, Inc. Incus, EAC External auditory canal, T Tegmen. (Image courtesy of Alex D. Sweeney, MD)

Conclusion

While the mechanism, diagnosis, and treatment of Ménière's disease are controversial, our patients with this debilitating condition deserve our efforts to manage them with our best understanding of the state of the art. Despite obvious limitations, patients can be reliably counseled that this condition can be managed successfully and the vast majority of patients are able to function well without a lifetime of disabling symptoms. A step-wise approach to treatment is usually best to avoid unnecessary morbidity related to aggressive management when simpler measures may suffice.

References

1. Harris JP, Alexander TH. Current-day prevalence of Meniere's syndrome. Audiol Neurootol. 2010;15(5):318–22.
2. Vrabec JT, Simon LM, Coker NJ. Survey of Meniere's disease in a subspecialty referral practice. Otolaryngol Head Neck Surg. 2007;137(2):213–7.
3. Minor LB, Schessel DA, Carey JP. Meniere's disease. Curr Opin Neurol. 2004;17(1):9–16.
4. Liu YF, Xu H. The intimate relationship between vestibular migraine and Meniere disease: a review of pathogenesis and presentation. Behav Neurol. 2016;2016:3182735.
5. Hallpike CS, Cairns H. Observations on the pathology of Meniere's syndrome: (section of otology). Proc R Soc Med. 1938;31(11):1317–36.
6. Merchant SN, Adams JC, Nadol JB Jr. Pathophysiology of Meniere's syndrome: are symptoms caused by endolymphatic hydrops? Otol Neurotol. 2005;26(1):74–81.
7. Salt AN. Regulation of endolymphatic fluid volume. Ann N Y Acad Sci. 2001;942:306–12.
8. Paparella MM, Kimberley BP. Pathogenesis of Meniere's disease. J Vestib Res. 1990;1(1):3–7.
9. Gibson WP, Arenberg IK. Pathophysiologic theories in the etiology of Meniere's disease. Otolaryngol Clin N Am. 1997;30(6):961–7.
10. Schuknecht HF. Meniere's disease: a correlation of symptomatology and pathology. Laryngoscope. 1963;73:651–65.
11. Ozeki H, Iwasaki S, Murofushi T. Vestibular drop attack secondary to Meniere's disease results from unstable otolithic function. Acta Otolaryngol. 2008;128(8):887–91.
12. Green JD Jr, Blum DJ, Harner SG. Longitudinal followup of patients with Meniere's disease. Otolaryngol Head Neck Surg. 1991;104(6):783–8.
13. House JW, et al. Meniere's disease: prevalence of contralateral ear involvement. Otol Neurotol. 2006;27(3):355–61.
14. Committee on Hearing and Equilibrium guidelines for the diagnosis and evaluation of therapy in Meniere's disease. American Academy of Otolaryngology-Head and Neck Foundation, Inc. Otolaryngol Head Neck Surg. 1995;113(3):181–5.
15. Lopez-Escamez JA, et al. Diagnostic criteria for Meniere's disease. J Vestib Res. 2015;25(1):1–7.
16. Neuhauser H, et al. The interrelations of migraine, vertigo, and migrainous vertigo. Neurology. 2001;56(4):436–41.
17. Radtke A, et al. Vestibular migraine: long-term follow-up of clinical symptoms and vestibulo-cochlear findings. Neurology. 2012;79(15):1607–14.
18. Neff BA, et al. Auditory and vestibular symptoms and chronic subjective dizziness in patients with Meniere's disease, vestibular migraine, and Meniere's disease with concomitant vestibular migraine. Otol Neurotol. 2012;33(7):1235–44.
19. Radtke A, et al. Migraine and Meniere's disease: is there a link? Neurology. 2002;59(11):1700–4.
20. Paparella MM, McDermott JC, de Sousa LC. Meniere's disease and the peak audiogram. Arch Otolaryngol. 1982;108(9):555–9.
21. Dobie RA, Snyder JM, Donaldson JA. Electronystagmographic and audiologic findings in patients with Meniere's disease. Acta Otolaryngol. 1982;94(1–2):19–27.
22. Young YH, Huang TW, Cheng PW. Assessing the stage of Meniere's disease using vestibular evoked myogenic potentials. Arch Otolaryngol Head Neck Surg. 2003;129(8):815–8.
23. Young YH, Wu CC, Wu CH. Augmentation of vestibular evoked myogenic potentials: an indication for distended saccular hydrops. Laryngoscope. 2002;112(3):509–12.
24. Sass K. Sensitivity and specificity of transtympanic electrocochleography in Meniere's disease. Acta Otolaryngol. 1998;118(2):150–6.
25. Arriaga MA, et al. Visually enhanced vestibulo-ocular reflex: a diagnostic tool for migraine vestibulopathy. Laryngoscope. 2006;116(9):1577–9.
26. Nakashima T, et al. Visualization of endolymphatic hydrops in patients with Meniere's disease. Laryngoscope. 2007;117(3):415–20.
27. Sano R, et al. Contrast enhancement of the inner ear in magnetic resonance images taken at 10 minutes or 4 hours after intravenous gadolinium injection. Acta Otolaryngol. 2012;132(3):241–6.
28. Soto E, Vega R. Neuropharmacology of vestibular system disorders. Curr Neuropharmacol. 2010;8(1):26–40.
29. Luxford E, et al. Dietary modification as adjunct treatment in Meniere's disease: patient willingness and ability to comply. Otol Neurotol. 2013;34(8):1438–43.
30. Sajjadi H, Paparella MM. Meniere's disease. Lancet. 2008;372(9636):406–14.
31. Santos PM, et al. Diuretic and diet effect on Meniere's disease evaluated by the 1985 Committee on Hearing and Equilibrium guidelines. Otolaryngol Head Neck Surg. 1993;109(4):680–9.
32. Bertlich M, et al. Histaminergic H3-Heteroreceptors as a potential mediator of Betahistine-induced increase in Cochlear blood flow. Audiol Neurootol. 2015;20(5):283–93.
33. Dziadziola JK, et al. Betahistine increases vestibular blood flow. Otolaryngol Head Neck Surg. 1999;120(3):400–5.
34. Lacour M, et al. Betahistine in the treatment of Meniere's disease. Neuropsychiatr Dis Treat. 2007;3(4):429–40.
35. Fraysse B, et al. Betahistine dihydrochloride versus flunarizine. A double-blind study on recurrent vertigo with or without cochlear syndrome typical of Meniere's disease. Acta Otolaryngol Suppl. 1991;490:1–10.
36. James AL, Burton MJ. Betahistine for Meniere's disease or syndrome. Cochrane Database Syst Rev. 2001;2001(1):CD001873.
37. Derebery MJ, Berliner KI. Prevalence of allergy in Meniere's disease. Otolaryngol Head Neck Surg. 2000;123(1 Pt 1):69–75.
38. Derebery MJ, Berliner KI. Allergy and its relation to Meniere's disease. Otolaryngol Clin N Am. 2010;43(5):1047–58.
39. Gates GA, et al. Meniett clinical trial: long-term follow-up. Arch Otolaryngol Head Neck Surg. 2006;132(12):1311–6.
40. van Sonsbeek S, Pullens B, van Benthem PP. Positive pressure therapy for Meniere's disease or syndrome. Cochrane Database Syst Rev. 2015;2015(3):CD008419.
41. Syed MI, et al. Positive pressure therapy for Meniere's syndrome/disease with a Meniett device: a systematic review of randomised controlled trials. Clin Otolaryngol. 2015;40(3):197–207.
42. Pondugula SR, et al. Glucocorticoids stimulate cation absorption by semicircular canal duct epithelium via epithelial sodium channel. Am J Physiol Renal Physiol. 2004;286(6):F1127–35.

43. Lee JJ, et al. Steroid intracochlear distribution differs by administration method: systemic versus intratympanic injection. Laryngoscope. 2017;128:189.
44. Garduno-Anaya MA, et al. Dexamethasone inner ear perfusion by intratympanic injection in unilateral Meniere's disease: a two-year prospective, placebo-controlled, double-blind, randomized trial. Otolaryngol Head Neck Surg. 2005;133(2):285–94.
45. Silverstein H, et al. Dexamethasone inner ear perfusion for the treatment of Meniere's disease: a prospective, randomized, double-blind, crossover trial. Am J Otol. 1998;19(2):196–201.
46. Portmann G. The saccus endolymphaticus and an operation for draining the same for the relief of vertigo. 1927. J Laryngol Otol. 1991;105(12):1109–12.
47. Thomsen J, et al. Placebo effect in surgery for Ménière's disease. A double-blind, placebo-controlled study on endolymphatic sac shunt surgery. Arch Otolaryngol. 1981;107(5):271–7.
48. Pillsbury HC, et al. Endolymphatic sac surgery. The Danish sham surgery study: an alternative analysis. Otolaryngol Clin North Am. 1983;16(1):123–7.
49. Welling DB, Nagaraja HN. Endolymphatic mastoid shunt: a reevaluation of efficacy. Otolaryngol Head Neck Surg. 2000;122(3):340–5.
50. Lim MY, et al. Current evidence for endolymphatic sac surgery in the treatment of Meniere's disease: a systematic review. Singapore Med J. 2015;56(11):593–8.
51. Brinson GM, Chen DA, Arriaga MA. Endolymphatic mastoid shunt versus endolymphatic sac decompression for Ménière's disease. Otolaryngol Head Neck Surg. 2007;136(3):415–21.
52. Dandy W. The surgical treatment of Meniere's disease. Surg Gynecol Obstet. 1941;72:421–5.
53. McDonnell MN, Hillier SL. Vestibular rehabilitation for unilateral peripheral vestibular dysfunction. Cochrane Database Syst Rev. 2015;1:CD005397.
54. Greenberg SL, Nedzelski JM. Medical and noninvasive therapy for Meniere's disease. Otolaryngol Clin N Am. 2010;43(5):1081–90.
55. Wu IC, Minor LB. Long-term hearing outcome in patients receiving intratympanic gentamicin for Meniere's disease. Laryngoscope. 2003;113(5):815–20.
56. Cohen-Kerem R, et al. Intratympanic gentamicin for Meniere's disease: a meta-analysis. Laryngoscope. 2004;114(12):2085–91.
57. Shea PF, et al. Hearing results and quality of life after streptomycin/dexamethasone perfusion for Meniere's disease. Laryngoscope. 2012;122(1):204–11.
58. Graham MD. Bilateral Meniere's disease. Treatment with intramuscular titration streptomycin sulfate. Otolaryngol Clin N Am. 1997;30(6):1097–100.
59. Hillman TA, Chen DA, Arriaga MA. Vestibular nerve section versus intratympanic gentamicin for Meniere's disease. Laryngoscope. 2004;114(2):216–22.
60. Garcia-Ibanez E, Garcia-Ibanez JL. Middle fossa vestibular neurectomy: a report of 373 cases. Otolaryngol Head Neck Surg. 1980;88(4):486–90.
61. Linthicum FH, Alonso A, Denia A. Traumatic neuroma: a complication of transcanal labyrinthectomy. Arch Otolaryngol. 1979;105(11):654–5.
62. Buchman C, Adunka O. Translabyrinthine vestibular neurectomy. In: Brackmann DE, Shelton C, Arriaga MA, editors. Otologic surgery. Philadelphia: Elsevier; 2016. p. 397–407.
63. Silverstein H, Smouha E, Jones R. Natural history vs. surgery for Menière's disease. Otolaryngol Head Neck Surg. 1989;100(1):6–16.
64. Lustig LR, et al. Cochlear implantation in patients with bilateral Meniere's syndrome. Otol Neurotol. 2003;24(3):397–403.
65. Perkins E, et al. Simultaneous labyrinthectomy and cochlear implantation in unilateral Meniere's disease. Laryngoscope Investig Otolaryngol. 2018;3(3):225–30.
66. Villavisanis DF, et al. Cochlear implantation in Meniere's disease: a systematic review and meta-analysis. Laryngoscope. 2021;131(8):1845–54.
67. Desiato VM, et al. Cochlear implantation in patients with Meniere's disease: a systematic review. World Journal of Otorhinolaryngology. 2021;7(4):303–11.
68. Phillips JO, et al. Vestibular implantation and longitudinal electrical stimulation of the semicircular canal afferents in human subjects. J Neurophysiol. 2015;113(10):3866–92.
69. Della Santina C, Migliaccio A, Patel A. Electrical stimulation to restore vestibular function development of a 3-d vestibular prosthesis. Conf Proc IEEE Eng Med Biol Soc. 2005;7:7380–5.
70. Basura GJ, et al. Clinical practice guideline: Ménière's disease executive summary. Otolaryngol Head Neck Surg. 2020;162(4):415–34.
71. Cureoglu S, et al. Histopathology of Meniere's disease. Oper Tech Otolaryngol Head Neck Surg. 2016;27(4):194–204.

52 Autoimmune Inner Ear Disease

Jeffrey P. Harris and Hitomi Sakano

Background

Historical Perspective

One of the earliest identified syndromes of hearing loss, which we now attribute to autoimmune ear disease (AIED), was Cogan's syndrome, described by Cogan in a series of case reports beginning in 1945 [21–23, 81] characterizing a number of patients with nonsyphilitic progressive bilateral vestibuloauditory disorders associated with keratitis and other systemic symptoms. McCabe is credited as the first to link an autoimmune process with sensorineural hearing loss (SNHL) and to recommend treatment. In 1979, he proposed a new entity of autoimmune SNHL in a series of 18 patients with progressive bilateral hearing loss, bilateral vestibular dysfunction, responding to cyclophosphamide and dexamethasone therapy [75]. In the patients tested, a lymphocyte inhibition assay revealed a positive reaction to human inner ear proteins, consistent with an autoimmune etiology. Since then, progressive SNHL that is responsive to steroids has been referred to as AIED, although as we will discuss later in this chapter, not all AIED is steroid responsive.

The Ear Is Not Immunologically Privileged

It had previously been believed that the ear is immunologically privileged; however, studies in the 1970s and 1980s revealed that this belief is incorrect. The endolymphatic sac is contiguous with the endolymph of the cochlea, and work by Rask-Andersen and Stahle suggested that the endolymphatic sac may be the site of immunological processing. Their studies using electron microscopy revealed lymphocytes and macrophages within the intraluminal endolymphatic sac [85] (Fig. 52.1). Mogi et al. found that immunizing animals to egg albumin resulted in a rise in antibody concentration in perilymph that was three to four times higher than that seen in cerebrospinal fluid (CSF), and suggested that the source may be blood vessels of the perilymphatic space rather than CSF [77]. Harris et al. showed unequivocally that the inner ear was immunoresponsive, that local perilymph antibody response was specific to the antigen with which it

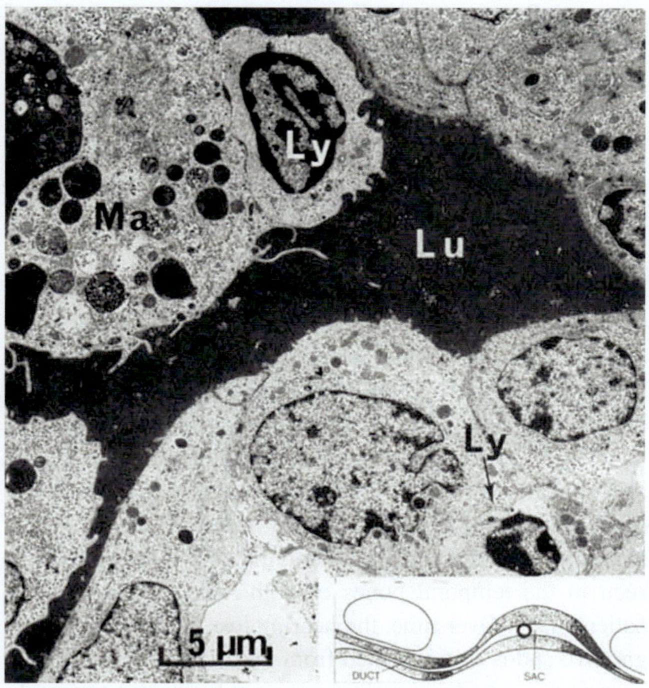

Fig. 52.1 Immune cells within the guinea pig endolymphatic sac. (Ma macrophage, Ly lymphocyte, Lu lumen of the endolymphatic sac). (Reproduced with permission from [85])

J. P. Harris (✉)
Department of Otolaryngology—Head and Neck Surgery, University of California San Diego Medical Center, San Diego, CA, USA

VA Healthcare System, San Diego, CA, USA
e-mail: jpharris@health.ucsd.edu

H. Sakano
Department of Otolaryngology—Head and Neck Surgery, University of Texas Southwestern Medical Center, Dallas, TX, USA

A. D. Sweeney et al. (eds.), *Haynes-Glasscock-Shambaugh Surgery of the Ear*, https://doi.org/10.1007/978-3-032-18264-7_52

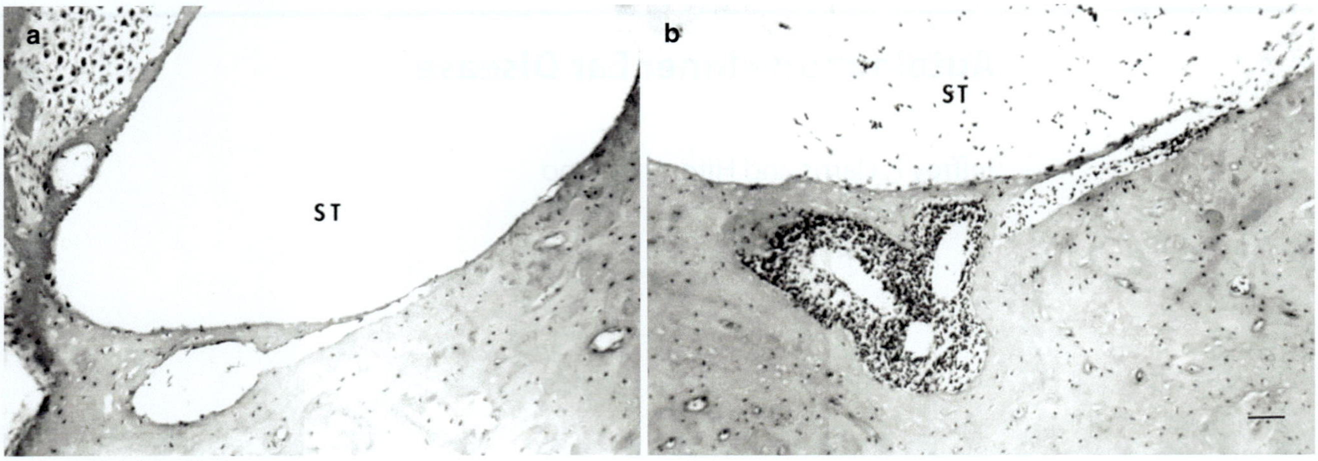

Fig. 52.2 (a) Collecting venule from the scala tympani joining the spiral modiolar vein within the modiolus below the basal turn from a normal guinea pig cochlea. ST—scala tympani. (b) Spiral modiolar vein with an adjoining collecting venule of the ST from the basal turn of a guinea pig cochlea undergoing secondary inner ear immune response to keyhole limpet hemocyanin. Immunoresponsive cells are accumulating in the perivascular space and streaming into ST. (Reproduced with permission from [43])

was challenged [38, 39, 41], and that the immune response seen in the inner ear is dependent on the presence of the endolymphatic sac [104]. The pathway of entry into the inner ear is predominantly through the spiral modiolar vein (Fig. 52.2) [31, 43]. Studies demonstrated that the spiral modiolar vein transforms into a high-endothelial venule expressing intercellular adhesion molecule-1 (ICAM-1) during this inflammatory process, which is consistent with the outpouring of inflammatory cells from general circulation into the scala tympani [100]. The cells can then proliferate, release inflammatory mediators, and initiate the series of changes that lead to hearing loss [43, 96, 100, 101]. Antigens introduced into the inner ear in a sensitized animal can result in hearing loss [40, 41, 70, 113].

Clinical Presentation

The true incidence of AIED is unknown, but it has been extrapolated to be less than 5/100,000 [107] and is the cause in <1% of sensorineural hearing loss (SNHL). It is characterized by progressive SNHL that can be unilateral, but often becomes bilateral. The timescale for hearing loss is weeks to months, a distinction from sudden SNHL, which occurs once and immediately. AIED hearing loss can fluctuate, and it is often difficult to distinguish from Ménière's disease. The similarity may reflect that endolymphatic hydrops can be seen in the temporal bones of both AIED and Ménière's patients [91]. Over time, the hearing loss is of AIED is progressive and is distinguished from presbycusis or hereditary hearing loss,which generally occurs gradually on a timescale of years. Although audiovestibular symptoms may be the only presenting symptom, the presence of other systemic autoimmune or autoinflammatory symptoms can aid in the diagnosis of AIED. These other symptoms may include rheumatoid arthritis, inflammatory bowel disease (IBD), vision loss, autoimmune thyroiditis (e.g., Hashimoto's disease) or renal disease, therefore, emphasizing the need to perform a thorough review of systems (Table 52.1).

Table 52.1 Autoimmune Hearing loss

Autoimmune hearing loss	
Vogt-Koyanagi-Harada syndrome	Uveitis, alopecia, periorbital depigmentation
Cogan's syndrome[a]	Interstitial keratitis, vasculitis
Susac's syndrome[a]	Encephalopathy, branch retinal artery occlusion
Systemic lupus erythematosus	Malar rash, nephropathy
Rheumatoid arthritis	Joint pain, fever, skin nodules
Granulomatosis with polyangiitis	Serous otitis media, nasal obstruction, subglottic stenosis, pulmonary nodule
Behçet's disease	Recurrent oral and genital ulcers, vasculitis
Systemic sclerosis	Xerostomia, sclerodactyly, CREST syndrome, Sjögren's syndrome
Inflammatory bowel disease	Bloody diarrhea, extraintestinal symptoms
Relapsing polychondritis	Perichondritis, arthritis
Temporal arteritis	Jaw claudication, temporal headache, blindness
Autoimmune thyroiditis	Fatigue, weight change, temperature dysregulation, heart arrhythmia, and skin, gastrointestinal and neurological symptoms

[a]Diagnosis requires inner ear involvement

Mechanism

Although it is unclear what triggers the autoimmune process, there is suggestion that autoantibodies may be produced in response to viral or bacterial infections as a result of molecular mimicry. In the case of Cogan's syndrome, Lunardi et al.

[69] suggested that a viral infection may lead to the production of autoantibodies. Through a random peptide library screen, they found that circulating autoantibodies in these patients recognizes a peptide (SGRDTSIQILWI) which they name "Cogan peptide." Interestingly, this peptide is similar to REOVIRUS III major core protein lambda 1 as well as autoantigens density-enhanced phosphatase-1 (DEP-1)/CD148 (expressed on endothelium) and connexin 26 (of the inner ear).

Several immune-mediated processes are associated with AIED. Consistent with the possibility that autoantibodies to ear antigens may be involved in the process of AIED, approximately 32% of patients with suspected AIED have sera that react to a 68 kDa inner ear protein on Western blotting [42]. Since then, the 68 kDa protein has since been determined to cross react with a heat shock protein (HSP70) [13], a ubiquitously expressed house-keeping protein. It is thought to be a result of a bystander effect of inflammation rather than a cause for hearing loss. It has nevertheless been a useful marker for AIED. Additional target proteins from inner ear (e.g., myelin protein P0, 27-30 kDa, 33-35 kDa, 45 kDa, 50 kDa, 58 kDa, 80 kDa) have been identified by immunoblotting with sera from patients with progressive SNHL [18, 19, 110, 114]. Relapsing polychondritis is associated with autoantibodies to collagen II and IV, which are also expressed in the inner ear [53].

T-cells may also play a role in AIED. Circulating T-cells recognizing inner ear antigens, including cochlin, a highly abundant inner ear protein, are more frequently found in AIED patients compared to controls [7]. In Vogt-Koyanagi-Harada syndrome, there is a T-cell mediated response to melanocyte antigens causing inflammation of the choroid. Interestingly, melanocytes are observed in the endolymphatic sac [37] and membranous labyrinth [117] and therefore it is not inconceivable that there is abnormal lymphocyte recognition of melanocyte antigens in the ear.

Endolymphatic hydrops can occur in AIED. In one study, half of AIED patients had abnormal electrocochleography results [16]. In a large series of 690 Ménière's patients, there is a higher rate of systemic autoimmune disease compared to the normal population [34]. Endolymphatic hydrops is observed in the temporal bones of AIED patients [91]. Tomiyama demonstrated that antigen challenge of the endolymphatic sac of sensitized animals will uniformly result in endolymphatic hydrops [103]. Others have shown that systemically immunizing animals with inner ear antigen also leads to this condition [15, 116]. In other cases, such as Granulomatosis with polyangiitis (GPA, historically known as Wegener's granulomatosis), there can be vasculitis in the cochlea, vestibule, and facial nerve (Fig. 52.3) [89]. Otopathology of Sjögren's syndrome reveals stria vascularis atrophy, IgG deposition in the basement membrane, and loss of spiral ganglion neurons [17]. In systemic lupus erythematosus (SLE), the most common findings are atrophy of the stria vascularis, loss of outer hair cells, and variable loss of spiral ganglion cells [32, 56, 95]. Fibrosis and bone deposition can also be seen (Fig. 52.4) [32]. Ultimately, inflammatory changes in the inner ear lead to fibrosis and osteoneogenesis [51, 52].

Animal models of AIED show infiltration of immune cells in the scala tympani, hemorrhage, perilabyrinthine fibrosis, osteoneogenesis (Fig. 52.5) and degeneration of

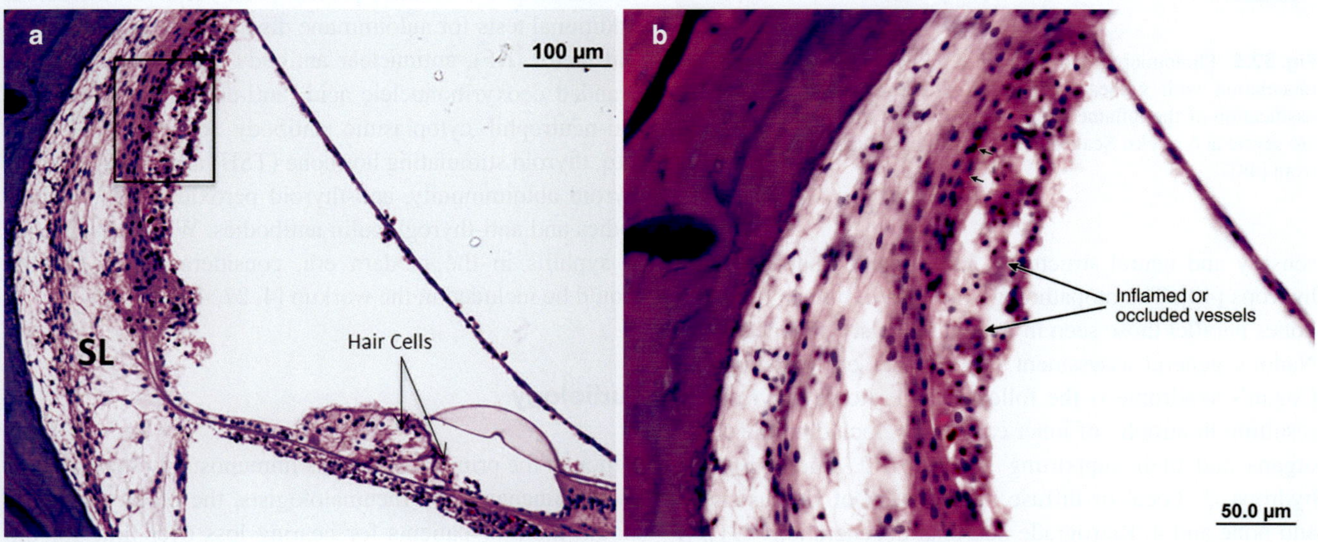

Fig. 52.3 Granulomatosis with polyangiitis. (left) The scala media in the basal turn of the cochlea. (right) Vessels in the stria vascularis and the spiral ligament were thickened and in some instances occluded (arrows). Punctate areas of hemosiderin deposition suggest prior hemorrhage (arrowheads). (Reproduced with permission from [89])

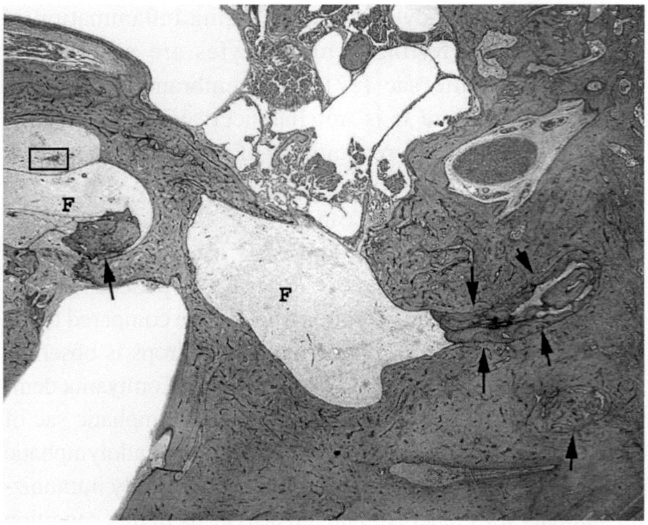

Fig. 52.4 There is new bone (arrows) and dense fibrous tissue (F) in the osseous labyrinth from the right ear of this patient with SLE. Note that there are no structures of the membranous labyrinth (hematoxylin-eosin, magnification, 310). (Reproduced with permission from [32])

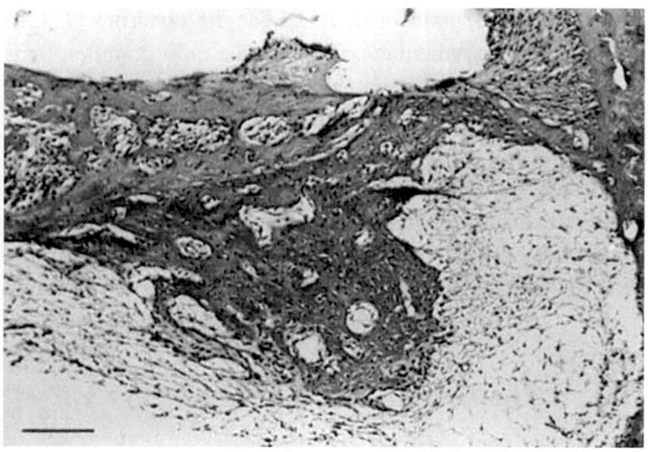

Fig. 52.5 Photomicrograph of a guinea pig cochlea 6 weeks following inoculation with guinea-pig-specific cytomegalovirus. Fibrosis and ossification of the inflamed perilymphatic scala that begin at 4 weeks are severe at 6 weeks. Scale bar, 120 µm. (Reproduced with permission from [44])

sensory and neural structures, and variable endolymphatic hydrops [40]. The otopathology findings in human temporal bones parallel those seen in animal models. Schuknecht and Nadol's general assessment of the inner ear pathology in Cogan's syndrome is the following: "1. Acute labyrinthitis resulting in atrophy of inner ear tissues, including the sense organs and their supporting structures, 2. Endolymphatic hydrops, 3. Focal or diffuse proliferation of fibrous tissue and bone and 4. Retrograde neuronal degeneration" [91]. It is possible that the exact mechanism of injury to the inner ear in AIED may be quite variable.

Testing

There Is Currently No Gold Standard Test to Diagnose AIED

Approximately 32% of patients with suspected AIED will have sera that react to a 68 kDa inner ear protein [42], corresponding to a heat shock protein (Hsp70) [13]. It is the basis for the OTOblot assay which is now marketed using purified bovine kidney Hsp70 protein. The sensitivity of this test in predicting steroid responsiveness has been reported to be approximately 50%, with a specificity ranging approximately 40–98% [13, 14, 50, 78]. A more recent retrospective study, however, reveals that its sensitivity and specificity in predicting steroid responsiveness in suspected AIED patients are not as high (54.5 and 42.9%, respectively) [73]. One study found that there was no correlation between seropositivity to Hsp70 and AIED [115]. The findings suggest that Hsp70 is not a reliable marker of AIED. Thus, the utility of immunoassay is limited since its commercialization from using inner ear antigen harvested from cow temporal bones to the use of purified Hsp70. The diagnosis of AIED should be suspected in bilateral and rapidly progressive hearing loss and those with co-existent systemic autoimmune disease, regardless of immunoassay results.

Serology

Infectious causes should be ruled out. Typically, patients are tested for syphilis, Lyme disease, and human immunodeficiency virus (HIV). A basic complete blood count (CBC) and inflammatory markers such as erythrocyte sedimentation rate (ESR) and C-reactive protein (CRP) should be ordered. Additional tests for autoimmune disorders include: rheumatoid factor (RF), antinuclear antibody (ANA), anti-double-stranded deoxyribonucleic acid (anti-dsDNA), cytoplasmic anti-neutrophil cytoplasmic antibody (c-ANCA), C3/C4, C1q, thyroid stimulating hormone (TSH) and if suspected of thyroid autoimmunity, anti-thyroid peroxidase (TPO) antibodies and anti-thyroglobulin antibodies. With a resurgence of syphilis in the modern era, consideration of syphilis should be included in the workup [4, 27, 46].

Audiology

Although the primary therapy is immunosuppression, which is often managed by rheumatologists, the otolaryngologist should monitor patients for hearing loss over time for the following reasons: 1. determine effectiveness of treatment, 2. determine relapse of disease potentially guiding the reinstatement of steroid treatment, and 3. determine need for hearing amplification or cochlear implantation. We recommend audiograms every 6 months or with sudden, perceived declines in hearing. It should be noted that this typically is not a medical emergency once the diagnosis of steroid responsiveness has been established as some of these patients will spontaneously undergo remission within several weeks without treatment. One cautionary note is that, in some individuals, steroid responsiveness becomes less effective over subsequent courses.

Imaging

Magnetic resonance imaging (MRI) is typically reserved for suspected autoimmune conditions that have central nervous system (CNS) manifestations such as with Susac's syndrome or neurosarcoidosis. Imaging is indicated for patients with asymmetric SNHL to rule out retrocochlear etiology such as a vestibular schwannoma at least once. However, it is not routinely suggested in patients with clear AIED and bilateral ear symptoms that appear in the course of their illness if an earlier MRI was negative.

Harris AIED Classification

Patients can be classified in the following general categories [73].

1. *Organ (ear)-specific*
   - Rapidly progressive bilateral SNHL
   - All age ranges, although middle age most common
   - No other clinical evidence of systemic autoimmune disease
   - Positive OTOblot (Western blot 68 kDa)
   - Negative serological studies (antinuclear antigen, sedimentation rate, rheumatoid factor, Clq binding assay among others)
   - Greater than 50% response rate to high-dose steroids
2. *Rapidly progressive bilateral SNHL with systemic autoimmune disease*
   - Rapidly progressive bilateral SNHL
   - Hearing loss often worst with flare of autoimmune condition
   - Other autoimmune condition is present (systemic lupus erythematosus, ulcerative colitis, polyarteritis nodosa, vasculitis, rheumatoid arthritis, and Sjögren's disease)
   - OTOblot might be positive or negative
   - Serological studies will be positive in accordance with the illness (i.e., antinuclear antigen high titers, rheumatoid factor positive, circulating immune complexes, thyroid autoantibodies)
   - Steroid responsive and might be managed in association with rheumatologists with targeted therapies for underlying illness
3. *Immune-mediated Ménière's disease*
   - Bilateral, fluctuating SNHL with vestibular symptoms that might predominate
   - Subset of patients with delayed contralateral endolymphatic hydrops or recent instability of better hearing ear in a patient with burned out Ménière's disease
   - OTOblot positive 37–58% might show presence of circulating immune complexes
   - Steroid responsive might require long-term immunosuppression due to relapses along with typical therapies for Ménière's disease
4. *Rapidly progressive bilateral SNHL with associated inflammatory disease (chronic otitis media, Lyme disease, and otosyphilis)*
   - Evidence of profound drop in hearing with long-standing chronic otitis media
   - Might show inflammation of the tympanic membrane and perforations
   - Hearing loss progresses despite treatment of the infectious agent (treponemal or rickettsial)
   - OTOblot negative, serological tests for the underlying disease might be positive—should be evaluated for granulomatous disease and vasculitis by biopsy if tissue is available
   - Steroid responsive and might require long-term immunosuppression along with appropriate antibiotics for the infectious condition.
5. *Immune-mediated SNHL with other discrete organ system disease (Cogan's syndrome, Granulomatosis with polyangiitis, and relapsing polychondritis)*
   - OTOblot negative, serology–(+) 55 kDa, type 2, 9 collagen antibodies, cANCA
   - Responds to high-dose steroids although becomes resistant over long term
   - Steroid resistant—often leads to cochlear implantation, especially Cogan's syndrome
6. *Nonimmune rapidly progressive SNHL (paraneoplastic syndrome)*
   - Young-elderly patients with idiopathic rapidly progressive bilateral SNHL leading to deafness
   - Severe ear pain, pressure, tinnitus, and some imbalance; OTOblot and all serology negative
   - Inciting event common; drug-related (oxycodone), paraneoplastic syndrome
   - No response to steroid or antiviral treatment and temporal bone studies have been unrevealing

Autoimmune Disorders with AIED [45]

Cogan's Syndrome

Cogan is credited with characterizing a syndrome of nonsyphilitic progressive bilateral vestibuloauditory disorders associated with keratitis [22, 23, 81]. Interstitial keratitis is a nonsuppurative inflammation of the corneal stroma, formerly synonymous with syphilis. There may be additional ocular findings such as uveitis, glaucoma, and retinal vasculitis. These patients are also likely to have systemic involvement such as vasculitis of the aorta, arthritis, renal involvement, skin nodules, and gastrointestinal complaints. Patients may have Menière's-like bilateral audiovestibular symptoms. Other disorders (e.g., syphilis, tuberculosis, chlamydia, sarcoid and GPA and polyarteritis nodosa) can also mimic Cogan's syndrome. The inner ear symptoms of this disorder are quite difficult to manage as they may be resistant to conventional treatments.

Vogt-Koyanagi-Harada Syndrome

The name of this syndrome is attributed to Alfred Vogt of Switzerland and to Koyanagi and Harada of Japan who independently described this disease [48]. The disease manifests with a prodrome of fever, headache, meningismus, nausea, vertigo, orbital pain, tinnitus, followed by granulomatous uveitis and blurry vision. The chronic stage of this syndrome may involve anterior uveitis, skin nodules, alopecia, and vitiligo. There is a very characteristic depigmentation around the eyes (Fig. 52.6). About 68% have audiovestibular symptoms, 46% with nystagmus, and 68% with documented SNHL. Of those with SNHL, 74% recovered their hearing over the long term [80]. There is an association with human leukocyte antigen (HLA) haplotypes (HLA-DR4, HLA-DR53, and HLA-DQ4) and with people of darker complexion.

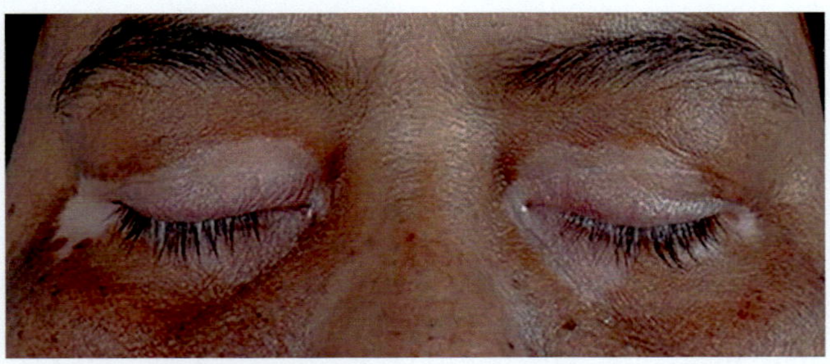

Fig. 52.6 Characteristic depigmentation around the eyes in Vogt-Koyanagi-Harada syndrome. (Reproduced with permission from [92])

Susac's Syndrome

A triad of encephalopathy, branch retinal artery occlusion (BRAO), and hearing loss was described by John Susac et al. [98]. It has also been referred to as SICRET (small infarctions of cochlear, retinal, and encephalic tissue) and RED-M syndrome (retinopathy, encephalopathy, deafness, and associated microangiography). The disease is attributed to autoimmune microangiopathy. MRI findings include T2 hyperintensities with a "snowball" appearance, usually involving the corpus callosum. Vision symptoms may include scintillating scotomas, which may lead one to erroneously diagnose migraines. Hearing loss is usually bilateral, low-to-mid frequency and can be episodic or fluctuating as in Ménière's disease. There are no consistent lab findings, but ESR and CRP may be elevated, and there may be an elevation of factor VIII, von Willebrand factor (vWF), and antiendothelial antibodies [99]. Treatment consists of oral and intravenous (IV) steroids, plasmapheresis, immunosuppressives (i.e., cyclophosphamide, azathioprine, methotrexate, interferon, intravenous immunoglobulin [IVIG]), and antithrombogenic treatments (aspirin, heparin, calcium channel blockers) [26, 61, 86].

Granulomatosis with Polyangiitis (GPA, Wegener's Granulomatosis)

A vasculitis of small vessels affecting many systems was formerly known as Wegener's granulomatosis. The name change was prompted by evidence that Wegener was a member of the Nazi party during World War II. This condition is well known to otolaryngologists, as 60% of GPA patients present with otologic manifestations (mixed hearing loss, serous otitis media, vertigo, facial nerve weakness). Other relevant ENT presentations include nasal masses, nasal obstruction, epistaxis, saddle nose, stridor, subglottic masses, and cough. Systemic symptoms include fevers, lethargy, ophthalmic symptoms (conjunctivitis, uveitis, retinal artery occlusion), renal failure, and pulmonary nodules. Although most hearing loss is mixed, it can be as high as 47% and reversible with early treatment [8, 62, 65, 76]. Biopsy yields necrotizing granulomatous inflammation with pauci-immune vasculitis in small- and medium-sized blood vessels. The key laboratory finding is positive anti-neutrophilic cytoplasmic antibodies (C-ANCA or PR3-ANCA).

Temporal Arteritis (Giant Cell Arteritis)

Temporal arteritis is a systemic inflammatory vasculitis involving medium-to-large vessels infiltrated by lymphocytes, macrophages, and multinucleated giant cells, which lead to luminal narrowing and ischemia. This disease commonly affects older adults with symptoms of headache and jaw claudication. ESR is elevated, and the diagnosis is generally made with biopsy and analysis of the temporal artery. Prompt diagnosis and treatment with steroids are important because up to 20% of patients develop bilateral vision loss. SNHL is rare, but it has been reported in 1–7% [47, 72]. In a small cohort [5], approximately 27% had measurable hearing improvement after 3 months of steroid treatment. About 88% had measurable vestibular dysfunction, a majority of whom had subjective improvement with treatment.

Behçet Disease

This multisystem disease is characterized by vasculitis resulting in recurrent oral and genital ulcers, erythema nodosum-like skin lesions, uveitis, superficial thrombophlebitis, and pulmonary aneurysm formation, first described in 1930 by Benediktos Adamantiades and in 1937 by the Turkish dermatologist Hulûsi Behçet [1, 10]. It often affects young males and is associated with HLA-B51. Pathology of oral and genital ulcers are exactly like aphthous ulcers (with infiltration of neutrophils and lymphocytes around vessels) [36]. Pathology is not specific and there is no blood test, thus diagnosis is made using clinical criteria. One study reported that 47% of patients had audiovestibular symptoms and 32% exhibited ⩾25 dB hearing level in at least two frequencies, usually in the high-frequency region [63].

Systemic Lupus Erythematosus

Systemic lupus erythematosus (SLE) is a multisystem disorder that is caused by autoantibodies and deposition of immune complexes. It has a 8-15x female preponderance [67]. Manifestations range from fever, polyarthralgia, anemia, pleurisy, pericarditis, endocarditis, scleritis, alopecia, malar rash, nephritis, oral ulcers, inflammatory bowel disease to neuropsychiatric syndrome. Otologic manifestations include chronic otitis media, vasculitis, and SNHL. Laboratory abnormalities include elevated ANA and ESR, and abnormal C3 and C4. More specific tests such as anti-smith, ssDNA, or false positive antiphospholipid tests may then be used. In one study, 67% of patients had audiovestibular symptoms including tinnitus (32%), vertigo (28%), and hearing loss (7%), and videonystagmography (VNG) abnormality was significantly more frequent (50%) than in controls (7.1%) [55].

Rheumatoid Arthritis

This is an autoimmune disorder resulting in inflammation and destruction of synovial tissues. Patients present with warm, swollen and tender joints, morning stiffness, fatigue, fever, and skin nodules. There is a strong familial and female tendency and HLA-DR4 association [30]. At least one positive test for rheumatoid factor (RF) or anti-citrullinated protein antibody (ACPA) is needed for diagnosis [112]. SNHL affects up to 36% of patients [35, 49, 58, 82, 102].

Relapsing Polychondritis

This is an inflammatory disease involving episodic inflammation of the cartilage of the ear, nose, upper respiratory tract, and joints. Patients may present with saddle nose, airway obstruction, auricular perichondritis, ocular symptoms, and polyarthritis. About 57% of patients have anti-type II and 62% have anti-type IV collagen antibodies [53]. Although both collagen types are associated with cartilage, they are expressed in the inner ear [54, 94]. There is no specific test for relapsing polychondritis, but CRP and ESR are often elevated in this condition.

Systemic Sclerosis (Scleroderma)

This is a rheumatic disease with autoantibodies to connective tissue, small vessel vasculopathy, and fibroblast dysfunction. Women in their 30–40 s are often affected. It has a heterogeneous manifestation of skin tightness, sclerodactyly, Raynaud's phenomenon, esophageal dysfunction, Sjögren's syndrome, interstitial lung disease, and cardiac and renal involvement. ANA is elevated. SNHL is found in 20–59% of patients [12, 59, 105].

Inflammatory Bowel Disease

Inflammatory bowel disease (IBD) includes Crohn's disease and ulcerative colitis. The former involves the small and large bowels with patchy lesions, sometimes transmural. The latter presents as continuous inflammatory lesions or ulcerations involving the mucosa of the colon and rectum. Symptoms include bloody diarrhea and abdominal pain, often affecting young females. Extraintestinal presentation may include uveitis, ankylosing spondylitis, vestibulopathy, and SNHL which can affect to as many as 57% [42, 57].

Thyroid Disease

Thyroid disease demonstrates significant association with cochleovestibular dysfunction [60]. Hearing loss and tinnitus are significantly higher among patients with hyperthyroidism (including Graves' disease) compared to controls [11, 111]. Approximately half of euthyroid patients with Hashimoto's thyroiditis exhibit subclinical vestibular dysfunction with abnormal vestibular evoked myogenic potential (VEMP) and caloric testing that is significantly elevated compared to control patients with multinodular goiter [20]. Studies have correlated thyroid autoantibodies with vestibular cochleovestibular dysfunction suggesting that circulating antibodies may cause inner ear damage [6, 20, 29, 97].

Treatment

Corticosteroids are an effective treatment for AIED. Fifty to seventy percent of patients initially respond well to steroids [16, 66, 79] but only 14% remain steroid responsive by 34 months [16]. Recommended treatment dosing for prednisone is 60 mg/day or (1 mg/kg) for at least 1 month or until symptoms stabilize before beginning a slow taper. Many respond initially but eventually develop resistance or relapse after the taper, and high-volume tinnitus has been reported as a sensitive predictor of imminent relapse [73]. If patients relapse, steroids are restarted. Intratympanic steroid injection is also an effective alternative, improving symptoms in 50% (15 of 30) of patients [73] and in 68.75% (6 of 11) of those who failed oral steroids and methotrexate [33]. Long-term steroid treatment has side effects of weight gain, hyperglycemia, immunodeficiency, acid reflux, peptic ulcer disease, hypertension, and psychiatric disturbances that may preclude its use [3, 45].

Alternative medications for steroid nonresponders include chemotherapies (methotrexate, cyclophosphamide, and azathioprine). AIED initially responds well to methotrexate, 53–70% [74, 88, 93]. However, a randomized controlled trial investigated methotrexate effectiveness in maintaining the hearing improvement by steroids [45]. Unfortunately, methotrexate was no better than placebo in maintaining hearing improvement subsequent to steroid treatment. Methotrexate is given at a dose of 7.5 mg/week initially and increased to 15 mg/week. It can be given in conjunction with or to follow steroid treatment. Toxicity includes myelosuppression, gastrointestinal ulcer, acute pneumonitis, diarrhea, and hepatic fibrosis. Routine CBC and hepatic labs are monitored.

Cyclophosphamide is an effective cytotoxic medication that was initially recommended by McCabe for the treatment of AIED. Efficacy can range from 33% to 50% [16, 64]. However, because of the significant risk of myelosuppression, risk for infection and malignancy, hair loss, and infertility, many people choose not to be treated with this agent. Dosing is started at 1 mg/kg/d and increased to 2 mg/kg/d. It is not recommended for children. Close monitoring with CBC, liver function testing, and urinalysis is needed. On rare occasions, this drug has been used with plasmapheresis [68].

Recently, biologic immunomodulators (i.e., antibodies that target the immune system) have been used for autoimmune ear disease [9, 87]. Biologics can target various pathways including tumor necrosis factor alpha (TNF-α), such as infliximab (Remicade®), adalimumab (Humira®), golimumab (Simponi®), and etanercept (Enbrel®); B-cells such as rituximab (Rituxan®); and interleukin-1β (IL-1β) such as anakinra (Kineret®). These biologics can suppress the immune system and increase the risk for infection and some may have local reactions at the site of injection. Their effects on AIED are actively being investigated: rituximab [25], infliximab [109], golimumab [28], and etanercept [24, 90] and anakinra (IL-1 inhibitor) [83, 108]. Interestingly, in steroid nonresponders, plasma IL-1β levels are elevated and promising results from an early efficacy trial show that anakinra (IL-1β inhibitor) had a 58% (7 of 12) hearing improvement rate in steroid resistant cases [83, 106, 108].

For patients who have not responded to treatment, one should search for causes of deafness that may be due to occult malignancies as can be seen with paraneoplastic syndromes as well as rare inflammatory illnesses such as neurosarcoidosis. In any case, if patients, with the guidance of their treating physicians, ultimately decide that treatment is too harmful to continue, they may go on to bilateral deafness. In such situations, the patients can be assured that they will still be candidates for cochlear implantation, which can be an excellent rehabilitative strategy in this setting [2, 71, 84].

Summary

AIED encompasses a wide variety of autoimmune disorders, and the mechanism of inner ear injury may be varied as well. Autoantibodies to the inner ear antigens are present in a subset of patients, but their presence is not necessarily correlated with the degree of hearing loss and is not a reliable indicator of AIED. Thus, there is debate as to whether AIED is a separate entity or if this is an immune-mediated inner ear disease. Nevertheless, autoimmune processes can damage the inner ear, which has been shown in both animal models and patient studies. There is no diagnostic test for AIED; therefore, the diagnosis should be suspected in bilateral asymmetric and rapidly progressive hearing loss and in patients with co-existent systemic autoimmune disease. Thus far, steroid treatment is the mainstay initial therapy for hearing improvement. This may be followed by other immunomodulators, and preliminary studies so far show promising results for biologic therapy in the treatment of AIED.

References

1. Adamantiades B. A case of relapsing iritis with hypopyon (in Greek). Archia Iatrikis Etairias; 1930. p. 586–93.
2. Aftab S, Semaan MT, Murray GS, et al. Cochlear implantation outcomes in patients with autoimmune and immune-mediated inner ear disease. Otol Neurotol. 2010;31:1337–42.
3. Alexander TH, Weisman MH, Derebery JM, et al. Safety of high-dose corticosteroids for the treatment of autoimmune inner ear disease. Otol Neurotol. 2009;30:443–8.
4. Amerson EH, Castillo Valladares HB, Leslie KS. Resurgence of syphilis in the US-USPSTF reaffirms screening guidelines. JAMA Dermatol. 2022;158:1241–3.
5. Amor-Dorado JC, Llorca J, Garcia-Porrua C, et al. Audiovestibular manifestations in giant cell arteritis: a prospective study. Medicine (Baltimore). 2003;82:13–26.
6. Arduc A, et al. "Evaluation of hearing functions in patients with euthyroid Hashimoto's thyroiditis." Endocrine. 2015;50(3): 708–714.
7. Baek MJ, Park HM, Johnson JM, et al. Increased frequencies of cochlin-specific T cells in patients with autoimmune sensorineural hearing loss. J Immunol. 2006;177:4203–10.
8. Bakthavachalam S, Driver MS, Cox C, et al. Hearing loss in Wegener's granulomatosis. Otol Neurotol. 2004;25:833–7.
9. Balouch B, Meehan R, Suresh A, et al. Use of biologics for treatment of autoimmune inner ear disease. Am J Otolaryngol. 2022;43:103576.
10. Behçet H. Über rezidivierende, aphthöse, durch ein Virus verursachte Geschwüre am Mund, am Auge und an den Genitalien. Dermatol Wochenschr. 1937;105:1152–7.
11. Berker D, et al. "Evaluation of hearing loss in patients with Graves' disease." Endocrine. 2012;41(1):116–121.
12. Berrettini S, Ferri C, Pitaro N, et al. Audiovestibular involvement in systemic sclerosis. ORL J Otorhinolaryngol Relat Spec. 1994;56:195–8.
13. Billings PB, Keithley EM, Harris JP. Evidence linking the 68 kilodalton antigen identified in progressive sensorineural hearing loss patient sera with heat shock protein 70. Ann Otol Rhinol Laryngol. 1995;104:181–8.
14. Bonaguri C, Orsoni JG, Zavota L, et al. Anti-68 kDa antibodies in autoimmune sensorineural hearing loss: are these autoantibodies really a diagnostic tool? Autoimmunity. 2007;40:73–8.
15. Bouman H, Klis SF, Meeuwsen F, et al. Experimental autoimmune inner ear disease: an electrocochleographic and histophysiologic study. Ann Otol Rhinol Laryngol. 2000;109:457–66.
16. Broughton SS, Meyerhoff WE, Cohen SB. Immune-mediated inner ear disease: 10-year experience. Semin Arthritis Rheum. 2004;34:544–8.
17. Calzada AP, Balaker AE, Ishiyama G, et al. Temporal bone histopathology and immunoglobulin deposition in Sjogren's syndrome. Otol Neurotol. 2012;33:258–66.
18. Cao MY, Gersdorff M, Deggouj N, et al. Detection of inner ear disease autoantibodies by immunoblotting. Mol Cell Biochem. 1995;146:157–63.
19. Cao MY, Dupriez VJ, Rider MH, et al. Myelin protein Po as a potential autoantigen in autoimmune inner ear disease. FASEB J. 1996;10:1635–40.
20. Chiarella G, et al. "Vestibular disorders in euthyroid patients with Hashimoto's thyroiditis: role of thyroid autoimmunity." Clin Endocrinol (Oxf). 2014;81(4):600–605.
21. Cogan D. Syndrome of nonsyphilitic interstitial keratitis and vestibuloauditory symptoms. Arch Opthalmol. 1945;33:144–9.
22. Cogan DG, Dickersin GR. Nonsyphilitic interstitial keratitis with Vestibuloauditory symptoms. A case with fatal Aortitis. Arch Ophthalmol. 1964;71:172–5.
23. Cogan DG, Sullivan WR Jr. Immunologic study of nonsyphilitic interstitial keratitis with vestibuloauditory symptoms. Am J Ophthalmol. 1975;80:491–4.
24. Cohen S, Shoup A, Weisman MH, et al. Etanercept treatment for autoimmune inner ear disease: results of a pilot placebo-controlled study. Otol Neurotol. 2005;26:903–7.
25. Cohen S, Roland P, Shoup A, et al. A pilot study of rituximab in immune-mediated inner ear disease. Audiol Neurootol. 2011;16:214–21.
26. Crawley BK, Close A, Canto C, et al. Susac's syndrome: intratympanic therapy for hearing loss and a review of the literature. Laryngoscope. 2009;119:141–4.
27. Darmstadt GL, Harris JP. Luetic hearing loss: clinical presentation, diagnosis, and treatment. Am J Otolaryngol. 1989;10:410–21.
28. Derebery MJ, Fisher LM, Voelker CC, et al. An open label study to evaluate the safety and efficacy of intratympanic golimumab therapy in patients with autoimmune inner ear disease. Otol Neurotol. 2014;35:1515–21.
29. Fattori B, et al. "Possible association between thyroid autoimmunity and Meniere's disease." Clin Exp Immunol. 2008;152(1): 28–32.
30. Firestein GS, Mcinnes IB. Immunopathogenesis of rheumatoid arthritis. Immunity. 2017;46:183–96.
31. Fukuda S, Harris JP, Keithley EM, et al. Spiral modiolar vein: its importance in viral load of the inner ear. Ann Otol Rhinol Laryngol Suppl. 1992;157:67–71.
32. Fukushima N, Fukushima H, Cureoglu S, et al. Hearing loss associated with systemic lupus erythematosus: temporal bone histopathology. Otol Neurotol. 2006;27:127–8.
33. Garcia-Berrocal JR, Ibanez A, Rodriguez A, et al. Alternatives to systemic steroid therapy for refractory immune-mediated inner ear disease: a physiopathologic approach. Eur Arch Otorhinolaryngol. 2006;263:977–82.
34. Gazquez I, Soto-Varela A, Aran I, et al. High prevalence of systemic autoimmune diseases in patients with Meniere's disease. PLoS One. 2011;6:e26759.
35. Goodwill CJ, Lord IJ, Jones RP. Hearing in rheumatoid arthritis. A clinical and audiometric survey. Ann Rheum Dis. 1972;31:170–3.
36. Gunduz O. Histopathological evaluation of Behcet's disease and identification of new skin lesions. Pathol Res Int. 2012;2012:209316.
37. Gussen R. Melanocyte system of the endolymphatic duct and sac. Ann Otol Rhinol Laryngol. 1978;87:175–9.
38. Harris JP. Immunology of the inner ear: response of the inner ear to antigen challenge. Otolaryngol Head Neck Surg. 1983;91:18–32.
39. Harris JP. Immunology of the inner ear: evidence of local antibody production. Ann Otol Rhinol Laryngol. 1984;93:157–62.
40. Harris JP. Experimental autoimmune sensorineural hearing loss. Laryngoscope. 1987;97:63–76.
41. Harris JP, Ryan AF. Immunobiology of the inner ear. Am J Otolaryngol. 1984;5:418–25.
42. Harris JP, Sharp PA. Inner ear autoantibodies in patients with rapidly progressive sensorineural hearing loss. Laryngoscope. 1990;100:516–24.

43. Harris JP, Fukuda S, Keithley EM. Spiral modiolar vein: its importance in inner ear inflammation. Acta Otolaryngol. 1990;110:357–65.
44. Harris JP, Heydt J, Keithley EM, et al. Immunopathology of the inner ear: an update. Ann N Y Acad Sci. 1997;830:166–78.
45. Harris JP, Weisman MH, Derebery JM, et al. Treatment of corticosteroid-responsive autoimmune inner ear disease with methotrexate: a randomized controlled trial. JAMA. 2003;290:1875–83.
46. Harris JP, Ciaranello AL, Tabb ES. Case 4-2022: a 55-year-old man with bilateral hearing loss and eye redness. N Engl J Med. 2022;386:583–90.
47. Hausch RC, Harrington T. Temporal arteritis and sensorineural hearing loss. Semin Arthritis Rheum. 1998;28:206–9.
48. Herbort CP, Mochizuki M. Vogt-Koyanagi-Harada disease: inquiry into the genesis of a disease name in the historical context of Switzerland and Japan. Int Ophthalmol. 2007;27:67–79.
49. Heyworth T, Liyanage SP. A pilot survey of hearing loss in patients with rheumatoid arthritis. Scand J Rheumatol. 1972;1:81–3.
50. Hirose K, Wener MH, Duckert LG. Utility of laboratory testing in autoimmune inner ear disease. Laryngoscope. 1999;109:1749–54.
51. Hoistad DL, Schachern PA, Paparella MM. Autoimmune sensorineural hearing loss: a human temporal bone study. Am J Otolaryngol. 1998;19:33–9.
52. Jenkins HA, Pollak AM, Fisch U. Polyarteritis nodosa as a cause of sudden deafness. A human temporal bone study. Am J Otolaryngol. 1981;2:99–107.
53. Joliat T, Seyer J, Bernstein J, et al. Antibodies against a 30 kilodalton cochlear protein and type II and IX collagens in the serum of patients with inner ear diseases. Ann Otol Rhinol Laryngol. 1992;101:1000–6.
54. Kalluri R, Gattone VH 2nd, Hudson BG. Identification and localization of type IV collagen chains in the inner ear cochlea. Connect Tissue Res. 1998;37:143–50.
55. Karatas E, Onat AM, Durucu C, et al. Audiovestibular disturbance in patients with systemic lupus erythematosus. Otolaryngol Head Neck Surg. 2007;136:82–6.
56. Kariya S, Kaya S, Hizli O, et al. Cochlear histopathologic findings in patients with systemic lupus erythematosus: a Human Temporal Bone Study. Otol Neurotol. 2016;37:593–7.
57. Karmody CS, Valdez TA, Desai U, et al. Sensorineural hearing loss in patients with inflammatory bowel disease. Am J Otolaryngol. 2009;30:166–70.
58. Kastanioudakis I, Skevas A, Danielidis V, et al. Inner ear involvement in rheumatoid arthritis: a prospective clinical study. J Laryngol Otol. 1995;109:713–8.
59. Kastanioudakis I, Ziavra N, Politi EN, et al. Hearing loss in progressive systemic sclerosis patients: a comparative study. Otolaryngol Head Neck Surg. 2001;124:522–5.
60. Kim SY, et al. "Association between Meniere's disease and thyroid diseases: a nested case-control study." Sci Rep. 2020;10(1): 18224.
61. Kleffner I, Ringelstein EB, Stupp N, et al. Neurological picture. Susac's syndrome: effective combination of immunosuppression and antiplatelet treatment. J Neurol Neurosurg Psychiatry. 2006;77:1335.
62. Kornblut AD, Wolff SM, Fauci AS. Ear disease in patients with Wegener's granulomatosis. Laryngoscope. 1982;92:713–7.
63. Kulahli I, Balci K, Koseoglu E, et al. Audio-vestibular disturbances in Behcet's patients: report of 62 cases. Hear Res. 2005;203:28–31.
64. Lasak JM, Sataloff RT, Hawkshaw M, et al. Autoimmune inner ear disease: steroid and cytotoxic drug therapy. Ear Nose Throat J. 2001;80:808–11, 815–6, 818 passim.
65. Lidar M, Carmel E, Kronenberg Y, et al. Hearing loss as the presenting feature of systemic vasculitis. Ann N Y Acad Sci. 2007;1107:136–41.
66. Loveman DM, De Comarmond C, Cepero R, et al. Autoimmune sensorineural hearing loss: clinical course and treatment outcome. Semin Arthritis Rheum. 2004;34:538–43.
67. Lu LJ, Wallace DJ, Ishimori ML, et al. Review: male systemic lupus erythematosus: a review of sex disparities in this disease. Lupus. 2010;19:119–29.
68. Luetje CM. Theoretical and practical implications for plasmapheresis in autoimmune inner ear disease. Laryngoscope. 1989;99:1137–46.
69. Lunardi C, Bason C, Leandri M, et al. Autoantibodies to inner ear and endothelial antigens in Cogan's syndrome. Lancet. 2002;360:915–21.
70. Ma C, Billings P, Harris JP, et al. Characterization of an experimentally induced inner ear immune response. Laryngoscope. 2000;110:451–6.
71. Malik MU, Pandian V, Masood H, et al. Spectrum of immune-mediated inner ear disease and cochlear implant results. Laryngoscope. 2012;122:2557–62.
72. Malmvall BE, Bengtsson BA. Giant cell arteritis. Clinical features and involvement of different organs. Scand J Rheumatol. 1978;7:154–8.
73. Matsuoka AJ, Harris JP. Autoimmune inner ear disease: a retrospective review of forty-seven patients. Audiol Neurootol. 2013;18:228–39.
74. Matteson EL, Fabry DA, Facer GW, et al. Open trial of methotrexate as treatment for autoimmune hearing loss. Arthritis Rheum. 2001;45:146–50.
75. Mccabe BF. Autoimmune sensorineural hearing loss. Ann Otol Rhinol Laryngol. 1979;88:585–9.
76. Mccaffrey TV, Mcdonald TJ, Facer GW, et al. Otologic manifestations of Wegener's granulomatosis. Otolaryngol Head Neck Surg (1979). 1980;88:586–93.
77. Mogi G, Lim DJ, Watanabe N. Immunologic study on the inner ear. Immunoglobulins in perilymph. Arch Otolaryngol. 1982;108:270–5.
78. Moscicki RA, San Martin JE, Quintero CH, et al. Serum antibody to inner ear proteins in patients with progressive hearing loss. Correlation with disease activity and response to corticosteroid treatment. JAMA. 1994;272:611–6.
79. Niparko JK, Wang NY, Rauch SD, et al. Serial audiometry in a clinical trial of AIED treatment. Otol Neurotol. 2005;26:908–17.
80. Noguchi Y, Nishio A, Takase H, et al. Audiovestibular findings in patients with Vogt-Koyanagi-Harada disease. Acta Otolaryngol. 2014;134:339–44.
81. Norton EW, Cogan DG. Syndrome of nonsyphilitic interstitial keratitis and vestibuloauditory symptoms; a long-term follow-up. AMA Arch Ophthalmol. 1959;61:695–7.
82. Ozturk A, Yalcin S, Kaygusuz I, et al. High-frequency hearing loss and middle ear involvement in rheumatoid arthritis. Am J Otolaryngol. 2004;25:411–7.
83. Pathak S, Goldofsky E, Vivas EX, et al. IL-1beta is overexpressed and aberrantly regulated in corticosteroid nonresponders with autoimmune inner ear disease. J Immunol. 2011;186:1870–9.
84. Quaranta N, Bartoli R, Giagnotti F, et al. Cochlear implants in systemic autoimmune vasculitis syndromes. Acta Otolaryngol Suppl. 2002;548:44–8.
85. Rask-Andersen H, Stahle J. Immunodefence of the inner ear? Lymphocyte-macrophage interaction in the endolymphatic sac. Acta Otolaryngol. 1980;89:283–94.
86. Rennebohm RM, Susac JO. Treatment of Susac's syndrome. J Neurol Sci. 2007;257:215–20.

87. Sakano H, Harris JP. Emerging options in immune-mediated hearing loss. Laryngoscope Investig Otolaryngol. 2019;4:102–8.
88. Salley LH Jr, Grimm M, Sismanis A, et al. Methotrexate in the management of immune mediated cochleovestibular disorders: clinical experience with 53 patients. J Rheumatol. 2001;28:1037–40.
89. Santos F, Salviz M, Domond H, et al. Otopathology of vasculitis in granulomatosis with polyangiitis. Otol Neurotol. 2015;36:1657–62.
90. Satoh H, Firestein GS, Billings PB, et al. Tumor necrosis factor-alpha, an initiator, and etanercept, an inhibitor of cochlear inflammation. Laryngoscope. 2002;112:1627–34.
91. Schuknecht HF, Nadol JB Jr. Temporal bone pathology in a case of Cogan's syndrome. Laryngoscope. 1994;104:1135–42.
92. Silpa-Archa S, Silpa-Archa N, Preble JM, et al. Vogt-Koyanagi-Harada syndrome: perspectives for immunogenetics, multimodal imaging, and therapeutic options. Autoimmun Rev. 2016;15:809–19.
93. Sismanis A, Wise CM, Johnson GD. Methotrexate management of immune-mediated cochleovestibular disorders. Otolaryngol Head Neck Surg. 1997;116:146–52.
94. Slepecky NB, Savage JE, Yoo TJ. Localization of type II, IX and V collagen in the inner ear. Acta Otolaryngol. 1992;112:611–7.
95. Sone M, Schachern PA, Paparella MM, et al. Study of systemic lupus erythematosus in temporal bones. Ann Otol Rhinol Laryngol. 1999;108:338–44.
96. Stearns GS, Keithley EM, Harris JP. Development of high endothelial venule-like characteristics in the spiral modiolar vein induced by viral labyrinthitis. Laryngoscope. 1993;103:890–8.
97. Sun X, Zhuang MS, Xiao ZW, Luo JQ, Long Z, Lan LC, Zhang HQ, Zhang GP. Autoimmune thyroiditis in patients with sudden sensorineural hearing loss. Laryngoscope Investig Otolaryngol. 2022;7:571–77.
98. Susac JO, Hardman JM, Selhorst JB. Microangiopathy of the brain and retina. Neurology. 1979;29:313–6.
99. Susac JO, Egan RA, Rennebohm RM, et al. Susac's syndrome: 1975-2005 microangiopathy/autoimmune endotheliopathy. J Neurol Sci. 2007;257:270–2.
100. Suzuki M, Harris JP. Expression of intercellular adhesion molecule-1 during inner ear inflammation. Ann Otol Rhinol Laryngol. 1995;104:69–75.
101. Takahashi M, Harris JP. Analysis of immunocompetent cells following inner ear immunostimulation. Laryngoscope. 1988;98:1133–8.
102. Takatsu M, Higaki M, Kinoshita H, et al. Ear involvement in patients with rheumatoid arthritis. Otol Neurotol. 2005;26:755–61.
103. Tomiyama S. Development of endolymphatic hydrops following immune response in the endolymphatic sac of the Guinea pig. Acta Otolaryngol. 1992;112:470–8.
104. Tomiyama S, Harris JP. The endolymphatic sac: its importance in inner ear immune responses. Laryngoscope. 1986;96:685–91.
105. Tosti A, Patrizi A, Veronesi S. Audiologic involvement in systemic sclerosis. Dermatologica. 1984;168:206.
106. Vambutas A, Davia DV. Biologics for immune-mediated sensorineural hearing loss. Otolaryngol Clin N Am. 2021;54:803–13.
107. Vambutas A, Pathak S. AAO: autoimmune and autoinflammatory (disease) in otology: what is new in immune-mediated hearing loss. Laryngoscope Investig Otolaryngol. 2016;1:110–5.
108. Vambutas A, Lesser M, Mullooly V, et al. Early efficacy trial of anakinra in corticosteroid-resistant autoimmune inner ear disease. J Clin Invest. 2014;124:4115–22.
109. Van Wijk F, Staecker H, Keithley E, et al. Local perfusion of the tumor necrosis factor alpha blocker infliximab to the inner ear improves autoimmune neurosensory hearing loss. Audiol Neurootol. 2006;11:357–65.
110. Veldman JE, Hanada T, Meeuwsen F. Diagnostic and therapeutic dilemmas in rapidly progressive sensorineural hearing loss and sudden deafness. A reappraisal of immune reactivity in inner ear disorders. Acta Otolaryngol. 1993;113:303–6.
111. Wang TC, et al. "Increased Incidence of Tinnitus Following a Hyperthyroidism Diagnosis: A Population-Based Longitudinal Study." Front Endocrinol (Lausanne). 2021;12:741719.
112. Wasserman AM. Diagnosis and management of rheumatoid arthritis. Am Fam Physician. 2011;84:1245–52.
113. Woolf NK, Harris JP. Cochlear pathophysiology associated with inner ear immune responses. Acta Otolaryngol. 1986;102:353–64.
114. Yamanobe S, Harris JP. Extraction of inner ear antigens for studies in inner ear autoimmunity. Ann Otol Rhinol Laryngol. 1993;102:22–7.
115. Yeom K, Gray J, Nair TS, et al. Antibodies to HSP-70 in normal donors and autoimmune hearing loss patients. Laryngoscope. 2003;113:1770–6.
116. Yoo TJ, Yazawa Y, Tomoda K, et al. Type II collagen-induced autoimmune endolymphatic hydrops in Guinea pig. Science. 1983;222:65–7.
117. Zechner G, Altmann F. Histological studies on the human endolymphatic duct and sac. Pract Otorhinolaryngol (Basel). 1969;31:65–83.

53 Dizziness in the Pediatric Patient

Henri Traboulsi

Introduction

The development of the inner ear and the vestibular system, common vestibular pathologies, treatment of vestibular conditions, and vestibular rehabilitation are detailed in other chapters of this book. This chapter will focus only on the most common conditions that are either only found exclusively in children or that have interesting and peculiar differences with the adult population. The history taking, physical exam, and vestibular testing in children do require special attention and will also be discussed in this chapter.

Assessment of the Pediatric with Dizziness or Imbalance

A. *History*:

Since children seldom complain of "dizziness," "vertigo," or "imbalance," they are often inappropriately labeled as being clumsy, and conditions pertinent to the vestibular system are often missed or misdiagnosed for years. History taking in children is very similar to adults, and questions about different organ systems need to be asked due to the variable symptomatology. Typical questions that apply to both groups include the nature of the symptoms, their duration, the frequency of the attacks, the presence of headaches, and triggers, such as standing or positional change. However, some information may be more relevant to children. For example, children with vestibular disorders may present with a learning disability due to difficulty reading in the presence of an inadequate vestibulo-ocular reflex (VOR). Inquiring about motor developmental milestones is also of the utmost importance, since it has been shown that children with motor developmental delays are at a higher risk of having vestibular deficits [1]. Children often have Eustachian tube dysfunction, leading to recurrent otitis media or chronic otitis media with effusions, which, according to many reports, is a common cause of imbalance in the pediatric population [2]. Similarly to adults, migraine and migraine variants most likely account for most cases of vertigo and imbalance in children [3]. Therefore, the clinician should ask about the presence of headaches, visual disturbances, a family history of migraine, and a past history of head tilting or torticollis (see benign paroxysmal torticollis of infancy [BPTI] below).

B. *Physical Exam*:

A detailed description of developmental reflexes is beyond the scope of this book. However, the failure of some reflexes to appear, or others to disappear, may indicate a vestibular or a central pathology. Examiners can familiarize themselves with a few (such as the Moro reflex, the Parachute reaction, and Doll's eyes response), which can be useful during a vestibular evaluation.

For infants and children who are too young to follow instructions, the evaluation of per-rotary or post-rotary nystagmus can be performed by simply spinning the child on a rotating stool. If the child is older, Frenzel or infrared goggles can be used to eliminate visual suppression. This is unnecessary in children younger than 6 months, who cannot suppress their VOR.

Positional testing, the head impulse test, Fukuda test, Romberg, head shake maneuver, and gait assessments are all helpful and can be performed in the pediatric population in the same manner as they are done in the adult population, provided they are old enough to follow instructions.

H. Traboulsi (✉)
Texas Children's Hospital Department of Surgery, Division of Otolaryngology, Houston, TX, USA

Bobby R. Alford Department of Otolaryngology—Head and Neck Surgery, Baylor College of Medicine, Houston, TX, USA
e-mail: hxtrabou@texaschildrens.org

A. D. Sweeney et al. (eds.), *Haynes-Glasscock-Shambaugh Surgery of the Ear*, https://doi.org/10.1007/978-3-032-18264-7_53

C. *Vestibular Screening in Children with Sensorineural Hearing Loss (SNHL)*:
The advent of cochlear implants has renewed our interest in vestibular impairments in children with SNHL, in view of the potential damage that implanting a cochlea may incur on the vestibule. This has become a particularly interesting topic now that bilateral implantation has become the standard of care for bilateral SNHL. We now realize that the incidence of vestibular impairment is very high, ranging between 20% and 70% [4–6], making vestibular dysfunction the most common comorbidity of congenital hearing loss. In comparison, QT abnormalities on electrocardiogram (EKG) screening are found in only up to 4% in children with congenital hearing loss [7]. Unfortunately, vestibular assessment is not routinely performed during the workup for SNHL in children. Since vestibular testing in children is not widely available, it has been suggested that screening for vestibular impairment through a simple protocol may help identify which children would benefit from more thorough vestibular testing. The following protocol is adapted by the cochlear implant program at the Hospital for Sick Children in Toronto [8]:
1. Inquire about gross motor developmental milestones:
As mentioned above, children with vestibular impairments have a high rate of delay in gross motor development [1]. More specifically, clinicians should inquire about the development of head control, sitting unsupported, and walking independently. Table 53.1 outlines the normal timelines for each of these milestones.
2. Age-appropriate assessment of balance skills:
The Bruininks Oseretsky Test of Motor Proficiency-2 (BOT2) has a balance subset which has been shown to be an effective screening tool in children with SNHL [9]. More specifically, the one-foot standing eyes open and eyes closed was found to be the most sensitive and specific. The expected performance of healthy children according to age is outlined in Table 53.2.
3. Assessment of horizontal semi-circular canal function:
This can be performed via the head impulse test, or, in young infants, with assessment of a pre-rotary or post-rotary nystagmus on a rotating stool, as described above.

Table 53.1 Normal ranges for the development of motor milestones

Motor milestone	Timeframe
Head control	3–4 months
Sitting unsupported	6–9 months
Walking independently	12–15 months

D. *Vestibular Testing*:
As opposed to common belief, vestibular testing *is* possible in the pediatric population. While vestibular testing does not provide a diagnosis, it provides information about the vestibular system, which, in conjunction with an accurate history and physical exam, helps the physician understand the pathology at hand. The invasive nature of some tests, expected poor patient cooperation, the lack of available pediatric testing centers, and the anticipation of uninterpretable results have rendered physicians reluctant to order vestibular testing in children [10]. Fortunately, vestibular tests now have some well-established normative data [11], and the number of pediatric vestibular programs are growing both on a national and international level. Clearly, not all tests can be performed at all ages and to all patients. Rather, pediatric vestibular programs typically establish a protocol that suggests a battery of tests depending on the patient's age group. In order to be successful, the program will have to choose the tests with the highest yield, and also start the battery with the better tolerated tests. As with audiologic testing, children are often unable to undergo all vestibular tests, and may need to complete testing on another day. In general, the main challenge of vestibular testing in children is to keep them engaged and comfortable. Consideration should be given to decorating labs in a child-friendly manner. Visual targets can be changed to colorful familiar characters.

Rather than describing the testing methods in detail, we will focus on the peculiarities of vestibular testing in children, with the differences from the adult population, and offer tips and directions on how to successfully administer these tests. Please refer to Table 53.3 for a suggestion on a vestibular battery according to age ranges.
1. *Oculomotor Testing/Videonystagmography (VNG)*:
VNG is used for oculomotor testing, positional testing, and calorics (see below). It is important to realize that children get distracted and fatigue more quickly than adults. Therefore, testers should prioritize testing that would provide the most useful information based on clinical suspicion and background. The principles of peripheral versus central causes of vestibular dysfunction are similar to those of adults.

Table 53.2 Expected one foot standing times according to age [9]

Age	Duration in seconds
30 months	1
36 months	2
4 years	5
5 years	10
>5 years eyes open	8
>5 years eyes closed	4

Table 53.3 Age considerations for vestibular testing in children

	Age range and considerations
Rotary chair	As of infancy. Chair modifications can be done as described in text
cVEMP	As of infancy
oVEMP	As of age 2 (before age 2, responses cannot be elicited)
VNG	As of age 3–5, also depends on appropriate goggle fitting
VHIT	As of age 4–7
Calorics	As of age 6–7. Otherwise poorly tolerated in younger children
CDP	As soon as children fit in the harness, at least age 4

CDP computerized dynamic posturography, *cVEMP* cervical vestibular-evoked myogenic potential, *oVEMP* ocular VEMP, *VNG* videonystagmography, *VHIT* video head impulse test

2. *Caloric Testing*:
As described in Chap. 13, caloric testing assesses the function of the ipsilateral horizontal canal. As in the adult population, air and water irrigations are administered in accordance with the preference of the physician and the audiologist, and both have advantages and disadvantages. They can both be performed in children; however, in view of the frequent presence of pressure equalizing tubes in children, water irrigations may be contraindicated. Another disadvantage of water irrigation is that the cessation of the test may require a momentary wait, in contrast with air irrigation where the stimulation can be abruptly stopped with the removal of the probe from the ear, if required. Otherwise, water irrigations can be quite successful with excellent results. In general, caloric testing is poorly tolerated in children younger than 5–7.
Tips and directions to successfully administer caloric testing in children are as follows:
   - Thoroughly explain the procedure to the child before testing.
   - Motivate the child, allowing to choose a prize after each irrigation.
   - Let the child feel the air from the probe, or touch the tubing for water irrigation before starting the test.
   - Have the child count to 60 (seconds), or sing songs during the irrigations.
   - Reduce irrigation time [12], and perform monothermal irrigations (warm preferably [13]), if needed.
3. *Rotary Chair Testing*:
Compared to caloric testing, rotary chair testing is relatively well tolerated, and has been considered the gold-standard vestibular test in children [12]. It is unaffected by the presence of middle ear disease, the presence of pressure equalizing tubes, or the size of the external auditory canals. However, the dark and confined nature of the test environment may cause young children to lose their alertness or to fall asleep during the test, and may cause stress or anxiety in older children.
To maximize head stabilization, modifications may need to be implemented for appropriate rotary chair testing in children. Some laboratories have attached car seats to their testing chairs with padded head restraints for immobilization. Another common option is to have a parent or a technician to hold the child on their lap [14].
Electronystagmography (ENG) is well tolerated in infants and young children and can be a good alternative to VNG, since dedicated pediatric goggles are not widely available. Also, a remote camera can be mounted to the chair to visualize the patients' eyes, which is particularly helpful in infants [15].
Adult normative data can sometimes be applied to children, but pediatric vestibular laboratories should develop their own normative data. It is important to recognize that children have mostly higher gains than adults [16, 17], and the gain decreases with age. Due to the progressive development of the velocity storage integrator, low-frequency phase angle in infants and children is often phase advanced compared to adult norms [18, 19]. Also, the slow development of the velocity storage integrator means that the time constant is not a good indicator of vestibular dysfunction in young children [20]. Symmetry can also be more variable than in adults.
Tips and directions to successfully administer rotary testing in children are as follows:
   - Use car seat with head restraints, or have child sit on parent's laps
   - Use remote camera for qualitative assessment of nystagmus in young children
   - Entertain children with video games, tablets, and projections between trials
4. *Video Head Impulse Test (VHIT)*:
Along with the vestibular-evoked myogenic potential (VEMP) testing, the VHIT test is a relative newcomer to the world of vestibular testing, and is generally child-friendly [21], since it is short, non-invasive, does not result in vertigo, and since children are not confined in a dark room. Fortunately, normative data has become more available in the literature [21–24]. The VHIT provides valuable information about the VOR for all six semi-circular canals, tested at a higher stimulus than the rotary chair.
While it is recommended that the tester achieves a peak head velocity of at least 150°/sec in adults, it appears that 100–150°/sec may be sufficient in children [25].
Although well tolerated in children, a commonly faced nuisance is goggle fitting since the currently available products are not specifically designed for children. The

manufacturers listed below are approved for use in the United States, along with a brief description on their use in children.

- Inter-acoustic EyeSeeCam: Can be used for younger children, and infants [23, 26].
- ICS impulse: Can fit the head of most children aged 3 and up, with the use of a cushion.
- Micromedical VHIT: Goggles are heavier and may not fit younger children.
- Synapsys VHIT: Approved by the FDA in 2025, this contact-free option relies on the presence of a camera positioned in front of the patient. This reduces slippage, discomfort, and motion artifacts, especially in uncooperative patients. It requires no calibration and can be used as early as 3 months of age.

Tips and directions to successfully administer VHIT in children are as follows:

- Explain why the goggles will have to be tightly fit.
- Avoid having children move their head during calibration by stimulating them with games, such as "count the dots." [15].
- Have children sit on parents' laps, or in a booster seat/high chair to have target at eye level.
- Use a colorful image or sticker (animals, or cartoon characters) as a visual target.

5. *Vestibular-Evoked Myogenic Potential (VEMP) Testing*:
   VEMP testing is not so different in children than in adults. However, the recommended positioning for adults may not be feasible in young children and infants. Modification is needed in order to encourage the child to contract their neck muscles.

   One of the main advantages of cervical VEMP (cVEMP) testing is that it can be administered early in infancy, as soon as infants can support their head, typically at about the age of 2–3 months (this might be delayed in the case of congenital vestibular impairment). Also, the test is reliable, child-friendly, non-invasive, and short. It has become an essential component of pediatric vestibular testing batteries. Some centers have used cVEMPs as a screening tool for vestibular impairments for children with hearing loss [27].

   In contrast, ocular VEMPs (oVEMP) responses start to appear at 2 years of age, and therefore cannot be tested for before that time. As with cVEMPs, children may need to be encouraged to look up with the help of toys, games, or videos on tablets.

   Tips and directions to successfully administer VEMPs in children are as follows:

   - Place cVEMP electrodes higher in the neck, as compared to adults, for young children [15].
   - For children younger than 6 years of age, have the child sit on a parent's lap, face to face. The parent will support the child's lower back, while an examiner holds the upper body back. EMG will provide feedback to the examiner while the child is encouraged to lift their neck [15]. Alternatively, the patient may be placed in the supine position with the upper body upon a sloping pillow [27].
   - For older children, they may be placed on a reclined table and asked to lift and rotate their head.
   - Use bone conduction stimuli if the presence of middle ear effusions (MEEs) is suspected, otherwise high threshold and low amplitude responses can be expected.

6. *Computerized Dynamic Posturography (CDP)*:
   CDP in children is done similarly to the adult population with the assessment of balance in the six described conditions. However, it appears that the visual and labyrinthine systems do not mature until later in childhood (as opposed to the proprioceptive system which is fully functional at the age of 6) and that children may not reach normal scores seen in the adult population until the age of 16 [28].

Vestibular Disorders

The presentation, workup, and management of many vestibular disorders are similar in the pediatric and the adult population, such as vestibular neuronitis, perilymphatic fistulas, or temporal bone trauma. Some entities are seen only in the pediatric population and will be described in detail below, such as congenital conditions or some of the migraine variants (BPTI, and RVC). Others can present in both the pediatric and adult population but with some interesting differences. Rather than describing these entities in their entirety, these differences in presentation and workup between children and adults will be discussed here only.

1. *Migraine and the Migraine Variants*:
   Similar to the adult population, migraine has been recognized as a major culprit in the world of pediatric vestibular disorders. A recent systematic review including 22 articles and 2726 cases concluded that migraine variants were the most common cause of vertigo in children [29]. The following migraine variants were reclassified and redefined in 2018 with the updated International Classification of Headache Disorders (ICHD) [30].
   - *Benign Paroxysmal Torticollis of Infancy (BPTI)*:
     BPTI is a condition in which infants, until the age of 3–4, have episodes of head tilting, imbalance, vertigo, often with irritability, pallor, or nausea and vomiting (Please see Table 53.4 for the diagnostic criteria as listed by the International Classification of Headaches disorders in 2018) [30]. Initially believed to be a form of labyrinthitis [31], BPTI is now considered a migraine variant due to the strong presence

Table 53.4 Diagnostic criteria of BPTI, adapted from ICHD, 3rd edition [30]

A. Recurrent attacks in a young child, fulfilling criteria B and C
B. Tilt of the head to either side, with or without slight rotation, remitting spontaneously after minutes to days
C. At least one of the following five associated symptoms or signs:
Pallor
Irritability
Malaise
Vomiting
Ataxia
D. Normal neurological examination between attacks
E. Not attributed to another disorder

Table 53.5 Diagnostic criteria of RVC [30]

A. At least five attacks fulfilling criteria B and C
B. Vertigo occurring without warning, maximal at onset and resolving spontaneously after minutes to hours without loss of consciousness
C. At least one of the following five associated symptoms or signs:
Nystagmus
Ataxia
Vomiting
Pallor
Fearfulness
D. Normal neurological examination and audiometric and vestibular functions between attacks
E. Not attributed to another disorder.

of a family history of migraine [32, 33], and the presence of associated symptoms that are frequently found in migraine attacks. Interestingly, some cases of BPTI have been linked to mutations in the *CACNA1A* gene, which is associated with familial hemiplegic migraine [34–36].

Recent URTIs, teething [37], and posture change [38] have been suggested as precipitating factors. Attacks typically last hours, up to 7 days, at intervals of days to months. Patients are asymptomatic between attacks, and physical examination is mostly normal. However, some published data have reported normal vestibular testing [32], while others have reported abnormalities in caloric testing [31], and rotary chair testing [39]. BPTI has been also linked to gross and fine motor developmental delays [32], and more recently to the presence of enlarged vestibular aqueduct (EVA) syndrome [40].

- *Recurrent Vertigo of Childhood (RVC)*:
  In 2021, the Committee for the Classification of Vestibular Disorders of the Bárány Society and the Migraine Classification subgroup of the International Headache Society introduced the new term "Recurrent Vertigo of Childhood", to replace "Benign Paroxysmal Vertigo of Childhood". RVC affects children in an older age group, typically from age 2 to 8. Attacks are characterized by a sudden onset of vertigo and imbalance, with or without nausea and vomiting. Hearing loss, ear pressure, tinnitus, and headaches are absent. As in BPTI, patients are asymptomatic between episodes, physical examination is normal between episodes, and results of vestibular testing have been variable, ranging from normal to complete canal paresis [39, 41–43].

  The diagnostic criteria of RVC are summarized in Table 53.5.
- *Vestibular Migraine*:
  The same committee mentioned above has also introduced "Vestibular Migraine of Childhood" (VMC) as well as "Probable Vestibular migraine of Childhood"(probable VMC). Unlike BPTI and RVC, vestibular migraine is definitely present in the adult population and is probably the most common cause of dizziness. In the pediatric population, vestibular migraine affects older children, mostly adolescents, and the presentation and management are very similar to adults, described in Chap. 61. Unfortunately, the literature suffers from a lack of dedicated studies for the treatment of migraine variants in children, and treatment trends are primarily based on the adult literature.
- As in all cases of migraine and migraine variants, treatment should be individualized and decided upon depending on the frequency and severity of the attacks. There are unfortunately no randomized controlled studies for the treatment of the vertigo-producing migraine variants in children. For acute abortive management of migraine attacks in children, a recent systematic review has reported that ibuprofen, prochlorperazine, and triptans are the most effective and safe agents to use [44]. Lifestyle changes and behavioral measures (such as sleep hygiene, and diet modifications) are also encouraged in children [45, 46]. For medical prophylaxis, topiramate, amitriptyline, propranolol [47], and cyproheptadine [48] are commonly used in children. Cognitive behavioral therapy [49] and biofeedback [50] have also been shown to be helpful.

2. *Benign Paroxysmal Positional Vertigo (BPPV)*:
   BPPV is more common in children than initially believed. In a recent study, Brodsky et al. published a series of 110 cases of children aged 5 to 19 with BPPV, which accounted to about 19.8% of patients seen for dizziness in a 5-year period [51]. About 80% of BPPV cases were associated with a "triggering incident," such as head trauma and migraine. Interestingly, compared to adults, it was reported that the proportion of horizontal, superior, and multiple semicircular canal involvement is much higher. In the adult population, low vitamin D levels have

been suggested to play a role in BPPV [52], but this relation has not been studied in the pediatric population.

Central Conditions Associated with Ataxia

There are many neurodegenerative diseases that are associated with imbalance and ataxia. Those that are exclusively associated with balance dysfunction without a constellation of other neurological symptoms are mostly genetic in origin. In general, symptoms begin to appear during childhood for autosomal recessive disorders, and during adulthood for autosomal dominant disorders. The most common conditions that can present in a pattern which may mimic other vestibular conditions are listed below. Given the potential for vestibular mimicry, it is important for an otolaryngologist to be familiar with the following.

The presence of these "mimickers" truly underlines the importance of a comprehensive history (including family history, full system review), an in-depth neurological exam, and a vestibular assessment with infrared or Frenzel goggles. Fortunately, many of the neurodegenerative and other neurological disorders can now be identified with widely available genetic panel testing.

1. *Friedreich's Ataxia (FA)*:
   FA is one the most common autosomal recessive ataxia disorders. Onset is around childhood or adolescence (mean of 10–15 years), and symptoms consist of gait and limb ataxia, spasticity, decreased proprioception, polyneuropathy, hearing loss, and other non-neurological conditions, such as cardiomyopathy and glucose intolerance [53]. All sensory systems are involved in FA; therefore, many diagnostic tests can be abnormal.
2. *Ataxia-Telangiectasia (AT)*:
   AT is also an autosomal recessive disorder. Patients may develop progressive ataxia (starting at an early age), oculo-cutaneous telangiectasias, immune deficiencies, and an increased risk of malignancies [53]. Oculomotor involvement is obvious with abnormal pursuits and saccades [15].
3. *Spinocerebellar Ataxias (SCAs)*:
   SCAs form a group of autosomal dominant conditions, which are almost invariably associated with cerebellar atrophy. The most common are type 2 and type 3. However, over 32 different types/genetic mutations have been identified. In addition to ataxia, other symptoms may include slow saccades, fasciculations, parkinsonism, vision loss, seizures, and tremors [53]. Several types of SCA may display a downbeat nystagmus on neutral gaze assessment [53].
4. *Episodic Ataxias (EAs)*:
   The episodic ataxias are also a group of autosomal dominant disorders, which, in contrast to SCAs or the other previously described conditions, display a constellation of symptoms that present episodically. EA is extremely important to recognize since they can mimic other peripheral disorders that are also present with episodic symptoms.
   - The most common type is *EA type 2*. As with BPTI and familial hemiplegic migraine, EA type 2 is associated with a mutation in the *CACNA1A* gene [54]. Patients typically present with an acute onset of ataxia, vertigo, nausea, and, often, with headaches, dystonia, or torticollis, which last hours to days. As such, EA type 2 can resemble migraine variants. Patients are essentially asymptomatic between episodes but most will eventually develop permanent cerebellar ataxia. A common finding, however, is the presence of a downbeat nystagmus even between episodes, when patients are asymptomatic [53]. Brain imaging may reveal cerebellar atrophy, and acetazolamide has been shown to decrease the frequency of the attacks [55].
   - *EA type 1* is less common, and the episodes are typically shorter, lasting seconds to minutes [53]. Patients may also develop neurologic symptoms such as seizures and cognitive decline. Patients are also typically asymptomatic between episodes but will often have muscle twitching and cramps [56].

Conditions Associated with Hearing Loss

1. *CHARGE Syndrome*:
   CHARGE syndrome is a genetic condition characterized by colobomas, heart defects, choanal atresia, growth retardation, developmental delay, genitourinary anomalies, and dysmorphic features. Hearing loss and vestibular dysfunction are also some of the most commonly recognized phenotypic features seen in CHARGE syndrome [57]. Commonly, the semi-circular canals are absent or dysmorphic. In addition to this anatomical factor, vestibular compensatory mechanisms may be affected (due to visual impairments, cerebellar and brainstem abnormalities), which put mechanisms patients with CHARGE syndrome at a considerable risk for delays in postural development and imbalance [58].
2. *Usher Syndrome*:
   There are three known types of Usher syndrome, all of which are associated with congenital hearing loss and retinitis pigmentosa and are transmitted in an autosomal recessive fashion. Patients with type 1 Usher syndrome have congenital severe-to-profound hearing loss with

vestibular areflexia, and retinitis pigmentosa which develops during the first decade of life [59]. As such, with hearing loss, vestibular and visual impairments, patients with type 1 Usher syndrome are at a substantial risk of developing significant imbalance and constraints in communication abilities. Patients with type 2 Usher syndrome have no vestibular impairment, and patients with type 3 Usher syndrome have progressive hearing loss and variable involvement of the vestibular system. Usher syndrome is an example where vestibular screening of patients with congenital hearing loss may help with an earlier diagnosis of a genetic condition, especially in view of the low sensitivity of routine ophthalmologic examinations at an early age for the detection of ocular problems in Usher syndrome.

3. *Enlarged Vestibular Aqueduct Syndrome (EVA)*:
   EVA is not a genetic condition in itself because it can be found in isolation. However, it can be found in association with other genetic conditions, such as CHARGE syndrome [58], Pendred syndrome [60], or branchio-oto-renal syndrome [61]. It has been suggested that vestibular organs may be damaged by the reflux of hyperosmotic fluid into the basal end of the cochlear duct, and that the resulting osmotic and chemical imbalances may cause damage or degeneration of vestibular cells [62]. Many patients with EVA may present with dizziness, vestibular hypofunction, or even BPPV [63].
4. *Middle Ear Effusions (MEEs)*:
   Acute and chronic otitis media with effusions are some of the most common conditions encountered in childhood. It has been postulated that the presence of middle ear effusions may cause vestibular impairment by causing changes in the composition of the inner-ear fluids, or by the transmission of pressure changes through the oval and round windows. It is not unusual for parents to report worsening in their children's balance during episodes of otitis media [64]. Indeed, some published data consider middle ear effusions to be the most common cause of dizziness in children [65]. Other studies have also reported long-term effects of middle ear effusions on balance and the vestibular system [2, 66].

Structural Central Nervous System Lesions

Physicians who evaluate patients with dizziness should be aware of the presence of lesions in the brain that can present with dizziness or imbalance. The signs and symptoms that indicate the presence of a central lesion in the adult population also apply to the pediatric population. Lesions in the brainstem, cerebellum, cerebellopontine angle, and cranio-cervical junction may all present with dizziness or disequilibrium.

The presence of a neoplasm should be suspected with a low threshold in children, since pediatric central nervous system (CNS) tumors are fairly common, and since the majority of them are infratentorial [67]. The discussion of arachnoid cysts, dermoid/epidermoid cysts, and vascular lesions is beyond the scope of this chapter, but these lesions can also be identified with a brain magnetic resonance imaging (MRI).

While present in about 0.3% of the general healthy population, a Chiari malformation should be suspected in children with imbalance, a down-beat nystagmus, and other symptoms such as speech/swallow difficulties. Chiari malformations can be congenital or secondary to increased intracranial pressure (ICP) later in childhood, and if symptoms are persistent or severe, can be decompressed with surgery [43].

Conclusion

The evaluation of a patient with dizziness can be puzzling due to the difficulty in describing symptoms and due to the long list of differential diagnoses that spans across several specialties. This is particularly true in the pediatric population where obtaining an accurate history is even more challenging, and where a physical exam and a vestibular assessment may require patience and expertise. Fortunately, the field of pediatric vestibular disorders is burgeoning, with more published data becoming available and with a growing number of dedicated pediatric vestibular laboratories and programs in the United States and across the globe.

References

1. Inoue A, Iwasaki S, Ushio M, et al. Effect of vestibular dysfunction on the development of gross motor function in children with profound hearing loss. Audiol Neurotol. 2013; https://doi.org/10.1159/000346344.
2. Pazdro-Zastawny K, Pośpiech L, Zatoński T. Long-term evaluation of the effect of middle ear effusion on the vestibular system in children. Int J Pediatr Otorhinolaryngol. 2018; https://doi.org/10.1016/j.ijporl.2018.03.015.
3. Gioacchini FM, Alicandri-Ciufelli M, Kaleci S, Magliulo G, Re M. Prevalence and diagnosis of vestibular disorders in children: a review. Int J Pediatr Otorhinolaryngol. 2014; https://doi.org/10.1016/j.ijporl.2014.02.009.
4. Licameli G, Zhou G, Kenna MA. Disturbance of vestibular function attributable to cochlear implantation in children. Laryngoscope. 2009; https://doi.org/10.1002/lary.20121.
5. Cushing SL, Gordon KA, Rutka JA, James AL, Papsin BC. Vestibular end-organ dysfunction in children with sensorineural hearing loss and cochlear implants: an expanded cohort and etiologic assessment. Otol Neurotol. 2013; https://doi.org/10.1097/MAO.0b013e31827b4ba0.

6. Buchman CA, Joy J, Hodges A, Telischi FF, Balkany TJ. Vestibular effects of Cochlear implantation. Laryngoscope. 2004; https://doi.org/10.1097/00005537-200410001-00001.
7. Chang RKR, Lan YT, Silka MJ, et al. Genetic variants for long QT syndrome among infants and children from a statewide newborn hearing screening program cohort. J Pediatr. 2014; https://doi.org/10.1016/j.jpeds.2013.11.011.
8. Cushing SL, Papsin BC. Cochlear implants and children with vestibular impairments. Semin Hear. 2018;39(3):305–20. https://doi.org/10.1055/s-0038-1666820.
9. Oyewumi M, Wolter NE, Heon E, Gordon KA, Papsin BC, Cushing SL. Using balance function to screen for vestibular impairment in children with sensorineural hearing loss and Cochlear implants. Otol Neurotol. 2016; https://doi.org/10.1097/MAO.0000000000001046.
10. Ciolek PJ, Kang E, Honaker JA, Woodson EA, Hopkins BS, Anne S. Pediatric vestibular testing: tolerability of test components in children. Int J Pediatr Otorhinolaryngol. 2018;113(July):29–33. https://doi.org/10.1016/j.ijporl.2018.07.009.
11. Maureen Valente L. Assessment techniques for vestibular evaluation in pediatric patients. In: Dizziness and vertigo across the lifespan; 2019. https://doi.org/10.1016/B978-0-323-55136-6.00004-6.
12. Fife TD, Tusa RJ, Furman JM, et al. Assessment: vestibular testing techniques in adults and children – report of the Therapeutics and Technology Assessment Subcommittee of the American Academy of Neurology. Neurology. 2000; https://doi.org/10.1212/WNL.55.10.1431.
13. Murnane OD, Akin FW, Lynn SG, Cyr DG. Monothermal caloric screening test performance: a relative operating characteristic curve analysis. Ear Hear. 2009; https://doi.org/10.1097/AUD.0b013e31819c3ec7.
14. Phillips JO, Backous DD. Evaluation of vestibular function in young children. Otolaryngol Clin N Am. 2002; https://doi.org/10.1016/S0030-6665(02)00062-2.
15. O'Reilly RC, Morlet T, Brodsky JR, Cushing SL. In: O'Reilly RC, Morlet T, Brodsky JR, Cushing SL, editors. Manual of pediatric balance disorders. 2nd ed. Plural Publishing; 2020.
16. Casselbrant ML, Mandel EM, Sparto PJ, et al. Longitudinal posturography and rotational testing in children three to nine years of age: normative data. Otolaryngol Head Neck Surg. 2010; https://doi.org/10.1016/j.otohns.2010.01.028.
17. Chan FM, Galatioto J, Amato M, Kim AH. Normative data for rotational chairs stratified by age. Laryngoscope. 2016; https://doi.org/10.1002/lary.25497.
18. Weissman BM, DiScenna AO, Leigh RJ. Maturation of the vestibulo-ocular reflex in normal infants during the first 2 months of life. Neurology. 1989; https://doi.org/10.1212/wnl.39.4.534.
19. Cioni G, Favilla M, Ghelarducci B, La Noce A. Development of the dynamic characteristics of the horizontal vestibulo-ocular reflex in infancy. Neuropediatrics. 1984; https://doi.org/10.1055/s-2008-1052354.
20. Clark DL, Cordero L, Bates J. Development of postrotatory nystagmus time constants. Acta Otolaryngol. 1984; https://doi.org/10.3109/00016488409107565.
21. Hamilton SS, Zhou G, Brodsky JR. Video head impulse testing (VHIT) in the pediatric population. Int J Pediatr Otorhinolaryngol. 2015; https://doi.org/10.1016/j.ijporl.2015.05.033.
22. Bachmann K, Sipos K, Lavender V, Hunter LL. Video head impulse testing in a pediatric population: normative findings. J Am Acad Audiol. 2018; https://doi.org/10.3766/jaaa.17076.
23. Hülse R, Hörmann K, Servais JJ, Hülse M, Wenzel A. Clinical experience with video head impulse test in children. Int J Pediatr Otorhinolaryngol. 2015; https://doi.org/10.1016/j.ijporl.2015.05.034.
24. McGarvie LA, MacDougall HG, Halmagyi GM, Burgess AM, Weber KP, Curthoys IS. The video head impulse test (vHIT) of semicircular canal function – age-dependent normative values of VOR gain in healthy subjects. Front Neurol. 2015; https://doi.org/10.3389/fneur.2015.00154.
25. Zhou G, Goutos C, Lipson S, Brodsky J. Range of peak head velocity in video head impulse testing for pediatric patients. Otol Neurotol. 2018; https://doi.org/10.1097/MAO.0000000000001793.
26. Wenzel A, Eck S, Hülse K, et al. Development of a new software and test setup for analyzing hVOR in very young children by vHIT. J Vestib Res Equilib Orientat. 2017; https://doi.org/10.3233/VES-170611.
27. Martens S, Dhooge I, Dhondt C, et al. Vestibular infant screening—Flanders: the implementation of a standard vestibular screening protocol for hearing-impaired children in Flanders. Int J Pediatr Otorhinolaryngol. 2019; https://doi.org/10.1016/j.ijporl.2019.02.033.
28. Hirabayashi S-i, Iwasaki Y. Developmental perspective of sensory organization on postural control. Brain Dev. 1995; https://doi.org/10.1016/0387-7604(95)00009-Z.
29. Davitt M, Delvecchio MT, Aronoff SC. The differential diagnosis of vertigo in children a systematic review of 2726 cases conclusions: although the most common causes of pediatric vertigo in. Pediatr Emerg Care. 2020; https://doi.org/10.1097/PEC.0000000000001281.
30. Headache Classification Committee of the International Headache Society. The international classification of headache disorders, 3rd edition. Cephalalgia. 2018;38(1):1–211. https://doi.org/10.1177/0333102417738202.
31. Snyder CH. Paroxysmal torticollis in infancy: a possible form of Labyrinthitis. Am J Dis Child. 1969;117(4):458–60. https://doi.org/10.1001/archpedi.1969.02100030460013.
32. Rosman NP, Douglass LM, Sharif UM, Paolini J. The neurology of benign paroxysmal torticollis of infancy: report of 10 new cases and review of the literature. J Child Neurol. 2009;24(2):155–60. https://doi.org/10.1177/0883073808322338.
33. Hadjipanayis A, Efstathiou E, Neubauer D. Benign paroxysmal torticollis of infancy: an underdiagnosed condition. J Paediatr Child Health. 2015;51(7):674–8. https://doi.org/10.1111/jpc.12841.
34. Roubertie A, Echenne B, Leydet J, et al. Benign paroxysmal tonic upgaze, benign paroxysmal torticollis, episodic ataxia and CACNA1A mutation in a family. J Neurol. 2008;255(10):1600–2. https://doi.org/10.1007/s00415-008-0982-8.
35. Giffin NJ, Benton S, Goadsby PJ. Benign paroxysmal torticollis of infancy: four new cases and linkage to CACNA1A mutation. Dev Med Child Neurol. 2002;44(7):490–3. https://doi.org/10.1017/S0012162201002407.
36. Vila-Pueyo M, Gené GG, Flotats-Bastardes M, et al. A loss-of-function CACNA1A mutation causing benign paroxysmal torticollis of infancy. Eur J Paediatr Neurol. 2014;18(3):430–3. https://doi.org/10.1016/j.ejpn.2013.12.011.
37. Drigo P, Giavonna C, Laverda AM. Benign paroxysmal torticollis of infancy: a case report. Brain Dev. 2000;22:169–72. https://doi.org/10.1016/S0387-7604(00)00099-1.
38. Cataltepe SU, Barron TF. Benign paroxysmal torticollis presenting as "Seizures" in infancy. Clin Pediatr (Phila). 1993;32(9):564–5. https://doi.org/10.1177/000992289303200913.
39. Brodsky J, Kaur K, Shoshany T, Lipson S, Zhou G. Benign paroxysmal migraine variants of infancy and childhood: transitions and clinical features. Eur J Paediatr Neurol. 2018;Vm:1–7. https://doi.org/10.1016/j.ejpn.2018.03.008.
40. Brodsky JR, Kaur K, Shoshany T, et al. Torticollis in children with enlarged vestibular aqueducts. Int J Pediatr Otorhinolaryngol. 2020; https://doi.org/10.1016/j.ijporl.2020.109862.
41. Basser LS. Benign paroxysmal vertigo of childhood. Brain. 1964;87(1):141–52.
42. Balatsouras DG, Kaberos A, Assimakopoulos D, Katotomichelakis M, Economou NC, Korres SG. Etiology of vertigo in children.

Int J Pediatr Otorhinolaryngol. 2007;71(3):487–94. https://doi.org/10.1016/j.ijporl.2006.11.024.
43. O'Reilly RC, Greywoode J, Morlet T, et al. Comprehensive vestibular and balance testing in the dizzy pediatric population. Otolaryngol Head Neck Surg. 2011;144(2):142–8. https://doi.org/10.1177/0194599810393679.
44. Patniyot IR, Gelfand AA. Acute treatment therapies for pediatric migraine: a qualitative systematic review. Headache. 2016; https://doi.org/10.1111/head.12746.
45. Kacperski J. Prophylaxis of migraine in children and adolescents. Pediatr Drugs. 2015; https://doi.org/10.1007/s40272-015-0125-5.
46. Millichap JG, Yee MM. The diet factor in pediatric and adolescent migraine. Pediatr Neurol. 2003; https://doi.org/10.1016/S0887-8994(02)00466-6.
47. Hershey AD, Powers SW, Coffey CS, Eklund DD, Chamberlin LA, Korbee LL. Childhood and adolescent migraine prevention (CHAMP) study: a double-blinded, placebo-controlled, comparative effectiveness study of amitriptyline, topiramate, and placebo in the prevention of childhood and adolescent migraine. Headache. 2013; https://doi.org/10.1111/head.12105.
48. Brodsky JR, Cusick BA, Zhou G. Evaluation and management of vestibular migraine in children: experience from a pediatric vestibular clinic. Eur J Paediatr Neurol. 2016;20(1):85–92. https://doi.org/10.1016/j.ejpn.2015.09.011.
49. Ernst MM, O'Brien HL, Powers SW. Cognitive-behavioral therapy: how medical providers can increase patient and family openness and access to evidence-based multimodal therapy for pediatric migraine. Headache. 2015; https://doi.org/10.1111/head.12605.
50. Blume HK, Brockman LN, Breuner CC. Biofeedback therapy for pediatric headache: factors associated with response. Headache. 2012; https://doi.org/10.1111/j.1526-4610.2012.02215.x.
51. Brodsky JR, Lipson S, Wilber J, Zhou G. Benign Paroxysmal Positional Vertigo (BPPV) in children and adolescents: clinical features and response to therapy in 110 pediatric patients. Otol Neurotol. 2018;39(3):344–50. https://doi.org/10.1097/MAO.0000000000001673.
52. AlGarni MA, Mirza AA, Althobaiti AA, Al-Nemari HH, Bakhsh LS. Association of benign paroxysmal positional vertigo with vitamin D deficiency: a systematic review and meta-analysis. European Archives of Oto-Rhino-Laryngology. 2018; https://doi.org/10.1007/s00405-018-5146-6.
53. Ashizawa T, Guangbin X. Ataxia. Contin (Minneap Minn). 2016;22:1208–26.
54. Strupp M, Zwergal A, Brandt T. Episodic Ataxia type 2. Neurotherapeutics. 2007; https://doi.org/10.1016/j.nurt.2007.01.014.
55. Jen JC, Wan J. Episodic ataxias. In: Handbook of clinical neurology; 2018. https://doi.org/10.1016/B978-0-444-64189-2.00013-5.
56. Baloh RW. Episodic ataxias 1 and 2. In: Handbook of clinical neurology; 2012. https://doi.org/10.1016/B978-0-444-51892-7.00042-5.
57. Choo DI, Tawfik KO, Martin DM, Raphael Y. Inner ear manifestations in CHARGE: abnormalities, treatments, animal models, and progress toward treatments in auditory and vestibular structures. Am J Med Genet Part C Semin Med Genet. 2017; https://doi.org/10.1002/ajmg.c.31587.
58. Abadie V, Wiener-Vacher S, Morisseau-Durand MP, et al. Vestibular anomalies in CHARGE syndrome: investigations on and consequences for postural development. Eur J Pediatr. 2000; https://doi.org/10.1007/s004319900409.
59. Mathur P, Yang J. Usher syndrome: hearing loss, retinal degeneration and associated abnormalities. Biochim Biophys Acta Mol basis Dis. 2015;1852(3):406–20. https://doi.org/10.1016/j.bbadis.2014.11.020.
60. Cremers CWRJ, Bolder C, Admiraal RJC, et al. Progressive sensorineural hearing loss and a widened vestibular aqueduct in Pendred syndrome. Arch Otolaryngol Head Neck Surg. 1998; https://doi.org/10.1001/archotol.124.5.501.
61. Stinckens C, Standaert L, Casselman JW, et al. The presence of a widened vestibular aqueduct and progressive sensorineural hearing loss in the Branchio-Oto-Renal syndrome. A family study. Int J Pediatr Otorhinolaryngol. 2001;59(3):163–72. https://doi.org/10.1016/S0165-5876(01)00473-6.
62. Everett LA. Targeted disruption of mouse Pds provides insight about the inner-ear defects encountered in Pendred syndrome. Hum Mol Genet. 2001; https://doi.org/10.1093/hmg/10.2.153.
63. Song JJ, Hong SK, Lee SY, et al. Vestibular manifestations in subjects with enlarged vestibular aqueduct. Otol Neurotol. 2018;39(6):e461–7. https://doi.org/10.1097/MAO.0000000000001817.
64. Casselbrant ML, Rubenstein E, Furman JM, Mandel EM. Effect of otitis media on the vestibular system in children. Ann Otol Rhinol Laryngol. 1995; https://doi.org/10.1177/000348949510400806.
65. Bower CM, Cotton RT. The spectrum of vertigo in children. Arch Otolaryngol Head Neck Surg. 1995;121:9110–915.
66. Jones NS, Prichard AJN, Radomskij P, Snashall SE. Imbalance and chronic secretory otitis media in children: effect of myringotomy and insertion of ventilation tubes on body sway. Ann Otol Rhinol Laryngol. 1990; https://doi.org/10.1177/000348949009900612.
67. Stiller CA, Nectoux J. International incidence of childhood brain and spinal tumours. Int J Epidemiol. 1994; https://doi.org/10.1093/ije/23.3.458.

Benign Paroxysmal Positional Vertigo

54

Peng You and Lorne S. Parnes

Introduction

Benign paroxysmal positional vertigo (BPPV) is the most common peripheral vestibular disorder and manifests as sudden, brief episodes of vertigo precipitated by certain head movements. The symptoms reflect inadvertent activation of the vestibular system causing an illusory sense of motion and characteristic nystagmus. In almost all cases, the diagnosis can be made by the history and physical exam, and in the majority, in-office treatment provides relief.

The clinical presentation was first described by Bárány in 1921 [1]. Dix and Hallpike further characterized the disorder in 1952 and coined the name benign paroxysmal positional vertigo [2]. While both authors mistook the pathophysiology for an otolith disorder, their clinical observations laid the foundation for our understanding today.

Epidemiology

Vertigo is a common presenting complaint with an estimated lifetime population prevalence between 3% and 10% [3]. Of patients with vertigo, 17–42% eventually arrive at a diagnosis of benign paroxysmal positional vertigo (BPPV) [4]. One European cross-sectional study estimated the lifetime prevalence of the disease to be 2.4% [5]. Elsewhere, a study in Japan found the incidence of BPPV to be 10.7–17.3 per 100,000 per year [6]. Though BPPV can affect patients of all ages, its peak onset is most commonly between the fifth and sixth decades of life [7]. Previous studies have also found women more likely to be affected, with a female to male ratio of 2-3 to 1 [7]. However, this gender difference is not observed in younger patients and those with an onset of BPPV following trauma [8].

Despite the prevalence of BPPV, there are frequent delays in its diagnosis and treatment [3]. A cross-sectional study of 100 elderly patients with non-balance-related chief complaints discovered a 9% rate of previously unrecognized BPPV [9]. Patients with BPPV may also face delays in diagnosis and treatment on the order of months [10]. These findings have prompted development of clinical practice guidelines [3] and underscored the importance of educating clinicians and trainees about this common inner ear disorder.

Pathophysiology

The vestibular system allows for the detection of head motion and position. The otolith organs (utricle and saccule) are sensitive to gravity and linear acceleration, whereas the semicircular canals detect angular acceleration. During rotational head motion, the endolymph of the semicircular canals aligning to the plane of movement lags due to inertia. The cupula, and its embedded hair cells, are forced to move in the opposite direction as the head movement. Depending on the canal, the deflection increases or inhibits the resting discharge rate of the corresponding hair cells and results in mechanotransduction. Once the movement of the endolymph normalizes, the cupula returns to its neutral location and the hair cell signals return to baseline. In the case of BPPV, aberrant signals from semicircular canals create an illusion of motion which results in the sensation of vertigo. Understanding this disease pathophysiology is important in the diagnosis of BPPV, interpretation of its physical findings, and rationale behind treatment strategies.

The two prevailing theories of BPPV's pathomechanism are canalithiasis and cupulolithiasis (Fig. 54.1). Canalithiasis attributes the etiology of BPPV to free-floating particles, known as canaliths, in the affected semicircular canal. On the

P. You · L. S. Parnes (✉)
Department of Otolaryngology-Head and Neck Surgery, Schulich School of Medicine and Dentistry, Western University, London Health Sciences Centre-University Hospital, London, ON, Canada
e-mail: Lorne.Parnes@lhsc.on.ca

A. D. Sweeney et al. (eds.), *Haynes-Glasscock-Shambaugh Surgery of the Ear*, https://doi.org/10.1007/978-3-032-18264-7_54

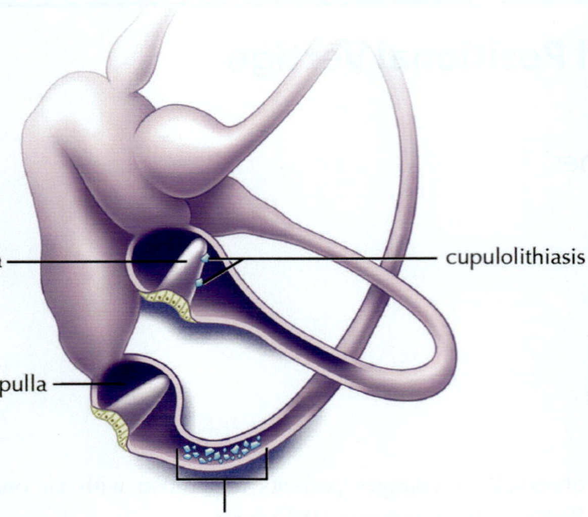

Fig. 54.1 Left inner ear. Demonstration of canalithiasis of the posterior canal and cupulolithiasis of the horizontal canal. (Reprinted with permission from Parnes et al. [14])

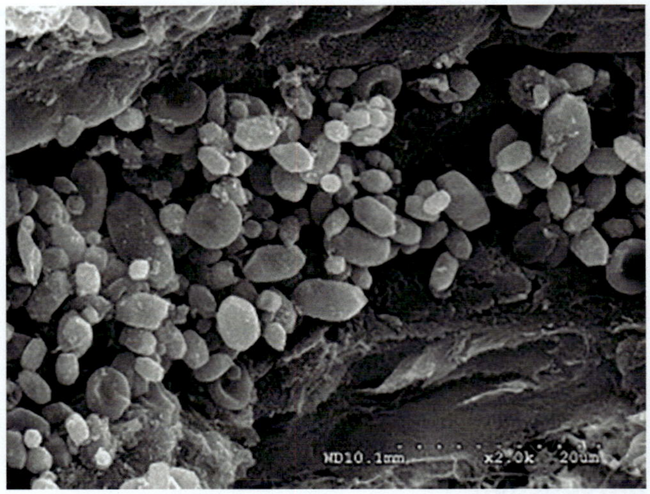

Fig. 54.2 Scanning electron micrograph image of otoconia within the posterior canal endolymphatic duct removed from a patient with intractable BPPV. (Image shown at 20000 magnification. Scale bar 20 micrometers. Reprinted with permission from Kao et al. [12])

other hand, cupulolithiasis refers to attachment of such canaliths to the affected canal's cupula. Both will cause abnormal signal modulation of the affected hair cells and ampullary nerves.

Consistent with the canalithiasis theory, endolymph particles were first demonstrated in vivo by Parnes and McClure in 1992 [11]. Recent examination of the particulate matter using scanning electron microscopy supports the hypothesis that the canaliths are broken off fragments from the utricular otolith membrane [12] (Fig. 54.2). Primary (idiopathic) BPPV is believed to be a function of age-related degenerative changes of the membrane's gel matrix, leading to detachment of canaliths [13]. By comparison, secondary BPPV is thought to be due to uncoupling of canaliths associated with closed head injury, otologic and non-otologic surgery, or inner ear diseases that lead to potential damage to the inner ear such as sudden sensorineural hearing loss (SNHL), Ménière's disease, vestibular neuritis, and even migraine [14].

While BPPV can affect each of the three semicircular canals, posterior canal BPPV is the most common variant (80–90%) [15]. In comparison, horizontal canal BPPV accounts for 10–20%, and a superior canal variant is seen in up to 3% of cases [15]. This discrepancy is due to the posterior canal being the most gravity-dependent part of the vestibular labyrinth. In contrast, the orientation of the superior and horizontal semicircular canals allows for particles to generally return to the utricle from natural head movements alone [14].

Within the affected semicircular canal, canaliths likely gather over time. They eventually reach a critical enough mass to create hydrodynamic drag from head movements

Table 54.1 Ewald's laws on vestibular physiology

Ewald's three laws
1. The axis of nystagmus parallels the anatomic axis of the semicircular canal that generated it
2. Utriculopetal endolymphatic flow evokes a stronger response than utriculofugal flow in the horizontal canal
3. Utriculofugal flow evokes a stronger response than utriculopetal flow in the vertical canals (anterior and posterior semicircular canals)

aligning with the affected canal. With the posterior canal affected, the first part of the Dix–Hallpike test induces utriculofugal endolymph and cupular deflection, which is an excitatory response [13] (Table 54.1). The associated vestibulo-ocular reflex culminates in contraction of the ipsilateral superior oblique and contralateral inferior rectus muscles. This results in deviation of the eyes downward and with torsion, moving the top pole of the eyes towards the uppermost ear (the slow phase of the nystagmus). The reflexive brainstem response produces a saccade in the opposite direction, accounting for the fast phase of nystagmus. It is during this mismatch of the visual and vestibular system that patients experience vertigo. When the canaliths reach their limit of descent, their drag force ceases and the cupula's elasticity returns it to the neutral position. This coincides with the cessation of the vertigo and nystagmus.

In horizontal canal BPPV, the resultant nystagmus is predominately horizontal [16]. The exact characteristic of the nystagmus varies depending on if the pathogenic mechanism is canalithiasis or cupulolithiasis.

In horizontal canal canalithiasis, canaliths are most often positioned in the long arm of the canal and relatively far from the ampulla [14]. As such, with the patient supine, head rota-

Table 54.2 Characteristic nystagmus associated with horizontal canal BPPV

	Direction of nystagmus	
Intensity of nystagmus	Apogeotropic	Geotropic
Stronger on the left side	Right cupulolithiasis	Left canalithiasis
Stronger on the right side	Left cupulolithiasis	Right canalithiasis

Table adapted from Parnes et al. [14]

tion toward the affected side creates utriculopetal endolymph flow and a stimulatory signal. This results in geotropic nystagmus (fast phase toward the ground). By comparison, turning the head away will result in ampullofugal flow, or an inhibitory response. However, this reversed direction nystagmus will remain geotropic given that the patient's head is now facing the opposite direction. In accordance with Ewald's second law, effects of stimulation are stronger than inhibition in the horizontal canal. Therefore, in horizontal canal canalithiasis, the direction that creates the stronger geotropic nystagmus is the affected side. On the other hand, horizontal canal cupulolithiasis causes geotropic cupular deflection and manifests as apogeotropic nystagmus (fast phase away from the ground). It commonly presents without latency during the provocative testing. Turning the head away from the affected side will create the stronger apogeotropic nystagmus (Table 54.2).

Diagnosis

History

Vertigo is an illusion of motion. In BPPV, the environment is perceived as spinning around relative to oneself or vice versa in the direction of the affected semicircular canal. It should be distinguished on patient history from other forms of "dizziness," such as disequilibrium and pre-syncope, as well as other causes of episodic vertigo such as Ménière's disease, migraine, and semicircular canal dehiscence. In patients with isolated BPPV, the cardinal symptom is sudden onset vertigo precipitated by specific head movements [2, 14]. Typical provocative movements include tilting the head to look up or down, getting up or down from the supine position, and most commonly rolling over in bed. The side to which the head is turned during a provocative roll in bed almost certainly coincides with the affected side in posterior canal BPPV. [17]

BPPV attacks occur in clusters, and it is common for patients to experience several attacks during the course of 1 day [18]. While the attacks of vertigo typically last less than 30 s, it may be accompanied by lingering, nonspecific imbalance and dizziness. On the other hand, vertigo caused by other disorders persists much longer. For instance, symptoms of Ménière's disease typically last hours, viral labyrinthitis or vestibular neuronitis days, and other central disorders can be associated with constant vertigo. As such, practitioners must be diligent in deciphering the duration of the vertigo itself.

Table 54.3 Differentiating features of BPPV versus central vertigo

	BPPV	Central vertigo
Duration of attack	Usually less than 30 s (longer in HC-BPPV)	Variable; usually longer than BPPV
Fatigability	Usual	Unusual
Nausea and vomiting	Rare; associated with intense nystagmus	Frequent even on single precipitating maneuver; not necessarily associated with intense nystagmus
Associated neurological signs and symptoms	None	Often cerebellar and other oculomotor signs; possibly none
Direction of nystagmus	Torsional/vertical (PC/AC-BPPV) and horizontal (HC-BPPV); compatible with the stimulated canal plane	Usually pure vertical (usually downbeat) or pure torsional
Mechanism	Canalithiasis or cupulolithiasis	Lesion of central vestibular/oculomotor pathways

Table adapted from Lee and Kim [13]. *AC* anterior canal, *PC* posterior canal, *HC* horizontal canal

While 50–70% of BPPV is idiopathic [14], practitioners should inquire about possible causes of secondary BPPV. The history should be mined for antecedent head trauma, viral infection/vestibular neuronitis, migraine, Ménière's disease, or otologic surgery. Clinicians should also be vigilant for central nervous system disorders that masquerade as BPPV [19] (Table 54.3). A complete history should, therefore, inquire about the presence of hearing loss, tinnitus, headaches, visual symptoms, or other sensory abnormalities. Moreover, patients should be assessed for risk of falls and resultant injury as a potential consequence of BPPV [3]. Few diseases mimic the brief, episodic positional change-induced vertigo seen in BPPV, and so any great departure from this pattern should prompt consideration of alternative or concurrent vestibular disease.

Diagnostic Maneuvers

For completeness, a full neurotologic examination should be conducted, which includes otoscopy, cranial nerve exam, cerebellar testing, and head impulse testing. Assessment should also identify older patients with neck, back, and hip problems as they will require special care during the diagnostic maneuvers. Clinicians should also be mindful of patients with vascular disease as the diagnostic maneuvers, and treatments, have the potential, albeit very rarely, to cause injury to the vertebral arteries.

The Dix–Hallpike maneuver is the definitive test for posterior canal BPPV. A diagnosis is made if the maneuver provokes an appropriate nystagmus [3]. When performed in office, it has an estimated sensitivity and specificity of 79–82% and 71–75%, respectively [20, 21]. The maneuver begins with the patient seated and head turned 45 degrees to the side being tested so as to isolate and vertically orient that side's posterior canal. The patient is then laid back into a supine position with the affected ear down (Fig. 54.3). Traditional teaching is to hang the head back over the edge of the bed, but this is not necessary for the Dix–Hallpike test alone and can, in fact, elicit a false positive response from the contralateral side.

The nystagmus evoked by the Dix–Hallpike maneuver in the head back position is almost pathognomonic (Table 54.4). The intensity of the nystagmus usually correlates with the severity of the vertigo experienced by the patient. Due to the inertia of the endolymph particles, the onset of the nystagmus is typically preceded by a brief latency (2–5 s). Once the particles migrate down to and stay in the more dependent position, the nystagmus and vertigo stop. The nystagmus usually lasts no more than 20 s and has a torsional and upbeating characteristic. The top pole of the eye beats towards the affected ear such that on the right, the fast phase torsional component (as seen by the examiner) beats counterclockwise, while it beats clockwise on the left. The nystagmus reverses directions when the patient is returned to the upright position. Lastly, the observed nystagmus will fatigue with repeated testing. This is believed to be due to dispersion of the particles, reducing their *en masse* effect.

In patients with positional vertigo and a negative Dix–Hallpike maneuver, horizontal canal BPPV should be considered [3]. The associated nystagmus is horizontal, has a shorter latency, and is less prone to fatigue [14, 22]. The most reliable way to diagnose horizontal BPPV is by a supine head roll maneuver, also referred to as the Pagnini-McClure or Pagnini-Lempert maneuver. [13] During the maneuver, the patient lies supine with a central head position. The head is then turned rapidly 45–60° to one side and the eyes are observed for nystagmus. The head is then returned to center and the same step is repeated on the contralateral side. Unlike the Dix–Hallpike test that isolates one posterior canal during testing, both horizontal canals are in play during supine head turns. The affected side is determined by comparing the nys-

Table 54.4 Nystagmus profile in posterior canal BPPV

Nystagmus profile	Mechanism
Latency	Inertia of canalith
Torsional and upbeat	Corrective activation of ipsilateral inferior oblique and contralateral superior rectus
Limited duration	Canalith reaches limit of descent and cupula resumes neutral position
Reversal nystagmus	Canalith mass moves in opposite direction, creating nystagmus in same plane but opposite direction
Fatigable	Dispersion of canaliths with movement

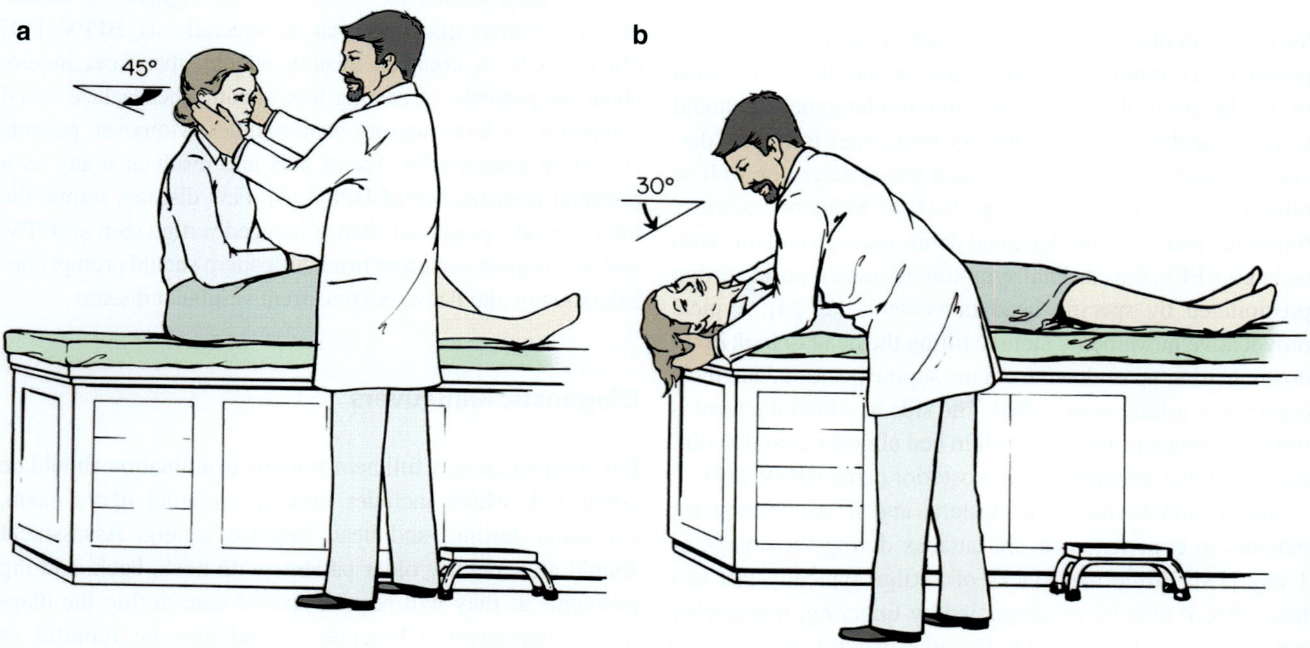

Fig. 54.3 Dix-Hallpike maneuver (right ear). (**a**) the patient is seated with head rotated at 45 degrees. (**b**) the patient is quickly lowered into supine position with the neck extended below the level of the table. With the head extended, the examiner observes the patient for nystagmus. (Reprinted with permission from Parnes et al. [14])

tagmus on each side and its direction (Table 54.2). Distinguishing between horizontal canal canalithiasis and cupulolithiasis is crucial as they are treated by different repositioning maneuvers.

Downbeating nystagmus during the Dix–Hallpike maneuver should raise suspicion for contralateral superior canal BPPV. Anatomically, the contralateral superior semicircular canal is coplanar with the ipsilateral posterior semicircular canal [23]. As such, the Dix–Hallpike maneuver tests for both entities. In a positive Dix–Hallpike exam of superior canal BPPV, the torsional component remains the same as for the posterior canal of the undermost ear, but the predominant nystagmus is downbeating [23].

Patients with a convincing history and characteristic nystagmus findings on provocative maneuvers are readily diagnosed with BPPV. Advanced electrophysiologic vestibular and auditory tests are rarely indicated for isolated BPPV. If concurrent symptoms and/or atypical findings raise suspicion for other or associated inner ear or posterior fossa abnormalities, further investigations should be arranged accordingly. For example, BPPV is not an uncommon sequela of superior vestibular neuronitis [14]. Patients with a history of severe constant vertigo for days that then transforms into positional vertigo may demonstrate abnormalities on tests of superior vestibular nerve function.

Nonsurgical Management

BPPV is an eminently treatable inner ear disease. It can be dangerous with its associated risk for falls and resultant injury, but mostly BPPV is a benign condition. Once the diagnosis is established, patients should be reassured to alleviate their fear of a more sinister illness. While BPPV carries a favorable prognosis, with nearly 25% of patients having spontaneous resolution by 1 month and up to 50% at 3 months [24], recurrence is common [25]. Education of the disease process is thus important to help patients anticipate and cope with possible relapses.

As the understanding of the disease improved, more antiquated treatments like rigorous in-patient physiotherapy [26] have given way to simple, effective in-office maneuvers. As such, while patient observation with follow-up is an option, it is not typically favored. Furthermore, treatment can help avoid discomfort and possible injury that may incur during episodes of vertigo [3]. With regard to pharmaceutical management, studies have shown labyrinthine sedatives to be less efficacious than repositioning maneuvers or vestibular training [27, 28]. Therefore, current evidence suggests clinicians should not routinely treat BPPV with vestibular suppressant medications.

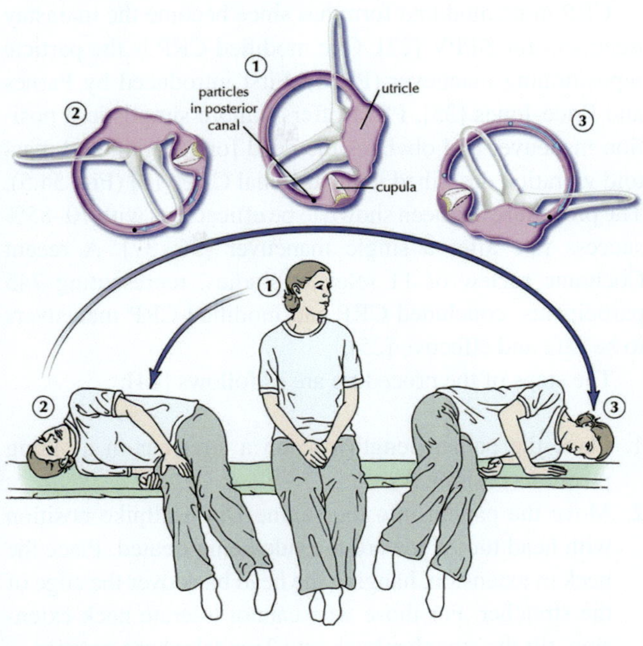

Fig. 54.4 Semont maneuver (right ear). The effect of the sequential movements on the labyrinth is depicted in the top panel. Transition from position 2 to 3 must be rapid. (Reprinted with permission from Parnes et al. [14])

Posterior Canal BPPV

In 1988, the French physical therapist Alain Semont and colleagues first described the liberatory maneuver, now known colloquially as the Semont maneuver [29]. The procedure was based on the cupulolithiasis theory with rapid, stepwise changes in head position aimed to free attached canaliths from the cupula (Fig. 54.4). The reported response rate of the Semont maneuver ranges from 70% to 90% with a recurrence rate of approximately 29% [30–32]. It has also been shown to be efficacious, safe, and advantageous compared to a sham-control [32]. Practically, because it has to be done rapidly, the Semont maneuver can be difficult to perform especially with elderly, obese, and infirm patients. But it offers the distinct advantage of not having to hyperextend the neck which may be appealing for patients with cervical spine or vascular conditions.

In the 1980s, John Epley was proposing a controlled set of head movements coined the canalith repositioning procedure (CRP), now known worldwide as the Epley maneuver. Based on the theory of canalithiasis, the procedure was engineered to return canaliths, under the influence of gravity, from the posterior semicircular canal back into the utricle from whence they came [14]. The procedure proved highly successful with Epley's original paper describing 100% resolution and 30% recurrence rate [33]. A subsequent systematic review showed CRP increases odds of resolution by 22–33 times compared to sham treatment [34].

CRP in its modified form has since become the mainstay treatment for BPPV [22]. One modified CRP is the particle repositioning maneuver (PRM). First introduced by Parnes and Price-Jones [35], PRM offers a more simplistic 3 position maneuver and obviates the need for sedation and mastoid vibration described in the original CRP [14] (Fig. 54.5). The procedure has been shown to be efficacious with 70–85% success rate after a single maneuver [36, 37]. A recent Cochrane review of 11 relevant studies, representing 745 participants, concluded CRP and modified CRP maneuvers to be safe and effective [25].

The steps of the procedure are as follows [14]:

1. Place the patient lengthwise on a stretcher in a sitting position (position A)
2. Move the patient into the supine Dix–Hallpike position with head turned toward the side being treated. Place the neck in extension, hanging the head back over the edge of the stretcher. For those who cannot tolerate neck extension, tilt the stretcher back into Trendelenburg position
3. Observe for presence of nystagmus
4. Maintain this position for 1–2 min (position B)
5. Turn the head 90° towards the opposite Dix–Hallpike position while keeping the neck in full extension (position C)
6. Continue to roll the patient another 90° until the head is diagonally opposite position B (position D). The change from position B, through C, into D, does not have to be rapid but should be done in less than 3–5 s in order to generate a nystagmus response
7. Observe for "secondary stage" nystagmus. If the particles continue moving in the same ampullofugal direction, that is, through the common crus into the utricle, this secondary stage nystagmus should beat in the same direction as the primary stage nystagmus.
8. This position is maintained for 30–60 s and then the patient sits up. With a successful maneuver, there should be no nystagmus or vertigo when the patient returns to the sitting position because the particles will have already been repositioned into the utricle.

To increase the success rate of PRM, practitioners should pay careful attention to the patient's nystagmus. Reversed or absent nystagmus at the second of a three-position PRM

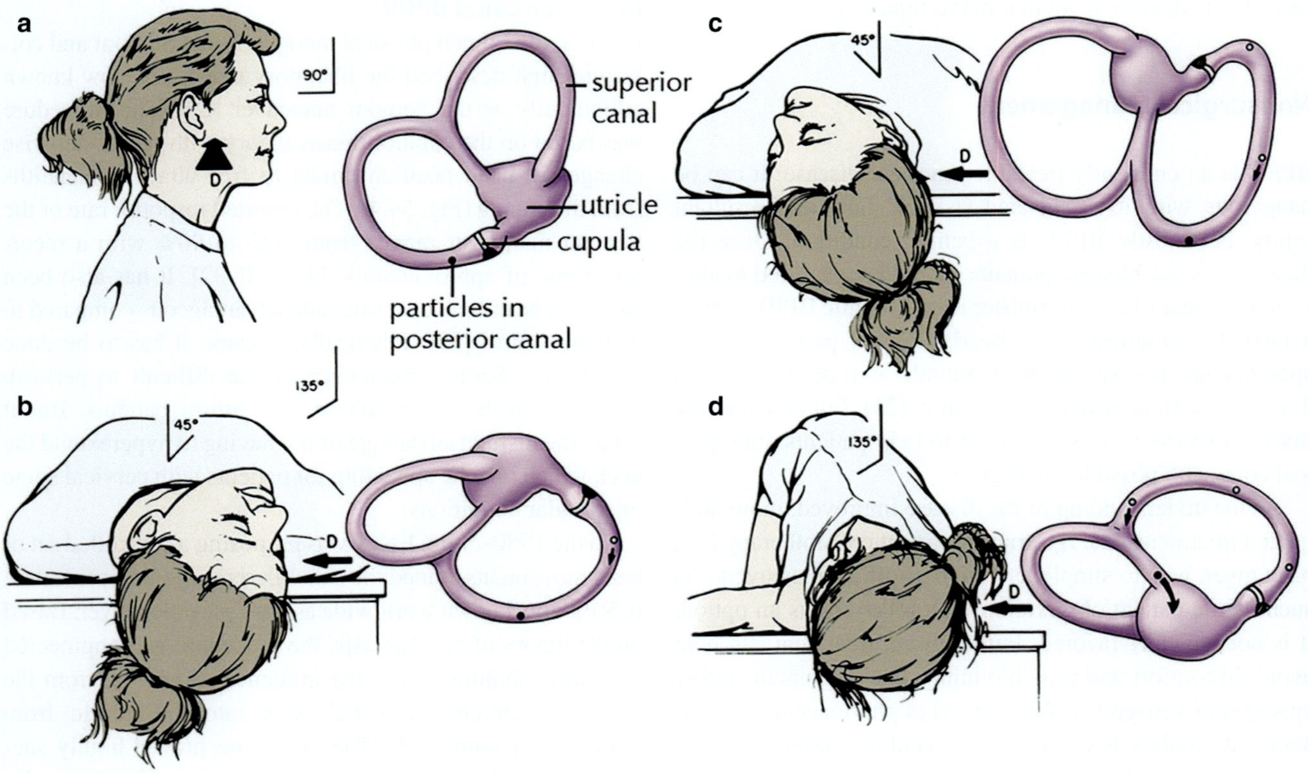

Fig. 54.5 Particle repositioning maneuver (right ear). Sequential movements and the corresponding position of the utricle and semicircular canals. (**a**) the patient is seated as viewed from the right side. (**b**) first step of particle repositioning maneuver and the same position assumed during normal Dix-Hallpike. This position is maintained for 1–2 minutes. (**c**) the patient's head is rotated toward the opposite side while the neck remains extended. (**d**) in a steady motion, the patient is rolled onto the opposite side. Position D is maintained for another 1 to 2 minutes before the patient sits up to position A. (Reprinted with permission from Parnes et al. [14]. Legend: D Direction of view of labyrinth, Dark circle Position of particle conglomerate, Open circle Previous position)

(Fig. 54.5c) or a reversed nystagmus in the sitting position at the conclusion of PRM (Fig. 54.5d) suggest that the canaliths have not been repositioned into the utricle [38]. In these scenarios, the PRM should be repeated. In comparison, post-treatment activity limitations, originally described by Epley, in hope of preventing canaliths from returning to the posterior canal have not been shown to be advantageous [39]. The use of mastoid vibration devices as an adjunct has also been contentious [40, 41]. In a retrospective study looking at a total of 168 patients, mastoid oscillation did not significantly enhance rate of success [40]. On occasion, oscillation may be helpful in cases resistant to conventional repositioning.

Follow-up after canal repositioning has not been standardized. A common follow-up interval is 1 month [3]. At the time of reassessment, patients should undergo Dix–Hallpike testing bilaterally. This helps determine the efficacy of the initial maneuver and accuracy of diagnosis. PRM should be repeated in the event of a positive repeat Dix–Hallpike maneuver.

Horizontal Canal BPPV

Several repositioning techniques are available for the treatment of horizontal canal BPPV. The treatment decision requires accurate assessment of the affected side and whether the presenting nystagmus is geotropic or apogeotropic. The former suggest canalithiasis and is more clinically responsive and well-studied [3].

To address the geotropic subtype, Lempert and Tiel-Wilck proposed a maneuver whereby patients roll in the plane of the semicircular canal [42]. This is referred to as the barbecue roll or barrel roll. Starting in a supine position, the head is first turned toward the affected ear. The head and body are then turned away from the affected side in 90-degree increments, holding each position for about 1 min until a full 360° rotation is completed. The patient is then returned to a seated position. Evidence shows this maneuver to have a variable success rate ranging from 50% to 100% [43, 44].

An alternative treatment for the geotropic subtype is the Gufoni maneuver [45]. The patient begins by lying sideways onto the unaffected side and then turning the head rapidly towards ground for 1–2 min before sitting up [45]. A randomized controlled trial showed comparable success between Gufoni (response rate of 60.9%) and barbecue roll (69.1%) [46]. In the event of apogeotropic nystagmus, the Gufoni maneuver begins with the patient lying sideways onto the affected side before turning the head rapidly toward the ground. Similarly, the patient holds the position for 1–2 min before sitting up. This maneuver, in addressing apogeotropic nystagmus, has been found to have a response rate of 73.1% [47].

Whereas the Gufoni maneuver depends on linear acceleration and positive inertia, Vannucchi's forced prolonged positioning relies on gravitational sedimentation [48]. In forced prolonged position, the patient assumes a lateral decubitus position on the unaffected side for 12 hours (affected side if nystagmus is apogeotropic). The original report showed a 90% resolution [48]. A prospective observational study found the effectiveness of forced prolonged position to be similar to that of Gufoni's maneuver after a single application (with success rates of 76 and 89%, respectively) [44].

Superior Canal BPPV

Superior canal BPPV is relatively rare (3%) and as such evidence on therapeutic management is limited. A systematic review identified Epley (or reverse Epley) and Yacovino as the most commonly published maneuver for superior canal BPPV, with a mean success rate of 75.9 and 78.8%, respectively [15]. The reverse Epley is effectively a PRM of the unaffected side, thus isolating the contralateral and affected anterior canal (beginning PRM with unaffected side in position Fig. 54.5a). In 2010, Li proposed a new technique for superior canal BPPV involving positional change in the sagittal plane [49]. The efficacy of the Li repositioning maneuver requires further research.

Special Considerations

Subjective BPPV describes patients with convincing clinical histories but no nystagmus during Dix–Hallpike testing [14]. Proposed theories for this include subclinical nystagmus, a fatigued response, and less severe BPPV that activate the sensation of vertigo but not the vestibulo-ocular reflex. Nevertheless, evidence suggests repositioning maneuvers in those with subjective BPPV are nearly as effective as they are for patients with objective BPPV [30, 50].

Repositioning maneuvers can be used to address both primary and secondary causes of BPPV. However, posttraumatic BPPV has a higher recurrence rate (57% in traumatic and 19% in idiopathic) and is more likely to be bilateral [51]. In the event of bilateral BPPV, the more symptomatic side should be treated first with plans to address the other side in follow-up. The contralateral side is not repositioned during the initial visit given theoretical risk of re-displacing the canaliths on the initially treated side.

Repositioning maneuvers are generally safe with few side effects. The most notable sequela is nausea, which is found in 16.7–32% of the cases [25]. In susceptible patients, prophylactic anti-emetics may be necessary. Canal conversion may occur in less than 5% of the cases when canaliths are displaced from the posterior canal into the horizontal canal during posterior canal particle repositioning [52]. In event of canal conversion, appropriate treatment of horizontal canal BPPV should ensue.

In instances of multiple failed repositioning maneuvers, a tertiary center referral should be considered [3]. Brandt-Daroff home exercises [26] can also be offered, though studies have shown it to be less efficacious than PRM or Semont maneuvers [53, 54]. Alternatively, patients unable to tolerate repositioning maneuvers may benefit from vestibular rehabilitation therapy under supervision.

Surgery

The majority of BPPV cases resolve either spontaneously or with appropriate repositioning maneuvers. As such, operative intervention is reserved for intractable cases. These patients fail to respond to repeated repositioning maneuvers or vestibular rehabilitation and experience severe, frequent symptoms that significantly impact quality of life. Ultimately, this is rare as less than 1% of BPPV patients require surgical intervention [55].

Preoperative testing should include audiometry given the operative risk of hearing loss. Vestibular testing of some kind, be it Electronystagmography (ENG), videonystagmography (VNG), or video head impulse test (VHIT), should be done to ensure normal vestibular function in the contralateral ear. Computed tomography (CT) of the temporal bone is helpful in defining the surgical anatomy and magnetic resonance imaging (MRI) may be used to rule out central lesions that may mimic BPPV. Currently, there are two main surgical techniques for intractable BPPV: singular neurectomy and posterior semicircular canal occlusion.

Singular Neurectomy

First popularized by Gacek, singular neurectomy is synonymous with posterior ampullary nerve transection [56]. It requires a trans-canal approach followed by exposure of the round window niche from its most anterior to posterior limits. Thereafter, the bony overhang covering the superior aspect of the round window niche is drilled away to expose the round window membrane. The singular canal is located 1–2 mm deep to the inferior round window membrane in the posterior one-third of the round window niche. The singular nerve is then exposed in its canal and transected with a pick or small right-angled hook. In doing so, the neurectomy eliminates the resting input from the affected posterior canal ampulla, creating a constant vestibular asymmetry. Secondary to this, patients will have immediate vertigo at rest with spontaneous torsional and downbeat (paralytic) nystagmus. Over time, compensation occurs by central adaptation which can be expedited by vestibular physiotherapy.

Singular neurectomy is technically difficult and has positive but variable results. While Gacek recently reported complete resolution of vertigo in 97% of patients [57], another large case series with 58 patients achieved 80% success rate [58]. The necessary surgical exposure places both the ampulla and vestibule at risk. As such, this procedure carries the potential risk of sensorineural hearing loss (SNHL) [59]. Smaller series reported complication rates of SNHL in 12%, 29%, 41% of cases among 8, 7, and 12 neurectomies, respectively [60–62]. By comparison, Gacek's updated series, summarizing 252 neurectomies, noted a 3.7% sensorineural hearing loss [57]. This illustrates the importance of operator experience as it relates to singular neurectomy.

Posterior Semicircular Canal Occlusion

Posterior semicircular canal occlusion serves as an easier and more reliable alternative surgical option [59]. Early experiments on guinea pigs by Parnes and McClure using brainstem auditory evoked responses showed no adverse effect on hearing with canal occlusion [63]. Armed with this understanding, in 1990, Parnes and McClure introduced posterior semicircular canal occlusion as treatment for intractable BPPV [64]. The procedure is based on the premise that obstruction of the posterior canal eliminates endolymph movement, effectively fixing the cupula. In doing so, the canal becomes unresponsive to head movement. While this creates a dynamic vestibular asymmetry, overtime central adaption relieves the initial postoperative imbalance.

Parnes and McClure initially performed the operation on two patients with pre-existing SNHL [64]. Postoperatively, the patients were vertigo free and maintained horizontal canal function shown by caloric responses. Subsequent case series showed posterior canal occlusion's effectiveness in abolishing BPPV while preserving hearing [65, 66]. A literature review by Leveque highlighted 97 reported cases of posterior semicircular canal occlusion in which 94 were symptom free postoperatively [59]. Moreover, when compared to singular neurectomy, posterior semicircular canal occlusion contained fewer risk and less technical challenges [59]. Parnes and Agrawal reported on 74 posterior canal occlusions in 68 patients with only one case of significant postoperative sensorineural hearing loss [67]. The delayed sudden hearing loss accompanied by a 7-day vertigo spell resulted in a working diagnosis of labyrinthitis.

Surgically, the posterior semicircular canal is accessed through a standard postauricular incision and mastoidectomy [67]. Following the limited mastoidectomy and identification of the posterior canal otic capsule, the bone is blue-lined. Thereafter, a 1 x 3 mm endosteal island is created with a 1 mm diamond burr (Fig. 54.6). A 90-degree pick is then used to remove the endosteal island and expose the perilymph, which is wicked or suctioned away with care to provide room for the canal plug. The plug, fashioned from dry mastoid cortex bone chips mixed with fibrinogen sealant, is gently but firmly inserted and packed tightly within the bony canal. Various alternative materials such as bone dust, or fas-

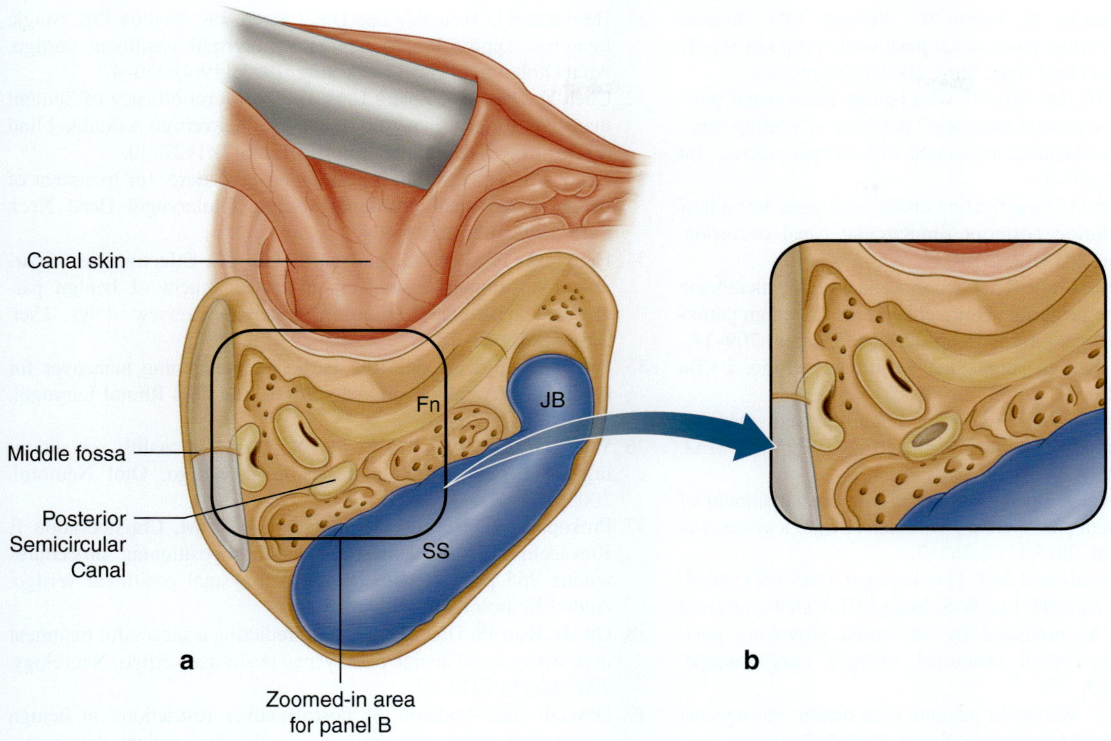

Fig. 54.6 Surgical exposure of posterior semicircular canal and creation of a fenestration. (**a**) A mastoidectomy has been performed. The relationship between the posterior semicircular canal and surrounding structures is demonstrated. (**b**) in a zoomed-in perspective, a small endosteal island has been created into the posterior semicircular canal, indicated by the asterisk. (Adapted from Parnes and Agrawal [67] Legend: JB Jugular bulb, SS Sigmoid sinus, Fn Facial nerve)

cia can also be used to occlude the canal. Bone wax may incite an inflammatory response in the inner ear and is best avoided. Lastly, the fenestra is covered with fascia and fibrinogen sealant. Reported variations in the technique include using the argon laser after "bluelining" the posterior canal [68] and use of the CO_2 laser to produce canal fibrous occlusions [69]. There are sporadic case reports of successful horizontal and anterior semicircular occlusion for treating the corresponding canal's intractable BPPV [70, 71].

Summary

Benign paroxysmal positional vertigo is a common disorder and presents with a characteristic history of brief, episodic, positional-provoked vertigo. The diagnosis can be established with a Dix–Hallpike maneuver for the posterior and anterior canals, or lateral head turns for the horizontal canal, and normally does not require additional ancillary testing. While often self-limiting, BPPV can have considerable impact on quality of life. Fortunately, understanding the pathophysiology of both canalithiasis and cupulolithiasis has allowed for the development of various repositioning techniques. Of these, the particle repositioning maneuver is a simple and effective way to treat posterior canal BPPV, the most common variant. For a small subset of patients with intractable BPPV, posterior canal occlusion is a relatively safe, straightforward, and highly efficacious procedure.

References

1. Barany R. Diagnose von Krankheitserscheinungen im Bereiche des Otolithenapparatus. Acta Otolaryngol Stock. 1921;2:434–7.
2. Dix MR, Hallpike CS. The pathology symptomatology and diagnosis of certain common disorders of the vestibular system. Proc R Soc Med. 1952;45(6):341–54.
3. Bhattacharyya N, Gubbels SP, Schwartz SR, et al. Clinical practice guideline: benign paroxysmal positional vertigo (Update). Otolaryngol Neck Surg. 2017;156(3_suppl):S1–S47.
4. Hanley K, O'Dowd T, Considine N. A systematic review of vertigo in primary care. Br J Gen Pract. 2001;51(469):666–71.
5. von Brevern M, Radtke A, Lezius F, et al. Epidemiology of benign paroxysmal positional vertigo: a population based study. J Neurol Neurosurg Psychiatry. 2007;78(7):710–5.
6. Mizukoshi K, Watanabe Y, Shojaku H, Okubo J, Watanabe I. Epidemiological studies on benign paroxysmal positional vertigo in Japan. Acta Otolaryngol Suppl. 1988;447:67–72.
7. Kim J-S, Zee DS. Clinical practice. Benign paroxysmal positional vertigo. N Engl J Med. 2014;370(12):1138–47.

8. Katsarkas A. Benign paroxysmal positional vertigo (BPPV): idiopathic versus post-traumatic. Acta Otolaryngol. 1999;119(7):745–9.
9. Oghalai JS, Manolidis S, Barth JL, Stewart MG, Jenkins HA. Unrecognized benign paroxysmal positional vertigo in elderly patients. Otolaryngol Head Neck Surg. 2000;122(5):630–4.
10. Fife D, FitzGerald JE. Do patients with benign paroxysmal positional vertigo receive prompt treatment? Analysis of waiting times and human and financial costs associated with current practice. Int J Audiol. 2005;44(1):50–7.
11. Parnes LS, McClure JA. Free-floating endolymph particles: a new operative finding during posterior semicircular canal occlusion. 1992. Laryngoscope. 2015;125(5):1033.
12. Kao WTK, Parnes LS, Chole RA. Otoconia and otolithic membrane fragments within the posterior semicircular canal in benign paroxysmal positional vertigo. Laryngoscope. 2016;90(March):709–14.
13. Lee S-H, Kim JS. Benign paroxysmal positional vertigo. J Clin Neurol. 2010;6(2):51–63.
14. Parnes LS, Agrawal SK, Atlas J. Diagnosis and management of benign paroxysmal positional vertigo (BPPV). CMAJ. 2003;169(7):681–93.
15. Anagnostou E, Kouzi I, Spengos K. Diagnosis and treatment of Anterior-Canal benign paroxysmal positional Vertigo: a systematic review. J Clin Neurol. 2015;11(3):262–7.
16. McClure JA. Horizontal canal BPV. J Otolaryngol. 1985;14(1):30–5.
17. Shim DB, Ko KM, Kim JH, Lee W-S, Song MH. Can the affected semicircular canal be predicted by the initial provoking position in benign paroxysmal positional vertigo? Laryngoscope. 2013;123(9):2259–63.
18. Kentala E, Pyykkö I. Vertigo in patients with benign paroxysmal positional vertigo. Acta Otolaryngol Suppl. 2000;543:20–2.
19. Shoman N, Longridge N. Cerebellar vermis lesions and tumours of the fourth ventricle in patients with positional and positioning vertigo and nystagmus. J Laryngol Otol. 2007;121(2):166–9.
20. Halker RB, Barrs DM, Wellik KE, Wingerchuk DM, Demaerschalk BM. Establishing a diagnosis of benign paroxysmal positional vertigo through the dix-hallpike and side-lying maneuvers: a critically appraised topic. Neurologist. 2008;14(3):201–4.
21. López-Escámez JA, López-Nevot A, Gámiz MJ, et al. Diagnosis of common causes of vertigo using a structured clinical history. Acta Otorrinolaringol Esp. 2000;51(1):25–30.
22. Hornibrook J. Horizontal canal benign positional vertigo. Ann Otol Rhinol Laryngol. 2004;113(9):721–5.
23. Balatsouras DG, Koukoutsis G, Ganelis P, Korres GS, Kaberos A. Diagnosis of single- or Multiple-Canal benign paroxysmal positional Vertigo according to the type of nystagmus. Int J Otolaryngol. 2011;2011:1–13.
24. Lynn S, Pool A, Rose D, Brey R, Suman V. Randomized trial of the canalith repositioning procedure. Otolaryngol Head Neck Surg. 1995;113(6):712–20.
25. Hilton M, Pinder D. The Epley manoeuvre for benign paroxysmal positional vertigo. Cochrane Database Syst Rev. 2014;12:1–38.
26. Brandt T, Daroff RB. Physical therapy for benign paroxysmal positional vertigo. Arch Otolaryngol. 1980;106(8):484–5.
27. Fujino A, Tokumasu K, Yosio S, Naganuma H, Yoneda S, Nakamura K. Vestibular training for benign paroxysmal positional vertigo. Its efficacy in comparison with antivertigo drugs. Arch Otolaryngol Head Neck Surg. 1994;120(5):497–504.
28. Sundararajan I, Rangachari V, Sumathi V, Kumar K. Epley's manoeuvre versus Epley's manoeuvre plus labyrinthine sedative as management of benign paroxysmal positional vertigo: prospective, randomised study. J Laryngol Otol. 2011;125(January):572–5.
29. Semont A, Freyss G, Vitte E. Curing the BPPV with a liberatory maneuver. Adv Otorhinolaryngol. 1988;42:290–3.
30. Haynes DS, Resser JR, Labadie RF, et al. Treatment of benign positional vertigo using the semont maneuver: efficacy in patients presenting without nystagmus. Laryngoscope. 2002;112(May):796–801.
31. Herdman SJ, Tusa RJ, Zee DS, Proctor LR, Mattox DE. Single treatment approaches to benign paroxysmal positional vertigo. Arch Otolaryngol Head Neck Surg. 1993;119(4):450–4.
32. Chen Y, Zhuang J, Zhang L, et al. Short-term efficacy of Semont maneuver for benign paroxysmal positional vertigo: a double-blind randomized trial. Otol Neurotol. 2012;33(7):1127–30.
33. Epley JM. The canalith repositioning procedure: for treatment of benign paroxysmal positional vertigo. Otolaryngol Head Neck Surg. 1992;107(3):399–404.
34. Helminski JO, Zee DS, Janssen I, Hain TC. Effectiveness of particle repositioning maneuvers in the treatment of benign paroxysmal positional vertigo: a systematic review. Phys Ther. 2010;90(5):663–78.
35. Parnes LS, Price-Jones RG. Particle repositioning maneuver for benign paroxysmal positional vertigo. Ann Otol Rhinol Laryngol. 1993;102(5):325–31.
36. White J, Savvides P, Cherian N, Oas J. Canalith repositioning for benign paroxysmal positional vertigo. Otol Neurotol. 2005;26(7):704–10.
37. Prokopakis E, Vlastos IM, Tsagournisakis M, Christodoulou P, Kawauchi H, Velegrakis G. Canalith repositioning procedures among 965 patients with benign paroxysmal positional vertigo. Audiol Neurotol. 2013;18(2):83–8.
38. Oh HJ, Kim JS, Han BI, Lim JG. Predicting a successful treatment in posterior canal benign paroxysmal positional vertigo. Neurology. 2007;68(15):1219–22.
39. Devaiah AK, Andreoli S. Postmaneuver restrictions in benign paroxysmal positional vertigo: an individual patient data meta-analysis. Otolaryngol Head Neck Surg. 2010;142(2):155–9.
40. Sargent EW, Bankaitis AE, Hollenbeak CS, Currens JW. Mastoid oscillation in canalith repositioning for paroxysmal positional vertigo. Otol Neurotol. 2001;22(2):205–9.
41. Li JC. Mastoid oscillation: a critical factor for success in canalith repositioning procedure. Otolaryngol Head Neck Surg. 1995;112(6):670–5.
42. Lempert T, Tiel-Wilck K. A positional maneuver for treatment of horizontal-canal benign positional vertigo. Laryngoscope. 1996;106(4):476–8.
43. Casani AP, Vannucci G, Fattori B, Berrettini S. The treatment of horizontal canal positional vertigo: our experience in 66 cases. Laryngoscope. 2002;112(1):172–8.
44. Korres S, Riga MG, Xenellis J, Korres GS, Danielides V. Treatment of the horizontal semicircular canal canalithiasis: pros and cons of the repositioning maneuvers in a clinical study and critical review of the literature. Otol Neurotol. 2011;32(8):1302–8.
45. Ciniglio Appiani G, Catania G, Gagliardi M. A liberatory maneuver for the treatment of horizontal canal paroxysmal positional vertigo. Otol Neurotol. 2001;22(1):66–9.
46. Kim JS, Oh S-Y, Lee S-H, et al. Randomized clinical trial for geotropic horizontal canal benign paroxysmal positional vertigo. Neurology. 2012;79(7):700–7.
47. Kim J-S, Oh S-Y, Lee S-H, et al. Randomized clinical trial for apogeotropic horizontal canal benign paroxysmal positional vertigo. Neurology. 2012;78(3):159–66.
48. Vannucchi P, Giannoni B, Pagnini P. Treatment of horizontal semicircular canal benign paroxysmal positional vertigo. J Vestib Res. 1997;7(1):1–6.
49. Li J, Li H. New repositioning techniques for benign paroxysmal positional vertigo: the Li repositioning manoeuvres. J Laryngol Otol. 2010;124(8):905–8.
50. Tirelli G, D'Orlando E, Giacomarra V, Russolo M. Benign positional vertigo without detectable nystagmus. Laryngoscope. 2001;111(6):1053–6.

51. Gordon CR, Levite R, Joffe V, Gadoth N. Is posttraumatic benign paroxysmal positional vertigo different from the idiopathic form? Arch Neurol. 2004;61(10):1590–3.
52. Herdman SJ, Tusa RJ. Complications of the canalith repositioning procedure. Arch Otolaryngol Head Neck Surg. 1996;122(3):281–6.
53. Amor-Dorado JC, Barreira-Fernández MP, Aran-Gonzalez I, Casariego-Vales E, Llorca J, González-Gay MA. Particle repositioning maneuver versus Brandt-Daroff exercise for treatment of unilateral idiopathic BPPV of the posterior semicircular canal: a randomized prospective clinical trial with short- and long-term outcome. Otol Neurotol. 2012;33(8):1401–7.
54. Soto Varela A, Bartual Magro J, Santos Pérez S, et al. Benign paroxysmal vertigo: a comparative prospective study of the efficacy of Brandt and Daroff exercises, Semont and Epley maneuver. Rev Laryngol Otol Rhinol (Bord). 2001;122(3):179–83.
55. Shaia WT, Zappia JJ, Bojrag DI, LaRouere ML, Sargent EW, Diaz RC. Success of posterior semicircular canal occlusion and application of the dizziness handicap inventory. Otolaryngol Head Neck Surg. 2006;134(3):424–30.
56. Gacek RR. Transection of the posterior ampullary nerve for the relief of benign paroxysmal positional vertigo. Ann Otol Rhinol Laryngol. 1974;83(5):596–605.
57. Gacek RR, Gacek MR. Results of singular neurectomy in the posterior ampullary recess. ORL J Otorhinolaryngol Relat Spec. 2002;64(6):397–402.
58. Silverstein H, White DW. Wide surgical exposure for singular Neurectomy in the treatment of benign positional Vertigo. Laryngoscope. 1990;100(7):701–6.
59. Leveque M, Labrousse M, Seidermann L, Chays A. Surgical therapy in intractable benign paroxysmal positional vertigo. Otolaryngol Head Neck Surg. 2007;136(5):693–8.
60. Pournaras I, Kos I, Guyot J-P. Benign paroxysmal positional vertigo: a series of eight singular neurectomies. Acta Otolaryngol. 2008;128(1):5–8.
61. Fernandes CM. Singular neurectomy in south African practice. S Afr J Surg. 1993;31(2):79–80.
62. Epley JM. Singular neurectomy: hypotympanotomy approach. Otolaryngol Head Neck Surg (1979). 1980;88(3):304–9.
63. Parnes LS, McClure JA. Effect on brainstem auditory evoked responses of posterior semicircular canal occlusion in guinea pigs. J Otolaryngol. 1985;14(3):145–50.
64. Parnes LS, McClure JA. Posterior semicircular canal occlusion for intractable benign paroxysmal positional vertigo. Ann Otol Rhinol Laryngol. 1990;99(5 Pt 1):330–4.
65. Parnes LS, McClure JA. Posterior semicircular canal occlusion in the normal hearing ear. Otolaryngol Head Neck Surg. 1991;104(1):52–7.
66. Agrawal SK, Parnes LS. Human experience with canal plugging. Ann N Y Acad Sci. 2001;942(519):300–5.
67. Parnes LS, Agrawal SK. Transmastoid semicircular canal occlusion for benign paroxysmal positional vertigo and other disorders. In: Brackmann D, Clough S, Arriag M, editors. Otologic surgery. 4th ed. Elsevier Health Sciences; 2015. p. 408–16.
68. Anthony PF. Partitioning of the labyrinth: application in benign paroxysmal positional vertigo. Am J Otol. 1991;12(5):388–93.
69. Antonelli PJ, Lundy LB, Kartush JM, Burgio DL, Graham MD. Mechanical versus CO_2 laser occlusion of the posterior semicircular canal in humans. Am J Otol. 1996;17(3):416–20.
70. Zhu Q, Liu C, Lin C, et al. Efficacy and safety of semicircular canal occlusion for intractable horizontal semicircular benign paroxysmal positional vertigo. Ann Otol Rhinol Laryngol. 2015;124(4):257–60.
71. Brantberg K, Bergenius J. Treatment of anterior benign paroxysmal positional vertigo by canal plugging: a case report. Acta Otolaryngol. 2002;122(1):28–30.

Vestibular Neuritis and Labyrinthitis

55

Renee M. Banakis Hartl, Hiroki Takeda,
and Samuel P. Gubbels

Introduction

Vestibular neuritis—a sudden loss of unilateral vestibular function—was first described as a clinical disorder by Dix and Hallpike in 1952 to distinguish the disorder from Ménière's disease [1]. Historically, the terms *vestibular neuritis* and *labyrinthitis* were used interchangeably; however, the terms are now used more specifically, with *vestibular neuritis* considered to be more appropriate for use describing a disorder limited to vestibular symptoms and *labyrinthitis* when auditory symptoms are present as well [2].

Vestibular Neuritis

Clinical Features

Classically, individuals with vestibular neuritis present with sudden or subacute onset of incapacitating vertigo that is often accompanied by nausea and vomiting, spontaneous nystagmus, and possibly postural imbalance. Patients may demonstrate a tendency to fall toward the affected side and may attempt to mitigate movement-induced worsening of symptoms by lying completely still. The vertigo in vestibular neuritis can last from 12 h up to a number of days or even up to two weeks with subsequent gradual resolution, though many individuals report non-vertiginous, balance-related dysfunction lasting up to several months after the resolution of acute vertiginous symptoms. Generalized unsteadiness, difficulty with quick movements or rapid turns, swaying while walking, or a generalized sense of feeling "off" are symptoms that may persist after the acute phase of vertigo has subsided.

While vestibular neuritis has been described as the second most common cause of vertigo seen in general practice [3], strong epidemiologic data is lacking. When examining emergency department visits, dizziness is the primary complaint for 3.3% of patients, and of those individuals, 5.6% are diagnosed with vestibular neuritis or labyrinthitis, which can be extrapolated to an annual incidence of 150,000 patients for these two diagnoses [4]. In specialized dizziness clinics, neuritis is estimated to account for 3–10% of diagnoses [3, 5, 6]. The incidence of vestibular neuritis was reported to be about 3.5 per 100,000 in a large Japanese population [7]. The same investigation described individuals with the diagnosis as being equally likely to be male or female and most likely to be between 40 and 50 years old [7].

Etiology

Historically, the term *idiopathic sudden vestibular paralysis* was used to describe vestibular neuritis due to lack of consensus regarding the underlying etiology of the disorder. In Dix and Hallpike's original description of the disease, they suggested that an infectious process affecting Scarpa's ganglion or the vestibular nerve itself was responsible for the symptoms of vestibular neuritis [1]. A vascular etiology has been suspected because the condition often spares the inferior division of the vestibular nerve, which is supplied by the posterior vestibular artery, while the superior division of the vestibular nerve is supplied by the anterior vestibular artery [8]. While an ischemic etiology is possible, no direct evidence for vascular insult has been shown histopathologically. Autoimmune disease has also been suggested as a possible underlying cause of vestibular neuritis [9, 10]. Several stud-

R. M. Banakis Hartl
Department of Otolaryngology—Head and Neck Surgery, University of Michigan School of Medicine, Ann Arbor, MI, USA

H. Takeda
Department of Otolaryngology—Head and Neck Surgery, University of Colorado School of Medicine, Aurora, CO, USA

Department of Otolaryngology—Head and Neck Surgery, Kumamoto University, Kumamoto, Japan

S. P. Gubbels (✉)
Department of Otolaryngology—Head and Neck Surgery, University of Colorado School of Medicine, Aurora, CO, USA
e-mail: samuel.gubbels@ucdenver.edu

A. D. Sweeney et al. (eds.), *Haynes-Glasscock-Shambaugh Surgery of the Ear*, https://doi.org/10.1007/978-3-032-18264-7_55

ies have described a viral etiology given the occurrence of some cases of vestibular neuritis around the same time within households or in association with upper respiratory infections [1, 2, 10]. More recently, there is increasing evidence in the literature to support viral reactivation as a possible etiology [11–17]. The suggested mechanism for herpes simplex virus type 1 (HSV-1) reactivation is similar to that described for idiopathic facial paralysis. Herpes simplex virus, type 1 (HSV-1) DNA has been identified in the human vestibular ganglion in postmortem histology [13–17], and mice with HSV-1 inoculation directed to the vestibular ganglion cells have demonstrated vestibular dysfunction [12].

Pathophysiology

Regardlessof the underlying etiology, the existence of resulting neural inflammation has been well-established. Higher levels of acute phase reactants—including plasma fibrinogen, C-reactive protein (CRP), lipoprotein, and D-dimer—support the presence of an acute inflammatory reaction in patients with vestibular neuritis [9]. Postmortem temporal bone histology in patients with the diagnosis demonstrate focal cellular degeneration in the vestibular nerve axons and geniculate ganglion—a pattern of atrophy similar to that seen following other viral diseases, such as mumps and measles [11, 14, 17]. These atrophic changes are typically sufficiently severe as to explain abnormalities seen on clinical tests of vestibular function [2].

Vestibular neuritis has been shown to preferentially affect the superior division of the vestibular nerve [8, 18–20], though distinct patterns of disease have been described according to the divisions of the nerve that are affected [20] (see Fig. 55.1). This predilection has been ascribed to anatomical differences between the channels for each branch of the vestibular nerve. In a study of 184 temporal bones, it was found that the lengths of the bony canals of the singular and inferior vestibular nerve were significantly shorter than that of the superior division. Additionally, the channel carrying the superior vestibular nerve and its vascular supply is sig-

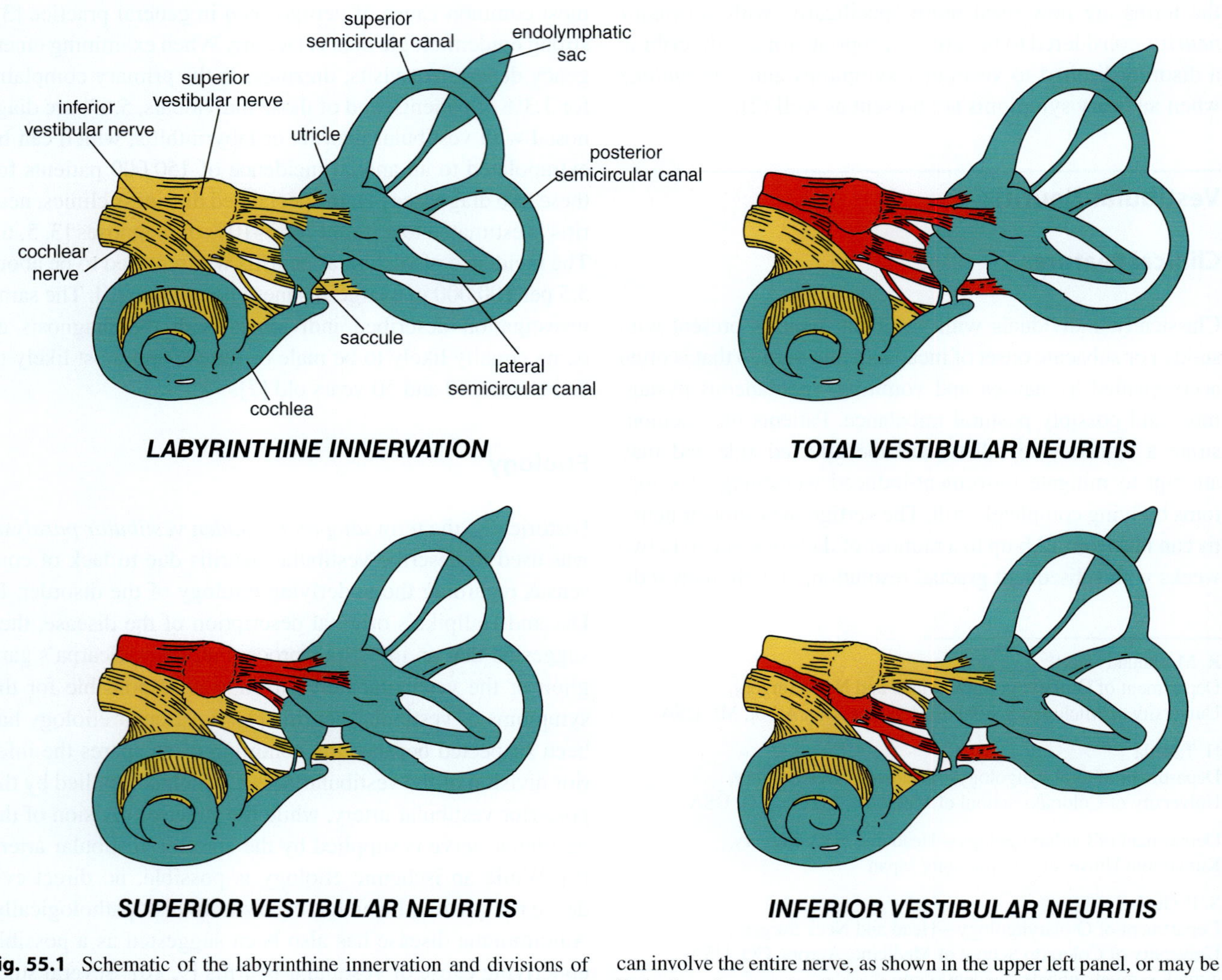

Fig. 55.1 Schematic of the labyrinthine innervation and divisions of the vestibular nerve. The superior vestibular nerve innervates the lateral and superior semicircular canals, as well as the utricle, while the inferior division innervates the posterior canal and saccule. Inflammation can involve the entire nerve, as shown in the upper left panel, or may be limited to the superior (lower left) or inferior (lower right) divisions. Limited superior nerve involvement is most common

nificantly narrower and contains more bony trabeculae [21, 22]. The anatomical variation suggests that the superior division may be more susceptible to mechanical or ischemic injury secondary to swelling or inflammation. It is also important to consider that the atypical presentation possible in neuritis limited to the inferior division, including atypical or absent patterns of nystagmus and normal caloric function, may lead clinicians away from the diagnosis of vestibular neuritis and ultimately underestimate its incidence [18].

Evaluation

As with all vestibular pathology, a complete and thorough physical exam is of the utmost importance in the workup for vestibular neuritis. In addition to a complete head and neck exam with a detailed cranial nerve exam, clinical exam should include cerebellar and gait assessment, as well as a complete neurologic evaluation.

Signs of unilateral vestibular hypofunction are readily apparent early in the course of the illness. These signs include a spontaneous nystagmus that can vary depending on the divisions of the nerve that are affected. When disease affects the superior division primarily, spontaneous nystagmus is present with horizontal and torsional slow components that are directed toward the ear with hypofunction. With disease of the inferior division, spontaneous nystagmus will be downbeating with a torsional component. The velocity of this nystagmus frequently increases in amplitude when patients look in the direction of the fast component. It can be suppressed by looking at a stationary object, whereas the torsional eye velocity (rotation about the line of sight) of the nystagmus is not affected by this maneuver. Early in the clinical course of the disease, spontaneous nystagmus may be present even with fixation, though it is better appreciated clinically with the removal of visual targets.

Bedside head impulse testing can be used as part of the complete head and neck evaluation to identify the presence of a unilateral vestibular weakness. A head thrust in the orientation of the canal planes may be useful in localization of the pathology to the superior or inferior divisions, though they may be more difficult to interpret. Quantitative head impulse testing may be useful to confirm the clinical exam; however, the study has shown that moderate unilateral vestibular deficits may be more difficult to detect with video head impulse test (VHIT) alone [23].

Additional Testing

Diagnostic testing, including videonystagmography (VNG), vestibular-evoked myogenic potential (VEMP) testing, and radiological evaluations, are rarely necessary to confirm the diagnosis of vestibular neuritis. In some patients, such as those with an atypical clinical course or incomplete recovery, diagnostic testing can be entertained and may provide findings supportive of the diagnosis or help in ruling out more insidious pathologies. When ordered, VNG can be used to document and quantify nystagmus, and may demonstrate a unilateral vestibular hypofunction on caloric testing, which is considered to be one of the primary findings in vestibular neuritis [20, 23, 24].

Cervical VEMP (cVEMP) responses are generally accepted as reflecting activity of the saccule and inferior vestibular nerve, and may be of limited utility given the low incidence of neuritis limited to the inferior division. Ocular VEMPs (oVEMPs) are hypothesized to reflect activity of the utricle and superior nerve, suggesting they may be helpful in diagnosing unilateral vestibular weakness due to neuritis. Indeed, some have suggested oVEMP testing can be used to differentiate between the affected subsites in vestibular neuritis [24, 25].

While routine audiometry is not necessary in patients without subjective hearing changes who present with the classic picture of vestibular neuritis, hearing is typically unaffected when audiometry is performed. A dedicated temporal-bone, high-resolution computerized tomography (CT) scan should be considered only for cases where temporal bone pathology is suspected. Similarly, magnetic resonance imaging (MRI) is warranted only in patients with atypical presentations, repetitive episodes, neurological findings, incomplete recovery, or when asymmetrical sensorineural hearing loss (SNHL) has been found on audiometry. Direct visualization of inflammation via isolated enhancement of the vestibular nerve with high-dose gadolinium contrast in a high-field strength MRI (3-Tesla) has been reported [26], but MRI is not recommended for this purpose alone. Additionally, though presence of elevated acute phase reactants has been shown in some patients [9], no serological testing is recommended as part of the standard workup.

Diagnosis

Three subtypes of vestibular neuritis have been proposed based on the results of newer vestibular tests, including the quantitative head impulse test, cVEMPs, and oVEMPs, which allow for the evaluation of the end organs individually. Figure 55.1 illustrates the subsites and resultant clinical subtypes.

The most common subtype is *superior vestibular neuritis*, and it presents with the most typical signs and clinical findings. Horizontal–torsional spontaneous nystagmus is present, with the slow phase in the direction of hypofunction. Head impulse test is positive in the direction of the involved lateral and/or superior semicircular canals. Unilateral vestibular hypofunction is confirmed by caloric weakness on the affected side. Ocular VEMP, when ordered, may be abnor-

Table 55.1 Vestibular function test results for the subtypes of vestibular neuritis

	Superior	Inferior	Complete
Spontaneous nystagmus	Horizontal or upbeating Torsional	Downbeating Torsional	Horizontal Torsional
Caloric testing	Unilateral weakness or absence	Normal	Unilateral weakness Or absence
Head impulse test: Superior canal	Abnormal	Normal	Abnormal
Head impulse test: Lateral canal	Abnormal	Normal	Abnormal
Head impulse test: Posterior canal	Normal	Abnormal	Abnormal
Cervical VEMP	Normal	Abnormal	Abnormal
Ocular VEMP	Abnormal	Normal	Abnormal

mal [24, 25], while cVEMP would be expected to be normal.

Inferior vestibular neuritis is the least common presentation, though the atypical presentation can make diagnosis more challenging and symptoms may be incorrectly attributed to central pathology [18, 20, 24]. Spontaneous nystagmus is characteristically downbeating and torsional. The head impulse test is positive in the orientation of the posterior canal, and cVEMPs are abnormal. Normal head impulse in the orientation of the lateral and superior canals, normal oVEMP testing, and the absence of unilateral weakness on caloric testing distinguish this presentation from superior neuritis.

Spontaneous nystagmus is most often horizontal and torsional in *complete vestibular neuritis*, with abnormal results of vestibular function testing mirroring that of both superior and inferior nerve disease. A summary of the test findings for each subtype can be found in Table 55.1.

Differential Diagnosis

No individual test can confirm the diagnosis of vestibular neuritis and it remains a diagnosis of exclusion. Patient history, especially symptom time course, physical exam, and audiometry (when hearing loss has been noted by the patient), will help in ruling out other peripheral vestibular disorders such as Ménière's disease, benign paroxysmal positional vertigo (BPPV), superior semicircular canal dehiscence syndrome, and perilymph fistula. Central disorders that may mimic vestibular neuritis include multiple sclerosis, cerebrovascular accident, and "pseudoneuritis" secondary to posterior fossa ischemic stroke. The vertigo and nystagmus in "pseudoneuritis" can be similar to that observed in vestibular neuritis. It is important that these be distinguished, as a stroke involving the inferior cerebellum can lead to swelling, brain stem compression, and death unless there is prompt neurosurgical intervention. One key distinguishing feature is the degree of postural instability. Patients with cerebellar hemorrhage or infarction are typically unable to walk and are very unstable when standing. Patients with vestibular neuritis, in contrast, are likely to have an unsteady gait, but can ambulate in general. Appropriate imaging such as a magnetic resonance imaging scan of the brain and posterior fossa should be obtained when there is suspicion that the symptoms may arise from an abnormality affecting the central nervous system.

Course

The acute phase of vestibular neuritis, characterized by severe intractable vertigo and imbalance, usually improves over the course of a few days up to a week. Typically, a generalized sense of imbalance can persist for weeks to months after the resolution of vertigo as the process of vestibular compensation takes place.

Recovery of balance reflexes following vestibular neuritis occurs through three mechanisms: spontaneous return of vestibular function in the affected ear (in about 50% of cases), vestibular compensation, and substitution of other sensory or motor strategies. Vestibular compensation is a process of neurological reorganization that allows recovery of balance after a unilateral vestibular lesion. Vestibular compensation will reliably occur in patients after vestibular neuritis unless the patient has developed an additional, fluctuating unilateral vestibular disorder (such as BPPV) or when centrally acting medications that slow vestibular compensation (such as anticholinergics) continue to be taken regularly after the vertigo phase of vestibular neuritis has resolved. An example of a substitution strategy includes the increased reliance on visual and proprioceptive information to maintain postural stability after loss of vestibular function.

Long-term follow-up of patients with vestibular neuritis has demonstrated a very low recurrence rate [6, 27], though there is suggestion that this population may be at higher risk for developing paroxysmal positional vertigo that is more difficult to treat [27].

Treatment

Treatment for vestibular neuritis is primarily supportive. For patients with intractable nausea and vomiting, antiemetic medication is recommended with intravenous rehydration as needed. Special populations, including children, elderly patients, pregnant patients, and those with underlying comorbid conditions may be more susceptible to dehydration and brief inpatient admission may be considered. The use of vestibular suppressant medication, including benzodiazepines, antihistamines, anticholinergic agents, antidopaminergic agents, and γ-aminobutyric acid–enhancing (GABAergic) agents, may also be considered, though prolonged use may delay central compensation. Given the proposed underlying etiology of viral reactivation, the use of both corticosteroids and antiviral medications has been suggested, though both remain controversial. While early administration of methylprednisolone was associated with improved vestibular function on caloric testing at 12-month follow-up in one placebo-controlled, double-blinded investigation, no shorter-term benefit of steroids has been shown [28–30]. Antivirals have not improved outcomes in any investigation [28].

Following resolution of the acute phase, treatment for neuritis is focused on vestibular rehabilitation in order to promote central compensation for any persistent unilateral vestibular weakness. During this time, exercise and activity are encouraged and the use of vestibular suppressant medication is discouraged. Though the degree of compensation expected for any individual patient may depend on factors such as age, residual vestibular function, disease severity, and patient motivation [31], clinical evidence suggests that rehabilitation is an effective treatment for improving patient function. Rehabilitation exercises focused on equilibrium training, fixation tasks, and active head movements should be encouraged.

Labyrinthitis

Clinical Features

Individuals with labyrinthitis often present similarly to patients with vestibular neuritis, with acute, severe incapacitating vertigo and imbalance; however, labyrinthitis is distinguished by the presence of hearing loss additionally. Hearing loss may vary in severity and configuration depending on the underlying etiology and pathophysiology. Other cochlear symptoms may include tinnitus, aural fullness, and otalgia. As in vestibular neuritis, the vertigo experienced by patients with labyrinthitis is often debilitating and associated with severe nausea and vomiting. Acute profound vertiginous symptoms generally last a few days, but unlike in vestibular neuritis, may demonstrate a waxing and waning pattern in severity.

The incidence and prevalence of labyrinthitis are difficult to report with certainty. According to one study, 37 of 240 patients presenting to a neurology clinic for the evaluation of positional dizziness were found to have neurolabyrinthitis [32]. Viral labyrinthitis most commonly affects individuals who are between 30 and 60 years of age, while bacterial disease can be seen at any age. Children under two years old are more susceptible to developing labyrinthitis secondary to meningitis [33–35].

Etiology

Inflammation of the labyrinth has been attributed to bacterial [36] or viral [37, 38] pathogens, infectious toxin byproducts [39], or autoimmune and inflammatory factors [40, 41]. Viral-mediated labyrinthitis is generally assumed to be the most common etiology, with symptoms being less severe than those seen in bacterial disease. Inner ear symptoms commonly present simultaneously or immediately following an infectious syndrome, such as an upper respiratory tract infection. Often, the temporal relation of the infection is the only clue to the viral nature of the disease, as there are typically no middle ear or obvious central nervous system findings. Viral pathogens known to potentially affect the inner ear include measles, mumps, cytomegalovirus (CMV), and herpes zoster, among others [37, 38, 42]. CMV is of particular relevance to the pediatric population, in which congenital infection has been shown to cause permanent vestibulocochlear dysfunction. Congenital disease typically occurs without symptoms during pregnancy and can result in mild-to-profound hearing loss in up to 17% of patients [43–45]. Early diagnosis with confirmatory bloodwork following birth and antiviral treatment has demonstrated promising early results for patients, but widespread clinical treatment trials are still ongoing [43, 46].

Bacteria known to cause middle ear infections and meningitis are those most commonly associated with labyrinthitis [36, 47]. *Haemophilus influenzae*, *Streptococcus pneumoniae,* and *Neisseria meningitidis* are associated with meningitis, while other pathogens typically seen in otitis media, can be causative, including the above as well as *Moraxella catarrhalis*, *Staphylococcus*, and other *Streptococcus* species [36, 47]. Bacterial disease may result from direct bacterial invasion of the labyrinth or through the passage of toxins and inflammatory mediators into the inner ear. Though bacterial labyrinthitis is a recognized complication of acute otitis media (AOM), it is far less common since the introduction of antibiotics. Meningitis remains a significant cause of permanent sensorineural hearing loss, ostensibly due to bacterial labyrinthitis [48–50].

Non-infectious inflammation of the inner ear may also cause a pattern of vestibular findings and hearing loss highly suggestive of labyrinthitis. The first description of a cohort of patients with steroid-responsive, idiopathic, progressive, bilateral sensorineural hearing loss introduced the possibility of autoimmune-mediated labyrinthine inflammation [40, 41].

Autoimmune inner ear disease (AIED) is rare, but may occur in isolation or in association with systemic inflammatory syndromes, such as granulomatosis with polyangiitis (GPA, formerly known as Wegener's granulomatosis) [51] or other autoimmune conditions. Though models of autoimmune inner ear disease have been challenging to develop, histology obtained from some animal models of AIED reveals patterns of inflammation that are similar to those seen in labyrinthitis resulting from viral and bacterial infections [52, 53].

Pathophysiology

There are two primary pathways for introducing pathogens into the labyrinth: *tympanogenic,* transmission via the middle ear space, and *meningogenic,* extension from the meninges to the inner ear in the setting of meningitis. Figure 55.2 illustrates the routes implicated in the pathogenesis of labyrinthitis.

Infection or inflammation of the middle ear space, mastoid antrum, or petrous apex can serve as the nidus of disease in *tympanogenic labyrinthitis* [36, 54, 55]. The extension of disease may occur directly, as in the case of a known fistulous connection between the middle and inner ear spaces, or indirectly, without a known connection between the spaces. Direct extension may result from an abnormal connection due to an erosion of the bony labyrinth from a cholesteatoma, a temporal bone fracture, or a planned entry into the labyrinth during otologic surgery, such as during a stapedotomy procedure. Without a known fistulous connection, an exact mechanism for spread of disease remains debated in the literature. The round window membrane has been proposed as a primary site for inflammatory spread [56–58]. Several temporal bone studies have shown evidence of direct bacterial and inflammatory cell spread through the round window membrane [36, 57, 59–61], though evidence for this pathway is conflicting. Thickening of the round window following otitis media has been found on temporal bone histology [57, 62], and animal studies have shown decreased bacterial invasion following such thickening; however, there is also evidence of increased permeability of the membrane to macromolecules [63]. Taken together, these data suggest that round window thickening may occur as a result of otitis media and assist in the prevention of direct bacterial spread, but may also increase passage of inflammatory macromolecules that may potentiate labyrinthine inflammation.

Other mechanisms have been proposed to explain the spread of tympanogenic disease in the absence of direct connection to the inner ear. Microscopic vascular channels transmitting infectious agents or septic emboli have been suggested [58], as well as the possibility of congenital perilymphatic fistula. No histologic or radiographic evidence has been found to date to support these alternative explanations.

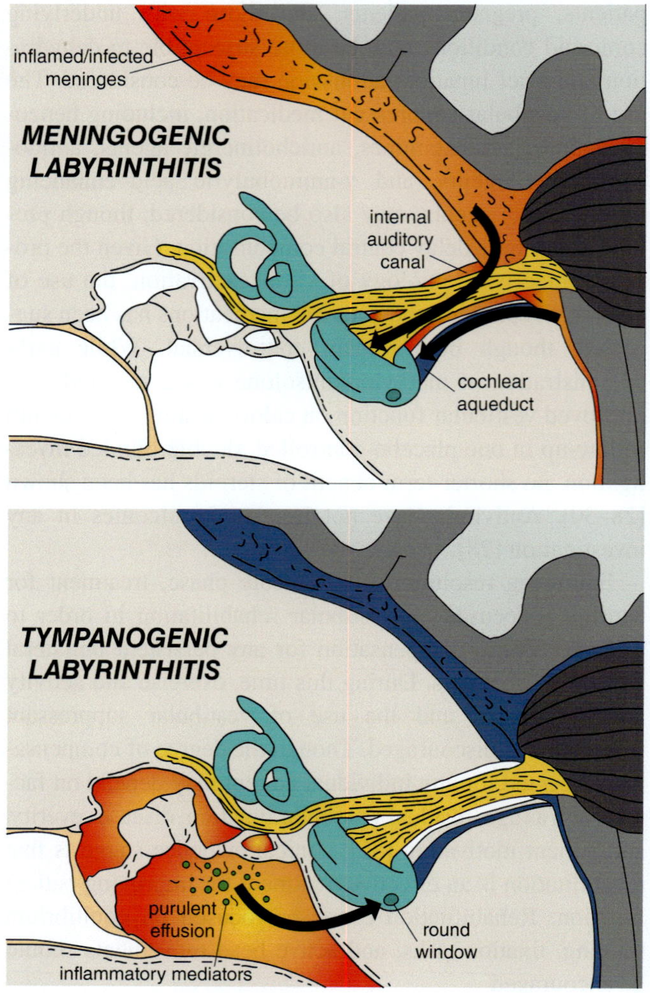

Fig. 55.2 Schematic of the pathways for labyrinthine infection and inflammation. Meningogenic labyrinthitis occurs in the setting of acute meningitis, with infection passing to the inner ear via the internal auditory canal and cochlear modiolus or the cochlear aqueduct, as shown in the upper panel. The lower panel illustrates the proposed pathway for tympanogenic labyrinthitis. Disease can extend directly via a labyrinthine fistula, often caused by a cholesteatoma or trauma, or infectious mediators may pass via the round window during an episode of acute otitis media

Up to 40% of patients who survive bacterial meningitis are found to have permanent sensorineural hearing loss [48–50], resulting from the spread of infection and inflammatory mediators directly to the inner ear [55, 60]. Both the cochlear modiolus and the cochlear aqueduct [34, 47] have been implicated in the pathway for so-called *meningogenic labyrinthitis.* The structure of the modiolus—permeated with multiple perineural and perivascular channels—lends itself to disease spread [34]. Several animal and human temporal bone studies have demonstrated that modiolar inflammation in patients with a history of meningogenic labyrinthitis supports this pathway of inflammation [34, 47]. Presence of

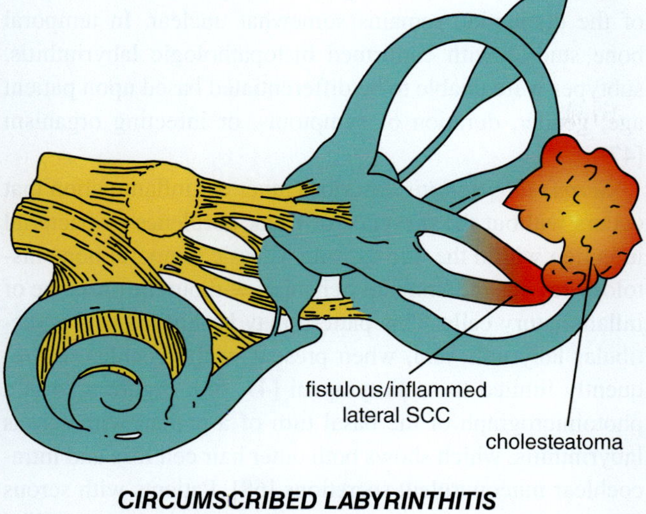

Fig. 55.3 Schematic of circumscribed labyrinthitis. Inflammation of the labyrinth—indicated by focal erythema in the diagram—is limited to a specific area. Frequently, circumscribed disease is seen following erosion of the lateral semicircular canal by a cholesteatoma, as pictured

inflammatory cells within the cochlear aqueduct was seen on a majority of specimens, presenting an alternative theory for disease spread in meningogenic disease [47].

While meningogenic labyrinthitis tends to result in a complete, diffuse inflammation of the membranous labyrinth, tympanogenic disease has been associated with both diffuse disease in some cases and in localized, limited inflammation in others. Localized disease has been described in the literature as *circumscribed labyrinthitis* [34, 64, 65]. This classification of labyrinthitis may be used to describe inflammation of specific and limited areas of the labyrinth, such as the membranous lateral semicircular canal when cholesteatomatous erosion of the bony canal has occurred. Fig. 55.3 illustrates a possible pattern of such an infection.

Evaluation

Classically, the presenting symptoms in patients with labyrinthitis will vary depending on the pathophysiology. Patients with tympanogenic labyrinthitis will have the clinical findings of labyrinthitis described above (vertigo and SNHL) in the setting of acute or chronic otitis media. Meningogenic labyrinthitis is typically discovered during or after a patient has developed meningitis with the classic and severe findings of fever, nuchal rigidity, photophobia, nausea, vomiting, and mental status changes. Since patients with meningitis are typically severely ill and often obtunded, the hearing loss and vertigo produced upon labyrinthine involvement may not become clinically apparent until the meningitis has resolved resulting in a delay in diagnosis of meningogenic labyrinthitis.

Otoscopy in tympanogenic labyrinthitis may typically reveal a bulging or erythematous tympanic membrane and middle ear purulence, or the classic findings of chronic otitis media including tympanic membrane perforation, purulent otorrhea, and/or cholesteatoma. Otoscopy in patients with meningogenic labyrinthitis is typically normal.

Audiometry in tympanogenic labyrinthitis demonstrates a unilateral (typically) mixed hearing loss with the asymmetric masked bone conduction thresholds confirming a sensorineural component due to labyrinthine involvement. In contrast, a pure, sensorineural hearing loss typifies meningogenic labyrinthitis and can involve one or both ears. The severity of the sensorineural loss in both types of labyrinthitis can vary in severity from mild-to-profound, typically with higher frequencies more severely affected.

Spontaneous nystagmus is frequently a presenting sign of labyrinthitis. It is most often beating in the direction of the unaffected ear, though patients may also demonstrate spontaneous nystagmus toward the infected ear during a brief initial period of disease. A recent review of patients with labyrinthitis secondary to acute otitis media revealed several patterns of spontaneous nystagmus, though the most common was direction-fixed toward the affected ear, which was postulated to be due to excito-toxic effects of inflammatory mediators on the afferent vestibular nerve fibers [66].

Additional Testing

As with vestibular neuritis, additional testing such as VNG and VEMP are not necessary to make the diagnosis in patients with clinically and audiologically apparent findings of labyrinthitis, whether tympanogenic or meningogenic. Vestibular testing may be performed in patients with labyrinthitis after their acute infectious process has been treated to evaluate the extent of labyrinthine dysfunction or in cases of incomplete recovery.

Similar to the workup for vestibular neuritis, imaging studies are not typically required for the diagnosis of labyrinthitis per se but can provide helpful adjuvant information regarding the inner and middle ear. When obtained, radiologic findings follow patterns of disease seen on postmortem histology, with tympanogenic disease more frequently associated with circumscribed inflammation limited to the basal turn of the cochlea, while diffuse labyrinthine involvement typifies meningogenic disease. MRI, when ordered, may demonstrate enhancement of the membranous labyrinth after administration of intravenous contrast. T1 sequences will show labyrinthine enhancement during the acute phase of labyrinthitis, and, in some cases, hyperintense T1 signals prior to the administration of contrast can suggest a secondary intralabyrinthine hemorrhage [67].

Computed tomography (CT) scan of the temporal bone is a helpful adjuvant for assessment of the bony structures of the middle and inner ear in cases of tympanogenic labyrinthitis. When cholesteatoma is present, CT can be particularly helpful to delineate the extent of disease and to demonstrate any extension into the otic capsule, which is important to identify given that definitive surgical treatment of the cholesteatoma will be needed. The role of CT scan for labyrinthitis in the setting of acute otitis media or chronic otitis media without cholesteatoma is less clear as it may not meaningfully impact treatment decisions.

Diagnosis

Two subtypes of labyrinthitis have been historically described based on the histopathologic findings associated with the disease. Post-mortem temporal bone studies have described the difference between these inflammatory patterns, but the distinction between the two can be difficult to make clinically [47], especially during the acute phase, and the utility of the distinction remains somewhat unclear. In temporal bone studies with confirmed histopathologic labyrinthitis, subtypes were unable to be differentiated based upon patient age, gender, duration of symptoms, or infecting organism [47].

Serous labyrinthitis describes inner ear inflammation that occurs without the presence of frank purulence or bacterial infection within the otic capsule. Classic temporal bone histology reveals inflammatory changes without the presence of inflammatory cells. This pattern may be limited to the vestibular labyrinth, and, when present in the cochlea, is frequently limited to scala tympani [47, 68]. Figure 55.4 is a photomicrograph of the basal turn of a patient with serous labyrinthitis, which shows both outer hair cell loss and intracochlear mucopurulent secretions [68]. Patients with serous disease often experience severe symptoms during the initial period of infection, but may be less likely to develop complete vestibular loss or profound permanent hearing changes.

Suppurative labyrinthitis is the frankly pyogenic infection of the inner ear that is histopathologically characterized by inflammatory changes and the presence of inflammatory

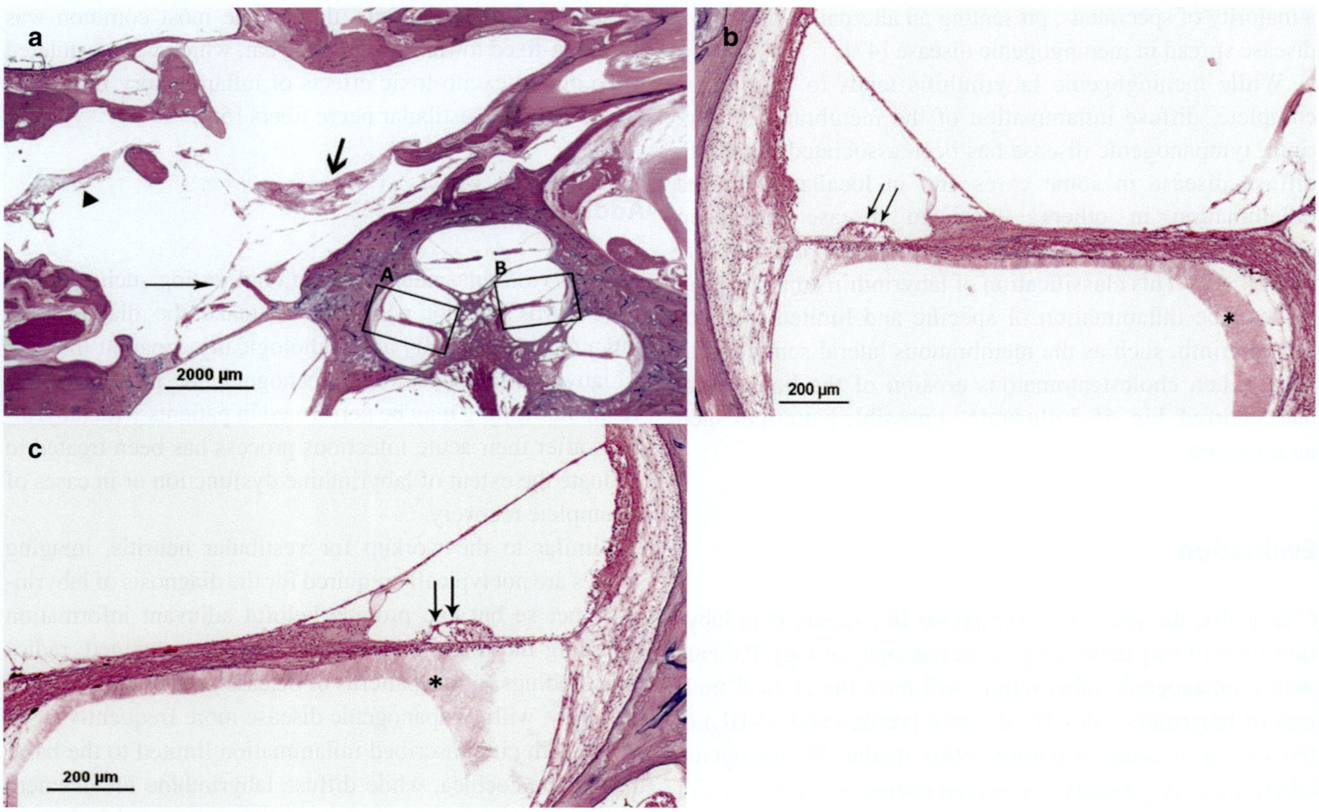

Fig. 55.4 Photomicrograph showing loss of outer hair cells (OHCs) in the temporal bone from an 18-year-old man with serous labyrinthitis. (**a**) Low-power image of upper basal turn and lower middle turn. Thick arrow = mucopurulent secretion; thin arrow = fibrous structure; arrowhead = fibrocystic structure. (**b**) Enlarged view of box A. Arrows = loss of OHCs. * serous labyrinthitis. (**c**) Enlarged view of box B. Arrows = loss of OHCs. * Serous labyrinthitis. Staining with hematoxylin-eosin (H&E). (Reprinted with permission from Kaya et al. [68])

cells and frank purulence in scala tympani, which may or may not extend to involve scala vestibuli and the vestibular labyrinth [34]. A small portion of cases with severe disease can demonstrate complete destruction of the organ of Corti [47], hair cell loss [47, 69], and atrophy of the stria vascularis [69]. Individuals with suppurative labyrinthitis are more likely to develop complete unilateral loss of vestibular function and unserviceable profound unilateral hearing loss.

Differential Diagnosis

The abrupt onset and time course of symptoms narrow the differential diagnosis to one of only a few peripheral vestibulopathies, including labyrinthitis, vestibular neuritis, Ménière's disease, and cerebello pontine angle (CPA) mass. The presence of cochlear symptoms will help to exclude the diagnosis of vestibular neuritis, and it is rare that a CPA mass would produce the abrupt onset, severe symptoms seen in labyrinthitis. If needed, an MRI may be utilized to rule out an underlying intracranial mass; however, the clinically evident meningitis or otitis media that lead to labyrinthitis make the diagnosis clear in most cases.

Course

The course of labyrinthitis is in many ways similar to that of vestibular neuritis, with an acute early phase of severe disabling vertigo, often associated with significant nausea and vomiting. The severe presenting vestibular symptoms can last days to weeks, but may be associated with a waxing and waning course during this time. There is some suggestion in the literature that serous disease is associated with milder symptoms and the severe, fulminant vertigo is more commonly seen in suppurative disease. This pattern may also be applicable to changes in hearing, with those who have suppurative disease more likely to experience a profound permanent hearing loss and those with serous disease more likely to have a partial hearing loss and show potential for some recovery. As in vestibular neuritis, after resolution of the acute phase of symptoms, patients may continue to experience persistent instability or disequilibrium for weeks to months. As mentioned above, labyrinthitis differs from vestibular neuritis in the presence of hearing loss with labyrinthitis that typically occurs coincident with the onset of vestibular symptoms and may or may not recover.

Labyrinthitis may be complicated by the development of *labyrinthitis ossificans,* which is a process of neo-osteogenesis that occurs after a delay of weeks to months [70] within the labyrinth after an initial period of acute inflammation [34, 71, 72]. It is more commonly associated with suppurative disease and is frequently a sequela of meningitis [60, 73], though it has occurred after tympanogenic disease and chronic otitis [74, 75]. After the initial infection associated with labyrinthitis, the acute inflammatory response results in fibrous changes within the perilymphatic spaces, including the deposition of fibroblasts, the development of granulation tissue, and the beginning of neovascularization [34]. This fibrous stage of inflammation is followed by an osseous stage, during which woven bone is deposited in a disorganized fashion throughout the inner ear. This bone is slowly resorbed, remodeled, and mineralized into dense lamellar bone [34, 76]; the pathogenesis underlying labyrinthitis ossificans may result in complete ossification of the cochlea in the most severe cases [71].

Treatment

Treatment of labyrinthitis varies depending on the etiology and pathophysiology of the disease. With viral disease, as in vestibular neuritis, treatment is primarily supportive. Treatment should avoid the use of vestibular suppressant medications that would prolong central compensation for any permanent loss in vestibular function. With severe vertigo or in special populations, hospitalization may be required to provide intravenous hydration and supportive care during the severe phase of the disease.

Treatment for bacteria-mediated disease will be directed by the underlying source of infection. In tympanogenic labyrinthitis due to acute otitis media (AOM), initial management includes oral antibiotics and possibly tympanostomy with culture of middle ear debris and ototopical antibiotic therapy in more severe cases. Depending on the status of the tympanic membrane, chronic otitis media without cholesteatoma may be managed similarly. Consideration should be given to combined ototopical and culture-directed oral or parenteral antibiotic therapy for patients with worsening clinical courses despite initial measures as above. If cholesteatoma is present, or in patients without cholesteatoma who are unresponsive to the measures above, a tympanomastoidectomy should be performed for removal of cholesteatoma (if present) and/or to reduce the middle ear and mastoid infectious burden [77–79]. While anti-inflammatory treatment with steroids may be of theoretical benefit in reducing the cochlear inflammatory response in tympanogenic disease, their use has not been well-validated in the literature to date for this indication [80].

The treatment of meningogenic labyrinthitis is directed towards the underlying meningitis with prompt administration of broad-spectrum parenteral antibiotics to prevent mortality and avoid systemic morbidities associated with meningitis. Narrowing of coverage directed to bacteria isolated on lumbar puncture in patients with meningitis follows the critical initial period of broad spectrum coverage with the total duration of parenteral antibiotic treatment ranging between four and eight weeks in general. Concurrent anti-inflammatory treatment with steroids is theorized to reduce the cochlear inflammatory response and has been shown in a recent Cochrane systematic review to improve hearing outcomes in high-income countries for patients with meningitis [81]. An important aspect of management in meningogenic disease when subjective hearing loss has become evident is the timely assessment of auditory function through inpatient bedside audiometric testing, auditory brainstem response testing, otoacoustic emission testing, or a combination of these tests. Early identification of a severe to profound hearing loss is of the utmost importance [48, 49]. Labyrinthitis ossificans may occur as early as three weeks following meningitis [70], and the presence of neo-osteogenesis may significantly complicate cochlear implantation, if deemed necessary. Early implantation in such cases may avoid less than favorable auditory outcomes associated with drill-out procedures or incomplete insertions that may be a consequence of cochlear ossification.

References

1. Dix MR, Hallpike CS. The pathology, symptomatology and diagnosis of certain common disorders of the vestibular system. Ann Otol Rhinol Laryngol. 1952;61(4):987–1016.
2. Schuknecht HF, Kitamura K. Vestibular neuritis. Ann Otol Rhinol Laryngol Suppl. 1981;90(1 Pt 2):1–19.
3. Neuhauser HK. Epidemiology of vertigo. Curr Opin Neurol. 2007;20(1):40–6.
4. Newman-Toker DE, Hsieh Y-H, Camargo CA, Pelletier AJ, Butchy GT, Edlow JA. Spectrum of dizziness visits to US emergency departments: cross-sectional analysis from a nationally representative sample. Mayo Clin Proc. 2008;83(7):765–75.
5. Guilemany JM, Martínez P, Prades E, Sañudo I, De España R, Cuchi A. Clinical and epidemiological study of vertigo at an outpatient clinic. Acta Otolaryngol. 2004;124(1):49–52.
6. Huppert D, Strupp M, Theil D, Glaser M, Brandt T. Low recurrence rate of vestibular neuritis: a long-term follow-up. Neurology. 2006;67(10):1870–1.
7. Sekitani T, Imate Y, Noguchi T, Inokuma T. Vestibular neuronitis: epidemiological survey by questionnaire in Japan. Acta Otolaryngol Suppl. 1993;503:9–12.
8. Fetter M, Dichgans J. Vestibular neuritis spares the inferior division of the vestibular nerve. Brain. 1996;119(Pt 3):755–63.
9. Greco A, Macri GF, Gallo A, et al. Is vestibular neuritis an immune related vestibular neuropathy inducing vertigo? J Immunol Res. 2014;2014:459048.
10. Bartual-Pastor J. Vestibular neuritis: etiopathogenesis. Rev Laryngol Otol Rhinol (Bord). 2005;126(4):279–81.
11. Richard C, Linthicum FH. Vestibular neuritis: the vertigo disappears, the histological traces remain. Otol Neurotol. 2012;33(7):e59–60.
12. Esaki S, Goshima F, Kimura H, et al. Auditory and vestibular defects induced by experimental labyrinthitis following herpes simplex virus in mice. Acta Otolaryngol. 2011;131(7):684–91.
13. Arbusow V, Derfuss T, Held K, et al. Latency of herpes simplex virus type-1 in human geniculate and vestibular ganglia is associated with infiltration of CD8+ T cells. J Med Virol. 2010;82(11):1917–20.
14. Gacek RR, Gacek MR. The three faces of vestibular ganglionitis. Ann Otol Rhinol Laryngol. 2002;111(2):103–14.
15. Theil D, Arbusow V, Derfuss T, et al. Prevalence of HSV-1 LAT in human trigeminal, geniculate, and vestibular ganglia and its implication for cranial nerve syndromes. Brain Pathol. 2001;11(4):408–13.
16. Arbusow V, Schulz P, Strupp M, et al. Distribution of herpes simplex virus type 1 in human geniculate and vestibular ganglia: implications for vestibular neuritis. Ann Neurol. 1999;46(3):416–9.
17. Baloh RW, Ishyama A, Wackym PA, Honrubia V. Vestibular neuritis: clinical-pathologic correlation. Otolaryngol Head Neck Surg. 1996;114(4):586–92.
18. Monstad P, Økstad S, Mygland Å. Inferior vestibular neuritis: 3 cases with clinical features of acute vestibular neuritis, normal calorics but indications of saccular failure. BMC Neurol. 2006;6:45.
19. Baloh RW. Clinical practice. Vestibular neuritis. N Engl J Med. 2003;348(11):1027–32.
20. Aw ST, Fetter M, Cremer PD, Karlberg M, Halmagyi GM. Individual semicircular canal function in superior and inferior vestibular neuritis. Neurology. 2001;57(5):768–74.
21. Gianoli G, Goebel J, Mowry S, Poomipannit P. Anatomic differences in the lateral vestibular nerve channels and their implications in vestibular neuritis. Otol Neurotol. 2005;26(3):489–94.
22. Goebel JA, O'Mara W, Gianoli G. Anatomic considerations in vestibular neuritis. Otol Neurotol. 2001;22(4):512–8.
23. Bartolomeo M, Biboulet R, Pierre G, Mondain M, Uziel A, Venail F. Value of the video head impulse test in assessing vestibular deficits following vestibular neuritis. Eur Arch Otorrinolaringol. 2013;271(4):681–8.
24. Magliulo G, Gagliardi S, Ciniglio Appiani M, Iannella G, Re M. Vestibular neurolabyrinthitis: a follow-up study with cervical and ocular vestibular evoked myogenic potentials and the video head impulse test. Ann Otol Rhinol Laryngol. 2014;123(3):162–73.
25. Walther LE, Blödow A. Ocular vestibular evoked myogenic potential to air conducted sound stimulation and video head impulse test in acute vestibular neuritis. Otol Neurotol. 2013;34(6):1084–9.
26. Karlberg M, Annertz M, Magnusson M. Acute vestibular neuritis visualized by 3-T magnetic resonance imaging with high-dose gadolinium. Arch Otolaryngol Head Neck Surg. 2004;130(2):229–32.
27. Mandalà M, Santoro GP, Awrey J, Nuti D. Vestibular neuritis: recurrence and incidence of secondary benign paroxysmal positional vertigo. Acta Otolaryngol. 2010;130(5):565–7.
28. Strupp M, Zingler VC, Arbusow V, et al. Methylprednisolone, valacyclovir, or the combination for vestibular neuritis. N Engl J Med. 2004;351(4):354–61.
29. Kim JC, Cha WW, Chang DS, Lee HY. The effect of intravenous dexamethasone on the nausea accompanying vestibular neuritis: a preliminary study. Clin Ther. 2015;37(11):2536–42.
30. Shupak A, Issa A, Golz A, Kaminer M, Braverman I. Prednisone treatment for vestibular neuritis. Otol Neurotol. 2008;29(3):368–74.
31. Magliulo G, Iannella G, Gagliardi S, Re M. A 1-year follow-up study with C-VEMPs, O-VEMPs and video head impulse testing in vestibular neuritis. Eur Arch Otorrinolaringol. 2015;272(11):3277–81.
32. Baloh RW, Honrubia V, Jacobson K. Benign positional vertigo: clinical and oculographic features in 240 cases. Neurology. 1987;37(3):371–81.
33. Thompson TL, Amedee R. Vertigo: a review of common peripheral and central vestibular disorders. Ochsner J. 2009;9(1):20–6.
34. Paparella MM, Sugiura S. The pathology of suppurative labyrinthitis. Ann Otol Rhinol Laryngol. 1967;76(3):554–86.
35. Druss JG. Pathways of infection in labyrinthitis: report of three different types. Arch Otolaryngol. 1929;9(4):392–403.
36. Altmann F, Waltner JG. Labyrinthitis following purulent infection of the middle ear: histopathologic studies. Arch Otolaryngol. 1945;42(2):93–109.

37. Karmody CS. Viral labyrinthitis: early pathology in the human. Laryngoscope. 1983;93(12):1527–33.
38. Lindsay JR. Viral labyrinthitis-histopathologic characteristics. Acta Otolaryngol. 1967;63(2–3):138–43.
39. O'Connor TP. Toxic labyrinthitis of nasopharyngeal origin. Laryngoscope. 1936;46(12):926–30.
40. Broughton SS, Meyerhoff WE, Cohen SB. Immune-mediated inner ear disease: 10-year experience. Semin Arthritis Rheum. 2004;34(2):544–8.
41. McCabe BF. Autoimmune sensorineural hearing loss. Ann Otol Rhinol Laryngol. 1979;88(5 Pt 1):585–9.
42. Beyea JA, Agrawal SK, Parnes LS. Transmastoid semicircular canal occlusion: a safe and highly effective treatment for benign paroxysmal positional vertigo and superior canal dehiscence. Laryngoscope. 2012;122(8):1862–6.
43. Grosse SD, Ross DS, Dollard SC. Congenital cytomegalovirus (CMV) infection as a cause of permanent bilateral hearing loss: a quantitative assessment. J Clin Virol. 2008;41(2):57.
44. Davis LE. Comparative experimental viral labyrinthitis. Am J Otolaryngol. 1990;11(6):382–8.
45. Stagno S, Pass RF, Dworsky ME, Alford CA. Congenital and perinatal cytomegalovirus infections. Semin Perinatol. 1983;7(1):31–42.
46. Kimberlin DW, Jester PM, Sánchez PJ, et al. Valganciclovir for symptomatic congenital cytomegalovirus disease. N Engl J Med. 2015;372(10):933–43.
47. Merchant SN, Gopen Q. A human temporal bone study of acute bacterial meningogenic labyrinthitis. Am J Otol. 1996;17(3):375–85.
48. Rodenburg-Vlot MBA, Ruytjens L, Oostenbrink R, Goedegebure A, van der Schroeff MP. Systematic review: incidence and course of hearing loss caused by bacterial meningitis: in search of an optimal timed Audiological follow-up. Otol Neurotol. 2016;37(1):1–8.
49. Karanja BW, Oburra HO, Masinde P, Wamalwa D. Prevalence of hearing loss in children following bacterial meningitis in a tertiary referral hospital. BMC Res Notes. 2014;7(1):138.
50. Worsøe L, Cayé Thomasen P, Brandt CT, Thomsen J, Østergaard C. Factors associated with the occurrence of hearing loss after pneumococcal meningitis. Clin Infect Dis. 2010;51(8):917–24.
51. Teszler CB, Williams MT, Belange G, Ayache D. Labyrinthitis related to Wegener granulomatosis: magnetic resonance imaging findings. Otol Neurotol. 2008;29(5):721–2.
52. García-Berrocal JR, Ramírez-Camacho R, Trinidad A, Zurita M, la Fuente de R, Lobo D. Controversies and criticisms on designs for experimental autoimmune labyrinthitis. Ann Otol Rhinol Laryngol. 2004;113(5):404–10.
53. Tomiyama S, Jinnouchi K, Ikezono T, Pawankar R, Yagi T. Experimental autoimmune labyrinthitis induced by cell-mediated immune reaction. Acta Otolaryngol. 1999;119(6):665–70.
54. Mysel P. LXXI Diagnosis and treatment of Labyrinthitis secondary to tympanic infection. Ann Otol Rhinol Laryngol. 194;51(3):761–73.
55. Cinelli AA. Clinical forms of labyrinthitis. Laryngoscope. 1938;48(3):157–67.
56. Engmér C, Laurell G, Bagger-Sjöbäck D, Rask-Andersen H. Immunodefense of the round window. Laryngoscope. 2008;118(6):1057–62.
57. Cureoglu S, Schachern PA, Rinaldo A. Round window membrane and labyrinthine pathological changes: an overview. Acta Otolaryngol. 2005;125(1):9–15.
58. Lumio JS. Contribution to the knowledge of Hematogenous Labyrinthitis. Acta Otolaryngol. 1949;37(1):80–4.
59. Dean LW, Wolff D. LVII. Pathology and routes of infection in Labyrinthitis secondary to middle ear otitis. Ann Otol Rhinol Laryngol. 1934;43:702–17.
60. Druss JG. Labyrinthitis secondary to meningococcic meningitis: a clinical and histopathologic study. Arch Otolaryngol. 1936;24(1):19–28.
61. Mackenzie GW. Suppurative labyrinthitis with report of cases. Ann Otol Rhinol Laryngol. 1927;36:1019–59.
62. Sahni RS, Paparella MM, Schachern PA, Goycoolea MV, Le CT. Thickness of the human round window membrane in different forms of otitis media. Arch Otolaryngol Head Neck Surg. 1987;113(6):630–4.
63. Schachern PA, Paparella MM, Hybertson R, Sano S, Duvall AJ. Bacterial tympanogenic labyrinthitis, meningitis, and sensorineural damage. Arch Otolaryngol Head Neck Surg. 1992;118(1):53–7.
64. Hilding DA, Kornfeld M, House WF. Circumscribed labyrinthitis. Laryngoscope. 1967;77(3):317–29.
65. Ruttin E. XLII. The pathology of Labyrinthitis. Ann Otol Rhinol Laryngol 1912;21(3): 557–580.
66. Kim C-H, Yang YS, Im D, Shin JE. Nystagmus in patients with unilateral acute otitis media complicated by serous labyrinthitis. Acta Otolaryngol. 2016;136(6):559–63.
67. Palacios E, Valvassori G. Hemorrhagic labyrinthitis. Ear Nose Throat J. 2000;79(2):80.
68. Kaya S, Tsuprun V, Hızlı Ö, Schachern PA, Paparella MM, Cureoglu S. Cochlear changes in serous labyrinthitis associated with silent otitis media: a human temporal bone study. Am J Otolaryngol. 2016;37(2):83–8.
69. Kaya S, Tsuprun V, Hizli Ö, Paparella MM, Cureoglu S. Quantitative assessment of Cochlear histopathologic findings in patients with Suppurative Labyrinthitis. JAMA Otolaryngol Head Neck Surg. 2016;142(4):364–9.
70. Nabili V, Brodie HA, Neverov NI, Tinling SP. Chronology of labyrinthitis ossificans induced by streptococcus pneumoniae meningitis. Laryngoscope. 1999;109(6):931–5.
71. Suga F, Lindsay JR. Labyrinthitis ossificans. Ann Otol Rhinol Laryngol. 1977;86(1):17–29.
72. Sugiura S, Paparella MM. The pathology of labyrinthine ossification. Laryngoscope. 1967;77(11):1974–89.
73. Xu HX, Joglekar SS, Paparella MM. Labyrinthitis ossificans. Otol Neurotol. 2009;30(4):579–80.
74. Lin H-Y, Fan Y-K, Wu K-C, Shu M-T, Yang C-C, Lin H-C. The incidence of tympanogenic labyrinthitis ossificans. J Laryngol Otol. 2014;128(7):618–20.
75. Suga F, Lindsay JR. Labyrinthitis ossificans due to chronic otitis media. Ann Otol Rhinol Laryngol. 1975;84(1 Pt 1):37–44.
76. Bloch SL, McKenna MJ, Adams J, Friis M. Labyrinthitis Ossificans: on the mechanism of Perilabyrinthine bone remodeling. Ann Otol Rhinol Laryngol. 2015;124(8):649–54.
77. Friesner I, Rosenwasser H. Treatment of labyrinthitis. Arch Otolaryngol. 1934;20(2):139–51.
78. Henninger LL. Differential diagnosis and treatment of acute labyrinthitis. Laryngoscope. 1913;23(7):781–6.
79. Shambaugh GE. XIII. When to operate on the labyrinth in labyrinth infection secondary to purulent otitis media. Ann Otol Rhinol Laryngol. 1913;22(2):303–7.
80. Heywood RL, Ifeacho SN, Narula AA. Effect of intratympanic steroid administration on sensorineural hearing loss associated with acute otitis media. J Laryngol Otol. 2016;130(6):532–5.
81. Brouwer MC, McIntyre P, Prasad K, van de Beek D. Corticosteroids for acute bacterial meningitis. Cochrane Database Syst Rev. 2015;12(9):CD004405.

Superior Semicircular Canal Dehiscence Syndrome

56

Benjamin T. Crane, Bryan K. Ward, and John P. Carey

Introduction

First described about 25 years ago, superior canal dehiscence syndrome (SCDS) [1] has well understood pathophysiology, and curative surgery is now regularly performed throughout the world [2–4]. The pathophysiology of SCDS is attributed to the presence of a "third mobile window" in addition to the normally present oval and round windows [5]. With this abnormal opening in the labyrinth at the superior semicircular canal, pressure entering the labyrinth via the stapes at the oval window is partially shunted away from the round window to a new, low impedance superior canal pathway. Bone conducted sound also now has a new route of entrance into the inner ear via the dehiscence.

Patients with SCDS often present clinically with sound-induced vertigo, oscillopsia (bouncing of vision), and decreased hearing thresholds for bone conducted sounds (i.e., conductive hyperacusis) while having increased thresholds for air conducted sounds. While the latter can lead to difficulty hearing external air conducted sound, it also causes heightened perception of bone conducted sound so patients can hear their pulse, eye movements, chewing, or footsteps and experience autophony. Dizziness and vertigo symptoms are also common and can be disabling. These symptoms include chronic disequilibrium as well as vertigo induced by loud sound or pressure changes [2, 6–8].

Diagnostic Evaluation

A thorough history is important for any patient presenting with complaints of dizziness. Patients with SCDS usually present with a primary complaint of either autophony or dizziness, although occasionally, isolated conductive hearing loss (CHL) [9] that can mimic otosclerosis is seen. Vertigo related to SCDS is usually brief and induced by loud sounds or pressure changes. Sound-induced dizziness or oscillopsia, otherwise known as Tullio phenomenon, is present in 90% of SCDS patients [8]. Pressure-induced vestibular symptoms, which often manifest with coughing or straining, are present in 73% of patients, with 67% exhibiting both pressure and sound-related symptoms [8]. Chronic disequilibrium may also be attributed to SCDS [10].

Auditory symptoms are common and may be present in 85% of SCDS cases [11]. Hyperacusis for bone-conducted sound [12, 13] is present in 52% [8]. Symptoms often include hearing one's pulse or eye movements. Autophony, defined as the patient's own voice sounding disturbing to them, is present in up to 60% of patients [8, 14].

Evoked eye movements in the plane of the superior canal are the hallmark clinical finding of SCDS [15, 16]. The eyes should be examined under Frenzel or video goggles to eliminate visual fixation. Tones at levels up to 110 dB normalized hearing level (nHL) should be delivered in one ear at a time. Sound-evoked eye movements were noted in 82% of SCDS patients [8]. Eye movements can also be induced with Valsalva maneuvers (75%) or pressure applied to the external auditory canal (45%). Depending on the type of stimulus either excitation or inhibition of the superior canal may occur (Fig. 56.1). Eye movements evoked by pressure or sound almost always occur in the superior canal plane (Fig. 56.2). If eye movements occur in another direction, the SCDS diagnosis should be questioned. In such a case, alternative diagnoses can include posterior canal dehiscence [17] or horizontal canal fistula [18]. Sound evoked rotation of the head in the superior canal plane can occur in 14% of patients.

The audiogram (Fig. 56.3) is an important part of the SCDS evaluation, and a minority of patients have only auditory symptoms [8, 9, 19, 20]. Conductive hearing loss (CHL) is often largest at lower frequencies [9, 19, 21], and bone conduction thresholds can be negative (conductive hyperacu-

B. T. Crane (✉)
University of Rochester School of Medicine, Strong Memorial Hospital, Rochester, NY, USA

B. K. Ward · J. P. Carey
Department of Otolaryngology—Head and Neck Surgery, Johns Hopkins University School of Medicine, Baltimore, MD, USA
e-mail: Bward15@jhmi.edu; jcarey@jhmi.edu

A. D. Sweeney et al. (eds.), *Haynes-Glasscock-Shambaugh Surgery of the Ear*, https://doi.org/10.1007/978-3-032-18264-7_56

sis). Because of the CHL and normal appearance of the ear, some patients with primarily auditory symptoms have been misdiagnosed as having otosclerosis [20]. Key differences between SCDS and otosclerosis in terms of clinical and audiologic findings include (1) conductive *hyperacusis* does not occur in otosclerosis and (2) the acoustic stapedial reflex, which is often normal in superior canal dehiscence, is generally absent in otosclerosis.

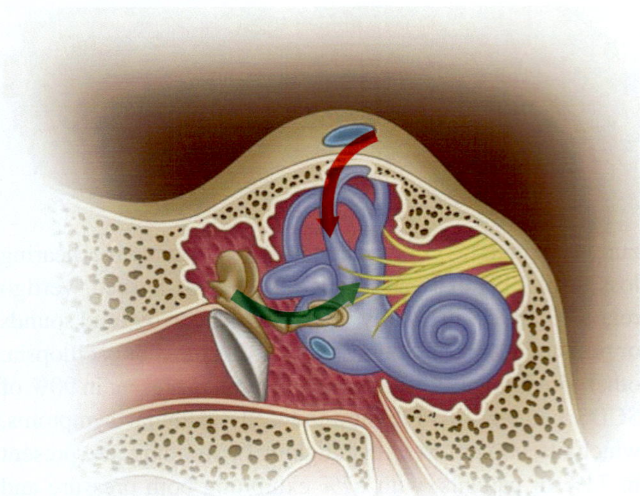

Fig. 56.1 Route of pressure changes causing stimulation of the superior canal ampulla in SCDS. Superior canal inhibition is caused by ampulopetal displacement of the cupula (red arrow) from negative external auditory canal pressure or glottic Valsalva maneuver, which transiently increases intracranial pressure. Superior canal excitation is caused by ampulofugal displacement of the cupula (green arrow) typically by positive external auditory canal pressure, nasal Valsalva, or sound. (Adapted from Diagnosis and Treatment of Vestibular Disorders. Eds. Babu. Schutt and Bojrab, Springer. 2019)

Vestibular evoked myogenic potential (VEMP) responses are enhanced in SCDS. The cervical VEMP (cVEMP) is measured from the sternocleidomastoid muscles using averaged electromyography in response to multiple loud clicks or tone bursts delivered to the ear. The reflex is thought to be activated by sound transmitted through the stapes footplate to the saccule and inferior vestibular nerve [22]. Decreased cVEMP thresholds are indicative of SCDS. For air-conducted 500 Hz tone bursts, for example, cVEMP thresholds were 80–95 dB sound pressure level (SPL) for 13 patients with SCDS (83.85 ± 1.40 dB SPL, mean ± SD), 20–30 dB lower than in normal control subjects (110.25 ± 1.28 dB SPL) [23]. It has been argued that cVEMP is better than 90% sensitive and specific for a superior canal dehiscence (SCD) [24] but sensitivity and specificity depend on the parameters used [25]. Ocular VEMP (oVEMP) similarly measures averaged electromyography in response to tone bursts delivered to the ear or sometimes forehead taps. The oVEMP reflex is thought to be activated by sound or vibration being transmitted via the utricle and superior vestibular nerve to the contralateral inferior oblique muscle [26, 27]. The amplitude of this excitatory potential is measured at surface recording electrodes placed beneath the eyes. Some centers prefer oVEMP to cVEMP because it is easily tolerated and may be a more sensitive and specific diagnostic test for SCDS than the cVEMP [28–30]. oVEMP testing can also be done quickly because it does not require finding the response threshold. As a result, oVEMP testing is becoming more widely available at aca-

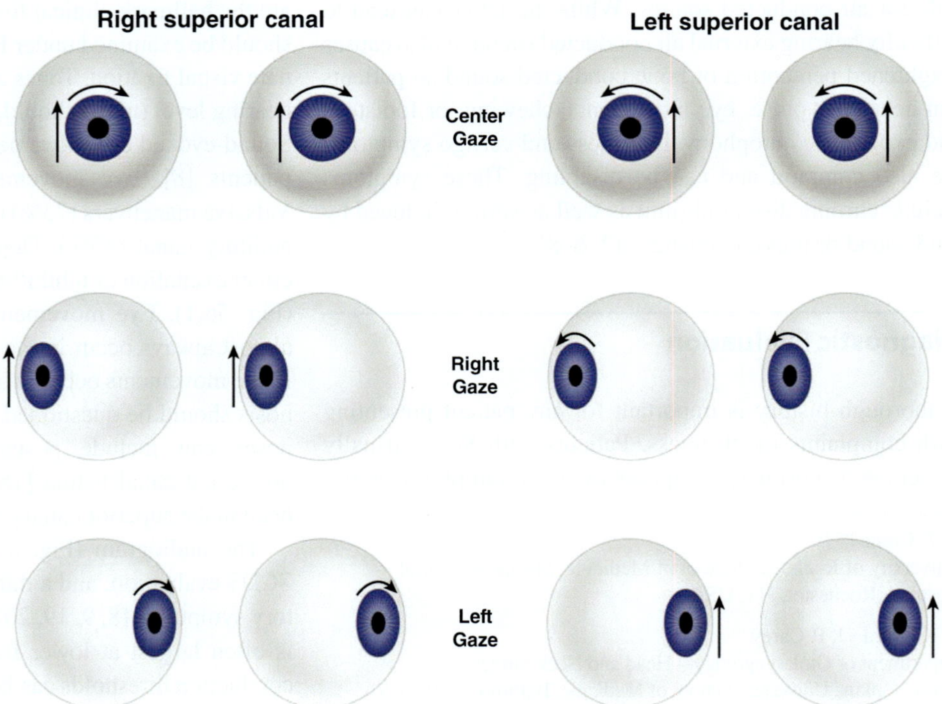

Fig. 56.2 The slow phase of nystagmus with superior canal excitation occurs in the plane of the superior canal regardless of gaze direction. There are both vertical and torsional components when the patient is looking directly ahead (center gaze). The components can be separated by having the patient look to the right or left during stimulation. (Adapted from Surgery of the Ear. Eds. Gulya, Minor, Poe. PMPH. 2010)

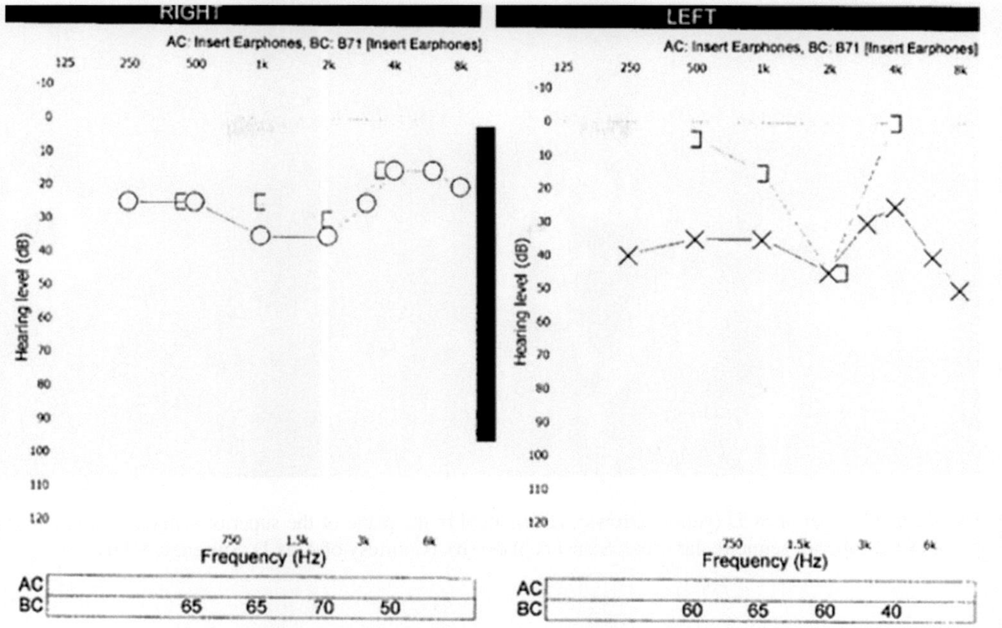

Reflex	Threshold (dB HL)					Decay (s)	
	500	1k	2k	4k	BBN	500	1k
R Ipsi	90	100	90				
L Ipsi	95	85	80				
R Contra	85	90	90				
L Contra	95	90	90				

Probe tone: 226 Hz

Fig. 56.3 Audiogram in a patient with left SCDS. Os and Xs represent air conduction and brackets represent bone conduction. There are negative bone conduction thresholds on the left relative to the right ear, and based on the bone threshold elevation at 2000 Hz, the patient was initially referred for the evaluation of "otosclerosis." The air–bone gap is largest at low frequencies, and reflexes are present (Courtesy of Alex D. Sweeney, MD)

demic centers. Despite their utility in diagnosing SCDS, these tests are poorly correlated with patient symptom severity [31].

The VEMP is not always measurable and is likely to be absent in those with previous middle ear surgery or conductive hearing loss due to ossicular dysfunction. Although the oVEMP can circumvent this problem using forehead taps [29], this version of the test is less commonly available. The VEMP threshold may also be decreased in other conditions such as enlarged vestibular aqueduct syndrome [32]. The use of VEMP can also differentiate SCDS from middle ear causes of conductive hearing loss in which VEMP responses should be absent [33].

Imaging of the temporal bone using computed tomography (CT) must show the absence of bone over the superior canal (SC) for SCDS to be considered (Fig. 56.4). If the SC appears surrounded with bone on CT, the diagnosis of SCDS is excluded; however, the appearance of a dehiscence on CT does not rule out thin bone covering the SC below the resolution of the scanner. Thus, CT is a highly sensitive test for SCD, but it is not specific [34] due to a high rate of false positives in conventional multi-detector scanners. In a review of temporal bone CT scans done in the general population 9% of scans had apparent SCD with one observer calling as many as 12% [35]. Many are likely false positives caused by the limits of resolving thin bone, since the incidence of SCD in a survey of temporal bones was only 0.7% [36]. However, due to the high risk of false positive findings and overestimation of dehiscence size [37], the diagnosis of SCD must never be based on a CT alone.

Magnetic resonance imaging (MRI) may suggest SCD [38]. The best images are heavily T2-weighted protocols (e.g., Constructive Interference in Steady State, or CISS) and reconstructed in the plane of the superior canal. However, even these protocols may have a high false positive rate, and CT is the better study for most evaluations. MRI may be useful postoperatively for evaluating the efficacy of previous canal plugging by assessing the fluid signal in the superior canal [39].

Overall, the diagnosis of SCDS should be based on CT imaging showing a dehiscence, symptoms consistent with a mobile third window, and at least one physiologic measure supporting the presence of a third mobile window. The diagnostic criteria for the diagnosis of SCDS [6] are shown in Table 56.1.

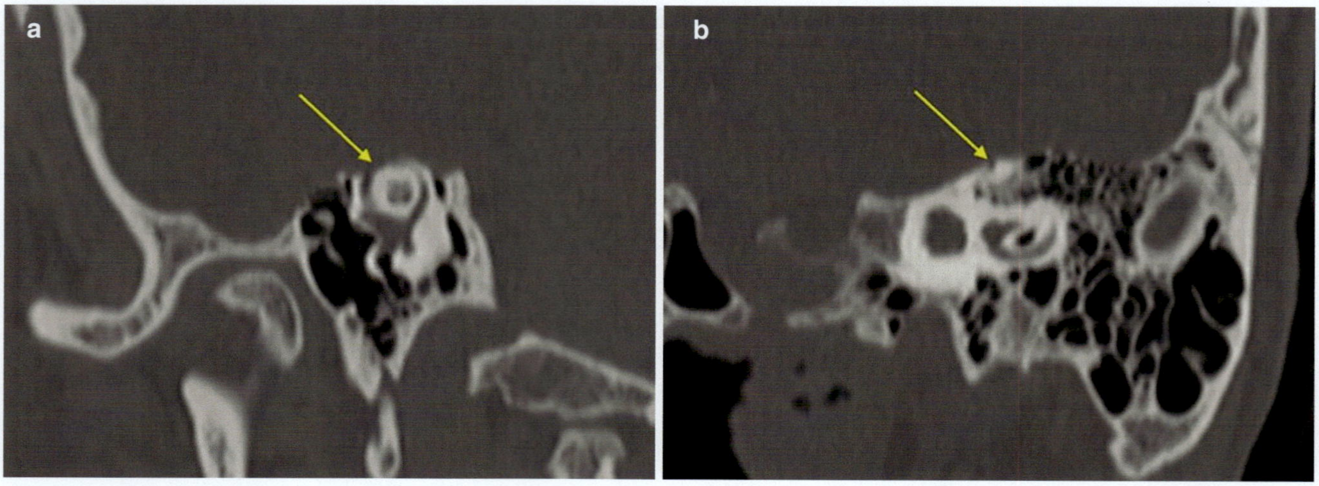

Fig. 56.4 CT scan of SCD (yellow arrows), reformatted in the plane of the superior semicircular canal, Pöschl plane (**a**) and orthogonal to the plane of the superior semicircular canal, Stenvers plane (**b**). (Courtesy of Alex D. Sweeney, MD)

Table 56.1 Bárány Society Criteria for superior semicircular canal dehiscence syndrome (SCDS) diagnosis

Diagnostic criteria for superior semicircular canal dehiscence syndrome
1. At least one of the following symptoms consistent with a third window lesion of the inner ear: 1. Bone conduction hyperacusis 2. Sound-induced vertigo and/or oscillopsia time-locked to the stimulus 3. Pressure-induced vertigo and/or oscillopsia time locked to the stimulus 4. Pulsatile tinnitus
2. At least one of the following diagnostic tests indicating a third mobile window of the inner ear: 1. Nystagmus characteristic of excitation or inhibition of the affected superior canal evoked by sound (Tullio phenomenon) or changes in middle ear pressure (Hennebert sign) or intracranial pressure 2. Low-frequency negative bone conduction thresholds on pure tone audiometry 3. Enhanced VEMP responses (low cervical VEMP thresholds or high ocular VEMP amplitudes)
3. High-resolution temporal bone CT imaging with multiplanar reconstructions demonstrating dehiscence of the superior canal
4. Not better accounted for by another vestibular disease or disorder

Adapted from Ref. [6]

Differential Diagnosis

Other common conditions can cause symptoms similar to SCDS, making it important to consider a differential diagnosis. When conductive hearing loss is present in a setting without trauma and with a normal otoscopic exam, SCDS should be considered along with otosclerosis. Autophony raises the possibility of a patulous Eustachian tube (PET), but SCDS can produce a similar sensation. Episodic vertigo evoked by intracranial or middle ear pressure changes could indicate a perilymphatic fistula, but SCDS should strongly be considered as an alternative diagnosis. We have seen several patients who have undergone previous surgical explorations for such presumed otological disorders, only later to be found to have SCDS.

The conductive hearing loss with SCDS often appears similar to otosclerosis because both occur in adulthood with a normal otoscopic exam [20]. The audiograms differ in that patients with SCDS often have negative bone conduction thresholds (Fig. 56.3), and if there is no previous history of middle ear surgery, the acoustic reflex is often intact.

Autophony is often the predominant symptom in patients with a patulous Eustachian tube (PET), [40] but it can also be the most disturbing symptom in SCDS [41]. One distinguishing feature is that patients with PET typically have autophony for their breath sounds (especially for nasal breathing), whereas patients with SCDS usually do not [40]. A history of vertigo and hyperacusis to bone conducted sound is atypical of a PET. The audiogram, VEMP, and CT will typically differentiate a PET and SCDS.

Perilymph fistula and fenestrations of other semicircular canals should be considered in the differential diagnosis of SCDS [42–44]. The diagnosis of perilymph fistula is most clear in the presence of recent stapes surgery, temporal bone fracture, or barotrauma injury. In these cases, acute vertigo is usually accompanied by sensorineural hearing loss. A fistula in the horizontal canal can be acquired in cases of cholesteatoma or prior mastoidectomy [45]. Spontaneous perilymph fistula is a controversial diagnosis, which if considered at all, should only be considered after all other possible causes are excluded [46].

The most common cause of spontaneous (non-positional) vertigo is vestibular migraine [47–50]. The migraine incidence is 17.6% of females and 5.7% of males [51], and approximately 25% of these report associated vertigo [52].

Migraine is much more common than SCDS, and inevitably symptoms in some patients with radiographically apparent SCD with non-specific symptoms may be better explained by migraine. Particularly challenging are those patients who have both SCDS and migraine [2, 53]. It may be difficult to determine if their sound sensitivity is due to one more than the other, for example. Their chronic disequilibrium may be related to migraine, or it may be due to the constant transmission of intracranial pressure pulsations through the dehiscence. The symptoms of SCDS could serve as triggers to exacerbate migraine in susceptible individuals. However, the neurotologist must also consider that failure to recognize and treat coexistent migraine can lead to disappointing results in SCDS surgery [50], as it can with other causes of vertigo. Optimization of migraine treatment is recommended prior to SCD surgery [2, 50, 53].

Operative Decision Making

The physician and patient must weigh the symptom severity against the risks and benefits of surgery. In the authors' experience, only a third of patients with SCDS elect to have surgery, with the remaining patients choosing to live with their symptoms or making lifestyle changes to avoid situations that exacerbate symptoms. Control of comorbid vestibular migraine has, in several cases, allowed patients to avoid surgery.

Most SCDS patients present to a neurotology clinic for dizziness or vertigo of variable severity. Some patients are disabled by their symptoms, and surgery is the only viable option for them to have an acceptable quality of life.

Autophony, or the abnormal sound of one's own voice, can be disabling. There is no medical treatment for autophony symptoms due to SCDS, as the sound transmission is via bone, not the Eustachian tube. Thus, for SCDS patients who are significantly disturbed by autophony, surgery is the only option for relief and has been shown to have a significant benefit [41, 54].

Conductive hearing loss is common in SCDS [9, 14, 55, 56], but it is often limited to low frequencies and one ear, so many patients do not have a significant disability from it. The risk of hearing loss progressing over time is also low [57, 58]. In most patients, the conductive hearing loss improves with surgery [55, 59]. However, plugging of SCD also carries a risk of hearing loss [60], which is greater in patients with prior ear surgery [55, 59]. Patients who have hearing loss as their primary symptom of SCDS should be encouraged to consider non-surgical options such as a hearing aid.

Although dizziness symptoms are often the motivation for surgery, imbalance symptoms may be worse during the immediate postoperative period. Symptoms improve as the patient adapts, and we typically prescribe vestibular rehabilitation. Benign paroxysmal positional vertigo (BPPV) has been reported in as many as 24% of cases [61] after plugging and can be treated with repositioning maneuvers. Plugging of the superior canal will cause loss of function due to hydrodynamic insufficiency of the canal [62, 63]. However, patients can adapt very well to this single-canal insufficiency, as low-frequency, low-acceleration head movements still generate useful inhibitory signals from the contralateral posterior canal.

Bilateral Dehiscence

About a quarter of individuals with SCDS have the appearance of bilateral SCD on high-resolution CT scan [64]. Fortunately, one side is usually responsible for most symptoms. In some cases, symptoms and signs can be elicited from both ears. In bilateral SCDS, every effort should be made to identify the more symptomatic ear and operate on that side first. In most cases, symptoms will either resolve after operating on the more symptomatic side or abate to the point that contralateral surgery is not required. Only 11% of patients with bilateral SCDS opt to have bilateral surgery [64]. We recommend the second side only be considered for plugging surgery after sufficient time for adaptation in the partial loss of vertical semicircular canal function, typically after six or more months have passed since the operation. Plugging of both superior canals significantly impairs the ability to sense downward head rotation in the vertical plane, so these patients are at risk of developing vertical oscillopsia during ambulation [64]. Patients with bilateral SCDS had worse symptom control than those with unilateral disease if one or both sides were treated [54].

Near Dehiscence

Although controversial, it is recognized that symptoms of SCDS can occur even if very thin bone remains over the superior canal [65]. In these cases, CT is often read as showing a dehiscence, and the patient can have other objective evidence of dehiscence including an air–bone gap on audiometry, increased oVEMP amplitude, and low cVEMP thresholds. Although these patients can benefit from surgery, caution is suggested as these patients have more residual symptoms and may have a higher rate of postoperative complications than patients with frank dehiscence [2], but they can, in some cases, benefit from surgery [66].

Operative Technique

The middle cranial fossa approach to superior canal dehiscence repair was described first [1] and is the technique detailed in the following paragraphs. Alternatively, a transmastoid approach to superior canal dehiscence repair has become popular. Advocates of the transmastoid approach have noted that it avoids a craniotomy, involves no temporal lobe retraction, and may lead to better stability of the canal plug. Moreover, most otolaryngologists are more familiar with mastoidectomy [67, 68]. The transmastoid approach was initially described after its use in two patients in 2001, and although these patients were relieved of vertigo symptoms, one patient experienced significant sensorineural hearing loss after surgery [69]. More recently, additional reports of transmastoid superior canal plugging have been published with both minimal morbidity and improvement in symptoms [2, 67, 68, 70–74].

The middle fossa approach has several advantages. The transmastoid approach does not allow direct confirmation of the dehiscence, and transmastoid plugging of a superior canal that was later found to be intact has been described [67]. The transmastoid approach may not be possible in patients with a low hanging dura or extensive tegmen dehiscences [67]. In the transmastoid approach, openings in the canal need to be created and plugging material must be advanced beyond these openings to be successful. Thus, the plug is placed closer to the sensory epithelia of the ampulla and the utricle. This may be more traumatic to these structures, risking disturbance of their baseline firing rates. Furthermore, opening the superior canal distal to the dehiscence may place the plug into the common crus, causing loss of sensory function of the posterior canal as well [63]. The transmastoid approach also creates a new dehiscence which can make it difficult to know the source if the patient develops residual symptoms later. Finally, the transmastoid approach requires drilling, irrigation, and suctioning on the bony canal. Once the canal is opened, these manipulations could contaminate or remove perilymph from the canal and cause collapse of the membranous labyrinth or serous labyrinthitis. To minimize this risk, a technique of plugging the canal while it remains submerged in a balanced salt solution has been described [72].

Round window plugging or reinforcement has been suggested as a treatment for SCDS [75, 76]. The procedure does not directly address the third window at the superior canal and some patients developed worse symptoms after this procedure [75]. A retrospective case review suggested that although some patients reported improvement in subjective symptoms such as autophony and vertigo, improvement in objective tests such as VEMP was rare and hearing was often diminished after the procedure [77]. Many of these patients require revision surgery via a transmastoid or middle fossa approach [78]. Long-term outcomes of round window reinforcement have been shown to be poor [79], and some surgeons who were initially advocates of the technique have now abandoned the procedure. Due to the concern over long-term outcomes and because it does not directly address the known pathophysiology of the disease, round window plugging is not widely employed [77, 80].

A transmastoid approach may be preferable in cases where the patient cannot tolerate a middle fossa surgery, or where the dehiscence cannot easily be accessed through the middle fossa—for instance, when the dehiscence is at the superior petrosal sinus [81, 82]. Some patients who have been symptomatic after a middle fossa approach have had relief of symptoms with revision surgery via a transmastoid approach [71]. It is difficult to directly compare outcomes via a transmastoid and middle fossa approach because of differences in relative indications between them.

For the middle fossa approach, the patient is usually positioned supine with the head turned 180° [83]. The incision is made from the helical root around the helix to a location over the external auditory canal, and then superiorly (Fig. 56.5). Temporalis fascia is harvested for later use in plugging the superior canal and for repair of any tegmen defects or cerebrospinal fluid leak that may occur (Fig. 56.6). Afterwards, the temporalis muscle is divided, and the area of the craniotomy is exposed.

The craniotomy should be centered over the superior canal, the external auditory canal is often a good landmark, but image-guided navigation can be used. The lower border of the craniotomy is placed just high enough to avoid the mastoid air cells. The width and height of the craniotomy should accommodate a middle fossa retractor, typically 3 cm wide by 4 cm high (Fig. 56.7). The craniotomy is opened by drilling troughs around the borders using a 4-mm burr. The dura should remain intact, and the bone flap removed and preserved in saline. The dura is further elevated from the edges of the craniotomy to allow retraction. The sharp edges of the craniotomy are removed using small Kerrison rongeurs, and the bone chips created in this process can be used as plugs for the superior canal.

The middle cranial fossa retractor is placed and used to gently elevate the dura off the middle fossa (Fig. 56.8). Dura here can be thin, especially if tegmen dehiscences are also present, and large cotton balls soaked in saline are a minimally traumatic means for the dural elevation. A hemostatic agent such as dry microfibrillar collagen (Avitene®) or gelatin powder (Gelfoam®) mixed as a paste with thrombin is

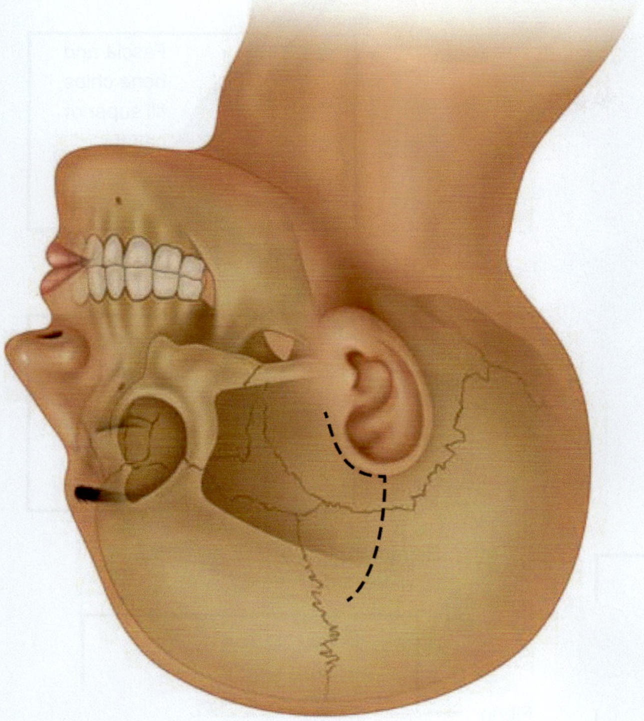

Fig. 56.5 Incision planning. (Adapted from Diagnosis and Treatment of Vestibular Disorders. Eds. Babu. Schutt and Bojrab. Springer. 2019)

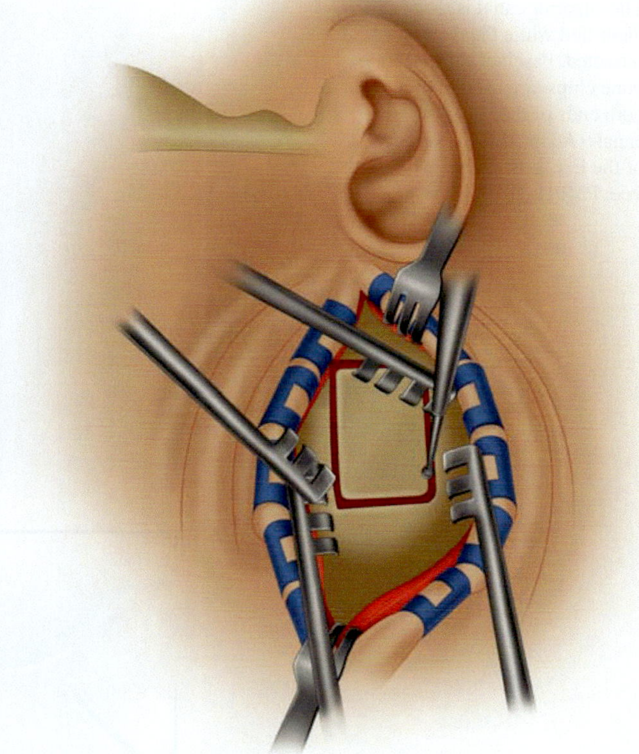

Fig. 56.7 Craniotomy. (Adapted from Surgery of the Ear. Eds. Gulya, Minor, Poe. PMPH. 2010)

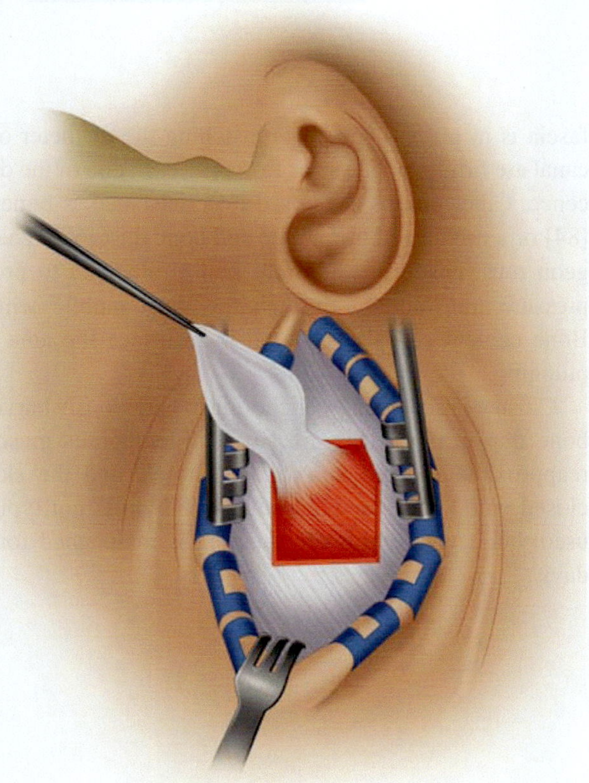

Fig. 56.6 Harvest of temporalis fascia after incision is opened and Raney clips are applied. (Adapted from Surgery of the Ear. Eds. Gulya, Minor, Poe. PMPH. 2010)

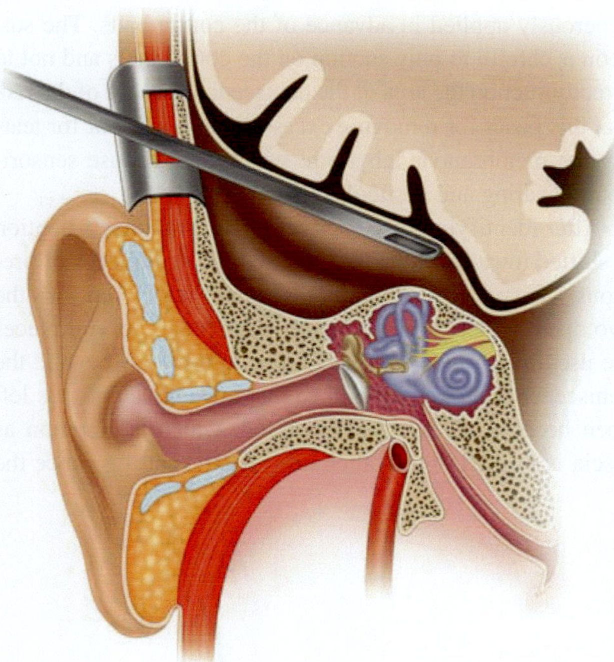

Fig. 56.8 Elevation of the dura using a middle fossa retractor to expose the superior canal. (Adapted from Diagnosis and Treatment of Vestibular Disorders. Eds. Babu. Schutt and Bojrab. Springer. 2019)

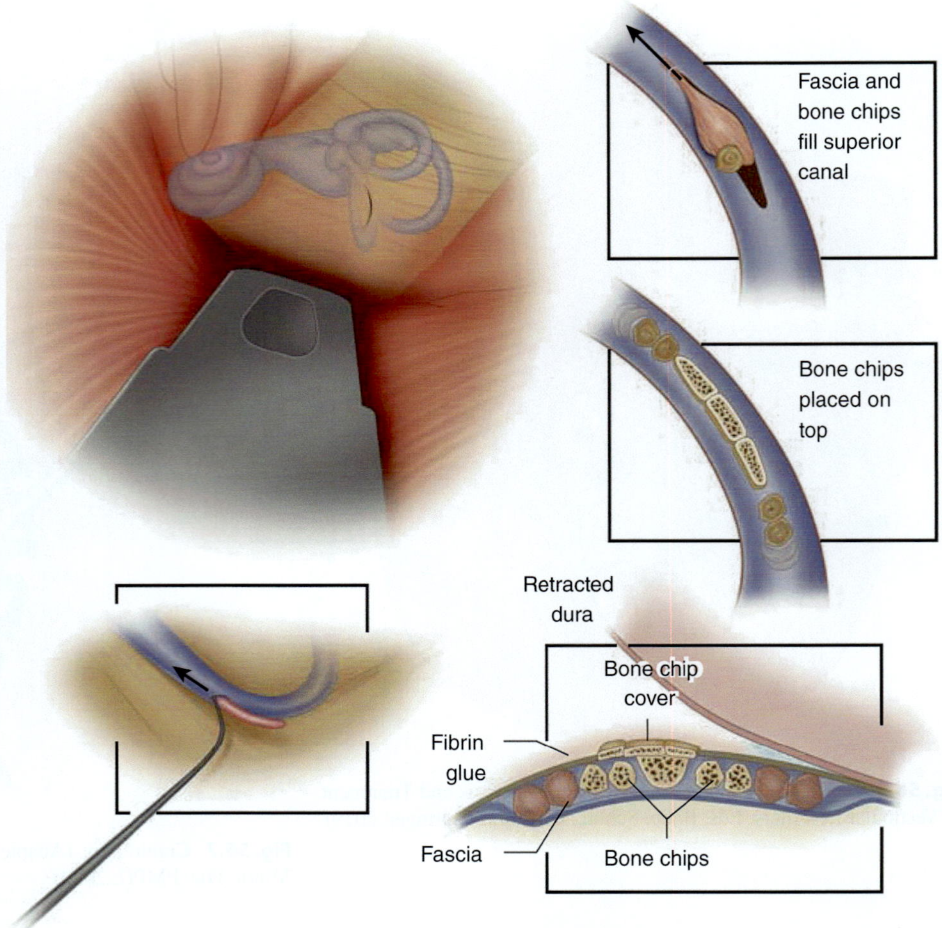

Fig. 56.9 Plugging of the superior canal dehiscence. The superior canal is identified while the dura is retracted. Fascia, followed by bone chips, are used to plug both ends of the superior canal. (Adapted from Surgery of the Ear. Eds. Gulya, Minor, Poe. PMPH. 2010)

generously applied in advance of the cotton balls. The surgeon is careful to only suction on the cotton balls and not to directly suction the area of the dehiscence because of the risk that this poses for removing excessive perilymph or for tearing the membranous labyrinth, which could cause sensorineural hearing and vestibular loss.

After identifying the superior canal dehiscence, attention is shifted towards plugging (Fig. 56.9). Small pieces of previously harvested temporalis fascia are gently slid into the two open lumens of the bony superior canal. Several pieces are used to advance the plugs a few millimeters beyond the dehiscence. Care must be taken that one end is not thus left open because its fascia is displaced, which is common as fascia is pushed in the other side. To prevent this, once the fascia is in place, bone chips matching the diameter of the canal are firmly lodged so as to "cork" each end of the dehiscence. Other groups have used materials such as bone wax [84] or a mixture of fibrin glue and bone dust [67]. The surgeon must ensure a watertight seal is obtained to prevent pressure transmission through the third mobile window. Bone cement can also be used to resurface the area after plugging.

Closure is achieved by anchoring the previously harvested bone flap in place (Fig. 56.10). The temporalis muscle is reapproximated with absorbable sutures, and the skin is closed with staples and/or sutures. A drain is not typically used, but a gentle pressure dressing is maintained for two days.

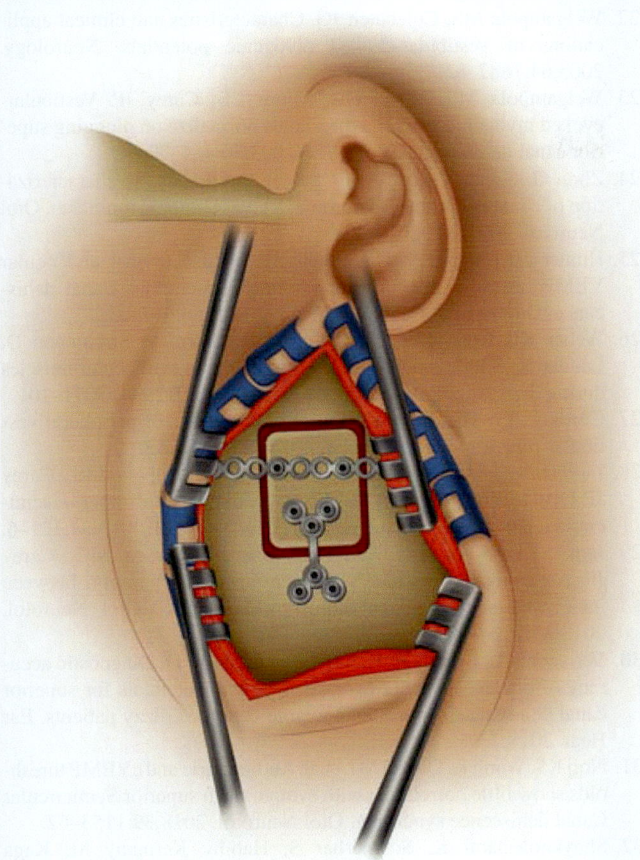

Fig. 56.10 Closure of the craniotomy. The bone flap is replaced using titanium plates. (Adapted from Diagnosis and Treatment of Vestibular Disorders. Eds. Babu. Schutt and Bojrab. Springer. 2019)

Postoperative Care

A monitored bed with neurological checks in the immediate postoperative period is recommended due to the epidural hematoma risk. Postoperative patients are treated with intravenous steroids which can be quickly tapered. Patients frequently experience nausea during the initial hours after surgery. This is best controlled using intravenous promethazine (Phenergan). Routine postoperative analgesics are sufficient to control the pain. If the patient is experiencing intense pain or if there is any change in mental status, an epidural hematoma may be the cause, and an immediate head CT should be considered. The typical hospitalization is usually at least overnight but can be as long as two or three days.

Long-Term Results

Most patients are extremely satisfied with the surgery, with studies supporting improvements in overall quality of life [74, 85], autophony [41], and dizziness symptoms [86]. Relief of dizzy symptoms has been documented by measuring the dizziness handicap inventory (DHI) [87] which improved by 26 points, with patients with more severe dizziness (DHI $\geq$ 30) improving by an average of 39 points [86]. Nearly all patients would recommend the surgery to others [54].

For some patients, autophony or hyperacusis for internal sounds is the primary reason for undergoing SCDS surgery and this is the most reported presenting symptom after dizziness [14]. Autophony is on average 89% improved immediately after surgery [41] and similar improvement is maintained long term [54]. Some autophony symptoms may take time to resolve due to fluid collecting in the middle ear after surgery.

The results for improving hearing with SCD surgery are gratifying if conductive hyperacusis is documented preoperatively. Dramatic results have been reported in some patients [88], but are uncommon. The air–bone gap that is present prior to surgery typically closes several months after surgery [59, 89] once any middle ear effusions or hemotympanum have resolved; however, patients can also experience hearing loss after SCD surgery. Two larger series found a mild (~10 dB) high-frequency sensorineural hearing loss in 25% of cases [59, 89] and profound hearing loss has been reported in 2.5% of cases [90]. In patients with previous middle cranial fossa or stapes surgery, one series found the risk of hearing loss was high [55]. A recent review found audiometric outcomes varied significantly among studies and although transmastoid and middle fossa approaches seem to be safe, subjective hearing improvement was not significant [91]. However, our own experience is that air–bone gaps, if present prior to surgery, are reduced after surgical plugging of the affected canal and that symptoms of conductive hyperacusis like autophony and pulsatile tinnitus are also ameliorated.

Summary

The diagnosis of SCDS is based on patient history, physical exam including eye movements in response to sound or pressure, and other supporting studies including the audiogram, VEMPs, and CT imaging. The spectrum and severity of SCDS symptoms vary significantly among individuals, and surgeons must carefully weigh the potential benefit of surgery against the risks and probability of success in each patient. A large fraction of patients with SCDS do not opt for surgery.

Both middle fossa and transmastoid approaches are reasonable treatments for SCDS. Patients generally experience an improvement in dizziness, autophony, and hyperacusis symptoms. Although there is often an improvement in hearing after surgery, this must be carefully weighed against the risk of hearing loss, which is more significant in patients who have had previous middle fossa or stapes surgery.

References

1. Minor LB, Solomon D, Zinreich JS, Zee DS. Sound- and/or pressure-induced vertigo due to bone dehiscence of the superior semicircular canal. Arch Otolaryngol Head Neck Surg. 1998;124:249–58.
2. Ward BK, Carey JP, Minor LB. Superior canal dehiscence syndrome: lessons from the first 20 years. Front Neurol. 2017;8:177.
3. Steenerson KK, Crane BT, Minor LB. Superior semicircular canal dehiscence syndrome. Semin Neurol. 2020;40:151–9.
4. Kontorinis G, Lenarz T. Superior semicircular canal dehiscence: a narrative review. J Laryngol Otol. 2022;136:284–92.
5. Rosowski JJ, Songer JE, Nakajima HH, Brinsko KM, Merchant SN. Clinical, experimental, and theoretical investigations of the effect of superior semicircular canal dehiscence on hearing mechanisms. Otol Neurotol. 2004;25:323–32.
6. Ward BK, van de Berg R, van Rompaey V, et al. Superior semicircular canal dehiscence syndrome: diagnostic criteria consensus document of the committee for the classification of vestibular disorders of the Barany Society. J Vestib Res. 2021;31:131–41.
7. Minor LB. Superior canal dehiscence syndrome. Am J Otol. 2000;21:9–19.
8. Minor LB. Clinical manifestations of superior semicircular canal dehiscence. Laryngoscope. 2005;115:1717–27.
9. Mikulec AA, McKenna MJ, Ramsey MJ, et al. Superior semicircular canal dehiscence presenting as conductive hearing loss without vertigo. Otol Neurotol. 2004;25:121–9.
10. Bigelow RT, Agrawal Y. Vestibular involvement in cognition: visuospatial ability, attention, executive function, and memory. J Vestib Res. 2015;25:73–89.
11. Yuen HW, Eikelboom RH, Atlas MD. Auditory manifestations of superior semicircular canal dehiscence. Otol Neurotol. 2009;30:280–5.
12. Watson SR, Halmagyi GM, Colebatch JG. Vestibular hypersensitivity to sound (Tullio phenomenon): structural and functional assessment. Neurology. 2000;54:722–8.
13. Brantberg K, Verrecchia L, Westin M. Enhanced auditory sensitivity to body vibrations in Superior Canal dehiscence syndrome. Audiol Neurootol. 2016;21:365–71.
14. Naert L, Van de Berg R, Van de Heyning P, et al. Aggregating the symptoms of superior semicircular canal dehiscence syndrome. Laryngoscope. 2017;127:118.
15. Cremer PD, Minor LB, Carey JP, Della Santina CC. Eye movements in patients with superior canal dehiscence syndrome align with the abnormal canal. Neurology. 2000;55:1833–41.
16. Grieser BJ, Kleiser L, Obrist D. Identifying mechanisms behind the Tullio phenomenon: a computational study based on first principles. J Assoc Res Otolaryngol. 2016;17:103–18.
17. Krombach GA, DiMartino E, Schmitz-Rode T, et al. Posterior semicircular canal dehiscence: a morphologic cause of vertigo similar to superior semicircular canal dehiscence. Eur Radiol. 2003;13:1444–50.
18. Sheehy JL, Brackmann DE. Cholesteatoma surgery: management of the labyrinthine fistula—a report of 97 cases. Laryngoscope. 1979;89:78–87.
19. Merchant SN, Rosowski JJ. Conductive hearing loss caused by third-window lesions of the inner ear. Otol Neurotol. 2008;29:282–9.
20. Halmagyi GM, Aw ST, McGarvie LA, et al. Superior semicircular canal dehiscence simulating otosclerosis. J Laryngol Otol. 2003;117:553–7.
21. Songer JE, Rosowski JJ. A mechano-acoustic model of the effect of superior canal dehiscence on hearing in chinchilla. J Acoust Soc Am. 2007;122:943–51.
22. Welgampola MS, Colebatch JG. Characteristics and clinical applications of vestibular-evoked myogenic potentials. Neurology. 2005;64:1682–8.
23. Welgampola MS, Myrie OA, Minor LB, Carey JP. Vestibular-evoked myogenic potential thresholds normalize on plugging superior canal dehiscence. Neurology. 2008;70:464–72.
24. Zhou G, Gopen Q, Poe DS. Clinical and diagnostic characterization of canal dehiscence syndrome: a great Otologic mimicker. Otol Neurotol. 2007;28:920–6.
25. Hunter JB, Patel NS, O'Connell BP, et al. Cervical and ocular VEMP testing in diagnosing superior Semicircular Canal dehiscence. Otolaryngol Head Neck Surg. 2017;156:917–23.
26. Weber KP, Rosengren SM, Michels R, Sturm V, Straumann D, Landau K. Single motor unit activity in human extraocular muscles during the vestibulo-ocular reflex. J Physiol. 2012;590:3091–101.
27. Curthoys IS. The interpretation of clinical tests of peripheral vestibular function. Laryngoscope. 2012;122:1342–52.
28. Zuniga MG, Janky KL, Nguyen KD, Welgampola MS, Carey JP. Ocular versus cervical VEMPs in the diagnosis of superior semicircular canal dehiscence syndrome. Otol Neurotol. 2013;34:121–6.
29. Janky KL, Nguyen KD, Welgampola M, Zuniga MG, Carey JP. Air-conducted oVEMPs provide the best separation between intact and superior canal dehiscent labyrinths. Otol Neurotol. 2013;34:127–34.
30. Verrecchia L, Brantberg K, Tawfique Z, Maoli D. Diagnostic accuracy of ocular vestibular evoked myogenic potentials for superior canal dehiscence syndrome in a large cohort of dizzy patients. Ear Hear. 2018;23
31. Noij KS, Wong K, Duarte MJ, et al. Audiometric and cVEMP thresholds show little correlation with symptoms in superior Semicircular Canal dehiscence syndrome. Otol Neurotol. 2018;39:1153–62.
32. Sheykholeslami K, Schmerber S, Habiby Kermany M, Kaga K. Vestibular-evoked myogenic potentials in three patients with large vestibular aqueduct. Hear Res. 2004;190:161–8.
33. Zhou G, Poe D, Gopen Q. Clinical use of vestibular evoked myogenic potentials in the evaluation of patients with air-bone gaps. Otol Neurotol. 2012;33:1368–74.
34. Crane BT, Minor LB, Carey JP. Three-dimensional computed tomography of Superior Canal dehiscence syndrome. Otol Neurotol. 2008;29:699–705.
35. Williamson RA, Vrabec JT, Coker NJ, Sandlin M. Coronal computed tomography prevalence of superior semicircular canal dehiscence. Otolaryngol Head Neck Surg. 2003;129:481–9.
36. Carey JP, Minor LB, Nager GT. Dehiscence or thinning of bone overlying the superior semicircular canal in a temporal bone survey. Arch Otolaryngol Head Neck Surg. 2000;126:137–47.
37. Tavassolie TS, Penninger RT, Zuniga MG, Minor LB, Carey JP. Multislice computed tomography in the diagnosis of superior canal dehiscence: how much error, and how to minimize it? Otol Neurotol. 2012;33:215–22.
38. Browaeys P, Larson TL, Wong ML, Patel U. Can MRI replace CT in evaluating semicircular canal dehiscence? AJNR Am J Neuroradiol. 2013;34:1421–7.
39. Sharon JD, Pross SE, Ward BK, Carey JP. Revision surgery for Superior Canal dehiscence syndrome. Otol Neurotol. 2016;37:1096–103.
40. Poe DS. Diagnosis and management of the patulous eustachian tube. Otol Neurotol. 2007;28:668–77.
41. Crane BT, Lin FR, Minor LB, Carey J. Improvement in autophony symptoms after superior canal dehiscence repair. Otol Neurotol. 2010;31:140–6.
42. Minor LB. Labyrinthine fistulae: pathobiology and management. Curr Opin Otolaryngol Head Neck Surg. 2003;11:340–6.

43. Chien WW, Carey JP, Minor LB. Canal dehiscence. Curr Opin Neurol. 2011;24:25–31.
44. Weinreich HM, Carey JP. Perilymphatic fistulas and superior semi-Circular Canal dehiscence syndrome. Adv Otorhinolaryngol. 2019;82:93–100.
45. Hakuba N, Hato N, Shinomori Y, Sato H, Gyo K. Labyrinthine fistula as a late complication of middle ear surgery using the canal wall down technique. Otol Neurotol. 2002;23:832–5.
46. Friedland DR, Wackym PA. A critical appraisal of spontaneous perilymphatic fistulas of the inner ear. Am J Otol 1999; 20:261–276; discussion 276–269.
47. Eggers SD. Migraine-related vertigo: diagnosis and treatment. Curr Pain Headache Rep. 2007;11:217–26.
48. Dieterich M, Obermann M, Celebisoy N. Vestibular migraine: the most frequent entity of episodic vertigo. J Neurol. 2016;263(Suppl 1):S82–9.
49. Lempert T, Olesen J, Furman J, et al. Vestibular migraine: diagnostic criteria. J Vestib Res. 2012;22:167–72.
50. Smetak MR, Cass ND, Manzoor NF, et al. Vestibular migraine confounds Management of Superior Canal Dehiscence Syndrome. Otol Neurotol. 2022;43:835–9.
51. Tepper SJ. A pivotal moment in 50 years of headache history: the first American migraine study. Headache. 2008;48:730–1.
52. Kayan A, Hood JD. Neuro-otological manifestations of migraine. Brain. 1984;107(Pt 4):1123–42.
53. Jung DH, Lookabaugh SA, Owoc MS, McKenna MJ, Lee DJ. Dizziness is more prevalent than autophony among patients who have undergone repair of superior canal dehiscence. Otol Neurotol. 2015;36:126–32.
54. Alkhafaji MS, Varma S, Pross SE, et al. Long-term patient-reported outcomes after surgery for Superior Canal dehiscence syndrome. Otol Neurotol. 2017;38:1319–26.
55. Limb CJ, Carey JP, Srireddy S, Minor LB. Auditory function in patients with surgically treated superior semicircular canal dehiscence. Otol Neurotol. 2006;27:969–80.
56. McEvoy TP, Mikulec AA, Armbrecht ES, Lowe ME. Quantification of hearing loss associated with superior semi-circular canal dehiscence. Am J Otolaryngol. 2013;34:345–9.
57. Patel NS, Hunter JB, O'Connell BP, Bertrand NM, Wanna GB, Carlson ML. Risk of progressive hearing loss in untreated superior semicircular canal dehiscence. Laryngoscope. 2017;127:1181–6.
58. Lookabaugh S, Niesten ME, Owoc M, Kozin ED, Grolman W, Lee DJ. Audiologic, cVEMP, and radiologic progression in Superior Canal dehiscence syndrome. Otol Neurotol. 2016;37:1393–8.
59. Ward BK, Agrawal Y, Nguyen E, et al. Hearing outcomes after surgical plugging of the superior semicircular canal by a middle cranial fossa approach. Otol Neurotol. 2012;33:1386–91.
60. Gioacchini FM, Alicandri-Ciufelli M, Kaleci S, Scarpa A, Cassandro E, Re M. Outcomes and complications in superior semicircular canal dehiscence surgery: a systematic review. Laryngoscope. 2016;126:1218–24.
61. Barber SR, Cheng YS, Owoc M, et al. Benign paroxysmal positional vertigo commonly occurs following repair of superior canal dehiscence. Laryngoscope. 2016;126:2092–7.
62. Janky KL, Zuniga MG, Ward B, Carey JP, Schubert MC. Canal plane dynamic visual acuity in superior canal dehiscence. Otol Neurotol. 2014;35:844–9.
63. Carey JP, Migliaccio AA, Minor LB. Semicircular canal function before and after surgery for superior canal dehiscence. Otol Neurotol. 2007;28:356–64.
64. Agrawal Y, Minor LB, Schubert MC, Janky KL, Davalos-Bichara M, Carey JP. Second-side surgery in superior canal dehiscence syndrome. Otol Neurotol. 2012;33:72–7.
65. Ward BK, Wenzel A, Ritzl EK, et al. Near-dehiscence: clinical findings in patients with thin bone over the superior semicircular canal. Otol Neurotol. 2013;34:1421–8.
66. Baxter M, McCorkle C, Trevino Guajardo C, et al. Clinical and physiologic predictors and postoperative outcomes of near dehiscence syndrome. Otol Neurotol. 2019;40:204–12.
67. Agrawal SK, Parnes LS. Transmastoid superior semicircular canal occlusion. Otol Neurotol. 2008;29:363–7.
68. Crovetto M, Areitio E, Elexpuru J, Aguayo F. Transmastoid approach for resurfacing of superior Semicircular Canal dehiscence. Auris Nasus Larynx. 2008;35:247–9.
69. Brantberg K, Bergenius J, Mendel L, Witt H, Tribukait A, Ygge J. Symptoms, findings and treatment in patients with dehiscence of the superior semicircular canal. Acta Otolaryngol. 2001;121:68–75.
70. Kirtane MV, Sharma A, Satwalekar D. Transmastoid repair of superior semicircular canal dehiscence. J Laryngol Otol. 2008:1–3.
71. Powell HR, Khalil SS, Saeed SR. Outcomes of transmastoid surgery for superior semicircular canal dehiscence syndrome. Otol Neurotol. 2016;37:e228–33.
72. Creighton F Jr, Barber SR, Ward BK, Sharon JD, Carey JP. Underwater endoscopic repair of Superior Canal dehiscence. Otol Neurotol. 2020;41:560.
73. Zhang L, Creighton FX Jr, Ward BK, Bowditch S, Carey JP. A cohort study of hearing outcomes between middle fossa craniotomy and Transmastoid approach for surgical repair of superior Semicircular Canal dehiscence syndrome. Otol Neurotol. 2018;39:e1160–7.
74. Allsopp T, Kim AH, Robbins AM, Page JC, Dornhoffer JL. Quality of life outcomes after transmastoid plugging of superior semicircular canal dehiscence. Am J Otolaryngol. 2020;41:102287.
75. Silverstein H, Kartush JM, Parnes LS, et al. Round window reinforcement for superior semicircular canal dehiscence: a retrospective multi-center case series. Am J Otolaryngol. 2014;35:286–93.
76. Nikkar-Esfahani A, Whelan D, Banerjee A. Occlusion of the round window: a novel way to treat hyperacusis symptoms in superior semicircular canal dehiscence syndrome. J Laryngol Otol. 2013;127:705–7.
77. Succar EF, Manickam PV, Wing S, Walter J, Greene JS, Azeredo WJ. Round window plugging in the treatment of superior semicircular canal dehiscence. Laryngoscope. 2017;128:1445.
78. Chemtob RA, Noij KS, Qureshi AA, Klokker M, Nakajima HH, Lee DJ. Superior Canal dehiscence surgery outcomes following failed round window surgery. Otol Neurotol. 2019;40:535–42.
79. Bunne M, Andersson H, Myhrum M. Long-term outcomes of round window reinforcement for superior Semicircular Canal dehiscence syndrome. Otol Neurotol. 2022;43:709–16.
80. Ahmed W, Rajagopal R, Lloyd G. Systematic review of round window operations for the treatment of superior Semicircular Canal dehiscence. J Int Adv Otol. 2019;15:209–14.
81. Schneiders SMD, Rainsbury JW, Hensen EF, Irving RM. Superior petrosal sinus causing superior canal dehiscence syndrome. J Laryngol Otol. 2017;131:593–7.
82. McCall AA, McKenna MJ, Merchant SN, Curtin HD, Lee DJ. Superior canal dehiscence syndrome associated with the superior petrosal sinus in pediatric and adult patients. Otol Neurotol. 2011;32:1312–9.
83. Andresen NS, Krishnan PS, Lin BM, Formeister E, Carey JP. Positioning for middle cranial fossa repair of superior Semicircular Canal dehiscence. Laryngoscope. 2023;133:1218–21.
84. Cheng YS, Kozin ED, Remenschneider AK, Nakajima HH, Lee DJ. Characteristics of wax occlusion in the surgical repair of Superior Canal dehiscence in human temporal bone specimens. Otol Neurotol. 2016;37:83–8.

85. Remenschneider AK, Owoc M, Kozin ED, McKenna MJ, Lee DJ, Jung DH. Health utility improves after surgery for Superior Canal dehiscence syndrome. Otol Neurotol. 2015;36:1695–701.
86. Crane BT, Minor LB, Carey JP. Superior Canal dehiscence plugging reduces dizziness handicap. Laryngoscope. 2008;118:1809–13.
87. Jacobson GP, Newman CW. The development of the dizziness handicap inventory. Arch Otolaryngol Head Neck Surg. 1990;116:424–7.
88. Wilkinson EP, Liu GC, Friedman RA. Correction of progressive hearing loss in superior canal dehiscence syndrome. Laryngoscope. 2008;118:10–3.
89. Niesten ME, McKenna MJ, Herrmann BS, Grolman W, Lee DJ. Utility of cVEMPs in bilateral superior canal dehiscence syndrome. Laryngoscope. 2013;123:226–32.
90. Xie Y, Sharon JD, Pross SE, et al. Surgical complications from Superior Canal dehiscence syndrome repair: two decades of experience. Otolaryngol Head Neck Surg. 2017;157:273–80.
91. Ossen ME, Stokroos R, Kingma H, et al. Heterogeneity in reported outcome measures after surgery in Superior Canal dehiscence syndrome-a systematic literature review. Front Neurol. 2017;8:347.

57 Idiopathic Facial Paralysis and Herpes Zoster Oticus

Bruce J. Gantz, Daniel Q. Sun, and Joseph P. Roche

Introduction

Of the multitude of causes of facial paralysis, Bell's palsy (idiopathic facial paralysis) and Ramsay Hunt syndrome (herpes zoster oticus) are two of the most common. Bell's palsy alone accounts for almost three quarters of all acute facial palsies. Although the diagnosis of Ramsay Hunt syndrome is generally obvious, a thorough evaluation and close follow-up are required to establish a firm diagnosis of Bell's palsy. This chapter discusses the pathology, pathophysiology, epidemiology, evaluation, and management of these common disorders.

Idiopathic Facial Paralysis

Epidemiology

Bell's palsy accounts for nearly three quarters of all acute facial palsies [1]. The incidence of Bell's palsy is 20–30 cases per 100,000 per year [2]. The median age is 40 years, but it can occur at any age [3]. The incidence is highest in patients older than 70 years and lowest in children younger than 10 years. The left and right sides are affected equally. Men and women are equally affected, but the incidence of Bell's palsy is higher in pregnant women (45 cases per 100,000).

B. J. Gantz
Department of Otolaryngology—Head and Neck Surgery, University of Iowa Hospitals and Clinics, Iowa City, IA, USA
e-mail: bruce-gantz@uiowa.edu

D. Q. Sun (✉)
Department of Otolaryngology—Head and Neck Surgery, University of Cincinnati, Cincinnati, OH, USA
e-mail: daniel-sun@uc.edu

J. P. Roche
Department of Otolaryngology—Head and Neck Surgery, University of Wisconsin, WI, Madison, USA
e-mail: jproche@wisc.edu

Clinical Presentation, Diagnosis, and Workup

The clinical presentation of Bell's palsy is well known; however, the clinician must exclude other causes of facial paralysis based on history and physical examination findings [4]. These include neoplasm, Ramsay-Hunt syndrome, necrotizing otitis externa, syphilis, Lyme disease, cerebrovascular accident, trauma, vasculitis, sarcoidosis, multiple sclerosis, Guillain-Barré syndrome, and Melkersson-Rosenthal syndrome. Patients describe an abrupt onset of unilateral paresis that occurs over 24–48 h. The paresis can progress over one–seven days to complete paralysis. Bilateral involvement, either simultaneously or consecutively, has been described [5]. Progressive weakness over weeks to months, repeated episodes of paralysis, and twitching of the facial muscles should not be considered symptoms of Bell's palsy. Other associated symptoms of hearing loss, vestibular symptoms, or other cranial nerve (CN) neuropathies also rule out the diagnosis of Bell's palsy.

On physical examination, the patient displays unilateral weakness or flaccid paralysis of all branches of the facial nerve. If forehead movement is normal, and there is strong eye closure and symmetric blinking, a central origin of paralysis should be suspected. The tympanic membrane should be of normal color and mobility. Careful bimanual palpation of the parotid gland should be performed to identify a deep lobe parotid neoplasm, which would rule out idiopathic facial weakness. Oral cavity examination may show loss of papillae on the ipsilateral tongue. Cranial nerve testing is normal with the exception of the involved CN VII. Serial examinations are essential; if some evidence of recovery is not noted within three to six months, an aggressive search for an underlying neoplasm should be undertaken.

Audiometric evaluation should reveal symmetric function except for an absent ipsilateral acoustic reflex. If unilateral hearing loss or acoustic reflex decay is present, further evaluation for retrocochlear pathology is necessary. If vestibular complaints are present, an electronystagmogram can be per-

A. D. Sweeney et al. (eds.), *Haynes-Glasscock-Shambaugh Surgery of the Ear*, https://doi.org/10.1007/978-3-032-18264-7_57

formed, and the diagnosis of Bell's palsy should be questioned. If the history and clinical presentation are highly suggestive of Bell's palsy, magnetic resonance imaging (MRI) and computed tomography (CT) are not routinely performed. High-resolution CT scans and MRI should be considered if patients have associated symptoms of otorrhea, vestibular complaints, and hearing loss at the time of presentation. Imaging can also be considered for surgical planning, if decompression is considered, or if symptoms persist or fluctuate in a manner distinct from the general expectations associated with Bell's palsy, as previously described. Our practice involves imaging for cases where surgical decompression is pursued and cases where persistent paralysis after six months is present. Serologic tests for Lyme disease (immunoglobulin G [IgG], immunoglobulin M [IgM]) are an important part of the workup for unexplained facial paralysis in endemic areas [6]. Serologic testing for antibodies to herpes simplex virus (HSV) or varicella zoster has provided some correlative evidence for a viral etiology in Bell's palsy, although laboratory investigations in general have not been found to provide clinically relevant data.

Electrophysiological testing is an important element of the diagnostic evaluation of facial paralysis and is discussed in detail in Chap. 13. The technique of electroneurography (ENoG), developed by Esslen [7], can distinguish the nerve fibers that have undergone Wallerian degeneration from fibers that are temporarily blocked (neurapraxia). ENoG testing is not performed until three–four days after the development of complete unilateral paralysis because Wallerian degeneration does not become apparent until 48–72 h after an acute injury to the nerve. ENoG testing is not performed when the patient exhibits paresis only. If the paresis progresses to total paralysis, ENoG testing is performed three days after the onset of total paralysis. Presence of voluntary movement four to five days after the onset of paresis indicates only minor injury, and complete recovery should be anticipated.

ENoG is most accurate when it is performed within three weeks of the acute injury. Patients exhibiting 90–100% degeneration or no response to electric stimulation must then undergo electromyography (EMG) testing to rule out early deblocking, which portends a favorable prognosis. Volitional EMG testing is *mandatory* if a surgical decompression is planned. If a facial paralysis has been slowly progressive over weeks to months, degeneration and regeneration of nerve fibers may co-occur within the nerve, resulting in similar dysynchronous discharge of evoked impulses and an inaccurate compound muscle action potential (CMAP) recording.

Pathology and Pathophysiology

Bell [8] first described a patient with a facial paralysis in 1821; subsequently, all patients with facial palsy of unknown etiology have come to bear his name. The etiology of this "idiopathic" disorder has become much clearer in recent years. Although first proposed in 1972 by McCormick [9], herpes simplex virus (HSV) has been identified as the disease vector only recently [10–12], and an animal model has been designed [13]. Murakami and associates [12] identified HSV type 1 (HSV-1) DNA fragments in perineural fluid in 11 of 14 patients undergoing facial nerve decompression. In this study, no control subjects had HSV-1 DNA in perineural fluid. Using polymerase chain reaction to analyze the saliva of patients with Bell's palsy, Furuta and colleagues [10] identified HSV-1 DNA in 50% of patients, which was significantly more often than in controls, a finding confirmed by other groups [14]. Polymerase chain reaction has also been used to isolate HSV-1 genomic DNA from the geniculate ganglion of a temporal bone in a patient who died during the acute phase of Bell's palsy [11].

Sugita and coworkers [13] proposed an animal model of Bell's palsy. Six days after inoculation of HSV-1 into the auricle or the tongue of mice, a temporary ipsilateral facial paralysis was identified that recovered spontaneously within three to seven days. Histopathologically, neural edema, vacuolar degeneration, and inflammatory cell infiltrate with associated demyelination or axonal degeneration were shown in the affected facial nerve and nucleus [15]. HSV-1 antigens were identified within the facial nerve, geniculate ganglion, and facial nucleus 6–20 days after inoculation [13]. Similar pathologic findings have been shown in rabbits after HSV-1 inoculation, but without the associated facial paralysis [16].

The histopathologic changes seen in autopsy specimens of patients who died with acute idiopathic facial paralysis have provided some insight into the underlying cellular mechanisms in Bell's palsy. Reddy and coworkers [17] found degeneration of the myelin sheath and axons, perivascular inflammation, and a phagocytic cell infiltrate in 10–30% of nerve fibers in a patient 17 days after the onset of an acute idiopathic facial paralysis. Fowler [18] found diffuse vascular engorgement throughout the intratemporal facial nerve and evidence of acute hemorrhage within the intracanalicular, labyrinthine, and geniculate portions of the facial nerve in a patient who died shortly after the onset of Bell's palsy. In examining an autopsy specimen of a patient who died 13 days after the onset of Bell's palsy, McKeever and colleagues [19] found a diffuse lymphocytic infiltration of the intratemporal facial nerve with ongoing myelin phagocytosis. They later re-examined the same specimen and noted the most pronounced lymphocytic infiltration of the nerve at the labyrinthine segment, findings that these authors believed were most consistent with an ongoing compression-type injury to the facial nerve.

Multiple reports have found that there seems to be evidence of constriction of the nerve at the meatal foramen in cases of Bell's palsy. In specimens examined during the acute phase of Bell's palsy, lymphocytic infiltration, perineural edema, and myelin degeneration have been noted [20]. In a nerve specimen examined one year after the diagnosis of Bell's palsy lymphocytic infiltration, perineural edema, and fibrotic changes were noted [21]. Intraoperative biopsy specimens of the greater superficial petrosal nerve from patients undergoing nerve decompression procedures for Bell's palsy have shown axonal demyelination and degeneration with lymphocytic infiltration [22]. Together, the histopathologic findings in Bell's palsy show demyelination and axonal loss with lymphocytic or phagocytic infiltration, findings that seem to be more pronounced at the labyrinthine segment of the facial nerve.

In considering this evidence, the pathogenesis of Bell's palsy becomes more apparent: a virally induced, inflammatory response that produces edema within the nerve. Fisch and Felix [22] first proposed that the facial nerve was entrapped at the meatal foramen as a result of neural edema. Intraoperative conduction studies have shown an electrophysiologic blockage at this site [23]. The constriction imposed produces a conduction block at first; however, with prolonged or increased constriction, ischemia results. Subsequently, Wallerian degeneration occurs, producing axonotmesis, neurotmesis or both. A spectrum of injury within the nerve from neurapraxia to neurotmesis may occur in Bell's palsy [18, 24]. The proportion of each of these types of injury determines the amount of facial function that returns when the acute phase of the disease subsides.

Medical Management

A review of the natural history of Bell's palsy shows that approximately 85% of patients begin to display some return of facial movement within three weeks of the onset of paresis [25]. The remaining 15% begin to improve three to six months after the onset of the disease. Most patients show a complete return of facial function, but 10–15% have residual unilateral weakness and develop secondary deformities of synkinesis, tearing, or contracture. In a study of over 1700 cases of Bell's palsy, Peitersen [1] found that 71% of patients regained normal function, 12% recovered to House-Brackmann (HB) II, 13% to HB III, and 4% to HB IV or V. No patient remained paralyzed. The risk of poor outcome (HB III or worse) is especially elevated in those presenting with complete paralysis. Peitersen showed that whereas 94% of patients presenting with paresis recovered to full function, only 61% who presented with complete paralysis did. Some motion returns in almost all individuals with Bell's palsy by six months. If no movement returns, a vigorous search for another etiology should begin anew.

The management of patients with Bell's palsy varies, depending on the type of specialist initially seeing the patient and on the training of the individual specialist. Figure 57.1 presents an overview of the management algorithm at our institution. Patients presenting within the first week of facial weakness with paresis are placed on steroid therapy (prednisone, 60–80 mg/day for 7 days) and an antiviral agent (valacyclovir, 500 mg three times per day for 10 days). If patients are seen 7–10 days after onset and motor function is stable or improving, medical treatment is unnecessary. Patients are instructed to return in one week for re-evaluation to deter-

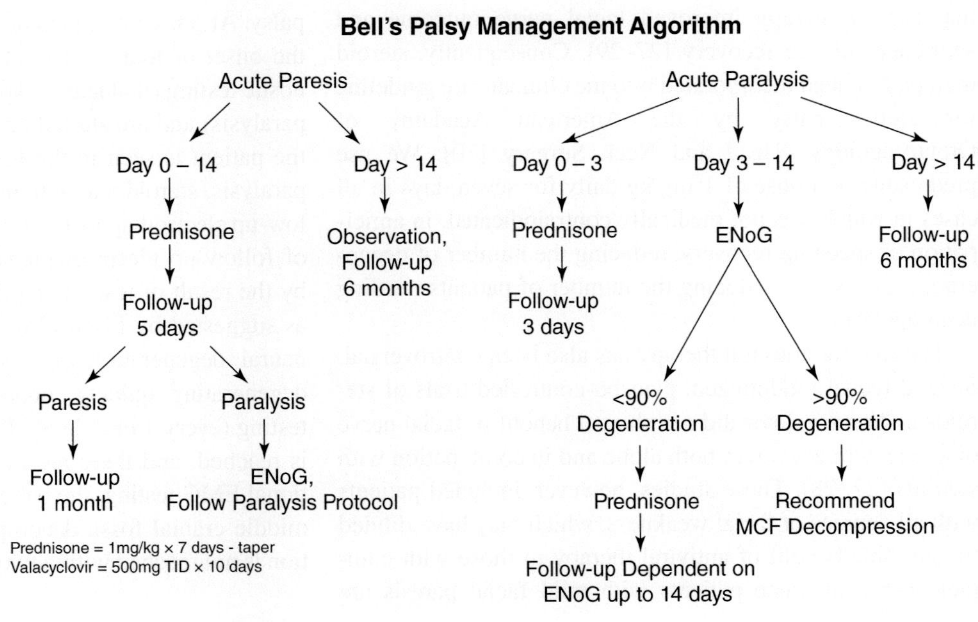

Fig. 57.1 Algorithm for the management of Bell's palsy. ENoG, electroneuronography; MCF, middle cranial fossa. (Reused with permission from Gantz et al. [38])

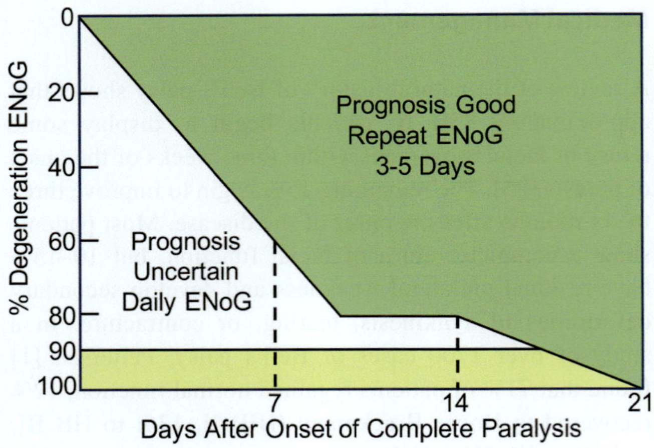

Fig. 57.2 Recommended electroneuronography (ENoG) testing schedule in acute facial paralysis. (Reused with permission from Gantz et al. [38]. Adaptation courtesy of Nathan R. Lindquist, MD and Ashley Reeb)

mine if neural degeneration has occurred. Electrodiagnostic testing is unnecessary as long as voluntary facial movement is present. If total paralysis occurs in the interim, the total paralysis protocol of Fig. 57.2 is followed. Stable or improving patients are seen in one month.

The use of steroids in Bell's palsy has been the subject of much debate but is now gaining increasing clinical acceptance. Many studies in the past were hindered by weaknesses such as lack of randomization, absence of blinding, retrospective design, and poor follow-up. As a result, little high-quality data were available. While a Cochrane review [26] in 2002 did not find a statistically significant benefit for steroid therapy, it was only able to identify three studies of adequate quality (117 patients total) and called attention to the lack of high-quality data in the field. Since then, several high-quality randomized controlled trials have been conducted and found that steroid therapy improved facial nerve outcome and shortened time to recovery [27–29]. Consequently, steroid therapy has been incorporated into the clinical care guideline for Bell's palsy by the American Academy of Otolaryngology—Head and Neck Surgery [30]. We use prednisone in a dose of 1 mg/kg daily for seven days in all cases in which it is not medically contraindicated, in anticipation of speeding recovery, reducing the number of degenerating axons, and reducing the number of patients needing decompression.

The role for antiviral therapy has also been controversial. Several recent randomized, placebo-controlled trials of steroids and/or acyclovir did not show a benefit in facial nerve outcome with acyclovir, both alone and in combination with steroids [27, 28]. These studies, however, included patients with all degrees of facial weakness, which may have diluted the possible benefit of antiviral therapy in those with complete paralysis since patients with mild facial paresis are known to have high rate of complete recovery regardless of any therapy. Furthermore, some have theorized that valacyclovir, with much greater bioavailability compared to acyclovir when taken orally, may be more effective in the treatment of Bell's palsy [31]. Evidence in favor of antiviral therapy includes a double-blind, randomized, controlled trial of acyclovir and prednisone versus prednisone alone that showed better results in the group receiving combination therapy [32]. This study documented poor facial function recovery in 23% of the prednisone-only group compared with 7% in the acyclovir-plus-prednisone group. In a systematic review for the American Academy of Neurology, Grogan and Gronseth [33] reported that patients who receive antiviral therapy in addition to steroids were 1.22 times as likely to have a good facial nerve outcome. In 2007, a multicenter, randomized, placebo-controlled, non-blinded study by Hato and colleagues [29] comparing steroids and antivirals with steroids alone found that the addition of valacyclovir improved the recovery rate from 89 to 96% in all cases of facial palsy and this benefit was most pronounced in the group with presenting with complete paralysis (from 75 to 90%). In 2015, a Cochrane review [34] pooled results from 10 trials that totaled 2280 patients and found a statistically significant benefit to antiviral therapy in combination with steroids compared to steroid therapy alone in the treatment of Bell's palsy (relative risk 0.61).

Perhaps just as important, no serious adverse effects have been documented in any study using antivirals in Bell's palsy. Furthermore, the number of patients with complete paralysis that need to be treated with antivirals in order to obtain one patient with improved recovery is relatively low, at 7 [31]. Also considering that a 10-day course of prednisone and 5-day course of valacyclovir may be relatively affordable [31], clinicians ought to strongly consider the addition of antivirals in the treatment of patients with Bell's palsy. At our center, patients presenting within one week of the onset of total unilateral paralysis undergo electrodiagnostic testing (if at least 3 days have passed since the onset of paralysis) and are started on prednisone and valacyclovir. If the patient is seen in the first three days after the onset of paralysis, steroid and antiviral therapy are initiated, and follow-up electrodiagnostic studies are arranged. The frequency of follow-up electrodiagnostic examinations is determined by the result of testing and the time interval after paralysis, as suggested by Fisch [35]. Patients exhibiting nearly 90% neural degeneration on ENoG examination, or who are degenerating quickly, undergo frequent electrodiagnostic testing (every 1 or 2 days). If greater than 90% degeneration is reached, and there are no motor unit potentials on volitional EMG testing, the patient is considered a candidate for middle cranial fossa decompression. When 90% degeneration is not reached within two weeks (14 days) after the onset of paralysis, no further electrodiagnostic studies need to be performed.

Patients seen for the first time more than two weeks after the onset of paralysis undergo EMG evaluation to determine if regeneration has begun. They are scheduled for a six-month follow-up to ensure that some motor function has returned. If no movement is evident at six months, it must be assumed that Bell's palsy was an incorrect diagnosis, and a search for another disease process is begun.

Surgical Management

Decompression of the facial nerve for Bell's palsy has been reported since the 1930s [36], and it is recommended in patients who exhibit greater than 90% degeneration on ENoG and no voluntary EMG activity within 14 days of the paralysis. Preliminary results suggested that early decompression of the labyrinthine, geniculate, and tympanic segments of the facial nerve through a middle cranial fossa approach improves recovery of severely degenerated cases [7], whereas decompression of the mastoid segment alone did not alter the natural history of the disease [37]. Gantz and associates [38] showed a statistically significant difference in facial nerve outcome when decompression is performed within two weeks of onset of the paralysis. The patients undergoing decompression exhibited HB grade I ($n = 14$) or II ($n = 17$) in 91% of cases; two patients had a grade III, and one patient had a grade IV outcome. There were no grade V or VI results in the surgical group. Patients who met surgical criteria but elected not to undergo surgery had a 58% chance of a poor outcome. Within the non-surgical group, 19 patients had a HB grade of either III or IV at seven-month follow-up. Recently, Cannon et al. [39] confirmed that facial nerve decompression is safe and efficacious. Five of fourteen patients ended up with a HB grade I, five ended up grade II, and the remaining four ended up grade III. While this study did not directly compare surgical to non-surgical patients, nevertheless it demonstrates that patients undergoing facial nerve decompression typically have good outcomes with low morbidity. This recent report reinforces the concept that those individuals with severe degeneration of the facial nerve, documented by objective ENoG, have better outcomes with decompression of the labyrinthine segment and meatal foramen of the fallopian canal.

Preoperative Preparation

The risks of middle fossa decompression of the facial nerve are discussed with the patient and include cerebrospinal fluid leak (4–6%), infection (1%), hearing loss (1%), dizziness (1%), intracranial hemorrhage (<1%), and aphasia (<1%). When the decision is made to proceed with surgical decompression, the procedure should be performed as soon as possible. Appropriate preoperative laboratory and imaging studies are obtained, along with a Stenvers projection plain radiograph of the temporal bone to identify the floor of the middle cranial fossa and superior semicircular canal. Cefazolin and dexamethasone are given before the skin incision and are continued for six doses.

General anesthesia and transoral endotracheal intubation are accomplished; thereafter, the bed is rotated 180 degrees for access (Fig. 57.3). Paralytic agents must be reversed before the skin incision. A urinary catheter is placed to monitor fluids and diuresis. Hair is shaved approximately 10 cm above and 5 cm behind the ear. The entire side of the head and face is prepared, and EMG needles are placed in the orbicu-

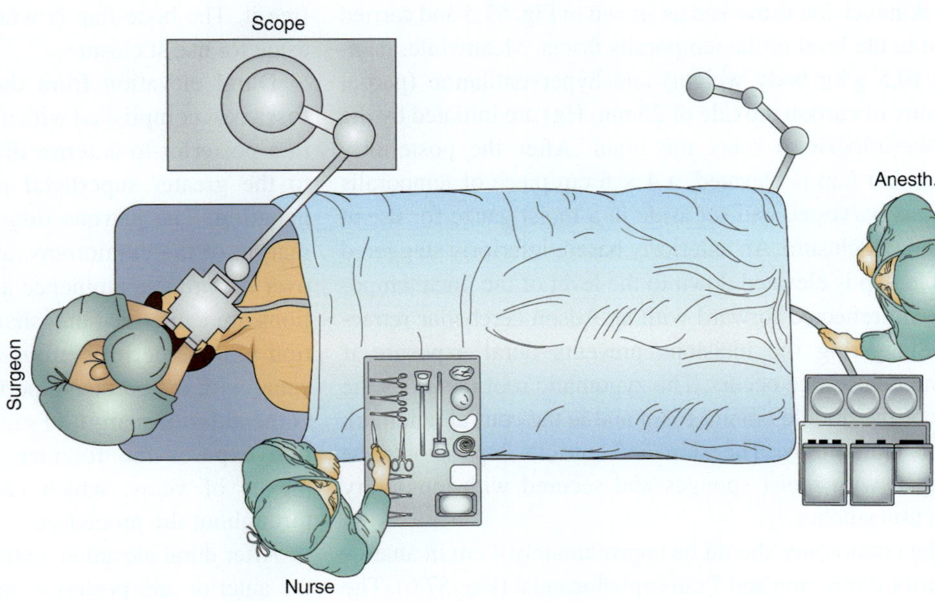

Fig. 57.3 Operating room setup for middle cranial fossa approach. (Adapted from Brackmann et al. [53])

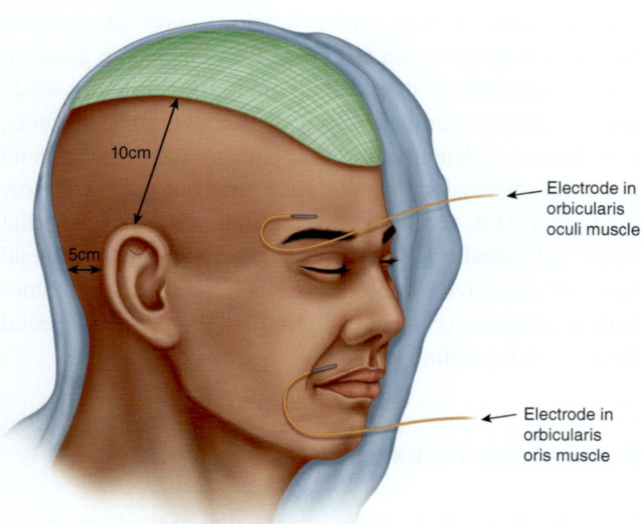

Fig. 57.4 Electrode placement for intraoperative electromyography. Draping is performed with exposure of the ipsilateral hemiface for visual monitoring of facial movement. (Adapted from Brackmann et al. [53])

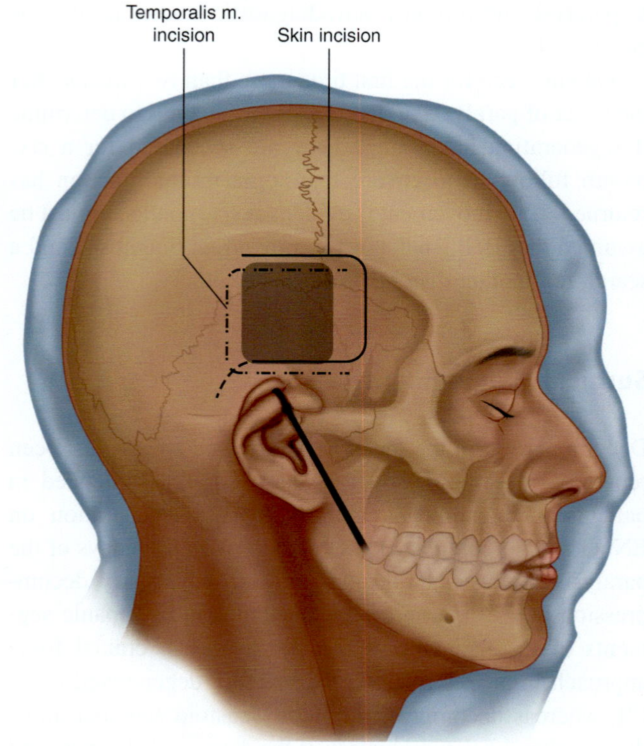

Fig. 57.5 A skin incision option for the middle cranial fossa approach. Mastoid exposure can be obtained by extending incision postauricularly, which is shown by the inferior extension of the skin incision line. An anteriorly based temporalis muscle flap is offset from the skin incision to keep suture lines from being directly in line. The location of the craniotomy is shaded. (Adapted from Brackmann et al. [53])

laris oculi and oris muscles (Fig. 57.4) for facial nerve monitoring. A clear drape is placed over the prepared area to allow visualization of the entire side of the face in the case of monitoring equipment failure. Standard auditory brainstem–evoked recording electrodes are placed in the right and left mastoid tips and the vertex and forehead (ground), and insert headphones are placed in both external auditory canals. The auditory brainstem response is monitored throughout the procedure.

Surgical Technique

The skin incision is marked as shown in Fig. 57.5 and carried down to the level of the temporalis fascia. Meanwhile, mannitol (0.5 g/kg body weight) and hyperventilation (partial pressure of carbon dioxide of 25 mm Hg) are initiated by the anesthesiologist to relax the brain. After the posteriorly based skin flap is elevated, a 4 × 6 cm piece of temporalis fascia is harvested and set aside in a moist gauze for use at the time of closure. An anteriorly based, inferiorly staggered muscle flap is elevated down to the level of the linea temporalis and reflected forward with an Adson cerebellar retractor. Staggering the incisions prevents dural exposure if wound dehiscence occurs. The zygomatic root identifies the floor of the middle cranial fossa and is the central landmark of the craniotomy. The skin and muscle flaps should be wrapped with moist sponges and secured with temporary retraction stitches.

The craniotomy should be approximately 4 cm in anteroposterior dimension and 5 cm cephalocaudal (Fig. 57.6). The anteroposterior margins must be kept parallel for stability of the middle cranial fossa retractor. The craniotomy can be created with either cutting burrs or a craniotomy saw. The bone flap should be elevated with care by use of a blunt dural elevator. Occasionally, the middle meningeal artery is embedded within the bone, requiring bipolar coagulation to free it. The bone flap is wrapped in a moist gauze and set aside for use at closure.

Dural elevation from the floor of the middle cranial fossa is accomplished with a Freer or joker elevator, always in a posterior-to-anterior direction, which prevents injury to the greater superficial petrosal nerve and geniculate ganglion. The petrous ridge is identified at the posterior margin of the craniotomy, and the dura is slowly elevated over the arcuate eminence and meatal plane. Dural reflections are cauterized and sharply transected to allow elevation to the anterior petrous ridge. The hiatus of the facial canal with the greater superficial petrosal nerve and artery is the anterior margin of elevation. Further anterior elevation exposes the foramen spinosum and the pterygoid plexus of veins, which can cause troublesome oozing throughout the procedure.

After dural elevation, cottonoid sponges can be placed at the anterior and posterior margins of the elevation to help

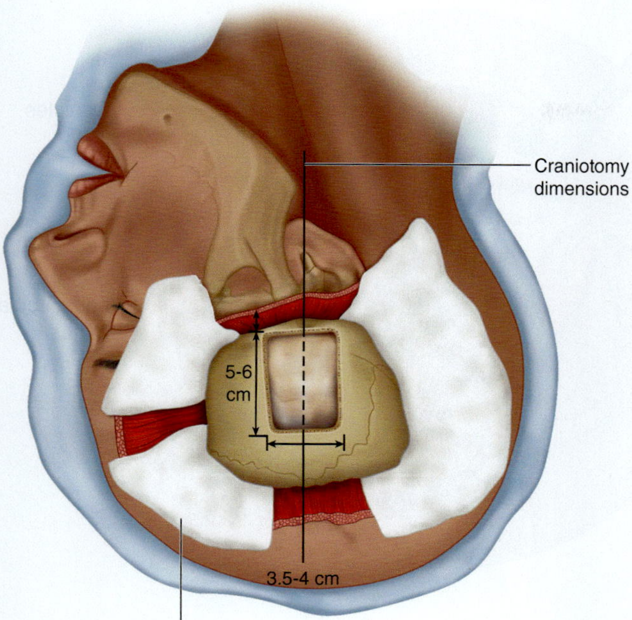

Fig. 57.6 Craniotomy for middle cranial fossa exposure. Inferior expansion of the craniotomy allows for more exposure during dural elevation. Vertical margins must be parallel for stability of the retractor. The craniotomy should be centered on the temporal root of the zygoma (dashed line). Placement of House-Urban middle cranial fossa retractor generally follows the exposure shown in this illustration and middle fossa dura elevation. (Adapted from Brackmann et al. [53])

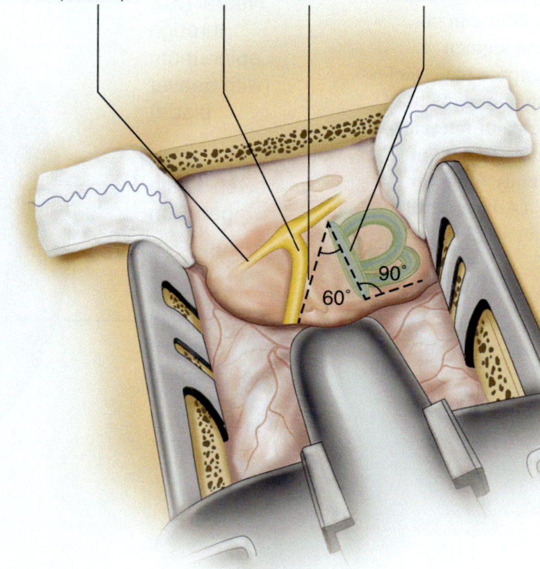

Fig. 57.7 Exposure of the superior semicircular canal blue line. The position of internal auditory canal (IAC) 60 degrees anterior to a line drawn through the blue line. The superior canal blue line almost always is perpendicular to the petrous ridge. (Adapted from Brackmann et al. [53])

retract the dura during placement of the self-retaining middle cranial fossa retractor (Fig. 57.6).

Before the bony exposure of the facial nerve, the Stenvers projection radiograph is re-examined to determine the depth of the superior semicircular canal in the temporal bone. The superior semicircular canal is the first structure to be located. When its blue line is identified, the remaining intratemporal structures have consistent anatomic locations. Landmarks of the middle cranial fossa floor can be quite subtle. The arcuate eminence may not be apparent and, in many instances, is not parallel with the superior semicircular canal. One consistent anatomic feature to remember is that the plane of the superior semicircular canal is almost always perpendicular to the petrous ridge (Fig. 57.7). If the arcuate eminence is not initially apparent, drilling is begun lateral to the superior semicircular canal, slowly removing the tegmen mastoideum with a moderate-sized diamond burr. The whitish color of the membranous temporal bone can be distinguished from the yellow, dense otic capsule bone of the superior canal. When the superior canal is identified, drilling in a parallel direction with the canal gradually exposes the blue line.

When the location of the superior canal is confirmed, an anterior line 60 degrees to the blue line locates the position of the internal auditory canal. The depth of the internal auditory canal varies, but drilling medially near the petrous ridge provides a safe route to the canal. Drilling laterally near the anterior ampulla of the superior semi-circular canal places the geniculate ganglion, labyrinthine segment of the facial nerve, and cochlea at risk. When the blue line of the internal auditory canal is exposed, bone is removed in a lateral direction until the vertical crest is found (Fig. 57.8). Bone can now be removed over the geniculate ganglion and tegmen tympani.

The labyrinthine segment of the facial nerve is the narrowest portion of the fallopian canal and lies in an anterosuperior plane from the vertical crest to the geniculate ganglion. A 1 mm diamond burr is used to remove bone over the labyrinthine segment, while the area directly anterior to the segment is closely observed for the blue line of the basal turn of the cochlea. The final layer of bone is removed from the labyrinthine, geniculate, and proximal tympanic segments of the facial nerve with thin, angled hooks and blunt microelevators. At this point, marked swelling of the nerve in the internal auditory canal, labyrinthine segment, geniculate ganglion, and proximal tympanic segments is usually observed. A dural ring at the meatal foramen is usually the point of greatest compression and this is opened with a 1.5 mm sharp hook or a disposable microscalpel (Beaver No. 59–10). The lysis of this constrictive band is critical in achieving full decompression of the labyrinthine segment.

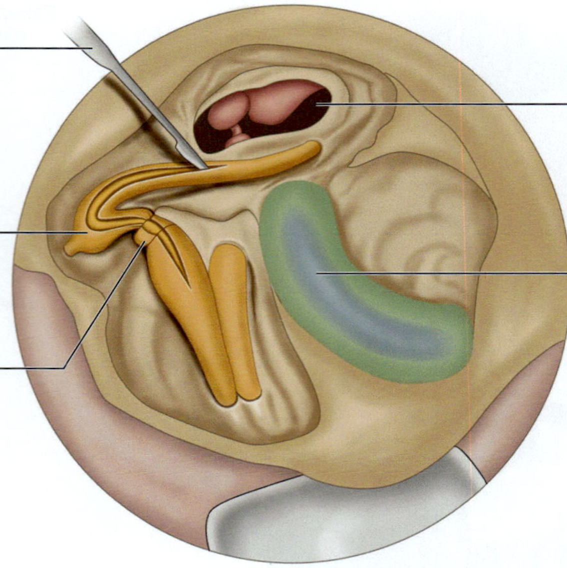

Fig. 57.8 Middle cranial fossa exposure of CN VII and surrounding anatomy. As is shown here, bone can be removed from tegmen tympani to expose the ossicles and the tympanic segment of CN VII. Edema of internal auditory canal segment of CN VII is frequently found in Bell's palsy. (Adapted from Brackmann et al. [53])

Intraoperative EMG is used to localize the region of the nerve conduction block. Direct stimulation of the most distal exposed tympanic segment of the nerve is performed with monopolar or bipolar microforceps. If the conduction block is medial to the point of stimulation, and the nerve is not completely degenerated, a motor unit potential is observed. Stimulating more medially toward the internal auditory canal fails to elicit a motor unit potential if the conduction block is at the meatal foramen. Even when ENoG shows 100% degeneration, motor unit potentials are often observed on intraoperative EMG, suggesting that there still exists nerve fibers capable of stimulation. Failure to generate a motor unit potential when the tympanic segment of the nerve is stimulated indicates that the nerve is completely degenerated with no conducting fibers remaining, or the site of conduction block is more distal. If the nerve appears normal in the tympanic segment while edema and erythema are present in the internal auditor canal segment, complete degeneration is suspected. However, if erythema and edema are apparent in the tympanic segment, a more distal block is suspected and a mastoidectomy decompression is then performed.

On completion of the decompression and confirmation of the site of the conduction block, the opened internal auditory canal is covered with a piece of temporalis muscle. The previously harvested temporalis fascia is placed over the opened floor of the middle fossa after bone waxing the opened mastoid air cells. The dural retractor is removed, and the anesthesiologist is asked to re-establish a normal partial pressure of carbon dioxide.

A corner of the craniotomy bone flap is harvested and placed superior to the fascia to prevent herniation of the temporal lobe dura into the attic and internal auditory canal. The temporal lobe is allowed to re-expand into the middle cranial fossa floor. The remainder of the craniotomy flap is placed on the dura, and the temporalis is closed, creating a watertight seal with interrupted absorbable sutures. Skin is closed with a deep layer of interrupted absorbable sutures and an outer layer of nylon absorbable sutures. A mastoid-type dressing is applied. No drains are used.

Postoperative Care

Postoperative care includes observation in the intensive care unit overnight, limitation of fluids (1500–1800 mL/day), dexamethasone (6 mg every 6 hours for 36 hours), cefazolin (1 g every 8 hours for 36 hours), routine neural checks, and limitation of analgesia to codeine. There is little postoperative pain, and narcotics stronger than codeine may mask intracranial complications. The patient is transferred to a routine postoperative floor the next morning, encouraged to begin ambulation, and started on a diet as tolerated. On postoperative day 3, and daily thereafter, observations for cerebrospinal fluid rhinorrhea are made by asking the patient to lean forward with the head between the knees. If cerebrospinal fluid rhinorrhea occurs, a spinal drain must be placed for four to five days. Following this regimen, only very rarely has a patient required surgical closure of the leak. Patients are usually discharged from the hospital on postoperative days 5–7. No intracranial complications, including intracranial hemorrhage, aphasia, or seizures, occurred in the Iowa series [38].

Limitations and Special Considerations

Dural elevation can be difficult, especially in patients older than 65 years. If a dural tear occurs, a temporalis fascia repair must be performed. Hearing loss can occur from contact of the rotating burr with an intact ossicular chain or by entrance into the cochlea or labyrinth. Vestibular dysfunction can occur in a similar fashion. If the bony labyrinth is violated, immediate placement of a small amount of bone wax may preserve auditory and vestibular function.

Correct positioning of the craniotomy and maintaining parallel vertical margins are essential. Meticulous hemostasis must be maintained with bipolar cautery, oxidized cellulose, and pressure. A dry surgical field is crucial for microscopic dissection of subtle landmarks and prevention of complications. If large apical air cells are opened, they must be plugged with temporalis muscle to prevent cerebrospinal fluid leakage.

In appropriately selected patients, facial nerve decompression offers a significant benefit for maximizing facial nerve outcomes [38]. The middle fossa approach is technically demanding and the anatomy of the middle cranial fossa floor is varied and presents some difficulty in identification of landmarks. The surgeon must have a precise knowledge of the three-dimensional anatomy of the temporal bone. Many hours in the temporal bone dissection laboratory are required to attain the delicate microsurgical skills necessary for this type of surgery. Therefore, the risk versus benefit analysis must be individualized not only to each patient but also to the experience level of each surgeon. For patients with complete paralysis who can tolerate middle fossa surgery and desire to proceed with surgical intervention, facial nerve decompression should be offered. Referral to a medical center with expertise in middle fossa surgery is warranted if these services are not available to the patient [40].

The American Academy of Otolaryngology—Head and Neck Surgery [30] has recently released guidelines for the management of Bell's palsy. The guidelines committee could not make a recommendation on whether decompression of the facial nerve was of value in Bell's palsy. This decision was made on the "non-randomized clinical trials and the equilibrium of the benefit and the harm." They also stated that "although the data supporting surgical decompression are not strong, there may be a significant benefit for a small subset of patients who meet eligibility criteria and desire surgical management." There were major differences of opinion on the committee with regard to surgical decompression. This difference of opinion derived from controversy regarding the strength of evidence (C level evidence vs. D level evidence.)

To date, three separate reports [35, 38, 39], employing similar measures to select patients for decompression of the facial nerve in Bell's palsy, suggest that the procedure is of value when it is limited to those with severe Wallerian degeneration, measured with the combination of ENoG and volitional EMG and surgical decompression includes the meatal foramen, labyrinthine segment, and geniculate ganglion. Unfortunately, it will be very difficult to accrue the necessary subject population to complete a randomized controlled study on an orphan-like disease patient population that would meet the criteria for surgical decompression. The Gantz et al. and Cannon et al. studies [38, 39] required 15 and 12 years, respectively, to accumulate the reported patient populations.

Herpes Zoster Oticus

Herpes zoster oticus refers to a syndrome of acute otalgia accompanied by a herpetic, vesicular rash. When accompanied by facial paralysis, the syndrome is known as Ramsay Hunt syndrome [41]. Ramsay Hunt syndrome is the second most common cause of facial paralysis (after Bell's palsy) and is induced by the reactivation of the varicella-zoster virus that remains latent in the geniculate ganglion after primary infection with chickenpox [42]. Classically, patients present with severe otalgia and unilateral facial paralysis. Vesicular eruptions may or may not be present initially, but they usually appear within three to five days of the paralysis. The vesicular lesions can appear on the concha, ear canal, postauricular skin, and tympanic membrane. Occasionally, the oral cavity, neck, and shoulder are also involved. The disease can affect other cranial nerves, including auditory, vestibular, trigeminal, glossopharyngeal, and vagus, prompting the name *herpes zoster cephalicus* [43].

Also in contrast to Bell's palsy, the symptoms are more severe, and the prognosis is worse in Ramsay Hunt syndrome. The frequency of complete neural degeneration of the facial nerve is substantially higher than with Bell's palsy, and complete recovery of facial motor function has ranged from 10 to 31% in several studies [44, 45]. Patients with auditory and vestibular dysfunction in addition to facial paralysis generally have a worse prognosis. In addition, patients with diabetes, hypertension, and advanced age have been reported to have a poorer prognosis in Ramsay Hunt syndrome [46].

The diagnosis of Ramsay Hunt syndrome is based on the history of otalgia, vesicular lesions or eschars, and facial paralysis. MRI shows enhancement of a large portion of the facial nerve, often the vestibular and cochlear nerves, the labyrinth, and the dura lining the internal auditory canal [47]. Imaging as part of routine evaluation is unnecessary. Electrodiagnostic studies have been unreliable in *herpes zoster oticus*.

The management of Ramsay Hunt syndrome has changed with the development of antiviral agents. The natural history of the disease was evaluated by Devriese and Moesker [45], who identified only a 10% rate of complete facial nerve recovery. Many studies have identified a superior recovery rate of 75% using a combination of steroids and antiviral agents [48–51]. The benefit of early initiation of steroid and antiviral treatment was clearly shown in a study by Murakami and colleagues [49], in which 75% of patients treated within three days of the onset had complete recovery, whereas only 30% of patients treated after seven days experienced a complete recovery. We have experienced similar successful results using intravenous acyclovir (10 mg/kg three times daily), oral acyclovir (800 mg five times daily), or oral valacyclovir (500 mg three times daily) for 10 days, in combination with a three-week (60–80 mg daily). Patients report rapid reduction in pain and occasionally experience return of facial movement during the medical therapy. Because of the presence of "skip" regions and diffuse neuritis of the facial nerve [52], surgical decompression of Ramsay Hunt syndrome is not recommended.

Summary

Bell's palsy is a clinical entity encountered with relative frequency by practitioners of many specialties. Before making the diagnosis of Bell's palsy, other causes of facial paralysis must be excluded through thorough history taking and physical examination. Bell's palsy and Ramsay Hunt syndrome seem to be due to viral etiologies, and seem to benefit from medical therapy with steroids and antiherpetic medications.

Electrodiagnostic testing in cases of Bell's palsy with complete paralysis is indicated and provides crucial information to guide surgical decision-making and patient counseling. In cases of Bell's palsy with greater than 90% degeneration on ENoG and absence of CMAP on EMG, middle fossa craniotomy with decompression of the labyrinthine, geniculate, and proximal tympanic segments of the nerve should be offered to patients without medical contraindications to an intracranial procedure. Familiarity with the anatomy of the middle cranial fossa is essential for the effective decompression of the facial nerve and avoidance of complications.

References

1. Peitersen E. Bell's palsy: the spontaneous course of 2,500 peripheral facial nerve palsies of different etiologies. Acta Otolaryngol Suppl. 2002;122:4–30.
2. Hauser WA, Karnes WE, Annis J, et al. Incidence and prognosis of Bell's palsy in the population of Rochester, Minnesota. Mayo Clin Proc. 1971;46:258–64.
3. Katusic SK, Beard CM, Wiederholt WC, et al. Incidence, clinical features, and prognosis in Bell's palsy, Rochester, Minnesota, 1968–1982. Ann Neurol. 1986;20:622–7.
4. Adour KK. Current concepts in neurology: diagnosis and management of facial paralysis. N Engl J Med. 1982;307:348–51.
5. Cwach H, Landis J, Freeman JW. Bilateral seventh nerve palsy: a report of two cases and a review. S D J Med. 1997;50:99–101.
6. Holland NJ, Weiner GM. Recent developments in Bell's palsy. BMJ. 2004;329:553–7.
7. E E. Electromyography and electroneurography. In: Fisch U, editor. Electromyography and electroneurography. Birmingham: Aesculapius; 1977. p. 93–100.
8. Bell C. On the nerves, giving an account of some experiments on their structure and function, which led to a new arrangement of the system. Philos Trans. 1821;111:398–424.
9. McCormick DP. Herpes-simplex virus as a cause of Bell's palsy. Lancet. 1972;1:937–9.
10. Furuta Y, Fukuda S, Chida E, et al. Reactivation of herpes simplex virus type 1 in patients with Bell's palsy. J Med Virol. 1998;54:162–6.
11. Burgess RC, Michaels L, Bale JF Jr, et al. Polymerase chain reaction amplification of herpes simplex viral DNA from the geniculate ganglion of a patient with Bell's palsy. Ann Otol Rhinol Laryngol. 1994;103:775–9.
12. Murakami S, Mizobuchi M, Nakashiro Y, et al. Bell palsy and herpes simplex virus: identification of viral DNA in endoneurial fluid and muscle. Ann Intern Med. 1996;124:27–30.
13. Sugita T, Murakami S, Yanagihara N, et al. Facial nerve paralysis induced by herpes simplex virus in mice: an animal model of acute and transient facial paralysis. Ann Otol Rhinol Laryngol. 1995;104:574–81.
14. Lazarini PR, Vianna MF, Alcantara MP, et al. Herpes simplex virus in the saliva of peripheral Bell's palsy patients. Braz J Otorhinolaryngol. 2006;72:7–11.
15. Liston SL, Kleid MS. Histopathology of Bell's palsy. Laryngoscope. 1989;99:23–6.
16. Carreno M, Llorente JL, Hidalgo F, et al. Application of the polymerase chain reaction to an experimental model of infection by herpes simplex virus type 1. Acta Otorrinolaringol Esp. 1998;49:15–8.
17. Reddy JB, Liu J, Balshi S, et al. Histopathology of Bell's palsy. Eye Ear Nose Throat Mon. 1966;45:62–6.
18. Fowler EP Jr. The pathologic findings in a case of facial paralysis. Acta Otolaryngol. 1963;56:113–25.
19. McKeever P, Proctor B, Proud G. Cranial nerve lesions in Bell's palsy. Otolaryngol Head Neck Surg. 1987;97:326–7.
20. Podvinec M. Facial nerve disorders: anatomical, histological and clinical aspects. Adv Otorhinolaryngol. 1984;32:124–93.
21. Jackson CG, Johnson GD, Hyams VJ, et al. Pathologic findings in the labyrinthine segment of the facial nerve in a case of facial paralysis. Ann Otol Rhinol Laryngol. 1990;99:327–9.
22. Fisch U, Felix H. On the pathogenesis of Bell's palsy. Acta Otolaryngol. 1983;95:532–8.
23. Gantz BJ, Gmur A, Fisch U. Intraoperative evoked electromyography in Bell's palsy. Am J Otolaryngol. 1982;3:273–8.
24. Proctor B, Corgill DA, Proud G. The pathology of Bell's palsy. Trans Sect Otolaryngol Am Acad Ophthalmol Otolaryngol. 1976;82:Orl70–80.
25. Peitersen E. Natural history of Bell's palsy. Acta Otolaryngol Suppl. 1992;492:122–4.
26. Salinas RA, Alvarez G, Alvarez MI, et al. Corticosteroids for Bell's palsy (idiopathic facial paralysis). Cochrane Database Syst Rev. 2002:Cd001942.
27. Sullivan FM, Swan IR, Donnan PT, et al. Early treatment with prednisolone or acyclovir in Bell's palsy. N Engl J Med. 2007;357:1598–607.

28. Engstrom M, Berg T, Stjernquist-Desatnik A, et al. Prednisolone and valaciclovir in Bell's palsy: a randomised, double-blind, placebo-controlled, multicentre trial. Lancet Neurol. 2008;7:993–1000.
29. Hato N, Yamada H, Kohno H, et al. Valacyclovir and prednisolone treatment for Bell's palsy: a multicenter, randomized, placebo-controlled study. Otol Neurotol. 2007;28:408–13.
30. Baugh RF, Basura GJ, Ishii LE, et al. Clinical practice guideline: Bell's palsy. Otolaryngol Head Neck Surg. 2013;149:S1–27.
31. Gilden DH, Tyler KL. Bell's palsy — is glucocorticoid treatment enough? N Engl J Med. 2007;357:1653–5.
32. Adour KK, Ruboyianes JM, Von Doersten PG, et al. Bell's palsy treatment with acyclovir and prednisone compared with prednisone alone: a double-blind, randomized, controlled trial. Ann Otol Rhinol Laryngol. 1996;105:371–8.
33. Grogan PM, Gronseth GS. Practice parameter: steroids, acyclovir, and surgery for Bell's palsy (an evidence-based review): report of the quality standards Subcommittee of the American Academy of neurology. Neurology. 2001;56:830–6.
34. Gagyor I, Madhok VB, Daly F, et al. Antiviral treatment for Bell's palsy (idiopathic facial paralysis). In: Cochrane Database Syst Rev; 2015. https://doi.org/10.1002/14651858.CD001869.pub9.
35. Fisch U. Surgery for Bell's palsy. Arch Otolaryngol. 1981;107:1–11.
36. Ballance C. A note on the operative treatment of facial palsy. Br Med J. 1932;1:787–8.
37. May M, Klein SR, Taylor FH. Idiopathic (Bell's) facial palsy: natural history defies steroid or surgical treatment. Laryngoscope. 1985;95:406–9.
38. Gantz BJ, Rubinstein JT, Gidley P, et al. Surgical management of Bell's palsy. Laryngoscope. 1999;109:1177–88.
39. Cannon RB, Gurgel RK, Warren FM, et al. Facial nerve outcomes after middle fossa decompression for Bell's palsy. Otol Neurotol. 2015;36:513–8.
40. de Ru JA, van Benthem PP, Janssen LM. All evidence is equal, but some is more equal than others. Otol Neurotol. 2010;31:551–3.
41. Sachs E Jr, House RK. The Ramsay hunt syndrome, geniculate herpes. Neurology. 1956;6:262–8.
42. Ikeda M, Hiroshige K, Abiko Y, et al. Impaired specific cellular immunity to the varicella-zoster virus in patients with herpes zoster oticus. J Laryngol Otol. 1996;110:918–21.
43. Adour KK. Otological complications of herpes zoster. Ann Neurol. 1994;35(Suppl):S62–4.
44. Devriese P. Herpes zoster causing facial paralysis. In: Fisch U, editor. Facial nerve surgery. Birmingham, AL: Aesculapius; 1977. p. 419–20.
45. Devriese PP, Moesker WH. The natural history of facial paralysis in herpes zoster. Clin Otolaryngol Allied Sci. 1988;13:289–98.
46. Yeo SW, Lee DH, Jun BC, et al. Analysis of prognostic factors in Bell's palsy and Ramsay hunt syndrome. Auris Nasus Larynx. 2007;34:159–64.
47. Brandle P, Satoretti-Schefer S, Bohmer A, et al. Correlation of MRI, clinical, and electroneuronographic findings in acute facial nerve palsy. Am J Otol. 1996;17:154–61.
48. Dickins JR, Smith JT, Graham SS. Herpes zoster oticus: treatment with intravenous acyclovir. Laryngoscope. 1988;98:776–9.
49. Murakami S, Hato N, Horiuchi J, et al. Treatment of Ramsay hunt syndrome with acyclovir-prednisone: significance of early diagnosis and treatment. Ann Neurol. 1997;41:353–7.
50. Stafford FW, Welch AR. The use of acyclovir in Ramsay Hunt syndrome. J Laryngol Otol. 1986;100:337–40.
51. Uri N, Greenberg E, Meyer W, et al. Herpes zoster oticus: treatment with acyclovir. Ann Otol Rhinol Laryngol. 1992;101:161–2.
52. Honda N, Yanagihara N, Hato N, et al. Swelling of the intratemporal facial nerve in Ramsay Hunt syndrome. Acta Otolaryngol. 2002;122:348–52.
53. Brackmann D, et al., editors. Otologic surgery. 4th ed. Elsevier; 2015.

Encephaloceles and Cerebrospinal Fluid Leaks

58

Nicholas L. Deep, Emily Kay-Rivest, and J. Thomas Roland Jr

Introduction

Cerebrospinal fluid (CSF) leaks are an uncommon condition but with an increasing incidence in recent years [1]. Due to their potentially life-threatening complications, CSF leaks necessitate prompt diagnosis and treatment. A CSF leak occurs when there is a dural tear and bony defect in a pneumatized portion of the skull base, allowing CSF to escape from the subarachnoid space and track extracranially. If the dural defect is large enough, an associated encephalocele or meningoencephalocele may be present [2]. The clinical presentation may be insidious and nonspecific, such as aural fullness and hearing loss due to a middle ear effusion, or patients may report clear drainage from their nose or ear [3]. In rare cases, meningitis may be the initial presentation [4]. While severe intracranial complications associated with CSF leaks and encephaloceles have decreased in the modern post-antibiotic era, the incidence of spontaneous CSF leaks has increased, largely in association with the rise in morbid obesity [5–8]. Cranial CSF fluid leaks may involve the anterior or lateral skull base, but for the purposes of this chapter, focus will be placed on lateral skull base CSF leaks.

We begin this chapter discussing the pathogenesis and causes of cranial CSF leaks, broadly classifying them into two main categories: (1) traumatic, which includes post-surgical and following head trauma and (2) nontraumatic or spontaneous CSF leaks. The subsequent section will discuss the diagnosis, with emphasis on spontaneous CSF leaks. The last section addresses treatment options and is subdivided into three sub-sections: treatment of spontaneous CSF leaks, prevention and management of postoperative skull base CSF leaks, and management of post-traumatic CSF leaks.

Pathogenesis

CSF Physiology

Cerebrospinal fluid is produced mainly by the choroid plexus (approximately 70%), at a rate of 0.25–0.6 mL/minute. Total volume of CSF is about 100–150 mL, and at any given time, about 40 mL of this volume is within the ventricular system of the brain. CSF is distributed throughout the brain and spinal cord via the subarachnoid space. Excess CSF is absorbed back into the bloodstream via structures called arachnoid granulations, which are located in the walls of the venous sinuses within the dura mater. Arachnoid granulations act as one-way valves that allow CSF to enter the bloodstream, while preventing blood from entering the subarachnoid

Supplementary Information The online version contains supplementary material available at https://doi.org/10.1007/978-3-032-18264-7_58.

N. L. Deep
Department of Otolaryngology—Head and Neck Surgery, Division of Otology and Neurotology, Mayo Clinic, Phoenix, AZ, USA
e-mail: deep.nicholas@mayo.edu

E. Kay-Rivest
Department of Otolaryngology—Head and Neck Surgery, McGill University, Montreal, QC, Canada
e-mail: emily.kay-rivest@mcgill.ca

J. Thomas Roland Jr (✉)
Department of Otolaryngology—Head and Neck Surgery, NYU Langone Health, New York, NY, USA
e-mail: J.Thomas.RolandJr@nyulangone.org

A. D. Sweeney et al. (eds.), *Haynes-Glasscock-Shambaugh Surgery of the Ear*, https://doi.org/10.1007/978-3-032-18264-7_58

space. Occlusion of a major venous sinus, therefore, is one of many causes that result in hydrocephalus (increased intracranial pressure) which in turn may precipitate a CSF leak. A normal CSF pressure is between 5 and 15 cm of water. A pressure of greater than 20 cm of water is considered abnormally high. Importantly, patients with an active CSF leak may have a CSF opening pressure that is falsely low.

Causes of Lateral Skull Base CSF Leaks

Cranial CSF leaks can be broadly classified as traumatic or nontraumatic/spontaneous (Fig. 58.1).

Traumatic

Traumatic CSF leaks represent 80% of all cases and are related to either head trauma or surgery (iatrogenic) [9, 10]. Cerebrospinal fluid leaks occur in 17% of temporal bone fractures and are more common with otic capsule-disrupting fractures compared to otic capsule-sparing fractures [11].

Following skull base surgery, CSF leaks are reported to occur in 5–10% of cases and may manifest as clear drainage from the incision (transcutaneous), from the nose (CSF rhinorrhea), or from the ear (CSF otorrhea) if the tympanic membrane has been violated [12, 13].

Nontraumatic or Spontaneous CSF Leaks

Spontaneous CSF leaks have an estimated incidence of 5/100,000 annually, with women being twice as likely to be affected as men. Spontaneous CSF leaks can be subdivided into high-pressure leaks that are associated with increased intracranial pressure (ICP) versus normal pressure leaks. In the cases of high ICP, continuous CSF pulsations progressively erode bone and eventually the dural membrane is breached leading to a direct connection between the subarachnoid space and the extracranial space [6, 14]. The fistula may originate from the middle or posterior fossa and may communicate with the middle ear, mastoid, or petrous apex.

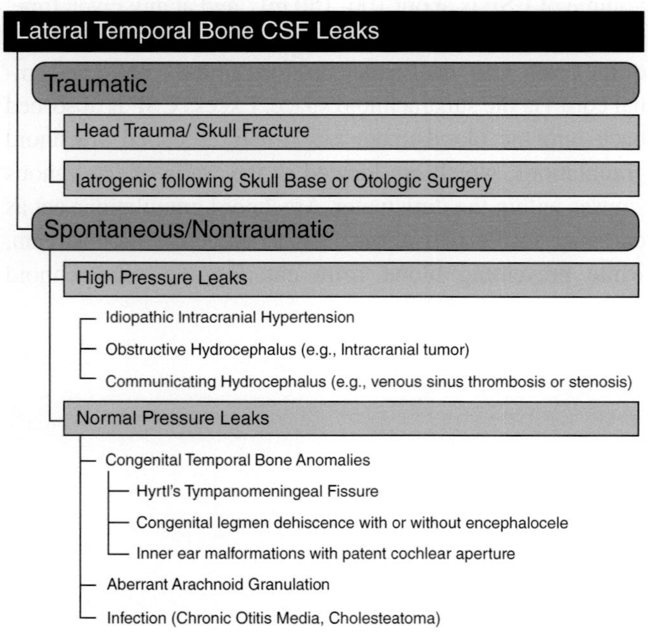

Fig. 58.1 Causes of lateral temporal bone CSF leaks

Patients with idiopathic intracranial hypertension (IIH), obesity, and obstructive sleep apnea are at risk of developing a spontaneous CSF leak. While the precise relationship between these clinical conditions is still being understood, it is thought that the increased intra-abdominal pressure in an obese patient leads to lower venous return and eventually higher intracranial pressure with consequent bone erosion [15]. Approximately 70–80% of spontaneous CSF leaks are due to idiopathic intracranial hypertension (IIH), largely attributable to the obesity epidemic [16]. In a study comparing the rates of CSF leak repair between 2002 and 2012, Nelson et al. found that there was no change in the rate of repair for iatrogenic or trauma-related CSF leaks; however, the rate of repair for spontaneous CSF leaks increased by 124% [8].

Other causes of high-pressure CSF leaks include intracranial tumors that result in obstructive hydrocephalus or dural sinus thrombosis (or stenosis) that results in communicating hydrocephalus. With these conditions, chronically elevated ICP accelerates bony breakdown and can lead to a CSF fistula.

Nontraumatic causes of normal pressure CSF leak include congenital cranial anomalies. Patients with a congenitally dehiscent tegmen or congenital middle ear encephalocele may present with a CSF leak. A patent Hyrtl's tympanomeningeal fissure has also been rarely reported. In a Hyrtl's fissure, there is failure of a connection between the subarachnoid space and hypotympanum to ossify in utero, leading to a persistent connection and CSF leak that bypasses the inner ear [17]. Other observed anomalies include an enlarged fallopian canal that allows CSF to leak into the middle ear adjacent to the facial nerve or anomalies of the stapes footplate [18–20]. Certain inner ear malformations are at higher risk of a CSF leak and meningitis, including those with a patent cochlear aperture (e.g., X-linked stapes gusher) [21]. The defective partition between the internal auditory canal (IAC) fundus and cochlea results in CSF coming into direct contact with the oval window and potentially erupting through the stapes footplate [22].

Aberrant arachnoid granulations may also potentiate a CSF leak. Arachnoid granulations are extensions of the arachnoid membrane that function as passive filters through which CSF drains into the dural venous sinuses. For an unknown reason, during development, some arachnoid granulations do not terminate in a venous sinus; rather they come to lie against a bony surface within the skull, presumably draining into the cancellous bone directly. Over time, the CSF pressure and pulsations can cause bone erosion and a CSF leak, especially if the bone being eroded is near a pneumatized part of the skull [23]. Aberrant arachnoid granulations most commonly involve the anterior and middle cranial fossa, but sometimes posterior fossa as well [24–26].

Lastly, tumors that directly invade the skull base or infections can result in a normal pressure CSF leak. Chronic festering otitis media or an expanding attic cholesteatoma may result in osteitis and bone erosion of the tegmen tympani with herniation of middle fossa contents and eventual CSF leak as the dura is breached [27].

Diagnosis

History

The diagnosis of a temporal bone CSF leak is largely guided by the clinical scenario. Spinal fluid leaks following skull base surgery or after head trauma resulting in a skull fracture are obvious and are often readily recognized after the patient presents with clear fluid from the nose, ear, or incision. On the other hand, patients with a spontaneous CSF leak may present more insidiously. The most common presenting symptoms in a patient with a spontaneous CSF leak are unilateral hearing loss, tinnitus, and ear fullness, occurring in 84% of patients [28]. Bilateral encephaloceles with CSF leaks can also occur in approximately 10% of cases, and this finding is more common in the setting of IIH [7, 14, 29]. The average age of a patient with a spontaneous CSF leak ranges from 45 to 63 years old and there is a slightly higher proportion of women affected compared to men [3, 5, 7, 14, 30]. Interestingly, the complaint of CSF rhinorrhea is uncommon in patients with spontaneous CSF leaks compared to patients who have recently undergone a skull base surgical procedure. Therefore, the diagnosis can potentially evade clinicians and go undiagnosed for years. Patients with a previously placed tympanostomy tube will present with persistent clear, persistent, odorless watery-type drainage that saturates their pillow at night. Such a history is uncommon in patients with chronic otitis media and should therefore alert the physician to a CSF leak. Tension pneumocephalus is uncommon but may be the presenting issue, particularly in a patient on continuous positive airway pressure (CPAP). In these cases, air enters the intracranial space through the bony defect, gets trapped and is allowed to accumulate [31, 32]. Uncommonly, patients may present with a history of recurrent meningitis, seizures or a brain abscess. The risk of meningitis depends on the etiology of the leak. For spontaneous CSF leaks, the average rate of meningitis is around 20%, but the reported incidence ranges widely from 6% to 58% [28, 33, 34].

Headaches, visual disturbances, and/or dizziness complaints may co-exist with a CSF leak and could suggest a diagnosis of IIH, especially in an obese patient with obstructive sleep apnea. Complaints of hearing of internal bodily sounds, such as pulsatile tinnitus, hearing footsteps or eyeball movements reverberating in the affected ear, and pressure- or sound-induced vertigo suggest a diagnosis of concomitant superior canal dehiscence.

Physical Exam

On otoscopic exam, the middle ear effusion is clear, in contrast with the amber color that is common in effusions due to Eustachian tube dysfunction. Since the fluid is clear and translucent, the middle ear may be mistaken for being well-aerated. Looking for an air bubble or meniscus signifying an air–fluid level is often the only clue on exam that confirms the presence of an effusion. Pneumatic otoscopy can also be a useful adjunct when assessing middle ear aeration. Audiometric testing can suggest the presence of retrotympanic fluid, and in this case, it usually shows a mild-to-moderate conductive hearing loss, with a type B (flat) tympanogram and normal volume. Nasopharyngoscopy is always performed in the setting of a unilateral middle ear effusion to assess for any masses obstructing the Eustachian tube.

With larger tegmen defects, brain herniation may occur. An encephalocele will look like a pale pulsatile mass in the superior aspect of the middle ear behind the tympanic membrane. The mass will increase in size with maneuvers that increase intracranial pressure such as Valsalva or jugular vein compression (Furstenberg sign). A high index of suspicion for an encephalocele is warranted in these cases and a biopsy is not performed until imaging can be done to rule out an encephalocele.

In cases where IIH is suspected, papilledema (often bilateral) may be identified on dilated fundoscopic examination. The most common profile of a patient who fits this diagnosis is a middle-aged, obese female.

A provocation test known as the Dandy maneuver can be done to reproduce the rhinorrhea and confirm diagnosis (Fig. 58.2). In this test, the patient leans forward with the head pointed down while performing a Valsalva against a closed glottis. The test is considered positive if clear fluid drips from the nostril. The side of the nostril from which the leakage occurs often corresponds to the side of the CSF leak. Consideration should be given to capturing the fluid as a specimen for analysis if fluid is produced.

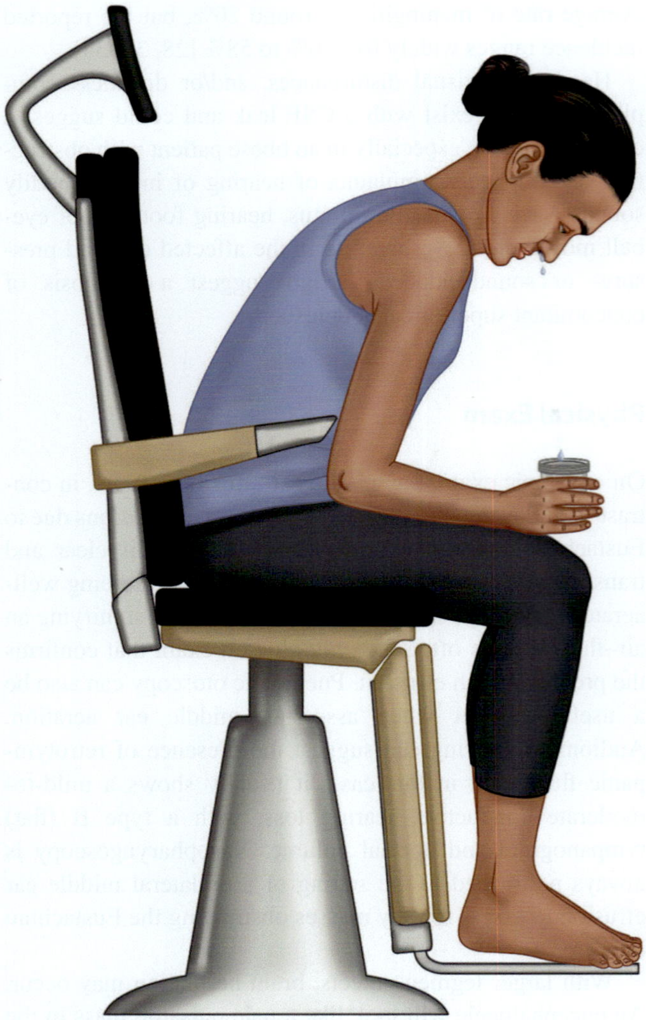

Fig. 58.2 The Dandy Maneuver is shown, which is a provocation test to attempt to reproduce CSF for collection and diagnosis. The patient leans forward and performs a Valsalva against a closed glottis which increases intracranial pressure. Fluid is captured into a specimen cup in case it will be sent for analysis. (Adapted from Mayo Clinic Media)

Labs

The gold standard confirmatory test for a CSF leak is a positive beta-2 transferrin study on the fluid sample [35]. Beta-2 transferrin is a protein that is only found in CSF and in certain fluids of the body such as perilymph of the inner ear and the aqueous and vitreous humor of the eye. It is not found in blood or other body fluids, making it a highly sensitive and specific marker for CSF.

Despite beta-2 transferrin being the gold standard confirmatory test, the authors of this chapter find that the history, physical exam, and imaging are sufficient to make the diagnosis. Patients who have undergone skull base surgery within the last three months are at risk of CSF leak, so testing for beta-2 transferrin is unnecessary as the diagnosis is assumed and further testing would only delay care. Similarly, in cases where the diagnosis of a spontaneous CSF leak is clear based on imaging and exam findings, the authors do not routinely perform a myringotomy to sample the fluid prior to surgical correction as this introduces the risk of infection.

If the diagnosis is uncertain, however, aspiration of the middle ear fluid may be performed and sent for beta-2-transferrin analysis. Placement of a tympanostomy tube is not recommended because this would lead to a persistent high-volume leak and would increase the risk of infection.

In patients with an intermittent leak, a beta-2 transferrin assay kit may be sent home with them to collect a fluid sample. Alternatively, a pledget study can be performed. This study involves placing a piece of cotton in the ear adjacent to a tympanostomy tube and additional pieces of cotton are placed in the left and right superior nasal cavity. The patient returns the next day and these cotton pledgets are removed and sent for beta-2 transferrin analysis.

Imaging

A high-resolution, thin-sliced temporal bone computed tomography (CT) is the best initial modality to detect the location of a lateral skull base defect. In cases of a CSF leak, the middle ear and mastoid are typically completely opacified, but bony septations are preserved septations of the mastoid air cells in the setting of a CSF leak (Fig. 58.3a). Sometimes, an encephalocele may be present without a CSF leak in the early stages of development suggesting the bone has resorbed but the dura is still intact (Fig. 58.3b). Close inspection is given to all potential sites of temporal bone CSF fistulas including the tegmen tympani (Fig. 58.3c), mastoid tegmen, posterior petrous bone adjacent to the mastoid, petrous apex, and other rare cranial anomalies (e.g., Hyrtl's tympanomeningeal fissure, facial nerve canal, and stapes). Approximately 20–40% of people have natural dehiscences of their skull base so looking for opacification of air cells adjacent to the dehiscent bone is necessary to confirm the site of the leak. Aberrant arachnoid granulations may be seen as bony pits along the middle fossa floor, and sometimes posterior petrous bone. Superior semicircular canal dehiscence can coexist in approximately 10–30% of patients with spontaneous CSF leaks and is also due to progressive erosion of the skull base floor (Fig. 58.3a**, arrow**) [29, 30, 36–38].

Magnetic resonance imaging (MRI) is helpful in showing encephaloceles with a high diagnostic yield around 75–90% [39, 40]. Coronal reformats of heavily weighted T2 sequences such as CISS (Siemens) or FIESTA (GE) are particularly helpful for identifying an encephalocele or site of CSF leak (Fig. 58.3d). An MRI is also helpful in looking for evidence of IIH, including a partially empty sella turcica, transverse venous sinus stenosis, flattening of the posterior globe, enhancement of the prelaminar optic nerves, prominent sub-

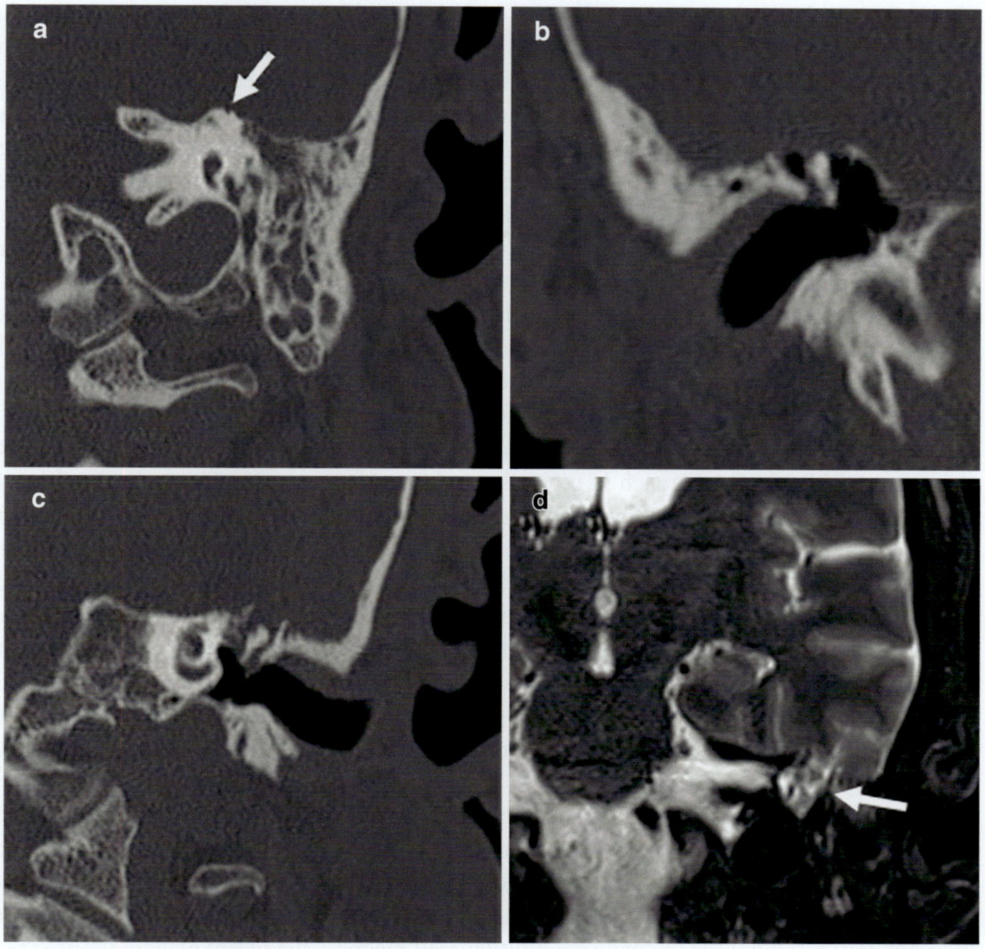

Fig. 58.3 (**a**) Coronal CT of a left ear demonstrating an opacified mastoid cavity with preserved bony septations of the mastoid air cells, compatible with a CSF leak. Note the white arrow which points to a dehiscent superior semicircular canal. (**b**) Coronal CT of the right ear in the same patient which demonstrates tegmen dehiscence with sagging of the temporal dura on the head of the malleus causing a conductive hearing loss. The area surrounding the ossicles are well-aerated suggesting the dura is intact and there is no active CSF leak. (**c**) Coronal CT of a left ear in the same patient demonstrating a more anterior slice through the middle ear which shows a tegmen tympani dehiscence with opacification surrounding the ossicles, consistent with a CSF leak. (**d**) High-resolution heavily T2-weighted coronal MRI demonstrating the encephalocele herniating into the middle ear

arachnoid space around the optics nerves, and vertical tortuosity of the optic nerves, among others [41]. The majority of patients with IIH and spontaneous CSF leak have an associated encephalocele, as opposed to CSF leak alone.

In patients with an intermittent leak, CT cisternography with intrathecal injection of a radiopaque material such as fluorescein can be performed to look for evidence of extravasation which identifies the site of the leak. However, for small or intermittent leaks, this study may lead to a false-negative. For this reason, this study is typically reserved for high-risk patients, such as those with a history of meningitis (particularly due to pneumococcus) or recurrent infections but without a localizing source of the CSF leak.

Treatment

Management of Spontaneous CSF Leaks

Indications

Patients with an encephalocele but without an active leak may be safely observed. However, any patient with an active CSF leak is recommended to undergo surgical repair given the risk of meningitis or other intracranial infection. Although some patients live with active leaks for years without complication, the authors aim to perform surgery within one to three months from diagnosis. There is limited evidence to support empiric antibiotics for patients with a spontaneous CSF leak without signs or symptoms of an active infection [34]. Antipneumococcal immunization is recommended, however [42].

For those with IIH, ophthalmology and neurology consultations are recommended to evaluate for papilledema, identify a visual field deficit, and initiate treatment (e.g., acetazolamide, weight loss, consideration for shunt). A lumbar puncture may be considered, but if the patient is actively leaking, the results of the test may underestimate the severity of the disease.

Choice of Approach

Careful review of the imaging will guide the surgical approach selection. The location of the defect with respect to the labyrinth is important as medial defects will require middle fossa exposure to correct, while defects lateral to the labyrinth can also be approached through a transmastoid route. The location with respect to the ossicles should be noted because defects located over the anterior epitympanum will require removal of the incus and malleus head to adequately expose via the transmastoid route, followed by an ossiculoplasty. While this is feasible, some surgeons may prefer to mitigate this by performing a middle fossa instead for anterior based defects.

Determining if there is a single well-defined defect versus multiple may also impact surgical approach. Patients with IIH, for example, often have multiple bony defects as opposed to a single well-defined fistula. Additionally, they are more likely to have an encephalocele in conjunction with their CSF leak as opposed to a CSF leak alone. For these reasons, a middle fossa approach is typically performed in patients with IIH because it allows broad exposure of the middle fossa floor for reconstruction.

Evaluating for a concurrent semicircular canal dehiscence should be identified prior to planning a middle fossa approach because inadvertent suctioning over a dehiscent superior canal during temporal lobe elevation can result in deafness. Likewise, identifying a dehiscent geniculate ganglion is also important if a middle fossa approach is planned due to the risk of injury to the facial nerve.

There are three surgical approaches that have been described: middle fossa craniotomy, transmastoid, and combined transmastoid-middle fossa. All of these have documented success rates of over 90% [43, 44]. Regardless of the approach taken, the goal is to achieve a multilayered reconstruction using both soft tissue to seal the leak, and a bony repair to prevent recurrent brain herniation. [43, 44] Below is a discussion of each approach, their indications and surgical technique.

Middle Fossa Approach

The middle fossa approach is suitable for larger (>1–2 cm diameter) tegmen defects, multifocal defects, medial defects (including over the petrous apex), or defects involving the anterior epitympanum (anterior to the head of the malleus). In patients with concurrent CSF leak and symptomatic superior canal dehiscence, the middle fossa approach offers a direct route to repairing both disorders.

The benefit of the middle fossa approach is gaining wide exposure to the skull base floor whereby the repair material can be laid down on top resurfacing the floor and sealing off the leak. The chief disadvantage of the middle fossa approach is that it requires a craniotomy with temporal lobe elevation. Although the elevation is extradural and typically does not require use of a retractor, the approach can be complicated in patients greater than 65 years old due to thin dura that is adherent to the middle fossa floor.

The operation for a middle fossa approach begins with a curvilinear incision above the ear. The larger "question-mark" style middle fossa incision that is commonly performed for tumor cases is typically not needed. The incision is taken down to the temporalis fascia. Fascia is harvested for later use. The temporalis muscle is then split vertically and bluntly spread. Cautery along the undersurface of the temporalis muscle is avoided to prevent injury to its vascular supply, which may lead to temporal wasting. The size and location of the temporal craniectomy are designed based on the circumstance. The bone flap is saved on the back table for later replacement. The temporal lobe dura is elevated from posterior to anterior until the bony defect and dural defect are encountered. A retractor is typically not needed for these cases.

If the patient has a concomitant superior semicircular canal dehiscence, the first step is to plug (or resurface) the canal in order to protect the inner ear from potential suctioning of the perilymph (Supplementary Video 58.1). Next, the stalk of the encephalocele is amputated using bipolar cautery at the level of the cranial base. The brain tissue within the herniated encephalocele is nonviable so separating it does not cause functional damage. After division, the viable brain retracts, and hemostasis inside the dura is confirmed. The encephalocele tissue is then carefully elevated out of the middle ear or mastoid.

Next, the dura is inspected and repaired. For small, focal dural defects a direct repair can be performed with 6–0 nylon suture. An extradural repair with dural substitute graft (e.g., Duragen®) is sufficient for most small defects and mitigates the risk of bleeding caused by intradural dissection. However, if the dural defect is large, an inlay dural substitute graft or temporalis fascia is placed.

Attention is then turned toward repair of the bony defect. There are a variety of materials that may be employed including temporalis fascia, cortical bone chips (taken as a full-thickness or split-thickness piece from the craniotomy flap), bone pâté, bone cement, cartilage, or a pedicled temporalis muscle flap. A multi-layered repair is often performed, such as the sandwich technique with fascia—bone—fascia (Fig. 58.4). If the heads of the ossicles are exposed, a collagen sponge (Gelfoam®, Pfizer Inc.) is placed into the epitympanum to prevent fixation of the ossicular chain. Temporalis fascia is first placed onto the bone to achieve a seal. Following this, a bone chip with a diameter larger than that of the defect is placed which functions to support the overlying dura and prevent recurrent herniation. Rigid fixation of the bone piece or use of bone cement can be considered to prevent lateral migration, although this is often not necessary (Supplementary Video 58.2). An additional larger piece of fascia is draped over the bone chip and covers the entire repair. Fibrin glue is helpful in holding the repair together, while the dura is laid back down.

In patients with IIH and multifocal defects or very thin at-risk areas, a wide area of the middle fossa floor is resur-

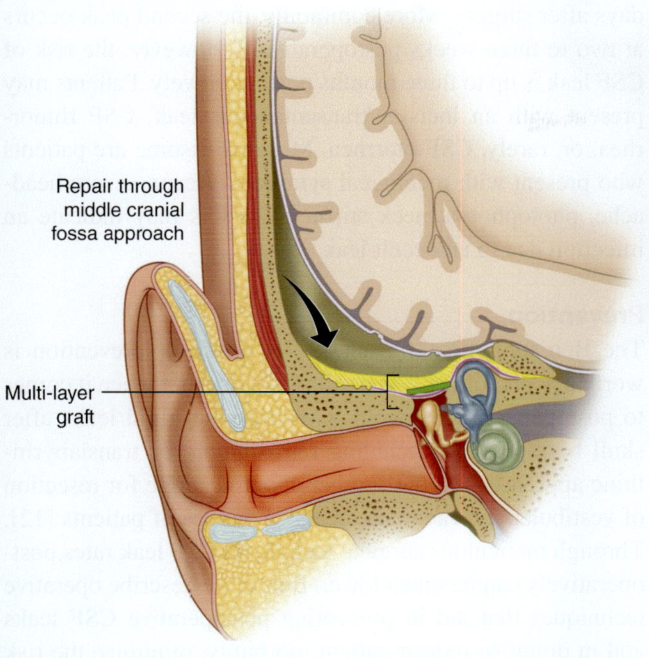

Fig. 58.4 Multilayered repair is commonly performed such as using fascia and bone taken from the craniotomy flap. (Adapted from Brackmann [49])

faced to prevent future CSF leaks. This can be achieved with temporalis fascia followed by cortical bone chips. Bone cement such as Hydroset® (Stryker Inc.)—which is less brittle and sets better in a wet environment compared to alternatives—can also be considered but use of any non-autologous material introduces the risk of infection and additional cost [45].

Placement of a lumbar drain at the time of surgery is controversial. The authors reserve the use of a lumbar drain to patients with a high-flow CSF leak such as those with IIH because these patients are at higher risk for failure. The lumbar drain is placed first to achieve satisfactory brain relaxation which allows easier temporal lobe elevation and access to the cranial defect. Postoperatively, the drain is left for two to three days to reduce the risk of a recurrent leak [44, 46]. Closure is performed in standard fashion. The bone flap is replaced and plated with titanium screws, followed by a multilayered closure.

Transmastoid Approach

The transmastoid approach can also be used for defects small or large, and for many neurotologists, this is the preferred method for repairing CSF leaks that are located lateral to the labyrinth. The approach is ideal for isolated defects located posterior to the epitympanum, such as defects involving the tegmen mastoideum or posterior fossa defects. Defects that involve the anterior epitympanum can also be approached transmastoid but require removing the incus and malleus

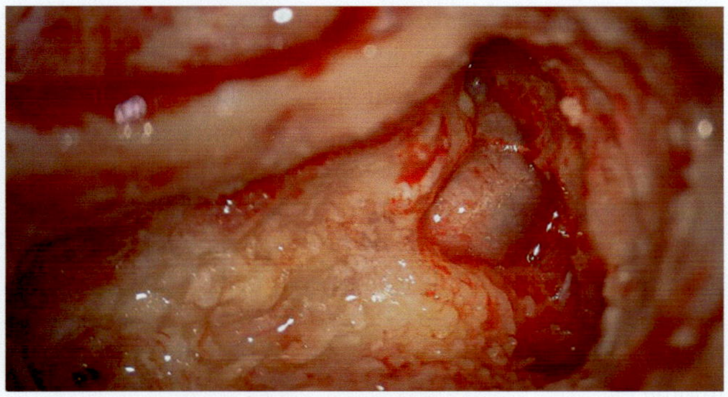

Fig. 58.5 Intraoperative view after left-sided mastoidectomy showing an encephalocele involving the epitympanum and located just medial to the head of the malleus and body of the incus

head in order to gain exposure. Following the repair, an incus interposition can be performed through the facial recess corridor at the same operation. Lastly, the transmastoid approach is also used after multiple failed repair attempts whereby a subtotal petrosectomy with blind sac closure of the ear canal and obliteration of the Eustachian tube is performed.

The benefit of the transmastoid approach is that it eliminates the need for a craniotomy and an intensive care unit (ICU) stay. It can be done outpatient in the vast majority of cases, which results in less morbidity and lower cost. In older patients and patients who are on anticoagulation for whom it is risky to come off, the transmastoid approach offers surgical repair of the CSF leak with lower risk. The primary disadvantage of the transmastoid approach is that the repair material must be pushed into the epidural space through the defect and then positioned securely onto the bony ledges, all without causing bleeding or undue trauma, which may be technically more challenging in certain cases.

The procedure is done through a standard postauricular incision. The lateral/cortical mastoid bone is removed in one piece and then thinned and fashioned to fit the shape and size that is needed for the bony reconstruction (Supplementary Video 58.3). The mastoidectomy is then completed down to the antrum until the bony defect is identified. If an encephalocele is present, it may look like a pale, blue-domed cyst emanating from superiorly (Fig. 58.5). Fascia is first placed through the defect and carefully tucked under the edges of the bone, while remaining extradural. Following this, the bone graft is carefully inserted through the defect and positioned onto the surrounding bone (Supplementary Video 58.2). The bone strip need not cover the entire defect because its primary function is to serve as a cantilever to support the overlying brain. Bone pâté is then used to fill the defect from the mastoid side and more fascia is used to achieve a seal. Larger CSF leaks with encephaloceles can also be treated with this approach (Supplementary Video 58.4).

Combined Transmastoid-Middle Fossa Approach

The combined transmastoid—middle fossa approach can also be performed. The craniotomy in these cases is often more limited. The advantage of this approach is that the repair material can be precisely placed over the defect via the craniotomy exposure while also inspecting and reinforcing the repair from below through the mastoid corridor. The primary disadvantage of this technique is that if the dural repair is insufficient, there is a risk that CSF may leak around the lateral aspect of the bone and directly into the mastoid and middle ear.

In the combined approach, a linear incision is made above the ear and curves postauricularly to provide access to the mastoid (Fig. 58.6a). Temporalis fascia is harvested and subsequently the temporalis muscle is split or reflected anteriorly exposing the cortex. A mastoidectomy is completed and the site of the encephalocele is encountered (Fig. 58.6b). Next, an otologic bur is used to create a middle fossa craniotomy, leaving a bridge of bone between the mastoid and the craniotomy. The temporal lobe dura can then be gently elevated, the encephalocele is amputated, and the dural and bony repair can be performed via the middle fossa exposure. The repair can be augmented from the mastoid side with bone pâté and fascia (Fig. 58.6c).

Management of Postoperative CSF Leaks Following Skull Base Surgery

Postoperative CSF leaks following skull base surgery occur in a bimodal distribution. The first peak is within the first few days after surgery. More commonly, the second peak occurs at two to three weeks postoperatively. However, the risk of CSF leak is up to three months postoperatively. Patients may present with an incision/transcutaneous leak, CSF rhinorrhea, or, rarely, CSF otorrhea. More worrisome are patients who present with meningeal symptoms (fever, severe headache, photophobia, neck stiffness) as this may indicate an infection due to an occult leak.

Prevention

The Benjamin Franklin adage "an ounce of prevention is worth a pound of cure" is particularly relevant when it comes to postoperative CSF leaks. Cerebrospinal fluid leaks after skull base surgery, including retrosigmoid or translabyrinthine approaches to the cerebellopontine angle for resection of vestibular schwannoma, occur in 5–10% of patients [12]. Through meticulous surgical technique, CSF leak rates postoperatively can be much lower. Below we describe operative techniques that aid in preventing postoperative CSF leaks and in doing so reduce patient morbidity, minimize the risk of meningitis, prevent revision surgery, shorten hospitalization, and expedite recovery.

For the translabyrinthine approach, prevention of CSF leak starts with skin incision. A single skin flap down to bone with a small stairstep is preferable to elevating a separate musculoperiosteal (Palva) flap. In the authors' experience, by the end of the case the Palva flap is contracted and severely dehydrated so it is unable to create a watertight closure for the deep layer. Elevating a separate Palva flap also creates a potential dead space between the Palva flap and the overlying adipose tissue. If this dead space fills with spinal fluid, it

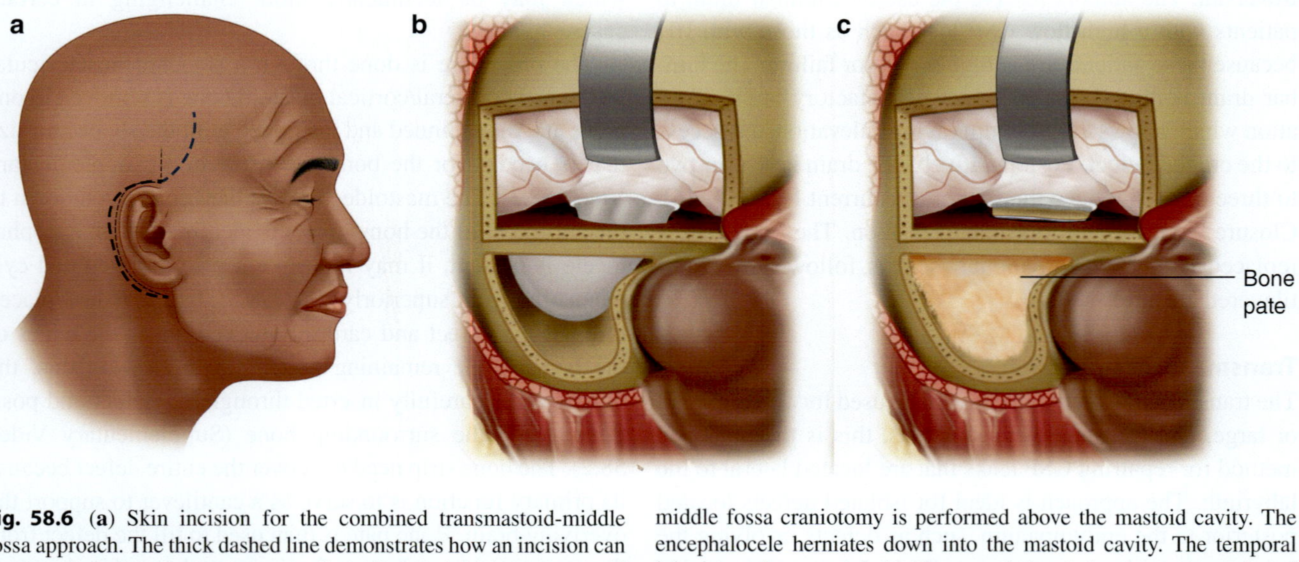

Fig. 58.6 (**a**) Skin incision for the combined transmastoid-middle fossa approach. The thick dashed line demonstrates how an incision can be staged during the surgery to allow for an initial transmastoid approach (black, thick dashed line) and a subsequent middle cranial fossa approach (blue, thick dashed line). A thin dashed line demonstrates an alternative incision that could be used for a limited middle fossa craniotomy in the setting of a smaller, posterior defect. (**b**) A middle fossa craniotomy is performed above the mastoid cavity. The encephalocele herniates down into the mastoid cavity. The temporal lobe is gently retracted. (**c**) The encephalocele has been resected, and repair through the middle fossa craniotomy has been performed. The repair has been augmented with bone pâté from through the mastoid. (Adapted from Driscoll and Oghalai [50])

may eventually work its way out of the incision. Elevating the skin flap as a single layer preserves the integrity of the deep musculoperiosteal tissue. The small stairstep creates an offset between the tissue layers which promotes tissue adhesion and prevents a direct route of spinal fluid out of the incision. During closure at the end of the case, this deep layer is reapproximated with 2–0 Vicryl® sutures in close approximation to achieve a watertight closure. Subsequently, the deep dermal layer is closed with 3–0 Vicryl® suture. The skin layer is closed with a 4–0 nylon in running locking fashion. In addition to meticulous incision opening and closure, blockage of any routes for CSF egress through the temporal bone is key. After tumor resection is complete, any exposed air cells around the IAC are sealed with bone wax. The posterior fossa dura is approximated with one or two stitches which act as a scaffold upon which strips of adipose tissue are placed like a "dumbbell" into the CPA. Next, the incus is removed and the Eustachian tube is packed with alternating pieces of muscle and Surgicel® using a House annulus elevator (gimmick). The middle ear is then obliterated with fat. If air cells of the facial recess are opened, bone wax is used to seal them. A piece of temporalis fascia is used to seal the antrum and cover the facial recess. Application of fibrin glue (Tisseel®, Baxter Inc.) is helpful in holding the repair in place and sealing off the middle ear in the early postoperative period. The mastoid is then packed with large pieces of adipose tissue. Fewer, large pieces of adipose tissue are preferable to multiple, small fragments.

For the retrosigmoid approach, an incisional leak is less common due to the thickness of the muscular tissue traversed during opening a retrosigmoid incision. However, spinal fluid may leak into the mastoid via posterior mastoid air cells which are opened during exposure when identifying the sigmoid sinus. It is our practice to wax these air cells after completing the craniectomy and again at the end of the case during closure as a double-check in case any of the wax dislodged during the case. Spinal fluid may also leak through exposed air cells around the IAC that were opened during intracranial drilling. When sealing air cells of the IAC after dissection, a small piece of bone wax is delivered to the area and compressed onto the bone with a small cottonoid. Adipose tissue is also used to fill the IAC bony defect and fibrin glue (Tisseel®) is applied. Lastly, the dural closure should be meticulous and watertight. Oftentimes, a temporalis fascia graft is incorporated into the dural closure and sutured as an inlay graft to achieve a watertight closure. To further seal the dural suture lines, a "pancake" of adipose tissue is placed on the dura. Following this, the bone flap is replaced and rigidly fixated with titanium screws. Filling the craniectomy defect with bone cement is an alternative method. Multilayered skin closure is then performed.

Postoperative Incisional/Transcutaneous CSF Leak

Patients presenting postoperatively with an incisional CSF leak are initially managed by over-sewing the wound. This is accomplished with a 4–0 nylon suture and taking large bites to recruit tissue and bring it together under tension. A mastoid pressure dressing is then applied to reduce the risk of a potential space from forming under the skin flap and filling with CSF. In rare circumstances, this initial treatment fails, and the patient should then be admitted to the hospital and a lumbar drain is placed for approximately five days to reduce pressure on the wound. The lumbar drain is set to match the rate of CSF production. The average production rate is 20 mL/hour. Pinning the lumbar drainage bag at the level of the patient's shoulder is a simple way to achieve this. To ambulate, the tubing is clamped. The patient will commonly have a headache while the lumbar drain is in place. Over drainage of CSF is to be avoided to reduce the possible complication of a subdural hematoma. If this fails, reoperation for internal sealing of CSF is required.

Postoperative CSF Rhinorrhea

Postoperative CSF rhinorrhea can occur if CSF percolates through the mastoid air cells and reaches the nasopharynx via the Eustachian tube. In some patients with a well-aerated temporal bone, spinal fluid may reach the Eustachian tube directly through communication of air cells around the IAC which are connected to peritubal air cells, thereby bypassing the middle ear and mastoid. Initial management involves placement of a lumbar drain for five days. If this fails, reoperation is necessary to seal all air cells that may communicate with the intracranial cavity. In cases that were performed via translabyrinthine approach or in any case where hearing has already been lost, a definitive approach is to obliterate the Eustachian tube. This is performed by opening up the incision and performing a subtotal petrosectomy with blind sac closure of the external auditory canal and packing of the Eustachian tube. Alternatively, a transcanal approach can be performed in which the skin of the external ear canal and tympanic membrane are resected, the Eustachian tube is packed with muscle or fascia, and the external meatus is overclosed [47]. In either method, the Eustachian tube packing should advance distal to the bony-cartilaginous junction to ensure any CSF leaking via peritubal air cells is also blocked. A final option is the endoscopic transnasal Eustachian tube obliteration. Since the Eustachian tube orifice in the nasopharynx is the final common pathway for CSF to drain, obliterating it should stop the leak.

Management of Post-traumatic CSF Leaks

In cases of head trauma resulting in spinal fluid otorrhea or rhinorrhea, stabilization of the patient is the priority. Spinal fluid leaks can often be managed concurrently with other neurological injuries. Unlike CSF leaks after skull base surgery, spinal fluid leaks after head trauma often resolve within five to seven days of conservative management with bed rest. Savva et al. reported that 26 of 29 patients with a CSF leak due to head trauma were successfully treated with conservative management alone, compared to 1 of 53 patients with post-surgical or spontaneous CSF leaks. However, if the leak persists despite conservative management, a lumbar drain may be necessary. Surgical repair can be considered if the leak persists after lumbar drainage and the patient is stable. Rates of meningitis with untreated CSF leaks following trauma may be as high as 29% [48].

Conclusion

Lateral skull base CSF leaks are either traumatic or spontaneous/nontraumatic. Traumatic CSF leaks due to a skull fracture or iatrogenic following surgery are more easily diagnosed, whereas spontaneous CSF leaks may present with more insidious symptoms, requiring the clinician to have a high degree of suspicion to diagnose. In recent years, there has been an increase in the occurrence of spontaneous CSF leaks, which coincides with the rise in both obesity and obstructive sleep apnea. Clinical history, physical examination, and high-resolution CT and MRI are usually sufficient to confirm the diagnosis, but beta-2 transferrin testing remains the gold standard for diagnosis and may be obtained if necessary. Although rare, CSF leaks should be treated to prevent the risk of meningitis or pneumocephalus. Antipneumococcal immunization is recommended. Management to stop the CSF leak and repair the bone is accomplished through a variety of approaches. The transmastoid approach is suitable for repairing defects small or large that are lateral to the labyrinth and has the benefit of sparing the patient a craniotomy with its associated risks and can often be performed on an outpatient basis. The middle fossa approach is ideal for defects medial to the labyrinth or over the anterior epitympanum, or in patients with multiple bony defects due to severe skull base erosion, such as in the setting of IIH. The combined transmastoid-middle fossa approach is popular among neurotologists as well since it combines the benefits of each approach. All approaches have a high success rate when multilayered closure is performed.

References

1. Wilson MN, Simon LM, Arriaga MA, Nuss DW, Lin JA. The management of spontaneous otogenic CSF leaks: a presentation of cases and review of literature. J Neurol Surg B Skull Base. 2014;75:117–24.
2. Eddelman DB, Munich S, Kochanski RB, et al. Repair of temporal bone defects via the middle cranial fossa approach: treatment of 2 pathologies with 1 operation. Neurosurgery. 2019;84:1290–5.
3. Gonen L, Handzel O, Shimony N, Fliss DM, Margalit N. Surgical management of spontaneous cerebrospinal fluid leakage through temporal bone defects—case series and review of the literature. Neurosurg Rev. 2016;39:141–50. discussion 150
4. Welge-Luessen A, Probst R. Spontaneous cerebrospinal fluid otorrhea in the posterior fossa as a rare cause of adult bacterial meningitis. Otolaryng Head Neck. 2004;130:375–7.
5. Kutz JW Jr, Tolisano AM. Diagnosis and management of spontaneous cerebrospinal fluid fistula and encephaloceles. Curr Opin Otolaryngol Head Neck Surg. 2019;27:369–75.
6. Stucken EZ, Selesnick SH, Brown KD. The role of obesity in spontaneous temporal bone encephaloceles and CSF leak. Otol Neurotol. 2012;33:1412–7.
7. LeVay AJ, Kveton JF. Relationship between obesity, obstructive sleep apnea, and spontaneous cerebrospinal fluid otorrhea. Laryngoscope. 2008;118:275–8.
8. Nelson RF, Gantz BJ, Hansen MR. The rising incidence of spontaneous cerebrospinal fluid leaks in the United States and the association with obesity and obstructive sleep apnea. Otol Neurotol. 2015;36:476–80.
9. Neely JG, Kuhn JR. Diagnosis and treatment of iatrogenic cerebrospinal fluid leak and brain herniation during or following mastoidectomy. Laryngoscope. 1985;95:1299–300.
10. Bani A, Gilsbach JM. Incidence of cerebrospinal fluid leak after microsurgical removal of vestibular schwannomas. Acta Neurochir. 2002;144:979–82. discussion 982
11. Brodie HA, Thompson TC. Management of complications from 820 temporal bone fractures. Am J Otol. 1997;18:188–97.
12. Selesnick SH, Liu JC, Jen A, Newman J. The incidence of cerebrospinal fluid leak after vestibular schwannoma surgery. Otol Neurotol. 2004;25:387–93.
13. Fishman AJ, Marrinan MS, Golfinos JG, Cohen NL, Roland JT Jr. Prevention and management of cerebrospinal fluid leak following vestibular schwannoma surgery. Laryngoscope. 2004;114:501–5.
14. Vivas EX, McCall A, Raz Y, Fernandez-Miranda JC, Gardner P, Hirsch BE. ICP, BMI, surgical repair, and CSF diversion in patients presenting with spontaneous CSF otorrhea. Otol Neurotol. 2014;35:344–7.
15. Allen KP, Perez CL, Kutz JW, Gerecci D, Roland PS, Isaacson B. Elevated intracranial pressure in patients with spontaneous cerebrospinal fluid otorrhea. Laryngoscope. 2014;124:251–4.
16. Schlosser RJ, Woodworth BA, Wilensky EM, Grady MS, Bolger WE. Spontaneous cerebrospinal fluid leaks: a variant of benign intracranial hypertension. Ann Otol Rhinol Laryngol. 2006;115:495–500.
17. Rich PM, Graham J, Phelps PD. Hyrtl's fissure. Otol Neurotol. 2002;23:476–82.
18. Ehmer DR Jr, Booth T, Kutz JW Jr, Roland PS. Radiographic diagnosis of trans-stapedial cerebrospinal fluid fistula. Otolaryngol Head Neck Surg. 2010;142:694–8.
19. Barcz DV, Wood RP 2nd, Stears J, Jafek BW, Shields M. Subarachnoid space: middle ear pathways and recurrent meningitis. Am J Otol. 1985;6:157–63.

20. Hipskind MM, Lindsay JR, Jones TD, Valvassori GE. Recurrent meningitis and labyrinthine gusher, related to congenital defects of the labyrinthine capsule and stapes footplate. Laryngoscope. 1976;86:682–9.
21. Eluvathingal Muttikkal TJ, Nicolasjilwan M. Congenital X-linked stapes gusher syndrome in an infant. A case report. Neuroradiol J. 2012;25:76–80.
22. Bluestone CD. Cochlear malformations, meningitis, and cochlear implants: what have we learned? Otol Neurotol. 2003;24:349–50.
23. Gacek RR. Arachnoid granulation cerebrospinal fluid otorrhea. Ann Otol Rhinol Laryngol. 1990;99:854–62.
24. Yew M, Dubbs B, Tong O, et al. Arachnoid granulations of the temporal bone: a histologic study of dural and osseous penetration. Otol Neurotol. 2011;32:602–9.
25. Gacek RR, Gacek MR, Tart R. Adult spontaneous cerebrospinal fluid otorrhea: diagnosis and management. Am J Otol. 1999;20:770–6.
26. Deep NL, Hoxworth JM, Stevens CJ, Link MJ, Driscoll CL, Wood CP. Giant posterior temporal bone arachnoid granulations: CT and MRI findings. Otol Neurotol. 2016;37:963–6.
27. Alberti PW, Dawes JD. Cerebrospinal otorrhoea in chronic ear disease. J Laryngol Otol. 1961;75:123–35.
28. Grinblat G, Dandinarasaiah M, Prasad SC, et al. Temporal bone meningo-encephalic-herniation: etiological categorization and surgical strategy. Otol Neurotol. 2018;39:320–32.
29. Yancey KL, Manzoor NF, Kelly PD, et al. Impact of obesity and obstructive sleep apnea in lateral skull base cerebrospinal fluid leak repair. Laryngoscope. 2020;130:2234–40.
30. Oh MS, Vivas EX, Hudgins PA, Mattox DE. The prevalence of superior semicircular canal dehiscence in patients with mastoid Encephalocele or cerebrospinal fluid otorrhea. Otol Neurotol. 2019;40:485–90.
31. Fairman HD, Brown NJ, Hallpike CS. Air embolism as a complication of inflation of the tympanum through the external auditory meatus. A clinico-pathological study of a fatal case. Acta Otolaryngol. 1968;66:65–71.
32. Cartwright MJ, Eisenberg MB. Tension pneumocephalus associated with rupture of a middle fossa encephalocele. Case report. J Neurosurg. 1992;76:292–5.
33. Thomeer HG, Schreurs C, van Doormaal TP, Straatman LV. Management and outcomes of spontaneous cerebrospinal fluid Otorrhoea. Front Surg. 2020;7:21.
34. Savva A, Taylor MJ, Beatty CW. Management of cerebrospinal fluid leaks involving the temporal bone: report on 92 patients. Laryngoscope. 2003;113:50–6.
35. Warnecke A, Averbeck T, Wurster U, Harmening M, Lenarz T, Stover T. Diagnostic relevance of beta2-transferrin for the detection of cerebrospinal fluid fistulas. Arch Otolaryngol Head Neck Surg. 2004;130:1178–84.
36. Kutz JW Jr, Husain IA, Isaacson B, Roland PS. Management of spontaneous cerebrospinal fluid otorrhea. Laryngoscope. 2008;118:2195–9.
37. Yancey KL, Manzoor NF, Haynes DS, Bennett ML, O'Malley M, Rivas A. Audiometric outcomes and middle ear disease following cerebrospinal fluid leak repair. Otolaryngol Head Neck Surg. 2020;162:942–9.
38. Allen KP, Perez CL, Isaacson B, Roland PS, Duong TT, Kutz JW. Superior semicircular canal dehiscence in patients with spontaneous cerebrospinal fluid otorrhea. Otolaryngol Head Neck Surg. 2012;147:1120–4.
39. Mostafa BE, Khafagi A. Combined HRCT and MRI in the detection of CSF rhinorrhea. Skull Base 2004; 14:157–162; discussion 162.
40. Breen JT, Edwards CR, Cornelius RS, et al. Utility of magnetic resonance imaging in differentiating cerebrospinal fluid leak from middle ear effusion. Otolaryngol Head Neck Surg. 2019;161:493–8.
41. Hendriks T, Thompson A, Boeddinghaus R, Tan HEI, Kuthubutheen J. Radiological findings in spontaneous cerebrospinal fluid leaks of the temporal bone. J Laryngol Otol. 2021;135:403–9.
42. Young N, Thomas M. Meningitis in adults: diagnosis and management. Intern Med J. 2018;48:1294–307.
43. Gioacchini FM, Cassandro E, Alicandri-Ciufelli M, et al. Surgical outcomes in the treatment of temporal bone cerebrospinal fluid leak: a systematic review. Auris Nasus Larynx. 2018;45:903–10.
44. Teachey W, Grayson J, Cho DY, Riley KO, Woodworth BA. Intervention for elevated intracranial pressure improves success rate after repair of spontaneous cerebrospinal fluid leaks. Laryngoscope. 2017;127:2011–6.
45. Ota T, Kamada K, Saito N. Repair of cerebrospinal fluid leak via petrous bone using multilayer technique with hydroxyapatite paste. World Neurosurg. 2010;74:650–3.
46. Doubi AO, Aljomah DS, Alhargan AO, Alfawwaz FS. The effect of lumbar drains on spontaneous cerebrospinal fluid leak repair. Neurosciences (Riyadh). 2018;23:281–5.
47. Friedman RA, Cullen RD, Ulis J, Brackmann DE. Management of cerebrospinal fluid leaks after acoustic tumor removal. Neurosurgery. 2007;61:35–9. discussion 39–40
48. Bernal-Sprekelsen M, Bleda-Vazquez C, Carrau RL. Ascending meningitis secondary to traumatic cerebrospinal fluid leaks. Am J Rhinol. 2000;14:257–9.
49. Brackmann D, Shelton C, Arriaga M, editors. Otologic surgery. 4th ed. Elsevier; 2015.
50. Driscoll CLW, Oghalai JS. Atlas of neurotologic and lateral skull base surgery. Springer; 2016.

Temporal Bone Trauma

59

Sagar Kansara, Akash Patel, and Alex D. Sweeney

Abbreviations

CSF	Cerebrospinal fluid
CT	Computed tomography
CTA	Computed tomography angiography
EAC	External auditory canal
IAC	Internal auditory canal
MRA	Magnetic resonance angiography
MRI	Magnetic resonance imaging
MRV	Magnetic resonance venography
TM	Tympanic membrane

Introduction

The consequences of temporal bone trauma exist on a wide spectrum of severity. In some locations, the bone simply serves as a shield for the central nervous system. However, in other areas, vital structures traverse through the temporal bone to connect the intracranial space and the neck, or, in the case of the cochleovestibular system, reside entirely within the bone; thus, trauma may have no functional significance or may have life-altering, disfiguring ramifications. Though there has been a relatively large amount of attention on this subject in the literature when compared to trauma in other areas of the skull base, uncertainty still remains regarding the optimal diagnostic and therapeutic algorithms for many patients in this setting. This chapter serves as a review of temporal bone trauma, with a particular focus on the evidence that is generally used to guide clinical decision-making.

Epidemiology of Temporal Bone Trauma

The demographic variables associated with temporal bone trauma can vary depending on the clinical environment, with specific differences noted between urban and rural settings [1–3]. However, it is relatively consistent across all reports that temporal bone injuries are more common in young, male patients [3, 4]. One of the largest reviews of such trauma comes from Brodie and Thompson, who reported on 820 fractures from a single institution. They identified a wide age range in affected patients (from 4 months to 87 years), though it was noted that most were between the ages of 11 and 30 years. Approximately 22% of patients were below the age of 17 years, and males represented 76% of cases. In terms of associated injuries, Schubl et al. reported on a series of patients in which 67% of patients with temporal bone fractures had additional fractures of the skull and 78% had an intracranial hemorrhage. These investigators also reported that concurrent facial bone and cranial vault fractures occurred in 34.5% and 24%, respectively, of temporal bone fracture patients [5]. Moreover, more than 90% of patients with temporal bone fracture have been found to have concomitant intracranial injury, and 9% cervical spinal injury [6]. Of note, bilateral fractures are found in as many as 10% of cases involving temporal bone trauma [7]. Reports on temporal bone trauma in the pediatric population have similarly identified a male predilection, though a bimodal age distribution has previously been reported by Lee et al. with peaks around 3 and 12 years of age [4]. Blunt force trauma, particularly as a consequence of motor vehicle accidents, appears to be the most common mechanism of temporal bone injury across age groups [1, 3, 4, 8, 9].

S. Kansara
Bobby R. Alford Department of Otolaryngology—Head and Neck Surgery, Baylor College of Medicine, Houston, TX, USA

A. Patel
Department of Neurosurgery, Baylor College of Medicine, Houston, TX, USA

A. D. Sweeney (✉)
Department of Otolaryngology—Head and Neck Surgery, Baylor College of Medicine, Houston, TX, USA
e-mail: alex.sweeney@bcm.edu

A. D. Sweeney et al. (eds.), *Haynes-Glasscock-Shambaugh Surgery of the Ear*, https://doi.org/10.1007/978-3-032-18264-7_59

Mechanisms of Temporal Bone Trauma

During the clinical evaluation of a patient with temporal bone trauma, it is important to consider the mechanism of injury. Oftentimes, a clinician involved in the care of a trauma patient is provided with relevant information before an involved patient presents for evaluation. Did the patient fall from a tree? Did a moving vehicle hit the patient? Was the patient stabbed with a knife? Was the patient shot with a firearm? A vast difference may exist between the expected degrees of injury in each of these scenarios, and these differences may influence management plans.

At the most fundamental level, trauma is caused by the transfer of energy from one structure to another. Laws of physics would thus dictate that the effects of trauma depend directly on both the mass of the structures involved and the amount of energy transferred, which is directly related to impact velocity. This simplified relationship between mass and velocity would suggest that not all temporal bone traumas are alike, and, consequently, that treatment planning and outcomes analysis cannot always be standardized for trauma. Though there are a multitude of variables that are relevant to trauma mechanism, a simple few essential elements are worth remembering. Primarily, most traumas can be categorized as blunt or penetrating, and, in the realm of penetrating trauma, as either "high-energy" or "low-energy" if energy is thought of as a function of velocity and mass [10]. Distinctions in velocity are generally relevant in terms of the offending object being handheld (e.g., knife—low velocity) or propelled by an explosive force (e.g., firearm—high velocity). Distinctions in mass and composition of a projectile are generally relevant in terms of origin (e.g., handgun, shotgun, rifle, or shrapnel) and the missile itself (e.g., shrapnel, birdshot, buckshot, solid bullet, or expanding bullet). Though categorizing trauma in these terms can be complicated, the importance of doing so becomes immediately apparent when simply considering that the most physically damaging aspects of high-energy penetrating trauma occurs beyond the direct path of a projectile due to cavitation [11]. When considering the patient scenarios from the preceding paragraph in this light, rather than saying that all patients simply suffered "temporal bone trauma," it would be perhaps more appropriate to say that the patient who is hit by a vehicle would be more likely to suffer "blunt trauma," the patient who was stabbed with a knife suffered "low-energy penetrating trauma," while the patient who was shot with a firearm, assuming the missile was a hollow-point bullet fired from a 9 mm pistol, could be said to have suffered a "high-energy penetrating trauma" from a handgun (Fig. 59.1). Though the complexity of this subject extends beyond the scope of this chapter, it is an important subject to consider in any discussion of temporal bone trauma as it provides an appropriate framework upon which therapeutic and diagnostic interventions as well as research can be based.

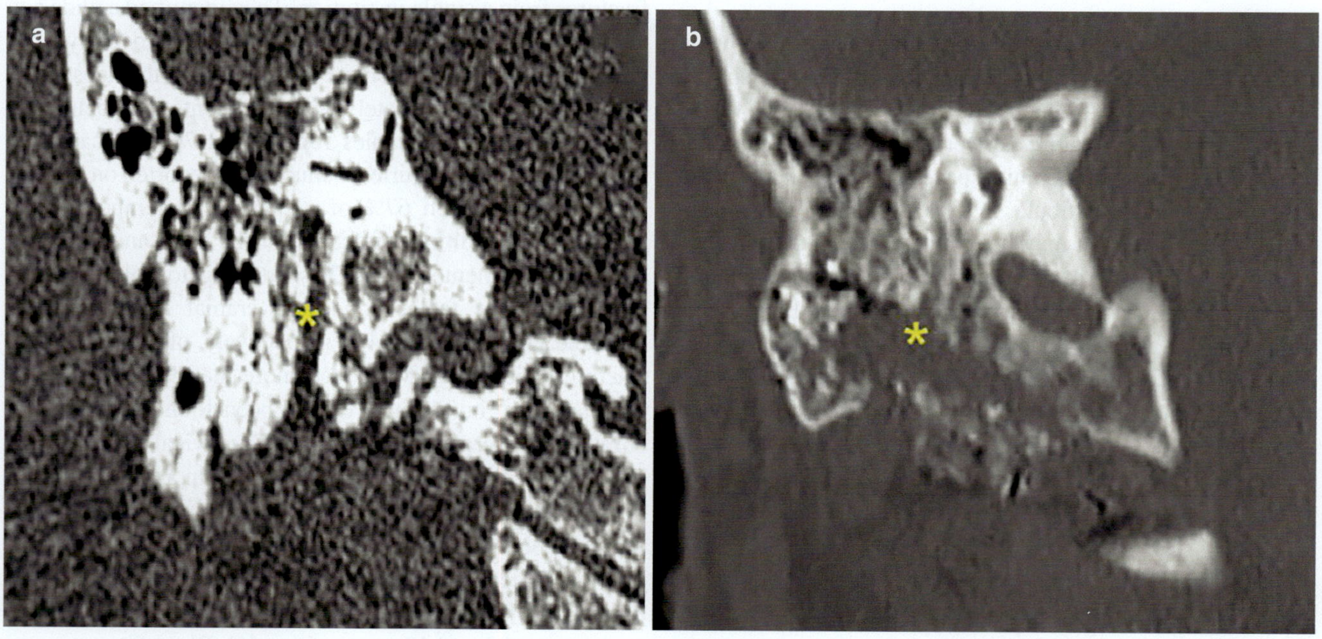

Fig. 59.1 Coronal view of CT scans from two different patients demonstrating traumatic facial paralysis from (**a**) low-energy blunt trauma and (**b**) high-energy penetrating trauma (gunshot wound). The * represents the site of injury to the facial nerve

Clinical Evaluation of Temporal Bone Trauma

Initially, trauma patients should be evaluated with respect to existing triage algorithms. The American College of Surgeons endorses the use of primary survey (airway, breathing, circulation, disability, exposure) to identify and treat potentially life-threatening conditions [12]. In this context, it is important to note that trauma to the temporal bone may be a less pressing aspect of the patient's initial evaluation. However, information from the first encounter, particularly a baseline assessment of facial nerve function, may ultimately prove valuable to the clinical decision-making as the patient recovers from more acute injuries.

A thorough history and physical examination is vital to the proper management of a trauma patient. Not infrequently, the initial clinical evaluation in this setting can be suboptimal compared to routine outpatient encounters: patients may be unable to participate in both questioning and physical exam, or more acute injuries could necessitate urgent interventions before an otologic assessment can occur. However, given the multitude of injuries that can be associated with temporal bone trauma, it is important to elicit any information regarding facial function, hearing loss, tinnitus, vertigo, otorrhea, and rhinorrhea. In some cases, particularly when a patient is mentally altered or obtunded, it may be necessary to consult with referring doctors or emergency personnel who had contact with the patient prior to their arrival.

The physical exam of a temporal bone trauma patient begins with an external survey of the areas surrounding the external ear and temporal bone. Specifically, a thorough head and neck examination should be performed in a systematic fashion. This includes an evaluation for external wounds, like what may be seen with the entry or exit of a penetrating trauma, as well as obvious bony deformities, crepitus, or an expanding hematoma. A pulsatile mass at the inferior aspect of the skull base with an audible bruit on auscultation could suggest vascular injury. Examination of the periorbital or postauricular areas may reveal ecchymosis (Raccoon or Battle sign, respectively) associated with a skull base fracture. An ocular exam should be performed to evaluate pupil reactivity and the extraocular movements at rest and with maximal effort. For example, a non-reactive pupil could indicate brain herniation, prompting urgent neurosurgical evaluation. If nystagmus is present, it is important to characterize it in terms of its directionality and fatigability.

Following an initial head and neck survey, the otologic exam is performed. The external ear may have been deformed by trauma in the form of laceration, contusion, hematoma, or avulsion, which can complicate analysis (Figs. 59.2 and 59.3). Otoscopy should be performed bilaterally to evaluate for soft tissue and bony injuries, foreign bodies, perforation of the tympanic membrane (TM), hemotympanum, or, in extreme cases, herniated intracranial contents. Pneumatic otoscopy can be helpful to assess the mobility of the TM, which may be impaired due to fluid in the middle ear. Additionally, pressure-induced nystagmus or vertigo may indicate the presence of a perilymphatic fistula (Hennebert's sign).

Another vital element of the otologic exam is an objective measure of auditory and vestibular function. Hearing loss has been reported as the most common subjective complaint following temporal bone injury, occurring in up to 40% of

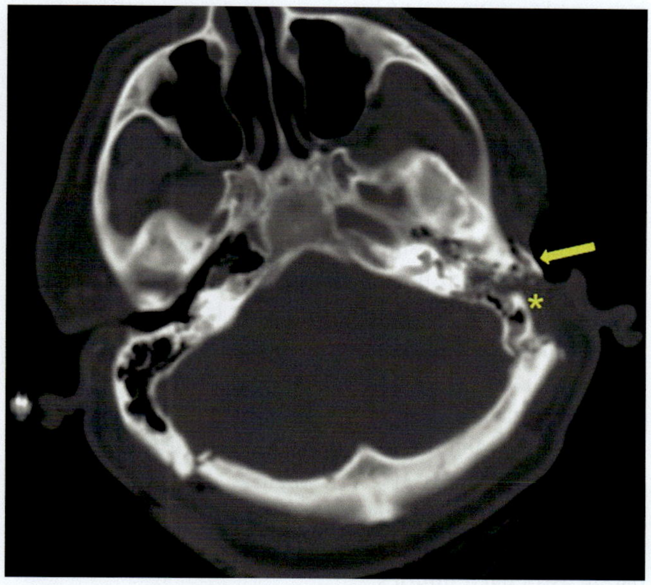

Fig. 59.2 Axial view of a CT scan demonstrating extensive blunt trauma to the temporal bone (*), which resulted in tissue avulsion and bone exposure (arrow)

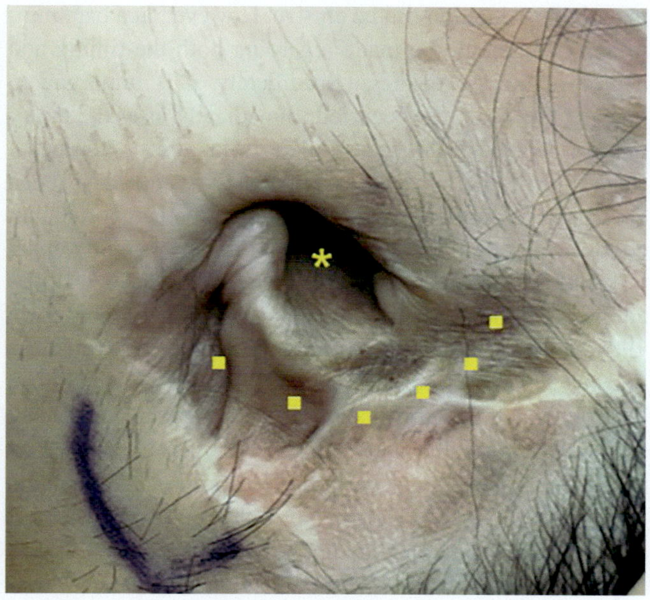

Fig. 59.3 Traumatic avulsion of a left auricle approximately 1 year following injury. The * marks the external auditory meatus. The dots represent the expected location of the auricle

those with a radiographically apparent fracture [13]. Prior to conventional audiometry, a tuning fork can be used to suggest the presence of a traumatic hearing loss. A Weber test that lateralizes to one side indicates an ipsilateral conductive hearing loss (CHL), as in the case of hemotympanum or ossicular discontinuity, or contralateral sensorineural hearing loss (SNHL), as in the case of temporal bone fractures involving the otic capsule. The Rinne test may help in distinguishing the two: if bone conduction is greater than air conduction, a CHL is the likely culprit. If air conduction is greater than bone conduction on both sides and the Weber test lateralized, an SNHL is likely. A focused neurologic exam and gait testing in cooperative patients are helpful adjuncts for evaluating vestibular function. Basic vestibular testing can generally be performed at the bedside, though caution should be exercised before performing any sort of physical manipulation of the head and neck to avoid exacerbating associated injuries.

Evaluation of the facial nerve deserves special mention in the evaluation of a patient with temporal bone trauma. Facial injuries are not uncommon after temporal bone trauma, though "best-practice" algorithms for diagnosis and management in this situation can be elusive. However, at a bare minimum, note should be made regarding both the timing and degree of facial weakness. Specifically, it is important to know if the weakness occurred immediately after the injury or in a delayed fashion, and if the weakness is complete. Regarding the latter, there are many tools that have been developed to standardize how facial function is reported, but choosing an optimal grading system remains a controversial task. House and Brackmann (HB) developed a scale that was adopted by the American Academy of Otolaryngology in 1985, which is arguably the most widely used [14]. Yet, it has become apparent over time that inter-observer variability can be problematic with this system [15–19]. A recent systematic review has suggested that both the Sunnybrook and Facial Nerve 2.0 systems are superior to the traditional HB system in this regard [17, 20]. Though the controversy of how to best quantify facial function may not be settled soon, it is at least imperative that clinicians who evaluate facial weakness consistently use the same validated scale for the sake of internal data validity.

Additional aspects from the history that may be useful in evaluation include the presence of cerebrospinal fluid (CSF) otorrhea or rhinorrhea. Brodie and Thompson reported that the incidence of CSF leak can be as high as 15% in temporal bone trauma, emphasizing the need to be vigilant in evaluating for this complication [3]. When a steady flow of fluid from the ear, nose, or an external wound is observed, the physical characteristics and quantity of the fluid should be noted. Additionally, the presence of a so-called "halo sign," or a clear ring surrounding a bloody central spot, should raise suspicion for a CSF fistula, though this finding is not considered to be particularly specific or sensitive [21]. In cases where the TM is intact, fluid may also be shunted to the Eustachian tube, passing into the oropharynx and oral cavity and resulting in a salty or bitter taste or clear rhinorrhea [9].

When considering the evaluation of a patient with temporal bone trauma, it is important for the otolaryngologist to understand the totality of the patient's management, as other injuries that are present may require more urgent operative intervention. When a thorough otologic exam is not initially possible due to concurrent injuries or a lack of patient cooperation, awareness of pending trips to the operating room can help to ensure that an opportunity for more extensive evaluation under anesthesia is not missed.

Diagnostic Workup

Utilizing diagnostic studies in a systematic fashion facilitates effective evaluation of temporal bone fractures. In most hospital-based patient encounters, the means to objectively assess the radiologic extent of a fracture, potential for vascular and intracranial injury, hearing loss, and facial weakness are present and should be pursued when available.

High-resolution computed tomography (CT) of the temporal bone remains the *sine qua non* of radiographic evaluation in this setting. When evaluating the temporal bone, an appropriate CT scan permits a clear assessment of the bony integrity of the temporal bone and its intrinsic structures. Ideally, a CT evaluation of the temporal bone would consist of a large-field axial perspective (2.5 mm thick with a 2.5 mm interval), zoomed right and left axial perspectives (0.625 mm with a 0.625 mm interval), and coronal, Poschl, and Stenvers perspectives (0.5 mm with a 0.5 mm interval). In general, the use of contrast for this particular study is usually not necessary in the absence of infectious or vascular complications. Unfortunately, a CT of this quality may not be included in the initial trauma evaluation, as concerns for intracranial, facial, and spinal injuries can take precedence, and the resolution of a CT of the brain performed to evaluate for intracranial bleeding is not sufficient to also evaluate for intratemporal pathology [22]. However, combination CT scans (i.e., CT head and CT face), which are often included in the initial trauma evaluation, can approach the sensitivity and specificity for intratemporal injuries of that achieved by CT temporal bones. Schubl et al. and Dempewolf et al. have both evaluated the need of a dedicated CT temporal bone in the setting of trauma and have suggested that a maxillofacial scan is sufficient for most cases, though vascular injuries may be better identified by the former [5, 23].

The classification of temporal bone fractures has received a considerable amount of attention. Historically, fractures were classified on the basis of their trajectory: either longitudinal or transverse [3, 13, 24]. Longitudinal fractures are felt to account for 70–90% of all temporal bone fractures and occur as a result of a blow to the temporoparietal region. Such fractures often begin at the external ear canal laterally and involve the bony canal and middle ear, extending anterior to the labyrinth, finally involving the petrous pyramid and middle cranial fossa medially. Facial nerve injury is less common with this type of fracture, though ossicular chain disruption is more commonly observed, resulting in persistent conductive hearing loss. Transverse fractures are felt to be less common. This fracture pattern occurs perpendicular to the axis of the petrous bone and can occur medially (resulting in injury to the cranial nerve [CN] VIII at the level of the internal auditory canal [IAC]) or laterally (resulting in injury to the bony labyrinth). These can be caused by frontal or occipital blows and can result in damage to the facial nerve and the vestibulocochlear apparatus, resulting in facial weakness, sensorineural hearing loss, tinnitus, and vertigo. Facial nerve injury in transverse fractures often occurs at the labyrinthine segment between the internal acoustic meatus and geniculate ganglion [9, 25, 26].

Classification of temporal bone fractures as described above is increasingly of historical significance. Many fractures of the temporal bone do not conform to these descriptions, a subject noted by Ghorayeb et al. in 1992 when recognizing that many patterns were actually "oblique" in trajectory [27]. Over time, descriptive schemes that favor clinical relevance over radiographic description have been emphasized. Specifically, involvement of the petrous temporal bone and otic capsule has become a more noteworthy radiographic finding. Using these paradigms, it is felt that clinical sequelae can be more accurately predicted. Ishman and Friedland reported that comparing fractures on such a basis proved to be clinically more useful than the traditional classification scheme; patients with petrous involvement were more likely to have a CSF leak, facial nerve injury, or SNHL [7]. Little and Kesser suggested that categorizing fractures as "otic capsule sparing" versus "otic capsule violating" had more clinical relevance in a series of 30 patients, and in another retrospective study, patients with otic capsule fractures were two times more likely to develop facial paralysis, four times more likely to develop CSF leak, and seven times more likely to experience profound SNHL [28, 29]. Dunklebarger et al. also demonstrated that this classification scheme is also appropriate for the pediatric population [30]. It is currently recommended that radiologic fracture description and categorization focus take these more recent findings into consideration.

Radiographic evidence of a fracture to the carotid canal or jugular foramen should prompt further investigation, especially in the context of hemorrhage or neurological defects. In general, CT or MRI (magnetic resonance imaging) angiography can be used in this scenario. Studies have clearly demonstrated the associated risk of carotid or vertebral artery injury when a fracture involves the canal or skull base foramen of one of these structures [31, 32]. However, the cost-effectiveness of dedicated vascular studies has been questioned in asymptomatic patients. A study by Resnick et al. demonstrated that of 230 patients with skull base fractures, 55 (24%) had carotid canal involvement on CT. Of these, 33 underwent some sort of angiography (MRI or CT). Only six of these patients (11% of those with carotid canal fractures) were found to have vascular injuries. These same six patients were also the only subjects in the study that exhibited clinical evidence of vascular injury in the form of transient ischemic attacks, severe epistaxis, for example. Thus, the authors concluded that CT evidence of carotid canal involvement may not be the best predictor of actual vascular injury [33]. Kahn et al. evaluated 105 patients with temporal bone trauma. Out of 12 carotid canal fractures seen on high-resolution CT, six patients underwent carotid angiography, which revealed one vascular injury in the only symptomatic patient (severe epistaxis) [34]. These studies would suggest that the pursuit of additional vascular imaging must be reviewed on a case-by-case basis to utilize resources most effectively.

High-resolution magnetic resonance imaging (MRI) of the skull base or internal auditory canal (IAC) can be a useful diagnostic adjunct in the setting of temporal bone trauma. Generally, MRI is sought in the setting of a suspected intracranial or peripheral neurologic injury. In many cases, the mechanism of the trauma and the initial assessment of an injury dictate when MRI should be performed. However, on rare occasions, it is noteworthy that blunt trauma can lead to cranial nerve injury in the absence of other intracranial findings and in a manner that does not correlate with a particular fracture pattern on CT. Specifically, abducens palsy has been noted following a temporal bone fracture, presumably due to shear injury and avulsion of the nerve [35]. Cases of injury to the cisternal facial nerve after temporal bone fracture have also been reported [36].

To objectively quantify hearing loss, an audiogram should be performed when possible. A tuning fork examination should always be utilized, but if a patient is appropriate for more extensive audiometric testing, a baseline post-traumatic assessment can be helpful in terms of both documentation and management. Brodie and Thompson suggested that nearly a quarter of patients with temporal bone fractures will report hearing loss, and in their review, 57% had SNHL, 21% CHL, and 22% mixed [3]. Otic capsule violating temporal bone fractures generally have some degree of SNHL or mixed hearing loss, whereas those that spare the otic capsule typically cause CHL [29]. It has also been suggested that the largest CHL is found in fractures involving the ossicular chain, and spontaneous improvement in the CHL is somewhat dependent on the other temporal bone subsites that are involved in the fracture [37]. The majority of patients with

CHL following temporal bone fracture experience spontaneous improvement with a significant closure of the air-bone gap within the months following trauma, presumably due to resorption of hemotympanum or spontaneous closure of TM perforation [38, 39]. However, a small portion of patients with persistent CHL will have ossicular chain pathology (fractures and discontinuity), persistent TM perforations, or post-traumatic cholesteatoma (Fig. 59.4). The prognosis is more guarded in cases of SNHL [3, 39]. Hearing outcomes in children are similar to those in adults after temporal bone fractures [40]. In any of these cases, the opportunity to follow audiometric testing over time could be valuable.

The presence of persistent rhinorrhea, otorrhea, or drainage from a fracture site should raise suspicion for CSF fistula. When possible, samples can be collected and sent for β_2-transferrin, though clinicians should be aware of the potential for falsely positive results [41]. Enzyme-linked immunosorbent assays (ELISA) for Dickkopf-related protein 3 (DKK3) have recently shown promise and should also be considered if clinically available [42]. The introduction of a clinically visible or radio-opaque contrast agent into the thecal sac can be helpful to confirm and localize a leak, though this manner of investigation is not without intrinsic risks. In some cases, high-resolution CT and MRI are often sufficient to localize the source of a CSF leak [43]. MR (magnetic resonance) cisternogram is also a relatively non-invasive method that can be useful in identifying both CSF and herniated brain tissue.

The diagnostic evaluation of facial injury also deserves specific mention. Over time, advances in imaging and neurophysiologic assessment have improved the clinical evaluation of facial injury. Initial analyses of facial dysfunction, such as those of Herbert Mayo and Charles Bell, were rooted in clinical observation, cadaveric anatomic dissection, and vivisection [44, 45]. In addition to diagnostic imaging, electrophysiologic testing has provided a potential opportunity to distinguish subclinical differences in an otherwise homogenous population of patients with facial paralysis. While these advances have allowed for the development of prognostic information for patients with idiopathic facial paralysis [46–48], the utility of such testing in the setting of trauma is yet to be validated.

Certainly, electromyography (EMG) is an effective tool to assess the presence or absence of reinnervation when complete facial paralysis persists over time. However, the use of electroneuronography (ENoG) to justify surgical intervention in patients with complete paralysis after trauma is a more controversial subject given the multitude of factors that should be also considered when formulating the management of a patient with traumatic facial paralysis, such as the mechanism of injury, the extent of injury, and the timing of paralysis onset after injury. Given that ENoG findings, at least, provide an objective assessment of dysfunction, it is felt that this information should be sought when available. However, ENoG data should be used with caution when weighing the risks and benefits of surgical intervention for traumatic facial paralysis. Generally speaking, ENoG is pursued in the setting of complete facial paralysis noted immediately following injury (i.e., not in the setting of *delayed* paralysis). The test is performed 72 h after injury to allow for Wallerian degeneration to occur but should be performed within the first 14 days following injury if possible. For most surgeons, an ENoG that supports surgical intervention is one that demonstrates at least 90% degeneration compared to the

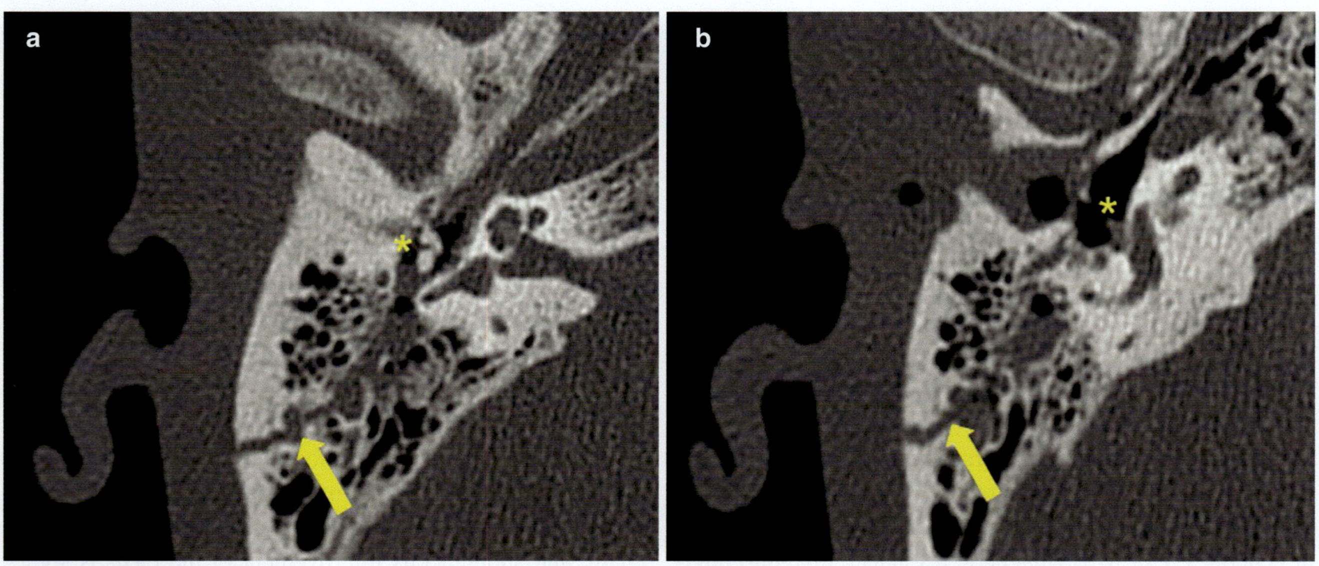

Fig. 59.4 Axial view of a CT scan from a patient with traumatic dislocation of the ossicular chain associated after temporal bone trauma. The causative fracture is demonstrated by the arrow. The malleus-incus joint (**a**) and the incus-stapes joint (**b**) have been affected (*)

non-injured side. Facial nerve electrodiagnostic testing is discussed in greater detail in Chap. 13.

Management

When considering the anatomy of the temporal bone, it is expected that many injuries can be managed expectantly. Generally, non-displaced fractures that do not involve a functional deficit or intracranial injury require no specific intervention and can be clinically followed. However, as described below, when complications do occur in this setting, formulating an evidence-based management plan can be a challenging endeavor.

Injury to the soft tissue overlying the temporal bone can be a complicating factor in the setting of temporal bone trauma. Some cases involve soft tissue avulsion or maceration that can leave bone exposed across a large surface area inside and outside the external ear canal. These situations may require a more urgent surgical intervention, particularly when an injury allows direct communication with a vascular or intracranial injury. Extreme cases may even require closure of the external auditory canal and/or free tissue transfer (Fig. 59.5). However, many cases do not involve such a dramatic soft tissue injury and, instead, may be limited to tissue lacerations in the external canal that correlate with fractures seen on CT. While many of these cases can be managed medically with steroid-containing otic drops and potentially even packing left in place for short periods of time in an attempt to deter stenosis, the formation of post-traumatic cholesteatoma and/or external canal stenosis should always be considered in the setting of soft tissue injuries, particularly given both the possibility that this entity can become a tremendous problem in and of itself, and given the possibility that this problem may take years to manifest (Fig. 59.6) [49–53]. Long-term clinical follow-up is recommended in the setting of external ear canal injuries.

As mentioned previously, most patients with CHL after temporal bone fracture make significant recovery. However, those with persistent CHL may have ossicular chain injury, post-traumatic cholesteatoma, or chronic TM perforation. A myriad of possible ossicular chain defects exist, including incudostapedial joint separation, incudomalleolar joint separation, incus dislocation, malleoincudal complex dislocation, and stapes dislocation. The incus, which has relatively less ligamental support, is particularly prone to ossicular dislocation. Incudostapedial joint separation is the most commonly seen ossicular anomaly after temporal bone trauma, followed by complete incus dislocation from its proximal and distal attachments [54]. Ossicular fractures are rare phenomena and are not as well characterized. When fractures do occur, they most commonly involve the long process of the incus, followed by the crura of the stapes [55]. Conductive hearing

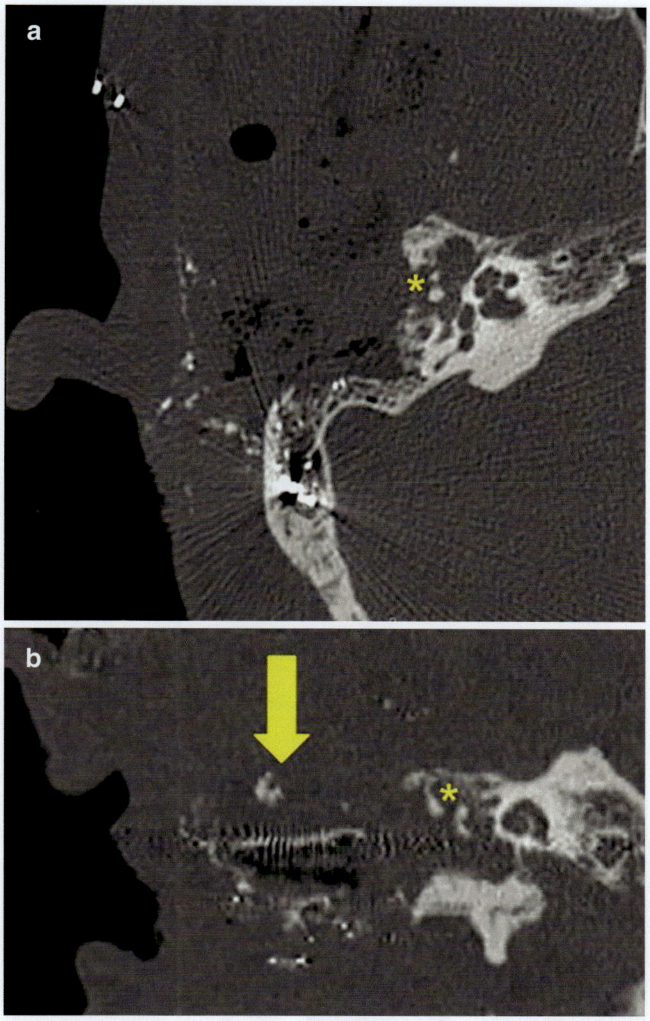

Fig. 59.5 Axial (**a**) and coronal (**b**) views of a CT scan demonstrating extensive destruction of the temporal bone in a patient who suffered a high-energy penetrating trauma. The * demonstrates the location of the ossicles. In (**b**), the arrow demonstrates the expected location of the tegmen. In a subsequent surgery, the temporal bone was cleared of squamous debris and obliterated with abdominal fat. The exposed brain parenchyma was left undisturbed, and the ear canal was overclosed

losses exceeding 30 dB that are present 2–3 months after the inciting event are highly suspicious for ossicular chain pathology [56]. Middle ear exploration and ossiculoplasty are best reserved for when inflammation from the initial trauma has resolved. The authors' preference is to wait 6 months after the initial trauma, although there are reports of ossicular chain reconstruction much earlier [56]. In isolated cases of ossicular chain disruption, near-closure of the air-bone gap is achievable.

In the rare case of stapes subluxation into the vestibule, intervention may be warranted more urgently, especially if a persistent perilymphatic fistula is suspected (Fig. 59.7). There have been reports of conservative management of traumatic stapedial subluxation in the literature that resulted in resolution of vestibular symptoms and improved hearing

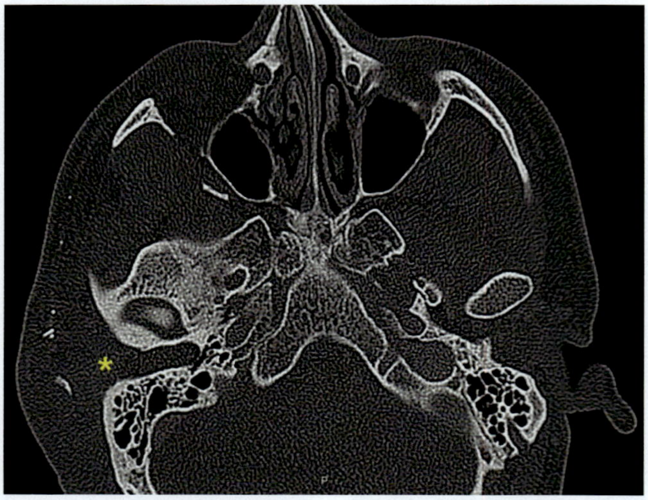

Fig. 59.6 Axial CT scan demonstrating an acquired cholesteatoma of the ear (*) canal and periauricular soft tissue 2 years after traumatic avulsion of the auricle

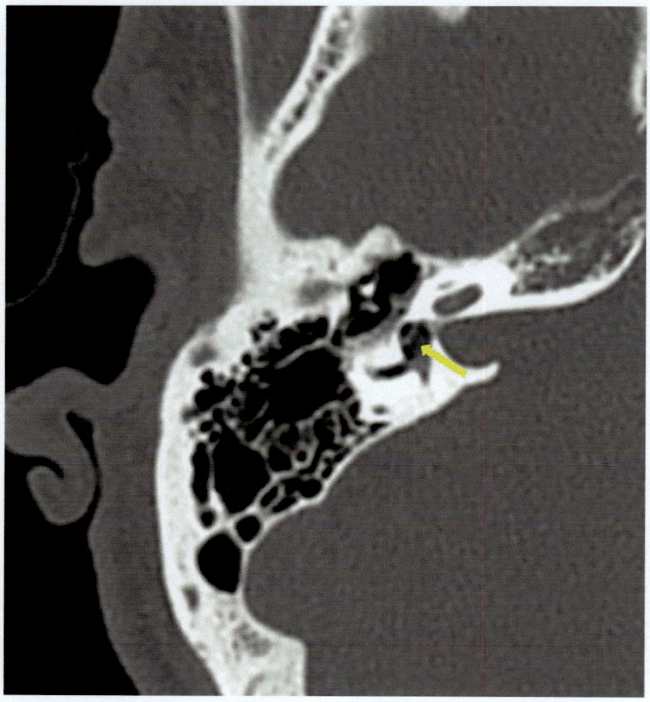

Fig. 59.7 Axial CT scan demonstrating depression of the stapes footplate and pneumolabyrinth (arrow) after temporal bone trauma

[57]. However, if vestibular symptoms and/or hearing worsen or do not improve, surgical exploration is warranted. If the stapes is easily accessible and is not significantly depressed into the vestibule, repair of any visualized oval window fistula and repositioning of the stapes can improve vestibular symptoms and potentially hearing. Stapedectomy is also a consideration when the stapes is dislocated [58]. Hearing loss may be a foregone conclusion in the setting of a stapes that is deeply depressed into the vestibule. In these challenging cases, surgical planning should depend primarily on the patient's symptomatology and preoperative findings with regard to hearing and vestibular function.

Damage to the cochlea or vestibular apparatus can result in both hearing loss and vertigo and can occur in the presence or absence of an evident fracture involving the inner ear (i.e., labyrinthine concussion). The medical management of sensorineural hearing loss after otic capsule violating temporal bone fractures generally involves the use of corticosteroids, though efficacy of this type of therapy is not well studied. For cases in which bilateral severe to profound SNHL persists, cochlear implantation is the hearing rehabilitation option of choice. Favorable outcomes are even possible in the setting of severe cochlear injury, provided a channel remains through which the implant can stimulate the auditory nerve [59]. It is noteworthy, however, that a unique set of challenges can face surgeons, patients, and audiologists when working with implants in this setting: particularly those that relate to the effects of concomitant brain injury after head trauma, and inadvertent stimulation of the facial nerve [60, 61]. Yet, hearing outcomes are generally better with implantation than any available alternative. Medina et al. recently evaluated the value of cochlear implantation for patients with bilateral hearing loss following head trauma. In a study of 14 patients with bilateral severe to profound SNHL as a result of temporal bone fracture, cochlear implantation resulted in useful open-set speech perception in all of the patients in the study. Interestingly, three of these patients had previous auditory brainstem implant, and cochlear implantation resulted in better auditory performance [62].

Vestibular symptoms are common but frequently self-limiting after temporal bone fractures [63]. Benign paroxysmal positional vertigo (BPPV) is not uncommonly seen after trauma, and management with repositioning exercises are generally expected to be curative. Acute vestibular injury can be a consequence of an otic capsule violating fracture, presumably due to direct damage to the vestibular end-organ. Central compensation generally occurs spontaneously, which leads to improvement in symptoms. Vestibular rehabilitation can accelerate recovery, though care must be taken to avoid inhibition of the compensatory process through the habitual use of vestibular suppressants. For cases involving persistent, disabling vertigo and profound SNHL, labyrinthectomy can be considered [64]. In cases of otic capsule sparing fractures, different mechanisms have been proposed to explain the presence of significant vestibular symptoms, labyrinthine concussions and delayed vestibular hydrops noteworthy among them [65].

The evidence-based management of facial nerve injury following temporal bone trauma is a complicated subject. Traditionally, questions that arise in this clinical setting regard the need for surgical decompression of the facial nerve, the timing of when that intervention should occur, and the use of systemic corticosteroids in the management of patients with facial weakness. Currently, the literature offers a plethora of observational evidence regarding the treatment of patients with traumatic facial paralysis. However, extrapolating the results of these prior works, and furthermore, performing a meta-analysis of the associated data, is made difficult by heterogeneity in data reporting. As referenced above, mechanism is an important factor to consider when formulating an algorithm for the management of traumatic facial paralysis. In the setting of high-energy penetrating trauma, complete transection of the nerve is more common, as is injury beyond the actual site of contact between a projectile and the nerve [66–68]. As such, the management of traumatic facial paralysis after a gunshot wound may be more likely to involve nerve grafting. In terms of blunt low-energy trauma, Nash et al. performed a systematic review in 2010 of facial paralysis in this setting [69]. In general, surgical interventions were not found to improve the outcome of facial function beyond what is achievable through observation, with or without steroids. In fact, in patients with complete facial paralysis, 57% of patients recovered normal facial function without a surgical intervention versus 21% of patients who underwent surgery. Furthermore, in patients with delayed onset paralysis, House–Brackmann grade I function was achieved in 80% of cases without surgical intervention versus 30% with surgery. This study also determined that the influence of steroids on the speed or degree of facial recovery after trauma is unclear based on the relevant literature. Moving forward, it seems fair to say that the utility of surgical decompression in treating traumatic facial paralysis is yet to be determined, though current evidence would suggest that surgical management is not always worthy of consideration. In the future, efforts to standardize data reporting for traumatic facial paralysis will hopefully clarify the optimal, evidence-based management strategy for this unfortunate subset of patients.

CSF fistula formation is another potentially serious complication of temporal bone trauma. Morbidity from CSF leaks is generally due to the risk of meningitis or pneumocephalus, and the goal of intervention in these cases is to mitigate the risk of these complications. When managing traumatic CSF fistula formation, the use of prophylactic antibiotics has been a topic of debate. A meta-analysis by Brodie in 1997 showed a significant reduction in the incidence of meningitis with antibiotic prophylaxis in patients with traumatic CSF leak [70]. However, subsequent meta-analyses have suggested that there is no clear benefit of prophylactic antibiotics in this setting [71]. A recent Cochrane database systematic review lent credence to the notion that antibiotics do not prevent meningitis in basilar skull fractures regardless of whether or not a CSF fistula is present [72]. Operative intervention is generally reserved for selected cases when the presence of a CSF fistula has been confirmed. Many CSF leaks close after trauma with only the use of conservative management in the form of antiemetics, head of the bed elevation, stool softeners, and antitussives [73]. Lumbar drains can also be useful in this setting to divert CSF flow away from the injury. However, in some cases, CSF drainage persists, and surgical management must be pursued. Once the location of the leak is identified, the optimal surgical approach depends on the patient's hearing status and the size and number of the defect(s). To approach a tegmen defect, transmastoid, middle fossa, or combined approaches are generally considered. The transmastoid approach can permit extracranial exploration of the injury as well as access to the middle ear, tympanic membrane, and Eustachian tube. Small tegmen defects (<2 cm) can generally be closed easily via this approach using a variety of different substrates. If the otic capsule has been destroyed by the injury and no potential remains for hearing rehabilitation, a translabyrinthine approach can also be used to access more medial aspects of the tegmen. If there is a large (>2 cm) or multifocal defect, a middle cranial fossa approach can also be used alone or in conjunction with the transmastoid approach, though the authors' preference is to use combined approaches to ensure both that the ossicular chain is visualized when retrieving herniated tissue from the perspective of the middle cranial fossa and that the flow of CSF into the mastoid and middle ear stops following repair [74–76]. The use of multiple substrates for closure of the fistula is generally recommended [77]. In recalcitrant cases, obliteration of the mastoid with fat, vascularized muscle, or bone pâté can be utilized, and when recovery of hearing is not anticipated, the middle ear and Eustachian tube can also be obliterated.

Vascular injury following temporal bone fractures is rare, but can be life-threatening. Potential complications include dissection, thrombosis, pseudoaneurysm, and hemorrhage, any of which may manifest as otorrhagia, epistaxis, hemorrhage through a laceration, cranial nerve palsy, or vision loss [78]. If hemorrhage or ischemia occurs from intratemporal carotid injury, angiography and endovascular stenting should be pursued [79]. Embolization or ligation can also be considered as a last resort, given the potential for cerebral ischemia. Injury to the middle meningeal artery is also seen in association with temporal bone trauma, and external bleeding through an open fracture or a contained epidural hematoma can result [80, 81]. Venous injury, if present, can often be managed conservatively. If it is severe enough to require intervention, ligation or intraluminal packing can be considered [34].

Emerging Considerations

When considering the complexity of temporal bone trauma, it is certain that more evidence is needed to define "best-practice" management paradigms in certain situations. Specifically, as described above, the optimal strategies for evaluating and treating of facial paralysis in this setting remain largely unclear. In one sense, it is fair to say that a randomized controlled trial (RCT) is needed to more conclusively address the question of whether or not surgical decompression is warranted in these cases. However, given the variety of factors that need to be taken into consideration in order to ensure a valid comparison between different management strategies, it may not be realistic to assume that an RCT is forthcoming. As such, when considering heterogeneity in data reporting as an obstacle to evidence-based care, a push toward standardization in data reporting, and the establishment of minimum reporting guidelines, will hopefully add internal and external validity to future work.

References

1. Waissbluth S, Ywakim R, Al Qassabi B, et al. Pediatric temporal bone fractures: a case series. Int J Pediatr Otorhinolaryngol. 2016;84:106–9.
2. Ort S, Beus K, Isaacson J. Pediatric temporal bone fractures in a rural population. Otolaryngol Head Neck Surg. 2004;131:433–7.
3. Brodie HA, Thompson TC. Management of complications from 820 temporal bone fractures. Am J Otol. 1997;18:188–97.
4. Lee D, Honrado C, Har-El G, Goldsmith A. Pediatric temporal bone fractures. Laryngoscope. 1998;108:816–21.
5. Schubl SD, Klein TR, Robitsek RJ, et al. Temporal bone fracture: evaluation in the era of modern computed tomography. Injury. 2016;47:1893–7.
6. Sun GH, Shoman NM, Samy RN, Cornelius RS, Koch BL, Pensak ML. Do contemporary temporal bone fracture classification systems reflect concurrent intracranial and cervical spine injuries? Laryngoscope. 2011;121:929–32.
7. Ishman SL, Friedland DR. Temporal bone fractures: traditional classification and clinical relevance. Laryngoscope. 2004;114:1734–41.
8. Wiet RJ, Valvassori GE, Kotsanis CA, Parahy C. Temporal bone fractures. State of the art review. Am J Otol. 1985;6:207–15.
9. Cannon CR, Jahrsdoerfer RA. Temporal bone fractures. Review of 90 cases. Arch Otolaryngol. 1983;109:285–8.
10. Stefanopoulos PK, Pinialidis DE, Hadjigeorgiou GF, Filippakis KN. Wound ballistics 101: the mechanisms of soft tissue wounding by bullets. Eur J Trauma Emerg Surg. 2017;43(5):579–86. https://doi.org/10.1007/s00068-015-0581-1.
11. Maiden N. Ballistics reviews: mechanisms of bullet wound trauma. Forensic Sci Med Pathol. 2009;5:204–9.
12. Advanced trauma life support (ATLS(R)): the ninth edition. J Trauma Acute Care Surg. 2013;74:1363–6.
13. Kamerer DB, Thompson SW. Middle ear and temporal bone trauma. In: Bailey BJ, editor. Head and neck surgery—otolaryngology. Philadelphia: Lippincott Williams & Wilkins; 2001.
14. Croxson G, May M, Mester SJ. Grading facial nerve function: House-Brackmann versus Burres-Fisch methods. Am J Otol. 1990;11:240–6.
15. Reitzen SD, Babb JS, Lalwani AK. Significance and reliability of the House-Brackmann grading system for regional facial nerve function. Otolaryngol Head Neck Surg. 2009;140:154–8.
16. Yen TL, Driscoll CL, Lalwani AK. Significance of House-Brackmann facial nerve grading global score in the setting of differential facial nerve function. Otol Neurotol. 2003;24:118–22.
17. Fattah AY, Gurusinghe AD, Gavilan J, et al. Facial nerve grading instruments: systematic review of the literature and suggestion for uniformity. Plast Reconstr Surg. 2015;135:569–79.
18. Coulson SE, Croxson GR, Adams RD, O'Dwyer NJ. Reliability of the "Sydney," "Sunnybrook," and "House Brackmann" facial grading systems to assess voluntary movement and synkinesis after facial nerve paralysis. Otolaryngol Head Neck Surg. 2005;132:543–9.
19. Vrabec JT, Backous DD, Djalilian HR, et al. Facial Nerve Grading System 2.0. Otolaryngol Head Neck Surg. 2009;140:445–50.
20. Henstrom DK, Skilbeck CJ, Weinberg J, Knox C, Cheney ML, Hadlock TA. Good correlation between original and modified House Brackmann facial grading systems. Laryngoscope. 2011;121:47–50.
21. Ray AM. Halo sign is neither sensitive nor specific for cerebrospinal fluid leak. Ann Emerg Med. 2009;53:288.
22. Aguilar EA 3rd, Yeakley JW, Ghorayeb BY, Hauser M, Cabrera J, Jahrsdoerfer RA. High resolution CT scan of temporal bone fractures: association of facial nerve paralysis with temporal bone fractures. Head Neck Surg. 1987;9:162–6.
23. Dempewolf R, Gubbels S, Hansen MR. Acute radiographic workup of blunt temporal bone trauma: maxillofacial versus temporal bone CT. Laryngoscope. 2009;119:442–8.
24. Travis LW, Stalnaker RL, Melvin JW. Impact trauma of the human temporal bone. J Trauma. 1977;17:761–6.
25. Lindeman RC. Temporal bone trauma and facial paralysis. Otolaryngol Clin N Am. 1979;12:403–13.
26. Harker LA, McCabe BF. Temporal bone fractures and facial nerve injury. Otolaryngol Clin N Am. 1974;7:425–31.
27. Ghorayeb BY, Yeakley JW. Temporal bone fractures: longitudinal or oblique? The case for oblique temporal bone fractures. Laryngoscope. 1992;102:129–34.
28. Dahiya R, Keller JD, Litofsky NS, Bankey PE, Bonassar LJ, Megerian CA. Temporal bone fractures: otic capsule sparing versus otic capsule violating clinical and radiographic considerations. J Trauma. 1999;47:1079–83.
29. Little SC, Kesser BW. Radiographic classification of temporal bone fractures: clinical predictability using a new system. Arch Otolaryngol Head Neck Surg. 2006;132:1300–4.
30. Dunklebarger J, Branstetter B, Lincoln A, et al. Pediatric temporal bone fractures: current trends and comparison of classification schemes. Laryngoscope. 2014;124:781–4.
31. York G, Barboriak D, Petrella J, DeLong D, Provenzale JM. Association of internal carotid artery injury with carotid canal fractures in patients with head trauma. AJR Am J Roentgenol. 2005;184:1672–8.
32. McKinney A, Ott F, Short J, McKinney Z, Truwit C. Angiographic frequency of blunt cerebrovascular injury in patients with carotid canal or vertebral foramen fractures on multidetector CT. Eur J Radiol. 2007;62:385–93.
33. Resnick DK, Subach BR, Marion DW. The significance of carotid canal involvement in basilar cranial fracture. Neurosurgery. 1997;40:1177–81.
34. Kahn JB, Stewart MG, Diaz-Marchan PJ. Acute temporal bone trauma: utility of high-resolution computed tomography. Am J Otol. 2000;21:743–52.
35. Azad TD, Veeravagu A, Corrales CE, Chow KK, Fischbein NJ, Harris OA. Abducens nerve avulsion and facial nerve palsy after temporal bone fracture: a rare concomitance of injuries. World Neurosurg. 2016;88(689):e685–8.
36. Corrales CE, Monfared A, Jackler RK. Facial and vestibulocochlear nerve avulsion at the fundus of the internal auditory canal in a child without a temporal bone fracture. Otol Neurotol. 2010;31:1508–10.

37. Kim SY, Kim YJ, Kim YH, Park MH. Audiologic patterns of otic capsule preserving temporal bone fracture: effects of the affected subsites. Clin Exp Otorhinolaryngol. 2016;9:206–11.
38. Tos M. Course of and sequelae to 248 petrosal fractures. Acta Otolaryngol. 1973;75:353–4.
39. Song SW, Jun BC, Kim H. Clinical features and radiological evaluation of otic capsule sparing temporal bone fractures. J Laryngol Otol. 2017;131:209–14.
40. Schell A, Kitsko D. Audiometric outcomes in pediatric temporal bone trauma. Otolaryngol Head Neck Surg. 2016;154:175–80.
41. Korem M, Ovadia H, Paldor I, et al. False negative beta-2 transferrin in the diagnosis of cerebrospinal fluid leak in the presence of Streptococcus pneumoniae. Laryngoscope. 2015;125:556–60.
42. Michaelides EM, Kuang H, Pieribone VA. Dickkopf-related protein 3 as a sensitive and specific marker for cerebrospinal fluid leaks. Otol Neurotol. 2016;37:299–303.
43. Mostafa BE, Khafagi A. Combined HRCT and MRI in the detection of CSF rhinorrhea. Skull Base. 2004;14:157–62; discussion 162.
44. Pearce JM. Sir Charles Bell (1774-1842). J R Soc Med. 1993;86:353–4.
45. Mayo H. Anatomical and Physiological Commentaries No. 1 (London: Thomas and George Underwood, 1822) & No. 2 (London: Thomas and George Underwood, 1823).
46. Gantz BJ, Rubinstein JT, Gidley P, Woodworth GG. Surgical management of Bell's palsy. Laryngoscope. 1999;109:1177–88.
47. Cannon RB, Gurgel RK, Warren FM, Shelton C. Facial nerve outcomes after middle fossa decompression for Bell's palsy. Otol Neurotol. 2015;36:513–8.
48. McAllister K, Walker D, Donnan PT, Swan I. Surgical interventions for the early management of Bell's palsy. Cochrane Database Syst Rev. 2011:Cd007468.
49. Sweeney AD, Hunter JB, Haynes DS, et al. Iatrogenic cholesteatoma arising from the vascular strip. Laryngoscope. 2017;127:698–701.
50. Vrabec JT, Chaljub G. External canal cholesteatoma. Am J Otol. 2000;21:608–14.
51. McKennan KX, Chole RA. Post-traumatic cholesteatoma. Laryngoscope. 1989;99:779–82.
52. McKennan KX, Chole RA. Traumatic external auditory canal atresia. Am J Otol. 1992;13:80–1.
53. Brookes GB, Graham MD. Post-traumatic cholesteatoma of the external auditory canal. Laryngoscope. 1984;94:667–70.
54. Bellucci RJ. Traumatic injuries of the middle ear. Otolaryngol Clin N Am. 1983;16:633–50.
55. Kollias SS. Temporal bone trauma. In: Lemmerling M, Kollias SS, editors. Radiology of the petrous bone. Berlin: Springer; 2004:49–58.
56. Wennmo C, Spandow O. Fractures of the temporal bone--chain incongruencies. Am J Otolaryngol. 1993;14:38–42.
57. Lao WW, Niparko JK. Assessment of changes in cochlear function with pneumolabyrinth after middle ear trauma. Otol Neurotol. 2007;28:1013–7.
58. Sarac S, Cengel S, Sennaroglu L. Pneumolabyrinth following traumatic luxation of the stapes into the vestibule. Int J Pediatr Otorhinolaryngol. 2006;70:159–61.
59. Morgan WE, Coker NJ, Jenkins HA. Histopathology of temporal bone fractures: implications for cochlear implantation. Laryngoscope. 1994;104:426–32.
60. Greenberg SL, Shipp D, Lin VY, Chen JM, Nedzelski JM. Cochlear implantation in patients with bilateral severe sensorineural hearing loss after major blunt head trauma. Otol Neurotol. 2011;32:48–54.
61. Espahbodi M, Sweeney AD, Lennon KJ, Wanna GB. Facial nerve stimulation associated with cochlear implant use following temporal bone fractures. Am J Otolaryngol. 2015;36:578–82.
62. Medina M, Di Lella F, Di Trapani G et al. Cochlear implantation versus auditory brainstem implantation in bilateral total deafness after head trauma: personal experience and review of the literature. Otol Neurotol 2014; 35:260–270.
63. Johnson F, Semaan MT, Megerian CA. Temporal bone fracture: evaluation and management in the modern era. Otolaryngol Clin North Am. 2008;41:597–618, x.
64. Benecke JE. Surgery for non-Meniere's vertigo. Acta Otolaryngol Suppl. 1994;513:37–9.
65. Ernst A, Basta D, Seidl RO, Todt I, Scherer H, Clarke A. Management of posttraumatic vertigo. Otolaryngol Head Neck Surg. 2005;132:554–8.
66. Maiman DJ, Cusick JF, Anderson AJ, Larson SJ. Nonoperative management of traumatic facial nerve palsy. J Trauma. 1985;25:644–8.
67. Shindo ML, Fetterman BL, Shih L, Maceri DR, Rice DH. Gunshot wounds of the temporal bone: a rational approach to evaluation and management. Otolaryngol Head Neck Surg. 1995;112:533–9.
68. McKennan KX, Chole RA. Facial paralysis in temporal bone trauma. Am J Otol. 1992;13:167–72.
69. Nash JJ, Friedland DR, Boorsma KJ, Rhee JS. Management and outcomes of facial paralysis from intratemporal blunt trauma: a systematic review. Laryngoscope. 2010;120(Suppl 4):S214.
70. Brodie HA. Prophylactic antibiotics for posttraumatic cerebrospinal fluid fistulae. A meta-analysis. Arch Otolaryngol Head Neck Surg. 1997;123:749–52.
71. Villalobos T, Arango C, Kubilis P, Rathore M. Antibiotic prophylaxis after basilar skull fractures: a meta-analysis. Clin Infect Dis. 1998;27:364–9.
72. Ratilal BO, Costa J, Pappamikail L, Sampaio C. Antibiotic prophylaxis for preventing meningitis in patients with basilar skull fractures. Cochrane Database Syst Rev. 2015;2015:Cd004884.
73. Prosser JD, Vender JR, Solares CA. Traumatic cerebrospinal fluid leaks. Otolaryngol Clin N Am. 2011;44:857–73, vii.
74. Carlson ML, Copeland WR 3rd, Driscoll CL, et al. Temporal bone encephalocele and cerebrospinal fluid fistula repair utilizing the middle cranial fossa or combined mastoid-middle cranial fossa approach. J Neurosurg. 2013;119:1314–22.
75. Sweeney AD, Carlson ML, Haynes DS, et al. A novel method for autograft placement during tegmen repair: the suture "pull-through" technique. Laryngoscope. 2015;125:323–5.
76. O'Connell BP, Hunter JB, Sweeney AD, et al. Outcomes of the suture "pull-through" technique for repair of lateral skull base CSF fistula and encephaloceles. Otol Neurotol. 2017;38:416–22.
77. Sanna M, Fois P, Russo A, Falcioni M. Management of meningoencephalic herniation of the temporal bone: personal experience and literature review. Laryngoscope. 2009;119:1579–85.
78. Duncan NO 3rd, Coker NJ, Jenkins HA, Canalis RF. Gunshot injuries of the temporal bone. Otolaryngol Head Neck Surg. 1986;94:47–55.
79. Cohen JE, Ben-Hur T, Rajz G, Umansky F, Gomori JM. Endovascular stent-assisted angioplasty in the management of traumatic internal carotid artery dissections. Stroke. 2005;36:e45–7.
80. Schneider RC, Boles R. Combined neuro-otologic and neurosurgical problems in head trauma. Laryngoscope. 1968;78:955–72.
81. Nadig AS, King AT. Traumatic extradural haematoma revealed after contralateral decompressive craniectomy. Br J Neurosurg. 2012;26:877–9.

Part VIII

Systemic Diseases Affecting the Audiovestibular System and Temporal Bone

60 Primary and Secondary Otalgia

Michael S. Harris, Jason A. Beyea, and Aaron C. Moberly

Introduction

Otalgia is a commonly encountered symptom in primary care offices, emergency departments, and otolaryngology clinics. Of the 2.2% of all emergency visits attributable to otologic diagnoses, almost all may present with otalgia as an isolated symptom or as part of a constellation of symptoms [1]. Otalgia may be primary, originating from a pathological process directly involving the pinna, external auditory canal (EAC), middle ear, inner ear, or skull base, or secondary, originating from elsewhere in the head and neck distant from the ear. This region's complex embryologic origin, as a juncture point between branchial and post-branchial tissue, is reflected in its complex and overlapping sensory innervation [2–4]. Contributions are made by cranial nerves V3 (EAC, tympanic membrane, middle ear), VII (concha, EAC), IX (middle ear), and X (concha, antihelix), and upper cervical nerve roots C2/C3, which give rise to the great auricular nerve and lesser occipital nerve. For this reason, referred pain from outside the ear is common, and subjective localization of the source of otalgia can be difficult.

M. S. Harris
Division of Otology and Neurotologic Skull Base Surgery, Department of Otolaryngology and Communication Sciences, Medical College of Wisconsin, Milwaukee, WI, USA

J. A. Beyea
Department of Otolaryngology, Queen's University School of Medicine, Kingston, ON, Canada

A. C. Moberly (✉)
Division of Otology and Neurotology, Department of Otolaryngology—Head and Neck Surgery, Vanderbilt University Medical Center, Nashville, TN, USA
e-mail: Aaron.C.Moberly@vumc.org

History and Physical Examination Considerations

Before discussing various etiologies responsible for primary or secondary otalgia, some characteristics of the pain, itself, and associated symptoms can be clinically informative. Continuous, acute onset, persistent pain is often associated with an infectious or inflammatory condition. Intermittent pain may be associated with a musculoskeletal condition that fluctuates, such as temporomandibular joint dysfunction. Deep, boring, unrelenting pain may raise suspicion for a malignant process.

Associated otologic symptoms typically point to a primary source of otalgia. Specifically, otorrhea, hearing loss, aural fullness, vertigo, and facial weakness suggest a primary otologic source of pain. In contrast, a paucity of associated otologic symptoms and symptoms distant from the ear suggest a secondary source of otalgia. These can include sinonasal complaints (nasal obstruction, rhinorrhea, epistaxis), upper aerodigestive symptoms (oral or pharyngeal sores or masses, bleeding, trismus, dysphagia, dysphonia, dyspnea, hemoptysis, or neck masses), or dental complaints (tooth pain, bruxism, temporomandibular joint clicking). Complaints suggestive of a systemic disease might also be elicited, typically associated with secondary sources of otalgia, including fevers, night sweats, or weight loss.

Primary Otalgia

Auricle

Etiologies of primary otalgia may be considered by progressing from the auricle medially. The auricle or pinna is composed of a framework of elastic cartilage overlaid by perichondrium and a thin layer of skin. Given its delicate composition and prominent location, the auricle is vulnerable to trauma or laceration, most commonly associated with

A. D. Sweeney et al. (eds.), *Haynes-Glasscock-Shambaugh Surgery of the Ear*, https://doi.org/10.1007/978-3-032-18264-7_60

human and animal bites (22%), motor vehicle collisions (17%), and burns [5]. The most frequent injury pattern includes the upper third of the auricle exclusively (41%), followed by the entire auricle (19%). Post-traumatic auricular hematoma can be a source of significant pain associated with perichondrial distension, which is relieved by incision, evacuation, and compressive dressing or sutured bolsters to prevent recurrence.

Noninfectious, inflammatory causes of otalgia localized to the external ear include perichondritis or relapsing polychondritis, benign entities characterized by diffuse, lobule-sparing edema and erythema that is typically responsive to systemic steroid therapy. Chondrodermatitis nodularis helicis may be encountered as an intensely tender nodule, most commonly seen on the helix or antihelix. Its etiology is incompletely characterized, but ischemic changes to underlying cartilage related to chronic pressure are suspected [6]. Biopsy is often indicated given similarity in appearance to cutaneous malignancies, in particular basal cell carcinoma and squamous cell carcinoma. Injection and/or topical steroid, pressure-relief, and surgical excision are commonly accepted therapies; photodynamic therapy and topical nitroglycerin are more recent treatments aimed at lowering post-treatment recurrence rates.

Infectious conditions of the auricle are typically accompanied by other signs and symptoms of infection that help differentiate them from noninfectious inflammatory etiologies. Recent history of trauma, burns, ear piercing, insect bite, or surgery may be elicited. Erysipelas (St. Anthony's Fire) or impetigo are causes of painful external ear infections affecting the dermis or hypodermis of the auricle, typically caused by *Streptococcus pyogenes* or *Staphylococcus aureus*, respectively. Bullae and golden crusting with erythema that does not spare the lobule distinguish erysipelas and impetigo from other benign entities. Treatment is oral antibiotics directed at these organisms.

External Auditory Canal

Progressing medially, the tissue composition of the EAC lends itself to a different complement of otalgia etiologies. Sebaceous and ceruminous glands, as well as vellus hair follicles, are found in the lateral cartilaginous third of the external auditory canal, while the medial two-thirds consist of thin skin directly overlying bone (Fig. 60.1a). Furuncles and carbuncles, typically caused by digital trauma or use of cotton-tipped swabs, may present as a painful pustular lesion

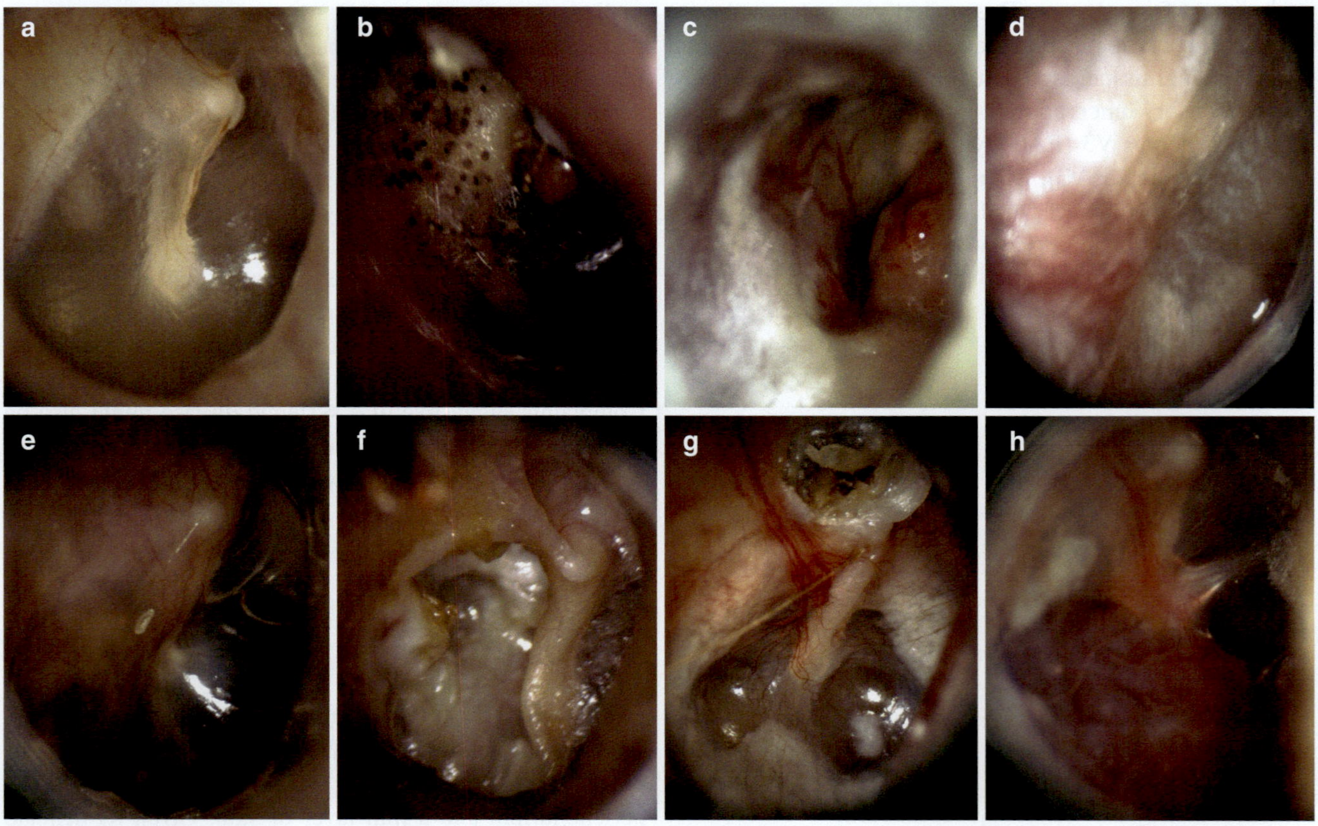

Fig. 60.1 Primary sources of right otalgia. For reference, (**a**) demonstrates normal right eardrum, (**b**) fungal chronic otitis externa with fungal hyphae, (**c**) malignant otitis externa with granulation at inferior external auditory canal, (**d**) acute otitis media, (**e**) otitis media with effusion, (**f**) mesotympanic cholesteatoma, (**g**) epitympanic cholesteatoma, and (**h**) glomus jugulare

in the lateral third of the ear canal and are typically successfully managed with warm compress, drainage, and oral antibiotic therapy. In the case of nonresponsive lesions or atypical history, the differential for a painful EAC mass must include less commonly encountered benign entities such as ceruminous gland adenomas or pleomorphic adenoma and malignancies including basal cell carcinoma, squamous cell carcinoma, adenoid cystic carcinoma, or ceruminous adenocarcinoma [7].

Cerumen obstruction or impaction and foreign bodies in the EAC may also present with otalgia and are among the most common ear-related reasons for physician visits [8]. Primary prevention and use of cerumenolytic agents, irrigation, or manual removal requiring instrumentation, ideally under otomicroscopic visualization, form the mainstay of management for symptomatic cerumen obstruction.

Acute otitis externa (AOE), or "swimmer's ear," is a common cause of exquisite otalgia that consumes significant time and resources [9–11]. Presenting symptoms of AOE include otalgia (70%), pain with mastication, otorrhea, pruritus (60%), aural fullness (22%), and acute hearing loss (32%). Otoscopy discloses purulence and canal edema, often precluding complete evaluation of the tympanic membrane. Tenderness can be elicited by touch of the tragus or even gentle manipulation of the pinna and can be out of proportion to physical exam findings, owing to edematous distension of the skin of the EAC. The clinician must maintain an appropriately broad differential diagnosis so as to distinguish AOE from clinical mimics with overlapping symptoms such as acute otitis media (AOM), cholesteatoma, or chronic otitis externa (COE) or less common, more worrisome entities such as malignancy of the EAC [10]. Likewise, recognition of complicating factors, in particular tympanic membrane perforation, retained foreign body, or presence of tympanostomy tubes, is important to ensure appropriate management. The most common pathogens responsible for AOE in North America are bacterial (98%) and polymicrobial: *Staphylococcus aureus* (10–70%), *Pseudomonas aeruginosa* (20–60%), and other Gram-negative organisms [12]. Treatment involves appropriate diagnosis, initial and sometimes serial ear cleanings under microscopy, and application of topical antimicrobial therapy empirically targeting commonly involved pathogens, most effectively in combination with ototopical steroids, which address the painful edema [13, 14]. Placement of an otowick is often necessary to ensure adequate delivery of topical medication. Modifications of behavioral risk factors that predispose to epithelial damage such as EAC instrumentation (e.g., Q-tip use, ear scratching) and medical factors that predispose to injury (e.g., dermatoses) or complicate wound healing are essential to prevent recurrence.

In contrast to AOE, COE is a painful and pruritic infectious process that may persist for months to years [15]. Recognizing and managing predisposing factors is imperative to the successful treatment of COE. Pruritus associated with dermatoses such as eczema, psoriasis, or seborrheic dermatitis may tempt the patient to perform trauma-inducing EAC instrumentation. Cerumen accumulation, local trauma, and trapped humidity accompanying hearing aid use can create an ideal milieu for pathogenic microorganisms. Unlike AOE, otomycosis is more commonly associated with COE (Fig. 60.1b). This may be due to disequilibrium of normal EAC pH associated with repeated topical antibiotic therapy. Strict dry ear precautions, topical antifungal therapy, acetic acid irrigation, and management of predisposing factors play key roles in treatment of COE. Medial canal fibrosis and secondary acquired canal stenosis with conductive hearing loss can result from long-term medically recalcitrant COE [16].

Malignant otitis externa (MOE), also known as skull base osteomyelitis, is an invasive infection of the soft tissues of the EAC and osteomyelitis of the temporal bone (Fig. 60.1c). It is a potentially life-threatening form of otitis externa, most often seen in elderly patients or immunodeficient individuals such as insulin-dependent diabetics [17, 18]. Granulation tissue along the floor of the EAC is a classic otomicroscopic finding that should raise suspicion for MOE, often in conjunction with cranial nerve deficits. *Pseudomonas aeruginosa* is the most commonly associated pathogen, although a high index of suspicion for nonpseudomonal agents should be maintained, in particular for patients without diabetes mellitus [19]. Under circumstances that are equivocal, biopsy is often required to rule out a malignant process.

The extension of the disease and management planning for MOE is defined by its imaging characteristics. Computed tomography (CT) and magnetic resonance imaging (MRI) have complementary utilities and typically should both be obtained. Temporomandibular joint erosion, tegmen involvement, infratemporal fossa destruction, and extension into the nasopharynx or intracranial compartment all portend poor prognosis [20]. Technetium-99m scans gauge extent of bony involvement in early disease. Gallium-67 scans are useful in monitoring disease through the course of treatment and in determining treatment duration. Treatment of MOE includes aggressive medical therapy in the form of risk factor management (specifically including normalization of blood glucose levels in diabetes) and ototopical and systemic antibiotics targeting *Pseudomonas*, or less common pathogens as directed by culture. Surgical debridement may be indicated for patients recalcitrant to medical therapy. MOE may progress to involve adjacent soft tissues and the skull base, meningitis, brain abscess, and death. This topic has been covered in Chap. 32.

Herpes zoster oticus (Ramsay Hunt syndrome, RHS) is a varicella-zoster mediated process, which typically presents with severe otalgia accompanied by erythematous, herpetiform lesions in the external auditory canal and pinna [21].

The diagnosis of RHS is suggested by facial paresis, vesicular lesions involving the concha, EAC, and hard palate, and vestibulocochlear symptoms. Relative to idiopathic facial nerve paresis or palsy (i.e., Bell's palsy), the prognosis for complete return of facial nerve function is poorer [22]. Treatment of RHS includes high-dose oral corticosteroid and antiviral therapy. This topic has been covered in Chap. 57.

Middle Ear and Temporal Bone

The tympanic space and middle ear contents host a variety of processes that may manifest with marked otalgia. Traumatic tympanic membrane perforation is associated with acute onset otalgia and may result from SCUBA or hyperbaric oxygen therapy-associated barotrauma [23, 24], blast injuries [25], slag burn injury [26], or instrumentation misadventures.

Acute otitis media (AOM) is the most common bacterial infection of childhood (Fig. 60.1d) [27]. Eustachian tube dysfunction from immature nasopharyngeal musculature, unfavorable orientation of the Eustachian tube, and the nascent nature of the immune system make AOM most common prior to two years of age. Other recognized risk factors include environmental allergy, recent viral upper respiratory infection, daycare attendance, as well as craniofacial malformations such as cleft palate and conditions associated with long-term Eustachian tube dysfunction, such as Down syndrome [28]. Otalgia from distension of the tympanic membrane and fever are the most common presenting symptoms. Otomicroscopy reveals an injected, bulging tympanic membrane often with loss of the light reflex in the anterior inferior quadrant. *Streptococcus pneumoniae*, *Haemophilus influenzae*, and *Moraxella catarrhalis* are the most frequently implicated organisms. It is important to discern AOM from otitis media with effusion (OME), which implies uninfected serous fluid in the middle ear (Fig. 60.1e) [29]. AOM and OME entities are distinguished by historical details and otomicroscopy. The latter more often is noted incidentally or alongside aural fullness and/or hearing loss, but otalgia is rare; exam discloses serous fluid, but erythematous bulging of the tympanic membrane is not seen.

Current management of AOM is directed by American Academy of Pediatrics (AAP) guidelines [30]. For children >6 months of age, who are not known to be inherently at "high risk" for complications of AOM (e.g., immunocompromised, inner ear malformations) and who have nonsevere unilateral AOM symptoms without otorrhea, can either be prescribed antibiotic therapy or offered an up-front period of observation based on joint decision-making with the parents/caregivers. The purpose of an observation period is to avoid the development of antibiotic resistance and medication-related complications such as diarrhea and allergic reaction. If observation is chosen, a mechanism for re-examination in 48–72 hours to assess for clinical improvement must be available. If clinical improvement is not apparent within 48–72 hours, oral antibiotic therapy is initiated with high-dose amoxicillin or amoxicillin-clavulanate, for beta-lactamase coverage.

When signs and symptoms of AOM persist beyond eight weeks, it is termed chronic otitis media (COM). When accompanied by middle ear effusion at the time of assessment, myringotomy with tympanostomy tube placement is indicated for recurrent or COM in order to provide middle ear ventilation, prevent painful tympanic membrane distension, lower the risk of spontaneous tympanic membrane perforation, and allow for delivery of ototopicals into the middle ear space, which is preferential to the use of oral antibiotic therapy [29]. Complications of untreated COM, infrequently encountered in developed countries since the introduction of antibiotics and tympanostomy tubes, include sigmoid sinus thrombosis, suppurative labyrinthitis, petrous apicitis, otitic hydrocephalus, meningitis, and intracranial abscess.

Petrous apicitis was once estimated to occur as a complication in one of every 300 cases of suppurative otitis media [31]. The constellation of abducens nerve paresis, severe retro-orbital pain, and otorrhea is known as Gradenigo syndrome. This complex is believed to be due to entrapment of the abducens nerve due to petrous apex inflammation as the nerve traverses Dorello's canal at the petrous tip. Management of petrous apicitis consists of culture-directed intravenous antibiotic therapy, often long-term, with surgery judiciously reserved for the infrequent scenario in which medical therapy is unsuccessful [32].

Acute mastoiditis is a clinical diagnosis defined by postauricular edema with obliteration of the postauricular sulcus, erythema, tenderness, and protrusion of the pinna [33]. Subperiosteal abscesses, such as Bezold abscess, where purulence accumulates medial to the attachment of sternocleidomastoid muscle, or Luc abscess, a subperiosteal collection in the temporal area, are infrequently encountered.

Chronic otomastoiditis and cholesteatoma (Fig. 60.1f, g) share pathophysiologic overlap and are the end stage of unremitting Eustachian tube dysfunction. Tympanic membrane retraction into the closed space of the middle ear prevents normal sloughing of squamous epithelium from the lateral face of the drum. Through direct expansion and osteolytic enzymatic influences of perimatrix, untreated cholesteatoma can have profound sequelae affecting hearing, facial nerve, and vestibular function. Cholesteatoma can progress to involve the tegmen and extend into the intracranial cavity. Otalgia, otorrhea, and subjective hearing loss are common presenting symptoms. Management is generally surgical, tailored to the extent and location of the patient's disease, and involves long-term management to ensure a safe, dry ear.

Less commonly, middle ear neoplastic processes may present with otalgia. These may include benign lesions such as paraganglioma (Fig. 60.1h) or middle ear adenoma. Otalgia can also result from direct extension of malignant processes with a cutaneous, temporal bone, parotid gland, or intracranial origin.

Secondary Otalgia

Secondary otalgia is defined as ear pain that takes its origin not from the ear itself, but rather from sources separate from the ear. A presumed underlying mechanism for referred pain is the neuronal convergence–projection theory, whereby multiple afferent sensory nerves join a shared neural pathway [34]. As a result of the intimate embryologic relationship among the ear and other structures of the head and neck, the sensory distribution of this part of the body is complex and overlapping [2–4]. Irritation of any of the distal sensory branches of cranial nerves V3, VII, IX, and X, or cervical roots C2 and C3 can result in perceived otalgia [35]. In the absence of local pathology, the physician must often look beyond the ear in search for the source of otalgia. Failure to do so may result in missed or delayed diagnoses of potentially life-threatening conditions.

Maxillofacial and Dental Sources

Maxillofacial and dental pathology are among the most frequent origins of referred otalgia [36, 37]. Inflammatory and infectious processes such as dental caries, abscesses, and periodontitis may be involved. Teething is an often-discussed source of perceived otalgia, although support for this etiology is limited and largely anecdotal [38]. Post-traumatic or pathologic facial fractures involving the mandible, maxilla, or zygoma with or without concomitant temporal bone fracture can generate pain referable to the ear. Similarly, otalgia may accompany neoplastic processes of dental and maxillofacial substrates such as keratocystic odontogenic tumor, ameloblastoma, or osteosarcoma.

Temporomandibular joint disorder (TMJD) is an extremely common cause of referred otalgia. Over half of patients known to have TMJD report ear pain [35]. The temporomandibular joint (TMJ) is a modified hinge synovial joint. Its articular surfaces consist of the glenoid fossa, the mandibular condyle head, and the articular tubercle of the temporal bone posteriorly. The articular disk of the TMJ is a fibrocartilaginous extension of the joint capsule, which lies between the articulating surfaces, dividing them into a superior compartment and an inferior compartment. The superior compartment, containing the disk, glenoid fossa, and articular tubercle, is associated with translational movement; the inferior compartment, containing the disk and condyle, is associated with rotational movement. The TMJ facilitates elevation, depression, protrusion, retrusion, and lateral movement of the mandible. A number of primary disorders can affect the TMJ including degenerative joint disease, and anterior disk displacement with reduction (full mouth opening not limited) or without reduction (full mouth opening limited).

Symptoms suggestive of TMJD include teeth clenching/grinding, dental malocclusion, audible or palpable popping or clicking with mouth opening or closing, and episodes of jaw locking open. Otalgia associated with TMJD from bruxism is usually worse in the morning and may radiate to the temporal region [39]. Signs suggestive of TMJD include TMJ tenderness to palpation, joint crepitus, tenderness of muscles of mastication, excessive dental facet wear, and restriction of TMJ range of motion. Risk factors for TMJ disorders include a history of blunt or penetrating jaw trauma, bruxism, jaw clenching, hard chewing, gum chewing, chronic stress/anxiety, poorly fit dentures, and dental malocclusion.

Most forms of TMJD may be successfully managed nonsurgically [40]. The treatment algorithm usually begins with behavioral measures. Cornerstones of this approach include patient education, stress/anxiety management, initiation of a soft diet, limited jaw movement (e.g., avoidance of gum chewing), joint massage, and application of warm compresses. In combination with behavioral measures, medical interventions may be used, such as nonsteroidal anti-inflammatory (NSAID) therapy, tricyclic antidepressants (TCAs), or botulinum toxin injection [41], unless otherwise contraindicated. Oral occlusal splints may be custom fit by a dentist, especially helpful when bruxism is a contributing factor. For more advanced management in cases of persistent pain refractory to conservative measures or complications such as joint ankylosis, referral to an oral-maxillofacial surgeon may be necessary.

Aerodigestive Tract and Neck

In any patient presenting with the complaint of otalgia without compelling signs or symptoms suggesting an otologic diagnosis, a neoplastic process of the aerodigestive tract must be thoroughly ruled out. Squamous cell carcinoma accounts for the majority of tumors of the aerodigestive tract, but benign and malignant salivary tumors, lymphoma, neuroendocrine tumors, or metastatic disease can all arise in this region and first present with otalgia. Occult malignancy in other regions of the head and neck may be associated with otalgia as well, including occult neck disease and lesions of the parapharyngeal space [42].

A history probing for risk factors for head and neck cancer should be performed including tobacco and alcohol consumption and history of prior radiation. Inquiry should be made regarding odynophagia, unintended weight loss, dysphonia, globus sensation, dysphagia, dyspnea, hemoptysis, or aural fullness. Special concern and evaluation for Eustachian tube obstructing nasopharyngeal pathology should be raised in the context of unilateral otalgia with or without effusion. Physical exam should consist of neck and thyroid gland palpation, oral and oropharyngeal inspection, and palpation of all mucosal surfaces (with removal of dentures), and nasopharyngoscopy or indirect laryngoscopy (mirror exam). Additional imaging, as appropriate, and referral are imperative for further work-up and definitive management of any patient with findings concerning for head and neck neoplasia.

Prior or ongoing chemoradiation therapy for primary lesions of the head and neck may also serve as an inciting factor for otalgia itself. Eustachian tube dysfunction associated with mucositis and/or nasopharyngeal edema can result in middle ear effusion resulting in aural fullness, conductive hearing loss, and otalgia. These symptoms may be mitigated by placement of myringotomy tubes, although timing of myringotomy tube placement is controversial, with the effusion often resolving following completion of radiation therapy [43]. More concerning, osteoradionecrosis of the temporal bone may result as a complication of radiation therapy, most commonly for primary lesions of the parotid gland, followed by the nasopharynx [44, 45]. Otorrhea, hearing loss, and otalgia are the most common symptoms. Dry ear precautions are recommended, and these patients often require regular follow-up for otomicrodebridement.

Non-neoplastic processes with origins in aerodigestive tract or neck that can occasionally be accompanied by or present with otalgia include inflammatory and infectious processes such as sinusitis, lymphatic adenitis, adenoiditis, tonsillitis and peritonsillar abscess, tonsilloliths, laryngopharyngeal reflux (LPR), or gastroesophageal reflux disease (GERD). Less common causes of referred otalgia include myofascial pain syndromes, cervical spine osteoarthritis, and Eagle syndrome. Eagle syndrome is associated with an elongated styloid process (>25 mm) or calcified stylohyoid ligament [46]. Symptoms of Eagle syndrome are generally nonspecific and may include otalgia, dysphagia, and shooting odynophagia. Clinical overlap may exist with neuralgias such as trigeminal or glossopharyngeal neuralgia. Eagle syndrome is often diagnosed incidentally by computed tomography findings. Treatment is intraoral or transcervical shortening of the styloid process [46, 47].

Summary

With the complex innervation of the ear and periauricular tissues, the underlying etiologies for both primary and secondary otalgia are numerous. Work-up of the patient with otalgia requires a thorough history and physical examination, along with adjunct diagnostic approaches where indicated. This thorough evaluation should ensure identification of the underlying otalgia etiology the majority of the time, or at least rule out sources of life-threatening disease.

References

1. Kozin ED, Sethi RK, Remenschneider AK, et al. Epidemiology of otologic diagnoses in United States emergency departments. Laryngoscope. 2015;125(8):1926–33.
2. Hollingshead WH. The ear. In: Hollingshead WH, editor. Anatomy for Surgeons Volume 1: The head and neck. 3rd ed. Philadelphia: Harper & Row Publishers; 1982. pp. 62–164.
3. Janfaza P, Nadol JB. Temporal bone and ear. In: Janfaza P, Nadol JB, Galla RJ, Fabian RL, Montgomery WW, editors. Surgical anatomy of the head and neck. Philadelphia: Lippincott, Williams & Wilkins; 2001. p. 430–2.
4. Adunka OS, Buchman CA. Anatomy of the temporal bone and adjacent structures. In: Otology, neurotology, and lateral skull base surgery: an illustrated handbook. New York: Thieme; 2010. p. 6–10.
5. Kolodzynski MN, Kon M, Egger S, Breugem CC. Mechanisms of ear trauma and reconstructive techniques in 105 consecutive patients. Eur Arch Otorhinolaryngol. 2016:1–6.
6. Shah S, Fiala KH. Chondrodermatitis nodularis helicis: a review of current therapies. Dermatol Ther. 2017;30(1) https://doi.org/10.1111/dth.12434.
7. Elsürer C, Senkal HA, Baydar DE, et al. Ceruminous adenoma mimicking furunculosis in the external auditory canal. Eur Arch Otorhinolaryngol. 2007;264(3):223–5.
8. Schwartz SR, Magit AE, Rosenfeld RM, et al. Clinical practice guideline (update). Otolaryngol Head Neck Surg. 2017;156(1):14–29.
9. Sanyaolu LN, Farmer SE. Acute otalgia and otorrhoea in primary care. BMJ. 2016;18(352):i844.
10. Rosenfeld RM, Schwartz SR, Cannon CR, et al. Clinical practice guideline: acute otitis externa. Otolaryngol Head Neck Surg. 2014;150(Suppl):S1–24.
11. Centers for Disease Control and Prevention. Estimated burden of acute otitis externa—United States, 2003-2007. MMWR Morb Mortal Wkly Rep. 2011;60:605–9.
12. Arshad M, Khan NU, Ali N, Afridi NM. Sensitivity and spectrum of bacterial isolates in infectious otitis externa. JCPSP. 2004;14(3):146–9.
13. Kaushik V, Malik T, Saeed SR. Interventions for acute otitis externa. Cochrane Database Syst Rev. 2010;(1):CD004740.
14. Amani S, Moeini M. Comparison of boric acid and combination drug of polymyxin, neomycin and hydrocortisone (polymyxin nh) in the treatment of acute otitis externa. J Clin Diagn Res. 2016;10(7):MC01–4.
15. Hajioff D, MacKeith S. Otitis externa. BMJ Clin Evid. 2015;2015:0510
16. Crosbie R, Chin A, Wardrop P. Combined meatoplasty and canalplasty for intractable chronic otitis externa: our experience of twenty cases with audiometric and patient-reported outcomes. Clin Otolaryngol. 2013;38:390–3.
17. Carfrae MJ, Kesser BW. Malignant otitis externa. Otolaryngol Clin North Am. 2008;41(3):537–49.
18. Sylvester MJ, Sanghvi S, Patel VM, Eloy JA, Ying Y. Malignant otitis externa hospitalizations: analysis of patient characteristics. Laryngoscope. 2017;127(10):2328–36. https://doi.org/10.1002/lary.26401.
19. Hobson CE, Moy JD, Byers KE, et al. Malignant otitis externa: evolving pathogens and implications for diagnosis and treatment. Otolaryngol Head Neck Surg. 2014;151(1):112–6.

20. Stevens SM, Lambert PR, Baker AB, et al. Malignant otitis externa: a novel stratification protocol for predicting treatment outcomes. Otol Neurotol. 2015;36(9):1492–8.
21. Valerio E, Cutrone M, Gentilomo C, et al. Ramsay Hunt syndrome. Pediatr Neurol. 2015;52(5):554–5.
22. Ryu EW, Lee HY, Lee SY, et al. Clinical manifestations and prognosis of patients with Ramsay Hunt syndrome. Am J Otolaryngol. 2012;33:313–8.
23. Carmichael ML, Boyev KP. Middle ear barotrauma causing transient facial nerve paralysis after scuba diving. Diving Hyperb Med. 2016;46(4):260–1.
24. O'Neill OJ, Weitzner ED. The O'Neill grading system for evaluation of the tympanic membrane: a practical approach for clinical hyperbaric patients. Undersea Hyperb Med. 2015;42(3):265–71.
25. Remenschneider AK, Lookabaugh S, Aliphas A, et al. Otologic outcomes after blast injury: the Boston Marathon experience. Otol Neurotol. 2014;35(10):1825–34.
26. Robertson MW, Morris DP. Welding injury to the ear: looking beyond the perforation. J Otolaryngol Head Neck Surg. 2011;40(2):E15–8.
27. Venekamp RP, Damoiseaux RA, Schilder AG. Acute otitis media in children. Am Fam Physician. 2017;95(2):109–10.
28. Prins-van Ginkel AC, Bruijning-Verhagen PC, Uiterwaal CS, van der Ent CK, Smit HA, de Hoog ML. Acute otitis media during infancy: parent-reported incidence and modifiable risk factors. Pediatr Infect Dis J. 2017;36(3):245–9.
29. Rosenfeld RM, Shin JJ, Schwartz SR, et al. Clinical practice guideline: otitis media with effusion executive summary (update). Otolaryngol Head Neck Surg. 2016;154(2):201–14.
30. Lieberthal AS, Carroll AE, Chonmaitree T, et al. The diagnosis and management of acute otitis media. Pediatrics. 2013 Mar;131(3):e964–99.
31. Myerson MC. Suppuration of the petrous pyramid: some views on its surgical management. Arch Otolaryngol. 1937;26(1):42–8.
32. Gadre AK, Chole RA. The changing face of petrous apicitis-a 40-year experience. Laryngoscope. 2018;128(1):195–201. https://doi.org/10.1002/lary.26571.
33. van den Aardweg MT, Rovers MM, de Ru JA, et al. A systematic review of diagnostic criteria for acute mastoiditis in children. Otol Neurotol. 2008;29(6):751–7.
34. Arendt-Nielsen L, Svensson P. Referred muscle pain: basic and clinical findings. Clin J Pain. 2001;17(1):11–9.
35. Charlett SD, Coatesworth AP. Referred otalgia: a structured approach to diagnosis and treatment. Int J Clin Pract. 2007;61(6):1015–21.
36. Taziki MH, Behnampour N. A study of the etiology of referred otalgia. Iran J Otorhinolaryngol. 2012;24(69):171–6.
37. Kim DS, Cheang P, Dover S, et al. Dental otalgia. J Laryngol Otol. 2007;121(12):1129–34.
38. Ingvarsson L. Acute otalgia in children - findings and diagnosis. Acta Paediatr Scand. 1982;71(5):705–10.
39. Kim SH. A case of bruxism-induced otalgia. J Audiol Otol. 2016;20(2):123–6.
40. Stepan L, Shaw CL, Oue S. Temporomandibular disorder in otolaryngology: systematic review. J Laryngol Otol. 2017;131(S1):S50–6.
41. Connelly ST, Myung J, Gupta R, et al. Clinical outcomes of Botox injections for chronic temporomandibular disorders: do we understand how Botox works on muscle, pain, and the brain? Int J Oral Maxillofac Surg. 2017;46(3):322–7.
42. Grosskopf CC, Kuperstein AS, O'Malley BW Jr, et al. Parapharyngeal space tumors: another consideration for otalgia and temporomandibular disorders. Head Neck. 2013;35(5):E153–6.
43. Shah JO, Herrera SJ, Roberts DB, Gunn GB, Gidley PW. Complications of tympanostomy tubes in head and neck cancer patients. Am J Otolaryngol. 2016;37(4):356–61.
44. Sharon JD, Khwaja SS, Drescher A, et al. Osteoradionecrosis of the temporal bone: a case series. Otol Neurotol. 2014;35(7):1207–17.
45. Phillips DJ, Njoku IU, Brown KD, Selesnick SH. Radiation-induced necrosis of the temporal bone: diagnosis and management. Otol Neurotol. 2015;36(8):1374–7.
46. Kumai Y, Hamasaki T, Yumoto E. Surgical management of Eagle's syndrome: an approach to shooting craniofacial pain. Eur Arch Otorhinolaryngol. 2016;273(10):3421–7.
47. Bahgat M, Bahgat Y, Bahgat A. Eagle's syndrome, a rare cause of neck pain. BMJ Case Rep. 2012;2012:bcr2012006278. https://doi.org/10.1136/bcr-2012-006278.

Vestibular Migraine: Diagnosis and Treatment

61

Adam M. Cassis and Stephen J. Wetmore

Introduction

Vestibular migraine (VM) is a frequent cause of dizziness that rivals (and likely surpasses) benign paroxysmal positional vertigo and vestibular neuritis in prevalence. VM has been reported to occur with a prevalence of almost 3% in the general population in the United States [1]. The occurrence of dizziness in patients with migraine has been known for over 50 years, but only recently has the relationship between migraine headache symptoms and migraine vestibular symptoms been recognized. Migraine, manifested by the characteristic headaches, is a very common disease that is present in 6% of males and 17% of females. Vestibular symptoms occur in approximately one-third of migraineurs but may not manifest for years. In a study by Neuhauser et al., migraine headaches preceded VM in 74% of the subjects. In fact, headache preceded vestibular symptoms by more than 5 years in 52% of subjects, and by more than 10 years in 26% [2]. Complicating the diagnosis of vestibular migraine is the fact that headache and vestibular symptoms frequently do not coincide; in fact, vestibular symptoms may occur years after the onset of migraine headaches, at a time when headache symptoms rarely occur. The diagnosis of vestibular migraine may be further obscured because of the wide variety of vestibular symptoms and the lack of a characteristic duration for these symptoms.

A. M. Cassis (✉)
Arizona Hearing and Balance, Chandler, AZ, USA
e-mail: acassis192@azvent.com

S. J. Wetmore
Department of Otolaryngology—Head and Neck Surgery, West Virginia University School of Medicine, Morgantown, WV, USA
e-mail: swetmore@hsc.wvu.edu

Diagnosis of Migraine

In order to make a diagnosis of vestibular migraine, clinicians should know how to differentiate migraine headaches from other causes of headaches. The Headache Classification Committee of the International Headache Society periodically publishes criteria that are used to diagnose the various types of migraine [3].

Migraine without aura, previously known as a common migraine, is the most common form of migraine. The diagnostic criteria are listed in Table 61.1. Keep in mind that only two of the four characteristics listed under criterion C are needed to make the diagnosis. For example, the criteria for migraine are met if a patient complains of multiple episodes of bilateral, moderately severe, pulsating headaches lasting 4–6 h that are associated with nausea. Migraine headaches are usually frontotemporal in location. In children and adolescents, migraine headaches are more often bilateral than in adults [3].

Migraine with aura, also known as classical migraine, consists of unilateral, fully reversible visual, sensory, or other central nervous system aura symptoms followed by headache and other associated migraine symptoms (Table 61.1). The aura most commonly consists of a visual disturbance, such as shimmering lights. Next in frequency are pins-and-needles sensations that can occur on one side of the body, face, or tongue. The aura is generally accompanied, or followed within 60 min, by headache. Sometimes, the aura will occur without a subsequent headache, and sometimes the typical migraine headache will occur without a preceding aura.

Migraine with brainstem aura is the current name for basilar migraine, basilar artery migraine, or basilar-type migraine (Table 61.1). The aura symptoms originate from the brainstem, but motor weakness is excluded in this classification. More than 50 years ago, Bickerstaff described vestibular migraine in 34 patients, most of whom were adolescent girls who had visual aura symptoms followed by vertigo, ataxia,

A. D. Sweeney et al. (eds.), *Haynes-Glasscock-Shambaugh Surgery of the Ear*, https://doi.org/10.1007/978-3-032-18264-7_61

Table 61.1 Selected migraine types. This table is adapted from the following

	Migraine without aura	Migraine with aura	Migraine with brainstem aura	Hemiplegic migraine	Vestibular migraine
Number of episodes	5	2	2	2	5
Duration	4–72 h	Nuanced–see characteristics below	Nuanced–see characteristics below	Nuanced–see characteristics below	5 min to 72 h
Must involve headache?	Yes	No	No	No	No
Characteristics	A. The headache must have two or more of the following: (a) Unilateral location (b) Pulsatile (c) Moderate or severe pain/intensity (d) Aggravation by or causing avoidance of routine physical activity B. The headache must have one or more of the following: (a) Nausea/vomiting (b) Photophobia and phonophobia	A. One or more fully reversible aura symptoms: (a) Visual (b) Sensory (c) Speech and/or language (d) Motor (e) Brainstem (f) Retinal B. Two or more of the following: (a) One symptom spread gradually over ≥5 min, and/or two or more symptoms occur in succession (b) Each individual aura symptom lasts 5–60 min (c) At least one aura symptom is unilateral (d) The aura is accompanied by a headache or followed by a headache within 60 min	A. Aura consisting of fully reversible visual sensory and/or speech/language symptoms B. No motor or retinal symptoms C. Two or more of the following brainstem symptoms (a) Dysarthria (b) Vertigo (c) Tinnitus (d) Hypacusis (e) Diplopia (f) Ataxia (g) Decreased level of consciousness D. Two or more of the following: (a) One symptom spread gradually over ≥5 min, and/or two or more symptoms occur in succession (b) Each individual aura symptom lasts 5–60 min (c) At least one aura symptom is unilateral (d) The aura is accompanied by a headache or followed by a headache within 60 min	A. Aura consisting of both fully reversible motor weakness and fully reversible visual, sensory and/or speech/language symptoms B. Two or more of the following: (a) One symptom spreads gradually over ≥5 min, and/or two or more symptoms occur in succession (b) Each individual aura symptom lasts 5–60 min and motor symptoms last <72 h (c) At least one aura symptom is unilateral C. The aura is accompanied by a headache or followed by a headache within 60 min	A. Must involve moderate to severe vestibular symptoms B. Current or previous history of migraine with or without aura according to the International Classification of Headache Disorders (ICHD) C. One or more migraine features with at least 50% of the vestibular episodes: (a) Headache with at least 2 of the following: one-sided, pulsation, moderate or severe pain intensity, aggravation by physical activity (b) Photophobia and phonophobia (c) Visual aura
Notes/comments	Symptoms must not be better explained by another ICHD diagnosis	Symptoms must not be better explained by another ICHD diagnosis	Symptoms must not be better explained by another ICHD diagnosis	Symptoms must not be better explained by another ICHD diagnosis.	Symptoms must not be better explained by another ICHD diagnosis. A "probable" vestibular migraine involves category (A) being fulfilled and only 1 of category (B) or (C) above being fulfilled

This table is adapted from the following:
Headache Classification Committee of the International Headache Society [3]
Lempert et al. [8]

dysarthria, paresthesias, and sometimes tinnitus, followed by typical migraine headaches [4]. The episodes were strikingly related to menstruation. For decades after the publication of this article, it was felt that dizziness associated with migraine was due to "basilar artery migraine." Migraine with brainstem aura is rare; although vestibular symptoms may occur in the aura phase of this entity, the vast majority of patients with vestibular migraine do not have migraine with brainstem aura.

Hemiplegic migraine is a form of migraine with aura that *includes* motor weakness (Table 61.1). A variant of this condition is **familial hemiplegic migraine,** in which at least one first- or second-degree relative has had episodes consistent with hemiplegic migraine. Vestibular migraine may occur in patients diagnosed with hemiplegic migraine, but at no greater incidence than what would be expected from the incidence of this variant.

Benign paroxysmal vertigo of childhood (BPV) is a disorder characterized by recurrent brief attacks of vertigo that occur without warning and resolve spontaneously. BPV is the most common cause of vertigo in children between the ages of 2–5 [5, 6]. Onset is often younger than age 4, and resolution usually occurs by ages 7–8 years [7]. Typically, the child suddenly feels frightened and describes a spinning sensation and cries, vomits, or staggers during an attack. A family history of migraine is common, and these children often develop classical migraine as they get older. Pediatric dizziness is discussed in more detail in Chap. 53.

Criteria for Diagnosing VM

Diagnosing VM has been a challenge for clinicians because, until recently, diagnostic criteria have been lacking. The characteristics of dizziness seen in patients with VM are more variable compared with almost all other types of dizziness in terms of frequency, duration, severity, and in the fundamental description of the character of the vestibular symptoms. In addition, the temporal relationship of migraine headaches and vestibular symptoms is quite variable and often inconsistent.

The lack of a clear definition of VM has hampered research in this important and common cause of dizziness. The Bárány Society, which represents the international community of basic scientists, otolaryngologists, and neurologists committed to enhancing research for this condition, put together a committee that formulated criteria for diagnosing VM. A consensus document of the Bárány Society and the International Headache Society that provided diagnostic criteria was published in 2012 [8]. This document separated the diagnosis into the following two categories: (1) vestibular migraine (Table 61.1), and (2) probable vestibular migraine (PVM) (Table 61.1). Basically, the diagnosis of VM requires a current or previous history of migraine *and* one or more migraine features associated with at least 50% of the vestibular events. The diagnosis of PVM requires only a current *or previous* history of migraine, *or* one or more migraine features, in 50% of the vestibular events. In other words, patients who have the required number of vestibular symptoms but who have only a history of migraine headaches can be diagnosed with PVM. In clinical practice, we frequently see patients who have nonspecific vestibular symptoms that do not fall into other vestibular entities and who have a history of migraine headaches that may have been quiescent for years. These patients can be diagnosed with PVM.

In 2013, the International Headache Society published the International Classification of Headache Disorders, third edition (beta version) [3]. Criteria for VM were published in the appendix, but the criteria for probable vestibular migraine were omitted.

The Bárány Society has described the vestibular symptoms to include spontaneous vertigo that could be either *internal* vertigo, a false sensation of self-motion, or *external* vertigo, a false sensation that the visual surround is moving [8]. Other forms of vertigo that may be associated with VM include positional vertigo occurring after a change in head position, visually induced vertigo brought on by a moving visual stimulus, and head-motion–induced vertigo. Vestibular symptoms may also consist of *dizziness with nausea,* characterized by a sensation of disturbed spatial orientation, but other forms of dizziness are excluded.

The duration of the vestibular symptoms ranges from 5 min to 72 h, but approximately 10% of patients have symptoms for only a few seconds; however, these vestibular symptoms recur with changes in head motion or visual stimulation, and in those patients, the episode includes the total period in which these short attacks occur.

The severity of vestibular symptoms is termed *moderate* when they interfere with but do not prohibit daily activities. *Severe* vestibular symptoms imply that daily activities cannot be continued.

Vestibular and auditory tests are not sufficiently specific to provide criteria for diagnosis. Cass et al. reported electronystagmographic findings in a cohort of 100 VM patients (2.2%) out of 4400 patients seen in a dizziness clinic [9]. Sixty-one percent had a normal test; the most common abnormalities were unilateral weakness in 18% and positional nystagmus in 13%. Audiometry showed normal hearing in 80 of 89 subjects (90%). Auditory fullness was present in 28%, 17% bilateral, and 11% unilateral. Tinnitus was reported in 26%.

Differentiating VM from Ménière's Disease

A prospective study of 78 patients with Ménière's disease (MD) compared with age- and sex-matched controls showed that the lifetime prevalence of migraine with or without aura was 56% compared to the rate of 25% in the control group [10]. Migrainous headaches occurred simultaneously with the major vestibular attacks of the Ménière's patients in 28% (22 of 78); half of these patients experienced headaches with all their Ménière's attacks, and half experienced headaches occasionally. In six patients, the headaches preceded the vertigo, but 16 patients stated that headaches occurred during or after the vertigo. Photophobia occurred during the Ménière's attack in 52% of patients, and aura in 10%. The authors of this study stated that the high prevalence of migraine in MD and the frequent occurrence of migrainous symptoms during Ménière's attacks could be explained by two possibilities: Either some of these patients actually have VM, or there is a pathophysiologic link between MD and migraine [10].

In 2012, Neff et al. reported a series of 147 patients with MD, VM, or both (MDVM) out of a cohort of 600 consecutive patients with complaints of vertigo, unsteadiness, or dizziness seen in a tertiary referral dizziness clinic [11]. Their diagnoses were based on the 1995 American Academy of Otolaryngology criteria for MD, the second edition of the International Headache Society for migraine, and the Neuhauser criteria for definite and probable VM, which are similar to the recently published report of the Bárány Society [8, 12, 13]. Fifty-five patients were diagnosed with definite or probable MD, 71 patients were diagnosed with definite or probable VM, and 21 patients met the criteria for both diagnoses and were placed in the MDVM group. Bivariate analysis showed that older age at onset and male sex favored MD. Most patients with MD reported that their dizzy spells lasted several hours, but just over one-third of the VM patients reported spells lasting several hours, with vertigo among VM patients ranging from seconds to days; hours-long spells were statistically associated with MD. Audiologic symptoms of fluctuating hearing loss, aural fullness, and tinnitus, and vestibular test abnormalities, such as head-shake–induced nystagmus and caloric asymmetries, were associated with MD but did not distinguish between MD and MDVM. Conversely, a history of moderate to severe headaches and photophobia during vestibular episodes was significantly associated with VM but did not differentiate between VM and MDVM. The only unique features of MDVM were a higher prevalence of a family history of vestibular symptoms and a greater perceived bilateral hearing loss than either MD or VM. Tinnitus and aural fullness were present in many of the patients in all three groups, although they tended to be higher for patients with MD. Although the rate of *bilateral* tinnitus was not different between VM and MD, the incidence of *bilateral* aural pressure was actually greater in VM than in MD (33% vs 19%). In summary, 28% of patients in this study with MD also had VM, and 23% of VM patients were also diagnosed with MD.

Differences in testing may have some ability to help distinguish between VM and MD. Abnormalities on the audiogram (initial/worst pure tone average, initial/change in discrimination, initial/worst hearing class) were more common in patients with MD. This would be expected as the diagnosis of MD depends on documented hearing loss. Caloric abnormalities were more likely to be observed with MD; however, the difference between MD and VM is much less than with audiometric findings. Therefore, we cannot simply differentiate the diagnosis based solely on caloric findings. Vestibular evoked myogenic potential (VEMP) testing (cervical VEMP and ocular VEMP) has been studied in this area as well. Regarding cervical VEMP testing, most studies show no difference between VM and MD; however, a few have noted that some MD patients have smaller amplitudes during 500 Hz tone burst testing. Likewise, ocular VEMP testing has demonstrated longer latencies and lower amplitudes on click testing. However, given the overall likelihood of abnormal VEMP testing in either condition, it should be considered a supplement to the clinical presentation [14].

Treatment of VM

Treatment of vestibular migraine can be challenging. The first challenge is establishing the diagnosis of VM. Although diagnostic criteria were recently established, the varied presentation and the intermittent and sometimes fluctuating symptoms may result in diagnostic hesitancy. Another challenge in treating VM is the varied intensity of the underlying symptoms. Some patients present with a mild chronic balance disturbance that can be tolerated and does not interrupt daily activity. These patients only require a diagnosis; no treatment is needed. Most patients, however, have bouts of severe vertigo and chronic vestibular symptoms that require intervention.

Due to what is perceived as a common pathophysiologic mechanism, we treat VM similarly to the treatment of migraine headaches. An individual approach to the treatment of VM is useful, considering the varying degrees of symptom severity, comorbid conditions, and patient treatment preferences. Various options for treatment are available for those with VM, and they are often combined until symptom control is achieved. Treatment may consist of dietary and lifestyle modifications (trigger avoidance), vitamins/supplements, pharmacotherapy (abortive and prophylactic), and/or physical therapy.

Trigger Avoidance

Similar to Ménière's disease, patients with VM may have triggers that need to be avoided (Table 61.2). The goal is for patients to identify their triggers, thus avoiding the catalyst

Table 61.2 Trigger foods

Caffeine
Alcohol
Aspartame
Dairy
MSG
Chocolate
Eggs
Citrus
Wheat
Nuts
Tomatoes
Onions
Corn
Apples
Bananas

Safe Foods: cooked vegetables, cooked/dried non-citrus fruits, rice, most condiments

Table 61.3 Supplements

Supplement	Dose
Magnesium	400 mg daily
Vitamin B2 (riboflavin)	400 mg twice daily
Coenzyme Q10[a]	100 mg daily-three times daily
Melatonin	3 mg every evening
Butterbur[a]	50 mg twice daily
Feverfew	250 mg daily

[a]Caution hepatic impairment/liver toxicity

that brings on migraine symptoms. Often, these come in the form of dietary triggers. Given the long list of migraine triggers, this dietary restriction can be challenging. Nonetheless, the severity of symptoms or the desire to avoid taking medications may be motivation enough for a patient to adhere to this regimen. Although there are various approaches to instituting a migraine diet, the following approach seems logical and straightforward. The diet is initiated with a two-week period of strict trigger avoidance, eating only foods deemed "safe." If symptoms improve, add back one trigger food at a time for 2 days (in abundance), starting with the least risky food, and assess for return of symptoms. If symptoms remain stable, it is likely a safe food; if symptoms return, then it is a trigger food and should be avoided. This regimen continues until dietary triggers have been fully established. An alternative or adjunctive technique is keeping a daily dietary and symptom journal to help identify triggers.

In addition to diet, other known triggers for migraine exist. Lack of exercise, poor sleep hygiene, hormonal disturbance, and stress can trigger a migraine episode. Routine exercise, regular sleep patterns, and strategies to relieve stress may improve the patient's symptoms. If a female patient has symptoms surrounding her menstrual cycle, discussion with her primary care physician about estrogen therapy may be beneficial.

Vitamins and Supplements

For many reasons, alternatives to traditional prescription medications are becoming more popular. As the desire for "naturopathic" medicine grows, it is helpful for the treating physician to be familiar with options to offer the patient. Various over-the-counter vitamins and supplements have been shown to be beneficial in preventing migraine (Table 61.3). Generally speaking, these supplements and vitamins are well tolerated, but some situations warrant precaution. Both Coenzyme Q10 (CoQ10) and butterbur have the potential for liver toxicity. Also, CoQ10 modulates cytochrome P450 enzymes in the liver and may have an effect on the patient's other medications.

Pharmacotherapy

Prescription medications for migraines come in two forms: abortive and prophylactic. The decision about which type of medication to prescribe depends on the symptoms of the individual patient. Those patients with infrequent episodes of vertigo may benefit from abortive medications, while those with frequent symptoms, symptoms of short duration, or chronic daily symptoms may benefit more from a prophylactic medication. A patient who suffers from two to three bouts of episodic vertigo a year, lasting hours to days, would be an ideal candidate for abortive medications. In this situation, the patient only needs relief from symptoms for a few days to weeks out of the year. Taking an abortive medication in this situation is a good option. Unfortunately, many patients with VM have frequent or chronic symptoms, or sometimes symptoms that are positional and/or very brief, for which a prophylactic medication makes more sense.

Abortive migraine medications usually consist of serotonin receptor agonists ("triptans") taken as soon as migraine symptoms appear. Few studies investigating the effectiveness of this class of medications in treating VM have been reported. To date, the only randomized, double-blinded, placebo-controlled drug trial for the treatment of VM was conducted by Neuhauser and colleagues in regard to treatment with zolmitriptan, a serotonin receptor agonist [15]. Although the response rate was higher with the study drug as compared with placebo, the study lacked power, and no conclusive evidence could be attained for the study. Another study by Bikhazi et al. found that headaches and vestibular symptoms responded well to sumatriptan [16]. Although retrospective in nature, a study investigating the effects of almotriptan on VM showed promise. It eliminated vertigo in 55% of patients in the acute phase, while 28% of patients had >50% reduction of vertigo, and 16% of patients experienced

<50% reduction in vertigo symptoms [17]. Various other reports have been published in which vestibular symptoms responded to other medications such as ergots, NSAIDs, and opiates.

As mentioned previously, most patients with VM who require pharmacologic intervention will need prophylactic medications. There are four distinct classes of medications used for migraine prophylaxis: beta blockers, calcium channel blockers, antidepressants, and neuroleptic medications (Table 61.4). How then does the treating physician decide on which medication to choose? Although a few of the medications in these classes are primarily used as migraine prophylactic medications, most of them have primary uses for conditions other than migraine. We often have the opportunity for a therapeutic two-for-one (e.g., treating VM with a beta blocker in a patient with hypertension or with a tricyclic antidepressant for a patient with depression). Also, each medication has a specific side effect profile, drug interactions, and contraindications. All this should be taken into account when providing treatment for the patient.

The following briefly describes each of the medications and the theory behind their use. For an extensive review of migraine prophylactic therapy, please refer to the articles by Buchanan and Ramadan [18, 19].

Beta Blockers

Beta blockers are commonly used to treat migraine headaches. In fact, this class of medications (e.g., propranolol, timolol) is one of the few medications that have received United States Food and Drug Administration (FDA) approval for the treatment of migraine headaches. These drugs prevent central sensitization by inhibiting norepinephrine release, antagonizing serotonin receptors, inhibiting nitric oxide synthase, and acting synergistically with N-methyl-D-aspartate (NMDA) receptors. Their primary use is for the treatment of hypertension, although they have been utilized in treating panic attacks, anxiety, and essential tremor. They should be avoided in patients with depression and diabetes mellitus. Contraindications for their use include congestive heart failure, Raynaud's disease, and asthma.

Recently, a placebo-controlled randomized controlled trial investigating the use of metoprolol (PROVEMIG trial) was completed, which did not demonstrate a reduction in vertigo compared with the control group, although it should be noted that the study was stopped early due to poor patient accrual (114 patients) [20].

Calcium Channel Blockers

Calcium channel blockers (CCB) have also been utilized in migraine prophylaxis, despite the lack of FDA approval specifically for that use. They block voltage-gated calcium channels that are thought to play a key role in migraine pathogenesis. Also, they prevent the release of calcitonin gene-related peptide (CGRP), which takes part in the inflammatory cascade in migraine pathophysiology. Verapamil is the most commonly prescribed CCB in the United States. Similar to beta blockers, their primary use is for hypertension, although they may be safer than beta blockers for patients with lung disease, such as asthma. Constipation is a

Table 61.4 Prophylactic drug therapy

Medication class	Medication	Trade name	Daily dose	Side effects	Contraindications
Beta blocker (BB)	Metoprolol	Toprol, Lopressor	25 mg to 100–400 mg	Fatigue, lightheadedness, diarrhea, unusual dreams, depression, blurry vision, sexual dysfunction, hair loss, bradycardia, cold hands/feet, hypotension	Asthma/COPD, heart failure, diabetes
	Propranolol	Inderal	40–240 mg		
Calcium channel blocker (CCB)	Verapamil	Calan, Verelan	120–480 mg	Constipation, hypotension, nausea, dizziness, headache, fatigue	Heart block
Tricyclic antidepressants (TCA)	Amitriptyline	Elavil	10–75 mg	Abdominal pain, blurry vision, dry mouth, dizziness, weight gain, sexual dysfunction, drowsiness, hypotension, dizziness, constipation, urinary retention	Monoamine Oxidase Inhibitor (MAOI) use, long QT interval on electrocardiography
	Nortriptyline	Pamelor			
Serotonin norepinephrine reuptake inhibitor (SNRI)	Venlafaxine	Effexor	37.5–225 mg	Headache, nausea, insomnia, weakness, dizziness, sexual dysfunction, dry mouth	Venlafaxine allergy, MAOI use, glaucoma
Neuroleptic	Topiramate	Topamax	50–100 mg	Mental fog, word finding difficulty, weight loss, paresthesias	None

common side effect. Other side effects include headaches and dizziness, with gingival hyperplasia being less common. They are contraindicated in patients with cardiac conduction abnormalities.

Antidepressants

This is a large class of medications, but the discussion will be limited to the most common medications used in migraine prophylaxis: tricyclic antidepressants (TCAs) and serotonin-norepinephrine reuptake inhibitors (SNRIs). TCAs have long been used in migraine prophylaxis, despite a lack of FDA approval for that use. They enhance antinociceptive neurons, inhibit serotonin receptors, modulate peripheral sensitization, and increase gamma-aminobutyric acid (GABA) levels. Amitriptyline (Elavil) and nortriptyline (Pamelor) are the two most commonly prescribed. In addition to depression, they are also used to treat neuropathic pain, anxiety, and panic disorder. Commonly experienced side effects are sexual dysfunction, weight gain, sedation, and orthostatic hypotension. TCAs are contraindicated in patients with certain cardiac conditions (long QT interval during electrocardiography) as well as in epileptics. SNRIs are a newer class of antidepressant medication that are gaining traction as an option for patients with VM. This class includes such medications as venlafaxine (Effexor), duloxetine (Cymbalta), and desvenlafaxine (Pristiq). Common side effects are drowsiness, sexual dysfunction, strange dreams, and anticholinergic side effects. The class as a whole has few contraindications, mainly concurrent monoamine oxidase inhibitor (MAOI) use.

Neuroleptics

The final class includes the neuroleptic medications that consist of valproic acid, lamotrigine, and topiramate. Although valproic acid works quite well in migraine prophylaxis, it requires routine monitoring because of potential life-threatening side effects, including hepatotoxicity and pancreatitis. In the authors' opinion, this medication should be prescribed and monitored by a neurologist familiar with its use. Lamotrigine acts by inhibiting glutamate secretion, a neurotransmitter associated with cortical spreading depression, a phenomenon that may be at least partially responsible for vestibular symptoms in VM. Topiramate blocks calcium channels and potentiates GABA. It also has carbonic anhydrase activity, similar to that of acetazolamide, which has been used in familial forms of migraine and ataxia. It carries FDA approval for the treatment of migraine. Common side effects include drowsiness, weight loss, paresthesia, somnolence, and cognitive blurriness ("brain fog").

Calcitonin Gene-Related Peptide (CGRP)-Targeted Therapies

Calcitonin gene-related peptide (CGRP) antagonists offer a promising targeted approach for vestibular migraine, supporting both prophylactic and acute abortive roles, particularly in refractory cases. A 2024 rapid systematic review and meta-analysis by Frosolini et al., including four studies and 99 patients, demonstrated significant symptom improvement with anti-CGRP monoclonal antibodies (erenumab, galcanezumab, fremanezumab), including reductions in monthly migraine days at 6 months and no severe adverse events—though limited by small samples, heterogeneous designs, and lack of randomized clinical trials [21]. Administered monthly or quarterly, these drugs may outperform conventional prophylactics in reducing dizziness handicap scores, vertigo frequency, and vestibular test abnormalities. For acute relief, smallmolecule gepants like rimegepant achieve rapid symptom freedom (headache, vertigo) within 2 hours.

Treatment Strategy

For most patients, some form of treatment is indicated. We suggest that all patients be counseled on the diagnosis of VM, which should improve treatment compliance. Likewise, patients should be aware of migraine triggers, both dietary and lifestyle, and take necessary steps to lower their migraine threshold. If the patient has non-debilitating symptoms or prefers avoiding drug therapy, a period of treatment with dietary and lifestyle modifications is reasonable before proceeding with drug therapy. Vitamins and/or supplements may be introduced at any time but may be a good first step into active treatment for VM, especially for those who desire nonprescription medications. These may be initiated individually or as multiple vitamin supplements from the suggested list. If these measures fail to adequately control symptoms, or for those patients presenting with severe symptoms, pharmacologic therapy may be needed. For those patients with symptoms lasting hours to days with few attacks a year, an abortive medication is likely a good starting point. Most patients, however, have clinical features that favor treatment with prophylactic medications, e.g., frequent spells of vertigo, symptoms lasting from seconds to minutes, patients with chronic symptoms, and those with a positional component to their dizziness. When instituting prophylactic therapy, one typically starts at the lowest dose, increasing every week or every other week until symptoms are controlled or until the maximal dose is reached. The duration of treatment with any one medication should be at least 3 months before a determination of benefit is made. During that time, the patient may experience vestibular symptoms that they may attribute to their medication as a side effect or medication intolerance but may in fact be due to VM. Side effects from medications are usually experienced upon starting the medication or during any escalation of the dose. In some individuals, more than one medication may be necessary to achieve symptom control.

Physical Therapy

Additionally, vestibular physical therapy (VPT) may have a role in treating VM. In general, the approach is desensitization and improving peripheral and central inputs to avoid aberrant/misguided neural input to the central nervous system. Some studies have shown a positive impact of physical therapy in the relief of vestibular symptoms in those with VM; however, this finding is not universal, and the role for VPT is not clearly understood in the setting of VM [22].

Miscellaneous

Botox®, or OnabotulinumtoxinA, is an FDA-approved treatment for chronic migraine headaches. Recently, Oh and colleagues published a longitudinal study on the effects of Botox type A injections on vestibular symptoms in those with VM [23]. They found that vertigo, headache, depression, and anxiety all improved at the 2-month follow-up. Interestingly, fMRI studies also showed changes in functional connectivity of the right superior temporal gyrus, which were believed to represent a normalization of cortical processing. Over time, Botox has been increasingly utilized as a prophylactic therapy for VM, particularly in patients refractory to oral preventives. Surmeli et. al. published a prospective, double-blind, randomized, placebo-controlled trial, demonstrating improvements in Dizziness Handicap Inventory, pain (visual analog scale), and Migraine disability assessment score (MIDAS) in the botox group compared to placebo (saline injection) [24]. These gains occurred without changes in objective vestibular tests (video head impulse test or vHIT, cervical vestibular evoked myogenic potential or cVEMP), suggesting Botox targets central sensitization and CGRP-mediated pathways rather than direct vestibular dysfunction. With a favorable safety profile mirroring chronic migraine use, quarterly Botox injections offer a systemic-alternative option in VM management.

There is also a host of other alternative, noninvasive treatment strategies that are focused on nerve stimulation. A noninvasive vagal nerve stimulator (nVNS) was recently approved for the treatment of acute migraine headaches. A retrospective review of this device utilized in the setting of acute VM demonstrated a reduction in vertigo symptoms [25]. In the future, devices such as these may be helpful for those who do not respond to traditional prescription medications or for those looking for non-pharmacologic interventions.

Conclusion

Despite the long history of vestibular symptoms associated with migraine sufferers, VM still remains a relatively new diagnosis, and the understanding of the pathophysiology continues to evolve rapidly. Although more physicians, including otolaryngologists, neurologists, and primary care physicians, are becoming aware of this entity, many patients are surprised to learn that their symptoms have a migraine etiology. VM may be the most common cause of vestibular symptoms in the general population; it is, therefore, crucial that we continue to study and investigate VM from the bench to the clinical setting. Our treatment of VM reflects our current understanding of basic migraine pathophysiology. In general, most patients respond to these treatments, and these treatments can be tailored depending on the severity of the dizziness.

References

1. Formeister EJ, Rizk HG, Kohn MA, Sharon JD. The epidemiology of vestibular migraine: a population-based survey study. Otol Neurotol. 2018;39(8):1037–44.
2. Neuhauser H, Radtke M, von Brevern M, et al. Migrainous vertigo: prevalence and impact on quality of life. Neurology. 2006;67:1028–33.
3. Headache classification Committee of the International Headache Society. The international classification of headache disorders, 3rd edition (beta version). Cephalalgia. 2013;33(9):629–808.
4. Bickerstaff ER. Basilar artery migraine. Lancet. 1961;277:15–7.
5. Li H. Diagnosis of vestibular migraine. In: Wetmore S, Rubin A, editors. Vestibular migraine. Switzerland: Springer; 2015. p. 11–22.
6. Gioacchini FM, Alicandri-Ciufelli M, Kaleci S, et al. Prevalence and diagnosis of vestibular disorders in children: a review. Int J Pediatr Otorhinolaryngol. 2014;78:718–24.
7. Cushing SL. Vestibular migraine in childhood. In: Wetmore S, Rubin A, editors. Vestibular migraine. Switzerland: Springer; 2015. p. 31–6.
8. Lempert T, Olesen J, Furman J, et al. Vestibular migraine: diagnostic criteria. Consensus statement of the Barany Society and the International Headache Society. J Vestib Res. 2012;22:167–72.
9. Cass SP, Furman JM, Ankerstjerne K, et al. Migraine-related vestibulopathy. Ann Otol Rhinol Laryngol. 1997;106:182–9.
10. Radtke A, Lempert T, Gresty MA, et al. Migraine and Meniere's disease: is there a link? Neurol. 2002;59:1700–4.
11. Neff BA, Staab JP, Scott D, et al. Auditory and vestibular symptoms and chronic subjective dizziness in patients with Meniere's disease, vestibular migraine, and Meniere's disease with vestibular migraine. Otol Neurotol. 2012;33:1235–44.
12. Committee on Hearing and Equilibrium guidelines for the diagnosis and evaluation of therapy for Meniere's disease. Otolaryngol Head Neck Surg. 1995;113:181–5.

13. Neuhauser H, Lempert T. Vestibular migraine. Neurol Clin. 2009;27:379–91.
14. Tabet P, Saliba I. Meniere's disease and vestibular migraine: updates and review of the literature. J Clin Med Res. 2017;9(9):733–44.
15. Neuhauser H, Radtke A, von Brevern M, Lempert T. Zolmitriptan for treatment of migrainous vertigo: a pilot randomized placebo-controlled trial. Neurology. 2003;60(5):882–3.
16. Bikhazi P, Jackson C, Ruckenstein MJ. Efficacy of antimigrainous therapy in the treatment of migraine-associated dizziness. Am J Otol. 1997;18(3):350–4.
17. Cassano D, Pizza V, Busillo V. P074.Almotriptan in the acute treatment of vestibular migraine: a retrospective study. J Headache Pain. 2015;16(Suppl 1):A114.
18. Buchanan TM, Ramadan NM. Prophylactic pharmacotherapy for migraine headaches. Semin Neurol. 2006;26(2):188–98.
19. Ramadan NM. Current trends in migraine prophylaxis. Headache. 2007;47(Suppl 1):S52–7.
20. Bayer O, Adrion C, Al Tawil A, et al. Results and lessons learnt from a randomized controlled trial: prophylactic treatment of vestibular migraine with metoprolol (PROVEMIG). Trials. 2019;20(1):813.
21. Frosolini, A. Lovato, A. Monoclonal antibodies targeting CGRP to treat vestibular migraine: a rapid systematic review and meta-analysis. Indian J Otolaryngol Head Neck Surg. 2024;76(4):3737–44.
22. Alghadir A, Anwer S. Effects of vestibular rehabilitation in the management of a vestibular migraine: a review. Front Neurol. 2018;9:440.
23. Oh SY, Kang JJ, Kim S, et al. A preliminary trial of botulinum toxin type A in patients with vestibular migraine: a longitudinal fMRI study. Front Neurol. 2022;13:955158.
24. Surmeli et al. Vestibular migraine: onabotulinum toxin effectivity, prospective-randomized study. Clin Neurol Neurosurg. 2025;254:108949.
25. Beh S, Friedman D. Acute vestibular migraine treatment with non-invasive vagus nerve stimulation. Neurology. 2019;93(18):e1715–9.

Persistent Postural-Perceptual Dizziness

62

Jeffrey P. Staab

Introduction

In 2017, persistent postural-perceptual dizziness (PPPD) was defined by an international panel of experts chartered by the Bárány Society and was entered into the International Classification of Vestibular Disorders (ICVD) [57]. A narrative definition was also included in the 11th edition of the International Classification of Diseases (ICD-11) [72]. A description of the evolution of PPPD from four previous concepts (phobic postural vertigo, space-motion discomfort, visual vertigo, and chronic subjective dizziness) was published shortly after its ICVD definition was finalized [15]. As listed in Table 62.1, the primary symptoms of PPPD are swaying or rocking (non-spinning) vertigo, unsteadiness, and non-vertiginous dizziness that are present most hours of the day, most days of the week, for at least 3 months (criterion A). These core symptoms are exacerbated by three factors: upright posture, active and passive movement, and exposure to environments with complex or moving visual stimuli (criterion B). PPPD may be precipitated by any condition that disrupts spatial orientation or interferes with normal balance functioning, including peripheral or central vestibular disorders, neurologic illnesses, other medical conditions, and episodes of high psychological distress (criterion C). A diagnosis of PPPD requires clinically distressing or impairing levels of symptoms, not just the presence of persistent dizziness (criterion D). PPPD also must be judged to be the best explanation for patients' symptoms, either alone or coexisting with other illnesses, after proper assessment of the differential diagnosis (criterion E). PPPD is not a diagnosis of exclusion. The diagnosis is made by carefully identifying (i.e., ruling in) the presence of all five criteria in patients' histories [15, 55, 57].

Various aspects of the definition of PPPD have been investigated since it was published in 2017. Yagi and colleagues [76] created the Niigata PPPD Questionnaire (NPQ), a 12-item self-report that measures patients' sensitivities to common activities that may exacerbate symptoms of the disorder (criterion B). In a factor analysis of the NPQ, Yagi et al. [76] identified a self-motion factor comprised of items related to upright posture and walking and a visual factor that included items related to exposure to complex or moving visual stimuli. The visual factor was the more sensitive and specific of the two for the full diagnosis of PPPD. Two other studies, both retrospective, examined the relative prevalence of triggering events for PPPD (criterion C). Habs et al. [20] and Waterston et al. [71] found results that were consistent with two cross-sectional studies of chronic subjective dizziness, one of the predecessors of PPPD [56, 59]. Illnesses caused by structural deficits of the peripheral or central vestibular system (most commonly benign paroxysmal positional vertigo or unilateral peripheral vestibulopathies, less commonly stroke) triggered PPPD (or CSD) in 21–25% of patients. Other neurologic precipitants included vestibular migraine (11–25% of patients), mild traumatic brain injury (3–15%), and dysautonomias (1–7%) and accounted for another 15–40% of patients. Various medical conditions with the potential to manifest dizziness, lightheadedness, or unsteadiness, such as paroxysmal cardiac dysrhythmias and metabolic illnesses, precipitated 3–11% of cases. Anxiety disorders, particularly panic and generalized anxiety disorders, were identified in 20–25% of patients in three of the studies [20, 56, 59], but in a substantially higher proportion of 42% of patients in the fourth study [71]. In clinical practice, specific precipitants may not be found in all cases, especially when patients' onset of vestibular symptoms is indistinct or when records of inciting events are unavailable or unclear.

J. P. Staab (✉)
Departments of Psychiatry and Psychology,
and Otorhinolaryngology—Head and Neck Surgery, Mayo Clinic,
Rochester, MN, USA
e-mail: staab.jeffrey@mayo.edu

A. D. Sweeney et al. (eds.), *Haynes-Glasscock-Shambaugh Surgery of the Ear*, https://doi.org/10.1007/978-3-032-18264-7_62

Table 62.1 Diagnostic criteria for persistent postural-perceptual dizziness (PPPD)

A. One or more symptoms of dizziness, unsteadiness, or non-spinning vertigo are present on most days for 3 months or more.
1. Symptoms last for prolonged (hours long) periods of time but may wax and wane in severity.
2. Symptoms need not be present continuously throughout the entire day.
B. Persistent symptoms occur without specific provocation, but are exacerbated by three factors:
1. Upright posture
2. Active or passive motion without regard to direction or position
3. Exposure to moving visual stimuli or complex visual patterns
C. The disorder is precipitated by conditions that cause vertigo, unsteadiness, dizziness, or problems with balance, including acute, episodic, or chronic vestibular syndromes, other neurologic or medical illnesses, or psychological distress.
1. When the precipitant is an acute or episodic condition, symptoms settle into the pattern of criterion A as the precipitant resolves, but they may occur intermittently at first and then consolidate into a persistent course.
2. When the precipitant is a chronic syndrome, symptoms may develop slowly at first and worsen gradually.
D. Symptoms cause significant distress or functional impairment.
E. Symptoms are not better accounted for by another disease or disorder.

Adapted from Staab et al. [57] with permission of Sage Publications, IOS Press and the authors

Epidemiology of PPPD

Two large clinical epidemiologic investigations conducted in university neurology clinics in China (N = 9200) [75] and Korea (N = 21,267) [28], and a smaller descriptive study from Croatia (N = 147) [1] reported a remarkably consistent point prevalence for PPPD of 19.0–21.8% among patients seeking consultations for vestibular and balance symptoms. A descriptive study from a general internal medicine clinic in Japan (N = 229) reported a point prevalence of 14.4%, also among patients presenting with chief complaints of dizziness [25]. In a subspecialty clinic in Canada designed specifically for patients with chronic dizziness (N = 292), a cross-sectional study found that PPPD was the sole diagnosis for 9.2% of referred individuals and coexisted with other illnesses in another 44.2% [60]. Thus, at all three levels of care (i.e., primary care, general neurology, and dedicated subspecialty clinics), PPPD was the most common diagnosis for patients presenting with chronic dizziness and one of the top three neuro-otologic diagnoses among all patients with vestibular and balance symptoms, along with benign paroxysmal positional vertigo and vestibular migraine.

These clinical epidemiologic studies found that PPPD affects adults across the lifespan. The average age of patients presenting for clinical care was the mid-50 s (range 53–59 years), and women outnumbered men by a ratio of 2:1 [1, 28, 75], which was consistent with previous investigations of patients with phobic postural vertigo [5] and chronic subjective dizziness [59]. PPPD also affects children and adolescents. A clinical epidemiologic investigation of patients presenting to a tertiary pediatric balance clinic in the USA (N = 1021) found that 7.3% were diagnosed with PPPD [70]. Patients in that study had an average age of 14.6 years (range 8–22 years), and girls outnumbered boys by a ratio of 5:1.

The incidence of PPPD among patients exposed to potentially precipitating events is not known, as prospective studies have not yet addressed this question. In a systematic review of ten retrospective and prospective investigations (total N = 552) that were conducted prior to PPPD being defined in 2017, Trinidade et al. [65] found that rates of chronic dizziness ranged from 7.5% to 53% (weighted mean of 26.3%) among individuals who experienced acute vestibular syndromes (mostly vestibular neuritis and benign paroxysmal positional vertigo). A retrospective study conducted by Kabaya et al. [27] using the 2017 definition of PPPD suggested that the true incidence may be at the lower end of that range. They reviewed medical records of 155 patients who presented to their tertiary neurotology clinic within 90 days of new-onset vestibular symptoms and found that eight (5.2%) developed PPPD over 18 months of follow-up. Seven of those eight patients met all diagnostic criteria for PPPD at the time of their initial evaluation except for the required 3-month duration of illness. Another 70 (45.2%) patients had elevated scores on the NPQ but did not report sensitivities across all three domains of the exacerbating factors of PPPD (i.e., upright posture, self-motion, and exposure to complex or moving visual stimuli). Only one of these patients developed PPPD during the follow-up period. Thus, sensitivities to self-motion and visual stimuli were quite common, reported by half of all patients who presented for evaluation of new-onset vestibular symptoms, but only those who experienced early sensitivities across all three domains of criterion B were at high risk of developing PPPD. This finding suggests that assessing exacerbating factors may be a means to identify individuals at risk for PPPD early in the course of illness.

Making the Diagnosis of PPPD

PPPD belongs at the top of the differential diagnosis for patients who present with chief complaints of chronic dizziness, unsteadiness, and swaying/rocking (non-spinning) vertigo. The first step in evaluating patients with this presentation is to inquire about the effects of upright posture, active and passive self-motion, and exposure to motion-rich environments (i.e., the exacerbating factors of criterion B) on their symptoms. Additional data from physical examinations, clinical and vestibular laboratory tests, or neuroimaging may be needed to identify precipitating or coexisting conditions and judge their current clinical state (e.g., compensation status of a previous peripheral vestibulopathy) and to determine if PPPD is the best diagnosis, either alone or with other conditions. If the presence or absence of PPPD cannot be determined from available clinical information, a period of prospective monitoring and reevaluation may be needed before rendering a final diagnosis [54, 55].

Three possible trajectories have been observed for the development of PPPD, depending on the nature of its precipitating events, as described in criterion C of its ICVD definition [57]. After an acute vestibular syndrome, such as a unilateral peripheral vestibulopathy (e.g., vestibular neuritis), symptoms of PPPD usually begin as the acute illness resolves, without an asymptomatic interval, as found by Kabaya et al. [27]. Following an episodic vestibular syndrome, such as benign paroxysmal positional vertigo, vestibular migraine, or panic disorder, symptoms of PPPD may begin in full after the initial attack or occur intermittently at first, eventually consolidating into a persistent pattern as attacks of the precipitating illness continue. Subsequent attacks of the episodic illness would then be superimposed on the chronic symptoms of PPPD. The most difficult clinical scenario is, fortunately, the least common. When the precipitant is a chronic illness, especially one that begins insidiously, such as a degenerative neurologic or otologic condition, gradually increasing generalized anxiety disorder, or slowly worsening orthostatic intolerance, hypersensitivity to visual stimuli may be the best indicator of the onset of PPPD. In patients with degenerative neurologic or otologic disorders or orthostatic intolerance, standing and walking, making quick head movements, and engaging in other forms of active or passive self-motion would be expected to exacerbate vestibular and balance symptoms. In contrast, exposure to complex or moving visual stimuli would not be expected to worsen symptoms when patients are seated and stationary. Thus, the presence of clinically significant hypersensitivity to visual stimuli during sedentary activities is a key differentiator in these clinical scenarios, indicating that PPPD has developed as a secondary complication of the underlying precipitant [15, 55, 57].

Two self-report questionnaires may aid the diagnostic work-up of PPPD, although neither one substitutes for properly obtained clinical histories, examinations, and test results. In their aforementioned study, Kabaya et al. [27] found that patients who scored 27 or higher on the NPQ within the first 90 days of incident vestibular symptoms were at high risk of developing PPPD over the next 18 months (sensitivity = 88%). However, the specificity of the NPQ was low at 52% when used for this purpose. Thus, the NPQ may be utilized as a screening tool during the early period of vestibular illnesses to identify patients at risk for PPPD, but prospective follow-up beyond 3 months is needed to confirm the diagnosis. For patients with chronic vestibular and balance symptoms, Graham et al. [19] found that patients who scored greater than 60 on the Dizziness Handicap Inventory (DHI) [26] were highly likely to have functional vestibular disorders, primarily PPPD, or psychiatric illnesses, primarily anxiety and depressive disorders, contributing to their morbidity, with or without coexisting structural neuro-otologic illnesses (specificity = 88%). On the other hand, patients who scored 30 or less were highly unlikely to have functional or psychiatric disorders (specificity = 98%). These results indicate that high or low DHI scores may be used to increase or decrease the likelihood of PPPD in the differential diagnosis of patients with chronic vestibular and balance symptoms, though a definitive diagnosis would require that patients' clinical histories meet all five criteria for the disorder. Future validation studies may establish the best way to use the NPQ and DHI to assess patients for PPPD.

Differential Diagnosis of PPPD

The differential diagnosis of PPPD was described in considerable detail in its defining document Staab et al. [57], which is part of the ICVD and available online, free of charge, at https://www.iospress.com/jvr-icvd. In working through the differential diagnosis, it is important to keep in mind that final diagnostic formulations should account for the full spectrum of patients' active vestibular and balance symptoms, whether due to PPPD, another chronic disorder, or a combination of illnesses [15, 54, 55]. Stumbling blocks include attributing persistent symptoms to previous acute illnesses that have resolved or remitted (e.g., a fully compensated acute peripheral vestibulopathy), diagnosing only an episodic condition in patients with chronic symptoms (e.g., Ménière's disease alone in patients with persistent hypersensitivity to visual stimuli), and failure to recognize commonly coexisting problems (e.g., PPPD and vestibular migraine). In patients with other chronic vestibular disorders, the diagnostic challenge is to determine if PPPD has developed as a comorbid condition. Finally, PPPD does not cause major alterations of gait, or repeated falls or near falls, so the presence of these symptoms or signs warrants consideration of structural, metabolic, and functional gait disorders and pre-syncope [54, 55].

Pathophysiological Mechanisms of PPPD

The first pathophysiological model of PPPD was adapted from hypotheses about mechanisms underlying its four predecessors and data derived from investigations of other patients who developed persistent dizziness following acute vestibular syndromes [15]. After the definition of PPPD was published in 2017, the initial model was updated with findings from studies of clinical phenomenology, physiological, and psychological variables, and alterations in brain functioning involving patients diagnosed specifically with the disorder [43, 54]. Revised models included five processes: (1) the presence of an anxiety diathesis that predisposed affected patients to have (2) high anxiety-related responses to precipitating events in the form of increased body vigilance and catastrophic worries about adverse outcomes, which in turn caused the normally short-term compensatory shifts in physiological functioning of (3) stiffened postural control and (4) visual dependence to persist long after the precipitating events resolved or remitted, thereby becoming pathological in nature in association with (5) altered activity and connectivity of brain networks that process information subserving spatial orientation and locomotion. Subsequent authors created second [8] and third-generation [55] models that incorporated ideas derived from Bayesian logic to account for the effects of prior experiences and changes in internal estimates of space and motion [8], and optimal control theory to explain suspected alterations in top-down control of posture and gait derived from misperceptions (overestimations) of self-motion [55].

1. *Anxiety-related Personality Traits*: Brandt and Dieterich [6] included the presence of obsessive-compulsive personality traits in their definition of phobic postural vertigo, and Godemann et al. [17] described dependent personality traits contributing to the development of chronic dizziness after acute vestibular syndromes. Complementing those studies, Tschan et al. [67] found that patients with higher resilience and a greater sense of coherence (personality traits associated with less likelihood of anxiety-related distress) had lower rates of chronic dizziness as a consequence of acute or episodic vestibular disorders. Building on those reports, two groups of investigators found that patients with chronic subjective dizziness had significantly higher levels of neurotic personality traits than patients with other vestibular disorders [9, 58] and healthy controls [9], and one group [78] found increased neuroticism in patients with PPPD. In contrast, data from a nationwide sample of patients with PPPD in the Republic of Korea found that levels of neuroticism and other personality traits were within population norms (Korean Balance Society Multicenter Working Group 2020. The characteristics of persistent postural-perceptual dizziness in Korea. XXXI Bárány Society Congress, Madrid, Spain, May 2022, poster FP1225). Furthermore, a systematic review of predictors of PPPD suggested that the presence of anxiety-related personality traits, such as obsessive-compulsive or dependent personality styles or neuroticism, may be more likely to predispose patients to the development of comorbid anxiety disorders in conjunction with PPPD than to PPPD itself, after precipitating events [65].
2. *Acute Body Vigilance and Negative Perceptions of Illness*: Attacks of vertigo may provoke higher levels of anxiety than other medical emergencies, especially when experienced for the first time [42]. Prospective studies conducted prior to 2017 of patients who developed chronic dizziness following vestibular neuritis or benign paroxysmal positional vertigo found that high anxiety occurring during and immediately after bouts of illness was a stronger predictor of subsequently developing persistent dizziness than severity of labyrinthine deficits [18, 21]. Two specific anxiety-related symptoms were associated with the onset of chronic dizziness, namely heightened body vigilance (i.e., conscious attention to sensations of dizziness and unsteadiness) and negative illness perceptions (e.g., worrisome thoughts about causes, consequences, and controllability of vestibular and balance symptoms). These results were replicated in a prospective study of 6-month outcomes of vestibular neuritis [11] and a pilot study of PPPD [64].
3. *Altered Control of Stance and Gait*: A consistent finding from research on phobic postural vertigo and chronic subjective dizziness was that patients with either predecessor of PPPD had stiffening of postural control manifested as higher frequency, lower amplitude adjustments to postural sway than normal individuals due to excessive co-contraction of lower leg muscles [29, 40] and a lower threshold than healthy volunteers for engaging closed-loop feedback to control stance [73]. In minimally challenging situations, a quiet stance is maintained largely through open-loop vestibulospinal reflexes. In more demanding circumstances, closed-loop control is engaged, which utilizes feedback from visual and proprioceptive inputs [73]. Patients with phobic postural vertigo were found to utilize high-demand postural strategies when standing quietly on the floor and when standing on foam, whereas normal individuals used high-demand strategies only in the more challenging condition of standing on foam [45, 52]. Stiffening of the lower body was observed to reduce overall postural stability in a portion of patients with chronic subjective dizziness who manifested increased upper body sway during static posturography [40] and in nearly all patients with PPPD during dynamic posturography (Sensory Organization Test conditions 5 and 6) [35]. Patients with phobic postural vertigo were also found to have slower mean gait speed, shorter mean stride length, wider base of support, and a fractional increase in duration of two-footed support during walking compared to normal individuals [51].
4. *Visual Dependence*: Visual dependence refers to the tendency to rely more strongly on visual than vestibular or somatosensory information for spatial orientation, even

when visual inputs are not the most accurate form of information available. Visual dependence may be measured by various tests that utilize tilted or moving backgrounds to confound visuospatial orientation tasks. In a prospective study, the combination of high body vigilance and visual dependence measured by the Rod and Disk Test within 48 hours of the onset of acute vestibular neuritis predicted the presence of PPPD-like chronic dizziness rather than asymptomatic recovery at 6-month follow-up [11]. In a cross-sectional study, patients with PPPD performed more poorly than healthy controls on the functional head impulse test [61].

5. *Changes in Brain Activity and Connectivity*: Multiple groups of investigators used structural and functional neuroimaging techniques to study brain morphology, activity, and connectivity in patients with PPPD or its predecessors. In five studies, investigators used task-related functional magnetic resonance imaging (fMRI) to compare patients to healthy controls, including sound-evoked vestibular stimulation in patients with chronic subjective dizziness [23] and visual motion stimuli in patients with PPPD [41, 46], phobic postural vertigo [44], and visual vertigo [48]. The latter study also used caloric irrigation [48]. In one study, researchers used task-related fMRI to compare brain responses to emotionally charged pictures (positive, neutral, or negative valence) in women with PPPD versus women who had recovered from other illnesses causing dizziness [69]. In four studies, researchers used resting state fMRI to compare patients with visual vertigo [68] or PPPD [31–33] to healthy controls. Investigators in one study used single-photon emission computerized tomography (SPECT) to compare patients with PPPD to healthy controls [37]. Research teams also used morphometric methods to investigate brain structure in patients versus healthy controls. One team used surface-based morphometry to study patients with PPPD [39]. Others used voxel-based morphometry to investigate patients with phobic postural vertigo [44] and PPPD [74]. Indovina and colleagues [24] summarized the results of these studies. After pooling results across the different patient populations and neuroimaging methods, they concluded that patients with PPPD had decreased local activity and functional connectivity in multimodal vestibular cortical areas (e.g., right posterior insula, parietal operculum, and surrounding regions) and reduced cortical folding and gray-matter volumes in those areas, though the cross-sectional design of the imaging studies precluded any conclusions about causal relationship between the structural and functional results. They also identified increased connectivity between the prefrontal cortex and primary visual and motor regions.
6. Predictive Processing (Use of Internal Estimates of Self-Motion and Prior Knowledge of Object Motion): Motion perception and spatial orientation often are considered to be the end result of central processing of vestibular, visual, and proprioceptive inputs. In actuality, there are many situations in which external stimuli contain ambiguous information about self and object motion. Examples include active versus passive self-motion, tilt with respect to gravity versus linear acceleration, and the trajectories of objects moving in the visual field. Physiologic studies in animals [12, 13] and humans [14] showed that these ambiguities are resolved by integrating internal predictions of self-motion and prior knowledge of typical movements of objects in the environment into the processing of vestibular, visual, and proprioceptive inputs. Furthermore, Arshad et al. [2] demonstrated that perception of space and motion relies on best estimates of their magnitudes derived from interhemispheric processing of relevant data rather than absolute indicators of these variables. Thus, perception of self and object motion is relative, not absolute, which could be another source of error in patients with functional vestibular disorders [3]. With these findings in mind, Castro et al. [8] included alterations in predictive processing of motion in their model of PPPD. Subsequent experiments lent credence to this idea by finding that patients with PPPD overestimate their own motion, including the magnitude of head roll tilt [77] and postural sway [49].
7. Optimal Control (Top-Down Influences on Locomotion): In addition to evidence about predictive processing and misperception of motion, two studies identified cognitive difficulties in patients with PPPD that cannot be explained easily by bottom-up processes. In one study, Breinbauer et al. [7] compared spatial navigation and spatial memory in patients with PPPD to patients with unilateral vestibular deficits and healthy controls using the virtual Morris Water Maze Test. Patients with PPPD performed worse than both comparison groups. In another study, Rizk et al. [47] measured self-reported cognitive symptoms such as momentary cognitive slips, absent-mindedness, and inattentiveness in patients with PPPD compared to patients with vestibular migraine, Ménière's disease, and benign paroxysmal positional vertigo using the Cognitive Failure Questionnaire. Again, patients with PPPD scored worse than patients in the comparison groups and also worse than population norms. This prompted Staab [55] to suggest that patients with PPPD use a top-down motor control scheme that optimizes stability over fluid locomotion. On top of the increased body vigilance, visual dependence, and stiffened postural control that occur acutely as proposed in first-generation models, Staab [55] hypothesized that patients with PPPD utilize a set of top-down commands driven by misperception of motion that prioritizes body stability in the immediate surroundings over fluid navigation through the larger world. The increased

cognitive effort associated with this top-down change comes at the expense of other cognitive tasks and perpetuates excessive overcontrol of stance, gait, and gaze, and heightened responses to motion of self and objects in the environment.

Treatment

Trinidade et al. [66] recently reviewed the literature on the treatment of PPPD. The three primary therapeutic interventions for PPPD were derived from treatments developed for its predecessors and include vestibular rehabilitation therapy (VRT), serotonin reuptake inhibitors, and cognitive behavioral therapy (CBT). These have not yet been tested in fully powered, randomized, controlled trials, but published retrospective reports, open-label studies, and early controlled trials that included patients specifically diagnosed with PPPD using 2017 criteria are increasing in size and sophistication.

A. *Vestibular Rehabilitation Therapy*: VRT was developed in the 1990s to treat patients with chronic dizziness [53]. A portion of patients in those early studies would likely have met criteria for PPPD. Thompson et al. [63] published the results of a retrospective review and telephone follow-up of 26 patients diagnosed with PPPD using a draft version of the ICVD criteria and found that nearly all patients valued education about the condition provided by experienced physical therapists, and 14 (56%) reported clinically significant benefits from individualized, self-paced, home-based, vestibular exercise programs. Nada et al. [38] reported a mean reduction of Dizziness Handicap Inventory (DHI) scores from 55 (high–moderate) to 36 (low–moderate) in a prospective study of 60 patients diagnosed with PPPD per the 2017 definition. This 19-point reduction in mean DHI scores exceeded the minimal clinically important difference (MCID) of 18 for that outcome measure [26]. Twenty-seven (45%) patients achieved endpoint scores less than 30 (mild) after 6 weeks of therapist-directed vestibular rehabilitation. Three other, smaller studies (N = 7–32) [10, 16, 62] reported mixed, though mostly positive, results from in-person, at-home, and online VRT strategies.

B. *Medication*: All six commercially available selective serotonin reuptake inhibitors (SSRIs) (fluoxetine, sertraline, paroxetine, fluvoxamine, citalopram, and escitalopram) and two of the five available selective serotonin and norepinephrine reuptake inhibitors (SNRIs) (venlafaxine and milnacipran) were included in at least one study of patients with chronic PPPD-like dizziness prior to 2017 (see Dieterich and Staab [15] for reviews, Table 62.2). These medications had roughly equal benefits and tolerability, with about 65% of all patients and 85% of patients who completed at least 8 weeks of treatment experiencing clinically meaningful reductions in symptoms (e.g., 50% decreases in DHI scores from the moderate–severe to mild–moderate range).

Table 62.2 Guidelines for use of serotonin reuptake inhibitors for PPPD

Medication	Starting dose[a]	Titration schedule	Final dose[b]
Sertraline	12.5–25 mg daily	25 mg q 2 wks	50–200 mg daily
Escitalopram	2.5–5 mg daily	5 mg q 2 wks	10–20 mg daily
Venlafaxine XR	37.5 mg daily	37.5 mg q 2 wks	75–225 mg daily

[a]The usual starting doses are 25 mg daily for sertraline or 5 mg daily for escitalopram. The lower doses may be best for patients who report being sensitive to medications

[b]Low-mid range doses are usually adequate for patients with uncomplicated PPPD. Higher doses may be needed for patients who have co-existing anxiety or depressive disorders

Two studies reported results of SSRI treatment of patients diagnosed specifically with PPPD. Min et al. [36] published a retrospective review of 197 patients with PPPD that they treated over a 3-year period with SSRIs (mostly escitalopram) with or without adjunctive low-dose benzodiazepines (mostly clonazepam). Their results mirrored the older studies in that 65% of all treated patients achieved clinically meaningful reductions in symptoms. Yu et al. [79] conducted an 8-week, two-arm, prospective study of 45 patients with PPPD treated with sertraline alone versus 46 patients treated with sertraline plus CBT. In the medication alone arm, the mean DHI scores decreased from 54 (moderate) to 26 (mild), exceeding the MCID. In the combined treatment arm, mean DHI scores decreased even more from 54 (moderate) to 15 (mild), despite the mean dose of sertraline being lower.

Typical dosing strategies for SSRIs and SNRIs start at one-half of the lowest therapeutic dose of the chosen drug for 1–2 weeks, followed by gradual titration into the middle of the therapeutic dose range [54, 55]. Based on clinical experience and published data from the predecessors of PPPD, any of the SSRIs or SNRIs may be used to treat PPPD, though three of them have been used most often. For sertraline, the starting dose is 25 mg daily with upward titration by 25–50 mg increments at 2-week intervals to reach a final dose of 50–100 mg daily. Further upward titration to as high as 200 mg daily may be undertaken, if needed and tolerated, especially for patients with coexisting anxiety or depressive disorders. For escitalopram, the starting dose is 5 mg daily, with a final dose of 10–20 mg daily for all patients. For venlafaxine extended release, the starting dose is 37.5 mg daily, titration increments are 37.5–75 mg at 2-week intervals, the final dose for uncomplicated PPPD is 75–225 mg daily, and doses up to 375 mg daily may be used for patients with coexisting psychiatric disorders. If patients do not tolerate a medication or fail to achieve at least a 50% reduction in symptoms, then they may be switched to another medication. Clinical experience suggests that effective medication should be continued for 1 year, at which time consideration may be given to tapering and discontinuing the medication slowly over a minimum of several weeks. If symptoms begin to reemerge during the slow taper, then another 6–12 months of treatment is indicated, possibly longer for patients with active medical or psychiatric illnesses that also contribute to dizziness.

C. *Psychotherapy*: Early studies of CBT produced nonsustained benefits for patients with phobic postural vertigo, but better results were obtained for chronic subjective dizziness (see Staab [54], for review). For patients with PPPD, Waterston et al. [71] reported results of a retrospective study of 150 patients that they treated with CBT over a 5-year period. Patients who completed a full course of CBT achieved a mean reduction in DHI scores from 50 (moderate) to 24 (mild), exceeding the MCID. In a prospective trial of 27 patients with PPPD, Kuwabara et al. [30] found that a 6-week program of acceptance and commitment therapy, a spin-off of CBT, combined with VRT reduced mean DHI scores from 49 (moderate) to 26 (mild) at 6-month follow-up, which was a large effect that exceeded the MCID.

Thus, there is growing evidence that VRT, SSRIs/SNRIs, and CBT-style psychotherapies produce roughly equal benefits for patients with PPPD, reducing symptoms by clinically meaningful amounts (≥50%) from moderate–severe to mild–moderate levels of dizziness-related handicap. Data from the prospective trial of Yu et al. [79] and other investigations of patients with functional forms of chronic dizziness, including PPPD [22, 34, 50], hint that combinations of these three interventions, particularly psychotherapeutic strategies added to VRT or medications, may produce better outcomes. Indeed, Axer et al. [4] reported that 305 patients with PPPD achieved sustained benefits through 6 months of follow-up from individualized combinations of these three modalities of treatment introduced during a week-long intensive outpatient program.

Conclusion

Persistent postural-perceptual dizziness (PPPD) was formally defined in 2017. Its definition is included in the International Classification of Vestibular Disorders and the International Classification of Diseases, 11th edition. Its prevalence in the general population is not yet known, but clinical epidemiologic studies have found that 20% of patients referred for dizziness to university- and hospital-based general neurology clinics and more than half referred to specialized dizziness and balance centers had PPPD, making it the most common cause of chronic dizziness in tertiary care and one of the top three diagnoses identified in adults seeking specialty consultation for vestibular symptoms, along with benign paroxysmal positional vertigo and vestibular migraine. A specific measure of PPPD has been created, the Niigata PPPD Questionnaire, with early results indicating that it may be helpful for screening patients with new-onset vestibular symptoms to identify those at risk of developing PPPD. The most recent models of pathophysiologic processes potentially underlying PPPD have incorporated data emerging from an expanding array of physiological, psychological, and neuroimaging investigations. They suggest that patients' misperception (overestimation) of their own motion may perpetuate a top-down, consciously focused, motor control strategy that emphasizes postural stability over smooth locomotion, resulting in overly controlled stance, gait, and gaze and heightened reactivity to self and object motion. Treatment strategies that were first developed for the precursors of PPPD have been investigated in retrospective and prospective studies of patients diagnosed with PPPD itself. Although fully powered, randomized, controlled trials have not yet been completed, available evidence supports the use of individualized combinations of vestibular rehabilitation, pharmacotherapy with SSRIs or SNRIs, and cognitive behavioral therapy to meaningfully reduce the morbidity of this highly prevalent and too often disabling disorder.

Acknowledgments Dr. Staab was supported by grant W81XWH1810760 from the U.S. Army Medical Research and Materiel Command via the Congressionally Directed Medical Research Program.

References

1. Adamec I, Meaški SJ, Skorić MK, Jažić K, Crnošija L, Milivojević I, Habek M. Persistent postural-perceptual dizziness: clinical and neurophysiological study. J Clin Neurosci. 2020;72:26–30.
2. Arshad Q, Ortega MC, Goga U, Lobo R, Siddiqui S, Mediratta S, Bednarczuk N, Kaski D, Bronstein A. Interhemispheric control of sensory cue integration and self-motion perception. Neuroscience. 2019;408:378–87.
3. Arshad Q, Saman Y, Sharif M, Kaski D, Staab JP. Magnitude estimates orchestrate hierarchical construction of context-dependent representational maps for vestibular space and time: theoretical implications for functional dizziness. Front Integr Neurosci. 2022;15:806940.
4. Axer H, Finn S, Wasserman A, Guntinas-Lichius O, Klingner CM, Witte OW. Multimodal treatment of persistent postural–perceptual dizziness. Brain Behav. 2020;10(12):e01864.
5. Brandt T. Phobic postural vertigo. Neurology. 1996;46:1515–9.
6. Brandt T, Dieterich M. Phobischer Attacken Schwankschwindel, ein neues Syndrom? Munch Med Wochenschr. 1986;28:247–50.

7. Breinbauer HA, Contreras MD, Lira JP, Guevara C, Castillo L, Ruëdlinger K, Muñoz D, Delano PH. Spatial navigation is distinctively impaired in persistent postural perceptual dizziness. Front Neurol. 2020;10:1361. https://doi.org/10.3389/fneur.2019.01361.
8. Castro P, Bancroft MJ, Arshad Q, Kaski D. Persistent postural-perceptual dizziness (PPPD) from brain imaging to behaviour and perception. Brain Sci. 2022;12:753.
9. Chiarella G, Petrolo C, Riccelli R, Giofrè L, Olivadese G, Gioacchini FM, Scarpa A, Cassandro E, Passamonti L. Chronic subjective dizziness: analysis of underlying personality factors. J Vestib Res. 2016;26(4):403–8.
10. Choi SY, Choi JH, Oh EH, Oh SJ, Choi KD. Effect of vestibular exercise and optokinetic stimulation using virtual reality in persistent postural- perceptual dizziness. Sci Rep. 2021;11(1):14437.
11. Cousins S, Kaski D, Cutfield N, Arshad Q, Ahmad H, Gresty MA, Seemungal BM, Golding J, Bronstein AM. Predictors of clinical recovery from vestibular neuritis: a prospective study. Ann Clin Transl Neurol. 2017;4:340–6.
12. Cullen KE. Vestibular processing during natural self-motion: implications for perception and action. Nat Rev Neurosci. 2019;20:348–63.
13. Cullen KE, Zobeiri OA. Proprioception and the predictive processing of active motion. Curr Opin Physiol. 2021;20:29–38.
14. Della Monache S, Indovina I, Zago M, Daprati E, Lacquaniti F, Bosco G. Watching the effects of gravity. Vestibular cortex and the neural representation of "visual" gravity. Front Integr Neurosci. 2021;15:793634.
15. Dieterich M, Staab JP. Functional dizziness: from phobic postural vertigo and chronic subjective dizziness to persistent postural-perceptual dizziness. Curr Opin Neurol. 2017;30(1):107–13.
16. Eldøen G, Kvalheim SE, Thesen T, Mygland Å, Ljøstad U, Bakke S, Holo MH, Løge I, Jonsbu E. Web-based vestibular rehabilitation in persistent postural-perceptual dizziness. Brain Behav. 2021;11(10):e2346.
17. Godemann F, Koffroth C, Neu P, Heuser I. Why does vertigo become chronic after neuropathia vestibularis? Psychosom Med. 2004;66(5):783–7.
18. Godemann F, Siefert K, Hantschke-Bruggemann M, Neu P, Seidl R, Ströhle A. What accounts for vertigo one year after neuritis vestibularis—anxiety or a dysfunctional vestibular organ? J Psychiatr Res. 2005;39:529–34.
19. Graham MK, Staab JP, Lohse CM, McCaslin DL. A comparison of dizziness handicap inventory scores by categories of vestibular diagnoses. Otol Neurotol. 2021;42(1):129–36.
20. Habs M, Strobl R, Grill E, Dieterich M, Becker-Bense S. Primary or secondary chronic functional dizziness: does it make a difference? A DizzyReg study in 356 patients. J Neurol. 2020;267:212–22.
21. Heinrichs N, Edler C, Eskens S, Mielczarek MM, Moschner C. Predicting continued dizziness after an acute peripheral vestibular disorder. Psychosom Med. 2007;69:700–7.
22. Herdman D, Norton S, Murdin L, Frost K, Pavlou M, Moss-Morris R. The INVEST trial: a randomised feasibility trial of psychologically informed vestibular rehabilitation versus current gold standard physiotherapy for people with persistent postural perceptual dizziness. J Neurol. 2022;269(9):4753–63.
23. Indovina I, Riccelli R, Chiarella G, Petrolo C, Augimeri A, Giofre L, Lacquaniti F, Staab JP, Passamonti L. Role of the insula and vestibular system in patients with chronic subjective dizziness: an fMRI study using sound-evoked vestibular stimulation. Front Behav Neurosci. 2015;9:334.
24. Indovina I, Passamonti L, Mucci V, Chiarella G, Lacquaniti F, Staab JP. Brain correlates of persistent postural-perceptual dizziness: a review of neuroimaging studies. J Clin Med. 2021;10(18):4274.
25. Ishizuka K, Shikino K, Yamauchi Y, Yanagita Y, Yokokawa D, Ikegami A, Tsukamoto T, Noda K, Uehara T, Ikusaka M. The clinical key features of persistent postural perceptual dizziness in the general medicine outpatient setting: a case series study of 33 patients. Intern Med. 2020;59(22):2857–62.
26. Jacobson GP, Newman CW. The development of the dizziness handicap inventory. JAMA Otolaryngol Head Neck Surg. 1990;116:424–7.
27. Kabaya K, Tamai H, Okajima A, Minakata T, Kondo M, Nakayama M, Iwasaki S. Presence of exacerbating factors of persistent perceptual-postural dizziness in patients with vestibular symptoms at initial presentation. Laryngoscope Investig Otolaryngol. 2021;7(2):499–505.
28. Kim HJ, Lee JO, Choi JY, Kim J. Etiologic distribution of dizziness and vertigo in a referral-based dizziness clinic in South Korea. J Neurol. 2020;267:2252–9.
29. Krafczyk S, Schlamp V, Dieterich M, Haberhauer P, Brandt T. Increased body sway at 3.5–8 Hz in patients with phobic postural vertigo. Neurosci Lett. 1999;259:149–52.
30. Kuwabara J, Kondo M, Kabaya K, Watanabe W, Shiraishi N, Sakai M, Toshishige Y, Ino K, Nakayama M, Iwasaki S, Akechi T. Acceptance and commitment therapy combined with vestibular rehabilitation for persistent postural-perceptual dizziness: a pilot study. Am J Otolaryngol. 2020;41(6):102609.
31. Lee J-O, Lee E-S, Kim J-S, Lee Y-B, Jeong Y, Choi BS, Kim J-H, Staab JP. Altered brain function in persistent postural perceptual dizziness: a study on resting state functional connectivity. Hum Brain Mapp. 2018;39:3340–53.
32. Li K, Si L, Cui B, Ling X, Shen B, Yang X. Altered spontaneous functional activity of the right precuneus and cuneus in patients with persistent postural-perceptual dizziness. Brain Imaging Behav. 2020a;14:2176–86.
33. Li K, Si L, Cui B, Ling X, Shen B, Yang X. Altered intra- and inter-network functional connectivity in patients with persistent postural-perceptual dizziness. NeuroImage Clin. 2020b;26:102216.
34. Limburg K, Radziej K, Sattel H, Henningsen P, Dieterich M, Probst T, Dale R, Lahmann C. A randomized controlled trial evaluating integrative psychotherapeutic group treatment compared to self-help groups in functional vertigo/dizziness. J Clin Med. 2021;10(10):2215.
35. McCaslin DL, Shepard NT, Hollman JH, Staab JP. Characterization of postural sway in patients with persistent postural-perceptual dizziness (PPPD) using wearable motion sensors. Otol Neurotol. 2022;43(2):e243–51.
36. Min S, Kim JS, Park HY. Predictors of treatment response to pharmacotherapy in patients with persistent postural-perceptual dizziness. J Neurol. 2021;268(7):2523–32.
37. Na S, Im JJ, Jeong H, Lee E-S, Lee T-K, Chung Y-A, Song I-U. Cerebral perfusion abnormalities in patients with persistent postural-perceptual dizziness (PPPD): a SPECT study. J Neural Transm. 2019;126:123–9.
38. Nada EH, Ibraheem OA, Hassaan MR. Vestibular rehabilitation therapy outcomes in patients with persistent postural-perceptual dizziness. Ann Otol Rhinol Laryngol. 2019;128(4):323–9.
39. Nigro S, Indovina I, Riccelli R, Chiarella G, Petrolo C, Lacquaniti F, Staab JP, Passamonti L. Reduced cortical folding in multi-modal vestibular regions in persistent postural perceptual dizziness. Brain Imaging Behav. 2019;13:798–809.
40. Ödman M, Maire R. Chronic subjective dizziness. Acta Otolaryngol. 2008;128:1085–8.
41. Passamonti L, Riccelli R, Lacquaniti F, Staab JP, Indovina I. Brain responses to virtual reality visual motion stimulation are affected by neurotic personality traits in patients with persistent postural-perceptual dizziness. J Vestib Res. 2018;28(5–6):369–78.
42. Pollak L, Klein C, Rafael S, Vera K, Rabey JM. Anxiety in the first attack of vertigo. Otolaryngol Head Neck Surg. 2003;128:829–34.
43. Popkirov S, Stone J, Holle-Lee D. Treatment of persistent postural-perceptual dizziness (PPPD) and related disorders. Curr Treat Options Neurol. 2018;20(12):50.
44. Popp P, Zu Eulenburg P, Stephan T, Bögle R, Habs M, Henningsen P, Feuerecker R, Dieterich M. Cortical alterations in phobic postural vertigo—a multimodal imaging approach. Ann Clin Transl Neurol. 2018;5:717–29.

45. Querner V, Krafczyk S, Dieterich M, Brandt T. Patients with somatoform phobic postural vertigo: the more difficult the balance task, the better the balance performance. Neurosci Lett. 2000;285:21–4.
46. Riccelli R, Passamonti L, Toschi N, Nigro S, Chiarella G, Petrolo C, Lacquaniti F, Staab JP, Indovina I. Altered insular and occipital responses to simulated vertical self-motion in patients with persistent postural-perceptual dizziness. Front Neurol. 2017;8:529.
47. Rizk HG, Sharon JD, Lee JA, Thomas C, Nguyen SA, Meyer TA. Cross-sectional analysis of cognitive dysfunction in patients with vestibular disorders. Ear Hear. 2020;41:1020–7.
48. Roberts R, Ahmad H, Patel M, Dima D, Ibitoye R, Sharif M, Leech R, Arshad Q, Bronstein A. An fMRI study of visuo-vestibular interactions following vestibular neuritis. NeuroImage Clin. 2018;20:1010–7.
49. San Pedro Murillo E, Bancroft MJ, Koohi N, Castro P, Kaski D. Postural misperception: a biomarker for persistent postural-perceptual dizziness. J Neurol Neurosurg Psychiatry. 2023;94(2):165–6.
50. Schmid DA, Allum JHJ, Sleptsova M, Gross S, Gaab J, Welge-Lüssen A, Schaefert R, Langewitz W. Effects of a program of cognitive-behavioural group therapy, vestibular rehabilitation, and psychoeducational explanations on patients with dizziness and no quantified balance deficit, compared to patients with dizziness and a quantified balance deficit. J Psychosom Res. 2018;105:21–30.
51. Schniepp R, Wuehr M, Huth S, Pradhan C, Brandt T, Jahn K. Gait characteristics of patients with phobic postural vertigo: effects of fear of falling, attention, and visual input. J Neurol. 2014;261:738–46.
52. Schniepp R, Wuehr M, Pradhan C, Novozhilov S, Krafczyk S, Brandt T, Jahn K. Nonlinear variability of body sway in patients with phobic postural vertigo. Front Neurol. 2013;4:115.
53. Shepard NT, Telian SA. Programmatic vestibular rehabilitation. Otolaryngol Head Neck Surg. 1995;112(1):173–82.
54. Staab JP. Persistent postural-perceptual dizziness. Semin Neurol. 2020;40(1):130–7.
55. Staab JP. Persistent postural-perceptual dizziness: review and update on key mechanisms of the most common functional neuro-otologic disorder. Neurol Clin. 2023;41(4):647–64.
56. Staab JP. Behavioural neuro-otology. In: Bronstein AM, editor. Oxford textbook of vertigo and imbalance. 2nd ed. Oxford, UK: Oxford University Press; 2025.
57. Staab JP, Eckhardt-Henn A, Horii A, Jacob R, Strupp M, Brandt T, Bronstein A. Diagnostic criteria for persistent postural-perceptual dizziness (PPPD): consensus document of the committee for the Classification of Vestibular Disorders of the Barany Society. J Vestib Res. 2017;27(4):191–208.
58. Staab JP, Rohe DE, Eggers SD, Shepard NT. Anxious, introverted personality traits in patients with chronic subjective dizziness. J Psychosom Res. 2014;76(1):80–3.
59. Staab JP, Ruckenstein MJ. Expanding the differential diagnosis of dizziness. Arch Otolaryngol Head Neck Surg. 2007;133:170–6.
60. Staibano P, Lelli D, Tse D. A retrospective analysis of two tertiary care dizziness clinics: a multidisciplinary chronic dizziness clinic and an acute dizziness clinic. J Otolaryngol Head Neck Surg. 2019;48:11.
61. Teggi R, Gatti O, Cangiano J, Fornasari F, Bussi M. Functional head impulse test with and without optokinetic stimulation in subjects with persistent postural perceptual dizziness (PPPD): preliminary report. Otol Neurotol. 2020;41:e70–5.
62. Teh CS, Abdullah NA, Kamaruddin NR, Mohd Judi KB, Fadzilah I, Zainun Z, Prepageran N. Home-based vestibular rehabilitation: a feasible and effective therapy for persistent postural perceptual dizziness (a pilot study). Ann Otol Rhinol Laryngol. 2023;132(5):566–77.
63. Thompson KJ, Goetting JC, Staab JP, Shepard NT. Retrospective review and telephone follow-up to evaluate a physical therapy protocol for treating persistent postural-perceptual dizziness: a pilot study. J Vestib Res. 2015;25(2):97–103.
64. Trinidade A, Harman P, Stone J, Staab JP, Goebel JA. Assessment of potential risk factors for the development of persistent postural-perceptual dizziness: a case-control pilot study. Front Neurol. 2021;21(11):601883.
65. Trinidade A, Cabreira V, Goebel JA, Staab JP, Kaski D, Stone J. Predictors of persistent postural-perceptual dizziness (PPPD) precipitated by peripheral vestibular disorders: a systematic review. J Neurol Neurosurg Psychiatry. 2023a;94(11):904–15.
66. Trinidade A, Cabreira V, Kaski D, Goebel JA, Staab JP, Popkirov S, Stone J. Treatment of persistent postural-perceptual dizziness (PPPD). Curr Treat Op Neurol. 2023b;25:281–306.
67. Tschan R, Best C, Beutel ME, Knebel A, Wiltink J, Dieterich M, Eckhardt-Henn A. Patients' psychological well-being and resilient coping protect from secondary somatoform vertigo and dizziness (SVD) 1 year after vestibular disease. J Neurol. 2011;258:104–12.
68. Van Ombergen A, Heine L, Jillings S, Roberts RE, Jeurissen B, van Rompaey V, Mucci V, Vanhecke S, Sijbers J, Vanhevel F, Sunaert S, Bahri MA, Parizel PM, Van de Heyning PH, Laureys S, Wuyts FL. Altered functional brain connectivity in patients with visually induced dizziness. NeuroImage Clin. 2017;14:538–45.
69. von Söhsten Lins EMD, Bittar RSM, Bazán PR, Júnior EA, Staab JP. Cerebral responses to stationary emotional stimuli measured by fMRI in women with persistent postural-perceptual dizziness. Int Arch Otorhinolaryngol. 2021;25:e355–64.
70. Wang A, Fleischman KM, Kawai K, Corcoran M, Brodsky JR. Persistent postural-perceptual dizziness in children and adolescents. Otol Neurotol. 2021;42(8):e1093–100.
71. Waterston J, Chen L, Mahony K, Gencarelli J, Stuart G. Persistent postural-perceptual dizziness: precipitating conditions, co-morbidities and treatment with cognitive behavioral therapy. Front Neurol. 2021;12:795516.
72. World Health Organization. ICD-11 for mortality and morbidity statistics (version 02/2022). AB320 Persistent Postural-Perceptual Dizziness; 2022. https://icd.who.int/browse11/l-m/en#/http://id.who.int/icd/entity/2005792829 Accessed 20 August 2022.
73. Wuehr M, Pradhan C, Novozhilov S, Krafczyk S, Brandt T, Jahn K, Schniepp R. Inadequate interaction between open- and closed-loop postural control in phobic postural vertigo. J Neurol. 2013;260(5):1314–23.
74. Wurthmann S, Naegel S, Steinberg BS, Theysohn N, Diener H-C, Kleinschnitz C, Obermann M, Holle D. Cerebral gray matter changes in persistent postural perceptual dizziness. J Psychosom Res. 2017;103:95–101.
75. Xue H, Chong Y, Jiang ZD, Liu ZL, Ding L, Yang SL, Wang L, Xiang WP. Etiological analysis on patients with vertigo or dizziness. Zhonghua Yi Xue Za Zhi. 2018;98(16):1227–30.
76. Yagi C, Morita Y, Kitazawa M, Nonomura Y, Yamagishi T, Ohshima S, Izumi S, Takahashi K, Horii A. A validated questionnaire to assess the severity of persistent postural-perceptual dizziness (PPPD): the Niigata PPPD Questionnaire (NPQ). Otol Neurotol. 2019;40:e747–52.
77. Yagi C, Morita Y, Kitazawa M, Nonomura Y, Yamagishi T, Ohshima S, Izumi S, Takahashi K, Wada Y, Kitahara T, Horii A. Head roll-tilt subjective visual vertical test in the diagnosis of persistent postural-perceptual dizziness. Otol Neurotol. 2021;42(10):e1618–24.
78. Yan Z, Cui L, Yu T, Liang H, Wang Y, Chen C. Analysis of the characteristics of persistent postural- perceptual dizziness: a clinical-based study in China. Int J Audiol. 2016;56:1–5.
79. Yu Y-C, Xue H, Zhang Y-X, Zhou J. Cognitive behavior therapy as augmentation for sertraline in treating patients with persistent postural-perceptual dizziness. BioMed Res Int. 2018:8518631.

Neurotologic Manifestations of Stroke

63

Abraham Jacob, Roksolyana Tourkevich, and Rihan Khan

Introduction

The World Health Organization defines "stroke" as a rapidly developing loss of brain function(s) due to disturbances of the blood supply to the brain. Also called cerebrovascular accidents (CVA), manifestations include ischemic cerebral infarction, intraparenchymal hemorrhage, and subarachnoid hemorrhage. Stroke is a major health problem worldwide, affecting three times as many people as breast cancer. Nearly one in five people in the United States suffers a stroke during their lifetime; approximately 750,000 people in the United States have a stroke each year; and about one-third of stroke victims die within a few months of their stroke. Only heart disease and cancer kill more people in the United States than stroke each year. Of those who survive, about 10% are able to return to their previous level of activity, about 50% regain enough function to return home and carry on with only limited assistance, and about 40% remain institutionalized or require significant assistance in caring for themselves [45]. The financial burden of stroke is substantial, with expenses totaling $65.5 billion in 2008, and costs are expected to rise as the population ages [49].

Stroke involving the vertebrobasilar system (Fig. 63.1) disrupts the posterior circulation and can cause neurotologic symptoms such as hearing loss, dizziness, and facial weakness. Differentiating peripheral (ear) from central (brain) lesions is critical to inform workup, treatment, and prognosis. The care of these patients is typically multidisciplinary, requiring input from neurologists, neuro-intensive care physicians, neurosurgeons, neurotologists, radiologists, audiologists, and neuro-rehabilitation specialists.

A. Jacob (✉) · R. Tourkevich
Center for Neurosciences, Tucson, AZ, USA
e-mail: ajacob@neurotucson.com

R. Khan
Department of Radiology, Dartmouth-Hitchcock Medical Center, Lebanon, NH, USA

A. D. Sweeney et al. (eds.), *Haynes-Glasscock-Shambaugh Surgery of the Ear*, https://doi.org/10.1007/978-3-032-18264-7_63

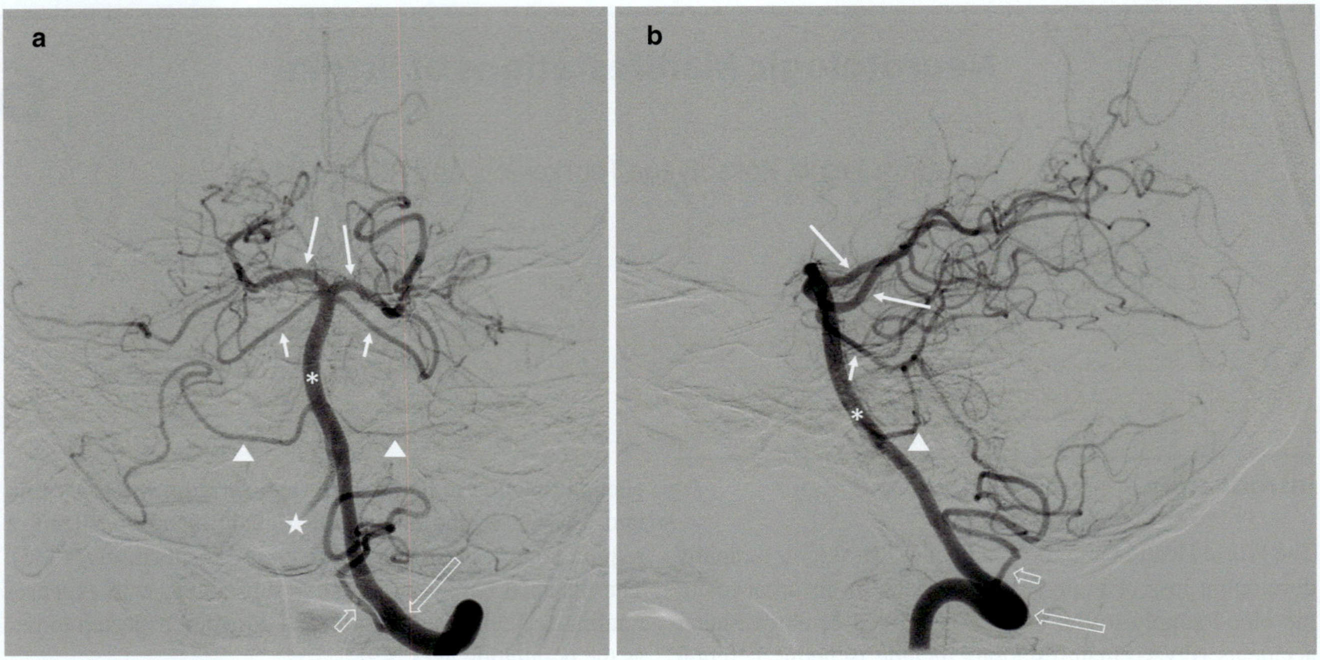

Fig. 63.1 Normal vertebrobasilar anatomy. Conventional angiogram (**a**) anterior to posterior and (**b**) lateral images show contrast opacifying the posterior circulation via a left-sided vertebral artery injection. Note the following normal arterial anatomy: long open arrow: left vertebral artery; short open arrow: left PICA arising from the left vertebral artery; asterisk: basilar artery; triangles: bilateral AICAs arising from the proximal basilar artery; short solid arrows: bilateral SCAs arising from the distal basilar artery just prior to its bifurcation; long solid arrows: bilateral Posterior Cerebral Arteries (PCA)s which are the terminal branches of the basilar artery; star: mild retrograde flash filling of the distal right vertebral artery

Peripheral Vascular Compromise

Hearing loss is one of the most common human sensory disabilities, impacting hundreds of millions of people worldwide. It is an especially prevalent health concern for the elderly, with between 40% and 50% of those over the age of 65 affected [36, 47]. Hearing loss is associated with communication difficulties, social isolation, and, more recently, with an increased risk of dementia [17, 33]. Dizziness is also highly prevalent. Recent data from the 2001 to 2004 National Health and Nutrition Examination Surveys, a cross-sectional survey of over 5000 American adults aged 40 years and older, estimated that 35% had vestibular dysfunction and a 12-fold increase in odds for falling [2, 41].

Anatomy and Physiology

The external ear, composed of the pinna and ear canal, funnels sound to the tympanic membrane while selectively amplifying high-frequency sounds due to the resonance characteristics of the concha (approximately 5300 Hz) and ear canal (approximately 3000 Hz). The middle ear helps match impedance between air and the fluid-filled cochlea through differences in surface area between the tympanic membrane and stapes footplate (20×) as well as lever effects of the ossicular chain. A traveling wave is generated along the cochlea's basilar membrane, depolarizing hair cells within the organ of Corti and thereby activating spiral ganglion auditory neurons within the cochlear modiolus. Spiral ganglion neurons collectively form the auditory portion of the vestibulocochlear (eighth cranial) nerve and project to the cochlear nucleus in the brainstem. Vascular insult to the cochlea or auditory nerve causes varying degrees of sensorineural hearing loss. The vestibular labyrinth is made up of three semicircular canals (sensitive to angular acceleration), two otolith organs (the utricle and saccule), and the endolymphatic sac (thought to be involved in fluid regulation within the inner ear). The vestibular system is integral to balance and posture by controlling vestibuloocular (image stabilization during head movement), vestibulocolic (head stabilization on the neck), and vestibulospinal (maintaining upright posture through trunk and lower extremity extensors) reflexes. Therefore, perturbation of the peripheral vestibular machinery results in vertigo and imbalance.

The arterial blood supply to the inner ear (Fig. 63.2) is provided by a single vessel, the internal auditory artery [4, 26, 53]. Though it sometimes emerges directly from the basilar artery and/or can be a branch of the posterior inferior cerebellar artery (PICA), it is a branch of the anterior inferior cerebellar artery (AICA) in 80% of people. In the internal auditory canal (IAC), the auditory nerve receives

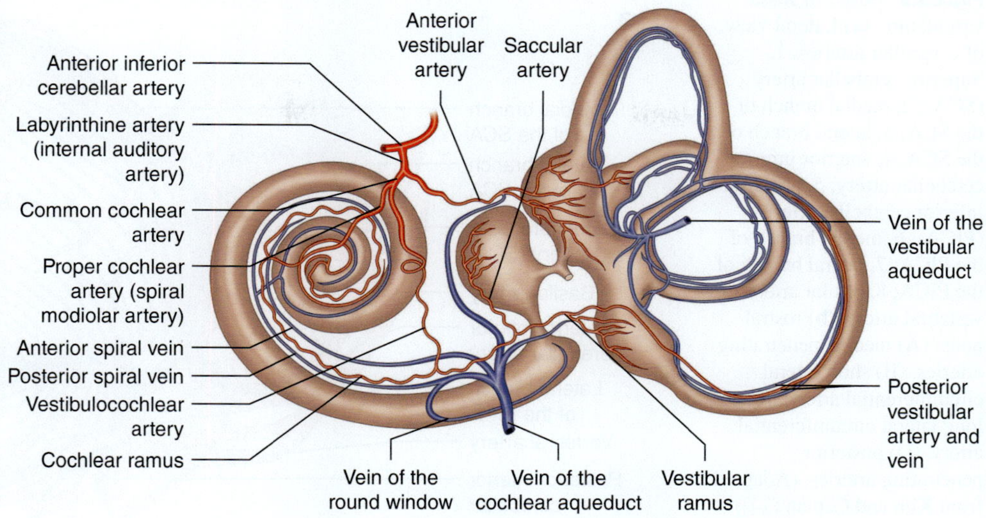

Fig. 63.2 Blood supply from the labyrinthine artery to the inner ear. (Adapted from Niparko [43])

collaterals from arteries supplying the dura mater and petrous bone. In the cerebellopontine angle, a network of anastomosing vessels from the AICA, PICA, and vertebral arteries provides the eighth cranial nerve with its blood supply [26, 37]. Entering the otic capsule through the internal auditory canal (Fig. 63.2), the labyrinthine artery first branches into the anterior vestibular artery and the common cochlear artery. The anterior vestibular artery supplies large areas of the superior and horizontal semicircular canals as well as the utricle. The common cochlear artery splits into the proper cochlear artery and the vestibulocochlear artery. The latter then branches into a cochlear ramus and the posterior vestibular artery. The proper cochlear artery supplies the apical portions of the cochlea. The posterior vestibular artery supplies the saccule and posterior semicircular canal, as well as smaller parts of the horizontal and superior canals.

Symptoms of Peripheral Vascular Injury

Lone occlusion of the labyrinthine artery is rare but can occur from arteriosclerosis in the vertebrobasilar system or as a result of an embolism [18]. The artery supplies both the cochlea and the vestibular labyrinth; therefore, obstruction of the main trunk or its terminal branches results in varying degrees of sudden unilateral hearing loss, tinnitus, and dizziness. The cochlea is more vulnerable to ischemia than the vestibular labyrinth [48, 50]. Transient experimental occlusion of the internal auditory artery produces complete cessation of auditory function within minutes, with irreversible degeneration of the cochlea [32]. The apical cochlear region is particularly vulnerable (reflected as low-frequency loss) while the vestibular end organ is most resistant [48, 50]. Labyrinthine infarction can be a marker for delayed AICA stroke. In a study by JS Kim and colleagues, 7.4% of patients with AICA territory infarction initially presented with symptoms of acute labyrinthitis [28].

Central Vascular Compromise

Cerebrovascular accidents can disrupt the central auditory pathways, resulting in several types of unilateral or bilateral hearing loss. These pathways are complex because information is not only relayed from the ear to the cortex but also has numerous interconnections that help decipher loudness, frequency, and temporal cues. Symptoms can be dramatic or subtle, sometimes requiring psychoacoustic and electrophysiological testing. Auditory dysfunction can go unrecognized, as patients may be critically ill or cognitively affected. Dizziness can manifest as true (spinning) vertigo, truncal instability, limb dysmetria, postural instability, gait abnormalities, or unsteadiness. Vertebrobasilar stroke often involves the ipsilateral cranial nerves along with crossed corticospinal signs. Cerebellar involvement is common, while sensory symptoms are typically ipsilateral for the face, but contralateral for the extremities. A unilateral Horner's syndrome can also occur. Taken together, a thorough history and exam help to formulate an appropriate differential diagnosis.

Anatomy: The Posterior Circulation (Fig. 63.3)

The vertebral artery (VA) originates as the first branch of the subclavian artery. Segment 1 extends from the subclavian to the fifth or sixth cervical vertebra, where the VA enters its transverse foramen. Segment 2 lies within the transverse foramina until C2, while Segment 3 traverses the suboccipital triangle to pierce the dura and becomes Segment 4.

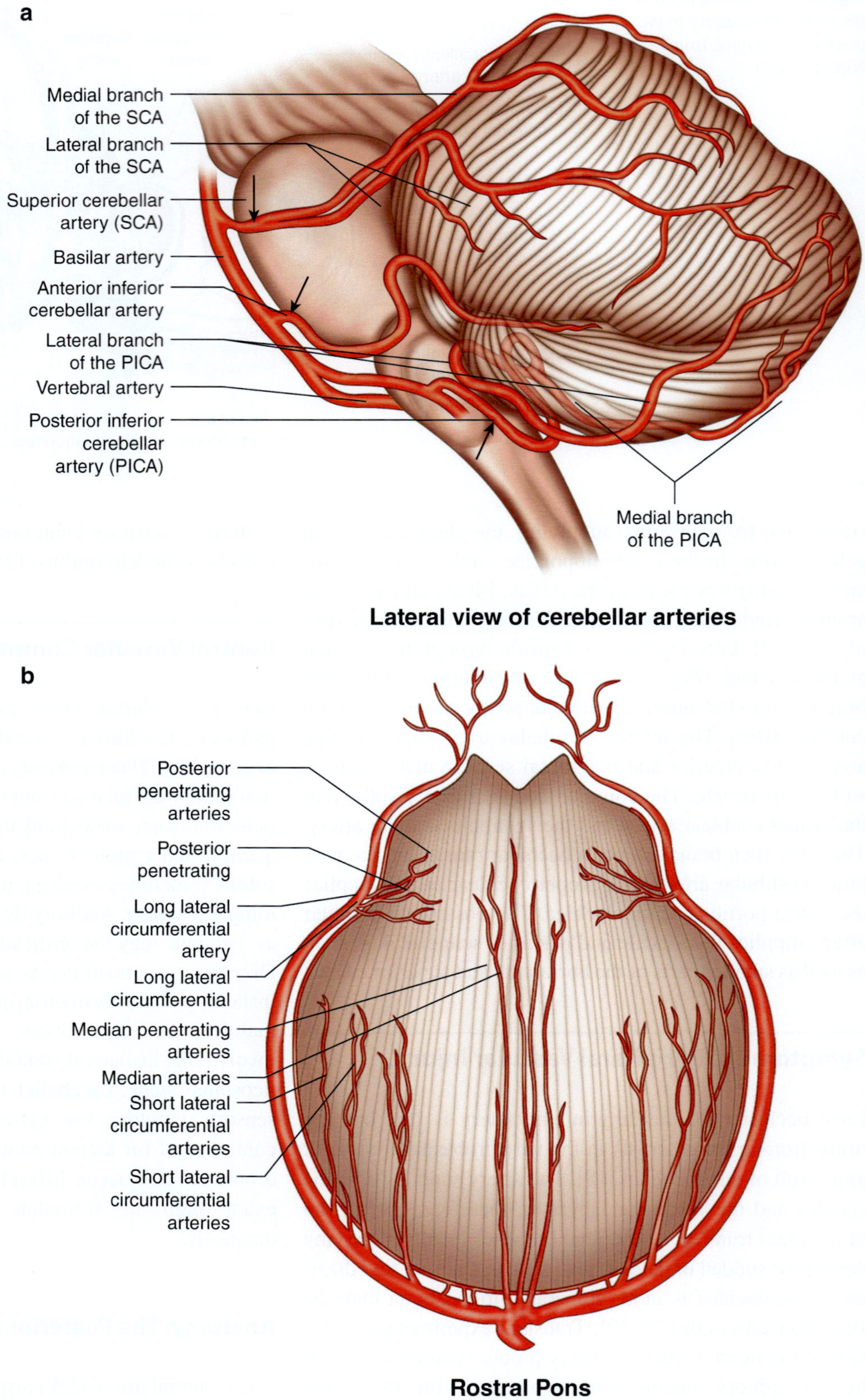

Fig. 63.3 Posterior fossa vasculature. (**a**) Lateral view of cerebellar arteries. 1, Superior cerebellar artery (SCA); 2, medial branch of the SCA; 3, lateral branch of the SCA; 4, anterior inferior cerebellar artery; 5, posterior inferior cerebellar artery (PICA); 6, medial branch of the PICA; 7, lateral branch of the PICA; 8, basilar artery; 9, vertebral artery. (**b**) rostral pons: (A) median penetrating arteries. (B) short lateral circumferential arteries. (C) long lateral circumferential artery. (D) posterior penetrating arteries. (Adapted from Kim and Caplan [24])

Though anatomic variations are common, the two vertebral arteries usually join at the pontomedullary junction to form the basilar artery (BA).

There are three paired long circumferential arteries supplying the brainstem/cerebellum, including the posterior inferior cerebellar artery (PICA), the anterior inferior cerebellar artery (AICA), and the superior cerebellar artery (SCA) (Fig. 63.3a). The PICA usually arises from the VA caudal to the roots of CN 9 and 10, encircles the medulla laterally, and has a complex course along the cerebellar tonsils. The PICA has two main terminal branches: a medial branch that supplies the dorsolateral medulla and the caudal/dorsomedial cerebellum, as well as a lateral branch that supplies the anterolateral cerebellum caudally. The AICA typically originates from the basilar artery and travels dorsally to supply the middle cerebellar peduncle, the flocculus, and portions of the anterior inferior cerebellum. The SCA arises from the rostral basilar artery and sends medial and lateral branches to the rostral cerebellum and the rostral pons. The brainstem parenchyma is primarily supplied by three groups of arterial perforators arising from the VA, BA, or any of the named branches described above (Fig. 63.3b). Paired median arteries penetrate the brainstem shortly after their takeoff and supply the paramedian, basal, and tegmental regions, while short lateral circumferential arteries supply the intermediate tegmentum and basal areas. The long lateral circumferential arteries (PICA, AICA, and SCA) supply the lateral tegmental regions of the brainstem; the labyrinthine artery supplies the cochlear nuclei. The superior olive and lateral lemniscus are supplied by short circumferential branches of the basilar artery, while the inferior colliculus obtains its blood supply from the superior cerebellar arteries. Thalamogeniculate arteries supply the medial geniculate body of the thalamus, and the middle cerebral arteries supply the auditory cortices/association areas.

Anatomy: The Brainstem

The brainstem (medulla oblongata, pons, and midbrain) contains ten pairs of cranial nerve nuclei (III–XII), the reticular formation (controlling consciousness, pain perception, and cardiopulmonary functions), as well as the fiber tracts from the cerebral cortex and spinal cord. Its dorsal median sulcus is continuous with the spinal cord, while dorsal columns on either side of the sulcus contain first-order sensory axons. These project to the nucleus gracilis and the nucleus cuneatus in the medulla, where axons decussate to form the medial lemniscus (second order neurons projecting to the thalamus). On the brainstem's ventral surface, pyramids (corticospinal motor projections) run on both sides of the ventral median fissure; these fibers cross in the caudal medulla as the pyramidal decussation.

Lateral to each pyramid lies the olive, which marks the inferior olivary nucleus. Along with the motor cortex, the sensory cortex, and the red nucleus, its crossed projections to the cerebellum influence equilibrium, balance, and deliberate movements. The upper third of the medulla contains the fourth ventricle, which is widest at the pontomedullary junction, where the foramen of Luschka is located. The cerebral aqueduct, which is a rostral continuation of the fourth ventricle, passes through the midbrain. The dorsal midbrain contains paired elevations, the superior and inferior colliculi, which house visual and auditory fibers, respectively. The ventral midbrain is dominated by the prominent crus cerebri, containing corticobulbar and corticospinal tracts. The ventral pons contains transverse pontocerebellar fibers that project to the contralateral cerebellar hemispheres via the middle cerebellar peduncles.

Along the floor of the fourth ventricle lie several lower cranial nerve nuclei. Medial to lateral, these include the hypoglossal nucleus, the dorsal nucleus of the vagus nerve (parasympathetic), and the vestibular nuclei. Ventromedial to the hypoglossal nucleus is the medial longitudinal fasciculus (MLF), connecting the vestibular nuclei to CN 3, 4, and 6 nuclei—essential to the vestibuloocular reflex (VOR). The dorsolateral aspect of the rostral medulla houses the inferior cerebellar peduncles and cochlear nuclei. Medial to the inferior cerebellar peduncle but ventral to the vestibular nuclei is the solitary nucleus and tract, which receives visceral afferents from CN 7, 9, and 10. Between this and the inferior olive is the nucleus ambiguus, motor to CN 9, 10, and 11. The trigeminal sensory nuclei and tracts, the rostral continuation of the spinal cord's dorsal horns, extend through much of the brainstem. Along the floor of the fourth ventricle in the pons lie the abducens nucleus, the facial motor nucleus, and the trigeminal motor nucleus. Cranial nerves 6 (abducens), 7 (facial), and 8 (vestibulocochlear) emerge at the pontomedullary junction, while the glossopharyngeal (CN9), vagus (CN10), and hypoglossal (CN12) nerves exit the ventrolateral medulla. CN11 has contributions from both the brainstem and spinal cord.

Anatomy: The Cerebellum

The cerebellum is connected to the midbrain, pons, and medulla by fiber tracts within the superior, middle, and inferior cerebellar peduncles, respectively. The cerebellum overlies the fourth ventricle and consists of two hemispheres joined by the midline vermis. Afferent projections to the cerebellum include the spinocerebellar fibers, the olivocerebellar fibers (from the inferior olive), the vestibulocerebellar fibers, and the pontocerebellar fibers. These enter via the peduncles and terminate either in the granular layer (mossy fibers), the Purkinje layer (climbing fibers), or in the deep cerebellar nuclei. Axons of Purkinje cells are the only axons that exit the cerebellar cortex, but most synapse on the deep cerebellar dentate, fastigial, globose, and emboliform nuclei. These deep nuclei also receive afferents from the pons, spinal cord, brainstem reticular formation, and vestibular nuclei; therefore, their efferent projections to the vestibular nuclei, the red nucleus, and the thalamus reflect a coordinated response to multiple inputs.

The flocculonodular lobe and the fastigial nucleus are involved in balance/equilibrium. They connect to the brainstem reticular formation and vestibular nuclei through the inferior cerebellar peduncle. A portion of the fastigial efferent system also contributes to the contralateral vestibulospinal and reticulospinal tracts; therefore, outputs from the fastigial nucleus are bilateral. The vermis/paravermis, along with the globose and emboliform nuclei, control muscle tone and posture. Afferent projections are ipsilateral, while efferents from the globose and emboliform nuclei project to the contralateral red nucleus via the superior cerebellar peduncle. Output (rubrospinal tract) from the red nucleus is also crossed. Lastly, the cerebellar hemispheres and the dentate nuclei control fine motor functions. Midline cerebellar lesions result in loss of postural control, while unilateral lesions of the cerebellar hemispheres cause ipsilateral incoordination of the arms (intention tremor) and gait instability without lower extremity weakness. Bilateral cerebellar lesions cause slurred speech (dysarthria), incoordination of both arms, and cerebellar ataxia (wide-based gait). Lesions involving the cerebellum can also cause nystagmus, typically made worse by gaze toward the side of the lesion.

Imaging of Acute Stroke

Though acute stroke imaging can be performed using either computed tomography (CT) or magnetic resonance imaging (MRI), CT is still the most commonly used modality. For the workup, a non-contrast head CT is obtained first, but this may be bundled with a CT angiogram (CTA) or CT perfusion scan (CTP) if necessary. A non-contrast head CT recognizes acute intracranial hemorrhage, which is a contraindication to the administration of thrombolytics. If no hemorrhage is found, signs of an acute infarction are then sought; for example, the presence of cytotoxic edema (Fig. 63.4), where edema blurs the gray-white matter junction. This edema may secondarily cause local mass effect, crowding the adjacent subarachnoid spaces. Sometimes, an arterial thrombus can be seen since the clot is denser than flowing blood within the vasculature. This is most common in the middle cerebral artery (MCA) and is known as the dense MCA sign; however, it can also be seen in the basilar artery. After the non-contrast head CT, a CTA may be obtained to look for arterial occlusion of a large proximal intracranial vessel (Fig. 63.5). A CTA of the neck is commonly performed in tandem (1) to evaluate the carotid and vertebral arteries, which may show a significant stenosis or plaque ulceration acting as a source for emboli, and (2) as an arterial map for a neurointerventionalist planning to perform catheter angiography. CT perfusion (CTP) studies can be obtained next to assess for an ischemic penumbra, which represents potentially salvageable brain tissue around the area of core infarct (Fig. 63.6). The main reference perfusion map for assessing core infarction is the cerebral blood volume (CBV) map. Barring abnormalities such as a cystic

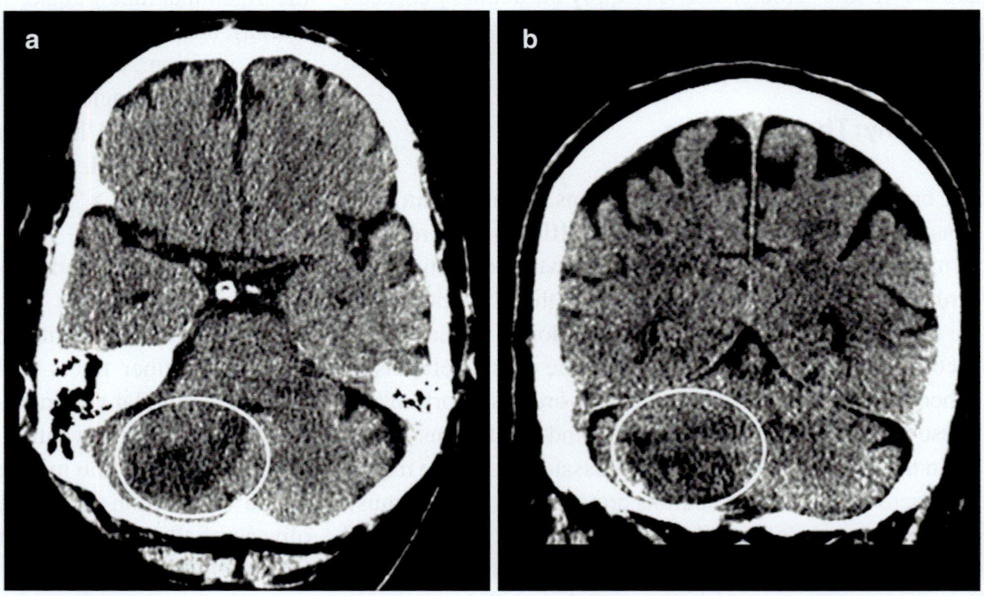

Fig. 63.4 Acute infarction on (**a**) axial and (**b**) coronal CT images. Cytotoxic edema from the infarct appears hypodense to the cerebellum. Note the involvement of both gray and white matter

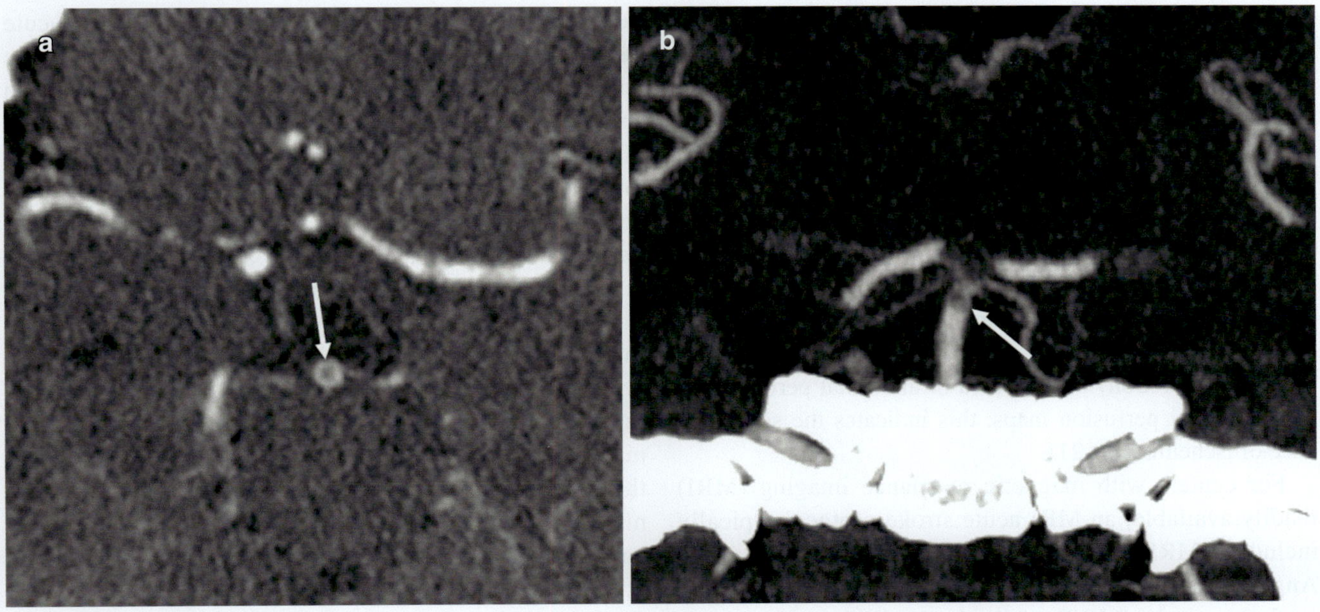

Fig. 63.5 Basilar tip thrombosis. Axial CTA image (**a**) shows contrast outlining central thrombus in the basilar artery, while the coronal CTA image (**b**) clearly shows thrombus at the tip of the artery

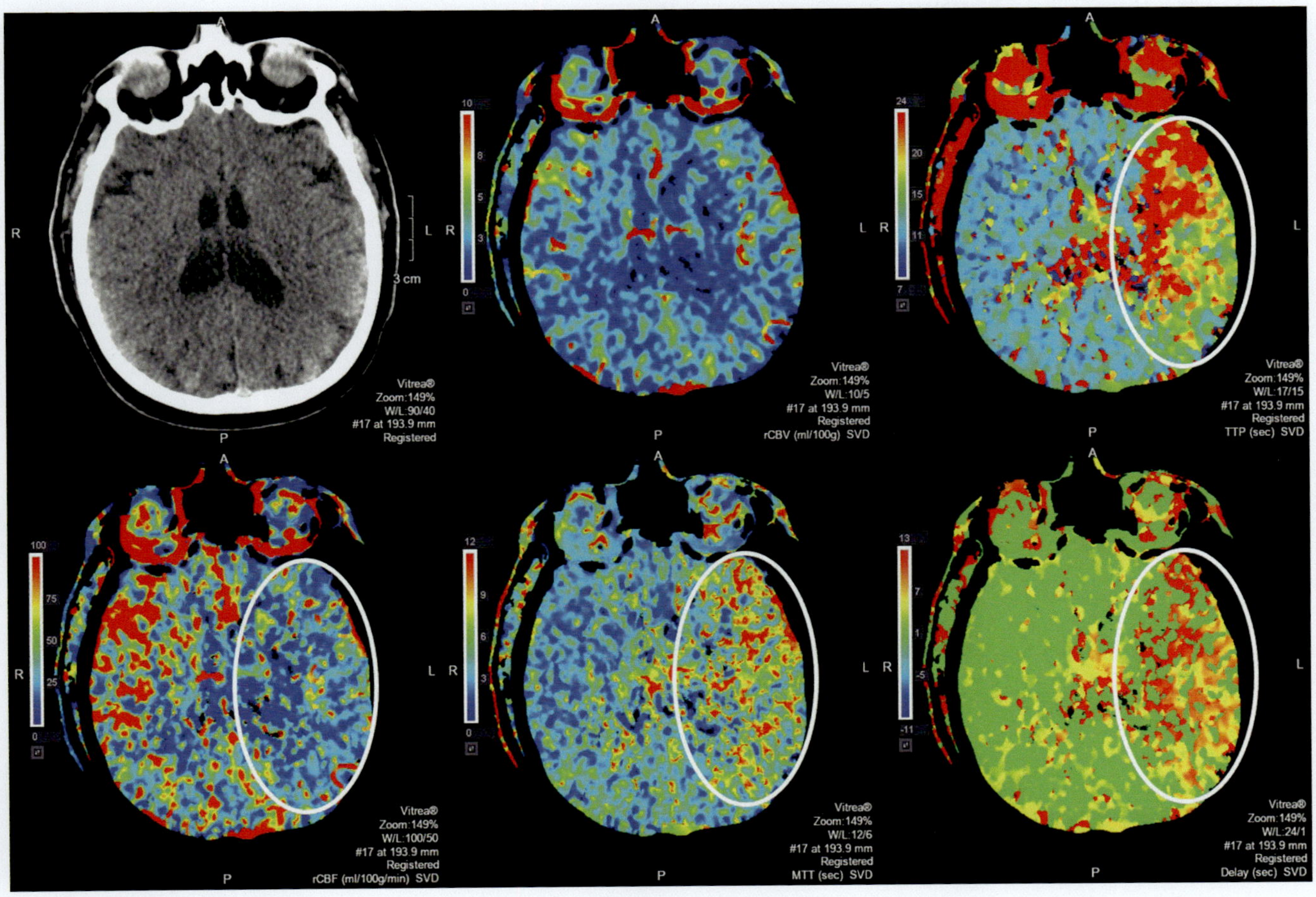

Fig. 63.6 CT perfusion of ischemia. CT perfusion images are in color. The rCBV map (center, upper image) shows normal, symmetric perfusion. The additional color perfusion maps show abnormal perfusion in the left middle cerebral artery territory. This pattern of normal rCBV with abnormal additional perfusion maps indicates ischemia

lesion or chronic infarct (which would have been seen on the non-contrast head CT), an area of low blood volume on the CBV map indicates the area of core infarction. The other perfusion maps measure specific elements of cerebral perfusion such as cerebral blood flow (CBF), mean transit time (MTT), and time to peak (TTP). If the area of abnormality on these maps is larger than the area of core infarction on the CBV map, the additional area around the infarct represents the ischemic penumbra. Should the area of abnormality on these maps be the same as the area on the CBV map, no ischemic penumbra is present. Alternatively, if there is normal CBV (no infarction) with an area of abnormal perfusion on the additional perfusion maps, this indicates the sole presence of ischemia [11, 21].

For centers with magnetic resonance imaging (MRI) readily available, an MRI acute stroke protocol typically includes MRI of the brain, Magnetic Resonance Angiography (MRA) of the head and neck, and an MR perfusion study (MRP) of the brain. With modern MRI scanners, a tailored acute stroke protocol can be performed in about 6 min, almost the same time as a CT/CTA/CTP protocol [40]. MR images with diffusion-weighted imaging sequences (DWI) show acute infarctions as bright. Since bright signal is not specific to acute infarction, this finding should be correlated with the apparent diffusion coefficient (ADC) map, in which an area of acute infarction will show dark signal. This pattern of infarction with bright DWI and dark ADC signal is known as restricted diffusion (Fig. 63.7). Certain processes, such as vasogenic edema, may show a bright signal on the DWI images and also a bright signal on the ADC map. In this case, the bright DWI signal is known as the T2 shine-through, which is not related to an acute infarction. If a non-contrast head CT is not performed, a gradient-recalled echo (GRE)–based MR sequence is imperative to assess for the presence of an acute intracranial hemorrhage where blood will appear black. MRA of the head and neck is used to assess intracranial/extracranial vascular stenosis or occlusion (Fig. 63.8). MRP, similar to CTP, is used to look for hypo-perfused brain tissue at risk surrounding the area of core infarct (Fig. 63.9). DWI is used as the reference sequence to assess core infarction, while perfusion maps such as relative cerebral blood flow (rCBF), MTT, TTP, and time-to-maximum (Tmax) are used to assess hypoperfusion [11].

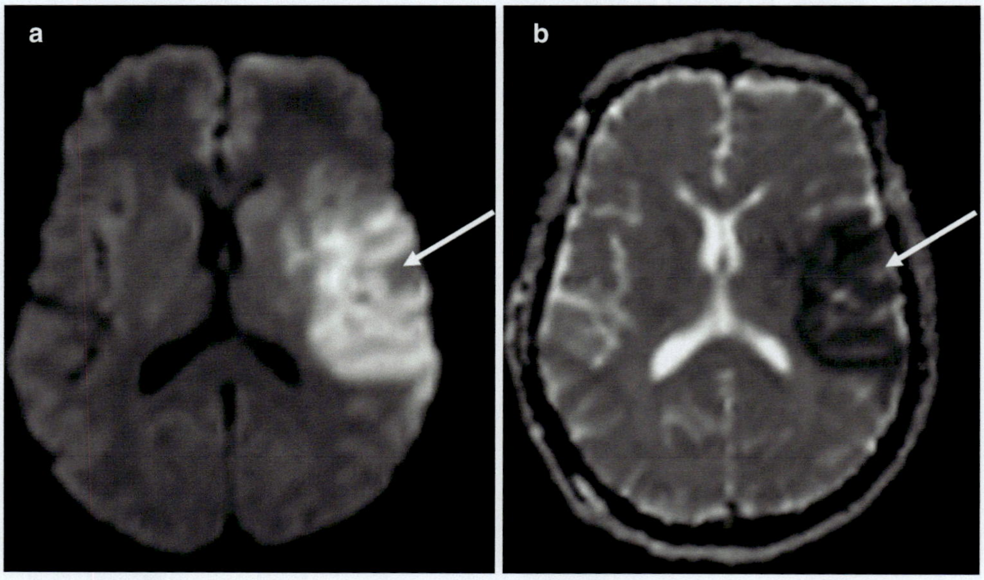

Fig. 63.7 Acute infarction on MRI DWI/ADC. DWI image (**a**) shows a bright signal in the area of acute infarction, which is confirmed as restricted diffusion with a corresponding dark signal on the ADC map (**b**)

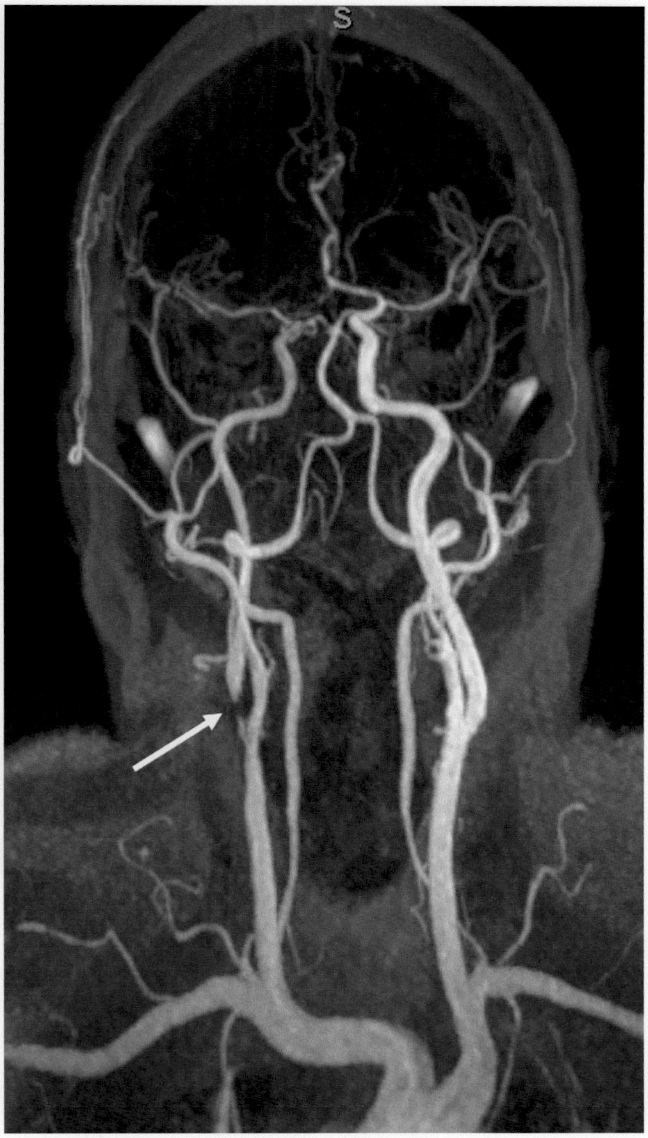

Fig. 63.8 Severe carotid stenosis. Contrast-enhanced MRA of the head and neck shows a string sign with near occlusion in the right carotid bulb

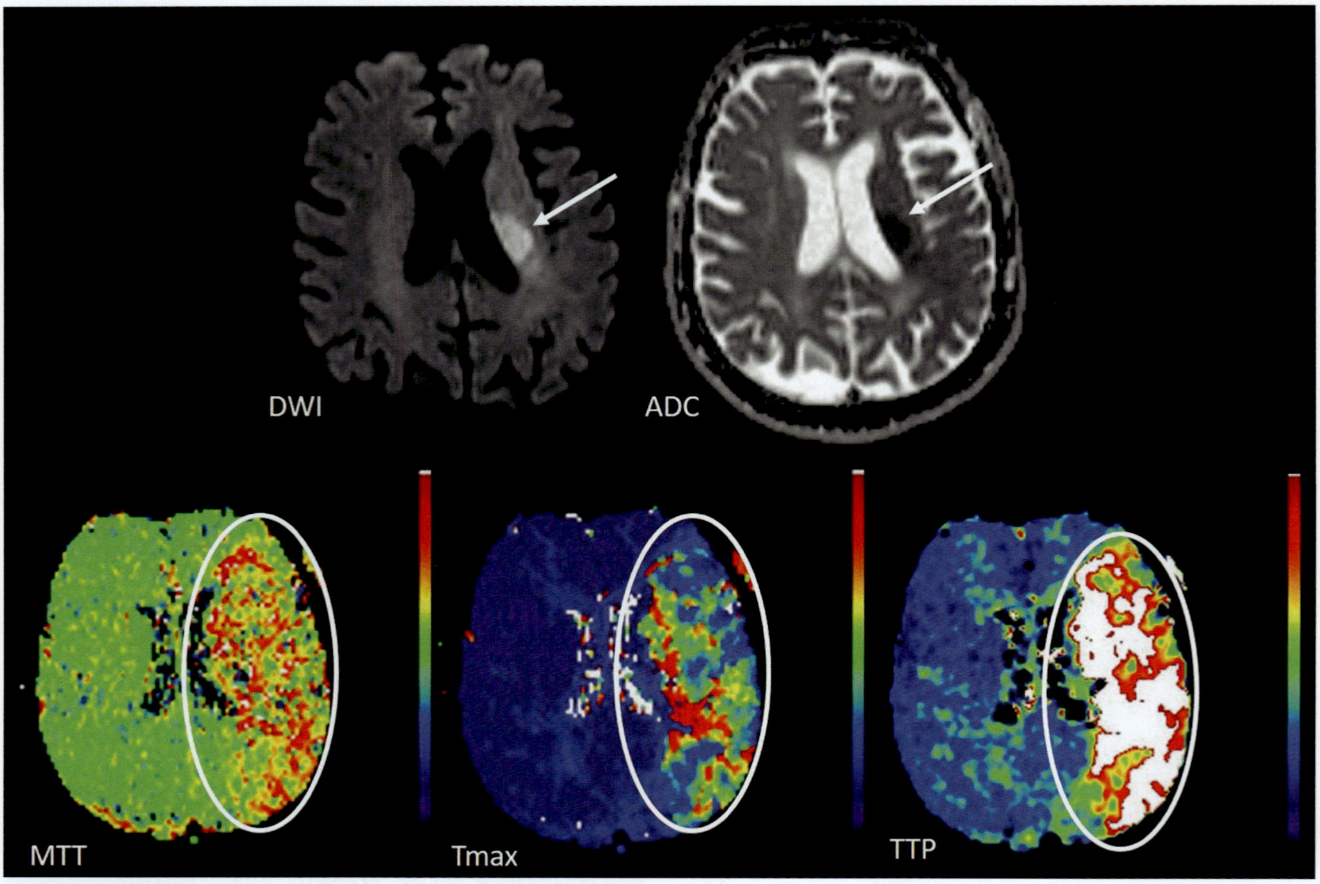

Fig. 63.9 MR Perfusion of the infarct and the surrounding brain at risk of infarction. MR perfusion images are in color. The DWI/ADC images show a small area of restricted diffusion, indicating the core infarction. The additional color perfusion maps show abnormal perfusion in the left middle cerebral artery territory well beyond the area of core infarction. This pattern indicates a sizable area of brain tissue at risk of infarction beyond the area of core infarct

Topographic Syndromes

Lateral Medullary Infarcts

Symptoms of lateral medullary infarction (Fig. 63.10) may be sudden or evolve over a period of days. Spinning vertigo occurs in approximately 60% of affected patients, and though this can sometimes improve or resolve, gait instability and imbalance can persist indefinitely [23]. Injury may involve the vestibular nuclei, vestibulospinal projections, the inferior cerebellar peduncle, spinocerebellar fibers, or the cerebellar parenchyma. Nausea and vomiting have a multifactorial etiology—vestibular, cerebellar, and injury to brainstem vomiting centers. Nystagmus is typically horizontal or torsional to the side opposite the infarct [15], while lateral gaze toward the lesion results in hypermetric saccades [13]. Injury to lemniscal fibers in the caudal medulla can cause ipsilateral paresthesias and extremity clumsiness [22]. Gait ataxia is more common than limb dysmetria [7] in these patients. Upper motor neuron type facial weakness is found in about 20% of patients [23], and Horner's syndrome occurs in up to 90% of patients. Two-thirds have dysphagia and hoarseness, but dysarthria is less common [23]. Sensory abnormalities are universal, including ipsilateral face and contralateral body, contralateral face and body, bilateral face and contralateral body, contralateral body only, and ipsilateral face only—based on involvement in the descending trigeminal tract, the ascending secondary trigeminal tracts, and the spinothalamic tracts [27].

Cerebellar Infarcts

The cerebellum has three main vascular territories: the SCA, AICA, and PICA. The SCA territory is the largest and supplies the entire surface of the superior cerebellar hemisphere, the ipsilateral superior vermis, the majority of the cerebellar deep white matter, and most of the dentate nucleus. The PICA supplies most of the posterior inferior cerebellar hemisphere and the ipsilateral cerebellum, while the AICA covers the inferolateral cerebellum. Occasionally, a vertebral artery will terminate in a common AICA–PICA trunk [10].

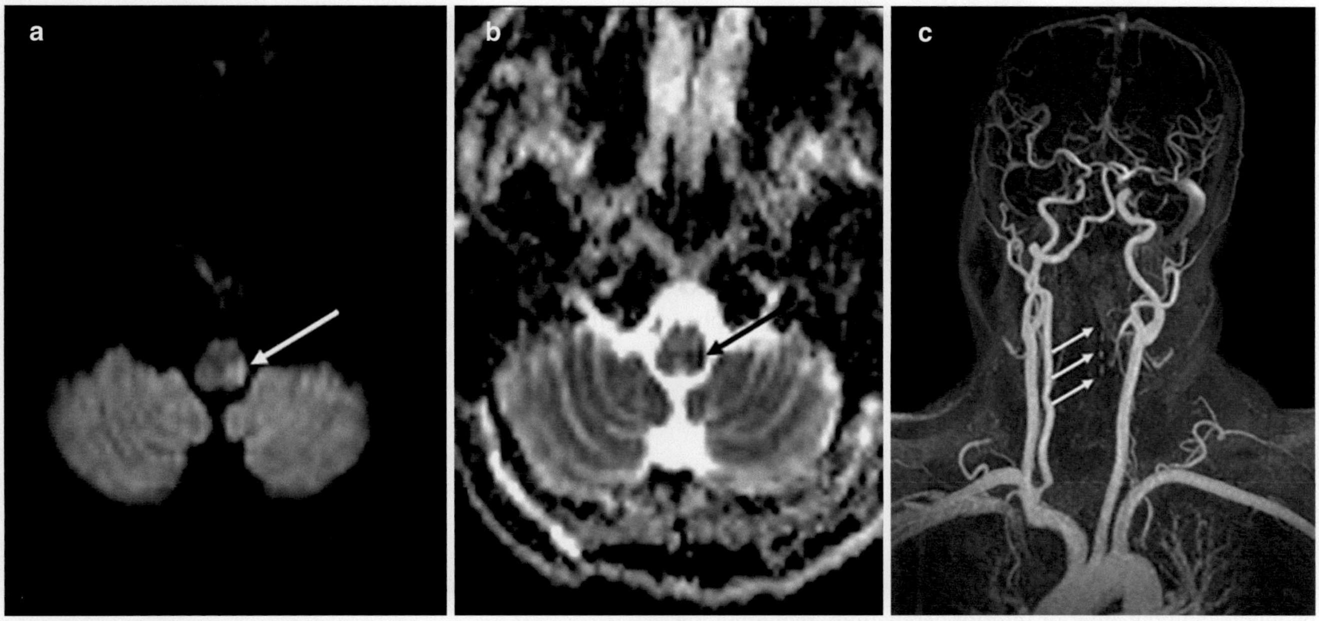

Fig. 63.10 Acute lateral medullary infarct. A pattern of restricted diffusion on the (**a**) DWI and (**b**) ADC images indicate acute infarction, in this case in the lateral medulla. (**c**) The source is an acute left vertebral artery dissection, which can be seen as faint interrupted contrast opacification in the mid to distal portion of the artery on the MRA

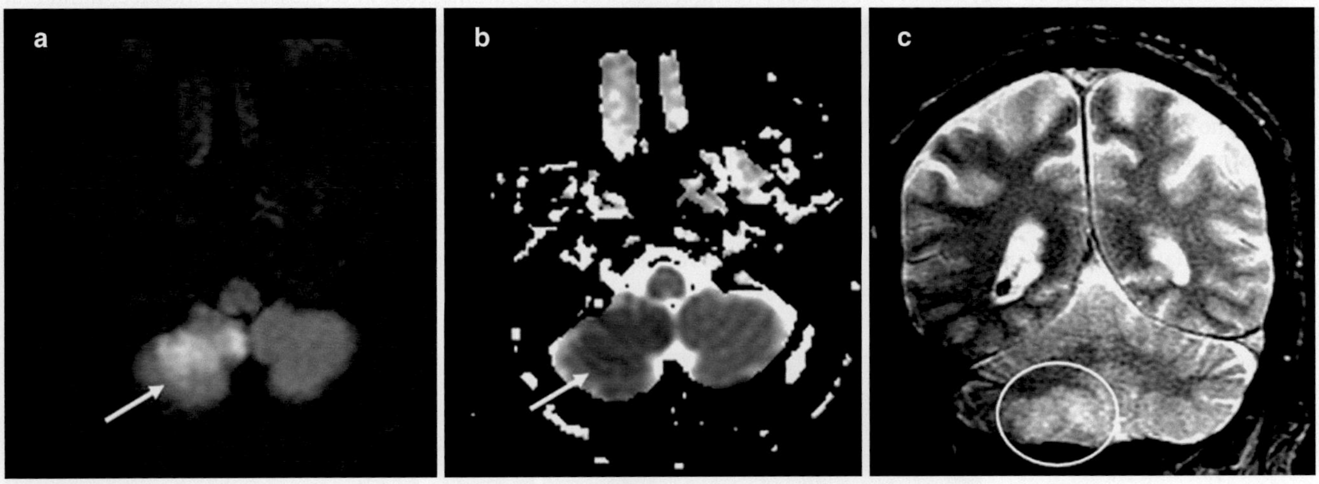

Fig. 63.11 Acute right PICA infarct. Acute infarction on the (**a**) DWI and (**b**) ADC images can be localized better on the coronal T2-weighted image (**c**), where associated edema is present (oval). The inferior and posterior cerebellar location localizes the infarct to the PICA territory

Cerebellar infarcts, arising from AICA, PICA, and/or SCA (superior cerebellar artery) disease, account for <5% of brain infarctions [5]. The most common symptoms are dizziness (vertigo is less common), nausea, and gait disturbance [34, 55]. Nystagmus is typically horizontal but can be vertical, bobbing, or complex. Dysarthria and limb clumsiness are important distinguishing signs of brainstem disease, while decreased consciousness may suggest impending tonsillar herniation. PICA infarcts with cerebellar compromise are most common (Fig. 63.11); partial territory PICA infarcts are more common than full territory infarcts; and medial territory infarcts outnumber lateral PICA infarctions [29]. Lateral PICA infarcts cause gait ataxia and limb ataxia. Medial PICA infarcts involving the uvulonodular vermis can present with isolated vertigo, mimicking vestibular neuritis; however, caloric testing in these patients is normal.

Posterior Inferior Cerebellar Artery (PICA) Infarcts

Sudden deafness due to a non-AICA territory infarction is associated with vascular compromise in the PICA distribution (Fig. 63.11). The labyrinthine artery usually originates from the AICA (80%), but can originate from the PICA (3%) or directly from the basilar artery (approximately 15%) [25]. PICA primarily supplies the dorsolateral medulla, the inferior part of the vestibular nuclear complex, the inferior cerebellar peduncle, and the posteroinferior cerebellum. Wallenberg's syndrome, first described in 1895 [56], accounts for about 2% of all patients admitted for acute stroke [44] and is associated with vertigo, ataxia, vomiting, diplopia, limb ataxia, ipsilateral Horner's syndrome, contralateral hemianesthesia, facial anesthesia, dysphagia, dysphonia, ocular tilt reaction, and spontaneous nystagmus.

Anterior Inferior Cerebellar Artery (AICA) Infarcts

The anterior inferior cerebellar artery supplies the inner ear, anterolateral regions of the caudal pons, the middle cerebral peduncle, and the anterior inferior cerebellum, including the flocculus. In 1943, Adams was the first to describe the neurotologic syndrome of AICA occlusion in which hearing loss was an early symptom [1]. Since that time, an acute ischemic stroke in the distribution of AICA is known to cause vertigo, sudden unilateral hearing loss, ipsilateral facial anesthesia and/or weakness, lateral gaze palsy, Horner's syndrome, cerebellar dysmetria, and occasionally contralateral body anesthesia. The most common mechanism of AICA infarction is an atheroma or thrombus in the parent basilar artery [1] near the AICA branch point. Interestingly, sudden hearing loss is common [16, 31, 46], present in up to 92% of AICA infarctions, and may be due to inner ear injury, auditory nerve compromise, or ischemia at the cochlear nucleus. Auditory disturbance has also been identified as a prodrome for AICA infarction [30, 35], and partial ischemia in the AICA territory can lead to an isolated acute auditory syndrome such as hearing loss and tinnitus [31]. Though rare, patients with vertebrobasilar insufficiency can also present with isolated dizziness. In a study by Fife and colleagues, these patients typically had atherosclerotic disease near the AICA branch point, likely resulting in transient ischemic attacks [14]. Because symptoms and signs of cerebellar infarction can be similar to this or even benign peripheral labyrinthine disorders, many patients with cerebellar infarcts may be overlooked unless specifically assessed by CT/MRI. Lee and colleagues, in their 2002 study, also found that when AICA is completely occluded, the joint brainstem and cerebellar signs are always present.

Superior Cerebellar Artery (SCA) Infarcts

Classical descriptions of SCA infarction (Fig. 63.12) describe ipsilateral limb ataxia, contralateral loss of pain and temperature sensation of the face, arm, leg, and trunk, ipsilateral Horner's syndrome, loss of expression in the face, unilateral or bilateral hearing loss, and contralateral fourth nerve palsy—most of these symptoms arising from injury to the upper pons and lower midbrain [9, 38]. Loss of hearing ability reflects damage to the lateral lemniscus. Interestingly, however, most patients do not have these symptoms; instead, they typically have signs of cerebellar dysfunction only. A recent study suggested that the most prominent clinical presentation in the medial SCA territory cerebellar infarction is severe gait ataxia with sudden falls or severe veering,

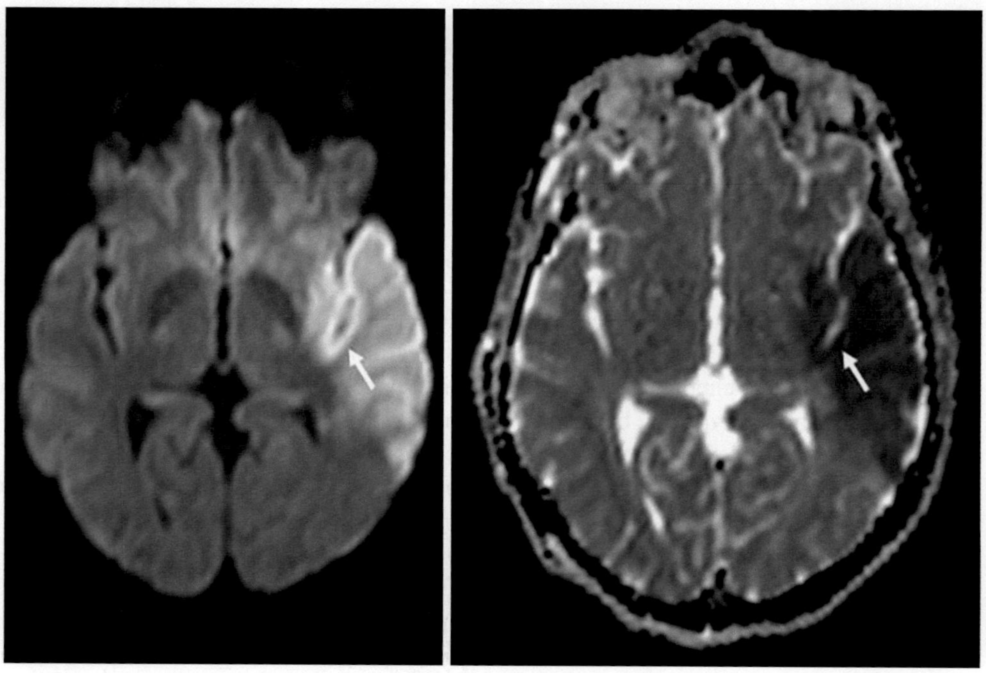

Fig. 63.12 Acute SCA infarcts. Seeing the temporal lobe (*), occipital lobe (triangle), and superior cerebellar peduncle (open arrow) in the plane all helps to localize this level to the upper cerebellum. The acute infarcts (solid arrows) are therefore in the SCA vascular territory

observed in 76% of patients [52]. Though rarer, SCA stroke may be impossible to distinguish from the more common partial AICA or PICA territory CVA. The superior cerebellum does not have many vestibular connections; therefore, cerebellar infarction in the region of the SCA is not often associated with vertigo [3, 19]. A low incidence of vertigo in SCA disease may be useful clinically to distinguish it from PICA or AICA cerebellar infarction.

Temporal Lobe Infarction

Central auditory disorders are characterized by cortical deafness and auditory agnosia. Cortical deafness is rare, requiring bilateral temporal lobe lesions, and only one case of acute, bilateral temporal lobe infarct has been reported [39]. More typically, the infarct involves one temporal lobe (Fig. 63.13) as a result of middle cerebral artery occlusion, causing symptoms such as hemiparesis and aphasia; then a second infarct on the contralateral side causes profound sensorineural hearing loss [6]. If the nondominant side suffers the first stroke, no auditory symptoms may be present. Some studies implicate gray matter damage as the source of cortical deafness, while others suggest that damage to the auditory radiations may contribute [12, 54]. For those suffering from cortical deafness, the extent of the temporal lobe infarct correlates with prognosis. Many patients recover their ability to recognize environmental sounds and tonality, but may have pure word deafness. Auditory agnosia refers to deficiencies in sound perception or identification in the context of intact hearing, cognitive functioning, and language. This can affect the isolated auditory domains. For example, verbal auditory agnosia is also known as pure word deafness, and amusia refers to deficits in music perception. The deficits may affect basic perception or interpretation of meaning [51].

Using HINTS (Head Impulse, Nystagmus, Test of Skew) to Differentiate Central from Peripheral Etiologies in Acute Vestibular Syndrome

Dizziness and vertigo account for about four million emergency department (ED) visits annually in the United States, and up to 15% have cerebrovascular causes [42, 57]. In patients having persistent dizziness, vertigo, or gait instability along with spontaneous nystagmus, a practitioner can utilize HINTS testing to distinguish peripheral from central lesions. This modality is a bedside option, quick/easy to perform, and provides useful clinical information. HINTS has been shown to be more sensitive than ABCD2 (risk stratification rule utilizing age, blood pressure, clinical features, duration of symptoms, and diabetes) and brain MRI with DWI sequences for diagnosing acute stroke of less than 48 h duration [20, 42].

Nystagmus must be present to use HINTS in the acute vestibular syndrome. Spontaneous vertical, horizontal, or pure-torsional gaze-evoked nystagmus can be seen with central lesions. However, unidirectional nystagmus following Alexander's law and mixed horizontal-torsional nystagmus are particularly characteristic of peripheral lesions.

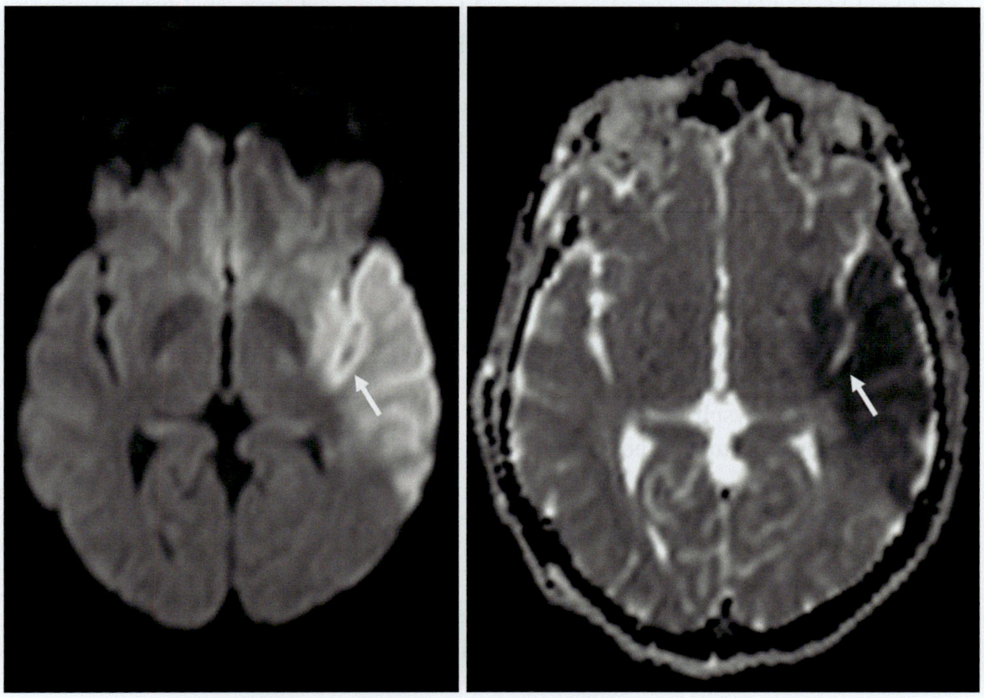

Fig. 63.13 Acute left temporal lobe infarct. This left temporal lobe infarct involves the cortex within the Sylvian fissure, including the area of Heschl's gyrus

Bedside head impulse testing (HIT) in **HI**NTS assesses the function of the semicircular canals, which initiate the vestibuloocular reflex. While a patient fixes on a target, the practitioner makes multiple, unpredictable, small-amplitude, high-frequency head rotations in the plane of the horizontal semicircular canals. The eyes should stay on the target during the bedside HIT. If the eyes initially move with the head during head impulse and then make a catch-up saccade back to the target, it is a positive HIT toward the side of the rapid head movement. Video HIT may be used instead if such equipment is readily available. Negative or normal HIT in acute vestibular syndrome usually suggests a central etiology. Positive or abnormal HIT is not always indicative of a peripheral lesion; exceptions include cases affecting the vestibular root entry zone, cranial nerve eight fascicle, or vestibular nucleus.

The test of Skew in HIN**TS** involves looking for vertical ocular misalignment due to static imbalance in the utriculo-ocular motor pathways. The test is performed by covering one eye for 1–2 s and then uncovering that eye while the other eye is covered quickly. The practitioner looks for a corrective refixation of the uncovered eye. Pronounced skew deviation would be seen with some central lesions.

The highest sensitivity component of the battery is the horizontal HIT, whereas skew deviation is the most specific part of the exam [8]. If any of the three sections of HINTS suggest a central localization (normal HIT, nystagmus not following Alexander's law, pronounced skew deviation), the practitioner must rule out central lesions. An urgent brain MRI with DWI sequences, along with MR angiography of the head/neck, is the next step. If MRI is contraindicated, consider CT perfusion with CT angiography of the head and neck. Should initial imaging not show a central lesion, consider repeating imaging tests after 72 h from the onset of symptoms [57].

A practitioner should also consider an anterior inferior cerebellar artery stroke in patients presenting with acute vertigo and hearing loss, along with a positive HIT. While MRI typically demonstrates posterior fossa ischemia, isolated labyrinthine ischemia is possible and would not be noted on MRI. Other components of the bedside exam for differentiating a stroke from peripheral vestibulopathy are head-shaking nystagmus (perverted, opposite to spontaneous, or with early reversal), saccadic ocular pursuit, hypo- or hypermetric saccades, hemiparesis, dysphagia, dysarthria, and inability to maintain an upright posture without support.

Conclusion

Strokes are difficult to diagnose as they often have complex multi-systemic manifestations. Peripheral audiologic and vestibular manifestations often involve acute and direct neurotology expertise. Central vascular compromise often requires neurology or neurosurgical interventions for diagnosis and treatment; neurotologists may be involved for the aural and vestibular components. A high index of suspicion must be kept with any patient presenting with spontaneous hearing loss or vertigo to avoid missing the diagnosis of stroke.

References

1. Adams RD. Occlusion of the anterior inferior cerebellar artery. Arch Neurol Psychiatry. 1943;49:765–70.
2. Agrawal Y, Carey JP, Della Santina CC, Schubert MC, Minor LB. Disorders of balance and vestibular function in US adults: data from the National Health and Nutrition Examination Survey, 2001-2004. Arch Intern Med. 2009;169(10):938–44.
3. Amarenco P, Hauw JJ. Cerebellar infarction in the territory of the superior cerebellar artery: a clinicopathologic study of 33 cases. Neurology. 1990;40:1383–90.
4. Axelsson A. The blood supply of the inner ear of mammals. In: Keidel WD, Neff WD, Ades HW, editors. Handbook of sensory physiology: auditory system. Berlin: Springer; 1974.
5. Bogousslavsky J, Van Melle G, Regli F. The Lausanne Stroke Registry: analysis of 1,000 consecutive patients with first stroke. Stroke. 1988;19:1083–92.
6. Brody RM, Nicholas BD, Wolf MJ, Marcinkevich PB, Artz GJ. Cortical deafness: a case report and review of the literature. Otol Neurotol. 2013;34(7):1226–9.
7. Caplan LR. Posterior circulation disease: clinical findings, diagnosis, and management. Boston: Blackwell Science; 1996.
8. Celebisoy N. Acute vestibular syndrome: clinical head impulse test versus video head impulse test. J Neurol. 2018;265(Suppl 1):44–7. https://doi.org/10.1007/s00415-018-8804-0. Epub 2018 Mar 5
9. Chaves CJ, Caplan LR, Chung CS, Tapia J, Amarenco P, Teal P, et al. Cerebellar infarcts in the New England medical center posterior circulation stroke registry. Neurology. 1994;44:1385–90.
10. Cormier PJ, Long ER, Russell EJ. MR imaging of posterior fossa infarctions: vascular territories and clinical correlates. Radiographics. 1992;12:1079–96.
11. Dehkharghani S, Andre J. Imaging approaches to stroke and neurovascular disease. Neurosurgery. 2017;80(5):681–700.
12. Engelien A, Silbersweig D, Stern E, et al. The functional anatomy of recovery from auditory agnosia. A PET study of sound categorization in a neurological patient and normal controls. Brain. 1995;118(Pt 6):1395–409.
13. Estanol B, Lopez-Rios G. Neuro-otology of the lateral medullary infarct syndrome. Arch Neurol. 1982;39:176–9.
14. Fife TD, Baloh RW, Duckwiler GR. Isolated dizziness in vertebrobasilar insufficiency: clinical features, angiography, and follow-up. J Stroke Cerebrovasc Dis. 1994;4(1):4–12.
15. Fisher CM, Karnes WE, Kubik CS. Lateral medullary infarction-the pattern of vascular occlusion. J Neuropathol Exp Neurol. 1961;20:323–79.
16. Gerace C, Pianura C. Sudden deafness without vertigo as a sole manifestation of AICA infarct. Neurol Sci. 2008;29(5):371–2.
17. Gurgel RK, Ward PD, Schwartz S, Norton MC, Foster NL, Tschanz JAT. Relationship of hearing loss and dementia: a prospective, population-based study. Otol Neurotol. 2014;35(5):775–81.
18. Huang MH, Huang CC, Ryu SJ, Chu NS. Sudden bilateral hearing impairment in vertebrobasilar occlusive disease. Stroke. 1993;24:132–7.

19. Kase CS, White JL, Joslyn JN, Williams JP, Mohr JP. Cerebellar infarction in the superior cerebellar artery distribution. Neurology. 1985;35:705–11.
20. Kattah JC, Talkad AV, Wang DZ, Hsieh YH, Newman-Toker DE. HINTS to diagnose stroke in the acute vestibular syndrome: three-step bedside oculomotor examination more sensitive than early MRI diffusion-weighted imaging. Stroke. 2009;40(11):3504–10. https://doi.org/10.1161/STROKEAHA.109.551234. Epub 2009 Sep 17
21. Khan R, Nael K, Erly W. Acute stroke imaging: what clinicians need to know. Am J Med. 2013;126(5):379–86.
22. Kim JS. Sensory symptoms in ipsilateral limbs/body due to lateral medullary infarction. Neurology. 2001;57:1230–4.
23. Kim JS. Pure lateral medullary infarction: clinical-radiological correlation of 130 acute, consecutive patients. Brain. 2003;126:1864–72.
24. Kim JS, Caplan LR. Vertebrobasilar disease. In: Grotta JC, et al., editors. Stroke: pathophysiology, diagnosis, and management. Elsevier; 2015.
25. Kim H-A, Lee H. Recent advances in understanding audiovestibular loss of a vascular cause. J Stroke. 2017;19(1):61–6. https://doi.org/10.5853/jos.2016.00857.
26. Kim H-N, Kim YH, Park IY, Kim GR, Chung IH. Variability of the surgical anatomy of the neurovascular complex of the cerebellopontine angle. Ann Otol Rhinol Laryngol. 1990;99:288–95.
27. Kim JS, Lee JH, Lee MC. Patterns of sensory dysfunction in lateral medullary infarction. Clinical-MRI correlation. Neurology. 1997;49:1557–63.
28. Kim JS, Cho KH, Lee H. Isolated labyrinthine infarction as a harbinger of anterior inferior cerebellar artery territory infarction with normal diffusion-weighted brain MRI. J Neurol Sci. 2009;278(1-2):82–4.
29. Kumral E, Kisabay A, Atac C, et al. Spectrum of the posterior inferior cerebellar artery territory infarcts. Clinical-diffusion-weighted imaging correlates. Cerebrovasc Dis. 2005;20:370–80.
30. Lee H, Cho Y-W. Auditory disturbance as a prodrome of anterior inferior cerebellar artery infarction. J Neurol Neurosurg Psychiatry. 2003;74(12):1644–8.
31. Lee H, Sohn S-I, Jung D-K, et al. Sudden deafness and anterior inferior cerebellar artery infarction. Stroke. 2002;33(12):2807–12.
32. Levine RA, Bu-Saba N, Brown MC. Laser-Doppler measurements and electrocochleography during ischemia of the guinea pig cochlea: implications for hearing preservation in acoustic neuroma surgery. Ann Otol Rhinol Laryngol. 1993;102:127–36.
33. Lin FR, Jeffrey Metter E, O'Brien RJ, Resnick SM, Zonderman AB, Ferrucci L. Hearing loss and incident dementia. Arch Neurol. 2011;68(2):214–20.
34. Macdonell RA, Kalnins RM, Donnan GA. Cerebellar infarction: natural history, prognosis, and pathology. Stroke. 1987;18:849–55.
35. Martines F, Dispenza F, Gagliardo C, Martines E, Bentivegna D. Sudden sensorineural hearing loss as prodromal symptom of anterior inferior cerebellar artery infarction. ORL. 2011;73(3):137–40.
36. Martini A, Castiglione A, Bovo R, Vallesi A, Gabelli C. Aging, cognitive load, dementia and hearing loss. Audiol Neurotol. 2014;19(suppl 1):2–5.
37. Mazzoni A. Internal auditory artery supply to the petrous bone. Ann Otol Rhinol Laryngol. 1972;81:13–21.
38. Mills CK. Preliminary note on a new symptom complex due to lesion of the cerebellum and cerebello-rubro-thalamic system, the main symptoms being ataxia of the upper and lower extremities of one side, and the other side deafness, paralysis of emotional expression in the face, and loss of the senses of pain, heat, and cold over the entire half of the body. J Nerv Ment Dis. 1912;39:73–6.
39. Musiek FE, Baran JA, Shinn JB, et al. Central deafness: an audiological case study. Int J Audiol. 2007;46:433–41.
40. Nael K, Khan R, Choudhary G, Meshksar A, Villablanca P, Tay J, Drake K, Coull BM, Kidwell CS. Six-minute magnetic resonance imaging protocol for evaluation of acute ischemic stroke: pushing the boundaries. Stroke. 2014;45(7):1985–91.
41. Neuhauser HK, Radtke A, von Brevern M, Lezius F, Feldmann M, Lempert T. Burden of dizziness and vertigo in the community. Arch Intern Med. 2008;168(19):2118–24.
42. Newman-Toker DE, Kerber KA, Hsieh YH, Pula JH, Omron R, Saber Tehrani AS, Mantokoudis G, Hanley DF, Zee DS, Kattah JC. HINTS outperforms ABCD2 to screen for stroke in acute continuous vertigo and dizziness. Acad Emerg Med. 2013;20(10):986–96. https://doi.org/10.1111/acem.12223.
43. Niparko J. Anatomy of the vestibular system. In: Flint PW, et al., editors. Cummings otolaryngology. Elsevier; 2014.
44. Norrving B, Cronqvist S. Lateral medullary infarction: prognosis in an unselected series. Neurology. 1991;41:244–8.
45. Paciaroni M, Agnelli G, Caso V, Bogousslavsky J, editors. Manifestations of stroke. Frontiers of Neurology and Neuroscience, Vol. 30. Basel: Karger; 2012.
46. Park JH, Kim H, Han HJ. Recurrent audiovestibular disturbance initially mimicking Meniere's disease in a patient with anterior inferior cerebellar infarction. Neurol Sci. 2008;29(5):359–62.
47. Peracino A. Hearing loss and dementia in the aging population. Audiol Neurotol. 2014;19(suppl 1):6–9.
48. Perlman HB, Kimura RS, Fernandez C. Experiments on temporary obstruction of the internal auditory artery. Laryngoscope. 1959;69:591–613.
49. Rosamond W, Flegal K, Furie A, et al. Heart disease and stroke statistics—2008 update: a report from the American Heart Association Statistics Committee and Stroke Statistics Committee. Circulation. 2008;117:e25–e146.
50. Schuknecht HF. Pathology of the ear. 2nd ed. Philadelphia, PA: Lea and Febiger; 1993.
51. Slevc LR, Shell AR. Auditory agnosia. Handb Clin Neurol. 2015;129:573–87.
52. Sohn SI, Lee H, Lee SR, Baloh RW. Cerebellar infarction in the territory of the medial branch of the superior cerebellar artery. Neurology. 2006;66:115–7.
53. Sunderland S. The arterial relations of the internal auditory meatus. Brain. 1945;68(1):23–7.
54. Tanaka Y, Kamo T, Yoshida M, Yamadori A. 'So-called' cortical deafness. Clinical, neurophysiological and radiological observations. Brain. 1991;114(Pt 6):2385–401.
55. Tohgi H, Takahashi S, Chiba K, Hirata Y. Cerebellar infarction: clinical and neuroimaging analysis in 293 patients. Stroke. 1993;24(11):1697–701.
56. Wallenberg A. Acute bulbar affection (Embolie der art. cerebellar post. inf. sinistra?). Arch f Psychiat Nervenkr. 1895;27:504–40.
57. Zwergal A, Dieterich M. Vertigo and dizziness in the emergency room. Curr Opin Neurol. 2020;33(1):117–25. https://doi.org/10.1097/WCO.0000000000000769.

Systemic Disorders Affecting the Temporal Bone

64

Jonathan L. Hatch and Theodore R. McRackan

Introduction

Systemic disorders that affect the temporal bone are numerous and diverse pathologies that may be idiopathic, autoimmune, infectious, neoplastic, or genetic. Often, the initial manifestations of these disorders are found within the head and neck, including the ear. This chapter aims to promote an understanding of the basic underlying pathophysiology of these disorders, as well as systemic and ear-specific symptoms. In addition, key audiometric data, radiographic findings, and serologic markers are discussed. Finally, medical and surgical treatment modalities are highlighted.

Neurosarcoidosis

Sarcoidosis is a disease that is manifested by a multisystem, granulomatous inflammation that most frequently affects the lungs; however, it may involve any organ system, including the skin, eyes, kidneys, and heart [1]. Sarcoidosis tends to affect younger adults, with the onset of symptoms occurring before the age of 50 years [2]. There is a higher incidence and mortality rate among African Americans as compared to other racial or ethnic groups [3]. There is also a female preponderance [4]. The pathogenesis of sarcoidosis is unknown, but several associations have been implicated, including pollens, small inorganic particles, pesticides, and certain molds [5, 6]. The role of genetic predisposition has also shown that certain HLA classes are more prone to the development of sarcoidosis, especially within certain environmental settings [7]. Clinical symptoms may manifest as fatigue, weight loss, night sweats, dyspnea, dry cough, rashes, iritis, keratoconjunctivitis, peripheral lymphadenopathy, and/or musculoskeletal complaints [8, 9]. The hallmark pathological finding in sarcoidosis is granuloma formation in the affected organ. The granuloma is composed of multinucleated giant cells and lymphocytes that are surrounded by compact areas of fibroblasts, mast cells, and extracellular matrix [10]. The immune response that leads to granuloma formation is then followed by a reparative phase that leads to fibrosis, and this sequence promotes pulmonary fibrosis and other end-organ tissue damage [11].

Neurosarcoidosis is a neurologic manifestation of sarcoidosis that is estimated to occur in 5–20% of cases [12, 13]. However, neurosarcoidosis may develop without systemic involvement in 10–30% of patients [14]. Neurologic involvement can be classified as either brain neurosarcoidosis or spinal cord neurosarcoidosis. Presenting symptoms may include fatigue, headache, cognitive decline, mood disorders, hearing loss, vertigo, seizures, cranial neuropathies, facial pain, and mass formation [15, 16]. Carlson et al. published a large multicenter retrospective study ($n = 305$) looking at skull base manifestations of neurosarcoidosis. In their study, they found that the average patient age was 47 years (12–77), with females (53%) being affected more predominantly than males. They also found that 60% of patients had cranial neuropathies, with the most commonly affected cranial nerves being optic, trigeminal, and facial. Involvement of the vestibulocochlear nerve manifested as hearing loss in 17% of patients. The average time from the onset of symptoms to the diagnosis of neurosarcoidosis was over 2 years [15]. Characteristic findings on MRI included enhancement of either meninges or cranial nerves, non-enhancing white matter lesions, and, less commonly, enhancing brain parenchyma masses [15, 18]. Interestingly, meningeal and cranial nerve involvement were correlated to patient symptoms in 64% of cases [18] (Fig. 64.1). Neurosarcoidosis can be a diagnostic challenge, as there are several other disease entities that can present similarly, and there are no laboratory tests that have been reliable [19]. Zajicek et al. proposed a classification system, which included the diagnosis of definite, probable, or possible for neurosarcoidosis [17]. This system was based upon exclusion of other more common diseases, positive serology (ACE levels, skin testing), posi-

J. L. Hatch (✉) · T. R. McRackan
Department of Otolaryngology—Head and Neck Surgery, Medical University of South Carolina, Charleston, SC, USA

A. D. Sweeney et al. (eds.), *Haynes-Glasscock-Shambaugh Surgery of the Ear*, https://doi.org/10.1007/978-3-032-18264-7_64

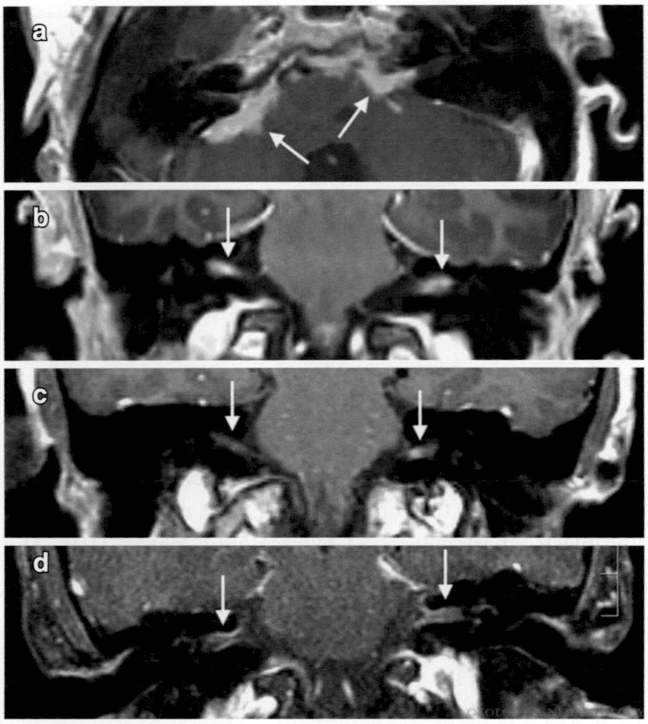

Fig. 64.1 Axial (**a**) and coronal (**b**) T1-weighted MRI with gadolinium demonstrating scattered subcentimeter enhancing nodules along the perimeter of the brain parenchyma. Axial (**c**) and coronal (**d**) MRI sequences demonstrating numerous subcortical enhancing lesions within the Virchow-Robin space. (Reprinted with permission from Carlson et al. [15])

tive CSF (ACE levels, protein ratios, lymphocytosis, or oligoclonal bands), or radiological findings as mentioned above. Currently, histological findings are the only definitive diagnostic test available [15, 17]. Treatment is primarily medical, for which the goal is amelioration of symptoms. This treatment often involves the use of corticosteroids, immunotherapeutics and immunobiologic agents [14, 20, 21]. Surgery is typically reserved for diagnostic biopsies and rehabilitation of cranial neuropathies [15].

Granulomatosis with Polyangiitis (Formerly Wegener's Granulomatosis)

Granulomatosis with polyangiitis (GPA) is an idiopathic disease that causes inflammation in small-to-medium-sized arteries, necrotizing granuloma formation within the respiratory tract, and necrotizing glomerulonephritis [22, 23]. Systemic symptoms may include fever, anorexia, and asthenia [24]. The estimated incidence is 5–10 cases per one million, with an equal distribution between males and females [24]. Caucasians have a higher prevalence rate compared to other demographic groups, and older individuals are more likely to be affected, with the peak incidence around 65 years [25, 26]. Several etiologic factors have been implicated, including infectious, pharmacologic, environmental, and genetic [24]. Prior to the availability of treatments for GPA, the mean survival time from diagnosis to death was 5 months. With appropriate treatment available, the median survival increased to over 20 years [27]. Diagnostic criteria have been established by the American College of Rheumatology, and a diagnosis is made when 2 or more of the following 4 criteria are met: (1) sinus involvement; (2) lung X-ray showing nodules, a fixed pulmonary infiltrate, or cavities; (3) urinary sediment with hematuria or red cell casts; and (4) histological granulomas within an artery or in the perivascular area of an artery or arteriole [28]. Currently, the key serologic test for diagnosis is the detection of anti-neutrophil cytoplasmic antibodies (c-ANCA). During acute disease flare-ups, the sensitivity and specificity of this serologic marker are 91% and 99%, respectively [29].

Granulomatosis with polyangiitis is of particular importance within the field of otolaryngology, as up to 95% of initial symptoms manifest within the head and neck [30]. Otologic manifestations of GPA are also frequent, with estimated prevalence ranging from 19% to 60% [31, 32]. Initial presenting symptoms involving the ear occur in approximately one-third of patients [33]. The most common site of otologic involvement is the middle ear, which may include unilateral or bilateral serous otitis media, and occasionally, purulent otitis media. Mastoiditis may also occur, and there have been case reports of bony destruction of the fallopian canal causing facial nerve palsy [34]. The middle ear disease process is thought to be mediated by Eustachian tube dysfunction from underlying sinonasal inflammation [35]. Inner ear involvement also occurs in up to one-third of patients and causes progressive sensorineural hearing loss along with tinnitus [36]. Vestibular involvement was initially thought to be a rare occurrence, but recent evidence suggests that ANCA-associated vasculitis, including GPA, may affect over 80% of patients in this manner [37, 38]. The presentation of vestibular involvement may be either acute or chronic. Acute involvement is more likely to be associated with sudden hearing loss, and chronic involvement is more likely to be associated with slowly progressive hearing loss [39]. Temporal bone history in patients with GPA found hemorrhage within the stroma of the semicircular canals and the spiral ligament of the cochlea. Vasculitis of the facial nerve and lymphocytic infiltration were also identified [40]. Within the head and neck, the most common site of involvement is sinonasal, which occurs in up to 85% of patients and may lead to soft tissue and bone destruction with resultant septal perforations, nasal obstruction, and nasal deformities [41].

Treatment is divided into two phases: induction and maintenance. The induction phase entails combination therapy involving corticosteroids and an immunologic modulating or suppressive agent, including rituximab, cyclophosphamide, or others [42]. Currently, there are several immunologic agents that are undergoing further study for use as either an induction or maintenance therapy [42, 43].

HIV

Human immunodeficiency virus (HIV) is a retrovirus that causes loss of CD4+ helper T cells, which leads to further dysregulation of antibody production through complex immunologic pathways [44, 45]. As the immune system declines to a point where the CD4+ cell count is less than 200/μl, the patient becomes susceptible to life-threatening infections, and the patient is then diagnosed with acquired immunodeficiency syndrome (AIDS) [46]. Initial presenting symptoms range widely from patients being asymptomatic to having patients with flu-like symptoms followed by a quiescent phase. It has been reported that approximately 80% of patients with HIV will have otolaryngologic manifestations [47, 48].

In a study of 968 patients with HIV, Prasad et al. found otologic involvement in 20% of patients, which included otitis media, otomycosis, and sensorineural hearing loss [48]. Another study found that otologic involvement affected 33% of patients, including tympanic membrane perforations, otitis externa, and acute otitis media. The same study found that sensorineural hearing loss was more severe in patients with more severe HIV [49]. Audiometric data have shown that HIV-infected adults had an approximately 34% higher rate of hearing loss (HL) using pure tone averages (PTA) of 0.5, 1, and 2 kHz >25 decibels (dB) compared to controls [50, 51]. Recently, Luque et al. found no statistically significant difference in overall PTA or hearing loss prevalence among patients with HIV and controls [52]. Further research is needed to delineate the relationship between hearing loss and HIV. It has also been demonstrated that HIV patients tend to experience significant disequilibrium or vertigo. Inner ear pathophysiology has been suggested to involve subepithelial elevation of the saccule and utricle neurosensory epithelium and inflammatory complex deposits within the endolymph [53]. Facial nerve palsy, either unilateral or bilateral, is up to 100-fold more common in HIV patients as compared to those without HIV [54, 55]. The mechanism of facial nerve palsy is thought to be idiopathic, viral reactivation (as in Ramsay Hunt syndrome), or intracranial masses leading to compression [56, 57]. Pediatric patients with HIV also have otologic manifestations with a much higher incidence as compared to their peers. In the largest study of pediatric patients ($n = 244$), Maro et al. found that these patients were more likely to have a history of ear drainage, imbalance, or dizziness, and abnormal tympanograms; however, there was no statistical difference with regard to PTA or auditory brainstem response (ABR) latencies. Interestingly, they found reduced magnitudes on distortion product otoacoustic emissions (DPOAE) at multiple frequencies [58].

Treatment for HIV involves combination therapy, termed a highly active antiretroviral therapy (HAART). HAART has been implicated in the past as a possible etiology for hearing loss through mitochondrial toxicity that could disrupt neural functioning, narrow the vasa nervorum, or reduce perfusion of the cochlea [59, 60, 61]. However, with the advent of newer HAART medications, these mechanisms and associations have been challenged. Current theories for hearing loss in HIV patients include an accelerated aging process with associated cognitive decline or dementia as compared to controls, which leads to hearing loss. It was found that the patient's age at baseline was significantly different among those with HIV and hearing loss as compared to those with normal hearing (54.4 vs. 44.9, $p < 0.01$, years). WRS was also worse in patients with advanced disease [52]. Treatment for HIV-related opportunistic infections (i.e., tuberculosis, multidrug-resistant bacteria, fungi, and viruses) or HIV-related malignancies (i.e., sarcomas, viral-mediated, hematologic) may also cause hearing loss [48, 62].

Syphilis

Syphilis is caused by the spirochete *Treponema pallidum* and can be transmitted either vertically from mother to fetus or, more commonly, through sexual contact. The incidence has steadily increased yearly in the United States and has been increasing throughout much of the world [63, 64]. Infection is divided into 3 stages: primary, secondary, and tertiary. Neurologic and audiovestibular involvement can occur in congenital, secondary, or tertiary stages [65]. From a 1978 paper by Zoller, 6% of patients presenting with sensorineural hearing loss have otosyphilis [66].

Otosyphilis may manifest as fluctuating hearing loss and/or episodic vertigo or disequilibrium. Congenital syphilis may present with hearing loss without vestibular involvement [67]. However, in secondary syphilis, patients may have sudden hearing loss along with tinnitus and some degree of vertigo [68]. Tertiary syphilis is the most well studied phase of the disease with regard to otologic involvement. Up to 90% of patients with tertiary syphilis will have hearing loss. The hearing loss is typically bilateral but may affect the ears asymmetrically [69, 70]. Syphilis is considered to be a "Great Mimicker" of other diseases, and this notion also applies to otosyphilis. Otosyphilis may present similarly to other more prevalent maladies of the ear, including Ménière's disease, autoimmune inner ear disease (AIED), perilymphatic fistula formation, and idiopathic sudden sensorineural hearing loss [65]. Alopecia syphilitica, which generally involves a patchy, non-scarring hair loss, can also be present. With proper treatment, otosyphilis-induced hearing loss may be reversible in up to one-third of patients, with preservation of the hearing at the time of treatment achieved in over 80% of patients [70, 71]. The following factors have been associated with hearing improvement: hearing loss for less than 5 years, fluctuating hearing loss, and age <60 years [71].

The pathogenesis of a *treponemal* infection involves endarteritis, which can also affect the cardiovascular system, resulting in syphilitic aortitis and aortic aneurysms [72]. This same process has been speculated to cause similar problems within the temporal bone, which lead to cochleovestibular symptoms. In otosyphilis, there is often a considerable delay from presentation to diagnosis. Common serologic testing is recommended for suspected cases. It requires the use of two tests:

1. *A non-treponemal test* (i.e., Venereal Disease Research Laboratory [VDRL] or Rapid Plasma Reagin [RPR])
2. *A treponemal test* (i.e., fluorescent treponemal antibody absorbed [FTA-ABS], the T. pallidum passive particle agglutination [TP-PA] assay, various enzyme immunoassays [EIAs]) [63].

RPR titers are particularly important to quantify the relevance of a "positive" result. Other tests, including a lumbar puncture, are needed to officially make the diagnosis of neurosyphilis, though empiric treatment can be pursued without an LP, depending on the clinical presentation and other serologic markers [65]. It is recommended that all patients with neurosyphilis also be screened for coinfection with HIV. Treatment of syphilis is dependent on the stage of the disease. For neurosyphilis, including otosyphilis, the CDC recommends high-dose IV aqueous crystalline penicillin G for 10–14 days [63].

Lyme Disease

Lyme disease is caused by *Borrelia burgdorferi* and other spirochete species. It is transmitted to humans through a reservoir tick host in the *Ixodes* genus. Lyme disease is found throughout the world, but it is classically described as a disease that affects people living in the northeastern and upper Midwest portions of the United States. The incidence has been increasing over time, with recent data estimating 300,000 new cases annually in the United States [73]. The stages of Lyme disease are divided into localized and disseminated. The initial presenting symptoms include a characteristic rash, erythema migrans, in up to 80% of patients. This rash usually resolves without treatment. Other symptoms may include arthritis, malaise, fever, headaches, or lymphadenopathy. In rare circumstances, a painless bluish-red nodule (borrelial lymphocytoma) may appear on the ear lobe or helix. This is more often found in children as compared with adults [74]. Only 3% of patients are believed to have neurologic involvement in this early stage [75]. However, of these patients, 7–10% may develop facial nerve palsy [76, 77]. In the disseminated stage of the disease, neurologic involvement, termed neuroborreliosis, is more common and may include cranial neuropathies (particularly facial nerve palsy), meningitis, radiculoneuropathy, and ocular problems [73]. With regards to facial nerve palsy, 16–23% of patients will continue to have residual effects, which may be more likely if prompt and thorough treatment is not given [76, 78, 79]. However, a recent study by Jowett et al. demonstrates that corticosteroid use in combination with antibiotic therapy was associated with a worse long-term facial function outcome [80]. Lyme disease has also been associated with sensorineural hearing loss. In a study of 165 patients with a diagnosis of sudden hearing loss, serology was positive for *B. burgdorferi* in 12% of cases [81]. It is estimated that the prevalence of hearing loss varies between 0% and 21% [82]. Unfortunately, consistent audiometric data are lacking concerning the type and degree of hearing loss in this patient population, making it unclear how significantly Lyme treatment improves hearing outcomes [81, 82].

The diagnosis of Lyme disease is made based on history and physical examination, followed by serologic testing. The latter utilizes an enzyme immunoassay, and if this is positive, a confirmatory IgM or IgG Western blot is performed. In cases of neurologic involvement, CSF studies are also indicated [73]. A clinical practice guideline by the Infectious Diseases Society of America has established treatment algorithms for both early and late stages, including neurological involvement. The latter includes intravenous ceftriaxone or doxycycline for 2–4 weeks [83].

Relapsing Polychondritis

Relapsing polychondritis is an autoimmune disorder that has an incidence of 3–4 per million and typically affects patients in the fourth and fifth decades of life [84, 85]. It is characterized by the presence of arthritis, cardiovascular disease (primarily valve incompetence), ocular inflammation, audiovestibular dysfunction, and damage to the cartilage frameworks of the auricle, nose, larynx, and lower airways. The latter are attributable to circulating antibodies and immune complex deposits in cartilaginous structures. Relapsing polychondritis can be slowly evolving or rapidly progressing. It is occasionally fatal [85]. Involvement of the auricular cartilage is estimated to occur in 20% of patients at the onset of the disease and in up to 90% as the disease progresses [86]. Pain, swelling, and purple discoloration that does not affect the lobule are frequently seen on examination. If this process is left untreated, auricular deformity may occur. Other manifestations of otologic involvement include otitis externa, chronic myringitis, Eustachian tube dysfunction, hearing loss, and tinnitus [87]. Associated hearing loss may either be conductive or sensorineural and affects up to 46% of patients [88]. Diagnostic criteria have been established and are based on histology and physical exam, including auricular, nasal, or laryngeal chondritis, and audiovestibular dysfunction [89, 90]. Medical management usually involves corticosteroids and other immunomodulatory agents.

Rheumatoid Arthritis

Rheumatoid arthritis (RA) is a systemic inflammatory autoimmune disorder that characteristically affects synovial joints but may also affect several other organ systems, including the lungs, the heart, and the eyes [91, 92]. The prevalence increases with age, and women are affected more than men. It is estimated that RA is present in 1–2% of the general population [93]. Hearing loss has been reported in RA, of which sensorineural hearing loss is most common (25–72% of patients) [94]. The pathogenesis of SNHL is postulated to be an autoimmune complex deposition within the cochlea, drug-induced toxicity related to treatment medications, and auditory neuropathy [95, 96]. Conductive and mixed hearing loss has also been demonstrated, and involvement of the synovial joints of the ossicular chain may result in fixation [91, 97]. Smaller studies have shown that RA may also affect the vestibular system [98, 99]. The diagnosis of RA is based on criteria created by a joint task force, which include physical exam findings and serologic testing [100]. Treatment involves combinations of corticosteroids, immunomodulatory agents, and other anti-inflammatory medications [101].

Histiocytosis

Langerhans cell histiocytosis (LCH) is a disease caused by the proliferation of Langerhans cells. It is relatively rare, affecting 1 in a million individuals, and it is most commonly seen in children and young adults [102]. There are three subtypes of LCH that were collectively and historically termed Histiocytosis X [103]. The three subtypes vary in their presentation from focal disease to systemic involvement, and cases can involve lytic lesions in the bones and disease in the lungs, liver, skin, pituitary gland, or other organ systems. Unifocal LCH, historically known as eosinophilic granuloma, is the least disseminated form of LCH. Hand–Schuller–Christian disease is a multifocal, unisystem manifestation of LCH. Of note, the *sella turcica* and the pituitary gland may be involved in one-third of patients, leading to exophthalmos and diabetes insipidus [104, 105]. Lastly, Letterer–Siwe disease is a multifocal, multisystem manifestation typically seen in young children with diffuse multiorgan involvement. This form of LCH generally has the worst prognosis [106]. In general, the skull is the most common site involved in this disease [107]. It is estimated that temporal bone involvement ranges from 8% to 61%. Manifestations of temporal bone involvement may include recurring otitis media, otitis externa, and bony masses. In a review of patients at the Mayo Clinic with temporal bone involvement, Modest et al. found that the most common presenting symptom was otorrhea, followed by postauricular swelling. An associated soft tissue mass can be found, and close to half of the patients have bilateral involvement. On examination, the most common finding was granulation tissue in the external auditory canal, followed by otitis media, conductive hearing loss, and EAC stenosis [108]. The diagnosis of LCH is often difficult to make, as there is no serologic testing that is both sensitive and specific. Imaging, including CT and MRI, is helpful in evaluating the extent of the disease. Histologic evaluation is needed to confirm the diagnosis, and multinucleated Langerhans cells, histiocytes, eosinophils, and characteristic Birbeck granules are seen. Whole-body imaging is recommended to evaluate the extent of the disease. Treatment may involve surgery for isolated disease, chemotherapy, radiation therapy, or a combination of these modalities, depending on the extent of the disease and organ involvement [108].

Paget's Disease

Paget's disease (osteitis deformans) of bone is a disorder that is characterized by abnormal bony remodeling that tends to affect people in their 40s–50s. The disease is the second most common bone disorder, following osteoporosis [109]. Bony remodeling may lead to multiple fractures and neurologic deficits [110]. Genetic predisposition, viral infections, and autoimmune disorders have been implicated in the pathogenesis of Paget's disease [111]. Most patients with Paget's disease are asymptomatic, but of those who have symptoms, skull base or temporal bone involvement can be seen in approximately 66% of cases. As a result of temporal bone involvement, audiovestibular dysfunction has been identified. Hearing loss is found in 30–50% of patients, and vertigo is seen in 25% [112–114]. The typical pattern of hearing loss is mixed, with a low-frequency conductive component and a high-frequency sensorineural component [112, 113]. Studies evaluating temporal bone specimens have found compression of the internal auditory canal, degeneration of the stria vascularis or spiral ligament, bony invasion of the otic capsule, and obliteration of the inferior cochlear vein in Cotugno's canal to be potential causes of the sensorineural loss [112, 113, 115, 116]. For conductive losses, fixation of the stapes, footplate fractures, and ossicular microfractures have been identified [112, 116]. Serologic and urine studies help in the diagnosis, but plain radiographs and bone scanning are more specific. CT and MRI are useful for evaluating complications, especially neurologic ones. Indications for medical treatment include active disease or hypercalcemia [117, 118]. Bisphosphonates are considered first line therapy [118]. Surgical treatment of hearing loss in Paget's disease has been described in case reports and includes stapes surgery and cochlear implants [119, 120].

Osteogenesis Imperfecta

Osteogenesis imperfecta (OI) is a connective tissue disorder that is caused by an autosomal dominant genetic mutation in COL1A1 or COL1A2 that results in either qualitative or quantitative defects in type 1 collagen production [121, 122]. There are four classically described types of OI, but more types are being discovered with a range of symptomatology. The defective collagen leads to bone fragility, which leads to fracture, blue sclera, joint laxity, triangular facies, scoliosis, and hearing loss. It is estimated that 45–80% of patients have hearing loss, which is a common symptom across all types of OI [123–126]. The hearing loss patterns can be sensorineural, conductive, or mixed. The causes of hearing loss are thought to be related to otosclerotic lesions that may affect any part of the otic capsule or internal auditory canal [127]. Other explanations for sensorineural hearing loss include atrophy of the stria vascularis and the hair cells, along with abnormal bone formation within the cochlea [128, 129]. Causes of conductive hearing loss also include idiopathic ossicular fractures, particularly in the stapes crura, and otitis media with effusion, which is more common in OI patients. The latter is believed to be the result of craniofacial abnormalities that lead to Eustachian tube dysfunction [130]. Otosclerosis is a prominent contributor to the conductive loss in OI patients. Abnormalities encountered in surgery include a fixed or thickened footplate, an obliterated footplate, and crura fractures [131, 132]. Stapes surgery in these cases has been considered to have inferior results compared to the general otosclerosis population in terms of postoperative air-bone gap closure within 10 dB (75–85% in OI compared to 90–95% in non-OI patients) [131–133]. However, in a recent study of 25 patients undergoing stapedotomy, Vincent et al. were able to show air-bone gap closure in 88% of patients [134], which contradicted prior reports of inferior results [131, 133]. Other treatments for hearing loss include hearing aids (conventional or bone anchored) and cochlear implants [129]. Treatment options globally for OI include bisphosphonates, hormone replacement, and potentially, gene therapy [135].

Fibrous Dysplasia

Fibrous dysplasia (FD) is a genetic disorder of bone metabolism that results in an abnormal or irregular pattern of immature bone and fibrous stroma [136, 137]. Due to the bony abnormalities, pain, and fractures are common symptoms. The disorder tends to affect the long bones, ribs, and craniofacial bones [136]. It affects both sexes equally and presents in childhood or early adulthood [138]. It has three subtypes: monostotic, polyostotic, and McCune–Albright syndrome. The latter classically presents with polyostotic lesions, café au lait spots, and endocrine dysfunction [139], and there is a risk of malignant transformation of the affected areas. In the latter situation, outcomes are generally poor [140].

Temporal bone involvement is seen in 25–70% of cases and is most commonly in the form of a monostotic lesion [141, 142]. In the largest study to date looking exclusively at cases of temporal bone involvement, Frisch et al. found that affected patients have hearing loss (conductive, sensorineural, and mixed), cosmetic deformities of the ear, ear canal stenosis, otitis media/externa, and cholesteatoma. The diagnosis of FD can be made based on plain radiographs or CT scans, which demonstrate a loss of corticomedullary boundaries, expansion of the bone involved, sclerosis or lucent areas, and a "ground glass" appearance [143–145]. However, there is a lack of correlation between symptoms and radiographic studies [143]. In general, treatment for FD is mainly conservative. Bisphosphonates have been used to help control symptoms. Surgery can have diagnostic value if radiologic findings are unclear. Also, surgery can be a useful measure when the extent of the disease obstructs the external auditory canal and causes cholesteatoma formation. There have been case reports of successful surgical outcomes after decompression of the internal auditory canal, tympanomastoidectomy, canaloplasty, and surgery has also played a role in cosmesis when lesions are deforming [143, 146].

Osteopetrosis

Osteopetrosis is a syndrome characterized by an abnormal bony resorption leading to bony enlargement and fragility. The latter are due to osteoclastic activity and marrow space obliteration [147]. As a result, affected patients may experience bony fractures, hematologic insufficiencies, nerve entrapment, and growth impairment. There are 3 forms of the disease, which can be either autosomal recessive or autosomal dominant: infantile (which carries the worst prognosis due to anemia and malignancy), intermediate, and adult [148]. The incidence of adult osteopetrosis is estimated to be 1:20,000, whereas infantile disease is much less common (1:240,000) [149].

Temporal bone involvement may result in a conductive loss from ossicular fixation or otitis media, sensorineural hearing loss, vertigo, and facial nerve entrapment leading to paralysis [150, 151]. The diagnosis of osteopetrosis is usually radiologic. Computed tomography shows characteristic findings of bony enlargement and sclerosis. Specific temporal bone findings include poor pneumatization of the mastoid air cells and middle ear cavity, and decreased diameter of the internal auditory canal [150, 152]. There have been case reports describing successful cochlear implantation in these patients [153]. Surgical decompression of the facial nerve has been described in the past, but complications are relatively common and outcomes are modest [154]. General treatment modalities include calcitriol, gamma interferon, corticosteroids (less preferred) and hematologic-modifying agents such as erythropoietin for anemia [155]. The only curative option for infantile osteopetrosis is bone marrow transplantation, which is a treatment modality that is limited to a subset of patients [156].

Conclusion

Though the temporal bone is a relatively small part of the human body, it is a relatively common site of disease. The potential for temporal bone manifestations of systemic disease (infectious, autoimmune, genetic and idiopathic) should inspire the otologic surgeon to be discerning when faced with abstract symptoms, atypical findings and recalcitrant pathology. The importance of multidisciplinary care in these cases cannot be overstated.

References

1. Iannuzzi MC, Rybicki BA, Teirstein AS. Sarcoidosis. N Engl J Med. 2007;357(21):2153–65.
2. Rybicki BA, Major M, Popovich J Jr, Maliarik MJ, Iannuzzi MC. Racial differences in sarcoidosis incidence: a year study in a health maintenance organization. Am J Epidemiol. 1997;145:234–41.
3. Baughman RP, Teirstein AS, Judson MA, et al. Clinical characteristics of patients in a case control study of sarcoidosis. Am J Respir Crit Care Med. 2001;164:1885–9.
4. Stern BJ, Krumholz A, Johns C, Scott P, Nissim J. Sarcoidosis and its neurological manifestations. J Arch Neurol. 1985;42:909–17.
5. Newman LS, Rose CS, Bresnitz EA, et al. A case control etiologic study of sarcoidosis: environmental and occupational risk factors. Am J Respir Crit Care Med. 2004;170:1324–30.
6. Kucera GP, Rybicki BA, Kirkey KL, et al. Occupational risk factors for sarcoidosis in African-American siblings. Chest. 2003;123:1527–35.
7. Rossman MD, Thompson B, Frederick M, et al. HLA-DRB1*1101: a significant risk factor for sarcoidosis in blacks and whites. Am J Hum Genet. 2003;73:720–35.
8. Pietinalho A, Ohmichi M, Lofroos AB, Hiraga Y, Selroos O. The prognosis of pulmonary sarcoidosis in Finland and Hokkaido, Japan. A comparative five-year study of biopsy-proven cases. Sarcoidosis Vasc Diffuse Lung Dis. 2000;17:158–66.
9. Wessendorf TE, Bonella F, Costabel U. Diagnosis of sarcoidosis. Clin Rev Allergy Immunol. 2015;49(1):54–62.
10. Zhang C, Chan KM, Schmidt LA, Myers JL. Histopathology of explanted lungs from patients with a diagnosis of pulmonary sarcoidosis. Chest. 2016;149(2):499–507.
11. Prasse A, Pechkovsky DV, Toews GB, et al. A vicious circle of alveolar macrophages and fibroblasts perpetuates pulmonary fibrosis via CCL18. Am J Respir Crit Care Med. 2006;173:781–92.
12. Nozaki K, Judson MA. Neurosarcoidosis. Curr Treat Options Neurol. 2013;15(4):492–504.
13. Segal BM. Neurosarcoidosis: diagnostic approaches and therapeutic strategies. Curr Opin Neurol. 2013;26(3):307–13.
14. Hoitsma E, Faber CG, Drent M, et al. Neurosarcoidosis: a clinical dilemma. Lancet Neurol. 2004;3:397Y407.
15. Carlson ML, White JR, Espahbodi M, et al. Cranial base manifestations of neurosarcoidosis: a review of 305 patients. Otol Neurotol. 2015;36(1):156–66.
16. Strub GM, Moore JE, Huang AT, Stevenson AW, Reiter ER. Chronic facial pain and Meckel cave masses as the initial presentation of neurosarcoidosis: a case report. Ear Nose Throat J. 2013;92(12):558–65.
17. Zajicek JP, Scolding NJ, Foster O, et al. Central nervous system sarcoidosis--diagnosis and management. QJM. 1999;92(2):103–17.
18. Shah R, Roberson GH, Curé JK. Correlation of MR imaging findings and clinical manifestations in neurosarcoidosis. AJNR Am J Neuroradiol. 2009;30(5):953–61.
19. Lynch JP 3rd. Neurosarcoidosis: how good are the diagnostic tests? J Neuroophthalmol. 2003;23:187Y9.
20. Pawate S, Moses H, Sriram S. Presentations and outcomes of neurosarcoidosis: a study of 54 cases. QJM. 2009;102:449Y60.
21. Ibitoye RT, Wilkins A, Scolding NJ. Neurosarcoidosis: a clinical approach to diagnosis and management. J Neurol. 2017;264:1023–8.
22. Wojciechowska J, Krajewski W, Krajewski P, Kręcicki T. Granulomatosis with polyangiitis in otolaryngologist practice: a review of current knowledge. Clin Exp Otorhinolaryngol. 2016;9(1):8–13.
23. Lutalo PM, D'cruz DP. Diagnosis and classification of granulomatosis with polyangiitis (aka Wegener's granulomatosis). J Autoimmun. 2014;48-49:94–8.
24. Stone JH; Wegener's Granulomatosis Etanercept Trial Research Group. Limited versus severe Wegener's granulomatosis: baseline data on patients in the Wegener's granulomatosis etanercept trial. Arthritis Rheum. 2003 Aug;48(8):2299–309.
25. Scott DG, Watts RA. Systemic vasculitis: epidemiology, classification and environmental factors. Ann Rheum Dis. 2000;59(3):161e3.
26. Lane SE, Watts R, Scott DG. Epidemiology of systemic vasculitis. Curr Rheumatol Rep. 2005;7(4):270e5.
27. Reinhold-Keller E, Beuge N, Latza U, de Groot K, Rudert H, Nolle B, et al. An interdisciplinary approach to the care of patients with Wegener's granulomatosis: long-term outcome in 155 patients. Arthritis Rheum. 2000 May;43(5):1021–32.
28. Leavitt RY, Fauci AS, Bloch DA, Michel BA, Hunder GG, Arend WP, et al. The American College of Rheumatology 1990 criteria for the classification of Wegener's granulomatosis. Arthritis Rheum. 1990 Aug;33(8):1101–7.
29. Rao JK, Weinberger M, Oddone EZ, Allen NB, Landsman P, Feussner JR. The role of antineutrophil cytoplasmic antibody (c-ANCA) testing in the diagnosis of Wegener granulomatosis. A literature review and meta-analysis. Ann Intern Med. 1995 Dec;123(12):925–32.

30. Srouji IA, Andrews P, Edwards C, Lund VJ. Patterns of presentation and diagnosis of patients with Wegener's granulomatosis: ENT aspects. J Laryngol Otol. 2007 Jul;121(7):653–8.
31. Langford CA, Hoffman GS. Rare diseases.3: Wegener's granulomatosis. Thorax. 1999;54:629–37.
32. Trimarchi M, Sinico RA, Teggi R, Bussi M, Specks U, Meroni PL. Otorhinolaryngological manifestations in granulomatosis with polyangiitis (Wegener's). Autoimmun Rev. 2013;12(4):501–5.
33. Nicklasson B, Stangeland N. Wegener's granulomatosis presenting as otitis media. J Laryngol Otol. 1982;96:277–80.
34. Takagi D, Nakamaru Y, Maguchi S, Furuta Y, Fukuda S. Otologic manifestations of Wegener's granulomatosis. Laryngoscope. 2002;112(9):1684–90.
35. Wierzbicka M, Szyfter W, Puszczewicz M, Borucki L, Bartochowska A. Otologic symptoms as initial manifestation of Wegener granulomatosis: diagnostic dilemma. Otol Neurotol. 2011;32:996–1000.
36. Gottschlich S, Ambrosch P, Kramkowski D, Laudien M, Buchelt T, Gross WL, et al. Head and neck manifestations of Wegener's granulomatosis. Rhinology. 2006 Dec;44(4):227–33.
37. Morita Y, Takahashi K, Izumi S, Kubota Y, Ohshima S, Horii A. Vestibular involvement in patients with otitis media with antineutrophil cytoplasmic antibody-associated vasculitis. Otol Neurotol. 2017;38(1):97–101.
38. Rasmussen N. Management of the ear, nose, and throat manifestations of Wegener granulomatosis: an otorhinolaryngologist's perspective. Curr Opin Rheumatol. 2001;13(1):3–11. [Review]
39. Erickson VR, Hwang PH. Wegener's granulomatosis: current trends in diagnosis and management. Curr Opin Otolaryngol Head Neck Surg. 2007 Jun;15(3):170–6.
40. Santos F, Salviz M, Domond H, Nadol JB. Otopathology of vasculitis in granulomatosis with polyangitis. Otol Neurotol. 2015;36(10):1657–62.
41. Lloyd G, Lund VJ, Beale T, Howard D. Rhinologic changes in Wegener's granulomatosis. J Laryngol Otol. 2002 Jul;116(7):565–9.
42. Guillevin L, Pagnoux C, Karras A, Khouatra C, Aumaître O, Cohen P, et al. Rituximab versus azathioprine for maintenance in ANCA-associated vasculitis. N Engl J Med. 2014 Nov;371(19):1771–80.
43. Lenert A, Lenert P. Current and emerging treatment options for ANCA-associated vasculitis: potential role of belimumab and other BAFF/APRIL targeting agents. Drug Des Devel Ther. 2015 Jan;9:333–47.
44. Pantaleo G, Graziosi C, Fauci AS. New concepts in the immunopathogenesis of human immunodeficiency virus infection. N Engl J Med. 1993;328(5):327–35.
45. Pantaleo G, Fauci AS. New concepts in the immunopathogenesis of HIV infection. Annu Rev Immunol. 1995;13:487–512.
46. 1993 revised classification system for HIV infection and expanded surveillance case definition for AIDS among adolescents and adults. MMWR Recomm Rep. 1992;41:1–19.
47. Jolles S, Kinloch de Loes S, Johnson MA, et al. Primary HIV-1 infection: a new medical emergency. BMJ. 1996;312:1243–4.
48. Prasad HK, Bhojwani KM, Shenoy V, Prasad SC. HIV manifestations in otolaryngology. Am J Otolaryngol. 2006;27(3):179–85.
49. Chandrasekhar SS, Connelly PE, Brahmbhatt SS, Shah CS, Kloser PC, Baredes S. Otologic and audiologic evaluation of human immunodeficiency virus-infected patients. Am J Otolaryngol. 2000;21(1):1–9.
50. van der Westhuizen Y, Swanepoel de W, Heinze B, Hofmeyr LM. Auditory and otological manifestations in adults with HIV/AIDS. Int J Audiol. 2013;52:37–43.
51. Torre P 3rd, Hoffman HJ, Springer G, Cox C, Young MA, et al. Hearing loss among HIV-seropositive and HIV-seronegative men and women. JAMA Otolaryngol Head Neck Surg. 2015;141:202–10.
52. Luque AE, Orlando MS, Leong UC, et al. Hearing function in patients living with HIV/AIDS. Ear Hear. 2014;35(6):e282–90.
53. Chandrasekhar SS, Siverls V, Chandra SH. Histopathologic and ultrastructural changes in the temporal bones of HIV infected human adults. Am J Otol. 1992;13:207–14.
54. Kim MS, Yoon HJ, Kim HJ, et al. Bilateral peripheral facial palsy in a patient with Human Immunodeficiency Virus (HIV) infection. Med J. 2006;47:745–7.
55. Belec L, Georges AJ, Vuillecard E, et al. Peripheral facial paralysis indicating HIV infection. Lancet. 1988;2:1421–2.
56. Goldani LZ, da Silva LF. Dora JM Ramsay Hunt syndrome in patients infected with human immunodeficiency virus. Clin Exp Dermatol. 2009;34:e552–4.
57. Chand V, Sweeney C, Agger WA. Mental neuropathy in patients with AIDS associated malignant lymphoma. Clin Infect Dis. 1997;24:521–2.
58. Maro II, Fellows AM, Clavier OH, et al. Auditory impairments in HIV-infected children. Ear Hear. 2016;37(4):443–51.
59. Lewis W, Dalakas MC. Mitochondrial toxicity of antiviral drugs. Nat Med. 1995;1:417–22.
60. Kujoth GC, Hiona A, Pugh TD, et al. Mitochondrial DNA mutations, oxidative stress, and apoptosis in mammalian aging. Science. 2005;309(5733):481–4.
61. Dai P, Yang W, Jiang S, et al. Correlation of cochlear blood supply with mitochondrial DNA common deletion in presbyacusis. Acta Otolaryngol. 2004;124(2):130–6.
62. Rubinstein PG, Aboulafia DM, Zloza A. Malignancies in HIV/AIDS: from epidemiology to therapeutic challenges. AIDS. 2014;28:453.
63. Syphilis. https://www.cdc.gov/std/tg2015/syphilis.htm. Updated July 27, 2016. Centers for Disease Control and Prevention.
64. Fenton KA, Breban R, Vardavas R, et al. Infectious syphilis in high income settings in the 21st century. Lancet Infect Dis. 2008;8:244Y53.
65. Phillips JS, Gaunt A, Phillips DR. Otosyphilis: a neglected diagnosis? Otol Neurotol. 2014;35(6):1011–3.
66. Zoller M, Wilson WR, Nadol JB Jr, Girard KF. Detection of syphilitic hearing loss. Arch Otolaryngol. 1978;104:63Y5.
67. Huges GB, Rutherford I. Predictive value of serologic tests for syphilis in otology. Ann Otol Rhinol Laryngol. 1986;95:250–9.
68. Morrison A. On syphilis and the ear: an otologist's view. Genitourin Med. 1992;68:420–2.
69. Steckelberg JM, McDonald TJ. Otologic involvement in late syphilis. Laryngoscope. 1984;94:753–7.
70. Yimtae K, Srirompotong S, Lertsukprasert K. Otosyphilis: a review of 85 cases. Otolaryngol Head Neck Surg. 2007;136(1):67–71.
71. Gliech LL, Linstrom CJ, Kimmelman CP. Otosyphilis: a diagnostic and therapeutic dilemma. Laryngoscope. 1992;102:1255–9.
72. Roberts WC, Barbin CM, Weissenborn MR, Ko JM, Henry AC. Syphilis as a cause of thoracic aortic aneurysm. Am J Cardiol. 2015;116(8):1298–303.
73. CDC, Division of Vector-borne Infectious Diseases. Lyme Disease. http://www.cdc.gov/ncidod/dvbid/lyme/index.htm. Accessed 17 Mar 2017.
74. Stanek G, Wormser GP, Gray J, Strle F. Lyme borreliosis. Lancet. 2012;379(9814):461–73.
75. Huppertz HI, Böhme M, Standaert SM, Karch H, Plotkin SA. Incidence of Lyme borreliosis in the Würzburg region of Germany. Eur J Clin Microbiol Infect Dis. 1999;18:697–703.
76. Kuehn BM. CDC estimates 300,000 US cases of Lyme disease annually. JAMA. 2013;310:1110.
77. Clark JR, Carlson RD, Sasaki CT, Pachner AR, Steere AC. Facial paralysis in Lyme disease. Laryngoscope. 1985;95:1341–5.
78. Halperin JJ. Nervous system Lyme disease. Infect Dis Clin N Am. 2015;29:241–53.

79. Kalish RA, Kaplan RF, Taylor E, Jones-Woodward L, Workman K, Steere AC. Evaluation of study patients with Lyme disease, 10–20-year followup. J Infect Dis. 2001;183:453–60.
80. Jowett N, Gaudin RA, Banks CA, Hadlock TA. Steroid use in Lyme disease-associated facial palsy is associated with worse long-term outcomes. Laryngoscope. 2017;127:1451–8.
81. Peltomaa M, Pyykkö I, Sappälä I, Viitanen L, Viljanen M. Lyme borreliosis, an etiological factor in sensorineural hearing loss? Eur Arch Otorhinolaryngol. 2000;257:317–22.
82. Peeters N, Van der Kolk BY, Thijsen SF, Colnot DR. Lyme disease associated with sudden sensorineural hearing loss: case report and literature review. Otol Neurotol. 2013;34(5):832–7.
83. Wormser GP, Dattwyler RJ, Shapiro ED, et al. The clinical assessment, treatment, and prevention of lyme disease, human granulocytic anaplasmosis, and babesiosis: clinical practice guidelines by the Infectious Diseases Society of America. Clin Infect Dis. 2006;43(9):1089–134.
84. Vitale A, Sota J, Rigante D, Lopalco G, Molinaro F, Messina M, et al. Relapsing polychondritis: an update on pathogenesis, clinical features, diagnostic tools, and therapeutic perspectives. Curr Rheumatol Rep. 2016;18:3.
85. Longo L, Greco A, Rea A, Lo Vasco VR, De Virgilio A, De Vincentiis M. Relapsing polychondritis: a clinical update. Autoimmun Rev. 2016;15(6):539–43.
86. Shimizu J, Oka H, Yamano Y, Yudoh K, Suzuki N. Cutaneous manifestations of patients with relapsing polychondritis: an association with extracutaneous complications. Clin Rheumatol. 2016;35:781–3.
87. Bachor E, Blevins NH, Karmody C, Kühnel T. Otologic manifestations of relapsing polychondritis. Review of literature and report of nine cases. Auris Nasus Larynx. 2006;33(2):135–41.
88. Cody DTR, Sones DA. Relapsing polychondritis: audiovestibular manifestations. Laryngoscope. 1971;81:1208–22.
89. McAdam LP, O'Hanlan MA, Bluestone R, Pearson CM. Relapsing polychondritis: prospective study of 23 patients and review of the literature. Medicine. 1976;56:193–215.
90. Damiani JM, Levine HL. Relapsing polychondritis. Laryngoscope. 1979;89:929–46.
91. Takatsu M, Higaki M, Kinoshita H, Mizushima Y, Koizuka I. Ear involvement in patients with rheumatoid arthritis. Otol Neurotol. 2005;26(4):755–61.
92. Emamifar A, Bjoerndal K, Hansen IM. Is hearing impairment associated with rheumatoid arthritis? A review. Open Rheumatol J. 2016;10:26–32.
93. Ruddy S, Harris ED Jr, Sledge CB, editors. Kelley's textbook of rheumatology. 6th ed. Philadelphia: WB Saunders; 2001.
94. Pascual-Ramos V, Contreras-Yáñez I, Rivera-Hoyos P, Enríquez L, Ramírez-Anguiano J. Cumulative disease activity predicts incidental hearing impairment in patients with rheumatoid arthritis (RA). Clin Rheumatol. 2014;33(3):315–21.
95. Ozcan M, Karakuş MF, Gündüz OH, Tuncel U, Sahin H. Hearing loss and middle ear involvement in rheumatoid arthritis. Rheumatol Int. 2002;22(1):16–9.
96. Poorey VK, Khatri R. Study of auditory function in rheumatoid arthritis. Indian J Otolaryngol Head Neck Surg. 2001;53(4):261–3.
97. Murdin L, Patel S, Walmsley J, Yeoh LH. Hearing difficulties are common in patients with rheumatoid arthritis. Clin Rheumatol. 2008;27(5):637–40.
98. Yilmaz S, Erbek S, Erbek SS, Ozgirgin N, Yucel E. Abnormal electronystagmography in rheumatoid arthritis. Auris Nasus Larynx. 2007;34(3):307–11.
99. Ferrara P, Modica A, Adelfio M, Salli L, Pappalardo A. Audiovestibular changes in patients with rheumatoid arthritis. Minerva Med. 1988;79:1043–7.
100. Aletaha D, Neogi T, Silman AJ, et al. 2010 Rheumatoid arthritis classification criteria: an American College of Rheumatology/European League Against Rheumatism collaborative initiative. Arthritis Rheum. 2010;62(9):2569–81.
101. Aletaha D, Funovits J, Keystone EC, Smolen JS. Disease activity early in the course of treatment predicts response to therapy after one year in rheumatoid arthritis patients. Arthritis Rheum. 2007;56(10):3226–35.
102. Howarth DM, Gilchrist GS, Mullan BP, Wiseman GA, Edmonson JH, Schomberg PJ. Langerhans cell histiocytosis: diagnosis, natural history, management, and outcome. Cancer. 1999;85:2278–90.
103. Lichtenstein L. Histiocytosis X; integration of eosinophilic granuloma of bone, Letterer-Siwe disease, and Schüller-Christian disease as related manifestations of a single nosologic entity. AMA Arch Pathol. 1953 Jul;56(1):84–102.
104. Scolozzi P, Lombardi T, Monnier P, Jaques B. Multisystem Langerhans' cell histiocytosis (Hand-Schuller-Christian disease) in an adult: a case report and review of the literature. Eur Arch Otorrinolaringol. 2004;261:326–30.
105. Mener DJ, Moskowitz HS, Stewart CM. Temporal bone involvement in Hand-Schuller-Christian disease. Otol Neurotol. 2015;36(3):e95–6.
106. Chu T, D'Angio GJ, Favara B, Ladisch S, Nesbit M, Pritchard J. The Writing Group of the Histiocyte Society. Histiocytic syndromes in children. Lancet. 1987;1:208–9.
107. Baumgartner I, von Hockstetter A, Baumert B, Luetolf U, Follath F. Langerhans' cell histiocytosis in adults. Med Pediatr Oncol. 1997;28:9–14.
108. Modest MC, Garcia JJ, Arndt CS, Carlson ML. Langerhans cell histiocytosis of the temporal bone: a review of 29 cases at a single center. Laryngoscope. 2016;126(8):1899–904.
109. Roodman GD, Windle JJ. Paget disease of bone. J Clin Invest. 2005;115:200–8.
110. Schuknecht HF. Pathology of the ear. 2nd ed. Philadelphia: Lea & Febiger; 1993.
111. Michou L, Collet C, Laplanche JL, Orcel P, Cornelis F. Genetics of Paget's disease of bone. Joint Bone Spine. 2006;73:243–8.
112. Lindsay JR, Suga F. Paget's disease and sensori-neural deafness: temporal bone histopathology of Paget's disease. Laryngoscope. 1976;86:1029–42.
113. Teufert KB, Linthicum F Jr. Paget disease and sensorineural hearing loss associated with spiral ligament degeneration. Otol Neurotol. 2005;26:387–91.
114. Davies DG. The temporal bone in Paget's disease. J Laryngol Otol. 1970;84:553–60.
115. Applebaum EL, Clemis JD. Temporal bone histopathology of Paget's disease with sensorineural hearing loss and narrowing of the internal auditory canal. Laryngoscope. 1977;87(10 Pt 1):1753–9.
116. Dimitriadis PA, Bamiou DE, Bibas AG. Hearing loss in Paget's disease: a temporal bone histopathology study. Otol Neurotol. 2012;33(2):142–6.
117. Lyles KW, Siris ES, Singer FR, Meunier PJ. A clinical approach to diagnosis and management of Paget's disease of bone. J Bone Miner Res. 2001 Aug;16(8):1379–87.
118. Singer FR, Bone HG 3rd, Hosking DJ, Lyles KW, Murad MH, Reid IR, et al. Paget's disease of bone: an endocrine society clinical practice guideline. J Clin Endocrinol Metab. 2014 Dec;99(12):4408–22.
119. Hamed AA, Fayad JN. Presence of otosclerosis and paget lesions in the same temporal bone. Otol Neurotol. 2009;30(8):1232–3.
120. Aoki M, Tanahashi S, Mizuta K, Kato H. Treatment for progressive hearing loss due to Paget's disease of bone – a case report and literature review. J Int Adv Otol. 2015;11(3):267–70.
121. Cole WG. The Nicholas Andry Award-1996. The molecular pathology of osteogenesis imperfecta. Clin Orthop Relat Res. 1997;343:235–48.

122. Cole WG. Advances in osteogenesis imperfecta. Clin Orthop Relat Res. 2002;401:6–16.
123. Pederson U. Hearing loss in patients with osteogenesis imperfecta. A clinical and audiological study of 201 patients. Scand Audiol. 1984;13:67–74.
124. Stewart EJ, O'Reilly BF. A clinical and audiological investigation of osteogenesis imperfecta. Clin Otolaryngol Allied Sci. 1989;14:509–14.
125. Kuurila K, Kaitila I, Johansson R, Grénman R. Hearing loss in Finnish adults with osteogenesis imperfecta: a nationwide survey. Ann Otol Rhinol Laryngol. 2002;111:939–46.
126. Hartikka H, Kuurila K, Körkkö J, et al. Lack of correlation between the type of COL1A1 or COL1A2 mutation and hearing loss in osteogenesis imperfecta. Hum Mutat. 2004;24:147–54.
127. Santos F, Mccall AA, Chien W, Merchant S. Otopathology in osteogenesis imperfecta. Otol Neurotol. 2012;33(9):1562–6.
128. Swinnen FK, De leenheer EM, Coucke PJ, Cremers CW, Dhooge IJ. Audiometric, surgical, and genetic findings in 15 ears of patients with osteogenesis imperfecta. Laryngoscope. 2009;119(6):1171–9.
129. Pillion JP, Vernick D, Shapiro J. Hearing loss in osteogenesis imperfecta: characteristics and treatment considerations. Genet Res Int. 2011;2011:983942.
130. Imani P, Vijayasekaran S, Lannigan FJ. Is it necessary to screen for hearing loss in the paediatric population with osteogenesis imperfecta? Clin Otolaryngol Allied Sci. 2003;28(3):199–202.
131. Garretsen TJ, Cremers CW. Ear surgery in osteogenesis imperfecta. Clinical findings and short-term and long-term results. Arch Otolaryngol Head Neck Surg. 1990;116(3):317–23.
132. Vincent R, Gratacap B, Oates J, Sperling NM. Stapedotomy in osteogenesis imperfecta: a prospective study of 23 consecutive cases. Otol Neurotol. 2005;26(5):859–65.
133. Shea JJ, Postma DS. Findings and long-term surgical results in the hearing loss of osteogenesis imperfecta. Arch Otolaryngol. 1982;108(8):467–70.
134. Vincent R, Wegner I, Stegeman I, Grolman W. Stapedotomy in osteogenesis imperfecta: a prospective study of 32 consecutive cases. Otol Neurotol. 2014;35(10):1785–9.
135. Harrington J, Sochett E, Howard A. Update on the evaluation and treatment of osteogenesis imperfecta. Pediatr Clin N Am. 2014;61(6):1243–57.
136. DiCaprio MR, Enneking WF. Fibrous dysplasia: pathophysiology, evaluation, and treatment. J Bone Joint Surg Am. 2005;87:1848–64.
137. Chapurlat RD, Orcel P. Fibrous dysplasia of bone and McCune-Albright syndrome. Best Pract Res Clin Rheumatol. 2008;22(1):55–69.
138. Fibrous Dysplasia Foundation. How rare is fibrous dysplasia? Available at: https://www.fibrousdysplasia.org/index.php?page516#12. Accessed 9 Apr 2017.
139. Albright F, Butler AM, Hampton A, Smith P. Syndrome characterised by osteitis fibrosa disseminata, areas of pigmentation and endocrine dysfunction, with precocious puberty in females. N Engl J Med. 1937;216:727–46.
140. Schwartz DT, Alpert M. The malignant transformation of fibrous dysplasia. Am J Med Sci. 1964;247:1–20.
141. Megerian CA, Sofferman RA, McKenna MJ, Eavey RD, Nadol JB Jr. Fibrous dysplasia of the temporal bone: ten new cases demonstrating the spectrum of otologic sequelae. Am J Otol. 1995;16:408–19.
142. Lustig LR, Holliday MJ, McCarthy FE, Nager GT. Fibrous dysplasia involving the skull base and temporal bone. Arch Otolaryngol Head Neck Surg. 2001;127:1239–47.
143. Frisch CD, Carlson ML, Kahue CN, et al. Fibrous dysplasia of the temporal bone: a review of 66 cases. Laryngoscope. 2015;125(6):1438–43.
144. Chong VF, Khoo B, Fan Y. Fibrous dysplasia involving the base of skull. Am J Roentgenol. 2002;178:717–20.
145. Lambert PR, Brackmann DE. Fibrous dysplasia of the temporal bone: the use of computerized tomography. Otolaryngol Head Neck Surg. 1984;92(4):461–7.
146. Morrissey DD, Talbot MJ, Schleuning AJ II. Fibrous dysplasia of the temporal bone: reversal of sensorineural hearing loss after decompression of the internal auditory canal. Laryngoscope. 1997;107:1336–40.
147. Stark Z, Savarirayan R. Osteopetrosis. Orphanet J Rare Dis. 2009 Feb;20(4):5.
148. el-Tawil T, Stoker DJ. Benign osteopetrosis: a review of 42 cases showing two different patterns. Skeletal Radiol. 1993 Nov;22(8):587–93.
149. Gerritsen EJA, Vossen JM, van Loo IHG, et al. Autosomal recessive osteopetrosis: variability of findings at diagnosis and during the natural course. Pediatrics. 1994;93:247–53.
150. Dozier TS, Duncan IM, Klein AJ, Lambert PR, Key LL Jr. Otologic manifestations of malignant osteopetrosis. Otol Neurotol. 2005;26:762–6.
151. Benecke JE Jr. Facial nerve dysfunction in osteopetrosis. Laryngoscope. 1993;103:494–7.
152. Abdel-aziz T, Upile T, Scholtz LU, Sudhoff HH. Osteopetrosis of the temporal bone. Otol Neurotol. 2012;33(6):e45–6.
153. Szymanski M, Zasławska K, Trojanowska A, Szymanska A, Zadrozniak M. Osteopetrosis of the temporal bone treated with cochlear implant. J Int Adv Otol. 2015;11(2):173–5.
154. Hamersma H. Total decompression of the facial nerve in osteopetrosis (marble bone disease-morbus Albers-Schonberg). ORL J Otorhinolaryngol Relat Spec. 1973;36:21–32.
155. Key L, Carnes D, Cole S, et al. Treatment of congenital osteopetrosis with high-dose calcitriol. N Engl J Med. 1984;310(7):409–15.
156. Mazzolari E, Forino C, Razza A, et al. A single-center experience in 20 patients with infantile malignant osteopetrosis. Am J Hematol. 2009;84(8):473–9.

65 Radiation Effects on the Ear and Temporal Bone

Paul W. Gidley

Introduction

Radiotherapy is a common modality to treat many head and neck cancers. The nasopharynx, oropharynx, and parotid are typical sites that often require radiotherapy. The central location of the temporal bone exposes it to receive some radiation dose, especially for these primary sites. Depending on the tumor location, target volume, and technique used, doses as high as 70 Gy may intentionally be delivered to portions of the temporal bone [65]. The success of treatment for these tumors means that more patients are outliving the cancer and are manifesting the long-term side effects of the radiotherapy and chemotherapy.

For some primary tumors, such as nasopharyngeal carcinoma, radiotherapy is a mainstay of therapy. While the methods of delivery and dosing have changed over time, the effects of radiation on the ear and temporal bone have been recognized for many years. The first cases of osteoradionecrosis were described independently by Ewing [35] and Phemister [107] in 1926. The first case of temporal bone osteoradionecrosis was described by Block in 1952 [18].

This chapter will examine the effects of radiation on the ear and temporal bone. Topics discussed will include changes in the ear canal, tympanic membrane, middle ear, and inner ear following radiotherapy. Serious complications, such as osteoradionecrosis, carotid blowout, and radiation-induced tumors, will be highlighted.

Radiation Fundamentals

Radiation uses electromagnetic particles to produce changes in DNA. Rapidly dividing cells are more sensitive to radiotherapy. Electrons, neutrons, protons, and photons have been used to treat cancers. Regardless of the particle used, the biophysical effect of radiation is DNA damage, which leads to cell death.

DNA damage can occur through either a direct or an indirect pathway. In the direct pathway, radiation damages DNA through high linear energy transfer. This leads to the breakdown of DNA and prevents cellular reproduction. Since the damage is done directly to DNA, the process is independent of oxygen. In the indirect pathway, radiotherapy produces free radicals principally from oxygen molecules. These free radicals then destroy DNA. As such, this pathway is dependent on oxygen, since it is the source of these free radicals. The effects of radiation manifest clinically at the tissue and organ level and are propagated by free radicals that cause tissue fibrosis and genomic instability [14].

Many different modalities for delivering radiation have been developed over time. The conventional external beam radiation therapy has largely been supplanted by newer forms. Computerized, 3-dimensional methods for calculating and delivering radiation dose to the target are currently used. Examples of such modalities are intensity modulated radiotherapy (IMRT) and intensity modulated proton therapy (IMPT). The ability to deliver a dose to a well-defined target and avoid radiation to sensitive targets (e.g., brainstem, salivary glands, etc.) are the main advantages of IMRT and IMPT over previous modes. Like their conventional counterparts, IMRT and IMPT are fractionated treatments, where a small daily dose (usually 2.0 Gy) is given over a period of time (e.g., Monday through Friday for 6 weeks) until the total prescription dose is delivered (in this example, 60 Gy).

While not frequently used for head and neck cancer, stereotactic radiosurgery is used for many intracranial tumors. This modality allows for a relatively large dose to be delivered to a very defined target at a single session while minimizing the dose delivered to surrounding tissues. Lastly, brachytherapy involves placing radioactive elements in contact with affected tissues and delivering a relatively high dose to the tissues over a short period of time.

P. W. Gidley (✉)
Department of Head and Neck Surgery, UT MD Anderson Cancer Center, Houston, TX, USA
e-mail: pwgidley@mdanderson.org

A. D. Sweeney et al. (eds.), *Haynes-Glasscock-Shambaugh Surgery of the Ear*, https://doi.org/10.1007/978-3-032-18264-7_65

Radiation Effects on Tissues

The effects of radiation on different tissues have been recognized since the development of radiotherapy. Ionizing radiation exerts its therapeutic effect by exploiting the differences in repair kinetics between neoplastic and normal cells [134]. These changes are typically dose-dependent, and the incidence of these effects rises with increasing dose. Dose tolerances have been studied and are used to guide the total dose given.

Radiation causes thinning of the skin, loss of fat and pigmentary changes in the skin.

Blood vessels are sensitive to radiotherapy. Radiotherapy causes endothelial cells to swell, blocking capillaries. Thickening of arteriolar walls can progress to intimal occlusion. The ultimate result of radiation damage to arteries is obliterative endarteritis. The true impact of vascular changes on blood flow and oxygen has not been measured, but these changes contribute to the pathophysiology of osteoradionecrosis [134]. These vascular changes occur within weeks of radiotherapy and at doses as low as 45 Gy [86].

Normal bone physiology depends on the balance of osteoblastic and osteolytic effects. Radiation damages osteocytes in a dose-dependent fashion, leading to empty lacunae and a lack of new bone formation. A dose as low as 30 Gy impairs osteoblastic cells, and a dose above 50 Gy kills osteoblastic cells [134], which upsets the balance of new bone formation and osteolysis. Osteolysis, thus, predominates. Osteolytic bone is replaced by fibrous connective tissue. In medullary bone, this leads to a loss of bone marrow.

The bones of the ear canal and temporal bone have some special features that make them particularly sensitive to the effects of radiation [109]. The ear canal is relatively superficial in location, and the skin covering the ear canal is quite thin, perhaps less than 2 mm. The ear canal has a relatively poor blood supply compared to other bones. The middle ear communicates with the upper aerodigestive tract, and this communication can lead to bacterial contamination. Lastly, the compact bone of the ear canal and temporal bone tolerates radiation poorly compared to cancellous bone.

Marx has proposed a “3-H theory” to explain the effects of radiation on bone [83]. This concept involves hypovascularity, hypoxia, and hypocellularity. Hypovascularity derives from vessel thrombosis and obliterative endarteritis. Hypoxia derives from the loss of an adequate blood supply and leads to cell death. Hypocellularity relates to the loss of cells, specifically the loss of osteoblasts. He advanced this theory to demonstrate that microorganisms play only a contaminant role in osteoradionecrosis and that trauma is only one mechanism of tissue breakdown leading to osteoradionecrosis.

A new theory proposed by Delanian and Lefaix emphasizes defective osteolysis and osteogenesis [32]. These defects lead to radiation-induced fibrosis and atrophy, which leads to necrosis. The end result of the changes induced by radiation is aseptic bone necrosis.

Time Line of Radiation Effects

The effects of radiation vary from the onset of treatment to late-stage effects. Early, in-treatment effects include erythema and desquamation of the skin. These skin effects are seen in the outer ear and ear canal. Hearing loss and imbalance usually start from 6 months to 2 years following treatment. Lastly, osteoradionecrosis and radiation-associated malignancies occur more than 4 years after treatment.

Otologic Effects of Radiation

The otologic effects of radiation can be studied from the outer ear, middle ear, and inner ear. As mentioned above, the outer ear and ear canal demonstrate acute effects from radiotherapy. Generally, these symptoms are mild and well tolerated. Skin care and the use of moisturizers are important. Erythema, desquamation, and pigmentary changes occur early in the course of radiotherapy, and these symptoms resolve over a few months once radiotherapy terminates.

Outer Ear and Ear Canal

During radiation, patients are instructed to use moisturizing ointments on the skin (e.g., Aquaphor®). Recently, Boswellia-based creams (frankincense) have been evaluated in a randomized controlled trial as an effective treatment to heal the skin changes from radiation in breast cancer patients [126].

Due to desquamation, the ear canal can accumulate keratin debris that requires cleaning. Patients should be admonished not to use cotton-tipped applicators (i.e., Q-tips®) in an attempt to clean out their ears. Some patients will need rather frequent debridements of the ear canals during and following treatment. Antibiotic eardrops are recommended when there are signs of infection. Ear wicks are avoided since they might abrade the ear canal. Oral antibiotics are generally not required. The ear canal changes will resolve within about 2 years of treatment completion. However, long-term effects of radiation therapy can result in loss of the outer ear (Figs. 65.1 and 65.2).

Within 2 months of radiotherapy, the loss of hair follicles and ceruminous glands occurs within the ear canal (Fig. 65.3). Thinning skin can lead to ulceration. The normal self-cleaning mechanism of the ear canal is also lost [3]. Late

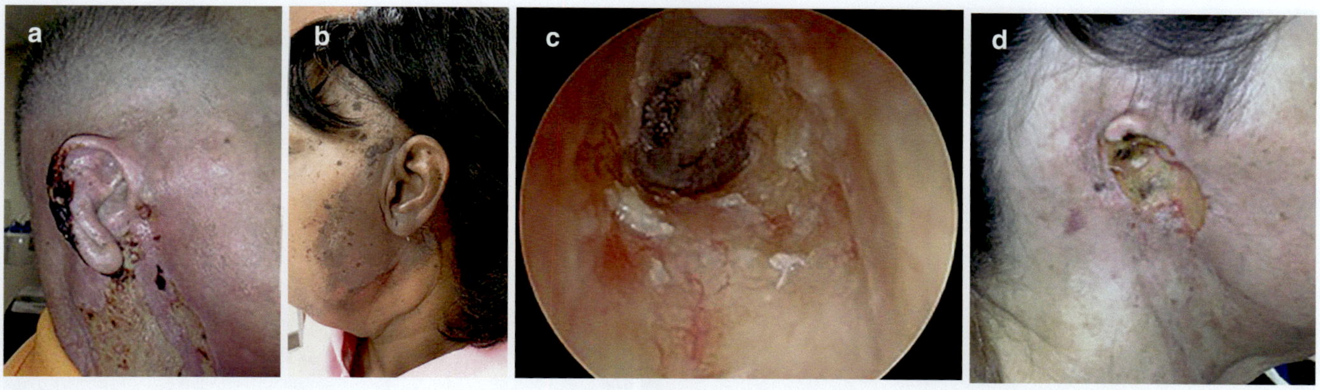

Fig. 65.1 Outer ear effects from radiotherapy. (**a**) Acute changes in the skin of the ear and neck during radiotherapy. (**b**) Pigmentary changes in the skin 2 weeks after finishing radiotherapy in this African American woman. (**c**) Left ear canal of the same patient as in (b), showing desquamation in the ear canal. (**d**) Long-term (10 years) effects of radiation causing loss of the outer ear. (©Used with permission, Paul W. Gidley, MD)

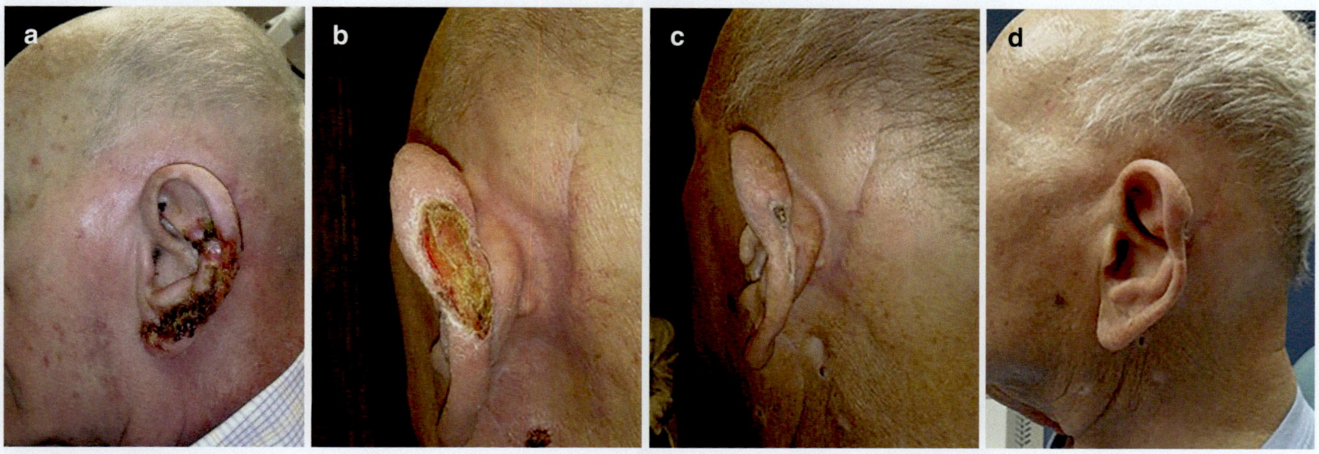

Fig. 65.2 Evolving effects of radiation on the outer ear. (**a**) Combined chemotherapy (weekly cisplatin) and radiotherapy (70 Gy by IMRT) in this 77-year-old man caused scabbing of the outer ear. (**b**) He later developed exposed cartilage of the helix about 4 months later. (**c**, **d**) At 1 year post-radiotherapy, his ear healed with local wound care and avoidance of picking. (©Used with permission, Paul W. Gidley, MD)

effects of radiotherapy on the ear canal involve atrophy of the skin and ulceration.

A decrease in wax secretion and a loss of self-cleaning can lead to a picture similar to keratosis obturans (Fig. 65.4). This keratin characteristically builds up in the anterior sulcus, and it can be quite painful to remove from the canal. Rubbing alcohol and hydrogen peroxide can be used to help soften and loosen this keratin debris, but care must be exercised to ensure that the tympanic membrane is not perforated [54].

Narrowing and scarring can occur within the ear canal, especially in the anterior sulcus [115, 122]. This scarring can produce a band between the ear canal and the tympanic membrane. These scarring effects produce conductive hearing loss (Fig. 65.5). Additionally, scarring can completely obscure and efface the tympanic membrane (Fig. 65.6). The treatment options might include tympanoplasty with canalplasty and a split-thickness skin graft, but this approach might run a significant risk of poor healing and hearing. Instead, either conventional or osseointegrated hearing aids might be a better option.

Middle Ear

In the middle ear, radiation causes inflammation of the mucosa with mucosal hypoplasia and loss of ciliary function. This mucosal swelling causes obstruction of the Eustachian tube. Inflammation produces transudation of sterile fluid and creates the clinical picture of serous otitis media, also called radiation otitis media (Fig. 65.7) [20, 96]. These middle ear changes are radiation dose-dependent, with more than 72% of patients developing serous otitis media with a radiation dose of 50 Gy or higher [21, 27, 95]. This radiation otitis

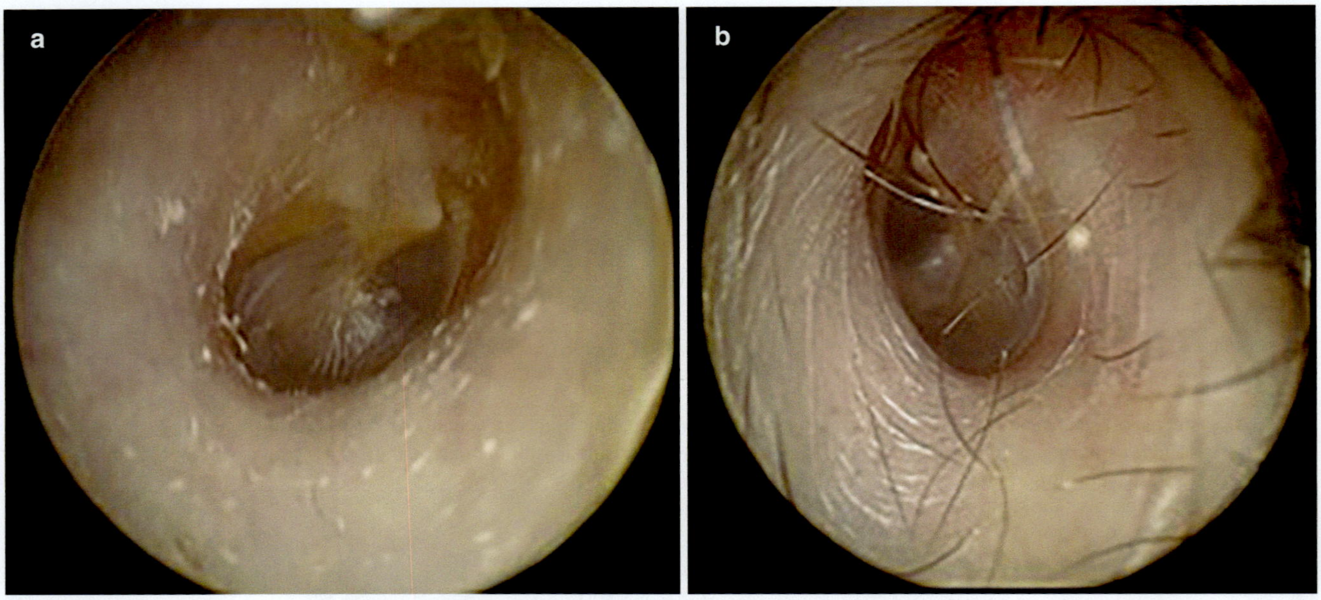

Fig. 65.3 Loss of hair follicles in the ear canal. (**a**) Irradiated right ear canal. (**b**) Normal left ear canal. (©Used with permission, Paul W. Gidley, MD)

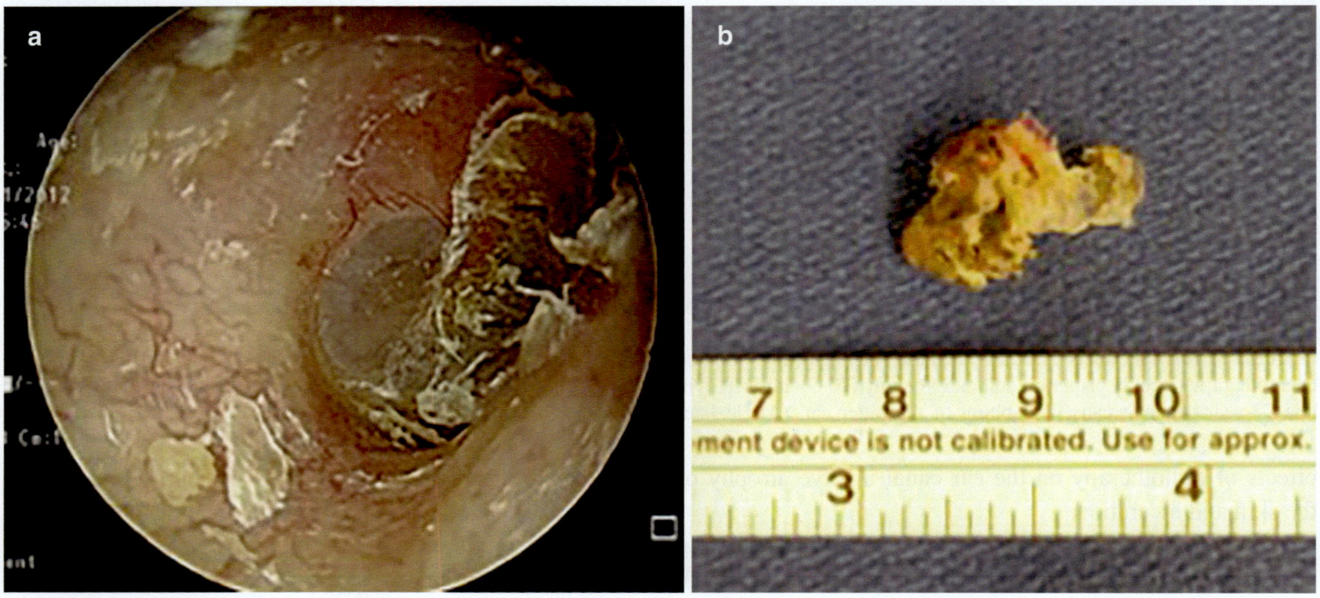

Fig. 65.4 Keratosis obturans. (**a**) Ear canal. (**b**) Keratin plug. (©Used with permission, Paul W. Gidley, MD)

media occurs in perhaps 40% of parotid cancer patients. The onset is usually within the first 6 weeks following radiotherapy. The tolerance dose for otitis media is 40 Gy. This otitis media will generally resolve with time. Nasal steroid sprays are often prescribed but lack any true evidence of clinical effectiveness. Myringotomy with or without a tube can be performed, but the potential risk of persistent perforation or chronic otorrhea might outweigh the benefit [96]. "Tincture of time" is probably the best medical strategy; the majority of patients with radiation otitis media will resolve within 3 months of treatment completion. Instructing patients on the Valsalva maneuver (pinch the nose, blow the nose, and swallow) helps to restore Eustachian tube patency.

Chronic otorrhea can occur in patients following radiotherapy (Fig. 65.8). The most common scenarios giving rise to this condition is myringotomy and tube before, during, or after radiotherapy. Frequently, the drainage is thin, stringy, or mucoid. The middle ear mucosa is often edematous and pale. This type of drainage does not stop with antibiotic drops. Keeping water out of the ear is helpful to minimize the risk of infection. The culture of this drainage can be helpful in deciding appropriate antibiotic drops.

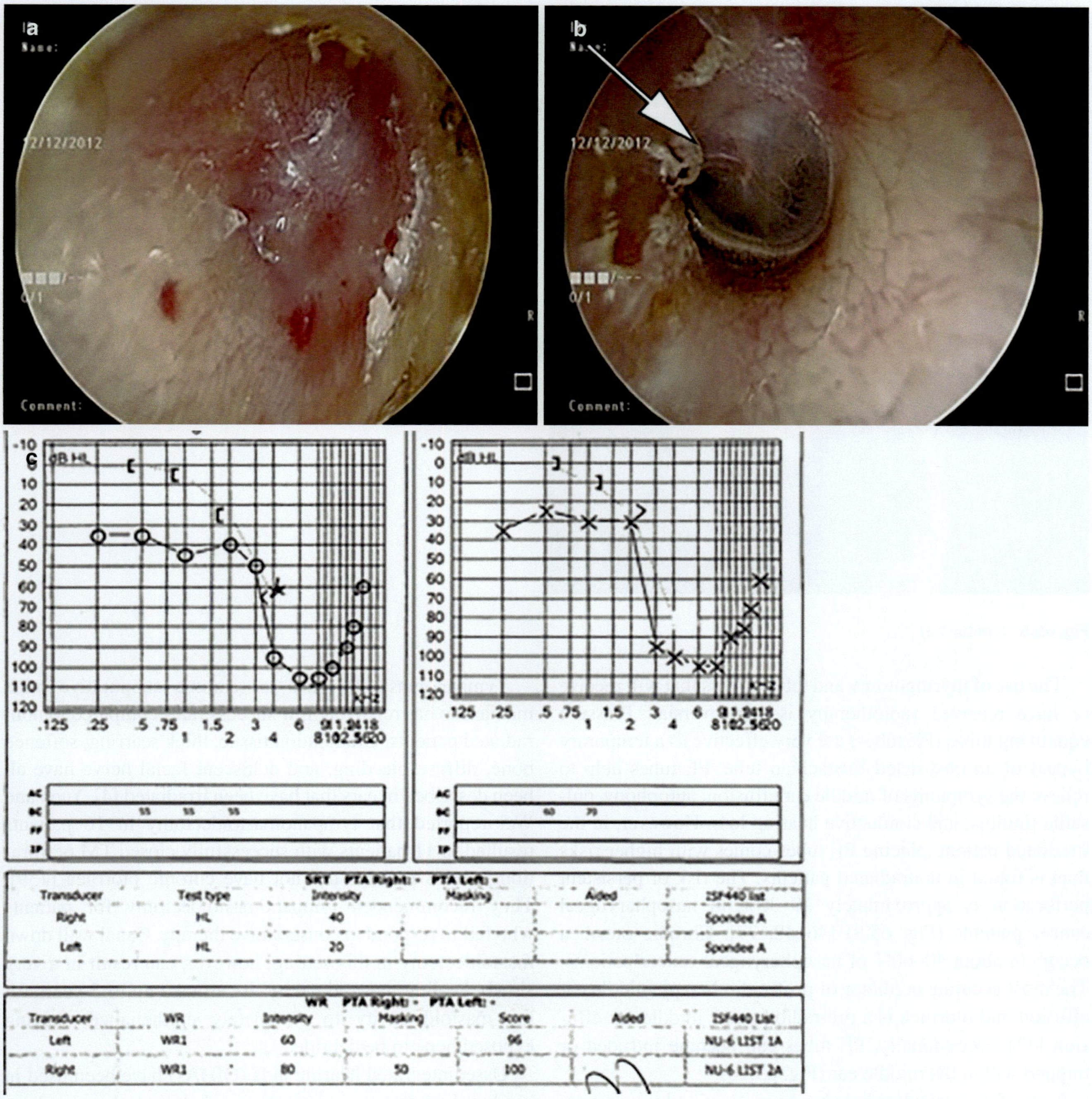

Fig. 65.5 Effacement of the tympanic membrane (TM) and scarring in the anterior sulcus. A 57-year-old man with a history of T4a N1 M0 SCCa in the right mandibular gingiva. Postoperative IMRT at a total dosage of 60 Gy. (**a**) Right ear canal and TM. (**b**) Left ear canal and TM (arrow points to scar band). (**c**) Audiogram. (**d**) CT scan at baseline prior to radiotherapy. (**e**) CT showing thickening of the right TM (arrow) and a normal aerated middle ear. (**f**) The left TM (arrow) is likewise thickened on CT. (©Used with permission, Paul W. Gidley, MD)

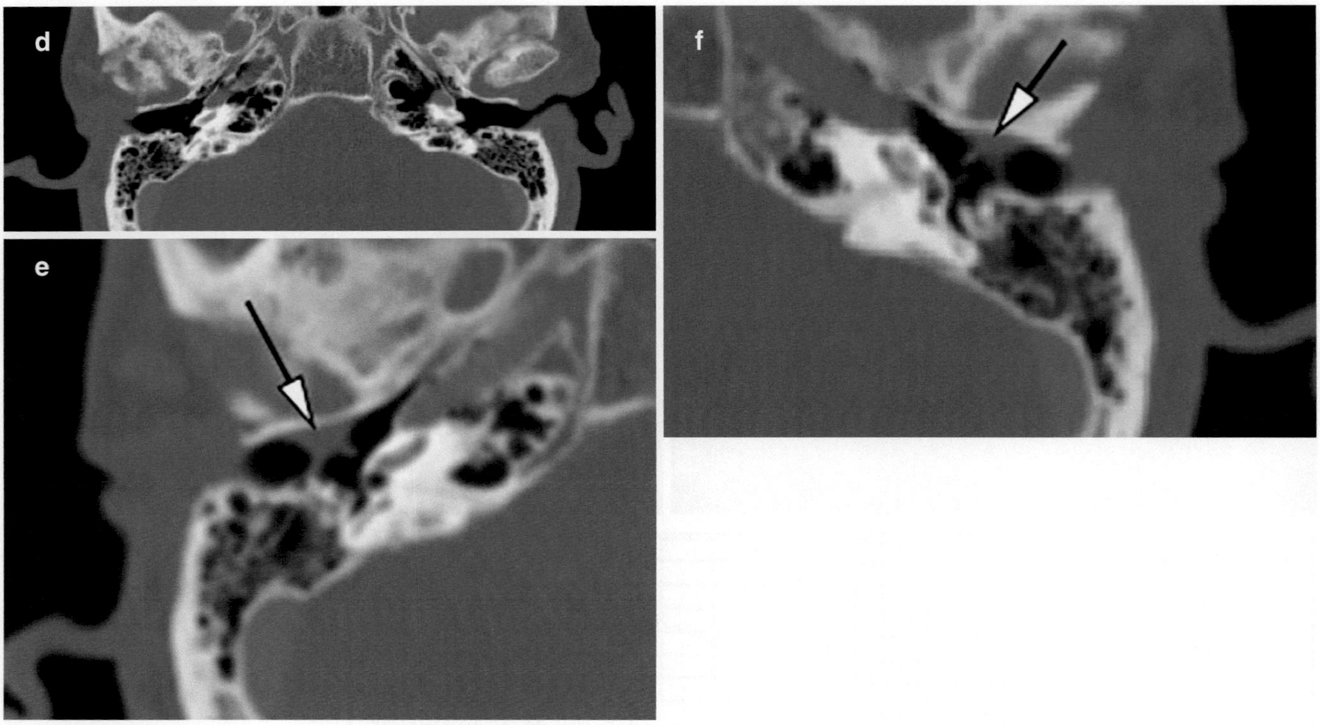

Fig. 65.5 (continued)

The use of myringotomy and tubes in ears that will receive or have received radiotherapy is controversial. Pressure equalizing tubes (PE tubes) are very effective as a temporary bypass of an obstructed Eustachian tube. PE tubes help to relieve the symptoms of middle ear effusion: autophony, pulsatile tinnitus, and conductive hearing loss. However, in the irradiated patient, placing PE tubes comes with higher risks than is found in nonradiated patients. The risk of persistent perforation is approximately 20–30% in nasopharyngeal cancer patients (Fig. 65.9) [46–48, 77]. Chronic otorrhea occurs in about 40–60% of nasopharyngeal cancer patients. The most accurate predictor of post-radiotherapy middle ear effusion and otorrhea is a pre-radiotherapy middle ear effusion [77]. Occasionally, PE tubes can become intruded or trapped within the middle ear (Fig. 65.10).

Loss of the ossicular chain has been described as a sequela of radiation to the temporal bone and is usually associated with ORN [40, 61, 112]. Gyorkey and Pollock were the first to describe this condition; their patient developed a central perforation after ossicular chain reconstruction [40]. Rotteveel et al. also caution about delayed healing in this setting [112].

Tympanoplasty in the irradiated ear has relatively poor outcomes. When the success rate for closure of uncomplicated tympanic membrane (TM) perforation might exceed 90% in a nonradiated ear, the rate of success of tympanoplasty in irradiated ears is only 50–60% [13, 51].

Tympanomastoidectomy for chronic suppurative otitis media also has relatively low success rates compared to nonradiated patients. Granulation tissue, thick scarring, softened bone, diffuse bleeding, and dehiscent facial nerve have all been described in ears that have been irradiated [4]. Yuen and Wei reported that tympanomastoidectomy in 16 patients resulted in 11 patients with successfully closed TM perforations, and 8 patients did not have chronic otorrhea [139]. They recommended tympanomastoidectomy for patients who fail to respond to conservative therapy. Canal wall down mastoidectomy in this setting, however, can result in a very slowly healing mastoid cavity. It can take up to 5 years for the mastoid cavity to completely epithelialize, leaving exposed bone to be debrided.

Osseointegrated hearing aids (OIHAs) have been used in head and neck cancer patients to rehabilitate hearing loss. This hearing loss could be either from surgical intervention, such as lateral temporal bone resection, or from the effects of chemoradiotherapy, as in the case of nasopharyngeal cancer patients.

In the largest series published to date on the use of OIHA for the rehabilitation of hearing from lateral temporal bone resection, Nader et al. identified that patients receiving implants before radiotherapy had better outcomes than patients who received the implant after radiotherapy [92]. Implants placed after radiotherapy had a significantly higher complication rate than those placed before radiotherapy. The

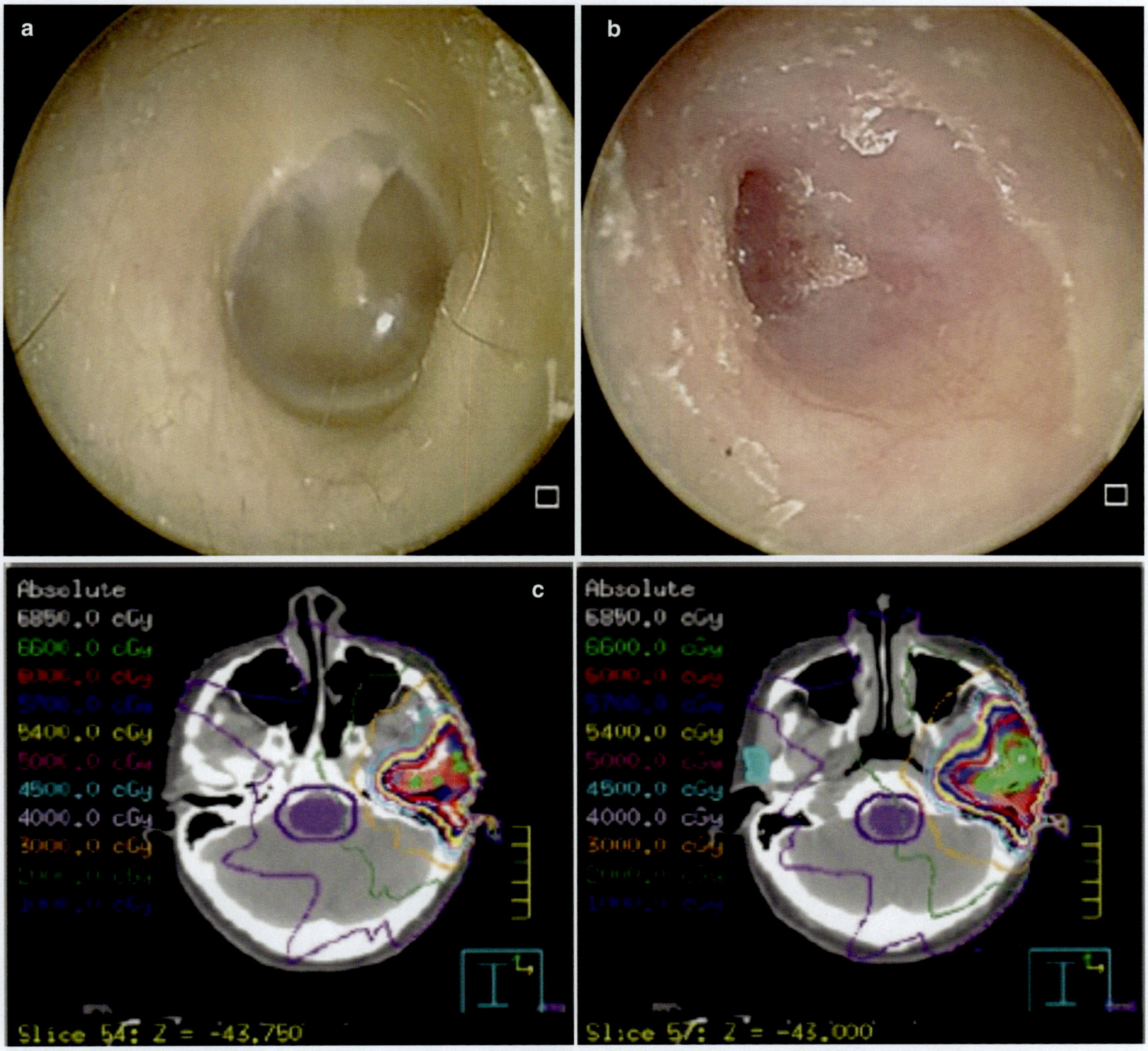

Fig. 65.6 Effacement of the tympanic membrane (TM). This 44-year-old woman had an acinic cell carcinoma of the left parotid gland, s/p left total parotidectomy and completed postoperative radiotherapy. (**a**) Normal right TM. (**b**) Completely effaced left TM. (**c**) Radiation treatment isodose lines. (**d**) CT scan showing thickened left TM (arrow). (**e**) Audiogram. (©Used with permission, Paul W. Gidley, MD)

implants were extruded in only two patients, and both patients received the implants after radiotherapy. Soo et al. described a series of 11 patients who had hearing loss following treatment for nasopharyngeal cancer and who could not wear conventional aids [123]. They reported that the OIHA improved subjective hearing clarity, reduced ear discharge, and increased patient satisfaction.

Inner Ear

In the inner ear, radiotherapy causes a dose-dependent, time-delayed sensorineural hearing loss (SNHL). The effects of radiotherapy on the inner ear are magnified when ototoxic chemotherapy, chiefly cisplatin, is administered either concurrently or sequentially.

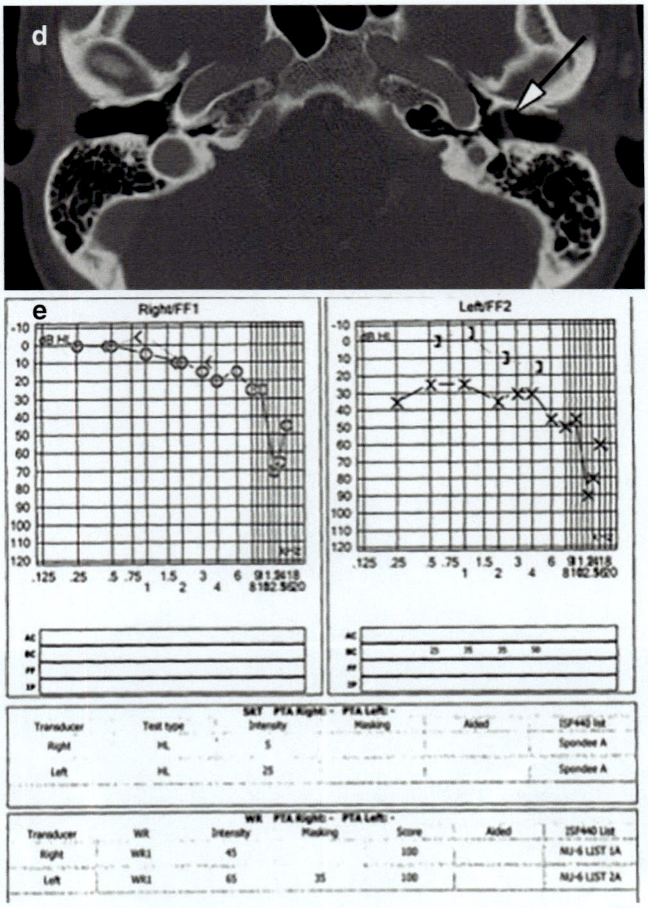

Fig. 65.6 (continued)

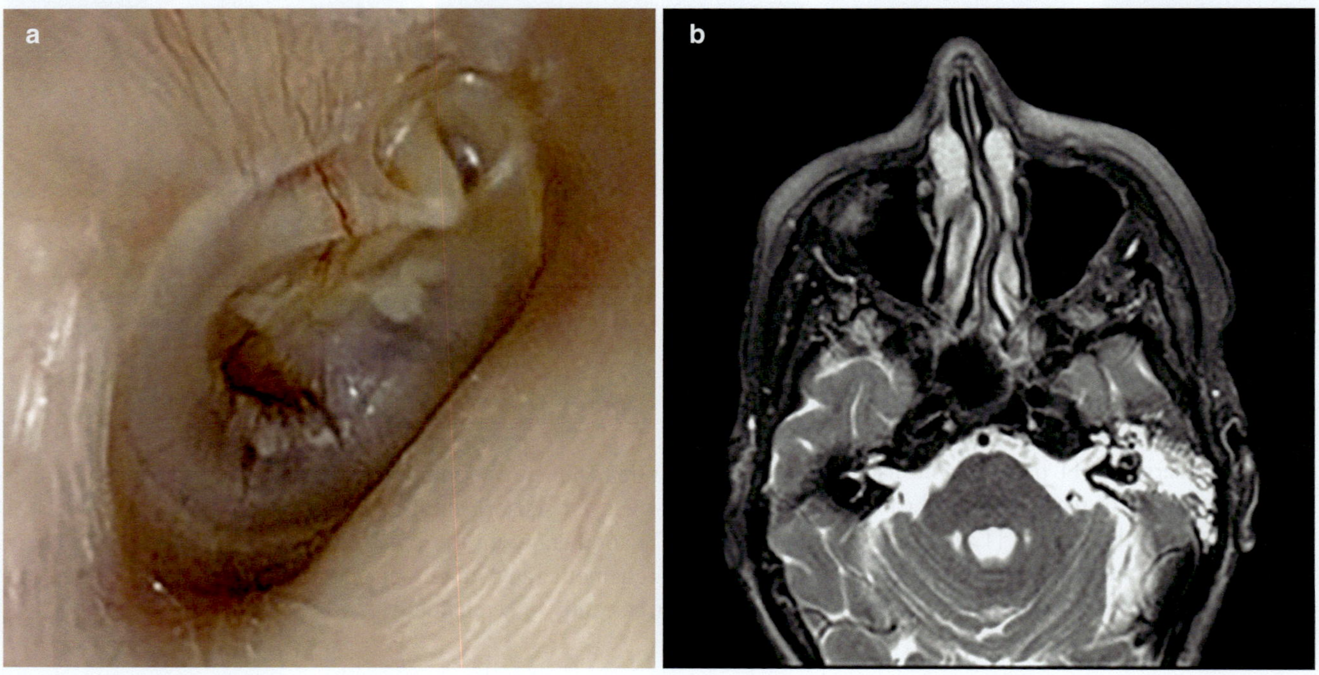

Fig. 65.7 This patient received IMPT for left parotid cancer (max cochlear dose = 24.9 Gy). (**a**) Serous otitis media. (**b**) MRI showing T2 hyper-intense signal 2 months after radiotherapy, consistent with radiation serous otitis media. (©Used with permission, Paul W. Gidley, MD)

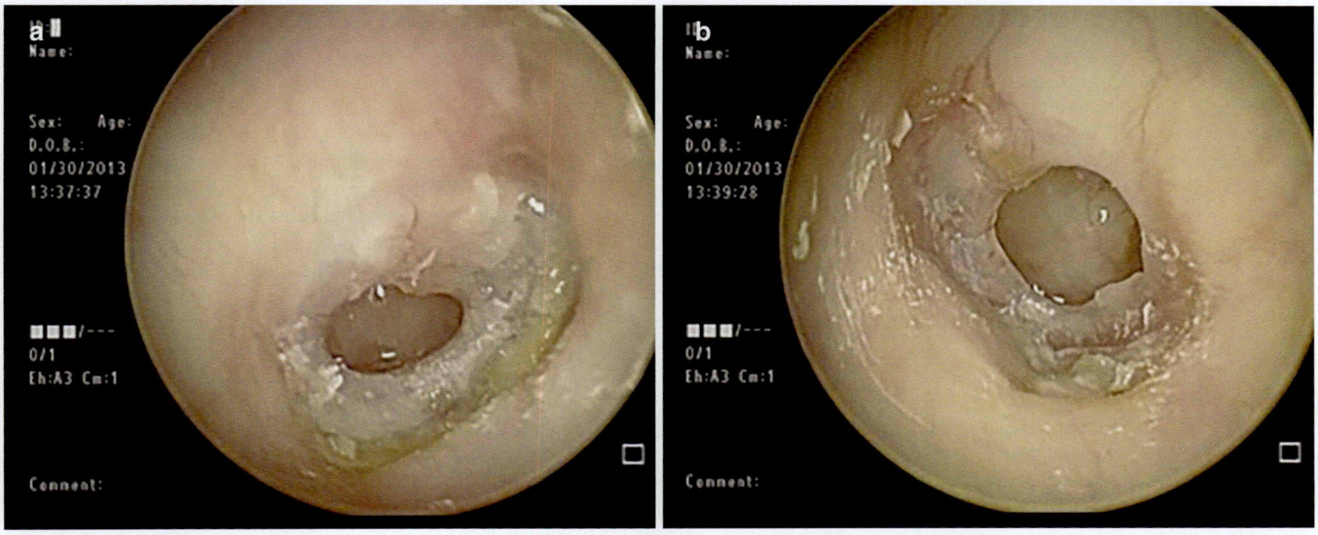

Fig. 65.8 Chronic TM perforation and otorrhea. This patient received chemoradiotherapy for nasopharyngeal carcinoma and had suffered chronic bilateral otorrhea. (**a**) Right ear (**b**) Left ear. (©Used with permission, Paul W. Gidley, MD)

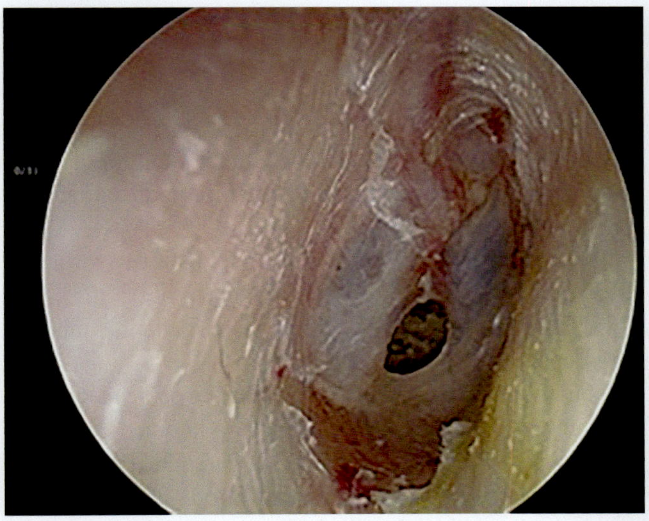
Fig. 65.9 Dry, persistent perforation in the right TM following induction chemotherapy and concurrent chemotherapy for nasopharyngeal cancer. He had a PE tube placed prior to radiotherapy. (©Used with permission, Paul W. Gidley, MD)

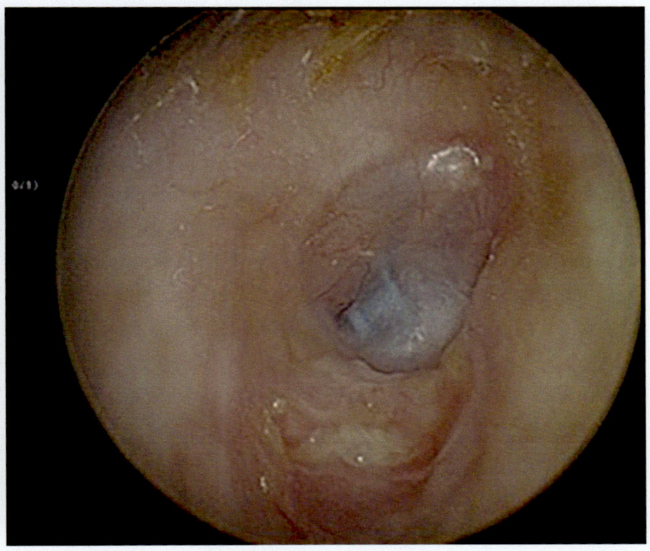
Fig. 65.10 An intruded PE tube was placed in the right TM following induction chemotherapy and concurrent chemoradiotherapy for nasopharyngeal carcinoma. (©Used with permission, Paul W. Gidley, MD)

The definition of significant hearing change varies among studies. Given that radiation can cause both conductive and sensorineural hearing loss, bone conduction (BC) levels are used to assess SNHL. The American Speech-Language-Hearing Association uses a shift of greater than or equal to 20 dB at any frequency or a shift of greater than or equal to 10 dB at 2 or more consecutive BC frequencies [10]. The Common Terminology for Criteria for Adverse Events version 4 uses a threshold shift of 15–25 dB averaged at 2 or more contiguous frequencies in at least one ear (Table 65.1) [1]. The incidence of SNHL with radiotherapy varies from 0% to 43% [124]. The incidence of SNHL with chemoradiotherapy ranges from 17% to 88% [124]. The incidence of SNHL is influenced by radiation dose to the cochlea, length of follow-up, baseline hearing level, age, and cisplatin dose [124].

Radiotherapy affects both inner and outer hair cells throughout the cochlea [49]. The cochlea is more sensitive to radiotherapy than the brain or the auditory nerve [19, 79]. The basal turn of the cochlea is particularly at risk. Histopathologic examination of the irradiated cochlea reveals damage to the organ of Corti and atrophy of the basilar membrane, spiral ligament, and stria vascularis [7, 49, 67, 115]. These changes are greater than what is seen in age-

Table 65.1 Common terminology for criteria for adverse events, version 4, ear and hearing

Adverse event	1	2	3	4
Hearing: patients with/without baseline audiogram and enrolled in a monitoring program	*Adults* enrolled in a monitoring program (on a 1, 2, 3, 4, 6, and 8 kHz audiogram): threshold shift of 15–25 dB averaged at 2 contiguous test frequencies in at least one ear *Adults* not enrolled in monitoring program: subjective change in hearing in the absence of documented hearing loss *Pediatric* (on a 1, 2, 3, 4, 6 and 8 kHz audiogram): threshold shift >20 dB at 8 kHz in at least one ear	*Adults* enrolled in a monitoring program (on a 1, 2, 3, 4, 6, and 8 kHz audiogram): threshold shift of >25 dB averaged at 2 contiguous test frequencies in at least one ear *Adults* not enrolled in monitoring Program: hearing loss but hearing aid or intervention not indicated; limiting instrumental ADL *Pediatric* (on a 1, 2, 3, 4, 6, and 8 kHz audiogram): threshold shift >20 dB at 4 kHz and above in at least one ear	*Adults* enrolled in a monitoring program (on a 1, 2, 3, 4, 6, and 8 kHz audiogram): threshold shift of >25 dB averaged at 3 contiguous test frequencies in at least one ear, therapeutic intervention indicated *Adults* not enrolled in monitoring Program: hearing loss with hearing aid or intervention indicated; limiting self-care ADL *Pediatric* (on a 1, 2, 3, 4, 6 and 8 kHz audiogram): hearing loss sufficient to indicate therapeutic intervention, including hearing aids; threshold shift >20 dB at 3 kHz and above in at least one ear, additional speech-language related services indicated	*Adults*: decrease in hearing to profound, bilateral loss (absolute threshold >80 dB HL at 2 kHz and above); non-serviceable hearing *Pediatric*: audiologic indication for cochlear implant and additional speech-language related services indicated
Hearing: Patients without baseline audiogram and not enrolled in a monitoring program	–	Hearing loss not requiring hearing aid or intervention (i.e., not interfering with ADL)	Hearing loss requiring hearing aid or intervention (i.e., interfering with ADL)	Profound, bilateral hearing loss (>90 dB)

Adapted from the National Cancer Institute Division of Cancer Treatment & Diagnosis (2010). Accessed on 10/13/2024. https://ctep.cancer.gov/protocoldevelopment/electronic_applications/ctc.htm#ctc_40

matched controls. Outer hair cell loss, mainly in the basal turn and sometimes in the middle turn, has been described. This finding would correspond to the high-frequency loss seen in these patients, particularly the 4 kHz frequency [7].

Degeneration of sensory and supporting cells occurs in the stria vascularis, spiral ligament, and basilar membrane [115]. The loss of spiral ganglion cells is especially prominent in the basal turn [67], and this loss might account for the primarily high-frequency sensorineural hearing loss following radiotherapy. Inner ear hemorrhages have been described within the scala media from the stria vascularis and compression of the endolymphatic space from perilymphatic edema [57, 60].

Cochlear hair cells do not divide; cell damage causes permanent loss of these cells. The mechanism of cell death may be related to reactive oxygen species (ROS), a p53 apoptotic pathway, or a p53-independent pathway. Dose-dependent production of ROS has been demonstrated at 1 hour postirradiation in a cochlear inner ear cell line [80]. ROS might explain the high-frequency loss seen in postirradiation patients, since outer hair cells in the basal turn have less antioxidant capacity than do cells in the apical turn. [114] On the basis of in vitro experiments, epithelial cells die as a result of apoptosis [80]. Cochlear hair cells are more susceptible to the damaging effects of radiation than are spiral ganglion cells of the eighth cranial nerve [135]. However, the direct damage of radiation on cochlear hair cells would produce a sudden hearing loss, and this does not explain the delayed and long latency period seen with radiation-induced sensorineural hearing loss [91].

The activation of p53 is a recognized pathway for apoptotic cell death and is a dose-dependent process [25]. The p53 activation starts 72 hours postirradiation and is dose-dependent.

Non-apoptotic pathways might include a p53-independent mechanism or caspase-independent programmed cell death mechanisms [79]. The sphingomyelin-ceramide pathway is a dose-dependent, p53-independent apoptotic pathway that is prominent in epithelial cells 24 hours following radiation-induced DNA damage.[58, 59] This pathway is not found in cochlear hair cells, but it is in vascular endothelial cells, which are found in the stria vascularis [100]. It is possible that vascular effects in the stria vascularis, combined with induced inflammatory changes from radiotherapy, account for the relatively long latency period seen with radiation-induced sensorineural hearing loss

It is difficult to tease apart age-related hearing loss from treatment-related hearing loss [125]. Both conditions may share a similar apoptotic pathway [78]. Williams et al. reported on 100 children with brain tumors [133]. They identified a 27% cumulative incidence of 20 dB or greater hearing loss in the speech range by the fifth year after radiotherapy. The cumulative incidence increases up to 50% within 9 years. None of these patients received chemotherapy. The mean radiation dose was 54 Gy (range 36–70 Gy), and the time to onset ranged from 14 months to 102 months (mean 49 months) [133].

A similar longitudinal study by Hua et al. reported a 14% incidence of hearing loss occurring within 3–5 years [52]. Hearing loss was found to be dose related, being low for 30 Gy or less and high for doses greater than 40–45 Gy. Hearing loss was greatest at 6–8 kHz.

Moeller et al. found that the use of proton beam radiation for childhood medulloblastoma resulted in a low risk of hearing loss at 1 year [87].

Theunissen et al. examined whether concomitant chemoradiation therapy produced progressive hearing loss and found a 21.6 dB increase from baseline in high frequencies (8–12.5 kHz) at short-term follow-up and a further 5 dB hearing loss at long-term follow-up [125]. This hearing loss is greater than what would be expected from aging only.

Li et al. prospectively studied 42 patients with nasopharyngeal carcinoma treated with radiotherapy only. After 1 month, the BC threshold at 8 kHz was statistically significantly increased [71]. The incidence of significant SNHL at 4 kHz was 12.5% at 1 month, 42% at 1 year, and 50% at 2 years.

Hearing loss starts at 4 kHz and higher frequencies, and the incidence of this hearing loss increased with time [124]. This hearing loss occurs within 1.5–2 years posttreatment [15, 47, 48].

The tolerance dose for the cochlea is quoted to be 60 Gy [34]. The rate of SNHL may be as high as 24–36% after radiation doses of 60 Gy [62, 84, 91]. The probability of hearing loss increased with doses above 40 Gy, and the clinical goal is to keep the cochlear dose below 30 Gy [50].

The incidence of SNHL in nasopharyngeal cancer patients is about 30% on average (range 0–57%), and this hearing loss generally occurs over the first 2 years following therapy [129]. Wei et al. compared hearing results between nasopharyngeal patients who received radiation alone versus chemoradiotherapy [132]. Hearing loss was more severe in the chemoradiotherapy group than in the radiotherapy group, especially in the high-frequency range. They found that hearing level is seriously damaged when the cochlear dose exceeds 46 Gy [132].

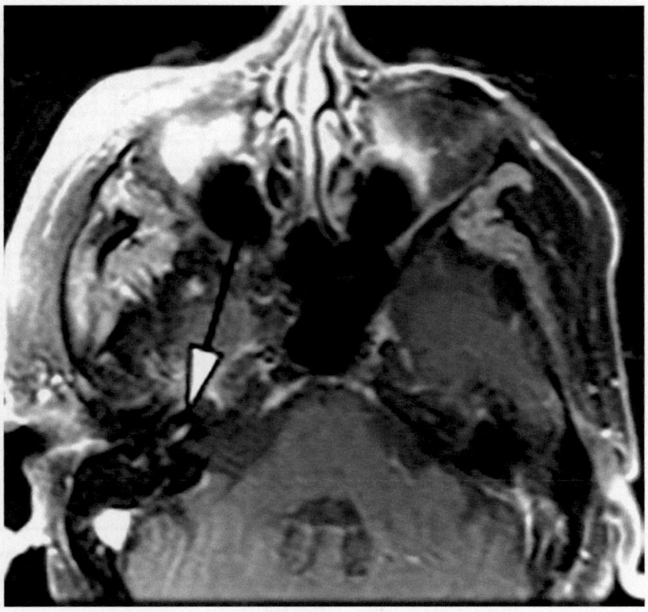

Fig. 65.11 T1 contrast-enhanced MRI showing enhancement of the basal turn of the right cochlea (arrow) after sudden hearing loss 5 years post-XRT for NPCa. (©Used with permission, Paul W. Gidley, MD)

Herrmann et al. showed, in a dose-effect analysis, a 50% incidence of significant SNHL (15 dB or greater change) with a dose of 20–25 Gy [44]. Other studies indicated an increased risk of SNHL when the cochlea received a total dose of at least 47–55 Gy [15, 23, 26, 106].

Sudden hearing loss has been described in this same population (Fig. 65.11), and it occurs in roughly 8% of patients [138]. Caution should be exercised in the use of intratympanic steroids since these have been associated with total or near-total tympanic membrane perforations in the postradiation setting [117].

The vestibular organs are thought to be more radioresistant than the cochlea [36]. Histologic examination of the vestibular system after radiotherapy shows normal semicircular canals [49]. Mechanisms to explain imbalance and dizziness with radiotherapy have been attributed to direct injury of the inner ear and radiotherapy-induced otitis media. Dizziness is thought to affect 25–30% of patients with radiotherapy to the temporal bone [120]. Caloric weakness has been reported in 9–36% of patients with irradiated temporal bones (Fig. 65.12) [55].

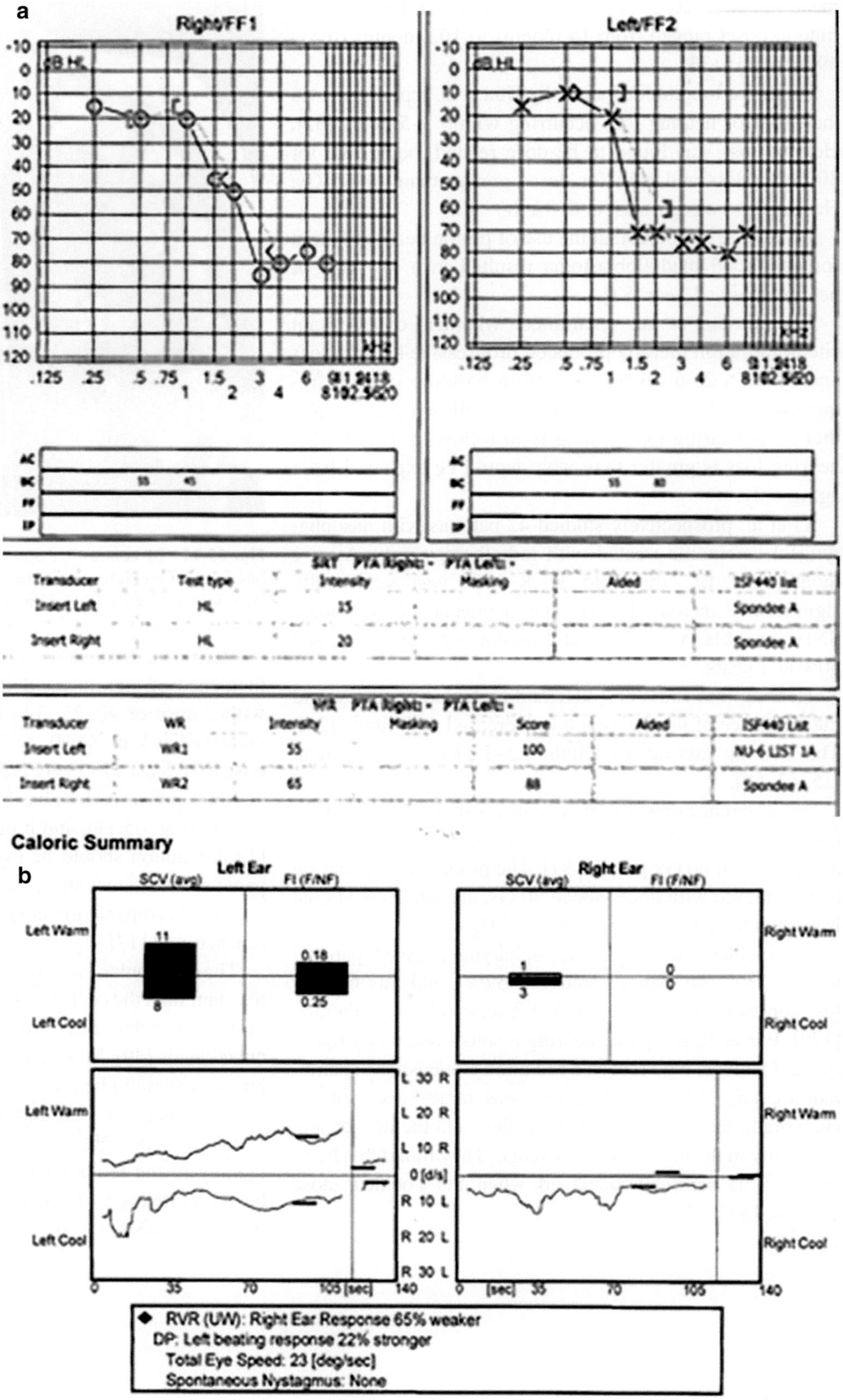

Fig. 65.12 Vestibular weakness following radiation to the parotid gland. This 77-year-old man with a history of metastatic squamous cell cancer of the skin, status post right parotidectomy and neck dissection, followed by PORT (60 Gy). He began to have balance problems about 6 months after completing his radiotherapy. (**a**) Audiogram. (**b**) VNG. (©Used with permission, Paul W. Gidley, MD)

Major Complications of Radiotherapy to the Temporal Bone

Several complications can arise many years after radiotherapy to the temporal bone. These complications can involve the bone, brain, or blood vessels of the temporal bone. These complications are considered major since they often require surgical or medical intervention to avoid serious injury or death.

Osteoradionecrosis

Osteoradionecrosis (ORN) is the most common major complication of radiotherapy to the temporal bone. The most common symptoms of ORN are crusting within the ear canal (100%), otalgia (91%), otorrhea (91%), hearing loss (73%), foul-smelling otorrhea (45%) and retroauricular fistula (9%) [43]). The pain is occasionally described as deep or boring and can be intractable [17]. The overall incidence of ORN of the temporal bone is elusive. Ang et al. report that ORN of the mandible occurs in 4–30% of patients undergoing head and neck radiation [6]. Morrissey et al. reported an 8.5% incidence of ORN of the temporal bone in a surgical database of 82 head and neck cancer patients [89]. All of these affected patients had a parotidectomy. In a separate study of patients who underwent parotidectomy with postoperative radiotherapy, Leonetti et al. reported a 2% incidence of localized ORN after parotidectomy alone, a 13% incidence after parotidectomy with mastoidectomy, and 0% incidence of ORN after parotidectomy with subtotal temporal bone resection [69].

ORN is a late reaction to radiation, and it is followed by a compensatory reparative fibrosis [115]. Many different organisms, both bacterial and fungal, can be cultured from the surface and not the center of necrotic bone, whereas in osteomyelitis, the infecting organism is always found in the center of bone [83].

The *sine qua non* of ORN is exposed bone in the ear canal (Fig. 65.13). As described by Ramsden et al., ORN can be divided into two types: localized and diffuse [109]. CT scanning can be helpful in discerning these two types and determining which patients might require surgical intervention. CT can demonstrate external canal erosions, mastoid effusion, mastoid coalescence, enhancing soft tissue, soft tissue gas, temporomandibular joint erosion, and abscess formation [5].

Localized ORN involves a disease that is limited to the ear canal. The average latency period for localized disease is 7–12 years, but exposed bone can be identified as early as 4 months after radiotherapy [5, 42, 43]. The most common location for exposed bone is in the floor of the canal.

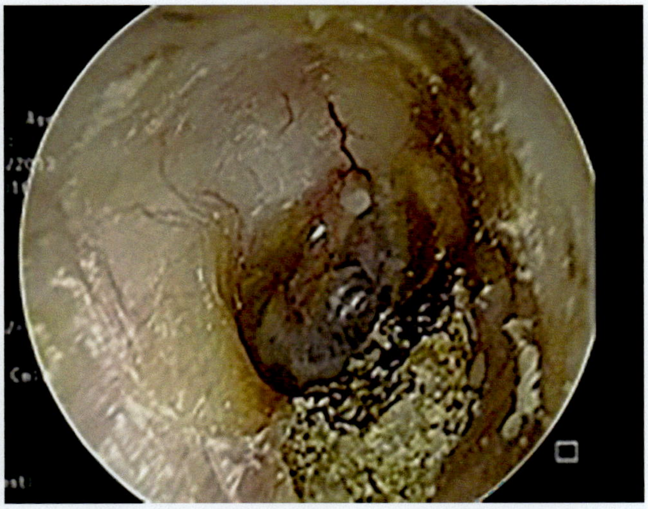

Fig. 65.13 Localized ORN in a nasopharyngeal cancer patient. (©Used with permission, Paul W. Gidley, MD)

Localized ORN is usually managed with ear cleaning to remove built-up keratin debris and crusts. Antibiotic drops, hydrogen peroxide, and vinegar–water irrigations can be used between cleanings to minimize bacterial overgrowth. Avoiding chronic use of antibiotic drops might help prevent the creation of resistant organisms [65]. The presence of biofilm in ORN has been postulated as an explanation for the recalcitrance of this disease process to antibiotic therapy [94].

In these patients, the granulation tissue and skin of the ear canal grow underneath the exposed bone. As this soft tissue builds up, it undermines the exposed bone. The bone can then be easily removed from the ear canal (Fig. 65.14). The process for complete healing and re-epithelialization can take several years. Hao et al. describe a group of 33 patients treated with sequestrectomy and HBO and found that this technique controlled the disease process in 77% of patients [42].

For localized ORN, operative intervention is usually not indicated. Skin grafts generally do not engraft due to the relatively poor blood supply of the ear canal. Hill et al. and Metselaar et al. have described using a postauricular skin flap for reconstruction of the ear canal for repair of ORN of the tympanic ring [45, 85]. They stress the fact that this flap comes from skin that has not been irradiated. A split temporalis muscle flap has also been described [127].

Diffuse ORN involves the temporal bone beyond the ear canal, usually including the mastoid (Fig. 65.15). The average latency period is 8 years. Diffuse ORN can create its own set of complications, including facial palsy, CSF leak, meningitis, brain abscess, carotid aneurysm, and sigmoid sinus thrombosis [17, 70, 72, 101, 119, 121]. By its very nature, diffuse ORN requires surgical intervention. Often, this surgi-

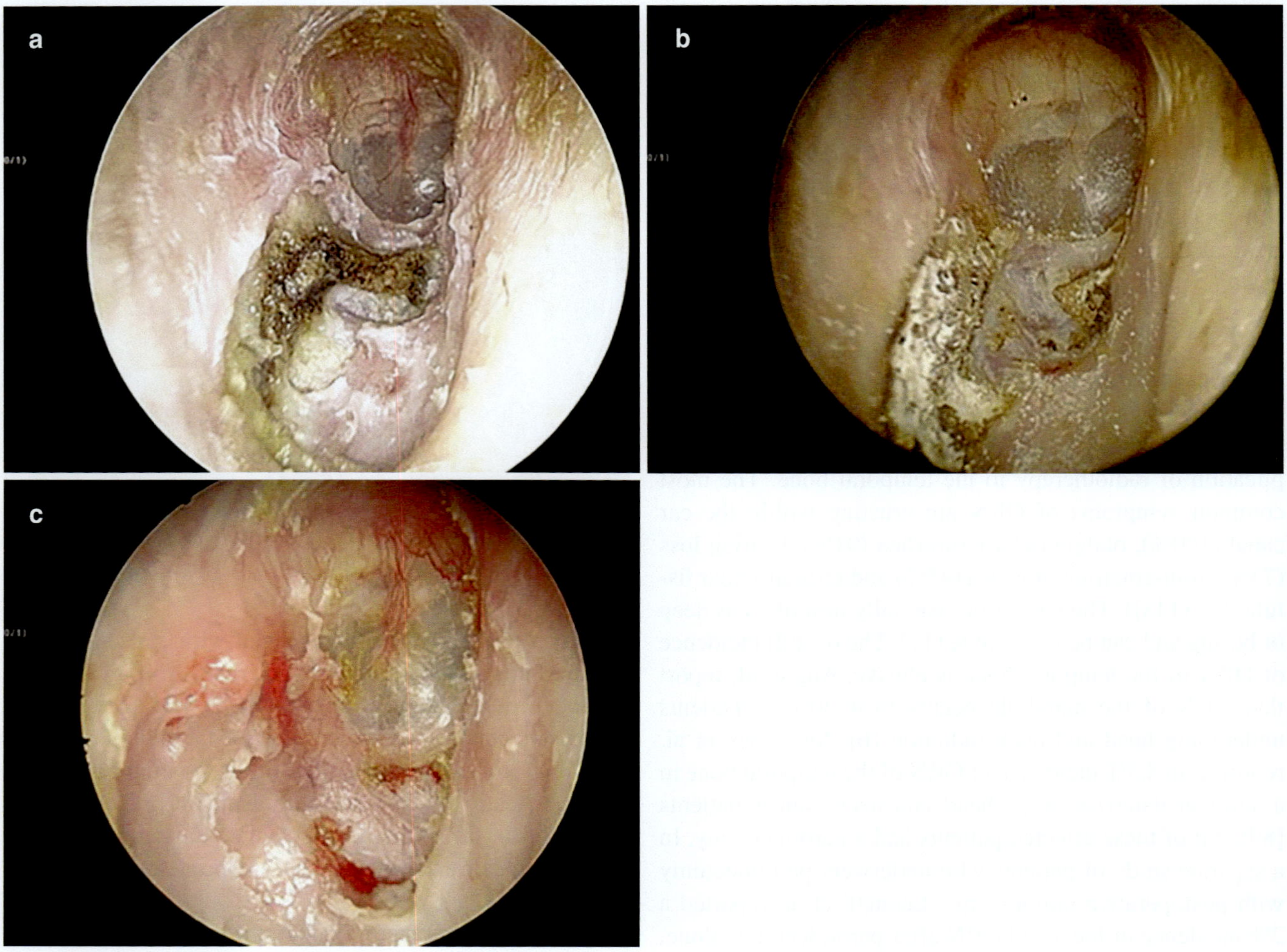

Fig. 65.14 Sequestrectomy of exposed bone from the ear canal. (**a**) The right ear canal of a woman who received radiotherapy for brain metastases of breast cancer. (**b**) One week later, following sequestrectomy. (**c**) 6 months later. (©Used with permission, Paul W. Gidley, MD)

cal intervention includes either mastoid obliteration, subtotal petrosectomy, or lateral temporal bone resection with closure of the ear canal [11, 39, 82, 98, 99, 119, 136]. Soft tissue coverage requires either a temporalis muscle flap or a microvascular free flap [6, 42].

A common feature of diffuse ORN is erosion of the posterior ear canal wall and the spread of disease into the mastoid air cells. Such a canal–mastoid fistula permits ear canal skin to penetrate into the mastoid (Fig. 65.16) [115]. Skin cannot exfoliate properly and accumulates in the airways. With time, this skin or cholesteatoma destroys the bone of the mastoid and can produce such complications as facial paralysis, meningitis, and sigmoid sinus thrombosis [115].

Lovin et al. conducted a review of 128 patients (145 temporal bones) with ORN at MD Anderson [76]. The most common primary tumor sites were periauricular skin (24%), parotid gland (22%), nasopharyngeal cancer (20%), and oral cavity (10%) [76]. The time from the end of radiotherapy to a diagnosis of ORN ranged from less than 1 year to 56 years, with a mean interval of 10 years. Age greater than 50 years at completion of radiotherapy was associated with an earlier diagnosis ($p < 0.001$). The time to development of ORN was not associated with the primary tumor location. The mean total dose to the primary was 61.8 Gy. In a subset of 58 patients, the mean cochlear dose was 40 Gy, the external canal dose of 49 Gy, and the mastoid dose of 47 Gy (unpublished data). Seventy-six percent (76%) had localized disease, and 24% had diffuse disease. Most patients (81%) were managed conservatively with periodic aural cleaning. Oftentimes, the epithelium of the ear canal undermines the exposed bone, and the dead bone can be curetted away. Only 28 patients required surgery, usually for diffuse ORN, canal–mastoid fistula, cholesteatoma, or Bezold's abscess. Surgery usually involves mastoid obliteration, subtotal petrosectomy, or lateral temporal bone resection. Risk factors associated with diffuse disease were diabetes, 3D-CRT, and periauricular skin primary [76].

Phillips et al. reported on 23 patients with ORN [108]. The most common tumor site was the parotid gland. The mean tumor dose was 58.2 Gy. The time interval was 2–48 years, with an average of 11 years. All patients in this series were managed conservatively with in-office debridement and antibiotic therapy.

Sharon et al. reported on 33 patients with ORN [118]. The parotid gland and nasopharynx were the most common primary tumor sites. The mean tumor dose was 62.6 Gy, with a mean dose to the temporal bone of 53 Gy and a mean dose to the tympanic bone of 65.2 Gy. The time interval was 1–22 years, with an average of 7.9 years. Surgery was performed in 18 out of 33 patients.

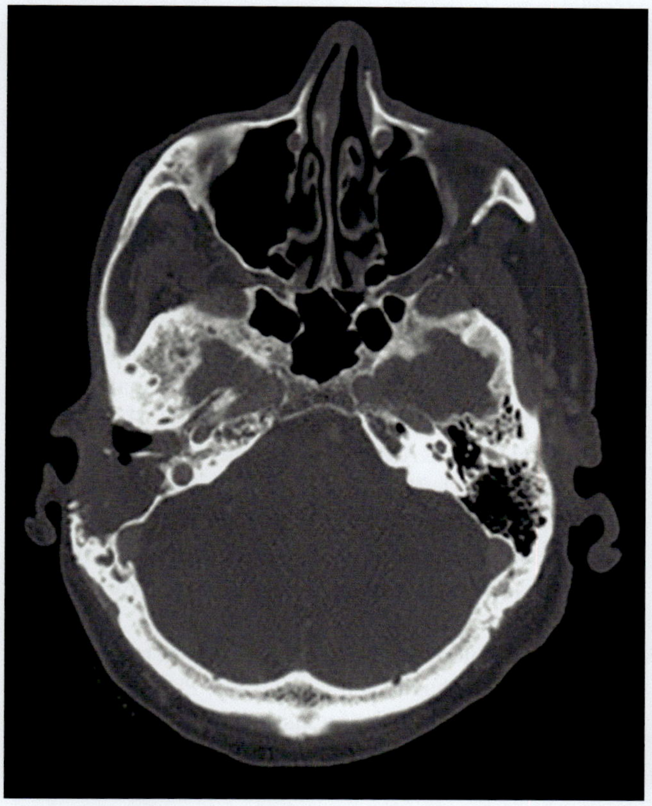

Fig. 65.15 Diffuse ORN 10 years after radiotherapy for parotid cancer. (©Used with permission, Paul W. Gidley, MD)

Nonsurgical management of ORN of the temporal bone has been described. Hyperbaric oxygen (HBO) treatment has been used by some groups in the management of ORN [6, 8, 9, 42, 43, 85, 93, 105, 113, 116, 128]. The reparative effect of HBO is through hyperoxygenation, which increases tissue oxygen levels, causes vasoconstriction without hypoxia, and increases antimicrobial activity [116]. HBO is not curative but might promote better wound healing. HBO is avoided in any patient with active cancer, since it might promote tumor growth.

A medical protocol for treating ORN of the jaw has been developed and tested in a randomized controlled trial [30–33, 110]. This protocol, developed for jaw ORN, has been applied to one case of temporal bone ORN [37]. This protocol, called PENTOCLO, has two phases. The first phase is an "antiseptic" phase using prednisone, amoxicillin/clavulanate, ciprofloxacin, and fluconazole for 2 weeks. The second phase uses pentoxifylline, vitamin E, chlodronate, ciprofloxacin, and prednisone (Table 65.2). This protocol achieves clinical and radiological regression of jaw ORN and a reduction in the need for major surgery [110].

A similar protocol called pentoxifylline–tocopherol (PENTO), since chlodronate is not available in the US, was used on 5 patients [75]. Four out of the five patients demonstrated a decrease in bone exposure over the study period (mean 302 days).

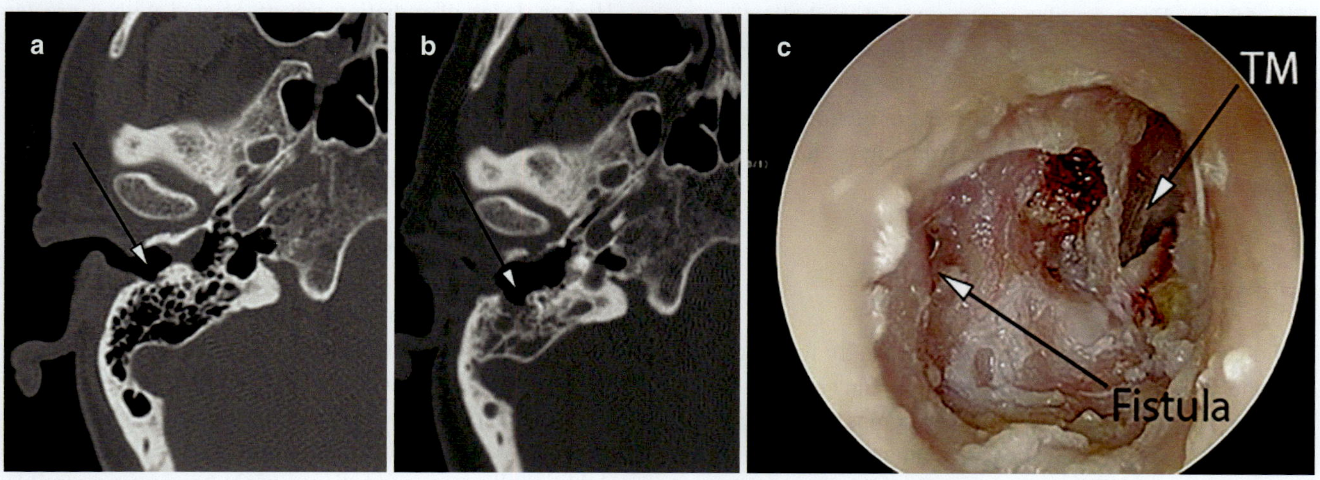

Fig. 65.16 Progression of ORN from ear canal fistula. (**a**) CT scan of right ear canal in a patient who received radiotherapy for Merkel cell carcinoma of the right cheek, showing a break in the ear canal bone (arrow). (**b**) CT scan taken 18 months later showing diffuse ORN and canal fistula (arrow). (**c**) Oto-endoscopic view at the same time as (b), showing canal fistula and TM. (©Used with permission, Paul W. Gidley, MD)

Table 65.2 PENTOCLO protocol for jaw ORN

Antiseptic treatment (2 weeks)		
Prednisone	20 mg	Daily
Amoxicillin/clavulanate	2 g/500 mg	Daily
Ciprofloxacin	1 g	Daily
Fluconazole	50 mg	Daily
PENTOCLO		
Pentoxifylline	400 mg	BID, 5 d/wk
Vitamin E	600 units	QAM, 5 d/wk
Vitamin E	400 units	QPM, 5 d/wk
Clodronate	1600 mg	Daily, 5 d/wk
Ciprofloxacin	1 g	On remaining 2 d/wk
Prednisone	20 mg	On remaining 2 d/wk

Sigmoid Sinus and Carotid Artery

Damage to the great vessels around the temporal bone can occur following radiotherapy. Lateral sinus thrombosis can occur without signs or symptoms of acute mastoiditis (Fig. 65.17). These patients present with daily headaches. While acute mastoiditis with lateral sinus thrombosis produces picket fence fevers, postradiation lateral sinus thrombosis can present without fever. Other symptoms, such as photophobia, phonophobia, and nausea or vomiting, can also be absent. Treatment is long-term anticoagulation. In the setting of acute infection and cholesteatoma, sigmoid sinus thrombosis has been treated with embolectomy and intraluminal packing [70].

Small, brief episodes of bleeding from the ear can herald impending carotid artery rupture [56]. Such "sentinel" bleeding episodes often occur in the setting of prior nasopharyngeal carcinoma. This is frequently associated with ORN of the temporal bone [66] or with recurrent nasopharyngeal carcinoma [63]. The key is to recognize these bleeding events as more than simply bloody show from abraded ear canal skin (Fig. 65.18). Endovascular treatment with embolization or coiling of the internal carotid artery is indicated to prevent a catastrophic hemorrhage [16, 28, 63, 66, 70]. Although this procedure can be associated with severe neurologic impairment such as hemiplegia [56], the alternative is exsanguination.

Temporal Lobe Necrosis

Radiotherapy to the temporal bone, especially for parotid or nasopharyngeal cancer, can produce brain necrosis in the temporal lobe [68, 90, 111, 130]. The symptoms of temporal lobe necrosis include headache, memory loss, and mood changes. CT and MRI show areas of cystic degeneration of the temporal lobe. Diffusion-weighted imaging is particularly useful to distinguish a brain abscess from necrosis [24]. Occasionally, such patients require a craniotomy to resect the dead brain (Fig. 65.19). Brain edema from temporal lobe necrosis has resulted in patient death [53].

Radiation-Associated Malignancy

Perhaps the most serious of these major complications is radiation-associated malignancy (RAM). Radiation-associated malignancies must satisfy certain criteria: (1) the tumor must arise in a location that was irradiated, (2) the tumor must be a different histologic type than the original tumor, and (3) there must be an interval period between radiation and the secondary tumor, usually more than 4 years [2, 22, 74, 102].

The pathophysiology of the development of RAM is poorly understood. Radiation-induced genomic instability and p53 mutations may contribute to their development [103, 104]. Typically, RAMs are sarcomas usually arising from bone and are generally high grade [104]. However, for the temporal bone, RAMs are either sarcomas or squamous cell carcinoma [12, 38, 73, 81]. In fact, squamous cell carcinomas are more frequent than sarcomas. In a series from MD Anderson on RAM, squamous cell carcinoma made up 76% of these tumors, while only 3 patients (24%) had sarcomas [64].

Typical symptoms of RAM in the temporal bone are otorrhea, otalgia, otorrhagia, and facial palsy. Physical examination can identify granulation tissue or frank malignancy (Fig. 65.20). The differential diagnosis includes chronic otitis media, cholesterol granuloma, primary tumor recurrence, metastatic tumor, and osteoradionecrosis [29, 131, 137]. In patients with a previous history of head and neck radiotherapy, these symptoms and an ear canal soft tissue mass should prompt a biopsy.

Higher doses of radiation are associated with a greater risk of the development of RAM. A total dose of 55 Gy or higher increases the risk of developing radiation-associated sarcomas [103]. Squamous cell carcinoma tends to develop in lower-dose radiation fields [97]. Since the EAC usually receives less than 50 Gy during treatment for nasopharyngeal, oropharyngeal, and parotid cancers, squamous cell carcinomas tend to predominate as the main RAM of the temporal bone.

RAM that arises in low-dose radiation fields tends to have a longer latency than sarcomas [41]. Lambert et al. reported an average latency period of 13 years (range 4–33 years). Other authors have reported similar mean latency periods (12.6–15.5 years) [2, 38, 73, 74, 81, 104].

Additionally, younger patients might be more susceptible to the tumorigenic potential of radiotherapy than older patients. This fact might account for a higher rate of sarcomas in younger patients than in older patients [64].

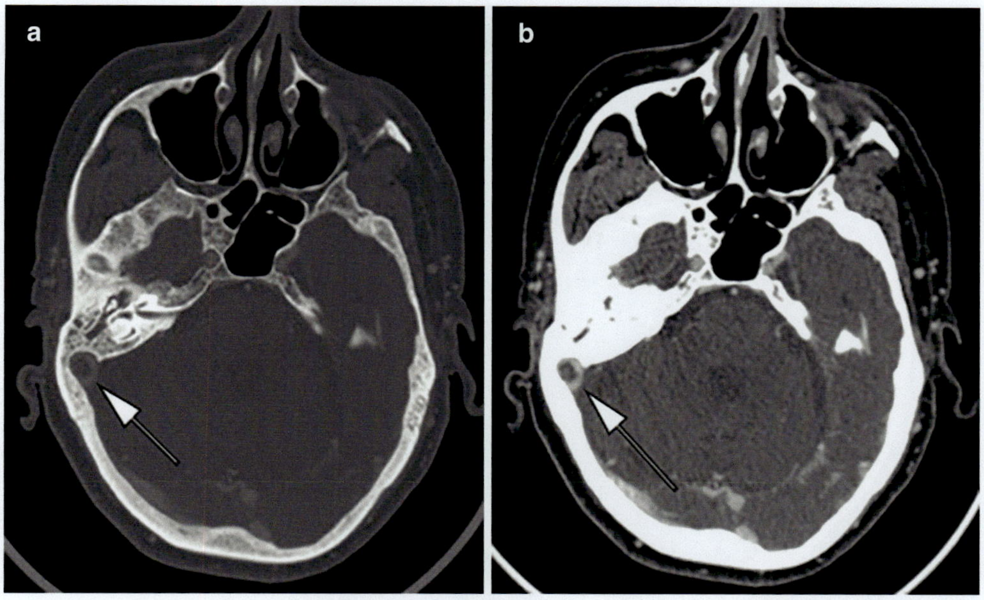

Fig. 65.17 Postradiation lateral sinus thrombosis (arrow). (**a**) Contrast-enhanced CT scan. (**b**) Contrast-enhanced MRI scan. (©Used with permission, Paul W. Gidley, MD)

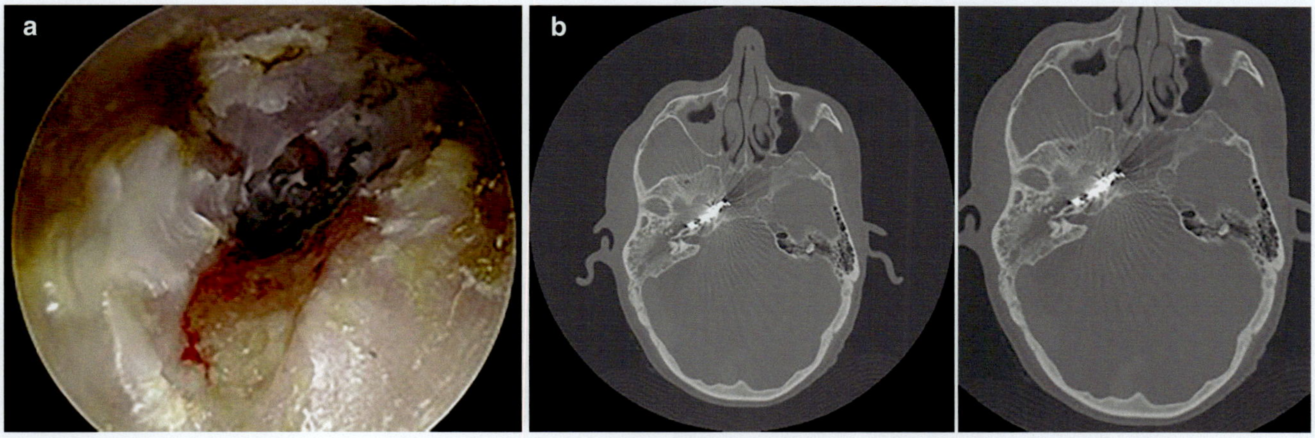

Fig. 65.18 Carotid artery rupture. This 57-year-old man had a history of squamous cell carcinoma of the right fossa of Rosenmuller. He was treated with concurrent chemotherapy (cisplatin 100 mg/M2) and radiotherapy (IMRT 70 Gy). Four years later, he presented with intermittent bleeding from the right ear. (**a**) Right ear canal, showing exposed bone and abraded canal skin. (**b**) He underwent endovascular coiling of the right internal carotid artery after a significant episode of otorrhagia. A CT scan shows the coils in the artery. (©Used with permission, Paul W. Gidley, MD)

Tumors that extend beyond the ear canal are more difficult to treat and have lower overall survival. This fact is true of all temporal bone cancers, and it is recognized in the Pittsburgh staging system for squamous cell carcinoma of the temporal bone [88]. Tumors limited to the ear canal (Pittsburgh stages 1 and 2) are effectively managed with lateral temporal bone resection. Once tumors extend beyond the ear canal, complete surgical excision becomes more difficult. The inability to obtain a frozen section on bone limits the ability to achieve negative margins. Indeed, in the study by Lambert et al., better outcomes were found in patients who were limited to the ear canal, older patients, and in cases with negative margins [64]. Higher staged tumors (Pittsburgh stage 3 or 4) are often treated with neoadjuvant chemotherapy followed by surgical resection. Reconstruction options for temporal bone resection can include either a temporalis muscle flap or a microvascular free flap. Since the temporalis muscle is often in the radiated field and since its blood supply might have been affected by prior surgery, microvascular free flaps are favored in this setting.

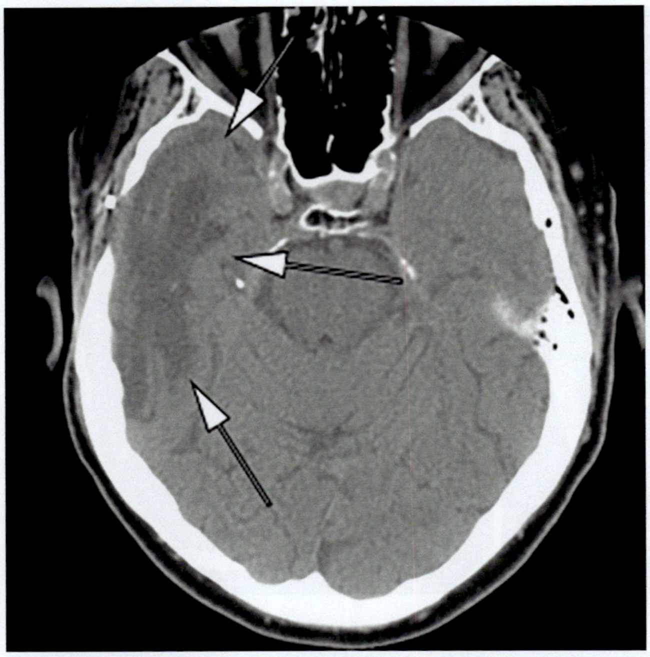

Fig. 65.19 Temporal lobe necrosis 4 years after postoperative radiotherapy for salivary duct carcinoma of the right parotid gland. Four years later, this patient developed diffuse ORN requiring lateral temporal bone resection. (©Used with permission, Paul W. Gidley, MD)

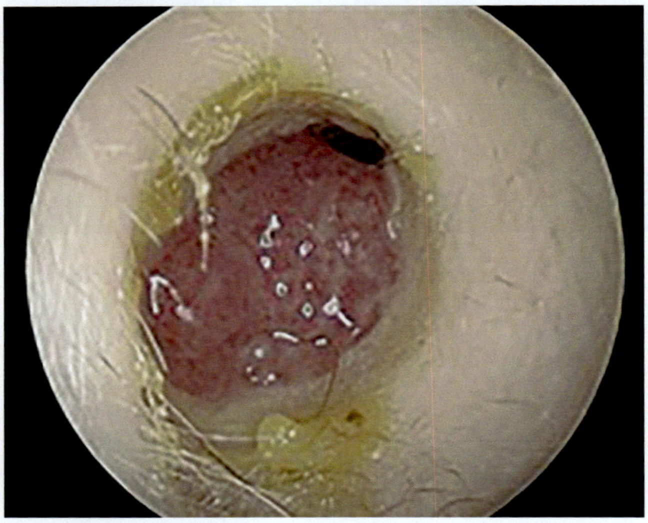

Fig. 65.20 Radiation-associated squamous cell carcinoma of the ear canal. (©Used with permission, Paul W. Gidley, MD)

Conclusion

While chemotherapy and radiotherapy can positively influence the survivability of head and neck cancer, they also introduce a risk for short- and long-term damage to the temporal bone and its related structures and functions. Healing impairment within a radiated field can be problematic when surgical treatment is pursued in this patient population, even in the setting of a relatively minor procedure such as a transtympanic injection. As the effects of radiotherapy evolve over time, a judicious and cautious management strategy is recommended, as is multidisciplinary care in the setting of infection or RAM.

References

1. 2010. Common Terminology Criteria for Adverse Events (CTCAE) Version 4.0. From https://evs.nci.nih.gov/ftp1/CTCAE/CTCAE_4.03_2010-06-14_QuickReference_8.5x11.pdf.
2. Abrigo JM, King AD, Leung SF, Vlantis AC, Wong JK, Tong MC, Gary M, Ahuja AT. MRI of radiation-induced tumors of the head and neck in post-radiation nasopharyngeal carcinoma. Eur Radiol. 2009;19(5):1197.
3. Adler M, Hawke M, Berger G, Harwood A. Radiation effects on the external auditory canal. J Otolaryngol. 1985;14(4):226–32.
4. Adunka OF, Buchman CA. Cochlear implantation in the irradiated temporal bone. J Laryngol Otol. 2007;121(1):83–6.
5. Ahmed S, Gupta N, Hamilton JD, Garden AS, Gidley PW, Ginsberg LE. CT findings in temporal bone osteoradionecrosis. J Comput Assist Tomogr. 2014;38(5):662–6.
6. Ang E, Black C, Irish J, Brown DH, Gullane P, O'Sullivan B, Neligan PC. Reconstructive options in the treatment of osteoradionecrosis of the craniomaxillofacial skeleton. Br J Plast Surg. 2003;56(2):92–9.
7. Asenov DR, Kaga K, Tsuzuku T. Changes in the audiograms of a nasopharyngeal cancer patient during the course of treatment: a temporal bone histopathological study. Acta Otolaryngol. 2007;127(10):1105–10.
8. Ashamalla HL, Ames JW, Uri A, Winkler P. Hyperbaric oxygen in the management of osteoradionecrosis. Med Pediatr Oncol. 1996;27(1):48–53.
9. Ashamalla HL, Thom SR, Goldwein JW. Hyperbaric oxygen therapy for the treatment of radiation-induced sequelae in children. The University of Pennsylvania experience. Cancer. 1996;77(11):2407–12.
10. American Speech-Language-Hearing Association. Audiologic management of individuals receiving cochleotoxic drug therapy [Guidelines]. ASHA; 1994. Available from: https://www.asha.org/policy/gl1994-00003/.
11. Bartoszewicz R, Bruzgielewicz A, Osuch-Wojcikiewicz E, Sokolowski J, Niemczyk K. Osteoradionecrosis of the temporal bone. Otolaryngol Pol. 2011;65(5 Suppl):85–92.
12. Beal DD, Lindsay JR, Ward PH. Radiation-induced carcinoma of the mastoid. Arch Otolaryngol. 1965;81:9–16.
13. Bennett M, Kaylie D, Warren F, Jackson CG. Chronic ear surgery in irradiated temporal bones. Laryngoscope. 2007;117(7):1240–4.
14. Bentzen SM. Preventing or reducing late side effects of radiation therapy: radiobiology meets molecular pathology. Nat Rev Cancer. 2006;6(9):702–13.
15. Bhandare N, Antonelli PJ, Morris CG, Malayapa RS, Mendenhall WM. Ototoxicity after radiotherapy for head and neck tumors. Int J Radiat Oncol Biol Phys. 2007;67(2):469–79.
16. Bien AG, Cress MC, Nguyen SB, Westgate SJ, Nanda A. Endovascular treatment of a temporal bone pseudoaneurysm presenting as bloody otorrhea. J Neurol Surg Rep. 2013;74(2):88–91.

17. Birzgalis AR, Ramsden RT, Farrington WT, Small M. Severe radionecrosis of the temporal bone. J Laryngol Otol. 1993;107(3):183–7.
18. Block E. Rontgenschadigung des Schkafenbeines. Z Hals Nas Ohrenheilkd. 1952;3:45–6.
19. Bohne BA, Marks JE, Glasgow GP. Delayed effects of ionizing radiation on the ear. Laryngoscope. 1985;95(7 Pt 1):818–28.
20. Borsanyi SJ. The effects of radiation therapy on the ear with particular reference to radiation otitis media. South Med J. 1962;55:740–3.
21. Brill AH, Martin MM, Fitz-Hugh GS, Constable WC. Postoperative and postradiotherapeutic serous otitis media. Arch Otolaryngol. 1974;99(6):406–8.
22. Cahan WG, Woodard HQ, Higinbotham NL, Stewart FW, Coley BL. Sarcoma in irradiated bone. Report of eleven cases. Cancer. 1948;1(1):3–29.
23. Chan SH, Ng WT, Kam KL, Lee MC, Choi CW, Yau TK, Lee AW, Chow SK. Sensorineural hearing loss after treatment of nasopharyngeal carcinoma: a longitudinal analysis. Int J Radiat Oncol Biol Phys. 2009;73(5):1335–42.
24. Chang S-C, Lai P-H, Chen W-L, Weng H-H, Ho J-T, Wang J-S, Chang C-Y, Pan H-B, Yang C-F. Diffusion-weighted MRI features of brain abscess and cystic or necrotic brain tumors: comparison with conventional MRI. Clin Imaging. 2002;26(4):227–36.
25. Chao C, Saito S, Anderson CW, Appella E, Xu Y. Phosphorylation of murine p53 at ser-18 regulates the p53 responses to DNA damage. Proc Natl Acad Sci USA. 2000;97(22):11936–41.
26. Chen WC, Jackson A, Budnick AS, Pfister DG, Kraus DH, Hunt MA, Stambuk H, Levegrun S, Wolden SL. Sensorineural hearing loss in combined modality treatment of nasopharyngeal carcinoma. Cancer. 2006;106(4):820–9.
27. Chen WC, Liao CT, Tsai HC, Yeh JY, Wang CC, Tang SG, Hong JH. Radiation-induced hearing impairment in patients treated for malignant parotid tumor. Ann Otol Rhinol Laryngol. 1999;108(12):1159–64.
28. Cheng K-M, Chan C-M, Cheung Y-L, Chiu H-M, Tang K-W, Law C-K. Endovascular treatment of radiation-induced petrous internal carotid artery aneurysm presenting with acute haemorrhage. A report of two cases. Acta Neurochir. 2001;143(4):351–6.
29. De Vos C, Gerard JM, Decat M, Gersdorff M. Metastatic renal cell carcinoma to the temporal bone: case report. B-ENT. 2005;1(1):43–6.
30. Delanian S, Chatel C, Porcher R, Depondt J, Lefaix J-L. Complete restoration of refractory mandibular osteoradionecrosis by prolonged treatment with a pentoxifylline-tocopherol-clodronate combination (PENTOCLO): a phase II trial. Int J Radiat Oncol Biol Phys. 2011;80(3):832–9.
31. Delanian S, Depondt J, Lefaix JL. Major healing of refractory mandible osteoradionecrosis after treatment combining pentoxifylline and tocopherol: a phase II trial. Head Neck. 2005;27(2):114–23.
32. Delanian S, Lefaix J. Complete healing of severe osteoradionecrosis with treatment combining pentoxifylline, tocopherol and clodronate. Br J Radiol. 2002;75(893):467–9.
33. Delanian S, Porcher R, Balla-Mekias S, Lefaix J-L. Randomized, placebo-controlled trial of combined pentoxifylline and tocopherol for regression of superficial radiation-induced fibrosis. J Clin Oncol. 2003;21(13):2545–50.
34. Emami B, Lyman J, Brown A, Cola L, Goitein M, Munzenrider J, Shank B, Solin L, Wesson M. Tolerance of normal tissue to therapeutic irradiation. Int J Radiat Oncol Biol Phys. 1991;21(1):109–22.
35. Ewing J. Radiation osteitis. Acta Radiol. 1926;6(1-6):399–412.
36. Gamble JE, Peterson E, Chandler JR. Radiation effects on the inner ear. Arch Otolaryngol. 1968;88(2):156–61.
37. Glicksman JT, Khalili S, Fung K, Parnes LS, Agrawal SK. Pentoxifylline-tocopherol-clodronate combination: a novel treatment for osteoradionecrosis of the temporal bone. Head Neck. 2015;37(12):E191–3.
38. Goh YH, Chong VF, Low WK. Temporal bone tumours in patients irradiated for nasopharyngeal neoplasm. J Laryngol Otol. 1999;113(03):222–8.
39. Guida RA, Finn DG, Buchalter IH, Brookler KH, Kimmelman CP. Radiation injury to the temporal bone. Am J Otol. 1990;11(1):6–11.
40. Gyorkey J, Pollock FJ. Radiation necrosis of the ossicles. AMA Arch Otolaryngol. 1960;71(5):793–6.
41. Hall EJ, Wuu C-S. Radiation-induced second cancers: the impact of 3D-CRT and IMRT. Int J Radiat Oncol Biol Phys. 2003;56(1):83–8.
42. Hao SP, Chen HC, Wei FC, Chen CY, Yeh ARM, Su JL. Systematic management of osteoradionecrosis in the head and neck. Laryngoscope. 1999;109(8):1324–7.
43. Hao SP, Tsang NM, Chang KP, Chen CK, Chao WC. Osteoradionecrosis of external auditory canal in nasopharyngeal carcinoma. Chang Gung Med J. 2007;30(2):116–21.
44. Herrmann F, Dorr W, Muller R, Herrmann T. A prospective study on radiation-induced changes in hearing function. Int J Radiat Oncol Biol Phys. 2006;65(5):1338–44.
45. Hill DS, Gaze MN, Grant HR. A simple reconstructive procedure for radiation-induced necrosis of the external auditory canal. J Laryngol Otol. 1998;112(12):1142–6.
46. Ho WK, Wei WI, Kwong DL, Sham JS, Au DK, Chua DT, Choy DT. Randomized evaluation of the audiologic outcome of ventilation tube insertion for middle ear effusion in patients with nasopharyngeal carcinoma. J Otolaryngol. 2002;31(5):287–93.
47. Ho WK, Wei WI, Kwong DL, Sham JS, Tai PT, Yuen AP, Au DK. Long-term sensorineural hearing deficit following radiotherapy in patients suffering from nasopharyngeal carcinoma: a prospective study. Head Neck. 1999;21(6):547–53.
48. Ho WK, Wei WI, Yuen AP, Hui Y, Wong SH. Otorrhea after grommet insertion for middle ear effusion in patients with nasopharyngeal carcinoma. Am J Otolaryngol. 1999;20(1):12–5.
49. Hoistad DL, Ondrey FG, Mutlu C, Schachern PA, Paparella MM, Adams GL. Histopathology of human temporal bone after cis-platinum, radiation, or both. Otolaryngol Head Neck Surg. 1998;118(6):825–32.
50. Honoré HB, Bentzen SM, Møller K, Grau C. Sensori-neural hearing loss after radiotherapy for nasopharyngeal carcinoma: individualized risk estimation. Radiother Oncol. 2002;65(1):9–16.
51. Hsu YC, Su CY. Tympanoplasty for chronic otitis media in post-irradiated nasopharyngeal carcinoma patients. Ann Otol Rhinol Laryngol. 2006;115(5):330–3.
52. Hua C, Bass JK, Khan R, Kun LE, Merchant TE. Hearing loss after radiotherapy for pediatric brain tumors: effect of cochlear dose. Int J Radiat Oncol Biol Phys. 2008;72(3):892–9.
53. Huang XM, Zheng YQ, Zhang XM, Mai HQ, Zeng L, Liu X, Liu W, Zou H, Xu G. Diagnosis and management of skull base osteoradionecrosis after radiotherapy for nasopharyngeal carcinoma. Laryngoscope. 2006;116(9):1626–31.
54. Jereczek-Fossa BA, Zarowski A, Milani F, Orecchia R. Radiotherapy-induced ear toxicity. Cancer Treat Rev. 2003;29(5):417–30.
55. Johannesen TB, Rasmussen K, Winther FO, Halvorsen U, Lote K. Late radiation effects on hearing, vestibular function, and taste in brain tumor patients. Int J Radiat Oncol Biol Phys. 2002;53(1):86–90.
56. John DG, Porter MJ, van Hasselt CA. Beware bleeding from the ear. J Laryngol Otol. 1993;107(2):137–9.
57. Kelemen G. Experimental defects in the ear and the upper airways induced by radiation. AMA Arch Otolaryngol. 1955;61(4):405–18.

58. Kim CS, Shin SO. Ultrastructural changes in the cochlea of the guinea pig after fast neutron irradiation. Otolaryngol Head Neck Surg. 1994;110(4):419–27.
59. Kolesnick R. The therapeutic potential of modulating the ceramide/sphingomyelin pathway. J Clin Invest. 2002;110(1):3–8.
60. Kovar M, Waltner JG. Radiation effect on the middle and inner ear. Pract Otorhinolaryngol (Basel). 1971;33(4):233–42.
61. Kveton JF, Sotelo-Avila C. Osteoradionecrosis of the ossicular chain. Am J Otol. 1986;7(6):446–8.
62. Kwong DL, Wei WI, Sham JS, Ho WK, Yuen PW, Chua DT, Au DK, Wu PM, Choy DT. Sensorineural hearing loss in patients treated for nasopharyngeal carcinoma: a prospective study of the effect of radiation and cisplatin treatment. Int J Radiat Oncol Biol Phys. 1996;36(2):281–9.
63. Lam HCK, Abdullah VJ, Wormald PJ, Van Hasselt CA. Internal carotid artery hemorrhage after irradiation and osteoradionecrosis of the skull base. Otolaryngol Head Neck Surg. 2001;125(5):522–7.
64. Lambert EM, Garden AS, DeMonte F, Roberts DB, Gidley PW. Radiation-associated malignancies of the ear canal and temporal bone. Laryngoscope. 2015;125(5):1198–204.
65. Lambert EM, Gunn GB, Gidley PW. Effects of radiation on the temporal bone in patients with head and neck cancer. Head Neck. 2016;38:1428–35.
66. Lau WYS, Chow CK. Radiation-induced petrous internal carotid artery aneurysm. Ann Otol Rhinol Laryngol. 2005;114(12):939–40.
67. Leach W. Irradiation of the ear. J Laryngol Otol. 1965;79(10):870–80.
68. Lee AW, Foo W, Chappell R, Fowler JF, Sze W, Poon Y, Law SC, Ng S, Tung SY, Lau W. Effect of time, dose, and fractionation on temporal lobe necrosis following radiotherapy for nasopharyngeal carcinoma. Int J Radiat Oncol Biol Phys. 1998;40(1):35–42.
69. Leonetti JP, Marzo SJ, Zender CA, Porter RG, Melian E. Temporal bone osteoradionecrosis after surgery and radiotherapy for malignant parotid tumors. Otol Neurotol. 2010;31(4):656–9.
70. Leonetti JP, Origitano T, Anderson D, Melian E, Severtson M. Intracranial complications of temporal bone osteoradionecrosis. Am J Otol. 1997;18(2):223-228; discussion 228-229.
71. Li JJ, Guo YK, Tang QL, Li SS, Zhang XL, Wu PA, Yang XM. Prospective study of sensorineural hearing loss following radiotherapy for nasopharyngeal carcinoma. J Laryngol Otol. 2010;124(1):32–6.
72. Lim BY, Pang KP, Low WK, Tan HM. CSF otorrhea complicating temporal bone osteoradionecrosis in a patient with nasopharyngeal carcinoma. Ear Nose Throat J. 2005;84(1):39–40.
73. Lim LH, Goh YH, Chan YM, Chong VF, Low WK. Malignancy of the temporal bone and external auditory canal. Otolaryngol Head Neck Surg. 2000;122(6):882–6.
74. Lo WC, Ting LL, Ko JY, Lou PJ, Yang TL, Chang YL, Wang CP. Malignancies of the ear in irradiated patients of nasopharyngeal carcinoma. Laryngoscope. 2008;118(12):2151–5.
75. Lovin BD, Choi JS, Lindquist NR, Phan J, Gidley PW, Nader ME. Pentoxifylline and tocopherol in the management of temporal bone osteoradionecrosis: a case series. Otol Neurotol. 2020;41(10):1438–46.
76. Lovin BD, Hernandez M, Elms H, Choi JS, Lindquist NR, Moreno AC, Nader ME, Gidley PW. Temporal bone osteoradionecrosis: an 18-year, single-institution experience. Laryngoscope. 2021;131(11):2578–85.
77. Low WK, Fong KW. Long-term post-irradiation middle ear effusion in nasopharyngeal carcinoma. Auris Nasus Larynx. 1998;25(3):319–21.
78. Low WK, Kong SW, Tan MG. Ototoxicity from combined Cisplatin and radiation treatment: an in vitro study. Int J Otolaryngol. 2010;2010:523976.
79. Low WK, Tan MG, Chua AW, Sun L, Wang DY. 12th Yahya Cohen Memorial Lecture: the cellular and molecular basis of radiation-induced sensori-neural hearing loss. Ann Acad Med Singap. 2009;38(1):91–4.
80. Low WK, Tan MG, Sun L, Chua AW, Goh LK, Wang DY. Dose-dependent radiation-induced apoptosis in a cochlear cell-line. Apoptosis. 2006;11:2127–36.
81. Lustig LR, Jackler RK, Lanser MJ. Radiation-induced tumors of the temporal bone. Am J Otol. 1997;18(2):230–5.
82. Ma KH, Fagan PA. Osteoradionecrosis of the temporal bone: a surgical technique of treatment. Laryngoscope. 1988;98(5):554–6.
83. Marx RE. Osteoradionecrosis: a new concept of its pathophysiology. J Oral Maxillofac Surg. 1983;41(5):283–8.
84. Merchant TE, Conklin HM, Wu S, Lustig RH, Xiong X. Late effects of conformal radiation therapy for pediatric patients with low-grade glioma: prospective evaluation of cognitive, endocrine, and hearing deficits. J Clin Oncol. 2009;27(22):3691–7.
85. Metselaar M, Dumans AG, van der Huls MP, Sterk W, Feenstra L. Osteoradionecrosis of tympanic bone: reconstruction of outer ear canal with pedicled skin flap, combined with hyperbaric oxygen therapy, in five patients. J Laryngol Otol. 2009;123(10):1114–9.
86. Milliat F, François A, Isoir M, Deutsch E, Tamarat R, Tarlet G, Atfi A, Validire P, Bourhis J, Sabourin J-C. Influence of endothelial cells on vascular smooth muscle cells phenotype after irradiation: implication in radiation-induced vascular damages. Am J Pathol. 2006;169(4):1484–95.
87. Moeller BJ, Chintagumpala M, Philip JJ, Grosshans DR, McAleer MF, Woo SY, Gidley PW, Vats TS, Mahajan A. Low early ototoxicity rates for pediatric medulloblastoma patients treated with proton radiotherapy. Radiat Oncol. 2011;6:58.
88. Moody SA, Hirsch BE, Myers EN. Squamous cell carcinoma of the external auditory canal: an evaluation of a staging system. Am J Otol. 2000;21(4):582–8.
89. Morrissey D, Grigg R. Incidence of osteoradionecrosis of the temporal bone. ANZ J Surg. 2011;81(12):876–9.
90. Mou YG, Sai K, Wang ZN, Zhang XH, Lu YC, Wei DN, Yang QY, Chen ZP. Surgical management of radiation-induced temporal lobe necrosis in patients with nasopharyngeal carcinoma: report of 14 cases. Head Neck. 2011;33(10):1493–500.
91. Mujica-Mota MA, Lehnert S, Devic S, Gasbarrino K, Daniel SJ. Mechanisms of radiation-induced sensorineural hearing loss and radioprotection. Hear Res. 2014;312:60–8.
92. Nader ME, Beadle BM, Roberts DB, Gidley PW. Outcomes and complications of osseointegrated hearing aids in irradiated temporal bones. Laryngoscope. 2015;126:1187–92.
93. Narozny W, Sicko Z, Kot J, Stankiewicz C, Przewozny T, Kuczkowski J. Hyperbaric oxygen therapy in the treatment of complications of irradiation in head and neck area. Undersea Hyperb Med. 2005;32(2):103–10.
94. Nason R, Chole RA. Bacterial biofilms may explain chronicity in osteoradionecrosis of the temporal bone. Otol Neurotol. 2007;28(8):1026–8.
95. Nishimura R, Baba Y, Murakami R, Baba T, Furusawa M, Ishikawa T, Ushio Y, Takahashi M. MR evaluation of radiation otomastoiditis. Int J Radiat Oncol Biol Phys. 1997;39(1):155–60.
96. O'Neill JV, Katz AH, Skolnik EM. Otologic complications of radiation therapy. Otolaryngol Head Neck Surg (1979). 1979;87(3):359–63.
97. Ondrey FG, Greig JR, Herscher L. Radiation dose to otologic structures during head and neck cancer radiation therapy. Laryngoscope. 2000;110(2 Pt 1):217–21.
98. Ou Y, Zheng Y, Chen S, Liu X, Xu Y, Huang X. Diagnosis and treatment on osteoradionecrosis of temporal bone in cases with nasopharyngeal carcinoma after radiotherapy. Lin Chuang Er Bi Yan Hou Ke Za Zhi. 2006;20(19):865–7.

99. Ou YK, Xu YD, Zheng YQ, Wu SN, Zhang SY, He XZ, Xu XJ. Surgical treatment of diffused osteoradionecrosis of temporal bone in cases with nasopharyngeal carcinoma after radiotherapy. Zhonghua Yi Xue Za Zhi. 2007;87(2):121–3.
100. Paris F, Fuks Z, Kang A, Capodieci P, Juan G, Ehleiter D, Haimovitz-Friedman A, Cordon-Cardo C, Kolesnick R. Endothelial apoptosis as the primary lesion initiating intestinal radiation damage in mice. Science. 2001;293(5528):293–7.
101. Park CW, Jin BJ, Jeong SW, Min HJ, Shin JH, Lee SH. CSF otorrhea resulting from osteoradionecrosis of the temporal bone in a patient with recurrent meningioma. Clin Exp Otorhinolaryngol. 2009;2(2):97–9.
102. Patel AJ, Rao VY, Fox BD, Suki D, Wildrick DM, Sawaya R, DeMonte F. Radiation-induced osteosarcomas of the calvarium and skull base. Cancer. 2011;117(10):2120–6.
103. Patel SG, See AC, Williamson PA, Archer DJ, Rhys Evans PH. Radiation induced sarcoma of the head and neck. Head Neck. 1999;21(4):346–54.
104. Patel SR. Radiation-induced sarcoma. Curr Treat Options in Oncol. 2000;1(3):258–61.
105. Pathak I, Bryce G. Temporal bone necrosis: diagnosis, classification, and management. Otolaryngol Head Neck Surg. 2000;123(3):252–7.
106. Petsuksiri J, Sermsree A, Thephamongkhol K, Keskool P, Thongyai K, Chansilpa Y, Pattaranutaporn P. Sensorineural hearing loss after concurrent chemoradiotherapy in nasopharyngeal cancer patients. Radiat Oncol. 2011;6:19.
107. Phemister D. Radium necrosis of bone. Am J Roentgenol. 1926;16:340.
108. Phillips DJ, Njoku IU, Brown KD, Selesnick SH. Radiation-induced necrosis of the temporal bone: diagnosis and management. Otol Neurotol. 2015;36(8):1374–7.
109. Ramsden RT, Bulman CH, Lorigan BP. Osteoradionecrosis of the temporal bone. J Laryngol Otol. 1975;89(9):941–55.
110. Robard L, Louis M-Y, Blanchard D, Babin E, Delanian S. Medical treatment of osteoradionecrosis of the mandible by PENTOCLO: preliminary results. Eur Ann Otorhinolaryngol Head Neck Dis. 2014;131(6):333–8.
111. Rottenberg DA, Chernik NL, Michael D, Ellis F, Posner JB. Cerebral necrosis following radiotherapy of extracranial neoplasms. Ann Neurol. 1977;1(4):339–57.
112. Rotteveel LJ, Siekman U, Linder TE. Incus necrosis after irradiation. Otol Neurotol. 2013;34(9):1699–702.
113. Rudge FW. Osteoradionecrosis of the temporal bone: treatment with hyperbaric oxygen therapy. Mil Med. 1993;158(3):196–8.
114. Rybak LP, Whitworth CA. Ototoxicity: therapeutic opportunities. Drug Discov Today. 2005;10(19):1313–21.
115. Schuknecht HF, Karmody CS. Radionecrosis of the temporal bone. Laryngoscope. 1966;76(8):1416–28.
116. Schweitzer VG. Hyperbaric oxygen management of chronic staphylococcal osteomyelitis of the temporal bone. Am J Otol. 1990;11(5):347–53.
117. Shapira Y, Telischi FF. Tympanic membrane breakdown after intratympanic injection of steroids in irradiated ears. Otol Neurotol. 2007;28(4):499–500.
118. Sharon JD, Khwaja SS, Drescher A, Gay H, Chole RA. Osteoradionecrosis of the temporal bone: a case series. Otol Neurotol. 2014;35(7):1207–17.
119. Sikand A, Longridge N. CSF otorrhea complicating osteoradionecrosis of the temporal bone. J Otolaryngol. 1991;20(3):209–11.
120. Singh I, Slevin NJ. Late audiovestibular consequences of radical radiotherapy to the parotid. Clin Oncol. 1991;3(4):217–9.
121. Small M, Hariri MA. Radio-necrosis of the temporal bone presenting as cerebellopontine angle lesion. J Laryngol Otol. 1990;104(5):423–5.
122. Smouha EE, Karmody CS. Non-osteitic complications of therapeutic radiation to the temporal bone. Am J Otol. 1995;16(1):83–7.
123. Soo G, Tong MC, Tsang WS, Wong TK, K. F. To, Leung SF, van Hasselt CA. The BAHA hearing system for hearing-impaired postirradiated nasopharyngeal cancer patients: a new indication. Otol Neurotol. 2009;30(4):496–501.
124. Theunissen EA, Bosma SC, Zuur CL, Spijker R, van der Baan S, Dreschler WA, de Boer JP, Balm AJ, Rasch CR. Sensorineural hearing loss in patients with head and neck cancer after chemoradiotherapy and radiotherapy: a systematic review of the literature. Head Neck. 2015;37(2):281–92.
125. Theunissen EA, Zuur CL, Bosma SC, Lopez-Yurda M, Hauptmann M, van der Baan S, de Boer JP, van der Molen L, Rasch CR, Dreschler WA, Balm AJ. Long-term hearing loss after chemoradiation in patients with head and neck cancer. Laryngoscope. 2014;124(12):2720–5.
126. Togni S, Maramaldi G, Bonetta A, Giacomelli L, Di Pierro F. Clinical evaluation of safety and efficacy of Boswellia-based cream for prevention of adjuvant radiotherapy skin damage in mammary carcinoma: a randomized placebo controlled trial. Eur Rev Med Pharmacol Sci. 2015;19(8):1338–44.
127. Veneman W, Metselaar RM, Koudstaal MJ, van der Wal KG. Osteoradionecrosis of the external auditory canal: three cases involving reconstruction with transposition of a split temporalis muscle flap. J Laryngol Otol. 2012;126(10):1022–6.
128. Vudiniabola S, Pirone C, Williamson J, Goss AN. Hyperbaric oxygen in the therapeutic management of osteoradionecrosis of the facial bones. Int J Oral Maxillofac Surg. 2000;29(6):435–8.
129. Wakisaka H, Yamada H, Motoyoshi K, Ugumori T, Takahashi H, Hyodo M. Incidence of long-term ipsilateral and contralateral ototoxicity following radiotherapy for nasopharyngeal carcinoma. Auris Nasus Larynx. 2011;38(1):95–100.
130. Wang PC, Tu TY, Liu KD. Cystic brain necrosis and temporal bone osteoradionecrosis after radiotherapy and surgery in a patient of ear carcinoma. J Chin Med Assoc. 2004;67(9):487–91.
131. Wang SZ, Li J, Miyamoto CT, Chen F, Zhou LF, Zhang HY, Yang G, Wang WF, Guo M, Ni XC, Wang L. A study of middle ear function in the treatment of nasopharyngeal carcinoma with IMRT technique. Radiother Oncol. 2009;93(3):530–3.
132. Wei Y, Zhou T, Zhu J, Zhang Y, Sun M, Ding X, Wang D, Li H, Li B. Long-term outcome of sensorineural hearing loss in nasopharyngeal carcinoma patients: comparison between treatment with radiotherapy alone and chemoradiotherapy. Cell Biochem Biophys. 2014;69(3):433–7.
133. Williams GB, Kun LE, Thompson JW, Gould HJ, Stocks RM. Hearing loss as a late complication of radiotherapy in children with brain tumors. Ann Otol Rhinol Laryngol. 2005;114(4):328–31.
134. Williams H, Davies A. The effect of X-rays on bone: a pictorial review. Eur Radiol. 2006;16(3):619–33.
135. Winther FO. X-ray irradiation of the inner ear of the guinea pig. Early degenerative changes in the cochlea. Acta Otolaryngol. 1969;68(1):98–117.
136. Xu YD, Ou YK, Zheng YQ, Zhang SY. Surgical treatment of osteoradionecrosis of the temporal bone in patients with nasopharyngeal carcinoma. J Laryngol Otol. 2008;122(11):1175–9.
137. Yang H, Zheng Y, Chen S, Liang M, Zhang Z, Xu Y, Liu X. Cholesterol granuloma of the middle ear in post-irradiated nasopharyngeal carcinoma patients. ORL. 2011;73(6):343–7.
138. Young Y-H, Lou P-J. Post-irradiation sudden deafness. J Laryngol Otol. 1999;113(09):815–7.
139. Yuen PW, Wei WI. Tympanomastoidectomy for chronic suppurative otitis media of irradiated ears of nasopharyngeal carcinoma patients. J Otolaryngol. 1994;23(4):302–4.

Part IX

Tumors of the Ear and Lateral Skull Base

Glandular Tumors of the External Auditory Canal and Middle Ear

66

Stanley Pelosi and Kiley Trott

Glandular Tumors of the External Auditory Canal

Overview

Glandular tumors of the external auditory canal (EAC) are rare neoplasms affecting the temporal bone. They arise from sebaceous and apocrine sweat glands, also referred to as ceruminal glands, within the dermis of the cartilaginous EAC [1]. They are estimated to represent 2.4% of all neoplasms affecting the temporal bone and can exhibit multiple histologies. Benign EAC neoplasms have most commonly been categorized as ceruminous adenoma, pleomorphic adenoma, and syringocystadenoma papilliferum. Malignant pathologies include adenoid cystic carcinoma, adenocarcinoma, and mucoepidermoid carcinoma. Glandular EAC tumors present as a mass within the ear canal, causing symptoms secondary to canal obstruction such as ear fullness, pain, hearing loss, and drainage. Treatment consists of surgical resection, with consideration of adjuvant treatment such as radiation, depending on the disease's biological profile.

Clinical Presentation

Clinical symptoms associated with glandular EAC neoplasms are typically nonspecific. Most commonly, tumors consist of a mass within the EAC that creates ear fullness, a pressure sensation, and/or hearing loss. The pattern of hearing loss detected on an audiogram is usually conductive in nature. Bloody otorrhea from the tumor may be a presenting symptom. Purulent drainage can also result from a superimposed ear infection, as reported in a case of pleomorphic adenoma and coexisting chronic otitis media [2]. Smaller tumors can be entirely asymptomatic and discovered incidentally. Pain is more likely to be suggestive of tumor invasiveness, although this symptom can be a feature of both benign and malignant pathologies [3]. Symptoms such as facial paralysis, paresthesia, or disequilibrium are rarely present and suggest biological aggressiveness and/or medial extension.

On gross inspection, tumors typically appear as an exophytic mass arising from the cartilaginous external auditory canal. Malignant tumors may exhibit clinical invasiveness of surrounding bone and/or soft tissue. Tumor appearance can otherwise vary significantly. A common description of ceruminous adenoma is a red-tan polypoid lesion [3], and this appearance is similar to pleomorphic adenoma [4]. Tumor sizes also vary, with most studies reporting an average tumor size upon diagnosis between 1 cm and 1.5 cm for both benign and malignant subtypes [1, 3].

There appears to be an overall greater number of malignant glandular EAC tumors than benign, although this finding may be secondary to reporting bias [1]. Benign tumors can affect a wide range of ages from adolescence to the elderly, but most commonly, they affect patients in middle age. The mean age of presentation for ceruminous adenomas has been reported to be 52–54 [3], while for pleomorphic adenoma, it is in the 40s [5]. Malignant glandular tumors tend to present slightly earlier in life, but they have a broad overall age incidence, ranging between 21 and 92 [6–8]. Conflicting reports exist as to whether a gender predominance exists for ceruminous gland neoplasms, and tumor subtype may be relevant to this consideration. One study suggested a slight gender predominance in females [1] for ceruminous carcinoma, while another noted that EAC pleomorphic adenomas tend to occur more commonly in males [3]. Because of the nonspecific symptoms, there is frequently

S. Pelosi (✉)
Department of Otolaryngology—Head and Neck Surgery, Long Island Jewish Medical Center, New Hyde Park, NY, USA
e-mail: spelosi@northwell.edu

K. Trott
Department of Otolaryngology—Head and Neck Surgery, Thomas Jefferson University School of Medicine, Philadelphia, PA, USA

A. D. Sweeney et al. (eds.), *Haynes-Glasscock-Shambaugh Surgery of the Ear*, https://doi.org/10.1007/978-3-032-18264-7_66

a delay in diagnosis, which has been reported as up to 52 months in ceruminous carcinoma [1].

Classification

The nomenclature and behavior of ceruminous gland neoplasms have historically been a source of controversy and confusion, due in part to their rarity, but also as a result of generic all-encompassing terminology. In the past, the term "ceruminoma" was used to describe both benign and malignant glandular tumors arising from the EAC. Wetli et al. later addressed the confusion in terminology by proposing a histopathology-based classification system for glandular tumors of the EAC [5]. They classified tumors into four categories: adenoma, pleomorphic adenoma, adenoid cystic carcinoma, and adenocarcinoma. The first two tumors were considered benign, and the latter two were considered malignant.

The use of the term ceruminoma is now discouraged and was excluded from the World Health Organization (WHO) classification system in 1991 [1, 9]. The WHO system is based on morphological instead of histogenetic analysis and is intended to allow for uniform reporting. Additional entities have been added to the main categories established by Wetli et al. [5] The benign category includes ceruminous adenoma, ceruminous pleomorphic adenoma, and ceruminous syringocystadenoma papilliferum. The malignant category includes ceruminous adenocarcinoma, ceruminous adenoid cystic carcinoma, and ceruminous mucoepidermoid carcinoma [1].

Pathogenesis

There are currently no known etiologic factors that have been identified to cause ceruminous adenomas, and work is still being performed to identify the cellular precursors to these tumors [3]. The WHO classification only identifies ceruminous adenoma and ceruminous adenocarcinoma as definitively arising from ceruminous glands [10]. The evidence supporting ceruminous glands as the cellular origin of glandular tumors of the EAC is based on several characteristics. For instance, there are cytological similarities between normal ceruminous glands and glandular tumors, and the tumors are located close to nonneoplastic glands, possibly with a transitional region. Moreover, there appears to be a correlation between the concentration of ceruminous glands in cartilaginous versus osseous portions of the EAC and tumor frequency at each respective site [11].

An accompanying explanatory note to the WHO classification system states that other glandular neoplasms, including pleomorphic adenoma, syringocystadenoma papilliferum, adenoid cystic carcinoma, and mucoepidermoid carcinoma, might also arise from ceruminous glands [11]. It is now generally accepted that, for pleomorphic adenomas of the EAC, the epithelial and mesenchymal elements within these tumors likely originate from myoepithelial cells, which in turn are known to exist within ceruminous glands [11]. Other theories, however, propose heterotopic salivary tissue as the site of origin for EAC pleomorphic adenoma, but this hypothesis has not been definitively proven [9].

Diagnosis

Diagnosis of EAC glandular tumors can be difficult, given nonspecific symptomatology and physical exam findings. Imaging findings may also be vague, but are useful for determining tumor location as well as the degree of expansion or invasion of adjacent tissues [2–4, 12]. A temporal bone computed tomography (CT) scan may show a homogeneous space-occupying mass within the EAC, potentially accompanied by inflammation in the middle ear and/or mastoid cells. Magnetic resonance imaging (MRI) will usually demonstrate homogeneous enhancement with contrast and can help to rule out any extension of parotid gland tissue or intracranial extension [4] (Fig. 66.1).

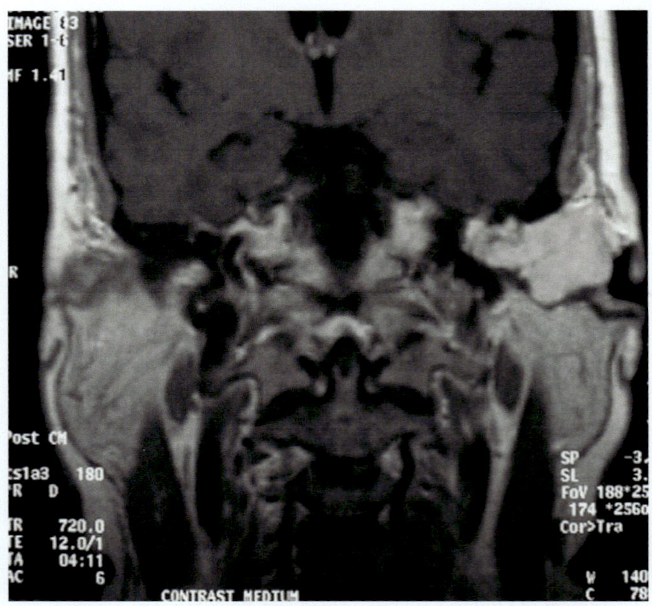

Fig. 66.1 MRI demonstrating homogeneous enhancement of an EAC glandular tumor. (Reprinted with permission from Elsevier: American Journal of Otolaryngology, 2008) [4]

Microscopy

Accurate pathologic diagnosis of EAC lesions can be difficult to achieve because biopsy specimens may be small and fragmented, increasing the likelihood of inadequate sample size or inability to analyze tumor margins. Thus, wide excisional biopsies are recommended for EAC lesions.

Ceruminous adenomas are well-differentiated neoplasms that demonstrate papillary proliferation of glands having structures and histology similar to normal ceruminous glands [3, 13]. Adenomas have two distinct cell layers, an inner luminal layer of epithelial cells and an outer layer of basal myoepithelial cells near the basement membrane [13]. The luminal cells show immunohistochemical reactivity to cytokeratin 7, and the basal myoepithelial cells react strongly to S-100, findings which are identical to normal cerumen glands [3].

Pleomorphic adenomas of the EAC are well-differentiated benign tumors defined by tubular, papillary, or nested structures typical of a normal cerumen gland [4]. Similar to the salivary gland tumor of the same name, it is a benign mixed tumor of glands that has undergone ceruminal differentiation with yellow-brown pigmentation within the cytoplasm [4]. Histologically, epithelial cells line the lumen of tubular structures surrounded by myoepithelial cells inside a mucoid matrix. Additionally, parotid tissue must be absent within the neoplasm to confirm a ceruminous pleomorphic adenoma versus an extension from a tumor in the parotid gland [3]. Finally, ceruminous syringocystadenoma papilliferum is the rarest of benign ceruminous neoplasms, and it can be identified by its papillary architecture accompanied by infiltration of inflammatory plasma cells (Fig. 66.2) [3, 14].

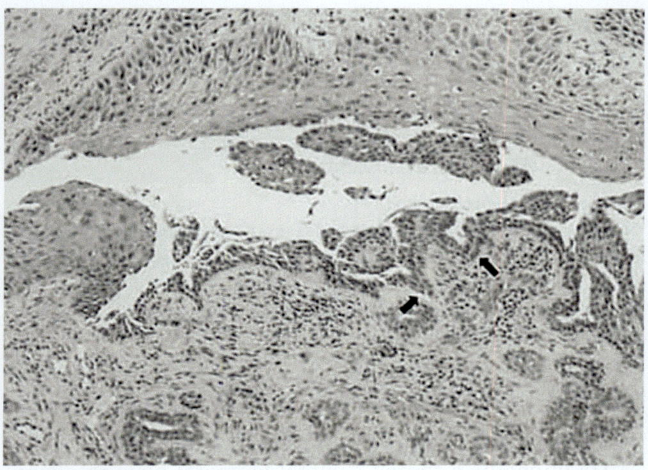

Fig. 66.2 Histopathology of benign glandular EAC tumors. Cystadenoma papilliferum. The upper portion of the lesion shows epidermal invagination with papillomatous projections (black arrows), which is compatible with findings of syringocystadenoma papilliferum (H&E, ×100). (Reprinted with permission from Cambridge University Press: The Journal of Laryngology and Otology, 2005) [14]

Malignant ceruminous tumors are more likely to demonstrate greater infiltration, perineural invasion, cellular pleomorphism, and prominent nucleoli when compared to benign ceruminous tumors in the EAC [1]. Ceruminous adenocarcinoma can show a spectrum of differentiation, from poorly- to well-differentiated lesions, which may be difficult to discern from benign ceruminous adenomas (Fig. 66.3a) [11]. Distinction from benign tumors is also complicated by the fact that benign ceruminous neoplasms can show a pseudoinfiltrative pattern as a result of hyalinized fibrosis [1, 3, 15]. In poorly differentiated adenocarcinomas, identifying a ceruminous origin can be aided by observing ceruminous glands within or adjacent to the tumor [1]. The cells within ceruminous adenocarcinoma resemble secretory cells, but they showcase a back-to-back gland arrangement and irregular configuration of the glands [5]. Also, the characteristic cerumen granules found within the cytoplasm of benign ceruminous glands are absent from malignant tumors [16]. A basal layer of myoepithelial cells, as found in normal ceruminous glands, can often be identified in ceruminous adenocarcinoma, and may be highlighted by the immunohistochemical myoepithelial and basal cell markers S100 and p63 (Fig. 66.3b) [1].

Ceruminous adenoid cystic carcinomas (ACC) can show cribriform, tubular, and solid patterns, just like their salivary counterparts. The former two patterns are most common and may be found within the same tumor. The hallmark Swiss cheese–like pattern can help in distinguishing ceruminous adenoid cystic carcinoma from ceruminous adenocarcinomas and mucoepidermoid carcinoma. More poorly differentiated cases may be predominated by solid regions, along with anaplastic cytologic findings [11]. Throughout the neoplasm are cylindrical structures with brightly eosinophilic connective tissue stroma around the epithelial cells. The basal myoepithelial cells typically have dark basophilic chromatin, a high nuclear-to-cytoplasmic ratio, and indistinct cell borders. A ceruminous origin can be confirmed by finding bilayered eosinophilic neoplastic cells and luminal cells with apocrine snouts [1].

Ceruminous mucoepidermoid carcinoma is a tumor with mucoid, epidermoid, and intermediate cellular components intermixed [1]. Dilated ducts or cysts filled with mucinous material can also be found within the tumor. The epidermoid cells have eosinophilic to clear cytoplasm. The intermediate cells have less cytoplasm than the epidermoid cells, with a higher nuclear-to-cytoplasmic ratio. There may also be mucocytes containing clear to foamy cytoplasm, which may compress the nucleus, creating a signet ring-like appearance. Alcian blue or mucicarmine stains can highlight these cells [1]. Dyskeratosis, keratin pearls, and intercellular bridges are typically not found in this neoplasm.

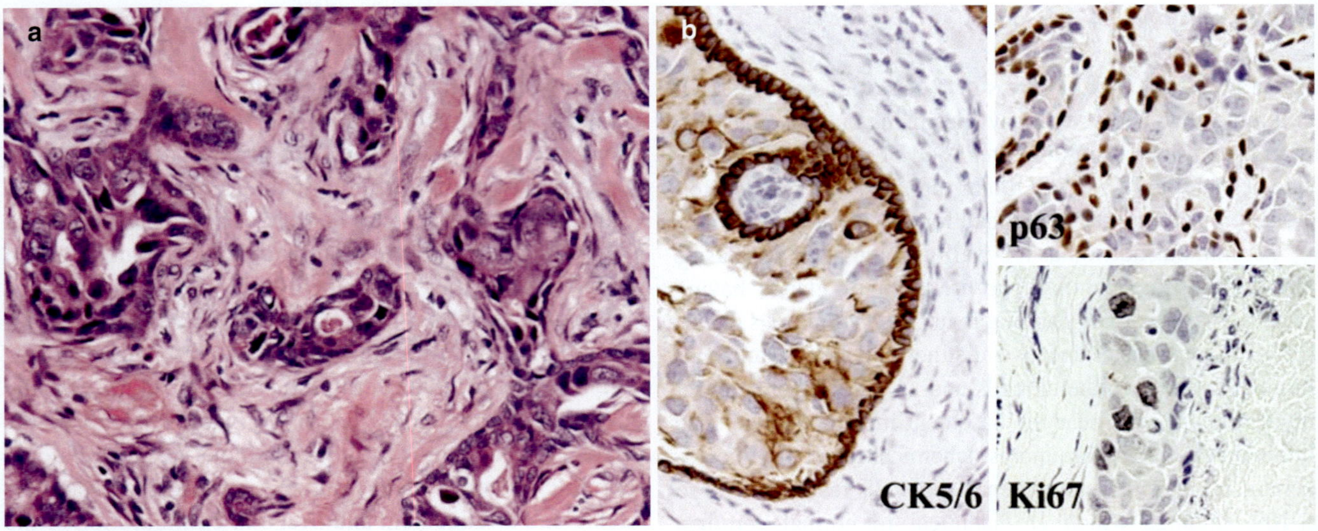

Fig. 66.3 Histopathology of ceruminous adenocarcinoma. (Reprinted with permission from Springer Nature [1]). (**a**) Microarchitecture showing irregular glands with biphasic cellular appearance and pleomorphism. (**b**) Immunohistochemical markers found in ceruminous adenocarcinoma

Treatment

Surgical resection is the mainstay of treatment for glandular EAC tumors. The extent of resection depends on tumor biology and the involvement of adjacent structures. For benign tumors confined to the external auditory canal and without bony erosion, a transcanal or endaural approach may be considered for tumor removal. Benign tumors that extend through the tympanic membrane require middle ear dissection, tympanic membrane repair, and potentially even ossicular reconstruction. Finally, those benign tumors with extension into the bony ear canal may benefit from modified radical mastoidectomy or lateral temporal bone resection.

Malignant EAC glandular tumors are more likely to cause erosion of bone and invasion of surrounding soft tissue. Because of the rarity of malignant glandular tumors, some authors have adapted guidelines for the extent of surgical resection from more common EAC malignancies, such as squamous cell carcinoma. The Pittsburgh staging system [17] for EAC squamous cell carcinoma is listed in Table 66.1 and categorizes tumor aggressiveness based on invasion of surrounding structures. Recommendations for the extent of surgical resection may be extrapolated from this staging system. For malignancies limited to the EAC without bony invasion, a sleeve resection can be employed, consisting of removal of the ear canal skin and cartilaginous EAC, followed by reconstruction with a skin graft. For larger tumors with invasion of the bony ear canal, en bloc resection can be accomplished with lateral temporal bone resection. Reconstruction in these cases is accomplished with ear canal overclosure and fat graft obliteration of the middle ear space, but if concurrent auriculectomy is necessary, locoregional or free transfer soft tissue flaps may be utilized.

Table 66.1 Pittsburgh staging system for external auditory meatus carcinoma

T status
T1—Tumor limited to the external auditory canal without bony erosion or evidence of soft tissue extension
T2—Tumor with limited external auditory canal bony erosion (not full thickness), or a radiographic finding consistent with limited (0.5 cm) soft tissue involvement
T3—Tumor eroding the osseous external auditory canal (full thickness) with limited (0.5 cm) soft tissue involvement, or tumor involving the middle ear and/or mastoid, or a patient presenting with facial paralysis
T4—Tumor eroding the cochlea, petrous apex, medial wall of the middle ear, carotid canal, jugular foramen, or dura, or with extensive (0.5 cm) soft tissue involvement
N status[a]
N0—No regional lymph node metastases
N1—Lymph node metastases present
M status[b]
M0—No distant metastases
M1—Distant metastatic disease present

Adapted from the reference [17]
[a]N status: Involvement of lymph nodes is a poor prognostic finding and automatically places the patient in an advanced stage (i.e., stage III (T1N1) or stage IV (T2, 3, and 4, N1) disease)
[b]M status: Distant metastasis indicates a very poor prognosis and immediately places the patient in the stage IV category

Traditionally, a formal subtotal temporal bone resection, whereby the labyrinth and/or cochlea are removed, but the petrous apex is preserved, has been recommended for malignant tumors that extend to the middle ear and mastoid cavity. Several authors, however, instead have suggested that the extent of temporal bone dissection at this level should be dictated only by involvement of surrounding structures, citing that formal subtotal resection may not provide a benefit to the patient's ultimate outcome while adding unnecessary morbidity [18, 19]. For malignant tumors with extension through the anterior ear canal wall, parotidectomy is employed, and in rare cases, this surgery may require exposure of the glenoid fossa and resection of the condyle. Finally, malignant tumors that invade critical structures such as the carotid artery, jugular foramen, or dura are generally considered unresectable, and in these cases, palliative treatments may be considered. Neck dissection is performed for patients with clinical evidence of metastatic spread to the neck, but elective neck dissection is not recommended by most authors.

It has been proposed that the extent of tumor resection should vary depending on tumor subtype. ACC has a propensity for perineural invasion and significant soft tissue invasion, and multiple authors have emphasized the importance of aggressive resection, which should, in most cases, include superficial parotidectomy along with temporal bone resection. In some patients, facial nerve sacrifice may be indicated [1, 6, 9, 20]. One report recommended a more aggressive approach to the management of ACC of the ear canal relative to SCC after finding that the only patient in their series who developed recurrence with negative margins had ACC [21].

Adjuvant radiation does not clearly have a role in benign tumors but does appear to have a role in malignant disease. Radiation is considered for patients with what are traditionally considered poor prognostic factors for malignancies of the head and neck, including positive margins [6] or other findings suggesting biological aggressiveness, including perineural invasion or significant bony destruction [20]. The dose of radiation employed is variable in the literature. Whether the potential benefit of radiation is dependent on tumor subtype is controversial. Traditionally, EAC ceruminous adenocarcinoma has been thought to be more radiosensitive than ACC [7, 9]. In contrast, Dong et al. [20] recommended adjuvant radiation for ACC based on its known benefit for ACC at other sites in the head and neck, and another author noted that a patient in their series with ACC and positive surgical margins underwent radiotherapy and was disease-free at 78 months after surgery [21]. Regardless of tumor subtype, the overall survival of patients with glandular EAC malignancies who receive radiotherapy appears similar to that of those who do not, and its primary role may be in palliation or delaying disease recurrence, without changing the ultimate incidence of recurrence [1].

Outcome/Prognosis

Prognosis is linked to underlying tumor biology. One series on ceruminous adenoma noted recrudescence in 4 of 40 patients with follow-up, 2 of which appeared to be true recurrence and 2 of which likely had residual disease after the first procedure [3]. For EAC pleomorphic adenoma, recurrence is also uncommon [22]. Malignant transformation of salivary gland pleomorphic adenoma is a well-described entity, but has not been reported for pleomorphic adenoma arising from the EAC [22].

Regarding malignant EAC tumors, long-term survival rates for ACC are substantially better than ceruminous adenocarcinoma, at a mean of 8.3 years for the former compared to 4.7 years for the latter. [1] However, the improved survival may be related to the propensity of ACC patients to develop later recurrences than those with adenocarcinoma, and it appears that a similar percentage of patients, roughly one-third, within each histologic subtype ultimately die from their disease [1]. Because of the potential for late recurrence, it is recommended that patients with ACC of the EAC be monitored for many years after their initial treatment.

Several factors suggesting a poorer prognosis for patients with glandular EAC malignancies have been proposed. Perzin et al. noted positive surgical margins, parotid gland involvement, bone extension, and perineural invasion to be poor prognostic indicators for ACC [6]. Multiple studies have also noted a high recurrence rate in glandular malignancies with parotid gland involvement at the time of initial surgery. One study suggested that a longer time from symptom onset to tumor diagnosis may lead to a poorer outcome [20], but this finding has not been substantiated in other studies [1].

Recurrent malignant disease may present locally or in distant metastatic sites. Metastases to the lung, kidney, and bone have been described. Lung metastases in ACC of the EAC can present many years after initial tumor treatment [23]. Cervical lymph node metastasis is only rarely reported for glandular EAC malignancies.

Glandular Tumors of the Middle Ear

Overview

Glandular tumors uncommonly present as middle ear masses. Middle ear adenoma was first described as a distinct pathologic entity by Hyams and Michaels in 1976 [24]. They described 20 middle ear neoplasms with glandular elements that did not resemble paraganglioma or salivary gland tumors. Shortly after, Derlacki and Barney (1976) described three cases with similar histopathology [25]. Middle ear carcinoid was initially described by Murphy et al. in 1980, who reported a middle ear tumor having histochemical and ultrastructural evidence of neuroendocrine differentiation [26]. Similarly behaving middle ear tumors have been given the designation of neuroendocrine adenoma [27, 28].

Controversy exists as to whether these labels actually represent a spectrum of one common pathologic entity [29] or whether middle ear adenoma and carcinoid are distinct biologic neoplasms [30, 31].

All glandular middle ear neoplasms are alike in that they have both epithelial and neuroendocrine elements. Two distinct patterns of immunohistochemical staining are present in these tumors: cytokeratin markers within the glandular components of the tumor and neuroendocrine markers in the stromal regions [29]. Electron microscopy of glandular tumors reveals ultrastructural features that reflect these different cell types.

Glandular middle ear tumors are generally benign, with well-differentiated histologic appearances and indolent local growth. More aggressive histologic patterns are sometimes observed, although it is unclear whether such features predict an increased risk of local invasiveness, recurrence, and/or metastasis. Cases have been described of locally invasive tumors that appear histologically benign, and conversely, there are reports of tumors with infiltrative/dysplastic cellular morphologies but lacking clinical invasiveness [25, 32]. The tumor's relative rarity, combined with uncertainties in classification and differences in biologic behavior, create difficulty in establishing rigid protocols for management of glandular middle ear tumors. Surgery is the recommended treatment strategy, with the surgical approach dictated by the extent of disease.

Clinical Presentation

Glandular middle ear tumors most commonly present as a nonspecific middle ear mass (Fig. 66.4). Tumors are not believed to have a gender preference [33], and the mean age of presentation is the fifth decade (range 14–80 years) [34]. Hearing loss is the most commonly reported symptom. A review of 94 previously published cases of middle ear glandular neoplasms described the following symptoms: hearing loss (86.3%), aural fullness (33%), tinnitus (27.6%), otalgia (15%), otorrhea (11.4%) and facial weakness (11%) [33]. Facial weakness has rarely been described in association with middle ear adenomas, and when present, is generally thought to result from local compression of a dehiscent nerve rather than nerve invasion [29, 35]. In comparison, actual infiltration of the facial nerve has been described in middle ear carcinoid [31].

Symptoms related to regional or even distant metastasis may be associated with glandular middle ear neoplasms. Middle ear carcinoid metastatic to the ipsilateral cervical lymph nodes has been described [36]. Systemic symptoms can occasionally be present in patients with carcinoid tumors, including diarrhea, abdominal cramps, skin flushing, and bronchoconstriction [37, 38].

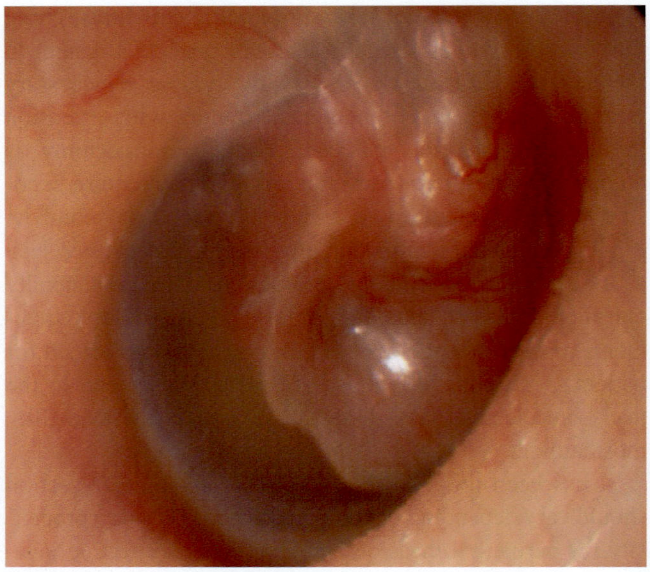

Fig. 66.4 Otomicroscopy of the right ear demonstrates a middle ear mass medial to an intact tympanic membrane

Diagnosis

The differential diagnosis of middle ear masses is extensive and includes both neoplastic, infectious, and rheumatologic diseases. Diagnosis is obtained by a combination of radiologic characteristics and tissue diagnosis.

Imaging

Both CT and MRI help to delineate tumor features and distinguish glandular tumors from other middle ear masses. CT demonstrates a nonspecific opacity centered in the middle ear cleft, which can extend to the tympanic cavity and mastoid (Fig. 66.5). The ossicles are generally embedded in the mass without bony erosion or destruction. Importantly, no characteristic differences between benign and malignant adenomatous middle ear tumors are detectable on CT.

MRI may be helpful in cases with extension to the posterior or middle cranial fossa [39, 40]. On MRI, tumors are isointense to hyperintense relative to white matter on T1-weighted images and avidly enhance with gadolinium administration. On T2-weighted images, tumors approximate the signal intensity of gray matter.

As previously noted, paraganglioma is an important consideration in the differential diagnosis of glandular middle ear tumors. Both glomus tympanicum and glandular middle ear tumors display strong enhancement on CT and MRI [41]. Temporal bone paragangliomas, however, are more likely to cause symptoms of pulsatile tinnitus, to be centered on the promontory in close proximity to Jacobson's nerve, and to exhibit a vascular blush on conventional angiography [41].

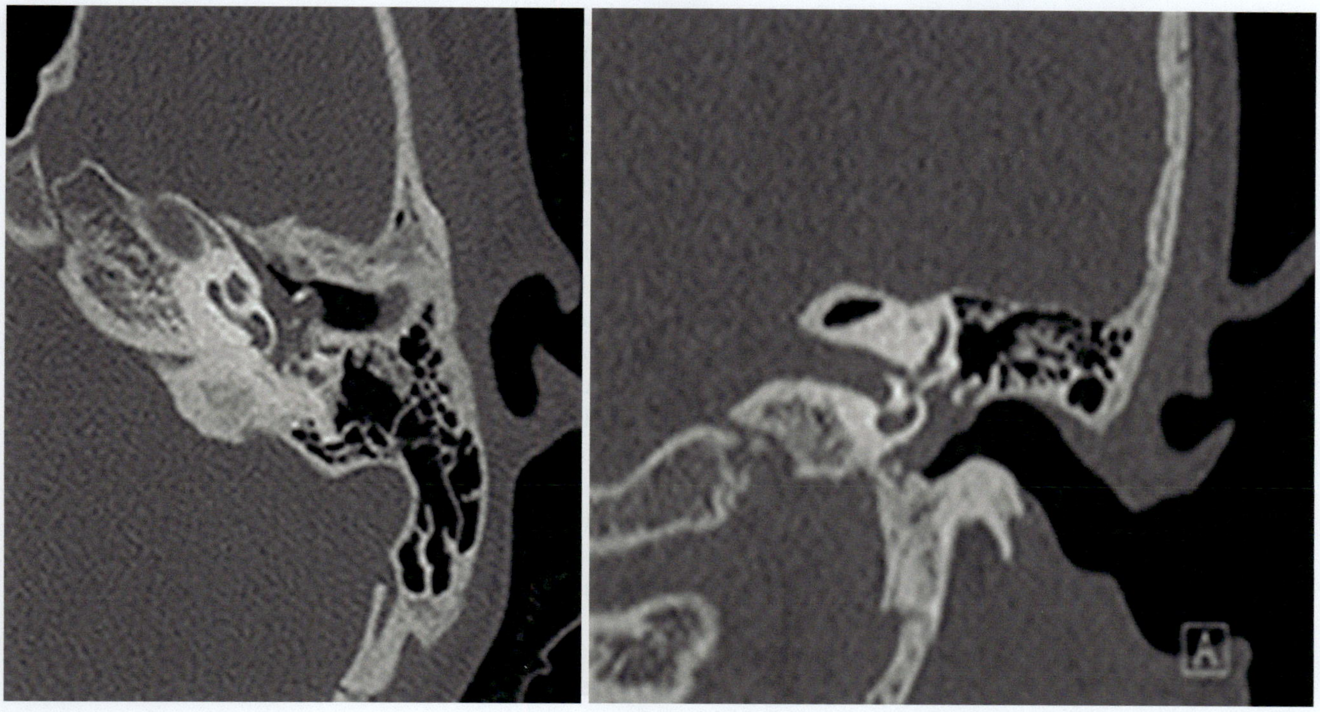

Fig. 66.5 Axial (**a**) and coronal (**b**) computed tomography images of a middle ear adenoma, demonstrating a nonspecific middle ear mass with ossicular chain involvement

In contrast, glandular middle ear tumors can occur anywhere in the middle ear space and have unimpressive conventional angiography findings.

Any temporal bone neoplasm extending to the middle ear should be considered in the differential diagnosis of glandular middle ear tumors. Facial schwannoma may be localized to the middle ear cavity but should appear contiguous with the fallopian canal, while glandular neoplasms are distinct. Ceruminous adenoma and pleomorphic adenoma may extend to the middle ear but are centered in the EAC. Meningiomas can occur as primary lesions in the temporal bone, but more commonly extend from the intracranial space. Jugular paragangliomas typically demonstrate erosion of the jugular bulb, and endolymphatic sac tumors are centered on the posterior petrous face. Finally, other nonneoplastic pathologies, including cholesteatoma, infection, and granulation tissue, can arise in association with middle ear tumors or rheumatologic processes like sarcoidosis, and should be considered in the differential diagnosis of middle ear masses.

The presence of a neck mass and/or systemic symptoms at the time of diagnosis should prompt evaluation for metastatic disease. This includes CT and/or MR imaging of the neck, chest, and abdomen. Octreotide scanning has an established role in the detection of metastatic disease for abdominal carcinoid tumors, but its role in carcinoid middle ear neoplasms is uncertain. A single case report in a patient with middle ear carcinoid employed the use of octreotide scanning to monitor for disease recurrence [42]. No studies have assessed the use of diagnostic and preoperative octreotide scanning for these tumors.

Pathogenesis

The precursor cell for glandular middle ear tumors is unclear. Early authors postulated an origin for middle ear adenoma from the surface epithelium mucosa [24, 25]. Another hypothesis is that middle ear adenomas develop from displaced or trapped embryonic rests of glandular cells in the middle ear mucosa [30], which may be of neural crest origin [29].

Other authors maintain that middle ear adenoma and neuroendocrine tumors are separate entities [43]. The middle ear does not normally contain cells with neuroendocrine features, such as enterochromaffin cells that normally give rise to carcinoid tumors in the lung and gastrointestinal tract, lending support to this argument. It has been proposed that an undifferentiated, pluripotent stem cell may give rise to a glandular middle ear tumor with both epithelial and neuroendocrine components [29].

Carcinoids are very rare in the middle ear and mastoid. The tumor occurs predominantly in the small intestine, and when these lesions develop in the head and neck region, the majority arise in the larynx [44, 45]. The first case of middle ear carcinoid was reported in 1980 [26], and as of 2005, a review had identified only 40 cases of documented middle ear carcinoid in the English literature [46]. Carcinoid has historically been considered a distinct neoplasm given its reported metastatic potential [31, 36, 47]. However, histologic analysis from several recent studies now suggests that middle ear adenoma and carcinoid may represent different stages of differentiation of the same tumor. Many authors currently view these tumors as a single primary low-grade glandular neoplasm, with more specific characterization based on immunohistochemical markers and the presence or absence of metastases [29, 33, 48].

Microscopy and Immunohistochemistry

Middle ear adenomas and carcinoid tumors may appear similar- or even indistinguishable—morphologically on light microscopy [49–51]. Tumor cells are often arranged in glandular spaces, trabeculae, festoons, ribbon-like patterns, anastomosing cords, and solid sheets [29]. There may be variability in predominant architectural patterns both between and within the same tumors. In both carcinoid and middle ear adenoma, the cells are described as cuboidal-to-columnar, uniform in size, with eosinophilic, finely granular cytoplasm. Light microscopy shows central or eccentrically located round-to-oval nuclei with finely dispersed chromatin, and they may have a plasmacytoid appearance [52]. Nucleoli are inconspicuous, and mitoses are rarely present. These characteristics are clearly distinguishable from other diagnostic considerations, such as paraganglioma, which contains richly vascularized stroma and a characteristic "zellballen" pattern.

Immunohistochemical staining for both middle ear adenoma and carcinoid has demonstrated very similar results [50, 52–54]. Both tumors are typically positive for some combination of epithelial, mesenchymal, and neuroendocrine markers, although the specific types vary between individual tumors. Glandular spaces commonly contain secretory product that stains with mucicarmine, periodic acid–Schiff, and Alcian blue [52]. Additionally, variable positivity for S-100, serotonin, glucagon, Leu-7, ACTH, and somatostatin has also been reported in each neoplasm subtype [29]. The individual tumor's architectural pattern may affect the location and degree of positivity of immunohistochemical staining. Cytokeratin has been most strongly identified in the cytoplasm of the glandular component and weakest in the solid component [54, 55], while neuroendocrine markers are most strongly identified in the trabecular, ribbon, and solid components [54, 56].

Immunohistochemical staining may be employed to differentiate glandular middle ear tumors from paraganglioma and other neuroendocrine tumors. Strongly positive keratin staining with the absence of S-100 protein positivity argues against a diagnosis of paraganglioma. Immunostaining for galanin may also be useful because carcinoid tumors are galanin-negative, while some paragangliomas have been found to be galanin-positive [47, 57].

Aggressive histologic subtypes of middle ear adenoma have been reported, but their true existence has been called into question due to their histologic and gross behavioral resemblance to endolymphatic sac tumors. Endolymphatic sac tumors were not recognized as a distinct biologic entity until 1989 [58]. They are biologically aggressive tumors that histologically contain neoplastic cells with adenomatous features arranged in papillary configurations. A number of clinical series predating this report have described aggressive middle ear "papillary adenoma" [59] or "adenocarcinoma," [60, 61] that caused significant bony destruction and facial nerve or posterior fossa involvement. The shared pathologic features and aggressive clinical presentation suggest that these aggressive tumors are more likely to be endolymphatic sac tumors than variants of middle ear adenoma.

Classification

A recent multi-institutional study proposed a staging system for middle ear adenomas (Table 66.2, Fig. 66.6) [62]. A T1 tumor is defined as a small adenoma confined to the middle ear space that does not envelope or strongly adhere to the ossicular chain. T2 tumors are separated into three subtypes: T2a fills the middle ear cleft and encases the ossicles, with or without ossicular bone erosion; T2b is a disease that also

Table 66.2 Overview of the staging system for middle ear adenomas

T status
T1—Tumor confined to the middle ear cavity that does not envelope or strongly adhere to the ossicular chain
T2a—Tumor fills the middle ear cleft and encases the ossicles with or without ossicular bone erosion
T2b—A T2a tumor that also extends into the mastoid
T2c—A T2a or T2b tumor that also extends through the tympanic membrane into the external auditory canal
T3—Tumor adheres to neurovascular structures such as the petrous ICA, facial nerve, sigmoid sinus, or dura
T4—Intradural tumor extension
N status
N0—No regional lymph node metastases
N1—Lymph node metastases present (commonly to the parotid and cervical lymph nodes)
M status
M0—No distant metastases
M1—Distant metastatic disease present (commonly to the bone, liver, and lungs)
S status
S0—Tumor is nonsecretory
S1—Hormone-secreting tumor (e.g., serotonin)

This table is adapted from reference [62]
Figure 66.6 also provides a pictorial reference of T staging

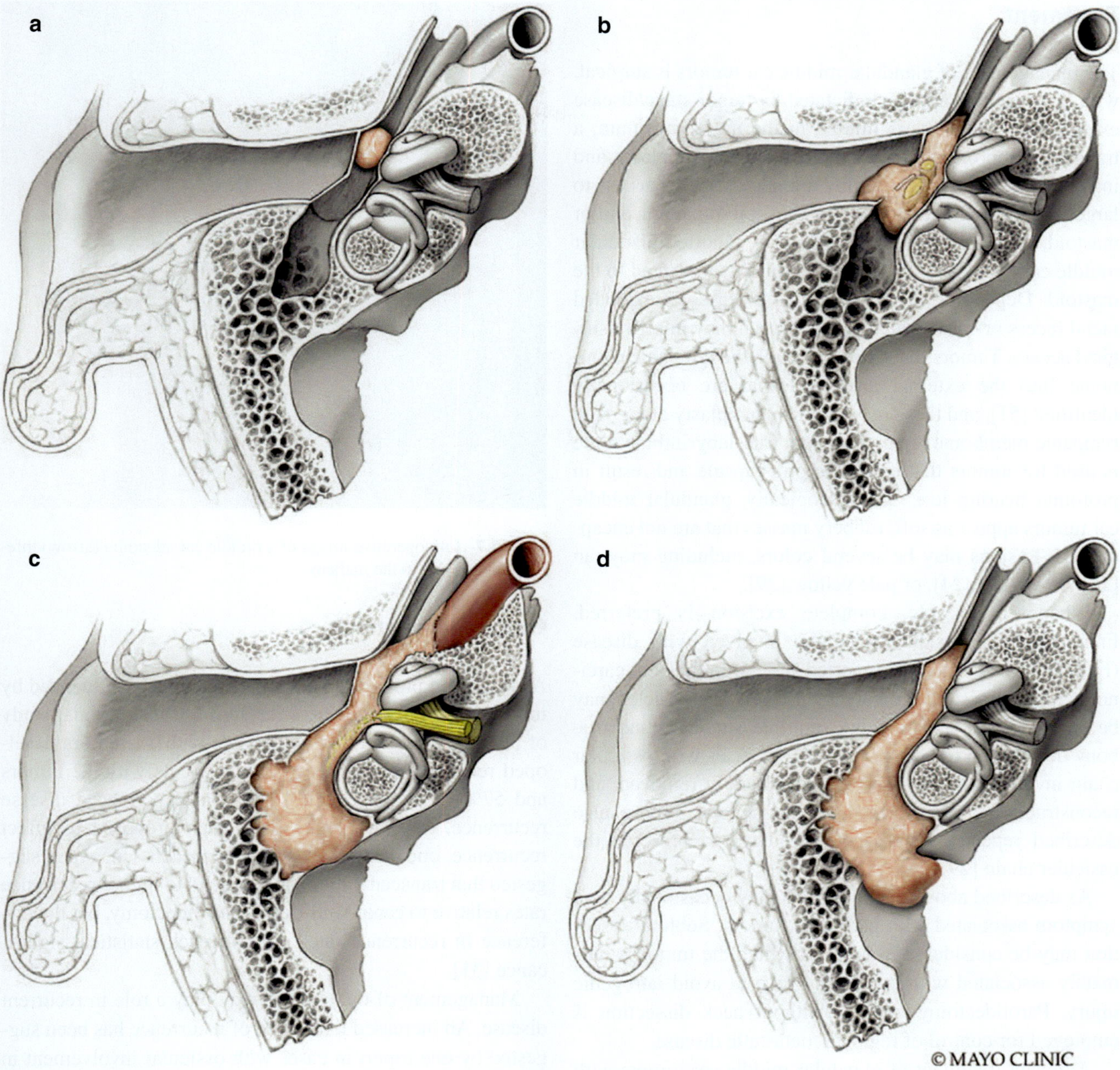

Fig. 66.6 A pictorial reference for T status in middle ear adenoma tumors. (From: Marinelli et al. [62]; used with permission of Mayo Foundation for Medical Education and Research, all rights reserved)

extends into the mastoid; and T2c is a T2a or T2b tumor that also extends through the tympanic membrane into the external auditory canal. A T3 tumor shows adherence to important neurovascular structures such as the carotid artery, facial nerve, sigmoid sinus, or dura. Intradural disease constitutes a T4 tumor. Nodal and distant metastases are defined by the presence or absence of metastatic disease and denoted by binary values (0 or 1). A secretory tumor is accounted for by the S-component of the staging system.

The staging system has been demonstrated to bear prognostic significance [62]. For instance, T3 tumors were significantly more likely to undergo subtotal or near-total resection compared with lower-staged tumors, owing to dense adherence to surrounding neurovascular structures such as the internal carotid artery and facial nerve ($p = 0.027$). Furthermore, T3 tumors were more likely to experience multiple recurrences, require adjuvant treatment, or develop permanent facial nerve weakness compared with lower-staged tumors. Finally, at the time of the last follow-up, no patients with T1 tumors developed recurrence, whereas 37% of patients with T2 tumors and 57% of patients with T3 tumors experienced disease recurrence.

Treatment

The management of glandular middle ear tumors is surgical, with the operative approach dictated by tumor stage/disease extent. For small tumors limited to the mesotympanum, a transcanal approach can be employed. Tympanoplasty and intact canal wall mastoidectomy are necessary for access to larger tumors with extension to the epitympanum and/or mastoid, as one review of 94 previously reported glandular middle ear neoplasms found 15% of tumors to extend to the mastoid. Depending on the extent of disease, an extended facial recess or canal-wall-down approach may improve surgical access. Tumors that extend through the tympanic membrane into the external auditory canal are occasionally identified [51], and these may require canalplasty along with tympanic membrane repair. Rarely, a translabyrinthine route is used for tumors that erode the otic capsule and result in profound hearing loss. Macroscopically, glandular middle ear tumors appear as soft, rubbery masses that are not encapsulated. Lesions may be several colors, including gray-tan [25], brown-red [24], or pale yellow [29].

Whenever possible, complete excision is preferred. Frequently, the ossicular chain is involved with disease (Fig. 66.7); Ramsey et al. reported 72% of middle ear carcinoids to have ossicular involvement [31]. The ossicles may be enveloped by a tumor, but multiple studies found true bony destruction to be rare [51, 63]. In cases with ossicular chain involvement, the ossicles are generally removed, and reconstruction is performed, although one report also described repeated debulking procedures to preserve the ossicular chain [29].

As described above, facial paresis may occasionally be a symptom associated with carcinoid tumors. Subtotal resection may be considered in cases in which the tumor is intimately associated with the facial nerve to avoid iatrogenic injury. Parotidectomy with or without neck dissection is employed for control of regional metastatic disease.

Adjuvant treatment of glandular middle ear tumors with radiation or chemotherapy is generally not recommended. Radiation has occasionally been previously described for the treatment of middle ear carcinoids, but it is not believed to improve control rates [31]. One report described metastatic spread following adjuvant radiation in a patient with a middle ear carcinoid [36].

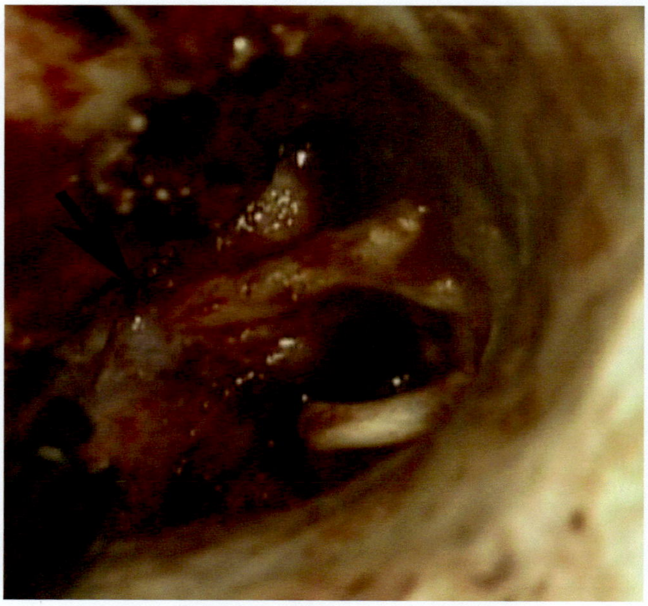

Fig. 66.7 Intraoperative image of a middle ear adenoma (arrow) inferior and anterior to the malleus

Outcome/Prognosis

As discussed previously, outcomes are largely influenced by tumor stage. For instance, a recent multi-institutional study of 32 patients found that no patients with T1 tumors developed recurrence, whereas 37% of patients with T2 tumors and 57% of patients with T3 tumors experienced disease recurrence. Several factors have been proposed to affect recurrence, one being the surgical approach. One study suggested that transcanal removal may lead to higher recurrence rates relative to canal-wall-down mastoidectomy, but the difference in recurrence rates did not reach statistical significance [31].

Management of the ossicles may play a role in recurrent disease. An increased likelihood of recurrence has been suggested by one report in cases with ossicular involvement in which the ossicular chain is not removed [29]. These findings were corroborated by another review, noting that in all patients with recurrence, the ossicular chain had been left intact at the initial surgery [33].

Whether intrinsic tumor biology affects recurrence rates is unclear. Of eight patients with recurrence in a series from Torske et al., moderate cellular pleomorphism was identified in two patients, and high cellularity was found in another two [29]. Similarly, metastatic disease is not necessarily associated with high-grade pathology. One study found that all cases of carcinoid recurrence were associated with well-differentiated neoplasms [31].

A few cases of metastatic primary middle ear carcinoid tumors have been reported. One report described a 64-year-old male with a 9-year history of a recurring middle ear neoplasm and ipsilateral cervical lymphadenopathy [36]. Another series presented two cases of primary middle ear carcinoid tumors with late recurrences and regional metastases [31]. To date, distant metastases from middle ear carcinoid tumors have not been reported, possibly secondary to their small relative size and the middle ear cavity's relative lack of vascularity [47].

Long-term follow-up is recommended for all patients with glandular middle ear tumors. No consensus exists regarding an optimal surveillance schedule, however. A reasonable strategy would be to use a clinical exam alone for benign lesions with limited disease at the time of initial surgery, while reserving a combination of otomicroscopy and CT/MRI to monitor for recurrence in more biologically aggressive tumors.

Conclusion

Glandular neoplasms of the middle ear and ear canal are rare, and this complicates the ability to synthesize best-practice treatment recommendations. However, the contemporary management of these tumors favors biopsy for accurate histologic diagnosis, and in many cases, surgical excision when possible. The use of adjuvant and neoadjuvant therapy is nuanced based on the specific pathology and extent of disease, and in all cases, close follow-up is recommended.

Acknowledgments The authors would like to thank Dr. David S Haynes (Department of Otolaryngology–Head and Neck Surgery, Vanderbilt University) for providing the images used in Figs. 66.5 and 66.7. Figure 66.4 was provided courtesy of Matthew Carlson, MD (Department of Otolaryngology–Head and Neck Surgery, Mayo Clinic). Shira Koss, MD, also provided a contribution to the content described in the section on the middle ear glandular tumors.

References

1. Crain N, Nelson BL, Barnes EL, Thompson LD. Ceruminous gland carcinomas: a clinicopathologic and immunophenotypic study of 17 cases. Head Neck Pathol. 2009;3(1):1–17.
2. Tsukahara K, Suzuki M, Tokashiki R, Motohashi R, Iwaya K. Pleomorphic adenoma of the external auditory canal complicated by hearing loss secondary to chronic otitis media. Auris Nasus Larynx. 2006;33(2):183–6.
3. Thompson LD, Nelson BL, Barnes EL. Ceruminous adenomas: a clinicopathologic study of 41 cases with a review of the literature. Am J Surg Pathol. 2004;28(3):308–18.
4. Markou K, Karasmanis I, Vlachtsis K, Petridis D, Nikolaou A, Vital V. Primary pleomorphic adenoma of the external ear canal. Report of a case and literature review. Am J Otolaryngol. 2008;29(2):142–6.
5. Wetli CV, Pardo V, Millard M, Gerston K. Tumors of ceruminous glands. Cancer. 1972;29(5):1169–78.
6. Perzin KH, Gullane P, Conley J. Adenoid cystic carcinoma involving the external auditory canal. A clinicopathologic study of 16 cases. Cancer. 1982;50(12):2873–83.
7. Pulec JL. Glandular tumors of the external auditory canal. Laryngoscope. 1977;87(10 Pt 1):1601–12.
8. Dehner LP, Chen KT. Primary tumors of the external and middle ear. Benign and malignant glandular neoplasms. Arch Otolaryngol. 1980;106(1):13–9.
9. Mills RG, Douglas-Jones T, Williams RG. 'Ceruminoma'--a defunct diagnosis. J Laryngol Otol. 1995;109(3):180–8.
10. Lassaletta L, Patrón M, Olóriz J, Pérez R, Gavilán J. Avoiding misdiagnosis in ceruminous gland tumours. Auris Nasus Larynx. 2003;30(3):287–90.
11. Mansour P, George MK, Pahor AL. Ceruminous gland tumours: a reappraisal. J Laryngol Otol. 1992;106(8):727–32.
12. Koyuncu M, Karagöz F, Kiliaçarslan H. Pleomorphic adenoma of the external auditory canal. Eur Arch Otorhinolaryngol. 2005;262(12):969–71.
13. Giuseppe M, Serena B, Sandro B, et al. Adenoma of the ceruminous gland (ceruminoma). Otol Neurotol. 2011;32(2):e14–5.
14. Lee CK, Jang KT, Cho YS. Tubular apocrine adenoma with syringocystadenoma papilliferum arising from the external auditory canal. J Laryngol Otol. 2005;119(12):1004–6.
15. Friedmann I. Pathological lesions of the external auditory meatus: a review. J R Soc Med. 1990;83(1):34–7.
16. Cankar V, Crowley H. Tumors of ceruminous glands: a clinicopathological study of 7 cases. Cancer. 1964;17:67–75.
17. Arriaga M, Curtin H, Takahashi H, Hirsch BE, Kamerer DB. Staging proposal for external auditory meatus carcinoma based on preoperative clinical examination and computed tomography findings. Ann Otol Rhinol Laryngol. 1990;99(9 Pt 1):714–21.
18. Moore MG, Deschler DG, McKenna MJ, Varvares MA, Lin DT. Management outcomes following lateral temporal bone resection for ear and temporal bone malignancies. Otolaryngol Head Neck Surg. 2007;137(6):893–8.
19. Gidley PW, Thompson CR, Roberts DB, DeMonte F, Hanna EY. The oncology of otology. Laryngoscope. 2012;122(2):393–400.
20. Dong F, Gidley PW, Ho T, Luna MA, Ginsberg LE, Sturgis EM. Adenoid cystic carcinoma of the external auditory canal. Laryngoscope. 2008;118(9):1591–6.
21. Chang CH, Shu MT, Lee JC, Leu YS, Chen YC, Lee KS. Treatments and outcomes of malignant tumors of external auditory canal. Am J Otolaryngol. 2009;30(1):44–8.
22. Haraguchi H, Hentona H, Tanaka H, Komatuzaki A. Pleomorphic adenoma of the external auditory canal: a case report and review of the literature. J Laryngol Otol. 1996;110(1):52–6.
23. Koopot R, Reyes C, Pifarré R. Multiple pulmonary metastases from adenoid cystic carcinoma of ceruminous glands of external auditory canal. A case report and review of the literature. J Thorac Cardiovasc Surg. 1973;65(6):909–13.
24. Hyams VJ, Michaels L. Benign adenomatous neoplasm (adenoma) of the middle ear. Clin Otolaryngol Allied Sci. 1976;1(1):17–26.
25. Derlacki EL, Barney PL. Adenomatous tumors of the middle ear and mastoid. Laryngoscope. 1976;86(8):1123–35.
26. Murphy GF, Pilch BZ, Dickersin GR, Goodman ML, Nadol JB Jr. Carcinoid tumor of the middle ear. Am J Clin Pathol. 1980;73(6):816–23.
27. Aquino BF, Chandra RK, Haines GK, Micco AG. Neuroendocrine adenoma of the middle ear. Otolaryngol Head Neck Surg. 2002;127(5):477–9.

28. Leong K, Haber MM, Divi V, Sataloff RT. Neuroendocrine adenoma of the middle ear (NAME). Ear Nose Throat J. 2009;88(4):874–9.
29. Torske KR, Thompson LD. Adenoma versus carcinoid tumor of the middle ear: a study of 48 cases and review of the literature. Mod Pathol. 2002;15(5):543–55.
30. Wackym AF, Friedman I. Unusual tumors of the middle ear and mastoid. In: tumors of the middle ear and temporal bone. Lippincott Williams and Wilkins; 2000. p. 128–45.
31. Ramsey MJ, Nadol JB Jr, Pilch BZ, McKenna MJ. Carcinoid tumor of the middle ear: clinical features, recurrences, and metastases. Laryngoscope. 2005;115(9):1660–6.
32. Pallanch JF, Weiland LH, McDonald TJ, Facer GW, Harner SG. Adenocarcinoma and adenoma of the middle ear. Laryngoscope. 1982;92(1):47–54.
33. Saliba I, Evrard AS. Middle ear glandular neoplasms: adenoma, carcinoma or adenoma with neuroendocrine differentiation: a case series. Cases J. 2009;2:6508.
34. Ayache S, Braccini F, Fernandes M, Homassin JM. Adenoma of the middle ear: a rare and misleading lesion. Otol Neurotol. 2002;23(6):988–91.
35. Krouse JH, Nadol JB Jr, Goodman ML. Carcinoid tumors of the middle ear. Ann Otol Rhinol Laryngol. 1990;99(7 Pt 1):547–52.
36. Mooney EE, Dodd LG, Oury TD, Burchette JL, Layfield LJ, Scher RL. Middle ear carcinoid: an indolent tumor with metastatic potential. Head Neck. 1999;21(1):72–7.
37. Farrior JB 3rd, Hyams VJ, Benke RH, Farrior JB. Carcinoid apudoma arising in a glomus jugulare tumor: review of endocrine activity in glomus jugulare tumors. Laryngoscope. 1980;90(1):110–9.
38. Latif MA, Madders DJ, Barton RP, Shaw PA. Carcinoid tumour of the middle ear associated with systemic symptoms. J Laryngol Otol. 1987;101(5):480–6.
39. Zan E, Limb CJ, Koehler JF, Yousem DM. Middle ear adenoma: a challenging diagnosis. AJNR Am J Neuroradiol. 2009;30(8):1602–3.
40. Maintz D, Stupp C, Krueger K, Wustrow J, Lackner K. MRI and CT of adenomatous tumours of the middle ear. Neuroradiology. 2001;43(1):58–61.
41. Bierry G, Riehm S, Marcellin L, Stierlé JL, Veillon F. Middle ear adenomatous tumor: a not so rare glomus tympanicum-mimicking lesion. J Neuroradiol. 2010;37(2):116–21.
42. Nikanne E, Kantola O, Parviainen T. Carcinoid tumor of the middle ear. Acta Otolaryngol. 2004;124(6):754–7.
43. Friedmann I. Middle ear adenoma. Histopathology. 1998;32(3):279–80.
44. Soga J, Ferlito A, Rinaldo A. Endocrinocarcinomas (carcinoids and their variants) of the larynx: a comparative consideration with those of other sites. Oral Oncol. 2004;40(7):668–72.
45. Ferlito A, Rinaldo A. The spectrum of endocrinocarcinomas of the larynx. Oral Oncol. 2005;41(9):878–83.
46. Chan KC, Wu CM, Huang SF. Carcinoid tumor of the middle ear: a case report. Am J Otolaryngol. 2005;26(1):57–9.
47. Ferlito A, Devaney KO, Rinaldo A. Neuroendocrine neoplasms of the larynx: advances in identification, understanding, and management. Oral Oncol. 2006;42(8):770–88.
48. Cruz Toro P, Domenech I, Clemente I, Farré A, Amilibia E. Neuroendocrine adenoma of the middle ear. Otol Neurotol. 2012;33(1):e7–8.
49. Mills SE, Fechner RE. Middle ear adenoma. A cytologically uniform neoplasm displaying a variety of architectural patterns. Am J Surg Pathol. 1984;8(9):677–85.
50. Manni JJ, Faverly DR, Van Haelst UJ. Primary carcinoid tumors of the middle ear. Report on four cases and a review of the literature. Arch Otolaryngol Head Neck Surg. 1992;118(12):1341–7.
51. Hosoda S, Tateno H, Inoue HK, Isojima G, Kondo S, Konishi T. Carcinoid tumor of the middle ear containing serotonin and multiple peptide hormones. A case report and review of the pathology literature. Acta Pathol Jpn. 1992;42(8):614–20.
52. Ribé A, Fernández PL, Ostertarg H, et al. Middle-ear adenoma (MEA): a report of two cases, one with predominant "plasmacytoid" features. Histopathology. 1997;30(4):359–64.
53. Ketabchi S, Massi D, Franchi A, Vannucchi P, Santucci M. Middle ear adenoma is an amphicrine tumor: why call it adenoma? Ultrastruct Pathol. 2001;25(1):73–8.
54. Paraskevakou H, Lazaris AC, Kandiloros DC, Papadimitriou K, Adamopoulos G, Davaris PS. Middle ear adenomatous tumor with a predominant neuroendocrine component. Pathology. 1999;31(3):284–7.
55. Stanley MW, Horwitz CA, Levinson RM, Sibley RK. Carcinoid tumors of the middle ear. Am J Clin Pathol. 1987;87(5):592–600.
56. Wassef M, Kanavaros P, Nemeth J, Adjamagbo H, Ba Huy PT. Amphicrine adenoma of the middle ear. Histological, immunohistochemical and ultrastructural study of a case. Ann Pathol. 1993;13(3):170–5.
57. Tadros TS, Strauss RM, Cohen C, Gal AA. Galanin immunoreactivity in paragangliomas but not in carcinoid tumors. Appl Immunohistochem Mol Morphol. 2003;11(3):250–2.
58. Heffner DK. Low-grade adenocarcinoma of probable endolymphatic sac origin a clinicopathologic study of 20 cases. Cancer. 1989;64(11):2292–302.
59. Gaffey MJ, Mills SE, Fechner RE, Intemann SR, Wick MR. Aggressive papillary middle-ear tumor. A clinicopathologic entity distinct from middle-ear adenoma. Am J Surg Pathol. 1988;12(10):790–7.
60. Fayemi AO, Toker C. Primary adenocarcinoma of the middle ear. Arch Otolaryngol. 1975;101(7):449–52.
61. Schuller DE, Conley JJ, Goodman JH, Clausen KP, Miller WJ. Primary adenocarcinoma of the middle ear. Otolaryngol Head Neck Surg. 1983;91(3):280–3.
62. Marinelli JP, Cass SP, Mann SE, et al. Adenomatous neuroendocrine tumors of the middle ear: a multi-institutional investigation of 32 cases and development of a staging system. Otol Neurotol. 2018;39(8):e712–21.
63. Hardingham M. Adenoma of the middle ear. Arch Otolaryngol Head Neck Surg. 1995;121(3):342–4.

Cutaneous Malignancies of the Pinna and External Auditory Canal

67

Joseph T. Breen and Myles L. Pensak

Introduction and Clinical Context

Malignant neoplasms of the skin are the most common of all cancers. Exposure to ionizing radiation in the form of ultraviolet (UV) light is the primary risk factor in fair-skinned individuals, and the prominent position of the pinna leads to its relatively high risk of harboring skin cancer [1]. In contrast, the external auditory canal (EAC) is anatomically protected from significant UV exposure. While this contributes to a far lower incidence of cutaneous malignancies at this site, cancers originating within the EAC typically mandate more radical treatment and are associated with a far higher risk of death from disease [2, 3]. Complex regional anatomy, the vital neural and vascular structures of the temporal bone, and aesthetic concerns lead to unique challenges in managing these tumors. Herein, the diagnosis and treatment of cutaneous malignancies of the pinna and EAC are reviewed. Glandular tumors and other primary temporal bone malignancies are discussed in subsequent chapters.

Anatomy

The pinna (auricle) is a skin-covered structure with an underlying framework of fibroelastic cartilage and perichondrium. The exception is the lobule, a fibrofatty appendage devoid of cartilage at the inferior aspect of the pinna. Hair follicles, sebaceous glands, and sudoriferous glands are distributed throughout the pinna. The concha and tragus funnel into the lateral portion of the EAC, which is similarly composed of elastic cartilage and overlying skin. The fissures of Santorini are variably present, vertically oriented defects in the anterior aspect of the cartilaginous EAC. These may have clinical relevance as a theoretical route of extension for infectious or neoplastic processes from the EAC into the parotid gland [4]. The medial two-thirds of the EAC is osseous, lined with thinner skin, and is sparsely populated by hair follicles and their appendages.

Cutaneous Malignancies: Overview and Epidemiology

Primary cutaneous malignancies can develop from any of the cell types that comprise the skin. Basal cell carcinoma (BCC) and squamous cell carcinoma (SCC) are frequently grouped together as "non-melanoma skin cancer" (NMSC) or as the now-preferred term of "keratinocyte carcinomas" (KC) due to their shared cellular lineage. Basal and squamous cell carcinomas of the skin are not formally reported or tracked by cancer registries, but an estimated 3.3 million individuals with KC were treated in the United States in 2012, far more than the total incidence of all other cancers combined [5]. The worldwide incidence of BCC has been estimated at 3–8%, and the average lifetime risk for a Caucasian to develop BCC approximates 30% [6, 7]. Estimates on BCC to SCC incidence ratios range from 4:1 to close to 1:1, with a more rapidly increasing incidence of SCC seen in recent years. Approximately 70–80% of KC occurs on the head and neck [8], with tumors involving the pinna accounting for 9–19% of KC [9]. Malignant melanoma of the external ear accounts for 7–20% of all melanomas affecting the head and neck, and 1–4% of all cutaneous melanoma [10–12].

The primary risk factor for the development of KC is exposure to ultraviolet (UV) radiation. Both UV-A (320–400 nm) and UV-B (280–320 nm) radiation can lead to DNA damage, suppression of cutaneous immunity, production of reactive oxygen species (ROS), inflammation, and

J. T. Breen
Department of Otolaryngology—Head and Neck Surgery, Mayo Clinic, Jacksonville, FL, USA
e-mail: breen.joseph@mayo.edu

M. L. Pensak (✉)
Department of Otolaryngology—Head and Neck Surgery, University of Cincinnati College of Medicine, Cincinnati, OH, USA
e-mail: myles.pensak@uc.edu

A. D. Sweeney et al. (eds.), *Haynes-Glasscock-Shambaugh Surgery of the Ear*, https://doi.org/10.1007/978-3-032-18264-7_67

cell dysregulation [13]. An examination of body distribution rates for all cutaneous malignancies suggests that SCC has the strongest correlation with UV radiation exposure. Based on these data, it is also posited that short duration and high intensity UV exposure earlier in life imparts specific risk for developing BCC or melanoma, whereas sustained and cumulative exposure is a stronger risk factor for SCC [8, 14]. Additional risk factors for KC include light-colored skin, increasing age, male gender, arsenic or other chemical and occupational exposures, radiation therapy, chronic inflammatory skin conditions, xeroderma pigmentosum (XP), nevoid basal cell carcinoma (Gorlin) syndrome, use of photochemotherapy (psoralen for eczema or psoriasis), immunosuppression, HPV infection, and smoking [15].

Immunosuppression after organ transplantation dramatically increases an individual's risk of developing skin cancer. The risk appears to be more significant for younger transplant recipients and increases with time since transplantation. For those receiving transplants prior to age 50, for example, there is up to a 200-fold increased risk by 6 years posttransplant when compared to age-matched controls [16]. Additionally, immunosuppressed patients have been shown to develop more aggressive tumors with higher rates of metastasis and lower rates of disease-free and overall survival [17, 18]. There appears to be a higher incidence of SCC than BCC in the immunosuppressed population [16]. Patients on calcineurin inhibitors (e.g., cyclosporine, tacrolimus) may be at particularly high risk for development of KC, and switching the immunosuppressive regimen to mTOR inhibitors (e.g., sirolimus, everolimus) may significantly decrease risk [19].

Clinical Evaluation

As with any otologic complaint, the history and physical examination are the first and most important steps in the evaluation of cancers involving the auricle and EAC. The history should include a review of previously treated skin cancers, other malignancies, exposure to carcinogens (including sun exposure), occupation, causes of immunosuppression, prior surgery or radiation in the region, and any other otologic diagnoses. The patient should be questioned regarding the lesion itself, including its duration, change in size or appearance, growth rate, or bleeding. Table 67.1 presents a review of the most common presenting symptoms for patients with temporal bone malignancies. Family history is important in cases of nevoid basal cell carcinoma (Gorlin) syndrome or xeroderma pigmentosum. Major medical comorbidities must be carefully reviewed to assess the patient's fitness for potentially extensive surgery.

The head and neck examination should be systematic and comprehensive, including careful inspection of the skin of the scalp, face, and neck. Binocular microscopy of the external auditory meatus, canal, and tympanic membrane is helpful in delineating the location and extent of the tumor. The skin of the bony portion of the EAC is generally thinner, is not hair-bearing, and will not be mobile with manipulation of the pinna [4]. Tumors originating on the pinna or cartilaginous EAC should be carefully assessed for medial extension involving the skin over the bony canal. The tumor should be manipulated to assess for fixation to underlying structures. The presence of trismus or malocclusion suggests invasion of the temporomandibular joint (TMJ) space. As with any neurotologic examination, cranial nerve assessment is essential. Facial weakness should be assessed as either being segmental or involving all divisions. Any cranial nerve dysfunction ipsilateral to the tumor is considered evidence of the tumor invading the nerve until proven otherwise [20]. The parotid and neck are carefully palpated to assess for direct invasion from the primary tumor or metastatic adenopathy.

Table 67.1 Most common signs and symptoms of EAC and temporal bone malignancies

Sign/symptom	Frequency at presentation (%)
Aural discharge	66
Otalgia	47
Hearing loss	37
Canal mass/lesion	35
Facial weakness	18
Bleeding	15

Data compiled from Pensak et al., Gidley et al., Zhang et al., Chi et al.

Differential Diagnosis

While the otologist/neurotologist most commonly focuses their examination on the structures of the ear and temporal bone medial to the pinna and EAC, they will often be called upon to assess abnormalities of the skin in the region. Ultimately, a biopsy should be pursued if there is any concern for malignancy. However, identification of skin neoplasms is enhanced by the ability to recognize stereotypical appearances of the most common malignancies and precancerous lesions.

Actinic Keratosis

Actinic keratoses (AKs) are the precursors to the majority of SCCs. The primary risk factor for their development is UV radiation exposure; hence, they are frequently located in the prominent and relatively exposed skin of the head and neck. They represent basal layer keratinocyte atypia that has not progressed to full-thickness involvement (SCC in situ) or extended into the dermis and beyond (SCC) [21]. Their characteristic appearance is rough and scaly. The rate of an individual lesion's transformation to SCC has been reported as between 0.025% and 16%. The average individual diagnosed with an AK harbors between 6 and 8 lesions [21].

Squamous Cell Carcinoma
Squamous cell carcinomas are classically papulosquamous, erythematous, hyperkeratotic, and ulcerated. The tumors may bleed easily with manipulation.

Basal Cell Carcinoma
Basal cell carcinoma typically has the appearance of a shiny or pearly papule with overlying telangiectasias. Tumors may have central umbilication or depression and rolled borders [22].

Malignant Melanoma
Malignant melanoma's typical appearance can be remembered by using the mnemonic ABCD: *A*symmetry in shape, *B*order irregularity, *C*olor variation, and *D*iameter greater than 6 mm. Lesions with any of these suspicious characteristics should be evaluated further by a full-thickness biopsy.

Merkel Cell Carcinoma
Merkel cells are bound to the terminal ends of sensory nerve fibers in the basal layer of the epidermis. Malignant transformation of these cells, likely related to the oncogenic Merkel cell polyomavirus, leads to the development of Merkel cell carcinoma. This rare and generally aggressive cancer can appear as a painless red/pink or blue/purple lesion that tends to grow rapidly. It most commonly occurs in sun-exposed sites and is more common in patients older than 50 with chronic immunosuppression [23, 24]. Information regarding its behavior when involving the pinna or EAC is limited to case reports or small series.

Non-epithelial Skin Cancers
The adnexal structures of the skin, including sebaceous or ceruminous glands, can generate malignancies involving the pinna and EAC. Ceruminous adenocarcinoma is a slow-growing and locally aggressive EAC tumor that may present as a painless nodular mass, variably ulcerated or covered by intact skin [25]. Adenoid cystic carcinoma (ACC) most commonly occurs in the salivary glands, but primary ACC of the EAC is occasionally seen. It has a significant propensity for perineural invasion (PNI), metastasis, and recurrence. Lesions may be painful [26]. Glandular carcinomas of the external auditory canal are more thoroughly reviewed in Chap. 66.

Sarcoma
Cutaneous angiosarcomas of the auricle are rare. They can appear as red-purple macular eruptions that might be mistaken for bruising with ill-defined borders. These aggressive lesions are associated with poor survival and propensity for metastasis. Kaposi's sarcoma is typically seen in immunosuppressed patients, most commonly among patients with acquired immunodeficiency syndrome (HIV/AIDS). These often present as red-purple or brown-red plaques or nodules [26].

Lymphoma and Other Lesions
Lymphoproliferative disorders involving the pinna can include primary cutaneous lymphoma, mycosis fungoides, *Borrelia burgdorferi* infection, reactions to ear piercings or other local trauma, and discoid lupus [27]. Clinical presentation is highly variable, and expert histopathological evaluation, including immunophenotyping, is mandatory for accurate diagnosis [28]. Other malignancies that can occur on the auricle include malignant fibrous histiocytoma, atypical fibroxanthoma, dermatofibrosarcoma protuberans, and metastatic disease.

Malignancies of the Pinna

Imaging

High-risk tumors of the pinna (diameter >2 cm or depth >2 mm, poorly differentiated, fixation to underlying structures, PNI, or lymphovascular invasion) should prompt consideration of imaging depending on the clinical situation. CT with contrast and positron emission tomography (PET) scanning can assess for regional or distant metastatic adenopathy. CT is the best study for assessing osseous invasion. MRI is of particular utility when there is extensive soft tissue involvement or when evidence of PNI is present [30].

Staging Tumors of the Pinna

The eighth edition of the American Joint Committee on Cancer (AJCC) Cancer Staging Manual and the Union for International Cancer Control (UICC) TNM (Tumor, Node, Metastasis) Classification of Malignant Tumors were published in 2016 [31]. Relevant staging systems for cutaneous malignancies are summarized in Tables 67.2 and 67.3. Notably, depth of invasion has been proven to be a significant prognostic factor for malignant melanoma. As such, it is staged with a system separate from that of KC, and depth of invasion factors prominently into the T stage.

Treatment for Malignancies of the Pinna

Medical
Topical application of 5-fluorouracil (5-FU) and imiquimod has been evaluated as both treatments for KC. In general,

Table 67.2 TNM classification for skin carcinoma of the head and neck

T stage				
TX—Primary tumor cannot be identified				
T0—No evidence of primary tumor				
Tis—Carcinoma in situ				
T1—Tumor 2 cm or less in greatest dimension				
T2—Tumor >2 cm and ≤4 cm				
T3—Tumor >4 cm or minor bone erosion or perineural invasion or deep invasion				
T4—Tumor with skull base or axial skeleton invasion including foraminal involvement and/or vertebral foramen involvement to the epidural space				
N stage				
N0—No regional lymph node metastasis				
N1—Metastasis in a single ipsilateral lymph node, 3 cm or less in greatest dimension without extranodal extension (ENE)				
N2—Metastasis described as: N2a—Metastasis in a single ipsilateral lymph node >3 cm but <6 cm without ENE N2b—Metastasis in multiple ipsilateral lymph nodes, none >6 cm, without ENE N2c—Metastasis in bilateral or contralateral lymph nodes, none >6 cm, without ENE				
N3a—Metastasis in a lymph node >6 cm in greatest dimension without ENE				
N3b—Metastasis in a lymph node >3 cm with ENE or multiple ipsilateral, or any contralateral or bilateral node(s) with ENE				
M stage				
M0—No distant metastasis				
M1—Distant metastasis				
Stage 0	Tis	N0	M0	The presence of skin involvement or soft tissue invasion with deep fixation/tethering to underlying muscle or adjacent structures or clinical signs of nerve involvement is classified as clinical extranodal extension
Stage I	T1	N0	M0	
Stage II	T2	N0	M0	
Stage III	T3 T1, T2, T3	N0 N1	M0 M0	
Stage IVA	T1, T2, T3, T4	N2, N3 Any N	M0 M0	
Stage IVB	Any T	Any N	M1	

Adapted from Ref. [31]

Table 67.3 TNM clinical classification for malignant melanoma of the skin

T stage				
TX—Primary tumor cannot be assessed				
T0—No evidence of primary tumor				
Tis—Melanoma in situ				
T1—Tumor 1 mm or less in thickness	*T1a—<0.8 mm, without ulceration* *T1b—<0.8 mm with ulceration or >0.8 mm and <1 mm, with or without ulceration*			
T2—Tumor >1 mm and <2 mm	*T2a—Without ulceration* *T2b—With ulceration*			
T3—Tumor >2 mm and <4 mm	*T3a—Without ulceration* *T3b—With ulceration*			
T4—Tumor >4 mm	*T4a—Without ulceration* *T4b—With ulceration*			
N stage				
N0—No regional lymph node metastasis				
N1—Metastasis in one regional lymph node (LN) or intralymphatic regional metastasis without nodal metastases	*N1a—Microscopic metastases* *N1b—Macroscopic metastases* *N1c—Satellite or in-transit metastasis without regional nodal metastasis*			
N2—Metastasis in 2–3 regional LNs or intralymphatic regional metastasis with nodal metastases	*N2a—Microscopic metastases* *N2b—Macroscopic metastases* *N2c—Satellite or in-transit metastasis with 1 regional nodal metastasis*			
M stage				
M0—No distant metastasis	Stage 0	Tis	N0	M0

(continued)

Table 67.3 (continued)

M1—Distant metastasis	Stage IA	T1a, T1b	N0	M0
M1a—Skin, subcutaneous tissue, or LNs beyond the regional LNs	Stage IB	T2a	N0	M0
M1b—Lung	Stage IIA	T2b, T3a	N0	M0
M1c—Other non-CNS sites	Stage IIB	T3b, T4a	N0	M0
M1d—CNS	Stage IIC	T4b	N0	M0
Suffixes for M category:	Stage III	Any T	N+	M0
(0) LDH not elevated	Stage IIIA	T1, T2a	N1a, N2a	M0
(1) LDH elevated	Stage IIIB	T1, T2a T2b, T3a	N1b, N1c, N2b N1, N2a, N2b	M0
	Stage IIIC	T1, T2, T3a T3b, T4a T4b	N2c, N3 N+ N1, N2	M0
	Stage IIID	T4b	N3	M0
	Stage IV	Any T	Any N	M1

Adapted from Ref. [31]

their use is relegated to superficial-type BCC, actinic keratosis, and SCC in situ (Bowen's disease). Widely ranging cure rates after courses lasting 6–12 weeks have been reported, with efficacy exceeding 90% for longer and more intense regimens treating superficial BCC using either agent [32, 33]. Efficacy of imiquimod for other lesions is generally lower, and it is not recommended for SCC. Adverse reactions are generally limited to local skin reactions.

Photodynamic therapy refers to the application of a photoactivating light to the lesion after an exogenous photosensitizer is administered. It is rarely employed for tumors isolated to the pinna. Response rates ranging from 75% to 97% using various regimens have been reported, with few studies providing longer-term follow-up [33].

Excellent cure rates of small KCs, including those involving the pinna, have been reported with cryosurgery, which uses liquid nitrogen to take affected tissue through rapid freeze/thaw cycles [34]. Electrodessication and curettage are techniques that similarly seek to destroy the tumor without formal excision. Five-year tumor control rates for all KCs are in excess of 95%, which nearly approaches that of Mohs micrographic surgery, which is often avoided around the ears, eyes, and nose due to relatively inferior aesthetic outcomes [35, 36].

Surgery

Malignancy of the pinna is a surgical disease. The goal of surgery is to completely remove the tumor with minimal disturbance to the appearance and function of the ear. The recommended margins for wide local excision vary. At least 4–5 mm margins are advocated for low-risk SCC, with larger (>2 cm), more invasive (>6 mm), or higher-risk tumors (poorly differentiated, perineural invasion) mandating at least 6 mm and perhaps up to 10 mm margins based on expert opinion [37]. Recommended margins for BCC vary from 4–5 mm for relatively low-risk lesions on the pinna up to 1.5 cm for larger (>3 cm) tumors [38]. Relatively high rates of incomplete excision, up to 13%, are reported for BCC of the ear managed by wide local excision. This leads some authors to recommend all KC in this region to be deemed high risk, mandating at least 6 mm margins with intraoperative margin analysis or Mohs micrographic surgery [39].

Mohs Micrographic Surgery

The primary advantage of Mohs micrographic surgery (MMS) is minimizing the size of the defect while providing excellent local control rates. Narrow excisions are permissible due to the circumferential margin analysis, which is a valuable feature for lesions of the pinna, where adequate cosmesis and function are important. Overall, the cure rates for auricular carcinomas are excellent with MMS, ranging from 92.3% to 94.7% at 5 years for SCC [40–43]. This compares favorably to non-Mohs modalities, with SCC control rates at approximately 84% at 5 years [43]. Though it requires significant specialized training, the cost-effectiveness of MMS has been demonstrated [44].

Surgery for Malignant Melanoma

In general, 1–2 cm resection margins are recommended for malignant melanoma (MM), with sentinel lymph node biopsy (SLNB) performed for lesions >1 mm in depth. MMS has been demonstrated as an effective technique for treating MM of the head and neck [45], though it is not yet considered standard of care for lesions of the pinna [11]. Margin analysis is a more challenging pathological exercise overall in MM than with KC. Overall survival of 85% at 5 years and 70–77% at 10 years has been reported with surgery for MM of the pinna [11].

Reconstruction

Techniques along the entire spectrum of reconstructive surgery are viable options after tumor removal. Healing by secondary intention, skin grafting, primary closure, local flaps, and prostheses might all be utilized, depending on the characteristics of the defect. Comprehensive review of these reconstructive options is beyond the scope of this chapter, however.

Radiation Therapy

Patients with malignancies of the pinna who refuse surgery or are medically unfit for surgery may be candidates for primary radiation therapy (RT). Radiation has the obvious additional benefit of avoiding potentially disfiguring surgery, though at considerably higher expense with longer treatment courses when compared to surgery. Silva et al. presented a series of 334 lesions involving the pinna. Two- and five-year control rates for BCC and SCC were 86.6% and 79.2%, respectively. Trends toward better early control rates were seen in the BCC group (93% vs. 82% at 2 years, 83% vs. 79% at 5 years), and tumors larger than 2 cm were significantly more likely to recur [9]. Caccialanza et al. reported on a series of 115 patients undergoing RT for incident or recurrent KC (99 BCC, 16 SCC) of the pinna. The 5-year cure rate was 78%, with all recurrences in the BCC group [46].

Radiation-induced malignancy (RIM) is a rare (between 0.4% and 1%) complication of RT, which typically develops 10–40 or more years after treatment for benign or malignant lesions [47, 48]. Outcomes with RIM are very poor, with 5-year survival estimates between 10% and 30% [49]. Other sequelae of radiation to the lateral skull base for malignancy include sensorineural hearing loss, osteoradionecrosis, and chronic otitis media [50]. Caution is recommended in applying RT to younger patients.

Regional Nodal Dissection

Overall, the metastatic risks of KC are low, but are higher for tumors on the pinna [51]. Regional metastases occur in approximately 5–18% of auricular SCCs and in 2–6% of BCCs. The nodal basins most at risk are the parotid and periauricular nodes, with the upper jugulodigastric nodes being less commonly involved [52, 53]. Recurrent disease, tumor size >2 cm, perineural or vascular invasion, poor differentiation, and Clark level ≥4 have been associated with higher risks of regional metastasis [54, 55]. Of those with metastatic cutaneous SCC, approximately 5–15% develop distant metastasis, which is associated with very low survival rates [56, 57]. Metastasis of BCC taken as a whole is a very rare event (0.0028–0.55%), though spread to bone, liver, lung, or skin (in-transit) accounted for 56% of all BCC metastases (regional or distant) in a large literature review [58].

Therapeutic neck dissection is recommended for patients with lymphadenopathy in the at-risk nodal basin or biopsy-proven regional metastasis. Elective lymph node dissection (ELND) (clinically N0) is more controversial for advanced KC. No prospective data exist to support its use. Many authors state that clinical judgment and the presence of several of the aforementioned risk factors may direct a surgeon toward ELND [59]. Elective parotidectomy to stage and treat the high-risk nodal basin within the gland has been evaluated, as well. Osborne et al. noted no occult metastases in their series of 19 patients with various high-risk auricular malignancies [60]. In contrast, Kadakia et al. reported a 37.5% (39/104) rate of occult parotid metastasis for auricular SCCs larger than 2 cm [61]. In the setting of parotid metastasis and a clinically N0 neck, a 20–27% rate of occult neck metastasis has been demonstrated for SCC. Most positive nodes will be located in level 2 or 3 of the neck for ear and anterior scalp primary tumors. Therefore, at least a selective neck dissection in this region is recommended if parotid metastasis is encountered [62, 63].

Sentinel lymph node biopsy (SLNB) is a minimally invasive procedure to remove the lymph node or nodal basin deemed most at risk for the development of regional metastasis. The node is identified by injection near the lesion of radiotracers or visible dyes, which travel to regional lymph nodes that are found with lymphoscintigraphy, handheld gamma probes, or intraoperative visualization. This procedure has found extensive use in the management of intermediate-thickness (1.20–3.50 mm) melanoma, and survival benefit with SLNB has been demonstrated in this group [64]. The role of SLNB in advanced KC is less clear, with some studies finding that it confers no survival advantage over watchful waiting [55].

Adjuvant Therapy

Adjuvant radiation therapy is indicated for advanced primary SCC (T3 or T4), in the setting of recurrence, and node-positive disease [65, 66]. It should also be considered for cases of substantial perineural invasion or positive margins [67]. Similar indications can be considered for advanced BCC, though data are even more limited. If advanced SCC is treated with adjuvant chemotherapy or chemoradiotherapy, platinum-based combination regimens are typically used, but data regarding efficacy are limited.

Recent years have seen the emergence of vismodegib, a targeted inhibitor of smoothened homologue (SMO), leading to inhibition of the Hedgehog signaling pathway, in the treatment of advanced BCC. Initial reports on tumor responsiveness are encouraging, but longer-term survival outcomes are pending.

Interferon alpha-2 (IFNα) has seen extensive use in the adjuvant setting for melanoma. This is most commonly utilized for stage IIB–III disease, where the survival impact is expected to be greatest [68]. Meta-analyses have shown improvement in overall and recurrence-free survival with adjuvant IFN [69, 70]. Other chemotherapy, immunotherapy, vaccine, and antiangiogenic agents have also been explored, but a discussion of their use is beyond the scope of this text.

Malignancies of the External Auditory Canal

Additional Imaging and Ancillary Testing

It is rare that physical examination alone will lead to a full understanding of an EAC malignancy's extent. For many surgeons, CT with intravenous contrast is the first-line imaging study. Subtle bone erosion is best defined by this modality, making CT an essential component of some tumor staging systems [71]. Additionally, information can be obtained regarding tumor extent, regional adenopathy, parotid involvement, and spread beyond the temporal bone. MRI with gadolinium can more clearly delineate the extent of the primary tumor when there is extratemporal extension or perineural spread. PET scanning is utilized in the staging and posttreatment surveillance of head and neck cancer, with particular utility in the detection of distant metastasis. In a selection of published surgical series of SCC of the EAC and temporal bone where the presence or absence of regional metastasis was reported, metastatic rates range from 0% to 22% [72–78], with a cumulative rate of 7.5% (22/293 patients). Metastasis of BCC is rarely reported, in keeping with the known behavior of this tumor type at other locations [79]. Distant metastasis of BCC or SCC also appears to be very rare. Given this pattern of tumor behavior, PET scanning or other cross-sectional imaging of the chest, abdomen, or pelvis is not typically pursued in the staging of epithelial malignancies of the EAC.

Staging

There is no universally accepted specific staging system for malignancies of the external auditory canal and temporal bone. The AJCC or UICC TNM classifications include language that upstages tumors that invade bone or the skull base. However, the anatomical complexities of the temporal bone make this level of detail inadequate for accurate risk stratification. The rarity of EAC malignancies impedes the development of staging systems based on high-level evidence, but multiple systems have been proposed. This proliferation of multiple staging systems often makes it difficult to pool published data into any meaningful meta-analysis or comparison between treatment strategies.

Many single-institution patient series with a variety of tumor types have been published, accompanied by unique staging systems, three of which are summarized in Tables 67.4, 67.5, and 67.6 [2, 80–84]. Some systems have been externally validated to a degree by use in a handful of published case series. Common features of these systems include increasing stage with medial invasion, extent beyond the temporal bone, intracranial invasion, and metastasis. Absolute tumor size is generally not factored into staging.

Table 67.4 Staging system proposed by Stell and McCormack [84]

T1	Tumor limited to the site of origin, that is with no facial nerve paralysis and no bone destruction
T2	Tumor extending beyond the site of origin indicated by facial paralysis or radiological evidence of bone destruction, but no extension beyond the organ of origin
T3	Clinical or radiological evidence of extension to surrounding structures (dura, base of the skull, parotid gland, temporomandibular joint, etc.)
TX	Patients with insufficient data for classification, including patients previously seen and treated elsewhere

Table 67.5 University of Cincinnati Grading System for temporal bone tumors [2]

Grade I	Tumor in a single site, <1 cm
Grade II	Tumor in a single site, >1 cm
Grade III	Transannular tumor extension
Grade IV	Mastoid or petrous air-cell invasion
Grade V	Periauricular or contiguous extension (extratemporal)
Grade VI	Neck adenopathy, distant anatomic site, or infratemporal fossa extension

Table 67.6 Staging system as proposed by Manolidis et al. [83]

Stage 1	Disease confined to the external auditory canal, including spread from auricular cancer.
Stage 2	Disease spread from the external auditory canal to one or more of the following: 1. Temporomandibular joint 2. Parotid 3. Infratemporal fossa
Stage 3	Disease spread from the external auditory canal to one or more of the following: 1. Middle ear 2. Mastoid 3. Facial nerve and fallopian canal
Stage 4	Disease spread to any one or more of the following: 1. Dura 2. Jugular bulb, sigmoid sinus 3. Carotid artery 4. Petrous apex extension

In 1990, Arriaga and colleagues first published the experience at the University of Pittsburgh in the staging and management of SCC of the external auditory meatus and canal [71]. Clinical staging utilizes preoperative CT scanning, which has been shown to correlate with histopathologic examinations [85]. This system follows a TNM format and was slightly modified in 2000 (Table 67.7) [73]. This has become the most widely utilized system in reporting results after treatment for temporal bone squamous cell carcinoma. As with all of the aforementioned staging systems, its validity in the staging of malignancies of other histologic types has not been thoroughly evaluated.

Table 67.7 Pittsburgh staging system for squamous cell carcinoma of the external auditory canal (2000) [73]

T stage			
T1—Limited to the EAC without bony erosion or evidence of soft tissue involvement			
T2—Limited to the EAC with bone erosion (not full thickness) or limited soft tissue involvement (<0.5 cm)			
T3—Erosion through the osseous EAC (full thickness) with limited (<0.5 cm) soft tissue involvement, or tumor involvement in the middle ear and/or mastoid			
T4—Erosion of the cochlea, petrous apex, medial wall of the middle ear, carotid canal, jugular foramen, or dura, or with extensive soft tissue involvement (>0.5 cm), such as involvement of the TMJ or styloid process, or evidence of facial paresis			
N stage			
N0—No regional nodes involved			
N1—Single metastatic regional node <3 cm in size			
N2a—Single ipsilateral node 3–6 cm in size			
N2b—Multiple ipsilateral metastatic lymph nodes			
N2c—Contralateral metastatic lymph node			
N3—Metastatic lymph node >6 cm in size			
M stage			
M0—No distant metastasis present			
M1—Distant metastasis present			
Stage I	T1	N0	M0
Stage II	T2	N0	M0
Stage III	T3 T1	N0 N1	M0 M0
Stage IV	T4 T2, T3, T4 any T any T	N0 N+ N2, N3 any N	M0 M0 M0 M1

Treatment for Malignancies of the External Auditory Canal

The rarity of ear canal malignancy has precluded the development of a treatment algorithm based on high-level evidence. The majority of the published data reviews the treatment of SCC, which is by far the most common EAC cancer (Table 67.8). There are several treatment paradigms that have evolved out of single-institution experiences, and the majority focus on surgery as the mainstay of therapy. The variability in location, extent, and invasiveness of malignancies involving EAC makes all modalities of anticancer therapy potentially viable. Chemoradiation therapy, primary radiotherapy, or palliative therapy may be considered for patients with significant medical comorbidities, tumors deemed unresectable (brain or internal carotid involvement), or distant metastasis.

Table 67.8 Malignancies of the temporal bone

Type	Number (%)
Epidermal	788 (80%)
Squamous cell carcinoma	640 (65%)
Basal cell carcinoma	132 (13%)
Malignant melanoma	16 (1.6%)
Glandular	132 (13%)
Adenoid cystic carcinoma	69 (7.0%)
Adenocarcinoma	36 (3.7%)
Other	27 (2.8%)
Sarcoma	29 (3%)
Rhabdomyosarcoma	9 (0.9%)
Other	20 (2.0%)
Other malignancies	32 (3.3%)
Total	981

Data compiled from Ref. [29] single institution studies of all temporal bone malignancies

Nonsurgical Treatment

Primary radiation therapy has been associated with limited success in curing ear canal and temporal bone malignancies, with several series demonstrating inferior outcomes for definitive radiation therapy when compared to radiation use in the adjuvant setting [86–88].

Recent years have seen increased use of definitive chemoradiotherapy (CRT) for SCC of the upper aerodigestive tract. Paralleling this trend, small case series reviewing the use of definitive or adjunctive CRT for advanced SCC of the EAC have appeared in the literature. A recent meta-analysis of these data reviewed 37 patients with advanced (estimated Pittsburgh stage T3/T4) disease treated by definitive CRT [89]. The reported 5-year survival was not significantly different from that of a collection of patients with T3/T4 disease who underwent subtotal or total temporal bone resection with or without adjuvant radiation therapy. Various chemotherapy regimens were utilized, including cisplatin, carboplatin, docetaxel, 5-FU, mitomycin, and topical bleomycin. In sum, the role of chemotherapy in the treatment of advanced SCC of the EAC is not established, but the authors suggest that definitive CRT may be a viable option.

Surgery for EAC Malignancies

Extent of Resection

The goal of surgery is complete tumor resection with functional preservation of structures not invaded or threatened by the cancer, if possible. Positive surgical margins have been associated with inferior disease-free and overall survival rates in advanced EAC malignancies [73, 90]. It follows, then, that the extent of surgery should be tailored to the extent of the tumor. Surgical strategies have been proposed based on several retrospective case series, but many controversies exist. It is unlikely that there will be clinical trials or higher-level evidence to clearly demonstrate a best treatment strategy in the near future. Decision-making ultimately relies on a thoughtful multidisciplinary evaluation and application of the available published data.

Lateral temporal bone resection (LTBR) is advocated by most surgeons for tumors that extend medial to the bony cartilaginous junction. Tumor extension into the middle ear (transannular carcinoma) and beyond may be managed by attempts at en bloc or piecemeal resection. Once the tumor extends beyond the confines of the external auditory canal, there is less of a physical barrier to impede its further growth. Several case series have demonstrated transannular spread (i.e., Pittsburgh T1/T2 vs. T3/T4 tumors) to be a negative prognostic factor in disease-free and overall survival [3, 73, 76]. The tumor may spread into the middle ear, mastoid, inner ear, facial nerve, parotid gland, temporomandibular joint, infratemporal fossa, and intracranial space [91]. For this reason, careful preoperative review of imaging studies is mandatory for developing a comprehensive surgical plan that is adaptable to intraoperative findings.

Tumors limited to the EAC can be resected en bloc without significant additional morbidity over a piecemeal resection, though this is not the case for more extensive tumors. Lewis described an en bloc subtotal temporal bone resection in 1983 [92], and Graham and colleagues first reported on the total en bloc temporal bone resection with lower cranial nerve and internal carotid artery sacrifice in 1984 [93]. Long-term survival data to demonstrate superiority or inferiority of these en bloc procedures compared to piecemeal techniques have never surfaced. In 1987, Kinney and Wood advocated an approach to advanced tumors that began with LTBR and removed the more medial portions of the tumor in a piecemeal fashion with preservation of the carotid artery, reporting a 72% (5/7 patients) overall survival rate at an undefined time period for tumors with "limited" extent beyond the EAC and 45% (5/11 patients) survival for those with "extensive" disease [80]. Most of the larger series published since then have utilized some permutation of this approach [2, 3, 73, 81, 94].

Facial weakness in the setting of temporal bone carcinoma imparts a grave prognosis regardless of management strategy [95]. Nevertheless, if invasion is evident clinically or intraoperatively, segmental nerve resection to negative margins is indicated. However, there is no evidence to support the sacrifice of an intact facial nerve in cases of tumor spread to the middle ear or mastoid. Survival is similarly dismal for patients with carotid canal involvement. Given the significant potential morbidity with carotid sacrifice and the unproven survival benefit trade-off, experienced surgeons tend to view these tumors as inoperable or elect to radiate the component involving the carotid [96, 97].

Surgical Techniques

Sleeve Resection

Relatively small tumors confined to the cartilaginous outer third of the EAC can be managed by sleeve resection, which refers to a wide local excision of the tumor, optionally excising the underlying cartilage. The area can be reconstructed with a split-thickness skin graft or left to heal by secondary intention. The term is also used to describe the removal of the skin overlying the bony ear canal and potentially the tympanic membrane, but we do not advocate its use in this fashion for malignant lesions. Zhang et al. reported a high rate of margin positivity and recurrence using sleeve resection for Pittsburgh T1 or T2 malignancies when compared to patients who underwent LTBR and superficial parotidectomy [98].

Lateral Temporal Bone Resection

First described by Conley and Novak in 1960, lateral temporal bone resection refers to the removal of the entire external auditory canal, tympanic membrane, malleus, and incus, typically in an en bloc fashion (Fig. 67.1) [99]. A large postauricular incision, with anterior reflection of the auricle after transecting the external auditory meatus lateral to the tumor, is often utilized. An additional option is a preauricular incision that extends into the temporal scalp and bifurcates around the meatus. This is carried around the lobule to be incorporated into a modified Blair parotidectomy incision that can extend into the neck. Finally, tumors that involve significant portions of the pinna and periauricular skin will mandate a large excision defect, from which extensions can provide adequate access to the temporal bone.

A wide cortical mastoidectomy with an extended facial recess approach is performed. The incudostapedial joint is divided. The mastoid tip may be removed. To remove the specimen en bloc, bony corridors must be created between the ear canal and the surrounding temporal bone. The first of these passes superior to the ear canal, lateral to the epitympanum, and inferior to the middle fossa floor until the glenoid fossa is reached. The second passes inferior to the ear canal, lateral to the facial nerve, jugular bulb, and carotid artery, and through the tympanic bone until the glenoid fossa and parotid fascia are encountered. The extended facial recess approach comprises the posterior portion of the medial bony dissection. The remaining osseous attachment is the anterior wall of the middle ear. This is either divided with an osteotome or fractured by applying anterior pressure. Care must be taken to ensure that all keratinizing epithelium is removed if the fracture occurs lateral to the annulus. The ear canal specimen is now free of all osseous attachments and can be either dissected from its soft tissue attachments to the parotid gland and temporomandibular joint capsule or kept attached to these structures for an en bloc removal of more extensive tumors.

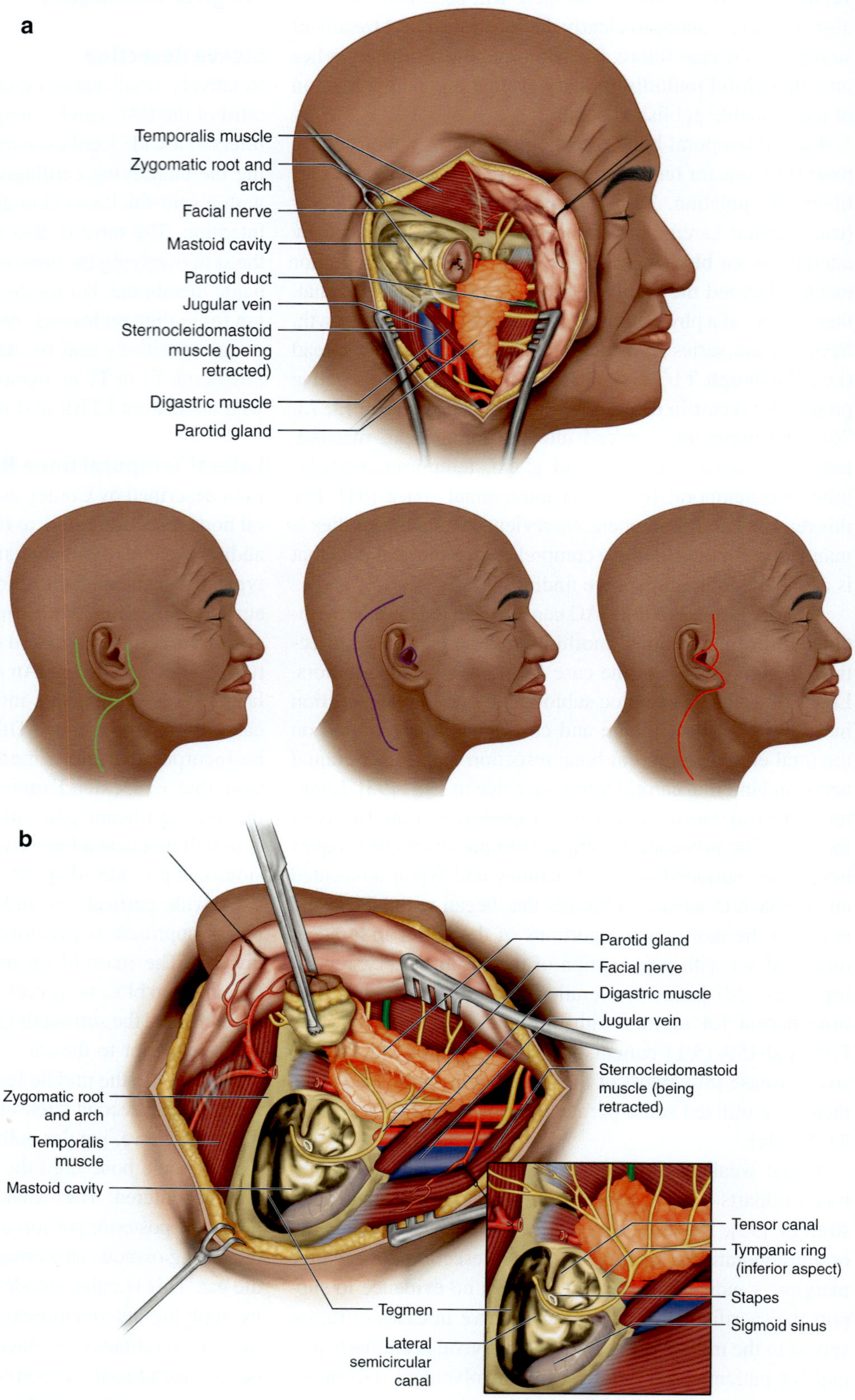

Fig. 67.1 Lateral temporal bone resection: (**a**) Anterior and posterior flaps are developed to expose the mastoid, parotid gland, and facial nerve at the stylomastoid foramen after initial exposure and mastoidectomy. A variety of different incisions can be used to perform a lateral temporal bone resection, depending on case-specific circumstances, and 3 different examples are shown here. (**b**) Surgical view at a point where the external auditory canal and tympanic membrane have been mobilized en bloc with the superficial parotid gland, and at a subsequent point when these mobilized structures have been removed. (Adapted from Glasscock and Shambaugh's *Surgery of the Ear*. 6th Ed. Eds. Gulya, Minor, Poe. PMPH. 2010)

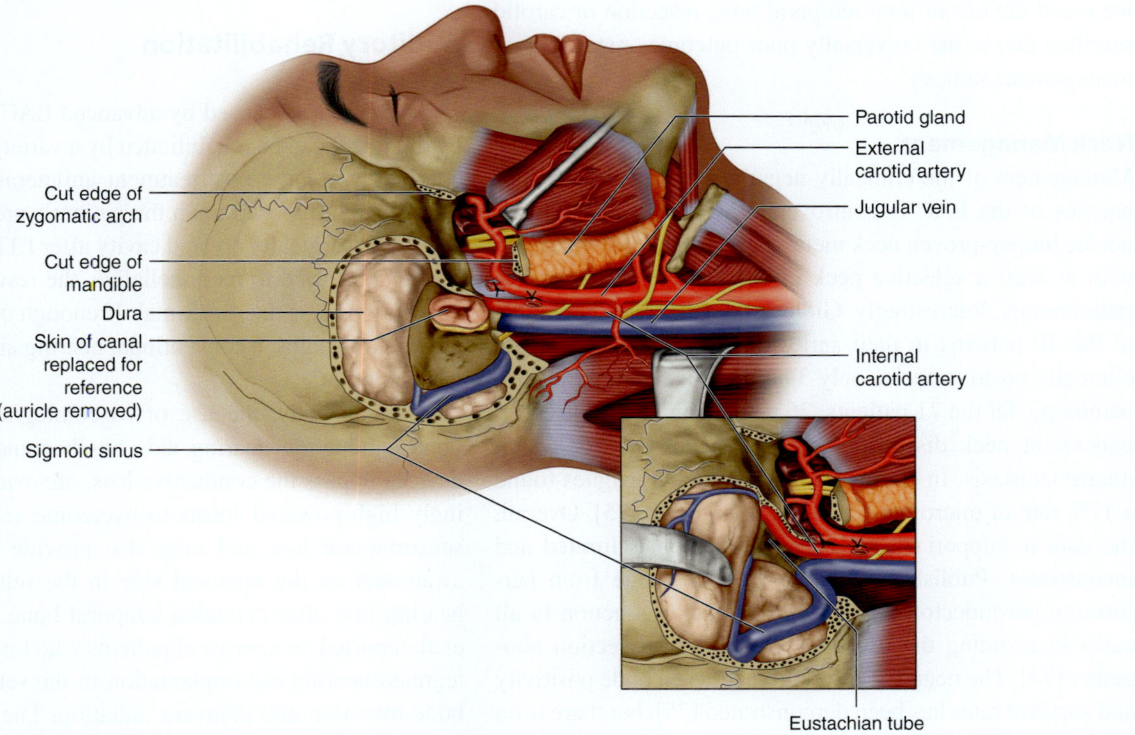

Fig. 67.2 Subtotal temporal bone resection: In the larger illustration, the major neurovascular structures of the neck have been identified. The ascending ramus of the mandible is removed, and a subtotal parotidectomy with facial nerve sacrifice has been performed. The common carotid artery is isolated, and the branches of the external carotid artery are sacrificed. The posterior and middle fossa dura are exposed, though the posterior and middle fossa bone plates are still present, as is the ear canal specimen. In the smaller illustration, the middle fossa and posterior fossa bone plates, as well as the ear canal, have been largely removed. The internal carotid artery has been exposed throughout its intratemporal course. The Eustachian tube will subsequently be obliterated. (Adapted from Glasscock and Shambaugh's *Surgery of the Ear*. 6th Ed. Eds. Gulya, Minor, Poe. PMPH. 2010)

Modified Lateral Temporal Bone Resection

For tumors that extend into the middle or inner ear, the resection can then be extended medially for piecemeal removal. The otic capsule bone is dense and likely more resistant to tumor invasion than surrounding structures. We would not advocate removal of the cochlea or labyrinth for tumors extending to the middle ear without gross bony invasion. Medial margins can be dependent on the functional consequence of additional bone removal. For example, a tumor invading into the cochlea and grossly invading the facial nerve calls for a segmental nerve resection to microscopically negative margins and drilling away the cochlea and bony labyrinth, as no additional morbidity is imparted by removing the remainder of the compromised and nonfunctional inner ear. Posterior petrosectomy or skeletonization of the temporal lobe dura can be done to further extend the bony margins.

Subtotal Temporal Bone Resection

Traditionally, subtotal temporal bone resection entails an en bloc removal of the temporal bone lateral to the carotid artery (Fig. 67.2). To achieve this, a temporal craniotomy and neck exposure for division of additional muscular attachments and control of the great vessels are added to the postauricular and canal incisions as previously described. The internal auditory canal (IAC) is identified from above, and its contents are divided. The tegmen, sigmoid sinus, and posterior fossa dura anterior to the sigmoid sinus are all skeletonized, circumscribing the temporal bone contents. The Eustachian tube and facial nerve at the stylomastoid foramen are divided. The remaining bony attachment along the vertical face of the internal carotid artery is divided with a combination of drilling, osteotomes, and gentle rocking.

Total Temporal Bone Resection

The total en bloc resection of the temporal bone, including sacrifice of the internal carotid artery, was first described by Graham et al. in 1984 [93]. As the procedure mandates unilateral sacrifice of cranial nerves VII through XI and introduces risk for major cerebrovascular events with internal carotid artery and jugular vein ligation, the imparted morbidity can be extreme. The procedure can also be completed in a piecemeal fashion as an extension of the previously described modified LTBR. At the University of Cincinnati, we avoid the use of total temporal bone resection or carotid sacrifice due to the universally poor outcomes regardless of management strategy.

Neck Management

Management of the clinically negative (N0) neck in malignancies of the EAC is controversial. Clinically positive or needle biopsy-proven neck metastases are typically managed with at least a selective neck dissection and postoperative radiotherapy. Interestingly, Gidley and colleagues noted that of the 10 patients in their series of SCC of the EAC with clinically positive necks, only 3 had positive nodes on histopathology. Of the 71 patients, 26 patients in that same series underwent neck dissection, with no occurrence of occult micrometastasis. In contrast, Mazzoni and colleagues found a 17% rate of micrometastasis in the N0 neck [75]. Overall, the data to support elective neck dissection is limited and inconsistent. Published recommendations range from performing parotidectomy and selective neck dissection in all cases to avoiding the use of elective neck dissection altogether [74]. The negative correlation between node positivity and survival rates has been demonstrated [75], but there is no published evidence that elective neck dissection is associated with superior outcomes. If neck status can drive decisions to recommend adjuvant therapy, there may be utility in performing the procedure as a staging exercise. Finally, if free tissue transfer is utilized for reconstruction, the additional morbidity of node removal when the neck is being dissected for access to vessels may be minimal.

Adjuvant Treatment

For advanced SCC of the EAC and temporal bone, the use of adjuvant radiation has been recommended by many investigators [2, 3, 74, 100], with evidence supporting its use for tumors at Pittsburgh stage T2 and above [3, 73]. The presence of adverse features, such as perineural invasion, positive margins, or nodal metastasis, will also strengthen the case for adjuvant therapy.

Stereotactic radiosurgery has not been thoroughly studied in the treatment of cutaneous EAC and temporal bone malignancies. Potential indications for its use include microscopically positive intracranial or skull base margins (particularly with perineural spread along cranial nerves) or unresectable recurrence in the setting of prior multimodality therapy.

As previously discussed in the management of advanced malignancies of the pinna, adjuvant chemotherapy for EAC cancer is reserved for the highest-risk disease. It has been utilized for patients with residual disease, T4 tumors, and distant metastases. Typically, platinum-based therapies are used for SCC and BCC, with the emerging option of vismodegib being a consideration for advanced BCC. There is no evidence to date demonstrating the efficacy of adjuvant chemotherapy in improving survival.

Auditory Rehabilitation

The hearing loss caused by advanced EAC malignancies or by treatment can be rehabilitated by a variety of means. Most commonly, a large posttreatment unilateral conductive loss will be superimposed upon the patient's pre-treatment hearing. If the surgically created cavity after LTBR is not obliterated and allowed to reepithelialize, the resultant conductive loss may be less than maximal. If enough of the structure of the pinna remains, a conventional hearing aid might be a feasible solution.

More recently, the use of osseointegrated implants for bone conduction hearing aids has become popular. These devices bypass the conductive loss, are available in increasingly high-powered forms to overcome various degrees of sensorineural loss and may also provide enhanced sound awareness on the operated side in the setting of complete hearing loss after extended temporal bone resection. Nader et al. reported on a series of patients who underwent osseointegrated hearing aid implantation in the setting of temporal bone resection and adjuvant radiation. The rate of implant-related complications (typically local skin reactions) was higher than that of a non-irradiated cohort overall. However, no adverse outcomes were noted in patients who were implanted at the time of tumor resection and then underwent adjuvant radiation, with second-stage abutment placement typically performed 6 months later [101].

Outcomes

Survival rates for cutaneous malignancies of the EAC and temporal bone have improved modestly over time, potentially owing to refinements in surgical technique and application of adjuvant therapy. The previously discussed evolution in staging systems makes it difficult to compare outcomes reported over time, but the improvements in overall survival could also be partially related to tumor diagnosis at earlier stages, when survival rates are clearly better. These outcomes are summarized in Table 67.9 [3, 72–74, 76, 77, 86, 102–105].

Future Considerations

Immunotherapy has become a promising treatment consideration for advanced cutaneous squamous cell carcinomas of the head and neck [106]. A number of different immunotherapeutic drugs have been investigated, and evidence suggests that there may be some role for their use as salvage or neoadjuvant agents [107, 108]. Specifically, in the realm of temporal bone cancer, hope is emerging that immunotherapy

Table 67.9 Selection of published survival rates for malignancies of the EAC and temporal bone

					Overall survival (%)									
					Stage I		Stage II		Stage III		Stage IV		Combined	
Author	Year	*n*	Pathology	Treatment modalities	2 y	5 y	2 y	5 y	2 y	5 y	2 y	5 y	2 y	5 y
Austin	1994	22	SCC	S, RT, S + RT		66	100[a]		50[a]		50[a]		64[a]	
Testa	1997	79	SCC, BCC, AC	S, S + RT, RT		100		77		45		16		52
Zhang	1999	33	SCC	S, S + RT, RT	100[b]	100[b]	100[b]	100[b]	83	69	46	20	70	41
Pfreundner	1999	27	SCC, ACC, MEC, S	S, S + RT	100[b]	86[a]	100[b]	86[b]	100	50	50	41	78	61
Moody	2000	32	SCC	S, S + RT	100		80		50		7		47	
Duro	2007	34	SCC, BCC, ACC, AC, MM	S, S + RT, PC		87[b]		87[b]		21[c]		21[c]		49
Moore	2007	35	SCC, BCC, ACC, AC	S, S + RT	100[b]	100[b]	100[b]	100[b]	67[c]	54[c]	67[c]	54[c]		77
Bibas	2008	17	SCC	S, S + RT, CRT			100	100	40[c]	40[c]	40[c]	40[c]	53	47
Kunst	2008	28	SCC	S, S + RT	85[b]	85[b]	85[b]	85[b]	64[c]	46[c]	64[c]	46[c]	75	64
Gidley	2010	71	SCC	S, S + RT, S + CRT, RT, CRT, PC	84	66	54	27	42[c]	28[c]	42[c]	28[c]	56	38
Chi	2011	72	SCC	S, S + RT	100	100	100	67	58	21	43	14	61	36

Stage-specific survival is reported for studies adhering to the Pittsburgh staging systems as outlined by Arriaga et al. or Moody et al. [71, 73]
S surgery, *RT* radiation therapy, *CRT* Chemoradiation therapy, *PC* palliative care, *SCC* squamous cell carcinoma, *BCC* basal cell carcinoma, *AC* adenocarcinoma, *ACC* adenoid cystic carcinoma, *S* sarcomas (chondrosarcoma, adenocarcinoma, rhabdomyosarcoma, spindle cell sarcoma, angiosarcoma), *MM* malignant melanoma, *MEC* mucoepidermoid carcinoma
[a]A 3-year survival was reported
[b]Stage I and Stage II reported in aggregate
[c]Stage III and Stage IV reported in aggregate

may be able to reduce the need for potentially disfiguring surgery [109].

Summary

Cutaneous malignancies in humans are very common but present many unique challenges when they involve the pinna or external auditory canal. The tumor type, location, and inherent features have a far more significant impact on outcomes than most treatment decisions. Early-stage disease tends to be curable with surgery alone, but involvement of the ear is a high-risk feature in and of itself, often prompting aggressive multimodality therapy. As evaluation and treatment paradigms become more uniform, data regarding rare tumors will hopefully lead to a clearer picture of ideal management strategies and better outcomes.

References

1. Soyer HP, Rigel DS, Wurm EM. Actinic keratosis, basal cell carcinoma and squamous cell carcinoma. In: Bolognia J, Jorizzo JL, Schaffer JV, editors. Dermatology. 3rd ed. Elsevier; 2012. p. 1773–93.
2. Pensak ML, Gleich LL, Gluckman JL, Shumrick KA. Temporal bone carcinoma: contemporary perspectives in the skull base surgical era. Laryngoscope. 1996;106(10):1234–7.
3. Gidley PW, Roberts DB, Sturgis EM. Squamous cell carcinoma of the temporal bone. Laryngoscope. 2010;120(6):1144–51.
4. Gulya AJ. Anatomy of the temporal bone with surgical implications. 3rd ed. CRC Press; 2007.
5. Rogers HW, Weinstock MA, Feldman SR, Coldiron BM. Incidence estimate of nonmelanoma skin cancer (keratinocyte carcinomas) in the US population, 2012. JAMA Dermatol. 2015;151(10):1081–6.
6. Roewert-Huber J, Lange-Asschenfeldt B, Stockfleth E, Kerl H. Epidemiology and aetiology of basal cell carcinoma. Br J Dermatol. 2007;157(Suppl. 1):47–51.
7. Sánchez G, Nova J, Rodriguez-Hernandez AE, et al. Sun protection for preventing basal cell and squamous cell skin cancers. Cochrane Database Syst Rev. 2016;7:CD011161.
8. Franceschi S, Levi F, Randimbison L, La Vecchia C. Site distribution of different types of skin cancer: new aetiological clues. Int J Cancer. 1996;67(1):24–8.
9. Silva JJ, Tsang RW, Panzarella T, Levin W, Wells W. Results of radiotherapy for epithelial skin cancer of the pinna: the Princess

Margaret Hospital experience, 1982-1993. Int J Radiat Oncol Biol Phys. 2000;47(2):451–9.
10. Jahn V, Breuninger H, Garbe C, Moehrle M. Melanoma of the ear: prognostic factors and surgical strategies. Br J Dermatol. 2006;154(2):310–8.
11. Jones TS, Jones EL, Gao D, Pearlman NW, Robinson WA, McCarter M. Management of external ear melanoma: the same or something different? Am J Surg. 2013;206(3):307–13.
12. Byers RM, Smith JL, Russell N, Rosenberg V. Malignant melanoma of the external ear. Review of 102 cases. Am J Surg. 1980;140(4):518–21.
13. Mounessa J, Qin R, Dunnick CA, Dellavalle RP. Chemoprevention of keratinocyte carcinomas: an updated review. Am J Clin Dermatol. 2016;17(5):475–84.
14. Corona R, Dogliotti E, D'Errico M, et al. Risk factors for basal cell carcinoma in a Mediterranean population: role of recreational sun exposure early in life. Arch Dermatol. 2001;137(9):1162–8.
15. American Cancer Society. Basal and squamous cell skin cancer risk factors. https://www.cancer.org/cancer/basal-and-squamous-cell-skin-cancer/causes-risks-prevention/risk-factors.html. Published May 10, 2016. Accessed 26 Apr 2017.
16. Moloney FJ, Comber H, O'Lorcain P, O'Kelly P, Conlon PJ, Murphy GM. A population-based study of skin cancer incidence and prevalence in renal transplant recipients. Br J Dermatol. 2006;154(3):498–504.
17. Manyam BV, Gastman B, Zhang AY, et al. Inferior outcomes in immunosuppressed patients with high-risk cutaneous squamous cell carcinoma of the head and neck treated with surgery and radiation therapy. J Am Acad Dermatol. 2015;73(2):221–7.
18. Martinez J-C, Otley CC, Stasko T, et al. Defining the clinical course of metastatic skin cancer in organ transplant recipients: a multicenter collaborative study. Arch Dermatol. 2003;139(3):301–6.
19. PhD LW, BA SJ, BS KAMP, MD BCL, MD JC. Skin cancer in organ transplant recipients: more than the immune system. J Am Dermatol. 2014;71(2):359–65.
20. Jackson CG, Glasscock ME, Hughes G, Sismanis A. Facial paralysis of neoplastic origin: diagnosis and management. Laryngoscope. 1980;90(10 Pt 1):1581–95.
21. Ratushny V, Gober MD, Hick R, Ridky TW, Seykora JT. From keratinocyte to cancer: the pathogenesis and modeling of cutaneous squamous cell carcinoma. J Clin Invest. 2012;122(2):464–72.
22. Brodland DG. Diagnosis of nonmelanoma skin cancer. Clin Dermatol. 1995;13(6):551–7.
23. Spurgeon ME, Lambert PF. Merkel cell polyomavirus: a newly discovered human virus with oncogenic potential. Virology. 2013;435(1):118–30.
24. Heath M, Jaimes N, Lemos B, et al. Clinical characteristics of Merkel cell carcinoma at diagnosis in 195 patients: the AEIOU features. J Am Acad Dermatol. 2008;58:375–81.
25. Jan J-C, Wang C-P, Kwan P-C, Wu S-H, Shu H-F. Ceruminous adenocarcinoma with extensive parotid, cervical, and distant metastases: case report and review of literature. Arch Otolaryngol Head Neck Surg. 2008;134(6):663–6.
26. Devaney KO, Boschman CR, Willard SC, Ferlito A, Rinaldo A. Tumours of the external ear and temporal bone. Lancet Oncol. 2005;6(6):411–20.
27. Swick BL, Baum CL, Venkat AP, Liu V. Indolent CD8+ lymphoid proliferation of the ear: report of two cases and review of the literature. J Cutan Pathol. 2011;38(2):209–15.
28. Olsen EA. Evaluation, diagnosis, and staging of cutaneous lymphoma. Dermatol Clin. 2015;33(4):643–54.
29. Elston DM, Stratman EJ, Miller SJ. Skin biopsy: biopsy issues in specific diseases. J Am Acad Dermatol. 2016;74(1):1–16; quiz17–8.
30. Humphreys TR, Shah K, Wysong A, Lexa F, MacFarlane D. The role of imaging in the management of patients with nonmelanoma skin cancer: when is imaging necessary? J Am Acad Dermatol. 2017;76(4):591–607.
31. Brierley JD, Gospodarowicz MK, Wittekind C. TNM classification of malignant tumours. Wiley; 2016.
32. Raasch B. Management of superficial basal cell carcinoma: focus on imiquimod. Clin Cosmet Investig Dermatol. 2009;2:65–75.
33. Bahner JD, Bordeaux JS. Non-melanoma skin cancers: photodynamic therapy, cryotherapy, 5-fluorouracil, imiquimod, diclofenac, or what? Facts and controversies. Clin Dermatol. 2013;31(6):792–8.
34. Kuflik EG, Gage AA. The five-year cure rate achieved by cryosurgery for skin cancer. J Am Dermatol. 1991;24(6 Pt 1):1002–4.
35. Chren M-M, Linos E, Torres JS, Stuart SE, Parvataneni R, Boscardin WJ. Tumor recurrence 5 years after treatment of cutaneous basal cell carcinoma and squamous cell carcinoma. J Invest Dermatol. 2013;133(5):1188–96.
36. Galles E, Parvataneni R, Stuart SE, Linos E, Grewal S, Chren M-M. Patient-reported outcomes of electrodessication and curettage for treatment of nonmelanoma skin cancer. J Am Acad Dermatol. 2014;71(5):1026–8.
37. Stratigos A, Garbe C, Lebbe C, et al. Diagnosis and treatment of invasive squamous cell carcinoma of the skin: European consensus-based interdisciplinary guideline. Eur J Cancer. 2015;51(14):1989–2007.
38. Bumsted RM, Ceilley RI, Panje WR, Crumley RL. Auricular malignant neoplasms. When is chemotherapy (Mohs' technique) necessary? Arch Otolaryngol. 1981;107(11):721–4.
39. Luz FB, Ferron C, Cardoso GP. Surgical treatment of basal cell carcinoma: an algorithm based on the literature. An Bras Dermatol. 2015;90(3):377–83.
40. Mohs F, Larson P, Iriondo M. Micrographic surgery for the microscopically controlled excision of carcinoma of the external ear. J Am Acad Dermatol. 1988;19(4):729–37.
41. Silapunt S, Peterson SR, Goldberg LH. Squamous cell carcinoma of the auricle and Mohs micrographic surgery. Dermatologic Surg. 2005;31(11 Pt 1):1423–7.
42. Niparko JK, Swanson NA, Baker SR, Telian SA, Sullivan MJ, Kemink JL. Local control of auricular, periauricular, and external canal cutaneous malignancies with Mohs surgery. Laryngoscope. 1990;100(10 Pt 1):1047–51.
43. Rowe DE, Carroll RJ, Day CL. Prognostic factors for local recurrence, metastasis, and survival rates in squamous cell carcinoma of the skin, ear, and lip. Implications for treatment modality selection. J Am Dermatol. 1992;26(6):976–90.
44. Cook J, Zitelli JA. Mohs micrographic surgery: a cost analysis. J Am Dermatol. 1998;39(5 Pt 1):698–703.
45. Bricca GM, Brodland DG, Ren D, Zitelli JA. Cutaneous head and neck melanoma treated with Mohs micrographic surgery. J Am Acad Dermatol. 2005;52(1):92–100.
46. Caccialanza M, Piccinno R, Kolesnikova L, Gnecchi L. Radiotherapy of skin carcinomas of the pinna: a study of 115 lesions in 108 patients. Int J Dermatol. 2005;44(6):513–7.
47. Sale KA, Wallace DI, Girod DA, Tsue TT. Radiation-induced malignancy of the head and neck. Otolaryngol Head Neck Surg. 2004;131(5):643–5.
48. Lustig LR, Jackler RK, Lanser MJ. Radiation-induced tumors of the temporal bone. Am J Otol. 1997;18(2):230–5.
49. Mark RJ, Poen J, Tran LM, Fu YS, Selch MT, Parker RG, Postirradiation sarcomas. A single-institution study and review of the literature. Cancer. 1994;73(10):2653–62.
50. Lambert EM, Gunn GB, Gidley PW. Effects of radiation on the temporal bone in patients with head and neck cancer. Eisele DW, ed. Head Neck. 2016;38(9):1428–35.

51. Veness MJ, Porceddu S, Palme CE, Morgan GJ. Cutaneous head and neck squamous cell carcinoma metastatic to parotid and cervical lymph nodes. Head Neck. 2007;29(7):621–31.
52. Lee D, Nash M, Har-El G. Regional spread of auricular and periauricular cutaneous malignancies. Laryngoscope. 1996;106(8):998–1001.
53. Bumpous J. Metastatic cutaneous squamous cell carcinoma to the parotid and cervical lymph nodes: treatment and outcomes. Curr Opin Otolaryngol Head Neck Surg. 2009;17(2):122–5.
54. Brougham NDLS, Dennett ER, Cameron R, Tan ST. The incidence of metastasis from cutaneous squamous cell carcinoma and the impact of its risk factors. J Surg Oncol. 2012;106(7):811–5.
55. Krediet JT, Beyer M, Lenz K, et al. Sentinel lymph node biopsy and risk factors for predicting metastasis in cutaneous squamous cell carcinoma. Br J Dermatol. 2015;172(4):1029–36.
56. Alam M, Ratner D. Cutaneous squamous-cell carcinoma. N Engl J Med. 2001;344(13):975–83.
57. Brunner M, Veness MJ, Ch'ng S, Elliott M, Clark JR. Distant metastases from cutaneous squamous cell carcinoma--analysis of AJCC stage IV. Head Neck. 2013;35(1):72–5.
58. Wysong A, Aasi SZ, Tang JY. Update on metastatic basal cell carcinoma: a summary of published cases from 1981 through 2011. JAMA Dermatol. 2013;149(5):615–6.
59. Martinez J-C, Cook JL. High-risk cutaneous squamous cell carcinoma without palpable lymphadenopathy: is there a therapeutic role for elective neck dissection? Dermatologic Surg. 2007;33(4):410–20.
60. Osborne RF, Shaw T, Zandifar H, Kraus D. Elective parotidectomy in the management of advanced auricular malignancies. Laryngoscope. 2008;118(12):2139–45.
61. Kadakia S, Saman M, Gordin E, Marra D, Ducic Y. The role of parotidectomy in the treatment of auricular squamous cell carcinoma. Otolaryngol Head Neck Surg. 2015;152(6):1048–52.
62. O'Brien CJ, McNeil EB, McMahon JD, Pathak I, Lauer CS. Incidence of cervical node involvement in metastatic cutaneous malignancy involving the parotid gland. Head Neck. 2001;23(9):744–8.
63. Ebrahimi A, Moncrieff MD, Clark JR, et al. Predicting the pattern of regional metastases from cutaneous squamous cell carcinoma of the head and neck based on location of the primary. Head Neck. 2010;32(10):1288–94.
64. Morton DL, Thompson JF, Cochran AJ, et al. Final trial report of sentinel-node biopsy versus nodal observation in melanoma. N Engl J Med. 2014;370(7):599–609.
65. Skulsky SL, O'Sullivan B, McArdle O, et al. Review of high-risk features of cutaneous squamous cell carcinoma and discrepancies between the American Joint Committee on Cancer and NCCN Clinical Practice Guidelines in Oncology. Head Neck. 2017;39(3):578–94.
66. Veness MJ, Morgan GJ, Palme CE, Gebski V. Surgery and adjuvant radiotherapy in patients with cutaneous head and neck squamous cell carcinoma metastatic to lymph nodes: combined treatment should be considered best practice. Laryngoscope. 2005;115(5):870–5.
67. Mendenhall WM, Amdur RJ, Hinerman RW, Cognetta AB, Mendenhall NP. Radiotherapy for cutaneous squamous and basal cell carcinomas of the head and neck. Laryngoscope. 2009;119(10):1994–9.
68. Agha A, Tarhini AA. Adjuvant therapy for melanoma. Curr Oncol Rep. 2017;19(5):36.
69. Mocellin S, Lens MB, Pasquali S, Pilati P, Chiarion Sileni V. Interferon alpha for the adjuvant treatment of cutaneous melanoma. Mocellin S, ed. Cochrane Database Syst Rev. 2013;29(6):CD008955.
70. Mocellin S, Pasquali S, Rossi CR, Nitti D. Interferon alpha adjuvant therapy in patients with high-risk melanoma: a systematic review and meta-analysis. J Natl Cancer Inst. 2010;102(7):493–501.
71. Arriaga M, Curtin H, Takahashi H, Hirsch BE, Kamerer DB. Staging proposal for external auditory meatus carcinoma based on preoperative clinical examination and computed tomography findings. Ann Otol Rhinol Laryngol. 1990;99(9 Pt 1):714–21.
72. Bibas AG, Ward V, Gleeson MJ. Squamous cell carcinoma of the temporal bone. J Laryngol Otol. 2008;122(11):1156–61.
73. Moody SA, Hirsch BE, Myers EN. Squamous cell carcinoma of the external auditory canal: an evaluation of a staging system. Am J Otol. 2000;21(4):582–8.
74. Kunst H, Lavieille J-P, Marres H. Squamous cell carcinoma of the temporal bone. Otol Neurotol. 2008;29(4):549–52.
75. Mazzoni A, Danesi G, Zanoletti E. Primary squamous cell carcinoma of the external auditory canal: surgical treatment and long-term outcomes. Acta Otorhinolaryngol Ital. 2014;34(2):129–37.
76. Chi F-L, Gu F-M, Dai C-F, Chen B, Li H-W. Survival outcomes in surgical treatment of 72 cases of squamous cell carcinoma of the temporal bone. Otol Neurotol. 2011;32(4):665–9.
77. Austin JR, Stewart KL, Fawzi N. Squamous cell carcinoma of the external auditory canal. Therapeutic prognosis based on a proposed staging system. Arch Otolaryngol Head Neck Surg. 1994;120(11):1228–32.
78. Nyrop M, Grøntved A. Cancer of the external auditory canal. Arch Otolaryngol Head Neck Surg. 2002;128(7):834–7.
79. Lo JS, Snow SN, Reizner GT, Mohs FE, Larson PO, Hruza GJ. Metastatic basal cell carcinoma: report of twelve cases with a review of the literature. J Am Dermatol. 1991;24(5 Pt 1):715–9.
80. Kinney SE, Wood BG. Malignancies of the external ear canal and temporal bone: surgical techniques and results. Laryngoscope. 1987;97(2):158–64.
81. Shih L, Crabtree JA. Carcinoma of the external auditory canal: an update. Laryngoscope. 1990;100(11):1215–8.
82. Spector JG. Management of temporal bone carcinomas: a therapeutic analysis of two groups of patients and long-term followup. Otolaryngol Head Neck Surg. 1991;104(1):58–66.
83. Manolidis S, Pappas D, Doersten Von P, Jackson CG, Glasscock ME. Temporal bone and lateral skull base malignancy: experience and results with 81 patients. Am J Otol. 1998;19(6 Suppl):S1–S15.
84. Stell PM, McCormick MS. Carcinoma of the external auditory meatus and middle ear. Prognostic factors and a suggested staging system. J Laryngol Otol. 1985;99(9):847–50.
85. Arriaga M, Curtin HD, Takahashi H, Kamerer DB. The role of preoperative CT scans in staging external auditory meatus carcinoma: radiologic-pathologic correlation study. Otolaryngol Head Neck Surg. 1991;105(1):6–11.
86. Zhang B, Tu G, Xu G, Tang P, Hu Y. Squamous cell carcinoma of temporal bone: reported on 33 patients. Head Neck. 1999;21(5):461–6.
87. Sarkar SK, Rashid MA, Patra NB, Goswami J. Evaluation of results of radiotherapy alone vs combined surgery and post-operative radiotherapy in carcinoma external auditory canal-10 years review. Indian J Otolaryngol Head Neck Surg. 2005;57(4):312–4.
88. Gandhi AK, Roy S, Biswas A, et al. Treatment of squamous cell carcinoma of external auditory canal: a tertiary cancer centre experience. Auris Nasus Larynx. 2016;43(1):45–9.
89. Takenaka Y, Cho H, Nakahara S, Yamamoto Y, Yasui T, Inohara H. Chemoradiation therapy for squamous cell carcinoma of the external auditory canal: a meta-analysis. Eisele DW, ed. Head Neck. 2014;37(7):1073–80.
90. Essig GF, Kitipornchai L, Adams F, et al. Lateral temporal bone resection in advanced cutaneous squamous cell carcinoma: report of 35 patients. J Neurol Surg B Skull Base. 2013;74(1):54–9.
91. Leonetti JP, Smith PG, Kletzker GR, Izquierdo R. Invasion patterns of advanced temporal bone malignancies. Am J Otol. 1996;17(3):438–42.

92. Lewis JS. Surgical management of tumors of the middle ear and mastoid. J Laryngol Otol. 1983;97(4):299–311.
93. Graham MD, Sataloff RT, Kemink JL, Wolf GT, McGillicuddy JE. Total en bloc resection of the temporal bone and carotid artery for malignant tumors of the ear and temporal bone. Laryngoscope. 1984;94(4):528–33.
94. Breau RL, Gardner EK, Dornhoffer JL. Cancer of the external auditory canal and temporal bone. Curr Oncol Rep. 2002;4(1):76–80.
95. Higgins TS, Antonio SAM. The role of facial palsy in staging squamous cell carcinoma of the temporal bone and external auditory canal: a comparative survival analysis. Otol Neurotol. 2010;31(9):1473–9.
96. Gidley PW. Managing malignancies of the external auditory canal. Expert Rev Anticancer Ther. 2009;9(9):1277–82.
97. Barrs DM. Temporal bone carcinoma. Otolaryngol Clin N Am. 2001;34(6):1197–218–x.
98. Zhang T, Li W, Dai C, Chi F, Wang S, Wang Z. Evidence-based surgical management of T1 or T2 temporal bone malignancies. Laryngoscope. 2012;123(1):244–8.
99. Conley JJ, Novack AJ. The surgical treatment of malignant tumors of the ear and temporal bone. Part I. Arch Otolaryngol. 1960;71:635–52.
100. Moffat DA, Wagstaff SA, Hardy DG. The outcome of radical surgery and postoperative radiotherapy for squamous carcinoma of the temporal bone. Laryngoscope. 2005;115(2):341–7.
101. Nader M-E, Beadle BM, Roberts DB, Gidley PW. Outcomes and complications of osseointegrated hearing aids in irradiated temporal bones. Laryngoscope. 2016;126(5):1187–92.
102. Testa JR, Fukuda Y, Kowalski LP. Prognostic factors in carcinoma of the external auditory canal. Arch Otolaryngol Head Neck Surg. 1997;123(7):720–4.
103. Pfreundner L, Schwager K, Willner J, et al. Carcinoma of the external auditory canal and middle ear. Int J Radiat Oncol Biol Phys. 1999;44(4):777–88.
104. Duro DL, Pendás JLL, Nieto CS. Primary tumours of the external auditory canal. Our experience in 34 patients. Acta Otorrinolaringológica Española (English Edition). 2007;58(1):20–4.
105. Moore MG, Deschler DG, Mckenna MJ, Varvares MA, Lin DT. Management outcomes following lateral temporal bone resection for ear and temporal bone malignancies. Otolaryngol Head Neck Surg. 2007;137(6):893–8.
106. Ferrarotto R, Amit M, Nagarajan P, et al. Pilot phase II trial of neoadjuvant immunotherapy in locoregionally advanced, resectable cutaneous squamous cell carcinoma of the head and neck. Clin Cancer Res. 2021;27(16):4557–65.
107. Kim EY, Ruiz ES, DeSimone MS, et al. Neoadjuvant-intent immunotherapy in advanced, resectable cutaneous squamous cell carcinoma. JAMA Otolaryngol Head Neck Surg. 2024;150(5):414–20.
108. Mehta NK, Li AR, Nguyen SA, et al. Immune checkpoint inhibitors for advanced cutaneous squamous cell carcinoma: a systematic review with meta-analysis. Target Oncol. 2021;16(6):743–52.
109. Shi MW, Huang J, Sun Y. Neoadjuvant immunotherapy of head and neck squamous cell carcinoma: expecting its application in temporal bone squamous cell carcinoma. Curr Med Sci. 2023;43(2):213–22.

Supplementary Reading

Allanson BM, Low TH, Clark JR, Gupta R. Squamous cell carcinoma of the external auditory canal and temporal bone: an update. Head Neck Pathol. 2018;12(3):407–18. https://doi.org/10.1007/s12105-018-0908-4. Epub 2018 Aug 1. PMID: 30069837; PMCID: PMC6081282.

Bhardwaj P, Tanenbaum ZG, Nguy PL, Jay AK, Dimopoulos YP, Hoa M. A rare presentation of primary cutaneous low-grade neuroendocrine tumor of the external auditory canal. Otol Neurotol. 2021;42(9):e1353–7. https://doi.org/10.1097/MAO.0000000000003260. PMID: 34224550.

Chan MP, Flack AB, Grisel JJ, Harms PW, McHugh JB. Microsecretory adenocarcinoma of the ear canal: novel cutaneous analog of a salivary gland neoplasm. Am J Dermatopathol. 2022;44(11):855–8. https://doi.org/10.1097/DAD.0000000000002270. Epub 2022 Jul 28. PMID: 35925564.

Schachtel MJC, Gandhi M, Bowman JJ, Porceddu SV, Panizza BJ. Epidemiology and treatment outcomes of cutaneous squamous cell carcinoma extending to the temporal bone. Head Neck. 2022;44(12):2727–43. https://doi.org/10.1002/hed.27185. Epub 2022 Sep 9. PMID: 36082824; PMCID: PMC9826480.

Tympanic and Jugular Paragangliomas

68

Enrique R. Perez, Zachary G. Schwam,
and George B. Wanna

Introduction

Paragangliomas originate in the body's paraganglia, which are naturally occurring nonneuronal structures found in close proximity to sympathetic ganglia as well as to the aorta and its main branches [1]. Paragangliomas have had multiple designations over the years as our understanding has evolved, including non-chromaffin paragangliomas, chemodectomas, glomerocytomas, receptomas, glomus tympanicum, glomus jugulare, and tympanic body tumors [2]. Paragangliomas can be classified as adrenal or extra-adrenal, with the former being named a pheochromocytoma and located within the adrenal medulla. While there are several paraganglia throughout the body, the ones of most interest to the skull base surgeon are the jugulotympanic paraganglia, which give rise to tympanic (also known as glomus tympanicum) and jugular (also known as glomus jugulare) paragangliomas that are now grouped under the JTP umbrella term. Despite the use of this umbrella term, however, it is important to note that tympanic and jugular paragangliomas arise from paraganglion cells in distinct locations within the lateral skull base, and as such, are approached differently from the perspective of staging and management, as discussed later in this chapter. Macroscopically, paraganglia resemble lobulated, ovoid bodies up to 1.5 mm in diameter and are sometimes visible on the promontory. Paragangliomas in this region often appear as highly vascular, encapsulated masses. Both histopathologic and molecular studies have demonstrated expression of angiogenic growth factors such as vascular endothelial growth factor (VEGF) and platelet-derived endothelial cell growth factor (PD-ECGF) [3–5]. Blood supply to the tumor is variable and depends on location and size; consistent sources include the ascending pharyngeal, occipital, external, and internal carotid, and vertebral arteries [6].

Characteristic microscopic features of paragangliomas are clusters of epithelioid chief cells arranged in "Zellballen" (German for "balls of cells") with supporting sustentacular cells. Chief cells are of neural crest origin and are recognized as part of the diffuse neuroendocrine system (DNES), which includes other neuroendocrine cell lines such as the thyroid parafollicular cells and adrenal pheochromocytes [7]. These cellular clusters are intimately associated with webs of small blood vessels, which account for these tumors' hypervascularity [8]. Compared to normal paraganglia tissue, tumors demonstrate a higher ratio of chief to sustentacular cells, resulting in a highly vascular, smaller stromal space. Endothelial cell deficiencies in the vessel walls often lead to the formation of sinusoidal blood spaces [2].

Metabolic Activity of HNPGs

Head and neck paragangliomas (HNPGs) secrete functionally significant catecholamines in only 1–3% of cases, but up to 30% of HNPGs produce dopamine [9–11]. Unlike adrenal medullary tissue, HNPGs lack phenylethanolamine-N-methyl transferase, an enzyme used to convert norepinephrine to epinephrine [12]. Nevertheless, it is good clinical practice to inquire about signs and symptoms of excessive catecholamine secretion, as they can affect perioperative management decisions. If discovered, synchronous lesions (particularly pheochromocytoma) at other high-risk sites must be ruled out [9]. Signs of excessive catecholamine secretion include palpitations, arrhythmia, headaches, excessive perspiration, nausea, and pallor, and usually have norepinephrine levels 3–5 times the upper limit of normal. While there are no clear guidelines as to when to order plasma or urine noremetanephrine and vanillylmandelic acid, it is good practice to acquire such studies when working up HNPGs, particularly in the face of familial or multifocal disease. Biochemical workup should also include plasma methoxytyramine, a dopamine metabolite, even though ele-

E. R. Perez · Z. G. Schwam · G. B. Wanna (✉)
Department of Otolaryngology—Head and Neck Surgery, Icahn School of Medicine at Mount Sinai, New York, NY, USA
e-mail: gwanna@nyee.edu

A. D. Sweeney et al. (eds.), *Haynes-Glasscock-Shambaugh Surgery of the Ear*, https://doi.org/10.1007/978-3-032-18264-7_68

vated levels will not change management. If surgical resection is to be attempted on an epinephrine- or norepinephrine-secreting lesion, the same perioperative protocol for pharmacologic blockade employed in pheochromocytoma surgery is used. We advocate for resection of synchronous, epinephrine- or norepinephrine-secreting lesions prior to addressing the JTP.

Genetics of HNPGs

While often sporadic, HNPG may be due to a germline mutation in up to one-third of patients [13]. Patients with germline mutations tend to be younger at the age of first diagnosis (36.2 years versus 50.2 years), more often have multiple paragangliomas, and are more likely to have malignant lesions [14]. There are four paraganglioma syndromes, which are summarized in Table 68.1. The most important mutations for the otolaryngologist are those in the succinate dehydrogenase subunits B and D (SDHB and SDHD, respectively), which play important roles in the tricarboxylic acid cycle and normal mitochondrial function [13]. Patients with germline mutations in SDHD are known to have multiple HNPGs in addition to lesions elsewhere, while those with SDHB mutations have a much stronger propensity to metastasize; recent data, however, suggest that metastatic risk in SDHB-mutated HNPG is no higher than in sporadic cases [9]. Patients with SDH*x* mutations are also at increased risk of renal cell carcinoma, papillary thyroid cancer, neuroblastoma, and breast cancer [13]. HNPGs are a component of von Hippel–Lindau (VHL) syndrome [15], but this is an exceedingly rare scenario.

Table 68.1 Clinical features of the paraganglioma syndromes and their associated succinyl dehydrogenase subunit mutations

Tumor syndrome	Gene	Inheritance pattern	Defining characteristics	Malignancy rate
PGL1	SDHD	A_D, possible maternal imprinting [13]	91–98% develop HNPG, 60–79% develop multiple HNPG, 16–21% develop pheochromocytoma and extra-adrenal lesions [13]	8% [98]
PGL2	SDHAF2	A_D	70–91% have multiple HNPG without lesions outside the head and neck [99–101]	0% [13]
PGL3	SDHC	A_D	Low tumor penetrance (12–25%). Usually single HNPG, but multiple HNPG 19–31%. Lesions outside the head and neck uncommon [13, 14, 102]	Rare
PGL4	SDHB	A_D	Pheochromocytoma 18–28%, 52–84% extra-adrenal lesions, 27–31% HNPG. Usually solitary lesion [98, 102–106]	13–41%

Abbreviations: A_D Autosomal dominant, *HNPG* head and neck paraganglioma, *PGL* paraganglioma syndrome, *SDH* succinate dehydrogenase

Clinical Presentation

JTPs are slow growing and most commonly present during the fourth or fifth decade of life, afflicting women significantly more than men. Originating from paraganglia on the tympanic plexi of Jacobson's and Arnold's nerves or the adventitia of the jugular bulb, these tumors spread along tracts of least resistance, including mastoid and petrous air cells, neurovascular foramina, and the Eustachian tube [16]. As they grow, JTPs can infiltrate the otic capsule, carotid canal, posterior fossa plate, mastoid, and external auditory canal (EAC). Even the internal auditory canal (IAC) can serve as a route of spread. The most common mode of intracranial extension is via the pars nervosa of the jugular foramen into the cerebellopontine angle [17] (Fig. 68.1).

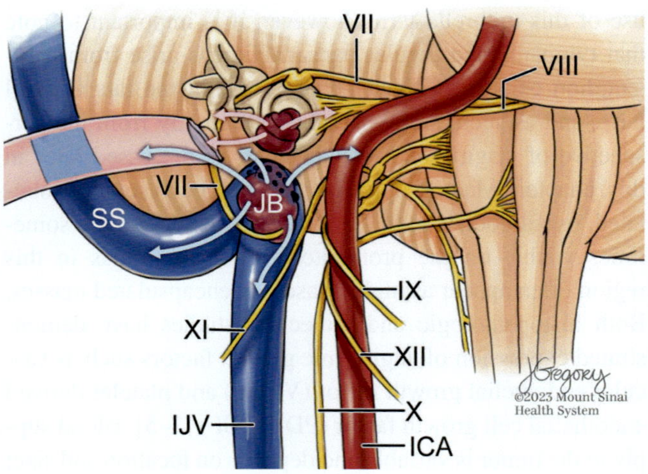

Fig. 68.1 Oblique view of the relevant neurovascular anatomy and routes of spread for tympanic and jugular paragangliomas. Lesions in this area may spread to the middle ear, mastoid, external auditory canal, neck, and into the cerebellopontine angle. (Printed with permission from ©Mount Sinai Health System). Abbreviations: IJV internal jugular vein, JB jugular bulb, SS sigmoid sinus, VII facial nerve, VIII vestibulocochlear nerve, IX glossopharyngeal nerve, X vagus nerve, XI accessory nerve, XII hypoglossal nerve

Using physical and radiologic findings, JTPs can be classified according to the modified Fisch–Mattox [18] (Table 68.2) and Glasscock–Jackson [19] (Table 68.3) stag-

Table 68.2 Modified Fisch-Mattox classification

Class	Definition
A	Tumors confined to the middle ear.
A1	Tumor margins clearly visible on otoscopic examination.
A2	Tumor margins not visible on otoscopy. Tumors may extend anteriorly to the Eustachian tube and/or to the posterior mesotympanum.
B	Tumors confined to the tympanomastoid cavity without destruction of the bone in the infralabyrinthine compartment of the temporal bone.
B1	Tumors involving the middle ear with extension to the hypotympanum.
B2	Tumors involving the middle ear with extension to the hypotympanum and the mastoid.
B3	Tumors confined to the tympanomastoid compartment with erosion of the carotid canal.
C	Tumors extending beyond the tympanomastoid cavity, destroying the bone of the infralabyrinthine and apical compartments of the temporal bone, and involving the carotid canal.
C1	Tumors with limited involvement of the vertical portion of the carotid canal.
C2	Tumors invading the vertical portion of the carotid canal.
C3	Tumors with invasion of the horizontal portion of the carotid canal.
C4	Tumors reaching the anterior foramen lacerum.
D	Tumors with intracranial extension.
De1	Tumors up to 2 cm dural displacement.
De2	Tumors with more than 2 cm dural displacement.
Di1	Tumors up to 2 cm intradural extension.
Di2	Tumors with more than 2 cm intradural extension.
Di3	Tumors with inoperable intradural extension.
V	Tumors involving the vertebral artery.
Ve	Tumors involving the extradural vertebral artery.
Vi	Tumors involving the intradural vertebral artery

Adapted from reference [18]

Table 68.3 Glasscock–Jackson staging system for temporal bone glomus/paraganglioma tumors

Tumor class	Tympanicum/tympanic	Jugulare/jugular
I	Limited to promontory	Involves the jugular bulb, middle ear, and mastoid
II	Completely fills the middle ear cavity	Extends under the internal auditory canal May have intracranial extension
III	Completely fills the middle ear Extends into the mastoid	Extends into the petrous apex May have intracranial extension
IV	Completely fills the middle ear Extends into the mastoid or through the tympanic membrane May involve the carotid artery	Extends into clivus or infratemporal fossa May have intracranial extension

Adapted from reference [19]

ing systems to aid in surgical planning and the standardization of outcomes reporting.

Although often locally aggressive, JTPs are rarely clinically malignant. As there is no consensus on histologic criteria for defining malignancy, these tumors are considered malignant upon demonstration of metastatic foci in locoregional lymph node basins and in other areas of the body not known to normally harbor paraganglial tissue [20]. It is estimated that <4% of JTP are malignant, but metastases to the lymph nodes, liver, lung, skeleton, and spleen have been documented [20, 21]. In contrast to JTPs, nearly 19% of vagal paragangliomas are considered malignant and will often demonstrate functionally significant catecholamine secretion and a more rapidly progressive course [20, 22].

Diagnosis

The most common presenting symptoms of JTPs are pulsatile tinnitus and/or hearing loss. The tumor may encapsulate and erode the ossicular chain or invade the cochlea, causing conductive, sensorineural, or mixed hearing losses. Tumors that have traversed the tympanic membrane and involve the EAC may present with bloody otorrhea. Lower cranial neuropathies involving the glossopharyngeal, vagus, accessory, and hypoglossal nerves may present with dysphagia, dysphonia, aspiration, shoulder weakness, and dysarthria. Facial nerve (FN) palsy is uncommon, and when present, portends a poor outcome. In very advanced cases, brainstem compression and obstructive hydrocephalus are possible [19]. As these tumors are usually slow growing, neurological symptoms may go unnoticed, and patients may compensate over time.

On physical exam, a red, pulsatile EAC or retrotympanic mass is often seen, as in Fig. 68.2 [23, 24]. While the boundaries of a tympanic paraganglioma may be visualized if it is small (as in Fig. 68.3), in the case of jugular paragangliomas, one can often only see the tip of the tumor jutting out into the hypo- and/or mesotympanum (Fig. 68.4). Differentiating tympanic from jugular paragangliomas is only possible with imaging, and it is critical to consider a broad differential diagnosis that includes an aberrant petrous carotid artery, meningioma, (meningo) encephalocele, schwannoma, and hemangioma.

Biopsy of a presumed JTP to confirm a likely diagnosis is not warranted, and in fact, is recommended against. Transcanal biopsy of any of these lesions can lead to significant bleeding and make for a disastrous clinic visit. Furthermore, without appropriate imaging in hand, one risks the rare and catastrophic situation of biopsying an aberrant petrous segment of the internal carotid artery.

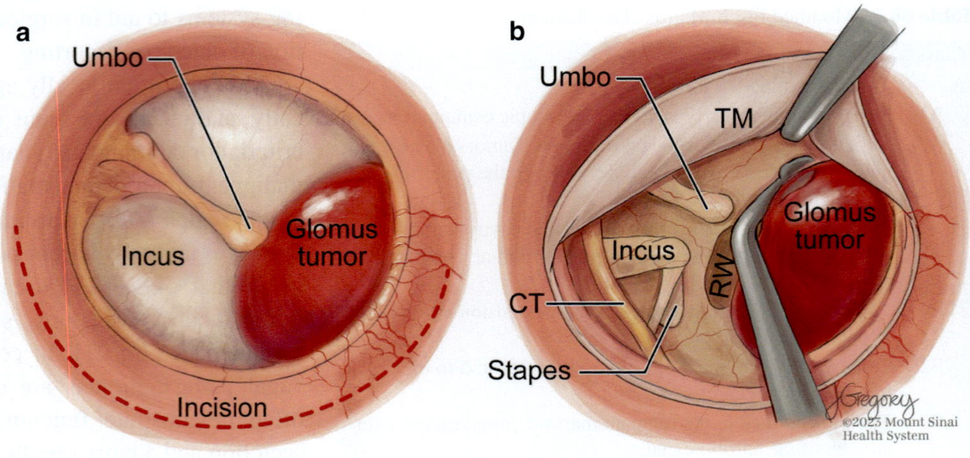

Fig. 68.2 This is a transcanal view of a right ear with a small tympanic paraganglioma centered on the promontory. The dashed line marks the incision, and the tympanomeatal flap is lifted. Once isolated on its pedicle, a right-angled instrument is used to sweep behind it and extract it en bloc. (Printed with permission from ©Mount Sinai Health System). Abbreviations: CT chorda tympani, TM tympanic membrane

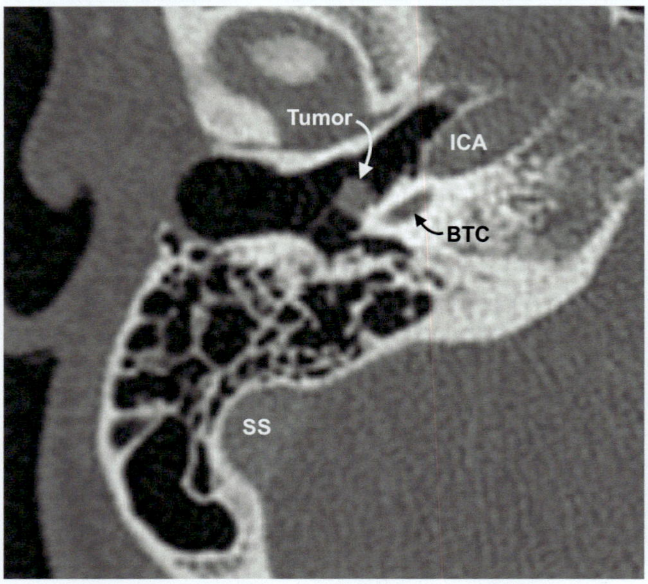

Fig. 68.3 An axial cross section of a right CT temporal bone shows a small tympanic paraganglioma on the cochlear promontory. Such a lesion is readily resectable using a transcanal approach. Abbreviations: BTC basal turn of cochlea, ICA internal carotid artery, SS sigmoid sinus

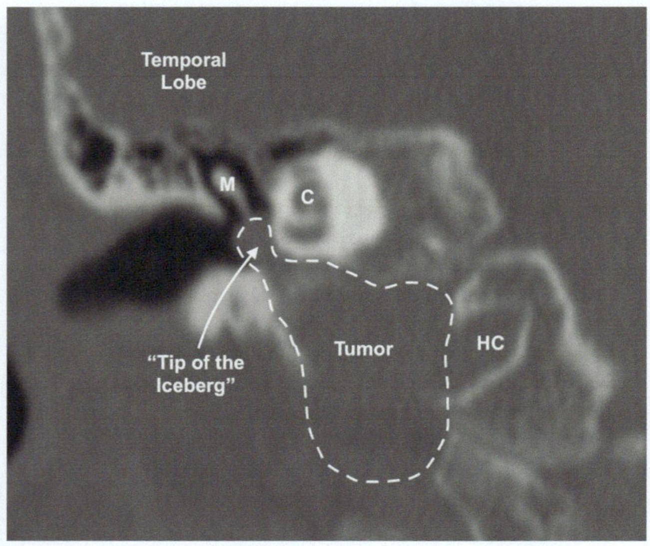

Fig. 68.4 This coronal cross section of a CT temporal bone demonstrates a large tumor in the jugular foramen with a small projection into the hypotympanum; this is the so-called "tip of the iceberg," and all one sees with looking transcanal. Abbreviations: C cochlea, HC hypoglossal canal, M malleus

Imaging

CT of the temporal bone is often one of the first studies ordered after a presumptive diagnosis of JTP. Differentiating a large tympanic paraganglioma from a jugular one is often done by examining the caroticojugular spine; if eroded, the lesion is likely a jugular paraganglioma (Figs. 68.5 and 68.6). CT is an excellent modality for determining the relationships of the tumor to the petrous carotid, Eustachian tube, and middle/posterior fossae [16]. Magnetic resonance imaging (MRI) is best used for defining relationships to critical neurovascular structures and delineating involvement of the neck and intracranial cavity (Figs. 68.7, 68.8, 68.9, and 68.10). JTPs are usually intermediate in signal on both T1- and T2-weighted MRI and enhance intensely after gadolinium administration. Lesions >2 cm often show intratumoral flow voids, giving them the pathognomonic "salt-and-pepper" appearance [25] (Fig. 68.11). The presence of flow voids can help distinguish JTPs from schwannomas, which typically enhance homogeneously and may dumbbell through the jugular foramen [24]. MR angiography and venography (MRA, MRV) can help further elucidate great vessel involvement [25]. Similar findings can be noted with CT angiography or venography, albeit with less soft tissue definition.

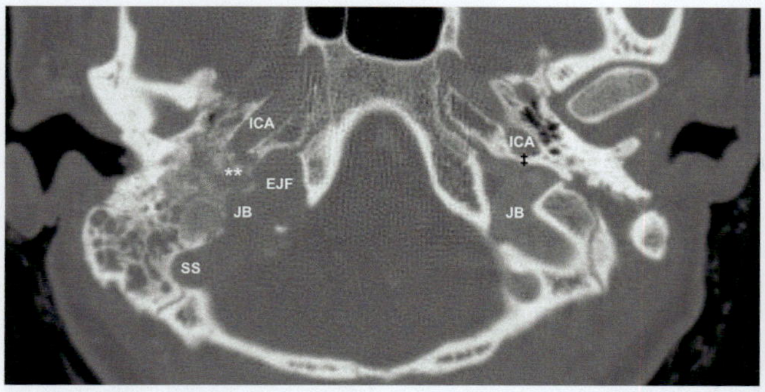

Fig. 68.5 This axial CT of the temporal bone allows easy comparison between the tumor (right) and normal (left) sides. On the right, the jugular bulb loses its definition and clearly expands the jugular foramen. The caroticojugular spine is mottled on the tumor side (**) compared to the crisp definition on the left (‡). Abbreviations: EJF expanded jugular foramen, ICA internal carotid artery, JB jugular bulb, SS sigmoid sinus

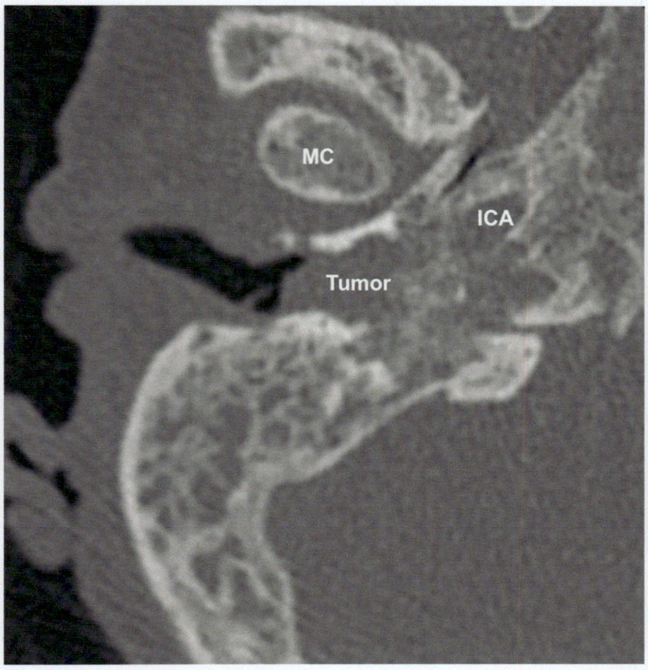

Fig. 68.6 This axial CT shows a tumor in the external auditory canal with erosion of the bone surrounding the internal carotid artery. This patient presented with aural bleeding. Abbreviations: ICA internal carotid artery, MC mandibular condyle

Nuclear medicine has also played a large role in the workup of JTP; radionuclide scintigraphy imaging exploits the expression of somatostatin type 2 receptors by paragangliomas and other neuroendocrine tumors (Fig. 68.12) [26]. Octreotide and DOTATATE, both somatostatin analogs, can be coupled to radioligands to perform whole-body scans to screen patients for multifocal disease. Octreotide scans have also been used to detect recurrent or residual disease posttreatment with a relatively high sensitivity and specificity [27].

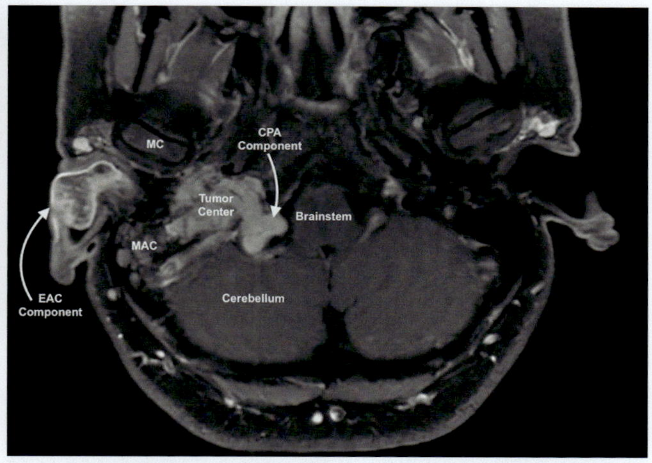

Fig. 68.7 Axial T1 with contrast. A large jugular paraganglioma is centered on the right jugular foramen and extends into the external auditory canal and cerebellopontine angle. The mastoid air cells are opacified. Abbreviations: CPA cerebellopontine angle, EAC external auditory canal, MAC mastoid air cells, MC mandibular condyle

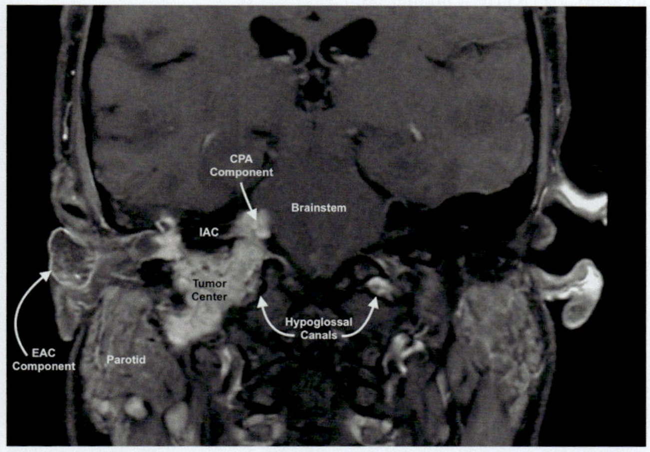

Fig. 68.8 A coronal view of the same patient with a right-sided jugular paraganglioma seen in the previous figure. The ear canal and CPA components are easily seen. The hypoglossal canal is eroded. Abbreviations: CPA cerebellopontine angle, EAC external auditory canal, IAC internal auditory canal

In recent years, positron-emitting radiotracers (PET) have been combined with CT to achieve high-resolution scans that are capable of detecting even subcentimeter lesions. ^{18}F-fluorodihydroxyphenylalanine (^{18}F-DOPA) is a radiolabeled dopamine precursor that targets cells with catecholamine biosynthesis. Together with ^{68}Gallium-radiolabeled somatostatin analogs, the sensitivity and specificity for parasympathetic tumor detection and multifocal disease (as found in patients with SDHD mutations) are >90%. These two modalities are, however, less suited to detecting sympathetic tumors [28–36]. Tumors associated with SDHB mutations, however, are often better visualized with ^{18}F-fluorodeoxyglucose (^{18}F-FDG) PET/CT, which targets

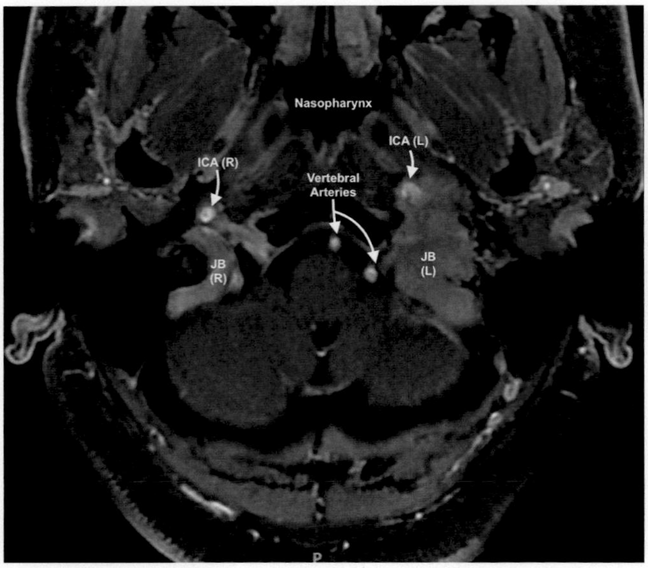

Fig. 68.9 This left-sided lesion is centered on the jugular foramen and has a 180-degree carotid encasement. Abbreviations: ICA (L) left internal carotid artery, ICA (R) right internal carotid artery, JB (L) left jugular bulb, JB (R) right jugular bulb

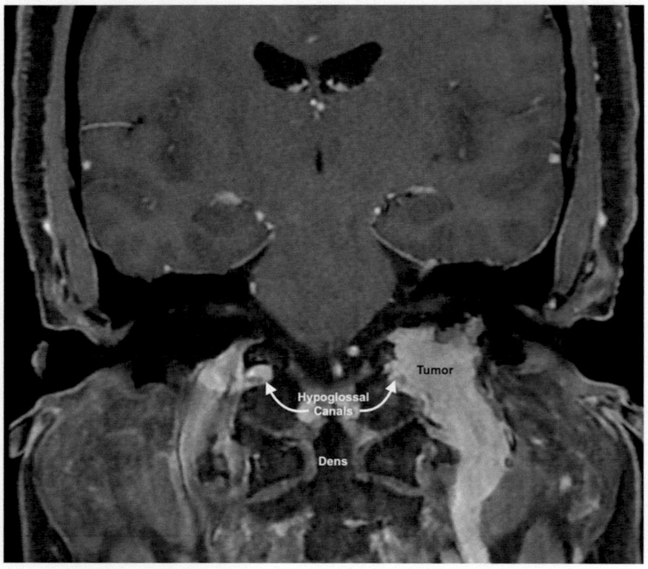

Fig. 68.10 A coronal view of the same tumor shows extension into the neck and involvement of the adjacent hypoglossal canal

the augmented glycolytic metabolism of these lesions [25]. Regardless of the isotope, imaging should include everything from the skull base through the pelvis.

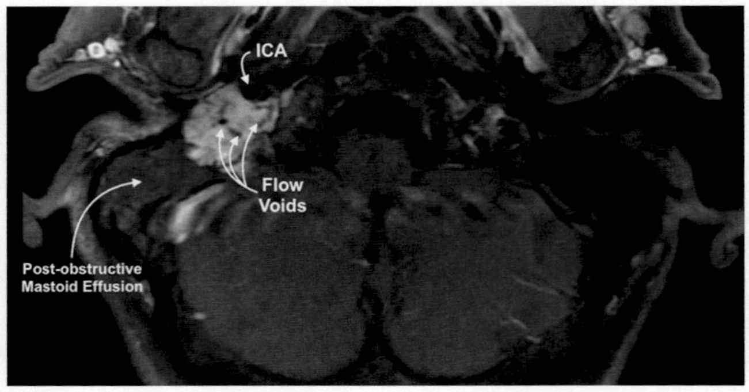

Fig. 68.11 This right-sided jugular paraganglioma has characteristic flow voids, which give tumors >2 cm their pathognomonic "salt-and-pepper" appearance. Enhancement distinguishes a tumor from a simple post-obstructive effusion in the mastoid air cells. Abbreviations: ICA internal carotid artery

Preoperative diagnostic angiography with tumor embolization is an important adjunct in the surgical treatment of all Fisch class C, D, and large class B JTP (Fig. 68.13). Such a study will identify and ideally occlude the relevant tumoral feeding vessels, ideally leading to less intraoperative bleeding [25]. When performed in the 1–2 days preceding surgery, the revascularization phenomena seen with longer intervals are largely avoided [37]. While embolization with various substrates has proven effective for JTPs over the years [37–39], it is not without risk. There are reports of temporary and permanent cranial neuropathies as a result of a shared blood supply between the tumor and the vasa nervorum of the cranial nerves. As a result, the rate of new facial nerve palsy has been reported as high as 36.8% [40]. A thorough pre- and post-embolization cranial nerve exam is recommended; if a new cranial neuropathy is found, it is the surgical team's decision as to whether it is best to wait for recovery or proceed with resection. Balloon occlusion testing should be performed if carotid sacrifice or bypass is at all contemplated. While internal carotid sacrifice is not recommended in the vast majority of cases due to the attendant risk of catastrophic stroke, having the knowledge that one can likely safely sacrifice the carotid if catastrophic bleeding is encountered is valuable information. That said, the results of such testing may not accurately reflect the body's physiologic response to abrupt hypoperfusion; the false-negative rate of balloon occlusion testing is reported to be up to 10% [41].

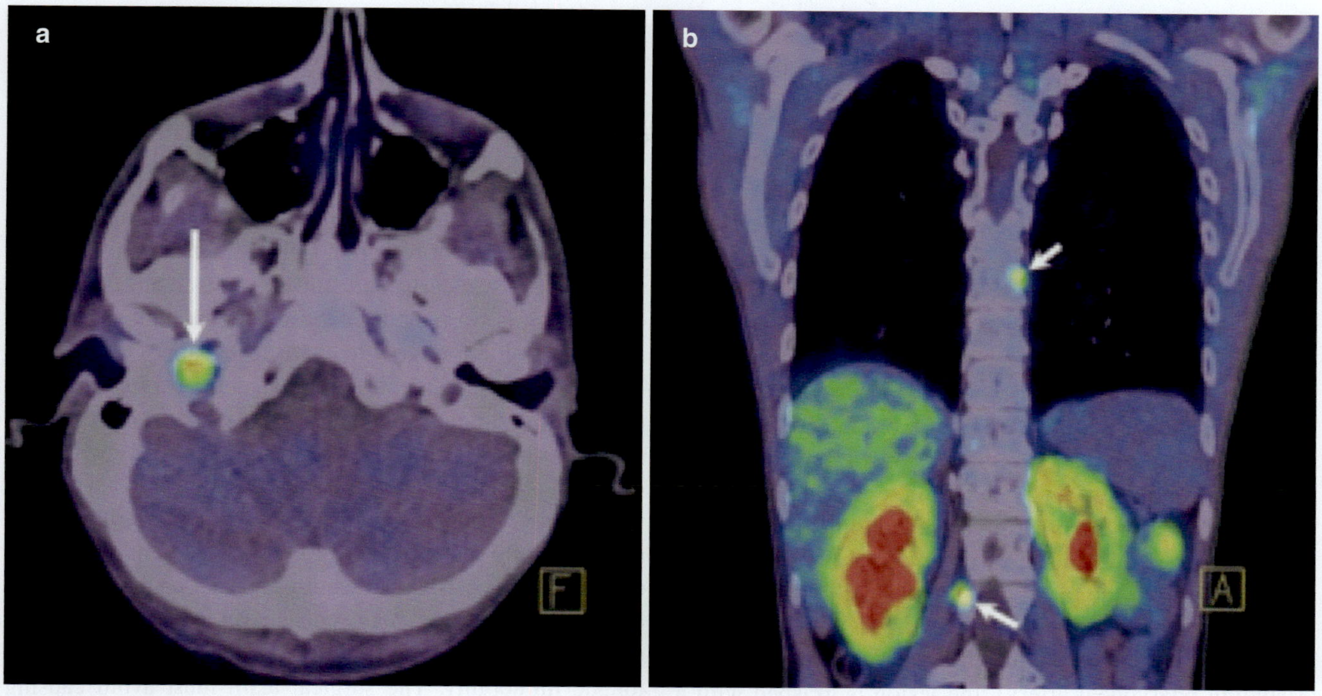

Fig. 68.12 Fusion CT/⁶⁸Gallium-DOTATATE PET imaging showing focal uptake in the (**a**) right jugular foramen (arrow) and (**b**) thoracolumbar vertebrae (arrows) consistent with a metastatic jugular paraganglioma

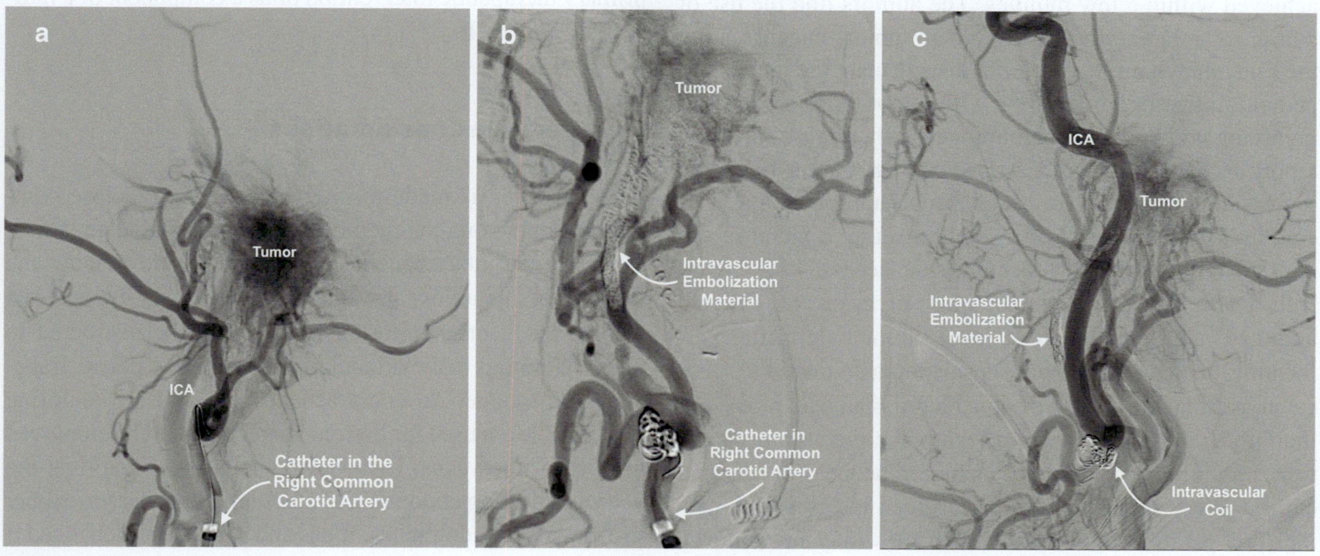

Fig. 68.13 (**a**) This is a right-sided jugular paraganglioma undergoing preoperative diagnostic angiogram with embolization. The catheter is in the right common carotid artery with several feeding vessels off the external carotid artery system. (**b**) This shows the same tumor after instillation of intravascular embolization material with a resultant decrease in vascularity. (**c**) After using embolization material as well as intravascular coils, the tumor is distinctly less vascular compared to the initial diagnostic angiogram. Abbreviations: ICA internal carotid artery

Surgical Resection

Tympanic Paragangliomas

Gross total resection (GTR) is the ideal for tympanic paragangliomas as surgical management can achieve 92% long-term tumor control with a rather low incidence of complications [42]. While staging systems and algorithms can be informative [16, 23], the success of the operation will depend on gaining adequate exposure to accommodate tumor size and being able to dissect it from critical surrounding structures.

Smaller tumors limited to the promontory are often removed via a transcanal approach; endoscopic resection has been described [43–45] and is the preferred technique by the authors for its superior visualization (Fig. 68.2). A microbipolar is often used to preemptively coagulate the tumor away from the facial nerve, and small cottonoids are used to elevate the lesion from the surrounding bone. Once isolated on its pedicle (often the tympanic branch of the ascending pharyngeal artery), the lesion is grasped with a cup forceps or pulled out with a right-angle pick. Once removed, there is often a rush of blood; the tympanic cavity is packed off with cottonoids, and hemostasis is often achieved within a few minutes. The authors find the use of a laser to be largely ineffective. With tumors encapsulating the ossicular chain, we prefer to disarticulate the incudostapedial joint before proceeding with tumor removal. Lesions involving the tympanic membrane usually require resecting a portion thereof to avoid early bleeding. Larger tympanic tumors may necessitate a postauricular approach, mastoidectomy to access antral or mastoid disease, a facial recess approach for selective retrotympanic access, or a canal-wall-down tympanomastoidectomy in cases of external auditory canal erosion. If residual tumor is left after performing canal-wall-down tympanomastoidectomy, ear canal overclosure should be considered if all squamous epithelium from the ear canal and tympanic membrane can be removed. The facial nerve, cochlea, and petrous internal carotid artery should never be sacrificed in cases with normal preoperative function. The ossicles may be removed for access, with hearing rehabilitation in these patients achieved with modern ossicular chain reconstructive and tympanoplasty techniques or via bone conduction hearing implants.

Jugular Paragangliomas

Treatment of jugular paragangliomas requires a more nuanced, multidisciplinary approach that requires the establishment of certain surgical goals and a certain degree of restraint. While it is tempting to try for GTR in every case, there is often a cost in the way of cranial neuropathies or unnecessary blood loss. A new pharyngeal hypoesthesia with high vagal paralysis can lead to dysphagia, aspiration, and a breathy voice, which can be devastating. While new cranial neuropathies occur in 30–33% with observation alone [18, 46, 47], this must be compared to new cranial neuropathy rates post-resection, which can be >50% depending on tumor extent and degree of resection [48–50]. Resection should be avoided in the elderly and unwell, and an initial trial of observation is warranted for those patients without a pressing indication for surgery to characterize tumor growth [24, 46, 47, 51–55]. Large lesions that demonstrate steady or rapid growth, impinge upon critical structures, or have brainstem compression should be addressed surgically with consideration for planned subtotal resection with lower cranial nerve preservation to avoid unnecessary morbidity in the neurologically intact patient [46, 54]. Treatment of multifocal head and neck disease requires special consideration, as bilateral lower cranial nerve palsies can lead to an insensate pharynx, aspiration, the need for tracheostomy, or complete tongue immobility. The surgical team must avoid causing devastating bilateral cranial neuropathies. Other treatment modalities such as radio- and systemic therapy will be discussed later in this chapter and should be considered as the primary therapeutic intervention or as a component of a multimodal approach.

Perioperative Considerations

If the decision is made to intervene surgically, close communication among the members of the surgical team is necessary. In the intact patient, it is informative to monitor the facial, glossopharyngeal, vagus, accessory, and hypoglossal nerves; the neuromonitoring team should be instructed to place electrodes in the orbicularis muscles, soft palate, trapezius, and tongue. An endotracheal tube with a monitoring electrode, often used for thyroid surgery, should be employed to monitor the vagus. It should be noted, however, that the neuromonitoring endotracheal tubes tend to be larger-caliber than standard endotracheal tubes and should be exchanged if prolonged intubation is expected. While neurosurgeons often prefer the use of a Mayfield skull clamp, having the head fixed may complicate the cervical exposure. There is potential for heavy blood loss; as such, communication with the anesthesia team and blood bank is necessary to ensure the proper blood products are readily available. While there are reports of using a cell salvage system in the bloodiest cases [56], it is important to avoid such situations altogether. In the case of multifocal disease, as can be found in patients with SDHD mutations, we recommend the up-front resection of catecholamine-secreting lesions first, before treating the head and neck. In the rare case of a catecholamine-secreting head and neck lesion, non-selective and non-competitive α_1- and α_2-adrenoceptor blockade is typically started in the 7–14 days leading up to surgery, with the primary goal being normotension [57, 58]. Dopamine-secreting tumors, however, do not require special antihypertensive protocols as they are unlikely to affect perioperative hemodynamics [59].

Infratemporal Fossa Type A (ITFA) and Facial Bridge Techniques

As with tympanic paragangliomas, the approach used for jugular paraganglioma tumor resection depends on the extent of the tumor. Most jugular paragangliomas require a combined transcervical-transtemporal approach in order to get vascular control and access the jugular foramen at the skull base. While the smallest of jugular paragangliomas may be approached transcanal or transmastoid if debulking or subtotal resection is planned, we will be discussing the formal infratemporal fossa approaches as described by Fisch in the 1980s [60, 61] with modifications for a facial bridge technique [62] (Figs. 68.14 and 68.15).

The patient is positioned supine with the head turned away. A small shoulder roll is placed to augment the cervical exposure. An incision approximately 3–4 cm away from the postauricular crease begins just above the anterior auricle, goes postauricular, and is brought into a cervical neck crease. A skin and soft tissue flap is raised in the plane just superficial to the temporalis fascia. A posteriorly based periosteal flap is then made, and the ear canal is transected and overclosed using standard techniques. We prefer to do this at the start of the case, as it can be rather tedious and best not left for last. The neck is opened, and subplatysmal flaps are raised inferiorly and superiorly after ligating the external jugular vein and transecting the great auricular nerve. The sternocleidomastoid (SCM) and digastric are skeletonized as in standard neck dissection techniques, and the internal jugular vein (IJV), internal/external carotid arteries (ICA/ECA), and cranial nerves X–XII are isolated and traced toward the skull base. Vascular loops with mini-

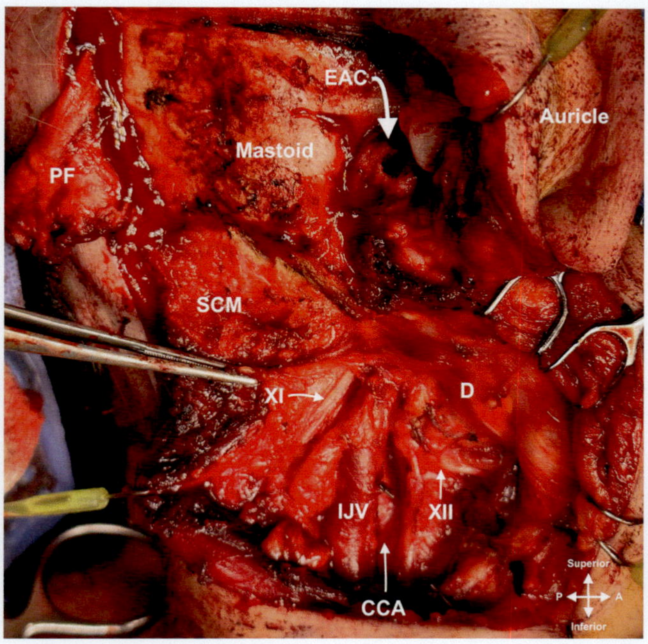

Fig. 68.14 Right infratemporal fossa approach demonstrating the necessary cervical exposure. The mastoid is exposed and the ear canal transected and overclosed. The periosteal flap is reflected posteriorly, and the sternocleidomastoid is separated from the mastoid and reflected back. The internal jugular and carotid arteries are exposed, and cranial nerves X–XII are traced proximally to the skull base. The digastric is later split and the styloid removed. Abbreviations: CCA common carotid artery, D digastric, EAC external auditory canal, IJV internal jugular vein, PF periosteal flap, XI accessory nerve, XII hypoglossal nerve

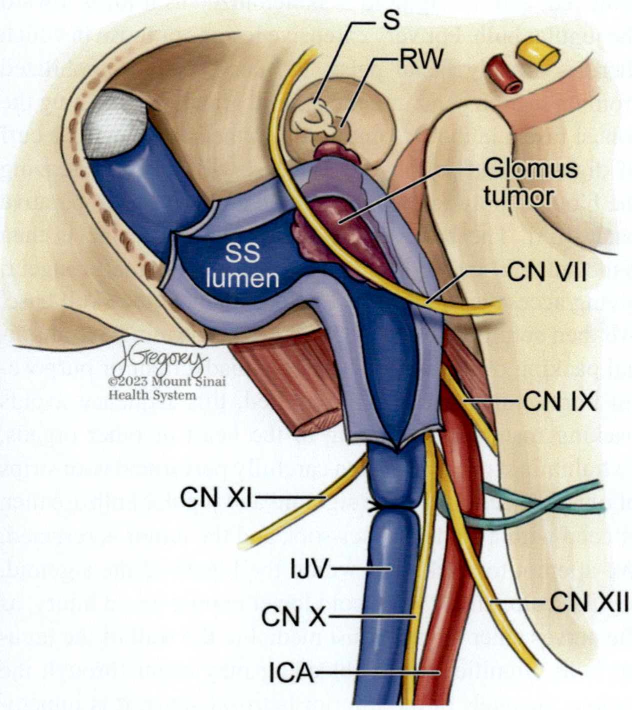

Fig. 68.15 An infratemporal fossa approach with the facial bridge technique is illustrated. A canal-wall-down mastoidectomy has been performed, extraluminal packing performed on the proximal sigmoid, the internal jugular vein ligated, and the sigmoid and jugular bulb opened to reveal a jugular paraganglioma with a small hypotympanic extension. The digastric has been divided and the styloid process removed. A vascular loop is around the internal carotid artery for proximal control. The course of the more distal internal carotid artery is shown. For an infratemporal fossa type B or C dissection requiring more distal carotid exposure, the mandibular condyle and zygomatic arch are removed, and the middle meningeal artery and the third branch of the trigeminal nerve are transected. Printed with permission from ©Mount Sinai Health System. Abbreviations: CN cranial nerve, RW round window, S stapes, IJV internal jugular vein, JB jugular bulb, SS sigmoid sinus, VII facial nerve, VIII vestibulocochlear nerve, IX glossopharyngeal nerve, X vagus nerve, XI accessory nerve, XII hypoglossal nerve

mal tension are placed around the IJV and ICA for vascular control. The SCM is then detached from the mastoid tip, and the digastric is split.

Attention is then turned to the temporal bone. A large canal-wall-down mastoidectomy is performed, leaving significant bone stock on the proximal 1.5–2.0 cm of sigmoid sinus so that extraluminal packing can be performed later. The incus and malleus are removed, and the stapes is left in place. All squamous epithelium of the ear canal and tympanic membrane must be removed to avoid the development of a cholesteatoma in an overclosed cavity. The vertical segment of the facial nerve is identified and traced into the stylomastoid foramen, leaving a thin shell of bone proximal to the fascia. When possible, we prefer to perform a facial bridge technique wherein the nerve is not mobilized. After identifying the sigmoid and digastric ridge through the mastoid, the mastoid tip is removed. Retrofacial air cells are removed, and the sigmoid is skeletonized as it turns toward the jugular bulb. For very extensive lesions or those in which there is already facial palsy, the nerve is now mobilized from its second genu into the parotid gland. Maintaining the robust fascia in the stylomastoid foramen and leaving a cuff of digastric and stylohyoid muscles will aid in preserving the blood supply to the facial nerve and limit postoperative palsy [63]. The bone of the caroticojugular spine is then removed, and the styloid is removed with a small rongeur, giving access to the ICA just before it enters the skull base. We then suture-ligate the IJV before performing extraluminal packing of the sigmoid; in case inadvertent or purposeful intraluminal packing is required, this sequence avoids packing material embolizing to the heart or other organs. Extraluminal packing is then carefully performed with strips of oxidized cellulose. The sigmoid and jugular bulb are then opened with a blade and scissors, and the tumor is resected. We attempt to work only within the lumen of the sigmoid, jugular bulb, and IJV to avoid lower cranial nerve injury, as the nerves enter the neck just medial to the wall of the jugular bulb. Significant back-bleeding may occur through the venous channels of the inferior petrosal sinus; it is imperative not to pack this area too tightly, as cranial nerve damage may occur. After resection, the periosteal flap, SCM, and temporalis are used to close the defect. We will often use either the temporalis muscle or the temporoparietal fascia rotational flap to eliminate the dead space over the great vessels in the skull base. When harvesting the temporoparietal fascia flap, a superior extension of the incision is often necessary anteriorly, and raising of the flap done from the outset as the plane of dissection is just under the skin's hair follicles. A drain is placed in the neck, and a multilayer closure is then performed.

Techniques for More Extensive Lesions

To obtain access to the petrous apex, clivus, pterygopalatine fossa, intrapetrous ICA, and nasopharynx, a more extended infratemporal fossa approach is required, typically Fisch Type B or C (ITFB and ITFC, respectively). Mobilization of the facial nerve is not required for isolated anterior disease, but long-segment mobilization from the geniculate ganglion to the stylomastoid foramen may be required, depending on disease extent, and is expected to have worse facial outcomes. In addition to the standard ITFA approach, the mandibular condyle is resected, the zygoma downfractured, and the middle meningeal artery and V3 are transected in an ITFB approach. Clearing these structures allows the surgeon to trace the ICA and achieve distal control. To access the pterygopalatine fossa, sphenoid sinus, and nasopharynx as in an ITFC, the pterygoid muscles are cleared from the pterygoid plates, and the petrous ICA is traced further distally. While not routinely recommended, some surgeons recommend stenting of the ICA to reduce the risk of vascular injury [64]. Generally, it is wise to have appropriate personnel from vascular and neurosurgery available for vascular bypass in the event of an intraoperative ICA injury.

Intracranial portions of the tumor may be treated at the time of initial resection or staged depending on location and likelihood of persistent cerebrospinal fluid (CSF) leak. Retrosigmoid, translabyrinthine, transcochlear, far lateral, and middle fossa approaches may be utilized depending on tumor location and neurologic status. The authors prefer to stage the intracranial component to avoid a CSF leak into the neck. Dural defects may be closed primarily or with the use of allo- or autografts such as fascia, abdominal fat, acellular dermal matrix, or vascularized tissue in the form of pedicle flaps or free flaps. The Eustachian tube obliteration is performed routinely to avoid CSF rhinorrhea.

Surgical Outcomes

Despite refined microsurgical techniques, one of the largest series looking at outcomes in 152 patients with jugular paragangliomas (57.9% Glasscock–Jackson Class III and IV tumors) demonstrated locoregional control in 85% of cases over a mean follow-up time of 54 months [48]. Major complications such as death, CSF leak, stroke, and carotid injury were rare (1–3%). Tumor recurrence was found in 4.9% and developed late (mean, 8.17 years).

Subtotal resection with observation or radiation of the residual tumor has recently gained traction in functionally intact patients. In 12 intact patients with Glasscock–

Jackson class III and IV jugular paragangliomas undergoing planned subtotal resection, no patients sustained long-term cranial neuropathies. Average residual tumor volume was 27.7% of the preoperative size, and with an average follow-up of 44.6 months, there was no subsequent tumor growth in 66.7%. When residual volumes were less than 20% of the preoperative volume, no tumor growth was encountered [54]. It is possible that achieving a critical level of devascularization from a subtotal resection can render residual disease dormant. This strategy lends itself to the possibility of planned limited resection followed by adjuvant radiosurgery [65]; preliminary outcomes of combining these strategies for the treatment of JTP in elderly patients indicate favorable results regarding tinnitus, hearing, and CN status [65].

Rehabilitation of Functional Deficits Following Surgery

Rehabilitation of cranial neuropathies is an important component in the management of JTP, as new-onset neuropathy or worsening of baseline preoperative dysfunction are not uncommon. If the facial nerve is mobilized, some degree of postoperative weakness is expected. Even if full function is expected to return, early and aggressive treatment of lagophthalmos is advocated to avoid exposure keratopathy and corneal abrasion. Artificial tears, ophthalmic lubricant, and the use of a humidification bubble chamber are conservative alternatives to lid-loading procedures. Other static and dynamic facial nerve reanimation procedures may be performed in consultation with a facial plastic surgeon and are beyond the scope of this chapter (see Chap. 24). For those with vocal cord paralysis, vocal fold medialization via injectables or implants, along with concurrent adjunctive procedures, can aid in phonation and avoid aspiration [65–68]. Hearing is generally rehabilitated with a bone conduction hearing implant once the ear is overclosed, with special circumstances requiring other devices.

Radiation

In an effort to strike a balance between locoregional control and treatment morbidity, radiotherapy has emerged as a major modality in treating jugular paragangliomas. It is used practically to arrest growth, as reductions in tumor volume rarely exceed 25% [18]. Early studies utilized fractionated external beam radiation (EBRT) for primary and salvage treatment, demonstrating high locoregional control rates of 86–100% [69–71]. EBRT soon gave way to stereotactic radiosurgery (SRS), which achieved similar outcomes using lower biological doses with steeper gradients, resulting in less collateral damage to surrounding normal structures [72, 73]. Single-fraction SRS is considered most effective in tumor diameters <3 cm, and a 2018 meta-analysis demonstrated locoregional and symptom control rates of 92% and 93%, respectively, with only an 8% complication rate [74]. Similarly, both large multi-institutional and smaller series have demonstrated high efficacy rates with low complication rates [75–82]. In one large multi-institutional series, cranial neuropathies were found to improve in 11%, and new ones developed in 15% [75]. We advocate the use of radiation in poor surgical candidates as well as in those with recurrent or residual disease after resection. Unfortunately, the literature is underpowered to show definitive differences between gross total resection (GTR), subtotal resection (STR), STR + SRS, and primary SRS. However, using the data available in the form of two large meta-analyses, which do not control for tumor size, primary SRS was found to have the highest locoregional control rate (Table 68.4) [83, 84].

Table 68.4 Demographics (a) and pooled estimates of the rates of tumor control (b) after different treatment modalities for jugular paragangliomas

(a)					
	Treatment				
	GTR (*n* = 351)	STR (*n* = 82)	STR + SRS (*n* = 97)	SRS (*n* = 339)	*p*-value
Sex (M:F)	188:163	68:14	50:47	139:200	<0.001
Mean age (years)	45	53	59	58	0.014
Mean tumor size (cm)	–	–	2.0	2.6	NS
Fisch class					<0.001
A	9%	14%	0%	0%	–
B	9%	14%	0%	4%	
C	63%	43%	91%	39%	
D	19%	29%	9%	57%	
Mean length follow-up	88	72	96	71	<0.01

(b)	
Treatment	Rate (95% CI)
STR	69% (57–82%)
GTR	86% (81–91%)
STR + SRS	71% (58–83%)
SRS	95% (92–99%)

Adapted from reference [83]

Abbreviations: *GTR* gross total resection, *STR* subtotal resection, *SRS* stereotactic radiosurgery, *NS* not significant

Systemic Therapies

Systemic treatment plays a limited role in the management of JTP and is primarily reserved for those patients with metastases and high tumor burden. While beyond the scope of this chapter, targeted radionuclide therapy, chemotherapy, and tyrosine kinase inhibitors may be used for extensive lesions and should be overseen by an experienced multidisciplinary team [28, 85–97].

Observation

A wait-and-scan observation strategy for the management of jugular paragangliomas has gained significant traction in recent years, while tympanic lesions are almost always resected unless there are extenuating circumstances. Patients with jugular lesions foregoing treatment for various reasons were closely monitored to establish tumor growth rates and to determine an optimal observation strategy. Jansen and colleagues reviewed 11 JTP observed for a period of at least 1 year and noted that 55% of the tumors demonstrated radiologic progression, with a median growth rate of 0.8 mm per year [46]. It is important to note that this series did not specify whether the tumors were jugular or tympanic in origin and that nearly 80% of their cohort had hereditary, multifocal disease. It is also important to call attention to the small sample size and the growth rate being within the margin of error of test-retest reliability.

In one of the largest series reviewing an observation strategy for 23 Fisch class C and D jugular paragangliomas for a minimum period of 3 years, Prasad and colleagues demonstrated that 65% of tumors remained stable or regressed in size over a median follow-up of 61 months [18]. Tumors growing less than 3 mm per year were deemed slow growing, and 88% of those demonstrating radiologic progression fit this category. Interestingly, these data may also be used to infer that part of the high tumor control rates attributed to radiation treatment may, in fact, be biased by a disease process that often demonstrates little to no tumor growth [18]. That said, 7 patients in their cohort (30%) developed new-onset lower cranial neuropathies during the observation period.

Carlson and colleagues corroborated these results by reporting on 16 GJ tumors managed with primary observation. Of the 12 lesions with serial imaging and a median follow-up of 57.6 months, 7 (58%) remained stable while the rest demonstrated volumetric radiologic growth (>20% increase). Median growth rate for the growing tumors was 0.8 mm/year. Combining these data with those of Prasad and colleagues, only 3/39 observed patients eventually required treatment [47]. The limited data available regarding cranial nerve outcomes for observation show that they are comparable to those for SRS and better than those for GTR, albeit with potentially lower rates of locoregional control. Some degree of selection bias in these reports is likely present, as they feature predominantly older patients who may harbor more indolent disease, which may not be generalizable to a younger population with more aggressive disease.

Conclusion

Treatment of JTPs requires a nuanced treatment algorithm, an experienced multidisciplinary team, and appropriate restraint. While once popular, radical resection with neurologic compromise has given way to planned subtotal resection with functional preservation techniques and the use of adjuvant therapies.

References

1. Moncure AC, Goodman ML. Case records of the Massachusetts General Hospital. Weekly clinicopathological exercises. Case 14-1975. N Engl J Med. 1975;292:741–5.
2. Gulya AJ. The glomus tumor and its biology. Laryngoscope. 1993;103:7–15.
3. Jyung RW, LeClair EE, Bernat RA, Kang TS, Ung F, McKenna MJ, Tuan RS. Expression of angiogenic growth factors in paragangliomas. Laryngoscope. 2000;110:161–7.
4. Guild SR. A hitherto unrecognized structure, the glomus jugularis, in man. Anat Rec. 1941;79:28.
5. Guild SR. The glomus jugulare, a nonchromaffin paraganglion, in man. Ann Otol Rhinol Laryngol. 1953;62:1045–71.
6. Gaynor BG, Elhammady MS, Jethanamest D, Angeli SI, Aziz-Sultan MA. Incidence of cranial nerve palsy after preoperative embolization of glomus jugulare tumors using onyx. J Neurosurg. 2014;120:377–81.
7. Pearse AG. The diffuse neuroendocrine system: historical review. Front Horm Res. 1984;12:1–7.
8. Brown JS. Glomus jugulare tumors revisited; a ten-year statistical follow-up of 231 cases. Laryngoscope. 1985;95:284–8.
9. Richter S, Qiu B, Ghering M, et al. Head/neck paragangliomas: focus on tumor location, mutational status and plasma methoxytyramine. Endocr Relat Cancer. 2022;29:213–24.
10. Darr R, Pamporaki C, Peitzsch M, et al. Biochemical diagnosis of phaeochromocytoma using plasma-free normetanephrine, metanephrine and methoxytyramine: importance of supine sampling under fasting conditions. Clin Endocrinol. 2014;80:478–86.
11. Rao D, Peitzsch M, Prejbisz A, et al. Plasma methoxytyramine: clinical utility with metanephrines for diagnosis of pheochromocytoma and paraganglioma. Eur J Endocrinol. 2017;177:103–13.
12. Blanchet EM, Martucci V, Pacak K. Pheochromocytoma and paraganglioma: current functional and future molecular imaging. Front Oncol. 2012;6(1):58.
13. Boedeker CC, Hensen EF, Neumann HP, et al. Genetics of hereditary head and neck paragangliomas. Head Neck. 2014;36:907–16.
14. Burnichon N, Rohmer V, Amar L, et al. The succinate dehydrogenase genetic testing in a large prospective series of patients with paragangliomas. J Clin Endocrinol Metab. 2009;94:2817–27.

15. Gaal J, van Nederveen FH, Erlic Z, et al. Parasympathetic paragangliomas are part of the von Hippel–Lindau syndrome. J Clin Endocrinol Metab. 2009;94:4367–71.
16. Sanna M, Fois P, Pasanisi E, Russo A, Bacciu A. Middle ear and mastoid glomus tumors (glomus tympanicum): an algorithm for the surgical management. Auris Nasus Larynx. 2010;37:661–8.
17. Spector GJ, Sobol S, Thawley SE, Maisel RH, Ogura JH. Panel discussion: glomus jugulare tumors of the temporal bone. Patterns of invasion in the temporal bone. Laryngoscope. 1979;89:1628–39.
18. Prasad SC, Mimoune HA, D'Orazio F, Medina M, Bacciu A, Mariani-Costantini R, Piazza P, Sanna M. The role of wait-and-scan and the efficacy of radiotherapy in the treatment of temporal bone paragangliomas. Otol Neurotol. 2014;35:922–31.
19. Jackson CG, Glasscock ME 3rd, Harris PF. Glomus tumors: diagnosis, classification, and management of large lesions. Arch Otolaryngol. 1982;108:401–10.
20. Mediouni A, Ammari S, Wassef M, Gimenez-Roqueplo AP, Laredo JD, Duet M, Tran Ba Huy P, Oker N. Malignant head/neck paragangliomas. Comparative study. Eur Ann Otorhinolaryngol Head Neck Dis. 2014;131:159–66.
21. Davis JM, Davis KR, Hesselink JR, Greene R. Malignant glomus jugulare tumor: a case with two unusual radiographic features. J Comput Assist Tomogr. 1980;4:415–7.
22. Druck NS, Spector GJ, Ciralsky RH, Ogura JH. Malignant glomus vagale: report of a case and review of the literature. Arch Otolaryngol. 1976;102:634–6.
23. Carlson ML, Sweeney AD, Pelosi S, Wanna GB, Glasscock ME 3rd, Haynes DS. Glomus tympanicum: a review of 115 cases over 4 decades. Otolaryngol Head Neck Surg. 2015;152:136–42.
24. Wanna GB, Sweeney AD, Haynes DS, Carlson ML. Contemporary management of jugular paragangliomas. Otolaryngol Clin N Am. 2015;48:331–41.
25. Corrales CE, Fischbein N, Jackler RK. Imaging innovations in temporal bone disorders. Otolaryngol Clin N Am. 2015;48:263–80.
26. Telischi FF, Bustillo A, Whiteman ML, Serafini AN, Reisberg MJ, Gomez-Marin O, Civantos FJ, Balkany TJ. Octreotide scintigraphy for the detection of paragangliomas. Otolaryngol Head Neck Surg. 2000;122:358–62.
27. Bustillo A, Telischi FF. Octreotide scintigraphy in the detection of recurrent paragangliomas. Otolaryngol Head Neck Surg. 2004;130:479–82.
28. Jha A, Taieb D, Carrasquillo JA, et al. High-specific-activity-(131) I-MIBG versus (177)Lu-DOTATATE targeted radionuclide therapy for metastatic pheochromocytoma and paraganglioma. Clin Cancer Res. 2021;27:2989–95.
29. Janssen I, Blanchet EM, Adams K, et al. Superiority of [68Ga]-DOTATATE PET/CT to other functional imaging modalities in the localization of SDHB-associated metastatic Pheochromocytoma and Paraganglioma. Clin Cancer Res. 2015;21:3888–95.
30. Janssen I, Chen CC, Taieb D, et al. 68Ga-DOTATATE PET/CT in the localization of head and neck paragangliomas compared with other functional imaging modalities and CT/MRI. J Nucl Med. 2016;57:186–91.
31. Archier A, Varoquaux A, Garrigue P, et al. Prospective comparison of (68)Ga-DOTATATE and (18)F-FDOPA PET/CT in patients with various pheochromocytomas and paragangliomas with emphasis on sporadic cases. Eur J Nucl Med Mol Imaging. 2016;43:1248–57.
32. Han S, Suh CH, Woo S, Kim YJ, Lee JJ. Performance of (68) Ga-DOTA-conjugated somatostatin receptor-targeting peptide PET in detection of pheochromocytoma and paraganglioma: a systematic review and meta-analysis. J Nucl Med. 2019;60:369–76.
33. Gild ML, Naik N, Hoang J, et al. Role of DOTATATE-PET/CT in preoperative assessment of phaeochromocytoma and paragangliomas. Clin Endocrinol. 2018;89:139–47.
34. King KS, Chen CC, Alexopoulos DK, et al. Functional imaging of SDHx-related head and neck paragangliomas: comparison of 18F-fluorodihydroxyphenylalanine, 18F-fluorodopamine, 18F-fluoro-2-deoxy-D-glucose PET, 123I-metaiodobenzylguanidine scintigraphy, and 111In-pentetreotide scintigraphy. J Clin Endocrinol Metab. 2011;96:2779–85.
35. Amodru V, Romanet P, Scemama U, et al. Tumor multifocality with vagus nerve involvement as a phenotypic marker of SDHD mutation in patients with head and neck paragangliomas: a (18) F-FDOPA PET/CT study. Head Neck. 2019;41:1565–71.
36. Treglia G, Cocciolillo F, de Waure C, et al. Diagnostic performance of 18F-dihydroxyphenylalanine positron emission tomography in patients with paraganglioma: a meta-analysis. Eur J Nucl Med Mol Imaging. 2012;39:1144–53.
37. Murphy TP, Brackmann DE. Effects of preoperative embolization on glomus jugulare tumors. Laryngoscope. 1989;99:1244–7.
38. Valavanis A. Preoperative embolization of the head and neck: indications, patient selection, goals, and precautions. AJNR Am J Neuroradiol. 1986;7:943–52.
39. Ladner TR, He L, Davis BJ, Yang GL, Wanna GB, Mocco J. Initial experience with dual-lumen balloon catheter injection for preoperative onyx embolization of skull base paragangliomas. J Neurosurg. 2016;124:1813–9.
40. Persky MS, Setton A, Niimi Y, Hartman J, Frank D, Berenstein A. Combined endovascular and surgical treatment of head and neck paragangliomas--a team approach. Head Neck. 2002;24:423–31.
41. Linskey ME, Jungreis CA, Yonas H, Hirsch WL Jr, Sekhar LN, Horton JA, Janosky JE. Stroke risk after abrupt internal carotid artery sacrifice: accuracy of preoperative assessment with balloon test occlusion and stable xenon-enhanced CT. AJNR Am J Neuroradiol. 1994;15:829–43.
42. Forest JA III, Jackson CG, McGrew BM. Long-term control of surgically treated glomus tympanicum tumors. Otol Neurotol. 2001;22:232–6.
43. Fermi M, Ferri G, Bayoumi Ebaied T, Alicandri-Ciufelli M, Bonali M, Badr El-Dine M, Presutti L. Transcanal endoscopic management of glomus tympanicum: multicentric case series. Otol Neurotol. 2021;42:312–8.
44. Kaul VF, Filip P, Schwam ZG, Wanna GB. Nuances in transcanal endoscopic surgical technique for glomus tympanicum tumors. Am J Otolaryngol. 2020;41:102562.
45. Killeen DE, Wick CC, Hunter JB, Rivas A, Wanna GB, Nogueira JF, Kutz JW Jr, Isaacson B. Endoscopic management of middle ear paragangliomas: a case series. Otol Neurotol. 2017;38:408–15.
46. Jansen JC, van den Berg R, Kuiper A, van der Mey AG, Zwinderman AH, Cornelisse CJ. Estimation of growth rate in patients with head and neck paragangliomas influences the treatment proposal. Cancer. 2000;88:2811–6.
47. Carlson ML, Sweeney AD, Wanna GB, Netterville JL, Haynes DS. Natural history of glomus jugulare: a review of 16 tumors managed with primary observation. Otolaryngol Head Neck Surg. 2015;152:98–105.
48. Jackson CG, McGrew BM, Forest JA, Netterville JL, Hampf CF, Glasscock ME 3rd. Lateral skull base surgery for glomus tumors: long-term control. Otol Neurotol. 2001;22:377–82.
49. Moe KS, Li D, Linder TE, Schmid S, Fisch U. An update on the surgical treatment of temporal bone paraganglioma. Skull Base Surg. 1999;9:185–94.
50. Fayad JN, Keles B, Brackmann DE. Jugular foramen tumors: clinical characteristics and treatment outcomes. Otol Neurotol. 2010;31:299–305.
51. Alvarez-Morujo RJ, Ruiz MA, Serafini DP, Delgado IL, Friedlander E, Yurrita BS. Management of multicentric paragangliomas: review of 24 patients with 60 tumors. Head Neck. 2016;38:267–76.

52. Moore MG, Netterville JL, Mendenhall WM, Isaacson B, Nussenbaum B. Head and neck paragangliomas: an update on evaluation and management. Otolaryngol Head Neck Surg. 2016;154:597–605.
53. Sniezek JC, Netterville JL, Sabri AN. Vagal paragangliomas. Otolaryngol Clin N Am. 2001;34:925–39.
54. Wanna GB, Sweeney AD, Carlson ML, Latuska RF, Rivas A, Bennett ML, Netterville JL, Haynes DS. Subtotal resection for management of large jugular paragangliomas with functional lower cranial nerves. Otolaryngol Head Neck Surg. 2014;151:991–5.
55. Lloyd S, Obholzer R, Tysome J, Group BC. British skull base society clinical consensus document on management of head and neck Paragangliomas. Otolaryngol Head Neck Surg. 2020;163:400–9.
56. Esper SA, Waters JH. Intra-operative cell salvage: a fresh look at the indications and contraindications. Blood Transfus. 2011;9:139–47.
57. Berends AMA, Kerstens MN, Lenders JWM, Timmers H. Approach to the patient: perioperative Management of the Patient with Pheochromocytoma or sympathetic Paraganglioma. J Clin Endocrinol Metab. 2020;105:dgaa441.
58. Buitenwerf E, Osinga TE, Timmers H, et al. Efficacy of alpha-blockers on hemodynamic control during pheochromocytoma resection: a randomized controlled trial. J Clin Endocrinol Metab. 2020;105:2381–91.
59. Van Der Horst-Schrivers AN, Osinga TE, Kema IP, Van Der Laan BF, Dullaart RP. Dopamine excess in patients with head and neck paragangliomas. Anticancer Res. 2010;30:5153–8.
60. Fisch U. Infratemporal fossa approach for glomus tumors of the temporal bone. Ann Otol Rhinol Laryngol. 1982;91:474–9.
61. Fisch U. Infratemporal fossa approach for lesions in the temporal bone and base of the skull. Adv Otorhinolaryngol. 1984;34:254–66.
62. Pensak ML, Jackler RK. Removal of jugular foramen tumors: the fallopian bridge technique. Otolaryngol Head Neck Surg. 1997;117:586–91.
63. Leonetti JP, Brackmann DE, Prass RL. Improved preservation of facial nerve function in the infratemporal approach to the skull base. Otolaryngol Head Neck Surg. 1989;101:74–8.
64. Piazza P, Di Lella F, Bacciu A, Di Trapani G, Ait Mimoune H, Sanna M. Preoperative protective stenting of the internal carotid artery in the management of complex headand neck paragangliomas: long-term results. Audiol Neurootol. 2013;18:345–52.
65. Willen SN, Einstein DB, Maciunas RJ, Megerian CA. Treatment of glomus jugulare tumors in patients with advanced age: planned limited surgical resection followed by staged gamma knife radiosurgery: a preliminary report. Otol Neurotol. 2005;26:1229–34.
66. Mok P, Woo P, Schaefer-Mojica J. Hypopharyngeal pharyngoplasty in the management of pharyngeal paralysis: a new procedure. Ann Otol Rhinol Laryngol. 2003;112:844–52.
67. Netterville JL, Jackson CG, Civantos F. Thyroplasty in the functional rehabilitation of neurotologic skull base surgery patients. Am J Otol. 1993;14:460–4.
68. Netterville JL, Civantos FJ. Rehabilitation of cranial nerve deficits after neurotologic skull base surgery. Laryngoscope. 1993;103:45–54.
69. Cole JM, Beiler D. Long term results of treatment for glomus jugulare and glomus vagale tumors with radiotherapy. Laryngoscope. 1994;104:1461–5.
70. Larner JM, Hahn SS, Spaulding CA, et al. Glomus jugulare tumors. Long-term control by radiation therapy. Cancer. 1992;69:1813–7.
71. Carrasco V, Rosenman J. Radiation therapy of glomus jugulare tumors. Laryngoscope. 1993;103:23–7.
72. Hu K, Persky MS. Treatment of head and neck paragangliomas. Cancer Control. 2016;23:228–41.
73. Pollock BE. Stereotactic radiosurgery in patients with glomus jugulare tumors. Neurosurg Focus. 2004;17:E10.
74. Shapiro S, Kellermeyer B, Ramadan J, Jones G, Wiseman B, Cassis A. Outcomes of primary radiosurgery treatment of glomus jugulare tumors: systematic review with meta-analysis. Otol Neurotol. 2018;39:1079–87.
75. Sheehan JP, Tanaka S, Link MJ, et al. Gamma knife surgery for the management of glomus tumors: a multicenter study. J Neurosurg. 2012;117:246–54.
76. Eustacchio S, Trummer M, Unger F, Schrottner O, Sutter B, Pendl G. The role of gamma knife radiosurgery in the management of glomus jugular tumours. Acta Neurochir Suppl. 2002;84:91–7.
77. Sheehan J, Kondziolka D, Flickinger J, Lunsford LD. Gamma knife surgery for glomus jugulare tumors: an intermediate report on efficacy and safety. J Neurosurg. 2005;102:241–6.
78. Sharma MS, Gupta A, Kale SS, Agrawal D, Mahapatra AK, Sharma BS. Gamma knife radiosurgery for glomus jugulare tumors: therapeutic advantages of minimalism in the skull base. Neurol India. 2008;56:57–61.
79. Lior U, Rotem H, Uzi N, Roberto S. LINAC radiosurgery for glomus jugulare tumors: retrospective – cohort study of 23 patients. Acta Neurochir. 2020;162:839–44.
80. Wegner RE, Rodriguez KD, Heron DE, Hirsch BE, Ferris RL, Burton SA. Linac-based stereotactic body radiation therapy for treatment of glomus jugulare tumors. Radiother Oncol. 2010;97:395–8.
81. Hurmuz P, Cengiz M, Ozyigit G, et al. Robotic stereotactic radiosurgery in patients with unresectable glomus jugulare tumors. Technol Cancer Res Treat. 2013;12:109–13.
82. Patel AK, Rodriguez-Lopez JL, Hirsch BE, Burton SA, Flickinger JC, Clump DA. Long term outcomes with linear accelerator stereotactic radiosurgery for treatment of jugulotympanic paragangliomas. Head Neck. 2021;43:449–55.
83. Ivan ME, Sughrue ME, Clark AJ, Kane AJ, Aranda D, Barani IJ, Parsa AT. A meta-analysis of tumor control rates and treatment-related morbidity for patients with glomus jugulare tumors. J Neurosurg. 2011;114:1299–305.
84. Guss ZD, Batra S, Limb CJ, Li G, Sughrue ME, Redmond K, Rigamonti D, Parsa AT, Chang S, Kleinberg L, Lim M. Radiosurgery of glomus jugulare tumors: a meta-analysis. Int J Radiat Oncol Biol Phys. 2011;81:e497–502.
85. Taieb D, Jha A, Treglia G, Pacak K. Molecular imaging and radionuclide therapy of pheochromocytoma and paraganglioma in the era of genomic characterization of disease subgroups. Endocr Relat Cancer. 2019;26:R627–52.
86. Satapathy S, Mittal BR, Bhansali A. Peptide receptor radionuclide therapy in the management of advanced pheochromocytoma and paraganglioma: a systematic review and meta-analysis. Clin Endocrinol. 2019;91:718–27.
87. Huang H, Abraham J, Hung E, et al. Treatment of malignant pheochromocytoma/paraganglioma with cyclophosphamide, vincristine, and dacarbazine: recommendation from a 22-year follow-up of 18 patients. Cancer. 2008;113:2020–8.
88. Averbuch SD, Steakley CS, Young RC, et al. Malignant pheochromocytoma: effective treatment with a combination of cyclophosphamide, vincristine, and dacarbazine. Ann Intern Med. 1988;109:267–73.
89. Niemeijer ND, Alblas G, van Hulsteijn LT, Dekkers OM, Corssmit EP. Chemotherapy with cyclophosphamide, vincristine and dacarbazine for malignant paraganglioma and pheochromocytoma: systematic review and meta-analysis. Clin Endocrinol. 2014;81:642–51.
90. Asai S, Katabami T, Tsuiki M, Tanaka Y, Naruse M. Controlling tumor progression with cyclophosphamide, vincristine, and Dacarbazine treatment improves survival in patients with metastatic and Unresectable malignant Pheochromocytomas/Paragangliomas. Horm Cancer. 2017;8:108–18.

91. Deutschbein T, Fassnacht M, Weismann D, Reincke M, Mann K, Petersenn S. Treatment of malignant phaeochromocytoma with a combination of cyclophosphamide, vincristine and dacarbazine: own experience and overview of the contemporary literature. Clin Endocrinol. 2015;82:84–90.
92. Tanabe A, Naruse M, Nomura K, Tsuiki M, Tsumagari A, Ichihara A. Combination chemotherapy with cyclophosphamide, vincristine, and dacarbazine in patients with malignant pheochromocytoma and paraganglioma. Horm cancer. 2013;4:103–10.
93. Jawed I, Velarde M, Darr R, et al. Continued tumor reduction of metastatic pheochromocytoma/paraganglioma harboring succinate dehydrogenase subunit B mutations with cyclical chemotherapy. Cell Mol Neurobiol. 2018;38:1099–106.
94. Baudin E, Goichot B, Berruti A, et al. First international randomized study in malignant progressive pheochromocytoma and paragangliomas (FIRSTMAPPP): an academic double-blind trial investigating sunitinib. Ann Oncol. 2021;32:S621–5.
95. O'Kane GM, Ezzat S, Joshua AM, et al. A phase 2 trial of sunitinib in patients with progressive paraganglioma or pheochromocytoma: the SNIPP trial. Br J Cancer. 2019;120:1113–9.
96. Hadoux J, Favier J, Scoazec JY, et al. SDHB mutations are associated with response to temozolomide in patients with metastatic pheochromocytoma or paraganglioma. Int J Cancer. 2014;135:2711–20.
97. Perez K, Jacene H, Hornick JL, et al. SDHx mutations and temozolomide in malignant pheochromocytoma and paraganglioma. Endocr Relat Cancer. 2022;29:533–44.
98. Van Hulsteijn LT, Dekkers OM, Hes FJ, Smit JW, Corssmit EP. Risk of malignant paraganglioma in SDHB-mutation and SDHD-mutation carriers: a systematic review and meta-analysis. J Med Genet. 2012;49:768–76.
99. Hao HX, Khalimonchuk O, Schraders M, et al. SDH5, a gene required for flavination of succinate dehydrogenase, is mutated in paraganglioma. Science. 2009;325:1139–42.
100. Bayley JP, Kunst HP, Cascon A, et al. SDHAF2 mutations in familial and sporadic paraganglioma and phaeochromocytoma. Lancet Oncol. 2010;11:366–72.
101. Kunst HP, Rutten MH, de Mönnink JP, et al. SDHAF2 (PGL2-SDH5) and hereditary head and neck paraganglioma. Clin Cancer Res. 2011;17:247–54.
102. Neumann HP, Bausch B, McWhinney SR, Freiburg-Warsaw-Columbus Pheochromocytoma Study Group. Germ-line mutations in nonsyndromic pheochromocytoma. N Engl J Med. 2002;346:1459–66.
103. Neumann HP, Erlic Z, Boedeker CC, et al. Clinical predictors for germline mutations in head and neck paraganglioma patients: cost reduction strategy in genetic diagnostic process as fall-out. Cancer Res. 2009;69:3650–6.
104. Pasini B, Stratakis CA. SDH mutations in tumorigenesis and inherited endocrine tumours: lesson from the phaeochromocytoma-paraganglioma syndromes. J Intern Med. 2009;266:19–42.
105. Erlic Z, Rybicki L, Peczkowska M, et al. Clinical predictors and algorithm for the genetic diagnosis of pheochromocytoma patients. Clin Cancer Res. 2009;15:6378–85.
106. Boedeker CC, Neumann HPH, Maier W, Bausch B, Schipper J, Ridder GJ. Malignant head and neck paragangliomas in SDHB mutation carriers. Otolaryngol Head Neck Surg. 2007;137:126–9.

Non-paraganglioma Jugular Foramen Tumors

69

Andrew J. Thomas, Mana Espahbodi, Clough Shelton, and Richard K. Gurgel

Abbreviations

ADC	Apparent Diffusion Coefficient
CN	Cranial Nerve
CPA	Cerebellopontine Angle
CT	Computed Tomography
HL	Hearing Loss
JF	Jugular Foramen
MRI	Magnetic Resonance Imaging
SCM	Sternocleidomastoid
WBRT	Whole Brain Radiotherapy

Overview

The jugular foramen (JF) is a skull base foramen (more accurately, a canal) located between the temporal and occipital bones. The JF has important relationships with intracranial and extracranial structures; these anatomic relationships account for the clinical symptoms of lesions of the JF and create critical considerations in the management of patients with JF tumors. Bordering the JF anteriorly is the internal carotid artery, superiorly the otic capsule, posterolaterally the facial nerve, and posteromedially the posterior fossa. Compartmentalization of structures within the JF is variable, but is categorized into the anteromedial *pars nervosa,* comprised of cranial nerve (CN) IX and the inferior petrosal sinus [1], and the posterolateral *pars vascularis*, made up of CN X, CN XI, and the jugular bulb [1–3]. In addition to these structures coursing along the JF, Jacobson's nerve (the tympanic branch of CN IX) and Arnold's nerve (the auricular branch of CN X) branch off their respective parent nerves within the course of the foramen. Any JF tumors and treatments for such may impact the structures surrounding and within the JF. Accurate diagnosis and appropriate management are imperative for optimizing outcomes.

Jugular paragangliomas (formerly glomus jugulare tumors) are the most common primary tumors of the JF; they represent approximately 60–80% of tumors of the JF and are discussed in greater detail in Chap. 68 [4–6]. Of the non-paraganglioma, primary JF tumors, the most common are JF schwannomas and meningiomas, discussed in greater detail in Chap. 76, which represent approximately 3–4% and 1% of all intracranial schwannomas and meningiomas, respectively. Less commonly, metastatic disease can occur in the JF. In this chapter, we specifically focus on the primary non-paraganglioma JF tumor types of schwannoma, meningioma, and metastatic disease. For each of these tumor types, we describe epidemiology, clinical presentation, and diagnosis, as well as treatment specific to each. Chordomas and chondrosarcomas, which may also involve the jugular foramen, are covered in Chap. 79. The clinical presentation of JF tumors is often nonspecific to the tumor type and results from local effects of the tumor at the JF, though there are some suggested tumor-specific differences in the relative incidence of presenting lower CN deficits and otologic symptoms. Signs and symptoms may include those of neuropathies of the facial, vestibulocochlear, and lower CNs. We do not discuss secondary, non-paraganglioma JF tumors such as endolymphatic sac tumors, plasmacytomas, and Langerhans cell histiocytosis, which may grow into the JF but do not originate within it [7].

Our discussion of diagnosis focuses on imaging characteristics of the different tumors, as imaging is critical in differentiating JF tumors. Computed tomography (CT) and magnetic resonance imaging (MRI) are both necessary for evaluation [8, 9]. Complementing features of the bony anatomy on CT imaging and the soft-tissue detail of MRI provide an informative picture of the JF tumor type, its extension

A. J. Thomas · M. Espahbodi · C. Shelton · R. K. Gurgel (✉)
Department of Otolaryngology—Head and Neck Surgery, University of Utah School of Medicine, Salt Lake City, UT, USA
e-mail: Mana.Espahbodi@hsc.utah.edu; Richard.Gurgel@hsc.utah.edu

A. D. Sweeney et al. (eds.), *Haynes-Glasscock-Shambaugh Surgery of the Ear*, https://doi.org/10.1007/978-3-032-18264-7_69

beyond the JF, including potential vascular involvement (MRI), and assist in preoperative planning [4]. When obtaining imaging of JF lesions, we recommend obtaining noncontrast CT scans with axial, 1.0 mm or thinner sections, in bone algorithm (maximum edge enhancement), with coronal reconstruction. For MRI, we recommend axial and coronal imaging, 4 mm or thinner sections, with T1- and T2-weighted sequences, gadolinium-enhanced T1-weighted sequences with fat saturation, and diffusion-weighted sequences to allow for calculation of apparent diffusion coefficient (ADC) values. We find fat saturation to be particularly useful for evaluating bone marrow involvement, as may be the case for JF tumors that extend into the petrous apex and clivus. Thin contrast sequences can be crucial for identifying perineural spread of the tumor and involvement of neural foramina of the skull base [4]. It is also important to evaluate the patency of the contralateral venous system and the presence of venous occlusion on the ipsilateral side. Ligation of a partially patent ipsilateral venous system in the presence of a small contralateral system may lead to postoperative intracranial hypertension.

Treatment options are reviewed by tumor type as well. In general, the options for each tumor type include observation, surgical resection, and stereotactic radiotherapy. Outcomes of treatment, including recurrence rates and CN outcomes, vary by tumor type [10].

Jugular Foramen Schwannomas

Epidemiology

Lower CN schwannomas in the JF represent only 2.9–4% of all intracranial schwannomas and 1% of all types of temporal bone lesions [8, 11]. The incidence of JF schwannomas is greater in women than men (roughly double the incidence); diagnosis is usually made in middle age (average age of 37 years), and it is exceedingly rare for these tumors to be diagnosed at less than 20 years or greater than 70 years of age [12]. When schwannomas present in early life (at less than 20 years of age), a diagnosis of neurofibromatosis type 2 should be strongly considered [11].

Presentation

As is the case with all JF lesions, the presentation of JF schwannomas is dependent on the particular anatomic involvement of the tumor. The most common presenting symptoms of JF schwannomas are hearing loss (HL), tinnitus, and swallowing difficulties, followed in incidence by headache and then dizziness/vertigo [13]. Consistent with the incidence of these presenting symptoms, the most common presenting CN deficits are also reported to be IX and X, followed by VIII [14]. In contrast to paragangliomas, non-paraganglioma tumors have a lower incidence of tinnitus at presentation [6]. JF schwannomas may be primarily intracranial, extracranial, or span the JF and have both intracranial and extracranial extension ("dumbbell" lesions). The extent of JF involvement likely correlates with the degree of lower CN deficits, and patients with a primarily intracranial mass and limited JF involvement may present with the nonspecific symptoms of HL, tinnitus, and vertigo, without additional findings to clinically suggest JF involvement (e.g., no lower CN deficits) [12]. Unlike jugular paragangliomas, otologic examination is unlikely to demonstrate any mass or specific middle ear findings [8].

All types of JF lesions may present with neuropathies of CNs V–XII; the lower CNs IX–XI, which traverse the jugular foramen, are most commonly involved, and audiovestibular dysfunction may result as well [4]. CN deficits related to JF tumors are most often attributed to paragangliomas, as they are the most common tumor at this location, though non-paraganglioma JF tumors may present similarly [12]. These *JF syndromes* may result from lesions anywhere along the course of the lower CNs from the brainstem to their site of innervation. Therefore, these particular findings may also be seen in pathology outside of the JF, such as stroke, trauma, and infectious processes, such as abscess formation [12]. In addition to the constellation of signs/symptoms seen with dysfunction of CN IX–XI, which is termed *JF syndrome* or *Vernet's syndrome*, the addition of CN XII involvement is termed *Posterior Lacerocondylar (Collet-Sicard) syndrome*, and the addition of XII and the sympathetic chain is termed *Posterior Retropharyngeal (Villaret's) syndrome*.

Imaging Characteristics

On CT imaging, characteristic bony changes are suggestive of a diagnosis of JF schwannoma: smooth-corticated margin of bone without invasion into the marrow is usually seen, as schwannomas grow slowly and gradually expand (Fig. 69.1) [6, 15]. This pattern contrasts with the bony invasion often seen with JF meningiomas and jugular paragangliomas. On MRI, the characteristic imaging findings of schwannomas include T1 isointensity, T2 hyperintensity, and T1 post-gadolinium avid enhancement (Fig. 69.2) [15]. The absence of flow voids that are seen with paragangliomas and the absence of dural tails that are seen with meningiomas also help distinguish JF schwannomas. The permeative-destructive osseous changes associated with paraganglioma (Fig. 69.3), which are described further in Chap. 15 as well as Chap. 68, are not seen in JF schwannomas. Because schwannomas arise from the Schwann cells of the peripheral nerve sheath, they generally grow as circumscribed and elongated masses,

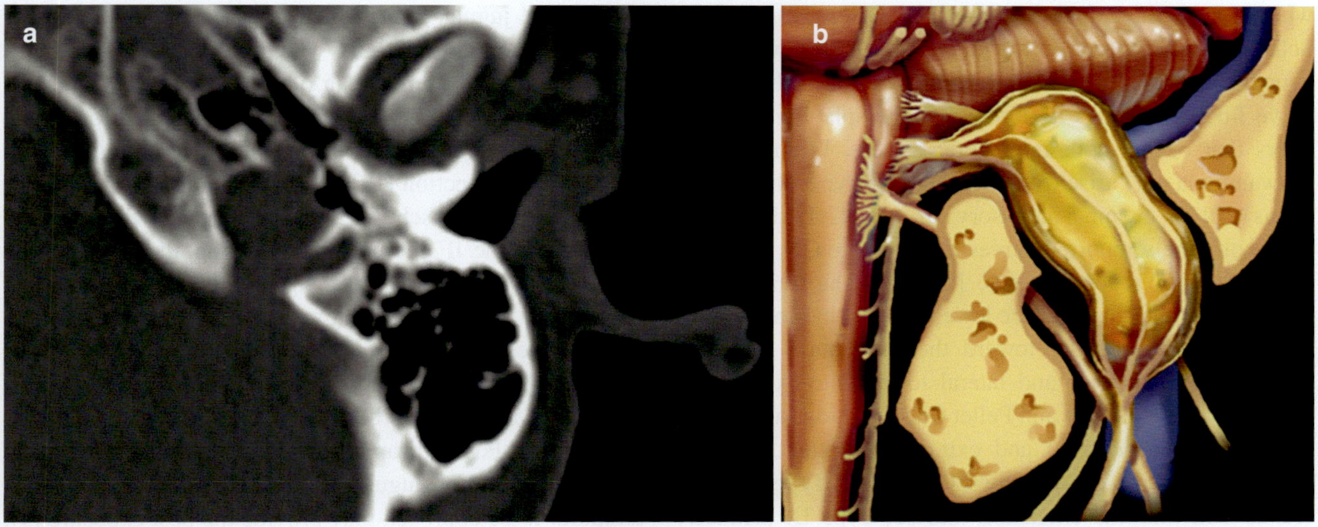

Fig. 69.1 CT (**a**) in the axial plane with a bone algorithm and illustration (**b**) in the coronal plane showing smooth scalloped surgical margins of a slow-growing benign nerve sheath lesion, which causes gradual enlargement of the jugular foramen—consistent with a jugular foramen schwannoma. (Image **b** reproduced from Imaging in Otolaryngology by H. R. Harnsberger and R.K. Gurgel with permission from Elsevier)

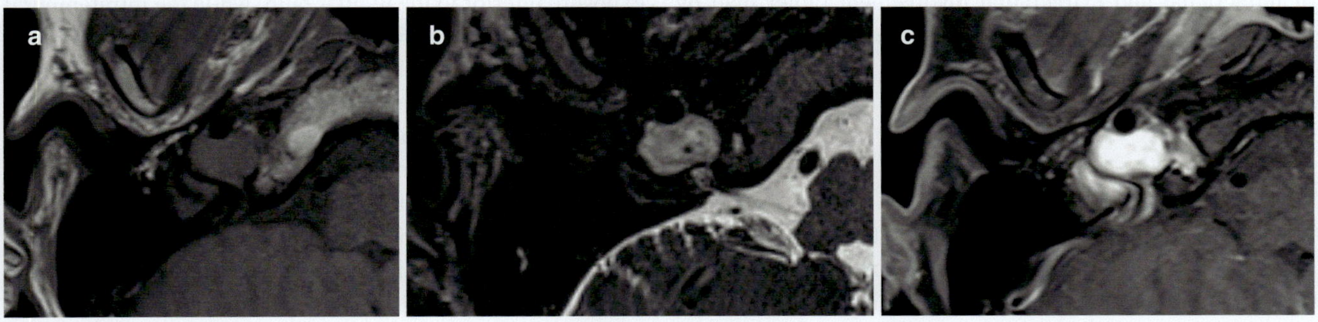

Fig. 69.2 A right lower cranial nerve schwannoma involving the jugular foramen on axial MRI, isointense on Axial T1 without contrast (**a**), hyperintense on heavily weighted T2 (**b**), and avid enhancement on T1 post-contrast with fat saturation (**c**)

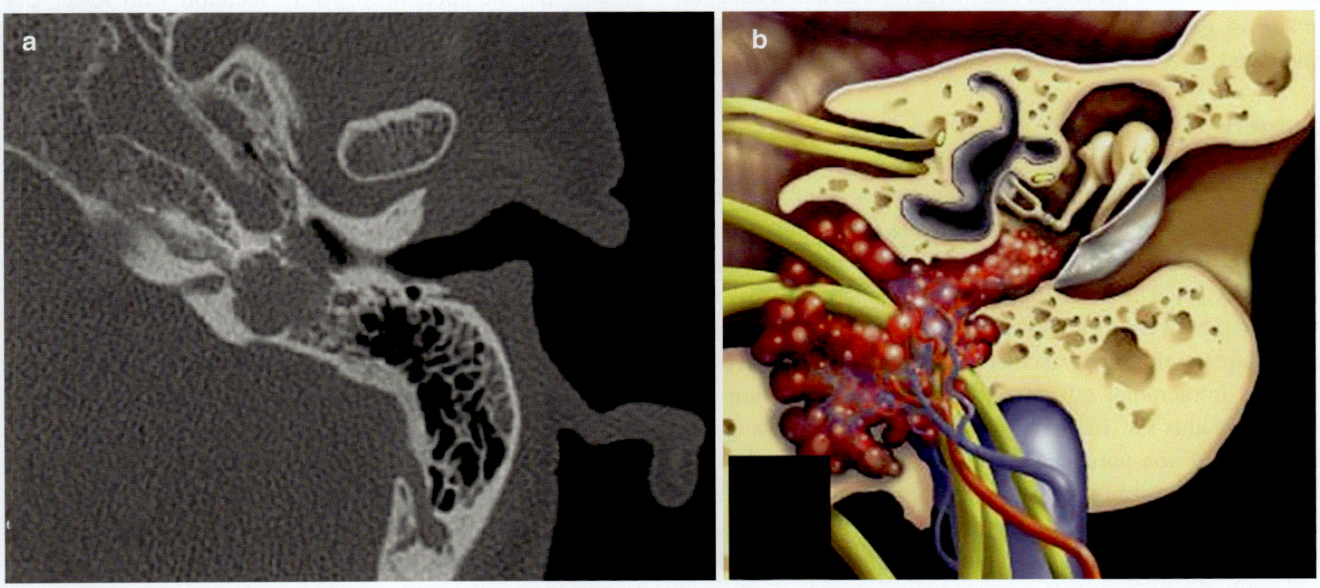

Fig. 69.3 Axial CT (**a**) with a bone algorithm and illustration (**b**) in the coronal plane of permeative changes characteristic of a jugular foramen paraganglioma. (Image **b** reproduced from Imaging in Otolaryngology by H. R. Harnsberger and R.K. Gurgel with permission from Elsevier)

which follow the course of the involved CN [12]. Because Schwann cells comprise the nerve sheath, schwannomas generally push the intact nerve away without splaying the nerve fibers, which is in contrast to the splaying of nerve fibers that occurs with intraneural tumors. Within the JF, schwannoma may arise from the glossopharyngeal (CN IX), vagus (CN X), or spinal accessory nerve (CN XI), though the most commonly reported nerves involved are CN IX and X (up to 90% of reported cases) [15, 16]. The tumors then extend along the course of the lower CN as they slowly grow superiorly and medially toward the intracranial posterior fossa, and/or posterior and lateral toward the extracranial carotid space. The Kaye and Pellet Classifications are used to describe the intracranial and extracranial extent of these tumors [17, 18]. Kaye describes Types A–C: Type A: intracranial and minimal extension into JF, Type B: primarily within JF, Type C: primarily extracranial with minimal in JF or intracranial [17]. Later, Pellet described Type D: both intracranial and extracranial components extending from JF (dumbbell shape) [18]. However, for clarity, we will refer to these tumors throughout the chapter by describing the extent of intracranial and extracranial involvement rather than by the Kaye and Pellet classification scheme.

Treatment

Observation

The age of the patient and the size/growth of the tumor are important considerations in treatment planning. Observation of schwannomas and meningiomas may be the most appropriate strategy for management in older patients with small tumors and in patients who are unable to undergo surgery or stereotactic radiation. With observation by MRI imaging, the rate of growth of the lesion can be monitored and a decision made to proceed with surgery or stereotactic radiation if indicated.

Surgery

The key principles of approaching JF schwannomas and any JF tumor are to obtain the best exposure for controlling neurovascular structures and performing the maximum extent of tumor resection possible, while causing the least amount of morbidity [9]. The most appropriate approach for a given JF tumor depends on its location and extent, relationships with important neighboring vascular and neurologic structures, as well as intracranial effects of brainstem compression and hydrocephalus [9, 10]. One key difference in the surgical treatment of non-paraganglioma JF tumors compared to the approach to paraganglioma tumors is that the benign tumors of the JF, such as schwannomas, are less likely to invade venous structures, whereas paragangliomas are more likely to invade the lumen of the sigmoid sinus, jugular bulb, and the internal jugular vein, which may require ligating these venous structures. Without vascular invasion, the non-paraganglioma JF tumors can often be resected with a less extensive approach, including the recent application of the endoscope, to improve exposure while decreasing drilling and surgical dissection [19].

For intracranial schwannomas associated with minimal extension to the JF and preserved hearing, the retrosigmoid craniotomy approach is advantageous for gaining excellent exposure of the cerebellopontine angle (CPA) while preserving the internal auditory canal and hearing function [8, 9, 20]. Drawbacks to this approach are the higher associated rates of postoperative headache and cerebrospinal fluid (CSF) leak. For schwannomas that are primarily located within the JF, a transjugular approach or Fisch type A infratemporal fossa approach may provide the best exposure [9]. Facial nerve rerouting or the fallopian bridge technique can be used to improve exposure and preserve the facial nerve, but results in some degree of facial nerve weakness postoperatively [21]. For schwannomas that are primarily extracranial, the transcondylar or far lateral approaches allow exposure inferior to the jugular bulb, while the infratemporal fossa approaches provide excellent exposure lateral and anterior to the jugular bulb. In addition to the exposure provided to the extracranial portion of the tumor within the JF and temporal bone, the infratemporal fossa approach also allows for access to intracranial extension in the posterior fossa [8]. Multiple combined approaches may be appropriate for some lesions, such as the dumbbell-shaped schwannomas, which may require both infratemporal and posterior fossa approaches [8, 9].

Surgical Complications

Complications from surgery for non-paraganglioma JF tumors may be specific to the JF location with lower CN deficits or injury to surrounding structures, or may be general complications associated with neurotologic procedures and the particular operative approach, such as cerebrospinal fluid (CSF) leak and infection/meningitis. Neurologic deficits result from injury to nerves coursing through or neighboring the JF and en route to the surgical approach (CN VII, VIII, IX, X, XI, XII, sympathetic chain). Of these neurologic injuries, the most common early complication seen in JF tumor procedures is vocal cord paralysis from CN X dysfunction, which may occur postoperatively in up to 25–33% of cases; the most common late complications usually result from other lower CN dysfunction and produce symptoms such as speech and swallowing dysfunction (IX, X) or shoulder problems (CN XI) [13]. These procedures are associated with a small mortality risk (likely less than 1%), though due to the rarity of mortality from these proceduresand the rarity of non-paraganglioma JF tumors, the actual incidence is difficult to determine [22]. CSF leak may occur in 3.9–6.6% of cases of jugular foramen tumor resection, which is similar to the risk associated with these surgical approaches, rather than being specific to non-paraganglioma JF tumors [13]. Avoiding CSF leak by meticulous closure and attention to this possible complication is important in general for these surgical approaches, and potential methods of reducing CSF leak risk include strong dural closure, use of fat graft to fill the dead space of the resulting defect, or even the use of local and free flap reconstruction when necessary [13, 17]. Postoperative lumbar drains are rarely needed in infratemporal fossa approaches with dural opening, but can be utilized in high-risk cases and in the management of postoperative CSF leaks. The extensive removal of skull base bone and dissection of the neck creates a skull base defect that can be difficult to control with fat packing.

Extent of Resection

Complete surgical resection is the goal for JF schwannomas, though unacceptable morbidity and individual patient factors may limit or preclude surgical resection. A more conservative approach is generally tolerated in schwannoma surgery due to the decreased risk of recurrence (compared to meningioma). Conservative near-total resection may also be advisable to reduce morbidity and risk of postoperative CN deficits. In one series, a more conservative approach to JF schwannoma resection decreased postoperative CN deficits without significantly increasing the risk of recurrence (5.7% recurrence rate in the gross total tumor resection group compared to 10.7% in the group with more conservative resection aimed at preserving the pars nervosa, $p = 0.36$) [23]. Similar to vestibular schwannomas, JF schwannomas with posterior fossa extension may also impact the facial nerve and cause facial nerve dysfunction: Postoperative facial weakness has been reported in 20–25% of patients [12]. If subtotal resection is necessary or surgery must be avoided, stereotactic radiation is a reasonable treatment option for JF schwannomas [23, 24].

Follow-Up

Patients also require long-term follow-up with clinical exams and imaging by MRI to monitor for recurrence, which may take years to detect due to the slow growth of schwannomas. There is no specific rule for the frequency or duration of follow-up for these patients; we titrate the follow-up schedule and imaging to the extent of the initial resection, as well as tumor growth on follow-up imaging. For patients with a known remaining gross tumor (subtotal resection), we recommend surveillance for the rest of the patient's life with MRI imaging intervals adjusted for tumor growth. We perform imaging every year for the first few years, then if there is no significant growth of the tumor, we extend the interval to every 2–3 years, and after a sustained period of no growth, we will then extend the imaging interval to every 5 years.

Radiotherapy

Stereotactic radiotherapy has a greater amount of demonstrated utility in the literature on vestibular schwannoma, though more recently, there has been increasing evidence of utility in treating JF schwannomas [23, 24]. In the case of vestibular schwannoma, radiotherapy has been associated with good short-term tumor control and minimal adverse CN outcomes [25]. For JF schwannomas, there similarly appear to be promising results, including 5-year progression-free survival of 89% in a cohort of 117 patients, of whom 48% were treated with stereotactic radiation as primary therapy and 52% had previously undergone a surgical resection [26]. Another study reported an 82% rate of progression-free survival in 92 patients treated with stereotactic radiation (55% were treated with stereotactic radiation as primary therapy, and 45% had previously undergone subtotal surgical resection) [27]. Stereotactic radiation is most appropriate for small or medium-sized JF schwannomas without any brainstem mass effect, or for those patients who are unable to tolerate surgery. The outcomes for stereotactic radiation are encouraging, with low rates of CN dysfunction and other morbidity, high rates of tumor control, and even reversal of CN neuropathies in up to two-thirds of patients [14, 23]. However, the length of follow-up is relatively limited (10 years). Radiotherapy without surgery may actually result in improvement in lower CN function (average of 20% of neuropathies improved in one series); 47% of cases with no surgical treatment and 21% of all cases with or without prior surgical resection had improvement in lower CN function at 16 months postradiation [22]. In another series of 56 patients who had primary stereotactic radiation and 61 with adjuvant therapy after prior resection, two-thirds of patients demonstrated improvement in lower CN dysfunction after radiotherapy [26]. Radiotherapy for lateral skull base tumors is covered in detail in Chap. 81. Since the goal of radiation is to prevent tumor growth, we recommend using stereotactic radiation only after tumor growth has been demonstrated on serial imaging, as true growth (indication for further treatment) is difficult to assess after radiation.

Recurrence

Jugular foramen schwannomas are less likely to recur than meningiomas; a 7.4% (6 / 81) recurrence rate is reported after surgical resection for JF schwannomas [23]. Although there appears to be a trend toward increased recurrence in patients who underwent subtotal resection followed by stereotactic radiation rather than complete resection, this was not significant, and there was a significant reduction in postoperative neuropathies with this treatment [23]. These limited data, specific to JF schwannoma, would suggest that the slight potential increase in recurrence with subtotal resection is outweighed by reduced morbidity. This finding is contrary to our knowledge about vestibular schwannoma, where the approximately 3–11% rate of recurrence for gross total and near-total resection is increased to about 32–53% depending on the extent of subtotal resection [25, 28].

Cranial Nerve Outcomes

JF schwannomas are associated with a higher preoperative incidence of CN dysfunction, but a lower (approximately 15–22.2%) rate of postoperative CN dysfunction, compared with paragangliomas and meningiomas [4, 12, 13, 29, 30]. One explanation for postoperative CN dysfunction is a facial nerve paresis that is usually temporary and may result from transposition of the nerve [31]. As transposition can often be avoided for JF schwannomas, this rate of paresis may be reduced relative to other tumor types [32].

Jugular Foramen Meningiomas

Epidemiology

JF meningiomas are rare; these tumors represent only 0.7–4% of all posterior fossa meningiomas and are less common JF tumors than paragangliomas or schwannomas [20, 33]. Posterior fossa meningiomas are already unusual as they only represent up to 10% of intracranial meningiomas. JF meningiomas occur more commonly in females and are more likely to be diagnosed in the fourth or fifth decade of life [12].

Presentation

Presenting features of JF meningioma are nonspecific and most often include HL, lower CN dysfunction, and/or a middle ear mass. In contrast to JF schwannomas, the meningiomas appear more likely to present with lower CN deficit symptoms, such as difficulty swallowing or changes in voice, but they seem to have a decreased incidence of HL at presentation [6]. Single lower CN neuropathy is a common presentation, and is more likely than neuropathy of multiple lower CNs [12]. Conductive HL may result from a tumor extending into the middle ear. Conductive HL from meningioma surrounding the ossicles without causing destruction of the ossicles is a characteristic finding in meningiomas involving the middle ear [34].

Imaging Characteristics

Meningiomas are often described by "dural tails," which result from the "en plaque" spread of the tumor along the dura [15, 35]. These are solid and well-circumscribed extraparenchymal tumors that often demonstrate adjacent, sclerotic bone with increased density on CT (Fig. 69.4). Primary JF meningiomas originate within the JF and are generally more infiltrative with centrifugal growth, resulting in both intraosseous extension and limited expansion of the JF [4]. Although there may be irregular erosion of the bony cortex with JF meningiomas, the amount of JF expansion associated with meningiomas is markedly less than that of schwannomas; this feature aids in distinguishing these tumors [7]. In general, JF meningiomas result in the "permeative-sclerotic" changes of bone, in contrast to the "permeative-destructive" changes associated with JF paragangliomas (compare Fig. 69.4 to Fig. 69.3) [7, 15]. MRI usually demonstrates strong, homogeneous gadolinium enhancement and a "dural tail"; T1 and T2 sequences do not show flow voids (in contrast to the paraganglioma) (Fig. 69.5) [4, 34]. Mass extension into the JF without bony expansion or infiltration has been the standard pattern of growth associated with meningiomas that secondarily grow into the JF and do not originate within it [15].

Treatment

Observation

Observation of meningiomas, like schwannomas, is a reasonable option, particularly for those patients who cannot tolerate surgery or are elderly with small tumors. Meningiomas are also slow growing and require long-term follow-up by exam and serial MRIs.

Surgery

A JF meningioma that is primarily intracranial may be exposed by posterior approaches such as the retrosigmoid approach, which has the potential for hearing preservation. Large meningiomas in the posterior fossa with poor preoperative hearing can be effectively treated through a translabyrinthine approach, which also provides good exposure to the jugular foramen. Meningiomas with more extensive infratemporal involvement or cervical extension are treated through an infratemporal fossa approach. An infratemporal fossa approach with facial nerve routing allows excellent control of vascular structures, direct visualization of lower CNs, and a large corridor for tumor removal. Regardless of the particular approach, it is recommended that a complete resection be attempted due to a high associated recurrence rate [36].

Radiotherapy

Stereotactic radiation for JF meningiomas is a primary treatment option that may be appropriate for patients who are unable to undergo surgery, and as adjunctive therapy if a complete resection is not possible or there is growth of the tumor when monitored on postoperative MRI [4]. Local con-

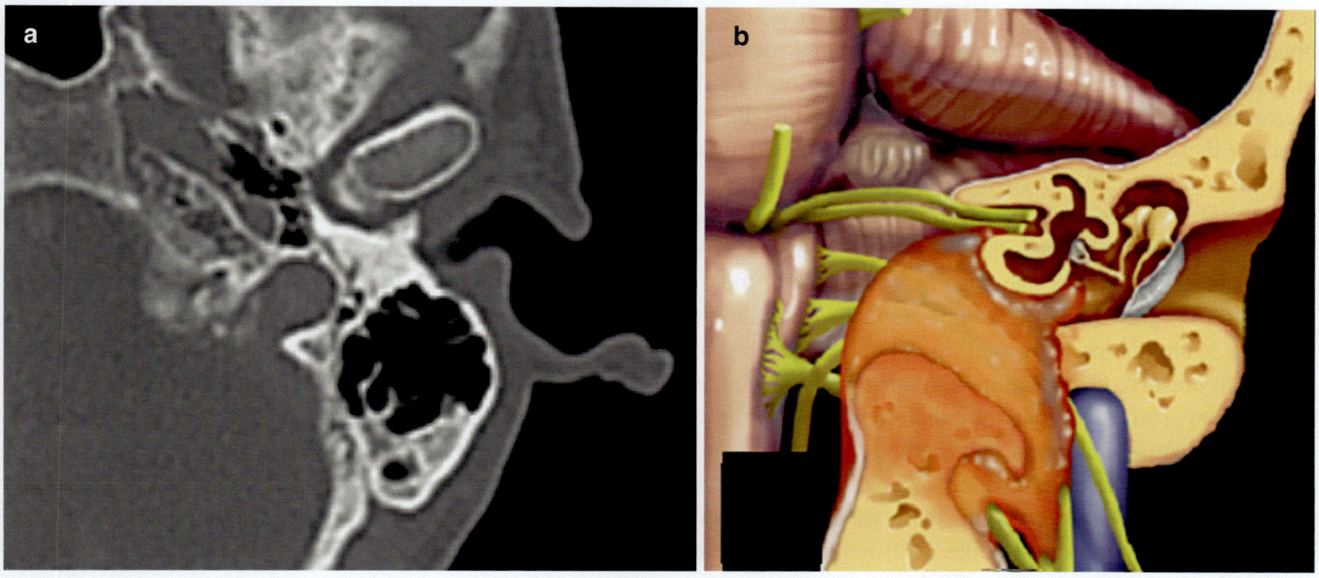

Fig. 69.4 CT (**a**) in the axial plane with a bone algorithm and illustration (**b**) in the coronal plane of hyperostotic changes found adjacent to a jugular foramen meningioma. (Image **b** reproduced from Diagnostic Imaging: Head and Neck, first edition by H. R. Harnsberger et al. with permission from Elsevier)

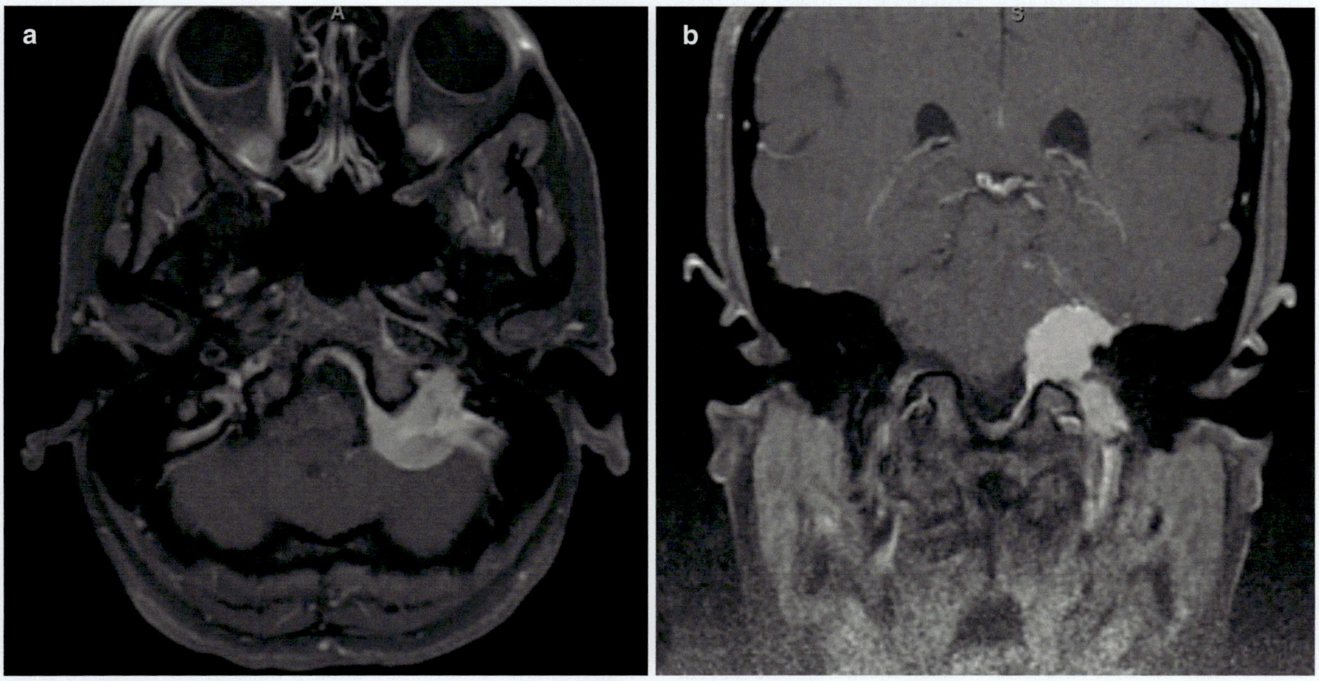

Fig. 69.5 MRI T1 post-contrast with fat saturation showing an avidly enhancing extra-axial mass with dural tails involving the left jugular foramen and cerebellopontine angle in an axial (**a**) and coronal (**b**) plane, consistent with a jugular foramen meningioma. No flow voids are seen within the tumor on T1 and T2 sequences (in contrast to a jugular foramen paraganglioma)

trol rates of 92–100% have been reported after stereotactic radiation for skull base meningiomas; an incidence of associated permanent CN deficits is reported as 1.6–9.8%, and usually less than 5% for any CN toxicity [37]. Stereotactic radiation may also be useful as adjuvant therapy after subtotal resections, though it is recommended that this be reserved specifically for cases of documented growth of residual tumor on postoperative MRI surveillance in order to reduce unnecessary radiation-related morbidity.

Recurrence

JF meningiomas are associated with a higher recurrence rate of 25% after 5 years [4, 36]. Though a more complete resection is also associated with a reduction in this risk of recurrence, a complete resection, including removal of associated bone and dura (Simpson grade I), of intracranial meningiomas is associated with a 5-year recurrence rate of 4%. The increased overall recurrence rate may be related to the tendency of these tumors to invade surrounding bone and, therefore, be less amenable to gross total resection. Attempts at gross total resection, including potentially involved bony margins, may be performed to decrease this recurrence risk, but stereotactic radiation may also be considered if there is postoperative growth of the tumor remnant on follow-up imaging. Subtotal or near-total resection should be performed to preserve CN function with postoperative monitoring for growth with MRI and radiotherapy if there is interval growth of the residual tumor. This method has been shown to be successful in a series of 6 patients who underwent retrosigmoid intradural tumor resection; there were no new lower CN deficits after surgery, and 50% (3/6) required radiotherapy 8–12 months after surgery, which was effective in causing tumor shrinkage or control [38].

Cranial Nerve Outcomes

The 50–60% incidence of new postoperative lower CN dysfunction is greatest for JF meningiomas, relative to paragangliomas (18.9–30%) and JF schwannomas (15–22.2%) [4, 12, 13, 29, 30]. A series of 13 JF meningiomas reported 46.1% HB I or II function postoperatively [35]. CN outcomes after radiotherapy depend on the dose of radiation delivered [37].

Metastatic Lesions

Epidemiology

Temporal bone and intracranial metastasis are surprisingly common occurrences in patients with malignant neoplasms: intracranial metastasis is seen in 15–35% of cancer patients [39, 40], and 22.2% of patients with neoplasms believed to be nondisseminated disease have been found on post-mortem temporal bone histology to have temporal bone metastasis [41]. For systemic malignancy, it is estimated that metastatic disease may involve the skull base, including the JF, in approximately 4% of cases [42]. Primary prostate, thyroid, breast, kidney, and lung malignancies have all been found to metastasize to the JF [43–46].

Presentation

Metastatic disease results in a more rapid development of symptoms and lower cranial neuropathies compared to the other JF tumors discussed in this chapter, and metastatic disease is the most common cause of the multiple lower CN deficits associated with *JF syndrome* [42, 47]. Aside from the more rapid symptom development related to more aggressive tumor behavior, the signs and symptoms of metastatic tumors to the JF are similar, and the types of associated presenting features and neurologic deficits can be found in our earlier discussion of JF.

Imaging Characteristics

On CT, destructive changes of the skull base are seen (Fig. 69.6). These marrow-replacing changes to the osseous surroundings of the JF are also particularly evident on the T1 MRI sequence (Fig. 69.6). Metastases from primary sites such as renal and thyroid carcinoma may appear similar to paragangliomas on MRI (Fig. 69.7) and CT, aside from the particularly aggressive and destructive growth of metastatic lesions. This growth pattern is distinct from the slow growth typically seen for other tumor types, and the predictable growth along the path of least resistance through the JF seen with paragangliomas [47]. Diffusion-weighted MRI sequences and calculation of ADC values may be of utility in distinguishing metastatic lesions from other JF tumor types.

Treatment

Observation

Observation or whole brain radiation therapy (WBRT) are options for patients with metastatic JF tumors who are not surgical candidates.

Surgery

Single JF metastatic tumors are likely to respond best to surgical excision, though disease elsewhere or unacceptable surgical morbidity is likely to preclude many cases of JF metastatic tumors from being appropriate operative candidates [39].

Radiotherapy

For metastatic disease to the JF, WBRT is often recommended with or without surgical excision. Limited data prevent us from making any strong recommendations specific to JF metastatic tumors. A standard dose of 30 Gy in 10 fractions daily has been suggested [48]. Although likely inferior to surgical management, there is a potential role for primary stereotactic radiation therapy for isolated metastatic JF tumors [49, 50].

Chemotherapy

If the primary lesion is known to be sensitive to chemotherapy, this can often be included in the treatment paradigm. Moreover, since malignant lesions that are metastatic to the JF have likely spread elsewhere in the body, systemic chemotherapy or immunotherapy may offer the best palliative treatment.

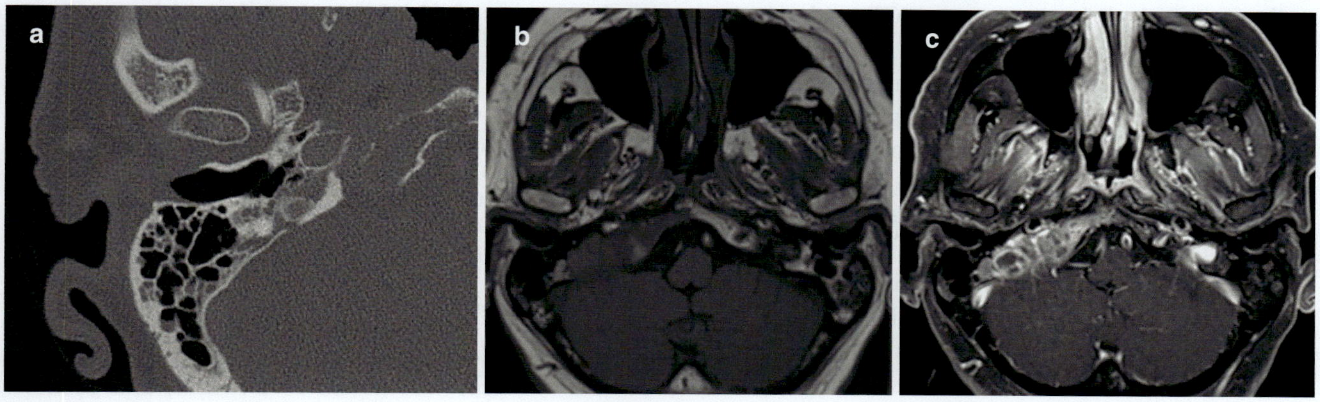

Fig. 69.6 CT findings with metastatic lesions often reflect the aggressive and destructive nature of the metastatic disease. Axial bone algorithm CT demonstrates destructive changes of the bone surrounding the right jugular foramen due to metastatic melanoma (**a**). Corresponding, axial T1-weighted MRI without fat saturation demonstrates marrow replacement (**b**); axial T1-weighted MRI post-contrast with fat saturation demonstrates a cystic, septated, and enhancing mass (**c**)

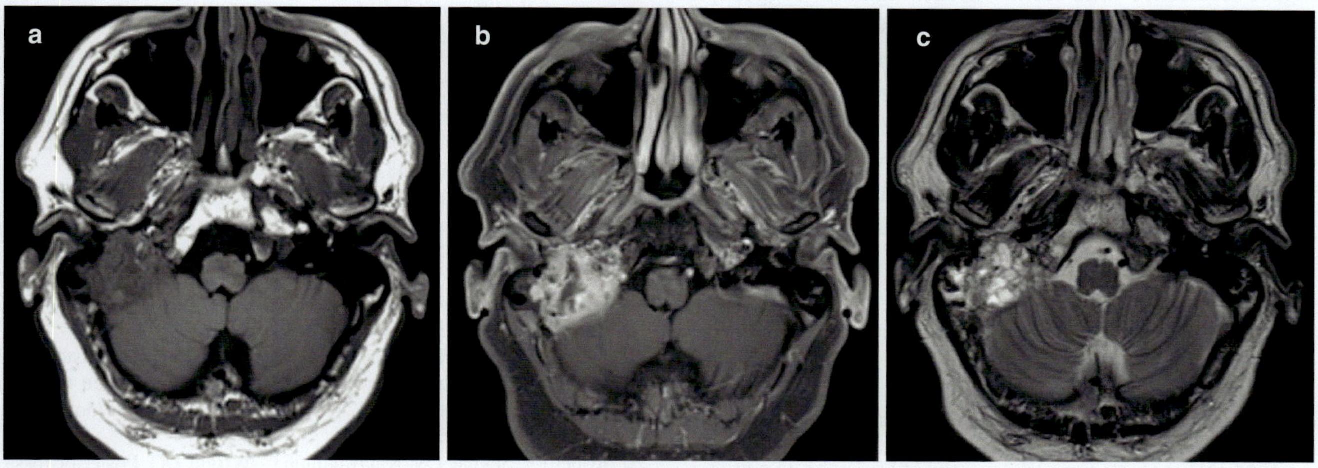

Fig. 69.7 MRI findings of a right jugular foramen metastasis from renal cell carcinoma. Axial MRI shows the following: (**a**) T1 without fat saturation demonstrates low signal intensity with flow voids, (**b**) T1 post-contrast with fat saturation shows avid enhancement, (**c**) T2 demonstrates hyperintensity with flow voids. Notice the similarities in these imaging characteristics to those seen in paraganglioma

Cranial Nerve Outcomes

Lower CN dysfunction of rapid onset is associated with metastatic disease to the JF, likely related to the rapid local growth and destruction seen with metastatic tumors at this location [42, 47]. Postoperative outcomes are unclear, but unlikely to be promising given how locally destructive these tumors are. Doses of approximately 60 Gy to CNs are associated with a 5% rate of dysfunction, and therefore it is recommended to keep radiation doses below 60 Gy to minimize this risk in the treatment of metastatic tumors to the JF [51].

Summary

Non-paraganglioma JF tumors are a rare group, which include schwannomas, meningiomas, chordomas, chondrosarcomas, and metastatic disease originating from the JF. Of these rare tumors, the JF schwannomas and meningiomas are most common. Presentation of all JF tumors is often similar, as it is related to the anatomy of the JF; presenting signs and symptoms may include deficits of the lower CNs, hearing loss, tinnitus, facial weakness, and/or a middle ear mass. The incidence of preoperative lower CN deficit is highest for JF schwannomas, then meningiomas; both have a higher incidence of preoperative lower CN dysfunction than paragangliomas of the JF. However, the incidence of postoperative lower CN dysfunction is highest for meningiomas, then paraganglioma, followed by schwannoma. Metastatic disease to the JF is associated with the highest incidence of multiple preoperative CN deficits and, therefore, is most likely to result in a lower CN syndrome, which includes at least dysfunction of CN IX, X, and XI. As clinical features are often indistinct and variable, imaging is paramount for diagnosis. Both CT and contrasted MRI should be obtained to optimally evaluate both bony structures (CT) and soft tissues (MRI). All of the non-paraganglioma JF tumors, with the exception of metastatic disease, are generally slow growing, and observation is reasonable for appropriate patients (older, unable to tolerate surgery, asymptomatic small tumors). Surgical treatment has traditionally been the preferred modality, though there is growing and promising evidence for stereotactic radiation therapy for the treatment of JF tumors (with the exception of metastatic disease). The optimal approach to microsurgical resection of these tumors depends on a number of patient- and tumor-specific factors, but the most JF-specific anatomic consideration is the extent of intracranial and extracranial involvement of the tumor. Adjuvant stereotactic radiation improves tumor control after subtotal or near-total resection, provides optimal CN outcomes, and may decrease the dose of radiation required. The role of radiation therapy varies by tumor type and behavior; higher recurrence rates seen with meningiomas suggest particular utility of adjuvant radiation for these tumors, though it is often advisable to reserve adjuvant radiation as needed for growth of residual tumor or recurrence. For all tumor types, a long duration of follow-up, including MRI, is recommended as surveillance for tumor growth and recurrence, though intervals of examination and imaging may be progressively extended if there is no recurrent tumor or no growth of residual tumor.

References

1. Rhoton AL Jr, Buza R. Microsurgical anatomy of the jugular foramen. Research Support, U.S. Gov't, P.H.S. J Neurosurg. 1975;42(5):541–50. https://doi.org/10.3171/jns.1975.42.5.0541.
2. Van Loveren HR, Sing Liu S, Pensak ML, Keller JT. Anatomy of the jugular foramen: the neurosurgical perspective. Oper Tech Otolaryngol Head Neck Surg. 1996;7(2):90–4.
3. Inserra MM, Pfister M, Jackler RK. Anatomy involved in the jugular foramen approach for jugulotympanic paraganglioma resection. Review. Neurosurg Focus. 2004;17(2):E6.
4. Gilbert ME, Shelton C, McDonald A, et al. Meningioma of the jugular foramen: glomus jugulare mimic and surgical challenge. Laryngoscope. 2004;114(1):25–32. https://doi.org/10.1097/00005537-200401000-00004.
5. Moffat DA, Hardy DG. Surgical management of large glomus jugulare tumours: infra- and trans-temporal approach. J Laryngol Otol. 1989;103(12):1167–80.
6. Guinto G, Kageyama M, Trujillo-Luarca VH, Abdo M, Ruiz-Than A, Romero-Rangel A. Nonglomic tumors of the jugular foramen: differential diagnosis and prognostic implications. World Neurosurg. 2014;82(6):1283–90. https://doi.org/10.1016/j.wneu.2014.07.013.
7. Szymanska A, Szymanski M, Czekajska-Chehab E, Szczerbo-Trojanowska M. Non-paraganglioma tumors of the jugular foramen – growth patterns, radiological presentation, differential diagnosis. Neurol Neurochir Pol. 2015;49(3):156–63. https://doi.org/10.1016/j.pjnns.2015.04.003.
8. Wilson MA, Hillman TA, Wiggins RH, Shelton C. Jugular foramen schwannomas: diagnosis, management, and outcomes. Laryngoscope. 2005;115(8):1486–92. https://doi.org/10.1097/01.mlg.0000172196.76865.a1.
9. David CA. Preoperative planning and surgical approaches to tumors of the jugular foramen. Oper Tech Neurosurg. 2005;8(1):19–24.
10. Thomas AJ, Wiggins RH 3rd, Gurgel RK. Nonparaganglioma jugular foramen tumors. Review. Otolaryngol Clin N Am. 2015;48(2):343–59. https://doi.org/10.1016/j.otc.2014.12.008.
11. Samii M, Babu RP, Tatagiba M, Sepehrnia A. Surgical treatment of jugular foramen schwannomas. J Neurosurg. 1995;82(6):924–32. https://doi.org/10.3171/jns.1995.82.6.0924.
12. Kryzanski JT, Heilman CB. Clinicopathologic features of jugular foramen tumors. Oper Tech Neurosurg. 2005;8(1):6–12.
13. Fayad JN, Keles B, Brackmann DE. Jugular foramen tumors: clinical characteristics and treatment outcomes. Otol Neurotol. 2010;31(2):299–305. https://doi.org/10.1097/MAO.0b013e3181be6495.
14. Suri A, Bansal S, Singh M, Mahapatra AK, Sharma BS. Jugular foramen schwannomas: a single institution patient series. J Clin Neurosci. 2014;21(1):73–7. https://doi.org/10.1016/j.jocn.2013.02.029.
15. Macdonald AJ, Salzman KL, Harnsberger HR, Gilbert E, Shelton C. Primary jugular foramen meningioma: imaging appearance and differentiating features. Case Reports Review. AJR Am J Roentgenol. 2004;182(2):373–7. https://doi.org/10.2214/ajr.182.2.1820373.
16. Song MH, Lee HY, Jeon JS, Lee JD, Lee HK, Lee WS. Jugular foramen schwannoma: analysis on its origin and location. Otol Neurotol. 2008;29(3):387–91. https://doi.org/10.1097/MAO.0b013e318164cb83.
17. Kaye AH, Hahn JF, Kinney SE, Hardy RW Jr, Bay JW. Jugular foramen schwannomas. Case Reports. J Neurosurg. 1984;60(5):1045–53. https://doi.org/10.3171/jns.1984.60.5.1045.
18. Pellet W, Cannoni M, Pech A. The widened transcochlear approach to jugular foramen tumors. J Neurosurg. 1988;69(6):887–94. https://doi.org/10.3171/jns.1988.69.6.0887.
19. Samii M, Alimohamadi M, Gerganov V. Endoscope-assisted retrosigmoid infralabyrinthine approach to jugular foramen tumors. Case Reports. J Neurosurg. 2016;124(4):1061–7. https://doi.org/10.3171/2015.3.JNS142904.
20. Roberti F, Sekhar LN, Kalavakonda C, Wright DC. Posterior fossa meningiomas: surgical experience in 161 cases. Surg Neurol. 2001;56(1):8–20; discussion 20–1
21. Pensak ML, Jackler RK. Removal of jugular foramen tumors: the fallopian bridge technique. Otolaryngol Head Neck Surg. 1997;117(6):586–91.
22. Martin JJ, Kondziolka D, Flickinger JC, Mathieu D, Niranjan A, Lunsford LD. Cranial nerve preservation and outcomes after stereotactic radiosurgery for jugular foramen schwannomas. Clinical Trial. Neurosurgery. 2007;61(1):76–81 ; discussion 81. https://doi.org/10.1227/01.neu.0000279726.90650.6d.
23. Sedney CL, Nonaka Y, Bulsara KR, Fukushima T. Microsurgical management of jugular foramen schwannomas. Neurosurgery. 2013;72(1):42–6; discussion 46. https://doi.org/10.1227/NEU.0b013e3182770e74.
24. Cavalcanti DD, Martirosyan NL, Verma K, et al. Surgical management and outcome of schwannomas in the craniocervical region. J Neurosurg. 2011;114(5):1257–67. https://doi.org/10.3171/2010.5.JNS0966.
25. van de Langenberg R, Hanssens PE, van Overbeeke JJ, et al. Management of large vestibular schwannoma. Part I. Planned subtotal resection followed rjr: radiological and clinical aspects. J Neurosurg. 2011;115(5):875–84. https://doi.org/10.3171/2011.6.JNS101958.
26. Hasegawa T, Kato T, Kida Y, et al. Gamma knife surgery for patients with jugular foramen schwannomas: a multiinstitutional retrospec-

tive study in Japan. J Neurosurg. 2016;125(4):822–31. https://doi.org/10.3171/2015.8.JNS151156.
27. Kano H, Meola A, Yang HC, et al. Stereotactic radiosurgery for jugular foramen schwannomas: an international multicenter study. J Neurosurg. 2018;129(4):928–36. https://doi.org/10.3171/2017.5.Jns162894.
28. Milligan BD, Pollock BE, Foote RL, Link MJ. Long-term tumor control and cranial nerve outcomes following gamma knife surgery for larger-volume vestibular schwannomas. Case Reports. Review. J Neurosurg. 2012;116(3):598–604. https://doi.org/10.3171/2011.11.JNS11811.
29. Lustig LR, Jackler RK. The variable relationship between the lower cranial nerves and jugular foramen tumors: implications for neural preservation. Review. Am J Otol. 1996;17(4):658–68.
30. Ramina R, Neto MC, Fernandes YB, Aguiar PH, de Meneses MS, Torres LF. Meningiomas of the jugular foramen. Case Reports. Neurosurg Rev. 2006;29(1):55–60. https://doi.org/10.1007/s10143-005-0415-4.
31. Coscarella E, Tummala RP, Morcos JJ. Infratemporal fossa approaches to the jugular foramen. Oper Tech Neurosurg. 2005;8(1):25–30.
32. Cokkeser Y, Brackmann DE, Fayad JN. Conservative facial nerve management in jugular foramen schwannomas. Case Reports. Am J Otol. 2000;21(2):270–4.
33. Sanna M, Bacciu A, Falcioni M, Taibah A, Piazza P. Surgical management of jugular foramen meningiomas: a series of 13 cases and review of the literature. Case Reports Research Support, Non--U.S. Gov't Review. Laryngoscope. 2007;117(10):1710–9. https://doi.org/10.1097/MLG.0b013e3180cc20a3.
34. Hamilton BE, Salzman KL, Patel N, et al. Imaging and clinical characteristics of temporal bone meningioma. AJNR Am J Neuroradiol. 2006;27(10):2204–9.
35. Toyama C, Santiago Gebrim EM, Brito R, Bento RF. Primary jugular foramen meningioma. Case Reports. Otol Neurotol. 2008;29(3):417–8. https://doi.org/10.1097/MAO.0b013e31815882ba.
36. Molony TB, Brackmann DE, Lo WW. Meningiomas of the jugular foramen. Otolaryngol Head Neck Surg. 1992;106(2):128–36.
37. Combs SE, Ganswindt U, Foote RL, Kondziolka D, Tonn JC. State-of-the-art treatment alternatives for base of skull meningiomas: complementing and controversial indications for neurosurgery, stereotactic and robotic based radiosurgery or modern fractionated radiation techniques. Review. Radiat Oncol. 2012;7:226. https://doi.org/10.1186/1748-717X-7-226.
38. Ito S, Saegusa T, Ozawa Y, et al. Function-preserving multimodal treatment for jugular foramen meningiomas. J Neurol Surg B Skull Base. 2019;80(3):239–43. https://doi.org/10.1055/s-0038-1668137.
39. Mintz A, Perry J, Spithoff K, Chambers A, Laperriere N. Management of single brain metastasis: a practice guideline. Curr Oncol. 2007;14(4):131–43.
40. Paek SH, Audu PB, Sperling MR, Cho J, Andrews DW. Reevaluation of surgery for the treatment of brain metastases: review of 208 patients with single or multiple brain metastases treated at one institution with modern neurosurgical techniques. Neurosurgery. 2005;56(5):1021–34; discussion 1021–34
41. Gloria-Cruz TI, Schachern PA, Paparella MM, Adams GL, Fulton SE. Metastases to temporal bones from primary nonsystemic malignant neoplasms. Research Support, Non-U.S. Gov't. Research Support, U.S. Gov't, P.H.S. Arch Otolaryngol Head Neck Surg 2000;126(2):209–14.
42. Hayward D, Morgan C, Emami B, Biller J, Prabhu VC. Jugular foramen syndrome as initial presentation of metastatic lung cancer. J Neurol Surg Rep. 2012;73(1):14–8. https://doi.org/10.1055/s-0032-1301406.
43. Balasubramaniam S, Deshpande RB, Misra BK. Gamma knife radiosurgery in jugular foramen endolymphatic sac adenocarcinoma. Case Reports. J Clin Neurosci. 2009;16(5):710–1. https://doi.org/10.1016/j.jocn.2008.07.086.
44. Thomas AJ, Wiggins RH 3rd, Gurgel RK. Metastatic renal cell carcinoma masquerading as jugular foramen paraganglioma: a role for novel magnetic resonance imaging. Ann Otol Rhinol Laryngol. 2017;126(8):606–10. https://doi.org/10.1177/0003489417714487.
45. Ciavarro G, Bozzetti F, Falcioni M. Jugular foramen metastasis from lung cancer: a case of "a mass without his syndrome". J Int Adv Otol. 2019;15(3):469–71. https://doi.org/10.5152/iao.2019.6540.
46. Aydin I, Sayyahmelli S, Pyle M, Baskaya MK. Gross total resection of a jugular foramen thyroid medullary metastasis via a transjugular transsigmoid approach. J Neurol Surg B Skull Base. 2018;79(Suppl 5):S424–s425. https://doi.org/10.1055/s-0038-1669970.
47. Caldemeyer KS, Mathews VP, Azzarelli B, Smith RR. The jugular foramen: a review of anatomy, masses, and imaging characteristics. Radiographics. 1997;17(5):1123–39. https://doi.org/10.1148/radiographics.17.5.9308106.
48. Tsao MN, Lloyd N, Wong RK, et al. Whole brain radiotherapy for the treatment of newly diagnosed multiple brain metastases. Meta-Analysis Research Support, Non-U.S. Gov't Review. Cochrane Database Syst Rev 2012;4:CD003869. https://doi.org/10.1002/14651858.CD003869.pub3.
49. Nieder C, Grosu AL, Gaspar LE. Stereotactic radiosurgery (SRS) for brain metastases: a systematic review. Radiat Oncol. 2014;9(1):155. https://doi.org/10.1186/1748-717X-9-155.
50. Yomo S, Hayashi M. A minimally invasive treatment option for large metastatic brain tumors: long-term results of two-session gamma knife stereotactic radiosurgery. Radiat Oncol. 2014;9:132. https://doi.org/10.1186/1748-717X-9-132.
51. Hauptman JS, Barkhoudarian G, Safaee M, et al. Challenges in linear accelerator radiotherapy for chordomas and chondrosarcomas of the skull base: focus on complications. Int J Radiat Oncol Biol Phys. 2012;83(2):542–51. https://doi.org/10.1016/j.ijrobp.2011.08.004.

Endolymphatic Sac Tumors

70

Cameron C. Wick, Nauman F. Manzoor, Maroun T. Semaan, Cliff A. Megerian, and Sarah E. Mowry

Introduction

Endolymphatic sac tumors (ELST) are slow-growing, locally aggressive, low-grade malignancies that originate from the epithelium of the endolymphatic duct and sac. The classification of adenomatous tumors arising from the temporal bone has undergone many changes. A brief review of those name changes and classification schemes shows how we arrived at the current understanding of ELST pathophysiology. It also explains the nearly 300% increase in ELST publications from 2000–2010 compared to 1984–1999 [1].

The origin of adenomatous tumors in the temporal bone has long been a source of investigation. In 1957, Johnstone et al. recognized that adenomas and adenocarcinomas of the external auditory canal originated from apocrine glands of the canal, thus coining the term "ceruminoma" [2]. The origin of primary adenomatous tumors within the middle ear cleft continued to be debated. Some authors hypothesized that aberrant ceruminous glands were responsible, while others thought the tumors arose from native middle ear mucosa [3, 4].

In 1988, Gaffey et al. recognized a particularly aggressive variant of "low-grade papillary adenocarcinoma" in the temporal bone that exhibited hypervascularity and local invasion with bony destruction [5]. The following year, a series with 20 cases had similar papillary architecture that was centered along the posteromedial petrous bone, which led to the name "adenocarcinoma of the endolymphatic sac (AES)" [6]. This was the first report to suggest that aggressive adenomatous tumors of the temporal bone originated from endolymphatic sac epithelium. A prior study from 1984 had incidentally found a small adenomatous lesion during decompression surgery for Ménière's disease, but the correlation between that small tumor contained within the sac and larger, aggressive variants was not made [7].

Still, proof that these tumors did not originate as adenocarcinomas of the middle ear, metastases, or choroid plexus tumors continued to be debated [8–12]. In 1995, Megerian et al. found eight specimens from the Massachusetts Eye and Ear Infirmary's temporal bone collection that were consistent with aggressive papillary tumors of the temporal bone. All patients had sensorineural hearing loss (SNHL), and many had a Ménière's-like presentation. One patient, a 48-year-old male with von Hippel-Lindau syndrome (VHL), was believed to have had metastatic renal cell carcinoma to the left temporal bone, but upon further analysis, this tumor was more consistent with a local, aggressive papillary lesion. Fortuitously, in this patient's contralateral temporal bone, a small *de novo* lesion within the endolymphatic sac was also identified and was histologically identical to the destructive lesion on the contralateral side [13]. The importance of this study was threefold. First, it validated that the epithelium of the endolymphatic sac was capable of producing a low-grade papillary tumor with potential for local expansion and an insidious outcome. Secondly, it gave merit to the proposed renaming scheme of "endolymphatic sac tumors." [14] Finally, it suggested that patients with VHL are predisposed to ELST.

Follow-up studies further confirmed ELST as a unique entity from choroid plexus tumors, despite very similar appearances on hematoxylin and eosin staining. The distinction was that choroid plexus pathology stains strongly for transthyretin (prealbumin), while ELST does not [15]. The modern discovery of ELST has enabled appreciation of its natural history, associations with other diseases, development of a staging classification system, and improved outcomes.

C. C. Wick · M. T. Semaan · C. A. Megerian · S. E. Mowry (✉)
Department of Otolaryngology—Head and Neck Surgery, University Hospitals Cleveland Medical Center, Cleveland, OH, USA
e-mail: Sarah.Mowry@UHhospitals.org

N. F. Manzoor
Department of Otolaryngology—Head and Neck Surgery, Virginia Commonwealth University, Richmond, VA, USA

A. D. Sweeney et al. (eds.), *Haynes-Glasscock-Shambaugh Surgery of the Ear*, https://doi.org/10.1007/978-3-032-18264-7_70

Clinical Presentation

ELSTs are rare tumors, and the true incidence is unknown. Sporadic ELST are more common than those associated with VHL. Sporadic ELSTs have been diagnosed over a wide age range (15–77 years), with the mean age between 40 years and 50 years [16, 17]. There is no gender predilection for sporadic cases [13].

Cochleovestibular dysfunction is the most common presenting symptom. Most patients will have some degree of SNHL (86–100%) and tinnitus (71–89%). Asymmetric complaints are common [16–18]. The degree of SNHL does not always correlate with tumor extension. A sudden hearing loss may occur in up to 43% of patients and is thought to be from intralabyrinthine hemorrhage, which leads to inflammation and neural degeneration. Gradual SNHL is hypothesized to be from secondary endolymphatic hydrops or direct otic capsule invasion [19–21]. Vertigo and aural fullness are present in 70% and 37% of patients, respectively [17, 21]. The presentation of SNHL, tinnitus, aural fullness, and vertigo mimics Ménière's disease and may delay diagnosis [13, 22, 23]. This point illustrates that Ménière's disease is a diagnosis of exclusion, and imaging to exclude lesions like ELST is a necessary part of the workup [24, 25].

Other cranial neuropathies may also accompany ELST, depending on where the tumors extend. Facial nerve weakness is seen in 5–43% of cases [1, 17, 21]. Trigeminal and glossopharyngeal neuropathies have also been reported. Slow tumor progression accounts for an average delay between symptom onset and radiologic tumor detection of 10 years [13]. From its origin at the posteromedial aspect of the temporal bone, ELST most commonly spreads posteriorly into the cerebellopontine angle. With significant brain stem compression, headache and hydrocephalus may develop. Lateral extension via the middle ear and mastoid is the next most common pathway and may involve the facial nerve or produce symptoms that mimic chronic otitis media and Eustachian tube dysfunction [1, 26]. ELSTs have even eroded through the middle ear cleft and been diagnosed as an external auditory canal mass. Superior extension through the semicircular canals and into the middle fossa can also contribute to imbalance. Finally, anterior extension along the petrous ridge with invasion of the clivus, cavernous sinus, or sphenoid sinus can result in death [18, 27]. There have been no reports of distant hematogenous metastasis, although "drop metastasis" to the spinal column, causing lower extremity paralysis have been reported [28, 29]. Additionally, cerebrospinal fluid cytology has revealed large epithelioid cells in a patient with a known ELST that were consistent with prior cytological ELST descriptions [30, 31].

Association with von Hippel-Lindau Syndrome

VHL was first described in the early twentieth century by the German ophthalmologist Eugene von Hippel and the Swedish pathologist Arvid Lindau [32]. VHL is an autosomal dominant multisystem syndrome characterized by both central nervous system (CNS) and visceral lesions. The CNS lesions include retinal and craniospinal hemangioblastomas and ELST. The visceral lesions include renal cell carcinoma, renal or pancreatic cysts, pheochromocytomas, extra-adrenal paragangliomas, pancreatic neuroendocrine tumors, and cystadenomas of the epididymis and broad ligament [33].

In contrast to sporadic tumors, VHL-associated ELST present earlier with a mean age of 22 years at the time of diagnosis and have a 2:1 female predominance. The VHL incidence is 1 in 39,000 individuals, and the penetrance is high, approaching 90% [33, 34]. Those afflicted with VHL have between a 3.6% and 16% chance of developing a unilateral ELST, with most reports indicating the risk is between 11% and 16% [35–38]. Among the patients with VHL-associated ELST, the risk of having bilateral disease is between 14% and 30% [35–37, 39, 40].

Von Hippel-Lindau syndrome is the result of a mutated *VHL gene*. Since its discovery in 1988, multiple mutations have been described, ranging from deletions to missense mutations [41]. Germline mutations account for 95% of individuals affected by VHL, and the majority (60–70%) carry a missense mutation [42]. The *VHL* locus is on the short arm of chromosome 3 (3p25.5) and encodes the VHL protein (pVHL) [43].

pVHL functions as a tumor suppressor through the E3 ubiquitin ligase complex. This protein complex targets the degradation of Hypoxia Inducible Factor (HIF)1-alpha. Normally, patients have two copies of the wild-type (normal) *VHL* allele. Those with VHL have one mutated allele; therefore, when the wild-type allele is inactivated (loss of heterozygosity), the patient becomes susceptible to VHL-related tumors (tumorigenesis). (Table 70.1) [33, 42]. HIF regulates angiogenesis and cell metabolism. In the hypoxic state, HIF

Table 70.1 von Hippel-Lindau-related tumors

Central nervous system tumors	Visceral tumors
Retinal hemangioblastoma Craniospinal hemangioblastoma Endolymphatic sac tumors	Renal cell carcinoma Renal or pancreatic cysts Pheochromocytomas Extra-adrenal paragangliomas Pancreatic neuroendocrine tumors Cystadenomas (epididymis/broad ligament)

is down-regulated to allow an increase in vascular endothelial growth factor (VEGF), erythropoietin (EPO), EPO receptor, transferrin, and angiopoietin. In VHL, HIF is not down-regulated in certain organs, creating an environment for the growth of highly vascular tumors [44–46].

Histology

ELST are low-grade, locally infiltrative, highly vascular, poorly circumscribed neoplasms. They are grossly described as polypoid lesions. On light microscopy, they have two distinct patterns: papillary and follicular. The papillary pattern refers to cuboidal or low columnar epithelial cells arranged in papillary projections (Fig. 70.1). In contrast, the follicular pattern is cystic with spaces that contain proteinaceous material reminiscent of a thyroid follicle, but thyroglobulin stains are negative. Some tumors may display both features [6, 13, 19]. The differential diagnosis includes middle ear adenoma, adenocarcinoma, paraganglioma, choroid plexus papilloma, adenoid cystic carcinoma of the ceruminal gland, and metastatic adenocarcinoma (thyroid and kidney) [15, 47]. Cytology is rarely necessary, but if obtained, intratumor cystic contents and CSF samples have been described as epithelial cell clusters with papillary features, foamy macrophages, and blood [29, 30].

Immunohistochemical staining helps differentiate ELST from the other pathologies on the differential. The endolymphatic sac is a neuroectoderm-derived structure; therefore, ELST are cytokeratin and vimentin-positive. The majority stain positive for S-100 as well. Differentiating from paraganglioma may be aided by the chromogranin-negative immunohistochemical profile of ELST. Choroid plexus tumors are distinctly transthyretin positive, whereas ELST are negative. ELST are thyroglobulin negative, a feature that helps to differentiate them from metastatic thyroid cancer. The staining patterns are summarized in Table 70.2 [15, 16, 47–50].

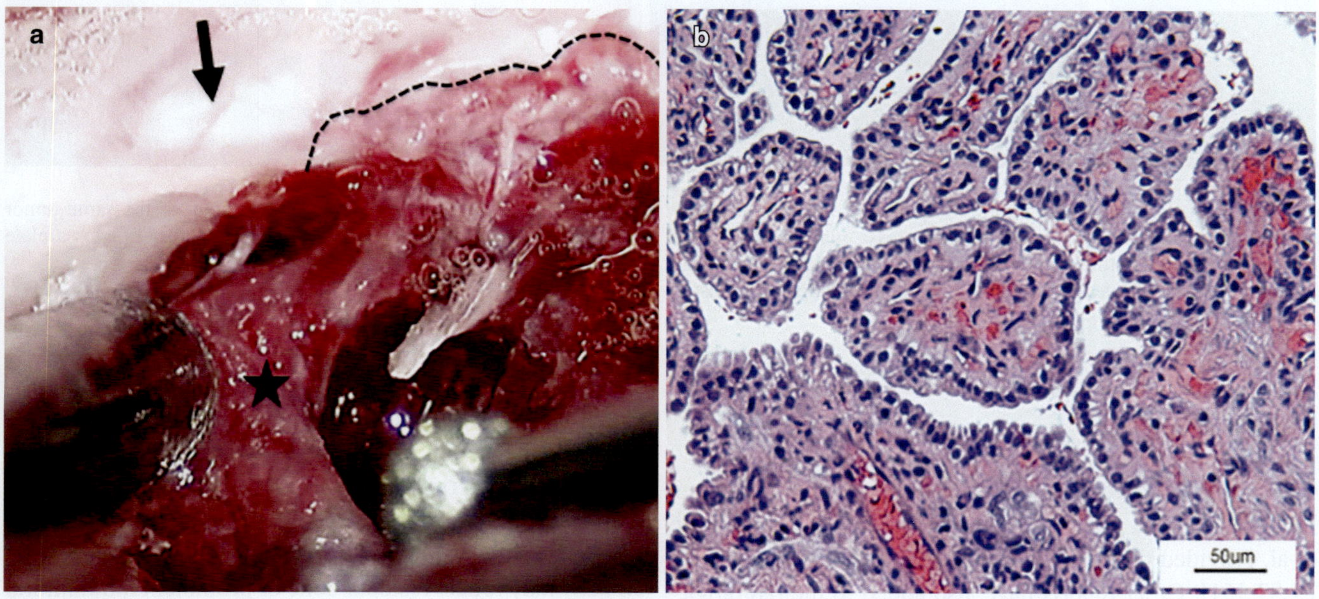

Fig. 70.1 (**a**) Intraoperative photo from a left translabyrinthine approach for endolymphatic sac tumor (ELST) resection. The vascular, polypoid, and poorly circumscribed tumor (star) is being resected from the retrofacial space. Tumor has eroded (dashed line) into the fallopian canal (arrow). (**b**) Low-power light microscopy of the same tumor depicts a papillary pattern with common cystic areas lined by cuboidal epithelial cells disposed in a fibrous, vascular stroma

Table 70.2 Endolymphatic sac tumor differential diagnosis and immunohistochemical stains

IHC Target	ELST	Paraganglioma	Thyroid metastasis	Renal cell metastasis	Ceruminoma	Choroid plexus adenoma
Cytokeratin	+	–		+	++	*Variable*
Vimentin	+		+	+		±
S-100	±			+	+	±
Transthyretin	–					±
Thyroglobulin	–		+	–		
Chromogranin	–	+		–		

ELST endolymphatic sac tumor, *IHC* immunohistochemical

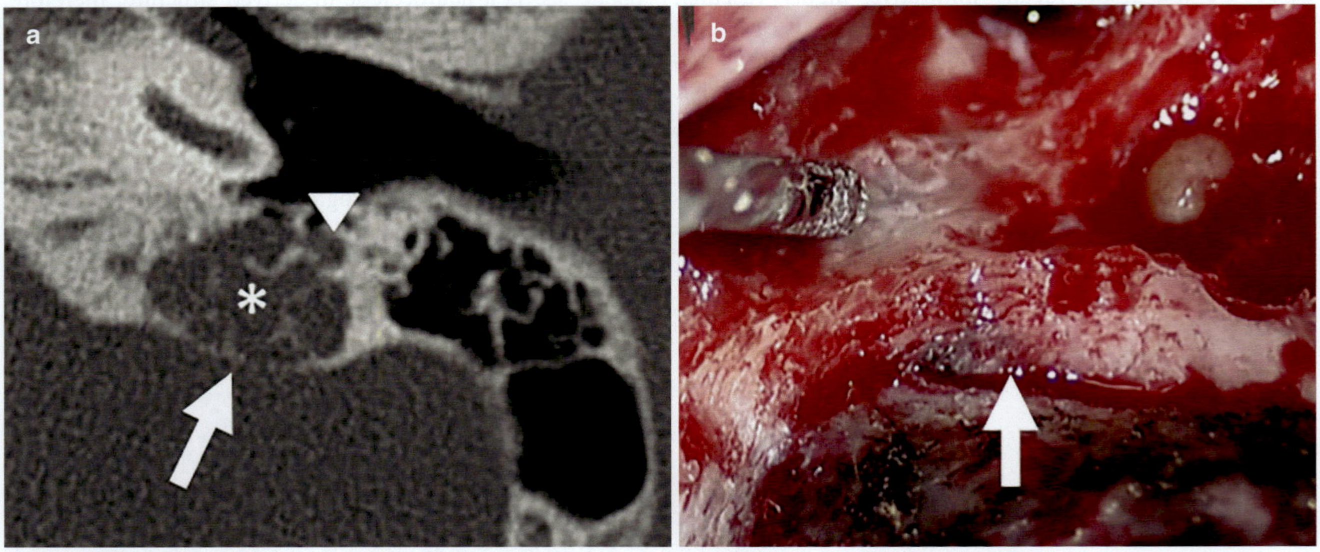

Fig. 70.2 (**a**) Computed tomography without contrast of the left temporal bone shows erosion of the posterior fossa plate (arrow) with extension into the mastoid cavity (asterisk) and effacement of the facial nerve (arrowhead). Note the intratumor central spiculations and posterior rim calcification. (**b**) An intraoperative view of the same tumor demonstrates the gross appearance of the eroded posterior fossa plate (arrow)

Imaging

Characteristic radiographic findings can help to diagnose ELST and aid in preoperative planning. In 1997, Mukherji et al. provided the first comprehensive radiologic review of ELST [51]. Other reports have also added to the radiologic profile [52–54].

Computed tomography (CT) shows bone erosion centered over the endolymphatic sac at the posteromedial temporal bone. Its highly vascular nature manifests as intense enhancement with contrast. Prominent intratumor (central) spiculations and posterior rim calcification are often seen (Fig. 70.2). These tumors often widen or erode the endolymphatic duct as well. On magnetic resonance imaging (MRI), ELST show heterogeneous foci of low and high signal intensity on T1- and T2-weighted sequences. The hyperintense areas on non-contrasted T1-weighted MRI are due to intraparenchymal hemorrhage and subsequent deposition of methemoglobin, hemosiderin, and cholesterol crystals. Intralabyrinthine hyperintensity without contrast suggests an intralabyrinthine hemorrhage, even in radiographically small or undetectable tumors. Intralabyrinthine hemorrhage can also be seen on fluid-attenuated inversion recovery (FLAIR) sequences, which correlate with sudden SNHL [55]. Hypointense areas on MRI may reflect residual bone or prominent intratumoral calcifications. With gadolinium contrast, the tumors will demonstrate heterogeneous enhancement and, if large enough, may have flow voids analogous to those seen with paragangliomas (Fig. 70.3) [53, 54]. New imaging modalities, like ^{68}Ga DOTATATE PET/CT, may take advantage of differential surface protein expression. This octreotide derivative binds to somatostatin receptors on the cell membrane, which are expressed on ELST cells and other neuroendocrine tumors [57].

Angiography can be both diagnostic and therapeutic for ELST. The blood supply for the endolymphatic duct arises from either the inferior tympanic artery, which is a branch of the ascending pharyngeal artery; a dural branch of the stylo-

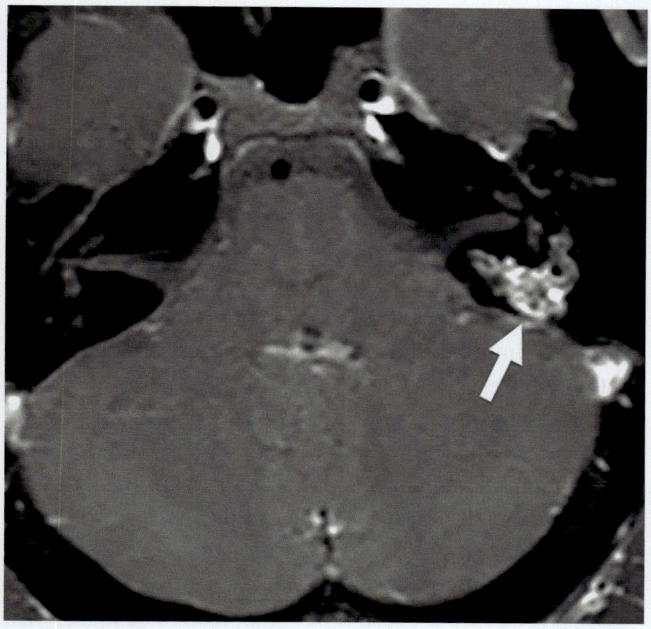

Fig. 70.3 Axial T1-weighted magnetic resonance imaging with contrast demonstrates heterogeneous enhancement in the left mastoid region (arrow). On the T1-weighted images, the "salt and pepper" appearance caused by flow voids or intratumor calcifications can make endolymphatic sac tumors difficult to distinguish from paragangliomas, particularly if the jugular bulb is involved

mastoid artery; or a branch from the posterior auricular artery. If angiography confirms that a main feeding vessel arises from the external carotid circulation, then preoperative embolization can greatly assist the surgical efforts [51]. The radiographic differential diagnosis for ELST includes paragangliomas (glomus jugulare or glomus tympanicum), choroid plexus tumors, ceruminoma, metastasis (particularly thyroid or renal cell), eosinophilic granuloma, meningioma, arachnoid granulation, aneurysmal bone cyst, plasmacytoma, or a primary bone tumor [15, 16, 48–50, 54, 58, 59].

Staging and Surveillance

In 2004, a retrospective analysis of 149 ELST led to an anatomical classification system, the Bambakidis and Megerian grading system for ELST [16]. This grading scheme also provides surgical treatment options based on the extent of tumor invasion and hearing status (Table 70.3) [16, 60]. The review by Bambakidis et al. found that ELST in patients with VHL tend to be diagnosed at a lower grade compared to sporadic tumors (grade 1, 40% versus 25%; $p < 0.05$). Routine radiographic surveillance in VHL likely accounts for earlier detection and hence lower-grade tumors. The lower grade of VHL-associated ELST reflects the more frequent use of MRI for routine surveillance of patients with VHL.

Table 70.3 Grading and treatment system for endolymphatic sac tumors

Grade	Tumor extent	Surgical options
I	Confined to temporal bone, middle ear cavity, and/or external auditory canal	Hearing preservation with retrolabyrinthine transdural approach
II	Extension into posterior fossa	Extended retrolabyrinthine transdural approach; approach with labyrinthectomy if hearing poor[a]
III	Extension in posterior fossa and middle cranial fossa	Subtemporal craniotomy with petrosectomy[a]
IV	Extension to clivus and/or sphenoid wing	Staged anterior and posterior fossa techniques[a]

Derived from Bambakidis et al. [16]

[a]Preoperative embolization for grades II–IV and postoperative stereotactic radiosurgery for postoperative residual disease may be adjunctive

Currently, there are no established guidelines for VHL surveillance or early detection of VHL-associated ELST. Institutional practices vary and should be tailored to the patient's overall tumor burden. Subjective hearing changes should prompt immediate audiometric testing and consideration of repeat imaging. MRI sequences with thin slices through the internal auditory canal are useful to detect early disease [37]. Patients with VHL carry between an 11% and 16% risk of having a unilateral ELST. Those with a VHL-associated ELST have an approximately 30% risk of having bilateral disease. Subclinical disease may also be present before a tumor is radiographically visible [16, 35]. Support for microscopic foci and subclinical disease comes from a report that found 65% of ears in patients with VHL had SNHL, even though only 6% showed evidence of a tumor [35]. If the disease is stable, MRI repeated on an annual or biennial basis is advised and is often driven by other more common VHL-related tumors, like craniospinal hemangioblastomas. Genetic testing for all ELST patients is advised but is particularly important for patients and family members with VHL [33, 37]. Whether the ELST is sporadic or VHL-associated, early diagnosis and lower tumor grades offer greater potential for hearing preservation, less morbid treatment, and disease eradication.

Treatment

Surgery

The mainstay of ELST management remains complete surgical excision. Surgical approaches have evolved with new knowledge regarding the tumor's natural history and growth patterns. For the appropriately sized tumor (Grade I and some Grade II), a hearing preservation approach may be attempted. The approach, termed the retrolabyrinthine-transdural approach, enables removal of the tumor with both sides of the dural sleeve and preservation of the inner ear [20, 39].

The retrolabyrinthine-transdural approach begins with the patient in a supine position. Hair is shaved, but head frame placement is not necessary. Facial nerve monitoring is used, and paralytics are avoided. Using an extended postauricular incision, a mastoidectomy is performed with identification of the horizontal semicircular canal and facial nerve. The jugular bulb is skeletonized, as are the tegmen mastoideum and sinodural angle. All pre-sigmoid bone covering the posterior fossa dura is then removed, and the posterior semicircular canal is blue-lined. This exposure should facilitate visualization of the hypervascular endolymphatic sac and tumor. The endolymphatic duct is followed with a diamond drill under the posterior semicircular canal toward the vestibule. The tumor is removed by cutting away the posterior fossa dura along with a margin around the diseased endolymphatic sac and duct (Figs. 70.4 and 70.5). After the resection, the antrum and any open-air cells are sealed with bone wax and can be covered with temporalis fascia. A dural substitute and abdominal fat seal the dura. Additional reinforcement with a tissue sealant can help prevent cerebrospinal fluid leaks.

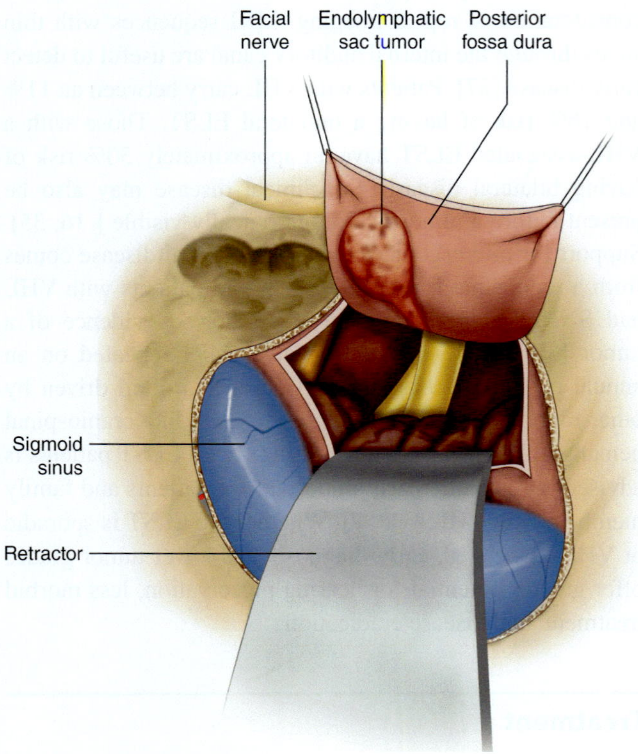

Fig. 70.4 Illustration of a left retrolabyrinthine-transdural approach for resection of an endolymphatic sac tumor (ELST). This hearing preservation approach for Grade I and some Grade II tumors allows complete resection of the endolymphatic sac and duct, including their medial wall. The posterior semicircular canal is visualized to avoid labyrinthine injury. (Adapted from Megerian et al. [37])

Prior to the description of the retrolabyrinthine-transdural approach, a more limited transmastoid approach had been advocated. The transmastoid approach involves a cortical mastoidectomy with removal of the posterior petrous plate. The endolymphatic sac is then peeled from the inner dural sleeve rather than complete resection of the involved dura. While this may prevent a larger opening into the posterior fossa and limit cerebrospinal fluid leakage, it risks inadequate tumor resection [39]. Similarly, a posterior fossa (retrosigmoid) approach leaves the outer dural sleeve intact and lacks direct visualization of the posterior semicircular canal during tumor dissection [20, 39]. Therefore, in small tumors with serviceable hearing, the preferred approach is retrolabyrinthine-transdural. If the patient has non-serviceable hearing, a translabyrinthine approach is advised.

Lesions that are a Grade II or higher tend to be highly vascular, putting them at risk for significant intraoperative bleeding. Preoperative embolization should be considered in these situations. Exposure of larger lesions is usually adequate through the translabyrinthine approach. Pronounced anterior tumor extension may require the use of combined approaches: subtemporal transpetrosal, transotic, or infratemporal fossa. Likewise, posterior or inferior intracranial tumor extension may benefit from a retrosigmoid approach. In cases that present with non-serviceable hearing, or cases in which the approach sacrifices hearing, a cochlear implant may be considered as long as the cochlea and cochlear nerve are intact. This situation is particularly relevant for VHL-associated ELST that have a higher rate of bilateral disease [61–64].

The rarity of these tumors prevents large case series, and to date, there have been no systematic reviews or meta-analyses. Therefore, outcomes data are largely derived from institutional experiences and limited case reports. The House Ear Clinic published its single institutional experience with surgical management of ELST in 2013 [17]. They reported on 18 patients, all treated with microsurgical techniques for tumors with a mean size of 2.4 cm. Total resection was possible in 17 of 18 (94%) tumors, and after a mean follow-up of 67 months, 16 patients (89%) remained disease-free. Most patients had significant hearing loss prior to surgery, but the two candidates with serviceable hearing maintained it following a retrolabyrinthine-transdural approach. Good preoperative facial function was present in 13 of 18 patients (72%), and all but two of them maintained it. Excluding CN VII and VIII injuries, the most common complications involved lower cranial nerve damage (CN IX, X, or XII) in 4 patients (22%). Additionally, there were 3 cerebrospinal fluid leaks and 2 cases of hydrocephalus. In reviewing the literature, the

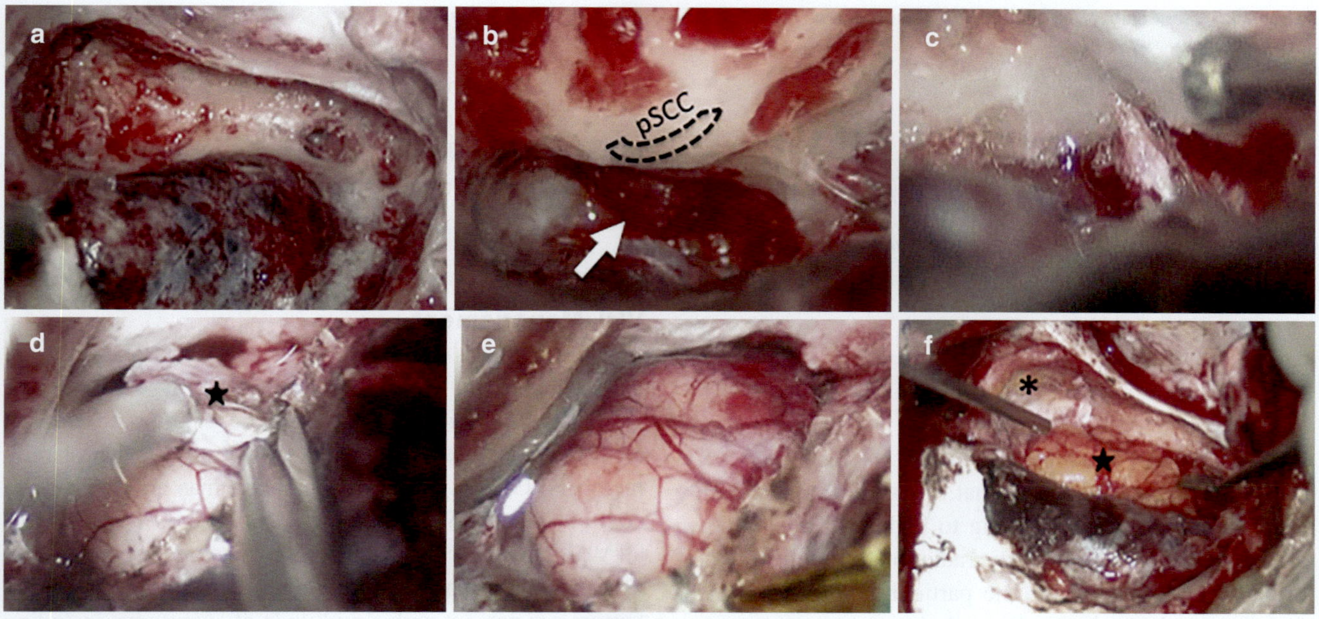

Fig. 70.5 Intraoperative pictures from a right-sided retrolabyrinthine-transdural hearing preservation approach for resection of an endolymphatic sac tumor (ELST). (**a**) A cortical mastoidectomy is performed with removal of bone over the sigmoid sinus and posterior fossa dura. (**b**) ELST (arrow) is seen inferior and medial to the posterior semicircular canal (pSCC, dashed line). (**c**) The endolymphatic duct is drilled out under the pSCC to expose the operculum. (**d**) The endolymphatic sac, duct, and posterior fossa dura are excised *en bloc* (star). (**e**) After resection, the cerebellum and posterior fossa are exposed. (**f**) Reconstruction is performed with a dural substitute (not pictured), abdominal fat (star), fascia (asterisk) to block the antrum, and tissue sealant (not pictured). Bone wax is also used to seal any potential air cell tracts

authors concluded that the overall ELST surgical complication rate was 26%.

Other authors have reported variable oncologic outcomes using microsurgical techniques for ELST, with more favorable reports in recent years. The overall rate of disease eradication among 102 surgically resected ELST tumors was 86.3% [1, 6, 17, 40, 56, 65–68]. The results are summarized in Table 70.4.

The best approach to preserve hearing in grade I ELST remains to be determined. The retrolabyrinthine-transdural approach is advantageous for good visualization of the posterior semicircular canal, thus preventing inadvertent violation of the labyrinth. With regard to resecting both dural leaflets of the endolymphatic sac, Megerian et al. recommended this approach because it enables excellent visualization of the labyrinthine structures as well as visualization of the posterior petrous bone [39]. The drawback of the retrolabyrinthine-transdural approach is the need to repair the dura with abdominal fat or other mechanisms. Ultimately, no single approach is required for successful hearing preservation [17, 39, 61].

Table 70.4 Microsurgical results for endolymphatic sac tumors

Author (year)	Patients	Mean F/U (months)	Tumor control
Heffner (2009)	16	61	11 (69%)
Luff (2002)	3	60	3 (100%)
Rodrigues (2004)	7	69	6 (86%)
Doherty (2007)	3	32	3 (100%)
Bae (2008)	4	33	3 (75%)
Kim (2013)	33[a]	50	30 (91%)
Carlson (2013)	11	63	10 (91%)
Husseini (2013)	7[b]	84	6 (86%)
Friedman (2013)	18	67	16 (89%)
	102		88/102 (86.3%)

[a]Kim et al. [40] reported on 31 consecutive patients who had 33 distinct endolymphatic sac tumors

[b]The lone recurrence in Husseini et al. [1] occurred 13 years after the original resection

Radiation

The role of radiation for the management of ELST remains controversial. Overall, the reported radiotherapy tumor control rate is 61% (22 of 36), but the small reports have considerable heterogeneity that warrants further discussion. Experience with external beam radiation (EBRT) has shown particularly poor tumor control, with 53% (10 of 19) patients demonstrating tumor growth after therapy [6, 13, 18, 27, 40, 56, 69–71]. Three deaths have also been attributed to poor tumor control after EBRT or an adverse event during EBRT treatment [13, 18, 27]. Stereotactic radiation techniques have shown more promise with a tumor control rate of 75% (12 of 16 patients) [13, 40, 56, 72–77]. The literature lacks standardization of stereotactic radiation techniques, fractionations, and dosages. The radiotherapy results for ELST are summarized in Table 70.5.

Table 70.5 Summary of external beam versus stereotactic radiosurgery outcomes

	External beam radiation	Stereotactic radiosurgery	
Tumor control	9	14	SRS tumor control was 30.4% better (CI −4.4% to 54.7%)
Treatment failure	10	4	
	Tumor control: 47.4%	*Tumor control*: 77.8%	

Adapted from Wick et al. Case Series and Systematic Review of Radiation Outcomes for Endolymphatic Sac Tumors. *Otol Neurotol.* 2018;39(5)

Radiation has been reserved for ELST in poor surgical candidates, focal recurrences that risk significant morbidity if resected, and those unwilling to undergo surgery. When radiation is utilized, stereotactic radiation techniques are preferred. Superiority of any one particular stereotactic technique has not been shown. Overall, there are few case series regarding the use of primary radiotherapy or adjuvant therapy and little long-term data regarding tumor control exists. Furthermore, no consensus regarding the need for fractionation or total dose exists. Further studies in this area are needed [56].

Radiation may play a role in the management of recurrent tumors. Two patterns of ELST recurrence have been previously suggested: recurrence after gross total resection and recurrence after subtotal resection [18, 56]. Gross total ELST resections have very good long-term control, with the infrequent recurrences limited to focal disease. Those limited, focal recurrences are often amenable to surgical resection. Planned adjuvant radiation therapy is not advised if a gross total resection is achieved. Stereotactic radiation may be considered as an alternative to surgical resection for focal recurrences. Subtotal ELST resections have a greater propensity for sizable or multifocal recurrences. In this situation, planned adjuvant radiation can be considered to help with tumor control, but the physicians and patients should be aware of the limitations of the currently reported data.

Chemotherapy

There is no data to support a therapeutic role for chemotherapy in the management of ELST. However, further characterization of the molecular makeup of these tumor cells may provide opportunities for targeted immunotherapy agents in the future.

VHL Management

The management of patients with VHL is complex and requires multidisciplinary care. Genetic testing is advised for all patients afflicted with VHL and for any of their family members. Craniospinal hemangioblastomas are much more common than ELST, presenting in between 60% and 90% of all VHL patients [33]. The common location for craniospinal hemangioblastomas is the cerebellum. These benign, vascular tumors can present with a multitude of symptoms, including death, depending on their size and location. Studies on the natural history of VHL-associated hemangioblastomas have shown that 49% will grow in the course of a 5-year period. The growth cycle is unpredictable, with 42% demonstrating a saltatory pattern, while 47% have an exponential pattern. The presence of a peritumoral cyst increases the likelihood of symptomatic growth to 75% over 3 years [33, 78]. In addition to the CNS tumors, patients with VHL need to be screened for adrenal and extra-adrenal paragangliomas, neuroendocrine tumors, and renal cell carcinoma. A sampling of the CNS and visceral VHL-associated tumors is depicted in Fig. 70.6.

In rare cases of bilateral deafness from either the ELST or their treatment, cochlear implantation remains a viable option for hearing rehabilitation as long as the cochlea and cochlear nerve can be preserved [61–64, 79]. In patients with known bilateral tumors, cochlear implantation should be considered in the ear undergoing the first surgical resection if a hearing preservation surgery cannot be performed. The risk of hearing loss in the contralateral ear is high with or without treatment. Placement of a cochlear implant in the first ear, if possible, would allow the patient time to acclimate to the

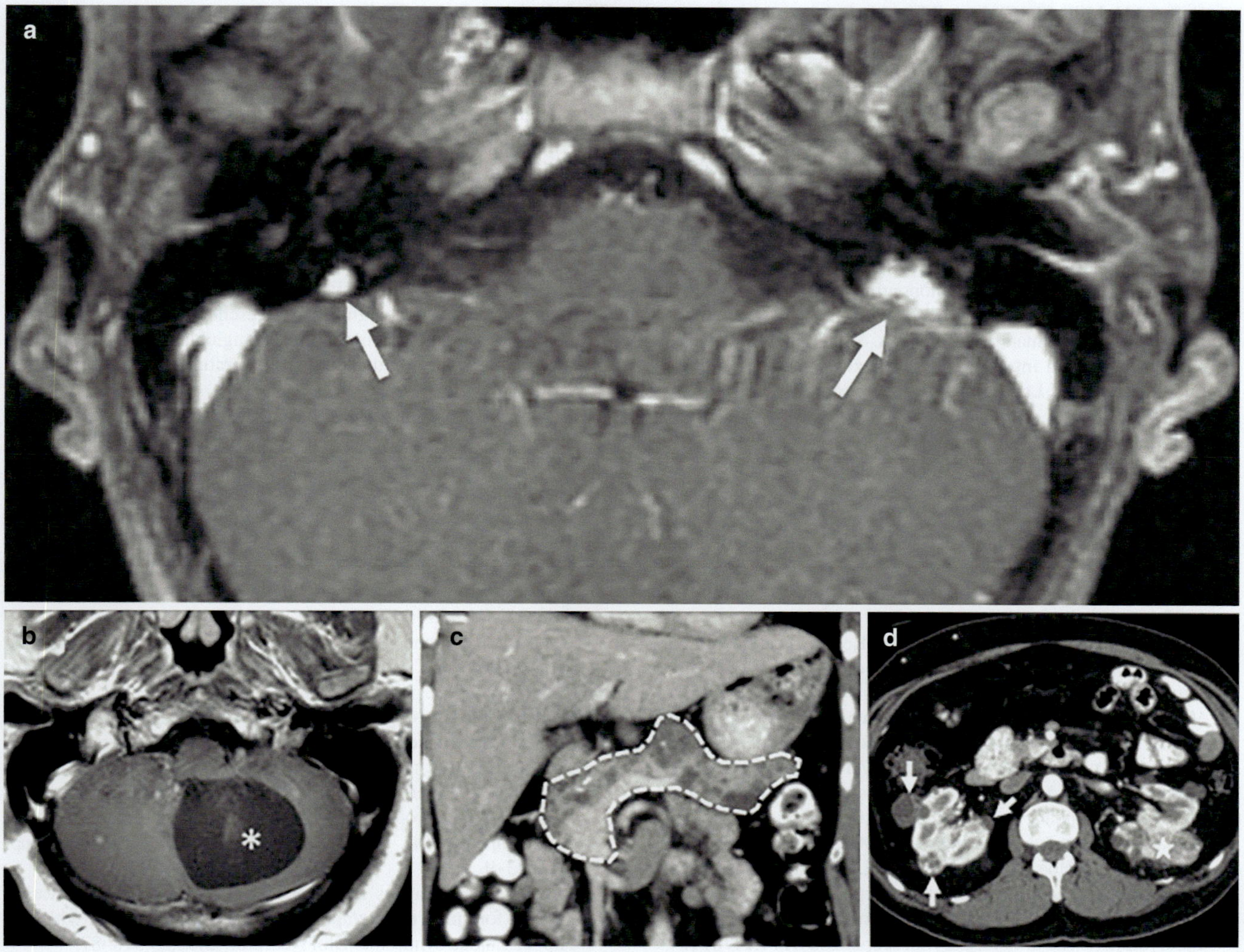

Fig. 70.6 Tumors associated with von Hippel-Lindau disease (VHL) as seen on T1-weighted magnetic resonance imaging (MRI) with contrast. (**a**) Axial slices illustrate bilateral endolymphatic sac tumors (arrows). The tumor on the left was previously shown in Fig. 70.2a. (**b**) A peritumoral cyst (asterisk) may accompany cerebellar hemangioblastomas (not shown). (**c**) Coronal slices depict a cystic pancreas (dashed lines). (**d**) Axial slices show multiple renal cysts (arrows) on the right and renal cell carcinoma (star) on the left

implant and prevent the patient from enduring a period of profound deafness.

Conclusion

The ELST is a slow-growing, locally aggressive neoplasm that originates from the epithelium of the endolymphatic sac and duct. Disease progression can lead to profound SNHL, posterior fossa invasion, brainstem compression, drop metastasis, and eventual death. Early diagnosis with MRI enables the most options for successful surgical management, including hearing preservation through the retrolabyrinthine-transdural approach. Surgical management remains the mainstay of treatment. External beam radiation has dismal tumor control rates, and while stereotactic radiation techniques show promise, the limited data prevent its routine use. The association between ELST and VHL has increased our knowledge of this rare tumor and may provide new therapeutic options in the future.

References

1. Husseini ST, Piccirillo E, Taibah A, Paties CT, Almutai T, Sanna M. The Gruppo Otologic experience of endolymphatic sac tumor. Auris Nasus Larynx. 2013;40:25–31.
2. Johnstone JM, Lennox B, Watson AJ. Five cases of hidradenoma of the external auditory meatus: so-called ceruminoma. J Pathol Bacteriol. 1957;73:421–7.
3. Harrison K, Cronin J, Greenwood N. Ceruminous adenocarcinoma arising in the middle ear. J Laryngol Otol. 1974;88:363–8.
4. Hyams VJ, Michaels L. Benign adenomatous neoplasm (adenoma) of the middle ear. Clin Otolaryngol. 1976;1:17–26.

5. Gaffey MJ, Mills SE, Fechner RE, et al. Aggressive papillary middle ear tumor: a clinicopathologic entity distinct from middle ear adenoma. Am J Surg Pathol. 1988;12:790–7.
6. Heffner DK. Low-grade adenocarcinoma of probable endolymphatic sac origin: a clinicopathologic study of 20 cases. Cancer. 1989;64:2292–302.
7. Hassard AD, Boudreau SF, Cron CC. Adenoma of the endolymphatic sac. J Otolaryngol. 1984;12:213–6.
8. Castleman B, McNeely BU. Case records of the Massachusetts General Hospital: case 47-1966. N Engl J Med. 1966;275:950–9.
9. Naguib MG, Chou SN, Mastri A. Radiation therapy of a choroid plexus papilloma of the cerebellopontine angle with bone involvement. J Neurosurg. 1981;54:245–7.
10. Blamires TL, Friedmann I, Moffat DA. Von Hippel Lindau disease associated with an invasive choroid plexus tumor presenting as a middle ear mass. J Laryngol Otol. 1992;106:429–35.
11. Poe DS, Tarlov EC, Thomas CB, et al. Aggressive papillary tumors of the temporal bone. Otolaryngol Head Neck Surg. 1993;108:80–6.
12. Pollak A, Bohmer A, Spycher M, et al. Are papillary adenomas endolymphatic sac tumors? Ann Otol Rhinol Laryngol. 1995;104:613–9.
13. Megerian CA, McKenna MJ, Nuss RC, et al. Endolymphatic sac tumors: Histologic confirmation, clinical characterization, and implication in von Hippel-Lindau disease. Laryngoscope. 1995;105:801–8.
14. Li JC, Brackmann DE, Lo WW, et al. Reclassification of aggressive adenomatous mastoid neoplasms as endolymphatic sac tumors. Laryngoscope. 1993;103:1342–8.
15. Megerian CA, Pilch BZ, Bahn A, McKenna MJ. Differential expression of transthyretin in papillary tumors of the endolymphatic sac and choroid plexus. Laryngoscope. 1997;107:216–21.
16. Bambakidis NC, Megerian CA, Ratcheson RA. Differential grading of endolymphatic sac tumor extension by virtue of von Hippel-Lindau disease status. Otol Neurotol. 2004;25(5):773–81.
17. Friedman RA, Hoa M, Brackmann DE. Surgical management of endolymphatic sac tumors. J Neurol Surg B. 2013;74:12–9.
18. Hansen MR, Luxford WM. Surgical outcomes in patients with endolymphatic sac tumors. Laryngoscope. 2004;114:14701474.
19. Lonser RR, Kim HF, Butman JA, et al. Tumors of the endolymphatic sac in von Hippel-Lindau disease. N Engl J Med. 2004;350:2481–6.
20. Kim HF, Butman JA, Brewer C, et al. Tumors of the endolymphatic sac in patients with von Hippel-Lindau disease: implications for their natural history, diagnosis, and treatment. J Neurosurg. 2005;102:503–12.
21. Butman JA, Kim HF, Baggenstos M, et al. Mechanism of morbid hearing loss associated with tumors of the endolymphatic sac in von Hippel-Lindau disease. JAMA. 2007;298(1):41–8.
22. Ong YK, Chee NW, Hwang PY, Goh J. Endolymphatic sac tumour: a rare cause of recurrent vertigo. Singapore Med J. 2006;47(7):627–30.
23. Raghunandhan S, Vijaya Krishnan P, Murali S, Anand Kumar RS, Kameswaran M. Endolymphatic sac tumour: a neoplastic cause for Ménière's syndrome. Indian J Otolaryngol Head Neck Surg. 2014;66(S1):S352–5.
24. Committee on Hearing and Equilibrium. Committee on Hearing and Equilibrium guidelines for the diagnosis and evaluation of therapy in Ménière's disease. Otolaryngol Head Neck Surg. 1995;13:181–5.
25. Goebel JA. 2015 Equilibrium committee amendment to the 1995 AAO-HNS guidelines for the definition of Ménière's disease. Otolaryngol Head Neck Surg. 2016;154:403–4.
26. Mishra G, Sharma Y, Padhya C, Parikh B, Gupta M. Endolymphatic duct papillary tumour: captured undercover of complicated chronic otitis media. Indian J Otolaryngol Head Neck Surg. 2013;65(S3):S662–4.
27. Poletti AM, Dubey SP, Barbo R, et al. Sporadic endolymphatic sac tumors: its clinical, radiological, and histological features, management and follow-up. Head Neck. 2013;35:1043–7.
28. Bambakidis NC, Rodrique T, Megerian CA, et al. Endolymphatic sac tumor metastasis to the spine: case report. J Neurosurg Spine. 2005;3:68–70.
29. Tay KY, Yu E, Kassel E. Spinal metastasis from endolymphatic sac tumor. AJNR Am J Neuroradiol. 2007;28:613–4.
30. Bynum JP, Bishop J, Ali SZ. Cerebrospinal fluid cytology of an endolymphatic sac tumor. Diagn Cytopathol. 2015;43:339–42.
31. Murphy BA, Geusubger KR, Bergman S. Cytology of endolymphatic sac tumors. Mod Pathol. 2001;14:920–4.
32. Bamps S, Van Calenbergh F, De Vleeschouwer S, et al. What the neurosurgeon should know about hemangioblastoma, both sporadic and in von Hippel-Lindau disease: a literature review. Surg Neurol Int. 2013;4:145–54.
33. Schunemann V, Huntoon K, Lonser RR. Personalized medicine for nervous system manifestations of von Hippel-Lindau disease. Front Surg. 2016;3:1–5.
34. Neumann HP, Wiestler OD. Clustering of features of von Hippel-Lindau syndrome: evidence for a complex genetic locus. Lancet. 1991;337:1052–4.
35. Manski TJ, Heffner DK, Glenn GM, et al. Endolymphatic sac tumors: a source of morbid hearing loss in von Hippel-Lindau disease. JAMA. 1997;277(18):1461–6.
36. Choo D, Shotland L, Mastroianni M, et al. Endolymphatic sac tumors in von Hippel-Lindau disease. J Neurosurg. 2004;100:480–7.
37. Poulsen ML, Gimsing S, Kosteljanetz M, et al. von Hippel-Lindau disease: surveillance strategy for endolymphatic sac tumors. Genet Med. 2011;13(12):1032–41.
38. Bausch B, Wellner PM, et al. Characterization of endolymphatic sac tumors and von Hippel-Lindau disease in the International Endolymphatic Sac Tumor Registry. Head Neck. 2016;38(suppl 1):E673–9.
39. Megerian CA, Haynes DS, Poe DS, et al. Hearing preservation surgery for small endolymphatic sac tumors in patients with von Hippel-Lindau syndrome. Otol Neurotol. 2002;23:378–87.
40. Kim HJ, Hagan M, Butman JA, et al. Surgical resection of endolymphatic sac tumors in von Hippel-Lindau disease: findings, results, and indications. Laryngoscope. 2013;123:477–83.
41. Seizinger BR, Rouleau GA, Ozelius LJ, et al. von Hippel-Lindau disease maps to the region of chromosome 3 associated with renal cell carcinoma. Nature. 1988;332:268–9.
42. Lonser RR, Glenn GM, Walther M, et al. von Hippel-Lindau disease. Lancet. 2003;361:2059–67.
43. Maher ER, Neumann HP, Richard S. von Hippel-Lindau disease: a clinical and scientific review. Eur J Hum Genet. 2011;19:617–23.
44. Kawahara N, Kume H, Ueki K, et al. VHL gene inactivation in endolymphatic sac tumor associated with von Hippel-Lindau disease. Neurology. 1999;53:208–10.
45. Kaelin WG. Molecular basis of the VHL hereditary cancer syndrome. Nat Rev Cancer. 2002;2:673–82.
46. Vanharanta S, Shu W, et al. Epigenetic expansion of VHL-HIF signal output drives multiorgan metastasis in renal cancer. Nat Med. 2013;19:50–6.
47. Devaney KO, Ferlito A, Rinaldo A. Endolymphatic sac tumor (low-grade papillary adenocarcinoma) of the temporal bone. Acta Otolaryngol. 2003;123(9):1022–6.
48. Gopal P, Parker JR, Debski PJC Jr. Choroid plexus carcinoma. Arch Pathol Lab Med. 2008;132:1350–4.
49. Truong LD, Shen SS. Immunohistochemical diagnosis of renal neoplasms. Arch Pathol Lab Med. 2011;135:92–109.
50. Giuseppe M, Serena B, Sandro B, et al. Adenoma of the ceruminous gland (ceruminoma). Otol Neurotol. 2011;32:e14–5.

51. Mukherji SK, Albernaz VS, Lo WWM, et al. Papillary endolymphatic sac tumors: CT, MR imaging and angiographic findings in 20 patients. Radiology. 1997;202:801–8.
52. Lo WWM, Applegate LJ, Carberry JN, et al. Endolymphatic sac tumors: radiologic appearance. Radiology. 1993;189:199–204.
53. Mukherji SK, Castillo M. Adenocarcinoma of the endolymphatic sac: imaging features and preoperative embolization. Neuroradiology. 1996;38:179–80.
54. Patel N, Wiggins RH, Shelton C. The radiologic diagnosis of endolymphatic sac tumors. Laryngoscope. 2006;116:40–6.
55. Lee JI, Yoon RG, Lee JH, et al. Prognostic value of labyrinthine 3D-FLAIR abnormalities in idiopathic sudden sensorineural hearing loss. AJNR Am J Neuroradiol. 2016;37:2317–22.
56. Carlson ML, Thom JJ, Driscoll CL, et al. Management of primary and recurrent endolymphatic sac tumors. Otol Neurotol. 2013;34:939–43.
57. Papdakis GZ, Millo C, Sadowski SM, Bagci U, Patronas NJ. Endolymphatic sac tumor showing increased activity on ^{68}Ga DOTATATE PET/CT. Clin Nucl Med. 2016;41:783–4.
58. Alkonyi B, Gunthner-Lengsfeld T, Rak K, Nowak J, Solymosi L, Hagen R. An endolymphatic sac tumor with imaging features of aneurysmal bone cysts: differential diagnosis considerations. Childs Nerv Syst. 2014;30(9):1583–8.
59. Sweeney AD, Hunter JB, Rajkumar SV, Lane JI, Jevremovic D, Carlson ML. Plasmacytoma of the temporal bone, a great imitator: report of seven cases and comprehensive review of the literature. Otol Neurotol. 2017;38:400–7.
60. Megerian CA, Semaan MT. Evaluation and management of endolymphatic sac and duct tumors. Otolaryngol Clin N Am. 2007;40:463–78.
61. Schipper J, Maier W, Rosahl SK, et al. Endolymphatic sac tumors: surgical management. J Otolaryngol. 2006;35(6):387–94.
62. Belal A. Is cochlear implantation possible after acoustic tumor removal? Otol Neurotol. 2001;22:497–500.
63. Boccio CM, Raffo GM, Parsini C. Cochlear implantation in a bilateral endolymphatic sac tumor patient. A case report. Int J Pediatr Otorhinolaryngol. 2007;71:1803–7.
64. Jagannathan J, Lonser RR, Stanger RA, et al. Cochlear implantation for hearing loss associated with bilateral endolymphatic sac tumors in von Hippel-Lindau disease. Otol Neurotol. 2007;28:927–30.
65. Luff DA, Simmons M, Malik T, Ramsden RT, Reid H. Endolymphatic sac tumours. J Laryngol Otol. 2002;116:398–401.
66. Rodrigues S, Fagan P, Turner J. Endolymphatic sac tumors: a review of the St. Vincent's hospital experience. Otol Neurotol. 2004;25:599–603.
67. Doherty JK, Yong M, Maceri D. Endolymphatic sac tumor: a report of 3 cases and discussion of management. Ear Nose Throat J. 2007;86:30–5.
68. Bae CW, Cho YH, Chung JW, Kim CJ. Endolymphatic sac tumors: report of four cases. J Korean Neurosurg Soc. 2008;44:268–72.
69. Feghali JG, Levin RJ, Llena j, Bradley MK, Kantrowitz AB. Aggressive papillary tumors of the endolymphatic sac: clinical and tissue characteristics. Am J Otol. 1995;16:778–82.
70. Patel PC, Pellitteri PK, Ream CL, Martin JS, Szymanski MB. Aggressive papillary tumor of the temporal bone: delayed extensive recurrence following radiation therapy. Skull Base Surg. 1997;7:45–8.
71. Gupta R, Vaidhyswaran AN, Murali V, Kameswaran M. Endolymphatic sac papillary carcinoma treated with surgery and post-operative intensity-modulated radiotherapy: a rare case report. J Cancer Res Ther. 2010;6:540–2.
72. Ferreira MA, Feiz-Erfan I, Zabramski JM, Spetzler RF, Coons SW, Preul MC. Endolymphatic sac tumor: unique features of two cases and review of the literature. Acta Neurochir. 2002;144:1047–53.
73. Hashimoto M, Yokota A, Urasaki E, Imada H, Yamamoto H. Surgical treatment of endolymphatic sac tumor with adjunctive stereotactic radiation therapy-case report. Neurol Med Chir (Tokyo). 2004;44:595–9.
74. Balasubramaniam S, Deshpande RB, Misra BK. Gamma knife radiosurgery in jugular foramen endolymphatic sac adenocarcinoma. J Clin Neurosci. 2009;16:710–1.
75. Cheng X, Qin S, Wang X, Li P, Shrestha B, Wang W. Gamma knife treatment of an endolymphatic sac tumor: unique features of a case and review of the literature. Neurol India. 2011;59:608–11.
76. Kunzel J, Agaimy A, Hornung J, et al. Sporadic endolymphatic sac tumor – a diagnostic and therapeutic challenge. Int J Clin Exp Pathol. 2014;7:1641–2646.
77. Ünçüncü Kefeli A, Yilmaz M, Sengoz M, Peker S. Gamma knife radiosurgery for tumors of the endolymphatic sac. Turk Neurosurg. 2014; https://doi.org/10.5137/1019-5149.JTN.13345-14.0. [Epub ahead of print].
78. Ammerman JM, Lonser RR, Dambrosia J, Butman JA, Oldfield EH. Long-term natural history of hemangioblastomas in patients with von Hippel-Lindau disease: implications for treatment. J Neurosurg. 2006;105:248–55.
79. Kveton JF, Abbott C, April M, Drumheller G, Cohen N, Poe DS. Cochlear implantation after transmastoid labyrinthectomy. Laryngoscope. 1989;99:610–3.

Inner Ear Schwannomas

71

Brian A. Neff

Introduction

Inner ear schwannomas (IES) (formerly known as intralabyrinthine schwannomas) arise from progenitor Schwann cells within the distal inner ear labyrinth [1]. Tumors arising in this area are far less common than the typical vestibular schwannomas (VS) originating within the internal auditory canal (IAC) or cerebellopontine angle (CPA). First described by Mayer in 1917, IES has been found to be a more common diagnosis than was initially reported [2–4]. A recent epidemiology study by Marinelli et al. showed that the overall incidence rate of IES was 1.1 per 100,000 person-years. IES incidence also increased with age, with individuals aged 60 to 69 at 2.7 per 100,000 person-years, and for individuals ≥70 years old, it was 4.1 per 100,000 person-years. Lastly, they emphasized that spontaneous VS still had an incidence rate around four times greater than IES [5].

Prior to the advent of magnetic resonance imaging (MRI), these tumors were found exclusively at the time of autopsy or as an unexpected discovery during neurotologic surgery [6]. Due to their presentation overlap with Ménière's disease (MD) and idiopathic sudden sensorineural hearing loss (viral labyrinthitis), diagnosis can be delayed. The diagnosis of IES has become less challenging as magnetic resonance imaging (MRI) has become more available, but it still requires attention to image quality and the utilization of the correct MRI sequences in order to avoid incorrect or missed diagnoses [7].

Pathogenesis

Schwann cells occur in higher density within the IAC near the Schwann-glial junction; however, studies of pathologic specimens have shown that VS can occur anywhere along the course of the axons of the eighth cranial nerve [8–10]. It has been hypothesized that cochlear IES might originate in the more distal cochlear nerve fibers within the modiolus, where Schwann cell concentration is also high [3]. IES limited to the vestibule likely arises from Schwann cells located in the terminal branches of the vestibular nerves within the membranous labyrinth of the semicircular canals, utricle, or saccule.

IES can grow by extension into adjacent inner ear spaces along the path of least resistance, and therefore, it is unlikely that they will spread beyond the highly dense otic capsule. However, a tumor can easily spread throughout the labyrinth: from the cochlea to the vestibule to the semicircular canal and vice versa. Reports of tumor spreading to the middle ear by passing through the round window or displacing the stapes footplate within the oval window are relatively rare [11, 12]. Although not occurring frequently, a tumor may break through the cribriform plate located at the distal end of the IAC and then grow more proximally into the IAC toward the CPA.

Clinical Presentation

The average age for IES diagnosis is 49 (range 14–89), with no male–female predilection [3]. As alluded to previously, the overlap in IES symptoms with other more common neurotologic diseases, such as Ménière's disease, vestibular migraine, or labyrinthitis, can potentially delay the decision to obtain a diagnostic MRI. As the most common symptoms are hearing loss and vertigo, we examine these in greater detail in this section.

Early reports of the IES series demonstrated that nearly all patients initially presented with hearing loss [6, 7, 13]. In 2013, a large literature review examined 234 cases and reported a 99% rate of hearing loss, with the vast majority (87%) presenting with the American Academy of Otolaryngology–Head and Neck Surgery (AAO-HNS) Class D hearing [3, 14]. The pattern of hearing loss is variable and

B. A. Neff (✉)
Department of Otolaryngology—Head and Neck Surgery, Mayo Clinic, Rochester, MN, USA
e-mail: neff.brian@mayo.edu

A. D. Sweeney et al. (eds.), *Haynes-Glasscock-Shambaugh Surgery of the Ear*, https://doi.org/10.1007/978-3-032-18264-7_71

may not provide a means of discriminating these tumors from patients with Ménière's disease. IES presents with progressive, sudden, and fluctuating patterns of hearing loss. One case series found rates of 61% progressive loss, 32% sudden loss, and 7% fluctuating hearing loss [7]. Another literature review showed that fluctuating hearing loss occurred only 3% of the time for IES, while many IES patients (39%) were misdiagnosed with Ménière's disease [3].

Though there have been histologic reports of isolated neural damage at only the tumor site, potentially causing isolated frequencies of hearing loss, this presentation is not commonly seen with IES. The fact that many IES do not involve the cochlea (30%), yet 99% of patients report hearing loss, means that another pathophysiologic mechanism of hearing loss must exist. One hypothesis is that isolated tumors of the vestibule and semicircular canals still may cause hearing loss by either direct compression of the ductus reuniens or any other site along the pathway of endolymph flow toward the endolymphatic sac, thus leading to endolymphatic hydrops [7]. Others feel that the presence of abnormal metabolites or the interruption of potassium cycling within the tumor-containing labyrinth may directly damage or alter the function of the organ of Corti [15, 16].

Lastly, the clinician should be aware of the possibility of a mixed hearing loss occurring in a small subset of patients with IES. Stapes footplate fixation or displacement into the middle ear from extension of intracochlear tumors can occur [12, 17] (Fig. 71.1). Hamed and Linthicum captured an example of this in a temporal bone histology section of the cochlea and stapes footplate [18]. In this patient, a tumor was discovered filling the vestibule, primarily, but it had extended into the proximal scala vestibuli. The tumor extended along the superior vestibular nerve as far as its entry point into the IAC, but abruptly stopped at that point. Instead of growing into the IAC, stapes footplate dislocation into the middle ear had occurred. These examples of "inner ear" conductive hearing loss would appear as a mixed pattern on audiologic testing.

Patients with IES may describe variable vestibular symptoms, including spontaneous vertigo, motion-induced dizziness, and disequilibrium. Abnormal balance and unsteadiness were found to be more common than vertigo [3]. Vertigo has been reported in 59% of patients, and the vertigo was episodic in all but 1 patient, who described constant vertigo. The relatively high rate of episodic vertigo described by these patients, in addition to the near-uniform presence of sensorineural hearing loss (SNHL) and tinnitus, makes differentiating these lesions from Ménière's disease challenging.

The pathophysiologic mechanism to explain episodic vertigo is not definitively established. A greater rate of vestibular subsite involvement has been reported in patients presenting with vestibular symptoms, but vertigo can also occur with isolated cochlear lesions [3]. One report found that 26% (7/27) of patients with vertigo had isolated cochlear IES. A temporal bone study found that three of seven cochlear IES patients had histologic evidence of endolymphatic hydrops, and perhaps, this is the reason for vestibular symptoms in patients having isolated cochlear tumors [4].

Lastly, it should be noted that the percentage of patients with IES having vertiginous symptoms seems to be higher than that of patients with the more common VS of the IAC,

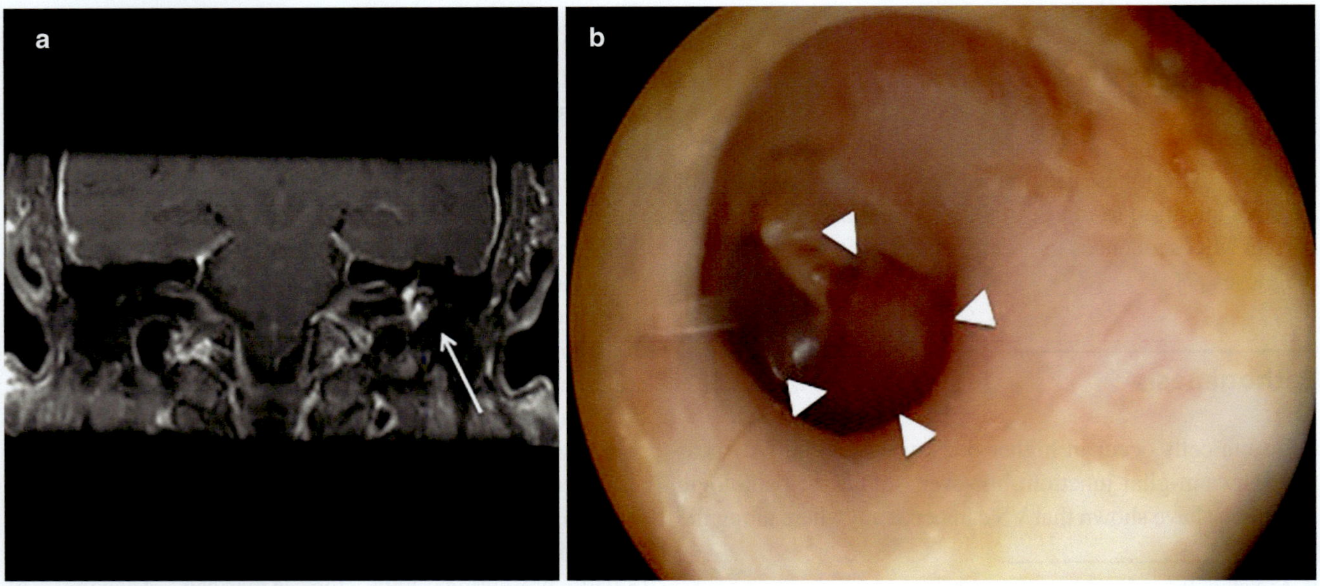

Fig. 71.1 PIES with extension through the round window into the middle ear, left ear (same patient for MRI and exam). (**a**) coronal T1-weighted MRI with gadolinium contrast showing PIES with middle ear extension (white arrow); (**b**) In office, 0° endoscopic view of left ear showing middle ear PIES with tympanic membrane contact (white arrowheads)

in whom the presentation is often disequilibrium without vertigo [6]. This might be because IES arises from a more distal site within the vestibular system. Distal vestibular damage might create abnormal or fluctuating neural input to the more proximal vestibular system, whereas an IAC schwannoma originating near Scarpa's ganglion might lead to a more stable, yet reduced, vestibular input to the brainstem.

Imaging

The diagnosis of IES is ultimately made with MRI in the context of the clinical presentation. Unfortunately, there are no pathognomonic clinical symptoms, physical exam findings, or audiologic criteria that will definitively suggest IES pathology. MRI is an integral test for preoperative localization and surgical planning, or as a method of following stable tumors. Early MRI reports describe a lack of normal fluid density on T2-weighted imaging, with corresponding enhancement seen on gadolinium-enhanced T1-weighted scans [19]. However, other specific MRI sequences are also important for accurate diagnosis. The standard 2D fast-spin T2 sequence, typically acquired at a slice thickness of 3 mm, may miss smaller tumors [3]. 3D imaging techniques that include constructive interference in a steady state (3D CISS) and variable flip angle 3D fast spin echo T2-weighted sequences (T2 SPACE), acquired at a 1 mm slice thickness or less, have become critical for evaluation of pathology involving the membranous labyrinth and inner ear [20]. At the authors' institution, we also employ variable flip angle 3D FSE T1-weighted sequences (T1 SPACE), which can be acquired at 0.6 mm sections through the labyrinth. Utilizing both the 3D T2-weighted sequences and fat-saturated post-gadolinium 3D T1-weighted images allows for precise localization of tumor margins [21]. Physicians evaluating for IES must make sure these sequences are performed because many routine MRI protocols may not include these sequences unless they are specifically requested.

Differential Diagnosis: Clinical and Radiographic

The clinical differential diagnosis of IES depends on whether the patient is presenting with complaints of hearing loss, disequilibrium, vertigo, or a combination of these symptoms. Ménière's disease, vestibular migraine, labyrinthitis, vestibular neuritis, autoimmune hearing loss, otosyphilis, and classic VS of the IAC or CPA are all considered. Typically, once MRI has been obtained, the clinician has to decide between possible diagnoses based on the appearance of an enhancing inner ear lesion. This list can generally be divided into primary enhancing lesions confined to the inner ear or enhancing lesions that extend to and include the inner ear. Labyrinthine hemorrhage is a relatively rare diagnosis that presents similarly to acute viral labyrinthitis (Fig. 71.2) in patients with concussive head trauma, patients with systemic diseases such as leukemia or sickle cell disease, or spontaneously in patients on anticoagulant therapy. Chronic labyrinthitis with or without ossification can result from bacterial meningitis in children and adults or from systemic autoimmune diseases that have a propensity to cause SNHL, such as ulcerative colitis, Crohn's disease, or granulomatosis with polyangiitis (GPA). All of these MRI abnormalities show a more diffuse inner ear enhancement without discrete borders. Alternatively, IES presents as a discrete enhancement with sharply margined borders on both contrast-enhanced T1-weighted, T2-SPACE, and 3D CISS sequences (Fig. 71.3).

There are several very rare case reports of primary tumors arising within the labyrinth. One such case reported a recurrent (or residual) cochlear IES after resection of an IAC VS [22]. A few intralabyrinthine lipomas have been reported, and these were diagnosed by suppression of tumor hyperintensity on fat-suppressed T1-weighted MRI sequences [23]. Another case report highlighted a traumatic neuroma following labyrinthectomy [24]. This patient had a remote history of Ménière's disease treated with labyrinthectomy and then later developed a more chronic disequilibrium. However, it is not entirely certain whether the traumatic neuroma was truly causative of the imbalance. Lastly, the author's institution has treated a patient who presented with unilateral deafness and an MRI showing a discrete inner ear lesion similar to an IES. However, the tumor showed atypical T1 hyperintensity without contrast and an extremely rapid growth rate, extending to involve the CPA. Surgical pathology confirmed the diagnosis of melanocytic schwannoma arising from the vestibule.

There are also rare instances where tumors or inflammatory lesions arise outside the inner ear but extend to involve the cochlea or vestibule. Meningiomas of the IAC, lymphoma, posttransplant lymphoproliferative disease (PTLD), endolymphatic sac tumors, paraganglioma, temporal bone sarcomas, inflammatory pseudotumor [25], and metastases can all present with unilateral SNHL and vestibular complaints. The MRI appearance of these lesions can be similar to a contrast-enhancing IES that has extended to involve the IAC or middle ear.

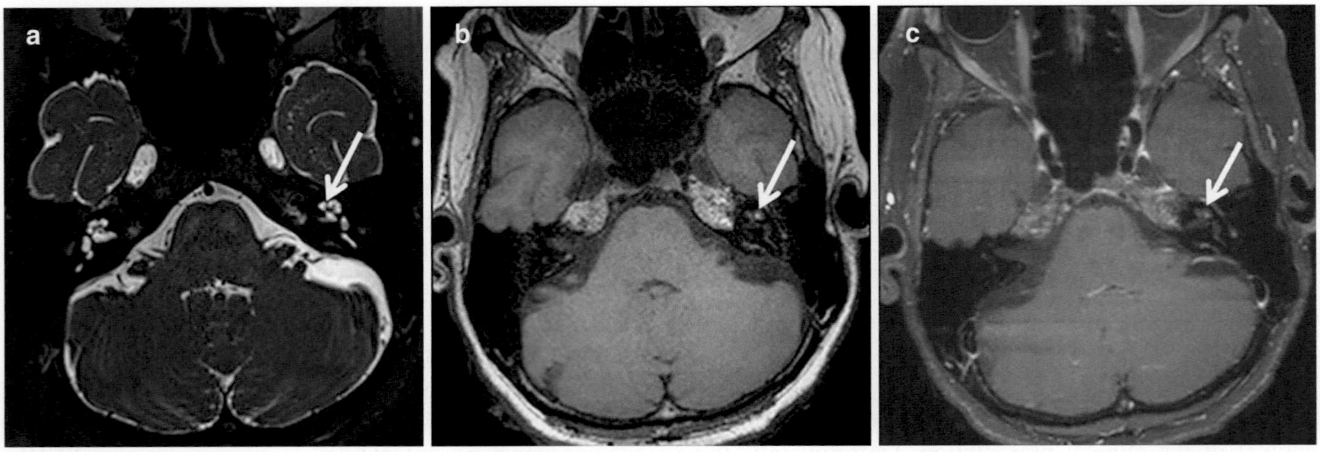

Fig. 71.2 Acute labyrinthitis with hemorrhage, left ear. (**a**) axial 3D fast spin echo T2-weighted image shows normal fluid signal within the inner ear and cochlea (arrow); (**b**) axial pre-contrast 3D fast spin echo T1-weighted image shows signal hyperintensity of the cochlea (arrow); (**c**) axial fat-saturated post-contrast 3D fast spin echo T1-weighted image demonstrates no substantial enhancement (arrow)

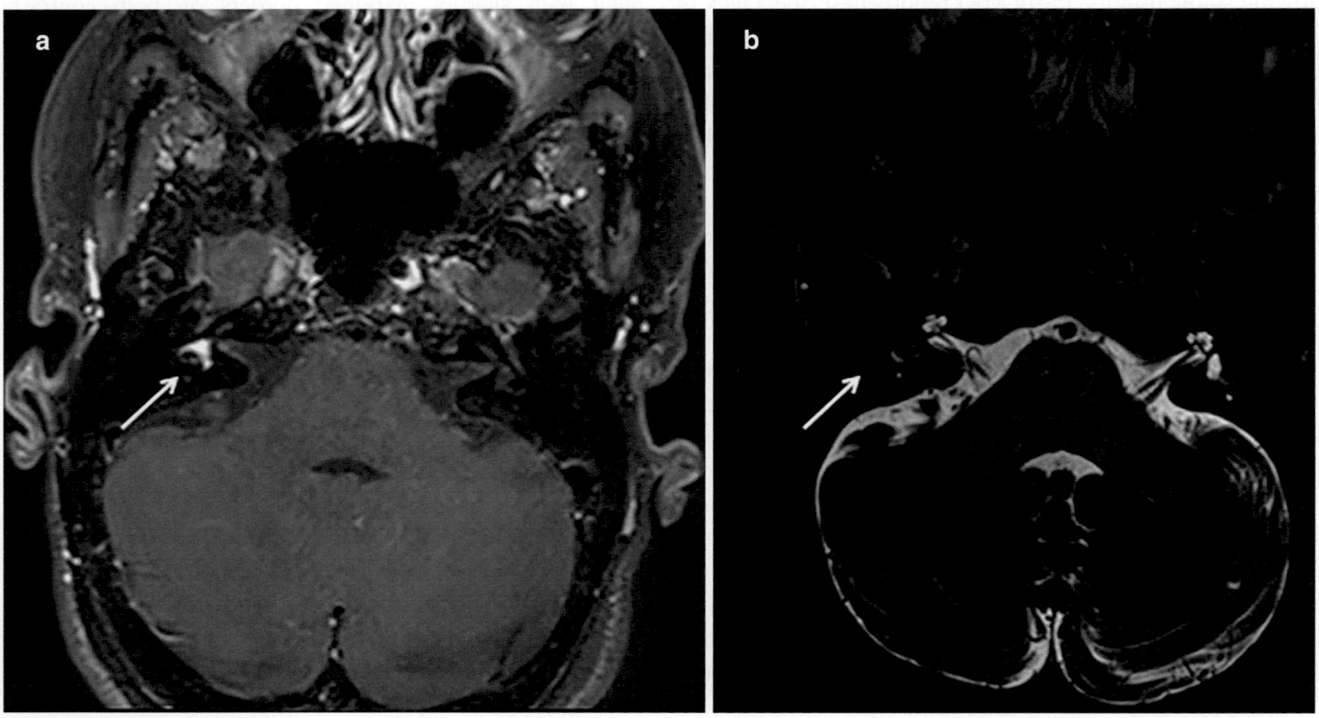

Fig. 71.3 Intralabyrinthine schwannoma, right cochlea. (**a**) axial post-contrast T1-weighted image demonstrates enhancement of the vestibule and lateral semicircular canal (white arrow); (**b**) variable flip angle 3D fast spin echo T2-weighted sequences (T2 SPACE) shows filling defect (hypointensity) within the bright vestibule fluid signal (white arrow)

Management and Outcomes

Management

The treatment approach for IES is dictated by patient symptoms, tumor size, and tumor location. Surgical indications for IES removal are intractable vertigo, growth into the IAC or middle ear, and uncertainty regarding diagnosis [1, 3, 6, 7, 12]. In other instances, when cochlear implantation is being considered, tumor resection is often performed simultaneously with cochlear implantation. Management options primarily include observation with serial MRIs versus surgical removal, with the approach dictated by tumor size and location. Excluding patients with concomitant IAC extension of their IES, there still has been very few reported patients who have received stereotactic radiosurgery for their IES [3, 7, 26, 27]. Until larger series are published, the author reserves this option primarily for those medically unfit to undergo surgery. There has also been a single report utilizing transtympanic steroid injections for an IES patient with sudden SNHL [28]. This patient experienced short-term hearing improvement until the inevitable, permanent, tumor-induced SNHL.

In a 2013 IES review, 53% of patients (109/189) were observed with serial MRI scans. Only 3% of observed patients went on to need surgical removal due to vestibular symptoms or significant tumor growth. This was despite MRI evidence of slow tumor growth in 52% of these patients. Interestingly, they found that in the observation group, 93% (55/59) had stable or improved vertigo, tinnitus, or unsteadiness [3]. These findings provide support for a more conservative approach to the management of these tumors.

When patients experience recurrent, severe vertigo or tumor growth into the IAC, CPA, or middle ear, treatment is required. Earlier removal of these tumors prior to extensive IAC involvement is likely to have less risk of postoperative facial paralysis [29]. The middle ear IES extension has also historically been an indication for tumor removal. The provided reasoning for this is that the tumor lacks a barrier to spread once it has reached the middle ear. This decision is probably sound in more quickly growing tumors, but it can be questioned in the majority of slow-growing tumors. The middle ear may provide slow-growing tumors with an increased area to expand asymptomatically without consequence. In general, the author removes tumors with middle ear extension through the oval window due to the proximity of the tympanic facial nerve. This allows tumor removal when facial nerve contact is at a minimum and may provide easier dissection and facial nerve preservation. Additionally, middle ear IES are also removed prior to significant Eustachian tube involvement, since this can add a degree of difficulty to complete tumor resection. Slow-growing tumors extending through the round window into the hypotympanum might be observed if they have not radiographically encroached upon the facial nerve.

Clinicians may rarely be faced with an IES patient experiencing severe vertigo without tumor growth or hearing loss. Transtympanic gentamicin injection could be done in these instances, especially if the patient did not wish to have surgery or was medically unfit for surgery. Patients should be counseled that this treatment does not prevent tumor growth, and any remaining hearing could be lost due to the injection.

Ultimately, the vast majority of patients requiring treatment will undergo surgical removal. It is helpful to have IES classification schemes in order to choose an appropriate surgical approach for the tumor location, and a revised scheme was published in 2024 [30]. It is important that patients understand that they will no longer have any hearing regardless of the surgical approach selected, although most patients with these IES present with non-serviceable hearing [3]. Patients with tumors isolated to the vestibular system (vestibule or semicircular canals) can effectively undergo tumor removal via a transmastoid labyrinthectomy. If there is an extension of a labyrinth IES into the IAC or CPA, the translabyrinthine approach provides adequate exposure for tumor resection. The older standard for cochlear IES resection was the transotic approach, regardless of whether there was tumor extension into the IAC. This would also provide adequate exposure for cochlear tumors involving the middle ear. The transotic approach requires over-closure of the external auditory meatus, packing of the middle ear, and Eustachian tube obliteration to prevent a CSF leak from the IAC through the resected basal cochlear modiolus (Fig. 71.4). However, current surgical approach selection is more tailored for tumors with less than total cochlear involvement (all 2½ turns), which can often be removed without a transotic approach. Case reports of transcanal, endoscopic transcanal [31], and transmastoid removal of small cochlear IES have been published. The transcanal approaches required broad TM elevation and bone removal around the annulus, with a cochleostomy done with or without the aid of endoscopic visualization. Although controversial as to the extent of possible safe tumor removal, all of these approaches are probably best preserved for small tumors isolated to the cochlear basal turn or middle turn IES on the shallow side of the modiolus. For the transmastoid approach, the authors describe a standard facial recess approach and enlarged cochleostomy for tumor removal [32]. This approach is best utilized for tumors involving the basal turn of the cochlea that do not "turn the corner" to involve the pars ascendens of the basal turn. Additionally, a few authors have published on techniques of tumor removal deep to the modiolus by multiple cochlear turn cochleostomies combined with push-through or pull-through tumor delivery techniques utilizing suture, Gelfoam®, or silicone stylet/dummy electrodes (a.k.a "pipe-cleaner" or "dental floss" technique). This has the advantage of potentially not disrupting or resecting the modiolus, but the disadvantage is that the tumor removal deep to the modiolus is not under direct visualization [33–35]. More recently, Plontke et al. have published several papers describing their combined transcanal–transmastoid approach for subtotal cochleoectomy with partial resection of the apical and middle turn modiolus for more extensive basal and middle turn tumors. This technique allowed the removal of the tumor from the basal and middle turns of the cochlea on the deep side of the modiolus. They achieved gross total tumor resection without sacrificing all of the spiral ganglion cells or getting a "routine" CSF leak that occurs with the classic transotic resection of the entire modiolus.

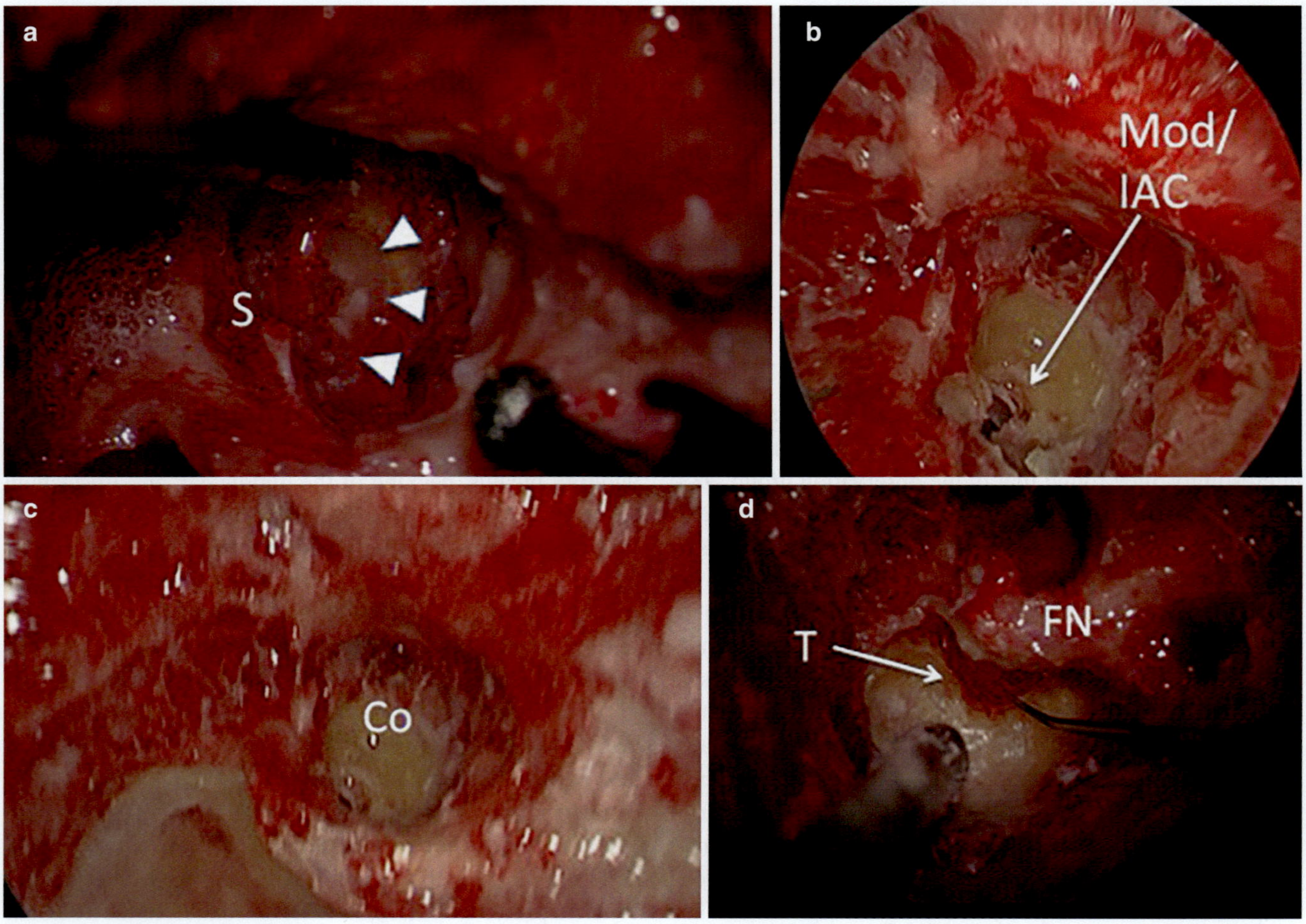

Fig. 71.4 Transotic resection of right IES involving the cochlea, vestibule, and distal IAC (Kennedy class- translabyrinthine IES). (**a**) The posterior external auditory canal wall has been removed to expose the middle ear and stapes (s). The cochlea has been opened to expose the tumor filling the basal turn of the cochlea (white arrowheads). (**b**) The entire cochlea has been opened, and the tumor has been removed from both sides of the basal and middle cochlear turns. The cochlear modiolus (mod) has been removed, and the distal IAC has been entered with egress of CSF. (**c**) Additional surgical view after the removal of the tumor and cochlea (Co). The facial ridge and the facial nerve are more easily visualized. (**d**) A labyrinthectomy has been performed, and a schwannoma tumor (T) is seen filling the vestibule deep to the facial nerve (FN)

With cochlea reconstruction utilizing lateral wall cartilage shims and cartilage island-perichondrium and bone pâté reconstruction of the lateral cochlear wall (otic capsule), they were able to simultaneously place a peri-modiolar cochlear implant in their patients [36, 37]. As an alternative, large cochlear IES tumors involving all of the cochlear turns (especially transmacular IES with IAC extension) may still require drilling across the entire modiolus, or a transotic approach, with the resultant CSF leak. The major disadvantage of the transotic approach is that without preservation of any of the modiolus, successful cochlear implantation is not possible. Lastly, although extensive cochlear tumor removal is possible with the transpromontory endoscopic approaches [38], these tumors are probably best managed with the subtotal cochleoectomy or transotic approach until further research shows a serious advantage to the endoscopic approach, and the incidence of complications, postoperative CSF leak, and complete tumor resection are found to be comparable.

Outcomes

To date, no operated patient has developed tumor recurrence after gross total IES excision, but long-term imaging follow-up was not available for many case series. One patient who underwent subtotal tumor removal required a second surgery due to residual tumor growth in the cochlea after an initial transotic approach [39]. Surgical excision of IES has resulted in vertigo resolution in many patients, although patient selection for surgery was not uniformly applied [6, 7]. Additionally, the utilization of standardized vestibular symptom definitions was also not performed. It is unlikely that spontaneous-onset vertigo was systematically distinguished from head-motion–induced vertigo, disequilibrium while walking, or constant dizziness present in all positions and activities. Spontaneous vertigo from tumor irritation would likely respond well to surgical vestibular ablation, whereas the latter chronic symptoms, which are indicative of poor central vestibular compensation, are unlikely to improve after surgery.

Complications after IES surgery are seemingly rare. Unfortunately, facial nerve outcomes are difficult to assess due to sporadic reporting practices in the literature. Postoperative facial nerve paresis or paralysis was an unusual complication seen in 4% (2/55) of surgical patients. One patient initially had House-Brackmann (HB) grade III/VI facial paresis that completely resolved by 1 year, and another patient had HB grade IV function 12 months postoperatively [6, 7]. There have been 3 cases of patients experiencing post operative CSF leak [40, 41]. One of these was managed conservatively, one had an unknown clinical course, and one underwent an operation upon the development of meningitis.

There are a few controversies regarding the management of IES. The first is regarding whether young patients (≤50 years old) with a slowly growing IES should undergo prolonged observation, even if they lack vestibular symptoms. As previously highlighted, many surgeons promote a wait and scan policy in all non-vertiginous IES patients, irrespective of age, because surgery will not offer any hearing or tinnitus improvement. On the other hand, even if growth is limited to 1 mm every 2–3 years, the tumor will likely run out of room within the inner ear and extend to the IAC at some point over the next 30–40 years. This would then need treatment in a more elderly patient group. Of course, treatment could be accomplished with stereotactic radiosurgery (SRS) with a subsequent unclear prognosis, but because of this likely need to treat within the patient's lifetime, surgery should probably be a treatment option discussed with the younger (≤50 years old), asymptomatic patient with a slowly growing IES. Moreover, even with conservative MRI follow-up schedules every 2–5 years, this is a large commitment of patient time and medical resources over the younger patient's lifetime.

The second controversy surrounding IES management is whether stereotactic radiosurgery should be considered a valid, first-line treatment option. There have been a few reports of SRS treatment for IES without IAC extension. One series reported treating 4 patients with IES not extending to the IAC with Gamma Knife radiosurgery (GKR). The marginal tumor dose was 12 Gy, with the mean maximum cochlea dose of 11.2 Gy. They did not have any tumor growth on the last MRI follow-up, although the MRI follow-up period was not defined, so one has to assume only short-term success [27]. The second small series of 5 patients was also treated with GKR to a marginal tumor dose of 12 Gy (cochlear dose not reported). All 5 patients had stable tumors at a mean MRI follow-up of 1.5 years. Additionally, they reported that one of their posttreatment patients had stable, serviceable hearing of Gardner-Robinson Class 2 with undefined follow-up of no more than 3.5 years [26]. Despite this very preliminary, promising hearing result, hearing preservation is probably not possible in the rare patient with serviceable hearing due to the high cochlear radiation dose, and SRS treatment should probably not be considered until AAO-HNS class D hearing levels are reached. The indications for SRS could potentially be similar for IES and IAC schwannomas, and this would include tumor growth on serial MRI scans, growth of the tumor to involve the IAC, and intractable spontaneous vertigo. Imbalance, constant dizziness, and motion-provoked vertigo are not good SRS (or surgical) indications since these are more likely to result from poor central compensation rather than an irritative tumor phenomenon. There is some hesitancy to recommend SRS to treat IES tumors causing spontaneous vertigo, since theoretically, the tumor that is causing abnormal vestibular input has not been removed. Surgical removal of IES tumors also accomplishes total vestibular ablation, which may allow patients better spontaneous vertigo control. These hypotheses have not really been well studied in the treatment of IES or standard vestibular schwannomas. Lastly, the risk-benefit analysis for IES tumors is different from that of standard IAC or CPA tumors. Complete microsurgical removal of IES tumors without IAC involvement is generally easily accomplished, and the risk of facial nerve morbidity is limited compared to standard vestibular schwannomas. Currently, SRS for the treatment of IES has been reserved for the medically infirm who cannot undergo surgical anesthesia. With the relative infrequency of these tumors, the slow growth, and the difficulty in measuring growth on serial scans, it is unlikely that a randomized, prospective trial comparing SRS, microsurgery, and observation will ever occur. Future systematic reviews will be needed to assist in defining the best treatment practices.

Hearing Rehabilitation

Increasingly, patients with unilateral, profound SNHL are finding significant benefit from cochlear implantation (CI). CI restores a degree of bilateral hearing that may help with sound localization and hearing in noise that cannot be provided by contralateral routing of signal (CROS) strategies [42]. Currently, in the United States, insurance companies are starting to approve cochlear implantation for single-sided deafness, but in these instances, reimbursement coverage standards for CI are very haphazardly applied or approved.

CI for unilateral sensorineural hearing loss is slowly becoming more mainstream, with consistent outcome studies to demonstrate benefit [43]. This is significant for patients with IES since most of these patients will have unilateral, profound SNHL in need of rehabilitation. Routine CI rehabilitation might also shift the current IES treatment paradigm away from observation to early stereotactic radiosurgery or surgical removal at a time when the tumor is at its smallest.

When considering CI and IES treatment, there are three overall treatment pathways: tumor resection with CI (simultaneous or delayed), stereotactic radiation treatment with subsequent CI, and placement of the CI without any tumor treatment. The latter two options may require placement of the CI through the tumor if the IES has an intracochlear location. Currently, there are many unanswered questions as to which approach is best applied to which patient, and which approach leads to the optimal CI hearing outcomes. Tumor location within the inner ear also likely has some importance to decision-making and cochlear implant outcomes. It is the author's preference to perform simultaneous labyrinthectomy and CI for tumors limited to the vestibule and semicircular canals. However, these patients can clearly be treated with stereotactic radiosurgery and CI or CI without tumor treatment. Although unproven to date, it can be hypothesized that these patients may have better CI outcomes than those with intracochlear IES due to the noninvolvement of the cochlear structures. Due to small numbers of patients treated with each modality, it is not clearly known which group will demonstrate the best long-term CI and tumor outcomes. Intracochlear IES should be considered as a distinct subgroup of patients when considering outcomes of various tumor treatment approaches and CI. There have now been a small number of reported cases with limited cochlear schwannomas involving only the proximal basal turn, which were resected with simultaneous successful CI placement after short-term follow-up [32, 44]. To date, tumor resection through an expanded cochleostomy or round window opening with simultaneous CI has been the authors' preferred approach. However, this same group of patients has not been systematically compared to similar small intracochlear IES groups having undergone stereotactic radiosurgery with CI or CI through the untreated tumor. Larger cochlear IES that fill most or all the cochlear turns may be difficult to remove while still maintaining enough cochlear spiral ganglion cells and distal cochlear nerve branches to ensure significant CI benefit. Although not tested to date, there is the same theoretical concern that stereotactic radiation may also damage the critical intracochlear cells and structures required for good cochlear implant performance. As referenced previously, Plontke et al. reported on subtotal cochleoectomy with cochlea reconstruction and simultaneous peri-modiolar CI placement in 16 of their patients. The short-term hearing results have been at least equivalent to those of their non-tumor CI patients, and hopefully, these results can be replicated at other institutions [36, 37]. There have only been a small number of cochlear IES treated with radiosurgery with successful short-term CI outcomes. In these few cases, the CI was placed after radiosurgery completion so that the CI did not negatively impact the precise treatment targeting plan needed for such radiation treatments [45]. Due to the small case numbers, conclusions cannot yet be drawn about how these CI outcomes compare to surgery with CI, or CI alone, through the untreated tumor. To this point, the author's center has reported 9 CI patients with stable, non-growing IES (SRS treated or observed) who have had a styleted CI placed through the soft intracochlear tumor. Preliminary outcomes over a relatively short follow-up period have shown benefit in 7 out of 9 patients with a median Consonant-Nucleus-Consonant (CNC) word score of 57% (range: 28–88%) [45].

Although it is becoming more common to perform CI at the time of primary tumor extirpation, it cannot be said that this is definitively superior to CI placement in a delayed fashion after tumor removal surgery. One of the current reasons for this delay is to allow a window of time for MRI follow-up to ensure that tumor residual or recurrence is not detected prior to placing a CI that may cause an obscuring artifact on these initial surveillance MRIs. Although this concern cannot be completely dismissed, there are several reports of successful MRI surveillance of resected IES with a CI in place. It does help if the internal receiver/stimulator implant body is placed more posterior and superiorly, and it requires specific MRI protocols to reduce image artifact [36, 46]. If CI placement were staged for any reason, the window of time for successful CI insertion is also not well established. Concern over delayed labyrinthitis ossificans development and subsequent implantation failure has been highlighted in case reports of patients who previously underwent labyrinthectomy [47]. Recently, 21 of 65 (32%) patients who were post-translabyrinthine VS resection were found to have partial or complete cochlear ossification by MRI at varying time points after surgery [48]. How quickly ossification develops in most patients is still not clear, but this suggests that simultaneous IES removal and CI should be performed if at all possible, or in those patients wishing to delay implantation, a CI depth gauge or obturator should be placed as a space holder until CI placement can be performed.

Conclusion

IES are uncommon tumors that were historically found either at the time of autopsy or unexpectedly during surgery for control of vertigo in patients thought to have Ménière's disease. Numerous retrospective case reports, case series, and literature reviews have increased our knowledge of these tumors. The routine use of high-resolution MRI has increased the likelihood of discovering these tumors and has subsequently increased their incidence. Armed with the knowledge of their clinical presentation and overlap with other neurotologic pathologies, as well as the imaging specifics required to visualize these tumors, clinicians will certainly decrease delays in diagnosis. Though a conservative "wait and scan approach" can be used for patients, operative or radiosurgical management is increasing, especially with the increasing application of CI for single-sided deafness. Like the more common IAC and CPA VS, future IES reports and meta-analyses need to help clarify comparative tumor control, symptom control, and CI hearing outcomes for wait and scan, primary stereotactic radiosurgery, and microsurgical resection.

References

1. Green J. Intralabyrinthine schwannoma. In: Tumors of the ear and temporal bone. Philadelphia: Lippincott Williams & Wilkins; 2000. p. 146–55.
2. Mayer O. Ein Fall von multiplen Tumoren in den Endansbreitungen des Akustikus. Z Ohrenheilk. 1917;75:95–113.
3. Van Abel KV, Carlson ML, Link MJ, et al. Primary inner ear schwannomas: a case series and systematic review of the literature. Laryngoscope. 2013;123(8):1957–66.
4. Dubernard X, Somers T, Veros K, et al. Clinical presentation of intralabyrinthine schwannomas: a multicenter study of 110 cases. Otol Neurotol. 2014;35:1641–9.
5. Marinelli JP, Lohse CM, Carlson ML. Incidence of intralabyrinthine schwannoma: a population-based study within the United States. Otol Neurotol. 2018;39:1191–4.
6. Neff BA, Willcox TO, Sataloff RT. Intralabyrinthine schwannomas. Otol Neurotol. 2003;24:299–307.
7. Kennedy RJ, Shelton C, Salzman KL, et al. Intralabyrinthine schwannomas: diagnosis, management, and a new classification system. Otol Neurotol. 2004;25:160–7.
8. Sterkers JM, Perre J, Viola P, et al. The origin of acoustic neuromas. Acta Otolaryngol. 1987;103:427–31.
9. Xenellis JE, Linthicum FH. On the myth of glial/Schwann junction (Obersteiner-Redlich zone): origin of vestibular nerve schwannomas. Otol Neurotol. 2003;24:1.
10. Roosli C, Linthicum FH, Cureoglu S, et al. What is the site of origin of cochleovestibular schwannomas. Audiol Neurotol. 2012;17:121–5.
11. Amoils CP, Lanser MJ, Jackler RK. Acoustic neuroma presenting as a middle ear mass. Otolaryngol Head Neck Surg. 1992;107:478–82.
12. Stoney PJ, Rurka J, Dolan E, et al. Acoustic neuroma presenting as a middle ear mass. J Otolaryngol. 1991;20:141–3.
13. Doyle KJ, Brackmann DE. Intralabyrinthine schwannomas. Otolaryngol Head Neck Surg. 1994;110:517–23.
14. Committee on Hearing and Equilibrium guidelines for the evaluation of hearing preservation in acoustic neuroma (vestibular schwannoma). American Academy of Otolaryngology–Head and Neck Surgery Foundation, Inc. Otolaryngol Head Neck Surg. 1995;113:179–80.
15. DeLozier HL, Gacek RR, Dana ST. Intralabyrinthine schwannoma. Ann Otol Rhinol Laryngol. 1979;88:187–91.
16. Miyamoto RT, Isenberg SF, Culp WM, et al. Isolated intralabyrinthine schwannoma. Am J Otol. 1980;1:215–7.
17. Hallpike CS. Stapes fixation by an intralabyrinthine 'seedling' neurofibroma as a cause of conductive deafness in a case of von Recklinghausen's disease. Acta Otolaryngol Suppl. 1963;183:62–5.
18. Hamed A, Linthicum F. Intralabyrinthine schwannoma. Otol Neurotol. 2005;26:1085–6.
19. Donnelly M, Daly C, Briggs R. MR imaging features of an intracochlear acoustic schwannoma. J Laryngol Otol. 1994;108:1111–4.
20. Lane JI, Witte RJ, Bolster B, et al. State of the art: 3T imaging of the membranous labyrinth. Am J Neuroradiol. 2008;29:1436–40.
21. Casselman JW, Kuhweide R, Deimling M, et al. Constructive interference in steady state-3DFT-MR imaging of the inner ear and cerebellopontine angle. Amer J Neuroradiol. 1993;14:47–57.
22. Green JD Jr, Beatty CW, Czervionke LF, et al. Intracochlear vestibular schwannoma: a potential source for recurrence after translabyrinthine resection. Otolaryngol Head Neck Surg. 2000;123:281–2.
23. Dahlen RT, Johnson CE, Harnsberger HR, et al. CT and MR imaging characteristics of intravestibular lipoma. Am J Neuroradiol. 2002;23(8):1413–7.
24. Linthicum FH, Alonso A, Denia A. Traumatic neuroma: a complication of transcanal labyrinthectomy. Arch Otolaryngol. 1979;105:654–5.
25. Tan B, Loh A, Yong TT, et al. Inflammatory pseudotumor of the endolymphatic sac: a case report. Am J Otolaryngol Head Neck Med Surg. 2013;34:574–8.
26. Massager N, Drogba L, Delbrouck C, et al. Gamma knife radiosurgery for intralabyrinthine schwannomas. J Radiosurg SBRT. 2011;1:237–45.
27. Tuleasca C, George M, Schiappacasse L, et al. Gamma knife radiosurgery for intravestibular and intracochlear schwannomas. Acta Neurochir. 2019;161:63–7.
28. Iseri M, Ulubil SA, Topdag M, et al. Hearing loss owing to intralabyrinthine schwannoma responsive to intratympanic steroid treatment. J Otolaryngol Head Neck Surg. 2009;38:E95–7.
29. Moffat DA, Parker PA, Hardy DG, et al. Factors affecting final facial nerve outcome following vestibular schwannoma surgery. J Laryngol Otol. 2014;128(5):406–15.
30. Plontke SK, Lloyd SKW, Freeman SRM, et al. Revised classification of inner ear schwannomas. Otol Neurotol. 2025;46:3–9.
31. Presutti L, Alicandri-Ciufelli M, Cigarini E, et al. Cochlear schwannoma removed through the external auditory canal by a transcanal exclusive endoscopic technique. Laryngoscope. 2013;123:2862–7.
32. Schutt CA, Kveton JF. Cochlear implantation after resection of an intralabyrinthine schwannoma. Am J Otol Head Neck Surg. 2014;35:257–60.
33. Aschendorff A, Arndt S, Laszig R, et al. Treatment and auditory rehabilitation of intralabyrinthine schwannoma by means of cochlear implants: English version. HNO. 2017;65(Suppl 1):46–51.
34. Sudhoff H, Scholtz LU, Gehl HB, et al. Quality control after intracochlear intralabyrinthine schwannoma resection and cochlear implantation. Brain Sci. 2021;11(9):1221.
35. Sudhoff H, Riemann C, Kim R, et al. A new device for the removal of cochlear schwannoma: a temporal bone study. Front Surg. 2023;10:1077407.
36. Plontke SK, Kösling S, Rahne T. Cochlear implantation after partial or subtotal cochleoectomy for intracochlear schwannoma removal-A technical report. Otol Neurotol. 2018;39:365–71.
37. Plontke SK, Fröhlich L, Wagner L, et al. How much cochlea do you need for cochlear implantation? Otol Neurotol. 2020;41(5):694–703.
38. Marchioni D, De Rossi S, Soloperto D, et al. Intralabyrinthine schwannomas: a new surgical treatment. Eur Arch Otorrinolaringol. 2018;275:1095–102.

39. Falcioni M, Taibah A, DiTrapani G, et al. Inner ear extension of vestibular schwannomas. Laryngoscope. 2003;113:1605–8.
40. Storrs LA. Acoustic neuromas presenting as middle ear tumors. Laryngoscope. 1974;84:1175–80.
41. Tran Ba Huy P, Hassan JM, Wassef M, et al. Acoustic schwannoma presenting as a tumor of the external auditory canal. Ann Otol Rhinol Laryngol. 1987;96:415–7.
42. Blasco MA, Redleaf MI. Cochlear implantation in unilateral sudden deafness improves tinnitus and speech comprehension: meta-analysis and systematic review. Otol Neurotol. 2014;35(8):1426–32.
43. Sladen D, Carlson ML, Dowling BP, et al. Early outcomes after cochlear implantation for adults and children with unilateral hearing loss. Laryngoscope. 2017;127(7):1683–8.
44. Kronenberg J, Horowitz Z, Hildesheimer M. Intracochlear schwannoma and cochlear implantation. Ann Otol Rhinol Laryngol. 1999;108:659–60.
45. Carlson ML, Neff BA, Sladen DP, et al. Cochlear implantation in patients with intracochlear and intralabyrinthine schwannomas. Otol Neurotol. 2016;37:647–53.
46. Francella S, Ariano M, Bevilacqua F, et al. Cochlear implantation in intralabyrinthine schwannoma: case series and systematic review of the literature. Audiol Res. 2023;13:169–84.
47. Chen DA, Linthicum FH Jr, Rizer FM. Cochlear histopathology in the labyrinthectomized ear: implications for cochlear implantation. Laryngoscope. 1988;98(11):1170–2.
48. Charlett SD, Biggs N. The prevalence of cochlear obliteration after labyrinthectomy using magnetic resonance imaging and the implications for cochlear implantation. Otol Neurotol. 2015;36:1328–30.

Facial Nerve Schwannoma

72

Nicholas L. Deep and Matthew L. Carlson

History

Facial nerve schwannomas (FNS) are slow-growing, benign neoplasms arising from the seventh cranial nerve. They may arise anywhere from the root-exit zone at the brainstem to the terminal branches of the extratemporal facial nerve. Sporadic cases of "facial neuromas" were first reported in the literature as early as 1930, when they were usually discovered incidentally during posterior fossa, temporal bone, or parotid surgery. However, it was not until 1969, when Jack Pulec, working at the Mayo Clinic, published a series of 11 facial nerve tumors and reviewed the literature of the previous 75 reported cases, that a greater understanding and awareness of these rare tumors came [1]. The natural history of FNS was unknown during these early years, and similar to other benign tumors of the skull base, a mere diagnosis served as an indication for aggressive surgery to achieve complete removal [2, 3].

In recent decades, advances in neuroimaging technology, particularly magnetic resonance imaging (MRI), have led to a greater number of patients being diagnosed with smaller, less symptomatic tumors. As a result, observation has taken a more prominent role in the management of FNS [4]. In addition, the advent of stereotactic radiosurgery (SRS) and less aggressive nerve preservation surgical techniques has expanded the treatment options for these benign tumors. Taken together with a larger number of patients being observed and a greater understanding of the natural history, a trend toward preserving neurologic function has taken precedence over disease eradication [5].

N. L. Deep
Department of Otolaryngology—Head and Neck Surgery, Division of Otology and Neurotology, Mayo Clinic, Phoenix, AZ, USA
e-mail: deep.nicholas@mayo.edu

M. L. Carlson (✉)
Department of Otolaryngology—Head and Neck Surgery, Mayo Clinic, Rochester, MN, USA
e-mail: carlson.matthew@mayo.edu

Epidemiology

Schwannomas are the most common tumors of the facial nerve, yet they are rare, with an incidence estimated at 0.8% according to cadaveric temporal bone studies [6]. To provide perspective, cerebellopontine angle (CPA) tumors account for approximately 10% of all intracranial neoplasms, and of all CPA tumors, 80–90% are vestibular schwannomas, while FNS account for only 1–2% [7–9]. Given the rarity of FNS, demographic information is limited to a handful of large case series and systematic reviews [4, 5, 10–14].

The incidence of FNS began to increase after the widespread adoption of MRI in the early 1990s, owing to its enhanced sensitivity for detecting these neoplasms. They are slow-growing tumors with a typical growth rate of around 1.5–2 mm/year, which closely matches the growth rate of other skull base schwannomas, including vestibular schwannomas [11, 15]. FNS most commonly present in the fourth or fifth decade of life, but have been reported in patients as young as 1 month old to as old as 81 years of age [10, 11, 13, 16]. There does not appear to be a strong gender predilection for FNS [10]. Patients with neurofibromatosis type 2 (NF2) are more likely to have an FNS compared with the general population, though the correlation is not as strong as is seen with vestibular schwannomas [17].

Histopathology

Schwannomas are benign tumors that grow eccentrically to the nerve fibers and result in damage by compressing the nerve trunk and adjacent structures. FNS are thought to be derived from the sensory fibers of the facial nerve, while other theories contend that they originate in the area of the geniculate ganglion due to embryologic diversity [13]. Proximal to the geniculate ganglion, the facial nerve is devoid of epineurium; however, distal to it, there is an ingrowth of connective tissue and separation into fascicles

A. D. Sweeney et al. (eds.), *Haynes-Glasscock-Shambaugh Surgery of the Ear*, https://doi.org/10.1007/978-3-032-18264-7_72

[14]. This finding has surgical implications, since the intracranial portion of the nerve is more delicate and more likely to be spread out in the presence of a tumor due to the absence of epineurium. Importantly, histologic studies have shown that, in approximately 65% of cases, the tumor pushes the nerve trunk to the periphery, but in the remaining patients, the nerve fibers are spread throughout the substance of the tumor [18]. For this reason, a blind biopsy of the tumor is not recommended. Alternatively, if the schwannoma appears to be arising from a more peripheral nerve fiber under high-powered magnification during surgery, it may be amenable to resection with preservation of the bulk of the facial nerve [19]. Classically, FNS have been described to contain "skip lesions" along the nerve based on radiographic evidence of multiple tumors along the nerve with normal-appearing intervening segments; however, on microscopic examination, there are often multiple discrete intraneural connections seen connecting the distant portions of the lesion [11, 18]. It is not uncommon for FNS to "dumbbell" through foramina. For example, an FNS tumor involving the distal internal auditory canal and the geniculate ganglion will usually contain a constriction point at the meatal foramen and the labyrinthine segment. Indeed, true radiologic skip lesions are rare and are not reported in most modern series. The exception to this finding is in the case of a severe phenotype of NF2, where multiple separate tumors may develop along multiple cranial nerves.

Histologically, two predominant patterns can be seen: Antoni A and Antoni B. Antoni A patterns are compact, cellular regions with elongated, uniform spindle cells and whirling or palisading nuclei aligned in rows (termed Verocay bodies). Antoni B areas are loose and less cellular regions with a spongy appearance. On immunohistochemistry, both normal and neoplastic Schwann cells express S-100, a calcium-binding protein and marker for nerve-derived tumors. Schwannomas are also vimentin-positive and epithelial membrane antigen (EMA)-negative.

Anatomical Locations

FNS may involve any portion of the facial nerve—from "pons to parotid"—and classically involve multiple contiguous segments. On average, two to three segments of the facial nerve are involved [12, 16]. The most common location for an FNS is the labyrinthine/geniculate segment of the facial nerve, which is involved in approximately 53% of cases (Fig. 72.1) [4, 5, 11, 15, 16, 20–22]. The internal auditory canal (IAC) and tympanic segments are the next most frequently involved sites (52% and 42%, respectively), since these segments are often implicated by direct extension from the tumor originating in the labyrinthine/geniculate area. The CPA, mastoid, and intraparotid segments are less frequently involved, at approximately 40%, 31%, and 15%, respectively. The actual percentage of IAC-CPA involvement may be higher, given that FNS isolated to this region are typically presumed to be vestibular schwannomas until proven otherwise [5, 11, 16, 21]. In fact, FNS may account for about 2% of supposed vestibular schwannomas [9]. Other areas that have been reported to be involved by FNS include the nervus intermedius, the greater superficial petrosal nerve, the nerve to the stapedius, and the chorda tympani [23–25].

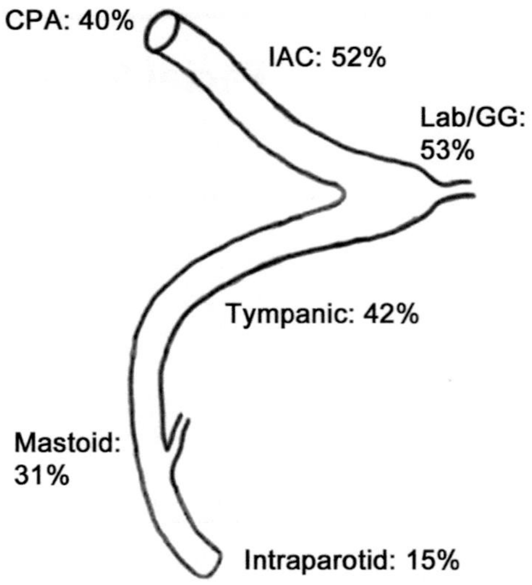

Fig. 72.1 Rate of involvement of each facial nerve segment. The labyrinthine/geniculate area is the most frequent site involved and appears to be the origin for many FNS. Therefore, as they grow to involve adjacent segments of the nerve, the IAC and tympanic segments are the next most frequently involved sites. However, FNS may originate from any segment of the facial nerve, and extend retrograde or anterograde to involve additional segments. (Percentages are based on the combined, non-redundant data from the largest case series, mostly performed in the post-MRI era [4, 5, 11, 15, 16, 21])

Clinical Evaluation

History

The presentation of FNS is widely variable and depends on the location of the tumor. Hearing loss and facial nerve symptoms (discussed below) are the most common presenting complaints. Other reported symptoms include tinnitus, imbalance, vertigo, pain, otalgia, headache, epiphora, parotid mass, dysgeusia, otorrhea, and xerostomia. Large tumors expanding in the CPA can affect adjacent cranial nerves such as CN V, causing facial numbness, and can result in brainstem compression, resulting in ataxia, hydrocephalus, and numerous other complaints (Table 72.1).

Table 72.1 Clinical manifestations

Symptom	Frequency (%)[a]
Hearing loss	50–79
Facial paralysis or spasms	50–60
Facial numbness	14–25
Tinnitus	13–60
Ear canal mass	10–15
Otalgia	10–15
Vertigo or imbalance	10–48
Otorrhea	2–6

[a]A range of reported frequency of symptoms according to the largest case series [4, 11, 14–16, 23]

Hearing Loss

Hearing loss is reported in 50–70% of patients with FNS at presentation, most of whom demonstrate a sensorineural (SNHL) pattern of loss [4, 11, 16, 23]. SNHL occurs with tumors involving the CPA, IAC, or labyrinthine segments and is due to compression of the cochlear nerve or erosion into the cochlea by the tumor. Conductive hearing loss occurs when the tumor involves the tympanic or mastoid segments, whereby it comes into contact with the ossicular chain or blocks mastoid air cell drainage patterns, resulting in a localized effusion. Rarely, a tumor involving the mastoid segment may expand into the external auditory canal, resulting in obstruction [26].

Facial Nerve Symptoms

Facial nerve symptoms, including paresis, spasm, synkinesis, and/or contracture, are present in over 50–60% of patients at presentation [10, 11]. Facial weakness is slowly progressive over weeks to months in over 80% of patients with FNS, unlike Bell's palsy, which occurs quickly over the course of one or 2 days [27, 28]. The remaining patients may have an abrupt onset, transient, or recurrent facial palsy, thereby masquerading as Bell's palsy [23]. However, the concomitant finding of asymmetric hearing loss in many patients with FNS is not typical of Bell's palsy. Unfortunately, a delay in diagnosis of up to 2–3 years is reported in many patients with FNS due to an initial misdiagnosis as Bell's palsy [11, 20, 27].

In modern series, approximately 50% of the patients have normal, House-Brackmann Grade (HB) I facial nerve function, 10–30% have mild-to-moderate facial nerve weakness (HB II–III), and the remaining patients have severe facial nerve function (HB IV–VI) at presentation [4, 5, 11, 14–16]. Since many patients will have normal function, it is critical to ask about a history of transient facial weakness, facial spasms, or twitching. Facial weakness and spasms are more common in tumors involving the intratemporal facial nerve course—particularly the labyrinthine, geniculate, or tympanic segments—since growth of the tumor within the bony confines of the fallopian canal results in neural compression and vascular plexus congestion, which leads to ischemia of the motor fibers [11, 13, 27]. In contrast, tumors involving the parotid gland and those predominantly within the CPA are less likely to present with facial paresis, since the tumor is surrounded by more distensible tissue and has less resistance during expansion [11, 13]. McMenomey et al. highlight the importance of location on facial nerve symptoms in their study, which showed that 0% of tumors (0/12) involving the CPA-IAC solely caused facial nerve dysfunction, while 83% of tumors (15/18) involving the more distal, intratemporal course of the facial nerve did present with facial weakness [13].

Physical Exam & Electrical Testing

On physical exam, facial nerve weakness and/or synkinesis may be evident. Otoscopy may reveal a pale, nonpulsatile middle ear mass in the upper two-thirds of the tympanic membrane (Fig. 72.2). Occasionally, the tumor may be seen within the external ear canal, particularly if the mastoid segment of the facial nerve is involved (Fig. 72.2b). An audiogram will confirm hearing loss, which will be sensorineural, conductive, or mixed in nature, depending on the location. In select cases, electrical testing may also be helpful in evaluating and monitoring facial nerve deficits. Evoked electromyography (EEMG) will show a prolonged conduction latency with or without a reduced amplitude if a tumor is present [29]. Since FNS expands slowly, electromyography (EMG) can show signs of degeneration (fibrillation) and regeneration (polyphasic potentials) simultaneously.

Office biopsy of these tumors is not recommended because intact nerve fibers can permeate the tumor and, if transected, facial paralysis may occur. In most cases, the diagnosis can be made based on a characteristic history, physical exam, and imaging findings, particularly when multiple contiguous segments are involved. In cases where the diagnosis remains uncertain, an operative biopsy can be performed by mapping the tumor surface and taking a small diagnostic sample in a region that does not evoke EMG activity with monopolar stimulation.

Radiology

Imaging plays a vital role in the diagnosis and management of FNS, and both CT and MRI serve important, complementary roles. Any patient with slowly progressive facial paralysis, recurrent ipsilateral paralysis, hyperkinesis, or asymmetric sensorineural hearing loss should undergo MRI to evaluate the full length of the facial nerve from the brainstem to the parotid. Multiple, contiguous segments of facial nerve involvement—evidenced by enlargement of the fallopian canal on CT and enhancement on post-contrast MRI—

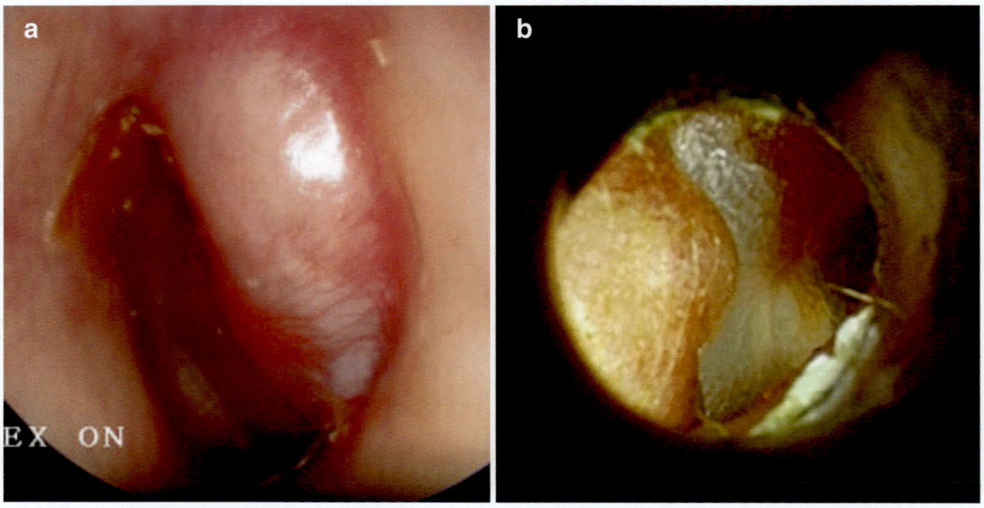

Fig. 72.2 Two examples of facial nerve schwannomas involving the middle ear and mastoid seen during otoscopy. (**a**) In the first example, a left-sided tumor is seen filling the posterior mesotympanum with lateral displacement of the tympanic membrane. (**b**) In the second example, a right-sided facial nerve schwannoma is seen displacing the posterior tympanic membrane and the medial bony canal wall. (Published with permission from Carlson et al. [11])

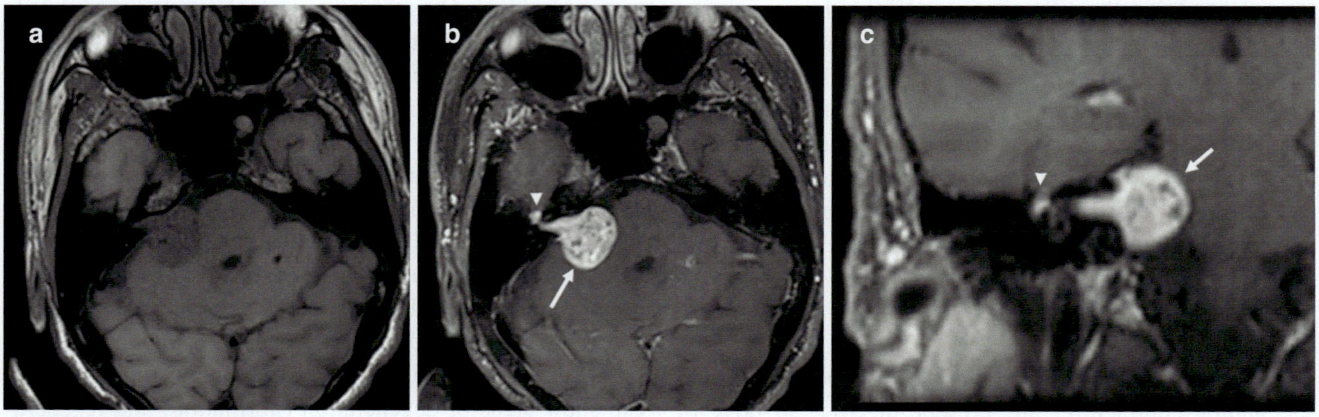

Fig. 72.3 (**a**) Pre-contrast T1 axial, (**b**) post-contrast T1 axial and (**c**) post-contrast T1 coronal MRI depicting a right-sided facial nerve schwannoma involving the cerebellopontine angle (white arrow), the internal auditory canal, and the geniculate ganglion (white arrowhead). Posterior fossa facial nerve schwannomas can be reliably distinguished from vestibular schwannoma only when there is radiological evidence of tumor extension into the labyrinthine segment or beyond

are nearly diagnostic for FNS. On MRI, schwannomas are hypointense or isointense relative to brain tissue on non-contrasted T1-weighted images and enhance following gadolinium administration (Fig. 72.3) [21]. When large, schwannomas can have heterogeneous densities or areas of microcystic or macrocystic degeneration, which most commonly occur in the parotid gland and the CPA [11].

Comparing facial nerve enhancement to the contralateral side is often used clinically as a measure to identify pathology. However, this technique should be used with caution because even normal facial nerves may enhance—occasionally asymmetrically as well—following contrast administration [30]. For this reason, CT can serve a complementary role when faced with equivocal enhancement patterns. On CT, an FNS will appear as a benign, expansile mass with smooth osseous widening of the fallopian canal rather than bony destruction (Fig. 72.4) [21]. As the tumor grows, it tends to spread longitudinally within the bony fallopian canal, resulting in a smooth fusiform bony expansion, which may be very subtle on imaging. Otic capsule erosion may be seen, and localized effusions may develop as mastoid air cell tracts become obstructed.

Differential Diagnosis

FNS has a wide differential, largely based on location. Broadly, these include vestibular schwannoma, meningioma, hemangioma, a paraganglioma tumor (including glomus faciale), traumatic neuroma, facial nerve neurofibroma, granular cell tumor, perineurioma, parotid tumors (e.g., pleomorphic adenoma, malignant parotid tumors with perineural spread), sarcoidosis/neurosarcoidosis, hypertrophic polyneuropathy, and metastatic disease (e.g., breast cancer, lung cancer, lymphoma). When limited to a single anatomic location, the diagnosis may be difficult to differentiate from other

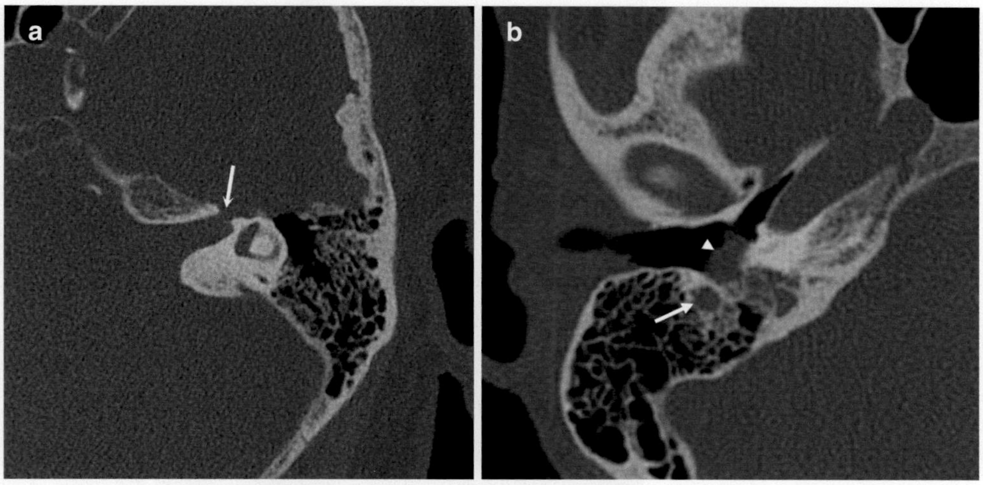

Fig. 72.4 (**a**) Temporal bone CT scan demonstrating a left facial nerve schwannoma involving the labyrinthine segment and resulting in the widening of the fallopian canal (arrow). (**b**) A different case depicting a right-sided facial nerve schwannoma is seen involving the tympanic (arrowhead) and mastoid (arrow) segments. Note the enlarged diameter of the fallopian canal within the mastoid

neoplasms common to the area, but when multiple segments of the facial nerve are involved, the diagnosis of FNS becomes significantly more apparent.

IAC-CPA Segments

The greatest diagnostic dilemma is often encountered with purely intracanalicular FNS or those growing into the CPA. Close attention to the presence of a "labyrinthine tail" (enhancement) will aid in accurately diagnosing an FNS over the more common vestibular schwannoma [21]. However, without evidence of labyrinthine involvement, these tumors are radiographically indistinguishable from a vestibular schwannoma (Fig. 72.5a). The reported misdiagnosis rate for FNS as vestibular schwannomas ranges from 20–64% [4, 11, 13, 21, 31, 32]. This is sensible given their similar clinical presentations. FNS isolated to the CPA-IAC present with SNHL and rarely with facial weakness, and likewise, <5% of patients with vestibular schwannomas present with facial weakness. Therefore, the diagnosis of a vestibular schwannoma is presumed based on probability [33, 34]. A high index of suspicion is necessary to diagnose an FNS. Clues that may alert the clinician to suspect a FNS include a history of transient facial weakness, twitching, or spasm. In the future, high-density diffusion tensor MRI may be valuable in the evaluation of CPA tumors by delineating the neural structures from which a tumor originates.

Meningiomas should also be considered in this location, since they share radiographic features with schwannomas. Classically, meningiomas are more eccentrically positioned relative to the IAC at the porus acusticus, have a broad dural tail, and less frequently extend into the IAC. However, meningiomas may occasionally originate in the IAC and extend laterally to involve the temporal bone, tracking along the cochlear or vestibular nerves and resulting in a wide invasion of the cochlea and vestibular apparatus [35, 36]. In rare cases, meningiomas have demonstrated intrafascicular spread along multiple, contiguous segments of the facial nerve, particularly in children with NF2, and appear radiographically indistinguishable from FNS [37, 38].

Labyrinthine/Geniculate Segments

FNS may resemble a "dumbbell" when the tumor extends from the IAC through the fundus and labyrinthine segment and into the geniculate fossa (or vice versa) (Fig. 72.3) [39]. It is important to differentiate these cases from a transmodiolar vestibular or cochlear schwannoma, which would be identified by its extension into the cochlea [39]. Alternatively, meningiomas intrinsic to the geniculate ganglion may grow into the IAC, giving rise to the same "dumbbell" appearance as an FNS [40]. For surgical planning purposes, it is important to carefully inspect for a cochlear fistula, which increases the risk of postoperative sensorineural hearing loss if present.

FNS primarily involving the geniculate ganglion appears as a round-to-oval focal enlargement of the geniculate fossa itself [12]. They have been reported to extend along the greater superficial petrosal nerve, giving a scalloped appearance to the adjacent bony petrous apex and presenting as a middle cranial fossa mass (Fig. 72.6) [41, 42]. Rarely, a large cystic tumor may involve the geniculate ganglion, mimicking a petrous apex cyst [11]. A geniculate ganglion hemangioma (GGH) can resemble an FNS of the geniculate fossa. GGH tumors are discussed in greater detail in Chap. 73, though classically, they have an amorphous honeycomb appearance with intratumoral calcifications on CT, which can be absent in 50% of cases [26, 43]. Therefore, other differentiating factors include the more heterogeneous enhancement on MRI for hemangiomas and the more irregular, poorly defined, "moth-eaten" appearance of the bony margins on CT versus the smooth bony margins of an FNS [21]. Even small hemangiomas can result in facial nerve weakness, which is uncommon for schwannomas.

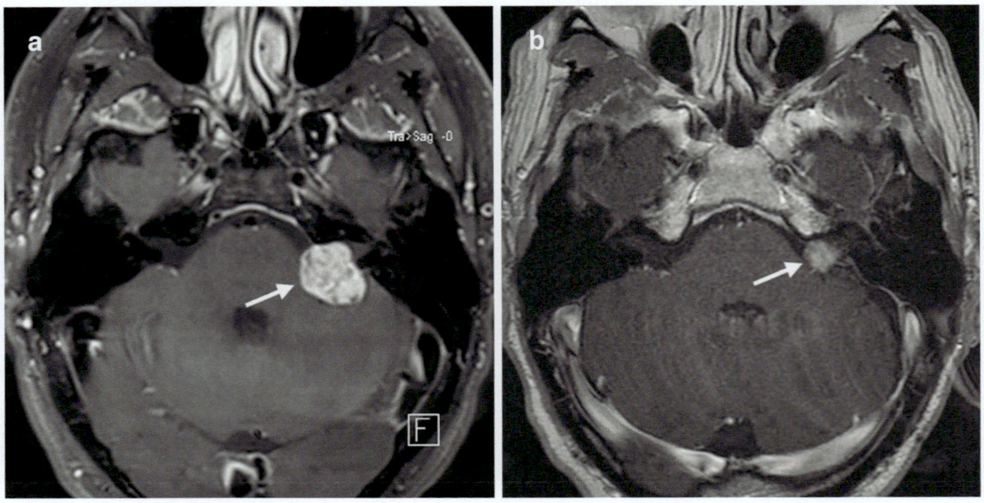

Fig. 72.5 (**a**) A left-sided 2.3 cm facial nerve schwannoma involving the cerebellopontine angle and the porus acusticus is seen. Without evidence of labyrinthine or middle ear involvement, this is radiologically presumed to be a vestibular schwannoma. (**b**) Following retrosigmoid craniotomy and subtotal resection, a 6-mm maximum dimension residual tumor is seen on postoperative MRI. (Published with permission from Carlson et al. [11])

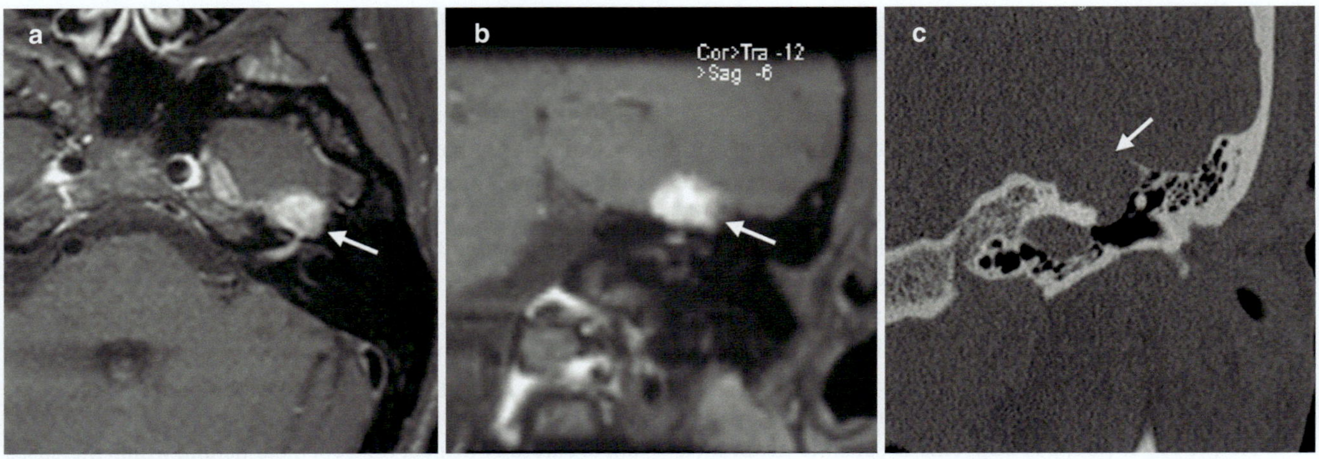

Fig. 72.6 (**a**) A left-sided facial nerve schwannoma involving the internal auditory canal, labyrinthine/geniculate, and tympanic segments of the facial nerve. Coronal (**b**) MRI and (**c**) CT demonstrate marked expansion with "autodecompression" of the geniculate portion of the tumor; however, tight narrowing persists at the meatal foramen. This patient experienced facial spasm without paresis over a 38-month course of observation with serial MRI. The white arrows indicate the portion of the left-sided facial nerve schwannoma that involves the geniculate ganglion and the middle fossa. (Published with permission from Carlson et al. [11])

Tympanic Segment

When the tympanic segment is involved, FNS appears as a middle ear mass that can result in smooth pressure erosion and displacement of the ossicular chain. Erosion into the lateral semicircular canal can be seen [12]. A cholesteatoma can yield similar radiographic findings on CT and may present clinically in the same way (e.g., conductive hearing loss, sudden or slowly progressive facial nerve weakness, a white mass behind an intact tympanic membrane); however, in contrast to FNS, cholesteatomas do not enhance on post-contrast MRI and do demonstrate diffusion restriction. Furthermore, most cholesteatomas have involvement of the tympanic membrane, evidenced by retraction or crusting, while FNS usually presents with an intact tympanic membrane.

A paraganglioma (glomus tympanicum) should also be considered in the setting of a fleshy middle ear mass, though in this case, otoscopy would usually demonstrate a more red, pulsatile mass. Even more rare is a paraganglioma of the facial nerve, which commonly presents with flow voids and facial paralysis, even with smaller tumors [44]. A middle ear adenoma could appear similar, but it does not usually extend into the facial canal [26].

A traumatic neuroma of the facial nerve may develop following head trauma and have similar radiographic findings [45]. However, the history of trauma immediately preceding the paralysis is a clue that the lesion is not a true neoplasm, but rather, a pseudotumor. During the normal regenerative process after a nerve is disrupted, the distal segment undergoes Wallerian degeneration, and the proximal segment sends regenerative axons into the distal endoneurial tubes, forming a small neuroma. Traumatic neuromas arise when there is a gap that cannot be bridged, which results in a proliferation of Schwann cells and misdirected growth of axons, which ultimately form a large neuroma that radiographically mimics an FNS or GGH [45].

Mastoid Segment

FNS involving the mastoid segment results in a widened fallopian canal, particularly when compared to the contralateral side (Fig. 72.4b). They may erode into the external auditory canal, resulting in symptoms of otitis externa or mimicking a canal cholesteatoma [26]. The tumor may also extend to involve the branch to the stapedius or chorda tympani nerves [23, 24]. As it expands, the tumor breaks through the thin-walled septations between mastoid air cells, giving rise to an irregular, destructive-appearing tumor margin, mimicking an invasive tumor such as a metastasis or perineural spread from a parotid or cutaneous malignancy [21].

An intraneural perineurioma is another rare, benign tumor that may clinically and radiographically masquerade as an FNS since it has been described to involve multiple segments of the intratemporal facial nerve, including the tympanic and mastoid segments [46, 47]. Due to the similarity in growth patterns and symptoms, differentiation is made on histopathology, where perineurial cell proliferation extending into the endoneurium and concentrically surrounding endoneurial capillaries and nerve fibers are seen [46, 48]. Perineuriomas stain positive for epithelial membrane antigen and negative for S-100 protein (in contrast to schwannomas) [49].

Extracranial Segments

Intraparotid FNS typically resembles a benign pleomorphic adenoma, both clinically and radiographically [26]. As a result, there is frequent misdiagnosis when the FNS is isolated to the parotid gland without extension into the mastoid. Tumor extension toward the stylomastoid foramen favors the diagnosis of a FNS over a pleomorphic adenoma; however, this presentation also mimics a malignant salivary tumor with perineural spread, such as adenoid cystic cancer, particularly in the setting of partial facial paresis. Since FNS within the parotid gland is not confined by bone, it can often develop large cystic components as they grow [11].

Management Overview

Historically, gross total resection (GTR) involving nerve sacrifice and reinnervation with a cable graft or nerve transfer was the standard management of FNS. However, over recent decades, there has been a growing trend toward conservatism in the treatment of benign skull base pathology, whereby the focus has shifted from complete tumor removal toward strategies that minimize long-term cranial nerve dysfunction [4, 5]. As a result, observation has taken a more prominent role, and alternative nerve-preserving techniques, including decompression, "nerve stripping," subtotal resection (STR), and GTR with nerve preservation, have been described. In addition, the use of stereotactic radiosurgery—which has had success in the treatment of vestibular schwannomas—has emerged as a viable treatment modality for FNS as well.

In the following section, each modality will be explored, and a simplified algorithm is presented (Fig. 72.7). However, in practice, the decision to proceed with observation, surgery, radiation, or multimodality therapy is highly nuanced and depends on several factors, including the tumor location, size, growth pattern, patient age, status of facial nerve function, hearing status, reconstructive efforts, and the patient's desires.

Observation

Observation with serial MRI surveillance has become increasingly utilized in the management of FNS because the natural history of these tumors is better understood, particularly in comparison with the outcomes of treatment. In the House Clinic series on FNS, 0 of the 27 tumors (0%) diagnosed prior to 1995 were observed, whereas 15 of the 52 tumors (28.8%) diagnosed after 1995 were initially observed, highlighting this trend toward conservatism [5]. Patients with FNS but without confirmed growth, those with normal or mild-to-moderate facial nerve weakness (HB I–III), and those without brainstem compression are good candidates for observation. Furthermore, elderly patients or the medically infirm with tumors that are unlikely to result in severe complications over their expected life span are good candidates for observation.

Perez et al. reported on 13 cases, which were observed with serial MRI over a mean follow-up of 5 years. Eight patients (62%) had stable facial nerve function, and 5 patients (38%) developed worsening facial weakness. However, of those 5 patients with deteriorating facial function, all except 1 patient maintained an HB II or III at last follow-up, which is as good or better than the results of nerve grafting [15]. Liu and Fagan reported on 10 patients who were observed over 10 years, and found that 80% maintained normal facial function [50]. Yang et al. reviewed 21 cases of FNS and found that 87% of patients maintained good facial nerve function (HB I–III) over the course of a 6.4-year follow-up. They also found that larger tumors (>1 cm) were observed to grow faster over the observation period [51]. In the Mayo Clinic series of 80 FNS diagnosed in the post-MRI era, 31 patients (39%) were initially observed, of which 29 presented with HB I–III and 2 presented with HB IV–VI. At last follow-up

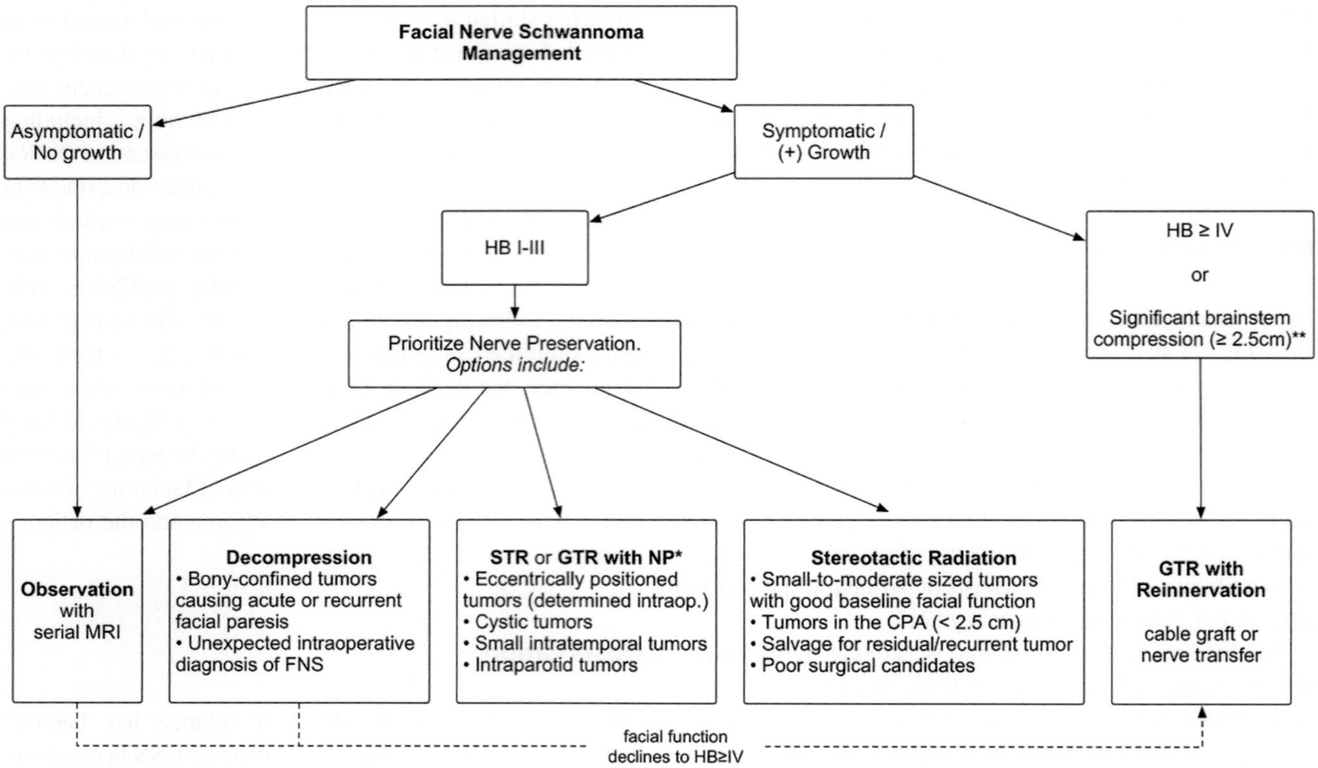

Fig. 72.7 A simplified management algorithm for facial nerve schwannomas. CPA cerebellopontine angle, GTR gross total resection, HB House-Brackmann Grade, NP nerve preservation, STR subtotal resection. *GTR with nerve preservation has been described in different ways by different authors, and may include "stripping surgery," [65, 66] "fascicle preservation surgery," [10, 63] or "shaving off" the tumor while preserving at least 50% of the nerve in continuity [14]. **In general, a tumor that is roughly 2.5 cm or greater in dimension within the CPA is not a candidate for SRS since posttreatment swelling may result in hydrocephalus

(median 33 months), 28 patients demonstrated HB I–III function, suggesting that only 1 patient suffered a decline in function to the point where surgical grafting would yield similar results [11].

These studies suggest that over half of the patients with asymptomatic FNS can be conservatively managed with serial MRI alone, thereby delaying or avoiding treatment altogether. This spares the patients the potential morbidity of surgery and allows them to maintain normal or near-normal facial nerve function for a longer period of time, which is better than what can be achieved with grafting. A caveat that deserves mention is that the mean follow-up time in these studies may be insufficient to foster a long-term understanding of slow-growing tumors like FNS. It is possible that, over a longer period of follow-up, more of these patients (especially young patients) in the observation cohort will require treatment as their tumors grow and become symptomatic.

Traditionally, surgical intervention is indicated after a patient's facial nerve function progresses to an HB III or IV, because facial nerve grafting would, at best, yield similar results. Occasionally, other considerations besides facial nerve function drive the decision to operate, including brainstem compression, cosmetic deformity from a large parotid lesion, or the risk of a labyrinthine fistula, which would result in deafness and dizziness. Over recent decades, the greater use of SRS (discussed below) and the use of nerve preservation microsurgical techniques have provided alternatives to earlier surgical intervention by potentially being able to halt tumor growth or prevent symptom onset or progression.

Stereotactic Radiosurgery

Growing experience with SRS has supported its role in the treatment of FNS. SRS for vestibular schwannomas has demonstrated success, with 10-year tumor control rates around 90% and a ≤1% incidence of facial nerve paresis [52]. Given the efficacy of SRS for vestibular schwannomas, its application for FNS was a natural extension, and preliminary studies have suggested that FNS responds to SRS in a similar fashion [53–55]. Radiation therapy comes in 3 different forms: Gamma Knife (GKS), Linear Accelerator/LINAC (including CyberKnife), and fractionated SRS. The goal of SRS is the prevention of long-term tumor growth (as opposed to removing the tumor), maintenance of neurologic function, and prevention of new neurologic deficits.

In 2015, McRackan et al. published a meta-analysis summarizing 11 studies including 45 patients with at least 2-years of follow-up. Using SRS, a 93.3% tumor control rate was found, which is defined as no growth or shrinkage of the tumor. The facial nerve function was stable in 66%, improved in 20.5%, and worsened in 12.8%. Of the patients with serviceable hearing prior to SRS, 64.3% had stable hearing, and 36.7% had worsened function after SRS. Carlson et al. reported on 11 patients with IAC or CPA tumors treated primarily with SRS and 2 patients treated with adjuvant SRS after STR. Nine of 11 patients (82%) treated primarily achieved tumor control [11].

Moon et al. reviewed 14 patients with FNS treated with GKS (13.2 Gy mean tumor margin dose), 5 of whom had already undergone STR [56]. Control of tumor growth was achieved in 100% of patients who were followed for longer than 2 years. Facial nerve function improved in 2 patients, remained unchanged in 9 patients, and worsened in 3 patients. In the 3 patients who experienced deteriorating facial nerve function, the onset was within 3 months of SRS, and the schwannomas involved bony-confined segments of the facial nerve (labyrinthine/geniculate segments). In addition, they demonstrated expansion with a loss of central enhancement on MRI at 6 months (Fig. 72.8). For this reason, the authors suggested the development of facial palsy after radiosurgery for FNS—which appears to be higher than in vestibular schwannoma treatment—might be due to mechanical damage to the facial nerve caused by the transient edema and expansion within the bony-confined temporal bone, which results in neuropraxia. The use of corticosteroids to control edema during the first several months after radiosurgery may help prevent and alleviate facial palsy [56]. With respect to hearing outcomes, all patients who had serviceable pretreatment hearing maintained their hearing at a useful level after treatment. The authors propose GKS as a good primary treatment option for patients with a small-to-medium-sized FNS when facial nerve function and hearing are relatively preserved [56].

Sheehan et al. reviewed the results of 42 patients treated at 8 separate centers that are part of the North American Gamma Knife Consortium [57]. Fifteen (36%) had prior STR; the mean marginal dose was 12.5 Gy, and the mean follow-up was 42 months. Tumor control was achieved in 90% of patients [57]. Preoperative facial nerve function was preserved in 38 of 42 patients (90%). Patients with pre-SRS facial function of HB I–III and those with smaller tumors (≤ 1 cm^3 in volume) were more likely to preserve pretreatment function, suggesting that upfront SRS may be the treatment of choice for small FNS, in addition to its use as an effective salvage treatment for residual/recurrent tumor that remains or progresses after resection. The authors found that temporary or permanent neurologic symptoms were avoided by keeping the tumor margin dose to 12.5 Gy or less [57]. Another multi-institutional retrospective study was published in 2016 by Hasegawa et al., who reviewed 42 cases of FNS treated at 10 separate medical centers affiliated with the Japan Leksell Gamma Knife Society [58]. Thirteen (31%) had prior microsurgery, the mean marginal dose was 12 Gy, and the median follow-up was 48 months. The actuarial 5-year progression-free survival rate was 92%. Facial function improved in 8 (19%) patients, remained unchanged in 29 (69%), and worsened in 5 (12%). In the 5 patients with facial nerve decline, 2 patients with pre-SRS HB I developed HB III, and 3 patients with pre-SRS HB II nerve function developed HB III (2 patients) or Grade IV (1 patient). These results suggest that even in those patients who do suffer facial nerve paresis, it is comparable to surgical outcomes with grafting. Of the 40 evaluated patients, hearing function

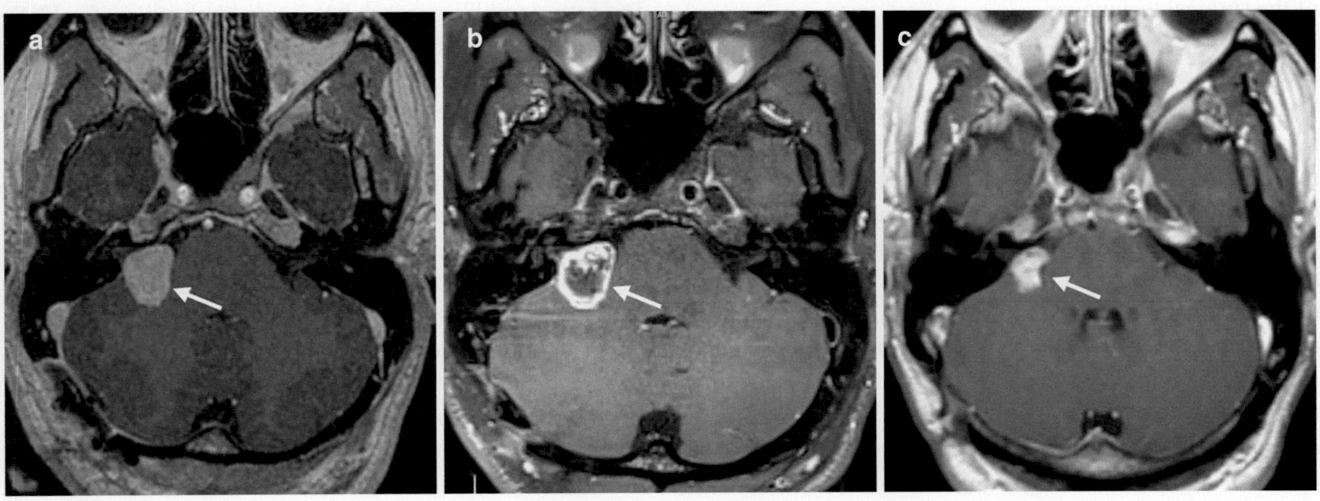

Fig. 72.8 (**a**) Two cm right-sided facial nerve schwannoma involving the cerebellopontine angle. (**b**) Six months after radiosurgery, the tumor has remained stable in size with loss of central enhancement consistent with tumor necrosis. (**c**) Twelve months after treatment, the tumor has shrunk in size compared with the pretreatment tumor volume. (Published with permission from Carlson et al. [11])

improved in 1 (3%) patient, remained stable in 35 (88%), and worsened in 4 (10%) [58].

Taken together, these data suggest that SRS may be indicated in a variety of cases, including primary treatment of small- to medium-sized tumors in patients with good facial function, adjuvant therapy after surgery if a remnant tumor begins to grow, or in elderly or medically infirm patients who are not good surgical candidates. On the other hand, SRS is generally contraindicated for large tumors (>2.5 cm) causing life-threatening brainstem and fourth ventricle compression. Such large tumors, even if not clinically symptomatic, can cause postoperative problems when there is swelling, which can lead to obstructive hydrocephalus requiring emergent intervention. Overall, preliminary results with SRS for FNS are very promising. Longer-term studies are needed to more adequately compare treatment outcomes to the more conventional surgical methods and to observation alone.

Microsurgery

Historically, microsurgical resection was the mainstay of treatment for any tumor involving the CPA or IAC. Though rates of surgery for benign skull base tumors have declined in recent decades, surgery remains an important part of the treatment algorithm. In general, patients with poor facial nerve function (HB IV–VI) or with evidence of brainstem compression may be best treated with GTR followed by reinnervation. However, for patients with normal-to-moderate facial nerve weakness (HB I–III), the indications for surgery are more nuanced and controversial. A variety of surgical techniques emphasizing nerve preservation have been described, including decompression, STR, and GTR with nerve preservation. In the following section, the various surgical approaches will be described, followed by a discussion of the surgical techniques.

Surgical Approaches

The full spectrum of neurotological surgical approaches is relevant to FNS, given its propensity to involve multiple segments of the facial nerve. The choice depends on the location of the tumor, the segments involved, the hearing status of the patient, and the reconstructive needs. The majority of FNS involve the intratemporal facial nerve course, but many extend intracranially and/or extracranially, and therefore, combined approaches may be necessary for complete exposure. For example, a tympanic segment FNS approached transmastoid may necessitate a middle fossa craniotomy to clear a positive margin more proximally or to access the proximal stump for nerve grafting. Furthermore, at the time of surgery, tumors may exhibit microscopic extension that is more extensive than predicted based on clinical and radiographic examination. For this reason, it is imperative that the surgeon is comfortable with exposing the entire course of the facial nerve because the ablative and reconstructive efforts may require extensive exposure.

The standard mastoidectomy approach can be used for tumors involving the vertical segment of the facial nerve, all the way to the stylomastoid foramen. An atticotomy and facial recess can be drilled to access the tympanic portion of the nerve. Often, the ossicular chain is displaced due to a tumor in the middle ear, in which case an ossiculoplasty may be performed.

Hearing status plays an important role in deciding the surgical approach for tumors that involve the geniculate ganglion, labyrinthine, IAC, or CPA segments. In patients with good hearing, a tumor that is centered around the geniculate ganglion (as is often the case) can be accessed via the combined transmastoid–middle fossa approach. The transmastoid approach allows the surgeon to remove a tumor that extends along the tympanic and vertical segments and provides a corridor below the dura and above the horizontal semicircular canal to access the geniculate ganglion. A middle fossa craniotomy (MCF) allows the surgeon to clear the nerve margin as the tumor extends along the labyrinthine and intracanalicular segments. This approach can also access tumors up to about 1 cm into the CPA. The MCF approach also provides access to a proximal stump of the nerve for nerve grafting. Mowry et al. reported that all patients who underwent the MCF approach retained serviceable hearing, and specifically, all patients maintained their preoperative word recognition scores of between 80% and 100% [59].

In patients without serviceable hearing, the translabyrinthine technique provides wide exposure to the entire length of the facial nerve from the brainstem to the stylomastoid foramen. Additionally, it provides the best access for facial nerve grafting. For large tumors involving the geniculate fossa, a transotic approach provides even greater exposure. The retrosigmoid approach has limited indications for FNS, especially because it is unable to access the labyrinthine segment of the facial nerve, which is frequently involved. The retrosigmoid approach may be preferred for tumors largely extending into the CPA with or without brainstem compression, particularly in patients with serviceable hearing. The retrosigmoid approach can access the CPA and IAC without violation of the otic capsule; however, distal stump neurorrhaphy cannot be feasibly performed if the tumor extends beyond the lateral third of the IAC.

Parotid tumors are approached through standard parotidectomy techniques, with identification of the main trunk of the facial nerve, followed by the branches distally. Often, intraparotid FNS are pedunculated off one of the peripheral branches of the facial nerve and are amenable to being "shaved off" without significant functional loss (Fig. 72.9) [60]. This is also made possible due to the redundant innervation provided by the extensive branching pattern within

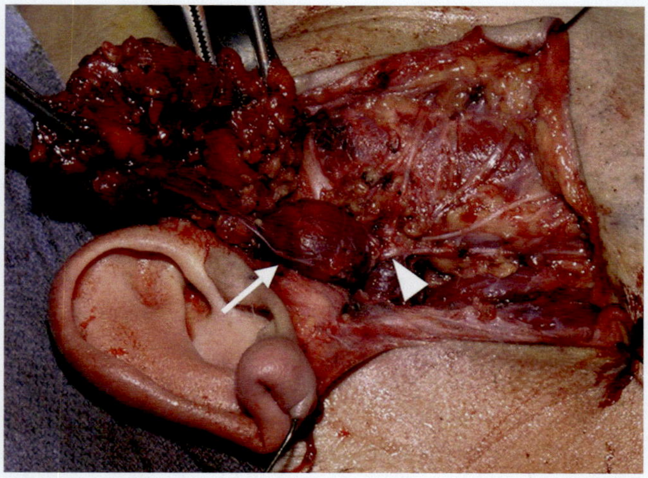

Fig. 72.9 A right-sided facial nerve schwannoma involving the stylomastoid foramen and proximal extratemporal facial nerve. Following a superficial parotidectomy, a pedunculated tumor (white arrow) with a relatively thin stalk can be seen tethered to the main trunk of the facial nerve (white arrowhead). In this case, the tumor could be completely resected, with recovery of normal postoperative facial nerve function. (Published with permission from Carlson et al. [11])

the parotid gland. If the tumor extends intratemporally, a mastoidectomy will also be required for complete tumor removal. In these cases, careful incision planning is required to avoid devascularizing the pinna.

Gross Total Resection with Reinnervation

Gross total resection (GTR) with excision of the facial nerve followed by reinnervation is the most definitive treatment for FNS. Young patients with large tumors and moderate-to-poor facial nerve function (HB ≥ IV) or patients with moderate brainstem compression (>2.5 cm) are good candidates [11]. Since this approach ensures an immediate postoperative HB VI followed by slow recovery to an HB III–IV at best, it is typically reserved for tumors that have already resulted in poor facial nerve function (HB ≥ IV) [5, 11].

In the House Clinic series of 79 patients, 37 patients (47%) underwent GTR with grafting or primary anastomosis. They found that 84% of patients achieved an HB III or IV after surgery with grafting [5]. In the Mayo Clinic series of 80 patients, 29 patients (36%) underwent surgical resection, and of these, 26 (90%) had a GTR followed by reinnervation (the remaining underwent STR). Over half of the patients were reanimated with an interposition nerve graft from the greater auricular or sural nerve. The remaining patients had nerve substitution procedures—such as facial-hypoglossal or facial-trigeminal nerve transfers—due to insufficient nerve stumps for grafting or due to a long duration of paralysis [11]. Sixty-two percent of patients achieved an HB III or IV at the last follow-up [11]. Though surgical resection resulted in poorer overall facial nerve function compared with the other treatment modalities, tumor resection with interposition grafting was the only treatment option that resulted in improved scores in patients with baseline moderate or severe facial paresis [11]. Through these studies, it is worth emphasizing that, while HB III is commonly cited as the most favorable outcome with GTR and cable grafting, there are many cases in which functional outcomes are worse.

Decompression

Several microsurgical techniques have evolved that emphasize functional preservation over curative resection. Among these is facial nerve decompression, which was popularized by Angeli and Brackmann in 1997 as a management option for patients with FNS and good baseline facial function [61]. Decompression involves the wide removal of bone from around the nerve to decompress the tumor and allow it to grow without causing neural compression and axonal injury. The goal of surgery is not to remove the tumor, but to “buy time” in which the tumor can continue to expand with less risk of facial nerve injury related to bony compression.

The approach for nerve decompression depends on the location of the tumor and the presumably compressed segment. For medial aspects of the intratemporal facial nerve, decompression can be performed via the middle fossa approach, whereby the nerve can be exposed from the porus acusticus to the cochleariform process. Alternatively, in patients without useful hearing, the translabyrinthine approach can also be performed, which has the additional advantage of decompressing the lateral segments of the nerve, distal to the cochleariform process. In the IAC, the nerve is skeletonized widely, and a blunt elevator is used to remove the final layer of overlying bone, which is less traumatic to the nerve. Next, the dura of the IAC is incised longitudinally, which allows the tumor to expand into the space created by the bone removal [61].

Tumors encased in bone (e.g., labyrinthine, geniculate segments) are most amenable to this technique, since facial nerve weakness is highest in these segments. Nerve decompression may be most appropriate for patients who experience an acute onset of facial paralysis, in addition to steroids. Also, patients with good facial nerve function who are unexpectedly diagnosed with an FNS intraoperatively may be decompressed instead of proceeding with tumor removal, the latter of which would guarantee an immediate poor facial nerve outcome. Small, asymptomatic tumors in patients with normal facial nerve function may also be candidates, but traditionally, these cases are simply observed with serial MRI studies or potentially may be considered for SRS, given the encouraging early experiences with this treatment modality. It is important to emphasize to patients who undergo decompression that continued surveillance will be required, and further treatment may be required in the future. Wilkinson et al. reported that of the 19 patients who underwent decompression, 2 patients later underwent resection, and 2 other patients underwent SRS [5].

Though the goal of decompression is to preserve facial function for a longer period of time, some series have found that long-term facial nerve outcomes between observation and decompression are similar. Specifically, Wilkinson et al. compared decompression ($n = 19$) with observation ($n = 9$), and at the last follow-up, all the patients in both groups with an HB grade of I or II retained at least a grade II [5]. In addition, there was no significant difference in hearing loss between the two groups [5]. A similar finding was reported by Carlson et al., whereby the HB grade was the same or improved in approximately 80% of patients in both the observation and decompression cohorts [11].

Subtotal Resection

Given the trend in recent years toward preserving cranial nerve function, STR or "debulking" has been described by some groups to treat patients with good preoperative facial nerve function in an effort to remove the mass effect caused by the tumor and thereby minimize the risk of declining facial nerve function in the future [13, 27]. During postoperative surveillance, if the residual tumor grows, it can be treated noninvasively with radiosurgery. Therefore, a post-treatment MRI within 6 months is important for establishing a baseline by which to monitor future growth (Fig. 72.5). However, performing a STR on a patient with good facial function (HB I–II) can be risky due to potential injury to nerve fascicles, which may run through the tumor [18]. Therefore, other groups recommend against STR, citing the uncertain and potentially suboptimal facial nerve outcomes that have been reported, including immediate postoperative HB IV through VI with only partial recovery later [5, 10, 13, 59].

In order to lower the risk of a poor facial nerve outcome, STR is performed using the intraoperative facial nerve monitor to guide dissection. Often, the plane between facial nerve fascicles and the tumor is indistinct, so the tumor surface is "mapped" using monopolar stimulation to ascertain whether a portion of the tumor can be safely excised. Short bursts of electrical activity on the nerve monitor are acceptable; however, if fibrillation potentials are produced, the dissection should be stopped.

Mowry et al. reported on 11 patients with preoperative HB I-II and FNS isolated to the IAC-CPA. By using the intraoperative facial nerve stimulator as a guide, they reported removing more than 80% of the tumor in 90% of patients. Upon long-term follow-up (>1 year), 8 patients (72.7%) maintained good function (HB I-II), but 3 patients (27.3%) developed poor function (HB $\geq$ III) [59]. In 2012, the Otology Group of Vanderbilt reported on 56 cases treated surgically, of which 8 underwent STR and were found to have a statistically significant decrease risk of having postoperative HB $\geq$4 compared with GTR. None of these patients had evidence of postoperative degradation of facial function, and 2 patients actually had improvement. In addition, over the 44.9-month average follow-up, none of the patients experienced growth of their residual tumor or required a second surgery [4]. In contrast, Li et al. reported that, although 93% of patients who underwent STR maintained good facial nerve function (HB I-II) initially, 4 patients (27%) demonstrated growth of the remnant tumor during the 7-year average follow-up, which was related to the amount of residual tumor volume left behind [62].

In summary, STR with the use of the intraoperative nerve monitor can achieve good facial nerve outcomes, particularly if the tumors are eccentrically located, but the results are not guaranteed and are often unpredictable. Furthermore, the likelihood of recurrent growth of the tumor remnant puts the facial nerve at risk again in the future. Lastly, a clinical dilemma arises when a patient awakens after STR with an HB VI. While the literature supports observing for 1 year to allow time to regain facial function, if it fails to recover, the patient will have suffered the morbidity of a "lost year" waiting for nerve recovery, as well as additional surgery to reanimate the face, which itself will likely yield poorer results due to the delay in reinnervation. For this reason, many centers advocate for waiting for declining facial function worse than HB III–IV prior to surgical intervention in the form of GTR with immediate reinnervation.

Gross Total Resection with Nerve Preservation

GTR with nerve preservation is the final and most surgically ambitious technique, which aims to achieve both goals of surgery: curative resection and preservation of facial function. Occasionally, the tumor arises from the nervus intermedius or is within the parotid gland, pedunculated from the nerve, making it resectable while preserving the motor branch of the facial nerve [11, 59]. However, in most cases, GTR with nerve preservation requires extensive microdissection to separate any fascicles that travel through the tumor, which occurs in over a third of the cases [18]. As an alternative, the tumor may be "shaved off" with the sacrifice of any fascicles that it contains [14]. The challenge is determining when this technique will result in better outcomes versus complete transection with grafting. Like STR, there is a degree of unpredictability in facial nerve outcomes due to nerve fibers that travel throughout the substance of the tumor [18]. This notion is highlighted by the case series by McMenomey et al., whereby 5 tumors were completely dissected free from the main trunk of the facial nerve, and of these, 4 patients obtained good outcomes (one with HB II, three with HB III). One patient had a HB V and ultimately underwent a hypoglossal–facial nerve transfer [13].

In 1995, Sataloff described the "fascicle preservation" technique for posterior fossa FNS, which can be particularly challenging since the facial nerve proximal to the IAC is devoid of the epineurium, making it especially fragile and without an obvious plane between the tumor and the perineurium of the facial nerve [10, 13, 27, 63, 64]. In Nadeau and Sataloff's review of the literature on posterior fossa FNS, they found that most tumors are not amenable to "nerve preservation" techniques, but when the schwannoma takes a more eccentric position along the nerve, this technique can result in better long-term facial nerve function (such as HB II) compared to nerve grafting because the anatomical continuity of the nerve is preserved [10].

In contrast to posterior fossa FNS, tumors within the distal IAC and temporal bone may be more amenable to nerve preservation since the facial nerve is more robust as it acquires a connective tissue sheath from the dura within the IAC. Perez et al. reviewed 5 patients who had good preoperative facial function (HB I–III) and intratemporal tumors that were amenable to complete resection with facial nerve preservation. There were no recurrences, and all patients retained stable facial nerve function (except 1 patient who went from an HB I to HB II) [15]. Lee et al. reported on 6 cases of FNS, all with HB I–II preoperative facial nerve function, and in 4 of 6 (66.7%), GTR with nerve preservation was achieved via a "stripping" technique. At the last follow-up, 2 of these patients had stable facial function, and the other 2 went from HB I to HB II [65]. Similarly, Sun et al. reviewed 18 cases of FNS, all with good baseline facial nerve function (HB I–III), and 11 (61%) were amenable to GTR with nerve preservation via a nerve "stripping" technique. In all cases, favorable facial nerve function was maintained [66]. In both of these studies, approximately 35% of tumors were determined intraoperatively not to be amenable to stripping, presumably due to nerve fascicles running through the tumor, and therefore, these tumors were treated with decompression instead, which also yielded favorable facial nerve outcomes.

Management Algorithm

A simplified management algorithm is presented in Fig. 72.7; however, in practice, the management of FNS must be tailored on an individualized basis, depending on several tumor and patient characteristics. Patients with large posterior fossa tumors ($\geq$2.5 cm), brainstem compressive symptoms, or severe facial weakness (HB $\geq$ IV) at presentation are typically best treated with upfront GTR with reinnervation. However, the majority of patients (60–80%) present with normal facial nerve function or mild-to-moderate weakness (HB I-III), and in these cases, an initial observation period for 6–12 months followed by repeat imaging is appropriate to determine if the tumor is actively growing or resulting in progressive symptoms. The natural history of these tumors suggests that 20–40% of patients undergoing observation will experience deterioration of facial nerve function. If new symptoms arise during the observation period, the decision to intervene and the timing of treatment is a matter of debate. To date, there is no clear consensus on the management of these rare tumors.

Patients who experience acute or recurrent facial paralysis during the course of observation are treated with steroids, and decompression of the facial nerve is considered, particularly if the tumor is located in a bony-confined area within the temporal bone (e.g., labyrinthine or geniculate segments). Removal of bone allows the tumor to expand into the surrounding space, which reduces the compression along the main nerve trunk and reverses neuropraxia.

SRS may also be considered for growing small- to medium-sized tumors in patients with good baseline facial function in an effort to halt further growth and progressive neurological deficits. Though some groups still advocate for STR or GTR with nerve preservation in patients with good baseline function, this strategy is used less commonly today, given the unpredictability of immediate facial nerve outcomes, the high likelihood of recurrent tumor growth after STR, and the low likelihood of being able to preserve a functional nerve during resection. Instead, surgery to remove the tumor is delayed until patients have progressed to or beyond an HB IV, since facial nerve grafting can achieve, at best, an HB III, and more commonly HB IV or worse [67]. This approach allows patients the opportunity to preserve neurological function over a longer period of time.

It is critical to intervene as soon as possible when a patient has progressed to HB IV, since the results of grafting are directly related to the duration of preoperative deficits, with the best results being achieved in patients with the shortest duration of preoperative facial weakness [67]. As the length of time of facial paralysis increases, greater nerve degeneration occurs. Over time, irreversible degenerative changes occur at the level of the facial nucleus, and atrophy of the innervated musculature is observed. Once this occurs, nerve interposition grafting is unable to recover useful function, and alternative facial reanimation techniques are required (*see below*) [61]. Therefore, augmenting serial MRI surveillance with serial electrical testing via EEMG can help detect subclinical nerve denervation (reduced amplitude, increased latency) caused by the expanding tumor [61]. Better postoperative results may be achieved when the nerve repair is performed before the compound action potential decreases by more than 50% [5].

If a patient undergoes STR or GTR with nerve preservation and postoperatively demonstrates HB VI facial function, a useful predictive model published by Rivas et al. can be used to determine the rate of facial function recovery in order to select candidates for reanimation surgery sooner than the traditional waiting period of 1 year [68]. In the study, the authors conclude that the rate of facial nerve recovery over the first 6 months after tumor resection is an early independent predictor of ultimate facial nerve recovery and function, predicting poor facial nerve recovery with 97% sensitivity and 97% specificity [68]. Though the study specifically involved patients who underwent vestibular schwannoma resection with facial nerve preservation, its results may have application in the management of patients who undergo FNS resection with nerve preservation. Therefore, if patients do not show recovery by 6 months, early intervention should be considered, since "time is muscle."

Management of an unexpected FNS that is intraoperatively diagnosed when performing surgery for a presumed vestibular schwannoma—which can occur in 1–2% of cases—can pose a unique challenge. A high index of suspicion is required to make the diagnosis intraoperatively. FNS should be suspected if there is great difficulty separating the facial nerve from the tumor, but the superior and inferior vestibular nerves appear to be easily separated. Also, if the large majority of the tumor surface appears to stimulate at a low threshold, this may serve as a clue to the tumor being an FNS. Indeed, a facial nerve that is dorsally displaced and splayed over a vestibular schwannoma is very rare. In cases when a preoperatively presumed vestibular schwannoma is discovered to be an FNS during surgery, it is the authors' preference to prioritize facial nerve function. In these cases, options include gross or subtotal resection, isolated decompression of the IAC without resection, or aborting the operation followed by observation with serial MRI or SRS. In smaller tumors with normal preoperative function, the authors generally advocate for a more conservative approach involving isolated IAC decompression, with or without postoperative SRS. In cases of larger tumors that result in significant brainstem compression, gross or subtotal resection is usually advisable regardless of facial nerve function. Ultimately, the decision should be made in a multidisciplinary fashion and on an individualized basis.

Facial Reanimation

Restoration of facial symmetry and function after tumor resection can present its own set of challenges. An in-depth analysis of management, surgical techniques and outcomes is discussed in Chap. 22. In general, patients who maintain anatomic continuity of the facial nerve regain better postoperative facial nerve function. When the nerve is transected for tumor removal, a combination of dynamic and static reanimation procedures can be performed to restore facial function. Dynamic function is best achieved by primary nerve repair via tension-free, direct end-to-end coaptation of the distal and proximal facial nerve segments, which can result in an HB III at best. However, this method requires a small gap of <1 cm and is rarely possible since most FNS involve multiple facial nerve segments. Additionally, rerouting of the facial nerve to gain length compromises the blood supply and may result in worse outcomes [10].

Therefore, nerve grafting with the greater auricular nerve or sural nerve is the next best option for providing a tension-free repair and is the most common technique employed. Ideally, grafting is performed as soon as possible to maintain continuity between the facial nucleus and facial musculature. The greater auricular nerve will provide up to 10 cm in length, while the sural nerve can provide up to 30 cm of nerve graft. With this method, an HB grade III (and more commonly HB IV) may be achieved, though results may be diminished if the native facial muscles are severely atrophied [69, 70]. Grafting of the intratemporal facial nerve is relatively reliable since the nerve has a robust layer of epineurium and resides within a secure and stationary position inside the temporal bone. In fact, sutureless coaptation techniques, such as fibrin glue, have produced results similar to suture neurorrhaphy with shorter operative times [10, 71]. In contrast, suture neurorrhaphy in the posterior fossa is notoriously difficult and requires a sufficient stump of nerve at the brainstem. Alternative methods of coaptation are being developed, such as Axogen Avance®, an allogeneic sural nerve graft (AxoGen, Inc., Alachua, FL), but long-term outcomes have not been well-established at this time.

When an insufficient nerve stump is left at the brainstem, nerve transfer procedures, including hypoglossal-to-facial or masseter-to-facial nerve transfers, are performed. Outcomes with nerve transfer are best when done within 1 to 2 years after loss of function. Occasionally, this procedure can be combined with a temporalis muscle transposition procedure for lower facial reanimation in order to provide a greater degree of symmetry. If the duration of facial paralysis is greater than 2 years, microvascular free flap reconstruction (e.g., serratus, gracilis) can be performed, as well as other static facial reanimation procedures.

The paralyzed eye should be reanimated through a separate procedure—usually an upper eyelid gold weight or lateral tarsal strip tarsorrhaphy—in order to prevent severe corneal exposure and risk of infection and blindness. This is especially critical in the setting of concomitant corneal hypoesthesia. It is therefore of utmost importance that the patient be educated about eye care, including the use of ointments, moisture chambers, and eye patches or sunglasses to protect the eye from wind or dust.

Conclusion

FNS are rare tumors that may arise from any segment of the facial nerve but most commonly involve the labyrinthine/geniculate segment and extend intracranially and/or throughout the intratemporal course of the facial nerve. Clinically, they exhibit a wide array of manifestations depending upon location and size, and therefore, require a high index of suspicion to properly diagnose. Since the advent of high-resolution imaging techniques, FNS are being diagnosed more frequently, and the natural history of these benign tumors is better understood. Despite the significant advances in modern microsurgical techniques, a trend has emerged toward functional preservation over curative resection. Therefore, observation has taken a more prominent role in the primary management of these tumors, since complete tumor removal generally results in an unacceptably high risk of permanent facial paralysis in patients with good baseline function. As experience grows, the role of SRS is also becoming better defined and may have several indications in the treatment of patients with FNS with good facial function in an effort to prevent functional decline. In patients with poor facial nerve function (HB ≥ IV) or brainstem compressive symptoms, surgery in the form of GTR with facial nerve interposition or donor nerve reinnervation usually affords durable tumor control and long-term HB grade III–IV function.

References

1. Pulec JL. Facial nerve tumors. Ann Otol Rhinol Laryngol. 1969;78(5):962–82.
2. Carlson ML, Habermann EB, Wagie AE, et al. The changing landscape of vestibular schwannoma management in the United States--A shift toward conservatism. Otolaryngol Head Neck Surg. 2015;153(3):440–6.
3. McRackan TR, Brackmann DE. Historical perspective on evolution in management of lateral skull base tumors. Otolaryngol Clin N Am. 2015;48(3):397–405.
4. McRackan TR, Rivas A, Wanna GB, et al. Facial nerve outcomes in facial nerve schwannomas. Otol Neurotol. 2012;33(1):78–82.
5. Wilkinson EP, Hoa M, Slattery WH 3rd, et al. Evolution in the management of facial nerve schwannoma. Laryngoscope. 2011;121(10):2065–74.
6. Saito H, Baxter A. Undiagnosed intratemporal facial nerve neurilemomas. Arch Otolaryngol. 1972;95(5):415–9.
7. Brackmann DE, Bartels LJ. Rare tumors of the cerebellopontine angle. Otolaryngol Head Neck Surg (1979). 1980;88(5):555–9.
8. Moffat DA, Saunders JE, McElveen JT Jr, McFerran DJ, Hardy DG. Unusual cerebello-pontine angle tumours. J Laryngol Otol. 1993;107(12):1087–98.
9. King TT, Morrison AW. Primary facial nerve tumors within the skull. J Neurosurg. 1990;72(1):1–8.
10. Nadeau DP, Sataloff RT. Fascicle preservation surgery for facial nerve neuromas involving the posterior cranial fossa. Otol Neurotol. 2003;24(2):317–25.
11. Carlson ML, Deep NL, Patel NS, et al. Facial nerve schwannomas: review of 80 cases over 25 years at Mayo Clinic. Mayo Clin Proc. 2016;91(11):1563–76.
12. Kertesz TR, Shelton C, Wiggins RH, Salzman KL, Glastonbury CM, Harnsberger R. Intratemporal facial nerve neuroma: anatomical location and radiological features. Laryngoscope. 2001;111(7):1250–6.
13. McMenomey SO, Glasscock ME 3rd, Minor LB, Jackson CG, Strasnick B. Facial nerve neuromas presenting as acoustic tumors. Am J Otol. 1994;15(3):307–12.
14. O'Donoghue GM, Brackmann DE, House JW, Jackler RK. Neuromas of the facial nerve. Am J Otol. 1989;10(1):49–54.
15. Perez R, Chen JM, Nedzelski JM. Intratemporal facial nerve schwannoma: a management dilemma. Otol Neurotol. 2005;26(1):121–6.
16. McMonagle B, Al-Sanosi A, Croxson G, Fagan P. Facial schwannoma: results of a large case series and review. J Laryngol Otol. 2008;122(11):1139–50.
17. Saada AA, Limb CJ, Long DM, Niparko JK. Intracanalicular schwannoma of the facial nerve: a manifestation of neurofibromatosis type 2. Arch Otolaryngol Head Neck Surg. 2000;126(4):547–9.
18. Hajjaj M, Linthicum FH Jr. Facial nerve schwannoma: nerve fibre dissemination. J Laryngol Otol. 1996;110(7):632–3.
19. Pulec JL. Facial nerve neuroma. Laryngoscope. 1972;82(7):1160–76.
20. Falcioni M, Russo A, Taibah A, Sanna M. Facial nerve tumors. Otol Neurotol. 2003;24(6):942–7.
21. Wiggins RH 3rd, Harnsberger HR, Salzman KL, Shelton C, Kertesz TR, Glastonbury CM. The many faces of facial nerve schwannoma. AJNR Am J Neuroradiol. 2006;27(3):694–9.
22. Shirazi MA, Leonetti JP, Marzo SJ, Anderson DE. Surgical management of facial neuromas: lessons learned. Otol Neurotol. 2007;28(7):958–63.
23. Lipkin AF, Coker NJ, Jenkins HA, Alford BR. Intracranial and intratemporal facial neuroma. Otolaryngol Head Neck Surg. 1987;96(1):71–9.
24. Biggs ND, Fagan PA. Schwannoma of the chorda tympani. J Laryngol Otol. 2001;115(1):50–2.
25. Kumon Y, Sakaki S, Ohta S, Ohue S, Nakagawa K, Tanaka K. Greater superficial petrosal nerve neurinoma. Case report. J Neurosurg. 1999;91(4):691–6.
26. Mundada P, Purohit BS, Kumar TS, Tan TY. Imaging of facial nerve schwannomas: diagnostic pearls and potential pitfalls. Diagn Interv Radiol. 2016;22(1):40–6.
27. Sherman JD, Dagnew E, Pensak ML, van Loveren HR, Tew JM Jr. Facial nerve neuromas: report of 10 cases and review of the literature. Neurosurgery. 2002;50(3):450–6.
28. Pillsbury HC, Price HC, Gardiner LJ. Primary tumors of the facial nerve: diagnosis and management. Laryngoscope. 1983;93(8):1045–8.
29. Fisch U, Esslen E. Total intratemporal exposure of the facial nerve. Pathologic findings in Bell's palsy. Arch Otolaryngol. 1972;95(4):335–41.
30. Gebarski SS, Telian SA, Niparko JK. Enhancement along the normal facial nerve in the facial canal: MR imaging and anatomic correlation. Radiology. 1992;183(2):391–4.
31. Fagan PA, Misra SN, Doust B. Facial neuroma of the cerebellopontine angle and the internal auditory canal. Laryngoscope. 1993;103(4 Pt 1):442–6.
32. Park HY, Kim SH, Son EJ, Lee HK, Lee WS. Intracanalicular facial nerve schwannoma. Otol Neurotol. 2007;28(3):376–80.

33. Malhotra PS, Sharma P, Fishman MA, et al. Clinical, radiographic, and audiometric predictors in conservative management of vestibular schwannoma. Otol Neurotol. 2009;30(4):507–14.
34. Lanman TH, Brackmann DE, Hitselberger WE, Subin B. Report of 190 consecutive cases of large acoustic tumors (vestibular schwannoma) removed via the translabyrinthine approach. J Neurosurg. 1999;90(4):617–23.
35. Nakamura M, Roser F, Mirzai S, Matthies C, Vorkapic P, Samii M. Meningiomas of the internal auditory canal. Neurosurgery. 2004;55(1):119–27; discussion 127–8.
36. Hamilton BE, Salzman KL, Patel N, et al. Imaging and clinical characteristics of temporal bone meningioma. AJNR Am J Neuroradiol. 2006;27(10):2204–9.
37. Deep NL, Gnagi SH, Carpentieri DF, Adelson PD, Weisskopf PA. Facial nerve meningioma: a cause of pediatric facial weakness. Otol Neurotol. 2017;38(3):e8–e12.
38. Singh KP, Smyth GD, Allen IV. Intracanalicular meningioma. J Laryngol Otol. 1975;89(5):549–52.
39. Salzman KL, Davidson HC, Harnsberger HR, et al. Dumbbell schwannomas of the internal auditory canal. AJNR Am J Neuroradiol. 2001;22(7):1368–76.
40. Magliulo G, Alla FR, Colicchio G, Trasimeni G. Geniculate ganglion meningioma. Skull Base. 2010;20(3):185–8.
41. Kienzle GD, Goldenberg MH, Just NW, Arbit E. Facial nerve neurinoma presenting as middle cranial fossa mass: CT appearance. J Comput Assist Tomogr. 1986;10(3):391–4.
42. Ginsberg LE, DeMonte F. Diagnosis please. Case 16: facial nerve schwannoma with middle cranial fossa involvement. Radiology. 1999;213(2):364–8.
43. Chung SY, Kim DI, Lee BH, Yoon PH, Jeon P, Chung TS. Facial nerve schwannomas: CT and MR findings. Yonsei Med J. 1998;39(2):148–53.
44. Frisch CD, Driscoll CL, Neff BA. Paraganglioma of the facial canal: a report of 2 cases and literature review. Am J Otolaryngol. 2014;35(6):800–5.
45. Snyderman C, May M, Berman MA, Curtin HD. Facial paralysis: traumatic neuromas vs. facial nerve neoplasms. Otolaryngol Head Neck Surg. 1988;98(1):53–9.
46. Hunter JB, Weidenheim KM, Lee AY, Dinces E. Intratemporal Intraneural Perineurioma of the facial nerve. Otol Neurotol. 2016;37(10):e414–6.
47. Li D, Schauble B, Moll C, Fisch U. Intratemporal facial nerve perineurioma. Laryngoscope. 1996;106(3 Pt 1):328–33.
48. Rodriguez FJ, Folpe AL, Giannini C, Perry A. Pathology of peripheral nerve sheath tumors: diagnostic overview and update on selected diagnostic problems. Acta Neuropathol. 2012;123(3):295–319.
49. Boyanton BL Jr, Jones JK, Shenaq SM, Hicks MJ, Bhattacharjee MB. Intraneural perineurioma: a systematic review with illustrative cases. Arch Pathol Lab Med. 2007;131(9):1382–92.
50. Liu R, Fagan P. Facial nerve schwannoma: surgical excision versus conservative management. Ann Otol Rhinol Laryngol. 2001;110(11):1025–9.
51. Yang W, Zhao J, Han Y, et al. Long-term outcomes of facial nerve schwannomas with favorable facial nerve function: tumor growth rate is correlated with initial tumor size. Am J Otolaryngol. 2015;36(2):163–5.
52. Watanabe S, Yamamoto M, Kawabe T, et al. Stereotactic radiosurgery for vestibular schwannomas: average 10-year follow-up results focusing on long-term hearing preservation. J Neurosurg. 2016;125(Suppl 1):64–72.
53. Kida Y, Yoshimoto M, Hasegawa T. Radiosurgery for facial schwannoma. J Neurosurg. 2007;106(1):24–9.
54. Litre CF, Gourg GP, Tamura M, et al. Gamma knife surgery for facial nerve schwannomas. Neurosurgery. 2007;60(5):853–9; discussion 853–9.
55. Madhok R, Kondziolka D, Flickinger JC, Lunsford LD. Gamma knife radiosurgery for facial schwannomas. Neurosurgery. 2009;64(6):1102–5; discussion 1105.
56. Moon JH, Chang WS, Jung HH, Lee KS, Park YG, Chang JH. Gamma knife surgery for facial nerve schwannomas. J Neurosurg. 2014;121(Suppl):116–22.
57. Sheehan JP, Kano H, Xu Z, et al. Gamma knife radiosurgery for facial nerve schwannomas: a multicenter study. J Neurosurg. 2015;123(2):387–94.
58. Hasegawa T, Kato T, Kida Y, et al. Gamma knife surgery for patients with facial nerve schwannomas: a multiinstitutional retrospective study in Japan. J Neurosurg. 2016;124(2):403–10.
59. Mowry S, Hansen M, Gantz B. Surgical management of internal auditory canal and cerebellopontine angle facial nerve schwannoma. Otol Neurotol. 2012;33(6):1071–6.
60. Gross BC, Carlson ML, Moore EJ, Driscoll CL, Olsen KD. The intraparotid facial nerve schwannoma: a diagnostic and management conundrum. Am J Otolaryngol. 2012;33(5):497–504.
61. Angeli SI, Brackmann DE. Is surgical excision of facial nerve schwannomas always indicated? Otolaryng Head Neck. 1997;117(6):S144–7.
62. Li Y, Liu H, Cheng Y. Subtotal resection of facial nerve schwannoma is not safe in the long run. Acta Otolaryngol. 2014;134(4):433–6.
63. Sataloff RT, Frattali MA, Myers DL. Intracranial facial neuromas: total tumor removal with facial nerve preservation: a new surgical technique. Ear Nose Throat J. 1995;74(4):244–246, 248–256.
64. Fenton JE, Morrin MM, Smail M, Sterkers O, Sterkers JM. Bilateral facial nerve schwannomas. Eur Arch Otorrinolaringol. 1999;256(3):133–5.
65. Lee JD, Kim SH, Song MH, Lee HK, Lee WS. Management of facial nerve schwannoma in patients with favorable facial function. Laryngoscope. 2007;117(6):1063–8.
66. Sun Y, Xing B, Han S, et al. Stripping surgery in facial nerve schwannomas with favorable facial nerve function. Am J Otolaryngol. 2015;36(4):513–6.
67. Falcioni M, Taibah A, Russo A, Piccirillo E, Sanna M. Facial nerve grafting. Otol Neurotol. 2003;24(3):486–9.
68. Rivas A, Boahene KD, Bravo HC, Tan M, Tamargo RJ, Francis HW. A model for early prediction of facial nerve recovery after vestibular schwannoma surgery. Otol Neurotol. 2011;32(5):826–33.
69. Stephanian E, Sekhar LN, Janecka IP, Hirsch B. Facial nerve repair by interposition nerve graft: results in 22 patients. Neurosurgery. 1992;31(1):73–6; discussion 77.
70. Kim CS, Chang SO, Oh SH, Ahn SH, Hwang CH, Lee HJ. Management of intratemporal facial nerve schwannoma. Otol Neurotol. 2003;24(2):312–6.
71. Knox CJ, Hohman MH, Kleiss IJ, Weinberg JS, Heaton JT, Hadlock TA. Facial nerve repair: fibrin adhesive coaptation versus epineurial suture repair in a rodent model. Laryngoscope. 2013;123(7):1618–21.

73 Geniculate Hemangioma

Nauman F. Manzoor, Sarah E. Mowry, Cliff A. Megerian, and Maroun T. Semaan

Introduction

Geniculate Ganglion Hemangiomas (GGH) are rare benign vascular malformations that arise along the course of the facial nerve. First described in 1969 by Pulec [1], these tumors are postulated to develop from the rich capillary plexus that surrounds the geniculate ganglion (GG) region, and hence, are extraneural in origin. The presence of this capillary plexus has been demonstrated in both animal and human temporal bone studies and is ten times denser around the GG region compared with the adjacent labyrinthine segment [2]. The anatomical location and presence of this plexus explain the clinical hallmarks of this rare entity (facial paralysis) and also have implications for surgical management.

The incidence of GGH was found to be 0.7% among 1430 tumors of the temporal bone in a retrospective study [3]. The majority of patients present in their 40s and 50s with facial paresis of varying degrees, and a minority will have additional cochlear dysfunction. In a recent systematic review of 120 patients, the mean age at presentation was 41.4 years, with 44% being female [4].

Originally termed "hemangiomas," there is mounting evidence that these lesions are not clonal proliferations of endothelial cells as seen in infantile hemangiomas. Benoit et al. used immunohistochemical methods to investigate the cellular origins of seven GGH. The tumors in their study did not harbor molecular markers of either infantile hemangiomas or lymphatic malformations, leading the authors to speculate that GGH are actually venous endothelial malformations [5]. However, the literature continues to use the older nomenclature, and as such, the term GGH will be used in this chapter.

Management of this rare condition has been controversial. However, a recent large case series with long-term follow-up and a systematic review of all reported cases [4, 6] have helped to mitigate some of these controversies. Notable differences are present in terms of clinical presentation, radiological appearance, and management when compared with primary facial nerve tumors, such as schwannomas, which are discussed in a different chapter.

Clinical Presentation

The clinical hallmark of GGH is facial nerve dysfunction. Facial nerve dysfunction in the form of paresis, paralysis, or hemifacial spasm is common even in small GGHs and is frequently disproportionate to the size of the malformation. Facial nerve dysfunction is postulated to be the result of "vascular steal" associated with the rich capillary plexus at the GG, leading to nerve ischemia. There is also a potential component of direct nerve compression in larger lesions.

The most common pattern of facial nerve dysfunction is progressive paralysis or hemifacial spasm, while some patients experience sudden paralysis or recurrent acute paralysis. Oldenburg et al. reported facial nerve dysfunction in 94% (113/120) of patients [4]. Of those, 42% of patients presented with progressive facial paralysis, and 18% presented with hemifacial spasm. Overall, the mean duration of preoperative facial nerve dysfunction was 27 months (range 1–132 months) with an average House-Brackmann (HB)

N. F. Manzoor
Department of Otolaryngology—Head and Neck Surgery, Virginia Commonwealth University, Richmond, VA, USA

S. E. Mowry · C. A. Megerian · M. T. Semaan (✉)
Department of Otolaryngology—Head and Neck Surgery, University Hospitals Cleveland Medical Center, Cleveland, OH, USA
e-mail: maroun.semaan@uhhospitals.org

A. D. Sweeney et al. (eds.), *Haynes-Glasscock-Shambaugh Surgery of the Ear*, https://doi.org/10.1007/978-3-032-18264-7_73

grade of 4.6. Similarly, Semaan et al. reported progressive facial nerve paralysis in 89% (16/18) of patients [6]. Facial twitching was present in 56% (10 / 18), and synkinesis was noticed in 17% (3/18) of patients. The duration of facial paralysis ranged from 2 months to 5 years. Sixty-two percent (11/18) presented with HB grade III or worse.

In a comparative study between GGH and GG schwannoma, 70% of patients with GGH presented with severe palsy (HB grade V and VI) compared to none in a GG schwannoma cohort, although the size of the schwannomas was significantly bigger than that of GGH (mean 16 mm versus 8 mm) [7]. These facial nerve symptoms are in contradistinction to Bell's palsy, which generally manifests with paralysis that develops suddenly (by definition, within 72 hours) and begins to improve within 3 weeks of onset. It is also unusual for Bell's palsy patients to have synkinesis or hemifacial spasm at presentation. The practitioner should thus have a high index of suspicion for another etiology in patients presenting with progressive palsy, hemifacial spasm, or failure to improve. Of course, insidiously worsening facial paresis should also raise concern for a malignant process with perineural invasion, and this possibility must be considered during the workup.

Symptoms related to cochlear dysfunction, such as hearing loss, are reported in 15–22% of patients at presentation [4, 6]. The presence of asymmetric sensorineural hearing loss should alert the physician to a possible cochlear fistula, which can arise with millimetric bony erosion, given the adjacent nature of the facial nerve and cochlea. Imaging should be closely reviewed in this clinical situation. Other symptoms, including disequilibrium, hyperacusis, and taste disturbance, are less common. Changes in lacrimation (dry eyes as well as hyper-lacrimation) have also been reported in some patients [4].

Radiographic Findings and Differential Diagnosis

Radiographic imaging can be used to differentiate between GGH and other lesions in the region of the GG [8]. The radiographic differential diagnosis includes facial nerve schwannoma, meningioma, congenital cholesteatoma, and perineural spread from parotid malignancy [9].

High-resolution CT scan (HRCT) findings of GGH include broadening and irregular expansion of the facial nerve canal adjoining the GG fossa, particularly the labyrinthine segment. Intralesional calcifications are very common. The edges of the fallopian canal may not appear sharp on HRCT, as these lesions tend to infiltrate and erode the bone around them (Fig. 73.1). In contrast, HRCT in the setting of a facial schwannoma shows a sharply delineated expansile lesion in the region of the GG without associated calcifications [10].

MRI findings of GGH include a lesion centered over the geniculate ganglion with an associated heterogeneous increase in signal intensity on T2-weighted images (Fig. 73.1). Different MRI protocols, including 2D fast spin echo (FSE) images as well as 3D FIESTA sequences, can be used, and these can identify 80–100% of GGH [11].

Other radiologic considerations relevant to the differential diagnosis of a facial tumor in this location include that a facial nerve schwannoma is typically described as a well-circumscribed, enhancing mass on a contrasted T1 sequence. Intralesional heterogeneity may be present, especially in larger lesions [10]. Congenital cholesteatoma does not enhance on post-contrast images, and in terms of perineural spread from an extratemporal malignancy, contiguous retrograde enhancement would likely be seen. In some cases, this enhancement can extend into the internal auditory canal.

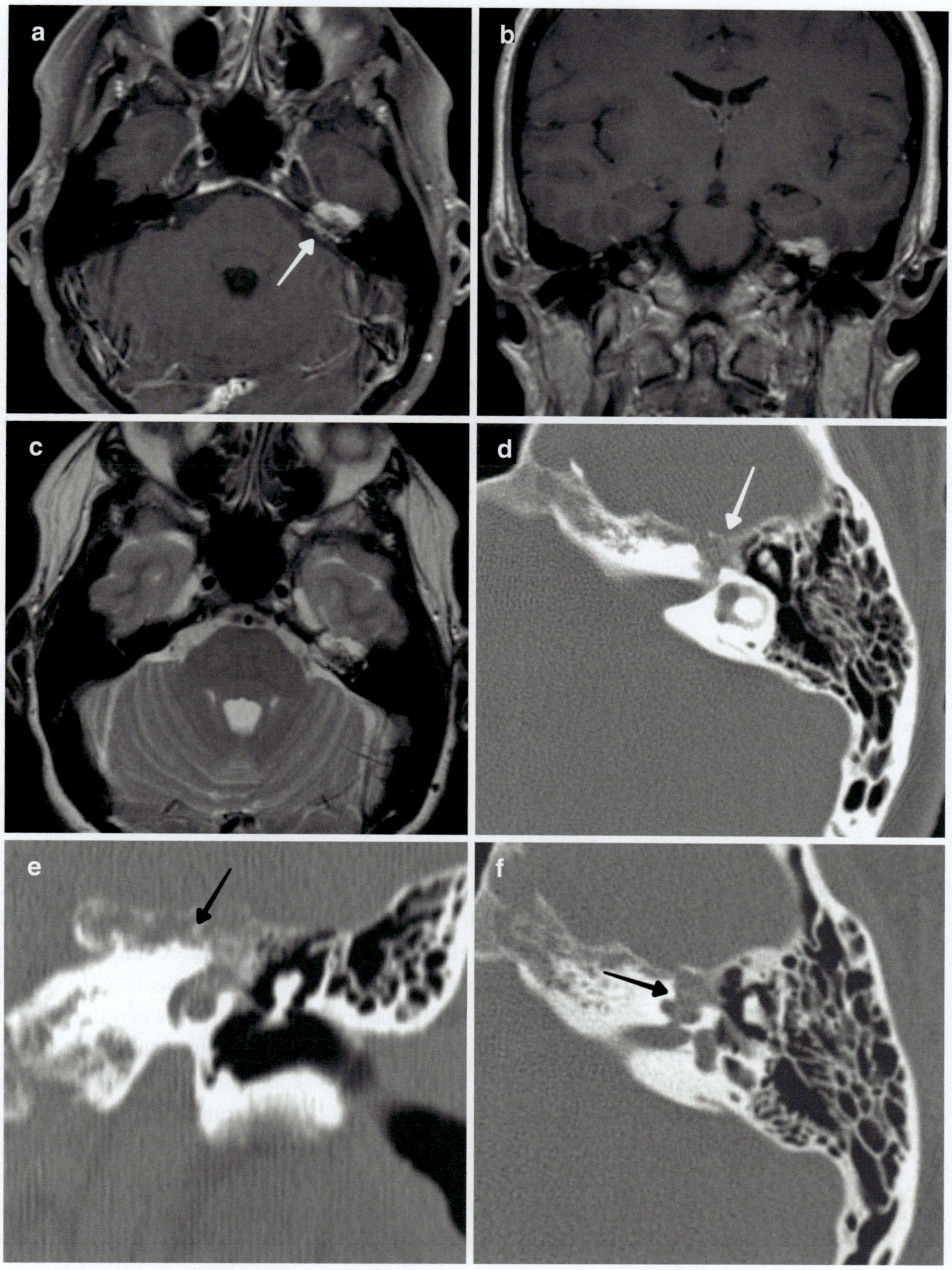

Fig. 73.1 Axial and coronal T1 post-contrast sequences show a lesion with enhancement (white arrow) centered over the left GG region with extension to the petrous apex (**a**, **b**). This lesion is also hyperintense on the T2 sequence (**c**). Axial CT scan shows a spiculated destructive lesion (white arrow) centered over the GGH (**d**) with radiographic evidence of otic capsule involvement (black arrow) (**f**). A coronal CT scan shows the medial extent of the lesion (black arrow) toward the petrous apex (**e**)

Adjunctive Testing

Electrical testing of the facial nerve can be useful in patients with complete facial paralysis at presentation. A complete discussion of electroneuronography (ENoG) and evoked electromyography (EEMG) is beyond the scope of this chapter. However, ENoG can be useful in evaluating the degree of neural degeneration. The degree of degeneration evaluated via ENoG may not be represented clinically by the patient's degree of paralysis. Semaan et al. identified patients with HB grade 1 or 2 facial movement; however, on ENoG, they had high degrees of degeneration [6]. This seeming incongruity may be explained by the fact that EEMG may demonstrate both fibrillation potentials and polyphasic action potentials simultaneously. This differential electrical activity is indicative of ongoing denervation and reinnervation and is particularly common in GGH patients.

Histopathology

Hematoxylin and eosin (H&E) staining demonstrates ectatic, irregularly shaped blood vessels with minimal smooth muscle in the vessel walls (Fig. 73.2a) [5]. The endothelial cells show expression of CD-34, which is a marker of vascular

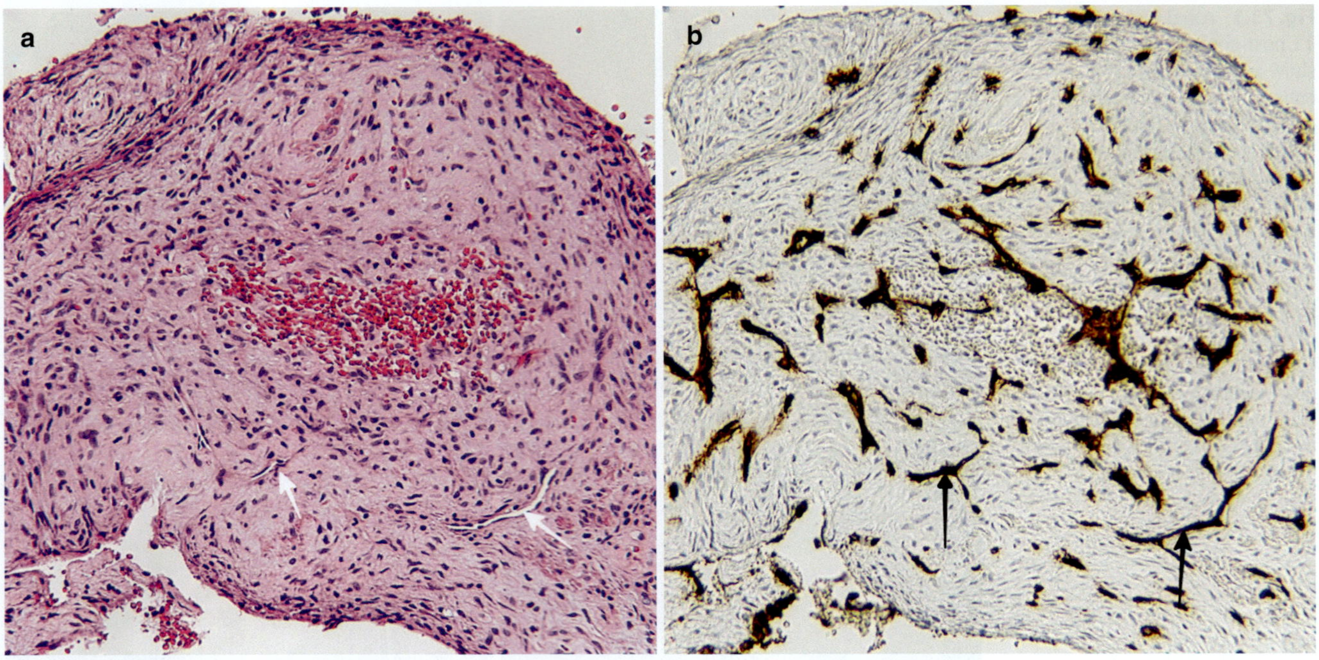

Fig. 73.2 Medium-power (Hematoxylin–eosin stain; original magnification: × 100) image showing irregular, dilated vascular spaces (white arrow), which have collapsed and are surrounded by cellular collagenous stroma (**a**). Immunohistochemistry for CD34 was positive (black arrow) in these structures and demonstrates numerous ectatic and collapsed vascular spaces interspersed with fibrous stroma (**b**)

endothelial cells (Fig. 73.2b). The growth may grossly appear spongy and compressible. Significant invasion of the surrounding bone may also give a granular appearance and feel to the tumor. Very few mitotic figures can be seen, consistent with a nonneoplastic etiology. As noted by Benoit et al., these malformations stain negatively for glucose transporter protein isoform 1 (GLUT1), podoplanin, and Lewis Y antigen, thus resembling a venous vascular malformation rather than a true hemangioma [5].

Management Strategies

Due to the rarity of GGH and the relatively high likelihood of facial weakness compared to other pathologies commonly managed in lateral skull base surgery, management can be controversial. Options include observation, subtotal resection (STR) with facial nerve decompression, gross total resection (GTR) with or without facial nerve transection and grafting. At present, there are no data on other modalities, such as stereotactic radiation or chemotherapy, in the treatment of GGH.

Observation alone has not been studied independently. Semaan et al. had 3 patients with normal hearing who declined surgery and hence constituted a nonsurgical cohort [6]. One of these patients had continued tumor growth and development of a cochlear fistula (but had no audiologic follow-up), and the other two patients did not have evidence of tumor growth over time. Oldenburg et al. reported on 7 patients who were observed and showed a progressive decline of facial nerve function [4]. Both authors concluded that observation alone is not recommended due to the unpredictability of tumor growth, complications related to the worsening of facial nerve function, and the possibility of otic capsule violation.

The surgical approach and degree of resection are guided by the degree and duration of facial nerve dysfunction and serviceable hearing. In some tumors, a cleavage plane can be dissected between the main trunk of the facial nerve and the tumor, allowing for preservation of facial nerve integrity. In other tumors, there is no plane between the tumor and the main trunk of the facial nerve, making GTR difficult without sacrificing the integrity of the facial nerve.

The middle cranial fossa (MCF) approach alone, or in combination with a transmastoid approach, has been widely reported for resection of these lesions with the intent of hearing preservation in relevant patients with serviceable acoustic hearing [4, 6, 7, 12]. In a majority of patients, complete or partial excision can be accomplished via an extradural MCF approach when serviceable hearing is still present [6]. Careful removal of diseased bone around the bony cochlear wall and the internal auditory canal (IAC) region to preserve hearing is paramount for hearing preservation. In cases where preoperative hearing is poor, a translabyrinthine approach can be used to extirpate the tumor. If there is an additional extent of the tumor into the petrous apex, an extended middle fossa (Kawase) approach can be utilized, as well.

When hearing preservation is a surgical goal, intraoperative identification of the cochlea is vital. Also, it is important that cochlear erosion, when present, is identified preoperatively on imaging. If the tumor is adherent to the cochlea or a cochlear fistula is identified, a STR may be prudent in order to prevent entrance into the cochlear duct, as the rate of recurrence after a STR of GGH is very low [6]. Such an approach will yield a higher likelihood of serviceable hearing postoperatively. In such a situation, patient counseling is paramount as it relates to the risk of hearing loss.

The decision to sacrifice or preserve the facial nerve is based on the preoperative functional status of the nerve and intraoperative findings. In cases with facial function of HB grade III or better prior to surgery, efforts should be made to remove the lesion while preserving the integrity of the nerve. There will be a subset of patients who have good preoperative facial function but no cleavage plane between the tumor and the nerve. In this smaller proportion of cases, the GGH can be resected, and the facial nerve can be grafted to reestablish continuity. Alternatively, facial nerve decompression without significant tumor removal can potentially preserve facial nerve function for as long as possible. In cases that involve long-term paralysis, facial nerve sacrifice, and other methods of facial reanimation should be considered.

Outcomes

Outcome data are limited, and because of limited sample sizes in relevant publications, a robust statistical analysis of various prognostic factors has not been carried out (Table 73.1) [4, 6, 7, 12, 13].

Facial Nerve Outcomes

Oldenburg et al. reported that the duration of preoperative facial nerve dysfunction and intraoperative preservation of nerve integrity were significantly better predictors of postoperative facial function. Specifically, a duration of facial nerve weakness less than 12 months in length was associated with significantly better preoperative (4.1 vs 5.1) and postoperative (2.9 vs 4.0) HB grades [4]. An ability to maintain nerve integrity also yielded significantly better postoperative HB grades (2.6 vs 3.9). However, neither the size of the GGH (<10 mm vs > 10 mm) nor the extent of the resection (STR vs GTR) was a statistically significant predictor of better postoperative HB grade. These results were also replicated in a study of 16 patients who were divided into cohorts based on duration of paralysis (<12-month vs > 12-month) and preservation of nerve continuity. Higher rates of nerve preservation were achieved in the shorter duration group, which also translated to a better postoperative HB grade [13].

In their series, Semaan et al. used a neural preservation approach in 11 patients. Of these, 73% (8/11) had postoperative recovery to HB grade I–II, while the remaining 3 patients recovered to HB grade III. In the 4 patients who had facial nerve resection and cable grafting, none improved to HB grade I–II [6]. Similarly, Oldenburg et al., in their case series of 8 patients, showed stable or improved facial nerve outcomes in patients with preserved neural integrity. In contrast, two

Table 73.1 Facial nerve and hearing outcomes among published studies examining geniculate ganglion hemangiomas

Authors	N	Size (mm)	Surgical approach	Extent of resection/ FN preservation	Facial nerve outcome (HB grade)	Hearing outcomes (fistula/hearing preservation)	Recurrence
Oldenburg et al.	8	8.5 (5–14)	MCF-TM = 5 MCF = 3	GTR = 4 STR = 4 FNP = 4 FNR-G = 4	FNP = 3 FNR-G = 5.5	Otic fistula = 0 Preservation = 87.5%	1 (no intervention)
Isaacson et al.	6	12 (10–15)	MCF-TM = 1 MCF = 5	GTR = 5 STR = 1 FNP = 1 FNR-G = 5	FNP = 3 FNR-G = 3.8	Otic fistula = 1 Preservation = 83.3%	None
Semaan et al.	18	9 (4–20)	MCF = 13 TL = 2	GTR = 10 STR = 5 FNP = 11 FNR-G = 4	FNP = 2.1 FNR-G = 4	Otic fistula = 2 Preservation = 64%	None
Lahlou et al.	10	8 (4–15)	MCF = 10	GTR = 10 STR = 0 FNP = 0 FNR-G = 10	FNP = N/A FNR-G = 3.4	Otic fistula = 1 Preservation = 94%	None
Wang et al.	16	NR	MCF-TM = 1 MCF = 14	GTR = 16 STR = 0 FNP = 7 FNR-G = 9	FNP = 2.4 FNR-G = 3.9	Otic fistula = 1 Preservation = 93.7%	None

Gross total resection (GTR), sub-total resection (STR), facial nerve preservation (FNP), facial nerve resection and grafting (FNR-G), middle cranial fossa-transmastoid (MCF-TM), middle cranial fossa (MCF), Translabyrinthine (TL), House-Brackmann (HB), not reported (NR)

patients in their series who had facial nerve grafting had follow-up >12 months, and both had HB grade VI function [4].

Hearing Outcomes

Semaan et al. discussed possible hearing loss in patients with GGH as it relates to the disease's natural history. They proposed three mechanisms: erosion into the otic capsule, vascular steal of end-arterial cochlear blood flow by the growing hemangioma, and extension of the lesion into the IAC, thereby compressing the vestibulocochlear nerve. While none of these mechanisms have been conclusively evaluated, intact pre-intervention hearing should prompt a surgeon to use an operative approach that will maximize the chances of hearing preservation. Though hearing loss is a risk of surgical intervention in these cases, it is reportedly an uncommon occurrence. Seven percent (8/120) of patients were reported to have hearing loss related to surgical intervention in a systematic review [4]. In Semaan et al., hearing remained unchanged in 64% (7/11) who had postoperative audiometric data available. Hearing deteriorated in 38% (4/11), and the latter included two patients who had profound hearing loss due to intraoperative identification of a fistula to the middle turn of the cochlea [6].

Recurrence

Postoperative recurrence is uncommon in patients who are surgically treated. None of the 15 patients treated surgically at the House Ear Clinic, either with a GTR or a STR approach, had recurrence detected on follow-up imaging [6]. These results were replicated in the study by Lahlou et al., in which no recurrence was noted in patients who had follow-up imaging [7]. In the series by Oldenburg et al., 1 patient treated with a STR approach had a 2 mm recurrence noted on imaging at 19 months [4]. This patient had a decline in their facial nerve function from HB grade II–III, as well. Synthesizing data from these studies suggests that, even in cases where the malformation is closely adherent to the nerve, a plane of dissection can often be developed. However, in cases where such a plane is identified, a STR approach can be used with a low likelihood of recurrence.

Conclusion

GGH are rare lesions of the facial nerve. Identification of these tumors requires a high index of suspicion. These lesions may be venous malformations capable of proliferation rather than true neoplasms; as such, they can often be treated successfully with a low risk of recurrence. Long-term facial nerve outcomes are dependent on pretreatment facial nerve function as well as the duration of paresis preoperatively.

References

1. Pulec JL. Facial nerve tumors. Ann Otol Rhinol Laryngol. 1969;78:962–82.
2. Balkany T, Fradis M, Jafek BW, Rucker NC. Hemangioma of the facial nerve: role of the geniculate capillary plexus. Skull Base Surg. 1991;1:59–63.
3. Mangham CA, Carberry JN, Brackmann DE. Management of intratemporal vascular tumors. Laryngoscope. 1981;91:867–76.
4. Oldenburg MS, Carlson ML, Van Abel KM, Driscoll CL, Link MJ. Management of geniculate ganglion hemangiomas: case series and systematic review of the literature. Otol Neurotol. 2015;36:1735–40.
5. Benoit MM, North PE, McKenna MJ, Mihm MC, Johnson MM, Cunningham MJ. Facial nerve hemangiomas: vascular tumors or malformations? Otolaryngol Head Neck Surg. 2010;142:108–14.
6. Semaan MT, Slattery WH, Brackmann DE. Geniculate ganglion hemangiomas: clinical results and long-term follow-up. Otol Neurotol. 2010;31:665–70.
7. Lahlou G, Nguyen Y, Russo FY, Ferrary E, Sterkers O, Bernardeschi D. Geniculate ganglion tumors: clinical presentation and surgical results. Otolaryngol Head Neck Surg. 2016;155:850–5.
8. De Foer B, Kenis C, Vercruysse JP, et al. Imaging of temporal bone tumors. Neuroimaging Clin N Am. 2009;19:339–66.
9. Magliulo G, Alla FR, Colicchio G, Trasimeni G. Geniculate ganglion meningioma. Skull Base. 2010;20:185–8.
10. Wiggins RH 3rd, Harnsberger HR, Salzman KL, Shelton C, Kertesz TR, Glastonbury CM. The many faces of facial nerve schwannoma. AJNR Am J Neuroradiol. 2006;27:694–9.
11. Yue Y, Jin Y, Yang B, Yuan H, Li J, Wang Z. Retrospective case series of the imaging findings of facial nerve hemangioma. Eur Arch Otorrinolaringol. 2015;272:2497–503.
12. Isaacson B, Telian SA, McKeever PE, Arts HA. Hemangiomas of the geniculate ganglion. Otol Neurotol. 2005;26:796–802.
13. Wang K, Chou H, Li Y. Facial nerve hemangiomas at geniculate ganglion: preservation of nerve integrity is correlated with duration of facial palsy. Am J Otolaryngol. 2015;36:264–7.

74 Sporadic Vestibular Schwannomas

John P. Marinelli, Ashley M. Nassiri, Michael J. Link, and Matthew L. Carlson

Introduction

Arising from Schwann cells in the vestibular division of the eighth cranial nerve, vestibular schwannomas constitute one of the most distinctive disorders in the field of neurotology and lateral skull base surgery over the past century [1]. Once referred to as acoustic neuroma, neurinoma, or neurilemmoma, some of history's most prominent neurologic and neurotologic surgeons gained their notoriety through advancing the treatment of vestibular schwannoma.

One of the earliest clinical reports of a patient with vestibular schwannoma was published by Sir Charles Bell in 1833 [2]. Shortly after the turn of the twentieth century, Harvey Cushing published one of his most famous works: *Tumors of the Nervus Acusticus and the Syndrome of the Cerebellopontine Angle* [3]. His discoveries reduced perioperative mortality from 80% to, eventually, less than 5%. In his book, he characterized the unique symptomatology of patients with vestibular schwannoma from that era:

> [It] can be gathered that the symptomatic progress of the average acoustic tumor occurs more or less in the following stages: First, the auditory and labyrinthine manifestations; second, the occipitofrontal pains with suboccipital discomforts; third, the incoordination and instability of cerebellar origin; fourth, the evidence of involvement of adjacent cerebral nerves; fifth, the indications of increase in intracranial tension with a choked disc (papilledema) and its consequences; sixth, dysarthria, dysphagia, and finally cerebellar crises and respiratory difficulties [3].

Neurosurgeon Walter Dandy built on Cushing's foundation with the development of the unilateral cerebellar approach. His decision to resect a portion of the cerebellum, disregard for the preservation of the facial nerve, and predilection to ligate the anterior inferior cerebellar artery highlight the therapeutic mentality of that era [4]. While studying novel techniques for the treatment of otosclerosis, otologist William F. House revisited the middle cranial fossa approach to the internal auditory canal in the early 1960s [5]. Soon thereafter, House realized that the translabyrinthine approach offered unique advantages in patients without serviceable hearing, and in 1964, he published a consecutive series of 47 patients who underwent microsurgical excision of vestibular schwannoma without a single report of fatality—a feat that had not been previously achieved [6]. Michael Glasscock and others were able to replicate House's results with frequent preservation of facial nerve function and minimal cerebellar trauma [7].

Temporally paralleling the advances made by House in the 1960s, Lars Leksell pioneered the advancement of stereotactic radiosurgery, and a patient with vestibular schwannoma was treated by Gamma Knife radiosurgery for the first time in 1976 [8, 9]. Over the years, substantial advances in microsurgical and radiosurgical techniques have minimized the morbidity of vestibular schwannoma management in the twenty-first century. Circa the early 2000s, several groups observed that not all tumors grow following diagnosis [10, 11], and some tumors that initially demonstrate growth do not continue to grow [12]. These findings inspired the use of observation (i.e., active surveillance) with serial imaging as a primary management modality, and published trends over time suggest that this strategy is being initially employed in the majority of new diagnoses [13, 14].

In the current chapter, a foundation for understanding vestibular schwannoma and its management is established. We emphasize the dramatic evolution in the epidemiology of vestibular schwannoma over the past half-century and its multiple implications on practice patterns. Next, patient presentation and diagnostic workup are discussed. Last, modern management paradigms are presented in light of the growing understanding of the natural history of vestibular schwannoma. Of note, other chapters provide a greater depth of dis-

J. P. Marinelli · A. M. Nassiri · M. L. Carlson (✉)
Department of Otorhinolaryngology—Head and Neck Surgery, Mayo Clinic, Rochester, MN, USA

M. J. Link
Department of Neurological Surgery, Mayo Clinic, Rochester, MN, USA

A. D. Sweeney et al. (eds.), *Haynes-Glasscock-Shambaugh Surgery of the Ear*, https://doi.org/10.1007/978-3-032-18264-7_74

cussion surrounding the genetics and molecular biology of vestibular schwannoma and associated disorders, such as neurofibromatosis type 2.

Evolution in Epidemiology and Its Implications

From the early 1900s through the 1960s, vestibular schwannoma incidence remained essentially unchanged, and patients commonly presented with very large tumors requiring urgent surgical intervention to alleviate life-threatening symptoms such as hydrocephalus or lower cranial nerve palsies [1]. However, the advent of computed tomography (CT) introduced a new era in the detection of vestibular schwannoma and foreshadowed modern detection capabilities of neuroimaging [13, 15]. By the mid-1980s, magnetic resonance imaging (MRI) was introduced into clinical practice, and the detection of smaller tumors of the cerebellopontine angle or even tumors confined entirely to the internal auditory canal became feasible [13, 14].

Stemming from these improved detection capabilities, in combination with a heightened understanding of the disease (e.g., screening patients with asymmetrical sensorineural hearing loss (SNHL) with MRI), the incidence of vestibular schwannoma rapidly rose throughout the 1980s, 1990s, and 2000s and has continued to increase throughout the twenty-first century [13, 14]. From a historical incidence around 1 per 100,000 person-years circa 1970, the modern incidence of sporadic vestibular schwannoma ranges between 3 and 5 per 100,000 person-years among all ages and about 20 per 100,000 person-years among those ≥70 years—an incidence comparable to Hodgkin's lymphoma and Parkinson's disease dementia [13, 14, 16–18]. Moreover, patients are now being diagnosed at older ages (median age in patients' early 60s) with smaller tumors that are oftentimes confined to the internal auditory canal and are just millimeters in their greatest diameter [13, 14].

The rising incidence of vestibular schwannoma is largely attributable to the increasingly widespread use of MRI and screening protocols for asymmetrical SNHL (Fig. 74.1). However, evidence suggests that improved detection alone may not fully account for the dramatic increase in incidence witnessed in recent years [19]. Several groups have suggested that environmental exposures, such as cell phone use or chronic noise exposure, may increase a person's risk for the development of vestibular schwannoma [20–22]. However, most of these reports are survey-based studies that are likely heavily influenced by recall bias. Moreover, several large objective case-control studies have failed to substantiate these associations [23–25]. As such, beyond a history of intracranial radiation, there are no widely accepted exposures that increase a person's risk of developing vestibular schwannoma.

Perhaps unsuspectingly, the rising incidence of vestibular schwannoma bears several clinically relevant implications.

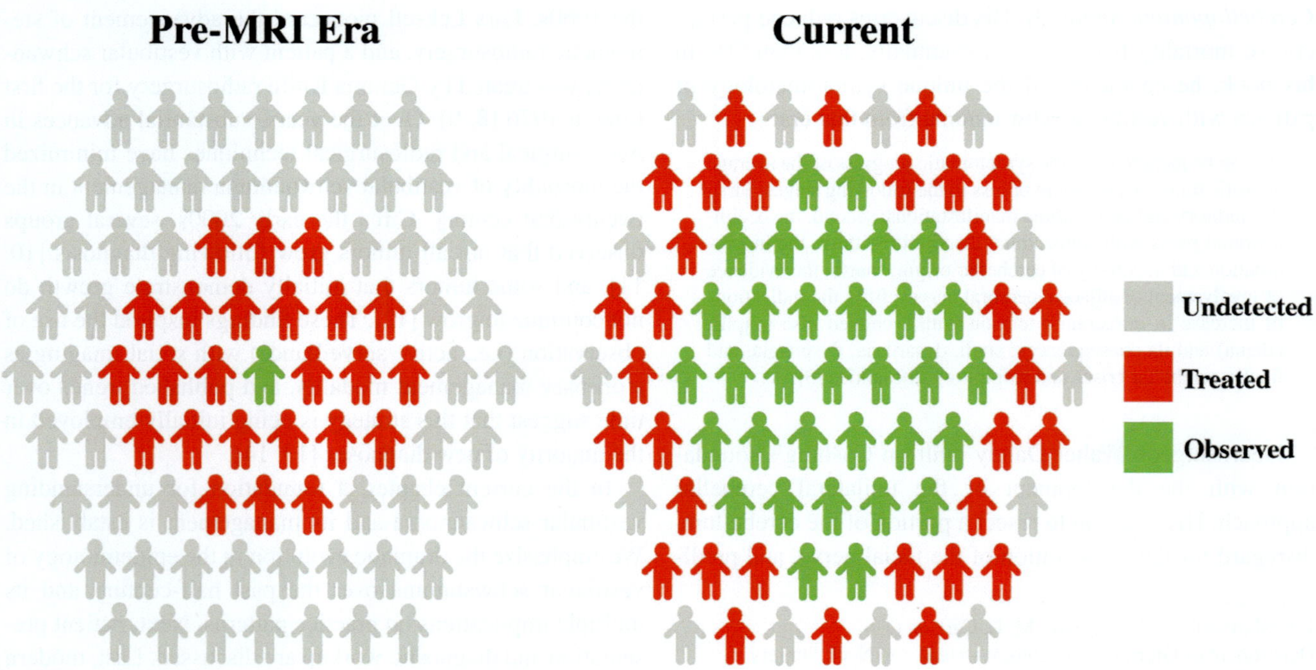

Fig. 74.1 Heightened detection of vestibular schwannoma as an explanation for the rising global incidence. Although more patients undergo observation than ever before, the detection rate has outpaced this transition, paradoxically leading to more tumors per capita treated than ever before. The concern for potential ongoing overtreatment of the disease is discussed in the section "Current Controversies and Challenges". (Used with permission from Carlson and Link [64])

First, since many tumors in the modern era undergo observation with serial imaging as their primary treatment modality, disease *prevalence* has risen considerably in recent years. Whereas the incidence rate of a disease encompasses the rate at which new cases are diagnosed in a population, the prevalence of a disease describes how many individuals within a population are living with the condition of interest. Because many patients in the modern era pursue watchful waiting with serial imaging as their primary treatment modality, they often live years without ever being "cured" (e.g., gross total resection), and disease prevalence accumulates over time. Strikingly, studies have shown that patients' risk of developing vestibular schwannoma throughout their lifetime exceeds 1 in 500, particularly in regions of the world that have elevated access to healthcare [26, 27]. Although commonly cited as a rare disease during patient counseling, disease prevalence estimates in this range render vestibular schwannoma not a "rare disease" legally within the United States and most countries around the world [28, 29]. Moreover, patients who would have lived their entire lives without knowledge of their disease just decades ago are now being diagnosed with increasing frequency. Since these patients are older with smaller tumors at the time of diagnosis, they most commonly pursue observation of their tumor with serial imaging. In this way, the dramatic evolution in the epidemiology of vestibular schwannoma over the past half-century suggests that the management of vestibular schwannoma in the twenty-first century will be largely characterized by "chronic disease management" rather than microsurgical or radiosurgical treatment.

Patient Presentation

Approximately 75% of patients with a vestibular schwannoma have asymmetrical sensorineural hearing loss (SNHL) [13, 30, 31]. Ipsilateral nonpulsatile tinnitus and associated imbalance, disequilibrium, or gait unsteadiness are the most common concomitant symptoms and are present in around 60% of patients [13, 30, 31]. Aural fullness often accompanies hearing loss, but symptoms of otalgia or otorrhea should be absent. Despite the widespread implementation of screening protocols for patients with asymmetrical SNHL, most patients experience a delay in diagnosis of several years [13, 30]. With the increasingly widespread use of MRI, the incidental diagnosis of vestibular schwannoma during the workup of other conditions has resulted in almost 25% of patients having no subjective symptoms at the time of diagnosis in the modern era [13, 32].

Less commonly, patients may experience sudden SNHL (present in about 2–8% of cases) or true episodic vertigo (<5–10% of cases) [13, 30, 33]. Although severe dizziness or vertigo is uncommon, its presence portends poor long-term quality of life outcomes [33, 34]. Other cranial nerve symptoms and mass effect (with or without hydrocephalus) are experienced in the minority of cases (<5% of new diagnoses) and are naturally associated with larger tumors with significant cerebellopontine angle tumor extension [13]. Of note, higher rates of other cranial nerve symptomatology may be observed in series from tertiary referral centers in the United States [30]. It is important to recognize, however, that referral bias renders presenting symptomatology in these cohorts not representative of the general vestibular schwannoma patient populace [35], and this distinction is important to consider when interpreting the existing literature. Notwithstanding, among the subgroup of patients with other cranial nerve involvement, trigeminal hypesthesia represents the most common other cranial nerve symptom. Facial nerve symptoms are uncommon but can occur in around 1–5% of cases, depending on the clinical setting [13, 30]. Given the infrequency of facial nerve symptoms in vestibular schwannoma, it is important to consider other potential pathologies, such as facial nerve schwannoma or malignancy, in patients presenting with facial nerve paresis. Secondary to early diagnosis and intervention, lower cranial nerve symptoms are relatively rare in the modern era and are found in association with less than 1% of new diagnoses [13].

A headache is commonly associated with vestibular schwannoma [36]. However, headache is also common in the general population, and its unrelated co-occurrence represents the majority of associations. For this reason, it is important to distinguish common headache disorders from headache associated with vestibular schwannoma secondary to tumor mass effect, with or without accompanying hydrocephalus. Large cerebellopontine angle tumors will often cause cerebellar compression with associated ataxia, intention tremor, or dysdiadochokinesis in up to 20% of these patients. Obstructive hydrocephalus occurs in vestibular schwannoma when large tumors induce significant compression of the fourth ventricle. Tumors of a sufficient size to cause hydrocephalus are rare in modern practice, and hydrocephalus is consequently observed in fewer than 1% of cases [13, 14].

Diagnosis

Audiometric Testing

Elucidated by patient history and tuning fork testing, any patient complaining of asymmetrical, gradual or sudden hearing loss should be further evaluated with formal audiometric testing. There exists no universally accepted definition of asymmetric SNHL. A widely used rule of thumb is that MRI should be obtained in patients with asymmetrical SNHL where the affected ear performs at least 10 dB worse across two contiguous frequencies or at least 15 dB in one frequency [37]. For speech audiometry, a word recognition score (WRS) that is at least 20% worse in the affected ear generally constitutes asymmetry. Interestingly, although tumor size typically correlates with patients' severity of hearing loss, it is not unheard of that patients with large vestibular schwannoma and substantial cerebellopontine angle extension can present with normal hearing thresholds and perfect word recognition scores.

It is well-known that retrocochlear pathology often disproportionally affects patients' speech discrimination compared to their pure-tone thresholds. A classic related phenomenon surrounds the idea of *rollover*, where patients' speech discrimination paradoxically worsens as the loudness increases in the setting of retrocochlear pathology. This observation is thought to stem from aberrant recruitment of axons damaged by the tumor. Of similar historical interest, stapedial reflex decay testing that demonstrates decay of the reflexive stiffening of the tympanic membrane to half-amplitude in five seconds or less is suggestive of retrocochlear pathology. In modern practice, however, these observations are of little clinical relevance as definitive screening with MRI is necessary in patients with confirmed asymmetric SNHL.

One critical concept surrounding audiometric assessments in vestibular schwannoma is the idea of "serviceable," or useful, hearing. The definition can vary by publication, but generally, many publications use a cutoff of ≥50 dB pure-tone average and ≥50% word recognition score as constituting "serviceable" hearing [38]. However, it is important to recognize that someone with perfect hearing in the contralateral ear often finds the affected ear to be of limited use, even when exceeding this ≥50% word recognition threshold. Substantiating this, a recent paper suggested that patients need at least 75% WRS to perceive hearing benefit [37]. Moreover, patients' word recognition is the primary driver of the utility of hearing in the affected ear, and studies have shown that anything less than perfect (i.e., 100% correct) word recognition is a poor prognosticator for maintaining useful hearing in the long term [38].

Vestibular Testing

Vestibular testing is not routinely used in the workup of patients presenting with asymmetrical SNHL or in patients with known vestibular schwannoma. Historically, the finding of decreased vestibular function on caloric testing in the affected ear had been implemented during the workup of vestibular schwannoma. However, given its relationship with the lateral semicircular canal and innervation only by the superior division of the vestibular nerve, it is not sufficiently sensitive to be used diagnostically in the modern era with widespread access to MRI. In more recent years, vestibular testing, such as vestibular evoked myogenic potentials (VEMP), has been used in an attempt to predict the nerve of origin of the tumor to aid in preoperative planning and counseling [39]. Although initial reports are promising, the utility of these studies in routine clinical practice remains controversial, and their use has not been widely adopted.

Neuroimaging

Historically, contrast-enhanced CT and other imaging modalities were used for tumor screening. Today, MRI represents the gold standard screening modality and is widely used across the globe. The prevalence of sporadic vestibular schwannoma in persons screened for asymmetrical SNHL with MRI is only around 3%. Thinly sliced, gadolinium-enhanced MRI of the internal auditory canals represents the preferred study and reliably detects tumors as small as 2 mm in their greatest diameter.

Vestibular schwannomas display several characteristic imaging features that enable clinical diagnosis alone without biopsy in the vast majority of cases (Fig. 74.2). These tumors are generally iso-to-hypointense to gray matter on pre-contrast T1-weighted MRI sequences and iso-to-hyperintense on T2-weighted sequences, and non-cystic tumors demonstrate uniform enhancement with gadolinium. Meningioma, the most common benign brain tumor, represents an important alternative diagnostic consideration in the workup of retrocochlear pathology, and vestibular schwannoma can be distinguished from these tumors by the observation that vestibular schwannomas are often isolated to the internal auditory canal or centered on the porus acusticus. Moreover, vestibular schwannomas do not generally exhibit prominent dural tails or hyperostosis of the underlying bone.

Particularly germane to understanding the literature surrounding treatment, it is important to understand how tumor size is defined within the context of vestibular schwannoma. Although the exact delineation varies by publication, small tumors are generally those with less than 1.5 cm of cerebellopontine angle extension, medium-sized tumors have between 1.5 and 2.5 cm of cerebellopontine angle extension, large tumors have between 2.5 and 3.5 cm, and giant tumors have >3.5 cm (Fig. 74.2). Of course, tumor size is not inherently categorical but occurs on a continuous spectrum; however, categorization such as this facilitates communication. Clinically, tumors are typically measured by taking the single greatest dimension of the cerebellopontine angle portion of the tumor in the axial imaging plane. Intracanalicular tumors (i.e., those without extension into the cerebellopontine angle) are typically measured along the axis of the internal auditory canal in the axial imaging plane and are often just several millimeters in size. Other linear or volumetric measurements exist largely for research purposes [40, 41].

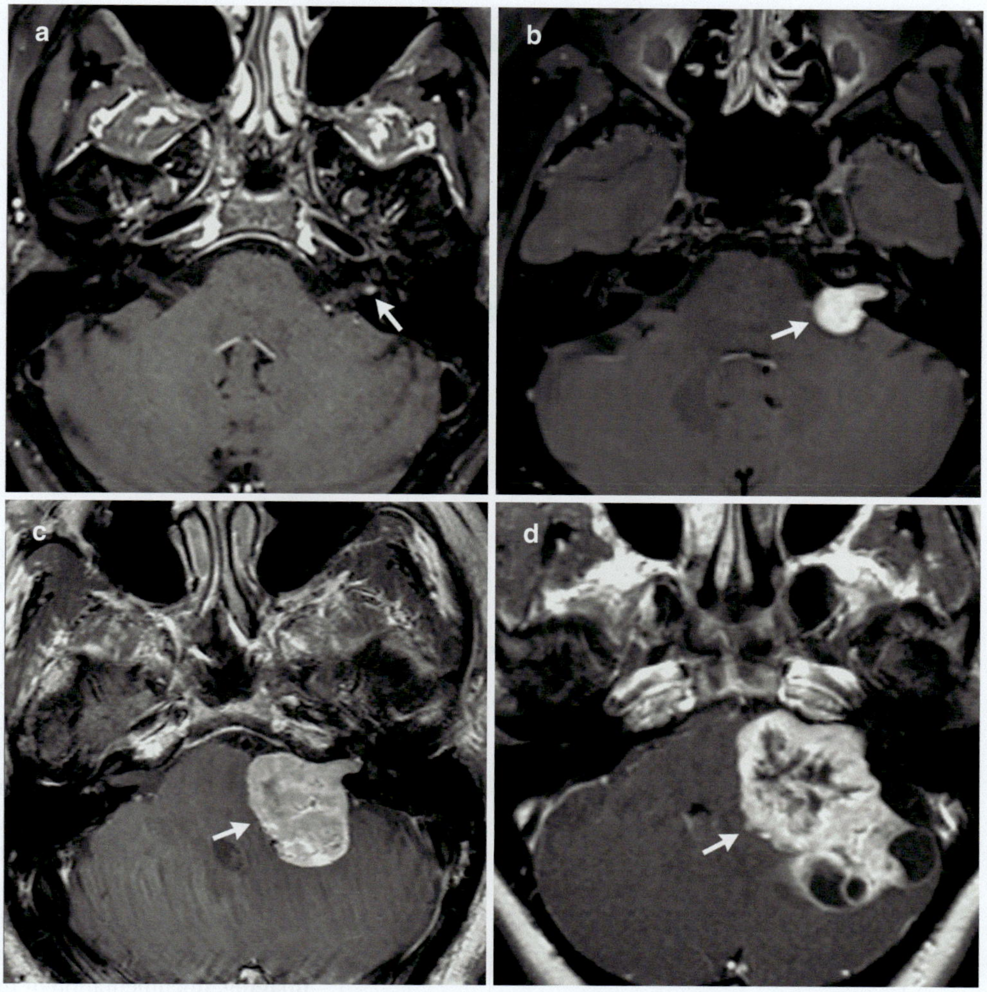

Fig. 74.2 Variations in the size of vestibular schwannomas at diagnosis. (Used with permission from Carlson and Link [64])

Management

Overview

Paralleling the improvements in medical technology and disease understanding, the management of vestibular schwannoma has evolved considerably in recent decades. Existing paradigms prioritize patients' quality of life and the minimization of morbidity. Understandably, studies have shown that the patients' quality of life nadir occurs with the diagnosis of their vestibular schwannoma [42].

Management options broadly include observation, radiosurgery, and microsurgery. The decision to pursue definitive treatment with either radiosurgery or microsurgery is predominantly a function of tumor size and patient symptomatology, although patient and provider preferences play a critical role as well. Given the widespread geographic variation in treatment patterns across the United States, it is recommended that patients seek advice from more than one provider (Fig. 74.3) [43]. Generally speaking, for small- and medium-sized tumors, patients' symptoms are largely not expected to improve following treatment. Instead, symptoms may influence treatment approach (e.g., pursuing a translabyrinthine approach in a patient with non-serviceable hearing), be prevented from getting worse (e.g., hearing preservation microsurgery), or rehabilitated following treatment (e.g., vestibular therapy and facial nerve reanimation procedures). Nonetheless, regardless of the treatment modality that is eventually pursued, large multicenter studies have shown that there exists little to no clinically meaningful differences in quality of life or patient satisfaction between the three overarching management modalities (Fig. 74.4) [42, 44]. Instead, factors such as ongoing dizziness and headache appear to be the predominant drivers of long-term quality of life [34].

Observation

Observation with serial imaging represents the most common, initially pursued treatment modality among new diagnoses of vestibular schwannoma in the general patient populace. Large population-based studies suggest that

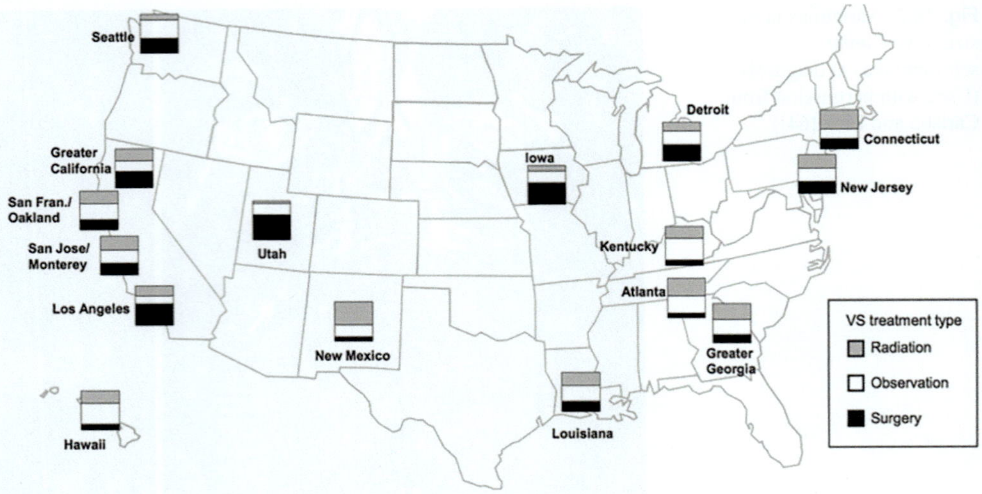

Fig. 74.3 National variation in initial management approach for patients diagnosed with sporadic vestibular schwannoma across the United States. (Used with permission from Carlson et al. [43])

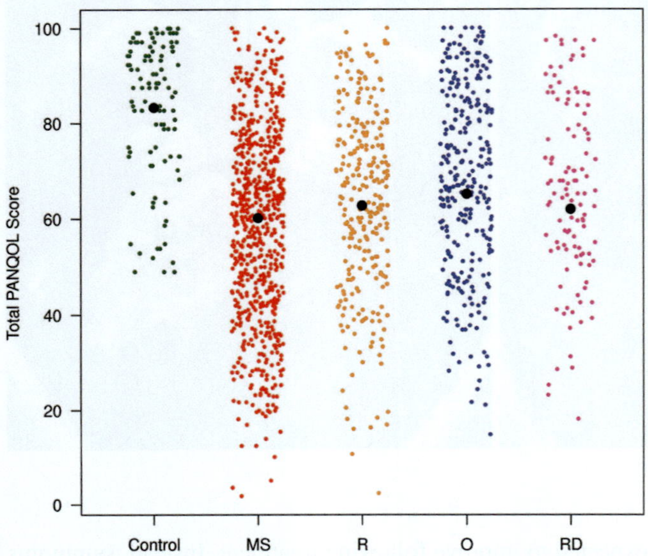

Fig. 74.4 Total Penn Acoustic Neuroma Quality of Life (PANQOL) scores for non-tumor controls and VS treatment groups. Adjusted means were 83, 60, 63, 65, and 62 (black dots) for the non-tumor control, microsurgery (MS), radiosurgery (R), observation (O), and recently diagnosed (RD) groups, respectively. (Used with permission from Chweya et al. [92])

around 70% of newly diagnosed patients pursue this option, citing lower invasiveness and lower risk as primary driving factors in their decision-making [13, 44, 45]. What is more, an initial period of observation of at least 6 months is associated with better quality of life and long-term patient satisfaction. This is likely secondary to the observational period, affording patients valuable time to come to terms with their new diagnosis and carefully consider their management options [44, 46]. Although referral bias renders the rate of observation lower among tertiary referral center cohorts in the United States, it is still initially pursued in more than 50% of cases [35, 47]. The theoretical basis for observation as a primary treatment modality stems from the realization that not all tumors continue to grow following diagnosis and that most tumors that grow do so at a slow rate of around 1–3 mm per year [10, 45]. At 10 years following diagnosis, about 45% of patients who presented with serviceable hearing retain their serviceable hearing during conservative management with observation [38].

Currently, there exists no widely adopted imaging schedule, but at many centers, an initial follow-up MRI is obtained at about 6 months after diagnosis. Assuming no detected tumor growth, MRIs are obtained yearly thereafter until 5 years post-diagnosis, after which patients undergo imaging every 2 years indefinitely to monitor for delayed tumor growth [48]. Beyond the period of observation with serial imaging, documentation of tumor growth (≥2-mm change in tumor size between serial scans) typically begets treatment at most centers in the United States. However, recent evidence has challenged this practice, demonstrating that tolerance of limited growth during observation up until a size threshold, whereby further tumor growth would predispose the patient to a disproportionally elevated risk of poor posttreatment outcomes, is justifiable and likely advantageous for most patients. This newer approach to observation management is termed "Size Threshold Surveillance" and is outlined at length elsewhere [49].

It is important to recognize that not all patients should be counseled to undergo observation with serial imaging following diagnosis. Patients with large tumors are almost always recommended to undergo microsurgery, and a delay in definitive therapy is avoided as much as possible. Many providers will also recommend upfront treatment of medium-sized tumors in patients with minimal symptoms in an effort to preserve functional hearing and avoid negative sequelae of further tumor growth, such as an increased risk of perioperative facial nerve morbidity. Age also plays a role, as younger patients are often healthier while also being at an elevated risk of future growth (more time left in life to experience growth); therefore, younger patients are often treated more aggressively than older adults. Nevertheless, decision-making must involve patient preference and acknowledgment that observation is linked with better quality of life metrics and excellent long-term patient satisfaction, regardless of the eventual treatment strategy pursued [44, 46].

Radiosurgery

Stereotactic radiation for the primary management of vestibular schwannoma has become a common practice in recent decades [13]. The avoidance of surgery and its attendant risks is often appealing to patients requiring definitive treatment. Techniques include single-session stereotactic radiosurgery (e.g., Gamma Knife®), hypofractionated (CyberKnife®) or conventionally fractionated radiotherapy, and proton beam therapy. Gamma Knife® stereotactic radiosurgery is currently used most commonly in the United States.

Overarchingly, radiosurgery in vestibular schwannoma aims to achieve long-term tumor control (i.e., cessation of further growth) while minimizing morbidity and maintaining existing neurologic function. Mechanistically, traditional radiotherapy science surrounding the treatment of malignancies and the cell survival curve do not immediately extend to the treatment of vestibular schwannoma, and the radiobiology of these tumors is incompletely understood [50]. Although around 40% of vestibular schwannomas demonstrate a radiographic phenomenon of "central necrosis" following radiosurgery, the majority of treated cases do not develop this finding, yet they still achieve long-term tumor control. Interestingly, the phenomenon of central necrosis appears to be unique to vestibular schwannoma and is not observed in comparable tumors such as meningioma or pituitary adenoma. Long-term tumor control rates of vestibular schwannoma approximate 90–95% of treated cases and are similar for both single-session stereotactic radiosurgery and fractionated stereotactic radiotherapy [51, 52]. Long-term patient satisfaction is excellent [44]. Since radiosurgery treatment can be completed in an outpatient, single-day session, it is often preferred over fractionated stereotactic radiotherapy out of convenience. Most centers recommend limiting the use of radiosurgery or radiotherapy in the primary management of vestibular schwannoma to tumors with less than 2.5 cm of cerebellopontine angle extension for optimal long-term tumor control and post-radiosurgery morbidity. Similarly, fast-growing tumors (>2.5 mm/year) may exhibit decreased responsiveness to radiosurgery [53].

Significant complications related to radiosurgery are rare. Given the close approximation of the cochlear nerve and cochlea to the tumor, these structures cannot be spared, and radiation-induced hearing loss results [54]. At 10 years following treatment, about 25% of patients will maintain serviceable hearing compared to 40–45% of those undergoing observation [55].

The risk of other cranial neuropathies is low and directly proportional to the radiation dose at the margin. Prior research demonstrated that margin doses less than 16 Gy significantly reduced cranial neuropathies, and most modern treatment plans use doses at the margin of about 12–13 Gy [56]. At this marginal dose, the risk of permanent post-radiosurgery facial nerve paresis is about 0.3% [56]. Trigeminal nerve dysfunction and secondary hydrocephalus are exceedingly rare in the management of small- to medium-sized tumors at modern radiation dosages [57]. Of note, post-radiosurgery tumor swelling is commonly observed and must not be mistaken for interval tumor growth in the immediate posttreatment period.

A common concern among patients surrounds the risk of malignant transformation of their tumor or the development of other brain tumors following stereotactic radiation. For context, the rate of spontaneous malignant transformation of sporadic vestibular schwannoma is estimated to be around 0.0014%, or 1.4 per 100,000 cases. The relative risk of malignant transformation increases approximately tenfold following radiosurgery; however, the absolute risk remains exceedingly low, estimated to be around 0.016% for sporadic vestibular schwannoma [58]. When including all brain neoplasms (e.g., meningioma and glioblastoma), the risk of developing other brain tumors at any site following radiosurgery is about 0.04% [59]. These rates should be viewed in the context of the comparable risk of perioperative mortality following a craniotomy [60].

Microsurgery

While conservative management of vestibular schwannoma has become more prominent in recent years, microsurgical resection represents a significant aspect of the treatment algorithm [61]. The multidisciplinary approach to patient care becomes paramount in this treatment modality, as preoperative planning, surgical resection, and postoperative management require a team-based approach for optimal patient outcomes. Certain situations, such as large tumors precipitating hydrocephalus, brain stem compression, or cerebellar edema, may necessitate upfront surgical resection. More commonly, however, patients can be effectively managed with more than one treatment option, and decision-making heavily relies on patient and multidisciplinary team preferences.

Compared to observation and radiosurgery, microsurgical resection is associated with increased convalescence and posttreatment complications. Nevertheless, microsurgical resection is the only option that offers the potential for complete "cure" with gross total resection. While a prospective analysis comparing three treatment groups did not identify significant differences in disease-specific overall quality of life (Fig. 74.4), patients who underwent microsurgery experienced a greater improvement in the anxiety domain [62]. This finding may be related to the psychological benefit of having been "cured" after complete tumor removal.

Overview of Surgical Approaches

Although the translabyrinthine, retrosigmoid, and middle fossa approaches are most commonly employed today, these approaches may be tailored or combined to improve surgical access to the tumor. This section will provide a broad overview of the three approaches (Fig. 74.5).

The translabyrinthine approach, first described in 1904 by Rudolf Panse, is a transmastoid, transtemporal approach that sacrifices the labyrinth to allow for access to the internal auditory canal (IAC) and cerebellopontine angle (CPA). Any residual preoperative hearing is inherently forgone in this approach; consequently, the translabyrinthine approach is largely used in patients without useful preoperative hearing.

The advantages of the approach include early identification of the facial nerve within the IAC, favorable position of the facial nerve relative to the tumor, and a broad access corridor reaching from the posterior fossa to the fundus of the IAC. In addition to hearing loss, the disadvantages include the length of time required to perform the approach, meaning that the tumor is encountered later in the surgery compared to the retrosigmoid and middle fossa approaches.

The retrosigmoid craniotomy, positioned posterior and inferior to the transverse-sigmoid sinus junction, permits unrestricted access to the posterior fossa and inferior CPA from the tentorium cerebelli to the foramen magnum. In patients with preoperative residual hearing, the retrosigmoid approach offers the potential for hearing preservation. The retrosigmoid approach is particularly advantageous for large vestibular schwannomas with significant ventral extension. While the IAC can be accessed through a retrosigmoid approach, all IAC drilling is intradural, and access to the fundus can be limited by the labyrinth. Traditionally, the retrosigmoid approach requires more cerebellar retraction and has been associated with increased postoperative headaches.

Finally, the middle fossa craniotomy allows for access to the IAC through the middle fossa corridor with retraction of the temporal lobe. This approach offers the potential for hearing preservation and exposes the length of the IAC from the porus acusticus to the fundus in most patients; however, access to the CPA is limited by the requirement to retract the temporal lobe, typically preventing access to tumors that have >1.0-cm CPA extension. While lateral IAC dissection with this approach is possible, the facial nerve is typically positioned between the surgeon and the tumor, requiring the surgeon to dissect around the facial nerve for tumor removal. The facial nerve position associated with this approach has been reported to result in poorer facial nerve outcomes when compared to the other two approaches; however, outcomes may be similar in experienced hands.

Complications

The risks of postoperative complications must be weighed against the benefits of surgical resection in each case. The risk of facial nerve paralysis is dependent on several factors, but tumor size remains the most consistent predictor of long-term facial nerve outcome. Published risk estimates range widely from 5% to 65% based on tumor size, although for tumors with ≤10 mm of CPA extension the risk is estimated to be 3–5% at high-volume centers [63–65]. Hearing loss remains a risk of surgery in patients undergoing hearing preservation surgery; the risk of early and delayed hearing loss is similarly dependent on several factors, including tumor size and location, surgical approach, and preoperative hearing level, and ranges broadly from 0 to 85% [61]. Other complications include infection, hydrocephalus, vascular complications, other cranial nerve neuropathy (dysphagia, dysphonia, diplopia, and facial hypesthesia), injury related to intraoperative positioning, fat graft donor site hematoma, long-term vestibulopathy, and headache. Complications associated with anesthetic drugs are less common, although patients should be counseled about these risks [61].

Postoperative Care

In the immediate postoperative period, patients are monitored for neurologic or hemodynamic decline in the neurologic intensive care unit. While postoperative complications are uncommon, rapid diagnosis and treatment are required to prevent devastating sequelae. Stable patients can generally be transitioned to a lower-acuity neurologic floor on the first postoperative day, where the surgical team can manage pain, encourage ambulation, and monitor for postoperative complications. An uneventful postoperative admission typically ranges from 3 to 4 days. However, infrequent, prolonged admissions are most commonly associated with persistent severe vestibulopathy that may require additional vestibular therapy in the hospital or admission to an inpatient rehabilitation facility.

Surgical Approach Selection

Much like the overall treatment decision-making, surgical approach selection depends on patient factors, tumor characteristics, temporal bone anatomy, and multidisciplinary team experience. In most cases, there exists more than one justifiable option, although prior multidisciplinary team experience may make one approach more desirable and successful over another [61].

Generally, tumor size and location, in conjunction with hearing status, are the chief considerations in determining the optimal surgical approach. If hearing preservation is feasible, a middle cranial fossa or retrosigmoid approach is selected. The authors reserve the middle fossa craniotomy

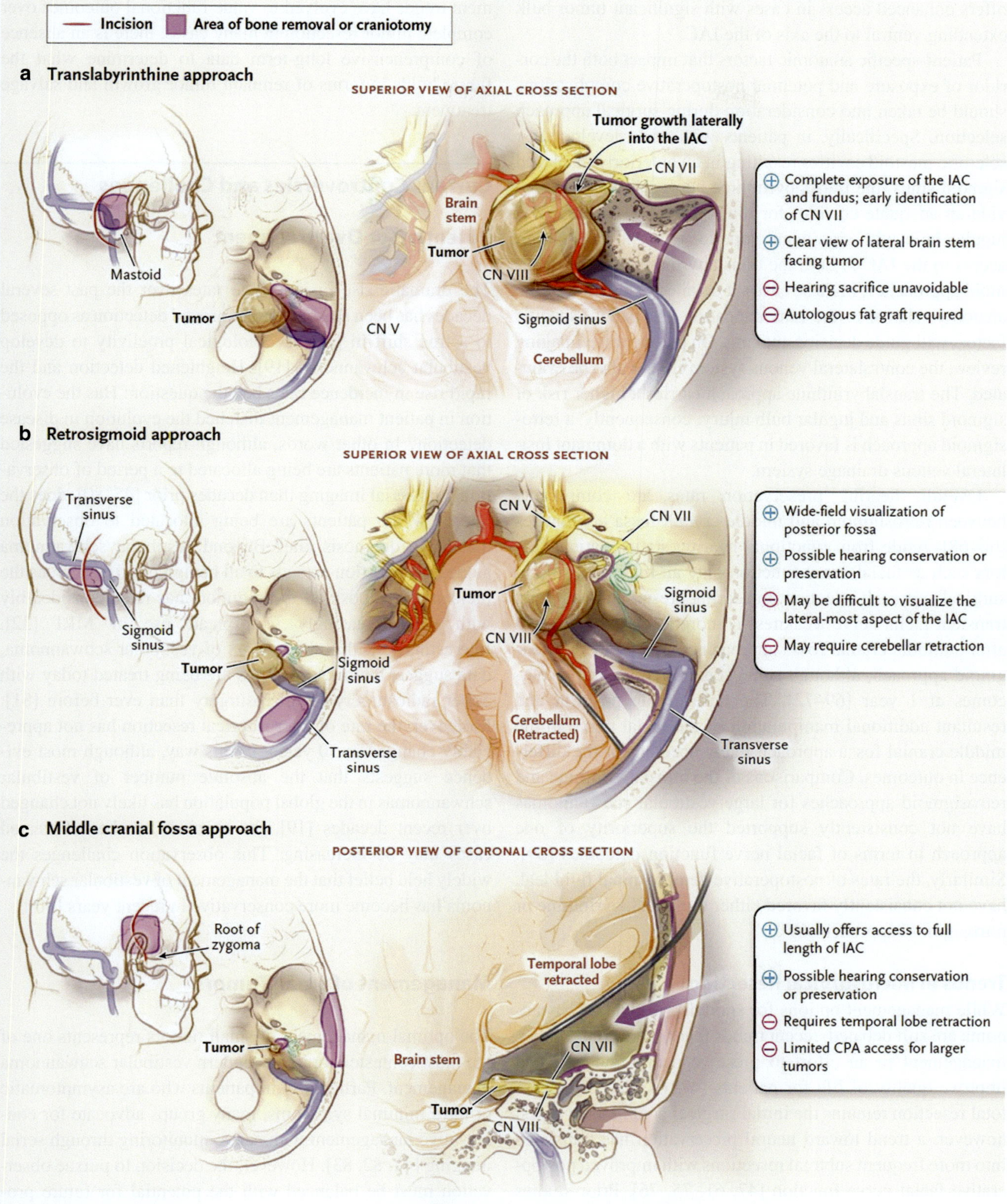

Fig. 74.5 Microsurgical approaches for the treatment of vestibular schwannomas. (Used with permission from Carlson and Link [64])

approach for patients with functional hearing and intracanalicular tumors in close proximity to the fundus. In some cases, intracanalicular tumors located in closer proximity to the porus acusticus may be resected with a retrosigmoid approach. In medium-sized tumors with functional hearing, the retrosigmoid approach is generally utilized. The translabyrinthine approach offers excellent exposure to the IAC and posterior fossa; however, the retrosigmoid approach offers enhanced access in cases with significant tumor bulk extending ventral to the axis of the IAC.

Patient-specific anatomic factors that impact both the corridor of exposure and potential postoperative complications should be taken into consideration during surgical approach selection. Specifically, in patients with underdeveloped or sclerotic mastoid cavities resulting in an anteriorly displaced sigmoid sinus, the translabyrinthine approach may not provide an adequate corridor for tumor resection. Similarly, a jugular bulb with significant superior extension may limit access to the IAC in both the translabyrinthine and retrosigmoid approaches; in these cases, a detailed evaluation of the anatomy relative to the tumor location and patient-specific factors will guide decision-making. On preoperative imaging review, the contralateral venous system should also be evaluated. The translabyrinthine approach carries a higher risk of sigmoid sinus and jugular bulb injury; consequently, a retrosigmoid approach is favored in patients with a dominant ipsilateral venous drainage system.

Overall, hearing preservation rates are comparable between retrosigmoid and middle cranial fossa approaches [66–68]. Aside from functional hearing status, patient factors such as facial nerve function play an important role in surgical approach selection. In hearing preservation surgery, transient facial nerve weakness is more frequently reported after a middle cranial fossa approach compared to a retrosigmoid approach, although some centers report similar outcomes at 1 year [69–72]. The unfavorable position and resultant additional manipulation of the facial nerve in the middle cranial fossa approach likely account for the difference in outcomes. Comparisons of the translabyrinthine and retrosigmoid approaches for large vestibular schwannomas have not consistently supported the superiority of one approach in terms of facial nerve function outcomes [69]. Similarly, the rates of postoperative cerebrospinal fluid leak have not consistently favored either the translabyrinthine or retrosigmoid approach [69].

Trends in Microsurgical Resection

While management options for sporadic vestibular schwannoma are still debated, recent trends favor more conservative management in an effort to preserve neural function and improve quality of life for patients [47, 61, 73, 74]. Gross total resection remains the initial surgical goal in most cases; however, a trend toward neural preservation has translated into more frequent subtotal resections with improved postoperative facial nerve function [47, 61, 75, 76]. Prior studies have compared recurrence rates between subtotal resection and gross total resection or near total resection, citing that recurrence rates are 11 times and 13 times more likely, respectively [77, 78]. Typically, tumor remnant growth can be treated with salvage radiosurgery, and recent studies show promising short-term tumor control rates [79]. While treatment trends have evolved to value functional outcomes over complete tumor resection in many cases, there is an absence of comprehensive long-term data to determine what the future holds in terms of remnant tumor growth and salvage treatment.

Current Controversies and Challenges

Potential for Overtreatment

The dramatic rise in incidence rates over the past several decades has been attributed to improved detection as opposed to a true shift in patients' biological proclivity to develop vestibular schwannoma [19]. Heightened detection and the rapid rise in incidence rates beg the question: Has the evolution in patient management matched the evolution in disease detection? In other words, although reports have suggested that more patients are being allocated to a period of observation with serial imaging than decades prior [45, 80], does the rate at which patients are being allocated to observation match the diagnosis rate? Beyond vestibular schwannoma alone, this question extends to all benign brain tumors, as the incidental diagnosis of these tumors has risen considerably with the increasingly widespread use of MRI [32]. Interestingly, within the context of vestibular schwannoma, data suggest that more patients are being treated today with either radiosurgery or microsurgery than ever before [81]. Moreover, the rate of microsurgical resection has not appreciably changed in 50 years. In this way, although most evidence suggests that the absolute number of vestibular schwannomas in the global population has likely not changed over recent decades [19], the absolute number of treated cases may be increasing. This observation challenges the widely held belief that the management of vestibular schwannoma has become more conservative in recent years [80].

Management of Small Tumors

The optimal management of small tumors represents one of the most contested topics in modern vestibular schwannoma management. Particularly in patients who are asymptomatic or have minimal symptoms, many groups advocate for conservative management with active monitoring through serial imaging [42, 82, 83]. However, the decision to pursue observation must be balanced with the potential for future progressive or sudden SNHL. Several groups advocate for early radiosurgery or microsurgery to preserve patients' functional hearing status [84–88]. For this reason, there is no accepted consensus on initial management strategy, and initial management is heavily influenced by both the physicians' and patients' preferences [74]. As a by-product, reported trends have shown that patients' initial management strategy significantly varies by geographic region within the United States [43]. Interestingly, a period of observation prior to definitive radiosurgical or microsurgical treatment has been shown to be associated with higher quality-adjusted life years regardless of the initial hearing status [89].

Intricately linked to the idea of overtreatment, most centers in the United States pursue definitive management with either radiosurgery or microsurgery following the detection of tumor growth [47]. However, growing evidence has challenged this paradigm, demonstrating saltatory growth patterns in sporadic vestibular schwannoma, where tumors may initially exhibit growth but can enter long and potentially indefinite periods of senescence [12]. A volumetric analysis of 361 tumors undergoing observation showed that up to 40% of patients who previously met the criteria for tumor growth demonstrated no further tumor growth at 5 years [90]. This observation is intuitive as patients with sporadic vestibular schwannoma necessarily *develop* their tumor (i.e., they were not born with their tumor), and it had to grow to the size detected at the time of diagnosis. Moreover, many providers advocate that patients should undergo an initial period of observation with serial imaging under the provision that if the tumor grows, it should be treated. In this way, this existing treatment paradigm presupposes a saltatory growth pattern of vestibular schwannoma and assumes that tumors may grow and eventually stop growing (or even spontaneously regress) [91]. Especially in light of the potential for overtreatment of patients, these observations suggest that continued conservative management—even despite documented tumor growth—is warranted in appropriately selected cases (e.g., older patients with slowly growing tumors, small vestibular schwannoma in an only-hearing ear, and patients with significant medical comorbidities). This approach that allows for some tumor growth during observation is termed "Size Threshold Surveillance" and is discussed at length elsewhere [49].

References

1. Ramsden RT. The bloody angle: 100 years of acoustic neuroma surgery. J R Soc Med. 1995;88(8):464P–8P.
2. Bell C. The nervous system of the human body. Washington, DC: Green; 1833.
3. Cushing H. Tumors of the nervus acusticus and the syndrome of the Cerebellopontile Ange. Philadelphia and London: W.B. Saunders Company; 1917.
4. Dandy WE. An operation for the total removal of cerebellopontine (acoustic) tumors. Surg Gynecol Obstet. 1925;41:29.
5. House WF. Surgical exposure of the internal auditory canal and its contents through the middle, cranial fossa. Laryngoscope. 1961;71:1363–85.
6. House WF. Transtemporal bone microsurgical removal of acoustic neuromas. Evolution of transtemporal bone removal of acoustic tumors. Arch Otolaryngol. 1964;80:731–42.
7. Glasscock ME 3rd, Hays JW. The translabyrinthine removal of acoustic and other cerebellopontine angle tumors. Ann Otol Rhinol Laryngol. 1973;82(4):415–27.
8. Bergstrom M, Greitz T. Stereotaxic computed tomography. AJR Am J Roentgenol. 1976;127(1):167–70.
9. Leksell L, Jernberg B. Stereotaxis and tomography. A technical note. Acta Neurochir (Wien). 1980;52(1–2):1–7.
10. Stangerup SE, Caye-Thomasen P, Tos M, Thomsen J. The natural history of vestibular schwannoma. Otol Neurotol. 2006;27(4):547–52.
11. Flint D, Fagan P, Panarese A. Conservative management of sporadic unilateral acoustic neuromas. J Laryngol Otol. 2005;119(6):424–8.
12. Ferri GG, Pirodda A, Ceroni AR, Fioravanti A, Calbucci F, Modugno GC. Management of growing vestibular schwannomas. Eur Arch Otorrinolaringol. 2013;270(7):2013–9.
13. Marinelli JP, Lohse CM, Carlson ML. Incidence of vestibular schwannoma over the past half-century: a population-based study of Olmsted County, Minnesota. Otolaryngol Head Neck Surg. 2018;159(4):717–23.
14. Reznitsky M, Petersen M, West N, Stangerup SE, Caye-Thomasen P. Epidemiology of vestibular schwannomas - prospective 40-year data from an unselected National Cohort. Clin Epidemiol. 2019;11:981–6.
15. Tos M, Stangerup SE, Caye-Thomasen P, Tos T, Thomsen J. What is the real incidence of vestibular schwannoma? Arch Otolaryngol Head Neck Surg. 2004;130(2):216–20.
16. Schwartz M, Fisher L. Incidence and clinical characteristics of acoustic neuroma in Beverly Hills. Skull Base. 2006;16(S 1):A040.
17. Kleijwegt M, Ho V, Visser O, Godefroy W, van der Mey A. Real incidence of vestibular schwannoma? Estimations from a National Registry. Otol Neurotol. 2016;37(9):1411–7.
18. Koo M, Lai JT, Yang EY, Liu TC, Hwang JH. Incidence of vestibular schwannoma in Taiwan from 2001 to 2012: a population-based National Health Insurance Study. Ann Otol Rhinol Laryngol. 2018;127(10):694–7.
19. Marinelli JP, Lohse CM, Grossardt BR, Lane JI, Carlson ML. Rising incidence of sporadic vestibular schwannoma: true biological shift versus simply greater detection. Otol Neurotol. 2020;41(6):813–47.
20. Moon IS, Kim BG, Kim J, Lee JD, Lee WS. Association between vestibular schwannomas and mobile phone use. Tumour Biol. 2014;35(1):581–7.
21. Deltour I, Schlehofer B, Massardier-Pilonchery A, et al. Exposure to loud noise and risk of vestibular schwannoma: results from the INTERPHONE international casecontrol study. Scand J Work Environ Health. 2019;45(2):183–93.
22. Cao Z, Zhao F, Mulugeta H. Noise exposure as a risk factor for acoustic neuroma: a systematic review and meta-analysis. Int J Audiol. 2019;58(9):525–32.
23. Aarhus L, Kjaerheim K, Heikkinen S, et al. Occupational noise exposure and vestibular schwannoma: a case-control study in Sweden. Am J Epidemiol. 2020;189:1342.
24. Schuz J, Steding-Jessen M, Hansen S, et al. Long-term mobile phone use and the risk of vestibular schwannoma: a Danish nationwide cohort study. Am J Epidemiol. 2011;174(4):416–22.
25. Roswall N, Stangerup SE, Caye-Thomasen P, et al. Residential traffic noise exposure and vestibular schwannoma - a Danish case-control study. Acta Oncol. 2017;56(10):1310–6.
26. Caulley L, Sawada M, Hinther K, Ko YI, Crowther JA, Kontorinis G. Geographic distribution of vestibular schwannomas in West Scotland between 2000-2015. PLoS One. 2017;12(5):e0175489.
27. Marinelli JP, Grossardt BR, Lohse CM, Carlson ML. Prevalence of sporadic vestibular schwannoma: reconciling temporal bone, radiologic, and population-based studies. Otol Neurotol. 2019;40(3):384–90.
28. Song P, Gao J, Inagaki Y, Kokudo N, Tang W. Rare diseases, orphan drugs, and their regulation in Asia: current status and future perspectives. Intractable Rare Dis Res. 2012;1(1):3–9.

29. Baldovino S, Moliner AM, Taruscio D, Daina E, Roccatello D. Rare diseases in Europe: from a wide to a local perspective. Isr Med Assoc J. 2016;18(6):359–63.
30. Matthies C, Samii M. Management of 1000 vestibular schwannomas (acoustic neuromas): clinical presentation. Neurosurgery. 1997;40(1):1–9; discussion 9–10.
31. Tos M, Charabi S, Thomsen J. Clinical experience with vestibular schwannomas: epidemiology, symptomatology, diagnosis, and surgical results. Eur Arch Otorrinolaringol. 1998;255(1):1–6.
32. Vernooij MW, Ikram MA, Tanghe HL, et al. Incidental findings on brain MRI in the general population. N Engl J Med. 2007;357(18):1821–8.
33. Andersen JF, Nilsen KS, Vassbotn FS, et al. Predictors of vertigo in patients with untreated vestibular schwannoma. Otol Neurotol. 2015;36(4):647–52.
34. Carlson ML, Tveiten OV, Driscoll CL, et al. What drives quality of life in patients with sporadic vestibular schwannoma? Laryngoscope. 2015;125(7):1697–702.
35. Saba ES, Marinelli JP, Lohse CM, Link MJ, Carlson ML. Quantifying tertiary referral center bias in vestibular schwannoma research. Otol Neurotol. 2020;41(2):258–64.
36. Carlson ML, Tveiten OV, Driscoll CL, et al. Risk factors and analysis of long-term headache in sporadic vestibular schwannoma: a multicenter cross-sectional study. J Neurosurg. 2015;123(5):1276–86.
37. Sweeney AD, Carlson ML, Shepard NT, et al. Congress of Neurological Surgeons systematic review and evidence-based guidelines on otologic and audiologic screening for patients with vestibular schwannomas. Neurosurgery. 2018;82(2):E29–31.
38. Hunter JB, Dowling EM, Lohse CM, et al. Hearing outcomes in conservatively managed vestibular schwannoma patients with serviceable hearing. Otol Neurotol. 2018;39(8):e704–11.
39. Piras G, Brandolini C, Castellucci A, Modugno GC. Ocular vestibular evoked myogenic potentials in patients with acoustic neuroma. Eur Arch Otorrinolaringol. 2013;270(2):497–504.
40. Monsell EM. Committee on hearing and equilibrium guidelines for the evaluation of hearing preservation in acoustic neuroma (vestibular schwannoma). Am Acad Otolaryngol Head Neck Surg. 1995;113(3):179–80.
41. Lees KA, Tombers NM, Link MJ, et al. Natural history of sporadic vestibular schwannoma: a volumetric study of tumor growth. Otolaryngol Head Neck Surg. 2018;159(3):535–42.
42. Carlson ML, Tveiten OV, Driscoll CL, et al. Long-term quality of life in patients with vestibular schwannoma: an international multicenter cross-sectional study comparing microsurgery, stereotactic radiosurgery, observation, and nontumor controls. J Neurosurg. 2015;122(4):833–42.
43. Carlson ML, Glasgow AE, Grossardt BR, Habermann EB, Link MJ. Does where you live influence how your vestibular schwannoma is managed? Examining geographical differences in vestibular schwannoma treatment across the United States. J Neuro-Oncol. 2016;129(2):269–79.
44. Carlson ML, Tveiten OV, Lund-Johansen M, Tombers NM, Lohse CM, Link MJ. Patient motivation and long-term satisfaction with treatment choice in vestibular schwannoma. World Neurosurg. 2018;114:e1245–52.
45. Stangerup SE, Caye-Thomasen P. Epidemiology and natural history of vestibular schwannomas. Otolaryngol Clin N Am. 2012;45(2):257–68, vii.
46. Carlson ML, Tombers NM, Kerezoudis P, Celda MP, Lohse CM, Link MJ. Quality of life within the first 6 months of vestibular schwannoma diagnosis with implications for patient counseling. Otol Neurotol. 2018;39(10):e1129–36.
47. Carlson ML, Link MJ, Wanna GB, Driscoll CL. Management of sporadic vestibular schwannoma. Otolaryngol Clin N Am. 2015;48(3):407–22.
48. Macielak RJ, Patel NS, Lees KA, et al. Delayed tumor growth in vestibular schwannoma: an argument for lifelong surveillance. Otol Neurotol. 2019;40(9):1224–9.
49. Marinelli JP, Lohse CM, Carlson ML. Introducing an evidence-based approach to wait-and-scan management of sporadic vestibular schwannoma: size threshold surveillance. Otolaryngol Clin North Am. 2023; 56(3):445–57. https://doi.org/10.1016/j.otc.2023.02.006.
50. Yeung AH, Sughrue ME, Kane AJ, Tihan T, Cheung SW, Parsa AT. Radiobiology of vestibular schwannomas: mechanisms of radioresistance and potential targets for therapeutic sensitization. Neurosurg Focus. 2009;27(6):E2.
51. Chung WY, Liu KD, Shiau CY, et al. Gamma knife surgery for vestibular schwannoma: 10-year experience of 195 cases. J Neurosurg. 2005;102(Suppl):87–96.
52. Liu D, Xu D, Zhang Z, Zhang Y, Zheng L. Long-term outcomes after Gamma Knife surgery for vestibular schwannomas: a 10-year experience. J Neurosurg. 2006;105(Suppl):149–53.
53. Pollock BE. Management of vestibular schwannomas that enlarge after stereotactic radiosurgery: treatment recommendations based on a 15 year experience. Neurosurgery. 2006;58(2):241–8; discussion 241–248.
54. Jacob JT, Carlson ML, Schiefer TK, Pollock BE, Driscoll CL, Link MJ. Significance of cochlear dose in the radiosurgical treatment of vestibular schwannoma: controversies and unanswered questions. Neurosurgery. 2014;74(5):466–74; discussion 474.
55. Carlson ML, Jacob JT, Pollock BE, et al. Long-term hearing outcomes following stereotactic radiosurgery for vestibular schwannoma: patterns of hearing loss and variables influencing audiometric decline. J Neurosurg. 2013;118(3):579–87.
56. Pollock BE, Driscoll CL, Foote RL, et al. Patient outcomes after vestibular schwannoma management: a prospective comparison of microsurgical resection and stereotactic radiosurgery. Neurosurgery. 2006;59(1):77–85; discussion 77–85.
57. Milligan BD, Pollock BE, Foote RL, Link MJ. Long-term tumor control and cranial nerve outcomes following gamma knife surgery for larger-volume vestibular schwannomas. J Neurosurg. 2012;116(3):598–604.
58. Seferis C, Torrens M, Paraskevopoulou C, Psichidis G. Malignant transformation in vestibular schwannoma: report of a single case, literature search, and debate. J Neurosurg. 2014;121(Suppl):160–6.
59. Patel TR, Chiang VL. Secondary neoplasms after stereotactic radiosurgery. World Neurosurg. 2014;81(3–4):594–9.
60. Samii M, Matthies C. Management of 1000 vestibular schwannomas (acoustic neuromas): surgical management and results with an emphasis on complications and how to avoid them. Neurosurgery. 1997;40(1):11–21; discussion 21–13.
61. Carlson ML, Link MJ. Vestibular Schwannomas. N Engl J Med. 2021;384(14):1335–48.
62. Carlson ML, Barnes JH, Nassiri A, et al. Prospective study of disease-specific quality-of-life in sporadic vestibular schwannoma comparing observation, radiosurgery, and microsurgery. Otol Neurotol. 2021;42(2):e199–208.
63. Gurgel RK, Dogru S, Amdur RL, Monfared A. Facial nerve outcomes after surgery for large vestibular schwannomas: do surgical approach and extent of resection matter? Neurosurg Focus. 2012;33(3):E16.
64. Falcioni M, Fois P, Taibah A, Sanna M. Facial nerve function after vestibular schwannoma surgery. J Neurosurg. 2011;115(4):820–6.
65. Bloch O, Sughrue ME, Kaur R, et al. Factors associated with preservation of facial nerve function after surgical resection of vestibular schwannoma. J Neuro-Oncol. 2011;102(2):281–6.
66. Sameshima T, Fukushima T, McElveen JT Jr, Friedman AH. Critical assessment of operative approaches for hearing preservation in small acoustic neuroma surgery: retrosigmoid vs middle fossa approach. Neurosurgery. 2010;67(3):640–4; discussion 644–645.

67. Hillman T, Chen DA, Arriaga MA, Quigley M. Facial nerve function and hearing preservation acoustic tumor surgery: does the approach matter? Otolaryngol Head Neck Surg. 2010;142(1):115–9.
68. Phillips DJ, Kobylarz EJ, De Peralta ET, Stieg PE, Selesnick SH. Predictive factors of hearing preservation after surgical resection of small vestibular schwannomas. Otol Neurotol. 2010;31(9):1463–8.
69. Ansari SF, Terry C, Cohen-Gadol AA. Surgery for vestibular schwannomas: a systematic review of complications by approach. Neurosurg Focus. 2012;33(3):E14.
70. Mangham CA Jr. Retrosigmoid versus middle fossa surgery for small vestibular schwannomas. Laryngoscope. 2004;114(8):1455–61.
71. Irving RM, Jackler RK, Pitts LH. Hearing preservation in patients undergoing vestibular schwannoma surgery: comparison of middle fossa and retrosigmoid approaches. J Neurosurg. 1998;88(5):840–5.
72. Colletti V, Fiorino F. Middle fossa versus retrosigmoid-transmeatal approach in vestibular schwannoma surgery: a prospective study. Otol Neurotol. 2003;24(6):927–34.
73. Strasnick B, Glasscock ME 3rd, Haynes D, McMenomey SO, Minor LB. The natural history of untreated acoustic neuromas. Laryngoscope. 1994;104(9):1115–9.
74. Carlson ML, Van Gompel JJ, Wiet RM, et al. A cross-sectional survey of the North American Skull Base Society: current practice patterns of vestibular schwannoma evaluation and management in North America. J Neurol Surg B Skull Base. 2018;79(3):289–96.
75. Gurgel RK, Theodosopoulos PV, Jackler RK. Subtotal/near-total treatment of vestibular schwannomas. Curr Opin Otolaryngol Head Neck Surg. 2012;20(5):380–4.
76. Akinduro OO, Lundy LB, Quinones-Hinojosa A, et al. Outcomes of large vestibular schwannomas following subtotal resection: early post-operative volume regression and facial nerve function. J Neuro-Oncol. 2019;143(2):281–8.
77. Nakatomi H, Jacob JT, Carlson ML, et al. Long-term risk of recurrence and regrowth after gross-total and subtotal resection of sporadic vestibular schwannoma. J Neurosurg. 2017;133:1–7.
78. Jacob JT, Carlson ML, Driscoll CL, Link MJ. Volumetric analysis of tumor control following subtotal and near-total resection of vestibular schwannoma. Laryngoscope. 2016;126(8):1877–82.
79. Troude L, Boucekine M, Montava M, Lavieille JP, Regis JM, Roche PH. Adjunctive gamma knife surgery or wait and scan policy after optimal resection of large vestibular schwannomas: clinical and radiologic outcomes. World Neurosurg. 2018;118:e895–905.
80. Carlson ML, Habermann EB, Wagie AE, et al. The changing landscape of vestibular schwannoma management in the United States--a shift toward conservatism. Otolaryngol Head Neck Surg. 2015;153(3):440–6.
81. Marinelli JP, Grossardt BR, Lohse CM, Carlson ML. Is improved detection of vestibular schwannoma leading to overtreatment of the disease? Otol Neurotol. 2019;40(6):847–50.
82. Breivik CN, Nilsen RM, Myrseth E, et al. Conservative management or gamma knife radiosurgery for vestibular schwannoma: tumor growth, symptoms, and quality of life. Neurosurgery. 2013;73(1):48–56; discussion 56–47.
83. Quesnel AM, McKenna MJ. Current strategies in management of intracanalicular vestibular schwannoma. Curr Opin Otolaryngol Head Neck Surg. 2011;19(5):335–40.
84. Maniakas A, Saliba I. Microsurgery versus stereotactic radiation for small vestibular schwannomas: a meta-analysis of patients with more than 5 years' follow-up. Otol Neurotol. 2012;33(9):1611–20.
85. Regis J, Carron R, Park MC, et al. Wait-and-see strategy compared with proactive Gamma Knife surgery in patients with intracanalicular vestibular schwannomas. J Neurosurg. 2010;113(Suppl):105–11.
86. Maniakas A, Saliba I. Conservative management versus stereotactic radiation for vestibular schwannomas: a meta-analysis of patients with more than 5 years' follow-up. Otol Neurotol. 2012;33(2):230–8.
87. Flickinger JC, Kondziolka D, Niranjan A, Lunsford LD. Results of acoustic neuroma radiosurgery: an analysis of 5 years' experience using current methods. J Neurosurg. 2001;94(1):1–6.
88. Niranjan A, Mathieu D, Flickinger JC, Kondziolka D, Lunsford LD. Hearing preservation after intracanalicular vestibular schwannoma radiosurgery. Neurosurgery. 2008;63(6):1054–62; discussion 1062–1053.
89. Morrison D. Management of patients with acoustic neuromas: a Markov decision analysis. Laryngoscope. 2010;120(4):783–90.
90. Marinelli JP, Lees KA, Lohse CM, et al. Natural history of growing sporadic vestibular schwannoma: an argument for continued observation despite documented growth in select cases. Otol Neurotol. 2020;41(9):e1149–53.
91. Huang X, Caye-Thomasen P, Stangerup SE. Spontaneous tumour shrinkage in 1261 observed patients with sporadic vestibular schwannoma. J Laryngol Otol. 2013;127(8):739–43.
92. Chweya CM, et al. Disease-specific quality of life in vestibular schwannoma: a national cross-sectional study comparing microsurgery, radiosurgery, and observation. Otolaryngol Head Neck Surg. 2021;164(3):639–44. https://doi.org/10.1177/0194599820941012. Epub 2020 Jul 21.

NF2-Related Schwannomatosis

75

Nicholas A. Dewyer, Dunia Abdul-Aziz,
and D. Bradley Welling

Introduction

NF2-related schwannomatosis (SWN) (formerly known as neurofibromatosis type 2, or NF2) is a genetic disorder that is characterized by the development of multiple central and peripheral nervous system tumors [1]. Bilateral vestibular schwannomas (VS) are the hallmark of this condition, though multiple meningiomas, other cranial nerve schwannomas, and ependymomas are also commonly seen. NF2 is a progressive, debilitating disease that presents many challenges in its management. In this chapter, we will discuss the relevant aspects of NF2 for otologists and cranial base surgeons.

Genetics and Epidemiology

NF2 is an autosomal dominant condition that results from mutations in the *NF2* gene, located on the long arm of chromosome 22. About half of the patients with this disorder inherit it from an affected parent, and half develop *de novo* mutations [2]. The *NF2* gene codes for the protein merlin (also called schwannomin), which is a tumor suppressor protein notably found in Schwann cells. Loss of function of merlin leads to overly rapid Schwann cell growth and proliferation and a failure of contact inhibition, producing the tumors characteristic of NF2. Although NF2 is inherited in an autosomal dominant pattern, two defective copies of the *NF2* gene are required for tumor formation. If inherited from a parent, one pathogenic variant is present on one of the alleles of every cell type. A "second hit" in the non-inherited allele occurs in all NF2 patients to allow expression of the disease phenotype. Multiple types of mutations have been identified throughout the *NF2* gene in patients with NF2.

NF2 has an estimated general prevalence of 1 in 25,000–60,000 persons [2–4]. In data from tumor registries in northwest England, for example, the prevalence is 1 in 56,000, and the birth incidence is 1 in 33,000 [3]. Over 50% of their cases were *de novo* mutations. Asian and African ethnicities appear to have a lower prevalence. A recent study from Japan estimates the prevalence at one in six million [5]. In sub-Saharan Africa, NF2-associated vestibular schwannomas accounted for only 0.16% of all intracranial tumors, unlike in North America, where vestibular schwannomas account for 8–10% [6]. In the UK, the annual incidence rate is estimated to be 1 in 2,355,000, which extrapolates to 140 new cases each year in the United States [2].

Clinical Presentation, Diagnosis, and Natural History

Symptoms of NF2 most commonly present in the late teens or early 20s, though there are wide ranges of symptom severity and age of onset. Adult patients tend to present with symptoms of VS, which are most frequently hearing loss, tinnitus, aural fullness, and/or disequilibrium. The presentation and management of sporadic VS are discussed in Chap. 74. Bilateral VS presents severe challenges to patients with NF2 (Fig. 75.1). About one-fifth of patients with NF2 present under the age of 15 years, and they tend not to present with eighth nerve dysfunction but with visual loss, seizures, myelopathy, cutaneous schwannomas, foot drop, or facial mononeuropathy from other tumors [3]. Meningiomas and ependymomas are also frequently identified in patients with NF2.

N. A. Dewyer
Department of Otolaryngology—Head and Neck Surgery, University of Arizona College of Medicine, Tucson, AZ, USA

D. Abdul-Aziz · D. B. Welling (✉)
Department of Otolaryngology—Head and Neck Surgery, Massachusetts Eye and Ear and Massachusetts General Hospital, Boston, MA, USA

Department of Otolaryngology—Head and Neck Surgery, Harvard Medical School, Boston, MA, USA
e-mail: brad_welling@meei.harvard.edu

A. D. Sweeney et al. (eds.), *Haynes-Glasscock-Shambaugh Surgery of the Ear*, https://doi.org/10.1007/978-3-032-18264-7_75

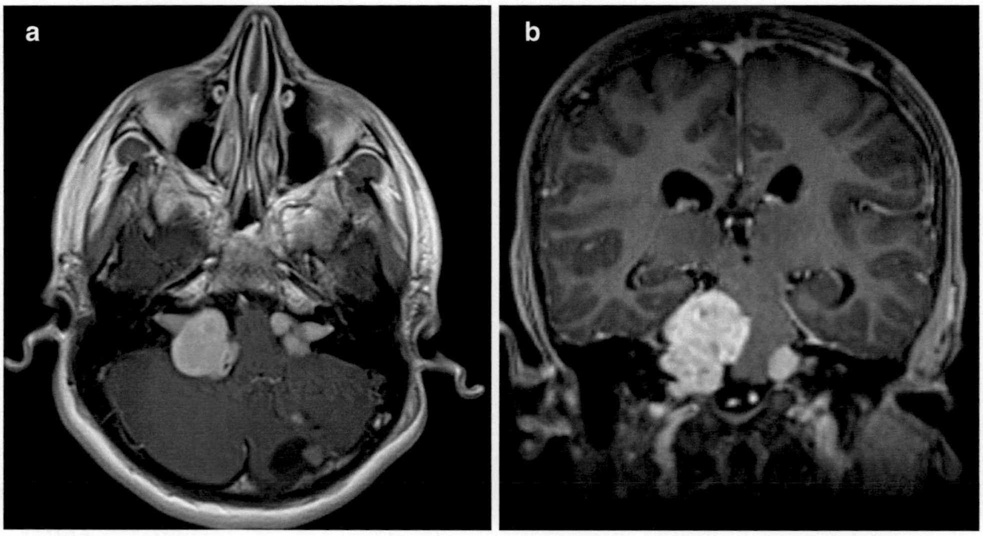

Fig. 75.1 Contrast-enhanced T1-weighted MRI of a patient with NF2 and bilateral vestibular schwannomas in the axial (**a**) and coronal (**b**) planes. (Courtesy of Alex D. Sweeney, MD)

The updated criteria for NF2 incorporate clinical features and genetic testing, with a focus on using molecular data to differentiate NF2 from other schwannomatosis (SWN) conditions. It is likely that continued refinement of these new criteria will be necessary as investigators study the diagnostic properties of the revised criteria and identify new genes associated with SWN. In the revised nomenclature, the term "neurofibromatosis 2" has been retired to improve diagnostic specificity [1].

Genetic testing for patients with a suspected NF2 diagnosis reveals a mutation in *NF2* as high as 72% in simplex cases (first member of a family) [7–11]. However, it is reported that up to one-third of patients with diagnosed NF2 and no family history carry the mutated allele in only a small proportion of their cells [8, 12, 13]. Genetic testing of blood cells in these mosaic individuals may not yield a mutation, as too few cells carry the mutant allele. In these individuals, genetic testing of tumor cells is much more likely to identify a mutation. A moderate correlation between the severity of the genotype and phenotype has been established, with missense mutations and mosaics having potentially milder phenotypes and more severe truncation mutations [14–16]. Genetics and tumor biology are discussed in detail in Chaps. 8 and 10, respectively.

Magnetic resonance imaging (MRI) with gadolinium enhancement and fine cuts through the brain and temporal bone is the gold standard for the detection and monitoring of intracranial tumors, including VS. Spinal or whole-body MRI should be considered to look for tumors of the spine and peripheral nerves at the initial screening if NF2 appears to be present on the cranial imaging. T2-weighted images without gadolinium have been used as a low-cost alternative to contrasted imaging for following growth patterns in unilateral sporadic schwannomas. Because of the multiplicity of tumors frequently associated with NF2, however, and the increased ability to detect new tumors, gadolinium-enhanced scans are routinely used for following tumor progression.

A full audiological assessment should be performed. Older texts advocate for the routine use of brainstem auditory evoked response (BAER), as abnormalities may be an early indicator of a VS; however, MRI is now widely available and has excellent resolution, frequently able to detect tumors as small as 1–2 mm, so BAER for VS detection is not necessary. Ophthalmological examination should be performed to assess for cataracts and other visual disorders.

When a new diagnosis of NF2 is made, the patient should be referred to a center that has expertise in the management of patients with this rare disease. High-volume centers may offer improved treatment outcomes for cranial nerve–sparing procedures and reduced complication rates. Also, collective research opportunities are enhanced.

The prognosis for patients with NF2 varies greatly between individuals, though affected family members often have a similar disease severity. In general, as more tumors arise and grow, neurological deficits accumulate and cause progressive symptoms. Bilateral deafness commonly occurs, and when blindness occurs as well, patients are particularly debilitated. Dysphonia, dysphagia, seizures, paralysis, and brainstem compression can occur. Patients with NF2 have reduced lifespans, with deaths often occurring in the twenties and thirties for patients with severe multi-tumor disease and in the sixties to eighties for patients with less severe disease [17, 18].

Genetic Screening and Counseling

A full discussion of genetic screening and counseling for NF2 is beyond the scope of this text, but key points are presented here. Identification of a pathogenic variant in an NF2 patient allows for genetic screening and counseling of family mem-

Table 75.1 Aggregate rates of reported tumor control and hearing preservation in NF2 patients by treatment modality. (Adapted from reference [26]). Tumor control is defined as no recurrence in the microsurgery group and no change or regression in the other groups. Hearing preservation is defined as no change or an improvement in the Gardner–Robertson hearing grade. Data are shown with the mean follow-up time

	Observation	Hearing preservation microsurgery	Stereotactic radiotherapy	Bevacizumab
Tumor control	67% (4.1 years)	56% (4.2 years)	96% (4.5 years)	86% (1.9 years)
Hearing preservation	70% (4.7 years)	52% (4.2 years)	45% (2.9 years)	93% (1.3 years)

bers. Determining whether or not a family member has NF2 allows for specific counseling and cessation of screening imaging studies and exams if the family member is found not to have NF2. Additionally, prenatal or preimplantation testing can be done for an embryo if a parent has known NF2. As there is no cure for NF2 at present, a thorough discussion with informed consent should occur among the treating physician, a genetic counselor with expertise in NF2, and at-risk asymptomatic family members prior to genetic testing.

Treatment of Vestibular Schwannomas in NF2

Clinical decision-making in the management of NF2 is complex. The overarching goal of management is to help the patient maintain maximal quality of life for as long as possible. Management decisions for VS in NF2 specifically focus on preserving hearing and facial nerve function while preventing symptomatic brainstem compression from massive tumors. Meningiomas are frequently observed, with surgical removal or debulking reserved for massive, symptomatic tumors.

There are four treatment modalities available for NF2 VS: observation, surgery, stereotactic radiotherapy, and systemic medical therapy with bevacizumab (Avastin).

Tumor control and hearing preservation rates for the various treatment modalities are summarized in Table 75.1.

Observation

NF2-associated VS can demonstrate variable and often unpredictable growth patterns. When NF2-associated VS are initially identified, our preferred initial treatment is dependent on a number of factors. Most VS grow slowly, and a few may even spontaneously decrease in size [17]. In these cases, avoiding active treatment may provide benefit to the patient's quality of life by prolonging hearing. Observation consists of a follow-up MRI 6 months after the initial diagnosis and then yearly thereafter. Although MRI with high-resolution T2 sequences and without gadolinium is adequate to monitor sporadic VS [19], MRI with gadolinium should be used in NF2 patients because it is more likely to reveal additional new tumors that may arise. If hearing preservation is a consideration, audiograms should be obtained yearly or upon a subjective change in hearing.

Consideration to move from observation to active treatment should occur if an observed tumor is clearly demonstrating growth on serial MRIs, a patient has bilateral VS and wishes to have one tumor resected in an attempt to preserve hearing, a tumor is causing neurological symptoms other than eighth cranial nerve dysfunction (e.g., facial paresthesias from fifth nerve compression), or a tumor is large and symptoms of brainstem compression are present or expected with tumor growth.

Although controversial, a special circumstance that could challenge the notion of initial observation occurs when a patient with normal hearing is found to have small vestibular schwannomas that are optimal for hearing preservation surgery. The most favorable tumor of this sort is small in size, originates on the superior vestibular nerve, and does not fill the lateral fundus of the internal auditory canal, in our experience. If the hearing is successfully preserved, then contralateral VS tumor removal may be considered. If, however, hearing is not preserved in the initial ear, the contralateral tumor is left in place and monitored for growth until such a time that hearing is lost or brainstem compression warrants tumor removal. If the cochlear nerve is preserved during tumor surgery, but acoustic hearing is lost, subsequent cochlear implantation may also be possible [20, 21].

Microsurgical Treatment of NF2 VS

Surgical treatment for VS is covered in detail in Chap. 74. The goal of surgery in both sporadic and NF2-related VS is to preserve neurological function and maximize quality of life. Microsurgery may be preferred if the tumor has demonstrated growth, has resulted in poor speech discrimination, is causing additional neurological symptoms such as facial nerve weakness or paresthesias, or is causing a shift of the brainstem from pressure, which may result in hydrocephalus. Depending on the patient's age, health, symptoms, and the extent of the tumor, a decision should be made about performing a gross total resection (GTR) versus a subtotal resection (STR). It is oftentimes more difficult to resect NF2 VS because the tumors may be multifocal and wrap around or invade the facial nerve, whereas sporadic VS are typically unifocal with the facial nerve running along their surface

[22]. Subtotal resection, however, faces a higher likelihood of recurrence. Facial nerve outcomes after microsurgery in NF2 compared to sporadic VS are worse, specifically with fewer patients maintaining House–Brackmann 1 functionality [23]. Some facial nerve weakness may result from primary seventh nerve schwannomas. Recurrence after resection is possible from residual tumor or new foci of tumor, and therefore, serial MRIs are recommended on at least a yearly schedule.

Rates of hearing preservation following hearing preservation surgery for NF2 VS are difficult to define due to patient, disease, and treatment heterogeneity and indications for attempting such a procedure. It does seem that better preoperative hearing, smaller tumors, younger patient age, and subtotal resection make hearing preservation more likely. Microsurgery with hearing preservation for small tumors with good preoperative hearing has been reported in 42–63% of cases [24, 25]. It is also important to note that, even if hearing is initially preserved, it may progressively decline following intervention, whether or not tumor recurrence occurs [26, 27].

Despite these challenges, experienced surgeons are often able to achieve gross total removal with good facial nerve outcomes and low recurrence rates in carefully selected patients with growing tumors [28].

Stereotactic Radiotherapy for NF2 VS

Stereotactic radiotherapy (SR) for VS is discussed in detail in Chap. 81. NF2 VS have demonstrated response to SR, with tumor control rates from 75% to 80% [26, 27, 29].

A concern about SR for NF2 VS, particularly in younger patients with longer expected lifespans after treatment, is the malignant transformation of a VS following SR. Malignant transformation of a VS after SR is rare; however, about half of the reported cases of malignant change are in patients with NF2 despite many more patients undergoing SR for sporadic VS [27]. This suggests that there is an increased risk of malignant degeneration of NF2 VS after SR. The overall risk for malignant change in sporadic VS following radiation is on the order of 1 in 1000 patients and is not higher than those with untreated tumors [30]. In NF2, the risk is 4.7%, which represents a 40-fold increase compared to nonirradiated NF2 VS [31].

Long-term hearing preservation rates for NF2 tumors treated with SR are reported to be 20–57% [26, 27]. Fractionated SR has been touted to offer better rates of hearing preservation than single-dose regimens [26], although no solid clinical evidence is available to support this premise.

The ideal tumor for SR is a growing VS that is not abutting the brainstem in an older patient. SR is also useful as a salvage therapy for a growing residual tumor following surgery. Because some swelling of the tumor is expected following radiation treatment, radiation should not be used when the brainstem compression is on the threshold of compromising cerebrospinal fluid (CSF) flow.

Systemic Medical Therapy for NF2 VS

Bevacizumab (Avastin) is a humanized monoclonal antibody against vascular endothelial growth factor (VEGF) that was developed and approved for the treatment of various malignancies and is currently the only effective medical therapy available for NF2 VS. Bevacizumab may be considered for tumors where surgery or radiation may result in high morbidity. Clinical trials have demonstrated efficacy in both halting and, potentially, reversing tumor progression and hearing loss in patients with disease not amenable to other treatments [26, 27, 32–34]. Bevacizumab is administered as an intravenous infusion every 3 weeks. Side effects of bevacizumab include hypertension, proteinuria, elevated liver enzymes, irregular or termination of menstruation, fatigue, infection, and bleeding [35]. The main drawbacks to bevacizumab therapy are the need for continued regular intravenous infusions and the side effects. Hypertension and proteinuria occur in up to 50% of patients on treatment within 2 years [35, 36]. Also, following termination of bevacizumab, tumor growth may rebound to a growth rate similar to the pretreatment rate.

Hearing Rehabilitation in NF2

Deafness is the most common and one of the more disabling symptoms of NF2. It may be caused by VS or their treatment. Hearing loss tends to occur postlingually, so patients often have not learned to use sign language. As a result, many patients are interested in surgical hearing rehabilitation by cochlear implant (CI) or auditory brainstem implant (ABI). CI and ABI are discussed in detail in Chaps. 19, 20, 21, and 22.

ABI has been the most commonly performed method of hearing rehabilitation for bilateral deafness in NF2. An ABI is ideally placed at the time of tumor resection, either via translabyrinthine or retrosigmoid craniotomy. A systematic review published in 2017 reports that only 12% of NF2 patients with an ABI achieve open-set word recognition [26]. However, patients with an ABI also report benefit beyond what is measured with standard audiological test batteries and, specifically, that the ABI acts as an aid to lip reading.

CI for NF2 has been less commonly performed, and data should be interpreted with caution because of the small numbers of patients utilizing this modality. There are a few scenarios in NF2 where CI can be considered to rehabilitate

Table 75.2 Aggregate hearing rehabilitation results in patients with NF2. Word recognition scores were determined in quiet without lip reading

	CI with stable VS	CI with irradiated VS	CI after failed HP surgery	CI after CNSTL	ABI
Proportion of users (%)	100 (*n* = 5)	95 (*n* = 17)	86 (*n* = 14)	69 (*n* = 11)	87 (*n* = 358)
Word recognition score (%)	69 (*n* = 5)	49 (*n* = 13)	42 (*n* = 21)	38 (*n* = 16)	12 (*n* = 247)

Adapted from reference [25]

CI cochlear implant, *VS* vestibular schwannoma, *HP* hearing preservation, *CNSTL* cochlear nerve–preserving translabyrinthine surgery, and *ABI* auditory brainstem implant

poor hearing: (1) stable, untreated tumor; (2) irradiated tumor; and (3) after failed hearing preservation surgery with cochlear nerve preservation. Hearing preservation surgery includes middle cranial fossa and suboccipital approaches, but recently, a translabyrinthine approach has also been utilized for CI. Data on rates of use and function are presented in Table 75.2 [26]. These data suggest that, in general, if a CI can be used, it is expected to provide better speech recognition than an ABI and that speech recognition with CI is better in untreated than in treated tumors. Additionally, for VS patients undergoing CI, evidence suggests that those who have been observed or who have had radiosurgery have had better CI outcomes than those who had microsurgical resection [37]. It is the senior author's experience that hearing perception with electrical stimulation may be absent in the first month after surgery, but it may recover by the third month after surgery. Therefore, testing in a delayed fashion may be useful in decision-making.

Summary

Clinical decision-making in NF2 is challenging. Patients will likely benefit from referrals to centers that have considerable experience in providing specialized multidisciplinary care for NF2. Treatment decisions should be focused on minimizing neurological symptoms and maximizing quality of life. For VS in NF2, one of the most complex decisions is whether to intervene early or to observe small tumors until hearing is lost. Early hearing preservation surgery should not be excluded unless the patient cannot be treated at a center with deep surgical experience. Surgical treatment should be performed prior to facial paralysis or symptomatic brainstem compression. Decisions about the timing and modality of intervention must be tailored to each patient's individual situation. Radiation may present an increased risk of malignant change in patients with a preexisting tumor suppressor mutation and should be avoided if at all possible. Hearing rehabilitation is an essential component of NF2 treatment. ABI is often helpful as an aid for lip reading, but open-set speech discrimination is infrequently obtained. CI has demonstrated much better auditory results when the cochlear nerve is kept intact. Overall, more effective treatments are needed for NF2, as each current option carries with it its own set of risks and benefits. Specifically, improved targeted treatments and direct treatment of NF2 with gene replacement therapy represent the goals of current research efforts.

References

1. Plotkin SR, Messiaen L, Legius E, Pancza P, Avery RA, Blakeley JO, et al. Updated diagnostic criteria and nomenclature for neurofibromatosis type 2 and schwannomatosis: an international consensus recommendation. Genet Med. 2022;24(9):1967–77. https://doi.org/10.1016/j.gim.2022.05.007. Epub 2022 Jun 9.
2. Evans DG, Huson SM, Donnai D, Neary W, Blair V, Teare D, et al. A genetic study of type 2 neurofibromatosis in the United Kingdom. I. Prevalence, mutation rate, fitness, and confirmation of maternal transmission effect on severity. J Med Genet. 1992;29(12):841–6.
3. Evans DG, Howard E, Giblin C, Clancy T, Spencer H, Huson SM, et al. Birth incidence and prevalence of tumor-prone syndromes: estimates from a UK family genetic register service. Am J Med Genet A. 2010;152A(2):327–32.
4. Uhlmann EJ, Plotkin SR. Neurofibromatoses. Adv Exp Med Biol. 2012;724:266–77.
5. Iwatate K, Yokoo T, Iwatate E, Ichikawa M, Sato T, Fujii M, et al. Population characteristics and progressive disability in neurofibromatosis type 2. World Neurosurg. 2017;106:653–60.
6. Ohaegbulam S, Okwunodulu O, Ndubuisi C, Mezue W, Chikani M, Nkwerem S, et al. Vestibular schwannoma appears to be very rare in a region of sub-Saharan Africa. Surg Neurol Int. 2017;8:171.
7. Baser ME, Friedman JM, Wallace AJ, Ramsden RT, Joe H, Evans DG. Evaluation of clinical diagnostic criteria for neurofibromatosis 2. Neurology. 2002;59(11):1759–65.
8. Evans DG, Ramsden RT, Shenton A, Gokhale C, Bowers NL, Huson SM, et al. Mosaicism in neurofibromatosis type 2: an update of risk based on uni/bilaterality of vestibular schwannoma at presentation and sensitive mutation analysis including multiple ligation-dependent probe amplification. J Med Genet. 2007;44(7):424–8.
9. Evans DG. Neurofibromatosis 2 [Bilateral acoustic neurofibromatosis, central neurofibromatosis, NF2, neurofibromatosis type II]. Genet Med. 2009;11(9):599–610.
10. Kluwe L, Nygren AO, Errami A, Heinrich B, Matthies C, Tatagiba M, et al. Screening for large mutations of the NF2 gene. Genes Chromosomes Cancer. 2005;42(4):384–91.
11. Wallace AJ, Watson CJ, Oward E, Evans DG, Elles RG. Mutation scanning of the NF2 gene: an improved service based on meta-PCR/sequencing, dosage analysis, and loss of heterozygosity analysis. Genet Test. 2004;8(4):368–80.
12. Evans DG, Wallace AJ, Wu CL, Trueman L, Ramsden RT, Strachan T. Somatic mosaicism: a common cause of classic disease in tumor-prone syndromes? Lessons from type 2 neurofibromatosis. Am J Hum Genet. 1998;63(3):727–36.
13. Kluwe L, Mautner VF. Mosaicism in sporadic neurofibromatosis 2 patients. Hum Mol Genet. 1998;7(13):2051–5.
14. Evans DG, Trueman L, Wallace A, Collins S, Strachan T. Genotype/phenotype correlations in type 2 neurofibromatosis (NF2): evidence for more severe disease associated with truncating mutations. J Med Genet. 1998;35(6):450–5.
15. Parry DM, MacCollin MM, Kaiser-Kupfer MI, Pulaski K, Nicholson HS, Bolesta M, et al. Germ-line mutations in the neuro-

fibromatosis 2 gene: correlations with disease severity and retinal abnormalities. Am J Hum Genet. 1996;59(3):529–39.
16. Ruttledge MH, Andermann AA, Phelan CM, Claudio JO, Han FY, Chretien N, et al. Type of mutation in the neurofibromatosis type 2 gene (NF2) frequently determines severity of disease. Am J Hum Genet. 1996;59(2):331–42.
17. Wilding A, Ingham SL, Lalloo F, Clancy T, Huson SM, Moran A, et al. Life expectancy in hereditary cancer predisposing diseases: an observational study. J Med Genet. 2012;49(4):264–9.
18. Lawson McLean AC, Rosahl SK. Growth dynamics of intracranial tumors in patients with neurofibromatosis type 2. World Neurosurg. 2017;98:152–61.
19. Williams JC, Carr CM, Eckel LJ, Kotsenas AL, Hunt CH, Carlson ML, et al. Utility of noncontrast magnetic resonance imaging for detection of recurrent vestibular schwannoma. Otol Neurotol. 2018;39(3):372–7.
20. deTorres AT, Brewer CC, Zalewski CK, King KA, Walker R, Scott GC, et al. Audiologic natural history of small volume cochleovestibular schwannomas in neurofibromatosis type 2. Otol Neurotol. 2018;39(3):357–64.
21. Kelly EA, Levine S, Gravel KE, Hart DL, Huang T. Utilization of nerve integrity monitor for promontory stimulation testing prior to cochlear implant. Otol Neurotol. 2018;39(2):e60–2.
22. Sobel RA. Vestibular (acoustic) schwannomas: histologic features in neurofibromatosis 2 and in unilateral cases. J Neuropathol Exp Neurol. 1993;52(2):106–13.
23. Moffat DA, Lloyd SK, Macfarlane R, Mannion R, King A, Rutherford S, et al. Outcome of translabyrinthine surgery for vestibular schwannoma in neurofibromatosis type 2. Br J Neurosurg. 2013;27(4):446–53.
24. Friedman RA, Goddard JC, Wilkinson EP, Schwartz MS, Slattery WH 3rd, Fayad JN, et al. Hearing preservation with the middle cranial fossa approach for neurofibromatosis type 2. Otol Neurotol. 2011;32(9):1530–7.
25. Slattery WH 3rd, Brackmann DE, Hitselberger W. Hearing preservation in neurofibromatosis type 2. Am J Otol. 1998;19(5):638–43.
26. Lloyd SKW, King AT, Rutherford SA, Hammerbeck-Ward CL, Freeman SRM, Mawman DJ, et al. Hearing optimisation in neurofibromatosis type 2: a systematic review. Clin Otolaryngol. 2017;42(6):1329–37.
27. Maniakas A, Saliba I. Neurofibromatosis type 2 vestibular schwannoma treatment: a review of the literature, trends, and outcomes. Otol Neurotol. 2014;35(5):889–94.
28. Tysome JR, Macfarlane R, Durie-Gair J, Donnelly N, Mannion R, Knight R, et al. Surgical management of vestibular schwannomas and hearing rehabilitation in neurofibromatosis type 2. Otol Neurotol. 2012;33(3):466–72.
29. Chung LK, Nguyen TP, Sheppard JP, Lagman C, Tenn S, Lee P, et al. A systematic review of radiosurgery versus surgery for neurofibromatosis type 2 vestibular schwannomas. World Neurosurg. 2018;109:47–58.
30. Carlson ML, Glasgow AE, Jacob JT, Habermann EB, Link MJ. The short-term and intermediate-term risk of second neoplasms after diagnosis and treatment of unilateral vestibular schwannoma: analysis of 9460 cases. Int J Radiat Oncol Biol Phys. 2016;95(4):1149–57.
31. Baser ME, Evans DG, Jackler RK, Sujansky E, Rubenstein A. Neurofibromatosis 2, radiosurgery and malignant nervous system tumours. Br J Cancer. 2000;82(4):998.
32. Blakeley JO, Ye X, Duda DG, Halpin CF, Bergner AL, Muzikansky A, et al. Efficacy and biomarker study of bevacizumab for hearing loss resulting from neurofibromatosis type 2-associated vestibular schwannomas. J Clin Oncol. 2016;34(14):1669–75.
33. Plotkin SR, Stemmer-Rachamimov AO, Barker FG 2nd, Halpin C, Padera TP, Tyrrell A, et al. Hearing improvement after bevacizumab in patients with neurofibromatosis type 2. N Engl J Med. 2009;361(4):358–67.
34. Plotkin SR, Merker VL, Halpin C, Jennings D, McKenna MJ, Harris GJ, et al. Bevacizumab for progressive vestibular schwannoma in neurofibromatosis type 2: a retrospective review of 31 patients. Otol Neurotol. 2012;33(6):1046–52.
35. Morris KA, Golding JF, Blesing C, Evans DG, Ferner RE, Foweraker K, et al. Toxicity profile of bevacizumab in the UK Neurofibromatosis type 2 cohort. J Neuro-Oncol. 2017;131(1):117–24.
36. Slusarz KM, Merker VL, Muzikansky A, Francis SA, Plotkin SR. Long-term toxicity of bevacizumab therapy in neurofibromatosis 2 patients. Cancer Chemother Pharmacol. 2014;73(6):1197–204.
37. Dornhoffer JR, Haller T, Lohse CM, Driscoll CLW, Neff BA, Saoji A, Link MJ, Carlson ML. Cochlear implant outcomes between patients with sporadic and neurofibromatosis type 2-associated vestibular schwannoma. Otol Neurotol. 2023;44(8):791–7.

Cerebellopontine Angle and Internal Auditory Canal Meningiomas

76

Peter J. Morone and Reid C. Thompson

Introduction

Meningiomas represent 15–30% of all primary intracranial brain tumors, are located within the cerebellopontine angle (CPA) 5–10% of the time, and are the second most common neoplasm found within the CPA [1]. As meningiomas grow and reach larger sizes in the CPA, they can extend to involve surrounding structures such as the internal auditory canal (IAC). However, some meningiomas originate solely within the IAC and subsequently grow into the CPA, yet these are rare and occur less than 2% of the time [2]. While meningiomas can arise anywhere intracranially, those that take their origin in and around the IAC represent a series of unique management and surgical challenges to neurosurgeons and neurotologists. It is important to understand the unique anatomic relationships in this area. Moreover, it is important to recognize and consider the individual clinical and radiographic variables in each patient when developing a treatment recommendation.

Meningiomas are most prevalent in patients ranging from 40 to 60 years of age and are two times more frequent in women compared to men. Their annual incidence is 6 per 100,000 person-years. Generally, their etiology is sporadic, though they have been reported to occur after radiation treatment, with latencies ranging from 19 to 35 years [3]. Additionally, patients with neurofibromatosis type 2 have a higher propensity to develop meningiomas and often present with multiple lesions [4, 5].

Pathology

Meningiomas are derived from meningothelial—or arachnoid cap—cells and are generally dural-based, solitary masses. Meningiomas have distinctive microscopic characteristics such as whorls of tight, multilayered cells and psammoma bodies, which are composites of dystrophic calcification (Fig. 76.1). Common immunohistochemical markers in meningiomas include epithelial membrane antigen (EMA), vimentin, cytokeratin, and S100 [6]. Approximately 72% of meningiomas have loss of heterozygosity for chromosome 22.

Based upon their severity, meningiomas are classified by the World Health Organization (WHO) as either grade I, grade II, or grade III. Grade I tumors grow slowly, are noninvasive, and cause symptoms secondary to the compression of surrounding structures. Grade II tumors have variable growth rates and may invade the surrounding brain parenchyma. Grade III tumors are the most aggressive and invasive and

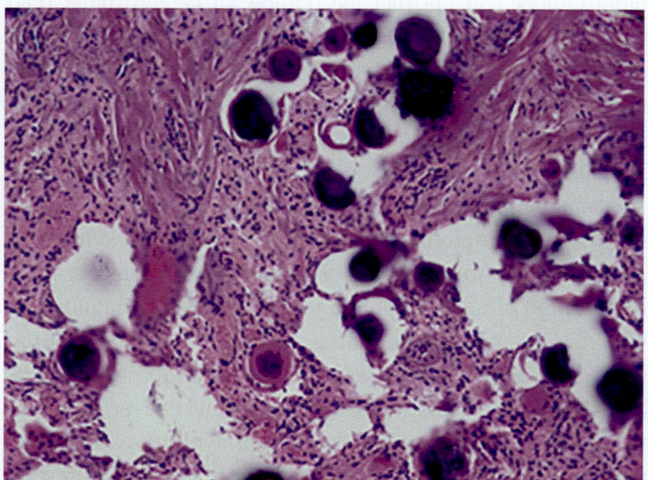

Fig. 76.1 A Hematoxylin & Eosin (H&E)-stained section shows a meningioma with multiple, large psammoma bodies. Original magnification: 200×

P. J. Morone (✉) · R. C. Thompson
Department of Neurological Surgery, Vanderbilt University Medical Center, Nashville, TN, USA
e-mail: peter.morone@vanderbilt.edu; reid.thompson@vanderbilt.edu

A. D. Sweeney et al. (eds.), *Haynes-Glasscock-Shambaugh Surgery of the Ear*, https://doi.org/10.1007/978-3-032-18264-7_76

Table 76.1 WHO-grade meningioma characteristics

WHO grade I	WHO grade II	WHO grade III
≤3 mitoses per ten high-power fields	≥4 mitoses per ten high-power fields	≥20 mitoses per ten high-power fields
And	*Or*	*Or*
No brain invasion *Subtypes:* meningothelial, fibrous, transitional, angiomatous, microcystic, secretory, metaplastic, lymphoplasmacyte-rich, psammomatous	Three of the following characteristics: High cellularity Cells with increased nucleus:cytoplasm ratio Prominent nucleoli Necrosis Brain invasion *Subtypes:* choroid, clear cell	Malignant features resembling carcinoma, melanoma, or sarcoma Necrosis, which is frequent but not required *Subtypes:* rhabdoid, papillary

WHO World Health Organization

have characteristics of other malignant tumors. A hallmark is the invasion of the adjacent brain, and in some instances, these tumors may metastasize to the lung, liver, bone, and lymph nodes. See Table 76.1 for further grade-based characteristics and subtypes of meningioma.

Diagnosis

Symptoms associated with CPA-IAC meningiomas depend largely upon their location and growth rate. Tumors that originate within the IAC may first present with hearing loss and tinnitus, while tumors that originate within the CPA may present with cranial neuropathies and symptoms associated with brainstem and cerebellar compression. See Table 76.2 for descriptions of common presenting symptoms based upon the lesion location and the compression of cranial nerves (CNs). Since most meningiomas grow slowly, they may reach relatively large sizes prior to diagnosis and cause multiple, nonspecific symptoms. Conversely, faster-growing lesions may cause more specific symptoms and may be diagnosed sooner. Occasionally, large tumors will obstruct the outflow of cerebrospinal fluid (CSF) from the fourth ventricle. This results in hydrocephalus and may cause patients to present with symptoms of high intracranial pressure, such as confusion, lethargy, emesis, and papilledema. The development of brainstem and/or cerebellar edema is a hallmark of a progressively enlarging or biologically aggressive tumor and is an important indication for treatment.

Given meningioma's multitude of presenting symptoms and its ability to mimic other pathologies, clinicians must have a high clinical suspicion to make an early diagnosis of CPA-IAC meningiomas. Thus, a complete medical evaluation of the patient is necessary, including a thorough history and detailed neurological examination, whenever a patient presents with hearing loss, tinnitus, or symptoms of cranial nerve dysfunction. When any of these findings are present, clinicians should have a low threshold to obtain a magnetic resonance imaging (MRI) scan, which is the most sensitive modality for diagnosing meningiomas and has the ability to identify relatively small tumors [7].

Table 76.2 Presenting symptoms based upon the lesion location

Lesion location	Symptom
CN IV	Vertical diplopia
CN V	Decreased sensation to the face, corneal drying, decreased salivation, weakness in mastication
CN VI	Medial eye deviation with the inability to look laterally
CN VII	Complete or partial paralysis of the face, hemifacial spasm, hyperacusis, impaired sense of taste
CN VIII	Positional vertigo, tinnitus, hearing loss
CN IX, X, XI	Dysphagia, dysarthria, aphonia
CN XII	Dysarthria, deviation of the tongue toward the affected side
Cerebellar and brainstem compression	Gait ataxia, dysarthria, nystagmus, respiratory difficulty, abnormal vital signs
Hydrocephalus	Confusion, lethargy, emesis, bladder incontinence, visual loss with papilledema

CN cranial nerve

General Features

CPA-IAC meningiomas are dural-based, encapsulated neoplasms with distinct margins. They generally range between 1 and 8 centimeters in size. Seventy-five percent have a hemispherical appearance and a broad base that faces the posterior petrous wall. Twenty percent present with bone invasion and hyperostosis of the adjacent petrous bone. Five percent appear as an ovoid mass that can resemble a vestibular schwannoma.

Computed Tomography

On a non-contrast computed tomography (CT) scan, 30% of meningiomas appear isodense, while 70% appear hypodense. Twenty-five percent of meningiomas contain calcification, which either appears homogenous or as speckled, small masses throughout the tumor. When reviewing a potential meningioma on a CT scan, it is important to view the bone-only windows to assess for the presence of hyperostosis and deformity of adjacent bone—such as flaring of the IAC or erosion of the petrous apex. On a contrast CT scan, 90% of meningiomas demonstrate strong, uniform enhancement, while the other 10% contain scattered areas of enhancement.

Magnetic Resonance Imaging

On a T1-weighted MRI, meningiomas appear isointense or minimally hyperintense compared to the gray matter, and areas of calcification appear hypointense. On a T2-weighted MRI, meningiomas have large signal heterogeneity and range from hypointense to isointense compared to the gray matter, making the T2-weighted sequence relatively nonspecific for diagnosis. However, the T2 sequence is helpful when evaluating CSF-vascular cleft spaces, where pial blood vessels appear as flow voids between the tumor and the brain parenchyma (Fig. 76.2). Evaluating these vascular relationships to the tumor is important in surgical planning, as they can guide the operative trajectory and boundaries of safe surgical resection. The T2-weighted sequence is also useful in evaluating peritumoral edema, which, if present, may signify a more aggressive and higher-WHO-grade meningioma [8]. On a T1-weighted sequence with contrast, 95% of meningiomas appear as homogeneously enhancing masses (Fig. 76.3), yet 5% of large lesions demonstrate heterogeneous enhancement. Most CPA-IAC meningiomas are centered along the posterior petrous wall, and 60% have associated dural thickening, which is generally referred to as a dural tail. Interestingly, the dural tail, in most cases, represents reactive rather than neoplastic change.

Angiography

Meningiomas with robust vascular supply have a classic "sunburst" appearance when visualized using diagnostic cerebral angiography, which is a result of larger dural vessels supplying the tumor center and smaller pial vessels supplying the tumor rim. Additionally, there is occasionally prolonged vascular "strain" into the venous phase of the angiogram, which can result in the appearance of arteriovenous shunting.

Imaging Recommendations

Currently, the most sensitive imaging modality for diagnosing CPA-IAC meningiomas is MRI. We recommend obtaining a brain MRI with T1- and T2-weighted images and, specifically, with T1 gadolinium-contrast sequences. Additionally, it is useful to obtain thin-section axial and coronal T1-weighted sequences with contrast to evaluate a meningioma's relationship to the IAC. If bone hyperostosis or invasion is suspected after reviewing MR images, it is rea-

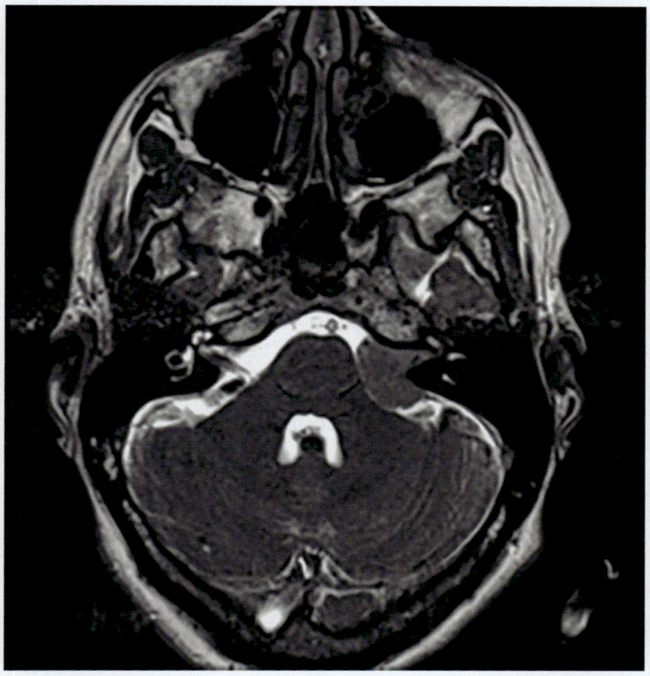

Fig. 76.2 Axial view of a T2-weighted MRI without contrast demonstrates a left cerebellopontine angle mass that appears iso/hypointense. On this MRI sequence, the cerebrospinal fluid space can be adequately visualized between the tumor border and the brainstem

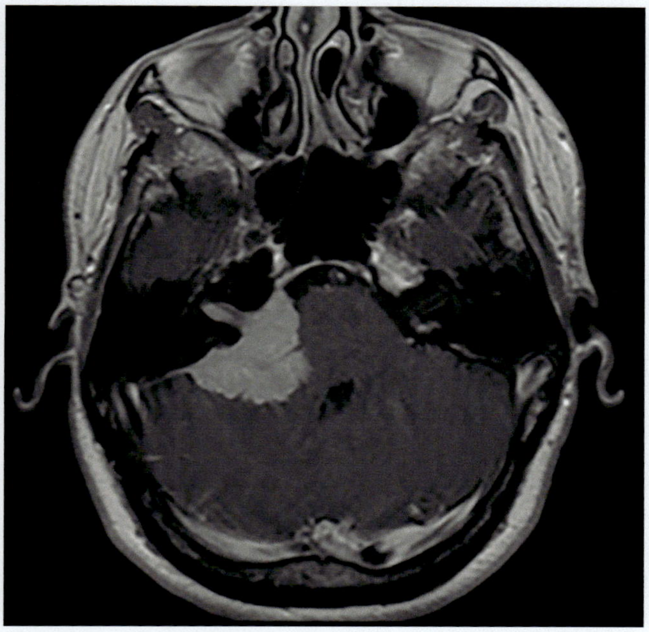

Fig. 76.3 Axial view of a T1-weighted MRI with contrast demonstrates a dural-based, homogeneously enhancing mass located within the right cerebellopontine angle that extends into the internal auditory canal

Table 76.3 Meningioma vs. vestibular schwannoma MRI characteristics

	Meningioma	vs.	Vestibular Schwannoma
Characteristic			
Origin	CPA; posterior portion of the petrous bone; may grow into the IAC[a]		IAC, may grow out of the IAC into the CPA
IAC appearance	Anatomic; no flaring[a]		Flaring of the porus acusticus
Vector of spread	May extend into the middle craniotomy fossa		Does not extend into the middle cranial fossa
Appearance with contrast	Dural tail and thickening		No dural thickening

[a]Rarely, meningiomas originate from the dura within the IAC (<2%). In these instances, both types of lesion may appear identical, and only a pathological specimen will yield a diagnosis

MRI magnetic resonance imaging, *CPA* cerebellopontine angle, *IAC* internal auditory canal

sonable to obtain a non-contrast CT scan, which yields more information about the bone and tumor relationship. In general, we do not evaluate CPA-IAC meningiomas with diagnostic cerebral angiography since tumor vasculature can be sufficiently visualized on T2-weighted MRI.

Differential Diagnosis

When evaluating a potential CPA-IAC meningioma, other lesions should also be considered in the differential diagnosis, including vestibular schwannoma, trigeminal/facial schwannoma, sarcoidosis, leptomeningeal metastasis, primary meningeal lymphoma, and a nonneoplastic cyst. Often, a CPA-IAC meningioma may appear almost identical to a vestibular schwannoma, making the ability to distinguish between these two entities challenging [9]. See Table 76.3 for imaging characteristics that help differentiate meningioma from vestibular schwannoma.

Treatment Options

There are three treatment options for meningiomas located within the CPA-IAC: observation, stereotactic radiation, or microsurgical resection. Each option has distinct advantages and disadvantages, and the treatment decision depends upon the location of the tumor, growth trajectory of the tumor over time, size of the tumor, degree of brainstem compression, symptoms associated with the tumor, and patient-specific characteristics, including age and overall health.

Observation

Often, meningiomas are asymptomatic and discovered incidentally, especially as brain MRI is increasingly used as a diagnostic tool for patients with multiple neurological complaints. When evaluating a patient with an incidental CPA-IAC meningioma, the surgeon should take into account the tumor's history and growth rate. In several studies, authors found that skull base meningiomas had a growth rate of 0.71[10]–1.20[11] cm^3/year. However, in one recent study of 38 skull base meningiomas, only 40% had any growth, while the other 60% remained stable in size [10]. Currently, there is no sufficient evidence to accurately predict growth rates based upon patient presentation and a tumor's radiographic appearance. Yet several tumor characteristics such as size (>25 mm), peritumoral edema, and the absence of calcification have been cited as factors that increase the risk of tumor growth [11]. Ultimately though, until we obtain a better understanding of the biology of meningiomas, predicting growth risk factors and growth rates of a meningioma for individual patients will remain an uncertain art that necessitates serial imaging.

In our practice, we monitor all patients with asymptomatic CPA-IAC meningiomas and only pursue stereotactic radiation or microsurgical resection if the tumor grows or becomes symptomatic. Typically, after the initial diagnosis, we obtain a follow-up MRI at 4–6 months to exclude rapidly growing tumors. Thereafter, we obtain annual MRI scans if the tumor remains stable. Generally, if yearly MRI scans show limited growth or stability and the patient is clinically stable, the window or frequency for reimaging can gradually be expanded. Most meningiomas will show incremental yearly growth, though instances of accelerated growth do occur, thus necessitating continued ongoing periodic surveillance imaging once the diagnosis has been made.

Stereotactic Radiosurgery

Over the past several years, the incidence of stereotactic radiosurgery has increased. While it is not curative, the goal of stereotactic radiosurgery is to temporize the patient's clinical symptoms and prevent tumor growth.

Advantages of treating CPA-IAC meningiomas with stereotactic radiosurgery include the following: decreased operative time, leading to decreased hospitalization time and costs; fewer complications compared to microsurgical resection; and its usefulness when patients are poor surgical candidates, such as the elderly or patients with multiple medical comorbidities. Disadvantages of stereotactic radiosurgery include the non-curative nature of this modality, the potential for radiation-related complications, and the possibility of radiation-induced malignancy [12–14].

Long-term patient outcomes following stereotactic radiosurgery for CPA-IAC meningiomas are unknown. A recent, multicenter study comprising 675 patients with posterior fossa meningiomas that underwent stereotactic radiosurgery concluded that 65% had no change in outcome, 27% had improved outcomes, and 8% had worse outcomes [15]. However, the mean follow-up time was only 5 years. Another study that included 74 patients with CPA meningiomas and had a median follow-up time of approximately 3 years demonstrated that 58% had unchanged symptoms, 31% had improvement, and 11% had worsening outcomes [16]. Unfortunately, at the present moment, these follow-up lengths are insufficient to make conclusions regarding the long-term efficacy of stereotactic radiosurgery. However, more informative results should be obtained over the next 10–20 years as patients continue to undergo this type of treatment.

Currently, we advocate the use of stereotactic radiosurgery or fractionated radiotherapy in the following situations: (1) as the sole therapy in a patient with progressive neurological symptoms, who is judged to be a poor surgical candidate; (2) after subtotal resection of a meningioma if the risk of repeat surgery outweighs the benefits or if the tumor had accelerated growth preoperatively; and (3) after resection of a malignant meningioma.

We typically recommend fractionated radiotherapy for the treatment of large (>3–4 cm), inoperable IAC region meningiomas rather than a single dose of stereotactic radiosurgery to avoid potential radiation toxicity [17]. Ultimately though, the decision to pursue stereotactic radiosurgery vs. fractionated radiotherapy should only be made after discussion with a radiation oncologist; the nuances of these radiation techniques are outside the scope of this chapter.

Microsurgical Resection

Microsurgical resection is the only definitive curative treatment for meningiomas. The extent of resection is most commonly classified using the Simpson Scale, which was developed in 1957, and describes meningioma resection using a five-category system (Table 76.4) [18]. The recurrence rate for Simpson Grade 1 resection is approximately 9%, and the recurrence rate increases as the grade increases. For example, the recurrence rate for a Simpson Grade 5

Table 76.4 Simpson grading system[a]

Grade	Description
I	Complete tumor removal with associated dural attachment and abnormal bone
II	Complete tumor removal with coagulation of the abnormal dura
III	Complete tumor removal without coagulation of abnormal dura or resection of bone
IV	Partial tumor removal
V	Simple decompression of the tumor

[a]Modified from Simpson [18]

resection is 100%. Interestingly, Al-Mefty et al. described a Simpson Grade 0 resection, which included gross total resection and the removal of a two-centimeter dural margin around the tumor's base. While this study of 37 patients was limited to only supratentorial meningiomas, the recurrence rate was 0% over a 5-year follow-up period [19]. Simpson grade aside, the goal of any surgical resection should always be the safest, most comprehensive resection possible, given that the degree of resection in these cases is associated with the likelihood of recurrence-free survival and resolution or stabilization of their presenting neurological symptoms.

Normally, a retrosigmoid craniotomy is sufficient for the exposure and resection of CPA meningiomas. However, depending upon surgeon preference and the amount of tumor extension into the IAC, meningiomas can also be safely resected via a translabyrinthine approach, although this sacrifices patient hearing [20]. While the procedural steps of a retrosigmoid craniotomy are beyond the scope of this chapter, several operative nuances are listed below. First, when performing the craniotomy, it is necessary to expose the transverse and sigmoid sinus and, for larger tumors, the presigmoid dura. This allows the sigmoid sinus to be retracted laterally after the dura is opened, which increases the operative corridor to the CPA and may obviate the need for fixed retraction on the cerebellum. Second, it is important to take time to open CSF cisternal spaces to allow for brain relaxation before beginning the tumor dissection and removal. Third, after the tumor has been adequately exposed, the dural attachment to the tumor, typically located along the posterior pyramid, should be coagulated and ultimately divided. Coagulation of the surrounding dura is a critical initial step that will help devascularize the tumor, as most CPA meningiomas receive their blood supply from the dura. Fourth, once the base of the tumor is devascularized, the tumor should be internally debulked. The tumor capsule should be coagulated and then sharply incised, and tumor debulking should occur until the tumor edges can be safely dissected from the surrounding brainstem, vascular structures, and cranial nerves. Often, the superior cerebellar artery is located superior and medial, the anterior inferior cerebellar artery is located medial, and the posterior inferior cerebellar artery is located inferior and medial to the tumor. Additionally, the posterior fossa cranial nerves have rather consistent relationships to CPA meningiomas. Cranial nerves IV and V are often displaced superiorly and medially; cranial nerves VI, VII, and VIII are usually pushed anteriorly; and cranial nerves IX through XII are usually pushed inferiorly. Facial nerve monitoring is critically important, and one should make certain that nerve VII is not aberrantly located along the visible tumor capsule prior to coagulating or entering the capsule. Variability in the relationship between the facial nerve and CPA-IAC tumors is dependent on the dural origin and growth trajectory of the meningioma at the opening of the IAC in the CPA. As the tumor is removed in a piecemeal fashion, each of these cranial nerves should be identified and protected. Fourth, once the tumor is completely removed, any remaining dura should be coagulated and resected, and hyperostotic bone should be removed with a drill.

Meningiomas located primarily within the IAC can be accessed via a middle fossa, translabyrinthine, or retrosigmoid approach [21]. Approach selection depends upon the surgeon's preference, the size of the tumor, and the patient's preoperative hearing status. The middle fossa approach is generally preferred for smaller tumors (1–1.5 cm) and when hearing preservation is desired [22]. The middle fossa approach spares the otic capsule and offers superior access to the fundus of the IAC, making it an ideal choice for tumors with lateral IAC extension. The translabyrinthine approach, while useful in resecting tumors of larger sizes, violates the otic capsule and sacrifices hearing. Therefore, it should generally be employed when preoperative hearing is no longer useful to the patient or when hearing preservation is not a realistic goal of the surgery. An advantage of the translabyrinthine approach is that it allows the greatest extent of the facial nerve to be exposed, allowing the surgeon to safely identify the nerve as it travels from the brainstem through the temporal bone. Specifically, the labyrinthine segment of the nerve can quickly be identified if the interface between the cisternal segment and the tumor is not clear.

Complications

As with any surgery, complications encountered in surgery for CPA-IAC meningiomas are inevitable. However, the incidence of complications can be significantly reduced by performing a thorough preoperative evaluation, having both an in-depth understanding of posterior fossa anatomy and a focus on meticulous microsurgical technique.

Intraoperative Complications

Cranial Nerve Injuries

Cranial nerve injuries are best prevented by identifying the cranial nerves during tumor dissection, which can be accomplished by understanding where they exit the brainstem and their course through the posterior fossa. Often, prior to entering the tumor capsule and debulking, the cranial nerves can be identified, dissected away from the tumor capsule, and protected. To aid in cranial nerve identification, we commonly monitor the facial nerve, CN VII, via the "Nerve Integrity Monitor," or NIM, which measures the nerve's electromyographic response when stimulated. Additionally, in cases where hearing preservation is important, we also routinely monitor CN VIII using brainstem auditory evoked responses (BAERs), where the latency of peak V is considered the best indicator for signaling damage to the cochlear nerve [23].

Bleeding

It is paramount to maintain meticulous hemostasis throughout the entirety of the surgery, from skin incision until the tumor is completely resected. Maintaining hemostasis not only improves patient outcomes and reduces the length of hospital stay but also allows the surgeon to recognize critical anatomic structures during dissection and protect them from injury. During the retrosigmoid and translabyrinthine approaches, the mastoid emissary vein may be encountered as the bone is drilled. Bleeding from the mastoid emissary vein can be handled using two maneuvers: (1) If the vein is found first in the bone, the surgeon can place bone wax over it and continue drilling. This process can be continued until the dura is exposed (2). If the vein is first identified along the dura as it drains into the sigmoid sinus, it can be eliminated using bipolar electrocautery. As drilling continues, the transverse and sigmoid sinuses should be encountered and exposed. Occasionally, a small tear in the sinus can occur, which can lead to heavy venous bleeding. This bleeding should quickly be controlled to prevent a venous air embolism and can be accomplished by immediately placing a large piece of Gelfoam® over the sinus and gently compressing it with a cottonoid. This technique alone is often adequate to stop further bleeding, as the dura over the sinus is usually too thin to suture and placing a stitch risks intraluminal sinus occlusion. After tumor exposure, prior to debulking, it is important to cauterize the tumor capsule and control capsular vessels. If *en passage* vessels adjacent to the capsule are encountered, they should be carefully dissected and gently moved aside. As the tumor is debulked, it is important to control bleeding from the tumor bed using bipolar electrocautery. To assist with hemostasis during tumor debulking, cotton balls—soaked in thrombin—can be placed in the resection cavity, as these can absorb blood, tamponade active bleeding, and improve visualization of the surrounding anatomy. During tumor dissection, one must preserve the surrounding posterior fossa vasculature, such as the superior cerebellar, anterior inferior cerebellar, and posterior inferior cerebellar arteries. Also, it is important to preserve draining veins that enter the inferior or superior petrosal sinuses. Cauterizing these veins can potentially lead to venous infarction, which usually presents several days after surgery and can lead to intracranial hemorrhage and increased intracranial pressure.

Cerebellar Edema and Hydrocephalus

Cerebellar edema, secondary to increased intracranial pressure, may be present when tumors reach large sizes. This edema can lead to the phenomenon of cerebellar herniation when the posterior fossa dura is initially opened but can be reduced by employing a few techniques. First, prior to dural opening, mannitol (1 gram per kilogram) should be administered to the patient. Second, when approaching the tumor through a retrosigmoid craniotomy, a small slit in the inferior aspect of the dura should be opened first, prior to the full dural opening. After making this initial dural incision, the surgeon can use a malleable brain retractor to retract the cerebellum and access the lateral cerebellomedullary cistern, which can be entered, allowing for aspiration of CSF. This maneuver lowers the intracranial pressure, relaxes the cerebellum, and allows for adequate tumor exposure.

Another cause of intraoperative cerebellar swelling is obstructive hydrocephalus. Obstructive hydrocephalus may be present preoperatively when the tumor compromises outflow through the ventricular system. However, obstructive hydrocephalus may also occur during surgical resection if blood products block CSF outflow from the fourth ventricle via the foramina of Luschka and Magendie. If intraoperative hydrocephalus is suspected, an emergent external ventricular drain may be inserted into the lateral ventricle by passing it through a burr hole, referred to as Keen's point, located 3 cm above and 3 cm posterior to the pinna of the ear [24].

In a worst-case scenario, when there is so much cerebellar swelling that the CSF cisterns are inaccessible and CSF cannot be released, some cerebellar tissue may be resected to prevent cerebellar herniation.

Postoperative Complications

Intracranial Hemorrhage

Several steps can be taken to mitigate the risk of intracranial hemorrhage in the postoperative period. After tumor resection, obvious sources of bleeding should be handled with bipolar electrocautery. However, bleeding from smaller, unidentifiable vessels can be controlled by lining the resection cavity with a hemostatic agent, such as thrombin-soaked Gelfoam®, and letting it sit in place for several minutes. After the hemostatic agent is removed, the resection cavity should be copiously irrigated to ensure that hemostasis has been achieved prior to closure. After the wound is closed, the systolic blood pressure should generally be kept less than 140 mmHg during extubation and for the following 24 hours.

Once the patient is extubated, a basic neurological examination should be performed, and the patient should be monitored with consecutive neurological examinations every hour for the next 24 hours. If there is any unexpected neurological deficit or if the patient fails to properly awaken, an emergency non-contrast head CT should be performed. If a posterior fossa hemorrhage is present, the surgeon should return to the OR immediately to remove the clot. Occasionally in this scenario, it is prudent to delay replacement of the craniotomy bone flap until a later date to allow for additional swelling, and we typically cover the cerebellum with a collagen dural substitute as a layer of protection. If hydrocephalus is present, which may be secondary to the hemorrhage, an emergent external ventricular drain should be placed via Kocher's point [25, 26].

Cerebrospinal Fluid Leak

It is always best to preemptively prevent a CSF leak by carefully and thoroughly waxing all exposed air cells, including in the IAC as well as the mastoid. However, a CSF leak may occur in the postoperative period via several routes: direct drainage through a dehiscence in the surgical site, direct drainage into peri-incisional soft tissue through a dural dehiscence but beneath an intact surgical site (a pseudomeningocele), or drainage into the temporal bone manifesting. In the case of the latter, CSF can collect beneath an intact tympanic membrane and remain visible on otomicroscopy, it can pass through a defect in the tympanic membrane as otorrhea, or it can pass through the Eustachian tube and drain out of the nose as rhinorrhea. A CT of the head is important to rule out hydrocephalus as a cause of the leak. If CSF is noted to be draining through the wound incision, but the wound looks otherwise healthy, the wound can be oversewn with a locking nylon suture. Often, this technique bolsters the wound and is sufficient to resolve the leak. In general, if CSF rhinorrhea or otorrhea occurs in the immediate postoperative period and in the absence of hydrocephalus, it is our practice to return to the OR to locate and seal the leak—this situation often arises due to unobliterated air cells. In this situation, a direct approach solves the problem, and a lumbar drain is unnecessary. If there is the presence of a tense pseudomeningocele underneath the incision or a persistent leak despite oversewing the wound or direct repair, the patient may benefit from the placement of a lumbar drain. A CT of the head should always be obtained first to be sure that there is no contraindication for placing a lumbar drain.

By draining 15–20 milliliters of CSF per hour for a period of 3–5 days, a lumbar drain allows CSF to be diverted away from the incision, potentially allowing it to heal. Prior to removal, the drain should be clamped for a minimum of 24 hours, and the incision should be monitored for the presence of a CSF leak or a pseudomeningocele. If a CSF leak is present during the drain clamping trial, the drain should be reopened and continued for several more days. Ultimately, if the CSF leak does not resolve with a lumbar drain, a ventriculoperitoneal shunt may need to be placed to provide permanent CSF diversion.

Since a patient with a CSF leak has a much higher risk of developing meningitis [27], symptoms of fever, headache, photophobia, or nuchal rigidity should be treated with concern. To rule out meningitis, CSF should be obtained via a lumbar puncture and sent for cell counts, glucose, protein, gram stain, and cultures. If the patient appears clinically ill, broad-spectrum intravenous antibiotics should be started prior to obtaining results of the CSF analysis, and the patient should be admitted to the hospital. Additionally, if the patient presents with symptoms concerning for infection, a contrast head CT scan should be obtained to rule out the presence of an intracranial abscess.

Summary

Meningiomas arising at the level of the IAC in the CPA present several unique management and surgical challenges for neurosurgeons and neurotologists. We believe that many patients can be managed conservatively—with close clinical and radiographic follow-up. Both radiation and microsurgery play important roles in the treatment of these specific meningiomas, and it is important to individualize therapy based on the clinical and radiographic features of each patient's tumor.

References

1. Friedmann DR, Grobelny B, Golfinos JG, Roland JT Jr. Nonschwannoma tumors of the cerebellopontine angle. Otolaryngol Clin N Am. 2015;48(3):461–75.
2. Nakamura M, Roser F, Mirzai S, Matthies C, Vorkapic P, Samii M. Meningiomas of the internal auditory canal. Neurosurgery. 2004;55(1):119–27; discussion 127–128.
3. Pollock BE, Link MJ, Stafford SL, Parney IF, Garces YI, Foote RL. The risk of radiation-induced tumors or malignant transformation after single-fraction intracranial radiosurgery: results based on a 25-year experience. Int J Radiat Oncol Biol Phys. 2017;97(5):919–23.
4. Pathmanaban ON, Sadler KV, Kamaly-Asl ID, et al. Association of Genetic Predisposition with Solitary Schwannoma or meningioma in children and young adults. JAMA Neurol. 2017;74:1123.
5. Agnihotri S, Suppiah S, Tonge PD, et al. Therapeutic radiation for childhood cancer drives structural aberrations of NF2 in meningiomas. Nat Commun. 2017;8(1):186.
6. Boulagnon-Rombi C, Fleury C, Fichel C, Lefour S, Marchal Bressenot A, Gauchotte G. Immunohistochemical approach to the differential diagnosis of meningiomas and their mimics. J Neuropathol Exp Neurol. 2017;76(4):289–98.
7. Saloner D, Uzelac A, Hetts S, Martin A, Dillon W. Modern meningioma imaging techniques. J Neuro-Oncol. 2010;99(3):333–40.
8. Gao K, Ma H, Cui Y, Chen X, Ma J, Dai J. Meningiomas of the cerebellopontine angle: radiological differences in tumors with internal auditory canal involvement and their influence on surgical outcome. PLoS One. 2015;10(4):e0122949.
9. Calzada AP, Go JL, Tschirhart DL, Brackmann DE, Schwartz MS. Cerebellopontine angle and intracanalicular masses mimicking vestibular schwannomas. Otol Neurotol. 2015;36(3):491–7.
10. Hashimoto N, Rabo CS, Okita Y, et al. Slower growth of skull base meningiomas compared with non-skull base meningiomas based on volumetric and biological studies. J Neurosurg. 2012;116(3):574–80.
11. Oya S, Kim SH, Sade B, Lee JH. The natural history of intracranial meningiomas. J Neurosurg. 2011;114(5):1250–6.
12. Lall RR, Lall RR, Smith TR, et al. Delayed malignant transformation of petroclival meningioma to chondrosarcoma after stereotactic radiosurgery. J Clin Neurosci. 2014;21(7):1225–8.
13. Novotny J Jr, Kollova A, Liscak R. Prediction of intracranial edema after radiosurgery of meningiomas. J Neurosurg. 2006;105(Suppl):120–6.
14. Mathiesen T, Kihlstrom L, Karlsson B, Lindquist C. Potential complications following radiotherapy for meningiomas. Surg Neurol. 2003;60(3):193–8. discussion 199-200
15. Sheehan JP, Starke RM, Kano H, et al. Gamma Knife radiosurgery for posterior fossa meningiomas: a multicenter study. J Neurosurg. 2015;122(6):1479–89.
16. Park SH, Kano H, Niranjan A, Flickinger JC, Lunsford LD. Stereotactic radiosurgery for cerebellopontine angle meningiomas. J Neurosurg. 2014;120(3):708–15.
17. Biau J, Khalil T, Verrelle P, Lemaire JJ. Fractionated radiotherapy and radiosurgery of intracranial meningiomas. Neurochirurgie. 2018;64(1):29–36. https://doi.org/10.1016/j.neuchi.2014.10.112.
18. Simpson D. The recurrence of intracranial meningiomas after surgical treatment. J Neurol Neurosurg Psychiatry. 1957;20(1):22–39.
19. Kinjo T, al-Mefty O, Kanaan I. Grade zero removal of supratentorial convexity meningiomas. Neurosurgery. 1993;33(3):394–9; discussion 399.
20. Ansari SF, Terry C, Cohen-Gadol AA. Surgery for vestibular schwannomas: a systematic review of complications by approach. Neurosurg Focus. 2012;33(3):E14.
21. Laudadio P, Canani FB, Cunsolo E. Meningioma of the internal auditory canal. Acta Otolaryngol. 2004;124(10):1231–4.
22. Peng KA, Wilkinson EP. Optimal outcomes for hearing preservation in the management of small vestibular schwannomas. J Laryngol Otol. 2016;130(7):606–10.
23. Bozorg Grayeli A, Refass A, Smail M, et al. Diagnostic value of auditory brainstem responses in cerebellopontine angle tumours. Acta Otolaryngol. 2008;128(10):1096–100.
24. Keen WW. Surgery of the lateral ventricles of the brain. Lancet. 1890;136(3498):553–5.
25. Muirhead WR, Basu S. Trajectories for frontal external ventricular drain placement: virtual cannulation of adults with acute hydrocephalus. Br J Neurosurg. 2012;26(5):710–6.
26. Hildebrandt G, Surbeck W, Stienen MN. Emil Theodor Kocher: the first Swiss neurosurgeon. Acta Neurochir. 2012;154(6):1105–15. discussion 1115
27. Magliulo G, Sepe C, Varacalli S, Fusconi M. Cerebrospinal fluid leak management following cerebellopontine angle surgery. J Otolaryngol. 1998;27(5):258–62.

Lateral Skull Base Epidermoids

77

Stephen P. Cass, Emily Ambrose, Emily Bacalao, and Samy Youssef

Introduction

Lateral skull base epidermoids are an uncommon but important group of congenital tumors that can involve the petrous portion of the temporal bone, diploic cranial bone, or, more commonly, the intradural, subarachnoid compartment of the skull base, particularly within the cerebellopontine angle (CPA) [1]. Intradural epidermoids grow slowly and spread along the subarachnoid spaces on the basal brain, frequently involving cranial nerves and vessels [2]. While these tumors are histologically benign, arising from ectopic embryonic rests of epithelial cells, they may reach large sizes and become adherent to critical structures [2]. They are associated with a high rate of cranial nerve dysfunction as well as recurrent growth following surgery [3]. Epidermoids are composed of stratified, keratinizing squamous epithelium lying on a collagen/connective tissue basement membrane. They enlarge by the accumulation of desquamating keratin debris, along with breakdown products of keratin, including cholesterol crystals and focal calcification [1, 2, 4]. These tumors do not have a specific blood supply but tend to deform bone, compress the brain, and insinuate along and in between vessels and cranial nerves as they enlarge over time. Because they arise from the ectopic epithelium, they do not display neoplastic growth rates; instead, they enlarge at a linear growth rate expected of the skin [5]. Epidermoids can be differentiated from dermoids, which contain additional adnexal elements of the skin, such as sweat or sebaceous glands, hair, or hair follicles. Dermoids are found in the body's midline, whereas epidermoids are generally found lateral to the midline [2].

S. P. Cass (✉) · E. Ambrose · E. Bacalao
Department of Otolaryngology—Head and Neck Surgery, University of Colorado Anschutz Medical Campus, Aurora, CO, USA
e-mail: Stephen.Cass@ucdenver.edu

S. Youssef
Department of Neurosurgery, University of Colorado Anschutz Medical Campus, Aurora, CO, USA

A. D. Sweeney et al. (eds.), *Haynes-Glasscock-Shambaugh Surgery of the Ear*, https://doi.org/10.1007/978-3-032-18264-7_77

Primary petrous bone epidermoids are rare, congenital tumors that can be distinguished from the far more common cholesteatoma of the middle ear and mastoid. Cholesteatoma is also a keratinizing squamous epithelial cyst, but the term cholesteatoma is typically used for an acquired lesion, most commonly arising in relation to chronic ear infection or tympanic membrane retraction or perforation. Petrous bone cholesteatoma refers to a subset of cholesteatoma that involves the petrous bone, and in practice, primary epidermoids of the petrous bone and petrous bone cholesteatoma are frequently lumped together in most surgical series and classified by the involved portions of the petrous bone [6–9].

Clinical Manifestations and Diagnosis

The clinical manifestations and diagnosis of lateral skull base epidermoids depend on the location of the lesion. Generally, these tumors fall into two groups: cranial (petrous apex/temporal bone and diploic cranial lesions) and intracranial (intradural) lesions.

Petrous Bone Epidermoids

Primary epidermoids of the petrous bone are rare, congenital tumors that arise from aberrant embryonic epithelium. They often present with longstanding and progressive symptoms, most commonly including hearing loss, facial nerve dysfunction (spasms and paresis), dizziness, tinnitus, or headache [9–11]. Extensive primary petrous bone epidermoids may be difficult to distinguish from acquired petrous bone cholesteatoma [9]. Most primary petrous bone epidermoids are found either incidentally or during an investigation into hearing loss, headache, or new cranial nerve dysfunction [9]. Diagnosis is made using both computed tomography (CT) and magnetic resonance imaging (MRI), and the differential diagnoses for lesions of the petrous apex include cholesterol granuloma, mucocele, chondrosarcoma, and asymmetric bone marrow. The imaging characteristics of these lesions are summarized in Table 77.1. An example of an epidermoid tumor involving the anterior petrous bone is shown in Fig. 77.1 and an epidermoid involving the posterior petrous bone in Fig. 77.2.

Intradiploic Cranial Epidermoids

Intradiploic cranial epidermoids are rare and present most commonly with soft tissue swelling over the cranium. The differential diagnoses for diploic or cranial bone lesions include epidermoid tumor, giant cell reparative granuloma, small cell tumor, meningioma, and metastatic carcinoma [12]. Imaging characteristics of these lesions are shown in Table 77.2.

Intradural Epidermoids

Intradural epidermoids of the posterior fossa commonly present in the third to fifth decades of life with cranial nerve dysfunction or headache [13]. Specifically, asymmetric sensorineural hearing loss, unilateral tinnitus, dizziness or imbalance, facial nerve spasms or paresis, trigeminal nerve distribution pain or numbness, and headache are frequently seen [1, 14, 15]. These symptoms may wax and wane over time but tend to progress. A relatively recent single-center review of 47 CPA epidermoids identified 40% of patients with facial or auditory dysfunction and 57% with headache. Lower cranial nerve dysfunction is less commonly reported. Cranial nerve dysfunction can be common even with small intradural epidermoid tumors and is thought to be related to direct neural irritation by keratin or irritative enzymes or related to direct neurovascular compression [9, 10]. The pattern of cranial nerve symptoms follows the growth pattern of the epidermoid, which can be variable. Specifically, tumors can extend ventrally into the prepontine space, across the midline into the contralateral CPA, posteriorly to the fourth ventricle and cerebellum, superiorly into the middle cranial fossa, or through the incisura to involve the parasellar cisterns.

MRI is the diagnostic modality of choice for posterior fossa lesions, and the imaging characteristics of common CPA lesions are shown in Table 77.3, along with an example of an MRI of a CPA epidermoid (Fig. 77.3). Signal intensity is often variable, depending on the relative lipid, cholesterol, and keratin composition of the tumor [16]. Proton density (PD) weighting highlights the structural heterogeneity of epidermoids [17]. Generally, T1-weighted images of epidermoids have low signal intensity, intermediate between that of brain and cerebrospinal fluid (CSF). On T2-weighted images, epidermoids often exhibit high signal intensity. Epidermoids typically do not show contrast enhancement on gadolinium administration [17]. Diffusion-weighted MRI is used as the imaging modality of choice in distinguishing epidermoids from other posterior fossa masses [18, 19]. In more recent literature, intracranial epidermoids have been distinguished as either black epidermoids or rarer white epidermoids based on MRI characteristics [16]. White epidermoids are described as hyperintense on T1-weighted imaging and hypointense on T2-weighted imaging, reversed features of the more common black epidermoid. White epidermoid tumors tend to have increased tumor adhesions to the surrounding structures, giving these lesions a higher risk of leaking epidermoid content during surgery, making early identification beneficial. Cystic contents often correlate with imaging characteristics of the MRI. Hyperintense T2 signal of "white" epidermoid cysts likely has hemorrhagic content, while a hypointense T2 signal likely has protein and more viscous content [16].

Table 77.1 CT and MRI characteristics of petrous apex lesions

Lesion	MRI (T1)	MRI (T2)	Enhancing	Expansile	CT
Cholesterol granuloma	Hyperintense	Hyperintense	No	Yes	Homogeneous or with hypointense, irregular debris
Cholesteatoma	Hypo-isointense	Hyperintense	No	Yes	Homogeneous
Mucocele	Hypointense-variable	Hyperintense	No	Yes	Homogeneous
Petrous apicitis	Hypointense	Hyperintense	Yes	No	Opacification and/or erosion of petrous air cells
Meningioma	Hypo-isointense	Hyper-isointense	Yes	Yes	Hyperostosis
Schwannoma	Low-isointense	Hyperintense	Yes	Yes	Can be cystic, smooth edges
Paraganglioma	Hypo/hyperintense "salt and pepper"	Hypo/hyperintense "salt and pepper"	Yes	No	Moth-eaten
Chondroma	Hypointense	Hyperintense	Variable	No	Lytic bone lesions, variable matrix calcification
Chondrosarcoma	Hypo-isointense	Hyperintense	Yes	No	Heterogeneous with rings of calcifications
Endolymphatic sac tumor	Hyperintense-variable	Variable	Yes	No	Bony erosion, calcifications
Metastases	Isointense	Isointense	Yes	No	Focal bony destructive
Trapped fluid	Hypo-hyperintense	Hyperintense	No	No	Pneumatized petrous apex

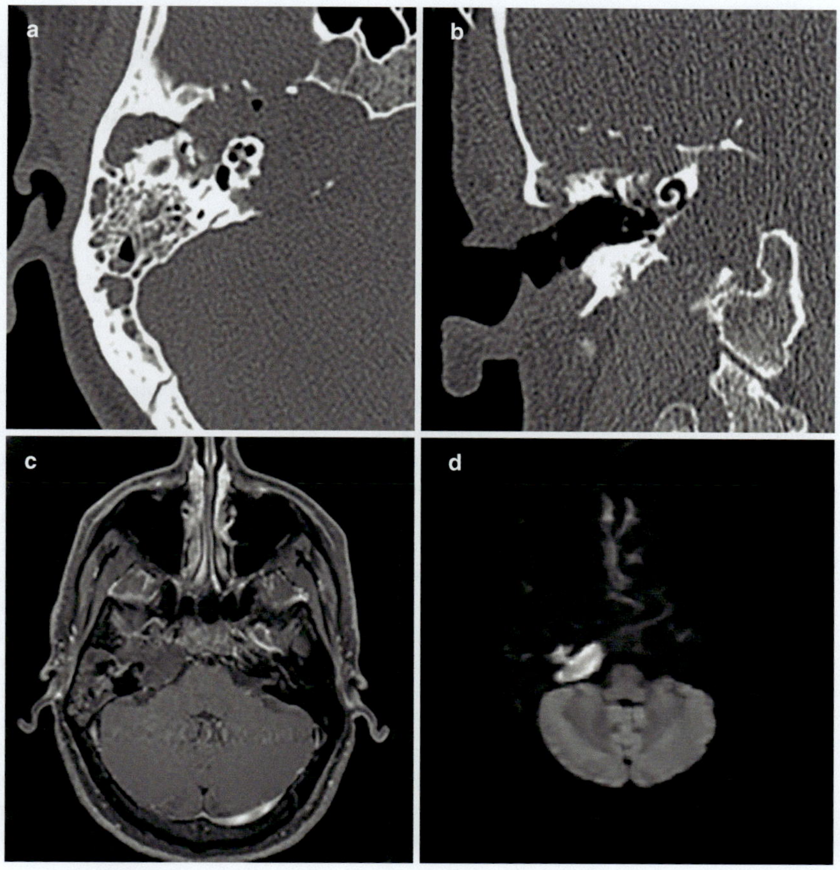

Fig. 77.1 A large epidermoid of the right petrous apex shown on computed tomography axial (**a**) and coronal (**b**) views. An axial view of a T1-weighted MRI (**c**) shows no significant enhancement in a hypointense lesion, which appears to have restricted diffusion (**d**)

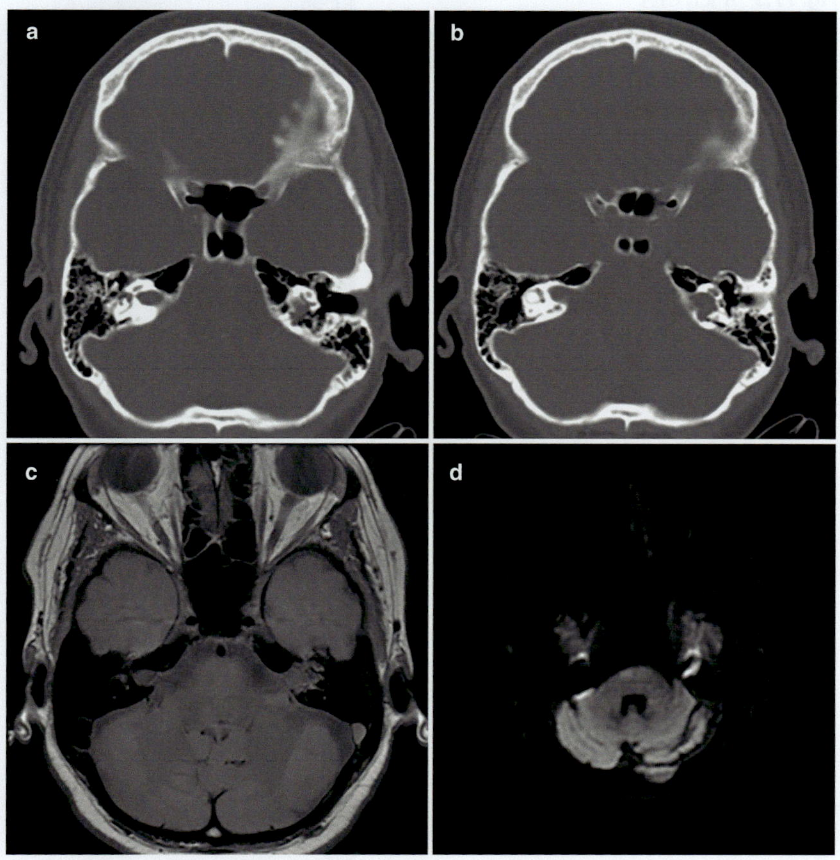

Fig. 77.2 A small epidermoid of the petrous apex shown eroding into the left cochlea on axial views of a computed tomography (**a** and **b**). An axial view of a T1-weighted MRI (**c**) shows the lesion to be hypointense, and it appears to have restricted diffusion (**d**)

Table 77.2 CT and MRI characteristics of cranial diploic lesions

Lesion	MRI (T1)	MRI (T2)	Enhancing	Expansile	CT
Epidermoid cyst	Isointense	Iso-hyperintense	No	Yes	Sclerotic, scalloped
Dermoid cyst	Variable	Variable			Heterogeneous, thick-walled with calcifications
Fibrous dysplasia	Hypointense	Variable	Yes	Yes	Ground glass
Osteoma	Hypointense	Variable	No	Yes	Sclerotic lesion, preservation of diploe
Hemangioma	Hypo-isointense	Hyperintense	Yes	Yes	Osteolytic, "sunburst," or "honeycomb" trabecular pattern
Eosinophilic granuloma	Hypointense	Hyperintense	Yes	No	Osteolytic, "button sequestrum"
Osteosarcoma	Hypointense- variable	Hypo-hyperintense	Yes	No	Osteolytic

Table 77.3 MRI characteristics of posterior fossa lesions

Lesion	MRI (T1)	MRI (T2)	Enhancing
Cholesterol granuloma	Hyperintense	Hyperintense	No
Epidermoid-black White	Hypo-isointense Hyperintense	Hyperintense Hypointense	No
Mucocele	Hypointense-variable	Hyperintense	No
Petrous apicitis	Hypointense	Hyperintense	Yes
Meningioma	Hypo-isointense	Iso-hyperintense	Yes
Schwannoma	Hypo-isointense	Hyperintense	Yes
Paraganglioma	Hypo/hyperintense "salt and pepper"	Hypo/hyperintense "salt and pepper"	Yes
Chondroma	Hypointense	Hyperintense	Variable
Chondrosarcoma	Hypo-isointense	Hyperintense	Yes
Endolymphatic sac tumor	Hyperintense-variable	Variable	Yes
Metastases	Isointense	Isointense	Yes
Trapped fluid	Hypo-hyperintense	Hyperintense	No
Hemangioma	Hypo-isointense	Hyperintense	Yes
Arachnoid cyst	Hypo-isointense	Hyperintense	Yes

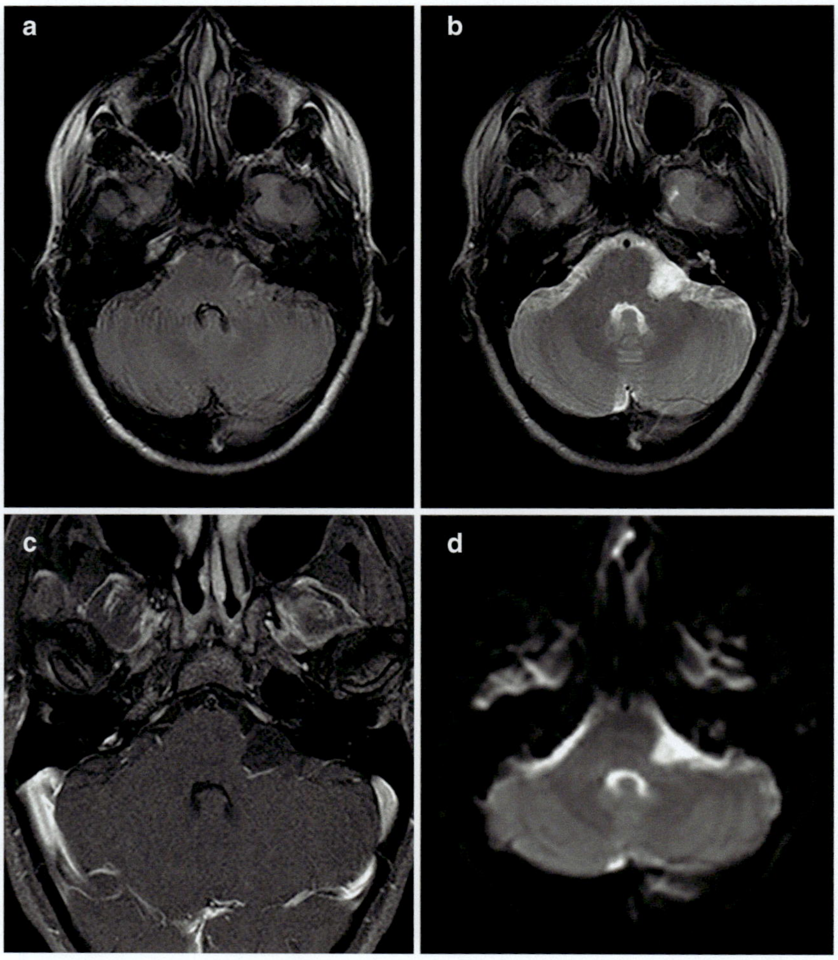

Fig. 77.3 A left CPA epidermoid shown on axial MRI. The lesion is iso/hypointense on T1 (**a**), hyperintense on T2 (**b**), non-enhancing on a post-gadolinium image (**c**), and diffusion restricting (**d**)

Management

The management of lateral skull base epidermoids includes both observation with active surveillance and surgical excision. There is no primary role for radiation therapy or chemotherapy. Epidermoids are occasionally found incidentally and may be observed if small and asymptomatic or if the patient is medically infirm. However, close surveillance is required, as patients often develop cranial nerve symptoms and require intervention over time [20]. Surgery is indicated when there is new or progressive cranial nerve dysfunction, headache or hydrocephalus, or progressive tumor growth threatening neurological dysfunction. As noted below, surgical resection can be effective in alleviating many symptoms, especially headache, dizziness, and irritative cranial nerve dysfunction involving the facial and trigeminal nerves. Sensorineural hearing loss rarely improves once present.

Surgical Technique

Petrous Bone Epidermoids

Gross total surgical removal of petrous bone epidermoids is optimal, as regrowth invariably follows subtotal removal. Surgical planning can be complex because the approach is based on the exact location, size, and extent of the epidermoid [8–10, 21, 22]. Preexisting hearing levels, involvement of vascular structures, and cranial nerve function, especially the facial nerve, are particularly relevant considerations. A variety of surgical approaches can be considered, including transmastoid, translabyrinthine, transcochlear, transotic, middle cranial fossa, and infratemporal fossa approaches. Occasionally, these approaches can be combined. Hearing preservation is not always possible in these cases, though it is an appropriate goal of treatment when the disease can be accessed without destroying the otic capsule [21, 23]. Classification systems for extensive primary and acquired temporal bone cholesteatomas, developed first by Fisch and Mattox [7] and modified by Moffat [9] and Sanna [8], are useful for conceptualizing and individualizing the surgical approach. When subtotal removal is necessary for a lesion within the temporal bone, a decision is required regarding whether to attempt exteriorization of the residual cyst or close off the ear and monitor for growth over time. As noted above, MRI using diffusion-weighted imaging is used to track residual epidermoid for growth over time.

Intradural Epidermoids

Gross total resection (GTR) is the goal of surgical intervention in the setting of an intracranial epidermoid; however, the cyst capsule may become firmly adherent to neurovascular structures, thus making complete surgical resection challenging. While translabyrinthine and transcochlear approaches have been described, the workhorse to assess these tumors has been and continues to be the retrosigmoid approach, which provides access to the posterior fossa from the tentorium to the foramen magnum [24]. Surgical technique involves decompression of cyst contents followed by removal of the non-adherent portions of the cyst capsule. Microdissectors and suction are usually adequate to evacuate the cyst contents. We use methylprednisolone mixed with warm lactated Ringer's solution in a 500 mg/500 ml ratio for irrigation of the surgical field in order to minimize the risk of chemical meningitis caused by the spill of the cyst content to the cerebrospinal fluid in the basal cisterns. Firm adhesion of the tumor capsule to vascular structures, cranial nerves, or the brain stem is the most common cause of incomplete resection. Applying the keyhole endoscopic–assisted microsurgery concept to posterior fossa epidermoid surgery has been particularly beneficial [25–27]. Compared with the microscope, endoscopes provide a wide angle of view, superb illumination, and an increased depth of focus, even with high magnification. After microsurgical removal of the contents of the cyst and dissection of the cyst capsule, a series of 0–30-degree-angled endoscopes can be introduced into the CPA to provide an enhanced direct visualization of the medial extent of the capsule to the brain stem and critical neurovascular structures while minimizing cerebellar retraction. Continuous irrigation is very important to overcome the heat at the tip of the endoscope. Bimanual dissection of the medial capsule can be performed with a combined microscopic/endoscopic view, with the endoscope fixed in a holder or held by an assistant. A firmly adherent capsule should be left in place in order to avoid catastrophic vascular or neural complications from damaging critical neurovascular structures.

Outcomes

Petrous Bone Epidermoids

Table 77.4 summarizes several recent surgical series of petrous bone cholesteatoma. Hearing loss is frequently a presenting symptom and rarely improves following surgery.

Table 77.4 Outcomes of petrous bone epidermoids

Author	# of patients	Approach	Recurrence rate (%)	Hearing	Facial nerve	Postoperative complications
Danesi et al. (2016) [22]	81 (congenital vs. acquired not specified)	TL 37/81 SP 22 MCF 14	26%	*Pre-op* 42/81 anacusis 38/81 moderate HL *Post-op* 75/81 anacusis	*Pre-op* FN Nl 15/81 FN HB VI 56/81 *Post-op* FN Nl 13/81	Not reported
Kim et al. (2014) [23]	31 (congenital vs. acquired not specified)	TM 15/31 TL 7 TC 5 SP 4	3.2%	*Pre-op* Deafness 9/31 Mixed HL 20/31 *Post-op* Deafness 20/31	*Pre-op* FN Nl 20/31 *Post-op* FN Nl 19/31	12.9% Wound infection 3.2% Vertigo
Senn et al. (2011) [21]	21 (5 recurrent)	MSP 21/21	19%	*Pre-op* Profound HL 4/21 Moderate HL 17/21 *Post-op* Profound HL 8/21 Hearing improved 8/21	*Pre-op* FN Nl 15/21 *Post-op* FN Nl 19/21	Not reported
Aubry et al. (2010) [11]	28 (5 congenital and 23 acquired; 17 recurrent)		29%	*Pre-op* Profound HL 15/28 Moderate HL 12/28 *Post-op* Profound HL 23/28	*Pre-op* FN Nl 18/28 *Post-op* FN Nl 18/28 6/12 with pre-op dysfunction improved	Transient FN weakness 22% CN XII dysfunction 7% CN X dysfunction 4% Hemiparesis 4%
Moffat et al. (2008) [9]	43 (10 recurrent)	SP 25/43 TT 7 TO 4 MF 2 TC 1	3.5%	*Pre-op* Significant HL 95%	*Pre-op* FN Nl 21/43 *Post-op* FN Nl 20/21 7 with nerve repair 2 with static reanimation	9.3% CSF leak 2.3% Seizure 2.3% Wound infection
Grayeli et al. (2000) [6]	19 (congenital vs. acquired not specified)	TO 9/19 MF 8 SP 1 RL 1	11%	*Pre-op* Deafness 13/19 *Post-op* Deafness 16/19	*Pre-op* FN Nl 7/19 *Post-op* FN Nl 11/19	CSF leak 11% CN IX injury 5%

TL translabyrinthine, *TO* transotic, *SP* subtotal petrosectomy, *MCF* and *MF* middle cranial fossa, *TM* transmastoid, *TC* transcochlear, *TT* transtemporal, *RS* retrosigmoid, *FN* facial nerve, *HB* House Brackmann grade, *NL* normal, *CN* cranial nerve, *CSF* cerebrospinal fluid leak

Facial nerve weakness is also a frequent presenting symptom. When preoperative facial nerve function is normal, most of the time, it remains normal after surgery. When preoperative facial nerve function is abnormal, some improvement in function is possible in some cases but may require nerve repair techniques or facial reanimation procedures [9, 21, 23]. Recurrence rates can vary considerably, and lifelong surveillance is generally suggested. Surgical complications are generally uncommon and reflect the surgical approach utilized.

Intradural Epidermoids

Treatment outcomes of intradural and CPA epidermoids are summarized in Table 77.5. Preoperative cranial neuropathies are often present, including facial weakness, facial hypoesthesia, dizziness, hearing loss, and dysphagia [28]. Surgical intervention can be undertaken to alleviate compressive and irritative cranial neuropathy, though hearing loss does not typically improve following removal of the epidermoid [29, 30]. That being said, hearing preservation is frequently possible surgically, and the literature suggesting as much would encourage the employment of a hearing preservation approach when possible [24]. Yawn et al. noted that all patients with preoperative facial weakness recovered function after the surgery, and only one patient experienced new facial weakness [20]. Kobata et al. demonstrated postoperative improvement in 30 patients with either trigeminal neuralgia or hemifacial spasm arising in association with an epidermoid [31]. Transient cranial neuropathies are also not uncommon after surgical resection [31].

Recurrence rates are highly variable for epidermoids, and the likelihood of recurrence may depend on the extent of resection, though there is some controversy around this subject. The likelihood of recurrence may be lower if a gross total resection is achieved, and when operating on a recurrent tumor, a gross total resection is less likely [1, 32]. However, given the infiltrative nature of epidermoid tumors, total resection can be difficult without causing additional morbidity. When radical resection is not feasible, subtotal resection is a valid alternative that offers good intermediate-

Table 77.5 Outcomes of intracranial epidermoids

Author	Number of patients	Extent of resection (%)	Recurrence rate (%)	Mean time to recurrence (yrs)	Postoperative complications
Yawn et al. (2016) [20]	47	GT-46 NT-13 ST-41	8 (GT-2%)	4.4	21% chronic pain 10% CSF leak 8% hypoesthesia 8% infection 8% hearing loss 3% aseptic meningitis 3% facial weakness
Czernicki et al. (2016) [3]	17	–	29.4	9	23.5% facial weakness 5.9% hearing loss 5.9% facial hypoesthesia
Aboud et al. (2015) [1]	26-*de novo* 8-recurrent	*De novo* GT-73 Recurrent GT-17	*De novo* 15.4 Recurrent 41.7	*De novo* 10.1 Recurrent 4.5	*De novo* 34.6% cranial neuropathy 15.4% CSF leak 3.5% seizure 3.5% death Recurrent 33.3% cranial neuropathy 16.7% hydrocephalus 8.3% CSF leak
Tuchman et al. (2014) [26]	12 (6 recurrent)	GT-15.3 NT-38.5 ST-46.2	–	–	30.8% aseptic meningitis 30.8% hearing loss 30.8% hypoesthesia 23.1% facial weakness
Gopalakrishnan et al. (2013) [32]	50	GT-62 NT-26 ST-12	44.7 (n = 38)	9.3	30% facial weakness 12% hearing loss
Miller et al. (2012) [24]	18 (2 recurrent)	–	11.1	–	11.1% facial weakness 11.1% hearing loss 5.6% CSF leak 5.6% meningitis
Kato et al. (2010) [15]	24 (4 recurrent)	–	16.7	9.5	12.5% hydrocephalus 4.2% facial hypoesthesia
Safavi-Abbasi et al. (2008) [29]	12 (3 recurrent)	GT-75	0	N/A	8.3% CSF leak 8.3% facial weakness 8.3% hydrocephalus
Schiefer et al. (2008) [14]	24	GT-54.2 NT-25 ST-20.8	25	6.2	41.7% hearing loss 12.5% facial weakness 8.3% aseptic meningitis 8.3% subdural hygroma 4.2% CSF leak 4.2% delayed hydrocephalus 4.2% exposure keratitis
Kaylie et al. (2005) [35]	10	GT-80	10	–	80% hearing loss 30% facial weakness 30% headache 10% seizures 10% earlobe necrosis 10% temporal lobe abscess
Meng et al. (2005) [30]	24	GT-54.2 NT-37.5 ST-8.3	–	–	37.5% hypoesthesia 25% hearing loss 16.7% facial weakness 12.5% aseptic meningitis
Darrouzet et al. (2004) [27]	7	GT-71.4	0	N/A	42.9% hearing loss 28.6% facial weakness 14.3% aseptic meningitis
Schroeder et al. (2004) [25]	8 (2 recurrent)	GT-37.5	0	N/A	12.5% facial weakness 12.5% hypoesthesia 12.5% hearing loss

(continued)

Table 77.5 (continued)

Author	Number of patients	Extent of resection (%)	Recurrence rate (%)	Mean time to recurrence (yrs)	Postoperative complications
Akar et al. (2003) [13]	28	GT-75 ST-25	7.1 (GT-0%)	6	28.6% hearing loss 21.4% facial weakness 17.9% hydrocephalus 10.7% aseptic meningitis
Kobata et al. (2002) [31]	30	GT-56.7	6.7	7	30% hearing loss 23.3% facial weakness 10% hypoesthesia 6.7% aseptic meningitis
Sakamoto et al. (2021) [33]	54 (congenital vs. acquired not specified)	LSO 97.8 ATP 89.3 CTP 97.3 ATP + LSO 96	3.7	5.2	5.5% CSF leak 1.8% CN IV deficit (transient) 9.3% CN V deficits 7.4% CN VI deficit (transient) 5.6% CN VII 9.3% CN VIII
Sellier et al. (2022) [28]	56	GTR 14 STR 61 PR 23	46	5.2	7.2% hearing loss 3.6% facial weakness 12.5% aseptic meningitis 7.1% hydrocephalus 5.4% cerebral ischemia 5.4% infield hematoma 0.54% septic meningitis 5.4% CSF leakage 3.6% coma 1.8% death

to-long-term outcomes, some of which indicate that recurrence probability is not always predictable with the extent of resection [3, 14, 20, 28, 31, 33]. Due to the slow-growing nature of these tumors, recurrence can become clinically evident over the course of decades, necessitating vigilant and long-term follow-up [5, 32, 33].

Postoperatively, there are a variety of complications worth considering after intracranial epidermoid resection. The rates of aseptic meningitis and hydrocephalus are particularly noteworthy in published literature. Aseptic meningitis has been reported in as many as 30% of cases [26]. Previous analysis of this association has suggested that the irritative nature of cyst contents, and keratin in particular, could be responsible [4]. The incidence of hydrocephalus and CSF leakage may be elevated for a similar reason, given that inflammation may inhibit CSF absorption [1, 2]. In addition to tumor recurrence, rare malignant transformation of these tumors into squamous cell carcinoma has been reported [34–36]. While overall survival is poor, radiation in addition to surgery may improve median survival in these patients [34].

Conclusions

Lateral skull base epidermoids are generally histologically benign lesions that have a low probability of malignant transformation. However, they can be problematic in terms of dysfunction in—and adherence to—associated structures. In growing lesions or those that are clearly symptomatic, surgical resection is a mainstay of management. GTR is preferred, though not always possible, and given the possibility of insidious growth in residual tumor, posttreatment follow-up should be vigilant and lifelong.

References

1. Aboud E, Abolfotoh M, Pravdenkova S, Gokoglu A, Gokden M, Al-Mefty O. Giant intracranial epidermoids: is total removal feasible? J Neurosurg. 2015;122(4):743–56.
2. Berger MS, Wilson CB. Epidermoid cysts of the posterior fossa. J Neurosurg. 1985;62(2):214–9.
3. Czernicki T, Kunert P, Nowak A, Wojciechowski J, Marchel A. Epidermoid cysts of the cerebellopontine angle: clinical features and treatment outcomes. Neurol Neurochir Pol. 2016;50(2):75–82.
4. Cherian A, Baheti NN, Easwar HV, Nair DS, Iype T. Recurrent meningitis due to epidermoid. J Pediatr Neurosci. 2012;7(1):47–8.
5. Alvord EC Jr. Growth rates of epidermoid tumors. Ann Neurol. 1977;2(5):367–70.
6. Grayeli AB, Mosnier I, El Garem H, Bouccara D, Sterkers O. Extensive intratemporal cholesteatoma: surgical strategy. Am J Otol. 2000;21(6):774–81.
7. Fisch U. Infratemporal fossa approach for extensive tumors of the temporal bone and base of skull. In: Silverstein HNN, editor. Neurological surgery of the ear. Birmingham, AL: Aesculapius; 1977. p. 33–53.
8. Sanna M, Zini C, Gamoletti R, et al. Petrous bone cholesteatoma. Skull Base Surg. 1993;3(4):201–13.

9. Moffat D, Jones S, Smith W. Petrous temporal bone cholesteatoma: a new classification and long-term surgical outcomes. Skull Base. 2008;18(2):107–15.
10. Axon PR, Fergie N, Saeed SR, Temple RH, Ramsden RT. Petrosal cholesteatoma: management considerations for minimizing morbidity. Am J Otol. 1999;20(4):505–10.
11. Aubry K, Kovac L, Sauvaget E, Tran Ba Huy P, Herman P. Our experience in the management of petrous bone cholesteatoma. Skull Base. 2010;20(3):163–7.
12. Arana E, Latorre FF, Revert A, et al. Intradiploic epidermoid cysts. Neuroradiology. 1996;38(4):306–11.
13. Akar Z, Tanriover N, Tuzgen S, Kafadar AM, Kuday C. Surgical treatment of intracranial epidermoid tumors. Neurol Med Chir (Tokyo). 2003;43(6):275–80. discussion 281
14. Schiefer TK, Link MJ. Epidermoids of the cerebellopontine angle: a 20-year experience. Surg Neurol. 2008;70(6):584–90; discussion 590.
15. Kato K, Ujiie H, Higa T, et al. Clinical presentation of intracranial epidermoids: a surgical series of 20 initial and four recurred cases. Asian J Neurosurg. 2010;5(1):32–40.
16. Loy LM, Aftab S, Ang YLS, Ding SLC, Ho CL. Intracranial "white" epidermoid tumours - An imaging approach and systematic review. Clin Imaging. 2022;91:1–8.
17. Kallmes DF, Provenzale JM, Cloft HJ, McClendon RE. Typical and atypical MR imaging features of intracranial epidermoid tumors. AJR Am J Roentgenol. 1997;169(3):883–7.
18. Tamilchelvan P, Boruah DK, Gogoi BB, Gogoi R. Role of MRI in differentiating various posterior cranial fossa space-occupying lesions using sensitivity and specificity: a prospective study. Cureus. 2021;13(7):e16336.
19. Henninger B, Kremser C. Diffusion weighted imaging for the detection and evaluation of cholesteatoma. World J Radiol. 2017;9(5):217–22.
20. Yawn RJ, Patel NS, Driscoll CL, et al. Primary epidermoid tumors of the cerebellopontine angle: a review of 47 cases. Otol Neurotol. 2016;37(7):951–5.
21. Senn P, Haeusler R, Panosetti E, Caversaccio M. Petrous bone cholesteatoma removal with hearing preservation. Otol Neurotol. 2011;32(2):236–41.
22. Danesi G, Cooper T, Panciera DT, Manni V, Côté DW. Sanna classification and prognosis of cholesteatoma of the petrous part of the temporal bone: a retrospective series of 81 patients. Otol Neurotol. 2016;37(6):787–92.
23. Kim MJ, An YS, Jang MS, Cho YS, Chung JW. Hearing and facial function after surgical removal of cholesteatomas involving petrous bone. Clin Exp Otorhinolaryngol. 2014;7(4):264–8.
24. Miller ME, Mastrodimos B, Cueva RA. Hearing preservation in management of epidermoids of the cerebellopontine angle: CPA epidermoids and hearing preservation. Otol Neurotol. 2012;33(9):1599–603.
25. Schroeder HW, Oertel J, Gaab MR. Endoscope-assisted microsurgical resection of epidermoid tumors of the cerebellopontine angle. J Neurosurg. 2004;101(2):227–32.
26. Tuchman A, Platt A, Winer J, Pham M, Giannotta S, Zada G. Endoscopic-assisted resection of intracranial epidermoid tumors. World Neurosurg. 2014;82(3–4):450–4.
27. Darrouzet V, Franco-Vidal V, Hilton M, et al. Surgery of cerebellopontine angle epidermoid cysts: role of the widened retrolabyrinthine approach combined with endoscopy. Otolaryngol Head Neck Surg. 2004;131(1):120–5.
28. Sellier A, Troude L, Baumgarten C, et al. Long-term surgical oncological and functional outcome of large petroclival and cerebellopontine angle epidermoid cysts: a multicenter study. Neurosurg Rev. 2022;45(3):2119–31.
29. Safavi-Abbasi S, Di Rocco F, Bambakidis N, et al. Has management of epidermoid tumors of the cerebellopontine angle improved? A surgical synopsis of the past and present. Skull Base. 2008;18(2):85–98.
30. Meng L, Yuguang L, Feng L, Wandong S, Shugan Z, Chengyuan W. Cerebellopontine angle epidermoids presenting with trigeminal neuralgia. J Clin Neurosci. 2005;12(7):784–6.
31. Kobata H, Kondo A, Iwasaki K. Cerebellopontine angle epidermoids presenting with cranial nerve hyperactive dysfunction: pathogenesis and long-term surgical results in 30 patients. Neurosurgery. 2002;50(2):276–85; discussion 285–276.
32. Gopalakrishnan CV, Ansari KA, Nair S, Menon G. Long term outcome in surgically treated posterior fossa epidermoids. Clin Neurol Neurosurg. 2014;117:93–9.
33. Sakamoto H, Kohno M, Matsushima K, Ichimasu N, Nakajima N, Yoshino M. Importance of appropriate surgical approach selection for radical resection of cerebellopontine angle epidermoid cysts with preservation of cranial nerve functions: our experience of 54 cases. Acta Neurochir. 2021;163(9):2465–74.
34. Hamlat A, Hua ZF, Saikali S, et al. Malignant transformation of intra-cranial epithelial cysts: systematic article review. J Neuro-Oncol. 2005;74(2):187–94.
35. Kaylie DM, Warren FM 3rd, Haynes DS, Jackson CG. Neurotologic management of intracranial epidermoid tumors. Laryngoscope. 2005;115(6):1082–6.
36. Chon KH, Lee JM, Koh EJ, Choi HY. Malignant transformation of an epidermoid cyst in the cerebellopontine angle. J Korean Neurosurg Soc. 2012;52(2):148–51.

Nonneoplastic Lesions of the Petrous Apex

78

Eric E. Babajanian and Neil S. Patel

Introduction

The petrous apex is the pyramidally shaped, medial portion of the petrous temporal bone (Fig. 78.1). Its boundaries are defined by the petrooccipital fissure medially, the petrosphenoidal fissure anteriorly, the inner ear laterally, and the posterior cranial fossa posteriorly. The superior boundary is the middle cranial fossa, while the inferior boundary is the inferior petrosal sinus and jugular bulb. The petrous apex is divided into a larger anterior portion and a smaller posterior portion by the internal auditory canal (IAC). The petrous apex may contain bone marrow and have variable degrees of pneumatization (symmetrically or asymmetrically).

The clinical presentation of pathologies involving the petrous apex is largely dependent on the involvement of adjacent structures. As such, it is difficult to reliably produce a diagnosis based on clinical findings alone. Symptoms that should prompt imaging evaluation of the petrous apex are varied. Some patients will present with generalized or focal headaches, prompting imaging that reveals a petrous apex lesion. While retro-orbital pain or deep otalgia may be related, it is generally thought that benign, non-expansile lesions of the petrous apex are not directly related to headache. Often, evaluation for a common otologic symptom yields a surprising finding in the petrous apex that then leads to additional investigation. Asymmetric mixed or sensorineural hearing loss is more commonly associated with nonneoplastic petrous apex lesions than with purely conductive hearing loss. Otorrhea is nonspecific, but it can be a symptom of a medial lesion affecting the middle ear. Dizziness, while inherently nonspecific, could be related to petrous apex pathology if a third window is created in the labyrinth or if the vestibulocochlear nerve is affected in the internal auditory canal.

Cranial neuropathy from nonneoplastic petrous apex lesions generally results from expansion and compression of regional nerves or coexistent pathologies that can result in nerve deficits (i.e., an extensive cholesteatoma with facial paralysis). The abducens nerve is most susceptible to localized petrous apex pathologies due to its location within Dorello's canal, bordered superiorly by the petrosphenoidal (Gruber's) ligament. Other regional cranial nerves, such as the trigeminal nerve or lower cranial nerves, are at a lower risk of dysfunction from the pathologies themselves but may be at significant risk if the lesion is treated surgically.

The workhorse imaging modalities for petrous apex lesions in general are computed tomography (CT) and magnetic resonance imaging (MRI). The specific signal characteristics are listed in the subsections below and compared in Table 78.1. Nuclear medicine studies using radioisotopes of gallium or technetium or radionuclide-tagged white blood cell imaging are only valuable in cases of skull base osteomyelitis affecting the petrous apex or central skull base.

This chapter describes the various nonneoplastic lesions that may be found in the petrous apex. These include pseudolesions, mucoceles, cholesteatomas, cholesterol granulomas, encephaloceles, and infections that can result in petrous apicitis or skull base osteomyelitis. The discussion of neoplastic lesions is beyond the scope of this chapter but may include benign lesions such as meningiomas, schwannomas, and paragangliomas, in addition to malignant lesions such as chondrosarcomas, chordomas, and metastases, all of which are discussed in other chapters. Relative to the rest of the temporal bone portions, the petrous apex is difficult to reach, given its deep position. Several approaches have been developed to access this area, which will also be described later in the chapter.

E. E. Babajanian
Spokane Ear, Nose and Throat, Spokane, WA, USA
e-mail: ebabajanian@spokaneent.com

N. S. Patel (✉)
Department of Otolaryngology—Head and Neck Surgery,
University of Utah, Salt Lake City, UT, USA
e-mail: neil.patel@hsc.utah.edu

A. D. Sweeney et al. (eds.), *Haynes-Glasscock-Shambaugh Surgery of the Ear*, https://doi.org/10.1007/978-3-032-18264-7_78

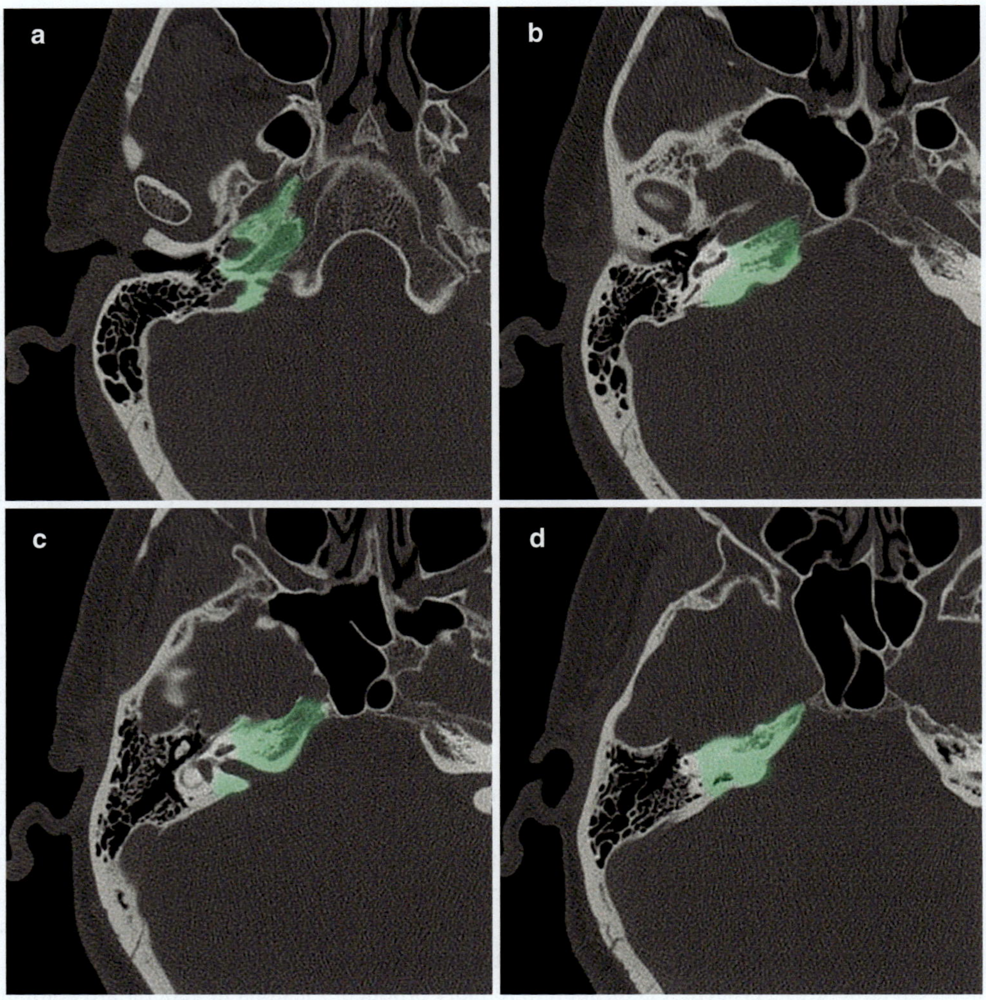

Fig. 78.1 Boundaries of the petrous apex on computed tomography at the level of (**a**) the jugular bulb, (**b**) cochlea, (**c**) internal auditory canal, and (**d**) superior semicircular canal

Table 78.1 Characteristics of petrous apex lesions

Lesion	Expansile	CT findings	MRI T1	MRI T2
Asymmetric pneumatization with fatty marrow	No	No bony remodeling	Hyperintense Suppressed on fat saturation	Hypointense
Effusion	No	No bony remodeling	Variable	Isointense to CSF
Mucocele	Yes	Cystic, smooth bony remodeling	Hypointense with post-gadolinium rim enhancement	Hyperintense
Cholesterol granuloma	Yes	Smooth bony remodeling	Hyperintense	Hyperintense
Cholesteatoma	Yes	Smooth bony remodeling	Hypointense	Hyperintense High diffusion restriction
Arachnoid cysts	Variable	Possible smooth bony remodeling	Hypointense	Isointense to CSF
Cephalocele	Yes	Possible smooth bony remodeling	Hypointense	Isointense to CSF
Petrous apicitis	No	Irregular bony remodeling	Hypointense with post-gadolinium rim enhancement	Hyperintense

Nonneoplastic Lesions of the Petrous Apex

Pseudolesions: Asymmetrical Pneumatization, Asymmetrical Marrow, and Effusion

Pseudolesions of the petrous apex refer to entities that are distinct and noteworthy on imaging but do not clearly correspond to pathologies requiring intervention. Pseudolesions are generally related to variable pneumatization of the petrous apex, which is present in up to 35% of patients [1] and can include asymmetric fatty marrow or a unilateral trapped effusion. Asymmetric pneumatization is reported in up to 7% of patients (Fig. 78.2). A trapped effusion that is T2 hyperintense to brain or isointense to cerebrospinal fluid (CSF) is generally innocuous unless there is clinical concern for a spontaneous or acquired cerebrospinal fluid fistula. In

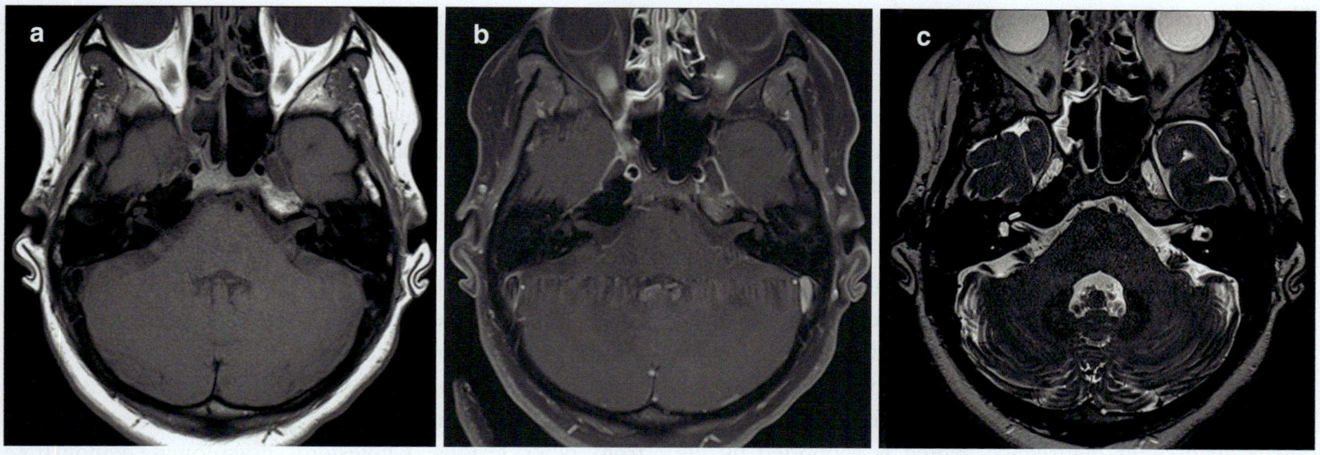

Fig. 78.2 Asymmetric pneumatization with fatty marrow of the left temporal bone. (**a**) T1-weighted image demonstrating signal isointense to fat, (**b**) gadolinium-enhanced T1-weighted image showing no contrast enhancement, and (**c**) heavily T2-weighted image showing signal isointense to brain

most of these cases, opacification of air cells elsewhere in the temporal bone or in the middle ear cavity is present.

Asymmetric fatty marrow within the petrous apex is a common incidental finding on head and neck imaging. This finding is important to identify, as it can sometimes lead to misdiagnosis or result in unnecessary further workup. Normal marrow contains a variable amount of fatty adipose tissue, which presents with similar signal characteristics as orbital fat on imaging. On MRI studies, fatty marrow will be hyperintense on T1-weighted sequences and somewhat hypointense on T2-weighted sequences. Fat saturation sequences can be useful in confirming the presence of fatty marrow.

Prior otitis media may result in unilateral, trapped petrous apex effusions due to the obstruction of drainage from the petrous air cells to the middle ear. Patients with this finding are typically asymptomatic unless there is an underlying active infectious process present. The latter would usually be evident with the use of contrast-enhanced MRI. On MRI, trapped fluid is generally hyperintense on T2-weighted images (similar to cerebrospinal fluid (CSF)) and with variable signal intensity on T1-weighted images. Proteinaceous trapped fluid can result in intermediate or high signal intensity on T1-weighted images. A unilateral trapped effusion is important to identify, as it can be mistaken for a cholesterol granuloma, which is discussed below. If high signal intensity on T2- and T1-weighted images is seen, further examination with CT is warranted to evaluate the expansile characteristics of the lesion or trabecular disruption, which will help distinguish a trapped effusion from a cholesterol granuloma [2]. It may also be prudent to obtain follow-up CT imaging over time to ensure that lesions with intermediate or high T1 signal intensity do not demonstrate continued expansion.

Mucocele

Mucoceles of the petrous apex are relatively uncommon lesions that may present as cystic lesions resulting from either obstructed ventilatory pathways or the inclusion of seromucinous tissue, leading to secretion retention [3]. Mucoceles can be expansile and locally destructive, leading to variable symptomatology depending on the size and location of the lesion. Described symptoms can include headache, dizziness, tinnitus, and/or hearing loss [3, 4]. The lining of a mucocele consists of thin, cuboidal epithelium producing mucous and may be inspissated in some instances. On CT imaging, mucoceles can appear similar to both cholesteatomas and cholesterol granulomas, as each may present with an expansile appearance. Mucoceles are cystic in appearance with sharp borders and potentially multiple loculations. Contrast enhancement is not generally seen within the mucocele, though the borders can be rim-enhancing. MRI can readily distinguish a cholesterol granuloma, but cholesteatomas and mucoceles may not be as easily differentiated. The MRI appearance of a mucocele can be variable, as it is determined by whether its contents are hydrated, proteinaceous, or inspissated [5]. Hydrated mucoceles usually present with low signal intensity on pre-contrast T1-weighted images, rim enhancement on post-contrast T1-weighted images, and uniformly high signal intensity on T2-weighted images [6]. Diffusion-weighted imaging is particularly useful, as cholesteatomas typically demonstrate high signal intensity due to restricted diffusion, while mucoceles or fluid-filled cysts of similar compositions do not [7].

Cholesterol Granuloma

Cholesterol granulomas are cyst-like lesions that form as a result of anaerobic metabolism of blood in a mucosalized space. A foreign body–like reaction is thought to occur as a result of a giant cell response to cholesterol crystals that are resistant to absorption [8]. Different hypotheses exist for why bleeding occurs in the petrous apex. One explanation is that the negative pressure from Eustachian tube dysfunction results in bleeding into a pneumatized and mucosalized space within the petrous apex, leading to an inflammatory response. Another potential explanation by Jackler and Cho is that there is exposed marrow to a pneumatized air cell secondary to osseous dehiscence, which is supported by the finding of osseous dehiscence in the contralateral petrous bone [9]. This explanation takes into account the notion that middle ear hemorrhage and hyperpneumatization of the temporal bone are rare in patients with Eustachian tube dysfunction and that pressure should be equalized once an air cell is filled with blood.

Cholesterol granulomas are the most common primary lesion found in the petrous apex, occurring up to ten times more often than petrous apex cholesteatomas [10]. Various symptoms can be associated with their presentation, including headache, retro-orbital pain or deep otalgia, hearing loss, dizziness, or ear pressure. Often, patients are asymptomatic, with lesions noted incidentally on imaging obtained for unrelated reasons. As with other lesions of the petrous apex, both CT and MRI studies are imperative for the diagnosis of cholesterol granulomas.

CT imaging demonstrates an expansile lesion with smooth surrounding bony erosion. CT angiography or venography may be indicated to evaluate for vascular compression if erosion into the carotid canal or jugular foramen is suspected. MRI is critical for differentiating cholesterol granulomas from other lesions. Cholesterol granulomas demonstrate high signal intensity on both T1- and T2-weighted images, distinguishing them from other petrous apex lesions (Fig. 78.3).

Management of cholesterol granulomas is dependent on the patient's symptoms at the time of presentation. Observation may be appropriate in asymptomatic or minimally symptomatic patients. Surveillance can be accomplished via interval MRI without gadolinium contrast so long

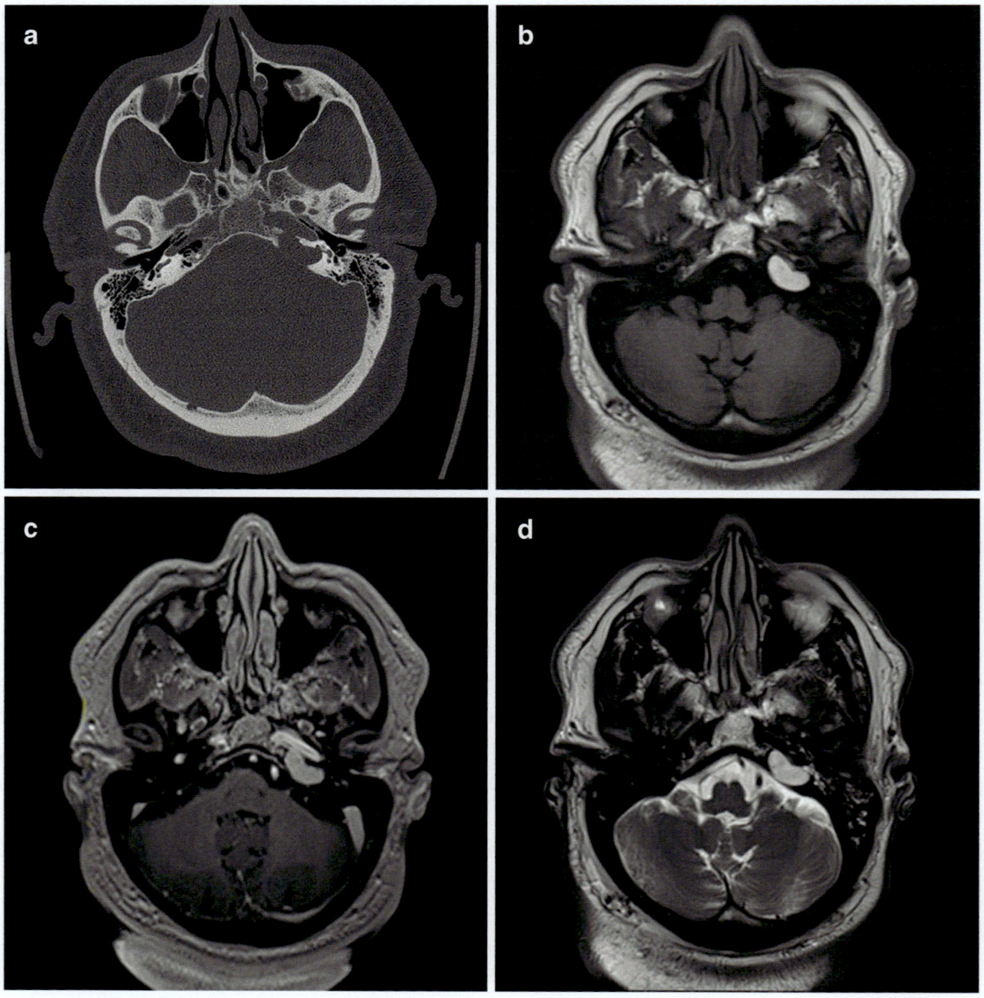

Fig. 78.3 Cholesterol granuloma of the left petrous apex. (**a**) CT demonstrating a smooth, scalloped appearance; (**b**) T1-weighted image; (**c**) gadolinium-enhanced T1-weighted image; and (**d**) T2-weighted image

as symptoms remain stable. CT imaging adds additional value in determining the degree of bony expansion or erosion and, as such, has value in monitoring disease progression, particularly when evaluating for the involvement of the carotid canal, labyrinth, or internal auditory canal. For symptomatic patients or those at risk for an impending complication with growth of the lesion, surgical management is appropriate. Operative intervention would entail marsupialization or excision. Marsupialization generally avoids the need for wide exposure of the lesion via craniotomy, though there is an increased risk for recurrence with this approach should an obstruction develop in the drainage tract [11]. Approaches to cholesterol granuloma drainage are described in more detail below.

Cholesteatoma

Cholesteatomas, or epidermoid cysts, in the petrous apex are generally considered to be congenital in origin, resulting from abnormal rests of epithelial tissue. These entities are discussed in Chap. 77. Acquired cholesteatoma is not common in the petrous apex, but aggressive lesions originating in the tympanomastoid cavity can result in extensive erosion of the petrous bone. While relatively uncommon overall, cholesteatomas account for up to 9% of all petrous apex lesions [12, 13]. The lining of a cholesteatoma (or "matrix") consists of stratified squamous epithelium. With desquamation of tissue within the cyst, keratinized debris accumulates, resulting in gradual expansion of the cyst and surrounding bony resorption. While these lesions are typically slow-growing and asymptomatic at first, enlargement can result in damage to nearby structures, resulting in symptoms such as hearing loss, dizziness, or cranial neuropathies [13]. Intradural extension of an epidermoid cyst can result in an uncommon but unique complication termed chemical meningitis, whereby the cyst contents create a sterile inflammatory meningitis. Bacterial meningitis could result as well but would more commonly be associated with an extensive infectious process involving the middle ear or ear canal. High-resolution CT imaging is essential to identifying the relationship of the lesion with the boundaries of the petrous apex, facial nerve, and labyrinth. A characteristic, clearly defined expansile lesion with smooth expansion of the surrounding bone is generally seen in these cases. As discussed earlier, MRI is particularly useful to differentiate cholesteatoma from other possible lesions (Fig. 78.4). Cholesteatomas have low signal intensity on T1-weighted images, high signal intensity on T2-weighted images, and high diffusion restriction on diffusion-weighted imaging [14], which distinguishes them from an arachnoid cyst. The absence of enhancement can be useful to distinguish a cholesteatoma from a benign bone tumor [3]. Complete resection of petrous apex cholesteatomas is challenging due to the involvement of surrounding neurovascular structures or the labyrinth. Serial postoperative imaging using MRI with diffusion-weighted imaging is necessary for surveillance, with the most common location for recurrence being the more medial petrous structures, including the labyrinthine portion of the facial nerve or the petrous carotid artery [15]. Often, multiple procedures are required in a patient's lifetime to debulk a cholesteatoma where the matrix is adherent to critical neurovascular structures.

Arachnoid Cysts and Cephaloceles

Arachnoid cysts are CSF-filled sacs that occur on the arachnoid membrane. Often incidentally discovered, these lesions rarely erode into the posterior aspect of the petrous apex [16]. CT imaging demonstrates scalloped bony erosion, and MRI demonstrates the exact same characteristics as CSF, with high signal intensity on T2-weighted images [17]. Arachnoid cysts often require no imaging follow-up unless there is risk of a CSF leak or new symptoms develop. Operative intervention is controversial for arachnoid cysts, as it is challenging to identify symptoms that are directly attributable to the lesion itself. If surgery is undertaken, fenestration of the cyst into a nearby cistern is favored over an attempt to "excise" the arachnoid membranes around it. Given that the overall volume occupied by CSF in these areas remains roughly the same, postoperative imaging may look quite similar to preoperative imaging, and patient symptoms should be used as a marker of a successful intervention. Extensive drilling should be avoided, as a CSF leak into the temporal bone could result.

Cephaloceles refer to cystic lesions that arise as a result of the herniation of intradural tissue. Within the petrous apex, these are rare entities that occur as a result of herniation via the posterolateral portion of Meckel's cave. While often asymptomatic, these may be the etiology of a spontaneous CSF leak [18]. CT imaging demonstrates smooth or scalloped bony erosion of the anterior petrous apex. On MRI, these lesions have the same characteristics as arachnoid cysts, but are often continuous with Meckel's cave, located in the anterior petrous apex (Fig. 78.5). Asymptomatic patients may be observed with serial imaging, but patients who present with CSF leaks should undergo operative intervention via a middle fossa approach to facilitate resurfacing and obliteration of the cyst cavity [17].

Petrous Apicitis

Petrous apicitis occurs as a result of the extension of otomastoiditis medially via pneumatized air cells to the petrous apex. This is a relatively rare infectious complication in the era of antibiotics, and the most common offending organisms

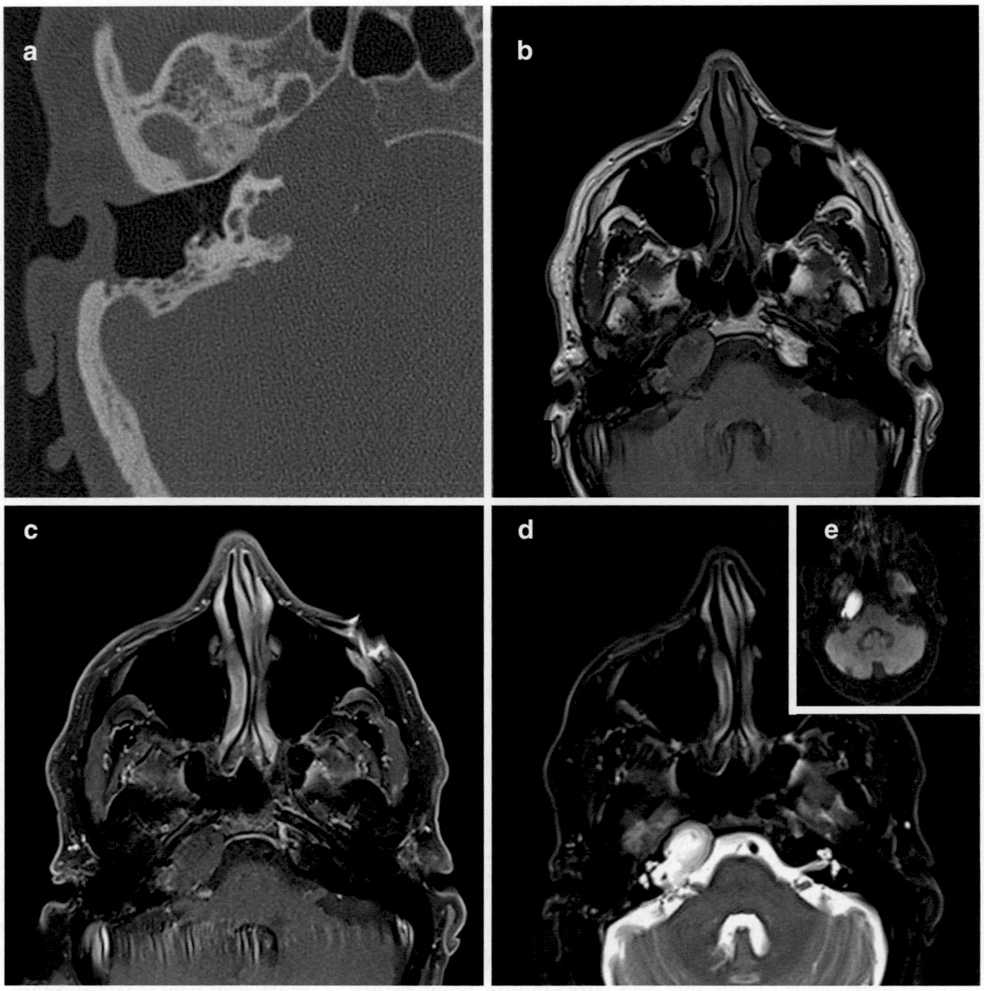

Fig. 78.4 Cholesteatoma (epidermoid cyst) of the right petrous apex. (**a**) CT imaging showing smooth bony expansion with destruction of the internal auditory canal and cochlea, (**b**) T1-weighted image, (**c**) gadolinium-enhanced T1-weighted image, (**d**) T2-weighted image, and (**e**) non-echo planar diffusion-weighted image showing diffusion restriction

are the same as those for acute otitis media [19]. Early in the process, purulent exudate fills the petrous apex. This may progress to cortical demineralization and bony resorption, which has the potential to spread into the adjacent marrow space, precipitating osteomyelitis of the petrous skull base. Complications of progressive infection include internal carotid vasospasm and/or arteritis, thrombophlebitis, sinus thrombosis, meningitis, and abscess formation [14].

The presentation of petrous apicitis is variable, with the most common symptoms being retro-orbital or facial pain in the trigeminal distribution, otorrhea, otalgia, and dizziness [20]. Gradenigo's triad refers to the combination of otorrhea, abducens palsy, and retro-orbital pain. While typically taught to be pathognomonic for petrous apicitis, Gradenigo's triad is only seen in 20% of patients [20].

CT imaging demonstrates opacification of the petrous apex with bony destruction akin to coalescent mastoiditis. MRI reveals a low signal intensity with rim enhancement on T1-weighted images and high signal intensity on T2-weighted images. Fluid-fluid levels may be present if there is purulence within the cavity.

Treatment for petrous apicitis typically involves parenteral antibiotic therapy and myringotomy with or without tympanostomy tube placement for aspiration culture and topical antibiotic delivery. Patients who fail to improve may require drainage of the petrous apex, though the risk-benefit analysis in this situation can be challenging if a drainage corridor is not readily apparent. Surgical approaches are described in detail below.

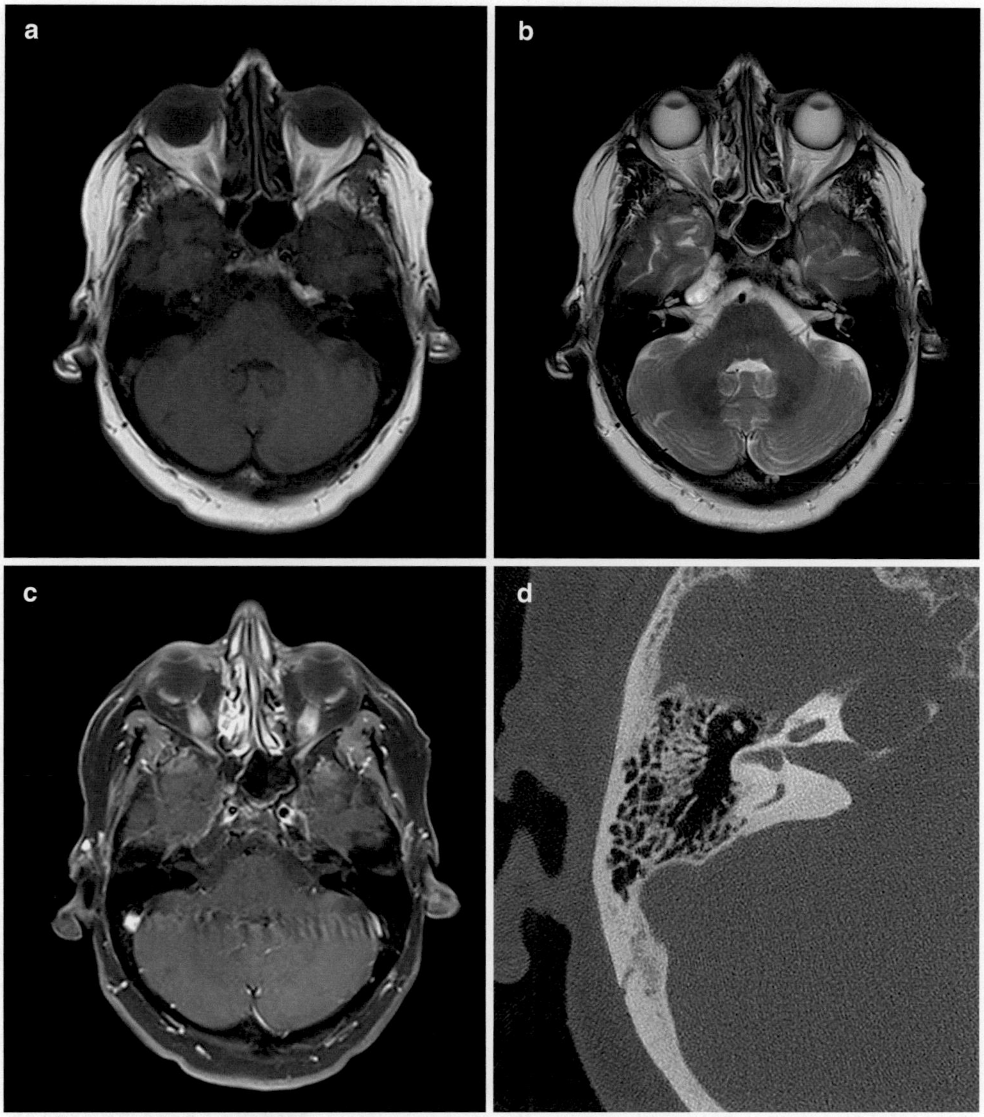

Fig. 78.5 Cephalocele of the right petrous apex. (**a**) T1-weighted image showing signal isointense to CSF and contralateral petrous apex with fat signal consistent with marrow, (**b**) T2-weighted image, (**c**) gadolinium-enhanced T1-weighted image, and (**d**) CT showing smooth boundaries without bony destruction

Approaches to the Petrous Apex

The petrous apex can be one of the most challenging structures to approach in otologic surgery. In some skull base pathologies, multiple surgical approaches exist and can be employed with similar results in a generalizable fashion. In the petrous apex, multiple approaches exist, but the approach selection needs to be carefully considered and individualized in light of multiple patient-specific factors. The optimal approach for accessing a petrous apex lesion is largely dependent on the following considerations:

- Present extent and natural history of the lesion
- Status and involvement of regional cranial nerves
- Preoperative hearing and vestibular function
- Patient age and medical comorbidities
- Side of lesion, as it pertains to the dominant or nondominant temporal lobe

Infralabyrinthine Approach

First described by Dearmin in 1937, the infralabyrinthine approach to the petrous apex allows exposure of a petrous apex lesion via the infralabyrinthine air cell tract and is the most commonly utilized approach for drainage of petrous apex lesions [21]. While this is a relatively direct approach to the anterior and inferior portions of the petrous apex, limitations include limited exposure through a relatively narrow corridor and the inability to remove the tissue lining of the lesion cavity. Given these limitations, it is not typically feasible to achieve gross total resection of a lesion, and rather, it can be a good approach to incise and drain an inferiorly located lesion. The infralabyrinthine approach preserves hearing, as neither the labyrinth nor the cochlea is entered. As such, it is a good option for patients with serviceable hearing who present with lesions that are amenable to drainage, such as cholesterol granulomas. The infralabyrinthine approach can be difficult—if not impossible—in patients with a high jugular bulb or posteriorly positioned carotid artery. Preoperative evaluation of imaging is imperative to determine whether the infralabyrinthine approach is feasible, as some patients may have a high jugular bulb in extremely close apposition to the inner ear structures. In some patients, the jugular bulb may be skeletonized and compressed to facilitate visualization and access to the lesion.

After performing a cortical mastoidectomy, the vertical segment of the facial nerve, sigmoid sinus, and jugular bulb are identified. The facial nerve serves as the anterior boundary of dissection, while the jugular bulb is the inferior border. Visualization and drainage aperture can be improved with bony decompression of the sigmoid sinus and removal of the bone over the posterior fossa to allow posterior retraction. The inferior portion of the posterior semicircular canal is skeletonized to delineate the superior border of the dissection, taking care not to expose the membranous portion of the canal. The infralabyrinthine retrofacial air cell tract can then be followed anteromedially toward the petrous apex, allowing for identification and drainage of the lesion.

Transcanal Infracochlear Approach

The transcanal infracochlear approach can be particularly useful for drainage of an inferior petrous apex lesion in patients with a high-riding jugular bulb that prohibits the previously described infralabyrinthine approach and is posteriorly oriented enough to create a corridor between it and the carotid artery [22]. As with the infralabyrinthine approach, the transcanal infracochlear approach is an approach best suited for patients with lesions amenable to drainage, as gross total resection is not feasible, given the relatively limited exposure. Advantages of this approach include a more direct route to the petrous apex and dependent drainage into an aerated portion of the middle ear near the Eustachian tube. Similar to the infralabyrinthine approach, neither the labyrinth nor the cochlea is entered as part of this approach, and as such, it can be used in patients with preserved hearing preoperatively. Limitations to this approach include the potential injury to the cochlea, carotid artery, and jugular bulb, and postoperative scarring can result in the obliteration of the drainage pathway. A high jugular bulb within the tympanic cavity can restrict the ability to perform this approach, though it may still be feasible in patients in whom a high jugular bulb obstructs the infralabyrinthine approach.

After raising a superiorly based tympanomeatal flap, the hypotympanum is exposed via drilling of the external canal bone anteroinferiorly. In order to prevent injury to the facial nerve, the chorda tympani can be followed inferiorly. With the round window serving as the superior border of dissection, air cells are removed inferior to the cochlea, exposing the course of the jugular bulb and the carotid artery, separated by the jugulocarotid spine. The jugular bulb serves as the inferior border of dissection and the posterior border of dissection (along with the facial nerve), while the carotid artery is the anterior border. Dissection is continued medially until the lesion is identified and drained. Some surgeons insert a small Silastic shunt to stent the tract open.

Transarcuate Approach

A rare approach to the petrous apex is the transarcuate approach, which allows access to the posterior petrous apex by following the air cell tract between the crura of the superior semicircular canal. This approach may also be utilized in patients with a non-pneumatized subarcuate area. Djalilian et al. determined that the mean anterior–posterior dimension of this intracrural space is 4.88 mm, while the superior–inferior dimension is 4.90 mm [23]. Similar to the transmastoid approach for treatment of superior semicircular canal dehiscence, the primary limiting factor for this approach would be a low-lying tegmen mastoideum. As the membranous labyrinth is not entered in this approach, hearing is generally preserved. Given the limited exposure attained, this approach is most suitable for drainage rather than resection, similar to what is described above.

After performing a cortical mastoidectomy, the tegmen mastoideum, sigmoid sinus, and lateral semicircular canal are identified. The labyrinth is skeletonized, followed by blue-lining of the superior semicircular canal. The intracrural space is then followed medially until the lesion is identified and drained.

Middle Fossa Approach

The middle cranial fossa serves as the superior boundary of the petrous pyramid, and thus, the middle fossa approach provides superiorly oriented access [24–26]. It is most often used for small vestibular schwannomas, superior canal dehiscence surgery, facial nerve lesions, or repair of CSF leaks or encephaloceles. For most lesions, the middle fossa approach is the only hearing-preserving means of resecting a lesion of the petrous apex. For instance, a cholesterol granuloma with serviceable hearing may be drained via lateral approaches, but resection of the cyst wall without violating the labyrinth may be most feasible through a middle fossa approach. The main disadvantage of this approach is temporal lobe retraction, which is contraindicated in elderly individuals or those with significant medical comorbidities, particularly if the lesion is left-sided. In addition, the carotid artery, Eustachian tube, internal auditory canal, and trigeminal nerve are all at risk during bone removal in the apex. Another disadvantage is that this approach may be suboptimal for lesions that are more inferior within the petrous apex.

The procedure begins with a temporal craniotomy that is centered two-thirds anterior to the coronal plane of the external auditory canal. Once the bone flap is removed, the lower edge of the craniotomy is lowered to the middle fossa floor, and the dura is meticulously elevated from posterior to anterior. Once the superior canal and the greater superficial petrosal nerve are identified, dissection of the dura is carried anteromedially until the trigeminal impression is encountered. Often, the middle meningeal artery is divided to provide greater dural elevation. After placing retractors, the bone of the petrous apex can be drilled until the lesion is encountered. A fat graft may be placed in the bony defect to mitigate the risk of a CSF leak or obliterate the space, but this is not required if the surrounding dura is intact.

Endoscopic Transsphenoidal Approach

Since Montgomery first described the transnasal transsphenoidal approach to the petrous apex in 1977, advances in endoscopic technique have allowed for a relatively direct approach to lesions located near the posterior wall of the sphenoid sinus [27]. Advantages to this approach include a reduced risk of injury to the facial nerve and inner ear contents, dependent drainage into the sinonasal system, and improved access to the inferior limits of the anterior petrous apex [28]. There is a relatively increased risk to the carotid artery, and this approach may not be feasible if the petrous portion of the carotid artery overlies the lesion medially. As the inner ear and middle ear conductive mechanisms are not exposed, hearing is preserved, and the risk of facial nerve injury is minimized with this approach. A particular advantage of this approach is the ability to open a relatively large drainage pathway that can be subsequently followed in the clinical setting.

After entering the sphenoid ostium via a transnasal or transethmoid approach, the ostium is enlarged inferiorly and medially. A posterior septectomy is performed, and the sphenoid mucosa is removed from the floor and back wall. The carotid artery defines the lateral border of dissection and is thus imperative to identify via intraoperative image-guided navigation and Doppler in order to avoid vascular injury. Image guidance can also be useful for preventing injury to the optic tract, cavernous sinus, and hypophysis. The posterior septal wall is then removed, and dissection is continued until the lesion is identified and drained.

Subtotal Petrosectomy

The term "subtotal petrosectomy" generally refers to a procedure in which most of the air cell tracts within the temporal bone are exteriorized. The subtotal petrosectomy approach with removal of the otic capsule allows complete exposure of the petrous apex, facilitating complete removal of lesions in this area [29]. It also permits access to the posterior fossa and the complete course of the intratemporal facial nerve by way of transotic or transcochlear techniques. Given the need for removal of the otic capsule in order to access the entire petrous apex from a lateral perspective, the primary disadvantage to this approach is that it can result in complete hearing loss and unilateral vestibulopathy. As a result, in the context of nonneoplastic lesions, this approach is most often used when the pathology has already resulted in significant destruction of the otic capsule (such as with a large epidermoid cyst). With wide exposure, gross total resection can frequently be achieved, if necessary.

The surgical approach begins with a canal wall down mastoidectomy, followed by removal of the supralabyrinthine, retrolabyrinthine, infralabyrinthine, and retrofacial air cells. At this point, the otic capsule is entered, and both the cochlea and bony labyrinth are removed. Transposition of the facial nerve can be performed, but in most instances, it is left in a fallopian bridge to avoid injury and facilitate identification if a future surgery is required. With the resulting wide exposure of the petrous apex, the lesion is then identified and excised using microsurgical techniques. The Eustachian tube is obliterated, the resulting cavity is obliterated with a fat graft, and the external auditory canal is closed.

Conclusion

The petrous apex is a relatively challenging region to access within the temporal bone, within which multiple neoplastic and nonneoplastic lesions may arise. As presenting clinical symptoms vary and depend on the location and extent of the offending lesion, imaging with MR or CT is imperative for diagnosis and surgical planning. As with any skull base lesion, patient factors, anticipated or extant progression, location, and status of the inner ear and facial nerve are the primary determinants of management. Access to the petrous apex can be achieved with a variety of transtemporal approaches, with the optimal choice being dependent on the location of the lesion and the goal of intervention.

References

1. Virapongse C, Sarwar M, Bhimani S, Sasaki C, Shapiro R. Computed tomography of temporal bone pneumatization: 1. Normal pattern and morphology. Am J Roentgenol. 1985;145(3):473–81.
2. Moore KR, Harnsberger HR, Shelton C, Davidson HC. 'Leave me alone' lesions of the petrous apex. Am J Neuroradiol. 1998;19(4):733–8.
3. Muckle RP, De la Cruz A, Lo WM. Petrous apex lesions. Am J Otol. 1998;19(2):219–25.

4. Memis A, Memis A, Alper H, Calli C, Ozer H, Ozdamar N. Petrous apex mucocele: high resolution CT. Neuroradiology. 1994;36(8):632–3.
5. Van Tassel P, Lee Y, Jing B, De Pena C. Mucoceles of the paranasal sinuses: MR imaging with CT correlation. Am J Roentgenol. 1989;153(2):407–12.
6. Larson TL, Wong ML. Primary mucocele of the petrous apex: MR appearance. Am J Neuroradiol. 1992;13(1):203–4.
7. Le BT, Roehm PC. Petrous Apex Mucocele. Otol Neurotol. 2008;29(1):102–3.
8. Kuruma T, Tanigawa T, Uchida Y, Tetsuya O, Ueda H. Large cholesterol granuloma of the middle ear eroding into the middle cranial fossa. Case Rep Otolaryngol. 2017;2017:1–5.
9. Jackler RK, Cho M. A new theory to explain the genesis of petrous apex cholesterol granuloma. Otol Neurotol. 2003;24(1):96–106; discussion.
10. Arriaga MA, Brackmann DE. Differential diagnosis of primary petrous apex lesions. Am J Otol. 1991;12(6):470–4.
11. Isaacson B. Cholesterol granuloma and other petrous apex lesions. Otolaryngol Clin N Am. 2015;48(2):361–73.
12. McGuire JK, Wasl H, Harris T, Copley GJ, Fagan JJ. Management of pediatric cholesteatoma based on presentations, complications, and outcomes. Int J Pediatr Otorhinolaryngol. 2016;80:69–73.
13. Reardon T, Turnow M, Elston S, Brown NJ, Koller GM, Sharma S, et al. Surgical management of petrous apex cholesteatomas in the pediatric population: a systematic review. Surg Neurol Int. 2022;13:494.
14. Chapman PR, Shah R, Cure JK, Bag AK. Petrous apex lesions: pictorial review. Am J Roentgenol. 2011;196(3 Suppl):WS26–37. Quiz S40-3.
15. Atlas MD, Moffat DA, Hardy DG. Petrous apex cholesteatoma: diagnostic and treatment dilemmas. Laryngoscope. 1992;102(12 Pt 1):1363–8.
16. Isaacson B, Coker NJ, Vrabec JT, Yoshor D, Oghalai JS. Invasive cerebrospinal fluid cysts and cephaloceles of the petrous apex. Otol Neurotol. 2006;27(8):1131–41.
17. Isaacson B, Kutz JW, Roland PS. Lesions of the petrous apex: diagnosis and management. Otolaryngol Clin N Am. 2007;40(3):479–519. viii
18. Sdano MT, Pensak ML. Temporal bone encephaloceles. Curr Opin Otolaryngol Head Neck Surg. 2005;13(5):287–9.
19. Gadre AK, Chole RA. The changing face of petrous apicitis-a 40-year experience. Laryngoscope. 2018;128(1):195–201.
20. Talmor G, Vakil M, Tseng C, Svider P, Ying M, Eloy JA. Petrous apicitis: a systematic review and case presentation. Otol Neurotol. 2022;43(7):753–65.
21. Dearmin RM. A logical surgical approach to the tip cells of the petrous pyramid. Arch Otolaryngol Head Neck Surg. 1937;26(3):314–20.
22. Giddings NA, Brackmann DE, Kwartler JA. Transcanal infracochlear approach to the petrous apex. Otolaryngol Head Neck Surg. 1991;104(1):29–36.
23. Lee A, Hamidi S, Djalilian H. Anatomy of the transarcuate approach to the petrous apex. Otolaryngol Head Neck Surg. 2009;140(6):880–3.
24. Diaz Day J. The middle fossa approach and extended middle fossa approach: technique and operative nuances. Neurosurgery. 2012;70(2 Suppl Operative):192–201.
25. Naguib MB, Aristegui M, Saleh E, Cokkeser Y, Landolfi M, Taibah A, et al. Surgical anatomy of the petrous apex as it relates to the enlarged middle cranial fossa approaches. Otolaryngol Head Neck Surg. 1994;111(4):488–93.
26. Lipschitz N, Kohlberg GD, Zuccarello M, Samy RN. Comprehensive review of the extended middle cranial fossa approach. Curr Opin Otolaryngol Head Neck Surg. 2018;26(5):286–92.
27. Montgomery WW. Cystic lesions of the petrous apex: transsphenoid approach. Ann Otol Rhinol Laryngol. 1977;86(4 Pt 1):429–35.
28. Van Gompel JJ, Alikhani P, Tabor MH, Van Loveren HR, Agazzi S, Froelich S, et al. Anterior inferior petrosectomy: defining the role of endonasal endoscopic techniques for petrous apex approaches. J Neurosurg. 2014;120(6):1321–5.
29. Coker NJ, Jenkins HA, Fisch U. Obliteration of the middle ear and mastoid cleft in subtotal petrosectomy: indications, technique, and results. Ann Otol Rhinol Laryngol. 1986;95(1 Pt 1):5–11.

Chordoma and Chondrosarcoma

79

Jamie J. Van Gompel, Garret W. Choby, Yuki Shinya, and Sukwoo Hong

Abbreviations/Acronyms

Gy	Gray
RTKs	Receptor tyrosine kinases
WHO	World Health Organization

Introduction

Principally due to their associated clival involvement, similar radiography, and confusion in initial pathology (a problem obviated by modern immunohistochemistry), chordoma and chondrosarcoma have been grouped together historically. Importantly, these two lesions differ significantly in their clinical outcomes. Both chondrosarcomas and chordomas are uncommon and constitute less than 1% of intracranial lesions [1, 2]. Both lesions pose a formidable challenge to operative as well as adjuvant treatment due to their proximity to critical cranial nerves, the brainstem, and the skull base vasculature. Due to the inability to obtain wide negative margins, both tumors have a propensity to recur locally. This is especially true when anatomic constraints force subtotal resection. Standard therapies for both tumors rely on the combination of maximal resection aimed at minimizing morbidity with postoperative high-dose radiation therapy. This approach may cure most low-grade chondrosarcomas and provides good long-term local control and quality of life in patients with chordoma and high-grade chondrosarcoma.

Chordomas are locally aggressive tumors with a malignant potential that are derived from notochord remnants. Chordoma has an incidence of 8.4 per ten million people in the United States [3]. It was first recognized in 1856 by Lushka, and concomitantly by Virchow in 1857, at autopsy as probably cartilaginous in origin [4, 5]. In 1958, Muller proposed that these tumors were derived from notochord rather than cartilaginous constituents [6]. Subsequently, the tumors were directly observed in the nucleus pulposus, incriminating their origin, and the term chordoma was utilized henceforth [7]. Chordomas occur in the axial skeleton where the notochord developmentally is located, and they are thought to represent retained notochordal cells that have degenerated. Their occurrence in the axial spine is thought of in terms of thirds, with a third arising in the skull base, spine, and sacrum, or 32%, 33%, and 29%, respectively. Although this appears to be somewhat evenly distributed relative to the total length of this axis, chordomas have a preponderance toward the ends of the developing notochord (clivus and sacrum). Moreover, other studies support a more caudal cranial distribution of cases with less axial spine involvement; however, this finding may represent referral bias [3]. As noted above, chordomas frequently recur locally despite aggressive surgical treatment. Although metastases do occur, these are uncommon and are not frequently found at initial presentation. There does appear to be a spectrum of disease associated with chordoma in that there is a dedifferentiated type, a common chordoma, a benign notochordal cell tumor

J. J. Van Gompel (✉)
Department of Neurologic Surgery, Mayo Clinic, Rochester, MN, USA
e-mail: Vangompel.jamie@mayo.edu

G. W. Choby
Department of Otolaryngology—Head and Neck Surgery, University of Pittsburgh, Pittsburgh, PA, USA

Department of Neurologic Surgery, University of Pittsburgh, Pittsburgh, PA, USA
e-mail: chobygw2@upmc.edu

Y. Shinya
Research Fellow in Neurosurgery and Otorhinolaryngology, Department of Neurologic Surgery, Mayo Clinic, Rochester, MN, USA
e-mail: Yuki.Shinya@mayo.edu

S. Hong
International Fellow in Neurosurgery and Otorhinolaryngology, Department of Neurologic Surgery, Mayo Clinic, Rochester, MN, USA
e-mail: Hong.Sukwoo@mayo.edu

A. D. Sweeney et al. (eds.), *Haynes-Glasscock-Shambaugh Surgery of the Ear*, https://doi.org/10.1007/978-3-032-18264-7_79

(BNCT) in other locations within the axial spine, and finally, an entity called ecchordosis physaliphora, which is also a remnant of the embryonic notochord. Ecchordosis physaliphora is an entity that is brachyury-positive and is thought to be less aggressive; it is typically found intradurally behind the clivus and anterior to the brainstem [8, 9]. Pathologically, ecchordosis physaliphora is virtually identical to chordoma, and the diagnosis often relies on radiographic features such as a lack of contrast enhancement and an associated bony stalk to the clivus [8, 9]. In a clinical context, however, these lesions are commonly smaller, and there is a complete lack of clival involvement, with the exception of a small bony attachment; however, this, in fact, may be posterior clival erosion, and these lesions frequently exhibit a benign clinical behavior [8, 9].

Chondrosarcomas are rare tumors of cartilaginous origin that may present as low-grade (WHO grade 1 or 2), which are considerably more common, or high-grade (WHO grade 3). A mesenchymal chondrosarcoma subtype also exists. Mesenchymal subtype and grade 3 tumors portend a worse prognosis [1, 2]. Interestingly, these tumors are much more common elsewhere in the body, given that only 1% of chondrosarcomas occur at the skull base [10]. There is still controversy as to the cell of origin in these tumors, though typically, they are thought to arise at a synchondrosis of the skull base, such as the spheno-occipital suture or petroclival suture, from either pluripotent mesenchymal cells or rests of cartilaginous cells remaining after endochondral ossification. Although clival involvement is frequent, most of these tumors generally present slightly eccentric to the midline, having arisen from a suture/fissure. However, with growth, they do frequently cross the midline [1, 2]. Sixty-six percent of skull base chondrosarcomas arise from the petro-clival fissure, an additional 28% percent from the clivus proper, and a further 6% from the sphenoethmoidal complex. [11] Chondrosarcomas are typically less aggressive than chordomas, are rarer, and very uncommonly metastasize [1, 2].

Presenting Characteristics

Chordoma

Chordomas are the most frequently encountered extradural clival tumors. The median age of presentation for skull base chordomas appears to be 60 years; however, there is a large range of presenting ages, which includes pediatric cases [3, 12–15]. Presenting symptoms are typically dictated by the location of the tumor and local compression. Currently, the most common presenting symptom in adults is diplopia; however, a substantial number of these tumors are detected on scans obtained for other reasons, such as headache or sinus problems. Upper clival chordomas commonly present with sixth-nerve palsies secondary to the tumor accessing the basilar venous plexus between the periosteal and parietal dural layers, producing a local compartment syndrome of Dorello's canal. However, other cranial neuropathies can be seen with cavernous sinus involvement, including third and, less commonly, fourth nerve palsies. Larger tumors can cause nasal obstruction as well as Eustachian tube dysfunction and may precipitate a sinus CT. Lower clival tumors can present with dysphagia due to mass effect or involvement of the hypoglossal canal or the jugular foramen. There are no known environmental risk factors for tumor development, nor is there evidence that exposure to radiation induces chordomas; however, these tumors are so uncommon that these associations are difficult to prove [1, 2]. There are no syndromes that chordomas appear to be associated with; however, brachyury, brachyury duplication, and tuberous sclerosis complex are being investigated with respect to genetic predisposition [1, 2, 16–18].

Chondrosarcoma

Of lesions of the clivus that are T2 hyperintense on MRI, about one in six will be chondrosarcoma, and the other five will typically be a chordoma. However, assessing the incidence of these tumors based on older literature is confounded by the fact that chordoma and chondrosarcoma were frequently combined, and chondrosarcoma may have been mistaken for chondroid chordomas. Presently, the latter distinction is more apparent due to the ability to stain for brachyury [1, 2]. The presenting characteristics for chondrosarcoma are similar to those stated above for chordomas. However, the former appears to have a slightly younger median age (40 s) at presentation [19]. Additionally, eccentric location gives chondrosarcoma slightly higher rates of cavernous sinus involvement, and as a result, associated diplopia is more frequent. Extension into the jugular foramen as part of the petroclival suture is more commonly seen in chordoma (Table 79.1) [19]. Although chondrosarcomas typically occur in isolation, unlike chordomas, they can be associated with Paget disease, Ollier disease, and Maffucci syndrome (in the setting of preexisting endochondroma) [11, 20].

Table 79.1 Petroclival chondrosarcoma staging system

Stage	Tumor size	Carotid involvement	Extent of disease
1	<2 cm		Limited to bone
2	2–4 cm		Posterior or middle fossa extension
3	>4 cm	>270-degree carotid encasement	
4	Any size, grade 3 tumor		Distant metastasis

Modified from Carlson et al. [19]

Imaging Characteristics

Chordomas

Classically, chordomas are described as hyperintense on T2-weighted MRI (Figs. 79.1 and 79.2) [21]. On T1-weighted images, they are somewhat heterogeneous, with a predominantly isointense-to-brain signal. [22] Gadolinium enhancement is variable, though classically, chordomas are enhancing lesions. Our own institutional data of over 30 skull base chordomas over 8 years demonstrated minimal enhancement in 45% (Fig. 79.2 is an example), normal enhancement in 30% (Fig. 79.1 is an example), and avid enhancement in 25%. Diffusion restriction was seen, though the bony interfaces of the skull base made this finding unreliable, and the reliability is worsened by stronger magnetic fields (3 T scanner vs. 1.5 T). Thirty percent demonstrated calcifications within the tumor, though this finding is typically not as extensive as is seen in chondrosarcomas. Dural transgression occurred 50% of the time at presentation in our series. In terms of anatomic localization, 80% demonstrated posterior clinoid involvement, 30% had occipital condylar involvement, and 70% had cavernous sinus involvement. The upper half of the clivus was involved in 95%, and the lower half of the clivus was involved in 30%.

Chondrosarcomas

Chondrosarcomas are similar to chordomas in that T2 hyperintensity is a hallmark (Fig. 79.3) [21]. CT typically demonstrates a calcified matrix within the tumor (Fig. 79.4), though some tumors have only minimal calcifications (Fig. 79.5). As stated previously, chondrosarcomas are more eccentric to the midline but are not intrinsically lateral skull base lesions. As noted above, chondrosarcomas have variable WHO grades from 1 to 3, but there are no imaging hallmarks to differentiate low- from high-grade tumors.

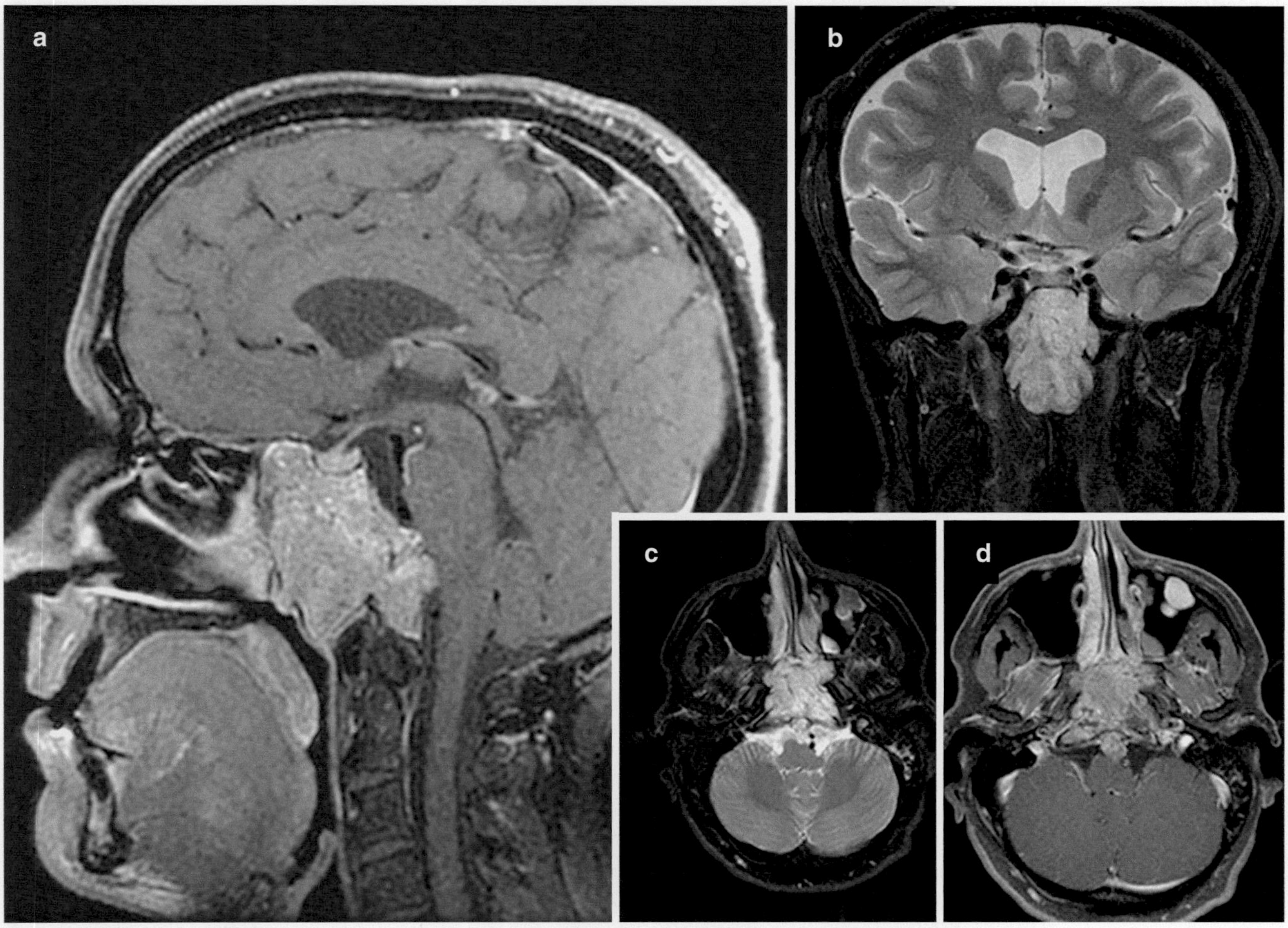

Fig. 79.1 Classic appearing midline whole clival chordoma. (**a**) Sagittal T1 with contrast, (**b**) coronal and (**c**) axial T2 images demonstrating the classic hallmark of chordomas is their T2 hyperintensity, and (**d**) axial contrast-enhanced T1 showing the minor dural transgression. Chordomas typically enhance on imaging

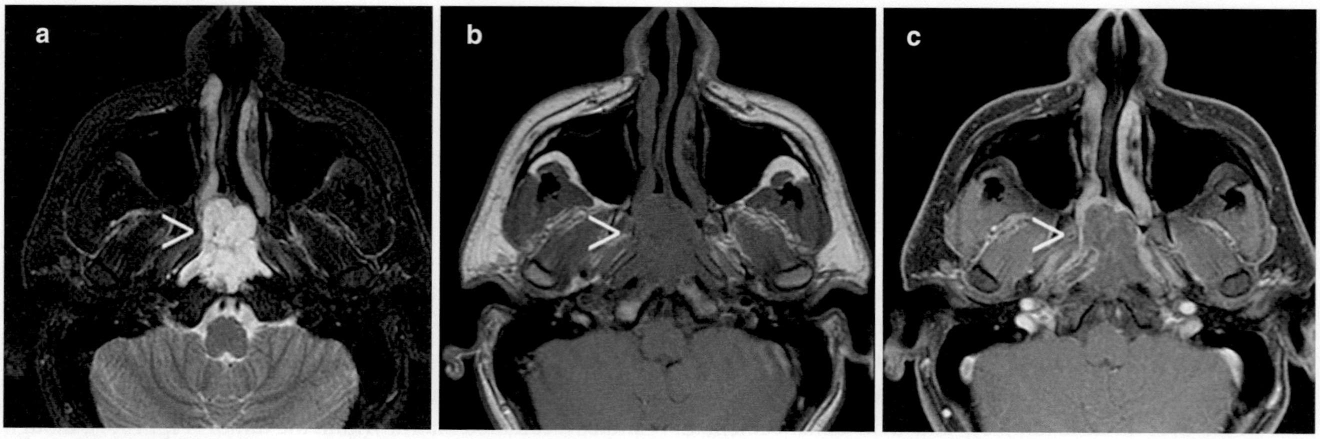

Fig. 79.2 Minimally enhancing chordoma: MRI with T2 hyperintense (**a**) mass (>), isodense to brain mass (>) on T1 (**b**). Interestingly, some chordomas take up very little contrast (**c**) compared to the example in Fig. 79.1

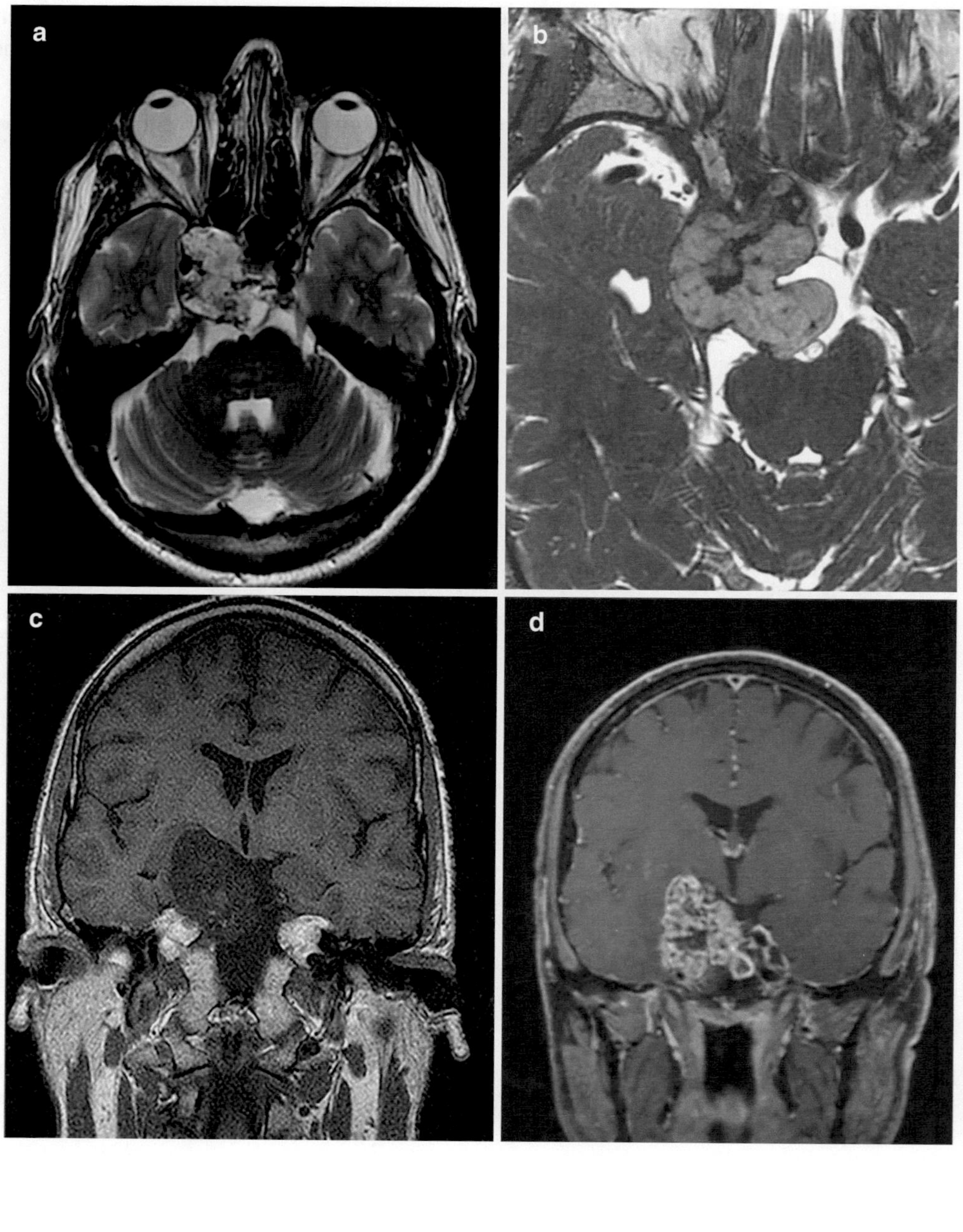

Fig. 79.3 Chondrosarcoma residing in the right petrous apex, petroclival fissure, and cavernous sinus: T2 axial (**a**) demonstrates the classic high T2 signal intensity. High-resolution cisternal imaging (**b**), such as fast imaging employing steady-state acquisition (FIESTA), is critical to understanding these lesions; here, the cisternal tumor clearly extends from the cavernous sinus to the cistern through the entry point of the third cranial nerve. Coronal T1 (**c**) and post-contrast T1 (**d**) demonstrate the heterogeneous and intense enhancement that is seen with these tumors

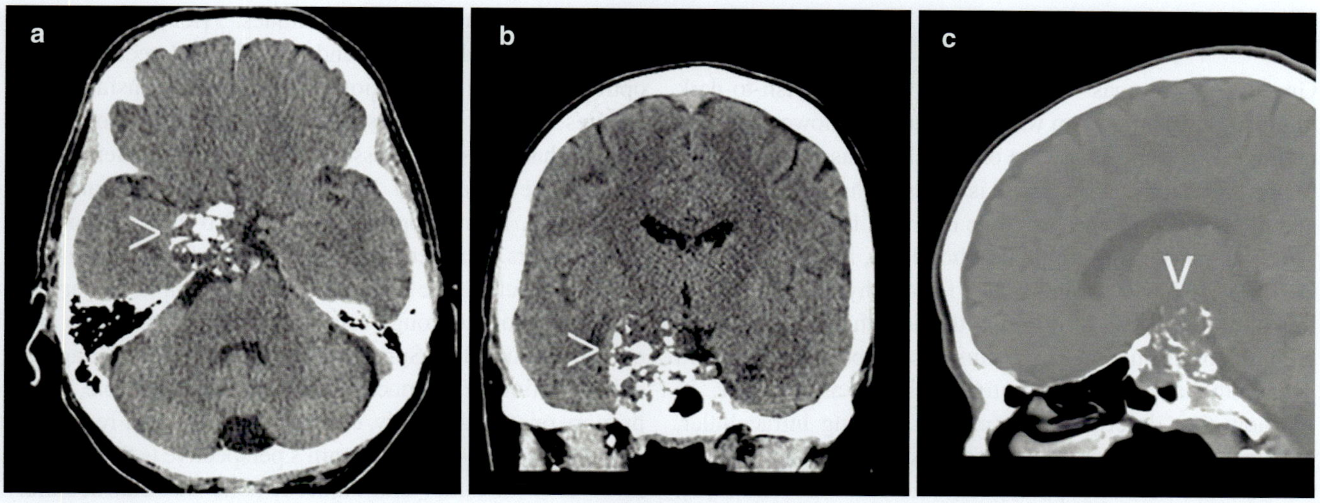

Fig. 79.4 CT example of a cavernous chondrosarcoma on axial (**a**), coronal (**b**), and sagittal (**c**) images. The chondrosarcoma (>) has a classic matrix within it, which is slightly less dense than the bone on CT. This matrix is not always present, as seen in Fig. 79.5

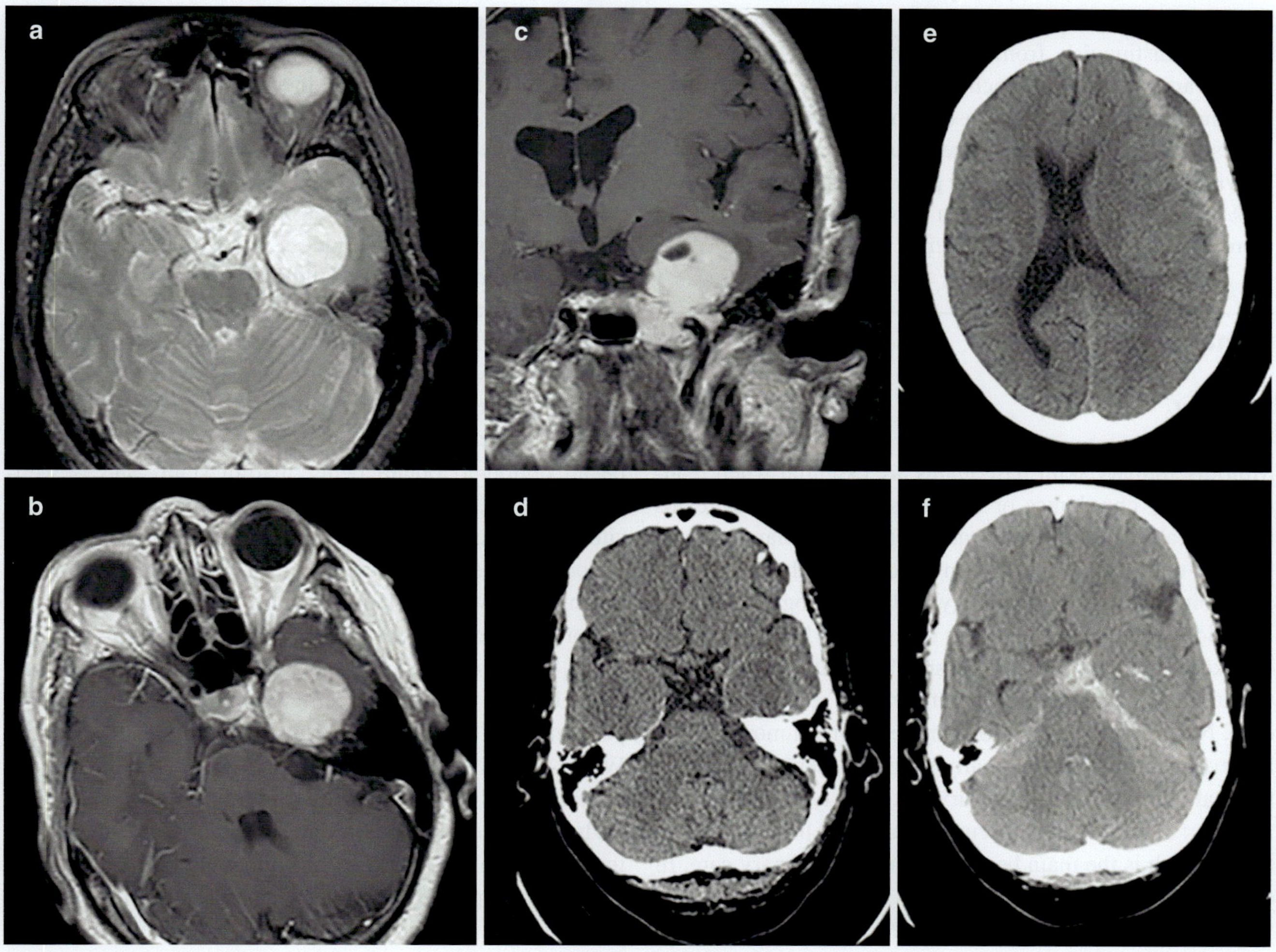

Fig. 79.5 Mesenchymal chondrosarcoma. This interesting tumor was T2 hyperintense (**a**) and avidly enhancing with contrast (**b**, **c**). It was watched for 3 years without progression in an elderly person. Note that the tumor does not have the typical chondroid matrix (**d**) and, therefore, was presumed to be a meningioma. The patient was transferred from an outside hospital with a subarachnoid hemorrhage, intratumoral hemorrhage, and mixed subdural hemorrhage from the tumor (**e**, **f**). This situation was suspicious for carotid involvement, and the patient was taken for a middle fossa craniotomy and resection with potential radial artery bypass of the carotid, which was not needed

Histologic Characteristics

Grossly, chordomas are lobulated and grayish-to-dark tumors. They can be firm with calcifications; however, in the authors' experience, they are often gelatinous and amenable to removal with suction. There is a subset that can be bloody and fibrous. Chordoma can come in one of three histological types: classical (conventional), chondroid, and dedifferentiated. [1, 2] They all stain positive for brachyury, which links this tumor to its cell of origin in the notochord and is now a hallmark of this tumor. These tumors stain positive for S-100 and epithelial membrane antigen (EMA) as well. [1, 2] Virchow first described this tumor as having intracellular, bubble-like inclusions, also known as physaliphorous cells, which are essentially pathognomonic for this tumor [5]. Unlike chondroid chordoma, chondrosarcomas are nonreactive for keratin and epithelial membrane antigen [1, 2]. Chondrosarcomas may have a gross appearance, much like chordomas, but more frequently, the former is firm and contains calcifications. Histologically, low-grade tumors are difficult to distinguish from chordoma, while higher-grade tumors are not. The mesenchymal subtype is considered to be a more aggressive chondrosarcoma [1]. The grading system is based on the degree of cellularity, atypia, and mitotic activity. In a large series of 200 patients, 51% were grade 1, 21% were grade 2, 29% were a mixed grade 1 and 2, and there were no grade 3 tumors seen [11].

Management

Surgery

Multidisciplinary skull base teams are essential when managing either chordomas or chondrosarcomas. These teams are typically composed of neurosurgery, otolaryngology, medical oncology, and radiation oncology, and participation also comes from endocrinology, ophthalmology, and rehabilitation specialists. Chordoma of the skull base can rarely be taken out *en bloc* unless it is small, which is in stark contrast to the sacrum or spine, where *en bloc* resection is standard. Nevertheless, the philosophy regarding tumor removal has evolved to an oncologically sound, piecemeal resection that balances function with survival. This type of resection requires intraoperative discussion among the skull base team, which is the main benefit of multidisciplinary care. In older literature, simple biopsy and intralesional curettage were performed for these tumors, often resulting in subtotal resection. This strategy was employed because approaching these tumors transnasally and in a minimally invasive manner was limited by the technology of the time. Moreover, high rates of postoperative cerebrospinal fluid (CSF) leak in these early endonasal series also limited enthusiasm for minimally invasive transnasal techniques. Prior to the modern era of endonasal surgery and vascularized reconstruction options, aggressive resection often required transfacial procedures, which, while still utilized in managing select tumors, had substantial associated morbidity. Alternatively, due to the associated morbidity of anterior transfacial approaches, lateral approaches were also used for some of these tumors. The recent advancement of skull base techniques to include the cultivation of endoscopic surgery has permitted more thorough removal of tumors with less postoperative morbidity. Some authors still advocate for aggressive resection of as much of the clivus as possible during primary or staged surgery, citing the frequency of recurrence as the reason [23–25]. Our team's perspective is that all bone involved with tumor and adjacent bone that can be safely removed should be; however, cavernous sinus involvement often precludes complete resection, and only a few authors advocate for carotid resection due to the high probability of morbidity. In turn, adjuvant radiation can be used to treat residual tumor. It should be noted that some surgical literature identifies relatively high rates of carotid injury, which may indicate that chordomas themselves locally invade the carotid artery, potentially leading to higher carotid artery injuries in the operating room. This may also be related to aggressive attempts at resection [26–28]. We advocate that skull base surgery teams have a clear plan to deal with intraoperative carotid bleeding and, in select cases, perform preoperative balloon occlusion studies in preparation for such a catastrophic vascular injury [27].

Lower clival tumors pose a unique predicament in that complete bony resection in this area may impart occipitocervical instability. In younger and healthier patients, however, complete resection with concomitant posterior fusion may be an option to obtain better margin status and is well-tolerated. [29] Typically, if the dura is not invaded, it is left in situ as a barrier. However, if there is dural transgression, we advocate for dural resection with a negative margin goal. Brainstem involvement is managed with resection of the tumor capsule, but obviously, brainstem margins are not taken. In cases of cranial nerve involvement, the hypoglossal nerve being a frequent concern, resection of a nerve is only performed if there is an opportunity for complete resection. We do not advocate bilateral hypoglossal sacrifice if there is bilateral involvement due to the morbidity associated with such a resection. The sixth cranial nerve is also frequently involved within Dorello's canal, though in such circumstances, we typically perform a decompression, resecting the tumor around the nerve but not the nerve itself. While the approach to each tumor is variable depending on its size and location, an anterior approach is favored in most cases since these tumors generally arise midline in the clivus. Lesions lateral to the cavernous sinus or the carotid artery will require a lateral approach in most circumstances. Advanced endoscopic approaches, such as the transpterygoid procedure, the extradural pituitary transposition (Fig. 79.6), the petrous apex approach (Fig. 79.7), and the far-medial approach (Fig. 79.8) can be employed to achieve complete resection of the tumor [30–32]. Although advantageous to use when available, a nasoseptal flap is not always necessary in closure. In some cases, the nasoseptal flaps are consumed by the tumor, and multilayered closure is still effective with fascia lata and fat (Fig. 79.9).

The most challenging hurdles encountered with endoscopic approaches to these tumors are defect closure and prevention of CSF leak. The use of a nasoseptal flap as part of a multilayered closure can be helpful in this regard. As noted above, a formidable challenge exists in cases where the nasoseptal flap cannot be harvested due to a previous operation or tumor involvement. Such cases may require a more classical multilayered closure (Fig. 79.9) or alternative local vascularized flaps, such as the inferior turbinate or lateral wall flap (Fig. 79.10).

The role for transoral approaches is limited to cases in which there is a low-riding odontoid relative to the hard palate. Transoral approaches do have a higher association with postoperative dysphagia when compared to endonasal approaches [33, 34]. Certainly, disease lateral to the carotid will require traditional lateral skull base approaches, such as anterior or posterior petrosectomy, as well as other transtemporal variants.

Lower clival tumors can also be reached by far- or extreme lateral approaches. Other open approaches remain necessary to address tumors lateral to the carotid arteries. Chondrosarcomas appear to be more indolent than chordomas, which may allow for a more conservative initial surgery. To that end, some very small tumors and other select cases may be addressed with observation. Furthermore, in select cases of chondrosarcoma where there is little to no preoperative growth, residual tumor in low-grade lesions can be observed closely without adjuvant treatment because local recurrence rates and metastatic potential are less than for chordoma. Ultimately, with either chordoma or chondrosarcoma, the surgical and adjuvant treatment plan should be tailored to each patient to optimize outcomes, with strong consideration of patient comorbidity and age. Also, as noted above, the role of multidisciplinary teams must be emphasized in determining nuances that may provide the best operative strategy at the lowest morbidity possible.

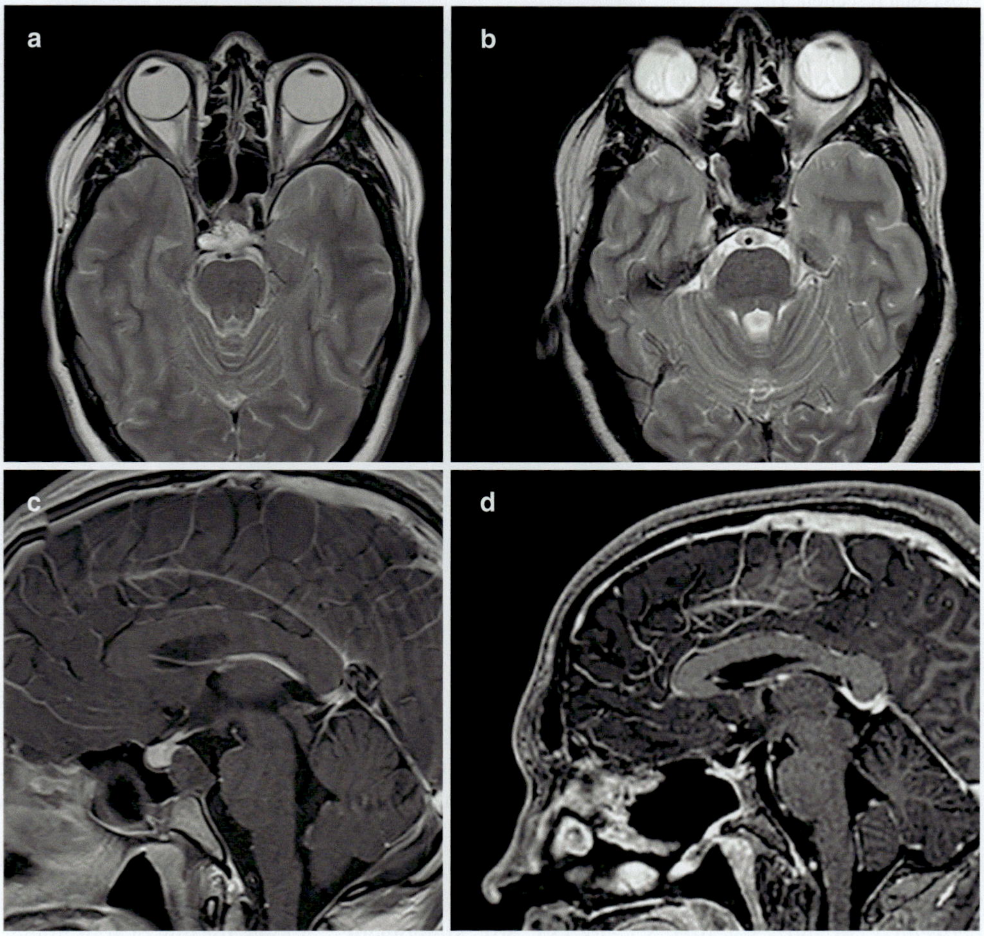

Fig. 79.6 Pre- (**a**, **c**) and postoperative (**b**, **d**) images of a chordoma, completely removed endoscopically with an interdural pituitary transposition

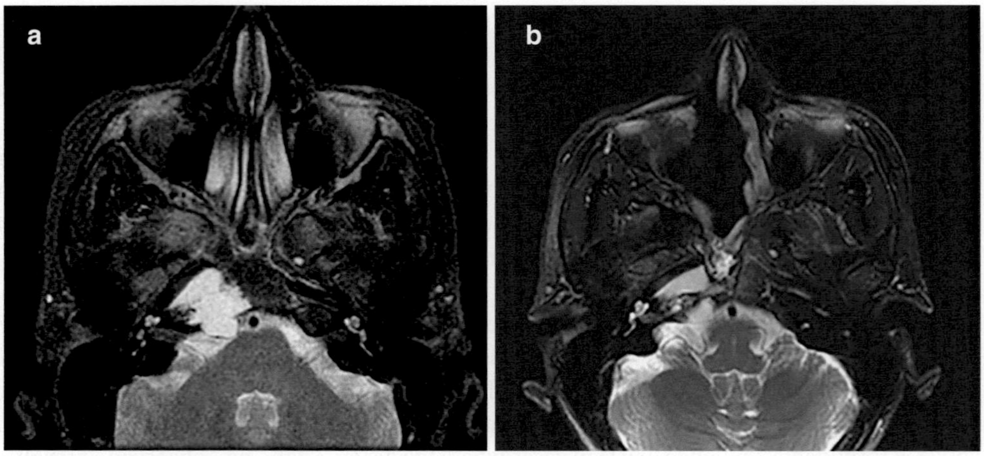

Fig. 79.7 Right petrous apex grade 1 chondrosarcoma observed for 5 years (**a**). The patient developed a sixth-nerve palsy and sought treatment. She underwent a subpetrous approach to the petrous apex (**b**), resulting in a subtotal resection and resolution of the sixth-nerve palsy. No growth has been noted for 3 years

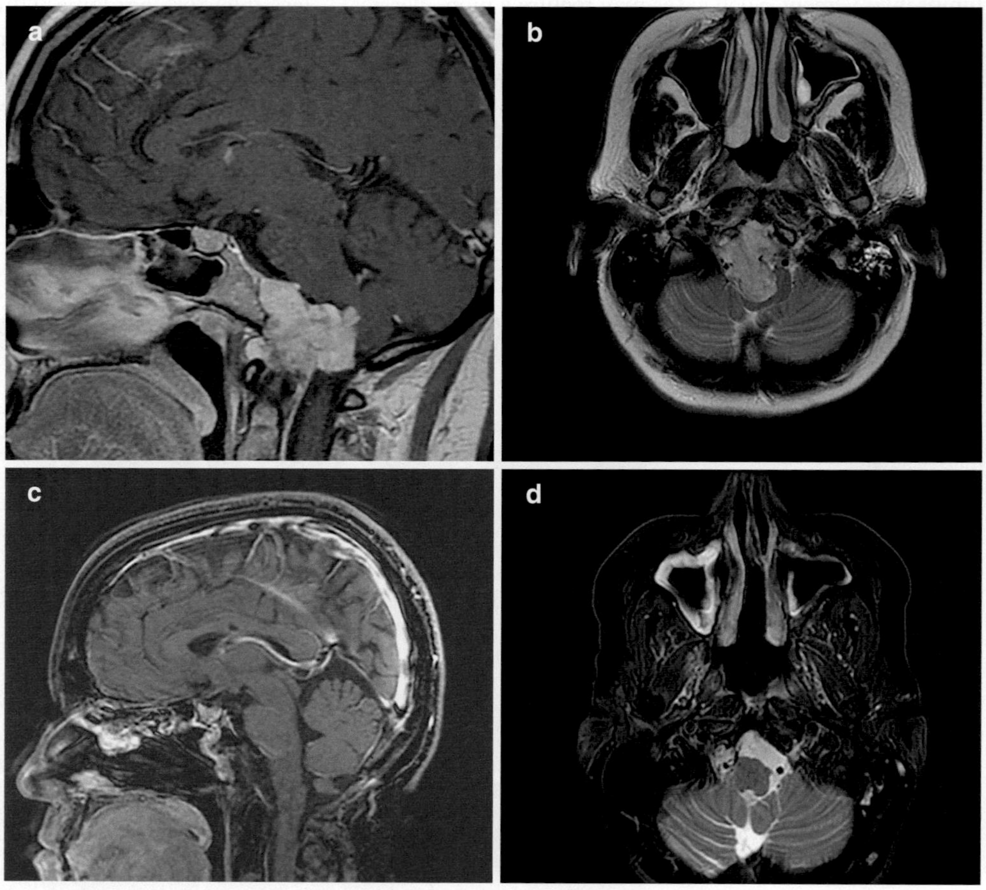

Fig. 79.8 Pre- (**a**, **b**) and postoperative (**c**, **d**) MRI T1 sequences with gadolinium contrast enhancement in the sagittal (**a**, **c**) and axial T2 (**b**, **d**) of a formidable lower-clivus chordoma requiring an endoscopic far-medial approach, followed by a far-lateral approach in a staged fashion, to achieve a gross total resection. The patient had no postoperative deficits

Radiation Therapy

The role of adjuvant radiation is a matter of debate; however, it is generally recommended after initial aggressive resection, especially with residual tumor. Controversy exists regarding the type of radiation that should be used. Conventional radiotherapy, with doses between 50 and 60 Gy, demonstrates poor local control rates, ranging between 17% and 23% after 5 years [35, 36]. Stereotactic fractionated radiation therapy at a median dose of 67 Gy appears to improve outcomes with 5-year local control rates at nearly 50% [37]. Currently, heavy particle and charged particle therapy are the most commonly recommended radiation treatments for chordoma and chondrosarcoma. Proton and carbon ion particle radiations have a theoretical advantage of higher doses delivered with less exit dose, which minimizes the radiation dose to the adjacent brainstem and allows for this overall higher treatment dose. However, pro-

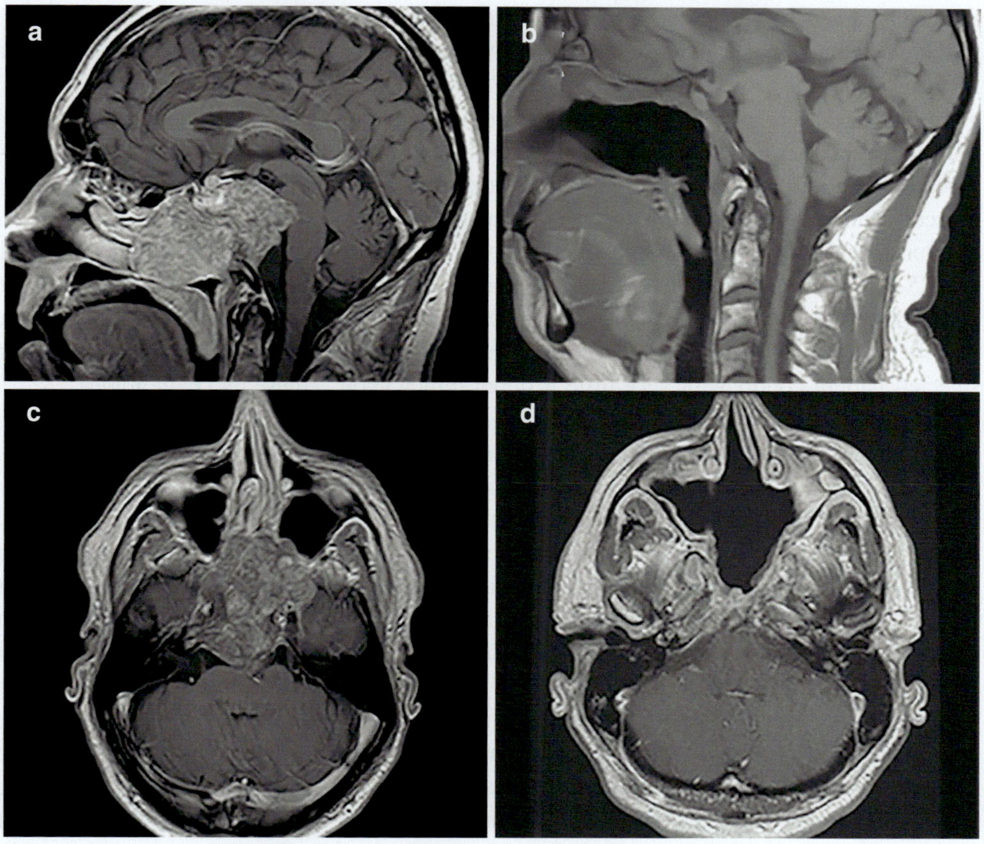

Fig. 79.9 Pre- (**a**, **b**) and postoperative (**c**, **d**) images of a large, 8-cm chordoma that underwent complete resection and classic multilayered closure without vascularized reconstruction. Classic closure was performed due to tumor contamination of the nasoseptal flaps. Sagittal preoperative T1 (**a**) and axial (**b**) perspectives with gadolinium contrast identify the contamination of the nasoseptal flaps and significant brainstem compression. Postoperative T1 sagittal (**c**) and axial perspectives with gadolinium contrast (**d**) demonstrate the skull base reconstruction. The patient is 3 years removed from resection and proton beam therapy without recurrence

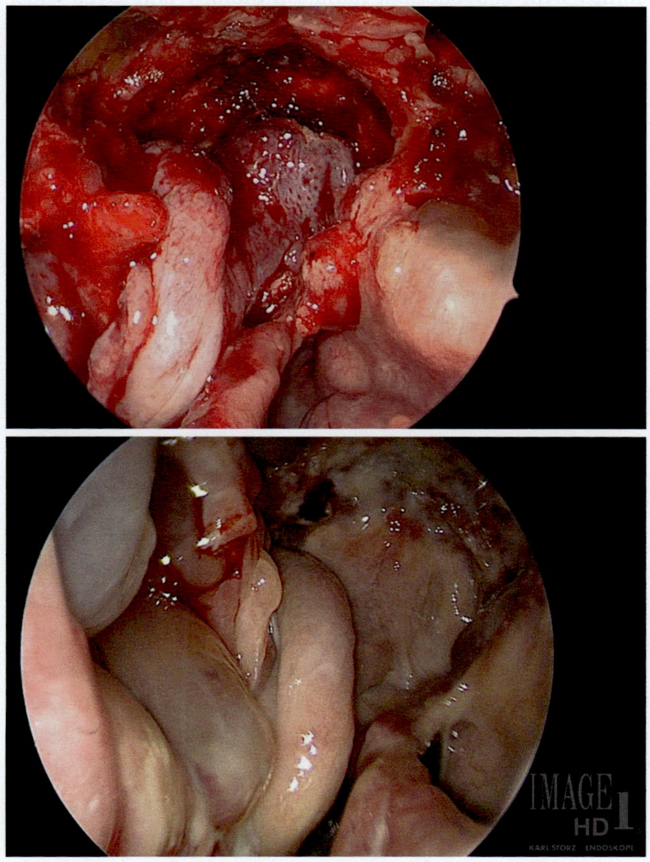

Fig. 79.10 Right-sided inferior turbinate/lateral wall flap utilization in a recurrent clival chordoma when previous surgery precluded the use of the nasoseptal flap. Harvest/placement in the operating room is noted in the upper pane, and healing in place 2 weeks after surgery is noted in the lower panel

ton beam can be 10 times more expensive than conventional radiation therapy, and it is not widely available to patients. As a result of the latter, patients frequently have to travel great distances to receive this therapy at the limited number of centers that offer it, which creates a large obstacle to widespread utilization. Regardless, proton beam treatment in its present form appears to have a survival advantage, with an approximate 50–84% progression-free survival at 5 years and 75–85% disease-specific survival at 5 years [38–44]. It should be noted that a confounder within relevant literature may be an overestimation of local control due to a highly selected patient cohort with very little residual tumor upon treatment. Carbon ion therapy is now available in Europe and Japan, and in addition to sharper radiation drop-off, heavy particle therapy may offer an additional advantage of biologic activity (called ablative) against tumors not traditionally responsive to photon-based radiation therapy [45–48]. Early results with carbon ion therapy demonstrate a local control rate of 70% at 5 years when used as an adjuvant to treat patients with residual tumors [45–48]. There appear to be similar toxicities between the modalities if the dose limitations are kept in mind. Intensity-modulated radiation therapy (IMRT) is frequently used in areas where particle therapy is not available and may offer a similar benefit; however, comparative outcomes have not been thoroughly investigated at this time. Most literature studying long-term outcomes with conventional radiation therapy employed older techniques that may not apply to current management. Finally, stereotactic radiosurgery (SRS) using Gamma Knife®, CyberKnife®, or other similar units certainly plays a role in primary radiation therapy for smaller tumors and adjuvant therapy for residual or recurrent disease. Previous studies evaluating SRS commonly indicated that a higher margin dose of ≥16 Gy would be required to achieve better tumor control. [49–52] Recently, the efficacy of high-dose SRS targeting the primary tumor sites was also reported. [53]

Chemotherapy

Due to the diversity of chemotherapeutic regimens used to control these tumors, little can be said of any one drug's efficacy. Typically, chemotherapy regimens are similar to those used in sarcoma and have shown little efficacy. Therefore, most chemotherapeutic regimens are currently used in a palliative fashion once surgical options are exhausted. Further, in cases of metastatic disease, chemotherapy is used to try to control the spread, though chondrosarcomas rarely metastasize, and as a result, it is infrequent that adjuvant chemotherapy is used with these patients. There is no data available at the time of this publication demonstrating a clear advantage of preoperative neoadjuvant therapy to improve surgical margins. Recently, there has been a revived enthusiasm in exploring molecular therapy for chordoma, as these tumors appear to have tyrosine kinase and related pathway mutations [54].

Patient Outcomes

As stated previously, the evaluation of chordomas and chondrosarcomas together in historical literature complicates the interpretation of outcome data. However, present data suggest that drastic differences are seen in the outcomes between these two pathologies.

Chordoma

If not treated, the natural history of chordoma is local progression with an average survival of approximately 18 months [55, 56]. While there is significant variance in outcomes with isolated surgical resection or radiation therapy alone, it is generally accepted that aggressive resection followed by postoperative adjuvant radiation therapy provides the best long-term outcomes. The median overall survival according to the most recent surveillance, epidemiology, and end results (SEER) results is 7.7 years, which dominates natural history outcomes [3]. Patients presenting under the age of 40 appear to have a better long-term survival (68%) at 10 years when compared to those older than 40 (43%) [3]. According to this data, elderly patients experience more aggressive disease [3]. Several reports have demonstrated that the extent of resection is directly proportional to long-term outcomes. For near-total or total resections, the 5-year overall survival is six times more when compared to subtotal resections (93% compared to 15%) [57]. There is also evidence to suggest that the quality of life in postsurgical patients is lower than the general population [58].

Chondrosarcoma

In chondrosarcoma patients, there is a clear survival advantage in patients who undergo resection when compared to observation [13]. However, it is interesting to note that some lower-grade lesions can be watched for years without progression, and therefore, a role exists for observation in select patients. Other important and favorable factors in survival analysis include female sex, smaller tumor size at presentation, and younger age at treatment, each being demonstrated in multivariate models from large series [13]. As already stated, WHO grade 3 and mesenchymal subtype pathology also portend a poorer prognosis [1]. Five- and 10-year mortality rates in the SEER database are reported at 87% and 68%, respectively, although when considering only low-grade chondrosarcomas, this number is considerably higher [13]. It should be noted that Carlson et al. proposed a simple petroclival chondrosarcoma system that appears to encompass important characteristics of these tumors that would guide the aggressiveness of treatment [19].

When these tumors demonstrate progression after initial treatment, they often show a slow but relentless local progression. Frequently, revision surgery can be performed with the goal of decompression for new deficits. Additionally, Gamma Knife treatment may be employed for local recurrences less than 3 cm in size [59]. Repeat palliative radiation may also be used and can halt progression temporarily. This is typically short-lived, however, and there is an increased incidence of radiation-induced complications. Although isolated in use, there are case reports of local ablation using either laser or cryotherapy. This may aid in palliative treatment, though the adoption of these modalities in the skull base has been limited. [60]

Molecular Profiling To date, numerous molecular genetic analyses have been reported for chordomas and chondrosarcomas.

Chordoma Several studies in the early 2000s reported chromosome abnormalities with a feature of more loss than gain (loss of 1p36, 7q33, and 9p21) associated with the development of chordoma [61–63]. Also, copy number alterations played an important role in chordoma [63]. In 2005, a gene expression signature of chordoma was first identified, reporting that the T-box transcription factor T (*TBXT*) brachyury was related to the embryonic structure of chordoma [64]. Other studies have also identified the important roles of brachyury in chordoma [16, 17, 65–67]. Moreover, after identifying driver mutations in chordomas, the *PI3K* pathway was found to be potentially significant in the development of chordoma, suggesting DNA methylation of tumor suppressor genes in chordoma [68–70]. Furthermore, recently, next-generation sequencing analysis for chordoma has significantly progressed [71–84]. According to the panel-based next-generation sequencing in chordoma, very low mutation rates of *KDR*, *KIT*, and *TP53* were shown; [71] chromatin regulatory genes, such as *SETD2* were frequently altered; and co-occurrence of alterations in both chromatin regulatory genes and *CDKN2A/2B* was common. [73] Additionally, whole-exome and whole-genome sequencing on chordoma exhibited a low-frequency mutation rate compared with other tumors; however, it revealed a novel gene fusion of *SMAD5–SASH1* [74], somatic duplications of *TBXT*, recurrent mutations of *PI3K* signaling genes, driver events in chromatin modeling genes, and nonrandom enrichment of truncating mutations in the lysosomal trafficking regulator protein [75]. In the dedifferentiated type, brachyury was completely lost, and the loss of *INI1/SMARCB1* was revealed, although it was expressed in the conventional and chondroid types [82]. In a multi-omics analysis, Meng et al. reported that the bone microenvironment was important in tumorigenesis [85]. Duan et al. also found six subclusters of chordoma cells, exhibiting properties of an epithelial-like extracellular matrix and stem cells with immunosuppression, a strong immunosuppressive effect exerted by regulatory T cells (Tregs) and M2 macrophages, and an enhanced tissue growth factor- beta (TGF-β) signaling pathway in tumor progression [83]. Williamson et al. detected features of single-copy losses affecting *SMARCB1*, hypomethylation of the *TBXT* promoter, overexpression of the brachyury tumor antigen and *CD274* (PD-L1), and $CD8^+$ T-cell, $CD79a^+$ B-cell, and plasma cell infiltration in a pediatric, recurrent, poorly differentiated chordoma patient [86]. Further genetic research with multiple techniques may contribute to individualized chordoma treatment strategies.

Chondrosarcoma

Several genetic alterations have been identified in isocitrate dehydrogenase (IDH) 1/2, tumor protein (TP) 53, mouse double minute 2 homolog (MDM2), cyclin-dependent kinase 4 (CDK4), and chromosome 8q24/10/11q22/13q14/17p13 [87]. Among those genetic abnormalities, those who had IDH 1 or 2 (1/2) mutations had worse overall survival than those with IDH wild type [88]. One thing to keep in mind is that the patients included in this study had chondrosarcoma in the extremities and axis (not exclusive to intracranial chondrosarcoma). One study on intracranial chondrosarcoma and chordoma showed IDH 1/2 mutations in 46% of chondrosarcoma and 0% of chordoma [89]. A gene fusion of YRPW motif 1 (HEY1) and nuclear receptor coactivator 2 (NCOA2) gene is recognized in mesenchymal chondrosarcoma [87]. These cytogenetic characteristics can be used to help make the diagnosis that lacks the typical histology features [90]. Based on these molecular features, studies on targeted therapies are underway, including the one for IDH 1 mutation inhibitor (ivosidenib, or AG-120) [87]. Its phase I study showed minimal toxicity and durable disease control [91].

Conclusions/Summary

Chordomas and chondrosarcomas represent locally aggressive tumors with many parallels in presentation, radiography, and pathology. Despite these similarities, differences in etiology, pathology, and prognosis are plentiful, and these differences should be considered in the management of each disease. In select circumstances, observation may be undertaken, though primary surgical resection, devised and executed in a multidisciplinary manner to minimize morbidity, is considered the current standard of care. Radiation therapy is often recommended regardless of the resection status. This recommendation is even stronger, however, in cases of residual tumor. Heavy ion radiation therapy is commonly recommended for postoperative adjuvant therapy, though access to this modality is limited, and more data are needed before it becomes the standard of care. There are few options beyond repeat resection or stereotactic radiation for salvage therapy, as chemotherapy is uncommonly used for these tumors. However, future targeted therapies may hold promise as an additional treatment tool.

References

1. Pathology and genetics of head and neck tumors. World Health Organization Classification of Tumours. International Agency for Research on Cancer: WHO Press; 2005.
2. Central nervous system. 4th ed. World Health Organization Classification of Tumours. International Agency for Research on Cancer: WHO Press; 2007.
3. Smoll NR, Gautschi OP, Radovanovic I, Schaller K, Weber DC. Incidence and relative survival of chordomas: the standardized mortality ratio and the impact of chordomas on a population. Cancer. 2013;119(11):2029–37. https://doi.org/10.1002/cncr.28032.
4. Luschka H. Die Altersveränderungen der Zwischenwirbelknorpel. Virchows Arch Pathol Anat. 1856;9:312–27.
5. Virchow R. Untersuchungen uber die entwickelung des schadelgrundes im gesunden und krankhafter zustande, und uber den einfluss derselben auf schadelform, gesichtsbildung und gehirnbau. G. Zeimer; 1857.
6. Müller H. Ueber das Vorkommen von Resten der Chorda dorsalis bei Mecschen nach der Geburt und uber ihr Verhaltnis zu den Gallertgeschwulsten am Clivus. Ztschr Rat Med. 1858;2:202–29.
7. Ribbert H. Ueber die Ecchondrosis physlifora sphenooccipitalis. Centralbl Allg Path Path Anat. 1894;5:457–61.
8. Ciarpaglini R, Pasquini E, Mazzatenta D, Ambrosini-Spaltro A, Sciarretta V, Frank G. Intradural clival chordoma and ecchordosis physaliphora: a challenging differential diagnosis: case report. Neurosurgery. 2009;64(2):E387–8; discussion E388. https://doi.org/10.1227/01.NEU.0000337064.57270.F0.
9. Iorgulescu JB, Laufer I, Hameed M, et al. Benign notochordal cell tumors of the spine: natural history of 8 patients with histologically confirmed lesions. Neurosurgery. 2013;73(3):411–6. https://doi.org/10.1227/01.neu.0000431476.94783.c6.
10. Bloch O, Parsa AT. Skull base chondrosarcoma: evidence-based treatment paradigms. Review. Neurosurg Clin N Am. 2013;24(1):89–96. https://doi.org/10.1016/j.nec.2012.08.002.
11. Rosenberg AE, Nielsen GP, Keel SB, et al. Chondrosarcoma of the base of the skull: a clinicopathologic study of 200 cases with emphasis on its distinction from chordoma. Am J Surg Pathol. 1999;23(11):1370–8.
12. Erdem E, Angtuaco EC, Van Hemert R, Park JS, Al-Mefty O. Comprehensive review of intracranial chordoma. Review. Radiographics. 2003;23(4):995–1009.
13. Jones PS, Aghi MK, Muzikansky A, Shih HA, Barker FG 2nd, Curry WT Jr. Outcomes and patterns of care in adult skull base chordomas from the Surveillance, Epidemiology, and End Results (SEER) database. J Clin Neurosci. 2014;21(9):1490–6. https://doi.org/10.1016/j.jocn.2014.02.008.
14. Menezes AH. Clival and craniovertebral junction chordomas. Comment World Neurosurg. 2014;81(5–6):690–2.
15. Tan NCW, Naidoo Y, Oue S, et al. Endoscopic surgery of skull base chordomas. J Neurol Surg Part B. 2012;73(6):379–86. https://doi.org/10.1055/s-0032-1321508.
16. Kelley MJ, Shi J, Ballew B, et al. Characterization of T gene sequence variants and germline duplications in familial and sporadic chordoma. Research Support, N.I.H., Extramural Research Support, N.I.H., Intramural Research Support, Non--U.S. Gov't Research Support, U.S. Gov't, Non-P.H.S. Hum Genet. 2014;133(10):1289–97. https://doi.org/10.1007/s00439-014-1463-z.
17. Pillay N, Plagnol V, Tarpey PS, et al. A common single-nucleotide variant in T is strongly associated with chordoma. Research Support, Non-U.S. Gov't. Nat Genet. 2012;44(11):1185–7. https://doi.org/10.1038/ng.2419.
18. Yang XR, Ng D, Alcorta DA, et al. T (brachyury) gene duplication confers major susceptibility to familial chordoma. Research Support, N.I.H., Intramural Research Support, Non-U.S. Gov't Research Support, U.S. Gov't, Non-P.H.S. Nat Genet. 2009;41(11):1176–8. https://doi.org/10.1038/ng.454.
19. Carlson ML, O'Connell BP, Breen JT, et al. Petroclival chondrosarcoma: a multicenter review of 55 cases and new staging system. Otol Neurotol. 2016;37(7):940–50.
20. Boorstein JM, Spizarny DL. Case report 476: chondrosarcoma of base of skull (CBS). Case reports. Skeletal Radiol. 1988;17(3):208–11.
21. Bag AK, Chapman PR. Neuroimaging: intrinsic lesions of the central skull base region. Review. Semin Ultrasound CT MR. 2013;34(5):412–35. https://doi.org/10.1053/j.sult.2013.08.004.
22. Doucet V, Peretti-Viton P, Figarella-Branger D, Manera L, Salamon G. MRI of intracranial chordomas. Extent of tumour and contrast enhancement: criteria for differential diagnosis. Neuroradiology. 1997;39(8):571–6.
23. Almefty K, Pravdenkova S, Colli BO, Al-Mefty O, Gokden M. Chordoma and chondrosarcoma: similar, but quite different, skull base tumors. Cancer. 2007;110(11):2457–67.
24. Al-Mefty O, Kadri PAS, Hasan DM, Isolan GR, Pravdenkova S. Anterior clivectomy: surgical technique and clinical applications. J Neurosurg. 2008;109(5):783–93. https://doi.org/10.3171/JNS/2008/109/11/0783.
25. Colli BO, Al-Mefty O. Chordomas of the skull base: follow-up review and prognostic factors. Neurosurgery. 2001;10(3):E1.
26. Fernandez-Miranda JC, Gardner PA, Snyderman CH, et al. Clival chordomas: a pathological, surgical, and radiotherapeutic review. Head Neck. 2014;36(6):892–906. https://doi.org/10.1002/hed.23415.
27. Gardner PA, Tormenti MJ, Pant H, Fernandez-Miranda JC, Snyderman CH, Horowitz MB. Carotid artery injury during endoscopic endonasal skull base surgery: incidence and outcomes. Neurosurgery. 2013;73(2 Suppl Operative):261–9; discussion 269–70. https://doi.org/10.1227/01.neu.0000430821.71267.f2.
28. Koutourousiou M, Gardner PA, Tormenti MJ, et al. Endoscopic endonasal approach for resection of cranial base chordomas: outcomes and learning curve. Neurosurgery. 2012;71(3):614–24; discussion 624–5. https://doi.org/10.1227/NEU.0b013e31825ea3e0.
29. Colli B, Al-Mefty O. Chordomas of the craniocervical junction: follow-up review and prognostic factors. J Neurosurg. 2001;95(6):933–43.
30. Fernandez-Miranda JC, Gardner PA, Rastelli MM, Jr., et al. Endoscopic endonasal transcavernous posterior clinoidectomy with interdural pituitary transposition. J Neurosurg. 2014;121(1):91–9. https://doi.org/10.3171/2014.3.JNS131865.
31. Fernandez-Miranda JC, Morera VA, Snyderman CH, Gardner P. Endoscopic endonasal transclival approach to the jugular tubercle. Case reports. Neurosurgery. 2012;71(1 Suppl

Operative):146–58; discussion 158–9. https://doi.org/10.1227/NEU.0b013e3182438915.
32. Van Gompel JJ, Alikhani P, Tabor MH, et al. Anterior inferior petrosectomy: defining the role of endonasal endoscopic techniques for petrous apex approaches. Comparative Study J Neurosurg. 2014;120(6):1321–5. https://doi.org/10.3171/2014.2.JNS131773.
33. Van Abel KM, Mallory GW, Kasperbauer JL, et al. Transnasal odontoid resection: is there an anatomic explanation for differing swallowing outcomes? Neurosurgery. 2014;37(4):E16. https://doi.org/10.3171/2014.7.FOCUS14338.
34. Van Gompel JJ, Morris JM, Kasperbauer JL, Graner DE, Krauss WE. Cystic deterioration of the C1-2 articulation: clinical implications and treatment outcomes. J Neurosurg Spine. 2011;14(4):437–43. https://doi.org/10.3171/2010.12.SPINE10302.
35. Romero J, Cardenes H, la Torre A, et al. Chordoma: results of radiation therapy in eighteen patients. Radiother Oncol. 1993;29(1):27–32.
36. Catton C, O'Sullivan B, Bell R, et al. Chordoma: long-term follow-up after radical photon irradiation. Radiother Oncol. 1996;41(1):67–72.
37. Debus J, Schulz-Ertner D, Schad L, et al. Stereotactic fractionated radiotherapy for chordomas and chondrosarcomas of the skull base. Int J Radiat Oncol Biol Phys. 2000;47(3):591–6.
38. Hug EB, Loredo LN, Slater JD, et al. Proton radiation therapy for chordomas and chondrosarcomas of the skull base. J Neurosurg. 1999;91(3):432–9. https://doi.org/10.3171/jns.1999.91.3.0432.
39. Weber DC, Rutz HP, Pedroni ES, et al. Results of spot-scanning proton radiation therapy for chordoma and chondrosarcoma of the skull base: the Paul Scherrer Institut experience. Int J Radiat Oncol Biol Phys. 2005;63(2):401–9. https://doi.org/10.1016/j.ijrobp.2005.02.023.
40. Matloob SA, Nasir HA, Choi D. Proton beam therapy in the management of skull base chordomas: systematic review of indications, outcomes, and implications for neurosurgeons. Br J Neurosurg. 2016;30(4):382–7. https://doi.org/10.1080/02688697.2016.1181154.
41. Castro JR, Linstadt DE, Bahary JP, et al. Experience in charged particle irradiation of tumors of the skull base: 1977-1992. Int J Radiat Oncol Biol Phys. 1994;29(4):647–55. https://doi.org/10.1016/0360-3016(94)90550-9.
42. Munzenrider JE, Liebsch NJ. Proton therapy for tumors of the skull base. Strahlenther Onkol. 1999;175(Suppl 2):57–63.
43. McDonald MW, Linton OR, Moore MG, Ting JY, Cohen-Gadol AA, Shah MV. Influence of residual tumor volume and radiation dose coverage in outcomes for clival chordoma. Int J Radiat Oncol Biol Phys. 2016;95(1):304–11. https://doi.org/10.1016/j.ijrobp.2015.08.011.
44. Iannalfi A, D'Ippolito E, Riva G, et al. Proton and carbon ion radiotherapy in skull base chordomas: a prospective study based on a dual particle and a patient-customized treatment strategy. Neuro-oncol. 2020;22(9):1348–58. https://doi.org/10.1093/neuonc/noaa067.
45. Schulz-Ertner D, Haberer T, Jakel O, et al. Radiotherapy for chordomas and low-grade chondrosarcomas of the skull base with carbon ions. Clinical Trial, Clinical Trial, Phase I Clinical Trial, Phase II. Int J Radiat Oncol Biol Phys. 2002;53(1):36–42.
46. Schulz-Ertner D, Karger CP, Feuerhake A, et al. Effectiveness of carbon ion radiotherapy in the treatment of skull-base chordomas. Int J Radiat Oncol Biol Phys. 2007;68(2):449–57.
47. Schulz-Ertner D, Nikoghosyan A, Didinger B, Debus J. Carbon ion radiation therapy for chordomas and low grade chondrosarcomas--current status of the clinical trials at GSI. Clinical Trial Clinical Trial, Phase I Clinical Trial, Phase II. Radiother Oncol. 2004;73(Suppl 2):S53–6.
48. Schulz-Ertner D, Nikoghosyan A, Thilmann C, et al. Carbon ion radiotherapy for chordomas and low-grade chondrosarcomas of the skull base. Results in 67 patients. Clinical Trial Comparative Study Evaluation Studies Research Support, Non-U.S. Gov't. Strahlenther Onkol. 2003;179(9):598–605.
49. Kim JH, Jung HH, Chang JH, Chang JW, Park YG, Chang WS. Gamma knife surgery for intracranial chordoma and chondrosarcoma: radiosurgical perspectives and treatment outcomes. J Neurosurg. 2014;121(Suppl):188–97. https://doi.org/10.3171/2014.7.GKS141213.
50. Koga T, Shin M, Saito N. Treatment with high marginal dose is mandatory to achieve long-term control of skull base chordomas and chondrosarcomas by means of stereotactic radiosurgery. J Neuro-Oncol. 2010;98(2):233–8. https://doi.org/10.1007/s11060-010-0184-y.
51. Hasegawa T, Ishii D, Kida Y, Yoshimoto M, Koike J, Iizuka H. Gamma Knife surgery for skull base chordomas and chondrosarcomas. J Neurosurg. 2007;107(4):752–7. https://doi.org/10.3171/JNS-07/10/0752.
52. Kano H, Iqbal FO, Sheehan J, et al. Stereotactic radiosurgery for chordoma: a report from the North American Gamma Knife Consortium. Neurosurgery. 2011;68(2):379–89. https://doi.org/10.1227/NEU.0b013e3181ffa12c.
53. Shinya Y, Hasegawa H, Shin M, et al. High dose radiosurgery targeting the primary tumor sites contributes to survival in patients with skull base chordoma. Int J Radiat Oncol Biol Phys. 2022;113(3):582–7. https://doi.org/10.1016/j.ijrobp.2022.02.024.
54. Akhavan-Sigari R, Gaab MR, Rohde V, et al. Expression of vascular endothelial growth factor receptor 2 (VEGFR-2), inducible nitric oxide synthase (iNOS), and Ki-M1P in skull base chordoma: a series of 145 tumors. Neurosurg Rev. 2014;37(1):79–88.
55. Eriksson B, Gunterberg B, Kindblom LG. Chordoma. A clinicopathologic and prognostic study of a Swedish national series. Research Support, Non-U.S. Gov't. Acta Orthop Scand. 1981;52(1):49–58.
56. Heffelfinger MJ, Dahlin DC, MacCarty CS, Beabout JW. Chordomas and cartilaginous tumors at the skull base. Cancer. 1973;32(2):410–20.
57. Ouyang T, Zhang N, Zhang Y, et al. Clinical characteristics, immunohistochemistry, and outcomes of 77 patients with skull base chordomas. World Neurosurg. 2014;81(5–6):790–7.
58. Diaz RJ, Maggacis N, Zhang S, Cusimano MD. Determinants of quality of life in patients with skull base chordoma. J Neurosurg. 2014;120(2):528–37. https://doi.org/10.3171/2013.9.JNS13671.
59. Kano H, Iyer A, Lunsford LD. Skull base chondrosarcoma radiosurgery: a literature review. Neurosurgery. 2014;61(Suppl 1):155–8. https://doi.org/10.1227/NEU.0000000000000382.
60. Kurup AN, Woodrum DA, Morris JM, et al. Cryoablation of recurrent sacrococcygeal tumors. J Vasc Interv Radiol. 2012;23(8):1070–5. https://doi.org/10.1016/j.jvir.2012.05.043.
61. Miozzo M, Dalpra L, Riva P, et al. A tumor suppressor locus in familial and sporadic chordoma maps to 1p36. Int J Cancer. 2000;87(1):68–72.
62. Kelley MJ, Korczak JF, Sheridan E, Yang X, Goldstein AM, Parry DM. Familial chordoma, a tumor of notochordal remnants, is linked to chromosome 7q33. Am J Hum Genet. 2001;69(2):454–60. https://doi.org/10.1086/321982.
63. Hallor KH, Staaf J, Jonsson G, et al. Frequent deletion of the CDKN2A locus in chordoma: analysis of chromosomal imbalances using array comparative genomic hybridisation. Br J Cancer. 2008;98(2):434–42. https://doi.org/10.1038/sj.bjc.6604130.
64. Henderson SR, Guiliano D, Presneau N, et al. A molecular map of mesenchymal tumors. Genome Biol. 2005;6(9):R76. https://doi.org/10.1186/gb-2005-6-9-r76.
65. Nibu Y, Jose-Edwards DS, Di Gregorio A. From notochord formation to hereditary chordoma: the many roles of Brachyury. Biomed Res Int. 2013;2013:826435. https://doi.org/10.1155/2013/826435.
66. Chen M, Wu Y, Zhang H, Li S, Zhou J, Shen J. The roles of embryonic transcription factor BRACHYURY in tumorigenesis and

progression. Front Oncol. 2020;10:961. https://doi.org/10.3389/fonc.2020.00961.
67. Gill CM, Fowkes M, Shrivastava RK. Emerging therapeutic targets in chordomas: a review of the literature in the genomic era. Neurosurgery. 2020;86(2):E118–23. https://doi.org/10.1093/neuros/nyz342.
68. Rinner B, Weinhaeusel A, Lohberger B, et al. Chordoma characterization of significant changes of the DNA methylation pattern. PLoS One. 2013;8(3):e56609. https://doi.org/10.1371/journal.pone.0056609.
69. Yu X, Li Z. Epigenetic deregulations in chordoma. Cell Prolif. 2015;48(5):497–502. https://doi.org/10.1111/cpr.12204.
70. Tu K, Lee S, Roy S, Sawant A, Shukla H. Dysregulated epigenetics of chordoma: prognostic markers and therapeutic targets. Curr Cancer Drug Targets. 2022;22(8):678–90. https://doi.org/10.2174/1568009622666220419122716.
71. Fischer C, Scheipl S, Zopf A, et al. Mutation analysis of nine chordoma specimens by targeted next-generation cancer panel sequencing. J Cancer. 2015;6(10):984–9. https://doi.org/10.7150/jca.11371.
72. Bell D, Raza SM, Bell AH, Fuller GN, DeMonte F. Whole-transcriptome analysis of chordoma of the skull base. Virchows Arch. 2016;469(4):439–49. https://doi.org/10.1007/s00428-016-1985-y.
73. Wang L, Zehir A, Nafa K, et al. Genomic aberrations frequently alter chromatin regulatory genes in chordoma. Genes Chromosomes Cancer. 2016;55(7):591–600. https://doi.org/10.1002/gcc.22362.
74. Sa JK, Lee IH, Hong SD, Kong DS, Nam DH. Genomic and transcriptomic characterization of skull base chordoma. Oncotarget. 2017;8(1):1321–8. https://doi.org/10.18632/oncotarget.13616.
75. Tarpey PS, Behjati S, Young MD, et al. The driver landscape of sporadic chordoma. Nat Commun. 2017;8(1):890. https://doi.org/10.1038/s41467-017-01026-0.
76. Bell AH, DeMonte F, Raza SM, et al. Transcriptome comparison identifies potential biomarkers of spine and skull base chordomas. Virchows Arch. 2018;472(3):489–97. https://doi.org/10.1007/s00428-017-2224-x.
77. Groschel S, Hubschmann D, Raimondi F, et al. Defective homologous recombination DNA repair as therapeutic target in advanced chordoma. Nat Commun. 2019;10(1):1635. https://doi.org/10.1038/s41467-019-09633-9.
78. Zhu GG, Ramirez D, Chen W, et al. Chromosome 3p loss of heterozygosity and reduced expression of H3K36me3 correlate with longer relapse-free survival in sacral conventional chordoma. Hum Pathol. 2020;104:73–83. https://doi.org/10.1016/j.humpath.2020.07.002.
79. Bai J, Shi J, Li C, et al. Whole genome sequencing of skull-base chordoma reveals genomic alterations associated with recurrence and chordoma-specific survival. Nat Commun. 2021;12(1):757. https://doi.org/10.1038/s41467-021-21026-5.
80. Mattox AK, Yang B, Douville C, et al. The mutational landscape of spinal chordomas and their sensitive detection using circulating tumor DNA. Neurooncol Adv. 2021;3(1):vdaa173. https://doi.org/10.1093/noajnl/vdaa173.
81. Wen X, Cimera R, Aryeequaye R, et al. Recurrent loss of chromosome 22 and SMARCB1 deletion in extra-axial chordoma: a clinicopathological and molecular analysis. Genes Chromosomes Cancer. 2021;60(12):796–807. https://doi.org/10.1002/gcc.22992.
82. Yepes S, Shah NN, Bai J, et al. Rare germline variants in chordoma-related genes and chordoma susceptibility. Cancers (Basel). 2021;13(11). https://doi.org/10.3390/cancers13112704.
83. Duan W, Zhang B, Li X, et al. Single-cell transcriptome profiling reveals intra-tumoral heterogeneity in human chordomas. Cancer Immunol Immunother. 2022;71(9):2185–95. https://doi.org/10.1007/s00262-022-03152-1.
84. Xu Z, Zhang L, Wen L, et al. Clinical and molecular features of sacrum chordoma in Chinese patients. Ann Transl Med. 2022;10(2):61. https://doi.org/10.21037/atm-21-6617.
85. Meng T, Huang R, Jin J, et al. A comparative integrated multi-omics analysis identifies CA2 as a novel target for chordoma. Neuro-Oncology. 2021;23(10):1709–22. https://doi.org/10.1093/neuonc/noab156.
86. Williamson LM, Rive CM, Di Francesco D, et al. Clinical response to nivolumab in an INI1-deficient pediatric chordoma correlates with immunogenic recognition of brachyury. NPJ Precis Oncol. 2021;5(1):103. https://doi.org/10.1038/s41698-021-00238-4.
87. Zając AE, Kopeć S, Szostakowski B, et al. Chondrosarcoma-from molecular pathology to novel therapies. Cancer. 2021;13(10):2390.
88. Lugowska I, Teterycz P, Mikula M, et al. IDH1/2 mutations predict shorter survival in chondrosarcoma. J Cancer. 2018;9(6):998–1005. https://doi.org/10.7150/jca.22915.
89. Arai M, Nobusawa S, Ikota H, Takemura S, Nakazato Y. Frequent IDH1/2 mutations in intracranial chondrosarcoma: a possible diagnostic clue for its differentiation from chordoma. Brain Tumor Pathol. 2012;29(4):201–6. https://doi.org/10.1007/s10014-012-0085-1.
90. Uneda A, Kurozumi K, Fujimura A, et al. Intracranial mesenchymal chondrosarcoma lacking the typical histopathological features diagnosed by HEY1-NCOA2 gene fusion. NMC Case Rep J. 2020;7(2):47–52. https://doi.org/10.2176/nmccrj.cr.2019-0123.
91. Tap WD, Villalobos VM, Cote GM, et al. Phase I study of the mutant IDH1 inhibitor ivosidenib: safety and clinical activity in patients with advanced chondrosarcoma. J Clin Oncol. 2020;38(15):1693–701. https://doi.org/10.1200/jco.19.02492.

Pediatric Temporal Bone Malignancies

80

Landon Massoth and Betty S. Tsai Do

Introduction

Malignant neoplasms of the temporal bone are uncommon in adults and are even rarer in the pediatric population. These neoplastic processes are often insidious and indistinct at the time of initial evaluation. Moreover, the management of these entities is complicated by variability in tumor histology (Table 80.1) and constraints of temporal bone anatomy. Soft tissue sarcomas are the most common malignancies of the pediatric temporal bone, with rhabdomyosarcoma (RMS) being the most frequently encountered. This chapter provides an overview of RMS, other soft tissue sarcomas, lymphoma, and malignant parotid tumor invasion of the temporal bone in children and reviews the key features of their evaluation and management.

Table 80.1 Malignant tumors of the temporal bone

Malignant tumors of the temporal bone
Adenocarcinoma
Adenoid cystic carcinoma
Burkitt lymphoma
Chondrosarcoma
Chordoma
Desmoid tumor/fibromatosis
Ewing sarcoma
Fibrosarcoma
Fibrous histiocytoma
Ganglioneuroblastoma
Granulocytic sarcoma
Hemangiosarcoma
Liposarcoma
Lymphoma
Osteosarcoma
Rhabdomyosarcoma
Squamous cell carcinoma

L. Massoth (✉)
Department of Otolaryngology—Head & Neck Surgery, University of Oklahoma Health Sciences Center, Oklahoma City, OK, USA

B. S. Tsai Do
The Permanente Medical Group, Kaiser Permanente, Walnut Creek, CA, USA
e-mail: Betty.x.tsaido@kp.org

Rhabdomyosarcoma

Overview

RMS is the most common soft tissue sarcoma of childhood and represents 4.5% of all pediatric malignancies. It primarily affects the head and neck area, in which 35–40% of RMS cases arise [1–4]. Site-specific involvement in the head and neck varies among studies. In the Intergroup RMS Study (IRS) IV, 7% of tumors arose in the soft tissues of the head and neck (oral cavity, oropharynx, larynx, and parotid), 9% in the orbit, and 25% in the parameningeal sites (nasal and paranasal cavities, middle ear and mastoid, parapharyngeal space, and pterygopalatine and infratemporal fossae) [2]. Lesions of the temporal bone, a parameningeal site, only account for approximately 4–7% of RMSs that occur in the head and neck. However, it is by far the most common type of pediatric temporal bone malignancy [5–7].

RMS has a bimodal age distribution, with a first peak of incidence between the ages of 2 and 6 years and a second peak of incidence between the ages of 10 and 18 years [8]. Overall, greater than 60% of all affected patients are younger than 10 years. For temporal bone RMS, an even larger proportion of patients are younger than 10 years old and are slightly more often male [7]. The majority of RMS cases arise sporadically. Yet cases may develop as a result of familial syndromes such as Li–Fraumeni syndrome, Beckwith–Wiedemann syndrome, neurofibromatosis type 1, Costello syndrome, pleuropulmonary blastoma, and Noonan syndrome [9].

RMS has an unclear etiology. It is largely held that these tumors occur as a consequence of regulatory disruption of skeletal muscle progenitor cell growth and differentiation. They are thought to arise from mesenchymal tissue rather than striated muscle, which explains why they may occur in areas such as the mastoid or middle ear where striated muscle is absent or scarce [10]. Today, RMS is divided histologically into three main variants: embryonal RMS, alveolar

A. D. Sweeney et al. (eds.), *Haynes-Glasscock-Shambaugh Surgery of the Ear*, https://doi.org/10.1007/978-3-032-18264-7_80

RMS, and pleomorphic RMS. Embryonal RMS is further subdivided into embryonal (conventional), botryoid, and spindle cell/sclerosing subtypes. The embryonal subtypes account for approximately 60–70% of all childhood RMS and account for 92% of middle ear RMS [2, 7].

Embryonal and alveolar variants have distinct molecular characteristics, which are used for diagnostic confirmation. Embryonal tumors often show loss of heterozygosity at chromosome 11p15, whereas a balanced translocation with fusion between the *FOXO1* gene on chromosome 13 and either the *PAX3* gene on chromosome 2 or the *PAX7* gene on chromosome 1 (*PAX3*– and *PAX7–FOXO1*) is associated with alveolar tumors. Identification of the variant of RMS is significant, as it impacts prognosis and treatment. Of these two main variants, the alveolar histology has been associated with a poorer prognosis. Therefore, current classification requires upstaging of tumors with alveolar pathology from low to intermediate risk [2, 11–13]. Additionally, growing insight into RMS biology has demonstrated that molecular features of tumors have prognostic significance. A recent clinical trial by the Children's Oncology Group (COG) demonstrated that the absence of the typical *PAX–FOXO1* fusion gene in alveolar RMS confers superior event-free survival and a similar prognosis to embryonal RMS [14].

RMS must be distinguished from other small, round-cell tumors of childhood, which is accomplished by identification of cross-striations characteristic of skeletal muscle or characteristic rhabdomyoblasts on light microscopy and immunohistochemistry stains to identify muscle-specific proteins [15]. These proteins include muscle-specific actin and myosin, desmin, myoglobin, Z-band protein, myogenin, and myoblast determination protein 1 (MyoD) (Fig. 80.1) [16]. Alveolar RMS is composed of small round cells in a dense configuration around septations that resemble pulmonary alveoli (Fig. 80.2). Embryonal RMS pathology is characterized by malignant cells that are spindle-shaped, with interspersed large rhabdomyoblasts and the absence of an alveolar pattern (Fig. 80.3).

RMS of the temporal bone commonly presents as a locally invasive, unresectable tumor that rarely metastasizes to regional lymph nodes but has a propensity for distant metastases. Tumors may spread by local destruction of tissue, by extension along nervous structures, by hematogenous spread to distant sites, and by lymphatic metastases. Regional lymph node spread is estimated to be between 5% and 20% for head

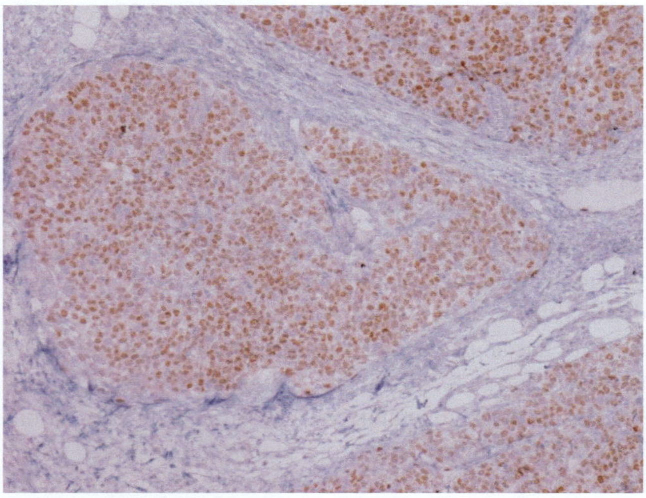

Fig. 80.1 Microscopic evaluation of rhabdomyosarcoma, alveolar type. This image demonstrates anti-myogenin labeling of the nuclei of rhabdomyoblasts. Myogenin is immunoreactive, establishing myogenic differentiation

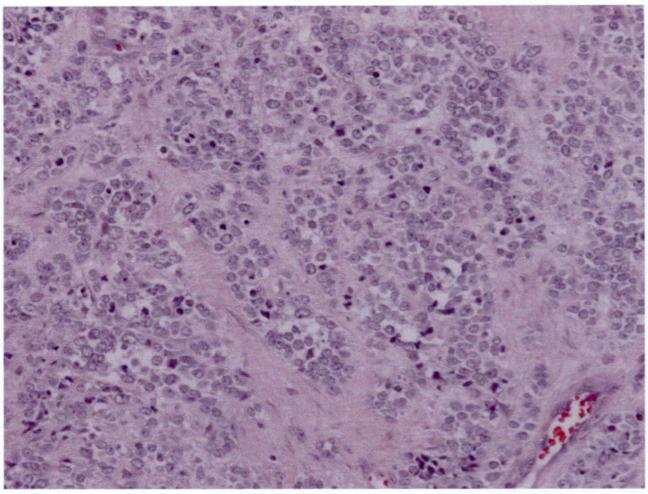

Fig. 80.2 Microscopic evaluation of rhabdomyosarcoma, alveolar type. This image demonstrates a small primitive blue cell tumor with small-to-medium-sized pleomorphic nuclei and scant cytoplasm, frequent mitoses, and apoptosis. Rhabdomyoblasts are not seen

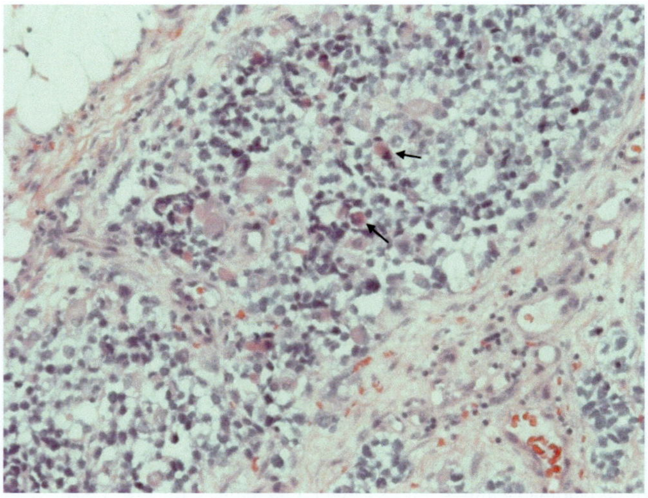

Fig. 80.3 Microscopic evaluation of rhabdomyosarcoma, embryonal type. This image demonstrates a neoplasm composed of primitive poorly differentiated mesenchyme containing rhabdomyoblasts (arrows) with bright eosinophilic cytoplasm and eccentric nuclei

and neck RMS. Raney et al. found regional metastatic disease to be rare in middle ear RMS, whereas nearly 14% of patients with parameningeal RMS have distant metastases at diagnosis [17, 18]. Hematogenous spread is more frequent than lymphatic spread due to the scarcity of lymphatic drainage of the temporal bone. The lung is the most frequent site of metastasis, but the skeletal system, brain, breast, liver, gastrointestinal system, and lymph nodes may also be sites of distant involvement [19]. Contiguous tumor extension is particularly worrisome because of its relationship with the skull base, cranial cavity, and the numerous vital structures in or near the temporal bone, including the sensory organs of hearing and balance, cranial nerves VII and VIII, the internal carotid artery, and the jugular bulb. RMS of the middle ear and mastoid readily spreads via the fallopian canal, round and oval windows, mastoid air cells, and Eustachian tube. The fallopian canal is the most vulnerable area medially in the middle ear, providing a potential pathway for direct tumor invasion to the internal auditory canal and posterior fossa [20, 21]. Additionally, the tumor may extend intracranially by erosion of the tegmen tympani and tegmen mastoideum into the middle cranial fossa. Vestibular or cochlear aqueducts are also a route of intracranial extension after invasion of the labyrinth. Invasion of the infratemporal fossa, nasopharynx, or neck can occur via tumor spread along the Eustachian tube [6].

Presentation

RMS of the temporal bone routinely mimics chronic otitis media at presentation, making early diagnosis difficult. The most common clinical manifestation of RMS of the middle ear is chronic otorrhea with polyp formation in the external auditory canal with or without facial nerve paresis. However, presentation varies based on the location of the tumor and the extent of disease. RMS involving the petrous temporal bone may have minimal ear-related symptoms and present with headache and cranial nerve palsies. Table 80.2 lists the most frequent signs and symptoms from several case series. Prat and Gray reviewed the signs and symptoms of 50 cases of RMS of the middle ear. Their findings included a mass in the region of the ear (56%), a polyp in the external auditory canal (54%), otorrhea (40%), bleeding (30%), otalgia (22%), and facial paresis (14%.) [22] Wiatrak and Pensak reviewed 12 cases of temporal bone RMS, and their findings of presenting complaints included a mass in the region of the ear (17%), a polyp in the external auditory canal (42%), otorrhea (50%), bleeding (8%), otalgia (17%), lymphadenopathy (8%) and facial paresis (50%) [6]. Durve et al. reviewed 14 cases and also noted a higher incidence of facial paresis (64%) and hearing loss (43%), accompanied by similar rates of otorrhea (64%), bleeding (43%), and aural polyp (64%) [23]. Other symptoms can include headache, tinnitus, vertigo, aural fullness, trismus, and cranial nerve V–XII palsies.

The nonspecific nature of the presenting symptoms often leads to prolonged medical management with antibiotic therapy and a delay in diagnosis. The delay from the onset of symptoms to diagnosis is considerable. Durve et al. reported a mean time interval of 21 weeks, and Sbeity et al. found a mean interval of 7 weeks from the onset of symptoms to diagnosis [23, 24]. Therefore, a diagnosis of a malignant process in a child presenting with chronic otorrhea with aural polyps or with bleeding, unresponsive to antibiotics, must be considered. Cranial nerve palsy, especially facial nerve paralysis, should raise the suspicion of such a lesion and be thoroughly investigated for the possibility of an underlying tumor. Biopsy is strongly recommended to rule out an underlying malignant process for pediatric patients with aural polyps or inflammatory granulation tissue in the setting of otitis media unresponsive to medical treatment.

Evaluation

In children with a suspected neoplasm of the temporal bone, the diagnostic evaluation begins with a detailed history and a thorough head and neck examination, including a complete neurotologic examination. Of particular importance is the assessment of the cranial nerves and the microscopic evaluation of the external auditory canal. Certain cranial nerve deficits may indicate the extent and location of the disease. Isolated paresthesia of the mandibular branch of the fifth cranial nerve or diplopia related to isolated sixth cranial nerve palsy can be encountered in tumor involvement confined to the infratemporal fossa or petrous apex, respectively. Ominous indicators of potential involvement of the orbital

Table 80.2 Presenting signs and symptoms of temporal bone rhabdomyosarcoma

Case series	Otalgia	Otorrhea	Bloody discharge	Hearing loss	Facial nerve palsy	Mass	Aural polyp	Lymph-adenopathy
Prat & Gray (*n* = 50)	22%	40%	30%	14%	14%	56%	54%	–
Durve et al. (*n* = 14)	43%	64%	43%	43%	64%	29%	64%	21%
Sbeity et al. (*n* = 6)	33%	16%	–	–	50%	33%	16%	17%
Wiatrak (*n* = 12)	17%	50%	8%	–	50%	17%	42%	8%
Raney (*n* = 24)	–	42%	–	–	58%	17%	83%	0%
Jaffe (*n* = 29)	–	69%	17%	–	52%	14%	55%	17%

apex or cavernous sinus include vision loss, diplopia, chemosis, and proptosis. Furthermore, lower cranial nerve deficits, such as dysphonia, dysphagia, or upper extremity and tongue weakness, may signal invasion of the hypoglossal canal or jugular foramen [25].

The next steps in evaluation include imaging studies of the primary site of involvement, biopsy to achieve a definitive diagnosis, and systemic baseline testing, including complete blood cell count, electrolyte panel, renal function tests, liver enzymes, and coagulation studies. Tissue biopsy is key to the diagnosis of RMS. As mentioned earlier, diagnosis is accomplished by the identification of rhabdomyoblasts and the use of immunohistochemistry (Fig. 80.1). Imaging of the suspected primary site is recommended prior to biopsy, given that these lesions can be secondarily infected, giving rise to falsely negative biopsies, and given the risk of inadvertent injury to adjacent structures such as the facial nerve, carotid, or jugular bulb.

Imaging the RMS of the temporal bone relies on the complementary nature of contrasted computed tomography (CT) and magnetic resonance imaging (MRI). High-resolution CT provides a better assessment of bone and bony erosion, whereas MRI provides a superior evaluation of soft tissue structures, including intracranial and neck contents, nerves, and the patency of the inner ear. Moreover, MRI can be helpful in delineating bone marrow invasion as well as for planning radiation therapy. On CT, RMS appears as a well-defined, homogeneous soft tissue mass in the middle ear, mastoid, or petrous temporal bone, accompanied by bony destruction (Fig. 80.4). It typically demonstrates mild contrast enhancement, similar to that of the adjacent muscle. On MRI, it has intermediate signal intensity on T1 and T2 sequences, with significant contrast enhancement. RMS is isointense relative to muscle and hypointense compared to fat on T1-weighted studies. It demonstrates a hyperintense signal relative to muscle on T2-weighted studies (Fig. 80.5) [26, 27]. Radiographic findings of RMS and other temporal bone malignancies described in this chapter are further detailed in Table 80.3. Of note, in younger children, it may be difficult to obtain radiographic studies without sedation or general anesthesia, which may create an opportunity for biopsy of readily accessible masses and otomicroscopy for the otherwise uncooperative patient.

Once the diagnosis of RMS is made, an extensive evaluation to determine the extent of the disease is performed. Further evaluations may include chest radiograph, CT scan of the chest and regional lymph nodes, bone scan, and bone marrow aspirate. Lumbar puncture is also needed to examine the cerebrospinal fluid (CSF) for the tumor when parameningeal sites such as the temporal bone are involved. Recently, positron emission tomography (PET) with fluorine-18-fluorodeoxyglucose (FDG) has been used to evaluate RMS and other sarcomas. However, the role of PET–CT in staging pediatric RMS has not been entirely established. Several recent studies have suggested that FDG PET has a relevant impact on therapy planning when compared with conventional imaging by more readily identifying nodal, bone, bone marrow, and soft tissue disease and more accurately allowing

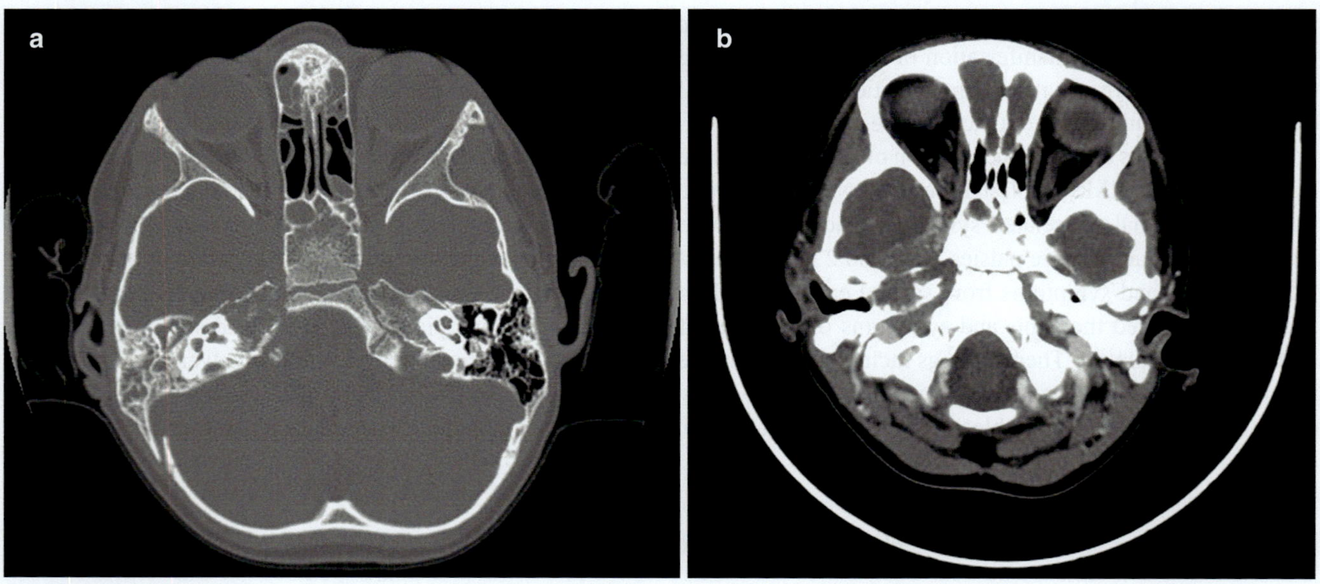

Fig. 80.4 Right temporal bone rhabdomyosarcoma. (**a**) Axial noncontrast CT of the brain shows a soft tissue mass involving the right petrous temporal bone with associated infiltrative bony destruction (arrow) and opacification of the right mastoid air cells and middle ear (arrowhead). (**b**) Axial CT of the brain with contrast demonstrates an enhancing soft tissue mass involving the right petrous temporal bone (arrow) and its extension into the middle cranial fossa

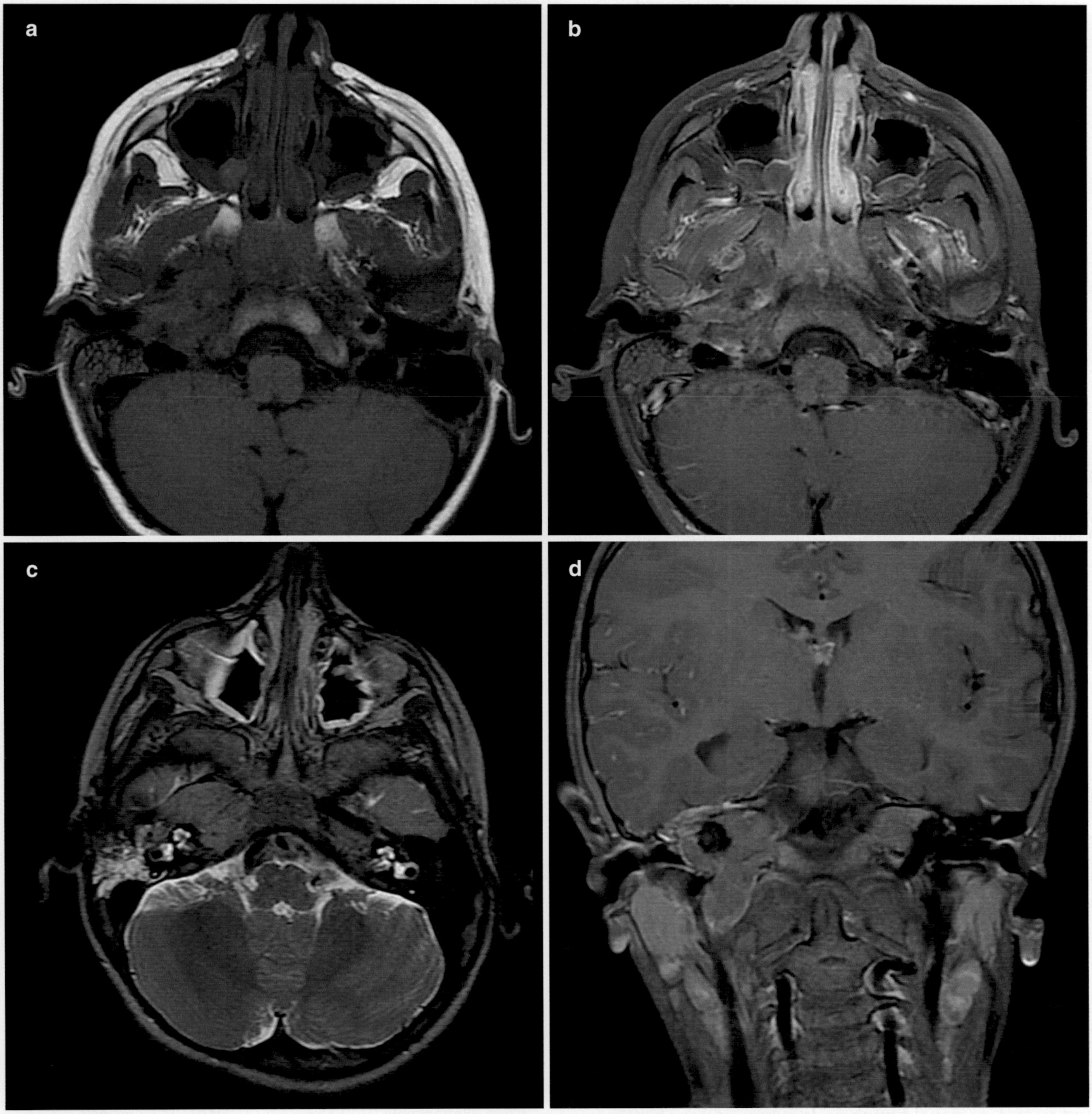

Fig. 80.5 Right temporal bone rhabdomyosarcoma. (**a**) Axial T1 MRI of the internal auditory canals shows an intermediate-intensity soft tissue mass of the right temporal bone (arrow) and opacification of the right mastoid air cells (arrowhead). (**b**) Axial T1 MRI with gadolinium of the internal auditory canal shows a heterogeneously enhancing soft tissue mass of the right petrous temporal bone. (**c**) Axial T2 MRI of the internal auditory canal shows a hyperintense right petrous temporal bone soft tissue mass as well as the associated T2 hyperintense mastoid effusion (arrowhead). (**d**) Coronal T1 MRI with gadolinium of the internal auditory canal shows dural enhancement superior to the soft tissue mass (arrow) and the limits of its inferior extension

Table 80.3 Imaging characteristics of malignant temporal bone tumors

	MRI			
Lesion	T1	T1 + Gd	T2	CT
Rhabdomyosarcoma	Isointense relative to muscle, hypointense relative to fat	Variable enhancement	Hyperintense	Well-defined, lytic bone destruction
Ewing sarcoma	Often hypointense	Heterogeneous enhancement	Hyperintense	Varying degrees of mineralization, aggressive periosteal reaction, homogeneous enhancement
Osteosarcoma	Intermediate intensity	Minimal or patchy to solid	Hyperintense	Bony destruction, matrix mineralization
Granulocytic sarcoma	Similar intensity to bone marrow	Mild enhancement	Isointense	Well-demarcated mass, expansile, lytic appearance
Lymphoma	Hypointense to muscle	Heterogeneous enhancement	Hyperintense to muscle	Homogenous mass, smooth borders

Gd gadolinium

for staging and restaging [28–30]. FDG PET may be sufficient to supplant bone scans for the evaluation of distant disease. Current Children's Oncology Group Soft Tissue Sarcoma (COG-STS) studies are collecting PET imaging data at baseline and during therapy to correlate with radiographic response by standard techniques [31].

Staging and Prognosis

Staging of rhabdomyosarcoma is complex. First, it involves assigning a pretreatment stage (Tables 80.4 and 80.5), followed by a surgical–pathologic clinical group (Table 80.6), and finally a risk group (Table 80.7). The surgical–pathologic clinical group and, subsequently, the pretreatment staging system were established by the Intergroup Rhabdomyosarcoma Study Group (IRSG) and are highly predictive of long-term outcomes [1, 2]. Of note, the IRSG later merged with the National Wilms Tumor Study Group and two large cooperative pediatric cancer treatment groups to form the Children's Oncology Group (COG). The current COG-STS protocol for rhabdomyosarcoma uses the tumor, node, metastasis (TNM)–based pretreatment staging system that incorporates the primary tumor site, the presence or absence of tumor invasion of surrounding tissues, tumor size, regional lymph node status, and the presence or absence of metastases. The surgical–pathologic groups are defined by the extent of disease, the amount of residual tumor after initial surgical resection, and the pathologic review. Following classification by stage and the surgical–pathologic group, a risk group is assigned. The risk group considers stage, surgical–pathologic group, and histology. Patients are classified for treatment protocol purposes as having a low risk (subsets A and B), intermediate risk, or high risk of disease recurrence. Data from IRS III, IV, and V (D-Series) provided rationale for this risk stratification [31]. Of note, the European Malignant Mesenchymal Tumor (MMT) committee of the International Society of Paediatric Oncology and the European Paediatric Soft Tissue Sarcoma Group (EpSSG) have used similar, clinically defined risk groups for treatment assignment, with the addition of early response and delayed resection as factors for the modification of treatment [32, 33].

Table 80.4 Rhabdomyosarcoma tumor staging definition of terms

Term	Definition
T1	Tumor confined to the organ or tissue of origin (noninvasive)
T2	Tumor extension beyond the organ or tissue of origin (invasive)
a	Tumor ≤5 cm in maximum dimension
b	Tumor >5 cm in maximum dimension
N0	No clinical regional lymph node involvement
N1	Clinical regional lymph node involvement
NX	Regional lymph nodes not examined; no information
M0	No metastatic disease
M1	Metastatic disease
Favorable site	Orbit; non-parameningeal head and neck; genitourinary tract other than kidney, bladder, and prostate; biliary tract
Unfavorable site	Any site other than favorable

Adapted from references [1, 2]

Table 80.5 Rhabdomyosarcoma Soft Tissue Sarcoma Committee of the Children's Oncology Group: pretreatment staging system

Stage	Sites of primary tumor	T stage	Tumor size	Regional lymph nodes	Distant metastasis
1	Favorable sites	T1 or T2	Any size	N0, N1, or NX	M0
2	Unfavorable sites	T1 or T2	a, ≤5 cm	N0 or NX	M0
3	Unfavorable sites	T1 or T2	a, ≤5 cm	N1	M0
			b, >5 cm	N0, N1, or NX	
4	Any site	T1 or T2	Any size	N0, N1, or NX	M1

Adapted from references [1, 2]

Table 80.6 Rhabdomyosarcoma Soft Tissue Sarcoma Committee of the Children's Oncology Group: surgical–pathologic group system

Group	Definition
I	Localized tumor, completely removed with microscopically clear margins and no regional lymph node involvement
II	Localized tumor, completely removed with:
IIA	Microscopic residual disease or
IIB	Regional disease with involved, grossly removed regional lymph nodes or
IIC	Regional disease with involved nodes, grossly removed but with microscopic residual and/or histological involvement of the most distal node from the primary tumor
III	Localized tumor, incompletely removed with gross residual disease after:
IIIA	Biopsy only or
IIIB	Subtotal resection
IV	Distant metastases present at diagnosis. This category includes:
IVA	Radiographically identified evidence of tumor spread or
IVB	Positive tumor cells in cerebrospinal fluid, pleural or peritoneal fluids, or implants in these regions

Adapted from references [1, 2]

Table 80.7 Rhabdomyosarcoma Soft Tissue Sarcoma Committee of the Children's Oncology Group: risk group classification

Risk group	Stage	Group	Histology
Low, subset 1	1, 2	I–II	Embryonal
	1	III (orbit)	Embryonal
Low, subset 2	1	III (non-orbit)	Embryonal
	3	I–II	Embryonal
Intermediate	2, 3	III	Embryonal
	1–3	I, II, III	Alveolar
High	4	IV	Embryonal or Alveolar

Adapted from references [1, 2]

RMS of the temporal bone is considered parameningeal in location, which is a prognostically unfavorable site. Therefore, from the outset, these lesions are at least stage II. Moreover, in a review of 179 patients with middle ear RMS enrolled into IRS I through IV, most tumors were not resected before chemotherapy and were, therefore, classified as group III. Nearly 12% of patients were found to have distant metastases at diagnosis. Also, tumors were locally invasive (T2), but the majority were small (<5 cm) and lacked nodal metastases (N0) [7]. Thus, temporal bone RMS is routinely considered intermediate- or high-risk in the risk group classification, with expected event-free survival rates of 50–70% and < 30%, respectively. Those with distant disease at presentation have a more favorable prognosis if they are between 1 and 10 years old and embryonal histology is present at diagnosis [7]. Moreover, Oberlin et al., in a review of pooled data of high-risk patients, found that those with less than two of the following risk factors had a much more favorable prognosis: age less than 1 or greater than 10 years old, unfavorable primary site, three or more sites of metastases, and bone or bone marrow involvement [34].

Management

Treatment of temporal bone RMS was, historically, aggressive surgical resection, which often resulted in significant morbidity without demonstrated survival benefit. Today, the successful management of newly diagnosed RMS in children relies on a multimodal approach adapted to specific clinical and pathologic prognostic factors. The combined use of systemic chemotherapy, with either surgery, radiation therapy (RT), or both, has improved survival overall significantly for children with RMS as well as those with lesions of the temporal bone despite their parameningeal location. In fact, for patients with middle ear RMS, the 5-year overall survival has dramatically improved from 33% in the early 1970s to 72% in the 1990s and even higher for those without base of skull involvement or intracranial extension [7, 35]. The information regarding these modalities as well as risk stratification have largely resulted from the findings of consecutive clinical trials and treatment protocols developed by large international cooperative groups, such as the IRSG and, subsequently, the COG-STS. The current standard treatment of temporal bone RMS is surgical biopsy for tissue diagnosis, followed by chemotherapy and RT for cure.

Surgery is a primary measure to achieve local control in RMS at many anatomical sites if surgical resection of the entire tumor can be performed without serious cosmetic or functional morbidity. Complete resection improves survival and reduces the requirements of adjuvant therapy and its associated comorbidities; however, for parameningeal disease, tissue biopsy is often all that is feasible because of the concern for disfigurement, injury to major cranial nerves, disability, and the high probability of incomplete resection. Importantly, there is also little evidence that debulking surgery improves outcomes, compared with biopsy alone [36]. Delayed primary excision of lesions has been evaluated for other, more accessible sites but has yet to be evaluated for middle ear or mastoid locations [37, 38]. Therefore, surgery is often limited today to biopsy alone for newly diagnosed temporal bone RMS, necessitating definitive radiation therapy for local control of the primary tumor following chemotherapy. Some authors, in the setting of an established craniofacial surgical team, recommend surgical excision in select cases, where complete excision with microscopically clear or only microscopic residual disease can be expected without significant morbidity [25, 39, 40]. This may involve a lateral or subtotal temporal bone resection, petrous apicectomy, or Fisch partial tympanomastoidectomy [25]. As mentioned earlier, regional lymph node metastases are uncommon, and prophylactic lymph node dissection is not recommended.

All children with RMS are recommended to receive chemotherapy, and the multi-agent regimens are tailored to the various prognostic groups listed previously. The results of the sequential IRS studies established vincristine, actinomycin D, and high-dose cyclophosphamide (VAC) as the foundation of chemotherapeutic management in these cases. Treatment outcomes for the low-risk and intermediate-risk groups have already dramatically improved with this intensive three-drug regimen, and current efforts have been directed at maintaining excellent outcomes while minimizing late complications as well as introducing new drugs. For certain subsets of low-risk patients, recent COG studies have maintained excellent outcomes with a shortened duration of therapy, including a modest dose of cyclophosphamide and a two-drug chemotherapy regimen [41]. For intermediate-risk patients, VAC remains the mainstay of the chemotherapy regimen. However, VAC alternating with cycles of vincristine and irinotecan (VI) is currently being investigated as a means to improve local control and the overall outcome for these patients [42]. For high-risk patients, unfortunately, treatment outcomes have not improved comparably to more favorable prognostic groups, and there is a need for novel treatment strategies. Recently, interval-compressed chemotherapy, use of the most active agents identified in previous studies, and use of irinotecan as a radiation sensitizer have improved long-term event-free survival in certain patients with metastatic RMS [43]. Future trials also plan to evaluate the addition of novel biologic agents with chemotherapy.

Within COG studies, RT can provide effective local control and is the mainstay of treatment for all patients with group II–IV RMS. In temporal bone RMS, conformal RT is often preferred because complete removal of these tumors is rare. Techniques to deliver radiation to the tumor while minimizing damage to normal tissue, such as three-dimensional conformal RT (3DCRT), intensity-modulated RT (IMRT), and proton beam therapy, are central to pediatric parameningeal radiation treatment. [44–46] Of interest, proton beam therapy has demonstrated improved normal tissue sparing when compared to IMRT for pediatric parameningeal RMS, but clinical outcomes related to this reduction remain unknown [47]. The treatment dose depends predominantly on the site, the histology, and the amount of residual disease. For parameningeal tumors, a minimum dose of 50.4 Gy is typically administered to the primary site, the adjacent meninges, and the region of intracranial extension, all with a 1.5-cm margin of normal tissue [35]. Patients with parameningeal disease and intracranial extension of the primary tumor do not require whole-brain irradiation or intrathecal therapy unless tumor cells are present in the CSF at diagnosis [35]. Recent COG protocols have investigated the timing of radiation, and data from the D9803 trial suggests that a delay of RT until 6–9 weeks of chemotherapy does not compromise outcomes for parameningeal tumors, even with bony skull base erosion or cranial nerve palsy [48].

In summary, contemporary multimodal therapy, including intensive multidrug chemotherapy regimens as well as tissue-sparing radiation modalities, has contributed to improved outcomes for temporal bone RMS. Although the role of surgery is largely restricted to tissue biopsy, certain cases of limited disease may allow for complete tumor removal, subsequent downstaging, and improved prognosis. It is our suggestion that eligible patients with RMS be enrolled in an active clinical research protocol to ensure that management is up-to-date and further our understanding of the disease, in general.

Ewing Sarcoma

Ewing sarcoma is an aggressive, malignant tumor that arises from the bone and primarily affects children and young adults. It is the second most common bone cancer in children, following osteosarcoma. However, it accounts for only 1% of all childhood cancers. While this neoplasm often involves the axial and appendicular skeleton, nearly a quarter develop in soft tissue, and between 1 and 6% of reported cases involve the skull [49]. It is more uncommon than RMS, and involvement of the temporal bone is exceedingly rare. Watanabe et al. reported in 1992 on 11 cases involving the cranium, only three of which involved the temporal bone [50]. Since that time, review of the literature demonstrates only a limited number of additional cases, a majority of which describe lesions of the petrous temporal bone [51–58]. Ewing sarcoma often presents as an expansile mass causing symptoms of increased intracranial pressure. In addition to headache, nausea, and vomiting, presentation may also be similar to those described for RMS, such as facial nerve palsy, hearing loss, otorrhea, or a temporal mass [53].

Evaluation for Ewing sarcoma, as well as the other tumors mentioned in this chapter, is similar to that described previously for RMS: CT, MRI, biopsy, and routine lab work. For Ewing sarcoma, lactate dehydrogenase (LDH) should also be included in serum chemistries because a normal level of this enzyme has been associated with a favorable prognosis. Imaging reveals an isodense, contrast-enhancing mass, which is typically a destructive osseous lesion with periosteal reaction. On MRI, the mass is hypointense on T1-weighted and iso- to hyperintense on T2-weighted images with heterogeneous contrast enhancement [59, 60]. Immunohistochemistry testing in Ewing sarcoma reveals vimentin and CD99 expression, and chromosomal translocation between chromosome 22 and chromosome 11 is frequently seen with fluorescence in situ hybridization (FISH) analysis.

As with RMS, multimodal therapy is the treatment of choice for temporal bone Ewing sarcoma. Current treatment paradigms favor primary induction chemotherapy, followed by surgery or RT and adjuvant chemotherapy. The chemotherapeutic agents commonly used include vincristine, doxorubicin, cyclophosphamide, etoposide, and ifosfamide. The best approach for local control, again, remains a matter of discussion. Tumors arising from the cranium may be amenable to complete excision. However, complete surgical resection of skull base lesions is often impossible without substantial morbidity. Thus, RT remains the preferred therapy in many cases, either as a primary mode of local control or as an adjuvant therapy in the setting of resection with positive margins.

Osteosarcoma

Osteosarcoma is the most common primary malignant bone tumor in children and adolescents. Most pediatric osteosarcomas arise in the appendicular skeleton, whereas craniofacial osteosarcomas are rare. These tumors represent fewer than 5% of cases and typically occur in older patients [61]. They are usually encountered in the mandible and, rarely, the temporal bone. Hadley et al., in 2014, described three cases of pediatric cranial osteosarcomas and identified only 35 previously reported cases involving the cranium and skull base in children. Less than one-third of the cases reported involvement of the temporal bone [62]. In most cases, the presentation of a primary lesion is simply a mass or swelling that enlarges over months and can be difficult to distinguish from a benign process.

Osteosarcoma is characterized by excessive immature bone production by malignant spindle cells. The World Health Organization organizes osteosarcomas into central (medullary) and surface (peripheral) tumors and recognizes several histological variants in each group. The most common pathologic group is conventional central osteosarcoma, which is further divided into osteoblastic, chondroblastic, and fibroblastic subtypes. Predisposing conditions include fibrous dysplasia, Paget's disease, Li–Fraumeni syndrome, and retinoblastoma. Additionally, ionizing radiation exposure is also associated with the development of osteosarcoma [63–65]. The general radiologic features are not specific and are dependent on the amount of osteoblastic and osteolytic activity of the tumor. CT and MRI have been reported to show a soft tissue mass with an aggressive pattern, the presence of bony destruction, and mineralization of the tumor. On MRI, osteosarcomas have been characterized as having intermediate signal on T1-weighted MR and hyperintensity on T2-weighted MR. However, varying signal intensity can be seen depending on the degree of mineralization, hemorrhage, and necrosis [66–68].

Osteosarcoma carries the worst prognosis of all temporal bone malignancies. Early studies reported a 5-year survival of 9% in patients of all ages, but more recent reports suggest that 5-year survival may be near 31% [69, 70]. Osteosarcoma of the head and neck metastasizes less frequently and less quickly compared to those in other sites of the body [71]. The most important prognostic factors are the presence of metastatic disease and the ability to completely resect the tumor [72]. Adequate surgical margins are of significant importance, as this tumor is relatively resistant to radiotherapy [73]. Therefore, complete resection is emphasized, in combination with cisplatin-based chemotherapy. When gross resection cannot be achieved, extensive resection coupled with adjuvant chemotherapy and radiation improves overall survival, local control, and disease-specific survival [74]. Furthermore, even in difficult-to-resect tumors, surgery is the treatment of choice for radiation-induced osteosarcoma, as these patients are typically not candidates to receive radiation of the previously irradiated field.

Non-rhabdomyosarcoma Soft Tissue Sarcomas

Non-rhabdomyosarcoma soft tissue sarcomas (NRSTS) are exceedingly rare in the temporal bone, and they include a heterogeneous group of tumors. The initial imaging and biopsies in patients with suspected NRSTS are the same as those of patients with RMS, and similar staging systems are used for both. Additionally, many of these sarcomas have high- and low-grade histological variants, which affect the disease presentation and outcome. Some of the NRSTS that have been reported to occur in the temporal bone of children and adolescents include chondrosarcoma, chordoma, fibrosarcoma, angiosarcoma, granulocytic sarcoma (chloroma), and liposarcoma [5, 75–77]. Successful treatment is again dependent on multimodal therapy. In contrast to temporal bone RMS, surgical resection is typically the primary mode of local control. In fact, pretreatment re-excision should be performed whenever it is uncertain whether the tumor was adequately excised [78]. Following wide local excision, patients receive systemic chemotherapy and/or RT. Ifosfamide and doxorubicin are considered to be the most active and among the most commonly used regimens in NRSTS [79]. Our recommendation is that patients with NRSTS be enrolled in clinical trials whenever possible to ensure that treatment is up-to-date, given the rarity of these tumors.

Among the aforementioned tumors, granulocytic sarcoma warrants further discussion. Traditionally known as chloroma because of its greenish hue, granulocytic sarcoma is an uncommon solid tumor composed of immature cells with myelogenous differentiation. It is encountered most frequently in the pediatric population and can be a manifestation of several myeloproliferative disorders, such as acute myelogenous leukemia (AML) [80]. Although rare in the head and neck region, granulocytic sarcomas of the orbit, face, maxilla, mandible, paranasal sinuses, and temporal bone have all been reported previously [76, 81–86].

The development of granulocytic sarcoma may herald the onset of leukemia or be the first sign of relapse or progression of disease in a patient previously diagnosed with leukemia. It is a locally aggressive and destructive lesion with a poor long-term prognosis, particularly for those patients with known leukemia [81]. On CT scan, this lesion is a well-demarcated mass with increased attenuation within a peripheral zone of enhancement. Lesions often have a lytic, rather than sclerotic, appearance. On MRI, granulocytic sarcomas demonstrate similar intensity to bone marrow on both T1- and T2-weighted sequences, as well as mild contrast enhancement [85, 87]. Recognition of this rare entity is important because the recommended course of treatment is the same therapeutic regimen used to treat AML rather than aggressive surgery. Specifically, treatment frequently involves chemotherapy and bone marrow transplantation, as well as radiotherapy for bulky or symptomatic lesions [88].

Lymphoma

Lymphoma, a neoplastic proliferation of monoclonal lymphoid cells, is the most common type of head and neck cancer encountered in children. Overall, lymphoma accounts for 10–15% of all childhood malignancies. The disease is subdivided into non-Hodgkin lymphoma (NHL) and Hodgkin lymphoma (HL). NHL makes up approximately 60% of all childhood lymphomas and predominates in terms of head and neck involvement [89]. Most cases in pediatric patients fall into one of the following three categories: mature B-cell NHL, lymphoblastic lymphoma, and anaplastic large cell lymphoma [90]. Of these forms, mature B-cell NHL comprises greater than 85% of all NHL diagnoses [91]. Although involvement of the temporal bone as a part of systemic lymphoma has been reported, primary involvement of the temporal bone is exceptionally rare. Only 24 cases have been reported in the literature since the initial description by Tucci et al. in 1992 [92–98].

The most common symptoms of primary lymphoma of the temporal bone are conductive hearing loss, otorrhea, otalgia, and cranial nerve deficits. However, facial nerve palsy is rare in lymphoma because the nerve sheath is resistant to tumor invasion [99]. Systemic symptoms such as night sweats and fever are also uncommon with disease localized to the temporal bone [94, 95]. Radiologically, lymphoma often appears as a homogeneous soft tissue density with smooth borders of the mastoid, middle ear, or internal or external auditory canal, with associated bony destruction, on high-resolution CT. On MRI, lymphoma is isointense to muscle on T1-weighted images and hyperintense to muscle on T2-weighted images and has heterogeneous contrast enhancement [92, 97, 100]. Biopsy and immunohistochemistry assist in diagnosis because it is difficult to differentiate between lymphoma and other neoplastic processes. Primary NHL of the bone in children requires both prompt systemic chemotherapy and local RT for successful disease control.

Parotid Tumors with Secondary Temporal Bone Invasion

Salivary gland tumors represent approximately 3% of all head and neck malignancies in the general population and less than 10% in children. The most commonly affected site among children is the parotid gland, accounting for 90% of lesions. Mucoepidermoid carcinoma and acinar cell carcinoma are the two most common malignant lesions afflicting the parotid gland in pediatric patients [101]. Of these two neoplasms, mucoepidermoid carcinomas tend to be more advanced in stage and are associated with a higher rate of nodal metastasis. However, high-grade tumors are infrequent in the pediatric population [102, 103]. Large parotid tumors can be locally invasive and involve the ear or temporal bone secondarily. In these rare instances, surgery remains the treatment of choice and consists of a superficial or total parotidectomy, combined with temporal bone resection. In addition, neck dissection is usually only recommended in cases of evident nodal metastasis [101, 104]. Adjuvant radiotherapy is considered for cases with widespread disease, positive surgical margins, perineural invasion, or aggressive histological features [104].

Conclusion

Pediatric temporal bone malignancies are rare. In general, the mainstays of treatment are nonsurgical, though there can be a role for surgical intervention as it relates to diagnostic biopsy and, in certain instances, complete surgical extirpation. Having a thorough understanding of the presentation, evaluation, and management of these tumors helps assist in earlier diagnosis and initiation of timely treatment.

Acknowledgments The authors would like to thank Elizabeth Gillies, MD, Associate Professor and Director of Surgical Pathology, University of Oklahoma Health Sciences Center, and Anthony Alleman, MD, Bob G. Eaton Chair in Radiological Sciences, University of Oklahoma Health Sciences Center, for their image contributions to this chapter.

References

1. Crist W, et al. The third intergroup rhabdomyosarcoma study. J Clin Oncol. 1995;13(3):610–30.
2. Crist WM, et al. Intergroup rhabdomyosarcoma study-IV: results for patients with nonmetastatic disease. J Clin Oncol. 2001;19(12):3091–102.
3. Maurer HM, et al. The intergroup rhabdomyosarcoma study-I. A final report. Cancer. 1988;61(2):209–20.
4. Maurer HM, et al. The intergroup rhabdomyosarcoma study-II. Cancer. 1993;71(5):1904–22.
5. Lyos AT, et al. Soft tissue sarcoma of the head and neck in children and adolescents. Cancer. 1996;77(1):193–200.
6. Wiatrak BJ, Pensak ML. Rhabdomyosarcoma of the ear and temporal bone. Laryngoscope. 1989;99(11):1188–92.
7. Hawkins DS, et al. Improved outcome for patients with middle ear rhabdomyosarcoma: a children's oncology group study. J Clin Oncol. 2001;19(12):3073–9.
8. Dasgupta R, Rodeberg DA. Update on rhabdomyosarcoma. Semin Pediatr Surg. 2012;21(1):68–78.
9. Ray A, Huh WW. Current state-of-the-art systemic therapy for pediatric soft tissue sarcomas. Curr Oncol Rep. 2012;14(4):311–9.
10. Merlino G, Helman LJ. Rhabdomyosarcoma--working out the pathways. Oncogene. 1999;18(38):5340–8.
11. Barr FG, et al. Examination of gene fusion status in archival samples of alveolar rhabdomyosarcoma entered on the Intergroup Rhabdomyosarcoma Study-III trial: a report from the Children's Oncology Group. J Mol Diagn. 2006;8(2):202–8.
12. Dumont SN, et al. PAX3/7-FOXO1 fusion status in older rhabdomyosarcoma patient population by fluorescent in situ hybridization. J Cancer Res Clin Oncol. 2012;138(2):213–20.
13. Koufos A, et al. Loss of heterozygosity in three embryonal tumours suggests a common pathogenetic mechanism. Nature. 1985;316(6026):330–4.
14. Skapek SX, et al. PAX-FOXO1 fusion status drives unfavorable outcome for children with rhabdomyosarcoma: a children's oncology group report. Pediatr Blood Cancer. 2013;60(9):1411–7.
15. Scrable H, et al. Molecular differential pathology of rhabdomyosarcoma. Genes Chromosomes Cancer. 1989;1(1):23–35.
16. Parham DM, et al. Immunohistochemical study of childhood rhabdomyosarcomas and related neoplasms. Results of an Intergroup Rhabdomyosarcoma study project. Cancer. 1991;67(12):3072–80.
17. Maurer HM. The intergroup rhabdomyosarcoma study: update, November 1978. Natl Cancer Inst Monogr. 1981;56:61–8.
18. Raney RB Jr, et al. Rhabdomyosarcoma of the ear in childhood. A report from the Intergroup Rhabdomyosarcoma Study-I. Cancer. 1983;51(12):2356–61.
19. Raney RB Jr, et al. Disease patterns and survival rate in children with metastatic soft-tissue sarcoma. A report from the Intergroup Rhabdomyosarcoma Study (IRS)-I. Cancer. 1988;62(7):1257–66.
20. Karatay S. Rhabdomyosarcoma of the middle ear. Arch Otolaryngol. 1949;50(3):330–4.
21. Myers EN, Stool S, Weltschew A. Rhabdomyosarcoma of the middle ear. Ann Otol Rhinol Laryngol. 1968;77(5):949–58.
22. Prat J, Gray GF. Massive neuraxial spread of aural rhabdomyosarcoma. Arch Otolaryngol. 1977;103(5):301–3.
23. Durve DV, et al. Paediatric rhabdomyosarcoma of the ear and temporal bone. Clin Otolaryngol Allied Sci. 2004;29(1):32–7.
24. Sbeity S, et al. Temporal bone rhabdomyosarcoma in children. Int J Pediatr Otorhinolaryngol. 2007;71(5):807–14.
25. Gluth MB. Rhabdomyosarcoma and other pediatric temporal bone malignancies. Otolaryngol Clin N Am. 2015;48(2):375–90.
26. Lee JH, et al. Rhabdomyosarcoma of the head and neck in adults: MR and CT findings. AJNR Am J Neuroradiol. 1996;17(10):1923–8.
27. Chevallier KM, et al. Differentiating pediatric rhabdomyosarcoma and langerhans cell histiocytosis of the temporal bone by imaging appearance. AJNR Am J Neuroradiol. 2016;37(6):1185–9.
28. Federico SM, et al. Comparison of PET-CT and conventional imaging in staging pediatric rhabdomyosarcoma. Pediatr Blood Cancer. 2013;60(7):1128–34.
29. Tateishi U, et al. Comparative study of FDG PET/CT and conventional imaging in the staging of rhabdomyosarcoma. Ann Nucl Med. 2009;23(2):155–61.
30. Volker T, et al. Positron emission tomography for staging of pediatric sarcoma patients: results of a prospective multicenter trial. J Clin Oncol. 2007;25(34):5435–41.
31. Malempati S, Hawkins DS. Rhabdomyosarcoma: review of the Children's Oncology Group (COG) Soft-Tissue Sarcoma Committee experience and rationale for current COG studies. Pediatr Blood Cancer. 2012;59(1):5–10.
32. Oberlin O, et al. Randomized comparison of intensified six-drug versus standard three-drug chemotherapy for high-risk nonmetastatic rhabdomyosarcoma and other chemotherapy-sensitive childhood soft tissue sarcomas: long-term results from the International Society of Pediatric Oncology MMT95 study. J Clin Oncol. 2012;30(20):2457–65.
33. Stevens MC, et al. Treatment of nonmetastatic rhabdomyosarcoma in childhood and adolescence: third study of the International Society of Paediatric Oncology--SIOP Malignant Mesenchymal Tumor 89. J Clin Oncol. 2005;23(12):2618–28.
34. Oberlin O, et al. Prognostic factors in metastatic rhabdomyosarcomas: results of a pooled analysis from United States and European cooperative groups. J Clin Oncol. 2008;26(14):2384–9.
35. Raney RB, et al. Treatment of children and adolescents with localized parameningeal sarcoma: experience of the Intergroup Rhabdomyosarcoma Study Group protocols IRS-II through -IV, 1978-1997. Med Pediatr Oncol. 2002;38(1):22–32.
36. Cecchetto G, et al. Biopsy or debulking surgery as initial surgery for locally advanced rhabdomyosarcomas in children?: the experience of the Italian Cooperative Group studies. Cancer. 2007;110(11):2561–7.
37. Rodeberg DA, et al. Delayed primary excision with subsequent modification of radiotherapy dose for intermediate-risk rhabdomyosarcoma: a report from the Children's Oncology Group Soft Tissue Sarcoma Committee. Int J Cancer. 2015;137(1):204–11.
38. Blatt J, et al. Delayed resection in the management of non-orbital rhabdomyosarcoma of the head and neck in childhood. Med Pediatr Oncol. 1997;28(4):294–8.
39. Daya H, et al. Pediatric rhabdomyosarcoma of the head and neck: is there a place for surgical management? Arch Otolaryngol Head Neck Surg. 2000;126(4):468–72.
40. Rodeberg DA, et al. Surgical principles for children/adolescents with newly diagnosed rhabdomyosarcoma: a report from the Soft Tissue Sarcoma Committee of the Children's Oncology Group. Sarcoma. 2002;6(4):111–22.
41. Walterhouse DO, et al. Shorter-duration therapy using vincristine, dactinomycin, and lower-dose cyclophosphamide with or without radiotherapy for patients with newly diagnosed low-risk rhabdomyosarcoma: a report from the Soft Tissue Sarcoma Committee of the Children's Oncology Group. J Clin Oncol. 2014;32(31):3547–52.
42. Hawkins DS, et al. Children's Oncology Group's 2013 blueprint for research: soft tissue sarcomas. Pediatr Blood Cancer. 2013;60(6):1001–8.
43. Weigel BJ, et al. Intensive multiagent therapy, including dose-compressed cycles of Ifosfamide/etoposide and vincristine/doxorubicin/cyclophosphamide, Irinotecan, and radiation, in patients with high-risk rhabdomyosarcoma: a report from the children's oncology group. J Clin Oncol. 2016;34(2):117–22.

44. Ladra MM, et al. Preliminary results of a phase II trial of proton radiotherapy for pediatric rhabdomyosarcoma. J Clin Oncol. 2014;32(33):3762–70.
45. Wolden SL, et al. Long-term results of three-dimensional conformal radiation therapy for patients with rhabdomyosarcoma. Cancer. 2003;97(1):179–85.
46. Lin C, et al. Effect of radiotherapy techniques (IMRT vs. 3D-CRT) on outcome in patients with intermediate-risk rhabdomyosarcoma enrolled in COG D9803--a report from the Children's Oncology Group. Int J Radiat Oncol Biol Phys. 2012;82(5):1764–70.
47. Ladra MM, et al. A dosimetric comparison of proton and intensity modulated radiation therapy in pediatric rhabdomyosarcoma patients enrolled on a prospective phase II proton study. Radiother Oncol. 2014;113(1):77–83.
48. Spalding AC, et al. The effect of radiation timing on patients with high-risk features of parameningeal rhabdomyosarcoma: an analysis of IRS-IV and D9803. Int J Radiat Oncol Biol Phys. 2013;87(3):512–6.
49. Buckley JD, et al. Epidemiology of osteosarcoma and Ewing's sarcoma in childhood: a study of 305 cases by the Children's Cancer Group. Cancer. 1998;83(7):1440–8.
50. Watanabe H, et al. Primary Ewing's sarcoma of the temporal bone. Surg Neurol. 1992;37(1):54–8.
51. Kawano H, et al. Primary pericranial Ewing's sarcoma on the temporal bone: a case report. Surg Neurol Int. 2016;7(Suppl 15):S444–8.
52. Nandi M, et al. Primary Ewing's sarcoma of the squamous part of temporal bone in a young girl treated with adjuvant volumetric arc therapy. J Cancer Res Ther. 2015;11(4):1015–7.
53. Kadar AA, et al. Ewing's sarcoma of the petrous temporal bone: case report and literature review. Skull Base. 2010;20(3):213–7.
54. Balasubramaniam S, et al. Primary Ewing's sarcoma of the petroclival bone. J Clin Neurosci. 2008;15(6):712–4.
55. Pfeiffer J, Boedeker CC, Ridder GJ. Primary Ewing sarcoma of the petrous temporal bone: an exceptional cause of facial palsy and deafness in a nursling. Head Neck. 2006;28(10):955–9.
56. Desai K, Goel A, Nadkarni TD. Primary petrous bone Ewing's sarcoma. Br J Neurosurg. 2000;14(2):143–5.
57. Kuzeyli K, et al. Primary Ewing's sarcoma of the temporal bone with intracranial, extracranial and intraorbital extension. Case Rep Neurosurg Rev. 1997;20(2):132–4.
58. Cherekaev VA, et al. Primary and metastatic Ewing sarcoma of the skull base - case reports and comparative analysis. Zh Vopr Neirokhir Im N N Bur. 2013;77(1):30–6; discussion 36.
59. Narayanan G, et al. Ewing's sarcoma of the cranial vault. J Neurosci Rural Pract. 2016;7(Suppl 1):S109–11.
60. Radhakrishnan R, Son HJ, Koch BL. Petrous apex lesions in the pediatric population. Pediatr Radiol. 2014;44(3):325–39; quiz 323–4.
61. Mirabello L, Troisi RJ, Savage SA. Osteosarcoma incidence and survival rates from 1973 to 2004: data from the Surveillance, Epidemiology, and End Results Program. Cancer. 2009;115(7):1531–43.
62. Hadley C, et al. Osteosarcoma of the cranial vault and skull base in pediatric patients. J Neurosurg Pediatr. 2014;13(4):380–7.
63. Ha PK, et al. Osteosarcoma of the head and neck: a review of the Johns Hopkins experience. Laryngoscope. 1999;109(6):964–9.
64. Kellie SJ, et al. Successful treatment of a radiation-associated extradural osteosarcoma with chemotherapy in an adolescent girl. Med Pediatr Oncol. 1989;17(6):514–9.
65. Gadwal SR, et al. Primary osteosarcoma of the head and neck in pediatric patients: a clinicopathologic study of 22 cases with a review of the literature. Cancer. 2001;91(3):598–605.
66. Murphey MD, et al. The many faces of osteosarcoma. Radiographics. 1997;17(5):1205–31.
67. Debnam JM, et al. Radiation-associated head and neck sarcomas: spectrum of imaging findings. Oral Oncol. 2012;48(2):155–61.
68. Bose B. Primary osteogenic sarcoma of the skull. Surg Neurol. 2002;58(3–4):234–9; discussion 239–40.
69. Caron AS, Hajdu SI, Strong EW. Osteogenic sarcoma of the facial and cranial bones. A review of forty-three cases. Am J Surg. 1971;122(6):719–25.
70. Shinoda J, et al. Primary osteosarcoma of the skull--a case report and review of the literature. J Neuro-Oncol. 1993;17(1):81–8.
71. Potter BO, Sturgis EM. Sarcomas of the head and neck. Surg Oncol Clin N Am. 2003;12(2):379–417.
72. Federman N, et al. The multidisciplinary management of osteosarcoma. Curr Treat Options in Oncol. 2009;10(1–2):82–93.
73. Marina N, et al. Biology and therapeutic advances for pediatric osteosarcoma. Oncologist. 2004;9(4):422–41.
74. Guadagnolo BA, et al. Osteosarcoma of the jaw/craniofacial region: outcomes after multimodality treatment. Cancer. 2009;115(14):3262–70.
75. Gadwal SR, et al. Primary chondrosarcoma of the head and neck in pediatric patients: a clinicopathologic study of 14 cases with a review of the literature. Cancer. 2000;88(9):2181–8.
76. Levy R, Shvero J, Sandbank J. Granulocytic sarcoma (chloroma) of the temporal bone. Int J Pediatr Otorhinolaryngol. 1989;18(2):163–9.
77. Borba LA, et al. Cranial chordomas in children and adolescents. J Neurosurg. 1996;84(4):584–91.
78. Chui CH, et al. Is reexcision in pediatric nonrhabdomyosarcoma soft tissue sarcoma necessary after an initial unplanned resection? J Pediatr Surg. 2002;37(10):1424–9.
79. Pervaiz N, et al. A systematic meta-analysis of randomized controlled trials of adjuvant chemotherapy for localized resectable soft-tissue sarcoma. Cancer. 2008;113(3):573–81.
80. Neiman RS, et al. Granulocytic sarcoma: a clinicopathologic study of 61 biopsied cases. Cancer. 1981;48(6):1426–37.
81. Alessi DM, et al. Granulocytic sarcomas of the head and neck. Arch Otolaryngol Head Neck Surg. 1988;114(12):1467–70.
82. Stack BC Jr, Ridley MB. Granulocytic sarcoma of the mandible. Otolaryngol Head Neck Surg. 1994;110(6):591–4.
83. Cankaya, H., S. Ugras, and I. Dilek, Head and neck granulocytic sarcoma with acute myeloid leukemia: three rare cases. Ear Nose Throat J. 2001;80(4):224–6, 228–9.
84. Nayak DR, et al. Granulocytic sarcoma of the head and neck: a case report. Am J Otolaryngol. 2001;22(1):80–3.
85. Lee B, et al. Granulocytic sarcoma of the temporal bone. AJNR Am J Neuroradiol. 2002;23(9):1497–9.
86. Prades JM, et al. Granulocytic sarcoma of the nasal cavity. Rhinology. 2002;40(3):159–61.
87. Noh BW, et al. Granulocytic sarcoma in the head and neck: CT and MR imaging findings. Clin Exp Otorhinolaryngol. 2009;2(2):66–71.
88. Roby BB, Drehner D, Sidman JD. Granulocytic sarcoma of pediatric head and neck: an institutional experience. Int J Pediatr Otorhinolaryngol. 2013;77(8):1364–6.
89. La Quaglia MP. Non-Hodgkin's lymphoma of the head and neck in childhood. Semin Pediatr Surg. 1994;3(3):207–15.
90. Swerdlow SH, et al. The 2016 revision of the World Health Organization classification of lymphoid neoplasms. Blood. 2016;127(20):2375–90.
91. Huang Z, Xu Z, Zhou Y. Chemotherapy alone versus chemotherapy followed by consolidative radiotherapy for limited-stage aggressive non-Hodgkin's lymphoma: a meta-analysis of randomized controlled trials. Cancer Radiother. 2013;17(8):736–43.
92. Vaid S, et al. Bilateral non-Hodgkin's lymphoma of the temporal bone: a rare and unusual presentation. Case Rep Otolaryngol. 2016;2016:2641876.

93. Sritharan N, et al. Primary non-Hodgkin lymphoma of the petrous temporal bone. Otol Neurotol. 2012;33(2):e11–2.
94. Jiang ZY, Saadia-Redleaf MI. Primary lymphoma of the temporal bone presenting as XIIth cranial nerve weakness. Ear Nose Throat J. 2011;90(3):125–7.
95. Tucci DL, Lambert PR, Innes DJ Jr. Primary lymphoma of the temporal bone. Arch Otolaryngol Head Neck Surg. 1992;118(1):83–5.
96. Li B, et al. Primary T-cell lymphoblastic lymphoma in the middle ear. Int J Pediatr Otorhinolaryngol. 2016;82:19–22.
97. Schmedes GW, Rizk HG, Lambert PR. Middle ear mass with facial weakness. Diffuse large B-cell lymphoma of the middle ear. JAMA Otolaryngol Head Neck Surg. 2015;141(1):89–90.
98. Santos Monton C, Garzon Guiteria MT. Radiological findings of a primary middle-ear lymphoma in a 8-year-old boy. Radiologia (Roma). 2015;57(3):268–70.
99. Saito H, Chinzei K, Furuta M. Pathological features of peripheral facial paralysis caused by malignant tumour. Acta Otolaryngol Suppl. 1988;446:165–71.
100. Choi HK, et al. Central skull base lymphoma in children: MR and CT features. Pediatr Radiol. 2008;38(8):863–7.
101. Allan BJ, et al. Malignant tumors of the parotid gland in children: incidence and outcomes. J Craniofac Surg. 2013;24(5):1660–4.
102. Vedrine PO, et al. Mucoepidermoid carcinoma of salivary glands in the pediatric age group: 18 clinical cases, including 11 second malignant neoplasms. Head Neck. 2006;28(9):827–33.
103. Hicks J, Flaitz C. Mucoepidermoid carcinoma of salivary glands in children and adolescents: assessment of proliferation markers. Oral Oncol. 2000;36(5):454–60.
104. Orvidas LJ, et al. Pediatric parotid masses. Arch Otolaryngol Head Neck Surg. 2000;126(2):177–84.

Stereotactic Radiosurgery and Radiotherapy for Lateral Skull Tumors

81

Christopher A. Schutt, Jeffery Jacob, and Seilesh Babu

History of Development

Lars Leksell pioneered stereotactic radiosurgery (SRS) as a professor at the Karolinska Institute. He was convinced that a more reliable method to reach deep intracranial structures was possible and began experimenting with guiding devices based on Cartesian coordinate systems. Over many years, this work led to the development of SRS. Interestingly, Leksell's main focus was the treatment of functional disorders, not tumors. His first device was fashioned in the 1950s to treat trigeminal neuralgia and consisted of an arch-centered platform with an attached orthodontic X-ray. After submitting the documentation of its use, it was rejected by a journal editor, stating that there was no such thing as SRS [1]. Though X-ray therapy showed promising results, Leksell knew that a different form of radiation was needed for improved penetration. He collaborated with a radiobiologist who specialized in proton beam and later investigated the use of linear accelerator technology, before producing his cobalt Gamma Knife® prototype in 1963 [1]. Acceptance of SRS was slow over the first 20 years of its use, and it was not until the 1990s that it was widely adopted for vestibular schwannoma. Since that time, SRS has become exceedingly popular, representing the primary treatment choice in 24% of patients diagnosed with vestibular schwannoma [2].

Radiobiology

SRS relies on high-energy photons produced by radioactive decay or an electric potential. Once inside the target tissue, the photons induce tumor cell death through a variety of pathways. Traditionally, emphasis has been given to the ability of radiation to create single- and double-strand DNA breaks, leading to necrosis or induced apoptosis after failed repair. More recently, radiation-induced damage to the endothelial cell layer of the tumor vasculature has been implicated in tumor control.

Methods of Delivery: Gamma Knife® and LINAC

Gamma Knife® functions by precisely locating a tumor within a three-dimensional (3D) coordinate system, referencing the target in defined stereotactic space and passing radiation through the target volume. All Gamma Knife® models consist of a spherical helmet possessing multiple collimators of cobalt focused at a geometric center. Conformation of radiation to the tumor's size is shaped by the use of multiple shots. Each shot consists of separate weights of radiation strategically placed at different locations within the tumor. As multiple sources of radiation are used, each extending from a noncoplanar location, individual beams consist of low-level radiation. However, summation at the geometric center allows for high levels of radiation to be present in the target tissue. Through this technique, radiation is accurately delivered at high doses with minimal radiation extending outside the target volume.

Gamma Knife Perfexion®, launched in 2006, represents the most commonly used system at major centers (Fig. 81.1). It consists of 192 ^{60}Co sources placed within a single collimator helmet. The patient is moved automatically through sequential shots, coordinated by the movement of the patient couch, firmly fixed to the stereotactic frame. The major improvement over model C, its predecessor, is the ability to treat lesions extending into the neck. Here, radiation may be delivered to the level of C2. Only intracranial lesions or those directly at the skull base could be treated with model C. More recently, the Gamma Knife® Icon has been introduced (Fig. 81.2). It offers the ability to perform mask-based

C. A. Schutt · S. Babu (✉)
Department of Neurotology, Michigan Ear Institute, Henry Ford Health System, Novi, MI, USA

J. Jacob
Department of Neurologic Surgery, Henry Ford Health System, Novi, MI, USA

A. D. Sweeney et al. (eds.), *Haynes-Glasscock-Shambaugh Surgery of the Ear*, https://doi.org/10.1007/978-3-032-18264-7_81

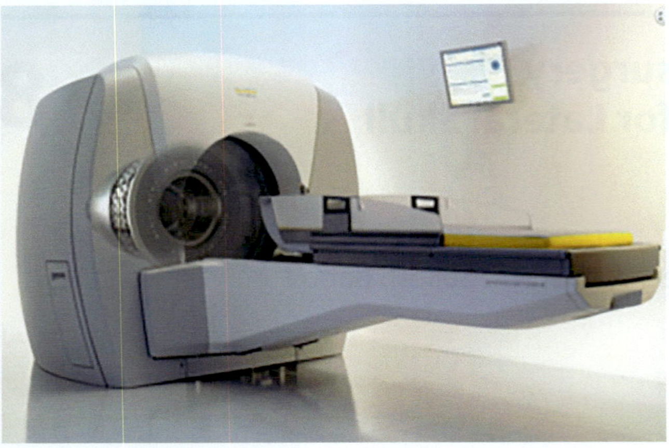

Fig. 81.1 Gamma Knife Perfexion® model. (Used with permission from Elekta)

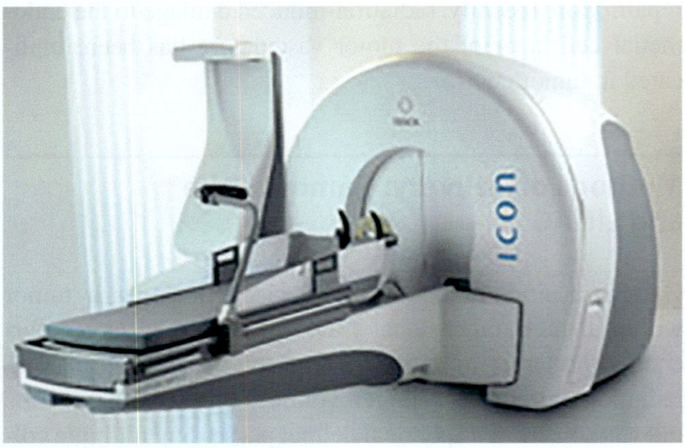

Fig. 81.2 Gamma Knife Icon® model. (Used with permission from Elekta)

treatments in addition to traditional frame-based delivery. When used in mask mode, a cone-beam CT is obtained before treatment and after the patient's movement to outline the cranial skeleton, establishing the stereotactic space. Though mask treatment holds appeal, it may not prove beneficial in the treatment of internal auditory canal (IAC) lesions where stereotactic frames are well-tolerated. Instead, this function may be better suited for other types of treatments, including fractionated therapy.

CyberKnife®, a linear accelerator (LINAC) alternative to Gamma Knife®, consists of a 6-MeV LINAC attached to a robotic arm. Radiation is delivered through sequential step-and-shoot motions. Between each shot, repeat images are obtained and compared to the pretreatment images to determine the location of the tumor and correct for patient motion. The dynamic nature of the robotic arm allows several advantages. First, radiation may reach the target through a possible 1600 separate paths, decreasing the amount of radiation received by non-pathologic peritumoral structures. Second, CyberKnife® may deliver radiation in a non-isocentric fashion. As CyberKnife® is not restrained by the merging of separate beams at a geometric core, it may provide improved radiation conformity to nonspherical tumors. Last, CyberKnife® is not limited to intracranial or high cervical targets, as it is a frameless technology.

Though differences exist in the workflow and unit features, no significant difference in clinical outcome has been proven during the comparison of CyberKnife® and Gamma Knife®. The choice of machine thus depends on the surgeon's preference and the availability within the practice.

Vestibular Schwannoma

Patient Selection and Counseling

The selection of treatment modality for vestibular schwannoma is a complex decision that must take into account factors related to the surgeon, the patient, the tumor, and its associated symptoms. During consultation, the treatment team, consisting of a neurotologist, neurosurgeon, and radiation oncologist, should discuss all treatment options, including microsurgery and observation.

Important patient characteristics to consider for treatment planning include medical comorbidities, age, and the psychological effect that the tumor has on an individual. Though medical comorbidities or age rarely preclude a patient from undergoing microsurgical excision, those who are infirm may benefit from the relative noninvasive nature of SRS. In addition, older patients have a relatively smaller potential to experience serious long-term complications, such as malignant transformation or late treatment failure. In contrast, younger patients may wish to avoid SRS, as the long-term effects of radiation are yet to be well-understood. The last patient characteristic that must be evaluated is the physiological effect that the tumor has on the patient. Some individuals deplore the idea of a craniotomy and are drawn to SRS. Others are psychologically unable to tolerate living with an intracranial mass and request surgical resection. This is compounded by the fact that SRS does not permit tissue diagnosis, thus leaving diagnostic ambiguity. Neither thought process is technically wrong, and both perspectives must be considered by the treating team.

The size and location of the tumor, in addition to auditory and vestibular function, should also be addressed with the patient. Reports of treating large vestibular schwannomas are becoming more common in the literature. No absolute cutoff has been established; however, many centers consider tumors that are 2.5–3 cm to represent the upper limit. Swelling after radiation typically results in a 20% enlargement of the tumor, but occasional increases up to 200% have been reported [3]. This type of growth may lead to brainstem compression and hydrocephalus in larger tumors, which can precipitate an emergency. Recently, several publications have encouraged subtotal resection with postoperative Gamma Knife® for this subset of patients [4]. The location of the tumor also plays an important role in modality selection. Medially based tumors may be associated with brainstem compression after SRS. Tumors at the fundus have worsened hearing outcomes secondary to higher cochlear doses and tumoral effects on the cochlea. Those already suffering from poor hearing or episodic vertigo may benefit from a microsurgical approach. Removal of fluctuating vestibular input through a translabyrinthine approach produces excellent vestibular outcomes after compensation [5].

Last, preoperative counseling should include the concept of radiation-associated tumors. This includes the development of new intracranial lesions and dedifferentiation of current benign tumors into malignancies [6, 7]. Due to the rarity of malignant transformation and follow-up limitations in extant literature, its true incidence is not known but is estimated at approximately 0.1% [8, 9]. This number is further confounded by ambiguity as to whether or not the malignancy arose after radiation through dedifferentiation or if the mass already represented a malignancy before treatment. Though reported rates of malignant transformation are low, the possibility of this outcome is significant, given that it occurs with a low probability of survival in the setting of what was originally a benign process.

Gamma Knife® Technique

Frame Placement

Appropriate placement of the stereotactic frame is crucial during Gamma Knife® treatment. It must be positioned properly to avoid collisions with the collimator cap and establish an accurate, stable stereotactic reference. Multiple combinations of anesthesia may be used to improve comfort, including lorazepam, midazolam, or fentanyl, followed by local anesthesia. The frame is first brought into position and temporarily stabilized through the help of ear bars, situated at 95–100 mm on the base ring. This location represents the center of the head frame and allows for a relative symmetry to be established. It is important for the frame to be centered on the tumor to avoid collisions with the collimator cap during treatment. For vestibular schwannoma, the frame should be adjusted to the side of the tumor to avoid contralateral collision. Likewise, in other posterior fossa tumors, the frame is shifted posteriorly to avoid anterior-based collisions. Titanium pins, which come in a variety of lengths, are first placed through insulated threads on the side of the tumor to define this important spatial relationship. Additional contralateral screws are then anchored to the skull, and the ear bars are removed. A firm engagement should be present, allowing the head and the frame to move as one unit. If movement of the frame occurs after imaging, it will significantly affect the accuracy, potentially leading to poor tumor coverage and complications resulting from treating tissue outside of the target volume. Alternative frame styles are made for patients who have undergone a previous craniotomy at the pin sites. These typically consist of a tri-pin mount.

To ensure that no collision occurs between the frame and the collimator during treatment, multiple measurements of the frame are taken. These measurements include the length of the screw extending past the frame post and the post lengths themselves. If 8–10 mm of screw exists beyond the frame, collision of the screw with the collimator cap may be possible, and a shorter version should be placed. However, if the screw is short and inserted within the post, the stability of the frame may be compromised and cause the frame to wobble. As an additional safety measure, a frame cap is placed over the frame. It represents the area of the collimator. If no collisions occur after its placement, it is unlikely for them to occur during treatment.

As a final safety check, skull geometry measurements are made through the use of a geometric helmet bubble with dipstick measurements. These are used to create a wire mesh that is directly compared to treatment imaging. If a good approximation of the two is present, it ensures that the imaging used for planning matches the patient.

Imaging (CT/MRI)

The accuracy of imaging directly influences the accuracy of treatment. As high-resolution 1-mm cuts are used in both CT and MRI modalities, the highest accuracy that can be quoted for Gamma Knife® therapy is 1 mm. Imaging starts with the placement of fiducial boxes. For vestibular schwannoma, only the lateral plates of the fiducial boxes are necessary, though anterior and posterior plates may improve stability. Fiducial boxes work by creating radiopaque markings at known locations within the images. From these, all points within the fiducial box may be assigned x, y, and z coordinates. This is the key principle of SRS. For CT scans, the radiopaque material used is an aluminum strip. MRI fiducials consist of tubes filled with dilute copper. Air bubbles must be checked for within the tube because they may cause inaccuracy in planning, requiring reimaging.

Though CT or MRI can technically be used in Gamma Knife® planning, MRI is preferred. Many treating centers obtain both to exploit their complementary characteristics. CT is fast and inexpensive and delivers highly accurate bony detail. However, it provides poor target resolution, leading to difficulty in determining the tumor extent. MRI compensates for this weakness by providing high resolution of the target

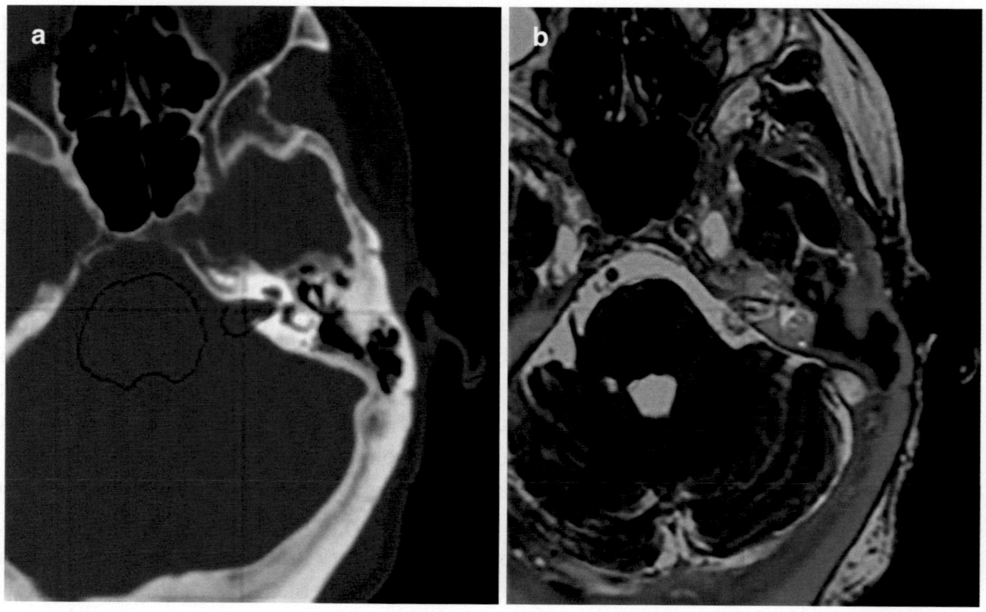

Fig. 81.3 Contoured imaging of the cochlea, labyrinth, brainstem, and vestibular schwannoma. (**a**) CT with excellent bony detail of the cochlea and labyrinth but poor target resolution of vestibular schwannoma. (**b**) MRI with exceptional definition of the tumor extent and the location of the brainstem

volume with decreased levels of metal artifact (Fig. 81.3). With either modality, Gamma Knife® programming requires high-resolution axial sequences with square pixels and low artifact.

Dose

Gamma Knife® treatment doses used for vestibular schwannoma have significantly decreased over time. Initial experiences used 18–20 Gy with excellent tumor control but unacceptably high rates of cranial neuropathies and poor short-term hearing outcomes. Currently, gradual dose escalation has led to a dose of 12–13 Gy being favored. Typically, radiation is given to the 50% isodose line. This indicates that the lowest level of radiation received by any point within the target volume is at least 50% of the maximal dose. The maximal dose delivered to a tumor receiving radiation to 12 Gy at the 50% isodose line is 24 Gy. This isodose percentage is chosen as it represents the steepest slope of radiation falloff, allowing high doses of radiation to be given, with minimal radiation extending outside the treatment volume.

Planning and Treatment

After image registration, both the tumor and the areas of potential risk, including the cochlea, labyrinth, and the brainstem, are contoured along their course (Fig. 81.3). This allows for the creation of 3D volumes, on which future statistical measures may be performed. In manual mode, multiple shots are placed by the treating physician at strategic locations within the target volume. Alternatively, inverse planning may be used. This function allows the formation of automated plans to be algorithmically calculated based on the treating physician's preference for tumor coverage and selectivity. In either manual or inverse planning modes, post-planning statistics should be run on established volumes. The tumor coverage should be evaluated to ensure that margins are adequately treated. In addition, the minimal dose that any volume of tumor receives should be greater than 9 Gy. After coverage is confirmed, selectivity should be evaluated to determine the conformation of radiation to the tumor's size and shape. Peritumoral areas may receive high levels of radiation if the plan exhibits poor conformity. In particular, the cochlea and brainstem should be evaluated for maximal and mean radiation dose. Cochlear doses of less than 4.2 Gy are currently thought to correlate with improved hearing outcomes, and brainstem doses of less than 12.5 Gy are well-tolerated [1]. After systematic evaluation, fine-tuning should occur with the movement of shots or radiation weighting or through the use of blocking until an appropriate plan is created (Fig. 81.4). The plan is then checked for potential collisions and is exported after agreement of the surgeon, radiation oncologist, and physicist. With current Gamma Knife® models, the patient is automatically moved through the treatment plan without the need for intervention.

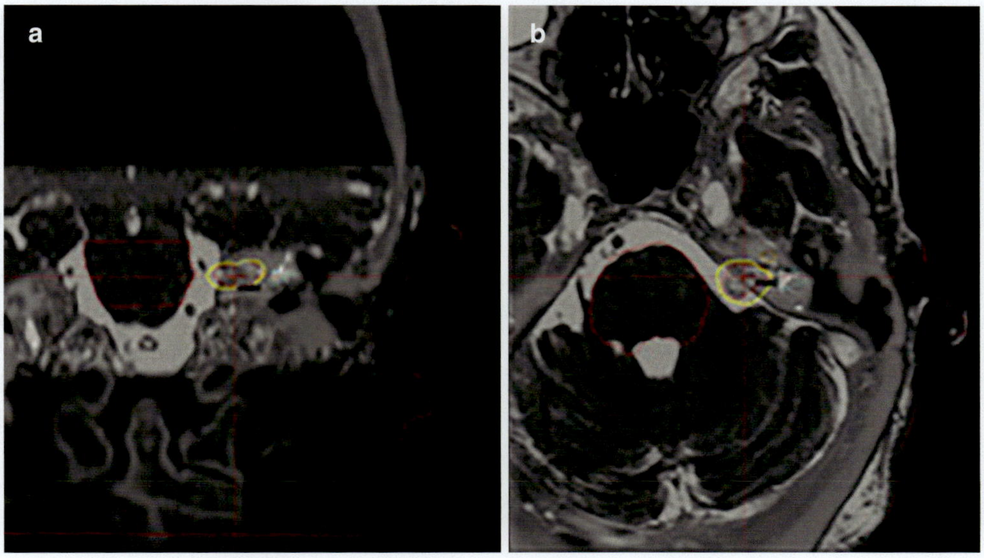

Fig. 81.4 Model Gamma Knife® plan for left vestibular schwannoma treated to 12.5 Gy to the 50% isodose line. (**a**) Coronal MRI. (**b**) Axial MRI

Outcomes

Tumor Control and Surveillance Imaging

An appropriate understanding of surveillance imaging after radiation is necessary to perform SRS. If not interpreted correctly, surgery or re-irradiation may be performed when not necessary, or failure may be missed. The most important aspect of surveillance imaging is serial examination with continued comparison of tumor volume.

Vestibular schwannomas undergo three post-SRS growth patterns. The first pattern, seen in 45–63% of patients, is an initial increase in size, followed by a regression in size. The average growth is 20% of the pretreatment size, with a peak increase occurring at approximately 6–9 months [3]. Patients may have increased rates of symptoms while tumor expansion is occurring. It is important to note that this does not represent failure in all cases. The second pattern of tumor growth, seen in 5–29% of tumors, is an increase in size, followed by stability. In Pollock's series, the median increase in tumor volume with stability was 105% of the pretreatment volume [3, 10, 11]. After reaching a growth plateau, these tumors tend not to show a second phase of growth, though a further long-term study is needed to rule out late failure. The last pattern of growth, exhibited by 2–8% of tumors, is continued growth, deemed an SRS failure. Importantly, tumor growth should be documented at 2–3 years after treatment to delineate true failure from transient swelling induced by central necrosis and inflammation [3, 10, 12].

On imaging, it is important for practitioners to understand that a transient loss of central enhancement will be seen in a majority of patients. This finding possibly represents apoptosis or necrosis. A lack of contrast enhancement will be present at 6 months in approximately 55% of patients, fading to 36% of patients at 1 year and a mere 5% at 3 years [13]. A return of enhancement should not be considered a failure necessitating further treatment.

The length of surveillance needed after radiation treatment for vestibular schwannoma has yet to be elucidated. A majority of tumors will show no further growth after stability, but late failures at 7 years or greater have been reported [13, 14]. Long-term surveillance in all patients is typically recommended until further data are available.

Hearing

Though often touted as a hearing preservation treatment, radiation damages the cochlear nerve and inner ear. The auditory pathway is injured through direct effect and secondary hypoxic compression of the cochlear nerve after tumor swelling. The cochlea is damaged from induced intracochlear hemorrhage [6]. When variables are analyzed, favorable hearing after SRS is associated with the presence of excellent pretreatment hearing, small tumor size, and low cochlear dose [15, 16].

True rates of hearing preservation continue to be unknown and are a point of contention among practicing physicians. Elucidation of this rate is hampered due to the poor standardization of the literature. Varying treatment protocols with different audiometric measures, including the neurotologic American Academy of Otolaryngology-Head and Neck Society (AAO-HNS) Hearing Guidelines and the neurosurgical Gardner–Robertson Hearing Scale, are used (Tables 81.1 and 81.2). In addition, a few studies include long-term audiometric data. This fact is important, as initial short-term data are inaccurate. Hearing loss after radiation includes both an initial acute drop, followed by a long progressive loss occur-

Table 81.1 AAO-HNS hearing guidelines

Class	Pure tone thresholds (dB)	Speech discrimination (%)
A	≤30 and	≥70
B	>30 and ≤ 50	≥50
C	>50	≥50
D	Any level	<50

Adapted from [17]

Table 81.2 Gardner–Robertson scale

Hearing grade	Pure tone average (dB)	Speech discrimination (%)
Grade I (good to excellent)	0–30	70–100
Grade II (serviceable)	31–50	50–71
Grade III (non-serviceable)	51–90	5–49
Grade IV (poor)	91-max	1–4

Adapted from [18]
If pure tone average and speech discrimination do not correlate, a lower grade is assigned

ring over many years [15, 19, 20]. This phenomenon is illustrated in Carlson's series of 44 patients with long-term follow-up undergoing SRS. Estimated rates of serviceable hearing after SRS at 1, 3, 5, 7, and 10 years were 80%, 55%, 48%, 38%, and 23%, respectively. The authors conclude that durable hearing preservation a decade after low-dose SRS was present in less than a quarter of patients [15]. In addition, the plot had a continued decreasing slope without a plateau, indicating that if patients were followed for a longer period, they may continue to have decreases in their serviceable hearing. However, to a lesser extent, long-term follow-up of patients undergoing retrosigmoid and middle fossa approaches or observation also shows a pattern of progressive loss after an initial preservation [21–24]. These studies highlight that there is currently no reliable way to treat vestibular schwannoma with long-term hearing preservation. Patients should be made aware of this reality during pretreatment discussions.

Facial Nerve

Facial nerve injury is one of the most common complications of SRS, occurring in 1–8% of patients [25–28]. The nerve is often within the treatment volume and receives relatively high levels of radiation. Histologically, radiation is seen to cause axonal degeneration, demyelination, and microvasculitis [29]. Initial changes sensitize the nerve to hypoxia, predisposing to paresis if additional tumor enlargement occurs. Decreasing the radiation dosage has been paramount in improving facial nerve outcomes, with increased risk of cranial nerve complications occurring at 15Gy or higher [26]. In a series of patients treated with 25 Gy, a third of the patients developed facial neuropathy [30]. When facial nerve function was compared in small-to-medium-sized tumors undergoing radiation at 12–13 Gy and matched controls undergoing microsurgery, radiation resulted in significantly improved posttreatment nerve function [31].

Separately, hemifacial spasm (HFS) may be present after SRS in 2% of patients treated for vestibular schwannoma. Distinct from other cranial neuropathies, it occurs near the two-year mark. In contrast, most facial paresis occurs between the sixth and ninth months [10]. The ideal management is watchful waiting, with symptomatic treatment, including carbamazepine. With this technique, HFS is often resolved without the finding of further growth of the tumor. Surgery at the time of HFS may result in disappointing facial nerve outcomes [10].

Hydrocephalus

Obstructive and communicating hydrocephalus can occur after Gamma Knife® treatment. The development of obstructive hydrocephalus occurs after tumor enlargement with compression of the ventricles and is associated with large or medially based tumors. Communicating hydrocephalus is thought to occur after SRS secondary to radiation-induced necrosis. This releases large levels of protein into the cerebrospinal fluid (CSF), impairing uptake at the level of the arachnoid [32, 33]. Overall rates of hydrocephalus after SRS have been reported at approximately 10% in small- and medium-sized tumors and 17% and 26% in tumors between 2.5 and 3 cm and larger than 3 cm, respectively. In comparison, rates of communicating hydrocephalus after surgical resection approximate 0.0008–0.68% [6, 34]. Treatment for hydrocephalus depends upon its severity and consists of conservative management, shunt placement, or endoscopic third ventriculostomy. In the aforementioned series evaluating Gamma Knife® in larger tumors, ventriculoperitoneal (VP) shunts were required in 18.5% of patients postradiation and were performed pretreatment in 8%. Due to these risks, some centers perform either a two-stage microsurgical resection or partial resection with post-operative Gamma Knife® in patients with larger tumors [35].

Tinnitus

For some patients, tinnitus may be the most disabling component of their vestibular schwannoma. It has been long known that observation leads to worsened tinnitus and that surgery may alleviate symptoms [36]. In a prospective trial comparing Gamma Knife® to translabyrinthine resection with sectioning of the cochlear nerve, surgery was found to be superior, with a 52% improvement compared to a 16% improvement in the Gamma Knife® group. In addition, 74% of those undergoing Gamma Knife® had a significant worsening of their tinnitus [37]. Increased tinnitus after Gamma Knife® is intuitive, as radiation causes direct damage to both the nerve and the cochlea proper. However, continued research is needed to clarify mixed reports in the literature [8].

Timing

When discussing treatment modalities with patients, the timing of intervention must also be addressed for small- and medium-sized tumors. National databases have shown a clinical shift toward conservative management [2]. However, clinical practice patterns do not always mirror the best practice, and a consensus has not been reached. Treatment with initial observation is supported by quality-of-life studies, which have shown that the diagnosis of vestibular schwannoma, not the specific treatment modality chosen, has a greater bearing on a patient's quality of life. As no difference exists, observation should occur until a tumor is proven to grow [38]. This is contrasted by separate papers, which support early intervention. In the evaluation of up-front Gamma Knife® versus a wait-and-see approach in intracanalicular tumors at 3, 4, and 5 years following diagnosis, the useful hearing preservation rates were 75%, 52%, and 41% in the observation group and 77%, 70%, and 64% in those receiving up-front SRS. In addition, 77% of those in the wait-and-see group had tumor growth. The conclusion was that up-front treatment should be given while hearing is still present, as an observational approach exposes the patient to elevated risks of tumor growth and degradation of hearing [39]. When all three modalities were compared in patients with small tumors and good hearing, it was suggested that early intervention with middle cranial fossa offered the best opportunity for hearing preservation and normal facial nerve function [40]. Further research with long-term follow-up will be needed to clarify this difficult clinical decision.

Special Considerations

Cystic Vestibular Schwannoma

Historically, cystic vestibular schwannomas have shown aggressive growth patterns and, thus, have required special considerations [41]. On average, they are larger than non-cystic tumors, have reduced facial nerve and hearing outcomes after microsurgical resection, and represent a risk factor for greater than 4 mm of growth a year [41–44]. In addition, SRS may itself induce cystic changes. Radiation scars the arachnoid tissue, creates micro-hemorrhage with secondary cavity formation, and increases vascular permeability, allowing for exudative collections of fluid to form [44–49].

As cystic vestibular schwannomas are rare, representing only 2.7–11.3% of all tumors, few studies discuss their treatment with SRS [50–53]. Those that do exist tend to show higher rates of failure in cystic tumors compared to solid tumors. In Delsanti's series of 54 patients with cystic schwannoma treated with radiosurgery, the failure rate was 6.4% compared to 2% found in solid tumors at a mean follow-up of 26 months [54]. Failure often requires salvage surgery in an irradiated field, possibly leading to worsened facial nerve outcomes [6, 55–60]. Secondary resection was seen in Pendl's series in three of six patients treated for cystic tumors with SRS due to progressive neurologic symptoms [50]. Recently, the Mayo Clinic published 20 cystic tumors treated with SRS, with a mean follow-up of 63 months, and solid and cystic tumors had equivalent rates of control [53]. This disparity demonstrates the need for further study with a standardization of cystic tumor classification. This type of study will be particularly important in determining the response of peritumoral cysts, which may represent a separate entity. Here, trapped arachnoid results in the collection of cystic fluid that may not be responsive to radiation treatment. In addition, peritumoral cysts lie near the 50% isodose line and receive less radiation than intratumoral cysts [53].

If tumor control rates of cystic vestibular schwannoma prove to be equivalent, treatment of these tumors with radiation may still require a guarded approach due to rare but potentially deadly complications. Several reports exist in the literature describing late enlargement of cystic schwannoma and intratumoral hemorrhage, resulting in mortality [50, 61]. Some radiotherapy centers continue to treat cystic schwannoma with caution, favoring microsurgery until more is known.

Neurofibromatosis Type 2

Neurofibromatosis type 2 (NF2) represents a challenging clinical entity. Patients tend to present at a young age with bilateral progressive disease. Currently, treatment options include observation, microsurgical resection, SRS, decompression, and systemic administration of vascular endothelial growth factor (VEGF) inhibitors. All options have their limitations, and treatment often ends with unsatisfactory results. The role of SRS in the treatment of NF2 has yet to be clarified. Only select centers use SRS for NF2 due to unique concerns for malignant transformation of tumors postradiation. Specifically, in contrast to what is discussed above, NF2 patients inherently have a mutation in a germline tumor suppressor, representing the first hit in a "two-hit" cancer model. It is thus postulated that SRS could provide the second hit, leading to malignancy. This concern is reflected in the findings that NF2 vestibular schwannoma has increased chromosomal abnormalities after radiation when compared to unirradiated tumors. Clinically, this finding is thought to render a 14× greater risk of transformation [62–64]. Finally, it is also worth noting that patients with NF2 tend to be young, and the effect of radiation is carried across their lifetimes.

Centers that use SRS for NF2 have shown favorable results. In 74 vestibular schwannomas across 62 patients and a mean follow-up of 53 months, control rates were 85%, 81%, and 81% at 5, 10, and 15 years. Serviceable hearing was preserved in 73% at 1 year, 59% at 2 years, and 48% at 5 years after SRS. Facial neuropathy occurred in 8% of tumors, trigeminal neuropathy occurred in 4%, and vestibular dysfunction occurred in 4% [65]. Further follow-up will be needed to ultimately determine rates of serviceable hearing, tumor control, and potential malignant transformation in this series. Until this data exists, many centers will continue to pursue conventional treatment.

Failure in Sporadic Vestibular Schwannoma

Though failure after SRS is rare, it represents a difficult dilemma in both pretreatment discussion of SRS versus microsurgical resection and in postradiation salvage treatment [3, 10, 12]. Historically, histologically, and intuitively, tumors that have previously been radiated can be difficult to dissect off of adjacent structures [56–58, 66, 67]. In the Gruppo Otologico experience of 19 patients treated with salvage surgery, they found a 93.3% rate of difficult dissection, defined as an absence of the peritumoral arachnoidal plane, abundant intraoperative bleeding, or excessive adherence to the brainstem, cerebellum, facial nerve, or trigeminal nerve. In particular, the tumor was adherent to the facial nerve in 86.6% of patients, the brainstem in 60%, the cerebellum in 46.6%, and the trigeminal nerve in 26.6% [6]. The difficult dissection translated into a clinical finding of worse facial nerve outcomes when compared to matched controls who had not previously received radiation [6]. Outcomes may also be affected by postradiation changes in the nerve, including the decreased ability for neural regeneration and impaired blood supply [58].

After obtaining similarly poor facial outcomes during salvage surgery, Friedman and colleagues at the House Ear Institute changed their microsurgical technique. Specifically, performing less aggressive surgery led to improved outcomes [58, 68]. In patients with a gross total resection, 21.7% had an unsatisfactory facial nerve outcome of a House–Brackmann (HB) grade V or VI, compared to only 7.1% in whom a partial resection was performed. At an average of 6 years of follow-up, no patient who received a partial resection had failed treatment. Though further long-term follow-up is necessary, techniques that place increased emphasis on facial nerve function in salvage surgery are appealing.

More recently, re-irradiation has been evaluated and may play a future role in the salvage treatment [69–72]. However, studies are limited in power and follow-up length. As such, our group continues to prefer microsurgical resection in this subpopulation. Our desire to treat these patients surgically is increased by the fact that by failing radiation once, these patients' tumors have already shown themselves to possess characteristics that may make them radio-resistant during a second treatment. In addition, tumors that continue to enlarge despite radiation therapy may harbor malignancy, which can only be proven at the time of resection.

Meningioma

Meningiomas are commonly seen by neurotologists within the cerebellopontine angle (CPA), posterior fossa, and the petroclival region. Pathologically, they arise from dural arachnoid cap cells and are often found incidentally on MRI. However, those located in the CPA may mimic vestibular schwannomas symptomatically. Radiographically, they are separated from vestibular schwannomas on MRI by their characteristic broad base, enhancing dural tail, and eccentric location in relation to the IAC. Calcification or hyperostosis may be seen on CT.

Radiosurgical treatment of meningioma mirrors techniques used for vestibular schwannoma. In elderly patients or in those who are asymptomatic, treatment is often deferred until growth is documented. Interestingly, meningiomas that show heavy calcification tend to be nongrowing instead of slow-growing. During dose planning, margins are typically treated at 11–13 Gy to the 50% isodose line. Unique to meningioma is the presence of an enhancing dural tail. The tail represents enhancing reactive dura and does not consist of a tumor. As such, multiple MRIs should be evaluated to ensure that the tail is not included in the treatment and that only the tumor is targeted. If this does not occur, radiation may be given needlessly.

The eccentric nature of CPA meningiomas creates surgical results that are dependent on the size and location of the tumor. In a large series of 347 CPA meningiomas treated with surgery, good tumor resection was possible, with Simpson grade I or II achieved in 86% of patients. In addition, House–Brackmann grade I or II facial nerve function was found in 89% of patients, with a 91% rate of hearing preservation [73]. The largest radiosurgery report, consisting exclusively of CPA meningioma, evaluated 177 patients through multicenter collaboration. Across the seven institutions, good tumor control was found with actuarial rates of progression-free survival at 5 and 10 years of 93% and 77%, respectively. Of these patients, 3.4% had worsened hearing, and 2.3% had facial weakness [74]. This report compares favorably to surgical options, indicating clear potential for the treatment of CPA meningioma with radiotherapy.

Facial Nerve Schwannoma

Facial nerve schwannomas represent a key pathology in which the use of SRS may hold large benefits over traditional facial nerve decompression or microsurgery with facial nerve grafting. As fascicles of the facial nerve run directly through the tumor in facial nerve schwannomas, surgery often requires complete transection of the nerve, resulting in poor facial nerve outcomes. Even with grafting, the best facial nerve outcome that can be expected is a House–Brackmann (HB) grade III, and this outcome is not a guarantee, being found in approximately 67% of patients [75]. Traditional treatment for these tumors has thus generally consisted of observation for patients with HB grade I or II function, surgical decompression for patients with HB grade II or III function, and tumor resection with grafting for individuals with HB grade IV or worse.

Though data on SRS is limited due to the rare occurrence of this type of tumor, it may represent the most favorable risk-benefit profile. A meta-analysis of SRS for facial schwannoma demonstrated no growth in 50%, growth in 6.7%, and size reduction (more than 2 mm in a linear direction or more than 20% of tumor volume) in 43.3% at 2 years of follow-up [76]. In this same meta-analysis, 39 patients were evaluated for pre- and postradiation facial nerve function, and 66.7% of patients showed no change in their HB score, 12.8% had a worsened HB score, and 20% reported an improved HB score. In regard to the hearing status, 26 patients had complete pre- and postradiation hearing data, with at least a 2-year follow-up. No patient had improved hearing after radiation. In the 14 patients who had serviceable hearing (AAO class A/B) before radiation, 64.3% showed no change in hearing class, and 36.7% had worsened hearing [76]. Early data presented shows that early SRS in patients with documented tumor growth is a reasonable first option for patients.

Paraganglioma

Paragangliomas have traditionally been addressed with gross total resection, during which cranial nerves were placed at risk. A shift toward less aggressive partial resection or SRS has occurred over time. Refined Gamma Knife® technology in both the Perfexion and Icon models allows improved access to the neck, facilitating the ability to treat this area. Dosing for paragangliomas typically utilizes 16–18 Gy to the 50% isodose line. Doses higher than 20 Gy should be avoided to prevent lower cranial neuropathy. Imaging for treatment planning should include both CT and MRI. Frame placement may prove challenging in tumors that extend to the level of C2. All target volumes must be positioned above the base ring of the head frame and sit within the fiducial box.

Numerous series, including a meta-analysis of jugular paraganglioma treated with Gamma Knife®, show excellent tumor control with limited lower cranial neuropathy [77]. This has led Gamma Knife® to become the first-line therapy for these tumors at many treatment centers. In a multicenter study, actuarial tumor control with Gamma Knife® was 88% at 5 years following SRS. New or progressive cranial neuropathy was noted in 15% of patients, and an improvement in cranial nerve deficits was observed in 11% of patients. Last, pulsatile tinnitus improved in 49% of patients who reported it at presentation [78]. The mixture of tumor control with lower cranial neuropathy found in Gamma Knife® treatment compares favorably with surgery. Even with experienced surgeons, injury to lower cranial nerves can range from 18.9% to 60% during this difficult surgery [79, 80]. In those who have pulsatile tinnitus as their main complaint, subtotal resection with or without adjuvant SRS may be considered.

Conclusions

Determining when and how to treat skull base tumors is complex. SRS represents an excellent addition to the treatment algorithm, generally offering a favorable side effect profile and good tumor control across multiple types of tumors. However, as with any relatively new technology, further research is needed to gain results of long-term follow-up. In particular, true rates of hearing preservation and tumor control will need to be clarified. Patients should be made aware of the risks and benefits related to the use of SRS as well as the alternatives, including microsurgery and observation. Each patient and each tumor is different, requiring tailoring of treatment options to individual needs and the use of a multispecialty team.

References

1. Dade Lunsford, L., Intracranial stereotactic radiosurgery. 2016, New York: Thieme.
2. Carlson ML, et al. The changing landscape of vestibular Schwannoma management in the United States–a shift toward conservatism. Otolaryngol Head Neck Surg. 2015;153(3):440–6.
3. Yu CP, et al. Sequential volume mapping for confirmation of negative growth in vestibular schwannomas treated by Gamma Knife radiosurgery. J Neurosurg. 2000;93(Suppl 3):82–9.
4. Gurgel RK, Theodosopoulos PV, Jackler RK. Subtotal/near-total treatment of vestibular schwannomas. Curr Opin Otolaryngol Head Neck Surg. 2012;20(5):380–4.
5. Godefroy WP, Hastan D, van der Mey AG. Translabyrinthine surgery for disabling vertigo in vestibular schwannoma patients. Clin Otolaryngol. 2007;32(3):167–72.
6. Husseini ST, et al. Salvage surgery of vestibular schwannoma after failed radiotherapy: the Gruppo Otologico experience and review of the literature. Am J Otolaryngol. 2013;34(2):107–14.

7. Tanbouzi Husseini S, et al. Malignancy in vestibular schwannoma after stereotactic radiotherapy: a case report and review of the literature. Laryngoscope. 2011;121(5):923–8.
8. Boari N, et al. Gamma Knife radiosurgery for vestibular schwannoma: clinical results at long-term follow-up in a series of 379 patients. J Neurosurg. 2014;121(Suppl):123–42.
9. Niranjan A, Kondziolka D, Lunsford LD. Neoplastic transformation after radiosurgery or radiotherapy: risk and realities. Otolaryngol Clin N Am. 2009;42(4):717–29.
10. Pollock BE. Management of vestibular schwannomas that enlarge after stereotactic radiosurgery: treatment recommendations based on a 15 year experience. Neurosurgery. 2006;58(2):241–8; discussion 241–8.
11. Delsanti C, et al. Morphological changes of vestibular schwannomas after radiosurgical treatment: pitfalls and diagnosis of failure. Prog Neurol Surg. 2008;21:93–7.
12. Pollock BE, Link MJ, Foote RL. Failure rate of contemporary low-dose radiosurgical technique for vestibular schwannoma. *Clinical article*. J Neurosurg. 2013;119(Suppl):840–4.
13. Delsanti C, et al. Changing radiological results, pitfalls and criteria of failure. Neurochirurgie. 2004;50(2–3 Pt 2):312–9.
14. Hasegawa T, et al. Long-term safety and efficacy of stereotactic radiosurgery for vestibular schwannomas: evaluation of 440 patients more than 10 years after treatment with Gamma Knife surgery. J Neurosurg. 2013;118(3):557–65.
15. Carlson ML, et al. Long-term hearing outcomes following stereotactic radiosurgery for vestibular schwannoma: patterns of hearing loss and variables influencing audiometric decline. J Neurosurg. 2013;118(3):579–87.
16. Watanabe S, et al. Stereotactic radiosurgery for vestibular schwannomas: average 10-year follow-up results focusing on long-term hearing preservation. J Neurosurg. 2016;125(Suppl 1):64–72.
17. Committee on hearing and equilibrium guidelines for the evaluation of hearing preservation in acoustic neuroma (vestibular schwannoma). American Academy of Otolaryngology-Head and Neck Surgery Foundation, INC. Otolaryngol Head Neck Surg. 1995;113(3):179–80.
18. Gardner G, Robertson JH. Hearing preservation in unilateral acoustic neuroma surgery. Ann Otol Rhinol Laryngol. 1988;97(1):55–66.
19. Hasegawa T, et al. Factors associated with hearing preservation after Gamma Knife surgery for vestibular schwannomas in patients who retain serviceable hearing. J Neurosurg. 2011;115(6):1078–86.
20. Roos DE, Potter AE, Zacest AC. Hearing preservation after low dose linac radiosurgery for acoustic neuroma depends on initial hearing and time. Radiother Oncol. 2011;101(3):420–4.
21. Chee GH, Nedzelski JM, Rowed D. Acoustic neuroma surgery: the results of long-term hearing preservation. Otol Neurotol. 2003;24(4):672–6.
22. Shelton C, et al. Hearing preservation after acoustic tumor removal: long-term results. Laryngoscope. 1990;100(2 Pt 1):115–9.
23. Friedman RA, et al. Long-term hearing preservation after middle fossa removal of vestibular schwannoma. Otolaryngol Head Neck Surg. 2003;129(6):660–5.
24. Stangerup SE, et al. Long-term hearing preservation in vestibular schwannoma. Otol Neurotol. 2010;31(2):271–5.
25. Flickinger JC, et al. Results of acoustic neuroma radiosurgery: an analysis of 5 years' experience using current methods. J Neurosurg. 2001;94(1):1–6.
26. Foote KD, et al. Analysis of risk factors associated with radiosurgery for vestibular schwannoma. J Neurosurg. 2001;95(3):440–9.
27. Miller RC, et al. Decrease in cranial nerve complications after radiosurgery for acoustic neuromas: a prospective study of dose and volume. Int J Radiat Oncol Biol Phys. 1999;43(2):305–11.
28. Prasad D, Steiner M, Steiner L. Gamma surgery for vestibular schwannoma. J Neurosurg. 2000;92(5):745–59.
29. Watanabe T, et al. Facial neuropathy due to axonal degeneration and microvasculitis following Gamma Knife surgery for vestibular schwannoma: a histological analysis. Case report. J Neurosurg. 2003;99(5):916–20.
30. Forster DM, et al. Radiosurgery: a minimally interventional alternative to microsurgery in the management of acoustic neuroma. Br J Neurosurg. 1996;10(2):169–74.
31. Golfinos JG, et al. A matched cohort comparison of clinical outcomes following microsurgical resection or stereotactic radiosurgery for patients with small- and medium-sized vestibular schwannomas. J Neurosurg. 2016:1–11.
32. Hayhurst C, Dhir J, Dias PS. Stereotactic radiosurgery and vestibular schwannoma: hydrocephalus associated with the development of a secondary arachnoid cyst: a report of two cases and review of the literature. Br J Neurosurg. 2005;19(2):178–81.
33. Bloch J, et al. Non-obstructive hydrocephalus associated with intracranial schwannomas: hyperproteinorrhachia as an etiopathological factor? Acta Neurochir. 2003;145(1):73–8.
34. Jeon CJ, et al. Communicating hydrocephalus associated with surgery or radiosurgery for vestibular schwannoma. J Clin Neurosci. 2010;17(7):862–4.
35. Porter RG, et al. Improved facial nerve outcomes using an evolving treatment method for large acoustic neuromas. Otol Neurotol. 2013;34(2):304–10.
36. Kameda K, et al. Effect of tumor removal on tinnitus in patients with vestibular schwannoma. J Neurosurg. 2010;112(1):152–7.
37. Park SH, et al. Change in tinnitus after treatment of vestibular schwannoma: microsurgery vs. Gamma Knife radiosurgery. Yonsei Med J. 2014;55(1):19–24.
38. Carlson ML, et al. Long-term quality of life in patients with vestibular schwannoma: an international multicenter cross-sectional study comparing microsurgery, stereotactic radiosurgery, observation, and nontumor controls. J Neurosurg. 2015;122(4):833–42.
39. Regis J, et al. Wait-and-see strategy compared with proactive Gamma Knife surgery in patients with intracanalicular vestibular schwannomas: clinical article. J Neurosurg. 2013;119(Suppl):105–11.
40. Meyer TA, et al. Small acoustic neuromas: surgical outcomes versus observation or radiation. Otol Neurotol. 2006;27(3):380–92.
41. Jian BJ, et al. Implications of cystic features in vestibular schwannomas of patients undergoing microsurgical resection. Neurosurgery. 2011;68(4):874–80; discussion 879–80.
42. Charabi S, et al. Cystic acoustic neuromas. Results of translabyrinthine surgery. Arch Otolaryngol Head Neck Surg. 1994;120(12):1333–8.
43. Paldor I, Chen AS, Kaye AH. Growth rate of vestibular schwannoma. J Clin Neurosci. 2016;32:1–8.
44. de Vries M, et al. Intratumoral hemorrhage, vessel density, and the inflammatory reaction contribute to volume increase of sporadic vestibular schwannomas. Virchows Arch. 2012;460(6):629–36.
45. Pollock BE, Brown RD Jr. Management of cysts arising after radiosurgery to treat intracranial arteriovenous malformations. Neurosurgery. 2001;49(2):259–64; discussion 264–5.
46. Park CK, et al. Microhemorrhage, a possible mechanism for cyst formation in vestibular schwannomas. J Neurosurg. 2006;105(4):576–80.
47. Yamamoto M, et al. Late cyst convolution after Gamma Knife radiosurgery for cerebral arteriovenous malformations. Stereotact Funct Neurosurg. 1998;70(Suppl 1):166–78.
48. Jacob JT, et al. Stereotactic radiosurgery in the management of vestibular schwannoma and glomus jugulare: indications, techniques, and results. Otolaryngol Clin N Am. 2015;48(3):515–26.
49. Shuto T, Matsunaga S. Two cases of cystic enlargement of vestibular schwannoma as a late complication following Gamma Knife surgery. J Clin Neurosci. 2016;33:239–41.

50. Pendl G, et al. Acoustic neurinomas with macrocysts treated with Gamma Knife radiosurgery. Stereotact Funct Neurosurg. 1996;66(Suppl 1):103–11.
51. Tali ET, et al. Cystic acoustic schwannomas: MR characteristics. AJNR Am J Neuroradiol. 1993;14(5):1241–7.
52. Charabi S. Acoustic neuroma/vestibular schwannoma in vivo and in vitro growth models. A clinical and experimental study. Acta Otolaryngol Suppl. 1997;530:1–27.
53. Frisch CD, et al. Stereotactic radiosurgery for cystic vestibular Schwannomas. Neurosurgery. 2016.
54. Delsanti C, Regis J. Cystic vestibular schwannomas. Neurochirurgie. 2004;50(2–3 Pt 2):401–6.
55. Pollock BE, et al. Vestibular schwannoma management: part II. Failed radiosurgery and the role of delayed microsurgery. J Neurosurg. 2013;119(Suppl):949–55.
56. Limb CJ, Long DM, Niparko JK. Acoustic neuromas after failed radiation therapy: challenges of surgical salvage. Laryngoscope. 2005;115(1):93–8.
57. Iwai Y, et al. Surgery after radiosurgery for acoustic neuromas: surgical strategy and histological findings. Neurosurgery. 2007;60(2 Suppl 1):ONS75–82; discussion ONS82.
58. Friedman RA, et al. Surgical salvage after failed irradiation for vestibular schwannoma. Laryngoscope. 2005;115(10):1827–32.
59. Nonaka Y, et al. Surgical management of vestibular schwannomas after failed radiation treatment. Neurosurg Rev. 2016;39(2):303–12; discussion 312.
60. Iwai Y, et al. Functional outcomes of salvage surgery for vestibular Schwannomas after failed Gamma Knife radiosurgery. World Neurosurg. 2016;90:385–90.
61. Ganslandt O, Fahrig A, Strauss C. Hemorrhage into cystic vestibular schwannoma following stereotactic radiation therapy. Zentralbl Neurochir. 2008;69(4):204–6.
62. Carlson ML, et al. Radiation-induced rhabdomyosarcoma of the brainstem in a patient with neurofibromatosis type 2. J Neurosurg. 2010;112(1):81–7.
63. Warren C, et al. Identification of recurrent regions of chromosome loss and gain in vestibular schwannomas using comparative genomic hybridisation. J Med Genet. 2003;40(11):802–6.
64. Baser ME, et al. Neurofibromatosis 2, radiosurgery and malignant nervous system tumours. Br J Cancer. 2000;82(4):998.
65. Mathieu D, et al. Stereotactic radiosurgery for vestibular schwannomas in patients with neurofibromatosis type 2: an analysis of tumor control, complications, and hearing preservation rates. Neurosurgery. 2007;60(3):460–8; discussion 468–70.
66. Lee DJ, et al. Clinical and histopathologic features of recurrent vestibular schwannoma (acoustic neuroma) after stereotactic radiosurgery. Otol Neurotol. 2003;24(4):650–60; discussion 660
67. Shuto T, et al. Microsurgery for vestibular schwannoma after Gamma Knife radiosurgery. Acta Neurochir. 2008;150(3):229–34; discussion 234.
68. Friedman RA, et al. A paradigm shift in salvage surgery for radiated vestibular schwannoma. Otol Neurotol. 2011;32(8):1322–8.
69. Liscak R, et al. Repeated treatment of vestibular schwannomas after Gamma Knife radiosurgery. Acta Neurochir. 2009;151(4):317–24; discussion 324.
70. Yomo S, et al. Repeat Gamma Knife surgery for regrowth of vestibular schwannomas. Neurosurgery. 2009;64(1):48–54; discussion 54–5.
71. Kano H, et al. Repeat stereotactic radiosurgery for acoustic neuromas. Int J Radiat Oncol Biol Phys. 2010;76(2):520–7.
72. Lonneville S, et al. Repeat Gamma Knife surgery for vestibular schwannomas. Surg Neurol Int. 2015;6:153.
73. Nakamura M, et al. Facial and cochlear nerve function after surgery of cerebellopontine angle meningiomas. Neurosurgery. 2005;57(1):77–90; discussion 77–90.
74. Ding D, et al. Gamma Knife radiosurgery for cerebellopontine angle meningiomas: a multicenter study. Neurosurgery. 2014;75(4):398–408; quiz 408.
75. Ozmen OA, et al. Outcomes of facial nerve grafting in 155 cases: predictive value of history and preoperative function. Otol Neurotol. 2011;32(8):1341–6.
76. McRackan TR, et al. Stereotactic radiosurgery for facial nerve schwannomas: meta-analysis and clinical review. Otol Neurotol. 2015;36(3):393–8.
77. Ivan ME, et al. A meta-analysis of tumor control rates and treatment-related morbidity for patients with glomus jugulare tumors. J Neurosurg. 2011;114(5):1299–305.
78. Sheehan JP, et al. Gamma Knife surgery for the management of glomus tumors: a multicenter study. J Neurosurg. 2012;117(2):246–54.
79. Wanna GB, et al. Contemporary management of jugular paragangliomas. Otolaryngol Clin N Am. 2015;48(2):331–41.
80. Fayad JN, Keles B, Brackmann DE. Jugular foramen tumors: clinical characteristics and treatment outcomes. Otol Neurotol. 2010;31(2):299–305.

82 Reconstruction of the Lateral Skull Base

Neil S. Patel, Matthew L. Carlson, and Jeffrey R. Janus

Introduction

Lateral skull base reconstruction following ablation of locally aggressive benign or malignant tumors of the external ear, temporal bone, or periauricular skin and soft tissues is difficult. Often, a complex defect involving the skin, soft tissue, and bone is generated that requires coverage of dura or brain, closure of a cerebrospinal fluid (CSF) leak, and protection of neurovascular structures in the temporal bone, infratemporal fossa, or upper neck. Reconstruction of the mandibular ramus and/or temporomandibular joint is also sometimes necessary. In addition, the ear, periauricular skin, and scalp offer minimal tissue laxity for primary closure. Many patients require postoperative radiation with or without chemotherapy, which will test the resiliency of the repair. The aesthetic and functional consequences of partial or total auricular loss can be quite severe as well, compelling the reconstructive surgeon to consider prosthetic rehabilitation and options for the resultant conductive or sensorineural hearing loss. This chapter reviews a classification of defects of the lateral skull base and associated soft tissues, discusses the considerations necessary for a durable reconstruction, and describes the most commonly utilized local, pedicled, and free tissue options.

N. S. Patel
Department of Otolaryngology—Head and Neck Surgery, University of Utah, Salt Lake City, Utah, USA

M. L. Carlson
Department of Otolaryngology—Head and Neck Surgery, Mayo Clinic, Rochester, MN, USA

J. R. Janus (✉)
Department of Otolaryngology—Head and Neck Surgery, Mayo Clinic, Jacksonville, FL, USA
e-mail: janus.jeffrey@mayo.edu

Defect Considerations

Extent of Temporal Bone Resection

Ablative procedures for tumors of the external auditory canal (EAC) and pinna that involve the temporal bone can be broadly categorized according to the anatomic unit extirpated. In reality, there is often significant overlap between these procedures based on the degree of tumor infiltration. These are discussed in detail in Chap. 67.

Lateral temporal bone resection (LTBR) involves the removal of the bony and cartilaginous external auditory canal. The external auditory meatus is everted and closed but may also be resected in continuity with portions of the auricle or surrounding soft tissues. The temporal bone defect is similar to that generated in a canal wall down mastoidectomy, with associated skin and soft tissue loss.

Subtotal temporal bone resection (STBR) involves the removal of the otic capsule (labyrinth and cochlea), with the fundus of the internal auditory canal serving as the medial boundary. Often, dissection extends into the hypotympanum and may require control of the proximal internal carotid artery and isolation and/or sacrifice of the sigmoid sinus. Dural exposure or resection is common, and they are potential sources of CSF leakage from the cochlear modiolus, internal auditory canal, middle fossa, or posterior fossa. In such cases, the facial nerve is often paretic preoperatively and is often sacrificed.

Total temporal bone resection (TTBR) extends the boundary of an STBR to include the petrous apex. Utilized for very advanced tumors, the exposure typically involves a combined approach with temporal craniotomy, infratemporal fossa exploration, mandibulotomy or mandibulectomy, and extensive soft tissue loss. The carotid artery and internal jugular vein may be sacrificed. Depending upon the extent of neck disease, compromise of vasculature may affect planned free tissue transfer and necessitate contralateral arterial donor and/or recipient vessel harvest.

A. D. Sweeney et al. (eds.), *Haynes-Glasscock-Shambaugh Surgery of the Ear*, https://doi.org/10.1007/978-3-032-18264-7_82

Auriculectomy

The external ear may require partial or complete resection for margin clearance in the case of cutaneous malignancies of the external auditory canal and conchal bowl. In some cases, skin and soft tissue resection that does not directly involve the auricle may compromise its vascular supply, leading to devitalization of the auricle and potential for delayed necrosis. Anatomic studies have demonstrated that the blood supply of the cephalic lateral (or anterior) portion of the auricle is from the superficial temporal artery, while the posterior surface is supplied by the postauricular artery [1]. Ligation of the external carotid artery during deep lobe parotidectomy, for example, would therefore deprive the auricle of both the major feeding vessels, in addition to the temporalis muscle. Ablation of tumors that directly extend from the parotid or infratemporal fossa or metastases to the temporal bone may compromise the underlying bony support of the auricle and result in a poor aesthetic result even if its intrinsic structure is unaffected.

Apart from oncologic considerations, it is important to assess the functional and aesthetic needs of the patient. Patients who wear glasses may benefit from preservation of even a small helical skin and cartilage remnant as opposed to total auriculectomy. If total auriculectomy is unavoidable, consideration should be given to staged placement of a bone- or skin-anchored auricular prosthesis. In cases where adjuvant radiotherapy will be needed, the authors generally prefer to delay osseointegrated screw placement for aural rehabilitation or auricular prosthesis until several months after the patient has completed radiotherapy. In most cases, the post-irradiated scalp and subcutaneous tissue are atrophic, and minimally invasive screw placement with a single 5-mm punch is performed to limit soft tissue complications. Furthermore, a two-stage procedure or delayed loading of the bone conduction implant (BCI) after a single-stage procedure should be considered in the setting of recipient post-irradiated bone.

Zygoma, Mandible, and Infratemporal Fossa

Anterior extension of cutaneous malignancies of the auricle or periauricular skin may require removal of the zygoma, lateral orbit, temporalis muscle, or malar eminence. The resultant loss of midfacial width or projection and temporal hollowing can generate a substantial aesthetic deformity. Medial tumor extension may involve the muscles of mastication, the mandibular division of the trigeminal nerve, or the mandible itself. Particularly in the context of prior or adjuvant radiation therapy, patients may experience significant trismus, malocclusion, or pain, all of which can compromise oral nutrition. In these situations, consideration should be given to bony reconstruction and functional mandibular reconstruction with free tissue transfer, which will be discussed later in this chapter.

Wound Considerations

Patient Factors

In contrast to patients with benign skull base tumors, those who undergo temporal bone resection for advanced cutaneous malignancies (the most common indication for these procedures) tend to be older and are more likely to have medical comorbidities that affect wound healing. Up to 55% of patients in large published series have undergone some form of prior treatment, including surgery, radiation, and/or chemotherapy [2]. A thorough preoperative history and examination is critical, with particular attention to the quality of tissues around the tumor site and scars of prior surgery, both ablative (i.e., prior neck dissection) and reconstructive (i.e., donor sites for reconstructive flaps).

Defect Location: Coronal and Axial Relationships

The geometry of skin and soft tissue defects plays a significant role when considering local and pedicled flap reconstruction. The authors consider the position of the external auditory canal (EAC) to demarcate "anterior" or "posterior" defects in the coronal plane, while the position of the zygomatic arch demarcates "superior" and "inferior" defects in the axial plane. "Posterior" defects include those where greater than 50% of the skin and soft tissue component of the lesion (or ablative defect) is centered posterior to the external auditory canal. "Anterior" defects involve those where the opposite is true. "Superior" defects are those where the cephalic portion of the defect extends beyond the level of the zygomatic arch, whereas "inferior" defects are located caudal to the zygomatic arch. Each position carries implications for the degree of skin laxity for primary closure; the arc of rotation for advancement or rotational skin and subcutaneous tissue flaps, pedicled muscle, or musculocutaneous flaps; and the position of donor site defects. Specific considerations will be discussed in subsequent sections on specific reconstructive options.

Dural Exposure

Regions of exposed dura overlying the temporal lobe or cerebellum following temporal bone resection must be addressed differently from partial-thickness defects of the temporal squama or occipital bone or simple periauricular soft tissue defects. In contrast to translabyrinthine craniotomy, for example, lateral skull base defects for skin or soft tissue malignancies tend to involve skin and soft tissue loss and secondary risk to the wound following prior or adjuvant radiation therapy. An otherwise uncomplicated surgical site infection in a patient with significant dural exposure could progress to an epidural abscess with subsequent intracranial sequelae. For these reasons, the authors advocate obliteration of the space generated by craniectomy defects, with or without the use of mesh cranioplasty, and vascularized tissue to separate the area from contaminated spaces such as the middle ear or pharynx. As a general rule, the authors prefer the use of autologous tissue to synthetic substrates (e.g., bone cement and titanium mesh) whenever feasible, given the greater risk of infection, extrusion, and pain, particularly following radiotherapy.

Dural Resection with Middle and/or Posterior Fossa CSF Leak

Tumors with gross dural invasion or those directly abutting the dura generally result in defects that communicate with the subarachnoid space. Temporal and subtemporal CSF leaks tend to be low-flow, while those involving the posterior fossa cistern tend to result in high-flow, high-pressure fistulae. While very small durotomies involving the posterior fossa may be treated in the same manner as those resulting from translabyrinthine craniotomy, for example, one must take into consideration the degree of skin or soft tissue loss and factors that may adversely affect wound healing.

Local Reconstructive Options

Primary Closure and Rotation Flaps

In complex defects of the lateral skull base, it is important to ensure that certain criteria are met to avoid postoperative wound dehiscence, infection, and exposure of critical structures when primary closure is attempted. Partial auriculectomy defects with limited bone removal are tempting to close primarily or with the aid of a cervicofacial rotation flap. As mentioned above, concomitant deep lobe parotidectomy or periauricular skin excision may render the blood supply to the auricle tenuous—particularly with regard to postoperative venous congestion. While collateral circulation from other sources may allow it to initially survive, consideration should be given to whether postoperative partial wound necrosis would lead to the exposure of the bone or critical neurovascular structures. Opting to use vascularized tissue to reinforce the area at the time of the initial operation may be advisable to surmount the rigors of radiation and/or tissue necrosis.

Free abdominal fat or composite dermal fat grafts are sometimes used to fill small bony defects in the temporal bone. Harvest is efficient with negligible donor site morbidity; however, significant delayed atrophy or fat necrosis may occur following radiation and must be considered. We advocate for their use in the obliteration of the middle ear space in temporal bone defects with small CSF leaks without a large dural defect. As it is not vascularized, it serves no role in secondary intention healing if necrosis of superficial skin and soft tissue occurs.

The cervicofacial and cervicothoracic rotation flaps are frequently used for auricular, periauricular, and facial defects. Advantages include low donor site morbidity, excellent color match, and efficient harvest and inset. When raised in a subcutaneous plane, the flap is a random-pattern flap that relies on a wide pedicle for viability. If raised in the plane deep to the superficial musculoaponeurotic system (SMAS) and platysma, the flap becomes an axial flap based on the transverse facial artery and perforators [3]. Recent work has shown a reduction in distal edge necrosis when using this technique [4]. The sub-SMAS plane is accessed in the same way as in parotidectomy; often, this has already been performed during tumor extirpation or clearance of the parotid and upper cervical nodal basin.

Temporalis Rotation Flap

The temporalis muscle takes its origin from the inferior temporal line, an arc that crosses the coronal suture spanning the frontal bone and a portion of the parietal bone. It inserts onto the coronoid process of the mandible and functions as a primary elevator and retractor of the mandible. Blood supply is derived from the anterior and posterior deep temporal arteries, which arise from the middle segment of the internal maxillary artery distal to the origin of the superficial temporal artery and proximal to the sphenopalatine foramen [5].

A preexisting incision can be extended above the temporal fossa. The origin of the muscle is then separated at the inferior temporal line. Carrying dissection in a subperiosteal plane along the squama temporalis can help prevent injury of nutrient vessels in the infratemporal fossa. Once released, the muscle can be rotated into the defect and secured to the surrounding periosteum and sternocleidomastoid muscle. To increase the arc of rotation, a zygomatic osteotomy or resection of the zygomatic arch can be performed. A split-thickness skin graft can be used to cover the exposed areas of the muscle, or the area can be allowed to heal by secondary intention (Fig. 82.1). The resultant donor site morbidity is minimal, though some degree of temporal hollowing does result. If profound, this temporal hollowing can be rectified with an abdominal dermal fat graft. Postoperative trismus can be avoided with jaw physiotherapy exercises.

Indications for the use of the temporalis muscle rotation flap include larger bony defects without substantial skin or soft tissue loss, soft tissue augmentation to support a cervicofacial rotation flap, and vascularized obliteration of a temporal bone defect with a small CSF leak. Contraindications

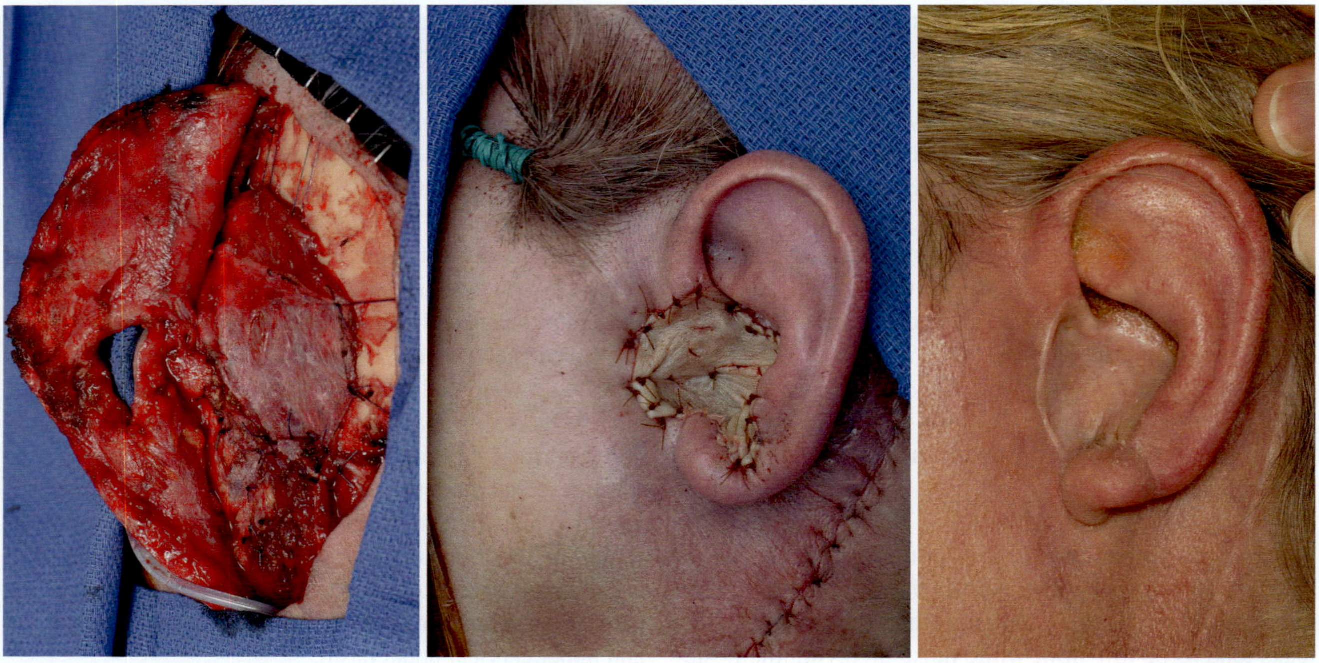

Fig. 82.1 Lateral temporal bone resection, parotidectomy, and neck dissection, reconstructed with temporalis muscle rotation flap (left panel) and split-thickness skin graft (center panel), with appearance at 4 months postoperatively (right panel)

to its use include prior radiation therapy, prior deep lobe parotidectomy, infratemporal fossa exploration, or sacrifice of the external carotid system during neck dissection.

Reported experience with the temporalis flap demonstrates a low incidence of wound complications. Hanasono et al. utilized the temporalis flap with or without a split-thickness skin graft in 26 patients who underwent LTBR and one patient who underwent TTBR. Two patients experienced wound dehiscence [6]. Among nine patients who underwent temporalis flap reconstruction, Patel et al. reported one wound complication necessitating revision closure [2]. Thompson et al. utilized the temporalis flap in 28 patients and reported 12 minor wound complications, including dehiscence, infection, hematoma, and stitch abscess [7].

Regional Reconstructive Options

Pectoralis Major Myocutaneous Flap

The pectoralis major muscle originates from the medial portion of the clavicle and sternum, six or seven superior costal cartilages, and the external oblique aponeurosis. It inserts onto the proximal anteromedial humerus and functions to adduct and medially rotate the upper arm. The pectoralis major myocutaneous flap (PMMF) is a pedicled flap based on the pectoral branch of the thoracoacromial trunk, which originates from the proximal portion of the axillary artery near the midclavicular line. The pedicle enters the deep surface of the pectoralis major muscle between the pectoralis major and minor muscles and can be readily palpated on flap elevation. The lateral and medial pectoral nerves innervate the pectoralis major muscle by piercing its deep surface. These must be divided to avoid muscular contraction with arm movements and permit gradual atrophy of the muscular component of the flap.

Since the original series by Ariyan [8], there have been several descriptions of the flap harvest technique for a variety of head and neck defects. Our approach is similar to that described by Jacono and Moscatello [9]. In men, an elliptical, vertically oriented skin paddle is outlined between the nipple and the sternum. To facilitate harvest, a skin incision is made from the cephalic end of the skin paddle to the axilla in a curvilinear fashion. In women, a similarly designed skin paddle can be utilized with an inframammary crease incision to access the lateral extent of the muscle and identify the pedicle. Prior to making the incision, a towel is used as a template to ensure that the caudal end of the skin paddle is able to reach the cephalic portion of the defect. Once subcutaneous flaps are raised, the edges of the skin paddle are sewn to the muscular fascia to prevent shear injury to musculocutaneous perforators. Elevation of the muscle on its deep surface proceeds in an inferior to superior direction between the pectoralis major and minor muscles. Attachments to the humerus are divided in all cases to facilitate rotation. A subcutaneous tunnel accommodating three to four fingerbreadths in the lower neck is created to transmit the flap to the periauricular region (Fig. 82.2).

Several modifications to the flap harvest technique have been described to facilitate increased reach to the lateral skull base and face. In their experience with eight patients, Resto et al. describe the inclusion of a cuff of the ipsilateral rectus sheath to suspend the muscle from residual temporalis fascia or pericranium, thereby mitigating tensile forces on the skin paddle itself. In cases where the cephalic aspect of the defect is still open secondary to insufficient reach, the temporalis muscle can be mobilized in the aforementioned manner and sutured directly to the pectoralis for superior defect coverage.

Advantages of the PMMF in lateral skull base reconstruction are numerous. The flap is robust and has a consistent, reliable pedicle that is rarely compromised during the ablative procedure. It offers sufficient soft tissue bulk to restore contour and a large skin paddle to close total auriculectomy defects. Many otolaryngologists are familiar with the harvest technique due to its ubiquitous use in laryngectomy, oropharyngectomy, and oral cavity reconstruction. The donor site can be closed primarily in most cases.

The primary disadvantage of the PMMF is its relatively limited reach. Defects posterior to the EAC and above the level of the zygoma are not ideal candidates for PMMF reconstruction. After transposition to the head, the caudal-most aspect of the skin paddle becomes the most cephalic portion, which coincidentally tends to be the highest tension portion of the reconstruction. Often, a segment of the skin paddle does not lie over the muscle; rather than relying on musculocutaneous perforators, this area takes on a random-pattern blood supply. In lighter-skinned individuals, color match tends to be suboptimal due to differential sun exposure to the face and chest. Patients with a higher proportion of adipose tissue in the flap may require subsequent debulking; however, this is common among other musculocutaneous or fasciocutaneous flaps as well.

Lower Island Trapezius

Originally described by Baek [10], the lower island trapezius flap is a workhorse of posterolateral skull, neck, and lateral skull base reconstruction. The trapezius muscle is a large fan-shaped muscle of the back that originates from the superior nuchal line, occipital protuberance, and spinous processes of C7 and all thoracic vertebrae and inserts on the clavicle, acromion, and spine of the scapula. Both the transverse cervical artery (a branch of the thyrocervical trunk) and the dorsal scapular artery (of variable origin but most commonly a branch of the subclavian artery) supply much of the muscle and overlying skin inferior to the scapular spine [11]. The spinal accessory nerve can be preserved to maintain the function of the shoulder.

Harvest of the flap is similar to the original description by Baek. We refer the reader to the article by Urken et al. for a detailed description of flap harvest that resembles our approach [12]. The rhomboid muscles should be preserved to avoid postoperative scapular "winging." To accomplish this, the dorsal scapular artery, emerging from between the rhomboid minor superiorly and rhomboid major inferiorly, must be divided to allow for adequate pedicle rotation to reach the auricular defects. Provided that the skin paddle overlies the trapezius muscle only and not the latissimus dorsi, it is safe to do so. The dorsal scapular artery can be preserved by dissecting it to the diastasis between the rhomboid minor and

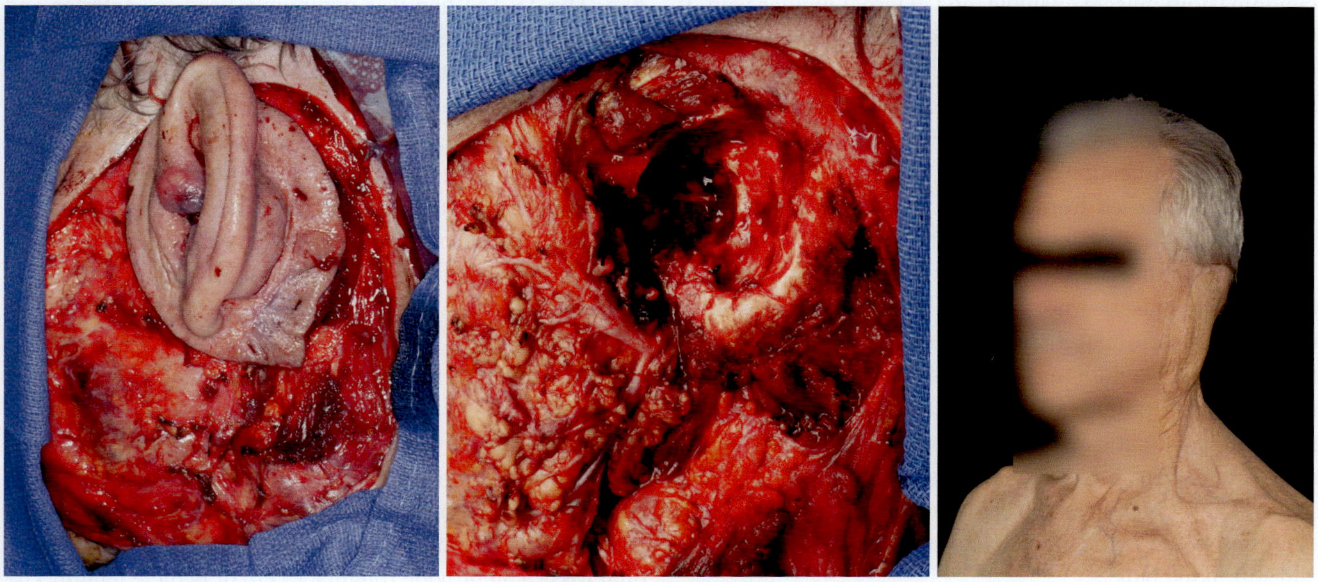

Fig. 82.2 Lateral temporal bone resection with total auriculectomy (left and center panel), reconstructed with pedicled pectoralis major myocutaneous flap, with appearance at 9 months postoperatively (right panel)

major muscles; myotomy of the rhomboid minor can provide additional pedicle length.

Advantages of the lower island trapezius flap include its reliable blood supply and tissue bulk for lateral skull base reconstruction. Donor site morbidity is low, and the site can be closed primarily. Its ability to reach auricular defects with posterior extension is unparalleled by other pedicled myocutaneous flaps. In contrast to the PMMF, an anterior chest incision is avoided, which may be preferable, particularly in female patients.

Disadvantages of the lower island trapezius flap are relatively few. The patient must be turned into a lateral decubitus position for harvest, which may result in compressive injuries of the contralateral brachial plexus or ulnar nerve. Also, simultaneous tumor ablation and harvest is not possible. Depending upon the extent of dissection, concomitant ipsilateral lateral neck dissection involving level IV may preclude its use due to ligation of the transverse cervical artery; we do not routinely sacrifice this vessel during neck dissection, however. Similar to the PMMF, color match is suboptimal.

Supraclavicular Island

The supraclavicular island flap has become increasingly popular for lateral face, neck, and ear reconstruction. Described originally by Lamberty, this thin, fasciocutaneous flap can be harvested quickly and can offer a large skin paddle to reconstruct partial or total auriculectomy defects with limited bony defects. As the name suggests, it is based on the supraclavicular artery, a consistent branch of the transverse cervical artery. The vessel is most easily identified in a space defined by the posterior border of the sternocleidomastoid muscle, clavicle, and external jugular vein. If the external jugular vein has been sacrificed previously, one may also find branches of the supraclavicular artery between the posterior belly of the omohyoid muscle near the clavicle and the trapezius muscle posteriorly. A handheld Doppler aids in its identification.

The flap is raised from a lateral-to-medial direction in a subfascial plane that initially overlies the deltoid muscle. Remaining in this plane posteriorly on the anterior edge of the trapezius muscle is not difficult; anteriorly, some authors describe subperiosteal dissection along the clavicle to protect the pedicle in this area [13, 14]. Once the pedicle is identified near the posterior border of the sternocleidomastoid muscle, a back-cut can be made to release the flap from the neck skin and facilitate rotation. A skin paddle up to 10 cm in width and 15 cm in length is reasonable. The distal portion can often be de-epithelialized and tucked into the defect to add soft tissue bulk.

Advantages of the supraclavicular island flap include its ease of harvest and good color match. Subsequent flap revision for contour irregularities is rare, given its thin nature. The flap can be de-epithelialized in its entirety to be used as fascial coverage of bony defects if primary skin closure is feasible. Donor site morbidity is minimal, and potentially exposed areas of the deltoid muscle can be left to heal by secondary intention or covered with a split-thickness skin graft.

Disadvantages are few and pertain mostly to situations where the supraclavicular island flap simply may not be the ideal reconstructive option. The thin nature of the flap renders it unsuitable for more substantial soft tissue defects. In myocutaneous flaps such as the PMMF, partial- or full-thickness skin necrosis may simply expose the underlying muscle that heals by secondary intention, often with a good color match. In contrast, loss of portions of a thin fasciocutaneous flap may result in bone or dural exposure. Also, as mentioned previously, the preservation and gentle handling of the transverse cervical vessels during cervical lymphadenectomy are paramount for the success of this flap.

Free Flaps

In some ways, free tissue transfer permits the greatest degree of reconstructive latitude with regard to lateral skull base defects. Specific flap considerations will be discussed in the sections that follow. In general, free flaps are utilized for large ablative defects, typically with total auriculectomy, that result in dural or brain exposure or CSF leak. At our institution, free flaps are used for nearly all tumors that have undergone previous treatment, particularly in cases of prior radiation therapy, where the vascularity and elasticity of locoregional options may be compromised.

A microvascular free flap of largely historical significance is the transverse rectus abdominis myocutaneous (TRAM) flap. The TRAM flap was commonly used for anterior and lateral skull base reconstruction due to its ample tissue bulk. To capture perforating vessels and the deep inferior epigastric artery pedicle, dissection is performed deep to the rectus fascia. As a result, the abdominal wall can be weakened, resulting in bulging or a hernia. This option has been replaced by the anterolateral thigh fasciocutaneous and latissimus dorsi myofascial or myocutaneous flaps, as these options result in significantly less donor site morbidity.

Radial Forearm Fasciocutaneous

The radial forearm fasciocutaneous flap (RFFF) is a stalwart of head and neck reconstruction for oral cavity, oropharyngeal, laryngopharyngeal, and skull base defects. This flap is based on the radial artery, which, when ligated in the antecubital fossa, can provide roughly 15 cm of pedicle length. The skin paddle can be of variable dimensions and can extend beyond the anterior surface onto the hair-bearing posterior surface without compromising viability. Both the venae comitantes and the more superficial cephalic vein may be harvested for venous drainage. For oral cavity or pharyngeal defects, harvesting the lateral antebrachial cutaneous nerve to create a sensate flap has been described; this is typically not necessary for lateral skull base reconstruction. Also, patients often develop some sensation passively without formal reinnervation [15]. In addition to the classic Allen's Test on clinical examination, we recommend a preoperative sonographic assessment of palmar arch collateralization to confirm ulnar flow to the radial aspect of the hand prior to radial artery harvest.

For a complete description of the harvest technique, we direct the reader to the method described by Urken et al. [16]. In brief, a rectangular incision with a "lazy S"–shaped para-midline forearm incision is fashioned, and dissection is carried to the plane between the paratenon of the forearm musculature and overlying fascia. The radial artery is ligated distally, and dissection is carried out in a distal-to-proximal direction. In the antecubital fossa, the branching of radial collateral arteries marks the limit of pedicle length, and it is divided and ligated at that point, in addition to venae comitantes. The forearm incision can be closed primarily, and the distal portion (area of skin paddle) is closed with a pie-crusted split-thickness skin graft, a vacuum-assisted closure device, and a rigid splint maintaining extension at the wrist. This is kept in place for 5 days.

As one of the most commonly used free microvascular flaps, the RFFF can be harvested quickly. Two-team harvest and ablation are feasible, and the arm can be closed and dressed, while a second team inserts the flap and performs microvascular anastomoses. Its thin, pliable nature provides good contour and rarely requires revision. However, its form factor is not ideal for deeper defects with substantial bone loss, dural exposure, or CSF leak. Lin and Lin describe a double-layer technique that employs a fat pad from the antecubital fossa to add soft tissue bulk when required [17]. Pedicle length depends on patient factors but can be up to 15 cm in length, permitting anastomosis to typical neck donor vessels.

Anterolateral Thigh Fasciocutaneous

The anterolateral thigh (ALT) fasciocutaneous flap is the most commonly utilized free flap for lateral skull base reconstruction at most centers. Its vascular pedicle takes its origin from the profunda femoris artery as the descending branch of the lateral femoral circumflex artery. Its versatility for soft tissue reconstruction is unparalleled due to the large skin paddle that can be harvested and the flexibility in the degree of soft tissue incorporated. Harvest of each type of ALT flap is well described by Wei et al. In brief, an ellipse of skin is outlined on the anterior thigh, with the midline of the long axis centered over the location of skin perforators identified by a handheld Doppler probe. Dissection is carried down to the tensor fascia lata until the perforators to the skin can be seen. If these are within the vastus lateralis muscle, dissection with a variable cuff of muscle can be performed, depending upon the characteristics of the defect. The pedicle is followed to the profunda femoris and is divided and ligated. The donor site can often be closed primarily, with vacuum-assisted closure devices or split-thickness skin grafts as adjuncts to closure.

The ALT flap can be harvested as virtually any combination of skin, fascia, fat, and muscle, rendering it extraordinarily versatile (Fig. 82.3). The pedicle is between 5 and 10 cm in length and, while not as long as the RFFF pedicle, typically accommodates anastomoses to donor vasculature in the neck. For most lateral skull base defects, the size of the flap permits primary closure of the donor site. Even when a substantial portion of the vastus lateralis muscle is included, the overall donor site morbidity is low. Perhaps the most significant disadvantage is the variability in vascular anatomy that can make harvest challenging. Shieh et al. summarized nine series (both anatomic and clinical) totaling over 350 flaps and found that there was little agreement among authors regarding the relative preponderance of septocutaneous or musculocutaneous perforators [18]. When a fasciocutaneous ALT flap is utilized in an obese patient, often the adipose component renders the flap bulky or irregular (particularly following radiation therapy), which may require debulking according to patient preference.

Fibula Osteocutaneous

Bony reconstruction for both aesthetic and functional rehabilitation can be considered for lateral skull base defects that involve the zygoma or mandible. Given the anatomic proximity of the ear canal and periauricular skin to the condyle, temporal and infratemporal fossae, and parotid nodal basin, direct or metastatic tumor extension to involve the mandible from condyle to angle can occur. Loss of the zygomatic arch with resultant loss of midfacial width may be a consideration in some patients. The fibula free flap (FFF) is an osteocutaneous flap based on the peroneal artery that can offer 10–15 cm of vascularized bone, with an associated skin paddle based on septocutaneous perforators. The bone can be contoured and segmented with angled osteotomies to reconstruct multiple segments of the mandible in direct continuity. The skin paddle is closely associated with the bone and, therefore, would not be suitable for large defects that are relatively far from the bone segment. Moore and Hamilton reported their experience with six patients who underwent hemimandibulectomy with the removal of the articular disk and all soft tissue within the condylar fossa. Soft tissue and muscle of the flap were placed in the condylar

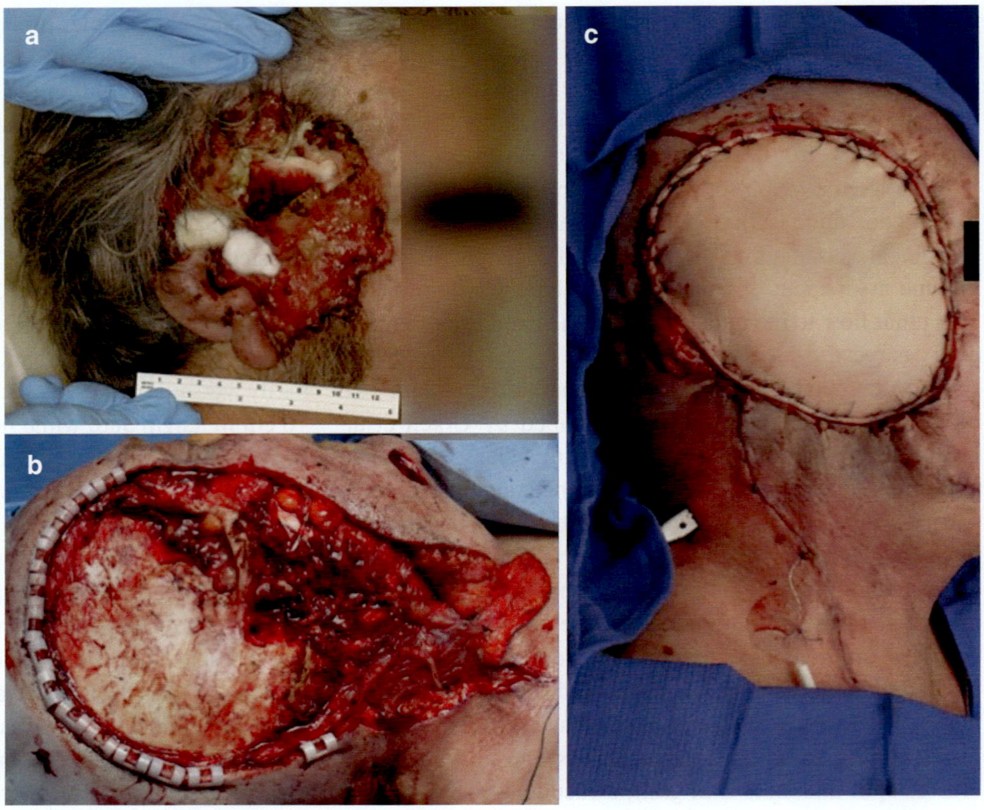

Fig. 82.3 (a–c) Anterolateral thigh flap for large total auriculectomy defect with a 12 × 12-cm skin and soft tissue defect. An edge of the defect can be left to epithelialize secondarily if closure is under tension

fossa prior to plating the bone to the native mandible. The neomandible remained in the glenoid fossa radiographically in all patients, and all were able to return to a normal or near-normal oral diet with no less than 4 cm of interincisal opening [19].

Subscapular System

There are a number of flaps based on the subscapular artery and its branches. Constituent tissue types include muscle-only (latissimus dorsi and serratus anterior), skin and fascia (scapular and parascapular), and bone (scapular tip and scapular border) and can frequently be harvested in continuity when applicable. Arterial anatomy is consistent without significant variation. In midfacial and oromandibular reconstruction, the amount and quality of bone offered with relatively minimal donor site morbidity make it an appealing option for reconstructing these complex three-dimensional defects. While the fibula osteocutaneous flap is generally preferred for mandibular ramus reconstruction, lower extremity atherosclerosis or extensive osteoporosis with concern for gait instability may make it unsuitable for harvest. Fortunately, the subscapular system tends to be spared from significant atherosclerotic disease, even in patients with advanced peripheral artery disease [20]. That said, substantial bony defects involving the zygoma and orbital rim, necessitating reconstruction that result from temporal bone malignancy extirpation, are rare. However, the latissimus dorsi muscle offers substantial soft tissue bulk and a long pedicle and is frequently used for scalp defects that may extend to include the periauricular soft tissues. Potential disadvantages include the inability to perform two-team surgery, the potential for scapular winging and postoperative shoulder dysfunction, and, particularly with latissimus harvest, the potential for donor site seroma or hematoma.

Conclusions

The complexity of lateral skull base defects renders this anatomic area quite challenging to reconstruct. The extent of skin and soft tissue loss must be considered alongside the potential for dural exposure or CSF leak to prevent costly wound complications. A multitude of patient factors should be considered to determine the availability of local, regional, or distant reconstructive options while taking into account functional and aesthetic demands that differ substantially among patients. Free tissue transfer has become a desirable primary option for many lateral skull base and facial defects and can be an efficient, robust reconstructive option in the modern era.

References

1. Henoux M, Espitalier F, Hamel A, et al. Vascular supply of the auricle: anatomical study and applications to external ear reconstruction. Dermatologic Surg. 2017;43:87–97.
2. Patel NS, Modest MC, Brobst TD, et al. Surgical management of lateral skull base defects. Laryngoscope. 2016;126:1911–7.
3. Schuster RH, Gamble WB, Hamra ST, et al. A comparison of flap vascular anatomy in three rhytidectomy techniques. Plast Reconstr Surg. 1995;95:683–90.
4. Jacono AA, Rousso JJ, Lavin TJ. Comparing rates of distal edge necrosis in deep-plane vs subcutaneous cervicofacial rotation-advancement flaps for facial cutaneous Mohs defects. JAMA Facial Plast Surg. 2014;16:31–5.
5. Cheung LK. The blood supply of the human temporalis muscle: a vascular corrosion cast study. J Anat. 1996;189(Pt 2):431–8.
6. Hanasono MM, Silva AK, Yu P, et al. Comprehensive management of temporal bone defects after oncologic resection. Laryngoscope. 2012;122:2663–9.
7. Thompson NJ, Roche JP, Schularick NM, et al. Reconstruction outcomes following lateral skull base resection. Otol Neurotol. 2017;38:264–71.
8. Ariyan S. The pectoralis major myocutaneous flap. A versatile flap for reconstruction in the head and neck. Plast Reconstr Surg. 1979;63:73–81.
9. Jacono AA, Moscatello AL. Pedicled myocutaneous flaps in head and neck surgery. Oper Tech Otolaryngol Head Neck Surg. 2000;11:139–42.
10. Baek SM, Biller HF, Krespi YP, et al. The lower trapezius Island myocutaneous flap. Ann Plast Surg. 1980;5:108–14.
11. Netterville JL, Wood DE. The lower trapezius flap. Vascular anatomy and surgical technique. Arch Otolaryngol Head Neck Surg. 1991;117:73–6.
12. Urken ML, Naidu RK, Lawson W, et al. The lower trapezius Island musculocutaneous flap revisited. Report of 45 cases and a unifying concept of the vascular supply. Arch Otolaryngol Head Neck Surg. 1991;117:502–11.
13. Hunt JP, Buchmann LO. The supraclavicular artery flap for lateral skull and scalp defects: effective and efficient alternative to free tissue transfer. J Neurol Surg Rep. 2014;75:e5–e10.
14. Emerick KS, Herr MW, Lin DT, et al. Supraclavicular artery Island flap for reconstruction of complex parotidectomy, lateral skull base, and total auriculectomy defects. JAMA Otolaryngol Head Neck Surg. 2014;140:861–6.
15. Vriens JP, Acosta R, Soutar DS, et al. Recovery of sensation in the radial forearm free flap in oral reconstruction. Plast Reconstr Surg. 1996;98:649–56.
16. Urken ML, Cheney M, Blackwell KE, Harris JR, Hadlock TA, Futran N. Atlas of regional and free flaps for head and neck reconstruction: flap harvest and insetting. Philadelphia: Wolters Kluwer Health/Lippincott Williams & Wilkins; 2011. p. 547.
17. Lin AC, Lin DT. Reconstruction of lateral skull base defects with radial forearm free flaps: the double-layer technique. J Neurol Surg B Skull Base. 2015;76:257–61.
18. Shieh SJ, Chiu HY, Yu JC, et al. Free anterolateral thigh flap for reconstruction of head and neck defects following cancer ablation. Plast Reconstr Surg. 2000;105:2349–57; discussion 58–60.
19. Moore EJ, Hamilton SS. Mandibular condyle reconstruction with fibula free-tissue transfer. Ear Nose Throat J. 2012;91:E18–24.
20. Brown J, Bekiroglu F, Shaw R. Indications for the scapular flap in reconstructions of the head and neck. Br J Oral Maxillofac Surg. 2010;48:331–7.

Index

A. D. Sweeney et al. (eds.), *Haynes-Glasscock-Shambaugh Surgery of the Ear*, https://doi.org/10.1007/978-3-032-18264-7

E

F

M

U

W

X

Y

Z

GPSR Compliance

The European Union's (EU) General Product Safety Regulation (GPSR) is a set of rules that requires consumer products to be safe and our obligations to ensure this.

If you have any concerns about our products, you can contact us on ProductSafety@springernature.com

In case Publisher is established outside the EU, the EU authorized representative is:

Springer Nature Customer Service Center GmbH
Europaplatz 3
69115 Heidelberg, Germany

Batch number: 10692884

Printed by Printforce, the Netherlands